PNEUMONIA
WITH SPECIAL REFERENCE TO
PNEUMOCOCCUS LOBAR PNEUMONIA

This volume is published as part of a long-standing cooperative program between the Harvard University Press and the Commonwealth Fund, a philanthropic foundation, to encourage the publication of significant scholarly books in medicine and health.

PNEUMONIA

WITH SPECIAL REFERENCE TO PNEUMOCOCCUS LOBAR PNEUMONIA

RODERICK HEFFRON, M.D.

A Commonwealth Fund Book

Harvard University Press
Cambridge, Massachusetts
London, England

Printed in the United States of America

Library of Congress Cataloging in Publication Data

Heffron, Roderick, 1901-
Pneumonia, with special reference to pneumococcus lobar pneumonia.

"A Commonwealth Fund book."
Reprint of the ed. published by the Commonwealth Fund, New York.
Bibliography: p.
Includes index.
1. Pneumonia. 2. Streptococcus pneumoniae.
I. Title. [DNLM: WC204 H461p 1939a]
RC771.H4 1979 616.2'41 78-10519
ISBN 0-674-67444-8

Second Printing, 1979

To GEORGE HOYT BIGELOW and
BENJAMIN WHITE
in memory of their outstanding service to public health, this book is affectionately and respectfully dedicated

FOREWORD TO THE SECOND PRINTING

NEARLY forty years have passed since this book was first published and it has been out of print for more than half of that time. That is a pity for, as the late Colin M. MacLeod predicted in his review for *Science* (v. 91, p. 73, 1940), Dr. Heffron's book has served for many years as the standard reference work, not only because of the great mass of observations which the author has sifted and correlated, but also because of his outlook on problems which, at that time, seemed to be far from solution.

The most pressing of those problems, according to MacLeod, was that of prophylaxis of pneumococcal pneumonias. The problem is now reasonably close to solution with the recent development, availability, and demonstrated efficacy of polyvalent pneumococcal polysaccharide vaccines. Much of the basis for these vaccines, and the early observations on their application and potential value, are presented in this book and in its companion volume, Benjamin White's *The Biology of Pneumococcus*. The greatest impetus for the development of the vaccine, in fact, came from Dr. MacLeod, and the successful application of the currently available vaccine is due to the persistent efforts of his former student and colleague, Dr. Robert Austrian.

The original publication of *Pneumonia* coincided with the advent of the new chemotherapeutic era and the earliest successful applications of sulfanilamide and its more effective derivatives. Some reference to the early use of these drugs, alone or in conjunction with antiserum therapy, are included in this book, but most aspects of therapy dealt with here relate to the development and use of type-specific antipneumococcal sera which, during the years when he was compiling this volume, were the primary concern of the author as Field Director of the Pneumonia Study and Service of the Massachusetts Department of Public Health.

Subsequent sulfanilamide derivatives, notably sulfadiazine, and later penicillin proved to be remarkably effective against pneumococci of all serotypes as well as against infections due to many other important bacterial pathogens. As a result, the therapeutic use of antipneumococcal sera was soon totally abandoned, as was the serotyping of pneumococci in all but a very few laboratories of clinical bacteriology, where such typing was usually limited to isolates from blood or purulent foci of infection. This resulted in the loss of skills, on the part of the laboratory workers and particularly of students and physicians on medical wards in the recognition of pneumococci, even in some of the best university teaching hospitals.

In more recent years there has been a new flurry of interest in the laboratory diagnosis of pneumococcal infections with the application of immunologic methods that were not available when Heffron's and White's books were published. For the most part this resulted in the rediscovery of much that was already known and referred to in these books. Many of the problems which recent workers encountered might well have been avoided had they been more thoroughly familiar with the earlier literature presented and analyzed in detail in these volumes.

While this book deals primarily and at greatest length with the most frequent and important disease caused by the pneumococcus, namely lobar pneumonia, it also covers the literature and all details of information available at the time on all varieties of pulmonary and extrapulmonary pneumococcal infections. Indeed, there is little of importance in the earlier clinical literature on pneumococcal infections which is not referred to, analyzed, classified, and cross-referenced in this volume.

For the medical student, clinical scholar, and particularly the specialist and clinical investigator in pulmonary medicine or in infectious disease, this volume should be indispensable in providing a most useful reference work, with its complete cross-reference index and bibliography of 1471 cited references to the literature. It should also be of interest even to the general practitioner of medicine. It should be most welcome in the many new medical schools, hospitals, and libraries which have been established since this book first became available and in any of the others that do not yet have it on their library's shelf. We should all be grateful to the Commonwealth Fund for its financial support in making this book again available.

MAXWELL FINLAND, M.D.
GEORGE RICHARDS MINOT PROFESSOR OF
MEDICINE, EMERITUS, HARVARD UNIVERSITY;
DISTINGUISHED PHYSICIAN, UNITED STATES
VETERANS ADMINISTRATION
JULY 1978

FOREWORD

THIS book is an outcome of the Massachusetts Pneumonia Study and Service, inaugurated by Dr. George H. Bigelow, conducted by the State Department of Public Health for the five years of 1931–35 and financed by the Commonwealth Fund. The success of this project in the state-wide extension of specific therapy of pneumococcus pneumonia was in large measure due to the enthusiasm and ability of Dr. Heffron, who served as Field Director.

The book is destined to fill an important place in the literature on pneumonia. It brings together in one place a comprehensive review of investigations dealing with the inciting agent, lesions produced, clinical aspects, factors influencing recovery, prevention, and treatment. It is especially valuable as a source of information concerning the results of specific therapy in large series of collected cases, including those observed during the Massachusetts Pneumonia Study and Service and the Continuing Program. The need for further investigation of special problems is pointed out.

Favorable results in the state-wide use in Massachusetts of specific therapy in the treatment of certain types of pneumococcus pneumonia have proved a useful example for other communities. The book contains helpful suggestions concerning the further extension of the use of antipneumococcic serum as a community project.

It is with profound satisfaction that I commend this book to the medical profession.

FREDERICK T. LORD

PREFACE

While the Massachusetts Pneumonia Study and Service was in progress, it was planned that one phase of the undertaking would be the publication of three books in which part of the experience resulting from the project would be recorded. The first volume, a handbook on *Lobar Pneumonia and Serum Therapy* by Dr. Frederick T. Lord and Dr. Roderick Heffron, was published by the Commonwealth Fund in 1936 and a revised edition entitled *Pneumonia and Serum Therapy* was published in 1938. The second publication, an exhaustive treatise on *The Biology of Pneumococcus: The Bacteriological, Biochemical, and Immunological Character and Activities of Diplococcus Pneumoniae* by Dr. Benjamin White, with the collaboration of Dr. Elliott S. Robinson and Dr. Laverne A. Barnes, was also published in 1938.

The present book, the third of the series planned, presents a comprehensive discussion of pneumonia with special reference to pneumococcus lobar pneumonia and measures for treatment. The more important findings resulting from the Massachusetts Pneumonia Study have been incorporated in the text. In the preparation of this volume much of the literature relating to pneumonia was reviewed and abstracted in detail. Most of the pertinent older literature deals with pneumonia in various of its anatomic forms, while bacteriologic diagnosis, when mentioned, is often considered only as a secondary matter. Therefore it has not always been possible to give as much emphasis to etiologic diagnosis as the importance of the subject makes desirable. The bibliography is not of course "complete"; the first three series of the *Index-Catalogue of the Library of the Surgeon-General's Office, United States Army,* give the titles of approximately ten thousand articles and books on the pneumococcus and pneumonia. However, it is believed that practically all the more important discussions through 1936 are referred to in the text and listed in the bibliography. Certain studies published since 1936 are also included.

Continued support by the Commonwealth Fund has made possible the preparation of this book. Grateful thanks are extended to the Fund for the foresight and vision that provided an opportunity to present a summary of the literature pertaining to such an important disease as pneumonia.

It was a great privilege, deeply appreciated, to work in collaboration with Dr. George Bigelow, who initiated the study of pneumonia in Massachusetts, and with Dr. Benjamin White, whose wisdom and enthusiasm were of inestimable aid. Men of outstanding ability and of unusual personal gifts as friends and as leaders, they did much to lessen the dread of pneumonia in the hearts of many people, and their death was a severe blow to the cause of public health. Fortune was kind in permitting me to work in close association with so distinguished a physician as Dr. Frederick T. Lord, whose keen insight, wide knowledge, and great interest in pneumonia have been a constant stimulus. I am grateful to him for reading the present manuscript and for valuable suggestions and sound advice.

To members of the Massachusetts Department of Public Health for their never-failing interest and cooperation I am deeply indebted: especially to Dr. Henry D. Chadwick, former Commissioner of Public Health of Massachusetts, for his kindness in providing invaluable assistance in the preparation of much of the manuscript and for placing at my disposal the records of cases treated in the Continuing Program in that state; to Dr. Gaylord W. Anderson, past Deputy Commissioner of Public Health of Massachusetts, for his similar assistance and confidence in the present undertaking; to Dr. Elliott S. Robinson, Director of the Antitoxin and Vaccine Laboratory, for many helpful suggestions; and to Miss Edith A. Beckler, Director of the State Bacteriologic Laboratory, for her wholehearted cooperation and assistance in matters pertaining to the typing of pneumococci. Grateful acknowledgment is made to the technicians in the bacteriologic laboratory, especially Miss Helen Gillette, Miss Florence Varley, Mrs. Patricia MacLeod, and Mrs. Olga Jewett; to Miss Angeline D. Hamblen for important aid in matters dealing with pneumonia death rates and in the statistical analysis of numerous series of figures; to Mrs. Gwennie Malcolm for secretarial help and aid in preparing many abstracts; to Miss Bessie Shack for her interest and valuable assistance in this same matter and for her care in checking the bibliography; and to Miss Dorothy Adams.

To Dr. Wilson G. Smillie, Dr. Lloyd D. Felton, Dr. Wheelan D. Sutliff, Dr. Maxwell Finland, Dr. Thomas Dublin, and many other friends and colleagues I extend cordial thanks for generous assistance on various occasions. Last but not least I wish to acknowledge my gratitude to my wife, Catharine Haman Heffron, for her understanding and cooperation in the long task now completed.

R. H.

41 East Fifty-seventh Street
New York, N. Y.
January 1939

CONTENTS

Foreword. *By Frederick T. Lord* ix
Preface xi
Introduction xv
I. Causative Organisms in Pneumonia; and Pneumonia not Due to Pneumococci 1
II. The Pneumococcus and Type Incidence in Pneumonia 18
III. Pathology of Lobar Pneumonia 90
IV. Aspects of Immunity 113
V. Experimental Pneumococcus Infections and Pathogenesis of Lobar Pneumonia 204
VI. Epidemiology 258
VII. Measures for the Prevention of Pneumonia 395
VIII. Symptoms of Lobar Pneumonia 484
IX. Physical Signs in Lobar Pneumonia 506
X. Clinical Varieties of Pneumonia and Association with Other Conditions 510
XI. Special Features in the Course of the Disease 526
XII. Complications: Incidence and Treatment 548
XIII. Diagnosis 612
XIV. Differential Diagnosis 648
XV. Prognosis 655
XVI. Recovery Factors and Duration of Immunity 728
XVII. General Therapeutic Measures 741
XVIII. Serum Treatment 805
XIX. Results of Serum Treatment 880
XX. Continuing Problems 921
Appendices 937
Bibliography 947
Index 1025

LIFE IS SHORT

AND THE ART LONG

THE OCCASION INSTANT

EXPERIMENT PERILOUS

DECISION DIFFICULT

Hippocrates

INTRODUCTION

Pneumonia has been known to man for centuries. Its symptomatology, though somewhat confused with that of pleurisy, and the methods of treatment prevalent in the fifth century before Christ were described by Hippocrates (644). Certainly the disease existed long before his time, for Ruffer (1142), using delicate histologic methods to examine Egyptian mummies, found in some of them evidence of pneumonia which had advanced to the stage of hepatization. These mummies were of a dynasty extant from 1250 to 1000 B.C. Well known to the Greeks, Romans, and Arabians (661), pneumonia has continued into modern times and, widely distributed, is at present a frequent cause of illness and one of the most common causes of death.

Pneumonia may be primary or secondary and the character of the lesion produced either patchy or massive. Patchy consolidations are typical of bronchopneumonia, while massive lesions are characteristic of lobar pneumonia. Confluent bronchopneumonia may be indistinguishable from lobar pneumonia. Any one of a number of organisms may cause acute inflammation of the lungs, but typical lobar pneumonia is nearly always caused by the pneumococcus. Although bronchopneumonia is often due to some other organism, the pneumococcus is usually the commonest invader found in this variety of pneumonia as well. The many types of pneumococci and other individual organisms which may give rise to pulmonary infection make it clear that pneumonia is not a single disease but a group of specific infections.

Our present clinical knowledge of pneumonia began largely with the excellent descriptions of Laënnec (755, 756). In 1819 and 1820 he described the pathologic changes and physical signs found during the course of the disease, advanced methods for distinguishing between this and other diseases of the chest, and for the first time made clear the clinical differentiation between pneumonia and pleurisy. Rokitansky (1104) in 1842 was apparently the first to distinguish lobar pneumonia from bronchopneumonia. In this early period investigations of pneumonia were few and chiefly of a clinical nature. Later, under the impetus of the discovery of bacteria and their possible relation to disease, a number of investigations of pneumonia and particularly of lobar pneumonia were begun. Gradually at first and then with increasing frequency bacteriologic studies of lobar pneumonia were made. The clinical type of study so prominent in the latter part of the last and in the early years of the present century gave way largely to bacteriologic and immunologic studies, the great value of which is only now becoming generally appreciated. In the meanwhile intensive research on the pneumococcus and the infections it produces is being continued in most parts of the civilized world.

Specialized and adapted for a parasitic life in man and in the higher animals, the pneumococcus has been found in many areas of the world and is doubtless present in all regions harboring such representatives of the animal kingdom. Normal man constitutes a vast reservoir of the organism, for a considerable proportion of all healthy individuals carry pneumococci in their nose and throat. In normal man in general the number of pneumococci appears to increase as a rising tide in temperate regions in the colder periods of the year and to recede again with the return of the sun. The frequency with which pneumonia occurs in such regions appears to parallel these changes.

A great many terms have been used for the identification of pneumonia. Among the older writers Wells (1400) in 1889 lists the synonyms for pneumonia as follows:

Peripneumonia
Pneumonia
Pneumonia vera
Peripneumonia notha
Peripneumonia catarrhalis
Pleuritis humida
Acute pneumonia
Lobar pneumonia
Acute lobar pneumonia
Primitive lobar pneumonia
Acute primitive diffuse pneumonia
Sthenic pneumonia
Croupous pneumonia
Acute croupous pneumonia
Croupous lobar pneumonia
Pneumonitis
Pleurisy and inflammation of the lungs
Lungenentzündung (lobäre)
Empresma pneumonitis
Simple legitimate pneumonia
Genuine fibrinous pneumonia
Acute asthenic exudative pneumonia
Pleuro-pneumonia
Pulmonia
Febris pneumonia
Lung fever
Pleuro-pneumonic fever
Pneumonic fever

Howard (661) gives the synonyms for lobar pneumonia as seen below:

Peripneumony
Peripneumonia vera
Febris peripneumonica
Febris pneumonica
Pneumonic fever
Pleuritis humida
Pleuro-pneumonia
Pneumonia
Croupous or fibrinous pneumonia
Acute or sthenic pneumonia

Acute lobar pneumonia
Congestion of the lungs
Inflammation of the lungs
Lung fever
Pulmonary fever

This investigator also gives German and French synonyms, as:

GERMAN

Fleier (North German)
Lungenentzündung, croupose Pneumonie
Pneumonitis, die genuine fibrinöse (lobäre) Pneumonie
(*Kruppösen Pneumonie* is also a German synonym)

FRENCH

Pneumonie lobaire
Fluxion de la poitrine
(*Pneumonie franche* is also a French synonym)

The *Manual of the International List of Causes of Death* for 1929 (1336), which is in current use, includes in the list under Diseases of the Respiratory System: 107. Bronchopneumonia (including capillary bronchitis); 108. Lobar pneumonia; and 109. Pneumonia, unspecified.

The titles listed in this classification under 107. Bronchopneumonia (including capillary bronchitis) are as follows:

(a) Bronchopneumonia includes

Aspiration pneumonia
Asthmatic pneumonia
Bronchial pneumonia
Bronchopleuropneumonia
Bronchopneumonia involving lobes
Bronchopulmonitis
Capillary pneumonia
Catarrhal inflammation of lung
  lung fever
  pneumonia
Chronic catarrhal pneumonia
Croupous bronchopneumonia
Deglutition pneumonia
Ether pneumonia
Infantile pneumonia
Inhalation pneumonia
Inspiration pneumonia
Insufflation pneumonia
Insular pneumonia
Lobular pneumonia
Membranous bronchopneumonia
Pleurobronchopneumonia
Pneumococcal bronchopneumonia
Septic bronchopneumonia
Typhoid bronchopneumonia
Vesicular pneumonia

(b) Capillary bronchitis includes

Acute capillary bronchitis
Capillary bronchitis
Chronic capillary bronchitis
Subacute capillary bronchitis
Suffocating bronchitis

The terms included under 108. Lobar pneumonia are:

Acute congestive pneumonia
  hepatization of lung
  inflammation of lung
  interstitial pneumonia
  pleuropneumonia
  pneumonia
  pneumonitis
  pulmonitis
Alcoholic pneumonia
  pneumonitis
Apex pneumonia
Apical pneumonia
Bilateral lobar pneumonia
  pleuropneumonia
  pneumonia
Central pneumonia
Circumscribed pneumonia
Congestive pneumonia
Consolidation of lung
Croupous pneumonia
Diplococcus pneumonia
Double pleuropneumonia
  pneumonia
Epidemic pneumonia
Fibrinous pneumonia
Fulminant pneumonia
Hepatization of lung
Hypostatic lobar pneumonia
Infectious pneumonia
Intermittent pneumonia
Lobar bronchopneumonia
Lobar pneumonia
Lung fever
Massive pneumonia
Migratory pneumonia
Organized pneumonia
Peripneumonia
Pleurolobar pneumonia
Pleuroperipneumonia
Pleuropneumonia
Pneumococcus pneumonia
Pneumonic fever
Pneumopleurisy
Pneumopleuritis
Solidifaction of lung
Splenopneumonia
True pneumonia
Unresolved pneumonia

The terms included under 109. Pneumonia, unspecified, are:

Adynamic pneumonia
Asthenic pneumonia
Cerebral pneumonia
Diffuse pneumonia
Fungoid pneumonia
Gangrenous pneumonia
Inflammation of chest
  lung
Latent pneumonia
Metastatic pneumonia
Pneumococcus infection (unqualified)
Pneumonia
Pneumonic congestion
Pneumonitis
Postoperative pneumonia
Progressive pneumonia
Pulmonitis
Senile pneumonia
Septic pleuropneumonia
  pneumonia
Suppurative pneumonia
Surgical pneumonia
Typhoid pneumonia

The terms this title (Pneumonia, unspecified) does not include and their numbers in the International List of Causes of Death are as follows:

Pneumonia: caseous (23) or bacillary (23), or any other synonym of tuberculosis of the lungs
Catarrhal pneumonia (107)
Interstitial pneumonia (114)
Pulmonary congestion (111)
Hypostatic pneumonia (111)
Pneumatosis (200)
Pneumococcemia (36)
Specific pneumonia (34)

For the purposes of this volume, discussion is confined primarily to lobar pneumonia, most cases of which are due to infection with pneumococci of some type. Concise descriptions of the disease are largely lacking. Perhaps the most satisfactory definition is that given by Lord (809). He states:

> Pneumonia due to the pneumococcus differs from pulmonary infection with other organisms in that it has an explosive onset, usual massive lung involvement, short course, abrupt termination and relatively rapid restoration of the involved area to normal.

At times, and whenever available, information relating to pneumonia in other forms is also included. The data presented relate chiefly to cases in adults; where cases in infants and children are included, mention of the fact is made. In nearly all instances, except as altered for some special purpose indicated in the text, the references cited are listed in chronologic order.

CHAPTER ONE

CAUSATIVE ORGANISMS IN PNEUMONIA; AND PNEUMONIA NOT DUE TO PNEUMOCOCCI

Causative Organisms in Pneumonia 1
Pneumonia Not Due to Pneumococci 3
Streptococcus Pneumonia 3
Friedländer's Bacillus Pneumonia 5
Influenza Bacillus (*Hemophylus influenzae*) Pneumonia 8
Staphylococcus Pneumonia 9
Mixed Infections 11
Miscellaneous Infections 16

CAUSATIVE ORGANISMS IN PNEUMONIA

THE careful investigation of several large series of cases of lobar pneumonia has revealed that nearly all cases are due to pneumococcus infection. Pneumococci were obtained from 95 per cent of 480 cases from which the etiologic agent could be isolated by Avery, Chickering, Cole, and Dochez (33) at the Hospital of the Rockefeller Institute for Medical Research in 1917. In 1926 Cecil, Baldwin, and Larsen (230) at the Bellevue Hospital, New York City, found pneumococci responsible for over 95 per cent of 2,000 cases. In addition, of 839 cases reported by Sutliff and Finland (1271) in 1933 from the Boston City Hospital, 98 per cent were caused by pneumococci. The findings in each of these series are summarized in Table 1. Almost all cases were in adults.

Of the combined total of 3,319 cases, 3,189, or 96.1 per cent, were due to the pneumococcus. Of the remaining 130 cases, 124 were attributed to infection by the streptococcus, Friedländer's bacillus, influenza bacillus, or staphylococcus, and the other 6 were reported as cases of mixed infection. Streptococci were found in only 2.8 per cent; Friedländer's bacilli in 0.5 per cent; and infections due to influenza bacilli and to staphylococci, and mixed infections accounted for 0.2 per cent each. It is extraordinary that organisms other than the pneumococcus so seldom cause lobar pneumonia.

Cole summarized the experience of the Hospital of the Rockefeller Institute for Medical Research with 1,517 cases of pneumonia of various varieties over a period of some sixteen years (298). This careful study embraced 1,172 cases of acute lobar pneumonia, 62 of which were of undetermined etiology, all the rest being attributed to pneumococci; and 345 cases of bronchopneumonia of varied etiology. It was found that cases of primary pneumonia due to organisms other than pneumococci were usually atypical and occurred in the form of bronchopneumonia with patchy consolidations. It is clear that if miscellaneous organisms do cause true lobar pneumonia, their incidence as the inciting factor in such cases has been small.

TABLE I. BACTERIOLOGIC CLASSIFICATION OF 3,319 CASES OF LOBAR PNEUMONIA

	PNEUMOCOCCUS CASES	STREPTOCOCCUS CASES	FRIEDLÄNDER'S BACILLUS CASES	INFLUENZA BACILLUS CASES	STAPHYLOCOCCUS CASES	MIXED INFECTION CASES	TOTAL CASES
Avery, Chickering, Cole, and Dochez (33)	454	8	3	6	3	6	480
Cecil, Baldwin, and Larsen (230)	1,913	76	8	1	2	–	2,000
Sutliff and Finland (1271)	822	10	6	–	1	–	839
Total	3,189	94	17	7	6	6	3,319
Per cent	96.1	2.8	0.5	0.2	0.2	0.2	100.0

Bullowa (190) reported the incidence of pneumococci and other organisms in a group of 4,416 cases of pneumonia (lobar pneumonia and bronchopneumonia together) in adults at the Harlem Hospital, New York City, studied over the period of July 1, 1928—June 30, 1936. In this series pneumococci were responsible for the pneumonia in 3,591 cases, or 81.3 per cent of the whole group. Cases due to other organisms, including mixed infections, numbered 825 and made up 18.7 per cent of the series. Nearly 10 per cent of all cases were due to streptococci, less than one per cent were due to staphylococci, and 1.1 per cent (50 cases) were due to Friedländer's bacilli. Mixed infections occurred in 121, or 2.7 per cent, of the cases, while in 88, or 2 per cent, the etiologic agent was not identified.

In the same report Bullowa (190) gave the incidence of pneumococci and other organisms in a series of 1,712 cases of pneumonia (lobar pneumonia and bronchopneumonia together) in infants and children over the eight-year period of 1928–1936. Pneumococci were found in 923 of the cases (53.9 per cent) and other organisms in 789 cases (46.1 per cent). A previous investigation of similar cases in infants and children was made by Nemir, Andrews, and Vinograd (931) over a period covering approximately five pneumonia seasons, from January 1931 to June 1935 at the Bellevue Hospital, New York City. Pneumococci were found in 796 of the 1,033 cases studied (77 per cent). When these two large series of cases in infants and children are combined, there is a total of 2,745 cases, of which 1,719, or 62.6 per cent, were due to pneumococci and 1,026, or 37.4 per cent, to other organisms.

PNEUMONIA NOT DUE TO PNEUMOCOCCI

Streptococcus Pneumonia

As already seen, the streptococcus has been reported responsible, under ordinary circumstances, for from 2 to 4 per cent of all cases of lobar pneumonia (33, 230, 1271). In most such cases hemolytic streptococci are found. It is probable, however, as Cecil, Baldwin, and Larsen (230) have stated, that in many instances where such organisms are found associated with lobar pneumonia the disease is initiated by the pneumococcus, and the streptococcus is simply a secondary invader. Both pneumococci and streptococci are frequently found together in such cases (1163, 969, 987, 1218). On the basis of clinical studies and necropsy observations it was determined that streptococcus pneumonia is usually (824, 969, 298, 259, 788), but not always (219), a bronchopneumonia. Attempts to produce experimental hemolytic streptococcus pneumonia in animals (monkeys, 126, and dogs, 772, 1292, 1328) have shown that, if pneumonia develops, it is of the diffuse bronchopneumonic type.

Streptococcus pneumonia is usually endemic but may become epidemic, as it did during the War (892, 219, 1163, 774, 298). Pathologic studies of such cases were made by various investigators (824, 219, 1250, 969). In most instances the lesion found in the lungs was a bronchopneumonia. The characteristic lesion varied from an interstitial bronchopneumonia with firm peribronchial nodes (MacCallum, 824, Cecil, 219) to more extensive lobular consolidations with subpleural abscesses and interstitial suppurative pneumonia (Opie, Blake, Small, and Rivers, 969, Cole, 298). In monkeys with experimental streptococcus pneumonia, Blake and Cecil (126) were able to duplicate these observations and found that the larger doses of organisms produced the more extensive lobular consolidations and tissue necrosis.

A great many streptococcus cases, apparently very similar to those referred to above, have occurred during the past decade among the African natives employed on the Witwatersrand Goldfields in South Africa where Lister and Ordman (788) regard the infection as probably secondary to some virus disease. Though streptococcus pneumonia is frequently secondary to some other acute illness, especially measles and influenza, it apparently may begin suddenly in individuals without previous illness (Amoss and Craven, 14). Negroes appear very susceptible to it (219, 788). A history of a previous upper respiratory infection may frequently be obtained (892, 298). At the time of onset pleural pain may or may not be present, and chill is frequently absent. The symptoms are usually severe with a high temperature, cherry-red cyanosis, prostration, hypotension, and evidence of a severe toxemia and a rapidly spreading process (892, 774, 298, 14). Bacteriemia is apparently not frequent (298, 219) but of very grave import if found (259, 190). Empyema may be found within a day or so of onset (892, 219) and is extremely common.

The lower lobes on either or both sides are attacked more frequently than other lobes (892). Chief among the lesions associated with the pneumonia is an intense reddening of the whole respiratory tract. In some, the larynx and adjacent structures may be involved with ulceration. While empyema is very common, pericarditis, peritonitis, sinusitis, and other focal lesions are not (824).

Though less frequent, cases due to non-hemolytic streptococci are milder and cause fewer empyemas than those due to hemolytic streptococci. Cecil (219) found only 10.9 per cent of 64 cases due to non-hemolytic streptococci developed empyema, whereas this complication occurred in 50 per cent of 118 cases due to hemolytic streptococci. The fatality rate of uncomplicated cases of non-hemolytic streptococcus pneumonia was 4.3 per cent. Among 53 cases of hemolytic streptococcus pneumonia without empyema there was a fatality rate of 11.3 per cent, as compared with a rate of 56.4 per cent for 55 cases due to this organism in which empyema was present. Observations of similar significance have been reported by other investigators (824, 1250, 774, 969, 298).

The general reported fatality rate of streptococcus pneumonia in adults has varied from 32.5 per cent among 346 cases (Miller and Lusk, 892) and 43 per cent in 83 cases (Cole, 298) to 54 per cent among 48 cases (Leopold, 774). In cases reported by Bullowa (190) the fatality rate of 191 cases due to streptococci of undetermined variety was 21 per cent (40 deaths); of 114 cases due to streptococcus *Alpha* 13.2 per cent (15 deaths); of 4 cases due to streptococcus *Gamma* 25 per cent; and of 99 cases due to streptococcus *Beta* 39.4 per cent (39 deaths). In children the fatality rate may be higher (821) or lower (1435, 190) than in adults. Bullowa (190) found a fatality rate of

27.6 per cent for 29 cases (8 deaths) in infants under two years of age and of 18.4 per cent for 38 cases (7 deaths) in older children with *Beta*-hemolytic streptococcus pneumonia. In cases due to streptococci of unidentified variety he also reported a fatality rate of 19.6 per cent for 183 cases (36 deaths) in infants under two years of age and of 1.3 per cent for 224 cases (3 deaths) in children over this age.

Numerous therapeutic agents have been used in streptococcus cases and in the past relatively little favorable effect was produced. Amoss, Persons, and Hansen-Prüss (15) and Amoss and Craven (14), however, report treating eight cases due to *Beta*-hemolytic streptococci with antistreptococcus horse serum with good results. Injections of the serum into the pleural cavity may have prevented the development of empyema in one case and been of benefit in the treatment of this complication in two others. Treatment with human immune blood or serum obtained from patients recovered from streptococcus infections may be used. The immuno-transfusion method of Lyons (822) may aid. Suitable donors are selected whose blood is shown by opsonic tests to contain antibacterial antibody and to facilitate phagocytosis of the streptococcus in question. Bullowa (190) advises the administration of as much as 100 cc. once or twice daily, of the serum of patients convalescent from scarlet fever. The recent introduction of sulfanilamide gives hope of much more satisfactory therapeutic results, at least in *Beta*-hemolytic streptococcus infections, than were formerly obtainable with other agents. Bullowa (190) has reported favorable results in some cases treated with sulfanilamide. The use of this preparation and its related compounds is described elsewhere (see pages 783–790).

Friedländer's Bacillus Pneumonia

Pneumonia due to Friedländer's bacillus is not often encountered. Of the 3,319 cases of lobar pneumonia listed in Table 1, only 17, or 0.5 per cent, were attributed to this organism. Over a period of sixteen years at the Hospital of the Rockefeller Institute for Medical Research, Cole (298) found only seven cases of Friedländer's bacillus pneumonia, and all of these presented signs of atypical consolidation. In a series of 5,000 pneumonias of all varieties at the Bellevue Hospital, New York City, Solomon (1217) found 32, or approximately 0.6 per cent, due to Friedländer's bacillus. In Bullowa's (190) series of 4,416 cases of pneumonia (lobar pneumonia and bronchopneumonia together) at the Harlem Hospital, New York City, 50, or slightly more than one per cent, were due to this organism. Heffron and

Varley (616) found *B. friedländeri* in only seven, or one per cent, of 716 specimens of sputum and other material obtained from patients with various kinds of respiratory disease. These figures suggest a much lower incidence than that reported by Belk (91) and Fremmel, Henrichsen, and Sweany (492) who, from a general review of the literature concerning this organism, state that its reported incidence in lobar pneumonia varies from 0.5 to 10 per cent. In a bacteriologic investigation of 100 cases of lobar pneumonia in India, Bhatnagar and Singh (100) found 13 due to Friedländer's bacillus. They also reported that the highest incidence of these cases occurred in summer. In the German epidemic described by Zander (1458) all of 411 cases occurred during the winter.

First isolated from patients with pneumonia in 1882 by Friedländer (500), this organism was subsequently shown to have an extraordinary similarity to the pneumococcus in many of its biologic and immunologic characteristics. Julianelle's studies indicate that, as with the pneumococcus, Friedländer's bacillus can be divided serologically into three specific types, referred to as Types A, B, and C, and a miscellaneous X group (695, 696, 697). The organism also may occur in type-specific, virulent, encapsulated forms or in species-specific, rough, avirulent, unencapsulated forms.

The virulent, encapsulated forms produce a soluble specific substance during their growth, and these substances, polysaccharide in nature, differ one from another and appear specific for the type by which they were produced. Further, this soluble substance has been found in the blood and urine of patients (Blake, 118) and animals (Julianelle, 697) infected with this organism. Its presence has also been detected in the sputum. At the Massachusetts State Bacteriologic Laboratory, using diagnostic serum for Friedländer's bacillus Type A, the Krumwiede test and Neufeld capsule-swelling technic of typing (see pages 629 and 625) have both been successfully applied, in the first instance to sputums from patients with pneumonia due to this organism, and in the second to the organism itself. Humoral agglutinins have been detected in the serum of a few patients at about the time of recovery (100).

The organism is a common inhabitant of the nasopharynx of persons with chronic sinusitis and some chronic lung lesions, such as tumors and bronchiectasis (807). Occasionally it is found mixed with pneumococci in the sputum of pneumonia patients and not uncommonly causes secondary pulmonary infection in such cases (807, 91, 492).

Though usually endemic, pneumonia due to Friedländer's bacillus has occurred in epidemic form. Zander (1458) described an outbreak in Germany during which 399 cases occurred in persons within a prison and 12 in others outside. The pulmonary lesion produced is usually atypical, though occasionally it may assume the lobar form. Lord (807) found this organism the only apparent cause of illness in 6 of 192 cases of lobar pneumonia coming to necropsy at the Massachusetts General Hospital. Belk (91), Olcott (966), and Bullowa (190) have likewise reported several necropsied cases of lobar pneumonia due to this organism. Still, from the discussion of Friedländer's bacillus pneumonia given by Fremmel and his associates (492), it is apparent that opinion is divided as to whether or not the organism can produce pneumonia in the lobar form. They reported that, pathologically, the most important findings were a pseudo-lobar consolidation due to a dense confluent bronchopneumonia and that true lobar consolidation was rare. In experimental animals infected with the organism, Lamar and Meltzer (757) produced what they regarded as a lobar type of pneumonia in dogs, while the consolidations obtained by Christie, Ehrich, and Binger (269) in dogs and by Hoyle (664) in mice were irregular and patchy.

In man the disease appears especially prone to occur in alcoholics around fifty years of age (492). The onset is generally sudden and without a chill. The infection is severe; the temperature is usually around 102° F.; and in cases with unmixed infections a moderate leucocytosis of 15,000 or less, with about 85 per cent polymorphonuclears, may be present, though normal counts, and even a leucopenia, are not uncommon (91, 492, 966). The course is irregular and, according to Fremmel and his co-workers, the diagnosis is made chiefly when the organism is found in the sputum, together with rareness of rales, and slight physical signs in an acutely ill patient (492). The usual absence of marked physical findings is attributed to the fact that, pathologically, the lesion resembles pulmonary engorgement rather than consolidation, and the lack of subcrepitant rales may be due to the extreme stickiness of the exudate filling the alveoli. Roentgenograms may show little early in the disease, but later frequently reveal thin-walled abscess cavities in the lung. The sputum is very tenacious, with little odor, and contains the organisms in large numbers. Blood cultures are occasionally positive (966, 100). Bullowa (190), however, reports bacteriemia in 63.5 per cent of cases either during the course of the illness or terminally. While the process may resemble lobar pneumonia and the course be somewhat similar, it usually terminates more abruptly. The prognosis is grave and death often occurs before the fourth day.

There is frequently much necrosis and destruction of lung tissue, leading to abscess formation. Lung abscesses were found in twelve of eighteen cases reported by Belk (91). In a few instances the lesion may assume a chronic nature and persist over weeks or months and at times be confused with pulmonary tuberculosis (310), though generally the temperature curve is more of the septic variety.

In its endemic form the fatality rate of Friedländer's bacillus pneumonia is high. In Cole's series of seven cases, 71 per cent died (298), as did over 92 per cent of thirteen cases reported by Bhatnagar and Singh (100). Of 39 cases given general medical treatment by Bullowa (190), death occurred in 32, or 82 per cent. The fatality rate of the epidemic form of the disease appears considerably lower, however, and was reported as 36 per cent among 399 cases in the prison epidemic studied by Zander (1458). Methods of nonspecific treatment have proved of little value. In some instances the use of a type-specific immune serum has been tried, though with no great success. In eleven serum treated cases reported by Bullowa (190) there were seven deaths (63.6 per cent).

Influenza Bacillus (Hemophylus influenzae) *Pneumonia*

The influenza bacillus rarely, if ever, causes true lobar pneumonia. Only 7, or 0.2 per cent, of the 3,319 cases in Table 1 were attributed to this organism, and details concerning these cases are lacking. Among eight cases due to this organism, reported by Cole (298), all showed atypical consolidations. Observations of similar significance have been reported by others (807, 788).

In both lobar pneumonia and bronchopneumonia the influenza bacillus is very commonly present in the sputum along with other organisms and most often is found in combination with the streptococcus or pneumococcus (969, 1108, 797, 230, 534). For years the influenza bacillus was regarded by many investigators as the etiologic agent responsible for the endemic, epidemic, and at times pandemic forms of influenza which were so often accompanied by severe pulmonary lesions, frequently leading to death (1304). Investigations in recent years have revealed that at least one form of the mild interpandemic diseases called influenza may be attributed to a filterable virus (1214, 479). It seems entirely possible that other forms of influenza will subsequently prove due to similar agents.

The influenza bacillus alone, however, is well known to be pathogenic for man, and in experimental animals may lead to a bronchopneumonia of variable severity, as was observed by Blake and Cecil (127, 234) in monkeys, and by Hoyle (664) in mice. In each instance repeated animal passage was necessary before the virulence of the test culture became sufficient to produce these lesions.

In monkeys with influenza bacillus pneumonia there was marked prostration and cough, an irregular temperature, and either leucopenia or no special change of the leucocyte count. Pathologically, acute sinusitis, tracheobronchitis, hemorrhagic edema of the lungs, bronchiolitis, and bronchopneumonia were found. In man the lesion may be more marked and produce a widespread injury to the mucosa and submucosa of the bronchi extending to the terminal bronchioles (119). Its intensity may vary from a catarrhal inflammation to actual necrosis and destruction of the bronchial walls leading to acute bronchiectasis. Bacteriemia is rare (259).

The fatality rate of pure influenza bacillus pneumonia is impossible to appraise, for in reported cases there is always the possibility that infection was initiated by some other organism or a filterable virus with the subsequent development of influenza bacillus pneumonia. The fatality rate of cases occurring in various military camps in this country during the influenza pandemic of 1917–1919 varied from 4 per cent to over 87 per cent and was highest early in the outbreak and thereafter gradually decreased (Lord, 807). Among the eight cases reported by Cole (298), none of which occurred during the influenza epidemic, one, or 12.5 per cent, died. During the War, convalescent serum was used for treatment, but its value was not proved (see page 812).

Staphylococcus Pneumonia

Of the 3,319 cases of lobar pneumonia listed in Table 1, only six, or 0.2 per cent, were attributed to the staphylococcus. It is not clear, however, that this organism can cause true lobar pneumonia, and the lesion produced is usually of the bronchopneumonic type (260, 969, 821, 1435, 298, 1067, 788). From a general review of the literature dealing with staphylococcus pneumonia, Reimann's findings suggest that about 7 to 9 per cent of all atypical pneumonias are due to this organism (1067). The organism usually present in these cases is the *Staphylococcus aureus*. Bronchopneumonia is produced in dogs (1364, 1328) and mice (664) suitably infected with this organism.

Staphylococcus pneumonias are likely to be secondary to other infections, especially respiratory, to follow operations, or to occur during the course of chronic debilitating diseases (260, 969, 298, 1067). Secondary pneumonia due to the organism may at times be the terminal event in the course of an ordinary pneumococcus lobar pneumonia and in some of these instances be responsible for an apparent failure of specific serum therapy. An extensive epidemic of atypical pneumonias, largely caused by the *Staphylococcus aureus,* occurred during the War at Camp Jackson, South Carolina. Chickering and Park (260) investigated the outbreak and reported 153 cases due to this organism. In 92 cases no other organism was present, while in the remainder influenza bacilli, pneumococci, or streptococci were also found.

The onset is usually (260), but not always (1067), insidious and without a chill and with a high fever. Prostration is marked, even early. The temperature is usually remittent, as is characteristic of staphylococcus infection elsewhere in the body, and sweats are variable. The general picture resembles a septicaemia. Cyanosis is marked and produces a peculiar cherry-red or indigo-blue color. Painful labored breathing is uncommon. The process tends to be diffuse, though not uncommonly dependent portions of the lungs, such as the lower lobes, are attacked. Physical examination and roentgenograms usually reveal little early, and, later, evidence of a diffuse involvement of the whole lung fields. The leucocyte count is variable, and normal or low counts are not infrequent. The course of five to ten days is rapid and generally shorter by a few days than that of ordinary pneumonia.

Chickering and Park (260) regard the character of the sputum as presenting the most typical feature of the disease. In their cases the sputum was usually purulent and of a dirty salmon pink, resembling "anchovy sauce," but in some instances was greenish-yellow or hemorrhagic. The appearance of the sputum, as well as the fact that it contains the organisms in large numbers, is of diagnostic importance. Bacteriemia is variable (260, 1067). Subcutaneous emphysema may occur (260).

Complications are not frequent, perhaps because the course is usually too short to permit their development. At necropsy, however, the lungs commonly show a confluent bronchopneumonia with multiple small scattered staphylococcus abscesses both in the parenchyma and just beneath the pleura. Empyema, pericarditis, endocarditis, otitis media, and meningitis may be present. In patients who survive, pulmonary abscess is almost the rule (259, 1067).

The prognosis of staphylococcus pneumonia in adults is usually poor. Only two of Chickering and Park's 153 cases recovered. Of Cole's (298) 19 cases, 13, or 68.4 per cent, died, as did 71 per cent of 7 cases reported by Chickering (259) in 1930. Death occurred in 55.6 per cent, or 15 of 27 cases studied by Bullowa (190). There were, however, only two deaths (33.3 per cent) among 6 cases observed by Reimann (1067). In infants and children the reported fatality rate has varied from 25 to 80 per cent (821, 1435, 190).

Immune antistaphylococcus horse serum and blood transfusions have been used in treatment with little or no apparent effect. Bullowa (190) considers intracutaneous injections of staphylococcus toxoid every third or fourth day may be of aid in non-bacteriemic cases.

Mixed Infections

Cases in which the possibility exists that two or more organisms are involved in the pneumonic process constitute an important group. Though instances of mixed infections have been reported by various observers in the past, few efforts were made to determine the relative significance of each of the organisms found (797, 821, 230, 298, 1321, 183). At times, however, in the course of special studies, occasional cases of mixed infection were carefully investigated (307, 969, 299, 238, 1272, 710, 188). In addition, the extensive investigations of Sutliff and Finland (1271), Finland and Winkler (468), Winkler and Finland (1429), and of Finland (445), who have combined clinical information with that obtained by bacteriologic, immunologic, and pathologic means, have thrown much light on this problem.

Under ordinary circumstances the nature of the organism causing infection in pneumonia is determined by examination of the sputum; or a throat culture, blood culture, or the urine, if sputum is not available (see pages 614–643). Various other means are also of use in establishing the identity of the etiologic agent responsible for the infection. During life or after death material may be removed for examination from an infected pleural cavity or from the lung by lung puncture or suction. At necropsy, cultures may be made from these areas, the blood, and other sources. And, finally, and occasionally of considerable importance, serum from convalescent patients may be tested against various organisms for agglutinins, precipitins, and bactericidal and mouse protective properties.

In any instance where multiple bacterial agents are obtained from the sputum or other sources from patients with pneumonia, it becomes necessary to determine, if possible, the role each plays in the infection. A true double infection may markedly affect the course of the illness, the expectancy of complications, the speed of application and efficacy of specific serum therapy in some instances, and at times practically extinguish the chances of recovery. In addition, in some instances, even though a single organism be isolated at first, subsequent study may show the patient to be infected with a different agent. Sutliff and Finland (1271) and Finland and Winkler (468, 469) made a comparison of the types of pneumococci found in the sputum in pneumonia and those isolated from other sources in the same patient, and of the antibody response of patients to infection with different types. Their results indicate "that certain types, such as Type I, II or V, are more apt to be etiologically significant than others, particularly Type III and certain of the types formerly classified in Group IV" (Finland, 445).

As suggested by Bullowa (183) and clearly shown by Finland (445), cases of mixed infection can be roughly classified into three groups: (a) those in which only one of the organisms found is causing the infection and the other or others are probably incidental; (b) those with concurrent infections in which more than one organism is producing a simultaneous invasion at the same or different sites; and (c) those with consecutive infections or superinfections where one invasion follows another in the same or different sites.

It will be appreciated that cases in the first of the above groups, in which only one of the organisms found is causing the infection, do not really represent mixed infections. Cases of pneumococcus pneumonia are frequently reported in this way, however, for unless they are intensively investigated from several angles it is often impossible to determine whether or not the other organisms present are involved in the infection. If the results of sputum examination alone were relied upon as evidence of a mixed infection, such cases would appear common, for two or more organisms may frequently be found in the sputum in pneumonia. This was recognized by Cecil, Baldwin, and Larsen (230), who analyzed 1,913 typed cases of pneumococcus lobar pneumonia to show the incidence of cases having a mixed flora in the sputum (see Table 2).

TABLE 2. PNEUMOCOCCUS LOBAR PNEUMONIA. NUMBER OF CASES AND NUMBER AND PERCENTAGE OF CASES WITH MIXED BACTERIAL FLORA IN THE SPUTUM, BY TYPE

	TOTAL CASES	CASES WITH MIXED FLORA *Number*	*Per cent*
Type I	644	119	18.4
Type II	368	87	23.6
Type III	268	64	23.9
Group IV	633	199	31.2
Total	1,913	469	24.5

From Cecil *et al.* (230)

Out of the total 1,913 cases, 469 or 24.5 per cent showed a pneumococcus plus some other organism present in the sputum. Occurrences of this nature were fewest among Type I cases (18.4 per cent) and most common among those due to pneumococci of Group IV (31.2 per cent). These investigators also noted that the incidence of cases with a mixed flora in their sputum was greater in some years than in others. In one winter only 11.5 per cent of the cases showed two or more organisms in the sputum, while in the following winter, during part of which influenza was prevalent in the community, over four times the proportion (52.7 per cent) of such occurrences was found.

The total group of cases of Cecil and his associates showing two or more organisms in the sputum was further divided to show the bacteria isolated (see Table 3). The most frequent combination of organisms found was a

TABLE 3. PNEUMOCOCCUS LOBAR PNEUMONIA CASES HAVING MORE THAN ONE ORGANISM IN THE SPUTUM. DISTRIBUTION BY BACTERIUM FOUND

ORGANISMS IN SPUTUM	NUMBER OF CASES
Pneumococcus and *B. influenzae*	330
Pneumococcus and hemolytic streptococcus	82
Pneumococcus, *B. influenzae,* and hemolytic streptococcus	28
Pneumococcus, *B. influenzae,* and non-hemolytic streptococcus	5
Pneumococcus, Type I and Type III	1
Pneumococcus, Type I and Group IV	4
Pneumococcus, Type III and Group IV	7
Pneumococcus and tubercle bacillus	4
Pneumococcus and Friedländer's bacillus	9
Total	470

From Cecil *et al.* (230)

pneumococcus in association with the influenza bacillus. This grouping was present in the sputum in 330 of the 470 cases tabulated. Others have also found the influenza bacillus frequently associated with either lobar pneumonia (534) or bronchopneumonia (797, 298). Studies over many years have shown, however, that the mere presence of various organisms in the sputum cannot be regarded as proof that they are necessarily involved in the pulmonary process.

Doubtless the incidental organisms found in the sputum are members of the group normally inhabiting the nasopharynx or at times associated with preceding infection of the upper respiratory tract (1181, 898, 1209, 1393, 732, 367, 1206, 1210, 301; see Pneumococcus Carriers, pages 342–378). The examination of indifferent specimens of sputum containing secretions from the mouth, nose, or throat, or of throat cultures carelessly obtained, frequently reveals such organisms. Occurrences of this nature doubtless account for numerous inconsistencies in the findings of sputum or throat culture examinations in which, in a single patient, pneumococci of one type are found in one sample and those of another in a different sample or in material from a different source (111, 1264, 1057, 445, 188). Cases in this group may show a pneumococcus of one type, such as Type III or one of the less common higher types, in the sputum at one examination and at repeated subsequent examinations of the sputum show only Type I or II. Or a pneumococcus of one type may be obtained from the sputum while cultures of the blood or material removed by lung puncture may show only pneumococci of another type (188), or examination of the patient's serum in convalescence may reveal that antibodies have developed against a type different from that found in the sputum (445). Repeated examinations of the sputum and urine and of serial blood cultures are an excellent and simple means of dealing with these cases, though at times a more intensive investigation will be necessary.

Unquestionably some of the cases reported by Cecil and his co-workers, listed in Table 2 as having a mixed bacterial flora in the sputum, did have a true mixed infection. Due to the nature of their report, it is not possible, however, to determine in what proportion of the cases this held true. In all, 24.5 per cent of their 1,913 cases showed a mixed flora in the sputum. Better evidence of the incidence of true mixed infections in pneumococcus pneumonia has been obtained by others who have carried out extensive studies for this purpose. Bullowa (183) reported that 56 or 3 per cent of 1,601 cases and Sutliff and Finland (1271) that 33 or 4 per cent of 822 cases had multiple infections. Finland (445) reported that among approximately 2,000 cases of pneumonia or pneumococcic infections there were 133 cases of pneumonia associated with the finding of a pneumococcus plus one or more other organisms. In 37 of these cases pneumococci of more than one type were present, including 4 cases with three types and 4 with pneumococci of two types plus some other organism. In the remaining 96 cases pneumococci of one type and one or more other organisms were found. In addition to these 133 cases, there were 9 others previously reported by Winkler and Finland (1429) whose serum in convalescence gave reactions indicating that their pneumonia was caused by a type of pneumococcus different from that isolated from the patient.

Returning again to the classification of cases of mixed infection mentioned above, the second group, or those with concurrent or simultaneous infections due to two or more organisms, may be mentioned. Proved cases of this variety, due either to pneumococci of two types or to a pneumococcus and some other organism, are rare. Finland (445) has called attention to these cases and has given a detailed report of two cases of this nature. In one, examination of the sputum and blood during life and cultures of the lung at necropsy showed the infection due to pneumococci of Types I and III. Bullowa (188) has reported a few cases which may be similar to this in that two types were obtained from the lung by lung puncture. In Finland's second case, the sputum showed Type VI pneumococci and Friedländer's bacilli, but only the latter organism was found in the blood. At necropsy, cultures of the heart's blood and the consolidated right lower lobe, as well as sections from this lobe, showed Friedländer's bacilli only. In the right middle lobe, however, which was also consolidated, pneumococci of Type VI were found in pure culture. In this case the different organisms were producing a simultaneous involvement in different sites.

The third group of mixed infections was that of super- or consecutive infections, where one invasion with one organism may be followed by another with a different organism in the same or different sites, as is also mentioned later (see pages 532–533). Cases of this nature were observed during epidemics of measles or influenza in some of the military camps during the War (307, 969). They may also occur in interepidemic periods and occasionally are responsible for the apparent failure of specific serum therapy of some cases of pneumococcus pneumonia (299, 238, 1299, 183, 1000, 1272, 710, 445, 813). These secondary infections are most frequently due to hemolytic streptococci, but occasionally to pneumococci of another type, or staphylococci, and less commonly to some other organism.

Finland (445) has reported several cases in this category, and, in three, considerable detail is given. One patient showed Type I pneumococci in the sputum at each of two examinations separated by a two-day interval. The pulmonary lesion extended, but the infection was apparently overcome with the aid of serum therapy. Parotitis developed. After a two-day period of considerable improvement, the patient again became seriously ill and died four days later. Blood cultures were repeatedly negative. At necropsy the parotid gland and involved portion of the lungs showed no pneumococci, but

Staphylococcus aureus was found in pure culture. A similar type of case with necropsy occurred during the Massachusetts Pneumonia Study (869). The second of Finland's cases was in a patient with Type VIII pneumonia who developed circulating antibodies against this organism. The lesion in the lobe originally involved was found to be resolving at necropsy, and patchy consolidation was present in one lobe on the opposite side. The lungs contained *Staphylococcus aureus* and hemolytic streptococci but no pneumococci. The third case in Finland's group recovered. Though only the right lower lobe was involved, this patient had two attacks of pneumonia separated by a few days. Type III pneumococci were found in the sputum in the first instance and, later, Type VII. In convalescence, circulating antibodies against both these types (those for Type III being found first) were demonstrated in the patient's serum.

It appears probable that in many cases superinfections, and possibly concurrent or simultaneous infections as well, arise from exogenous infection and are not simply the result of autoinfection due to a lowered resistance. Numerous cases supporting this view were studied by Opie, Blake, Small, and Rivers (969) during the War. Convalescent cases of lobar pneumonia due to one organism (mostly pneumococcus) in contact with cases due to another organism (usually streptococcus) frequently developed infection with the second organism and rapidly died. It would seem easier to prevent than to cure such cases.

Miscellaneous Infections

It has been the experience of workers investigating large series of cases of lobar pneumonia to encounter an occasional case from which the etiologic agent could not be isolated with the methods used or available. For example, in Cole's series of 1,172 cases 1,110 were attributed to pneumococcus infection, while the bacterial incitant of the remaining 62 cases was undetermined (298). In Bullowa's (190) group of 4,416 cases of pneumonia (lobar pneumonia and bronchopneumonia together) the etiology was unknown in 88, or 2 per cent of the cases. Whenever the procedures useful in etiologic diagnosis, mentioned above in connection with mixed infections, can be carefully applied, it should be possible to ascertain the nature of the infecting organism in practically every case (see also pages 614–645).

Pulmonary lesions of varying extent, though generally of the bronchopneumonic variety, are usual in psittacosis (807, 1139, 651) and are common in tularemia (1326, 575, 19, 1201). Pulmonary lesions may be associated with rheumatic fever, as will be seen later (see pages 652–653). Certain fungus diseases (in addition to those caused by bacteria), such as actinomycosis and torulosis, and infestation with some animal parasites may also cause pulmonary lesions of varying severity (376). These latter groups are well discussed by Lord (807) and Norris and Landis (961) and also by Castellani and Chalmers (217) in their *Manual of Tropical Medicine.**

* See also Reimann, H. A., *The Pneumonias,* Philadelphia, W. B. Saunders, 1938, 381 p., which was published subsequent to the preparation of this section.

CHAPTER TWO

THE PNEUMOCOCCUS AND TYPE INCIDENCE IN PNEUMONIA

The Pneumococcus 18
Biology 19
Morphology and Cultural Characteristics 20
Autolysis and Bile Solubility 20
Drying and Storage of Cultures 21
Toxin Production 21
Types and Their Identification 22
Cell Components 24
Pneumococcus Variants 26
Antigenicity 27
Proportion of Strains at Present Classifiable 29
World-wide Distribution of Pneumococcus Types 31
Type Incidence in Pneumonia 42
Types I, II, III, and Group IV 42
Incidence in Lobar Pneumonia 42
Variation of Incidence with Geographic Distribution 47
Types IV through XXXII 49
Causal Relation to Pneumonia 49
Incidence in Lobar Pneumonia 51
Incidence in Pneumococcus Pneumonia 54
Variation of Type Incidence in Lobar Pneumonia with Certain Factors other than Geographic Distribution 57
The Pneumococcus and Bronchopneumonia 67
The Pneumonias of Infants and Children 74
Commonest Types in Lobar Pneumonia and Bronchopneumonia 89

THE PNEUMOCOCCUS

In 1881 Pasteur (1002) in France and Sternberg* (1227) in this country almost synchronously, but quite independently, first isolated, cultured, and described the pneumococcus. Although the organism was first seen and studied by Sternberg, his results were not published until after those of Pasteur. The latter, in search of the etiologic agent of rabies, inoculated rabbits with the saliva of a child dead from that disease and produced what he called

* Afterward Surgeon General, United States Army.

a "sputum septicaemia." From the blood of these animals an organism was isolated and studied. Sternberg injected rabbits subcutaneously with saliva from himself and other normal persons and produced a similar type of infection. He likewise studied the organism obtained from the blood of rabbits so infected. The organism these workers isolated and described is now known as the pneumococcus or *Diplococcus pneumoniae.*

When first discovered, the organism was not known to be associated with disease in man. At that time, however, systematic studies were being carried on by various German investigators in search of the causative agent of pneumonia. In 1882 Friedländer (500) isolated an organism from eight cases of lobar pneumonia which he believed responsible for all pneumonias. The following year he published a paper in which he (501) termed this organism the "micrococcus of pneumonia." Subsequently, however, the organism was found responsible for only occasional cases of pneumonia and is now known as Friedländer's bacillus.

The intensive investigations of Fränkel (487, 488, 489) in 1884–1886 showed the true pneumococcus present in cases of lobar pneumonia. The confirmation of his findings by Weichselbaum (1396) in 1886 definitely established the pneumococcus as the usual cause of lobar pneumonia in man. Fränkel (488, 489) and others (1396, 1388) were also prompt to recognize that the pneumococcus might cause other infections, such as bronchopneumonia, pericarditis, endocarditis, otitis media, meningitis, and other localized lesions. A more detailed report of this early history has been given by Fränkel (488) and by Howard in the Oxford Monograph on the *Diagnosis and Treatment of Pneumonia* (661), and may also be found in the Medical Research Council (British), *System of Bacteriology* (556). Especially to be recommended is the historical discussion by White, with Robinson and Barnes (1417).

Biology

No attempt will be made here to give an exhaustive survey of the bacteriologic, immunologic, and chemical characteristics of the pneumococcus. These matters are discussed at length by White, with Robinson and Barnes (1417) in their monograph on *The Biology of Pneumococcus* from which information in this section is taken. The intention is to provide only such extracts of our knowledge of the pneumococcus as appear needed for an understanding of such matters as the epidemiology, pathogenesis, diagnosis, course, and treatment of pneumococcus pneumonia in man.

MORPHOLOGY AND CULTURAL CHARACTERISTICS. The pneumococcus (*Diplococcus pneumoniae*) is typically a lancet-shaped diplococcus, the contour making applicable the adjective "lanceolatus" used in some of its earlier names. There may be marked variation from this typical form even in smears of the same pneumococcus culture. Ordinarily the paired cocci occur singly or in short chains. Occasionally longer chains are found, particularly when the organism is grown in a fluid medium. Classically the pneumococcus is a Gram-positive organism, but occasional Gram-negative forms may be seen. Another characteristic of the organism, especially of virulent forms, is the presence of a well-defined capsule. In stained preparations this may often be seen as a clear area surrounding the diplococci. The capsule may be colored by the application of special staining methods. Further discussion of the capsule is deferred until later (see page 24).

Pneumococci are grown without difficulty at incubator temperatures of 36°–37° C. They will grow on a variety of media but are sensitive to moderate increases in acidity or alkalinity. The optimum reaction for growth is about pH 7.8, and the limiting hydrogen-ion concentration for initiating growth in ordinary media is within the range 7.0–8.3. It is characteristic of the organism that it grows in liquid media containing a sufficient amount of carbohydrate until the concentration of acid produced reaches pH 5.0, when growth ceases and the organism dies, the culture thus sterilizing itself. The possible relation of this to the occurrence of crisis in pneumonia is discussed later (see page 736).

Blood-agar plates are generally satisfactory for pneumococcus cultures and are frequently used, particularly as colonies on this medium are usually typical. Under ordinary conditions surface colonies appear as small, smooth, slightly raised flat discs which are whitish or colorless by reflected light. Examination of the growth by transmitted light shows little hemolysis and the colonies appear to be more or less green and surrounded by a greenish halo. After further incubation this greenish halo becomes brown and discolored. When grown in broth the pneumococcus usually produces uniform turbidity with some sedimentation of the organisms. The addition of small amounts of blood to broth media makes for more rapid and heavier growth. Small amounts of glucose also increase the quantity of growth but may cause early death of broth cultures because of the production of acid. Most stains of pneumococci ferment inulin.

AUTOLYSIS AND BILE SOLUBILITY. The solubility of the pneumococcus in bile affords one of the most satisfactory tests for distinguishing this organism from streptococci. The test may be carried out by adding whole bile or bile acids or their salts to a broth culture or suspension of the organisms. The addition of whole ox bile to pneumococcus cultures in a proportion of 1 to 500 should cause solution of true pneumococci within an hour at 37° C. If solution does not occur, there is grave doubt that the organism in question is a pneumococcus, for several investigators feel that organisms insoluble in bile, regardless of their cultural reactions, should not be classed as pneumococci.

The conditions which limit autolysis and bile solubility of this organism are apparently similar. Autolysis occurs to some extent in practically all pneumococcus cultures and is especially marked in old cultures. Enzymes are released by disruption of the cell which may hydrolyze proteins, especially peptones, and carbohydrates, and have a lytic action on fats. The possible relation of these actions to the process of resolution is discussed in the following chapter (pages 97–101).

DRYING AND STORAGE OF CULTURES. Pneumococcus cultures may be kept with little difficulty in a variety of ways. Virulent cultures may be injected into mice and small amounts of the heart's blood sealed in capillary tubes. The spleens of such mice may be collected aseptically, dried *in vacuo,* and stored in sealed tubes; or cultures of virulent or avirulent organisms may be frozen and dried *in vacuo* either in the recently devised Mudd-Flosdorf apparatus or by some of the older and simpler but probably less satisfactory methods.

TOXIN PRODUCTION. Although much effort has been expended in the search for a pneumococcus toxin, which has an obvious place in the clinical picture of pneumonia in the human subject, it is probable that no such substance has yet been isolated from pneumococci or from their growth products. This makes impossible any clear explanation of the more important symptoms occurring in this disease and, at present, the production of a true antitoxin for therapeutic purposes. Several of the substances isolated are, however, of sufficient interest to be worthy of mention. One of these, found in pneumococcus cultures, is the hemolysin for red blood cells of various animals. This hemolysin is inactivated by oxidation and therefore must be prepared under anaerobic conditions or be reduced if in the oxidized form. Though this substance was first described as an endocellular hemotoxin (Cole and Dochez 306, Cole 292), it is apparently an extracellular hemolysin and nontoxic (Cowan 328). No direct evidence has linked this hemolysin with the clinical picture of human pneumonia.

Another substance of interest is the purpura-producing substance which may be demonstrated by the injection of pneumococcus culture fluids into mice. This appears to be an autolytic product and may be demonstrated by the appearance of hemorrhages in the ears, feet, and tails of mice after injection with killed culture or with culture filtrates. Some preparations of SSS (see page 24), particularly the acetylated ones, also produce purpura. Anaerobically prepared autolysates of pneumococcus cultures contain substances (997, 1398) which, when suitably injected into animals, may cause skin necrosis, hemorrhagic edema of the lungs, and nephritis or nephrosis (115, 116, 114).

The fact that the more virulent the pneumococcus, the more likely it is to possess a large capsule, coupled with the fact that the capsule appears to be made up largely of a soluble polysaccharide, would suggest that this carbohydrate might have toxic properties. Although this carbohydrate is extremely important, as will be described later, it would appear that it does not possess any particular toxicity, for it may be injected into normal animals in fairly large amounts without ill effect. In man in small doses it has likewise proved benign.

TYPES AND THEIR IDENTIFICATION. The division of this species of bacteria into a number of different serologic types has made possible vastly important studies of pneumonia and other pneumococcus infections and their specific serum treatment. As early as 1899 Eyre and Washbourn (396) observed differences between pneumococcus strains in protection tests in animals. They concluded: "There exist varieties of the pneumococcus which at present can only be distinguished by the action of antipneumococcic serum." By virulence and opsonic tests Longcope and Fox (803) in 1905 divided pneumococci into two types.

The significance of these early findings was not fully appreciated, however, and it remained for Neufeld and Händel in Germany (936, 938) in 1909–1910 to show definite serologic differences between certain pneumococcus strains and to record the existence of at least two distinct groups of the organisms, one of which they regarded as a "typical" group. They likewise stated that there were perhaps several other separate groups as well. In 1913 Dochez and Gillespie (364) in New York City were able, by protection and agglutination tests, to subdivide pneumococci into four groups. Simultaneously and independently that same year, Lister (784) in South Africa reported the occurrence of several types or groups of pneumococci. He designated these as Groups A, B, C, D, and E (see page 30), and in general his findings were similar to those of Dochez and Gillespie.* As all strains within each of the first three groups identified by Dochez and Gillespie have been found immunologically identical, these groups are now designated as Type I, Type II, and Type III. These types are frequently referred to in foreign literature as the "American" types. It will be shown, however, that their distribution is essentially world-wide.

Dochez and Gillespie also recognized the existence of other types of pneumococci which did not belong to Type I, II, or III and which differed immunologically one from another. As none of these other types was encountered frequently, it seemed most convenient for descriptive purposes to place them together in a miscellaneous group and refer to them as Group IV pneumococci. For a while this fourth class was referred to as a type, but as this was misleading, the term has generally been discarded and the terms Group IV, X Group, or Unclassified Group have been generally adopted. The pneumococci in Dochez and Gillespie's Group I (Type I) corresponded to those in Neufeld and Händel's "typical" group. Group II (Type II) included the strain Neufeld and Händel designated the "Franz" strain. Group III (Type III) consisted of organisms of the *Pneumococcus mucosus* type, while Group IV included all other pneumococci.

In 1915 Avery (31) isolated pneumococci which resembled those of Type II but which presented certain atypical characteristics. These he divided into subgroups designated Types IIa, IIb, and IIx. In 1919 Stillman (1236) further subdivided these atypical Type II's into twelve types, referred to as Types IIa, IIb, IIc, and so forth. The problem of pneumococcus classification became further complicated, for in addition to the types described above by Avery and by Stillman, no less than seven or eight other workers and their associates, including Cooper, Mishulow, and Blanc (319), described several distinct types between 1916 and 1928. Few attempts were made, however, to gather representatives of all these types and to develop a uniform serologic classification until, at the suggestion of Park (987) in 1927, Cooper, Edwards, and Rosenstein (318) undertook such a task. Using pneumococci isolated by themselves and others, they segregated ten new types, designating them by the Roman numerals IV, V, VI, and so forth to XIII. Later Cooper, Rosenstein, Walter, and Peizer (320) added nineteen additional types to the list and correlated all the recently recognized types with those

* See also Appendix B, page 946.

previously described by other investigators. In all, then, Cooper and her associates have identified or reclassified twenty-nine types which were previously considered together as Group IV or Unclassified strains. These new types, in addition to the Types I, II, and III identified years ago, make a total of thirty-two well-recognized types at the present time. (Methods of pneumococcus typing are described elsewhere; see pages 620–641.)

Because of cross agglutination and cross protection between Types VI and XXVI and their respective serums, Cooper and her co-workers (320) have combined these and refer to them as Types VIa and VIb respectively or simply as Type VI. In addition, some workers consider Type XV and Type XXX identical. Except for this, the remainder of the types above Type III, which are referred to as the subtypes or higher types, appear to be separate and distinct and are, in the common sense of the term, apparently just as clearly "fixed types" as Type I, II, or III.

The classification of pneumococci into thirty-two serologic types, extensive as it is, obviously does not exhaust the possibility of there being still other types. The reports cited in a following section illustrate that pneumococci exist which cannot yet be identified as members of any generally recognized type (see page 29). In general, however, the number of such strains in Europe and North America appears to be small.

An interesting and important question is whether the various types are stable or are convertible from one type into another either in the body or under cultivation. It appears that such a change has been brought about by an involved laboratory procedure, but at the moment it is not clear that the pneumococcus can undergo this conversion under natural conditions in the animal body. Even the laboratory experiments which indicate that such conversion takes place are dependent upon changing a virulent pneumococcus of one type into a degraded avirulent pneumococcus and then, under the stimulus from a smooth virulent strain, inducing the production of a new capsular type-carbohydrate by the avirulent degraded organism.

CELL COMPONENTS. Of the various components of the pneumococcus cell which have been described in the literature, three deserve mention. These are the protein and the carbohydrate (C substance) of the cell body and the polysaccharide of the capsule, commonly called soluble specific substance or SSS. The somatic protein is apparently the same in all pneumococci whatever their type, virulence, or state of dissociation. As are other proteins, it is capable of stimulating antibody production in animals, and these antibodies are lacking in type-specificity, combining readily with pneumococci of the type homologous with or heterologous to that used in producing them. For our present purpose, little need be said of this protein and its antibodies, for no clear-cut relation of the protein to the symptoms of pneumonia has been established; nor does antiprotein serum display curative properties. The latter statement is based as much upon the fact that heterologous serums, necessarily containing antibody against the pneumococcal protein, are not of therapeutic value as upon direct experimental evidence.

Another constituent of the pneumococcus cell is a carbohydrate known as the C substance of Tillett and Francis (1312). Like the somatic protein, this carbohydrate is not type-specific nor is it associated only with virulent organisms. At the moment its importance in the pathology, symptomatology, and treatment of pneumonia is not understood.

The results of studies made in recent years of pneumococcal capsular polysaccharide are of tremendous importance to the whole field of immunology and immunologic chemistry. Specific polysaccharides have been isolated for several of the pneumococcus types and have been analyzed so that their chemical composition and structure are reasonably well defined. Each carbohydrate so far isolated is distinct and specific and there is every reason to believe that the same fact will hold true for each individual recognized type. It has been shown, furthermore, that the serologic differentiation of pneumococci into types is dependent upon these specific capsular polysaccharides.

Pneumococci owe their virulence at least in part to the content of the specific capsular polysaccharide. This is indicated by the fact that only virulent pneumococci produce considerable quantities of capsular carbohydrate during growth; and is demonstrated experimentally by the enhanced lethal effect when small amounts of homologous soluble specific substance are injected into animals along with living pneumococci of low virulence. The mechanism by which the carbohydrate aids the bacterium and injures the host is not fully understood, but it is known that the capsular polysaccharide will render pneumococcus antibody ineffective by combining with it (see also page 131).

The body fluids and at least some of the tissues of patients with pneumococcus infection contain demonstrable quantities of SSS. It has been found in the body fluids of patients with pneumonia as early as twelve hours after the initial chill and in some cases continued present up to fifty-eight days (Dochez and Avery, 363). The amount of SSS appearing in the urine varies with the patient and is of considerable prognostic importance, as will be seen later (see pages 693–695). Soluble specific substance has been found in the blood and consolidated lung. It has also been found in infected exudates and spinal fluids, sputum, and urine, where its presence may aid in rapidly determining the type of infection present (see pages 637–639).

PNEUMOCOCCUS VARIANTS. Mention was made above of the fact that virulent pneumococci may be converted into avirulent forms. Such a conversion is accompanied by a loss of type-specificity. This process of dissociation is accompanied by a number of changes in the growth characteristics of the organism. Colonies of the virulent and avirulent forms are reasonably distinctive on solid media. In broth the growth of dissociated avirulent pneumococci is also characteristic in that, instead of the uniform turbidity shown by the virulent organism, there is a pronounced tendency toward sedimentation. The virulent form is often referred to as the S form because its colony has a smooth, glistening appearance. The avirulent variant is called the R form because its colony has a roughened and dull surface. This phenomenon of a change in colonial type with an alteration in virulence is not confined to the pneumococcus but is apparently a general characteristic of bacteria. Studies of the enteric group of organisms, which includes the typhoid and colon bacilli among others, have suggested that the current designation of S and R applied to the pneumococci is perhaps an error and that a more accurate and complete classification would be to designate the form referred to above as S by the letter M meaning mucoid, and the form referred to above by the letter R by the letter S inasmuch as such terms fit in with the corresponding classification in the enteric group. There is also a third variant which is rightly designated as the R form. The concurrent use of these two nomenclatures presents the possibility of much confusion, but it is felt that in all probability the second scheme of terminology (M, S, and R) is in conformity with present-day knowledge and will be more generally used in the future.

The practical importance of pneumococcal variants in the study of human pneumonia is not clear. As suggested above, it is possible that pneumococci may change from one type to another by passing from the M form into the S or R form and then reverting to an M form of another type. This possibility has been demonstrated in certain laboratory experiments but has not been observed in the human host, nor in the animal body, except when certain steps of the process have been carried out in the test tube. Only in respect to the marked difference in virulence between these various forms of the same organism does dissociation appear to be of practical importance.

However, this question of virulence cannot be entirely dependent upon the particular form of pneumococcus involved, for it has been demonstrated that certain strains which are highly virulent for mice possess at the same time only a low grade of virulence for rabbits, although both animals are extremely susceptible to pneumococcal infection. It would thus appear that there is some as yet unknown factor which determines the virulence of bacterial species.

In a given culture some organisms may be in their fully virulent form and others may be in varying states of dissociation, and in consequence, if by repeated animal passage the culture becomes lethal in higher dilutions than at first, it will look as though the virulence of the culture had increased. On the other hand, if the culture initially used contained a large proportion of organisms in their fully virulent form, animal passage may produce little change, though the avirulent forms may disappear. This may explain many of the conflicting reports concerning the enhancement of virulence by animal passage.

The virulence of pneumococci isolated from human lesions has been studied chiefly in terms of their virulence for mice, a method which possesses possible sources of error. There appears to be, however, a general parallelism in the virulence for the two animal species, for those strains isolated from the obviously more severe human lesions, such as lobar pneumonia, are ordinarily more virulent for mice than are the cultures obtained from patients with terminal or post-operative pneumonia, conjunctivitis, or other pneumococcus infections. One would assume from this that the types most commonly encountered in cases of lobar pneumonia would be the most virulent; and the validity of this assumption has support in the experimental work of Whittle (1422) and of Gundel and Wasu (584).

ANTIGENICITY. The antigenic properties of pneumococci and of various pneumococcus derivatives are of importance in the preparation of therapeutic serums and in prophylactic immunization against pneumonia as well as in the development of natural immunity (see also page 133). This matter is extremely complicated, for it is involved in a mass of more or less conflicting evidence, particularly in respect to the antigenicity of the various pneumococcus constituents.

Both virulent and avirulent pneumococci are antigenic, but the action of the antibodies evoked in response to their injection is different. The most satisfactory antigen appears to be the unbroken cells, either alive or killed, of virulent pneumococci. Serums produced by the injection of such organisms into animals contain type-specific antibodies, including protective antibodies, in considerable amount. Avirulent pneumococci, even though used in the form of intact cells, are quite ineffective in producing a serum which will protect against infection with a virulent organism. Such serums contain species-specific but not type-specific antibodies.

A consideration of the antigenic effect of various fractions of the pneumococcus cell presents a confusing picture. The protein obtained from pneumococci will give rise to a serum similar to that obtained by the injection of intact avirulent organisms. In the earlier experiments, in some animals the injection of the specific capsular polysaccharide alone was not in any way effective, since no antibody appeared to be produced against it when it was injected apart from the pneumococcus cell. There is, however, definite evidence that an active immunity may be conferred on certain animal species, though not on others, by the injection of these carbohydrates even in the relatively crude and degraded forms in which they were first produced. Recent experiments dealing with forms of these complex sugars probably more like those actually present in the living pneumococcus cell suggest that these specific polysaccharides are more antigenic than was originally believed. As yet, however, there has been no evidence that the immunity produced even by these carbohydrates is of such high degree that serum from animals so immunized may be used for the passive protection of other animals or for the treatment of pneumonia in man. The manufacturer of therapeutic serums is therefore still dependent upon the use of whole pneumococci for the production of curative serum.

The problem of the prophylactic immunization of man against pneumonia is discussed in some detail in the section on prophylaxis (see pages 446–482). At this point, however, it may be said that the injection of pneumococcal vaccines will incite antibody formation in man. This has also been shown to occur following the injection of certain derivatives of the pneumococcus cell (Francis and Tillett, 485; Finland and Sutliff, 461; Francis, 478). Further, Felton's observations (424) suggest that a pneumococcus derivative may be both efficiently prepared and conveniently used for human immunization.

Observations concerning humoral antibodies homologous in type to the organism causing infection and their relation to pneumonia are discussed later.

Proportion of Strains at Present Classifiable

Whereas formerly, using only the diagnostic serums for Types I, II, and III, about one-third to one-half or more of pneumococcus strains remained unclassified, now, with serums for Types I through XXXII, it is possible to identify nearly all strains encountered. This is well illustrated by various reports from many places.

In New York, Cooper, Rosenstein, Walter, and Peizer (320) examined 414 strains of so-called Group IV pneumococci obtained from adults and children with lobar pneumonia and bronchopneumonia and found only a few they were unable to classify with serums for Types IV through XXXII. Raia, Plummer, and Shultz (1057), extending their previous study (1029), found that with serums for Types I through XXIV they were able, in 1929–1930, to classify all but 14.3 per cent of the strains isolated from 168 cases of pneumococcus pneumonia in children. Further, Webster and Hughes (1393), using serums for Types I through XXV, were able to type 97 per cent of about 500 strains of pneumococci obtained from normal persons. Results of similar significance were reported by Bullowa (183) and Bullowa and Wilcox (198). In an analysis of 2,058 cases of pneumococcus pneumonia in adults, the latter clearly demonstrated the steady decline from 1928 to 1933 in the number of cases due to unclassified pneumococci. Using serums for Types I to XXXII inclusive, they found in 1932–1933 that this group constituted but 3 per cent of their cases. Later Bullowa (188) reported that during 1933–1934 the number of unclassified strains had been further decreased so as to constitute only 1.2 per cent of his cases.

In Boston, Sutliff and Finland (1271) were able, with serums for Types I through XX, to type all but 13.4 per cent of the strains of pneumococci obtained from 1,264 patients with or without pneumonia. Finland (444) and Winkler and Finland (1429) state it is now possible to type nearly all strains of pneumococci. The experience of the recent Massachusetts Pneumonia Study (869) may also be cited. During that Study, carried out over a period of five years, more than 10,000 typings were done on sputums from patients with pneumonia and some other forms of respiratory disease in various laboratories throughout the state. At the central laboratory in Boston, where typing was carried out for all thirty-two types, 3,150 strains of pneumococci were encountered. Of these, 189 strains (6 per cent) were placed in the unclassified group. Some of these strains, however, died or were otherwise lost before typing was completed so that it is not clear that all of these were actually unclassifiable strains. There were, however, something less than a dozen strains which definitely proved to be other than Types I to XXXII inclusive, and confirmation of this was obtained from Cooper to whom cultures of these strains were sent.

In San Francisco, Kohl and Reitzel (734) studied pneumococci obtained from 142 patients with pneumonia and other infections with this organism. Only two strains of pneumococci were found which they could not identify with serums for Types I through XXXII.

In Canada, Brown (157), using serums for Types I through XXIX, typed strains recovered from 240 cases of pneumococcus pneumonia in adults and children. His report shows approximately 11 per cent of the strains from this group as unclassified.

In Germany, Gundel and Schwarz (582), using serums for Types I through XXXII, were able to type all but 3 of 133 strains isolated from persons with and without respiratory infections.

So far, only two reports encountered are at variance with the general trend of those cited above, in that these record a considerable proportion of strains which could not be identified as any of the types from I to XXXII inclusive. The first of these was from Great Britain where Christie (267), using serums for Types IV through XXXII, endeavored to determine the incidence of these types among 100 strains of pneumococci of Group IV. He was unable to identify 19 of 36 strains carried by healthy persons, 16 of 36 strains obtained from convalescent carriers (adults), and 12 of 28 strains isolated from patients with acute pneumococcus pneumonia. Of the total of 100 Group IV strains examined, 47 were apparently not strains of any of the types from IV through XXXII. The second report was from India where Napier and Dharmendra (924) typed pneumococci obtained from 45 cases of lobar pneumonia and 15 of bronchopneumonia in natives. Examinations were carried out for all thirty-two types, and in this group of 60 cases 53.3 per cent were found to be due to classifiable types and 46.6 per cent to other pneumococci, apparently for the most part two local types. As the above reports embrace observations on a rather limited number of strains of pneumococci, it is hoped that such investigations will be continued in Great Britain and in India and in other parts of the world as well.

At the South African Institute for Medical Research, Lister (784, 785) and Lister and Ordman (788) have identified eighteen types in addition to Types I, II, and III (the latter being referred to as Groups C, B, and E respectively in Lister's classification).* These are referred to as Groups A, D, F, G, and so forth. Elsewhere in Africa the existence of especially prevalent

* See also Appendix B, page 946.

types which were not Type I, II, or III has been described; one from the Belgian Congo (1376) and one from French Equatorial Africa (1349). In Australia a common local type other than Type I, II, or III has been identified by Penfold (1009). How many of these types might fall into Cooper's classification is unknown, but it is quite possible some do not, for Napier and Dharmendra (924) in India found one and possibly two other types which were common in Assam and failed to agglutinate in any of the serums (Types I through XXXII) supplied to them by Cooper.

World-wide Distribution of Pneumococcus Types

The presence of pneumococci of Types I, II, and III, and of Group IV isolated from persons with or without pulmonary infection has been reported in many parts of the world. In the United States, a survey of the available literature and personal communications reveals that the presence of such organisms has been reported from virtually every state east of the Mississippi River and from over one-half of those west of it. This is shown in the map on page 33 and in the following list of selected references which in many instances have been chosen because of the character of the report. In all, information is available from forty-one of the forty-eight states. Though relatively little typing appears to have been done in the western part of this country, it seems a foregone conclusion that pneumococci of various types are present in all states.

Source of selected reports indicating the presence of pneumococci of Types I, II, III, and Group IV in various states in this country

MAINE, NEW HAMPSHIRE, VERMONT, AND RHODE ISLAND
- Personal communications from a number of physicians

CONNECTICUT
- New Haven
  - Trask, O'Donovan, Moore, and Beebe (1321)
  - Blake (120)
  - Pepper (1010)
  - Bunim and Trask (201)
  - Blake, Howard, and Hull (128)
- Report of State Department of Health (313)

MASSACHUSETTS
- Boston
  - Alexander (9)
  - Locke, Thomas, and O'Hara (797)
  - Lyon (821)
  - McGuire (839)
  - Locke (793)
  - Rosenau, Felton, and Atwater (1111)
  - Powell, Atwater, and Felton (1048)
  - Finland (442)
  - Sutliff and Finland (1269)

MASSACHUSETTS
Boston (*cont.*)
Lord (809)
Finland and Sutliff (463)
Sutliff and Finland (1271)
Smillie (1206)
Smillie and Leeder (1210)
Sutliff and Finland (1272)
Finland and Sutliff (464)
Finland (445, 449)
Ayer (Camp Devens)
Spooner, Sellards, and Wyman (1222)
Spooner (1221)
Massachusetts Pneumonia Study
Bigelow (104)
Heffron (611)
Heffron and Varley (616)
Heffron and Anderson (614)
Beckler and MacLeod (86)
Anderson and Heffron (17)
Boston Health League Letter (142)
Lord and Heffron (813, 814)
Heffron and Robinson (615)

NEW YORK
New York City
Dochez and Gillespie (364)
Cole and Dochez (306)
Dochez and Avery (360)
Wollstein and Benson (1436)
Stillman (1234)
Pisek and Pease (1025)
Avery, Chickering, Cole, and Dochez (33)
Frissell and Famulener (503)
Thomas (1299)
Cecil and Larsen (236)
Conner (314)
Cecil and Baldwin (229)
Cecil, Baldwin, and Larsen (230)
Kessel and Hyman (713)

NEW YORK
New York City (*cont.*)
Bullowa, Rosenblüth, Park, and Cooper (195)
Park, Bullowa, and Rosenblüth (991)
Cecil and Sutliff (245)
Cole (298)
Cole (299)
Bullowa (175)
Plummer, Raia, and Shultz (1029)
Cecil and Plummer (238)
Webster and Hughes (1393)
Raia, Plummer, and Shultz (1057)
Shultz (1187)
Cecil and Plummer (239)
Bullowa (183)
Nemir (930) and co-workers (931)
Kereszturi and Hauptmann (710)
Bullowa and Wilcox (198)
Bullowa (186, 187, 188, 190)
Long Island (Camp Upton)
Cecil (219)
Tenney and Rivenburgh (1289)
Johnson City
Ryland (1144)
Other areas
Wadsworth (1365, 1366)
New York Pneumonia Study
Cecil (226)

NEW JERSEY
Tenafly (Camp Merritt)
Shorer, Clark, Sanderson, Dickson, and Huntoon (1163)
Ireland, Callender, and Coupal (675b)
Wrightstown (Camp Dix)
MacCallum (825)
Leopold (774)

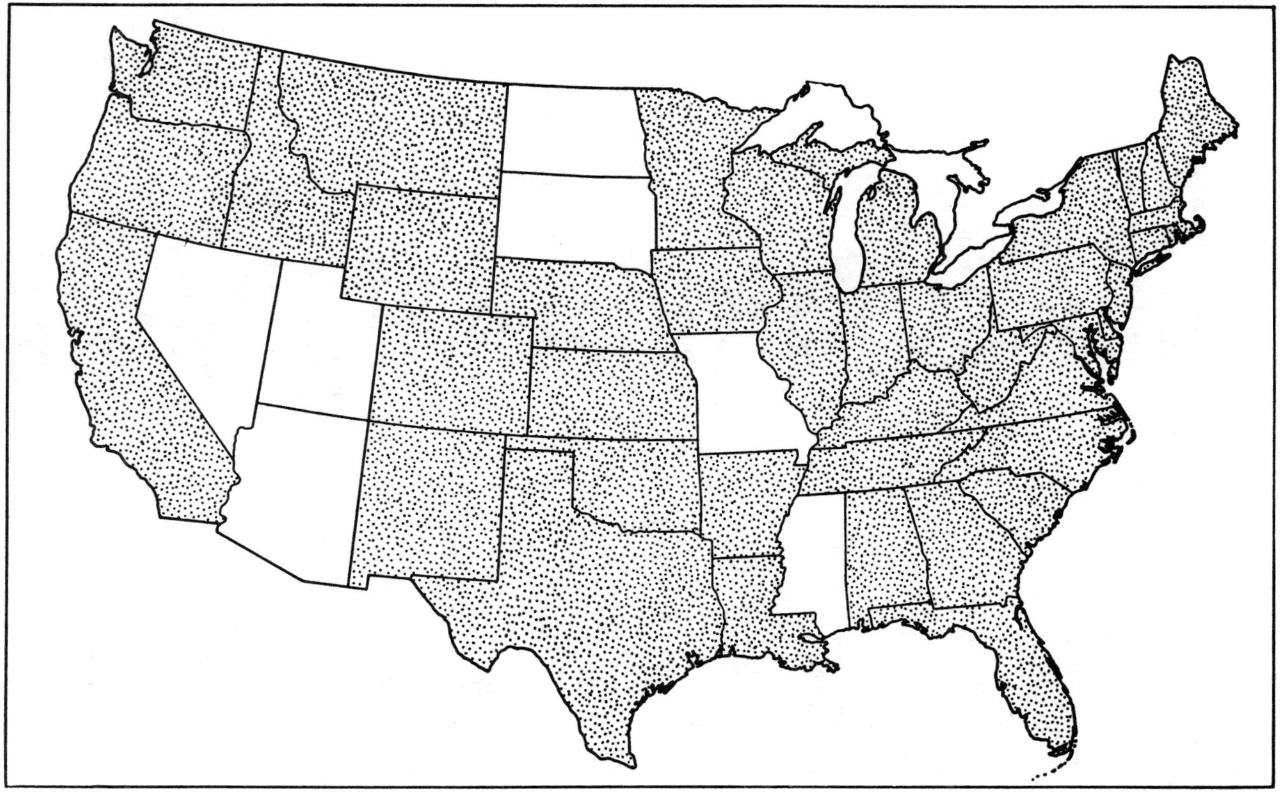

Map 1. States in which the available reports indicate pneumococci of Types I, II, III, and Group IV have been identified

PENNSYLVANIA
Philadelphia
Mitchell (899)
Jones (691)
Richardson (1079)
Richardson (1080)
Behrend and Cowper (90)
Bryn Mawr
Belk and Sharpe (93)
Sayre
Hamilton (592)
Pittsburgh
Hartman and Lacy (604)
McMeans (851)
Haythorn and Meller (607)

DELAWARE
Wilmington
Gay (personal communication)

MARYLAND
Camp Meade
Thomas (1295)
Baltimore
Clough (277)
Sydenstricker and Sutton (1282)
Bloomfield (134)
Sutton and Sevier (1277)
Bloomfield (136)
Bliss, McClaskey, and Long (133)

VIRGINIA
Petersburg (Camp Lee)
MacCallum (825)

WEST VIRGINIA
Charleston
Preston (personal communication)

NORTH CAROLINA
Durham
Personal correspondence

SOUTH CAROLINA
Columbia (Camp Jackson)
Park and Chickering (985)
Paris (Camp Sevier)
Vaughan and Schnabel (1351)
Spartanburg (Camp Wadsworth)
Birge and Havens (111)

GEORGIA
Macon (Camp Wheeler)
Cecil and Vaughan (246)
Atlanta (Fort McPherson)
Camac (211)

FLORIDA
Jacksonville (Camp Johnston)
Henson (634)

ALABAMA
Andalusia
Smillie and Caldwell (1209)

TENNESSEE
Memphis
Warr and Alperin (1385)

KENTUCKY
Louisville (Camp Taylor)
Hamburger and Fox (591)
Ireland, Callender, and Coupal (675b)

OHIO
Cincinnati
Benjamin, Blankenhorn, Ruegsegger, and Senior (94)
Chillicothe (Camp Sherman)
Friedlander, McCord, Sladen, and Wheeler (499)
Ireland, Callender, and Coupal (675b)

INDIANA
Indianapolis
Thornburg (personal communication)

MICHIGAN
- Detroit
  - Price (1051)
- Battle Creek (Camp Custer)
  - Blanton and Irons (130)

ILLINOIS
- Chicago
  - Mathers (872)
  - Quigley (1054)
  - Kelly and Gussin (709)
  - Bundesen (200)
  - Westlund (1412)
  - Jacobson (682)
  - Robertson, Graeser, Coggeshall, and Harrison (1086)
- Rockford (Camp Grant)
  - McClellan (828)

WISCONSIN
- Madison
  - Stovall (personal communication)

MINNESOTA
- Minneapolis
  - Blake (118)
  - Reimann (1068)

IOWA
- Des Moines (Camp Dodge)
  - Miller and Lusk (892)

ARKANSAS
- Little Rock (Camp Pike)
  - Small (1202)
  - Opie, Blake, Small, and Rivers (969)
  - Ireland, Callender, and Coupal (675b)

LOUISIANA
- Alexandria (Camp Beauregard)
  - McClelland (829)
- New Orleans
  - Chickering (258)

TEXAS
- Temple
  - Robinson (1099)
- El Paso (Mobilization Camp)
  - Nichols (952)
- Fort Worth (Camp Bowie)
  - Greenway, Boettiger, and Colwell (566)
- San Antonio (Fort Sam Houston)
  - Cole and MacCallum (307)
- Houston (Camp Logan)
  - Hall, Stone, and Simpson (588)
- Waco (Camp MacArthur)
  - Medalia and Schiff (879)

OKLAHOMA
- Tulsa
  - Goodman (personal communication)

KANSAS
- Camps Funston and Riley
  - Stone, Phillips, and Bliss (1251)
  - Opie, Blake, Small, and Rivers (969)

NEBRASKA
- Omaha
  - Russum (personal communication)

MONTANA
- Butte
  - Newman (personal communication)

IDAHO
- Boise
  - Craig-Sullivan (personal communication)

WYOMING
- Cheyenne
  - Zuckerman (personal communication)

COLORADO
Denver
Williams (personal communication)

NEW MEXICO
Deming (Camp Cody)
Lamb and Brannin (758)

CALIFORNIA
San Francisco
Kohl and Reitzel (734)
Palo Alto (Camp Fremont)
Brem, Bolling, and Casper (147)

CALIFORNIA (*cont.*)
Palo Alto (Camp Fremont) (*cont.*)
Ireland, Callender, and Coupal (675b)

OREGON
Portland
Robertson (personal communication)

WASHINGTON
Seattle (U. S. Naval Training Camp)
Henry (633)

In other countries where typing has been done, the presence of pneumococci of Types I, II, and III, and of Group IV has also been reported. The accompanying illustration (Map 2) shows the country of origin of the available pertinent reports. A list of selected references is also presented. From a consideration of the situation shown in Maps 1 and 2, it appears probable that pneumococci, at least of Types I, II, and III, and some strains of Group IV, occur in all parts of the world.

Source of selected reports indicating the presence of pneumococci of Types I, II, III, and Group IV in various countries throughout the world

North and South America

CANADA
Toronto
Brown (156)
Brown (157)
Montreal
Mills (897)
Howard (661)
Howard and Fullerton (663)

PUERTO RICO
San Juan
Suárez (1261)

VIRGIN ISLANDS
Smillie (cited by Cooper and her associates, 320)

PANAMA
Canal Zone
Clark (273)

North and South America (*cont.*)

ECUADOR
Crespo (cited by Gautier, 510)

CHILE
Santiago
Gonzalez (528)

ARGENTINA
Buenos Aires
Bachmann and Miravent (53a)

Europe

IRISH FREE STATE
Dublin
Moore (902)

ENGLAND
London
Armstrong (21)
Griffith (568)

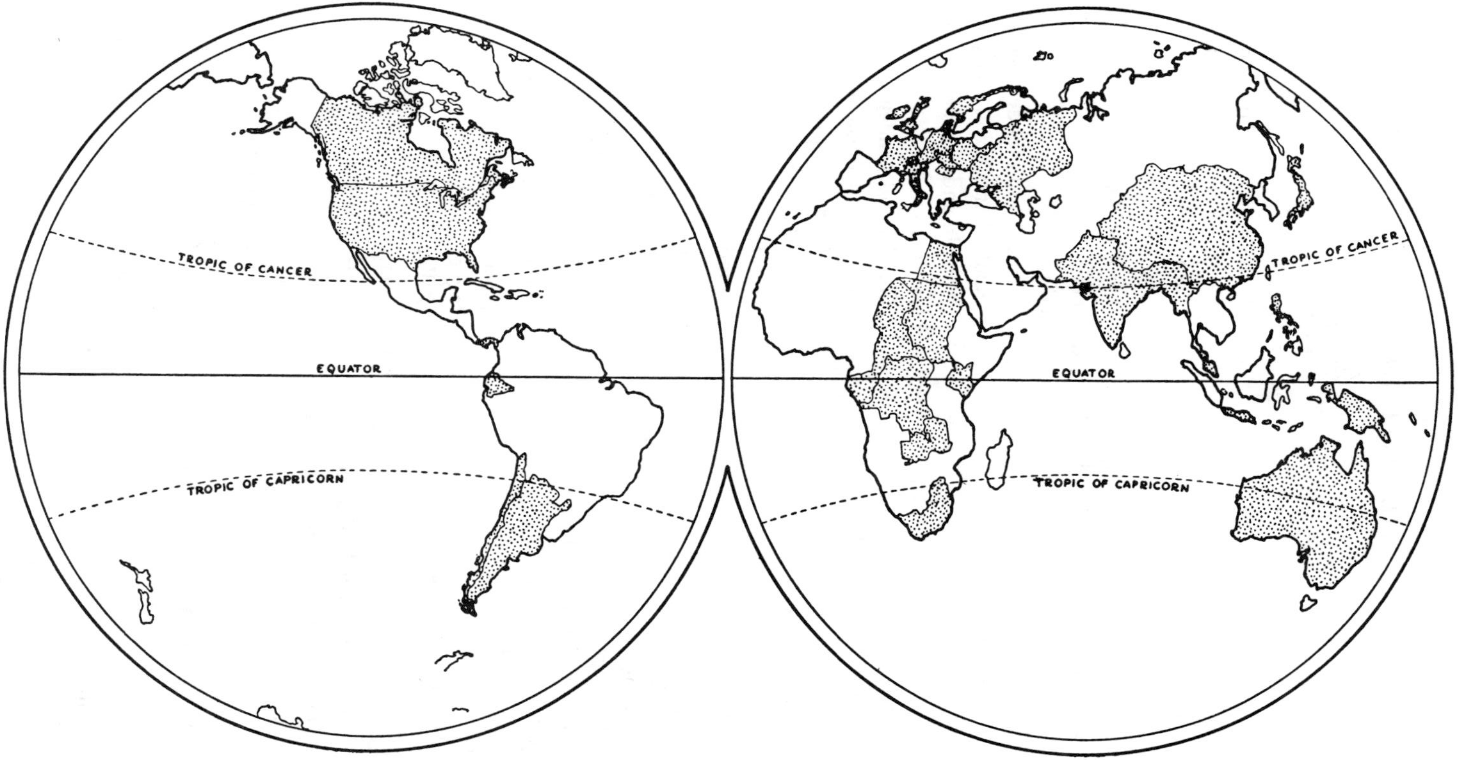

Map 2. Countries in which the available reports indicate pneumococci of Types I, II, III, and Group IV have been identified

Europe

ENGLAND

London (*cont.*)

Urquhart (1346)
Mallock (854)
Griffith (571)
Armstrong and Johnson (24)
Guy's Hospital Report (1145)
Davies, Hodgson, and Whitby (339)

Cambridge

Whittle (1422)

Liverpool

Glynn and Digby (520)

Manchester

Ferguson and Lovell (437)
Langley (765)
Langley (763)

Birmingham

Leys (779)

SCOTLAND

Glasgow

Grant (553)
Macgregor (837)
Blacklock and Guthrie (112)
Cruickshank (331)
Christie (267)

Edinburgh

McLachlan (844)
Alston and Stewart (13)

Aberdeen

Therapeutic Trials Committee of Medical Research Council (557)

NORWAY

Oslo

Thjötta and Hanneborg (1294)
Strøm (1252)

DENMARK

Copenhagen

Thomsen and Christensen (1303)
Christensen (264, 265)

Europe (cont.)

FRANCE

Paris

Nobécourt and Paraf (956)
Cotoni, Truche, and Raphael (324)

St. Nazaire

Feinblatt (406)

GERMANY

Berlin

Neufeld and Händel (936)
Neufeld and Händel (937)
Neufeld and Händel (938)

Heidelberg

Gundel and Linden (579)
Gundel and Wasu (584)
Gundel and Schwarz (582)
Gundel and Schwarz (581)
Gundel (578)
Gundel and Okura (580)

Leipzig

Becker (84)

Dresden

Hallermann and Kähler (589)

HUNGARY

Kramár and Gyüre (742)

CZECHOSLOVAKIA

Prague

Adler (5)

SWITZERLAND

Herzog (636)

ITALY

Rome

Pontano (1044)

Florence

Levi (775)

Siena

Marginesu and Corda (860)

RUSSIA

Moscow

Viktorow, Semzowa, and Oettinger (1353)

Europe (cont.)

POLAND

Warsaw

Przesmycki and his associates (1053)

Africa

EGYPT

Cairo

Gohar and Abboud (526)

ANGLO-EGYPTIAN SUDAN

Khartoum

Whitehead (1419)

FRENCH EQUATORIAL AFRICA

Brazzaville

Vaucel and Salaün (1349)

KENYA

Nairobi

Garnham and deSmidt (507)

BELGIAN CONGO

Elizabethville

Walravens (1376)

NORTHERN RHODESIA

N'dola

Ordman (971)

UNION OF SOUTH AFRICA

Johannesburg (the Rand)

Lister (784)
Lister (785)
Lister (786)
Ordman (970)
Lister and Ordman (788)
Peall (1007)

Far East

INDIA

Baluchistan

Malone (859)

Karachi

Bhatnagar and Singh (100)

Far East (cont.)

INDIA (*cont.*)

Punjab

Malone (857)

Madras

Cunningham, Cruickshank, and Ramakrishnan (334)

Calcutta

Napier and Dharmendra (924)

Assam

Napier and Dharmendra (924)

FEDERATED MALAY STATES

Kuala Lampur

Kingsbury (cited by Gautier, 510)

STRAITS SETTLEMENTS

Singapore

Allen (cited by Gautier, 510)

JAVA

Kirchner (720)

AUSTRALIA

Sydney

Tebbutt (1287)

Melbourne

Penfold (1009)
Patterson (1003a)
Patterson and Williams (1003b)
Webster (1394)

NEW GUINEA

Morgan (cited by Gautier, 510)

PHILIPPINE ISLANDS

Manila

Monserrat (900)

CHINA

Peiping

Wu and Chiu (1450)

JAPAN

Tokyo

Ishida (680)
Ishida, Nagai, and Saito (681)
Hirano (646)

TABLE 4. PNEUMOCOCCUS TYPES I–XXXII. DATA FROM SELECTED REPORTS SHOWING EXTENT OF TYPING, THE PLACE OF INVESTIGATION, AND THE GROUP SERVING AS CHIEF SOURCE OF THE ORGANISM

PLACE AND INVESTIGATOR	GROUP SERVING AS CHIEF SOURCE OF ORGANISM	TYPES FOR WHICH DIAGNOSTIC SERUM WAS AVAILABLE
New York City		
Cooper, Edwards, and Rosenstein (318)	pneumonia cases	I–XIII
Bullowa (175)	pneumonia cases	I–XVIII
Plummer, Raia, and Shultz (1029)	normals* and pneumonia cases	I–XIII
Park (987)	pneumonia	I–XXI
Webster and Hughes (1393)	normals	I–XXV
Raia, Plummer, and Shultz (1057)	normals and pneumonia cases	I–XXIV
Shultz (1187)	normals and pneumonia cases	I–XXIV
Cooper, Rosenstein, Walter, and Peizer (320)	normals and pneumonia cases	I–XXXII
Bullowa (183)	pneumonia cases	I–XXXII
Nemir (930)	pneumonia cases	I–XXII
Kereszturi and Hauptmann (710)	pneumonia cases	I–XXX
Bullowa and Wilcox (198)	pneumonia cases	I–XXXII
Bullowa (188)	pneumonia cases	I–XXXII
Bullowa (190)	pneumonia cases	I–XXXII
Nemir, Andrews, and Vinograd (931)	normals and pneumonia cases	I–XXXII
Massachusetts		
Heffron and Varley (616)	pneumonia cases	I–XXXII
Pneumonia Study (870, 615)	pneumonia cases	I–XXXII
Boston		
Sutliff and Finland (1271)	normals and pneumonia cases	I–XX
Smillie (1206)	normals and pneumonia cases	I–XIX
Smillie and Leeder (1210)	normals	I–XXXII
Finland (445)	pneumonia cases	I–XXXII
Sutliff and Steele (1276)	normals	I–XXXII
Finland (449)	normals and pneumonia cases	I–XXXII

* The term "normals" is used to include healthy persons, those with upper respiratory infections, or those with disease or infections elsewhere than in the respiratory tract.

TABLE 4 (*cont.*)

PLACE AND INVESTIGATOR	GROUP SERVING AS CHIEF SOURCE OF ORGANISM	TYPES FOR WHICH DIAGNOSTIC SERUM WAS AVAILABLE
Baltimore		
Bliss, McClaskey, and Long (133)	normals	I–XXXII
New Haven		
Bunim and Trask (201)	normals and pneumonia cases	I–XXXII
San Francisco		
Kohl and Reitzel (734)	normals and pneumonia cases	I–XXXII
Cincinnati		
Benjamin and associates (94)	pneumonia cases	I–XXXII
Canada		
Brown (157)	normals and pneumonia cases	I–XXIX
Virgin Islands		
Smillie, cited by Cooper and associates (320)	normals	I–XVIII
Great Britain		
Griffith, cited by Cooper and associates (320)	normals	"majority" of higher types
Christie (267)	normals and pneumonia cases	I–XXXII
Germany		
Gundel and Schwarz (582)	normals and pneumonia cases	I–XXXII
Gundel (578)	normals	I–XXXII
India		
Napier and Dharmendra (924)	pneumonia cases	I–XXXII

NOTE: For information relative to investigations in South Africa, see Appendix B, page 946.

Though less information is available concerning the occurrence of the higher types, Types IV to XXXII inclusive, throughout the world, it seems probable that they, too, are widely distributed. In this country the presence of various of these types has frequently been reported. In several instances their presence has been noted in other countries. Further, pneumococci of the types causing lobar pneumonia or bronchopneumonia have also been isolated from patients with other than pulmonary infections and from the mouths of normal individuals.

A selected list of the available reports, showing place of origin and character of the host, is given in Table 4.

TYPE INCIDENCE IN PNEUMONIA

Shortly after the classification of pneumococci into Types I, II, III, and Group IV by Dochez and Gillespie (364) in 1913, investigations were begun in various places to determine the frequency of these organisms as a cause of pneumonia. Many such studies have been made of lobar pneumonia but, except for a short period during the War when observations were carried out in a number of the military training camps in this country on several series of bronchopneumonia cases, which were mostly secondary to measles or influenza, relatively few studies have been made of the incidence of pneumococcus types in the ordinary bronchopneumonias of civilian life.

Types I, II, III, and Group IV

INCIDENCE IN LOBAR PNEUMONIA. Typing has been carried out on organisms obtained from a relatively large group of patients with pneumococcus lobar pneumonia. A compilation of the available reports is given in Table 5. Duplication has been avoided by omitting various series from this table. Also omitted are a few series of cases in patients of selected age groups and others in which cases of lobar pneumonia and bronchopneumonia are reported in combination. The series cited are believed to be almost exclusively adult cases. It is not possible in some reports to ascertain exactly the ages of the patients. It is known, however, that a few of the smaller groups do include, along with the findings in adults, those in a few cases in children. As the character of such reports precludes separation of the adult from the children's cases, these series have been included intact. It appears that the number of cases in children so included is small and thus has no special significance in altering the percentage type incidence in such a large group. The incidence of pneumococci of various types in the pneumonias of infants and children is dealt with separately later (see pages 74–89). For practical purposes Table 5 may be considered to represent findings in adults.

As far as known, but with certain notable exceptions, the great majority of cases in the American, Canadian, European, and Australian series in Table 5 were in white patients. The exceptions are in the American series. Two groups of cases were reported from the Harlem Hospital, New York (991, 188) where, Bullowa has stated,* approximately 85 per cent of the patients are of racial groups other than pure white. Most of them are Negroes. Many represent a mixture of various racial stocks including the white. It seems

* Personal communication.

TABLE 5. PNEUMOCOCCUS LOBAR PNEUMONIA CASES. NUMBER AND PERCENTAGE DISTRIBUTION BY LOCALITY, BY INVESTIGATOR, AND BY TYPE OF PNEUMOCOCCUS

SOURCE	PERIOD OF SURVEY	TOTAL CASES	TYPE I Number	TYPE I Per cent	TYPE II Number	TYPE II Per cent	TYPE III Number	TYPE III Per cent	GROUP IV Number	GROUP IV Per cent
United States										
New York										
Cole, Rockefeller Hospital (298)	1911–27	1,110	403	36.3	249	22.4	123	11.1	335*	30.2
Thomas, St. Luke's Hospital (1299)	1917–21	239	60	25.1	26	10.9	35	14.6	118	49.4
Conner, New York Hospital (314) ..	1920–22	90	23	25.6	9	10.0	9	10.0	49	54.4
Cecil and Plummer, Bellevue Hospital (239)	1920–31	4,310	1,384	32.1	991	23.0	477	11.1	1,458	33.8
Kessel and Hyman, Mt. Sinai Hospital (713)	1925–27	43	11	25.6	9	20.9	6	14.0	17	39.5
Park, Bullowa, and Rosenblüth, Harlem Hospital (991)	1926–28	793	223	28.1	124	15.6	85	10.7	361	45.5
Bullowa, Harlem Hospital (188)	1931–34	1,000	253	25.3	79	7.9	115	11.5	553	55.3
Boston										
Alexander, Peter Bent Brigham Hospital (9)	1913–17	104	25	24.0	22	21.2	12	11.5	45	43.3
Locke, Thomas, and O'Hara, City Hospital (797)	1919–20	293	105	35.8	66	22.5	45	15.4	77	26.3
Lyon, City Hospital (821)	1920–21	126	57	45.2	12	9.5	20	15.9	37	29.4
Smillie, various hospitals and private patients (1206)	1932–33	163	48	29.4	34	20.9	16	9.8	65	39.9
Finland, City Hospital (449)	1929–36	2,229	654	29.3	294	13.2	335	15.0	946	42.5

* Sixty-two cases Type II atypical included.

TABLE 5 (*cont.*)

SOURCE	PERIOD OF SURVEY	TOTAL CASES	TYPE I		TYPE II		TYPE III		GROUP IV	
			Number	*Per cent*	*Number*	*Per cent*	*Number*	*Per cent*	*Number*	*Per cent*
Philadelphia, Richardson (1080)	1913–17	409	117	28.6	87	21.3	34	8.3	171	41.8
Baltimore, Sydenstricker and Sutton (1282)	1917	62	24	38.7	4	6.5	–	–	34	54.8
Texas, Nichols (952)	1917	150	84	56.0	33	22.0	3	2.0	30	20.0
New Jersey, Shorer and associates (1163)	1917–18	101	31	30.7	15	14.9	18	17.8	37	36.6
Chicago, Quigley (1054)	1917–18	100	33	33.0	36	36.0	13	13.0	18	18.0
Louisiana, McClelland (829)	1918	113	33	29.2	11	9.7	5	4.4	64	56.6
Pennsylvania, Richardson (1079)	1919	46	7	15.2	5	10.9	2	4.3	32	69.6
Connecticut, Blake (120)	1921–31	606	194	32.0	79	13.0	122	20.1	211	34.8
Ohio, Benjamin, Blankenhorn, Ruegsegger, and Senior (94)	1935–37	485	156	32.2	52	10.7	50	10.3	227	46.8
Canada										
Montreal, Howard (661)	1927–29	149	17	11.4	25	16.8	10	6.7	97	65.1
Toronto, Brown (157)	1930	56	24	42.9	11	19.6	6	10.7	15	26.8
Puerto Rico										
San Juan, Suárez (1261)	1931	27	1	3.7	13	48.1	6	22.2	7	25.9
Europe										
Great Britain										
Liverpool, Glynn and Digby (520)	1921	96	44	45.8	22	22.9	2	2.1	28†	29.2
London, Mallock (854)	1920–21	67	24	35.8	10	14.9	2	3.0	31‡	46.3
London, Urquhart (1346)	1920–21	33	17	51.5	8	24.2	–	–	8	24.2
London, Griffith (571)	1920–27	278	95	34.2	67	24.1	15	5.4	101	36.3

† One case Type II atypical included.

‡ Fourteen cases Type II atypical included.

TABLE 5 (*cont.*)

SOURCE	PERIOD OF SURVEY	TOTAL CASES	TYPE I		TYPE II		TYPE III		GROUP IV	
			Number	*Per cent*	*Number*	*Per cent*	*Number*	*Per cent*	*Number*	*Per cent*
Europe										
Great Britain (*cont.*)										
Glasgow, Grant (553)	1922	38	12	31.6	23	60.5	2	5.3	1	2.6
Edinburgh, McLachlan (844)	1924–25	52	31	59.6	6	11.5	8	15.4	7	13.5
Manchester, Ferguson and Lovell (437)	1925–27	116	50	43.1	5	4.3	–	–	61	52.6
Edinburgh, Alston and Stewart (13)	1929–30	182	53	29.1	75	41.2	7	3.8	47	25.8
Glasgow, Macgregor (837)	1930–32	1,077	410	38.1	388	36.0	42	3.9	237	22.0
Manchester, Langley (763)	1931–33	292	158	54.1	67	22.9	4	1.4	63	21.6
London, Davies, Hodgson, and Whitby (339)	1932–33	137	55	40.1	13	9.5	20	14.6	49	35.8
Rest of Europe										
Irish Free State, Moore (902)	1923	110	36	32.7	25	22.7	7	6.4	42§	38.2
Norway, Thjötta and Hanneborg (1294)	1924	100	44	44.0	33	33.0	6	6.0	17	17.0
Denmark, Christensen (265)	1922–24	150	42	28.0	41	27.3	13	8.7	54	36.0
Germany, Hallermann and Kähler (589)	1930	66	18	27.3	21	31.8	23	34.8	4	6.1
Germany, Gundel and Linden (579)	1930–31	45	20	44.4	9	20.0	8	17.8	8	17.8
Germany, Becker (84)	1932–33	86	34	39.5	28	32.6	14	16.3	10	11.6
Switzerland, Herzog (636)	1924	57	15	26.3	14	24.6	22	38.6	6	10.5
Italy, Pontano (1044)	1922	27	14	51.9	6	22.2	3	11.1	4	14.8
Italy, Marginesu and Corda (860)	1923	44	16	36.4	5	11.4	6	13.6	17¶	38.6
Italy, Levi (775)	1933	85	25	29.4	21	24.7	16	18.8	23	27.1

§ Six cases Type II atypical included. ¶ Five cases Type II atypical included.

TABLE 5 (*cont.*)

SOURCE	PERIOD OF SURVEY	TOTAL CASES	TYPE I Number	TYPE I Per cent	TYPE II Number	TYPE II Per cent	TYPE III Number	TYPE III Per cent	GROUP IV Number	GROUP IV Per cent
Africa										
Anglo-Egyptian Sudan										
Whitehead (1419)	1927	27	8	29.6	3	11.1	2	7.4	14	51.9
Kenya, Garnham and deSmidt (507) ..	1930–31	55	4	7.3	1	1.8	1	1.8	49	89.1
Union of South Africa, Lister (786) ...	1913–17	148	32	21.6	24	16.2	2	1.4	90	60.8
Far East										
India										
Madras, Cunningham, Cruickshank, and Ramakrishnan (334)	1923–25	29	18	62.1	3	10.3	2	6.9	6	20.7
Karachi, Bhatnagar and Singh (100)	1935	87	43	49.4	21	24.1	5	5.7	18	20.7
Calcutta, Napier and Dharmendra (924)	1935	31	7	22.6	2	6.5	3	9.7	19	61.3
Assam, Napier and Dharmendra (924)	1935	45	4	8.9	1	2.2	1	2.2	39	86.7
China, Peiping, Wu and Chiu (1450) ..	1922–31	242	99	40.9	45	18.6	14	5.8	84	34.7
Straits Settlements, Singapore, Allen**	—	58	19	32.8	12	20.7	9	15.5	18	31.0
New Guinea, Morgan**	—	14	10	71.4	1	7.1	1	7.1	2	14.2
Australia										
Melbourne, Patterson (1003a)	1922	135	63	46.7	14	10.4	7	5.2	51	37.8
Grand total††		16,813	5,487	32.6	3,300	19.6	1,814	10.8	6,212	36.9

** Cited by Gautier (510) on *Tropical Pneumonia.*

†† Early compilation of data for this table showed a total of 14,869 cases with incidence figures as follows: Type I, 32.8 per cent; Type II, 20.6 per cent; Type III, 10.8 per cent; and Group IV, 35.8 per cent.

likely, in addition, that the small series from Baltimore (1282) and from Louisiana (829) may also represent largely cases in Negro patients. Essentially all the remaining cases in Table 5 (those reported from Africa and the Far East) were in natives of their respective countries.

Of the 16,813 cases listed in Table 5, Type I accounted for 5,487, or 32.6 per cent, and Type II for 3,300, or 19.6 per cent of the series. Even though the methods of typing used doubtless varied somewhat, as presumably did the intensity of search for pneumococci of the first two types, Type I and Type II together were responsible for 8,787, or 52.2 per cent of the cases. Failure to clearly differentiate typical from atypical strains of pneumococci of Type II may, in some instances, have increased the number of cases and consequently the proportion of those attributed to pneumococci of Type II. Pneumococci of Type III accounted for 1,814, or 10.8 per cent, and the remaining 6,212, or 36.9 per cent of the cases, were attributed to other pneumococci. These figures show a higher proportion of the cases due to Type I and Type II and a smaller proportion due to other types than was found by Wadsworth (1366) in his collected series of more than 30,000 cases. Unfortunately, the exact nature and source of his cases are not given.

VARIATION OF INCIDENCE WITH GEOGRAPHIC DISTRIBUTION. A review of the individual series listed in Table 5 shows that considerable variation of type incidence has been encountered in the same or different places. With the exception of a few series of substantial size from the United States and Great Britain, the groups are so small that the significance of their distribution is dubious. In general, and with a few marked exceptions, the incidence of Type I appears fairly high the world over. Type II shows great variation, even within the same country in some instances, and is usually, but not always, less commonly found than Type I. Type III likewise exhibits marked variability and in general is the least common of the first three types. A notable exception to this appears in some of the cases from Germany and Switzerland, and to a lesser extent from Italy, where Type III was reported as fairly common. Finally, pneumococci of Group IV also have shown great variability, even within the same country and at the same time (see also pages 57–67).

The total 16,813 cases include patients of various classes and racial groups from the temperate zones to the tropics. As so-called "racial" susceptibility or climatic factors may be of importance, it is advantageous for purposes of comparison to subdivide the series in Table 5 into groups depending upon certain geographic and climatic features.

In Table 6 a tabulation of cases has been made upon a geographic basis. Certain variations of type incidence are apparent. Type I and Type II together accounted for a larger proportion of the cases in Europe than elsewhere in the world. In the order of their combined frequency, these two types were responsible for 67 per cent of the cases in the European group, 56.4 per cent in the Far East–Australian group, 48.9 per cent in the American–Puerto Rican–Canadian group, and only 31.3 per cent of the cases in the African group. It appears that Types I and II account for over twice as many cases in Europe as in Africa. Though the number of cases in the African group (230 cases) is small as compared with that in the European group (3,138 cases), the difference in the incidence of Types I and II in these groups seems significant.*

TABLE 6. PNEUMOCOCCUS LOBAR PNEUMONIA CASES. PERCENTAGE DISTRIBUTION BY GEOGRAPHIC AREA AND BY TYPE

	TOTAL CASES	TYPE I	TYPE II	TYPES I AND II TOGETHER	TYPE III	GROUP IV
United States, Puerto Rico, and Canada ..	12,804	31.0	17.9	48.9	12.1	39.1
Europe	3,138	38.7	28.3	67.0	7.0	26.1
Africa	230	19.1	12.2	31.3	2.2	66.5
Far East and Australia	641	41.0	15.4	56.4	6.6	37.0
Total	16,813					

A division of the series in Table 5 on a basis of gross climatic differences is presented in Table 7. Pneumococci of Types I and II together accounted for more than one-half, or 52.6 per cent, of the 16,292 cases from the temperate zones. Though these types appear less frequent in cases in the tropical and subtropical zones, their importance even in those warm regions seems clear, for they were responsible for 43.5 per cent of 521 cases. Type III was less common in the tropical and subtropical group of cases and Group IV pneumococci more commonly found than in cases from the temperate zones. Finally, as the latter group of cases contains several large series and is about thirty-one times as large as the tropical and subtropical group, which is composed chiefly of a few small series of cases, not too much emphasis can be

* The standard deviation of the difference (35.7 ± 3.26) between the proportion of Type I and II cases in these groups is statistically significant.

placed upon any apparent differences in these groups at this time. In many respects it is remarkable that more marked differences between them are not apparent.

TABLE 7. PNEUMOCOCCUS LOBAR PNEUMONIA CASES. PERCENTAGE DISTRIBUTION BY CLIMATIC GROUP AND BY TYPE

	TOTAL CASES	TYPE I	TYPE II	TYPES I AND II TOGETHER	TYPE III	GROUP IV
Temperate zone	16,292	32.8	19.8	52.6	10.9	36.5
Tropical and sub-tropical zones*	521	28.0	15.5	43.5	6.1	50.3
Total	16,813					

* This group is comprised of the series listed in Table 5 from the following places: Puerto Rico, Suárez (1261); Africa, Anglo-Egyptian Sudan, Whitehead (1419); Kenya, Garnham and deSmidt (507); Union of South Africa, Lister (786); India, Cunningham and associates (334), Bhatnagar and Singh (100), Napier and Dharmendra (924), two series; and Straits Settlements, Allen, and New Guinea, Morgan, both cited by Gautier (510). The remaining series from Table 5 make up the large group of cases from the temperate zone.

Types IV through XXXII

CAUSAL RELATION TO PNEUMONIA. Certain characteristics of pneumococci of Types IV through XXXII and of conditions under which the organisms are frequently found have given rise to the question of their role in pneumonia of various forms. As will be seen later, pneumococci of the higher types commonly inhabit the nasopharynx of normal individuals. They are frequently found so associated with secondary and bronchopneumonia as to strongly suggest an etiologic relationship. Other studies have suggested that strains of most of the higher types are of low virulence. In addition, over a two-year period Gundel and his associates in Germany (584, 582) found nearly all cases of lobar pneumonia due to Type I or II and never found a case due to any of the types above Type III. In general this latter finding is in keeping with the situation revealed in Tables 5 and 6 that in lobar pneumonia in Europe Types I and II are more common and pneumococci above Type III less common than elsewhere.

A considerable body of information is now available, however, which would seem to indicate conclusively that pneumococci of many of the higher types can and do give rise to lobar pneumonia and to bronchopneumonia as well both in adults and in children. More than 400 strains of pneumococci of the higher types isolated from 397 adults and children with lobar pneumonia were examined by Cooper and her co-workers (318, 320). In more than 500 cases of lobar pneumonia in adults, Bullowa (175) found 122 cases due to pneumococci of Types IV through XVIII. Also, and of the greatest importance in this matter, were the results of intensive bacteriologic and immunologic studies of large groups of cases, as illustrated by the reports below. Sutliff and Finland (1271) found pneumococci of Types IV through XX responsible for 239 cases of lobar pneumonia. The results of sputum examination were confirmed in many of these cases by culturing the organisms from the blood and empyema fluids during life and from the heart's blood and lungs at necropsy. Subsequently Winkler and Finland (1429) investigated nine of the higher types* and showed that, during the course of lobar pneumonia or bronchopneumonia due to any one of these, patients developed humoral agglutinins and protective substances specific for the type homologous with that causing the infection and for no other types. Such antibodies could be specifically absorbed by pneumococci of the homologous but not heterologous types. The antigenic relationship of these higher types to pneumonia appeared similar to that of Types I, II, and III. Of like significance were the findings of Finland and Winkler (468, 469), who investigated the antibody response to infection with the immunologically related Types III and VIII, and Types II and V.

Bullowa and Wilcox's (198) study of more than 1,700 cases of pneumococcus pneumonia (lobar pneumonia and bronchopneumonia together), each of which was due to some type from I through XXXII, is also of importance in connection with the power of the pneumococcus to cause pneumonia. Pneumococci of the infecting type were isolated from the blood in cases due to twenty-three of these types. It may be noted, however, that bacteriemia in cases attributed to infection by the eight types, XI, XVI, XXII, XXVII, XXVIII, XXX, XXXI, and XXXII, was not demonstrated (see pages 555–556).

Further, Bullowa (188) found Types IV through XXXII responsible for 553 cases of pneumococcus lobar pneumonia in adults. In these patients the identity of the infecting organism was determined by several procedures. Typing was carried out on pneumococci obtained from one or more specimens of sputum, blood cultures, material obtained by lung suction (lung puncture), empyema fluids, spinal fluids, and necropsy cultures from the heart's blood and lungs.

* Types IV, V, VII, VIII, XII, XIV, XVII, XVIII, and XIX.

Finland's (449) findings in a series of 684 cases of pneumococcus pneumonia, examined at necropsy for pneumococci of the types from I through XXXII, are significant. In 339 of the cases with lobar pneumonia the six types most frequently encountered were Types I, III, II, V, VII, and VIII in the order named and were responsible for 83 per cent of the cases. In the whole series of 684 pneumonias no cases due to pneumococci of Type XV, XXV, XXX, XXXI, or XXXII were found at necropsy. As a consequence of the findings in these studies it is clear that pneumococci of probably a majority of the higher types (as well as those of Type I, II, or III) are able to give rise to pneumonia. With a few of the higher types, however, as the above data suggest, evidence is not available to indicate that organisms of those types may give rise to pneumonia. This seems particularly true of several of the types above Type XX. In either lobar pneumonia or bronchopneumonia the incidence of the different types may vary.

INCIDENCE IN LOBAR PNEUMONIA. Several series of cases are available from which an estimation may be made of the frequency of the higher types as a cause of lobar pneumonia in adults. Cooper and her collaborators (318, 320), using diagnostic serum for Types IV through XXIX, typed nearly 300 strains of pneumococci obtained from adult patients with lobar pneumonia. These cases and the series listed by Park and Williams (995) are doubtless from the same material and do not readily lend themselves to tabulation in the ordinary manner. It also seems likely that the series of 122 adult cases due to Types IV through XVIII reported by Bullowa (175) includes many of the 120 cases due to Types IV through XXI reported by Park (987). Further, Smillie (1206) determined the incidence of Types IV through XIX in 57 cases of lobar pneumonia. His series included some cases in children.

In Canada, Brown (157) determined the incidence of pneumococci of Types IV through XXIX in 72 cases of pneumonia. It is not clear that these were all lobar pneumonias. Lister (786) and Lister and Ordman (788), using Lister's classification, have reported the incidence of various of the types of pneumococci, other than those corresponding to Type I, II, or III, in more than 200 cases of lobar pneumonia in African natives. Napier and Dharmendra (924) typed two small groups of cases occurring in natives of India. In Calcutta, with serums for Type IV through at least Type XIV, four cases of Type VI were found, while pneumococci from fifteen other cases could not be classified. In Assam, eighteen cases could be classified with serums for Types IV through XXXII as follows: Type IV, four cases;

Types VIII, XIV, and XXV, two cases each; and Types VI, VII, X, XI, XVI, XVII, XVIII, and XXII, one case each. Twenty-one cases remained unclassified, and sixteen of these appeared due to two local types.

The above groups are of interest, but for various reasons no attempt will be made to tabulate them. There are three American series of considerable size, however, which can be combined to show the approximate incidence of the higher types in lobar pneumonia in adults. These are the series reported by Finland (449),* Bullowa (188), and Benjamin, Blankenhorn, Ruegsegger, and Senior (94), as shown in Table 8. For comparative purposes Type I, II, and III cases are included. Typing was carried out for all recognized types. There are 2,229 cases in Finland's series, 1,000 cases in Bullowa's series, and 484 in the group studied by Benjamin and his associates. Certain variations in the frequency with which some of the types were found are apparent. Most striking is the relatively small number of Type II and Type X cases and the large number of Type IV cases in Bullowa's series.

A certain few of the many types found in pneumonia are usually the commonest and are responsible for a large percentage of all cases. Cooper, Rosenstein, Walter, and Peizer (320) found that Types IV, V, VII, and VIII constituted 50 per cent of 278 Group IV strains isolated from 271 cases of lobar pneumonia in adults. These same types were also the most common in Bullowa's (175) early series of 122 cases of Types IV through XVIII. Brown (157), in 47 cases of "pneumonia" typed from IV through XXIX, found Types V, VII, and VIII accounted for 45 per cent of the group.

Reference to Table 8 shows, as Finland (449) pointed out for his series of 2,229 cases of pneumococcus lobar pneumonia, that of the higher types those of Types V, VII, and VIII were commonest. Together with Types I, II, and III, these six types were responsible for 79 per cent of his cases. In similar fashion Bullowa's (188) series shows that Types IV, V, VII, and VIII are the commonest of the higher types, and that together with Types I, II, and III these seven types accounted for 73.9 per cent of his 1,000 cases. Types I, II, III, V, VII, and VIII made up 76 per cent of the 484 cases in the series of Benjamin and his associates (94).

These three series combined total 3,713 cases. In this large group the six types most commonly encountered in pneumococcus lobar pneumonia, in the order of their frequency, were Types I, III, II, V, VIII, and VII, which together were responsible for 75.7 per cent of the total group of cases. Types

* This series includes 770 cases previously reported by Sutliff and Finland (1271).

TABLE 8. PNEUMOCOCCUS LOBAR PNEUMONIA CASES IN ADULTS REPORTED IN THE LITERATURE. NUMBER AND PERCENTAGE DISTRIBUTION BY TYPE

TYPE	FINLAND (449)	BULLOWA (188)	BENJAMIN AND ASSOCIATES (94)	TOTAL *Number*	TOTAL *Per cent*
I	654	253	156	1,063	28.6
II	294	79	52	425	11.4
III	335	115	50	500	13.5
IV	46	65	20	131	3.5
V	191	60	47	298	8.0
VI	28	29	9	66	1.8
VII	128	69	43	240	6.5
VIII	159	98	30	287	7.7
IX	30	25	8	63	1.7
X	37	8	2	47	1.3
XI	29	6	1	36	1.0
XII	38	14	13	65	1.8
XIII	13	8	–	21	0.6
XIV	51	45	6	102	2.7
XV	7	1	1	9	0.2
XVI	4	4	–	8	0.2
XVII	19	8	–	27	0.7
XVIII	38	24	6	68	1.8
XIX	19	16	10	45	1.2
XX	36	11	–	47	1.3
XXI	9	13	–	22	0.6
XXII	10	16	2	28	0.8
XXIII	2	3	1	6	0.2
XXIV	–	3	–	3	0.1
XXV	3	2	12	17	0.5
XXVII	1	2	–	3	0.1
XXVIII	–	9	2	11	0.3
XXIX	4	5	1	10	0.3
XXX	nr	2	nr	2	0.1
XXXI	3	3	–	6	0.2
XXXII	3	4	–	7	0.2
Unclassified	38*	nr	12	50	1.3
Total†	2,229	1,000	484	3,713	

nr = no record.

* In 35 instances typing was carried out only as far as Type XX.

† Early compilation of data for this table showed a total of 1,770 cases, of which 770 reported by Sutliff and Finland (1271) and due to pneumococci of the types from I through XX are, as earlier mentioned, included in Finland's (449) larger series here shown. The remaining 1,000 cases attributed to Types I through XXXII were those of Bullowa (188) as listed in the table.

IV, XIV, VI, XII, and XVIII, in that order, were next in frequency. It is seen that among the higher types, only Types V, VII, and VIII occurred in more than 5 per cent of the cases, and together these types accounted for 22.2 per cent of the 3,713 cases.

It is also apparent that in the series listed in Table 8 the types from I through VIII were by far the most common. They were responsible for 81 per cent of the 3,713 cases, while the remaining twenty-three types* from IX through XXXII accounted for only 19 per cent of the total. It appears, then, that pneumococci of the first eight types are responsible for about four-fifths of the cases of lobar pneumonia in adults.

INCIDENCE IN PNEUMOCOCCUS PNEUMONIA. Analyses of Type III and Type VIII infections have been presented by Finland and Sutliff (464) and of Type VIII and of Type XIV pneumonias by Bullowa (186, 187). Prior to Bullowa's report of the 1,000 cases (188) listed in Table 8, he found in adults with pneumococcus pneumonia (lobar pneumonia and bronchopneumonia together) that Type VIII accounted for 5.9 per cent of 2,067 cases and Type XIV for 2.6 per cent of 2,546 cases. The incidence of the remaining types in these latter groups of cases was not stated.

In a later study of type incidence in pneumococcus pneumonia (lobar pneumonia and bronchopneumonia together) Bullowa (190) at the Harlem Hospital, New York City, found that in a series of 3,591 cases† examined over the period of July 1928—June 1936, Types IV, V, VII, and VIII were the higher types most frequently encountered. These types occurred in 6.2 per cent, 7.9 per cent, 7.8 per cent, and 8.1 per cent, respectively, of the cases and together accounted for 30 per cent of the entire series. Type I was found in 23.7 per cent of the cases, Type II in 8 per cent, and Type III in 10.2 per cent. The seven types, Types I, II, III, IV, V, VII, and VIII, together accounted for 71.9 per cent of the cases.

Of some interest with respect to the frequency of occurrence of the higher types both in and around Boston (exclusive of the series reported by Finland [449] from the Boston City Hospital) and throughout the state, is the experience of the Massachusetts Pneumonia Study (869). During that Study typing was carried out at the central laboratory in Boston and in over sixty‡ other laboratories throughout the state. The sputums sent to these labora-

* Type XXVI cases are included in Type VI.

† This series includes Bullowa's cases of lobar pneumonia shown in Table 8.

‡ The number of typing laboratories was subsequently increased (615, 251, 6).

tories for examination came from patients with lobar pneumonia or with other forms of pneumonia or respiratory disease. In spite of the varied origin of such specimens, the results of typing pneumococci obtained from them lend added weight to the findings of others mentioned above. They also furnish additional evidence as to which types were most frequently the cause of respiratory disease throughout the whole state.

At the central laboratory in Boston specimens were examined for all thirty-two types of pneumococci. In the outlying laboratories typing was carried out for Types I, II, and III (and at times for Type V* also), and many cultures of strains found to be other than one of the first three types were sent to the central laboratory where they were typed out from Types IV through XXXII. The bulk of these cultures were sent to the central laboratory during the three winters of 1931–1932 to 1933–1934. Following that, due to an alteration of procedure, relatively few such cultures were received for examination. It is believed that the types found in these cultures may be regarded as representative of conditions throughout the state for that three-year period. Table 9 lists the findings in two groups of specimens. Group A represents the types found in specimens sent directly to the central laboratory from 1931 through 1935. Approximately 80 per cent of these came from patients residing in Boston or within a radius of about ten miles of it, and the remainder from more distant points in the state. Group B presents the types found in cultures of pneumococci sent from the outlying laboratories to the central laboratory, that is, types exclusive of Type I, II, or III. (For purposes of comparison, Types I, II, and III have been included in Group A.)

Of the 2,961 strains listed in Group A (Table 9), pneumococci of six types, namely Types I, II, III, V, VII, and VIII, were commonest and together made up 1,698 or 57.3 per cent of the group. Considering only the higher types in this table, some variation is apparent between their frequency in Group A and Group B. In the former the commonest types in the order of their occurrence are Types VIII, V, VII, XVIII, VI, and XIX, while in Group B Types VIII, VII, V, XIX, XVIII, and IV are the most frequent. In both groups, however, disregarding the order in which they occurred, Types V, VII, and VIII were the commonest. Thus these three types were the most frequent not only in Boston but over the remainder of Massachusetts as well and accounted for 732 or 32.4 per cent of the total 2,257 strains identified.

So far as the occurrence of certain of the higher types in pneumonia is con-

* Examination is now made for Types I, II, III, V, VII, and VIII in the outlying laboratories and in many instances for several other types as well.

TABLE 9. PNEUMOCOCCUS TYPES IV–XXXII ISOLATED FROM SPUTUM SPECIMENS AND CULTURES AT THE CENTRAL LABORATORY, BOSTON

TYPE FOUND	GROUP A *Sputums from Boston*	GROUP B *Cultures from outlying laboratories*	TOTAL *Number*	*Per cent*
I	534	–	–	–
II	140	–	–	–
III	439	–	–	–
IV	92	23	115	5.1
V	139	38	177	7.8
VI	106	19	125	5.5
VII	136	44	180	8.0
VIII	310	65	375	16.6
IX	95	17	112	5.0
X	50	18	68	3.0
XI	63	6	69	3.1
XII	33	6	39	1.7
XIII	50	12	62	2.7
XIV	61	14	75	3.3
XV	23	–	23	1.0
XVI	31	4	35	1.6
XVII	54	7	61	2.7
XVIII	117	24	141	6.2
XIX	98	31	129	5.7
XX	57	14	71	3.1
XXI	77	17	94	4.2
XXII	37	6	43	1.9
XXIII	49	7	56	2.5
XXIV	14	3	17	0.8
XXV	6	1	7	0.3
XXVI	–	–	–	–
XXVII	10	3	13	0.6
XXVIII	40	5	45	2.0
XXIX	38	10	48	2.1
XXX	35	8	43	1.9
XXXI	23	7	30	1.3
XXXII	4	–	4	0.2
Total	2,961*	409†	2,257‡	100.0

* There were, in addition, 189 strains of pneumococci which for various reasons remained unclassified. These are mentioned earlier in this chapter. There were also 1,190 other specimens examined which yielded no pneumococci, making a grand total of 4,340.

† In addition to these there were 312 cultures examined, some of which showed pneumococci, which were overgrown by contaminating organisms, died, or were otherwise lost in the process of examination and remained unclassified, and some of which showed no pneumococci.

‡ This does not include Type I, II, and III results in Group A.

cerned, the findings in lobar pneumonia and in pneumococcus pneumonia (lobar pneumonia and bronchopneumonia together) are all remarkably similar and their general significance seems clear. The reports from New York City (320, 175, 188, 190), Boston and the rest of Massachusetts (1271, 449, 1206, 869), Ohio (94), and Toronto, Canada (157), show that in the northeastern portion of the United States and a nearby section of southern Canada, from 1928 through 1936, pneumococci of Types V, VII, and VIII have been the most common of the higher types encountered in reported series of cases of pneumonia.

Types V, VII, and VIII also proved the commonest high types in a series of 111 cases of pneumococcus pneumonia reported from California (San Francisco) by Kohl and Reitzel (734). These cases were examined during 1934 and 1935 when typing was carried out for all thirty-two types. In this series of 111 cases Types V, VII, and VIII were found in 20 or 18 per cent and Types I, II, and III in 67 or 60.4 per cent of the cases. These six types together accounted for 78.4 per cent of the cases.

Variation of Type Incidence in Lobar Pneumonia with Certain Factors other than Geographic Distribution

MISCELLANEOUS FACTORS. Numerous factors appear to influence the frequency with which pneumococci of various types occur in lobar pneumonia. In connection with the discussion of the 16,813 cases listed in Table 5 (see page 43), it was earlier mentioned that geographic and gross climatic differences may affect type incidence. Types I and II accounted for more cases in Europe than elsewhere in the world and were more frequent in cases from the temperate than from the tropical zones.

But other factors than geographic and climatic must play a part, and experience has shown that the incidence of the various types is almost never the same in a given place in different years (360, 1234, 1299, 230, 571, 616, 1450, 331, 464, 557, 198, 734). The observations of Cecil, Baldwin, and Larsen (230) on 1,913 cases studied at the Bellevue Hospital, New York City, over a period of five winters may serve as an example to illustrate variations of this nature (see Table 10).

During different winters the incidence of Type I varied from 21 per cent to 45.2 per cent. Type II with a variation in incidence of from 15.9 to 20.6 per cent showed the smallest difference in the group. Type III varied from 7.9 to 17.2 per cent, and Group IV from 23.5 to 41 per cent. Such marked differences in the incidence of the various types in different years are apparently not always encountered, for Macgregor (837) reported finding relatively little variation in incidence among 1,077 cases studied in Glasgow. His study was confined to a more limited period, however, covering the years 1930 to 1932.

TABLE 10. PNEUMOCOCCUS LOBAR PNEUMONIA CASES IN ADULTS, NEW YORK CITY. PERCENTAGE DISTRIBUTION BY TYPE DURING FIVE SUCCESSIVE WINTERS

WINTER OF	TOTAL CASES	TYPE I	TYPE II	TYPE III	GROUP IV
1920–21	377	45.2	15.9	14.5	23.5
1921–22	534	33.7	18.1	15.7	32.5
1922–23	319	21.0	20.6	17.2	41.0
1923–24	275	30.9	20.0	16.0	33.0
1924–25	408	35.7	20.0	7.9	36.2
Total	1,913				

From Cecil *et al.* (230)

Variations in type incidence occur in the same year in different places, as is shown by many of the series previously listed in Table 5. Indeed, in different hospitals in a single community during the same year some variation of type incidence may be encountered.

Despite such variations, under ordinary conditions Types I and II are nearly always the two commonest types found. During the course of small epidemics, either of these or some other single type may prove unusually prevalent (see page 386).

It has long been recognized that in temperate climates the bulk of the cases of lobar pneumonia occurs over a period of a few months during winter and spring. Data on type incidence have come largely from the tabulation of such cases. While yearly differences in type incidence are easily demonstrable, as is the fact that in winter and spring, when pneumonia is most prevalent, the types most commonly causing lobar pneumonia are most frequently encountered (239, 464, 267, 734), yet adequate reports are lacking that clearly demonstrate the type incidence in a large series of cases occurring in summer. Smillie (1206), who typed 173 cases occurring in the course of a full year, reported that no one type was prevalent in only one month or one season, but rather there was a general distribution of the various types over the whole year. No considerable series of cases is available showing the incidence of the various types by months throughout the year. Finland and

Sutliff (464), however, have shown the monthly incidence of Types I, II, III, and VIII in cases of pneumococcus pneumonia for a period of over three years. Their findings illustrate that the months of highest incidence (winter and spring) were usually the same for all four types. In general, Type I and Type III showed a marked seasonal variation and were infrequent in mid-summer and far more frequent in late fall, winter, and spring. Type II was somewhat different in that, though it showed some seasonal variation, this was less striking than with the above two types and Type II tended to occur more uniformly throughout the year. Type VIII likewise showed a tendency to winter and spring prevalence but was frequently absent from cases occurring in summer. In some months an individual type showed a high incidence without a simultaneous and corresponding increase in the occurrence of other types. This was also observed in various places within Massachusetts during the course of the Massachusetts Pneumonia Study.

Lindau (783) has suggested that the incidence of the commoner types is the same in patients of the same social class residing in countries within the temperate zones. It is doubtful if satisfactory figures are available to prove or disprove this contention.

It is possible that there is some difference between the incidence of the various types in cases occurring in urban and in rural regions. Nearly all the 16,292 cases of pneumococcus lobar pneumonia from temperate zones, summarized in Table 7 (see page 49), were from urban communities. Pneumococci of Type I were found in 32.8 per cent, Type II in 19.8 per cent, Type III in 10.9 per cent, and Group IV in 36.5 per cent of the cases. In a small series of cases (46 cases) from rural Pennsylvania, Richardson (1079) found pneumococci of the first three types less often and of Group IV much more often than this. The percentage incidence of these organisms in his cases was as follows: Type I, 15.2; Type II, 10.8; Type III, 4.3; and Group IV, 69.6. In another series of 50 pneumococcus cases which occurred in a rural section of Alabama, Smillie and Caldwell's (1209) findings were much similar. In their series the percentage incidence was Type I, 14; Type II, none; Type III, 2; and Group IV, 84. The proportion of children in Richardson's series is not known, but in Smillie and Caldwell's series it must have been high, for the bulk of their cases were Group IV and most of these were children. Incidence figures very similar to this have been reported from Pittsburgh by McMeans (851). The source of his material, however, is not clear.

Though accurate figures to support the following view could not be obtained, the impression was gained during the course of the Massachusetts Pneumonia Study (869) that in the more rural areas the incidence of cases due to pneumococci of Types I and II was somewhat lower than in the urban areas. In one distinctly rural area, however, where sputum from essentially every case of lobar pneumonia (more than 70 cases) that occurred over a three-year period was examined bacteriologically, the incidence of pneumococci of the first three types and of Group IV was very similar to that shown above in Table 7.

In some districts of the state over a period of many months only a few cases of pneumonia occurred and these were due to pneumococci of Type III or Group IV. Then suddenly during the course of a few weeks a number of cases were encountered, most of which were due to Type I or, to a lesser extent, Type II. In other places the number and proportion of cases due to the various types were rather constant over a year or more, to be followed later by a rather abrupt increase of Type I, II, or Group IV cases with a concurrent apparent reduction in cases due to other types. Such variations appeared continuous and the incidence of the several types appeared to change during a single year or from year to year without obvious cause.

The appearance of influenza in a community may be followed by rapid and considerable changes in type incidence in lobar pneumonia (1221, 267).

VARIATION WITH AGE. The frequency with which pneumococci of the first three types occur in pneumococcus lobar pneumonia in adults generally shows certain characteristic variations depending upon the age of the patients. Among 585 cases in patients under thirty years of age, reported by Cecil, Baldwin, and Larsen (230), 246 or 42 per cent were Type I and 105 or 17.9 per cent were Type II. Including these cases, they found in 1,465 patients under fifty years of age that Type I accounted for 535 or 36.5 per cent and Type II for 280 or 12.2 per cent. In patients under fifty years of age Type I proved to be the commonest type found. In all, the above investigators reported the incidence of pneumococci of the first three types and Group IV in 1,867 cases in patients of various ages, as shown in Table 11.

Cases due to Type I were most common in young adults and accounted for 45.5 per cent of the cases in patients ten to twenty years of age. From here on, as age increased, the incidence of Type I decreased; and in patients over sixty years old this type accounted for but 20 per cent of the group. Nearly the reverse was true with Type III, however, for it accounted for only 5.9 per cent of the cases in patients ten to twenty years old; but in patients of greater age the incidence of this type progressively increased, and in the group over sixty years of age Type III was found in 33.7 per cent of the cases. In contrast to this variation of the incidence of Types I and III, the frequency of cases due to Type II and Group IV showed no special variation with the age of the patient.

TABLE 11. PNEUMOCOCCUS LOBAR PNEUMONIA: 1,867 CASES IN ADULTS OF VARIOUS AGES. NUMBER AND PERCENTAGE DISTRIBUTION BY TYPE

	10–20 YEARS		UNDER 30 YEARS		UNDER 40 YEARS	
	Cases	*Per cent incidence*	*Cases*	*Per cent incidence*	*Cases*	*Per cent incidence*
Type I	59	45.5	246	42.0	323	33.2
Type II	16	11.9	105	17.9	196	20.2
Type III	8	5.9	41	7.0	103	10.6
Group IV	51	38.0	193	32.9	348	33.6
	134	7.1	585	31.3	970	51.9

	UNDER 50 YEARS		OVER 50 YEARS		OVER 60 YEARS	
	Cases	*Per cent incidence*	*Cases*	*Per cent incidence*	*Cases*	*Per cent incidence*
Type I	535	36.5	92	22.8	32	20.0
Type II	280	12.2	82	23.9	22	13.7
Type III	166	11.3	97	24.1	54	33.7
Group IV	484	32.6	131	32.6	55	34.1
	1,465	78.4	402	21.5	163	8.5

From Cecil *et al.* (230)

There is essential agreement on the fact that Type I is the commonest type found in patients under fifty years old with pneumococcus lobar pneumonia and, further, that the great majority of Type I cases are in patients under this age (230, 238, 239, 120, 24, 1271, 1206, 779, 1272, 464, 557, 339). This latter point may be illustrated by dividing the cases in patients under and over fifty years of age, listed in Table 11, to show the proportion of those in each type that occurred in these age groups (see Table 12).

Of the total 1,867 cases, 1,465 or 78.5 per cent occurred in patients under fifty. Of the total number of cases in each type, the largest proportion occurred in patients under fifty years old; the percentages being Type I, 85.3; Type II, 77.3; Type III, 63.1; and Group IV, 78.7 per cent. Also, of the total number of cases in each type, Type III showed the largest proportion (36.9 per cent) in patients over fifty years of age.

TABLE 12. TYPE I, II, AND III AND GROUP IV LOBAR PNEUMONIA CASES IN ADULTS. NUMBER AND PERCENTAGE DISTRIBUTION BY AGE GROUP UNDER AND OVER FIFTY YEARS

	TOTAL CASES	UNDER 50 YEARS OF AGE		OVER 50 YEARS OF AGE	
		Cases	*Per cent incidence*	*Cases*	*Per cent incidence*
Type I	627	535	85.3	92	14.7
Type II	362	280	77.3	82	22.7
Type III	263	166	63.1	97	36.9
Group IV	615	484	78.7	131	21.3
Total	1,867	1,465	78.5	402	21.5

Compiled from Cecil *et al.* (230)

Of the 627 Type I cases in Table 12, 85.3 per cent occurred in patients under fifty. In a larger group of 1,380 Type I cases subsequently reported by Cecil and Plummer (239), 80 per cent were in patients aged ten to forty-nine years (see Table 13). It is obvious that most cases of Type I pneumonia occur in young people. In the series of Cecil and Plummer (Table 13) and of Sutliff and Finland (1271) more cases were in patients aged thirty to thirty-nine years than in any other age group. This was also true among 592 patients with Type I lobar pneumonia observed during the Massachusetts

TABLE 13. TYPE I AND TYPE II LOBAR PNEUMONIA CASES IN ADULTS. NUMBER AND PERCENTAGE DISTRIBUTION BY AGE GROUP

AGE IN YEARS	TYPE I *Cases*	TYPE I *Per cent incidence*		TYPE II *Cases*	TYPE II *Per cent incidence*	
10–19	94	6.8	80 per cent (10–49)	30	3.1	74.6 per cent (10–49)
20–29	325	23.6		165	16.8	
30–39	387	28.0		271	27.6	
40–49	298	21.6		266	27.1	
50–59	195	14.1		174	17.7	
60 and over	81	5.9		76	7.7	
Total	1,380			982		

From Cecil and Plummer (239)

Pneumonia Study (869). The average age of these latter patients was 34.3 years.

Though, as shown in Table 11, at the time of their report Cecil, Baldwin, and Larsen were unable to demonstrate any special variation in the occurrence of Type II cases with age, Cecil and Plummer (239) later, and with a larger group, found Type II closely resembled Type I in that it also was commonest in patients under fifty years of age. Further, of 982 Type II cases they found more cases in patients aged thirty to thirty-nine than in any other age group and that, in all, 74.6 per cent were in patients aged ten to forty-nine (see Table 13). Other investigators have likewise found the largest proportion of their Type II cases in patients under fifty years of age (120, 1271, 1206, 557). This was also true of 157 patients with Type II lobar pneumonia investigated during the Massachusetts Pneumonia Study (869). In this group the largest number of cases was in patients between the ages of forty and forty-nine years. Their average age, however, was 37.4 years, and this was somewhat higher than that of patients with Type I pneumonia as given above.

The age distribution by decades of patients with Type I and Type II pneumonia has been well shown by Cecil and Plummer (239; see Table 13). Their figures include the Type I and II cases listed in Table 11.

Type III was especially common in patients over sixty years of age in Cecil, Baldwin, and Larsen's series (Table 11). This high incidence of Type III among the older patients with pneumococcus pneumonia has also been reported by other workers and was especially emphasized by Blake (120), who found that approximately 70 per cent of his cases in patients over sixty years old had Type III infections. In addition, Blake (120), Sutliff and Finland (1271), Smillie (1206), Finland and Sutliff (464), and Davies, Hodgson, and Whitby (340) have found that most Type III cases were in their older patients. Of the 122 cases reported by Blake (120), 18 were in children. Omitting these, approximately 18 per cent of the remaining 104 cases were in patients ten to thirty-nine years of age, and 23 per cent in those from forty to fifty-four, while the balance or 58.6 per cent (61 cases) was in patients fifty-five years of age or over. Among 225 cases investigated by Finland and Sutliff (464) the largest proportion (58 per cent) was in patients forty to sixty-nine years old, and 11 per cent occurred in patients seventy or over. In all, the proportion of Type III cases in patients forty years of age or over was 60 per cent in the series of Cecil, Baldwin, and Larsen (determined from data in Tables 11 and 12), 69 per cent in Finland and Sutliff's group, and 81 per cent in Blake's series. Bullowa (186), however, did not find such a large percentage of Type III cases among his older patients, and most of his cases were in patients in their third and fourth decades of life. It is possible that this difference in age distribution shown by Bullowa's Type III cases is related to the fact that about 85 per cent of his patients are colored.

The age distribution of patients with pneumococcus Type V pneumonia was reported by Sutliff and Finland (1271). About two-thirds of 47 cases occurred in patients between the ages of twelve and forty-nine years. In other small groups of Type VII and VIII cases the majority were in patients between twenty and fifty-nine years old. In a subsequent study Finland and Sutliff (464) found that 64 per cent of 105 Type VIII cases occurred in patients thirty to fifty-nine years of age and 14 per cent in those sixty or over. The majority of Bullowa's (186) 122 Type VIII cases in adults occurred in patients between the ages of twenty and forty-nine years and were thus a somewhat younger group.

In the series of Sutliff and Finland (1271) mentioned above, the remaining cases, namely, those due to Types IV, VI, and IX to XX inclusive, were considered as a single group. These cases were most common in patients between the ages of twenty and fifty-nine years. Data giving the age distribution of patients with pneumonia due to other types of pneumococci are not yet available.

VARIATION WITH SEX. The 1,867 cases of pneumococcus lobar pneumonia in adults reported by Cecil and his associates (230), as listed in Table 11, were divided by the authors to show the distribution of cases in males and females due to pneumococci of Types I, II, III, and Group IV (see Table 14).

TABLE 14. PNEUMOCOCCUS LOBAR PNEUMONIA CASES IN MEN AND WOMEN. NUMBER AND PERCENTAGE DISTRIBUTION BY TYPE

	MALE		FEMALE	
	Cases	*Per cent incidence*	*Cases*	*Per cent incidence*
Type I	545	35.1	82	25.8
Type II	312	20.2	50	15.7
Type III	194	12.5	69	21.8
Group IV	499	32.2	116	36.6
Total	1,550		317	

From Cecil *et al.* (230)

Among men, Type I was more frequent (35.1 per cent) than among women (25.8 per cent). A similar, though less marked, difference in distribution between the sexes was shown by Type II cases. In women Type III cases were nearly twice as common (21.8 per cent) as in men (12.5 per cent), and Group IV cases slightly more common than in men.

The cases in Table 14 have been rearranged to show the proportion of those due to each type that occurred in males or females (see Table 15). Of the total 1,867 cases in Table 15, 1,550 or 83 per cent were in males. Of the 627 Type I cases, 86.9 per cent were in males, as were 312 or 86.2 per cent of the 362 Type II cases. Others have also found the largest proportion of Type I and Type II cases to occur in males (24, 1272). Observations of a similar nature were made during the Massachusetts Pneumonia Study (869), and of 599 Type I and 157 Type II cases, 69 and 80 per cent respectively occurred in males.

TABLE 15. TYPE I, II, AND III AND GROUP IV LOBAR PNEUMONIA CASES IN ADULTS. NUMBER AND PERCENTAGE DISTRIBUTION BY SEX

	TOTAL CASES	MALE		FEMALE	
		Cases	*Per cent incidence*	*Cases*	*Per cent incidence*
Type I	627	545	86.9	82	13.1
Type II	362	312	86.2	50	13.8
Type III	263	194	73.8	69	26.2
Group IV	615	499	81.1	116	18.9
Total	1,867	1,550	83.0	317	17.0

From Cecil *et al.* (230)

Of the total 263 Type III cases in Table 15, more than 73 per cent were in men. Nevertheless, a larger proportion of Type III cases (26.2 per cent) occurred in women than of cases due to any other type.

Blake (120), Finland and Sutliff (464), and Bullowa (186) likewise found that most of their Type III cases occurred in males. In addition, most of the Type VIII cases studied by Finland and Sutliff and by Bullowa were in males. The former also noted that among Type III pneumonias the incidence of cases in females increased and was highest among the oldest women, while the highest incidence of Type VIII cases in females occurred among younger women. In general, in Finland and Sutliff's series about twice as many females had Type III or VIII pneumonia as Type I or II.

VARIATION WITH AGE AND SEX. When both age and sex factors are considered, certain striking variations of type incidence appear. This was well shown by Cecil, Baldwin, and Larsen (230) in an analysis of their 1,867 cases (see Table 16).

TABLE 16. PNEUMOCOCCUS LOBAR PNEUMONIA: 1,867 CASES IN MEN AND WOMEN UNDER AND OVER FIFTY YEARS OF AGE. NUMBER AND PERCENTAGE DISTRIBUTION BY TYPE

	MEN UNDER 50 YEARS OLD		WOMEN UNDER 50 YEARS OLD	
	Cases	*Per cent incidence*	*Cases*	*Per cent incidence*
Type I	462	37.8	73	29.7
Type II	236	19.3	44	17.9
Type III	124	10.1	42	17.1
Group IV	398	32.5	86	35.1
Total	1,220		245	

	MEN OVER 50 YEARS OLD		WOMEN OVER 50 YEARS OLD	
	Cases	*Per cent incidence*	*Cases*	*Per cent incidence*
Type I	83	25.1	9	12.0
Type II	76	23.0	6	8.3
Type III	70	21.2	27	36.1
Group IV	101	36.6	30	41.6
Total	330		72	

From Cecil *et al.* (230)

Type I cases were more than three times as common in men under fifty as in women over this age (37.8 versus 12 per cent). A similar, though less striking, variation was shown by Type II cases (19.3 versus 8.3 per cent). In patients over fifty years of age, Type I cases were about twice as frequent in men (25.1 per cent) as in women (12 per cent) and Type II cases nearly three times as common in men (23 per cent) as in women (8.3 per cent). Most outstanding, however, was the finding in women over fifty years old of nearly four times the proportion of Type III cases (36.1 per cent) as in men under fifty (10.1 per cent). Type III caused about one out of every three cases in women over fifty. Group IV cases were also a little more common in the older women than in the younger men. In men under fifty Types I and II together accounted for 57.1 per cent of the cases, while in the group of older women 77.7 per cent of the cases were due to pneumococci of Type III and Group IV together.

The data in Table 16 may be rearranged to show the proportion of the cases of each type which occurred in the younger or older men and women (see Table 17).

TABLE 17. TYPE I, II, AND III AND GROUP IV LOBAR PNEUMONIA CASES IN ADULTS. NUMBER AND PERCENTAGE DISTRIBUTION BY SEX AND AGE GROUP UNDER AND OVER FIFTY YEARS

		UNDER 50 YEARS				OVER 50 YEARS			
		MEN		WOMEN		MEN		WOMEN	
	TOTAL CASES	*Number*	*Per cent*	*Number*	*Per cent*	*Number*	*Per cent*	*Number*	*Per cent*
Type I	627	462	73.7	73	11.7	83	13.2	9	1.4
Type II	362	236	65.2	44	12.2	76	21.0	6	1.7
Type III	263	124	47.1	42	16.0	70	26.6	27	10.3
Group IV	615	398	64.7	86	14.0	101	16.4	30	4.9
Total	1,867	1,220	65.3	245	13.1	330	17.7	72	3.9

Compiled from Cecil *et al.* (230)

Of the cases due to each type, by far the largest proportion was in men under fifty years of age: Type I, 73.7 per cent; Type II, 65.2 per cent; Type III, 47.1 per cent; and Group IV, 64.7 per cent. Among the 263 Type III cases 70 or 26.6 per cent occurred in the older men and 27 or 10.3 per cent were in the older women. Type III was the causative organism in the majority of cases in the older patients.

The Pneumococcus and Bronchopneumonia

The following discussion of the occurrence of pneumococci in bronchopneumonia deals primarily with cases in adults. The findings in cases in infants and children are given separately below. The pneumococcus is usually the commonest single invader in bronchopneumonia but is frequently found in combination with other organisms, such as streptococci, staphylococci, Friedländer's bacilli, influenza bacilli, and *Micrococcus catarrhalis* (797, 807, 1271, 661, 788). At times the mixture of organisms may be such as to render it impossible, without extensive immunologic studies, to determine which is responsible for the infection. Outbreaks due chiefly to streptococci have been described (see pages 3–5). Bronchopneumonia may be primary at any age, but in this form is commonest in young children and infants. It is frequently secondary to some other infection or to some debilitating disease and is especially liable to follow acute infectious diseases, such as measles and scarlet fever, and to be associated with epidemics of influenza.

The detailed investigations of Sutliff and Finland (1271), Winkler and Finland (1429), and of Finland and his colleagues (464, 468, 469, 456, 449) have demonstrated the etiologic relationship of pneumococci of many of the types, including a number of those above Type III, to pneumococcus bronchopneumonia. The organisms were isolated from the sputum, blood, or infected exudates during life and from the blood, lungs, and exudates after death. In addition, agglutinins and protective substances specific for the type causing the infection were demonstrated in many instances to appear or to increase in the blood at about the time of recovery.

PRIMARY BRONCHOPNEUMONIA. The frequency with which various organisms may be associated with primary bronchopneumonia has been studied by several investigators. The 1920 report of Locke, Thomas, and O'Hara (797) showed that in 164 such cases observed over a two-year period at the Boston City Hospital, pneumococci were found in 67. Streptococci of several varieties (chiefly hemolytic) were found in 46, staphylococci in 19, influenza bacilli in 44, and 53 were of unknown etiology. These organisms occurred either alone or with others in various combinations. In 1928 Cole (298) reported a series of 211 cases collected over a period of sixteen years at the Hospital of the Rockefeller Institute for Medical Research. These cases were divided as to the number caused by various organisms as follows: pneumococcus 39, streptococcus 83, staphylococcus 19, influenza bacillus 8, Friedländer's bacillus 7, question of *Bacillus mallei* one, mixed infection 26, and organism unknown 28. Of the total 211 cases the bacterial incitant was recognized in 183, and of these, pneumococci accounted for 21.3 per cent and streptococci for 45.4 per cent. The incidence of pneumococci was low in this series as compared with that above and with the 215 cases recently observed by Sutliff and Finland (1271) at the Boston City Hospital over a period of about three years. The latter found pneumococci which were identifiable as one or another of the types from Type I through Type XX in 140 or 65.1 per cent, and pneumococci of unknown type in 34 or 16 per cent of the cases. In all, pneumococci were responsible for 174 or 81 per cent of their cases, while the remaining 41 or 19 per cent were due to other organisms, among which hemolytic streptococci were found in 37, *Staphylococcus aureus* in 3, and Friedländer's bacillus in one.

The frequency with which the various types of pneumococci are found in bronchopneumonia approximately parallels the frequency with which they are carried in the mouths of normal persons, which suggests that chance may play a large part in these infections. As shown later, in the section on pneumococcus carriers (page 342), though normal individuals seldom carry pneumococci of Type I or II, they frequently carry those of Type III and commonly those of the higher types. In the 164 cases of Locke, Thomas, and O'Hara (797), which were apparently nearly all mixed infections, pneumococci were found as follows: Type I twice, Type II four times, Type III eighteen times, and Group IV forty-three times. They remarked on the scarcity of Types I and II in these cases and further reported that they had not seen a case of bronchopneumonia which had been shown pathologically to be due to either of these types. Sutliff and Finland (1271, 1272), Finland and Sutliff (464), and Finland (449), however, have reported several cases of Type I and II bronchopneumonia which were confirmed at necropsy. Pneumococci were found in only 39 of Cole's (298) 211 cases; in four instances they were of Type II, while the remainder were of Group IV.

For the accurate etiologic diagnosis of bronchopneumonia repeated examinations of the sputum and blood or of infected exudates or material removed by lung puncture should be carried out (see also page 614).

Of the available reports that lend themselves to tabulation, only a limited number, representing a relatively small group of cases, give the incidence of the types found in pneumococcus bronchopneumonia. These are shown in Table 18, where it is seen that of a total of 745 cases, Type I occurred in 42 or 5.6 per cent; Type II in 22 or 3 per cent; Type III in 112 or 15 per cent; and pneumococci of Group IV in 569 or 76.4 per cent. Types I and II together were responsible for 64 or 8.6 per cent of the cases, which is in marked contrast to their occurrence in lobar pneumonia, where they account for more than 50 per cent of the cases.

There are differences in the series listed in Table 18 which may be of importance in the interpretation of these figures. The American series of Finland (449)* is the largest and comprises 619 pneumococcus cases. In that series Type I occurred in 28 or 4.5 per cent and Type II in 15 or 2.4 per cent,

* Includes the series of 174 similar cases previously reported by Sutliff and Finland (1271).

TABLE 18. PNEUMOCOCCUS BRONCHOPNEUMONIA. NUMBER AND PERCENTAGE DISTRIBUTION OF 745 CASES BY TYPE*
(TYPES I, II, III, AND GROUP IV)

SOURCE	DATE	TOTAL CASES	TYPE I *Number*	TYPE I *Per cent*	TYPE II *Number*	TYPE II *Per cent*	TYPE III *Number*	TYPE III *Per cent*	GROUP IV *Number*	GROUP IV *Per cent*
United States										
Finland (449)	1937	619	28	4.5	15	2.4	99	16.0	477	77.1
Great Britain										
Grant (553)	1922	4	2	50.0	1	25.0	–	–	1	25.0
Germany										
Gundel and Linden (579)	1931	66	3	4.5	5	7.6	12	18.2	46	69.7
East Africa										
Garnham and deSmidt (507)	1931	17	3	17.6	–	–	1	5.9	13	76.5
India										
Napier and Dharmendra (924)	1935									
Calcutta		24	4	16.7	1	4.2	–	–	19	79.2
Assam		15	2	13.3	–	–	–	–	13	86.7
Total†		745	42		22		112		569	
Per cent		100.0	5.6		3.0		15.0		76.4	

* Some cases of secondary bronchopneumonia may be included in the series listed.

† Early compilation of data for this table showed a total of 300 cases distributed as follows: Type I, 6.3 per cent; Type II, 4.3 per cent; Type III, 14 per cent; and Group IV, 75.3 per cent.

the two types together accounting for only 6.9 per cent of the cases. As previously noted and as shown in Tables 5 and 6, Types I and II appear more common in Europe than in America in lobar pneumonia and, judging from the reports of Grant and of Gundel and Linden (Table 18), it is possible this same relation also holds in bronchopneumonia. The cases of Garnham and deSmidt (507) and of Napier and Dharmendra (924) listed in Table 18 occurred in natives of Africa and India within the tropics, and in these small groups the incidence of Type I appeared fairly high.

The incidence of the higher types in pneumococcus bronchopneumonia was studied by Finland (449). His series has been listed in Table 18, and in Table 19 is expanded to show the incidence of all the recognized types. The six commonest types found in this group of cases were, in the order of their frequency, Types III, VIII, X, XX, XVIII, and VII. Together these types accounted for 306 or 49.6 per cent of the total 619 cases. These were the only individual types occurring in 5 per cent or more of the cases.

TABLE 19. PNEUMOCOCCUS BRONCHOPNEUMONIA. NUMBER AND PERCENTAGE DISTRIBUTION OF 619 CASES BY TYPE* (TYPES I–XXXII)

TYPE	CASES *Number*	CASES *Per cent*	TYPE	CASES *Number*	CASES *Per cent*
I	28	4.5	XVII	20	3.2
II	15	2.4	XVIII	32	5.2
III	99	16.0	XIX	12	1.9
IV	18	2.9	XX	35	5.7
V	30	4.8	XXI	9	1.5
VI	30	4.8	XXII	10	1.6
VII	32	5.2	XXIII	3	0.5
VIII	68	11.0	XXIV	3	0.5
IX	12	1.9	XXV	2	0.3
X	40	6.5	XXVII	–	–
XI	18	2.9	XXVIII	4	0.6
XII	8	1.3	XXIX	4	0.6
XIII	12	1.9	XXXI	–	–
XIV	24	3.9	XXXII	1	0.2
XV	6	1.0	Unclassified	36†	5.9
XVI	8	1.3	Total	619	

From Finland (449)

* This series may include some cases of secondary bronchopneumonia.
† In 35 instances typing was carried out only as far as Type XX.

In addition to the foregoing series, the incidence of many of the higher types was determined in two small groups of cases by Napier and Dharmendra (924) in India. Typing was carried out at least as far as Type XIV in one group of twenty-four cases and for all thirty-two types in the other group of fifteen cases. Ten of the higher types were found present in these two series, namely, Types IV, V, VI, VIII, X, XI, XIII, XIV, XX, and XXI, each of which accounted for one or more cases; untyped pneumococci which accounted for several cases were also found.

Studying the relation of Type I, II, and III pneumococci to pneumonia, Trask, O'Donovan, Moore, and Beebe (1321) reported that in patients with Type I or II infections bronchopneumonia was rare, though with Type III infections pneumonia of this form was found in about one-third of their patients. Observations of similar significance were made by Finland and Sutliff (464) who studied Type III and Type VIII infections. They found that 21 per cent of their Type III and 30 per cent of their Type VIII infections were bronchopneumonias, while only 3 per cent of their Type I and 5 per cent of their Type II infections were diagnosed as bronchopneumonia.

SECONDARY BRONCHOPNEUMONIA. The bacteriology of secondary bronchopneumonia is confused. The presence of numerous organisms in such cases has been reported. In general, however, and in contrast to the usual situation in primary bronchopneumonia, streptococci are generally most prevalent. Pneumococci are next most frequently found. Such pneumococci as are present are seldom of Type I or II. While Type III is more frequent than Types I and II, the large majority are members of Group IV. The staphylococcus and influenza bacillus, and occasionally other organisms, may also be present.

During the War several thousand cases of secondary bronchopneumonia occurred in the military camps in this country, and efforts were made to investigate many of them bacteriologically. Though some of these cases followed outbreaks of scarlet fever (1295), many others followed epidemics of measles (307, 1202, 892, 591, 1251, 1351, 1295, 566, 969), and a far larger group were secondary to the epidemic of influenza prevalent in such camps during 1918–1919 (1222, 499, 147, 588, 130, 111, 825, 633, 758, 246, 985, 774, 969).

Greenway, Boettiger, and Colwell (566) and Opie, Blake, Small, and Rivers (969) gave a good account of the confused bacteriology of cases in military camps secondary to measles. The pathology of such cases was investigated by Cole and MacCallum (307) and by Opie, Blake, Small, and

Rivers (969). The latter, as well as MacCallum (825), also investigated the pathology of post-influenzal cases.

In one camp Lamb and Brannin (758) studied over 600 cases of post-influenzal bronchopneumonia. Their findings may be cited as fairly typical of this group. Sputum from 348 of these cases was examined bacteriologically. Pneumococci were obtained from 216 (62 per cent): Type I in 9, Type II in 7, Type III in 14, and Group IV in 186. Streptococci were obtained from 91 (26.1 per cent) and were hemolytic in 37 and non-hemolytic in 54. The remaining 41 cases (11.8 per cent) were of unknown etiology. The incidence of pneumococci as a group appears high in this series as compared with other series in which bacteriologic studies were made on cases at necropsy. In the latter, pneumococci were much less frequently found and streptococci were usually (111, 130, 406, 969), but not always (499), the most common.

A good example of the discrepancy between clinical studies and post-mortem findings was given by Birge and Havens (111). The percentage of various organisms found in the organs of 124 cases at necropsy was compared with the percentage found in the sputum of 60 of these cases during life (Table 20). As pneumococci of Group IV were found in 49.9 per cent of the sputums but in only 13.7 per cent of the cases at necropsy, it is obvious that their presence in the sputum means little as to the true nature of the infecting organism. In similar fashion, streptococci were found far more frequently in the organs at necropsy than in the sputum during life and, in all, streptococci were more common than pneumococci.

TABLE 20. SECONDARY BRONCHOPNEUMONIA. PERCENTAGE DISTRIBUTION OF VARIOUS ORGANISMS ISOLATED FROM THE ORGANS AT NECROPSY AND FROM SPUTUM DURING LIFE

	FROM ORGANS 124 CASES	FROM SPUTUM 60 CASES
Streptococcus (hemolytic)	48.3	25.0
Streptococcus (non-hemolytic)	11.3	6.6
B. influenzae	9.7	3.3
Pneumococcus Type I	0.8	3.3
Pneumococcus Type II	3.2	3.3
Pneumococcus Type III	12.1	8.3
Pneumococcus Group IV	13.7	49.9

From Birge and Havens (111)

Post-influenzal cases of bronchopneumonia were also investigated in various civilian hospitals (797, 807, 298, 1304), and in general the findings were similar to those cited above. When pneumococci were found, they were chiefly of types other than Type I or II.

The Pneumonias of Infants and Children

PNEUMONIA OF ALL FORMS. The pneumonias of infants and children (lobar, broncho, lobular, and so forth) may first be considered as a single group. Bacteriologic observations have been made on many such cases. Pneumonia of the lobar and broncho forms makes up approximately nine-tenths of all cases in infants and children, the remainder being due to less well-defined forms. As shown by the studies of investigators mentioned in the following discussion, pneumococci are responsible for most cases under ordinary conditions and are especially prevalent in cases of lobar pneumonia. In other varieties of pneumonia other organisms, especially streptococci, are also common. Mixed infection may occur, and at times two or more types of pneumococci may be present.

Material from several sources is available revealing the frequency with which pneumococci of various types have been found in the pneumonias of infants and children. Of special interest in this respect are observations on certain groups of cases in which typing was carried out for many of the higher types, with a consequent marked reduction in the proportion of cases due to unclassified pneumococci. In a series of 147 cases examined by Plummer, Raia, and Shultz (1029) at the Bellevue Hospital, New York City, during the winter of 1928–1929, when typing was carried out for Types I through XIII, pneumococci of Type VI were commonest among the classified strains and were found in 19 or 12.9 per cent of the cases (see Table 21). Types I and V in that order were next in frequency. During the second winter of their study, Raia, Plummer, and Shultz (1057) carried out typing for Types I through XXIV, and in 182 cases examined found Type XIV the most frequent, accounting for 20 or 10.9 per cent of the cases. The next most common were Types I, VI, VII, IV, and XVIII, as shown in Table 21.

Subsequently Smith (1212) reported that in a series of 1,033 cases from the same hospital, which presumably includes those in Table 21, Types I, XIV, and VI were most commonly found and accounted for 41 per cent of the group. Types XIX, V, and VII were likewise fairly common. This series is doubtless the same as that reported in some detail by Nemir, Andrews, and Vinograd (931) from the same hospital. Further description of this group is given below.

TABLE 21. PNEUMONIA IN INFANTS AND CHILDREN UNDER TWELVE YEARS OF AGE. NUMBER AND PERCENTAGE DISTRIBUTION OF 329 CASES BY ORGANISM FOUND*

ORGANISM	1928–1929 *Number of cases*	*Per cent*		1929–1930 *Number of cases*	*Per cent*	
Pneumococcus						
I	14	9.5		18	9.8	
II	3	2.0		6	3.2	
III	3	2.0		7	3.8	
IV	4	2.7		10	5.5	
V	9	6.1		8	4.4	
VI	19	12.9		16	8.7	
VII	5	3.4		11	6.0	
VIII	1	0.7		3	1.6	
IX	6	4.1		5	2.7	
X	–	–		1	0.6	
XI	–	–		6	3.2	
XII	1	0.7	81.6	–	–	75.2
XIII	2	1.3	per	–	–	per
XIV	nr	nr	cent	20	10.9	cent
XV	nr	nr		5	2.7	
XVII	nr	nr		4	2.2	
XVIII	nr	nr		10	5.5	
XIX	nr	nr		8	4.4	
XXI	nr	nr		1	0.6	
XXIII	nr	nr		3	1.6	
XXIV	nr	nr		2	1.1	
Unclassified	73	49.7		24	13.1	
Streptococcus viridans	2	1.3		11	6.0	
Hemolytic streptococcus	1	0.7		2	1.1	
Staphylococcus	4	2.7		1	0.6	
Total	147			182		

* The 1928–1929 series shows the findings of Plummer, Raia, and Shultz (1029), and the other series the findings of Raia, Plummer, and Shultz, as presented by the latter (1057). The two series include 254 cases of lobar pneumonia, 55 of bronchopneumonia, 7 of lobular pneumonia, and 13 cases of pneumonia of miscellaneous varieties.

nr = no record. Typing was not carried out for these types in 1928–1929.

In addition to these findings, Brown (157) in Canada observed two groups of pneumococcus pneumonias during the winters of 1930–1931 and 1931–1932. Typing was carried out for Types I through XXIX. In both groups, of 61 cases the first winter and 24 the second, Type I was the commonest, accounting for more than 20 per cent of the cases each winter. The types next in frequency in the first group were Types V and XXVI, and in the second group Types VII and XIX.

Bullowa (186), studying the incidence of certain types in pneumococcus pneumonia, found Type VIII in only 11 or 2.2 per cent of 500 cases over a period of five years at the Harlem Hospital, New York City. Type XIV, however, he found (187) over a five and one-half year period to be one of the commonest invaders of children and accounted for 85 or 16.1 per cent of 547 cases examined. He also found Type I to be about equally frequent, and that Types I and XIV together accounted for 31.3 per cent of the series.

In a subsequent report Bullowa (190) gave the type incidence in 1,712 cases of pneumonia (lobar pneumonia and bronchopneumonia) in infants and children seen at the Harlem Hospital during the period of July 1, 1928—June 30, 1936. This series, as well as that of 1,033 similar cases examined by Nemir, Andrews, and Vinograd (931), mentioned above, was referred to in Chapter I (see pages 2–3) where it was seen that together the series totalled 2,745 cases, of which 62.6 per cent were due to pneumococci and 37.4 per cent to other organisms. The types of pneumococci most commonly encountered, and in the order of their frequency in the total group of 2,745 cases, are shown in the accompanying summary.

Pneumococcus type	*Percentage distribution in 2,745 cases**
XIV	12.0
I	11.2
VI	7.7
XIX	3.9
V	3.6
IV	3.1
III	2.7
VII	2.1

* Earlier compilation of data from similar though smaller series of cases showed the types most commonly found to be Types I, XIV, VI, V, and VII in that order.

Together these eight types accounted for 1,271 or 46.3 per cent of the total 2,745 cases.

The frequency of occurrence of the different types varies markedly with the age of the patient. In infants and young children under two or three years of age, Type XIV appears to predominate (1057, 1212, 931, 190) and in Bullowa's series (187), mentioned above, this type accounted for about one-fifth of all cases, the majority of which occurred in males. It is of interest that in the group of 329 pneumonias reported by Plummer and Raia with Shultz (1029, 1057), listed in Table 21, only ten cases of Type III infection were found and all occurred in a group of 203 pneumonia patients under three years of age and none occurred in the older children. In older children Type I is commonest (1029, 1057, 1212, 187, 931, 190) and Types V, VII, and XIV are also frequent. Bullowa's observations (187) on 547 cases indicate that, as age increases, the incidence of Type XIV decreases, while that of Type I markedly increases. Of all strains of Type I encountered in cases in children, most have been obtained from those in the older age groups (1057, 680, 1053, 931, 190).

Various investigators have called attention to the low proportion of cases due to Types I, II, and III, and the high proportion due to Group IV pneumococci in the pneumonias of infants and children (1029, 987, 1057, 885, 112). With increasing age the proportion due to pneumococci of the first three types increases, however, with a consequent decrease in the number due to Group IV. Table 22 lists the pneumococcus cases (lobar pneumonia and bronchopneumonia together) reported by Nemir, Andrews, and Vinograd (931) divided by age groups. There are 445 cases each in the series in infants under two years of age and in the children from two to thirteen years of age. It is seen that as age increases the proportion of cases due to the

TABLE 22. PNEUMOCOCCUS PNEUMONIA (LOBAR PNEUMONIA AND BRONCHOPNEUMONIA TOGETHER) IN CHILDREN OF VARIOUS AGES. NUMBER AND PERCENTAGE DISTRIBUTION OF 890 CASES BY AGE GROUP AND TYPE*

AGE GROUP	TOTAL CASES	TYPE I		TYPE II		TYPE III		TYPES I, II, AND III	GROUP IV	
		Number	*Per cent*	*Number*	*Per cent*	*Number*	*Per cent*	*Per cent*	*Number*	*Per cent*
Under 2 years	445	26	5.8	1	0.2	15	3.4	9.4	393	88.3
2–13 years	445	116	26.1	27	6.1	22	4.9	37.1	280	62.9

From Nemir *et al.* (931)

* The series includes some cases in which organisms other than pneumococci were also present.

An earlier similar compilation of data on a smaller series of cases divided into age groups from birth to three years and from three to twelve years of age showed the incidence of Type I to rise from 4.2 per cent in the younger to 20.2 per cent in the older group. Together, Types I, II, and III were found in 11.1 per cent of the cases in the younger patients and in 25.2 per cent in the older patients.

first three types together increases from 9.4 per cent in the younger group to 37.1 per cent in the older group. Accompanying this increase there is a concurrent decrease in the proportion of cases due to pneumococci of Group IV (all other types) from 88.3 per cent for children in the younger group to 62.9 per cent for those in the older group.

Observations of a similar nature were reported by Blacklock and Guthrie (112). While Types I, II, and III were found in only 5.3 per cent of their 112 pneumonias in infants and children under three years of age, they accounted for 25 per cent of 28 cases in patients three to ten years old. The decreasing proportion of cases due to pneumococci of Group IV with increasing age was well shown by Menton, Bailey, and Debone (885), who studied necropsy cultures obtained from 131 pneumonias in infants and children. Pneumococci of Group IV were obtained from 82.6 per cent of the patients under two years of age, from 71.6 per cent of those two to six years old, and from 50 per cent of others six to fourteen years old.

TABLE 23. STRAINS OF PNEUMOCOCCUS ISOLATED FROM VARIOUS LESIONS IN CHILDREN OF DIFFERENT AGE GROUPS. NUMBER AND PERCENTAGE DISTRIBUTION BY TYPE

AGE GROUP IN YEARS	TOTAL STRAINS	TYPE I	TYPE II	TYPE III	GROUP IV	PER CENT TYPES I, II, AND III	
0 to 1	103	1	8	1	93	9.7	
1+ to 2	80	12	1	–	67	16.3	
2+ to 3	31	8	–	–	23	25.8	17.5 (0 to 5)
3+ to 5	38	12	1	–	25	34.2	
5+ to 9	31	20	–	–	11	64.5	65.0 (5+ to 13)
9+ to 13	9	5	1	–	3	66.7	
Total	292	58	11	1	222	24.0	

From Blacklock and Guthrie (112)

Striking additional evidence that Types I, II, and III (especially the first two) are found far more frequently in older than in younger children was provided by Blacklock and Guthrie (112). To illustrate this, they considered the pneumococci isolated from nearly 300 infants and children with all sorts of acute pneumococcus infections (pneumonia, empyema, otitis media, and so forth) as a single group (see Table 23).

The proportion of Types I, II, and III found gradually rose from 9.7 per cent in patients under one year old to 66.7 per cent in those between the ages of nine and thirteen years. Striking, too, is the fact that the first three types accounted for 17.5 per cent of the strains obtained from lesions in children under five years of age, while in others over this age but under thirteen years they were much more common and made up 65 per cent of the group. In addition, Type III was found only in the youngest individuals.

LOBAR PNEUMONIA. Many studies have been carried out to determine the incidence of pneumococci and other organisms in lobar pneumonia in infants and children. The available reports in which cases have been analyzed in a comparable manner, thus lending themselves to tabulation, are shown in Table 24. The individual groups of cases, mostly small and reported at various times from many places, include patients of different ages as indicated. Considerable variation in the incidence of cases due to pneumococci and other organisms is apparent. Of 697 cases, 630 or 90.4 per cent were caused by pneumococcus infection, while in the remaining 67 or 9.6 per cent no pneumococci were found. This percentage corresponds closely with the incidence of pneumococci in lobar pneumonia in adults (96.1 per cent, see Table 1, page 2). There is an appreciable difference between the two groups, however, in the frequency of occurrence of the various types of pneumococci as noted below.

Of the total 697 cases in Table 24, Part One, in which the general incidence of pneumococci in lobar pneumonia was demonstrated, Type I accounted for 155 or 22.2 per cent and was the commonest type found. Type II was considerably less frequent, occurring in only 52 or 7.5 per cent, and Type III was obtained from but 35 or 5 per cent of the cases. Pneumococci of Group IV were common, accounting for 388 or 55.7 per cent of the cases, while no pneumococci were obtained from the remaining 67 or 9.6 per cent. Though these latter two groups together accounted for 65.3 per cent of the cases, it is clear that pneumococci of Types I and II were fairly frequent, for considered together they were found in 29.7 per cent of the 697 cases. Types I, II, and III together accounted for 34.7 per cent of the cases.

Among the 826 cases of pneumococcus lobar pneumonia in Table 24, Type I was found in 185 or 22.4 per cent, Type II in 67 or 8.1 per cent, and Type III in 45 or 5.5 per cent, the three types together accounting for 36 per cent of the cases. The remaining 529 cases or 64 per cent were due to pneumococci of Group IV.

TABLE 24. LOBAR PNEUMONIA IN INFANTS AND CHILDREN. NUMBER AND PERCENTAGE DISTRIBUTION OF CASES BY TYPE

Part One. Lobar Pneumonia

REPORTED BY	AGE GROUP	TOTAL CASES	PNEUMOCOCCUS CASES					CASES HAVING NO PNEUMOCOCCI
			Type I	*Type II*	*Type III*	*Per cent Types I, II, and III*	*Group IV*	
Wollstein and Benson, 1916, New York (1436)	Under 4½ years	11	3	2	–	45.4	4	2
Pisek and Pease, 1916, New York (1025)	Under 6 years	31	9	11	1	67.7	7	3
Lyon, 1921–1922, Boston (821)	Under 12 years	73	14	2	7	31.5	36[a]	14
Webster, 1922–1923, Australia (1394)	"Children"	120	46	6	7	49.2	50	11
Westlund, 1924–1925, Chicago (1412)	Under 12 years	69	4	12[b]	2	26.1	42	9
Trask, O'Donovan, Moore, and Beebe, 1927–1929, New Haven (1321)	Under 12 years	96	36	5	10	53.1	33[c]	12
Ishida, 1927–1930, Japan (680)	Infants and children	31	9	7	2	58.1	12[d]	1
Plummer, Raia, and Shultz, 1928–1929, New York (1029)	Under 12 years	103	13	3	–	15.5	82[e]	5
Raia, Plummer, and Shultz, 1929–1930, New York (1057)	Under 12 years	151	17	4	6	17.9	114[f]	10
Blacklock and Guthrie, 1931–1932, Glasgow (112)	6 weeks to 13 years	12	4	–	–	33.3	8	–
Total		697	155	52	35	–	388	67
Per cent		100.0	22.2	7.5	5.0	34.7	55.7	9.6

TABLE 24 (*cont.*)

Part Two. Pneumococcus Lobar Pneumonia

REPORTED BY	AGE GROUP	TOTAL CASES	PNEUMOCOCCUS CASES				
			Type I	*Type II*	*Type III*	*Per cent Types I, II, and III*	*Group IV*
Cases cited in Part One		630	155	52	35	38.4	388
Mitchell, 1914–1916, Philadelphia (899)*	Average 2 years 3 months[g]	79	9	10	3	27.8	57
Locke, Thomas, and O'Hara, 1919–1920, Boston (797)*	Infants and children	42	11	5	4	47.6	22
Kereszturi and Hauptmann, 1931–1933, New York (710)*	2 months to 11 years	75	10	–	3	17.3	62[h]
Grand total		826	185	67	45	–	529
Per cent		100.0	22.4	8.1	5.5	36.0	64.0

[a] Includes 1 case Type IIa.
[b] Includes a few cases of Type IIa which, due to the character of the report, cannot be separated from those of Type II.
[c] Includes 3 cases Type IIa.
[d] Includes 3 cases Type IIa and 3 due to "rough" pneumococci.
[e] Typed through Type XIII.
[f] Typed through Type XXIV.
[g] Most patients were from six months to two years of age.
[h] Seventeen had infection due to mixed types. The remaining forty-five cases were typed through Type XXX.
* Cases from which no pneumococci were obtained were omitted from the reports.

In a few of the series in Table 24 typing was carried out for many of the higher types, and from these and other investigations of a similar nature it is possible to determine which of the types appear most commonly in cases of lobar pneumonia in infants and children (see Table 25). Among the 103 cases of Plummer, Raia, and Shultz (1029), Types I and VI were commonest and, respectively, accounted for 13 or 12.6 per cent and 9 or 8.7 per cent of the cases. Among 136 strains of Group IV pneumococci isolated from 126 cases, Cooper, Rosenstein, Walter, and Peizer (320) found Types VIa, XIV, and V were the commonest, being found 20, 17, and 16 times respectively. These three types, together with Types XV and XIX, which were next in frequency, accounted for 50 per cent of the strains found. The 151 cases of Raia, Plummer, and Shultz (1057) showed that Types XIV and I were commonest and, respectively, accounted for 18 and 17, or 11.2 per cent each, of the cases. Type VI with 14 cases and Type VII with 10 cases were next in frequency.

TABLE 25. LOBAR PNEUMONIA IN INFANTS AND CHILDREN. EXTENT OF TYPING AND COMMONEST TYPES OF PNEUMOCOCCI FOUND

REPORTED FROM NEW YORK CITY BY	TYPES EXAMINED FOR	TOTAL CASES	TYPES MOST COMMONLY FOUND
Plummer, Raia, and Shultz (1029)*	I–XIII	103	I, VI, V, IX
Cooper, Rosenstein, Walter, and Peizer (320)*	IV–XXIX	126	VIa, XIV, V, XV, XIX
Raia, Plummer, and Shultz (1057)	I–XXIV	151	XIV, I, VI, VII
Kereszturi and Hauptmann (710)	I–XXX	75	XIV, I, IV, VI, XIX
Nemir, Andrews, and Vinograd (931)†	I–XXXII	758	XIV, I, VI, V, VII, XIX
Total		1,213	

* There may be some duplication of cases in these series.
† Includes 276 cases previously reported by Nemir (930).

Among the 75 cases of Kereszturi and Hauptmann (710), Type XIV with 15 cases and Type I with 10 cases were the most frequent. Types IV, VI, and XIX with 4 cases each were next in order. These workers also observed that infection with Type XIV or Type I pneumococci was likely to result in lobar pneumonia. Bullowa (187) likewise noted the marked tendency of Type XIV to be associated with lobar pneumonia, even in infants less than a year old. Extending the observations of Raia and her colleagues, noted above, Nemir, Andrews, and Vinograd (931), at the same hospital, later examined an additional 758 cases. Types XIV, I, and VI were the three commonest types found and accounted respectively for 19.6 per cent, 17.8 per cent, and 9.3 per cent, or a total of 46.7 per cent of the whole series of cases.

From the foregoing reports based on extensive studies of 1,213 cases, it is seen that pneumococci of nine types, Types I, IV, V, VI, VII, IX, XIV, XV, and XIX, were reported as the most common in cases of lobar pneumonia in infants and children. Types XIV, I, VI, V, and VII, in approximately that order, were the most prevalent and accounted for nearly one-half of the cases.

As in most pneumonias in infants and children, the age of the patient is an important factor in relation to which types of pneumococci appear most frequently. Examining 63 strains of pneumococci from 57 infants and children under two years of age with lobar pneumonia, Cooper and her coworkers (320) found that, of the higher types, Types VIa and XIV were commonest, each being found eleven times. On the other hand, among 73 strains from 69 cases in older children the situation proved different, and Types V and VIa were commonest and were found fifteen and nine times respectively. Nemir's (930) observations are of similar significance. In 116 cases in infants she found Type XIV to be the predominating type and responsible for 39 or 33.6 per cent of these cases. Type VI was found next in frequency. In older children, however, Type I predominated and accounted for 52 or 32.5 per cent of 160 cases.

In general, as age increases, pneumococci of Types I, II, and III together become increasingly common in lobar pneumonia in children and tend to approach the incidence of these organisms in cases in adults. Under ordinary circumstances, however, this level is not reached. Nevertheless, Lyon (821) pointed out that these organisms may occur more frequently in such cases in children than is often appreciated. Trask, O'Donovan, Moore, and Beebe (1321) further emphasized the importance of these types in children's pneumonias and concluded that there was little difference between the incidence of the first three types in pneumococcus lobar pneumonia whether in children or in adults. Reference to some of the points made above and to certain of the series of cases listed in Table 24 furnishes some support for this contention. However, when the findings in the total 826 pneumococcus cases listed in that table are considered, it becomes necessary to alter this view, for only 297, or 36 per cent of the cases, were due to Type I, II, and III pneumococci together, whereas in adults (see Table 5, page 46) these types accounted for nearly twice as many, or 63 per cent of 16,813 cases (see Table 26). Pneumococci of Group IV were nearly twice as frequent (64 per cent) in cases in infants and children as in adults (36.9 per cent).

TABLE 26. PNEUMOCOCCUS LOBAR PNEUMONIA IN INFANTS AND CHILDREN AND IN ADULTS. PERCENTAGE DISTRIBUTION OF CASES BY TYPE

	TOTAL CASES	TYPE I	TYPE II	TYPE III	TYPES I, II, AND III	GROUP IV
Infants and children (Table 24)	826	22.4	8.1	5.5	36.0	64.0
Adults (Table 5)	16,813	32.6	19.6	10.8	63.0	36.9

BRONCHOPNEUMONIA. A tabulation of the available series of cases of bronchopneumonia in infants and children to show the incidence of cases attributed to pneumococci of Types I, II, III, and Group IV, and of cases from which no pneumococci were obtained, may be seen in Table 27. The series contains cases which occurred in many places in various years and in patients of various ages. Certain differences are apparent in the frequency with which some of the types were found. A relatively large proportion of the cases reported by Przesmycki and his collaborators were Type I. The series of Ishida shows many Type I and an especially large proportion of Type II cases. Little is known of the conditions under which the cases of these investigators occurred.

In 664 cases, pneumococci were obtained from 517 or 77.9 per cent, while the remaining 147 or 22.1 per cent yielded no pneumococci. The presence of pneumococci in nearly 78 per cent of these cases in infants and children is remarkably similar to their occurrence in some 81 per cent of cases of bronchopneumonia in adults, as reported by Sutliff and Finland (1271) (see page 69).

As shown in Table 27, among the 664 cases in which the general incidence of pneumococci was determined, Type I occurred in 32 cases or 4.8 per cent, Type II occurred in 64 cases or 9.6 per cent, Type III in 31 or 4.7 per cent, and pneumococci of Group IV in 390 or 58.7 per cent. Types I, II, and III together accounted for 19.1 per cent of the 664 cases. No pneumococci were found in 22.1 per cent of these cases of bronchopneumonia as compared with 9.6 per cent of cases of lobar pneumonia (see Table 24). Thus (as in adults) cases yielding organisms other than pneumococci are more often encountered in bronchopneumonia than in lobar pneumonia.

TABLE 27. BRONCHOPNEUMONIA IN INFANTS AND CHILDREN. NUMBER AND PERCENTAGE DISTRIBUTION OF CASES BY TYPE

Part One. Bronchopneumonia

REPORTED BY	AGE GROUP	TOTAL CASES	PNEUMOCOCCUS CASES *Type I*	*Type II*	*Type III*	*Per cent Types I, II, and III*	*Group IV*	CASES HAVING NO PNEUMOCOCCI
Wollstein and Benson, 1916, New York (1436)	Under 4½ years	36	3	4	–	19.4	21	8
Pisek and Pease, 1916, New York (1025)	Under 6 years	32	2	3	3	25.0	12	12
Lyon, 1921–1922, Boston (821)	Under 12 years	31	3	1	2	19.3	13[a]	12
Wollstein, 1921–1922, New York (1435)	3 years and under	87	3	7	–	11.5	54	23
Webster, 1922–1923, Australia (1394)	"Children"	17	1	–	–	5.9	10	6
Westlund, 1926, Chicago (1412)	Under 12 years	34	2	3	1	17.6	18	10
Trask, O'Donovan, Moore, and Beebe, 1927–1929, New Haven (1321)	Under 12 years	166	1	3	13	10.2	81	68
Ishida, 1927–1930, Japan (680)	Infants and children	102	13	39	9	59.8	37[b]	4
Plummer, Raia, and Shultz, 1928–1929, New York (1029)	Under 12 years	29	1	–	1	6.9	26[c]	1
Raia, Plummer, and Shultz, 1929–1930, New York (1057)	Under 12 years	26	1	2	1	15.4	19[d]	3
Blacklock and Guthrie, 1931–1932, Glasgow (112)	6 weeks to 13 years	104	2	2	1	4.8	99	–
Total		664	32	64	31	–	390	147
Per cent		99.9	4.8	9.6	4.7	19.1	58.7	22.1

TABLE 27 (*cont.*)

Part Two. Pneumococcus Bronchopneumonia

REPORTED BY	AGE GROUP	TOTAL CASES	PNEUMOCOCCUS CASES: *Type I*	*Type II*	*Type III*	*Per cent Types I, II, and III*	*Group IV*
Cases cited in Part One		517	32	64	31	24.6	390
Mitchell, 1914–1916, Philadelphia (899)*	Average 2 years 3 months	11	1	–	–	9.1	10
Przesmycki and associates, 1932, Warsaw, Poland (1053)*	6 months to 6 years	64	23	5	6	53.1	30
Kereszturi and Hauptmann, 1931–1933, New York (710)*	2 months to 11 years	30	–	1	–	3.3	29[e]
Total		622	56	70	37	–	459
Per cent		100.0	9.0	11.3[f]	5.9	26.2	73.8

[a] Includes 1 case Type IIa.
[b] Includes 19 cases Type IIa and 2 due to "rough" pneumococci.
[c] Typed through Type XIII.
[d] Typed through Type XXIV.
[e] Ten had infection due to mixed types. The remaining 19 cases were typed through Type XXX.
[f] Omitting Ishida's entire series of 98 pneumococcus cases, Type II accounted for 5.9 per cent of the remaining 524 cases due to pneumococci.
* Cases from which no pneumococci were obtained were omitted from the reports.

Comparing the findings in cases of pneumococcus lobar pneumonia in infants and children (Table 24) with those in bronchopneumonia (Table 27), certain differences are apparent (Table 28). The most marked difference is seen in the incidence of Type I, for in pneumococcus lobar pneumonia this type accounted for 22.4 per cent while in bronchopneumonia it was much less frequent and was found in only 9 per cent of the cases. The incidence of Types II and III in these cases seems to show differences of little significance. Types I and II considered together were found in 30.5 per cent of cases of lobar pneumonia and were less common in bronchopneumonia, where they made up 20.3 per cent of the cases. Omitting the cases of Ishida from the combined series shown in Table 27, the proportion of Type I and II cases drops to 14.1 per cent in bronchopneumonia. In all, Types I, II, and III together accounted for 36 per cent of the cases of lobar pneumonia and for a smaller proportion, or 26.2 per cent, of those with bronchopneumonia. The larger proportion of these types in lobar pneumonia appears due chiefly to the high incidence of Type I in that group. Pneumococci of Group IV were found less often (64 per cent) in lobar pneumonia than in bronchopneumonia (73.8 per cent).

TABLE 28. PNEUMOCOCCUS LOBAR PNEUMONIA AND BRONCHOPNEUMONIA IN INFANTS AND CHILDREN. PERCENTAGE DISTRIBUTION OF CASES BY TYPE

	TOTAL CASES	TYPE I	TYPE II	TYPE III	TYPES I, II, AND III TOGETHER	GROUP IV
Lobar pneumonia (Table 24)	826	22.4	8.1	5.5	36.0	64.0
Bronchopneumonia (Table 27)	622	9.0	11.3*	5.9	26.2	73.8

* Omitting Ishida's series, as mentioned in Table 27, this figure is 5.9 per cent.

Another interesting comparison may be made (Table 29). This concerns the incidence of Types I, II, III, and Group IV in cases of pneumococcus bronchopneumonia in infants and children (Table 27) and in adults (Table 18, page 70).

While Type I occurred in 9 per cent and Type II in 11.3 per cent of the cases of pneumococcus bronchopneumonia in infants and children, these types were less common in cases in adults and were found in 5.6 per cent and 3 per cent of the series. Type III, however, occurred in only 5.9 per cent of the cases in infants and children and was much more frequent in adults, being found in 15 per cent of the cases. Pneumococci of Group IV occurred about as commonly in cases in younger patients (73.8 per cent) as in older ones (76.4 per cent). Although the series of cases compared are small, there is considerable similarity in the incidence of the various types in the two groups.

TABLE 29. PNEUMOCOCCUS BRONCHOPNEUMONIA IN INFANTS AND CHILDREN AND IN ADULTS. PERCENTAGE DISTRIBUTION OF CASES BY TYPE

	TOTAL CASES	TYPE I	TYPE II	TYPE III	GROUP IV
Infants and children (Table 27)	622	9.0	11.3	5.9	73.8
Adults (Table 18)	745	5.6	3.0	15.0	76.4

In several series of cases of pneumococcus bronchopneumonia, typing has been extended to include varying numbers of the higher types. Among 37 Group IV strains obtained from 35 cases and typed from Type IV through XXIX, Cooper, Rosenstein, Walter, and Peizer (320) found pneumococci of Types VIa, XVIII, and XIX were the commonest, being found nine, four, and four times respectively in this group. Among the 29 cases of Plummer, Raia, and Shultz (1029), typed from I through XIII, Type VI with 8 cases and Type VII with 3 cases were the most frequent. In the same hospital the following winter with typing extended through Type XXIV, Type XVIII with 3 cases was the commonest of 26 studied (1057). Kereszturi and Hauptmann (710) carried out typing for Types I through XXX and in 30 cases investigated found Type XIX the commonest (7 cases) and Types XIV, XVIII, and XXII next in frequency (2 cases each).

Thus pneumococci of six types, Types VI, VII, XIV, XVIII, XIX, and XXII, have been commonest in cases of bronchopneumonia in infants and children. Though the number of cases on which these observations rest is small, it appears that Types VI, XIX, and XVIII, in about that order, are the most frequently encountered in cases of this nature.

In 23 cases in patients under two years of age Cooper and her associates (320) found Types VIa and XIX to be the commonest. Type VIa likewise proved commonest among 14 strains from 12 older children with bronchopneumonia. In infants Nemir (930) reported Type XIX the most frequent. Types XIV and VI were also common in her series.

Commonest Types in Lobar Pneumonia and Bronchopneumonia

From the foregoing it is clear that some types of pneumococci are more often associated with pneumonia under ordinary conditions than others. In Table 30 is shown a summary of data from Tables 5 (page 46), 8 (page 53), 19 (page 71), and 25 (page 82) and from the section above.

TABLE 30. PNEUMOCOCCUS LOBAR PNEUMONIA AND BRONCHOPNEUMONIA IN INFANTS AND CHILDREN AND IN ADULTS. TYPES OF PNEUMOCOCCI MOST COMMONLY FOUND

	TYPES MOST COMMONLY FOUND IN ORDER OF APPROXIMATE FREQUENCY
Lobar pneumonia	
Infants and children	XIV, I, VI, V, VII
Adults*	I, III, II, V, VIII, VII
Bronchopneumonia	
Infants and children	VI, XIX, XVIII
Adults*	III, VIII, X, XX, XVIII, VII

* Early compilation of smaller series of cases on which the incidence figures in adults are based revealed the types most commonly found to be Types I, II, III, VIII, VII, and V in lobar pneumonia and Types III, VIII, XVIII, X, V, and VII in bronchopneumonia.

In lobar pneumonia Types I, III, and XIV are most frequent, and in bronchopneumonia Types III, VI, VIII, and XIX. Some types, such as Types VI, XIV, and XIX, are found chiefly in the pneumonias of infants and children, while Types II, III, and VIII are found chiefly in cases in adults. In general, pneumococci of the types above Type X appear commoner in cases in infants and children than in adults.

In all, pneumococci of twelve types are listed in Table 30. Type VII appears three times; Types I, III, V, VI, VIII, and XVIII each appear twice; and Types II, X, XIV, XIX, and XX each appear once.

CHAPTER THREE

PATHOLOGY OF LOBAR PNEUMONIA

Incidence of Lobar Pneumonia in Necropsied Cases 90
Gross and Microscopic Pathology 91
Stages of Consolidation 92
Impairment of Pulmonary Circulation 95
Duration of Red and Gray Stages and Time of Maximum Consolidation 96
Resolution and Delayed Resolution 96
Termination in Fibrosis 101
Loeschcke's Views of the Pathology of Lobar Pneumonia 101
Relative Frequency of Stages of Consolidation Found at Necropsy 106
Lobes Involved in Pulmonary Lesion 107
Clinical Studies 107
Necropsy Data 109
Lesions Associated with Lobar Pneumonia 111

INCIDENCE OF LOBAR PNEUMONIA IN NECROPSIED CASES

Series of necropsied cases of lobar pneumonia have been analyzed by various investigators (399, 874, 882, 96, 406, 332, 449). Certain points in some of these series may be compared. Among a total of 2,791 necropsies at the Johns Hopkins Hospital covering a period of over seventeen years, Fabyan (399) found that an anatomical diagnosis of lobar pneumonia had been made in 195 or 7 per cent. At the City Hospital in Boston, Berry (96) reported that among 4,256 necropsies over a period of twenty-three years a diagnosis of lobar pneumonia was made in 400 or 9.4 per cent. The latter estimated that these 400 cases represented approximately one-eighth of the total deaths (3,000 deaths) from this disease believed to have occurred at that hospital during the period mentioned.

The proportion of all patients found at necropsy to have lobar pneumonia may vary considerably in the same or different countries. In the Philippine Islands, Cruz (332) reported lobar pneumonia present in 400 or 3.3 per cent of approximately 12,000 patients coming to necropsy over the eighteen-year period of 1908 to 1925; Gautier (510), however, reported that among 1,000 necropsies between 1910 and 1928 this disease was found in 33.3 per cent. Gautier also reported that the proportion of patients with lobar pneumonia was 9.5 per cent among 6,125 necropsies over a seven-year period at Singapore, 18 per cent among 4,806 necropsies over a twelve-year period in Panama, and 31.5 per cent among 149 necropsies during a single year in Honduras.

The sex distribution of the above cases reported by Fabyan, by Berry, and by Cruz was very similar. Combining these groups, there were 995 cases of lobar pneumonia which came to necropsy. Of these, the sex of the patient was known in 982, of which 708 or 72.1 per cent were male and 274 or 27.9 per cent were female.

The distribution of patients by age groups was given by both Fabyan and Berry, and their findings were again quite similar. Combining their two series, there were 595 necropsied cases of which the age was known in 570 (see Table 31). Of these 570 cases 423 or 74.2 per cent were in patients between the ages of twenty and sixty years.

TABLE 31. LOBAR PNEUMONIA AT NECROPSY. NUMBER AND PERCENTAGE DISTRIBUTION OF NECROPSIED CASES BY AGE GROUP

AGE GROUP IN YEARS	CASES *Number*	CASES *Per cent*	AGE GROUP IN YEARS	CASES *Number*	CASES *Per cent*
0–10	25	4.4	50–60	107	18.8
10–20	17	3.0	60–70	72	12.6
20–30	76	13.3	70–80	28	4.9
30–40	118	20.7	80 and over	5	0.9
40–50	122	21.4	Total	570	

From Fabyan (399) and Berry (96)

In addition to analyzing these cases by sex and age, Fabyan listed the proportion of white and Negro patients. Among 182 cases in which the race was known, 95 or 52.2 per cent were white and 87 or 47.8 per cent Negro.

The types of pneumococci most commonly found at necropsy after pneumococcus pneumonia are mentioned elsewhere (see page 51).

GROSS AND MICROSCOPIC PATHOLOGY

The lungs are the site of the chief anatomical lesions in lobar pneumonia. A part or the whole of one or more lobes may be involved by a diffuse inflammation resulting in the coagulation into a fairly cohesive mass of a hemorrhagic exudate filling the alveoli, adjacent terminal expansions of the bronchioles, and usually the smaller bronchioles as well. At necropsy the uninvolved portions of the lung collapse in the usual manner, while the affected portion remains distended and shows the imprint of the overlying bony structures on its surface. This appearance has given rise to discussion as to whether or not the involved lung is actually larger than normal. Though a century ago Laënnec (755) reported that the affected lung was not enlarged, it remains undecided whether the affected lobe is larger than normal, as some investigators believe (297, 807, 826, 661), or, as maintained by others, whether it is smaller than normal (323, 322). Grossly, the affected portion appears swollen, but never to the extent that it displaces the heart and mediastinum.

Other factors of gross appearance are somewhat dependent upon the stage of the disease at which the lung is examined. In nearly all cases there is involvement of the pleura over the affected portion, with a consequent loss of its natural gloss. This involvement may be limited in the very early and less often in the late stages to a slight roughening of the surface, possibly with a fine deposit of fibrin. In other instances it is usual to find a definite, and at times a thick, shaggy deposit of fibrin on the pleural surface. In nearly all cases there is a variable increase in the amount of fluid in the pleural cavity.

Stages of Consolidation

Laënnec (755) was possibly the first to divide the evolution of events in the pneumonic lung into three stages: engorgement, and red and gray hepatization. For descriptive purposes such a classification has many advantages. Some confusion has resulted from its adoption, however, as it is not always recognized that these terms refer simply to the various pathologic changes seen in a given part of the lung rather than in the lungs as a whole. The development of the pneumonic process follows a definite sequence and is such that it is rare to find the entire lesion at any single stage. Different sections of the lobe or lung may be involved at different times or develop at different rates, or the process may spread to the opposite lung. In consequence, the portion initially involved may be at one stage while, toward the periphery of the lesion or in areas developing more slowly or recently involved, other and younger stages of the lesion may be found. Generally, by studying different sections of the lung, all the stages can be observed. This situation has made it impossible to describe symptoms of the disease by which each of the three classical stages might be recognized clinically.

At necropsy it is rare to find any considerable section of the lung in the stage of engorgement alone. Areas of engorgement may be seen, however, in regions newly involved and at the periphery of older advancing lesions. In this stage the lung is heavier and more solid than normal but still crepitous. It is doughy to feel and pits on pressure. Laënnec (755) described the external color of the lung at this stage as of a livid or violet hue. On section the cut surface is livid or blue in color, and frothy serous blood-tinged fluid runs out. Microscopically, the lung shows great engorgement of the capillaries of the alveolar walls with swelling of the alveolar epithelium. The alveoli usually contain a variable amount of serous fluid, red blood cells, and desquamated epithelium. Much evidence points to the fact that this stage probably lasts only a few hours in the usual case and, due to the rapid outpouring of exudate, the lung soon acquires new characteristics—those of the second stage.

The stage of red hepatization is the earliest one commonly seen and reveals a more typical picture of lobar pneumonia. The lung no longer crepitates and in consistency and weight resembles liver. While excised portions of the lung in the stage of engorgement will float, parts in the second stage (or third stage) do not. The lung surface is dark red or reddish-brown in color. By this time a copious inflammatory exudate has filled the alveoli and become clotted. The cut or torn surface is dry and, due to the fibrinous clots plugging the alveoli which are forced forward as small granules by retraction of the elastic alveolar walls, the surface has a granular appearance. The involved area usually shows a clear line of demarcation and stands out prominently from other areas of the lung. The bronchi are reddened and, though not prominent, may show a variable amount of purulent exudate, while the smaller ones contain fibrin plugs. Fibrin is mostly found in the alveoli, and its amount decreases with an increase in the diameter of the air passages (798). On scraping the cut surface with a knife, it is possible to obtain a little reddish-brown viscid fluid containing some of the small granular masses from the alveoli. When the infection is due to pneumococci of Type III, the fluid is unusually viscid (807). The size of the granules, consisting of clotted alveolar contents, varies with the size of the alveoli, and the latter increase somewhat in size with the age of the patient (807).

Microscopically, the alveoli show some infiltration of their walls and capillary distention. Their lumen is filled with a coarse-meshed network of fibrin along with serum, many red blood corpuscles, organisms, polymorphonuclear and some mononuclear leucocytes, and desquamated epithelial cells. The fibrin bundles and threads of an alveolar network appear to twist themselves into a thin strand and pass, by the so-called "pores of Cohn," through the alveolar wall to join the fibrin network in the next alveolus. MacCallum (826) remarks that possibly the most distinctive thing about the exudate at this stage is its appearance of freshness and good state of preservation. The red blood cells appear fresh and clearly outlined, as do the leucocytes, which often by their content of pneumococci give evidence of phagocytosis. The presence of red cells and, to a lesser extent, of free hemoglobin, and the intense congestion of the blood vessels lend a deep reddish color to the tissue. The lymph vessels are frequently dilated and full of serum with some red cells, leucocytes, and fibrin.

Although the third stage is that of gray hepatization, it is common to find the lung in an intermediate condition and part red and part gray in color. Typically, the color in the third stage is gray, grayish-white, or grayish-yellow. The change in color from the red stage is not, of course, simultaneous in all parts of the involved area, and it is common for some areas to retain some redness. The lung appears enlarged and is dense, heavy, and friable. On section it is more moist than in the previous stage and, as the granular appearance is less distinct, not so rough. Fluid scraped from the surface is more turbid. Microscopically, the alveoli are found densely packed with cellular exudate consisting chiefly of leucocytes, especially polymorphonuclears. The leucocytes frequently show considerable numbers of ingested organisms. Their hemoglobin having been lost, only shadowy remnants are found of the numerous red cells present in the earlier stage. The fibrin network, so obvious before, now appears packed together, perhaps less in quantity, and much less distinct. The smaller blood vessels, and especially the capillaries of the alveolar walls, appear compressed and are no longer distended with blood. The lumen of some may be partially occluded by fibrin or thrombi. Occasionally a megalocaryocyte, swept from the bone marrow into the lung during the outpouring of leucocytes, may be found in the capillaries (826).

In general, at this stage the cells of the exudate show considerable degeneration. Their outlines are indistinct, they stain poorly and show fat droplets in their protoplasm. A yellowish pigment, probably hemosiderin, derived from the hemoglobin of the red cells is found in some. More desquamated epithelial cells are present, and these, too, show signs of degeneration and contain fat droplets and some granules of yellowish pigment. The appearance of this myriad of degenerating cells with their fat droplets and yellowish pigment, in conjunction with the generally anemic state of the lung, doubtless accounts for the grayish-yellow color of the lung.

Pneumococci present in the stage of red hepatization stain clearly and have the power of infecting rabbits when exudate from this stage is injected into them. In gray hepatization, however, the organisms appear degenerated, no longer stain clearly, and have largely lost their power to infect such animals (MacCallum, 826).

Impairment of Pulmonary Circulation

Studies to determine the extent of the impairment of circulation in the pneumonic lung have been made by various investigators. Following the intravenous injection of trypan blue vital stain into rabbits with pneumonia, Kline and Winternitz (729) found that little of the dye penetrated into the consolidated area. From this and other studies they reported that in pneumonia in both rabbits and man they found definite evidence of an impaired pulmonary circulation. They attributed this less to pressure exerted by the mass of alveolar exudate than to a widespread distribution of capillary fibrin thrombi which in man usually appeared uniformly distributed. In dogs with pneumonia Christie and his associates (269) and Wang and Van Allen (1378) also found evidence of an impaired circulation in the affected area. The latter injected Congo red into the bronchus of the affected lobe at varying intervals after infection and determined the time required for the dye to appear in the blood. A much longer interval was consumed before the dye appeared in the blood in dogs injected late, and in which consolidation was advanced, than in others injected only a few hours after the onset of their pneumonia.

It is highly probable that in man there is some impairment of the circulation through the affected lobe, though this may chiefly affect the smaller blood vessels. The occurrence during the gray stage of at least a relative ischemia in the affected portion may partially account for the lessened effectiveness of specific serum therapy during the latter stages, more especially after the third day, of the disease.

Robertson and his co-workers (1088) have considered the problem of an impaired circulation in pneumonia. In spite of the pathologic changes present, apparently sufficient blood circulates to protect the stroma of the lung, for otherwise abscesses and necrosis of the lung would occur far more frequently than they do. Injection of the blood vessels shows the capillaries still patent though they appear compressed by the exudate (694, 826). Hunnicutt and Sutliff (667) gave intravenous injections of concentrated antipneumococcic serum to three patients with extensive consolidations just prior to death. By serologic means at necropsy they were able to detect about the same concentration of horse serum in the consolidated lobes as in the normal lobes. Though the possibility of technical error was considerable, this finding is perhaps additional evidence that a functioning, if impaired, circulation is present during pneumonia.

Duration of Red and Gray Stages and Time of Maximum Consolidation

Under ordinary circumstances the red and gray stages of hepatization last approximately two to three days each. Roentgenographic observations on patients show that definite appearances of consolidation are usually present within twenty-four hours of the onset of the disease (552, 341, 128) and that for a period these progressively increase. The careful study of Graeser, Wu, and Robertson (552) of 40 patients, of whom 20 were seen within forty-eight hours of onset, illustrates that consolidation tends to become maximum between the third and the sixth day but fails to show a uniform rate of development. By the end of the third day consolidation is frequently so intense that the production of an artificial pneumothorax causes little, if any, collapse of the affected lobe (128). A detailed study of pathologic sections from 50 cases, however, led Loeschcke (798) to assume that the inflammatory process in the lung required only forty-eight hours to reach a stage of maximum consolidation.

Resolution and Delayed Resolution

Usually, several days after the development of the massive lesion of lobar pneumonia, the extraordinary changes of resolution begin. Cases in which the entire lesion is in the stage of resolution are seldom encountered at necropsy. As the process is patchy and irregular in its evolution (552), scattered areas of resolution may frequently be found (1095). Microscopically, the degeneration and disintegration of the cells and fibrin, which first became noticeable during gray hepatization, is now marked, and a general liquefaction of the exudate occurs. During this process the lung becomes softer and more friable. In two cases studied by MacCallum (826), the lungs became distinctly translucent and blood vessels were visible in the depths of the tissue. The granular formation of the alveolar masses disappears, and the lung becomes jelly-like and grayish or grayish-yellow in color. The cut surface is yellowish and wet, and on pressure exudes a creamy yellowish purulent fluid which may be of slimy consistency. With the gradual disappearance of the softened exudate, the lung again becomes crepitant and air-containing. Under ordinary circumstances, when this series of changes is completed, the lung gradually returns to its natural state and resumes its normal color and functions. This process usually takes some time, for several weeks are required before roentgenograms become clear (552, 341), and pathologically Robertson and Uhley (1095) found definite evidence of the previous pneumonia in three patients dying one to two months after recovery from this disease.

The problem of the disappearance of the exudate in resolution has been variously studied. Expectoration alone can account for the removal of only a fraction of the large amount of exudate present. Even in the absence of cough and expectoration, the exudate disappears. Absorption, then, must be the chief means of removing the exudate, which must first be prepared for this by extensive autolysis. Though the process is complex and not completely understood, some information is available which would appear to explain certain phases of the digestion of the exudate. Lord (807) states the work of Müller and Simon, which was later confirmed by Silvestrini and Flexner, suggested that autodigestion played an important part in resolution. It was found that autolysis occurred more rapidly and perfectly in portions of the lung in the gray than in the red stage of hepatization. The enzymes responsible for this autolysis appear largely derived from the leucocytes of the exudate, as Opie (968) and others have shown, and leucocytes make up a larger proportion of the exudate in the stage of gray than in the stage of red hepatization. Extracts of purulent sputum were found to have the power of digesting fibrin and albumin, but in pneumonia this power was absent from the sputum until after crisis. Opie also studied the enzymes and anti-enzymes found in inflammatory exudates. He demonstrated that serum from an inflammatory pleural exudate contained a substance (anti-enzyme) which had the power of inhibiting the action of the proteolytic ferments (enzyme) contained in the leucocytes present. The anti-enzyme is contained in the blood serum, from which it doubtless passes into the exudate.

In the evolution of the pneumonic process, there is an increase in the number of cells, a diminution in the amount of serum, and apparently some impairment of the local circulation. In consequence, biochemical changes reflected to only a limited extent in the body as a whole may take place in the involved region. Evidence is presented by Lord (805) suggesting that there is a local increase in the acidity, and similar observations have been made by Nakajima (922). A possible source of error in such determinations, however, is a postmortem increase in the acidity. Admixture with blood from the blood vessels, on the other hand, would tend to lower rather than increase the acidity. It is therefore desirable to devise a method for the determination during life of the hydrogen-ion concentration of the alveolar exudate alone without admixture with blood.

The destruction of the leucocytes and to a less extent of the pneumococci liberates enzymes which appear to be responsible for the digestion of the exudate (805, 806, 962, 922, 35, 36, 37, 556). As the acidity of the exudate increases, its enzymatic power increases (922) and the final stages of digestion progress most rapidly at a pH of about 5.2 to 6.3 (805). Apparently two enzymes liberated from leucocytes are importantly concerned in this action. The first of these has a proteolytic action in weakly alkaline or acid media which digests the coagulated serum and fibrin present. As the acidity increases, the activity of this first enzyme ceases, while that of the second is augmented. The second enzyme, which is also active during the proteolysis of the fibrin, splits the partially digested proteins (peptones) and reduces them to amino-acid nitrogen (805, 807). By this means, and possibly with the assistance of macrophages which appear to actively engulf and digest red and white blood cells as well as pneumococci at this stage (1095), the exudate may be digested. Following the absorption of the resultant products, the major part of resolution is completed. In rabbits, both the acidity and the enzymatic power of the lung return to normal as the lung regains its natural state (922).

Nye and Lord showed that in the balance between the cellular material of the exudate (with its contained enzyme) and serum (with its anti-enzyme), enzymatic action may be absent with more than about three parts of serum to one part of cells and active when less serum is present (806). Digestion of the alveolar walls does not occur because of the presence of serum in their capillaries protecting the stroma of the lung from enzyme action (806).

In addition to the foregoing, certain cellular changes have been found associated with resolution. Large mononuclear cells, variously described and named, have been found in the exudate during resolution in man (1049, 855, 826, 798, 1095), in monkeys (123), in dogs (1083, 286), and in rabbits (1014, 496). In man, Loeschcke (798) ascribed to these cells the function of ridding the alveoli of fibrin. However, the matter was first extensively studied by Robertson, Coggeshall, and Terrell (1083) and Coggeshall and Robertson (286) in dogs. These investigators observed that there occurred a marked swelling of the cells of the alveolar walls, producing a pronounced increase in their thickness. After reaching a certain size, the enlarged cells appeared to wander off into the exudate as active phagocytes, replacing the polymorphonuclear cells and assisting in the destruction and digestion of the cells and pneumococci present. While areas early in resolution showed few of these cells, other areas in later stages showed them in increasing numbers. Functioning as free histiocytes or macrophages, they became the predominant cells of the thinning exudate late in resolution. This phenomenon was termed the "macrophage reaction." Associated with the increasing proportion of macrophages in the exudate in late resolution there was a concurrent decrease in the number of pneumococci.

Extending these observations to man, Robertson and Uhley (1095) studied the lesions in ninety lobes of the lungs of forty patients dying at intervals of from six to twelve hours to two months after the onset of pneumococcus lobar pneumonia. Their findings were nearly identical with those previously described by Robertson and his associates in dogs. The first evidence of the macrophage reaction in man was an increase in the number of the large mononuclear cells in the alveolar walls. These subsequently became detached and wandered into the exudate as active phagocytes. The polymorphonuclears were gradually replaced, the total number of pneumococci and cells in the exudate diminished, the fibrin decreased, and open spaces began to appear in the air sacs. Though less easy to follow, the same general type of tissue cell reaction occurred in the lymph glands at the hilum of the lung. A swelling of the hilar glands in resolution was observed during life by roentgen-ray examination by Davies, Hodgson, and Whitby (341).

Though the appearance of the macrophage reaction was not confined to any one stage of the disease, it was only slightly in evidence before the fourth day and was common after that time. At about the tenth day the macrophage became the predominant cell of the exudate. Robertson and Uhley remark that "In no case was resolution observed in the absence of the macrophage reaction." Apparently this reaction precedes and always accompanies resolution. Wherever a well-developed macrophage reaction was present, pneumococci were few or absent; while in most lesions of all ages in which the exudate was composed chiefly of polymorphonuclear leucocytes, the organisms were numerous. The mobilization of macrophages may represent an immune response of the pulmonary tissue cells (1087, 1095; see pages 180–182).

Hickling (639) studied the relation of the monocytes in the peripheral blood to pneumonia in man and found that a monocytosis occurred which was usually greatest at about the time of crisis. He concluded that monocytes wandered into the lungs at this period to perform some function closely allied with resolution. However, large mononuclears of the macrophage type were rarely found in the pulmonary blood vessels in resolution (Robertson and Uhley, 1095). In cases ending fatally, the monocytosis did not develop (639, 1095) even though the macrophage reaction might be present (1095).

From the foregoing it is seen that resolution may be ascribed to the following factors: (a) autolysis of the exudate present, the polymorphonuclears being the chief source of ferment; (b) an increase in the local acidity within the consolidated area; (c) the ferment–anti-ferment balance (enzymes from leucocytes and organisms versus anti-enzymes of blood serum); and (d) the action of large mononuclear cells. The proliferation and detachment of the enlarged cells of the alveolar septa with their excursion into the exudate and the mobilization of monocytes in the peripheral blood stream may represent an immune response, but this is by no means certain at this time. If this view is correct, resolution appears primarily to be a local chemical phenomenon with some associated cellular changes. The latter may be of secondary importance or represent a second step in resolution. There is little reason to believe that both crisis and resolution are dependent upon the same factors. While resolution may begin before, during, or, as is more common, after crisis, not infrequently it fails to take place on a large scale and most of the involved area remains solid for days or weeks. In a very few cases resolution never occurs and scar tissue gradually replaces the exudate.

It would appear from the above that if the consolidated area should be deficient in leucocytes, insufficient enzyme may be present to cause rapid autolysis. Further, it should be possible to bring about the same slowing and inhibition of autolysis, and consequently resolution, if an excess of anti-enzyme (contained in serum) is present. Observations supporting this contention were made by Kline (726). By the intrabronchial injection of normal dog serum into dogs with pneumonia, he maintained an excess of serum (anti-enzyme) in their consolidated areas and in most instances was able to inhibit resolution. Pathologic examination of the lungs of these animals showed considerable areas of organization.

Clinically, when resolution is drawn out over a period of three weeks or more, it is usually considered delayed. Though the mechanism of delayed resolution is not clear, it seems likely that a disproportion between the number of leucocytes and other constituents present in the exudate is of great importance. The extent of the macrophage reaction in delayed resolution has not been determined (1095).

Termination in Fibrosis

In some instances resolution may be gradual but complete, while in others the exudate fails to be digested and thus cannot be removed by absorption. In such instances organization occurs. Granulation tissue from various points on the alveolar walls invades and gradually replaces the alveolar exudate with the result that after a few weeks the involved area becomes a contracted, dense, nearly airless mass of scar tissue which fills the alveoli. Epithelial cells tend to grow out from the alveolar walls and cover the new connective tissue, and though shrinkage of the fibrous tissue occurs, leaving some space for air (826), the function of the lung must remain markedly impaired.

As previously mentioned, by maintaining an excess of serum in the involved lobes of dogs with pneumonia, Kline (726) was able to delay resolution with the result that organization occurred. Wadsworth (1364) found organizing areas of considerable extent in dogs following pneumonia due to a mixed pneumococcus and staphylococcus infection. As organization was not seen in those animals infected with either of these organisms alone, the phenomenon suggests that mixed infection may play some part in the occurrence of organization. However, in monkeys with lobar pneumonia due to pneumococci alone, Blake and Cecil (123) always found scattered areas of organization in the lungs.

Haythorn and Meller's observations (607) on the relation of anthracosis to the occurrence of organizing lesions following pneumonia indicate that anthracosis, particularly in the more severe grades, leads to an increased incidence of organizing foci. The lungs of several hundred pneumonia patients were examined at necropsy and, whereas organization was found in only 2.6 per cent of patients with slight or mild anthracosis, the proportion with organization increased to 7 to 16.7 per cent in patients with the most marked anthracosis.

Loeschcke's Views of the Pathology of Lobar Pneumonia

The foregoing presents the classical stages of engorgement and red and gray hepatization which pathologists have long accepted as the orthodox view of the pathology of the disease. Essentially the same is true of the discussion of resolution, though an appreciation of the role of mononuclear cells in this process may be regarded, relatively speaking, as something "new." Discounting this latter point, the conception of the development and evolution of the inflammatory process in lobar pneumonia has changed little, if at all, for many years. In 1931, however, the conception was seriously challenged by Loeschcke (798). Superficially his views appear strikingly different from those previously held, but careful study of his observations brings to light fewer changes than at first expected. To be sure, some of his views do differ markedly from those presented above, but caution must be exercised to avoid mistaking changes in terminology for changes in pathologic observation or interpretation. Loeschcke's studies of human cases appear of sufficient importance to merit presentation in some detail.

Correlating the clinical with the pathologic features of fifty cases at necropsy, Loeschcke studied multiple sections of ninety lungs. The thoracic organs were removed in toto and, by the injection of formalin into the vascular tree, the lungs were hardened in the expanded state. Serial saggital sections were cut about two centimeters thick for gross study, and, by subdivision and further sectioning, one of the segments, usually toward the middle, was used for microscopic examination. Loeschcke's findings from the study of such preparations are summarized herewith.

Microscopically, in an extending process the periphery of the advancing zone of infiltration, which may be wide, showed much edema with a high content of pneumococci. Edema of similar extent also involved the septa and lymphatics of the interstitial tissues. Organisms were not found in these tissues until after they had appeared in the alveoli. Nearly everywhere within the involved area the bronchioles and bronchi showed an exudate containing pneumococci. In the vicinity of a pneumococcal exudate, congestion of dilated capillaries and the beginning of an emigration of leucocytes were always found, and this condition afforded a gradual transition to the next zone, in which the edema was characterized by desquamated alveolar epithelium and an increasing number of leucocytes. Cells of both these varieties showed evidence of phagocytosis. But few red blood cells were present at this time, and in places fibrin networks were beginning to form. The next step showed all the alveoli and their passages filled with masses of leucocytes, a few erythrocytes, and alveolar lining cells in a fine fibrin network. By this time pneumococci had largely disappeared and the capillaries, many of which had fibrin networks in their plasma, were mostly without blood. The alveolar exudate, rich in fibrin and leucocytes, also filled the bronchioles and bronchi as a solid coagulum. Later in this stage the leucocytes began to decrease, a process which was characteristic of the next stage.

Up to this point the widely expanded alveoli were filled with exudate and now a distinct shrinking of the fibrin occurs, separating it from the alveolar wall to which it appears attached only in places where fibrin threads extend into an adjacent alveolus through the pores of Cohn. In shrinking, the fibrin threads become more compact and draw together in close networks in which the threads appear crumpled. There is a progressive disappearance of leucocytes, but it is not clear that this is the result of autolysis. Thus far the process resembles ordinary blood clot formation and fibrin shrinkage, with the resultant expulsion of serum and cells.

Where previous to shrinkage the alveoli were overfilled, distended, and tense, the fibrin shrinkage is accompanied by a relaxation of the entire area and by a consequent refilling of the capillaries with blood. This accounts for the process observed in the stage of fibrin shrinkage, namely, that usually there is renewed bleeding into the alveoli, and this may be more pronounced than at the time of the original outpouring of cells. This may possibly be regarded as the hemorrhagic stage, for it is very evident, even on gross examination. At this point the bronchi free themselves of their exudate and the fibrinous bronchial discharge reappears in the sputum.

The alveolar fibrin, however, is now markedly shrunken and continues to become thicker and more solid. Its dissolution by ferments of leucocytic origin does not seem possible, for no leucocytes have been present in the alveoli for some time. Meanwhile, at the moment the fibrin begins to shrink, the linings of the alveoli begin to regenerate, and this process has long been completed by the time shrunken fibrin masses are found in all alveoli. The older the fibrin masses, the more completely they are covered with epithelium, for the alveolar lining grows over onto the fibrin at its points of attachment to the walls and soon entirely covers it. The alveolar epithelium appears to live on the fibrin masses much as cells do in a tissue culture. In due course the fibrin is gradually consumed, after which the cells degenerate. It is also probable that a part of the alveolar epithelium which is stripped from the walls at the beginning of the process does not degenerate but continues to live in the fibrin and contributes to its epithelization.

It appears, then, that Loeschcke regards the earliest phase of pneumonia as a stage of pneumococcic edema. Pneumococcus invasion of the lung results in hyperemia and a migration of leucocytes which phagocytize the organisms. The initial slightly hemorrhagic exudate causes a maximal distention of the alveoli, producing a local anemia. The alveolar exudate finally coagulates with precipitation of the fibrin. This stage, brought about by anemia and a high leucocyte count, is regarded as gray hepatization and represents the "crisis" of the illness. Sections showing a large number of leucocytes are regarded as representing the more acute phases of the disease rather than the less severe stages of "lysis," for leucocytes appear where pneumococci are present and begin to decrease with the disappearance of these organisms. Fibrin, as such, has no qualities of a nature to attract leucocytes. Resolution occurs by fibrin shrinkage and digestion by cells derived from the alveolar epithelium, with an accompanying refilling of the alveolar capillaries and often a hemorrhagic stage. As the fibrin clots become smaller, the networks, at first clear and compact, gradually become more and more indistinct.

A correlation was made of the microscopic picture with the gross findings in lungs prepared by the formalin hardening method. Grossly, the area of hyperemia and edema could be differentiated from that of the coagulated exudate, and the latter quickly passed into the next stage, that of fibrin precipitation. The section was then dominated by the gray-white color of the fibrin, which was accentuated by the anemic condition of the lung. This stage was referred to as gray hepatization. Following the fibrin shrinkage and re-expansion of the capillaries, hemorrhages appeared. Though not extensive, these were scattered and of varying intensity, the cut surface appearing spotted and often showing the appearance of red lines in the septa. Such hemorrhages gave the lung a different appearance from that of red hepatization, for in the latter stage there is diapedesis into edema-filled alveoli, resulting in an even distribution of the erythrocytes in the fluid, producing a basic dirty-red color. In the stage of fibrin shrinkage, however, hemorrhage occurred between the alveolar walls and the compact fibrin masses. As the blood surrounded but entered the fibrin only a little, it remained undiluted and retained an intensive red color. Hemorrhages of this nature, the refilling blood vessels, and the presence of red cells in the lymphatics appeared to account for the red stripes in the septa.

The final stage, that of fibrin disappearance, continues some time and is variable in appearance. At first the grayish-white color of the still relatively large fibrin thrombi dominates the picture. A reddish tint is added due to the refilling of the capillaries. The mixture of fibrin and blood fluctuates to the advantage of the latter, and the color becomes gray-red and then entirely red. Characteristic of the stage of fibrin disappearance, the exudate of this stage (which may perhaps be called red hepatization) and of the climax of fibrin shrinkage is firmly attached to the alveolar wall and is not easily expelled. The greater the fibrin shrinkage, the more the fibrin thrombi detach themselves, until they are attached merely by supporting threads.

To summarize, the stages of lobar pneumonia given by Loeschcke on the basis of these observations are:

1. The initial pneumococcic edema—edematous hyperemic lung;
2. Leucocytic and erythrocytic emigration—diffuse grayish-red lung;
3. Fibrin coagulation—gray hepatization (ischemic lung);
4. Fibrin shrinkage—gray hepatization with hemorrhages;
5. Fibrin disappearance—at first like stage 4, then followed by red hepatization; at the end, hypostatic-like congestion with very small well-detached fibrin thrombi.

Possibly the chief difference between this conception of the evolution of the lung lesion in lobar pneumonia and that previously given in this chapter is, as Loeschcke remarks, that he scarcely recognizes a stage of red hepatization prior to the gray one. Further, he finds that the narrow zone lying between the area of edema and that of gray hepatization is characterized by the emigration of red and white blood cells and is grayish-red or yellowish-red in color, but nearer to gray-yellow than to red. This zone is so narrow that the transition from the edematous area to the area of gray hepatization is almost direct. Red hepatization which takes in lobes or large lung areas is invariably not an early but a late stage of pneumonia and in point of time always occurs after gray hepatization. A stage of yellow or sometimes grayish-yellow hepatization, rich in leucocytes, always occurs before the stage of gray hepatization and should not be regarded, as previously, as a stage of lysis or resolution, for during lysis leucocytes are nearly entirely lacking. From a correlation of the pathologic and clinical data on numerous cases, it is assumed that the inflammatory process in the lungs requires only about forty-eight hours to reach the stage of gray hepatization with completed precipitation of the fibrin in the alveoli. Further, the fibrin may remain present without shrinking until the fifth day of the disease, but earlier shrinkage may occur. Evidences of fibrin shrinkage may be obtained from the fifth to the twenty-second day, when only small remnants remain.

If, as it may be, the general sequence of events in the lung in lobar pneumonia is actually that described by Loeschcke, it is somewhat surprising that it was not detected years ago. It is, however, becoming increasingly obvious that in both animals and man the initial response of the lung to pneumococcus infection is an extensive outpouring of edema fluid. This is further discussed in the following chapter (see page 255). In addition, in discussing the condition of the surrounding uninvolved lung found in nearly 200 cases of lobar pneumonia at necropsy, Fabyan (399) reported that the lung tissue was congested or edematous in 144 or 75.3 per cent, normal in only 8 or 4.1 per cent, dry in 6 or 3.1 per cent, and crepitant in 13 or 6.9 per cent. Normal lung tissue was found chiefly on the uninvolved side in patients with unilateral consolidations. Berry (96), studying the necropsy reports of 400 cases, found that the unaffected lung was described as congested or edematous in 167 or 41.8 per cent. Further, in 1913 Maynard (874) analyzed the findings in more than 500 necropsies of African natives with lobar pneumonia and found it impossible to correlate the duration of their illness with the stage of hepatization discovered at necropsy. He reported finding gray hepatization as early as one or two days and red hepatization as late as twelve days after the onset.

Loeschcke describes secondary hemorrhages occurring during the stages of fibrin shrinkage and disappearance. Somewhat analogous was the occasional finding in the latter stages of the process in dogs with lobar pneumonia of an increased engorgement of the alveolar capillaries with some secondary diapedesis, reported by Robertson, Coggeshall, and Terrell (1083). Further, as above mentioned, various workers have found large mononuclear cells present in the pneumonic exudate. The origin and precise function of such cells are still debatable, though from the reports above cited, especially those of Loeschcke and Robertson and his associates, it appears that cells of this nature may play an important role in the final clearing of exudate from the alveoli.

RELATIVE FREQUENCY OF STAGES OF CONSOLIDATION FOUND AT NECROPSY

Fabyan (399), Menetrier (882), Berry (96), and Cruz (332) have reported in various ways the stages of the consolidation found at necropsy; their combined cases number more than a thousand. Gray hepatization was the stage most commonly encountered. The findings in 400 cases at necropsy, as reported by Berry, appear typical in this respect and are given in Table 32. Gray hepatization alone was most common and was found 317 times, red and gray hepatization in combination was found 225 times, and red hepatization alone 212 times. Lungs in the stage of engorgement or resolution were not found.

TABLE 32. LOBAR PNEUMONIA AT NECROPSY. GROSS PATHOLOGIC CONDITION FOUND IN VARIOUS LOBES OF THE LUNGS IN 400 CASES

PATHOLOGIC STATE	NUMBER OF CASES
Red hepatization	212
Red and gray hepatization	225
Gray hepatization	317
Organizing pneumonia	2
Combination of above states	44
Abscess or gangrene	19
Infarct of lung	6

From Berry (96)

LOBES INVOLVED IN PULMONARY LESION

Clinical Studies

Lobar pneumonia more often attacks the right than the left lung (694, 1168, 26, 874, 255, 230, 830). The number and percentage distribution of the lesions by the lung involved is well shown by Juergensen's (694) series of 7,747 cases from two hospitals in Vienna (see Table 33). Though his report was made in 1875, there is no evidence in more recent literature of any important change in this connection.

TABLE 33. LOBAR PNEUMONIA. NUMBER AND PERCENTAGE DISTRIBUTION OF 7,747 CASES BY LUNG INVOLVED

LUNG INVOLVEMENT	CASES *Number*	CASES *Per cent*
Right lung alone	4,089	52.8
Left lung alone	2,902	37.5
Both lungs	756	9.8
Total	7,747	

From Juergensen (694)

Of the total 7,747 cases, 6,991 or 90.2 per cent had unilateral and 756 or 9.8 per cent had bilateral lesions. Of the whole series, involvement of the right lung was present in over one-half (52.8 per cent), of the left lung in over one-third (37.5 per cent), and of both lungs in a much smaller group (9.8 per cent). The frequency with which the various lungs were involved was very similar to that reported by Biach (101) in a series of 10,537 cases of "pneumonia." In the latter group the right lung was involved in 49 per cent of the cases, the left lung in 35 per cent, and both lungs in 15 per cent. A small number of the cases in Juergensen's series (Table 33) were doubtless included among those reported by Biach. It is not clear, however, that the latter's series included only cases of lobar pneumonia.

Maynard (874) studied several hundred cases of lobar pneumonia in African natives and reported that both right lung and bilateral involvements were more common in natives than in Europeans. That natives were less resistant to extension of the infection was suggested as a possible explanation of this.

Considering the frequency with which lobar pneumonia attacks the individual lobes of the lung, it is found that lesions of the lower lobe are the commonest and that the right lower lobe is usually, but not always, involved more often than the left lower lobe. The predominance of the disease on the right side and its common occurrence in the right lower lobe is, as Lord (807) remarks, believed to be owing to the larger size and straighter course of the bronchi in that region.

Though reports showing the involvement by lobes of typed cases of pneumococcus lobar pneumonia are scarce, Cecil, Baldwin, and Larsen (230) have presented their findings in 1,896 cases analyzed in this manner (see Table 34). Cases with involvement of the lower lobes, either on the right or left alone or both at once, made up nearly two-thirds (66.1 per cent) of the series. Of single lobe lesions, involvement of the left lower lobe was most common (505 cases or 26.6 per cent) and right lower lobe lesions were second in frequency (440 cases or 23.2 per cent). Infection of the right and left lower lobes was by far the most common of the double lobe lesions and was found in 308 or 16.3 per cent of the cases, while cases with two right lobes (8.1 per cent) or two left lobes (4.9 per cent) involved were found less often. Cases with three or four lobes involved were still less common.

Though not common, involvement of the upper lobes was nearly twice as frequent on the right (117 cases or 6.2 per cent) as on the left (68 cases or 3.6 per cent), and together apical lesions formed 9.8 per cent of the cases. This is a somewhat lower incidence of apical involvement than that (14.8 per cent) reported by Sears and Larrabee (1168) among 949 cases of "pneumonia" and that (14.2 per cent) found by Ashton and Landis (26) among 900 cases of lobar pneumonia. In neither of the latter series was the etiologic agent mentioned.

The frequency with which pneumococci of the first three types and Group

IV were found in the cases listed in Table 34 has been computed in per cent. No marked difference was found and about the same proportion of cases due to pneumococci of one type had lesions in the right lower, or middle, or upper, or left lower lobe, and so on, as that of another type. Thus the type of the infecting pneumococcus appears to have little relation to the lobe involved or to the extent of the infection.

TABLE 34. PNEUMOCOCCUS LOBAR PNEUMONIA. NUMBER AND PERCENTAGE DISTRIBUTION OF 1,896 CASES BY LOBES INVOLVED AND BY TYPE

TYPE	RIGHT LOWER	RIGHT MIDDLE	RIGHT UPPER	LEFT LOWER	LEFT UPPER	TWO RIGHT LOBES	TWO LEFT LOBES	THREE RIGHT LOBES	RIGHT AND LEFT LOWERS	THREE LOBES	FOUR LOBES
I	138	9	36	174	18	59	27	44	88	33	6
II	82	4	29	85	14	37	19	12	54	21	8
III	70	4	11	60	11	20	18	6	59	6	3
Group IV	150	11	41	186	25	38	29	10	107	22	12
Total	440	28	117	505	68	154	93	72	308	82	29
Per cent	23.2	1.5	6.2	26.6	3.6	8.1	4.9	3.8	16.3	4.3	1.5

From Cecil *et al.* (230)

Necropsy Data

The findings in series of necropsied cases have been variously analyzed by several investigators. Fabyan (399) reported the findings in 195 cases, Maynard (874) in 688 cases, Berry (96) in 400 cases, Feinblatt (406) in 139 cases, and Cruz (332) in 400 cases of lobar pneumonia. Menetrier's (882) report of 400 cases includes some data on cases of bronchopneumonia.

Unilateral involvement is the commonest and is found in from 56 to 80 per cent of the cases (399, 96, 332). Lesions are more often found in the right than in the left lung. Fabyan reported right lung involvement in four times as many cases as left lung involvement, and Berry and Cruz in twice as many cases. In these three series of necropsies together, data were available for 993 cases: the right lung was affected in 476 or 47.9 per cent, the left lung in 251 or 25.3 per cent, and both lungs were involved in 266 or 26.8 per cent. The number of bilateral involvements reported in this group of necropsies is nearly three times the number usually reported in clinical studies, a fact which suggests the seriousness of such lesions.

In Berry's (96) series of 400 cases, 210 had involvement of the right and 111 of the left lung, while the remainder (79 cases) had bilateral lesions. The total 321 cases with unilateral lesions have been divided to show the frequency of involvement of the various lobes of the lungs (see Table 35). Cases with involvement of all lobes on the right were most common (73 cases). Those with right upper lobe lesions (55 cases) were next in frequency, and those with lesions in both lobes on the left (54 cases) were nearly as common. Single lobe lesions were commoner in the right upper (55 cases) than in other lobes and, on the right, lower lobe lesions were much less frequent (32 cases). Lesions of the middle lobe alone were seldom found (7

TABLE 35. LOBAR PNEUMONIA AT NECROPSY. DISTRIBUTION OF 321 CASES BY LOBES OF RIGHT AND LEFT LUNG INVOLVED

LOBES INVOLVED ON RIGHT	NUMBER OF CASES	LOBES INVOLVED ON LEFT	NUMBER OF CASES
Upper	55	Upper	18
Middle	7	Lower	39
Lower	32	Both	54
Upper and middle	14		
Upper and lower	12		
Middle and lower	17		
All lobes	73		
Total	210		111

From Berry (96)

cases). On the left, lower lobe lesions were about twice as frequent (39 cases) as upper lobe lesions (18 cases). In general, cases with multiple lobe lesions or with upper lobe lesions on the right were common at necropsy.

In double pneumonia, with involvement of one or more lobes on each side, Fabyan (399) found the most frequent combination was infection of both lower lobes. In his series of 195 cases nearly one-half had some double involvement. In Berry's (96) group of 400 cases, however, double involvement was much less common, but of the cases with bilateral involvement most showed all lobes affected. The second commonest double lesion in both these series was infection of all the lobes on the right in combination with the lower lobe on the left.

Berry combined his cases to show the number of times any one lobe was involved. His figures show the right upper lobe was involved 204 times, the right lower 190 times, the left lower 160 times, the right middle 148 times, and the left upper lobe 110 times. Fabyan and Berry have both commented on the marked frequency with which involvement of the right upper lobe was found at necropsy. Their findings suggest that apical lesions on the right may have a more serious prognosis than lesions elsewhere. In general, however, lesions are found nearly as frequently at necropsy in the right lower as in the right upper lobe. Any lobe or any combination of lobes may be affected. The 400 cases analyzed by Berry were further divided to show the number of lobes involved in each instance. In this group infection was present in one lobe in 151 cases, in two lobes in 120 cases, in three lobes in 103 cases, in four lobes in 18 cases, and in all five lobes in 8 cases. In all, about one-third of these cases showed lesions in only one lobe, and in over two-thirds of the series (67.8 per cent) the infection was confined to one or two lobes.

LESIONS ASSOCIATED WITH LOBAR PNEUMONIA

Many of the lesions which occur in association with lobar pneumonia are briefly mentioned here. Others, and especially the more common and important of these, are discussed at length in the chapter on Complications (see page 548).

Some of the associated lesions may be caused by organisms different from those causing the pneumonia. These other organisms may be pneumococci of a different type, streptococci, staphylococci, or less often other bacteria. Occasionally a mixed or secondary infection due to such organisms may occur and give rise to various lesions, such as a second attack of pneumonia, or empyema, septicaemia, lung abscess, and the like. Infections of this nature usually produce a very severe illness and in experimental pneumonia in animals generally cause serious sequelae or death (1364, 1097, 1292). Their occurrence in man is frequently equally serious and at times may account for what appear to be failures of specific therapy (969, 1271, 1000, 470, 445, 446).

Bronchopneumonia has been found in another lobe in cases of lobar pneumonia at necropsy. In Fabyan's (399) series of 195 cases it was present in 18, or 9.2 per cent, and in Berry's (96) series of 400 cases it was found in 62, or 15.5 per cent. Interstitial pneumonia was present in an additional group of 5 of Fabyan's cases. In a series of 339 cases of pneumococcus lobar pneumonia examined at necropsy Finland (449) reported that one-sixth of all cases also showed areas of atypical consolidation in other portions of the lung.

As mentioned earlier in this chapter, some plugging of the smaller bronchi and bronchioles with fibrinous or purulent exudate may be found. Among 156 cases in which the condition of the bronchi was noted, Fabyan (399) reported the bronchi as injected in 87 per cent, containing pus in 20.5 per cent, plugged with fibrin in 5 per cent, dilated in 3.2 per cent, and normal in only 5 per cent. Observations similar to this have been reported by others (882, 96). A diffuse purulent bronchitis and tracheitis may occur, and Finland and Sutliff (464) found this especially common in cases having Type III pneumococcus infections. Bacteriemia, septicaemia, pleurisy with effusion, empyema, otitis media, mastoiditis, pericarditis, endocarditis, meningitis, and the like may occur.

The bronchial lymph glands are usually swollen (694). Among 70 cases at necropsy in which the state of these glands was mentioned, Fabyan (399) found them congested in 68 and normal in 2. Berry (96) also found enlargement of the bronchial glands in a number of cases. In Fabyan's (399) total group of 195 cases at necropsy, cardiac hypertrophy was found in 31, and in 37 others the heart weighed over 300 grams. Apparent cause for this enlargement was present in several instances, but in 34 or 17.3 per cent of the cases no cause other than the pneumonia could be found. Menetrier (882) reported finding occasional instances of cardiac dilatation in cases at necropsy, as did Berry (96). Among a total of 400 cases examined, the latter found cardiac hypertrophy in 98, dilatation in 6, and toxic changes of the myocardium in 15. As no other cause for these conditions could be found, Berry attributed them to the pneumonia.

Fabyan reported acute splenic tumor present in 74 or 37.9 per cent of his cases and liver necrosis in 10 or 5.1 per cent. In Berry's series an enlarged spleen was found in 192 or 48 per cent. He also reported finding acute myositis of the rectus abdominus muscle in 6 cases. Berry noted that "toxic" changes were most frequent and best seen grossly in the spleen, kidneys, liver, and heart, but on histological examination such changes were even more frequent in the adrenals and pancreas. Thomas and Parker (1298) studied such organs and considered the matter of toxic changes not associated with the actual presence of the infecting organism. The suggestion was made that these changes might be considered evidence of the action of a toxin. The possibility of a toxin of pneumococcus origin has already been discussed (see page 21). As Cruickshank (331) reported isolating pneumococci from the spleen as well as from the lung in all but one of twenty-four cases at necropsy, it is apparent that changes in organs *presumably* not associated with the presence of the infecting organism need careful study.

CHAPTER FOUR

ASPECTS OF IMMUNITY

Nature of Immunity 114
  Circulating Antibody 115
  Cellular Immunity 125
  Sensitivity of Tests for Immunity 127
  Correlation of Humoral Antibody with Immunity 127
  Substances Antagonistic to Antibody Action 131
  Specificity of Immunity 133
    Antigenicity of the Pneumococcus 133
    Type-specific and Species-specific Immunity 134
    Cross Immunity 135
    Non-specific Immunity 136
  Site of Antibody Formation and Unity of Function 136
Natural Immunity of Animals 137
Natural Immunity of Man 143
Mechanism of Natural Immunity 150
  Relation of Humoral Antibody to Natural Immunity 150
  Relation of Natural Humoral Antibody to Course and Outcome of Infection 153
  Relation of Natural Humoral Antibody to Pneumonia Morbidity 154
  Mode of Production of Natural Antibody 155
  Relation of Cellular Factors to Natural Immunity 157
Mechanism of Acquired Immunity 158
  Evidence of Altered Reactivity in Acquired Immunity 159
    Appearance of Humoral Antibody 159
    Variation in Antibody Response 161
    Increased Efficiency of Blood-clearing Mechanism 162
    Development of Ability to Immobilize Organisms and Localize Infection 164
    Prevention of Subsequent Infection and Alteration of Course 164
    Alterations in Skin Sensitivity 165
    Cellular Changes 167
  Relation of Humoral Antibody to Acquired Immunity 168
    Specific Antibody of the Rabbit and the Horse 172
  Relation of Humoral Antibody to Course and Outcome of Infection 173
  Host Factors and Physiologic Variables 177
  Local Lung Resistance 180

Relation of Hypersensitiveness and Allergy to Immunity 182
Factors Affecting Variations in Immunity 185
Animal Species 186
Genetic Factors 186
Age 186
Sex 192
Infecting Organism: Virulence and Type 193
Passage of Time 194
Immunization 196
Presence of Infection or Other Disease 199
Miscellaneous Factors 201

For the purpose of this book consideration must be given to certain aspects of the resistance of animals and of man to the pneumococcus. No attempt will be made to treat the matter exhaustively, for much of the problem is but little understood. In addition to the general discussion of immunity in this chapter, numerous references will be made to the subject in appropriate places in subsequent chapters.

Failure to take account of differences in the inherent capacity of various animals to respond to the administration of pneumococci or their derivatives, or failure to use identical materials in successive studies of the immune response has been responsible for more or less contradictory results in some experimental studies. Instead of attempting to correlate these divergences, an effort will be made to maintain emphasis on the more important positive findings. A detailed review of numerous aspects of immunity to the pneumococcus may be found in *The Biology of Pneumococcus,* by White, with Robinson and Barnes (1417).

NATURE OF IMMUNITY

Immunity to the pneumococcus appears to be dependent upon humoral factors in the form of antibodies, substances capable of reacting in various ways with pneumococci or their derivatives and which frequently can be isolated from the host and have been much investigated, and upon cellular factors inseparable from the host, which have been studied less extensively and are less well understood, but are hypothesized to explain the presence of immunity in the absence of demonstrable circulating antibody. Antibody commonly appears in the blood following either infection or immunization, at which time the resistance to reinfection by the experimental animal has been found to be enhanced. In consequence the presence of humoral antibody has been assumed to have a causal relation to immunity. Immunity is therefore frequently measured by qualitative and quantitative determinations of humoral antibody.

For the purpose of detecting the presence or absence either of antibody capable of reacting with pneumococci or their derivatives, or of cellular immunity, a number of *in vitro* and *in vivo* tests have been devised.

Circulating Antibody

Agglutinins, precipitins, opsonins or tropins, and bactericidal, protective, curative, neutralizing, immobilizing, and complement-fixing substances have been found in the blood of many immune individuals, as have substances which produce significant alterations in some of the biologic characteristics of pneumococci grown in contact with them. In some instances a slight antitoxic action has also been reported. At times the antibody demonstrable may exhibit only one or two of these functions. Formerly the view was held that the whole of the bacterial cell was involved in the combination of antigen and antibody. It appears now, however, that probably this is not so and that the reaction between the antibody of the surrounding fluids and the bacterial cell occurs at the surface of the latter and involves the surface antigens. A brief résumé will be given of some of the characteristics and qualities of antibodies, their significance, and the various conditions under which they have been demonstrated.

AGGLUTININS. Among the early workers who investigated the phenomenon of the gross agglutination of pneumococci in immune serum, Bezançon and Griffon (99), Neufeld (932), and Wadsworth (1360) may be mentioned. In recent years, more detailed studies (620) have shown that the process of agglutination is accompanied by an increase in cell volume, which may be due to the deposition of antibody upon the surface of the cell (689, 690), and depends upon the presence of certain lipoids in the serum (656). Under some circumstances the serum of either animals or man may contain type-specific or species-specific agglutinins, or both. Just as all the type-specific agglutinins may be removed from serums by their absorption with the specific capsular substance of pneumococci in the form of the acetyl polysaccharide (41), so their absorption with rough strains of this organism will remove the species-specific agglutinins (1063).

Agglutination tests have been used for the following purposes:

To identify types of pneumococci (938, 364, 784, 117, 1146, 1147, 196, 616)
To detect immune factors in the serum of
  Animals (932, 1360, 938, 748, 727, 168, 169, 1448, 531, 121, 41, 1135)
  Man (932, 1360, 1285, 1114, 937, 938, 1447, 295, 754, 118, 280, 1194, 815, 177, 459, 577, 1270, 121, 462, 12, 1429, 339)
To study variants of pneumococci (1256, 1063, 571, 344, 1393, 129, 345, 1004)

PRECIPITINS. Using solutions of pneumococci, Neufeld (932) and later Wadsworth (1360) demonstrated the presence of precipitins in immune serum. The latter also showed the presence of precipitins in the serum of some normal animals and of man.

Various studies of the precipitin reaction have been made (427, 626, 623, 624), and a mathematical expression of it has been devised (625). As with agglutination, the precipitin reaction in some immune serums is visibly demonstrable only in the presence of certain lipoids (656). Type-specific or species-specific precipitins or both may be present in some serums. While the former may be absorbed from the serum by the use of the acetyl polysaccharide or substances believed identical with it (392, 395, 41), species-specific precipitins may be removed by absorption with rough strains of pneumococci (1063).

The precipitin reaction has afforded a relatively simple means of studying and estimating the potency of immune serums (511, 427, 502, 1468, 626, 1347, 417, 601) and of determining the presence and specificity of various derivatives and growth products of pneumococci (511, 363, 617, 618, 46, 51, 44, 619, 1063, 41). The reaction has proved useful in the typing of pneumococci (363, 117, 32, 746, 1120, 616) and in pneumonia is of aid in following the urinary excretion of soluble specific substance, and has therefore proved of some prognostic value (33, 754, 118, 1054, 1321, 1010).

OPSONINS OR TROPINS AND BACTERICIDINS. Opsonins or tropins have been studied by many investigators. Substances in *normal* serum which alter bacteria in such a manner as to render them susceptible to phagocytosis were termed opsonins by Wright and Douglas (1442, 1443). Heating serum at 60° C. for fifteen minutes appeared to inactivate these substances. Neufeld and Rimpau (940, 941), however, found substances having a similar action in *immune* serums which were not inactivated by heating the serum as above described and termed them tropins.

The terms opsonin and tropin have been loosely used at times, with some resulting confusion. Recently the manner in which substances in serums prepare pneumococci for phagocytosis was reinvestigated by Ward and Enders (1383). These workers demonstrated that the same antibody may act either as an immune opsonin or an immune tropin and concluded that a single well-defined antibody, the anti-carbohydrate (anti-SSS) antibody, may be responsible for the phagocytic action of various normal and immune serums whether heated at 56° C. for thirty minutes or unheated. Though alone it was unable to cause phagocytosis and was not essential to the process, the presence of complement was found to greatly accelerate it. In view of these observations it was suggested that the term "tropin" be discarded, and that the term "opsonin" be reserved to designate the antibody in the serum, whether normal or immune, heated or not, which unites with the organism and leads to its phagocytosis. By opsonin, then, was meant any heat stable antibody which prepares bacteria for phagocytosis; and to facilitate subsequent discussion this terminology will be used throughout this book.

Many of Ward and Enders' experiments involved the use of soluble specific substance in its old form (presumably the deacetylated polysaccharide), and the findings suggested that in normal human serum a second heat stable antibody capable of preparing virulent pneumococci for phagocytosis might be present. However, subsequent studies by Enders and Wu (395), using A substance, which was identical with the new acetyl polysaccharide of Avery and Goebel (41), appeared to explain their earlier findings, and to confirm the view above cited that only a single well-defined antibody was present in normal or immune serum. The action of the opsonin in normal blood or immune serum can be largely eliminated by the absorption of this substance with acetyl polysaccharide, and the effect is type-specific (395).

Other studies of opsonic or tropic action have been made (1285, 1115, 1116, 936, 1254, 784, 1089, 1448, 1091), and in some instances observations were carried out on the serum of patients convalescent from lobar pneumonia (937, 1254, 388, 280, 5, 1194). Accurate quantitative measurements of opsonic or bacteriotropic action are difficult due to the possible variability in the distribution and vitality of the included living phagocytic cells which, of course, are essential to the test.

Tests devised to demonstrate the bactericidal or killing power of whole blood, plasma, or serum, or of serum-leucocyte mixtures have also been extensively used to investigate various phases of resistance to the pneumococcus. In these tests opsonins appear to play a significant role. The presence of both living organisms and living phagocytes is necessary, thus involving two variables and making the test somewhat difficult of control; in consequence, such tests can seldom be used for the quantitative determination of resistance. While in some instances the chief action noted has been a retardation of growth or multiplication, in others a definite and marked bactericidal action has been observed.

Neufeld and Rimpau (940), Dold (371), Wright, Morgan, Colebrook, and Dodgson (1445, 1446, 1447), Heist and Solis-Cohen (628), and Bull and Bartual (170) were among the first to study the bactericidal action of blood, plasma, or serum for pneumococci. Subsequent studies of the pneumococcidal power of various preparations were made by many workers beginning with Robertson, Sia, and Woo (1093) and Robertson and Sia (1089, 1090). These workers devised a new test using serum-leucocyte mixtures which might be incubated while being agitated in sealed tubes. Slight modifications of Robertson and Sia's test have been suggested (1096, 1451, 395).

Robertson and his associates have carefully investigated the immune properties of the blood and some of its constituents of many species of animals and of various groups of human beings before, during, or after infection or immunization, as will be mentioned below. Investigations of a similar nature have been carried out by other workers using whole blood after the addition of various anti-coagulants (1448, 174, 1274, 1275) or after defibrination (1379, 1382, 1270, 461, 462, 395). In the various preparations studied, bactericidal or growth-inhibiting power has been found dependent upon opsonization and upon phagocytosis with intracellular destruction of the organisms; and in preparations which lack either functioning opsonins or phagocytes, bactericidal action does not occur (371, 628, 170, 1089, 1439, 1189, 1448, 1091, 1097, 1379, 1086, 395). In fact this process is the only method thus far discovered by which the blood elements are able to kill pneumococci, and their death appears to occur within the phagocytic cells, the polymorphonuclear being the chief cell involved. While leucocytes must be present if pneumococci are to be killed, they seem to function equally well for this purpose whether obtained from susceptible or resistant individuals, even when infected with the homologous organism (1091, 1087), and the degree of resistance demonstrable in a given specimen of blood appears largely, if not wholly, determined by the concentration of opsonins in the serum. When solutions containing soluble specific substance are added to test preparations, the type-specific pneumococcidal-promoting properties of the serum are inhibited without apparent damage to the leucocytes (1189, 1091, 1379, 1382,

1383, 395). This nullifying action presumably results from the combination of the soluble substance with the opsonin, which renders the latter ineffective.

Bactericidal action is absent from normal and immune serum, and from plasma alone (1445, 1446, 1447, 1256, 628, 170, 1439, 1448). Though in 1911 Dold (371) obtained an extract of leucocytes which was bactericidal for pneumococci, Robertson and Sia (1091) in 1927 were unable to demonstrate that either leucocytes or extracts of them had any such action. In test preparations an optimum number of leucocytes is necessary, but doubling their number does not increase the bactericidal effect (1089, 1090, 1379, 1275); and, similarly, where immune serums are tested, an optimum amount is needed (1090, 1091, 1379), but the addition of more serum does not increase the effect (1090). In bactericidal tests the effect of both the leucocytes and the serum appears to be quantitative in nature.

By the application of the bactericidal test, Robertson and his associates have attempted to differentiate natural from acquired immunity in both animals and man. It was repeatedly observed that the unheated serum of many species of normal animals naturally resistant to pneumococcus infection, as well as a large proportion of normal human beings, possessed considerable pneumococcidal-promoting properties not present in identical samples of such serums *after* being heated at 56° C. for thirty minutes (1089, 1439, 1091, 1097, 1086, 1087); and while this property appeared in the serum of other individuals either as a result of active immunization or following pneumococcus infections, in this instance it was not destroyed by a similar application of heat (1090, 1097, 1194, 1087, 1088, 286). Thus, natural immune substances appeared heat labile and acquired immune substances heat stable. It remains doubtful, however, whether any clear-cut distinction between the quality of the antibody present in these two kinds of resistance can be demonstrated in all instances, as Robertson and Sia (1091) have pointed out, for not all natural opsonins are inactivated by heat, and heating the serum of the normal pig only partially reduced its opsonic effect. Robertson and his co-workers have also called attention to this difficulty in other reports (1097, 1087) and regard the differences observed in tests using heated or unheated serum as quantitative rather than qualitative in nature.

Though the immune factor of antipneumococcic serum, being an acquired factor, was not affected (1090) by heating such serum at 56° C. for thirty minutes prior to adding it to serum-leucocyte mixtures, Robertson, Sia, and Cornwell (1092) observed that in such preparations the pneumococcidal-promoting action was markedly influenced by the presence of a small amount of fresh normal serum. The addition of potent immune serum to normal serum-leucocyte mixtures conferred a marked pneumococcidal power on the preparation, which was absent, however, if the normal serum used was first inactivated by heat. The factor in fresh normal serum which activated immune serum was heat labile, seemed identical with complement, and appeared more necessary for the intracellular digestion of the organisms than for opsonization. Nevertheless, no appreciable impairment of the activating power was found in the serum of either animals or man during pneumococcus infections (1092, 1088).

Bactericidal tests with blood or serum have been carried out for the following purposes:

To determine the presence of antibody:
- In normal animals (371, 628, 170, 1089, 1439, 1189, 1448, 1091, 174, 483)
- In animals during or after immunization or infection (628, 170, 1090, 1448, 174, 1097, 1290, 1291, 1292, 286)

To study immunity in man:
- In his normal state (371, 1447, 1379, 1085, 1274, 1270, 461, 462, 551, 395)
- During or after pneumonia (371, 1194, 1275, 1094, 1382, 1086, 1087, 1088)

PROTECTIVE AND CURATIVE SUBSTANCES. The protective action of immune serum was first demonstrated by Klemperer and Klemperer (724). Among the other early workers who studied the properties of immune serum responsible for this action and the factors influencing the outcome of such tests, Eyre and Washbourn (396), Römer (1106), and Neufeld and Händel (936, 937) may be mentioned.

By the injection of immune serum into animals and the simultaneous or subsequent injection of living culture, the proportion protected from a fatal infection can be determined. Protection tests of this nature, however, are subject to the influence of several variables somewhat difficult of control. The tests are usually carried out in mice whose resistance may vary considerably according to their age, weight, breed, and the like. Of even greater importance apparently are the variables introduced by the use of living organisms, especially in relation to their virulence and power to produce neutralizing substances and their stage of growth (415, 416). In association with all these variables the action of the protective antibody in immune serum has been found to show certain characteristics in protection tests. Except within rather narrow limits the amount of serum required does not follow the law of multiple proportions (936, 937, 1330, 33, 540); there is a minimal amount of serum below which no protection can be demonstrated with a given amount of culture (1330), referred to as the limiting titer zone (540); there is also a limiting maximum amount of culture against which protection can be obtained, referred to as the *Schwellenwert* (936, 33, 540); and the failure of large amounts of horse antiserum to yield the protection readily obtained by the use of smaller amounts of such serum against standard doses of culture is referred to as the prozone effect (412, 540).

The protection test has been one of the most commonly used procedures to demonstrate the presence or absence of resistance. Despite the numerous variables which may affect the outcome, the test has proved of great value for quantitative determinations of resistance and, in consequence, has rendered essential aid in standardizing the potency of immune serums (396, 1106, 936, 308, 33, 407, 532, 412, 415, 416, 414, 1468, 601, 909, 537, 602, 721, 432). In addition, the protection test has been used to determine the presence of antibody in the serum:

Of animals:
- Normal (748, 168, 1089, 707, 1086, 1137)
- Subjected to infection (1388, 232, 1097, 531)
- Immunized (724, 1389, 936, 937, 748, 1330, 364, 750, 231, 240, 241, 242, 939, 1090, 243, 841, 888, 1126, 1127, 68, 532, 1310, 414, 699, 1240, 1370, 1241, 395, 1137, 77, 595)

Of man:
- Normal (936, 937, 205, 281, 577, 1270, 462, 12, 1429, 1138, 433)
- Actively immunized (228, 485, 459, 71, 72, 461, 1469, 478, 1135, 1138, 424)
- Recovering from pneumonia (1388, 937, 356, 784, 278, 61, 60, 1194, 815, 1275, 1094, 820, 468, 469)

The curative effect of immune serums in animals has been determined by their administration at various intervals after infection to rabbits (724, 981, 1363, 168, 531, 532, 1151, 1152, 536, 377), dogs (1363), guinea pigs (942), monkeys (233, 244), and mice (532, 1018, 909). In addition, the results obtained by the specific serum treatment of several thousand patients with pneumococcus pneumonia have demonstrated the curative value of such serums for man (see pages 880–918).

SUBSTANCES NEUTRALIZING SPECIFIC SOLUBLE POLYSACCHARIDE. There is a wealth of material available, as will be seen below (see page 131), attesting to the power of certain derivatives of pneumococci to combine with antibody in such a manner as to render the actions of the latter ineffective and indicating that this combining capacity depends chiefly, if not entirely, upon the amount of specific capsular polysaccharide which they contain or of substances regarded as identical with it. However, there is less direct evidence at hand indicating that antibody nullifies the inhibiting action of the soluble specific polysaccharide. Such evidence of this nature as is available is of importance, however, and strongly suggests that antibody does have a so-called "neutralizing" effect on the soluble substance.

Dochez and Avery (363) found that the urinary excretion of soluble specific substance in patients with pneumococcus Type I pneumonia often temporarily stopped during the treatment of such patients with antipneumococcic serum of homologous type and that the excretion of this substance was resumed after such treatment was discontinued. In some instances specific serum therapy has caused a complete cessation of the urinary excretion of soluble substance (33). Avery and his associates (51, 44) were the first to show that immune serum precipitated from solution specific soluble substance of homologous type. Using various procedures, other workers have demonstrated that serum from immunized animals (414, 1381), as well as that obtained late in their illness from patients with pneumonia (60, 1382), may exhibit neutralizing power. Because antibody and soluble specific substance appear mutually antagonistic, it is believed that one of the essential functions of type-specific antipneumococcic serum in assisting in overcoming pneumococcus infection is to combine with SSS and to counteract its inhibiting action or actions (33, 60, 195, 176, 444, 301, 546). From the observations of Blake (118) and of Pepper (1010) that agglutinins which develop during the course of pneumonia may be present in the blood of patients excreting soluble substance in their urine, it appears that the urinary excretion of the latter substance may persist even though some humoral antibody is present. In addition, specific soluble substance was found in the presence of circulating agglutinins in the blood of rabbits treated with specific serum after experimental intravenous infection with a strain of Type III pneumococci virulent for this animal (Drinker, Enders, Shaffer, and Leigh, 377).

SUBSTANCES WHICH IMMOBILIZE PNEUMOCOCCI. An important action of antibody was recently described by Rich (1077), who found that one of the specific properties of antibody was to assist in localizing infection. This finding was confirmed by Catron (218). Following the subcutaneous injection of pneumococci into rabbits or mice actively or passively immunized against the homologous type, an immediate immobilization of the organisms at the site of injection occurred that did not occur in control animals. A similar action was noted in animals injected with organisms previously sensitized with immune serum. The immobilizing action appeared to result from the adherence of the organisms to the surrounding tissue cells at the site of injection, was possibly assisted by the action of agglutinins, was independent of allergy, and occurred before any effective degree of inflammation developed, though inflammation when present presumably aided in keeping the infection localized. The immobilizing power was apparently directly proportional to the concentration of antibody.

SUBSTANCES PRODUCING IMPORTANT CHANGES IN PNEUMOCOCCI GROWN IN CONTACT WITH THEM. Various workers have observed and investigated many of the changes which occur in pneumococci grown in contact with the blood or serum of susceptible or resistant individuals (Pane, 981; Neufeld, 932; Wadsworth, 1360; and others, 1285, 362, 1256, 170, 570, 407, 1063, 1448, 571, 344, 129, 139, 1004). Pneumococci grown in contact with immune substances for the homologous organism rapidly develop significant alterations in many of their biologic characteristics which are either absent or develop only very slowly among strains not exposed to the influence of such substances during their growth. The growth of pneumococci in the serum of naturally susceptible animals, such as the rabbit (981, 1360, 139), is ample and diffuse, and at times large atypical forms may appear which Bordet (139) has termed "spherules."

In the presence of the serum of immunized rabbits growth also occurs but at a slower rate, and the organisms become matted together into a thin gray-white "skin" (981) or grow in the form of short chains clumped together with swollen capsules (981, 932, 1360), and this may occur even though ordinary antibodies are not demonstrable in such a serum (Wright, 1448). Growth in the presence of immune rabbit serum is not accompanied by the production of spherules (139). Alterations of growth characteristics, such as the production of short chains and clumps, may also occur apparently as a result of culturing pneumococci in contact with the serum of (a) various naturally resistant animals (1360, 170, 139), (b) immunized rabbits (570) and horses (1256, 170), and (c) man convalescent from pneumonia (1285). It is probable that such changes are brought about by the presence of antipneumococcal immune substances in the serums tested.

In addition to these gross changes, other and doubtless more important alterations occur in pneumococci grown in contact with specific antibody of homologous type. Substances are present in immune serum which specifically inhibit the proteolytic and glycolytic activities of the pneumococcus cell (Dochez and Avery, 362), and during the recovery of patients from pneumococcus lobar pneumonia such substances either appear for the first time or show a marked increase in the blood.

Further, several pronounced changes were shown to occur in pneumococci of Types I, II, and III grown in immune serums of homologous type, as was demonstrated by investigators such as Stryker (1256). The organisms became less agglutinable in serum for the homologous type and more agglutinable in serum of heterologous types, their virulence decreased, the power of capsule formation was lost, they developed a susceptibility to phagocytosis which was previously lacking, rabbits immunized with them produced antibodies more slowly than those immunized with strains not previously exposed to the action of such antibodies, and they absorbed agglutinins non-specifically from antipneumococcic serum. These important alterations in the biologic characteristics of the organisms occurred without the loss of their ordinary properties of being soluble in bile and capable of fermenting inulin and of reacting typically to the Gram stain.

Felton (407, 420) likewise has remarked upon the rapid loss of virulence which accompanies the growth of pneumococci in immune serum of homologous type. Other workers, such as Griffith (570, 571), Reimann (1063), Dawson (344), Blake and Trask (129), and Paul (1004), have observed that the growth of type-specific pneumococci in immune serum of the corresponding type results in changing organisms of the S form into those of the R form.

In the absence of leucocytes, pneumococci are not killed *in vitro* in the presence of specific antibody but under suitable circumstances may undergo significant alterations in many of their biologic characteristics.

MISCELLANEOUS ANTIBODIES. Circulating antibodies having actions different from those mentioned above have also been sought for. Complement-fixing antibodies were found present in immune serum (44, 264, 1448, 173, 414), but were absent from the serum of the normal pig (707), an animal which is considered to possess considerable natural resistance to the pneumococcus.

Though the curative properties of immune serums were early believed to be due to the action of contained antitoxins (724, 725, 1363), subsequent investigations have largely altered this view. The pneumococcus has never been shown to produce a true soluble exotoxin, though toxic substances having various properties have been obtained from cultures autolyzed in solutions of saline or bile (1117, 289, 290, 306, 292, 279, 50, 1118, 997, 115, 114, 328, 1398), from culture filtrates (683, 284), and by the acid extraction of an alkaline solution of the organisms (424). The investigation of some of these substances has shown that, while normal or immune horse serum has little if any effect in neutralizing their toxic properties (290, 306, 999, 1398), the serum of patients convalescent from pneumonia may neutralize them to a slight degree (683, 284). However, the immunization of animals with various of these toxic materials has evoked the production of antibodies having considerable neutralizing power for the respective antigen employed (997, 999, 998, 683, 114, 1398), and this action is usually species-specific and not type-specific. Antibodies having an essentially similar action were found in the serum of a limited number of children immunized with one of these toxic products (284).

Following the immunization of animals with one of these toxic substances, a so-called "antitoxic" serum was produced. While some investigators reported this serum to contain protective antibodies (998, 114), others were unable to show that it possessed either protective or curative value (1150, 989). The treatment of several patients having lobar pneumonia with an antitoxic serum was without demonstrable beneficial effect (Cecil, 223). Though the relation of any toxic substance thus far described to the outcome of natural pneumococcus infection is not clear, its effect is apparently but slight at the most.

Heterophile antigen has been found present in some pneumococci, and the properties of this antigen and the possible biologic significance of heterophile antibody in pneumococcus infection have been studied (55, 1047, 56, 57). Though the limited evidence available suggests that antibody of this nature may possibly have a bearing on the resistance of rabbits to pneumococcus infection, there is no evidence that heterophile antibody is importantly concerned in the resistance of man to the pneumococcus or in the course and outcome of lobar pneumonia in human subjects (457, 458).

Precipitins for C substance may be detected in the blood during the course of pneumococcus pneumonia in man (1312, 1313), but their significance is not understood.

Cellular Immunity

In addition to the tests for circulating antibodies mentioned above, other methods have been used to estimate resistance to the pneumococcus.

SURVIVAL OF INFECTION. The most direct method of determining resistance to the pneumococcus is to observe the course and outcome of infection with this organism. Pasteur (1002) in 1881 was the first to note differences in the resistance of animals subjected to experimental pneumococcus infection. Observations of a similar nature were subsequently made by Fränkel (487, 488) and a host of other workers. In many such instances little or no effort was made to determine the presence or absence of circulating antibody which may have aided in combating the infection. Additional studies have been carried out in animals, however, to determine the resistance to infection shown by individuals lacking demonstrable circulating antibodies. The results of such studies strongly suggest that resistance of a considerable degree may at times be present in the absence of humoral immunity. Numerous examples of the use of direct infection for determining resistance are mentioned in several of the following sections of this chapter, particularly in those dealing with the correlation of humoral antibody with immunity (page 127), acquired immunity (page 158), and immunization (page 196).

SKIN TESTS. The intradermal injection of autolysates or filtrates of pneumococcus cultures or of derivatives or extracts of this organism may at times give rise to skin reactions having various characteristics. Studies have been made of sensitivity or allergy in normal and actively and passively immunized animals and in those recovering from pneumococcus infection, as will be seen below (pages 165, 170, and 182). Additional similar studies have been made in both animals and man, and the findings correlated with the presence or absence of humoral antibodies and with the occurrence of resistance as manifested by recovery from infection (279, 841, 843, 1311, 485, 459, 486, 700, 461, 1270, 12, 477, 206, 595, 285).

As the materials used for skin testing have not always been identical in successive experiments, difficulty has been encountered in attempts to compare and interpret the results obtained. Nevertheless, under the proper conditions a typical wheal and erythema reaction to the intradermal injection of the specific capsular polysaccharide (SSS) would appear to be a definite indication of some cellular resistance. This reaction has been studied at various times by Tillett and Francis (1311, 485, 486, 477), Finland and Sutliff (459, 461, 1270), and Alston and Lowdon (12). While in normal man the reaction may be positive even in the absence of specific humoral antibody (459, 461, 1270) or negative in the presence of such substances (1311, 485, 459, 461, 477, 12), at the time of recovery from pneumococcus pneumonia a positive reaction apparently indicates the presence of both circulating antibody and active tissue resistance; and the absence of either of these factors results in a failure of the reaction to develop (1311, 485, 459, 477).

Sensitivity of Tests for Immunity

In the course of investigations of the circulating antibody of animals or man carried out before, during, or after immunization or infection, comparisons have been made of the relative value of the various tests employed for detecting the presence of humoral immune substances. In general, bactericidal, mouse protection, and agglutination tests have been most frequently used.

The bactericidal test has been found the most sensitive for detecting the presence of immune substances in the blood of normal man, and pneumococcidal power is frequently present in the blood or serum of many such individuals in the absence of protective or agglutinating power (1274, 1270, 462, 1383). Even in patients with pneumonia the bactericidal test appears superior to other tests for detecting the presence of antibody regarded as of natural origin (1094).

Though protective substance can be detected for a longer period than agglutinins in the blood of immunized rabbits (1241, 1245), it appears that in such animals the bactericidal test is the most delicate for determining the presence of acquired antibody, and substances which are destructive to virulent pneumococci or delay their growth appear earlier and persist longer than antibody having other actions and may be present in the absence of the latter (628, 1448).

In man, several investigators have found the mouse protection test the most sensitive for detecting the presence of type-specific antibody acquired as the result of infection or immunization (459, 462, 468). Though in some instances during the course of pneumonia, bactericidal power may develop earlier than protection, humoral immunity as measured by these two tests is usually roughly parallel (1275).

The skin test carried out with the specific capsular polysaccharide is regarded as a less sensitive indicator of antibody production in man than either the agglutination or the protection test (459).

Correlation of Humoral Antibody with Immunity

WHEN HUMORAL ANTIBODY IS PRESENT. Though the evidence is not yet conclusive, there is a large volume of data available indicating the existence of a direct correspondence between the presence of specific humoral antibody and the presence of active resistance to infection by pneumococci of homologous type. This relationship may be only a general one, however, and of greater significance in animals than in man. Though most of the available information concerning this matter is based upon studies of animals, there is some evidence at hand relating to man.

As will be seen below (page 137), experiments with normal animals of many species have revealed that they may be classified roughly into two groups, those resistant and those susceptible to infection with virulent pneumococci. In some instances at least, and where searched for, humoral antibody was usually found present in the blood of the various species of animals considered resistant but was not demonstrable in the blood of susceptible species. Comparative studies of the specific bactericidal power of the blood of many normally susceptible and resistant animals have revealed that the *in vitro* power of destroying virulent pneumococci or of retarding their growth corresponded closely with the animals' degree of resistance to infection with the homologous type of pneumococcus (170, 1439, 1091, 1085). Even susceptible animals may prove resistant to pneumococci of low virulence and show humoral antibody against such strains (628, 1439, 1189, 1097). Blake's (121) finding of a close correlation between the titer of species-specific agglutinins in the blood of the guinea pig, an animal which is relatively susceptible, and its ability to resist infection is also in accord with the point of view in question. Wadsworth (1360), however, was unable to find any correlation between the observed growth alterations of pneumococci cultured in the serum of various normal animals and the resistance of such animals to infection.

In some immunized animals the titer of specific antipneumococcal immune substances appearing in their blood and body fluids has been shown to parallel closely their acquired resistance for the strain of pneumococcus in question (785, 170, 939, 841, 888, 1126, 1448). Nevertheless, other observations have revealed that in occasional individual instances the possession by animals of acquired specific humoral antibody is not always a reliable index of their active resistance (532, 1370, 1245, 1136, 536).

There is no conclusive evidence that the presence in the blood following immunization or infection of any so-called "antitoxins" or heterophile antibodies necessarily indicates the presence of resistance in the host (see pages 124–125). From the limited data available there is likewise no evidence that the appearance of precipitins for C substance in the blood during pneumococcus infection is indicative of resistance, and such precipitins may be found in the blood during infections caused by any of several varieties of cocci which react positively to the Gram stain (1312, 1313).

In man, there is considerable evidence, both direct and indirect, that a relation exists between the presence of demonstrable humoral antibody at various ages and the incidence of pneumonia at those periods. The data at hand support the reasonable belief that at the extremes of life, when resistance is lowest, the incidence of pneumonia appears to be highest; while in the intervening period, when resistance is higher, the incidence of pneumonia is lower (see pages 186–192 and 299–307). Of course the operation of cellular immunity, which seemingly has an important relation to this whole matter, cannot be excluded here. In addition, the finding of specific humoral antibody for the homologous type in patients with pneumococcus lobar pneumonia at a time believed to be too early in the course of the disease to be the product of the infection is regarded as presumptive evidence that the disease can occur despite the presence of some circulating antibody (992, 223, 1379, 1275, 1094, 485). Likewise, the relation of natural and acquired specific humoral antibody to the course and outcome of pneumonia in man is such that it seems almost certain other factors must in many instances play an important part in the control and favorable termination of the illness (see pages 153–154, 173–177, and 728–737).

In consequence, as the exact relation of specific circulating antibody to the resistance of man is not clear, further investigation along these lines is needed.

WHEN HUMORAL ANTIBODY IS NOT PRESENT. In a broad way the presence of demonstrable humoral antibody may be regarded as evidence of the possession of a variable degree of resistance to infection. As humoral antibody is probably the product of biologic activities of important groups of cells within the body and may possibly become demonstrable in the blood only when an excess beyond that which becomes fixed in or upon other cells is present, the fact that many individuals have considerable resistance and yet show no circulating antibody is perhaps not surprising. There are numerous reports at hand of the occurrence of resistance in animals in the absence of humoral immune substances. Examples of this have been observed among normal cats (170) and young rats (1137) and after immunization or following recovery from infection among rabbits (628, 1448, 1309, 1097, 532, 1310, 699), rats (1136), dogs (286), and monkeys (231, 232, 240, 241, 242, 243).

Considerable individual variation has been encountered. It is also possible that the observed decrease in the incidence of pneumonia in immunized man which may occur in the absence of the development of demonstrable humoral antibody, as noted by Lister (785), may be the result of a similar phenomenon. Moreover, in many patients who have recovered from pneumococcus pneumonia it has not been possible to demonstrate humoral antibody by any of the methods usually employed for its detection (see pages 173–175). It thus seems clear that a considerable degree of resistance may be present in the absence of demonstrable circulating antipneumococcal immune substances.

The lack of humoral immunity may be more apparent than real in some instances in that negative reactions may be due to the use of an alien species for the test animal in procedures such as the protection test. Such an explanation is suggested by the inability of Goodner (532) and of Tillett (1310) to protect mice with immune rabbit serum. Yet because of negative results of *in vitro* opsonic and bactericidal tests in which the leucocytes used are derived from either the animal under test or from another of the same species, and because of the failure to find agglutinins, precipitins, or complement-fixing antibodies in some instances as well, it appears clear that no evidence of circulating antibody can be found in the blood of some resistant individuals.

Another factor which may account for the presence of resistance in the absence of humoral antibody is the always admitted possibility that the tests in use are not sufficiently delicate to reveal the presence of small amounts of immune substances. However, the observations of Robertson, Woo, Cheer, and King (1097) and of Coggeshall and Robertson (286) in relation to this matter appear of some importance. At various times Robertson and his associates have stressed certain differences in the humoral antibody content of the blood of naturally susceptible and resistant animals (see pages 137–143) and have noted that following recovery from infection, humoral antibody is usually present in resistant animals and is frequently absent in animals in the susceptible group until they have experienced repeated infections. This suggests that, while the mechanism involved in the control of humoral antibody in either instance is essentially similar, the difference lies in the animal species and in the group, whether resistant or susceptible, to which the individual belongs. The type of pneumococcus involved may have a bearing on this matter (1097). It is nevertheless clear that exceptions to the above generalization occur, for Coggeshall and Robertson (286) also found that specific humoral antibody appeared only inconstantly in the blood of the dog (a resistant animal) after recovery from experimentally induced pneumonia.

Substances Antagonistic to Antibody Action

Numerous studies have been made of substances, contained in or derived from virulent pneumococci, which inhibit the action of natural or acquired antibody and which, when injected into animals in the course of experimental infections, render a sublethal infection lethal. Substances of this nature were early designated as "virulins" by Rosenow (1116) and as "antiphagines" by Tchistovitch and Yourevitch (1286), though Strouse (1253) was unable to find evidence of their existence. Later Cole (295) observed that a soluble substance was present in infected exudates and in the blood of animals and man with pneumococcus infections which specifically inhibited or neutralized the antibody of antipneumococcic serum. The subsequent investigations of Dochez and Avery (363) and of Heidelberger and his associates (617, 618, 619), on the one hand, and of Felton and Bailey (426), Woo (1439), Sia (1189), and many additional workers, on the other, succeeded in establishing that this inhibiting substance is at least very similar to the specific capsular polysaccharide of the pneumococcus if not identical with it. Recent contributions of Avery and Goebel (41) and of Enders and Wu (395) also impressively favor this view.

The possibility that other substances which inhibit antibody action may also be present in pneumococci was suggested by Felton's (415, 416) finding that killed cultures contained a substance which may be different from the capsular polysaccharide and which specifically neutralized the protective antibody of immune serum. In addition, Goodner (535) observed that soluble specific substance was not necessary in some experimental infections in animals to give the effect of enhanced virulence which others mentioned below had reported from its use. He noted that the injection of autolysates of either virulent or avirulent strains of homologous or heterologous types along with live culture permitted a smaller dose of virulent Type III pneumococci to kill rabbits than was otherwise required. The factor which produced this virulence-enhancing effect was of an unknown nature and was not type-specific in its action. In this instance the autolysates apparently allowed a smaller number of pneumococci to do as much damage as ordinarily occurred from the use of a larger number without actually increasing the essential virulence of the culture used.

Aside from these observations by Felton and by Goodner, little is known of the antagonistic action of substances other than the specific capsular polysaccharide, and chief attention has been directed toward the latter. Because of the possible great importance of the specific polysaccharide both to the organism and to the infected host, considerable effort has been expended in the attempt to define its action. By virtue of its ability to combine with and precipitate the specific antibody and otherwise nullify its specific action, the specific capsular substance is regarded as having a so-called "neutralizing" power.

Various studies have demonstrated that the action of certain antibodies of natural or acquired origin may be partially or completely inhibited by the specific capsular polysaccharide or by substances now regarded as identical with it, and that such inhibition is type-specific. This has been shown for agglutinins (619, 476, 41), precipitins (619, 1380, 392, 1149, 476, 1382, 1151, 41), opsonins and bactericidins (426, 1439, 1189, 1091, 1379, 1380, 1195, 1382, 1383, 395, 546), and protective antibody (1380, 415, 416, 1149, 1151, 41, 395). The injection of slightly virulent pneumococci into animals along with a small amount of soluble specific substance or of a culture filtrate of homologous type results in an infection as severe as that produced by the use of highly virulent pneumococci alone. In effect the SSS injected appears to enhance the virulence of the culture used ten to one hundred times in mice (426) and 100,000 times in rabbits (1195).

It is presumably this same substance which in animals hinders the development of immunity by immunization (422, 1470) or, when injected following immunization, greatly reduces or eliminates the immunity produced (1470, 395). It appears that the host can absorb a limited amount of soluble specific substance without noticeable effect, but if more is present, the mechanism of resistance is definitely impaired. The means by which this is accomplished is not well understood. The results of bactericidal tests suggest that the specific inhibiting effect of soluble substance results from a neutralization of the sensitizing antibody (1189, 1380) rather than from any effect on the leucocytes concerned; and, as the organisms are not phagocytized, growth occurs. There is not complete agreement on this, however, for in studies involving the intraperitoneal infection of mice the soluble specific substance used appeared to inhibit the activity of the phagocytic cells present (546). In either type of experiment the presence of a large excess of specific antibody, and in some instances of substances such as heterologous serums, proteins, or lipoids, also appeared to have a decided retarding effect on phagocytic activity (1380, 546).

Specificity of Immunity

ANTIGENICITY OF THE PNEUMOCOCCUS. By experimental means early investigators, such as Eyre and Washbourn (396), Bezançon and Griffon (99), and Longcope and Fox (803), found differences between certain strains of pneumococci which suggested that there might be differences in the antigenic properties of these organisms. It was not until later, however, that definite evidence was obtained of the great complexity of the pneumococcus antigen. The facts that pneumococci may be divided into distinct serologic types (see page 22); that complex polysaccharides have been isolated from organisms of at least four of these types (617, 618, 619, 622), each having specific differences in its serologic behavior and chemical constitution; and that other substances which may be (424, 433) or are clearly different from these polysaccharides, such as nucleoprotein (43, 46, 51, 44, 1063), heterophile antigen (55, 1047, 57), and components of a toxic nature (289, 997, 999, 998, 683, 284, 114, 1398) have been obtained from them, all indicate the complexity of the antigenic structure of these organisms. It is not surprising, therefore, that antibodies having numerous actions may appear as the result of stimulation by such a complex material.

Great light was thrown on the structure of the pneumococcus cell by Avery and his co-workers (43, 46, 51, 44), who showed that the enveloping capsule of virulent forms is composed of the specific polysaccharide and that the cell body is made up of a complex nucleoprotein material. From the studies of these investigators and of Reimann (1063), it became clear that the antigenic properties of intact cells were quite different from those of disrupted cells. Under the proper conditions the intact cells gave rise to type-specific antibodies, while the use of solutions or extracts of disintegrated organisms or the use of rough forms produced only species-specific antibodies.

In general, the more closely the state of the organism used approaches that of the intact, vigorous, living, virulent cell, the greater is the type-specificity and adequacy of the immune response. The specific capsular polysaccharide appears to be the dominant antigen of the cell surface of intact virulent forms. By disrupting the integrity of the cell or by using rough degraded forms which have lost their capsule with its specific polysaccharide, the protein of the cell body beneath the capsule is exposed and exerts an antigenic action. This protein appears to act as the dominant surface antigen of avirulent rough pneumococci.

Under ordinary circumstances pneumococcus cultures contain intact cells of variable virulence and, in addition, some degraded cells and a certain amount of autolyzed material; and since it is practically impossible to separate these constituents from the whole organism, some cell protein is free to act as an independent antigen. Following immunization with such a mixture, the blood of animals contains both type-specific and species-specific antibody. The former reacts specifically only with pneumococci of homologous type or with the specific capsular polysaccharide derived from them and is frequently referred to as the anti-SSS or anti-carbohydrate antibody, while the latter reacts non-specifically with the protein of all pneumococci and with rough degraded strains which have lost their protective capsule and is termed the anti-P or anti-protein antibody.

Because a certain amount of autolysis occurs in all cultures, including those used for immunizing horses, ordinary therapeutic antipneumococcic serum, while containing a large amount of type-specific antibody, usually also contains some species-specific antibody. This may also be true of some diagnostic serums, and at times the content of anti-protein antibody may be sufficient to give rise to some cross agglutination.

While the nucleoprotein component of the organism gives the pneumococcus only species-specificity, the type-specificity of the organism and of the immunity induced by infection or by the immunization with the intact cells of virulent strains appears determined by the nature of the specific polysaccharide of the capsule. Goebel, with Avery and Babers (522, 524, 525, 523), has demonstrated that in conjugated polysaccharide-protein preparations, the configuration of the carbohydrate fraction of the molecule determines the specificity of the antibody response. At first regarded as a complex hapten or partial antigen having the power to combine with antibody of homologous type, though not itself antigenic (1465, 617, 46, 44), the specific capsular polysaccharide, or substances believed similar if not identical with it, was later found to be antigenic, to have the power of producing anaphylactic shock in guinea pigs passively sensitized with the serum of rabbits immunized against the homologous type (52, 392, 1369, 486, 595), and to stimulate the production of immunity in both animals (1012, 440, 1011, 1160, 1130, 1369, 1132, 1133, 422, 1470, 41, 424, 433) and man (485, 459, 461, 1469, 478, 424, 433, 425).

TYPE-SPECIFIC AND SPECIES-SPECIFIC IMMUNITY. Effective demonstrable immunity to the pneumococcus appears to be largely conditioned by the presence of type-specific antibody and hence to be dependent upon the action of such substance. Type-specific antibody has been found in the blood of many animals naturally resistant to pneumococcus infection (171, 1091, 1111, 1137, 707, 1195), and there is a probable correlation between the presence of such humoral antibody and the resistance of the individual as discussed earlier in this chapter. Though apparently little studied, at times species-specific anti-protein antibody has been detected in the serum of normal animals (344, 707), where its presence may be an indication of the possession of some active resistance (121). In immunized animals the presence of species-specific antibody appears to have little relation to the degree of immunity induced (46, 1309, 1310, 1245). Both type-specific (205, 281, 1379, 1274, 1085, 459, 1270, 1469, 462, 12, 551, 1429, 1094, 1138, 433) and species-specific (344, 121) antibody have been found in the blood of normal man.

In both animals and man the immunity resulting from infection or from immunization with a suitable antigen appears largely type-specific. It is probable, however, that, following infection or after immunization with ordinary vaccine, man as well as animals may develop some species-specific immunity in consequence of *in vivo* destruction of the organisms and the resultant liberation of antigenic material from within the cells. Species-specific humoral antibody (1311, 1321) and tissue sensitivity (1311) to pneumococcus protein have been demonstrated in patients convalescent from pneumonia, and what may be species-specific cellular immunity has been observed in immunized animals (1243, 1258).

The possible relation of heterophile antibody and of any so-called antitoxins to pneumococcus immunity has already been mentioned (see page 125). The action of these antibodies appears largely of a species-specific rather than of a type-specific nature. The relation of C substance (1312, 1313, 622) to pneumococcus immunity is not understood, and in animals the material is not antigenic.

CROSS IMMUNITY. In some instances, as a result of infection or immunization with a presumably suitable type-specific strain of pneumococci, specific immunity in the form of humoral antibody or of active resistance to infection may be found, not only for the homologous type, but occasionally, and to a slight degree, for heterologous types as well. This has been observed in mice (1243), rabbits (628, 173, 699), monkeys (231, 232), and man (1138). In other instances a certain amount of heterologous immunity has been produced by immunization with the specific capsular polysaccharide (461, 1470) or with derivatives obtained by Felton which have characteristics somewhat different from that substance (424, 433). The presence of overlapping groups in the antigens used, either alone or in combination with a reaction of the so-called anamnestic type, may assist in the development of such cross immunity.

NON-SPECIFIC IMMUNITY. The interesting studies of Tillett (1309, 1310) have shown that a non-specific form of immunity may be induced in rabbits by their immunization with pneumococci of heterologous types and R forms so long as the vaccine used contains formed cells. The active immunity produced was effective in the complete absence of type-specific antibody and appeared to have no relation either to the presence of species-specific antibody or to the variety of pneumococcus used for immunization. While the serum of rabbits possessing such immunity did not passively protect mice, it did protect other rabbits. The serum was most effective in protecting rabbits when the infecting organism was injected within a few hours of the administration of the serum. With whole blood, however, the protection was less marked in the early hours after it was administered and appeared most effective if the infecting dose was delayed twenty-four hours, when results were better than if serum alone was used.

The findings suggest that resistance under the conditions mentioned depends upon factors other than those operative in type-specific immunity or upon the same factors operating in a different way. The possibility that this form of immunity was due to an exaltation of the mechanism responsible for natural resistance in some instances was considered. The significant features of Tillett's observations were confirmed by Julianelle (699). The principles underlying immunity of this nature are not well understood.

Site of Antibody Formation and Unity of Function

No attempt will be made to discuss the numerous investigations carried out in the effort to determine the point of origin of antibodies, since little is yet known of the exact method of antibody production or of the precise cells and tissues involved in the process. Relatively little work has been done upon the antibodies of the pneumococcus, though the studies of Neufeld and Meyer (939) and of Meyer (888) should be mentioned.

Topley (1317) has reviewed this matter in some detail and states in summary:

The available evidence indicates that the cells of the reticulo-endothelial system, which are known to remove injected antigenic material from the blood and tissue fluids, play an essential part in the production of antibodies. Whether these cells themselves produce the antibodies in their final and complete form, or whether their rôle is confined to the temporary retention of antigen and its subsequent liberation in an altered or unaltered state, the actual synthesis of antibodies occurring elsewhere, cannot yet be determined. The present indications are that the part played by the reticulo-endothelial system is not confined to the retention and release of unaltered antigens.

The cells of the reticulo-endothelial system (25) that are presumably most concerned in the production of antibodies are the sessile histiocytes or macrophages of the endothelium of the capillaries of the liver (Kupffer cells), adrenals, and pituitary, and of the sinuses of the spleen, lymph vessels, and marrow, as well as the reticular cells of the spleen, lymphatic tissues and glands, and thymus and the like. The wandering histiocytes and macrophages are probably less important.

From the foregoing discussion, and particularly that in the section on neutralizing substances (page 121) and that dealing with substances antagonistic to antibody action (page 131), it appears that essentially all the actions of antibody, whether the latter is of natural or acquired origin, can be specifically inhibited by the specific capsular polysaccharide of the pneumococcus. This fact, together with the important observations of Felton (417), Ward and Enders (1383), Avery and Goebel (41), and Enders and Wu (395), which are of similar significance, strongly suggests that the anti-carbohydrate antibody may be the one essential serum factor responsible for the various actions of immune antibody. Except for the suggestion of Heidelberger and Kendall (625), so far little investigated, that there may be two antibodies present in immune serum which react with the specific soluble substance, most data at present available favor the view that the actions attributed to immune substances are the result of a single antibody, the anti-carbohydrate antibody, functioning in various ways depending upon the conditions present—a view which supports the unitarian conception of antibodies as advanced by Dean (348) and Zinsser (1460).

NATURAL IMMUNITY OF ANIMALS

Experience has shown that many species of animals, as well as man in general, possess variable degrees of natural immunity against the pneumococcus. Efforts to correlate the level of this immunity with the titer of the humoral antibody present have not always been successful. In consequence, it seems almost certain that cellular or other factors, as yet impossible to estimate or measure with accuracy, must play a significant role in natural immunity in many instances.

Observations are available on the relative resistance or susceptibility of several species of mammals and of two species of birds. Various procedures have been used in making these investigations. Studies have been made of the degree of phagocytosis occurring during pneumococcus infection, or of the amount of inflammation incited or the survival rate following infection, or of the pathology of the resulting lesion. Numerous tests for the detection of humoral antibody have also been carried out.

The results of these observations, when taken as a whole, are surprisingly uniform in indicating that with minor variations the animals investigated may be classed largely either in a susceptible or in a resistant group. To facilitate comparisons, the various animals concerning which information is at hand may be briefly considered in turn.

The Mouse

The mouse has long been known as one of the animals most susceptible to pneumococcus infection. Various workers, such as Friedländer (501), Fränkel (488), Tchistovitch (1284, 1285), Washbourn (1388), and others (936, 937, 938, 1360, 412, 415, 1159, 601, 218) have repeatedly demonstrated the susceptibility of the mouse to pneumococcus infection. Because of its great susceptibility, this animal has been extensively used for determinations of the protective antibody in various serums, as was earlier pointed out. Neither bactericidal substance (371, 170) nor substances stimulating the phagocytosis of pneumococci (1285) have been found in the serum of normal mice, and Wámoscher (1377) showed that the susceptibility of this animal is so complete that the injection into it of even a single pneumococcus may result in death. Strains of inbred mice, however, may exhibit individual responses to infection with pneumococci of various types, as shown by Webster and Clow (1392) and by Rake (1058), and some strains may be more resistant than others.

The Rabbit

Rabbits were apparently the first animals recognized as susceptible to pneumococcus infection and were used by Pasteur (1002) and by Sternberg (1227) in their original observations, which were the first studies made of this organism. The general susceptibility of rabbits was later demonstrated by Fränkel (487, 488), Tchistovitch (1284), and numerous others (932, 1360, 1285, 1361, 722, 1432, 508, 1448, 1229, 531, 532); and as the result of much work with this animal, Goodner and Stillman (548) have reported that about 98 per cent of rabbits show a complete lack of resistance to pneumococcus infection. The results of various tests, however, have revealed that this general susceptibility may vary considerably with the virulence of the strain of pneumococcus used (487, 488, 1285, 628, 1439, 1091, 1085, 1390); and, further, rabbits are generally less susceptible to strains of Type III than to many other types (1390), though some strains of this type are fully virulent for rabbits (1309, 539, 483, 377).

No evidence of agglutinins (932, 1360, 168), opsonizing and bactericidal substances (1285, 371, 628, 170, 1089, 1439, 1189, 1091, 1085), or protective substances (168, 707) for strains of virulent pneumococci, or of precipitins for solutions of such organisms (1360) was found in the blood or serum of normal rabbits, and organisms of this nature grow vigorously in rabbit blood (174, 139). However, substances having a growth-retarding or bactericidal action on strains of low virulence for the rabbit have been found in normal rabbit blood (628, 1439, 1189).

The Guinea Pig

The guinea pig has also been classed in the susceptible group, though apparently it is somewhat more resistant to pneumococcus infection than the rabbit and is able to withstand doses of the organism that are fatal to rabbits (1002, 501, 487, 488, 121, 139). As with other animals, the susceptibility of the guinea pig has been observed to vary with the virulence of the strain of the infecting organism (488). In some instances the blood or serum of guinea pigs was shown to contain substances which retarded the growth of virulent pneumococci (170) and agglutinated rough strains of the organism (344, 121), while in other instances little or no evidence of opsonins or bactericidal substances (1091, 1089) or of protective antibody (707) was found in their serum.

The Monkey

Monkeys constitute a mixed group of animals, some varieties appearing resistant and others somewhat susceptible to pneumococcus infection. During the course of extensive studies of experimentally induced and spontaneous pneumonia in monkeys carried out by Blake and Cecil (122, 123, 124, 125, 126, 127), Cecil and Blake (231, 232, 233, 234), and Cecil and Steffen (240), observations were made on the comparative resistance of three species of monkeys. It was concluded by the last mentioned workers that the *Macacus rhesus* monkey was the most resistant. Pneumonia of the interstitial or confluent variety rather than the lobar form was commonly produced in this animal. The *Cebus capucinus* monkey was regarded as occupying an intermediate position and only occasionally developed a true lobar lesion, while the Philippine monkey, *Macacus syrichtus,* appeared more satisfactory than the other two species and commonly developed a true lobar consolidation. Schöbl and Sellards (1162), however, did not find that *M. syrichtus* (*Pithecus philippinensis*) exhibited any extreme susceptibility to the pneumococcus. The view that *M. rhesus* and *C. capucinus* monkeys are endowed with considerable resistance to pneumococcus infection was corroborated by Stuppy, Falk, and Jacobson (1260).

Most estimations of the natural resistance of monkeys have resulted from studies of their active resistance to infection or of the variety of lesion produced by it, and direct observations on the presence or absence of humoral antibody in these animals are scarce. Robertson and his associates (1086), however, reported that, judging by the results of mouse protection tests, monkeys have slight or no demonstrable humoral immunity. In addition, Francis and Terrell (483) were unable to find bactericidal substance in the blood of the Java monkey (*Macacus cynomolgos*). Despite the possible significance of these negative tests, monkeys have sufficient resistance to localize pneumococcus infection; and under experimental conditions pneumonia may be produced in the normal monkey which more or less closely resembles the spontaneous lobar pneumonia of man (122, 123, 124, 232, 233, 240, 244, 1162, 483).

The Cat

Cats possess considerable resistance to the pneumococcus. Wadsworth (1360) found precipitins but no agglutinins in normal cat serum, and opsonins and growth-retarding or bactericidal substances have also been found in the serum of normal cats (170, 1089, 1189, 1091, 1097, 1290, 1291). Sia (1189) showed that the action of the growth-inhibiting or bactericidal substance in normal cat serum was type-specific and could be specifically inhibited by the addition of soluble specific substance to test preparations. In a few instances experimental pneumonia, which at times was of the lobar variety, has been produced in this animal (949, 1097).

The Dog

As was indicated by the early studies of Tchistovitch (1284, 1285) and of Wadsworth (1363), the dog also is a fairly resistant animal. In most instances the native resistance of the dog has proved sufficient to enable the animal to localize experimental pulmonary infections, with the result that under such circumstances pneumonia in the lobar form is usually produced (501, 757, 1363, 1437, 949, 726, 1364, 772, 269, 322, 632, 1290, 1291, 1292, 1083, 1084, 782, 286). The natural resistance of this animal has also aided in the localization of meningeal infections (1230).

Numerous efforts have been made to detect the presence of humoral antibody in the dog. Wadsworth (1360) found precipitins but no agglutinins, and Bull (169) neither agglutinins nor opsonins, though later Bull and Bartual (170) and Robertson and his co-workers (1089, 1091, 1292, 1086) demonstrated opsonins and growth-retarding or pneumococcidal-promoting substances in normal dog serum. By serial tests carried out before and during the course of infection in the dog, Terrell (1290, 1291) followed the changes in titer of serum agglutinins, opsonins, and bactericidal substances believed of natural origin.

The Rat

Ross (1131, 1137) has shown that the rat possesses varying degrees of natural resistance to pneumococci of Types II, III, IV, and VI and that protective substance against these types can frequently be found in normal rat serum. On the other hand, rats showed neither active resistance nor humoral antibody against pneumococci of Type I or of Type V.

The Pig

Robertson and Sia (1091), who found the serum of the pig to contain opsonins, have regarded this animal as resistant. The properties of normal swine serum were extensively studied by Kelley (707), who found it to contain agglutinins and protective substance. The titer of the latter varied and was highest against Type II, somewhat lower against Type I, and much lower against Type III. The agglutinin titer, however, did not parallel this and was greatest against Type III and least against Type I. By specific absorption with virulent pneumococci, protection for one type could be removed from the serum without reducing the protection for the other types. In addition, certain unusual findings were encountered. Normal pig serum appeared to possess no precipitins for the specific capsular polysaccharide; the addition of the latter either to the serum or to the culture used did not affect the protection this serum afforded; and the absorption of the normal serum with avirulent R pneumococci greatly reduced its protective power against Types I and II. In view of the present ideas of the nature of type-specificity, these findings appeared then and still appear unexplainable.

The Sheep

Normal sheep serum has been shown to contain growth-retarding (170) and opsonizing (1091) substances for the pneumococcus; and though no protective substance was found (707), the animal has been regarded as a member of the resistant group.

Animals of the Beef Group

The beef group of animals includes the bull, cow, and ox. These animals are presumably members of the resistant group, for, although protective substance may be absent from ox serum (707), agglutinins have been demonstrated in normal beef serum (932) and both agglutinins and precipitins (1360) in normal bullock serum.

The Horse

Normal horse serum has been shown to contain opsonins (1091, 1086, 139); and as the horse may occasionally have spontaneous pneumonia (1334) which at times may be of the lobar form (1086), it has been classed as a fairly resistant animal.

The Chicken

As first noted by Pasteur (1002) and later confirmed by Kyes (748), the chicken is a resistant animal. Though not always successful, numerous efforts have been made to show that the chicken possesses humoral antibody. In some instances neither agglutinin (748) nor protective substance (748, 707) was found in normal chicken blood, while in others clear evidence was obtained of the presence of protective substance (171) as well as of opsonin and bactericidal substance (170, 174, 1091). The protective substance of normal chicken serum was investigated by Bull and McKee (171), who showed it was effective against strains of pneumococci of Types I, II, and III, and certain other pneumococci now regarded as members of three of the higher types. In each instance the action of the protective antibody in the serum appeared type-specific, and the protection for one type could be specifically absorbed from the serum without apparent effect on the protection for the other types.

The Pigeon

Strouse (1253) called attention to the fact that pigeons are practically completely resistant to pneumococcus infection. He found but little phagocytosis in the exudate removed at intervals after intraperitoneal infection and presented impressive evidence that the resistance of the pigeon could be attributed to its high normal temperature (106.7° F.). Kyes (749), however, obtained ample evidence of *in vivo* phagocytosis following the intravenous injection of pneumococci into this animal. Though protective substance has not been demonstrated in the blood of the pigeon (1089, 707), humoral antibody in the form of opsonizing, growth-retarding, and bactericidal substances has been demonstrated in several instances (628, 170, 1091).

Summary

In summary, it is apparent that some species of animals possess little or no immunity against virulent pneumococci and that their blood contains little or no humoral antibody against such organisms, while other species are endowed with a relatively pronounced immunity against these organisms and the blood of such animals commonly contains considerable humoral antibody. The mouse and the rabbit are representative susceptible animals. Though its susceptibility may be less marked, the guinea pig presumably also belongs in this group. The monkey can scarcely be considered of great susceptibility, for it possesses considerable active resistance. The cat, dog, rat, horse, chicken and pigeon, and probably the pig, sheep, bull, cow, and ox as well, may be regarded as resistant animals.

NATURAL IMMUNITY OF MAN

As about one-half of normal people carry pneumococci in their upper respiratory tract at some time each year, it seems probable that, if man were not generally immune to this organism, the human race would have been extinct long ago. That man is able to localize pneumococcus infections and that approximately 75 per cent of the patients with pneumococcus lobar pneumonia are able to survive an infection of such severity are facts which likewise favor this view.

As cellular immunity is difficult or impossible of measurement, precise determinations of the natural immunity of man are concerned largely with qualitative and quantitative estimations of his circulating antibody. Sufficient evidence is at hand to indicate that a considerable proportion of normal persons possess circulating antibody against the pneumococcus. As with some of the lower animals, however, it is not clear that the absence of demonstrable humoral immunity in man may necessarily be regarded as evidence of susceptibility, and the immunity of the individual appears always to be much greater than is indicated by the level of his circulating antibody. In comparing the immunity of man with that of some of the lower animals, Wadsworth's (1363) findings indicate man to be more resistant than the rabbit; and though Robertson and his associates (1091) early regarded man as susceptible, after more extensive investigation it was concluded that man is about as immune as the dog (1086).

Humoral antibody having various actions has been demonstrated in the serum of normal man. Though Neufeld (932) failed to find agglutinins in human serum, Wadsworth (1360), Wright and his associates (1447), and others (1270, 461, 462, 12, 1429) have done so. Precipitins were demonstrated by Wadsworth (1360) and Zozaya and Clark (1469), and opsonins by Wright and Douglas (1443), Rosenow (1115, 1116), Ward and Enders (1383), and Enders and Wu (395). Protective substance was demonstrated by workers such as Neufeld (936, 937), Burhans and Gerstenberger (205), Clough (281), and many others (1274, 577, 1270, 461, 462, 12, 1429, 1138, 433). Growth-inhibiting or pneumococcidal-promoting substances were found by Dold (371), Bull and Bartual (170), Ward (1379), and numerous additional investigators (1274, 1085, 1094, 1270, 461, 462, 551, 1086, 395). Both Dawson (344) and Blake (121) observed the presence of species-specific agglutinins in normal human serum. In addition to these studies, determinations have been made of the skin sensitivity of normal man to pneumococci or to various fractions or derivatives of these organisms (635, 742, 459, 284, 1270, 12).

Humoral Antibody

The potency, specificity, and actions of the humoral antibody demonstrable in the blood of normal man have been extensively investigated by many workers (205, 281, 1379, 1274, 1085, 1094, 1270, 462, 551, 1429, 468, 1086, 1138, 433). Several of these studies were carried out in great detail, and no effort will be made here to report them in extenso; instead, as their significance is essentially similar, illustrative examples will be cited.

BACTERICIDAL SUBSTANCE. As previously mentioned, the bactericidal test has been found to be the most sensitive indicator of the presence of humoral immunity of natural origin (see page 127). It is clear from the observations of Ward (1379), Sutliff and Rhoades (1274), Robertson and his associates

(1085, 1094), Sutliff and Finland (1270), Finland and Sutliff (461, 462), Graeser and Harrison (551), and Robertson, Graeser, Coggeshall, and Harrison (1086), who have determined the pneumococcidal power of human blood or serum for pneumococci of several types, that a considerable proportion of normal individuals have varying amounts of bactericidal substance in their blood for various types of pneumococci. The action of this substance may be specifically inhibited by adding soluble specific substance to test preparations (see page 118). Where studies have been largely confined to determinations of killing power for Types I, II, and III, there has been

TABLE 36. NUMBER AND PERCENTAGE OF NORMAL PERSONS WHOSE BLOOD SHOWED PNEUMOCOCCIDAL ACTION, BY PNEUMOCOCCUS TYPE

	NUMBER OF PERSONS TESTED	PERSONS WHOSE BLOOD SHOWED PNEUMOCOCCIDAL ACTION*	
		Number	*Per cent*
Type I	72	21	29.2
Type II	67	54	80.6
Type III	58	28	48.4
Type V	72	48	66.7
Type VIb	71	67	94.4
Type VIII	72	66	93.1
Type IX	71	70	98.6

From Finland and Sutliff (462)

* Pneumococcidal action was considered to be present when 100 or more organisms were killed in 0.5 cc. of blood.

fairly general agreement that killing power was encountered least often for Type I, somewhat more frequently for Type III, and most commonly for Type II. Wide individual variations in the types killed have been noted, however, and killing power may be present for one or more types in the absence of this power for other types, and no apparent relation exists between the presence of killing power for one type and the presence of this power for any other type. Though in numerous instances this was as true for the immunologically related types, Types II and V and Types III and VIII, as for other unrelated types, it was noted that bactericidal action against each type tended to correlate slightly with the presence or absence of such action against all other types (462).

The report of Finland and Sutliff (462), who studied the incidence of killing power for strains of pneumococci of the eight types, Types I, II, III, V, VIa, VIb, VIII, and IX, among seventy-two persons, is one of the most detailed (see Table 36). In some instances tests were not carried out for all types; and, further, as the results with Type VIa were very similar to those with Type VIb, the former were not reported in detail.

The percentage of persons showing killing power in the blood against each type varied from 29.2 per cent against Type I to 98.6 against Type IX. The order of relative frequency of killing power for these types was, from the least to the greatest frequency, as follows: Types I, III, V, II, VIII, VI, and IX.

These same investigators also studied the quantitative killing power of the blood of the persons investigated for these same types (see Table 37). In some instances, as above, tests were not carried out for each of the types; and, also, as results with Type VIa were nearly the same as the results with Type VIb, only the latter were recorded.

TABLE 37. NUMBER AND PERCENTAGE OF NORMAL PERSONS WHOSE BLOOD SHOWED PNEUMOCOCCIDAL ACTION FOR VARIOUS NUMBERS OF PNEUMOCOCCI, BY PNEUMOCOCCUS TYPE

	NUMBER OF PERSONS TESTED	PERSONS WHOSE BLOOD SHOWED PNEUMOCOCCIDAL ACTION					
		FOR 0–10 DIPLOCOCCI		FOR 100–10,000 DIPLOCOCCI		FOR 100,000 OR MORE DIPLOCOCCI	
		Number	*Per cent*	*Number*	*Per cent*	*Number*	*Per cent*
Type I	72	51	70.8	19	26.4	2	2.8
Type II	67	12	17.9	39	58.2	16	23.9
Type III	58	30	51.7	26	44.8	2	3.4
Type V	72	24	33.3	42	58.3	6	8.3
Type VIb	71	4	5.6	26	36.6	41	57.7
Type VIII	72	6	8.3	46	63.9	20	27.7
Type IX	71	1	1.4	20	28.2	50	70.4

From Finland and Sutliff (462)

Individuals whose blood killed ten diplococci or less of any type were regarded as having no pneumococcidal substance present, and the percentage of persons in this group varied from 70.8 per cent in the case of Type I to only 1.4 per cent for Type IX. When individuals whose blood had killing power for 100,000 or more diplococci were grouped by types it was found that the number of individuals in each group was lowest for Type I, the next in order being Types III, V, II, VIII, VI, and IX, and the incidence of killing power was the same as in normal human blood. Thus pneumococci of the types against which killing power was least often encountered were killed by the blood in the smallest numbers, while pneumococci of the other types for which killing power was much more frequent were killed in the largest numbers.

PROTECTIVE SUBSTANCE. Humoral antibody in the form of protective substance against Type I, II, or III was demonstrated by Burhans and Gerstenberger (205) in the serum of 40 per cent of over fifty mothers and of 30 per cent of their newborn infants. In many instances the serum of both the mother and child showed protection against the same type or types, while occasionally protection was present only in the serum either of the mother or of the infant. Clough (281) studied the occurrence of protective substance in the serum of over twenty normal persons and found it present for Type I in four of twenty-two persons, for Type II in eight of eighteen persons, and for Type III in eleven of twenty-three persons. While it was usually slight in amount, it was sufficient in five instances to protect against from 1,000 to 100,000 lethal doses. Results very similar to this were obtained by Sutliff and Rhoades (1274) in twenty-seven persons and by Gundel (577), so far as Types I and II were concerned, in fifteen persons.

The studies of Sutliff and Finland (1270), Finland and Sutliff (461, 462), Alston and Lowdon (12), Winkler and Finland (1429), Ross (1138), and Felton, Sutliff, and Steele (433) on the occurrence of protective substance in the serum of normal man are all identical in general significance with those cited above. As with killing power, there is suggestive evidence that protective substance may be encountered least often for Type I, most often for Type II, with Type III occupying an intermediate position. However, among sixty-three persons Ross (1138) found protection for Type III more frequent than for either Type I or II. In a single serum, protection may be present for one or more types and absent for others. No correlation has been found between the presence of protective substance for one type and the presence of protective substance for another.

In normal man the general frequency of occurrence of protective substance is nearly always considerably less and its titer of a lower grade than the incidence and titer of bactericidal substance.

Finland and Sutliff (462) have presented data on the occurrence of protection against 100 or more lethal doses of pneumococci of the five types,

Types II, III, V, VIb, and VIII, in the serum of fifty-three persons, all of whom were included in their studies of bactericidal substance shown in Tables 36 and 37. At times the serum of some individuals was not tested against all five types (see Table 38). The proportion of these persons showing protection in their serum varied from 9.8 per cent against Type V to 42.6 per cent against Type VI. The order of the relative frequency of the finding of protection in the serum of this group of individuals against the types studied was, from the least to the greatest frequency, as follows: Types V, II, VIII, III, and VI. Except for Type III, the order of types is analogous to their order for blood pneumococcidal power as described above.

TABLE 38. NUMBER AND PERCENTAGE OF NORMAL PERSONS WHOSE SERUM SHOWED MOUSE PROTECTIVE SUBSTANCE, BY PNEUMOCOCCUS TYPE

	NUMBER OF PERSONS TESTED	PERSONS WITH PROTECTIVE SUBSTANCE IN THEIR SERUM	
		Number	*Per cent*
Type II	47	6	12.8
Type III	36	8	22.2
Type V	51	5	9.8
Type VIb	47	20	42.6
Type VIII	46	8	17.4

From Finland and Sutliff (462)

AGGLUTININS. Type-specific agglutinins have been found only irregularly in normal human serum. They were seldom present for Type I, II, or III, and in a few instances none were demonstrable for Type V or IX while small amounts were present for Types VIa, VIb, and VIII (1270, 461, 462, 12, 1429). When present, the titer of agglutinins has been low (usually about 1:2 to 1:4).

CORRELATION BETWEEN TESTS FOR ANTIBODY. Efforts have been made to correlate the results of tests for pneumococcidal and protective substances and for agglutinins. In a few instances normal human serums containing considerable type-specific protective substance caused no agglutination or phagocytosis of pneumococci of the homologous type (281). Apparently serums showing agglutinins also frequently show protection; and when antibodies causing either or both of these actions are present, killing power is almost always found (1274, 1270, 462, 1429). Occasional exceptions to this generalization have been encountered. By and large, pneumococcidal power has been found more often in the serum of normal man than humoral antibody having other actions.

Skin Sensitivity

The injection into the skin of whole cell vaccine or of various fractions or derivatives of pneumococci has occasionally been employed in an effort to estimate the immunity of normal man. While the occurrence of skin sensitivity in normal persons is largely regarded as evidence that the individual under test possesses some resistance in a broad sense, the varied nature of the substances used to elicit such reactions should be borne in mind, for such diversity may aid in explaining some discrepancies in the results obtained. As already pointed out, it is known that in normal man a positive skin reaction, at least to the specific capsular polysaccharide, may occur in the absence of demonstrable humoral immunity (see page 126).

As the majority of forty-nine normal individuals tested by Herrold and Traut (635) gave a positive skin reaction to the injection of filtrates and extracts of pneumococci and at the same time had no protective substance in their blood, these investigators regarded skin sensitivity as unrelated to demonstrable immunity. The above workers, as well as Kramár and Gyüre (742), who used whole cell vaccine, and Finland and Sutliff (459), who used the specific capsular polysaccharides of pneumococci of Types I, II, and III, found that a much higher proportion of *normal* persons gave positive skin reactions to the agent employed than did patients with pneumococcus pneumonia.

Coca (284) has regarded skin sensitivity to broth culture filtrates as evidence of resistance to the pneumococcus and has observed in a limited number of persons that, as with immunity to diphtheria, the number of immune adults was greater among a class of people represented by ward patients than among a class of people represented by physicians. This observation may well be significant. Sutliff and Finland (1270) determined the skin sensitivity of over forty persons to the acetic-acid-precipitable protein of four strains and the autolysates of three strains of pneumococci and observed that positive reactions occurred in the majority of these and that skin sensitivity to such products was markedly influenced by the age of the individual tested (see also pages 187–192).

In several instances studies were made of the skin sensitivity of normal individuals to the specific capsular polysaccharides of Types I, II, and III, some of the results of which, by the variations in the frequency of the skin response elicited against the different types, suggest the specificity of the reactions to these substances. Finland and Sutliff (459) carried out tests of this nature on twenty-four hospital patients having no history of pneumonia. In this group, typically positive immediate wheal and erythema reactions were encountered for Type I in four, for Type II in ten, and for Type III in none. Additional tests were carried out on seventy-two similar persons by Sutliff and Finland (1270). Definite positive reactions occurred for Type I in three, for Type II in thirteen, and for Type III in five. It appears from these studies that a positive skin reaction was more frequently obtained with the specific substance for Type II than with that for Type I or III. Among 281 other persons tested with the Type II capsular polysaccharide, Alston and Lowdon (12) observed skin sensitivity in 178 or 63 per cent.

Summary

In summary, it may be stated that man in general possesses considerable immunity to the pneumococcus. Judging by the results of various determinations, man's resistance is variable and may at any given time be different against pneumococci of different types.

MECHANISM OF NATURAL IMMUNITY

Relation of Humoral Antibody to Natural Immunity

As described as early as 1890, the infection of resistant animals, such as the dog (1284, 1285), with virulent pneumococci evokes an ample cellular response with evidence of phagocytosis not found under similar circumstances in susceptible animals such as the mouse or rabbit. For many years the somewhat unsatisfactory tests in use seldom showed evidence of any humoral immune substances in resistant animals. This led to the prevailing view, since outmoded, that natural immunity was the result of phagocytosis and depended upon certain fundamental characteristics of the leucocytes and other body cells and was perhaps but little related to the presence of circulating antibody. Much of this early work has been reviewed by Wadsworth (1362), Robertson and Sia (1089, 1091), Wright (1448), and White, with Robinson and Barnes (1417). It is of interest, as will be apparent from the following discussion, that as the result of studies carried out during the past decade or two, the natural immunity of resistant individuals has been largely attributed to the presence of circulating antibody. The situation has again changed, however, and now in the light of further work it has presumably been demonstrated that resistance may be present in the absence of humoral antibody which ". . . leaves no other alternative than to assume the existence of other unknown factors in the mechanism of natural resistance to the pneumococcus," as Robertson, Graeser, Coggeshall, and Harrison (1086) have so aptly stated.

The demonstration by the Klemperers (724) and others (396, 1106, 936) that the serum of immunized animals would protect other animals from infection early served to focus attention upon the problem of the relation of humoral antibodies to immunity to the pneumococcus. The observations of Heist and Solis-Cohen (628) gave further emphasis to this matter, for they found that the failure of pneumococci to grow in the whole uncoagulated blood of artificially immunized animals bore a direct relation to the degree of immunity established, and obtained evidence that the ability of a given strain of pneumococcus to grow in the blood of an animal was inversely proportional to the resistance of the animal for the organism in question. Findings of similar significance, though less definite, were reported by Bull and Bartual (170), who extended their studies to include observations on the blood of several of the naturally susceptible animals and of several resistant animals as well. From this study and that of Bull and McKee (171), it appeared probable that natural immunity could be attributed to the functioning of humoral elements, in the nature of opsonins, whose action was type-specific. The exact manner in which opsonins assisted in disposing of the organisms in the blood, however, was not clear.

The studies of Wright and his associates (1446), Heist and Solis-Cohen (628), and Bull and Bartual (170) all suggested, and those of Robertson and Sia (1089), Woo (1439), Sia (1189), Robertson and Sia (1091), and Robertson, Woo, Cheer, and King (1097) made it apparent that the death of the pneumococcus was not the simple result of the action upon it of some lethal substance in the body or blood; and it was clear that alone the serum of immunized or of naturally resistant animals would not kill the organism (1256, 170), but that the death of the pneumococcus resulted from phagocytosis and intracellular disintegration. This, in fact, is the only method so far demonstrated by which the host is able to kill the pneumococcus. While phagocytes, of course, are essential to the process, their mobilization prior to inducing experimental infection in susceptible animals (1253, 1159, 546) was not alone sufficient to produce evidence of immunity, nor did increasing their number above an optimum increase the number of organisms killed *in vitro* (1089, 1090, 1379, 1275).

Among others, Robertson and Sia (1089, 1091) demonstrated that the blood of resistant animals possesses destructive properties for virulent pneumococci which are lacking in the blood of susceptible animals. It was determined that these destructive properties were largely the result of the action of opsonins present in the blood of resistant animals which sensitized virulent organisms and stimulated phagocytosis and intracellular digestion. It seemed probable that variations in the natural immunity of different animals were due to variations in the concentration of these opsonins in their blood.

In test preparations involving the use of serum and leucocytes, satisfactory phagocytosis was obtained only when the organism was first sensitized with the serum of a resistant animal, the serum of susceptible animals proving of little or no value for this purpose. It apparently made no difference, however, whether the leucocytes used were derived from the blood of a susceptible or a resistant animal, providing the organisms had first been sensitized with the serum of an animal of the resistant group. The possibility that there might be cellular differences between the functional capacity of the leucocytes of a susceptible and of a resistant animal was considered, but no evidence was found to favor this view. An optimum concentration of both opsonins and leucocytes was essential for maximum phagocytosis (see pages 116–120).

The available evidence suggests that the immunity of naturally resistant animals and the action of their circulating antibodies, including opsonins, can be specifically impaired or inhibited by the presence of the specific capsular polysaccharide (see pages 131–132). It was pointed out above in the discussion of the natural immunity of animals and of man that humoral antibody has been found in the blood of man and of practically all species of animals regarded as resistant. In the latter instance, the monkey may be a possible exception, for while it is clear that several varieties of monkeys possess considerable active resistance to the pneumococcus, there is little or no evidence thus far that the animal possesses humoral immunity, at least in significant amounts demonstrable with the procedures used.

Various studies have indicated that the defense mechanism of relatively susceptible animals is very similar to, if not identical with, that possessed by highly resistant species (1285, 1253, 628, 170, 1439, 1448, 1091, 1097). The biologic reaction of susceptible animals to infection with strains avirulent for the species appears similar to the reaction evoked by the use of virulent strains in resistant animals; and, as earlier noted, humoral antibody for strains of avirulent pneumococci has been demonstrated in the blood of some susceptible animals. Robertson and his associates (1097) have pointed out that, in relation to the total resisting capacity of the body, the degree of potential pneumococcidal power resident in the blood suggests that it is an important, if not the chief, means of natural defense. Subsequent findings have necessitated some modification of this view.

Relation of Natural Humoral Antibody to Course and Outcome of Infection

If the immunity of some naturally resistant animals and of man could be ascribed solely to the presence of circulating antibody, it seems probable that such antibody would be absent from the blood of animals or man undergoing pneumococcus infection. It appears likely, however, that humoral antibody of natural origin specific for the infecting type may be present at the time of onset of pneumococcus lobar pneumonia in man and of pneumococcus infections including pneumonia in animals. Evidence for this is shown in the findings of the following investigators:

Findings in man: Park and Cooper (992); Cecil (223); Robertson, Terrell, Graeser, and Cornwell (1094); Francis and Tillett (485); Ward (1379); Sutliff and Rhoades (1275)

Findings in the cat and dog: Terrell (1290, 1291)

In addition, several studies have been made of the relation of humoral antibody regarded as of natural origin to the course and outcome of pneumococcus infection in both animals and man. During such infections in the cat and dog Terrell (1290, 1291) observed that in the presence of a generalized and overwhelming infection with early blood invasion there was a prompt and rapid decrease in the concentration of natural humoral antibody and that such antibody had disappeared from the circulation by the time of crisis. In other animals whose infections were better localized, humoral antibody was present all through the course, even though in some instances the infection ended fatally. The findings suggested that the chief function of humoral antibody of natural origin was to prevent blood invasion and that it had no effect on either the extension or the outcome of the infection.

In man with pneumococcus lobar pneumonia, Robertson, Terrell, Graeser, and Cornwell (1094) observed that, once the level of humoral antibody regarded as of natural origin underwent a marked decrease or disappearance, it did not increase again until shortly before or at the time of recovery. A suggestive relation was found between the titer of the humoral immune substances present and the occurrence of bacteriemia. When the killing power of the blood was well marked, bacteriemia was usually absent; but if this power was considerably decreased or lost, organisms appeared in the blood stream. It was suggested that natural humoral antibody assisted in localizing the infection in man and in destroying the organisms at the periphery of the lesion, thus retarding the spread and limiting or preventing invasion of the blood.

An extension of this work by Robertson, Graeser, Coggeshall, and Harrison (1086) showed, however, that there was no obvious relation between the concentration of natural pneumococcidal substances in the blood of man with pneumococcus pneumonia and the extension of the lesion in the lung, and that extension might occur whether or not killing power was present. Some alteration was also made in the previous views of these investigators concerning the relation of killing power to bacteriemia, for it was found that blood invasion occurred no more frequently in patients whose blood was without killing power than in those whose blood contained pneumococcidal substances. Nevertheless, there was still some correlation, though possibly not to a marked degree, between the titer of the killing power present and the presence or absence of bacteriemia. However, a marked decrease or loss of killing power from the blood was usually, but not always, followed by the appearance of bacteriemia. It was concluded that the presence of humoral antibody regarded as of natural origin bore no relation to the onset or spread or to the invasion of the blood or outcome of the illness in patients with pneumococcus lobar pneumonia and, in consequence, that natural immune bodies played only a minor role in the course of pneumonia. These observations, together with the appreciation that in some animals, as well as in occasional patients, successful localization and recovery from pneumococcus infection have occurred in the absence of demonstrable circulating humoral antibody regarded as of natural origin, made it necessary to assume that other factors might also be importantly concerned in the mechanism of natural resistance.

Relation of Natural Humoral Antibody to Pneumonia Morbidity

It was seen above that humoral antibody having type-specific action has been demonstrated in the blood of a considerable proportion of normal persons and that the level of such antibody at any given time may be different against pneumococci of different types, thus presumably rendering the individual more susceptible to some type or types than to others. While this suggests that a general relation might exist between the presence or absence of natural antipneumococcal humoral immunity and the inception of pneumococcus pneumonia, none has been found in the limited material available (1086). As pneumonia may occur in individuals who apparently possess considerable circulating antibody of natural origin specific for the type causing the infection, the role played by specific natural humoral immune substances in controlling the incidence of pneumonia in man is not clear.

Blake (121) has correlated the severity of experimental infections produced in guinea pigs with the presence or absence of natural circulating species-specific agglutinins in the blood of those animals, has determined the age incidence and type incidence of hospitalized patients with pneumococcus pneumonia, and has correlated such figures with the levels of species-specific agglutinins in the blood of nearly 900 normal persons of various ages. Results of his studies present suggestive evidence that the titer of species-specific agglutinins in normal man may be an index of the presence of active immunity to pneumococcus pneumonia. The findings indicated that immunity of a species-specific rather than of a type-specific nature might be operative in controlling the morbidity of pneumonia and suggested that the basic active resistance to pneumococcus infection is a broad antipneumococcal species immunity. Adequate confirmation of these observations is not at hand.

In respect to the possible influence of species-specific antibody in controlling the morbidity of pneumonia, the interesting observation of Dawson (344) may be mentioned. In the course of a study of the interconvertibility of R and S forms of pneumococci, he found that sufficient anti-R antibody may be present in normal human blood to cause the reversion *in vitro* of some strains of R pneumococci into S forms. Though the theoretical importance of this finding may be considerable, its practical significance at the moment is not clear.

Mode of Production of Natural Antibody

As Topley (1317) has pointed out, it seems probable that antibodies of natural origin may originate by one, or possibly more, of four mechanisms: (a) infection with the organism in question, (b) infection with a different organism having a common antigenic material component, (c) penetration into the tissues by way of the gastrointestinal tract or possibly other routes, such as the lungs or skin, of non-living antigenic material which evokes the production of antibodies having the active group in question, or (d) the normal functioning of the antibody-forming apparatus altogether apart from any specific stimulus of external origin.

In the case of the pneumococcus there is little direct evidence available concerning the possible mode of origin of natural antibodies. The development of such substances as the result of infections of a clinical or subclinical nature is a definite possibility. In this respect the presence of pneumococci in the nasopharynx of "healthy" carriers is probably of importance. Bloomfield (135) has presented evidence which suggests that organisms such as pneumococci which from time to time may be carried for considerable periods in the mouths of normal persons enter into a vital relationship with the tissue cells of the mouth. The failure to remove such organisms from the mouth by thorough and somewhat heroic cleansing procedures indicated their intimate association with the cells of the mucous membrane, the organisms presumably being harbored in crevices and gland orifices in this tissue from which a steady stream of them is discharged into the mouth. The fate of inanimate particles or organisms foreign to the normal oral flora which were introduced into the mouth and which lacked this biologic relationship was different, for they were rapidly removed by a similar cleaning process.

Neufeld and Etinger-Tulczynska (933) have demonstrated the occasional occurrence of a transient bacteriemia in normal mice, rabbits, and guinea pigs following a development of the carrier state as a result of the intranasal instillation of live pneumococci. In many animals the carrier condition persisted for several days or weeks. The carrier state in mice was followed by the development of considerable active immunity to intraperitoneal infection with pneumococci of the same type, the resistance being greatest in those animals having the most prolonged and luxuriant growth of the organism in the nose. These findings strongly suggest that the persistence of the carrier condition in animals is evidence of actual infection, a view which Webster and Hughes (1393) also hold for man. Neufeld and Etinger-Tulczynska also observed the development of immunity in mice subjected to the periodic intranasal instillation of killed pneumococci.

The development of resistance in the animals mentioned above may have been due to acquired antibody. However, the possibility that it was due, at least in part, to natural antibody cannot be excluded. Variation of the natural immunity of animals with age is discussed later.

In man, natural humoral immunity has been demonstrated to vary considerably with age; and, excluding any endowment of antibodies present at birth, natural resistance appears to be of a low order in the young and in the old as well and to be greatest in young and middle-aged adults (see pages 186–192). It is possible, and indeed probable, that at least a part of this resistance results from the frequent presence of pneumococci in the nose and throat of normal individuals. The finding of such organisms in the nasopharynx of infants within a period after birth ranging from two to four days (581) to eight (730) to twelve months (681) is evidence that contact with the pneumococcus begins at an early age, and there is ample evidence available that few if any individuals escape carrying this organism at some time (see pages 342–378). In a few instances Finland and Winkler (468, 469) and Winkler and Finland (1429) have demonstrated, in persons having mild upper respiratory infections such as the common cold, the presence of humoral antibody homologous in type with the pneumococcus present in the sputum. It is doubtless debatable whether such antibody may be considered of natural or acquired origin. Humoral antibody homologous in type with the pneumococcus isolated from the pharynx was also demonstrated by Finland and Tilghman (465) in the serum of a group of healthy carriers. In this instance, however, the evidence suggested that such antibody might be considered to be acquired.

A consideration of the data at hand and of the observations of Sutliff and Finland (1270), who have investigated and discussed certain aspects of this problem, leads to the conclusion that, while direct evidence such as that cited above suggests certain means by which natural antibodies may arise, it is not at all clear that other mechanisms may not also contribute to the origin of these substances.

Relation of Cellular Factors to Natural Immunity

The factors other than humoral antibody which appear operative in the natural immunity of many individuals are presumably those of a cellular nature inherent in the host. It seems clear that the importance of such factors in natural resistance must be considerable in many instances. While the matter appears to have been little studied, some evidence supporting this view is at hand.

From observations on the persistence of inspired bacteria in the lungs of normal mice, Stillman (1237) concluded that it was possible to depress host resistance by intoxicating such animals with alcohol. As determined by cultural methods, pneumococci disappeared from the lungs within four hours after subjecting normal mice to the inhalation of sprayed cultures, and only 3 per cent died of pneumococcus septicaemia. In other mice similarly treated but also intoxicated with alcohol, such organisms persisted in the lungs for as long as twenty-four hours and more than 40 per cent died of septicaemia. Alcoholic intoxication appeared to alter the natural defense mechanism sufficiently to allow the inspired organisms to invade the body in large enough numbers to produce death by septicaemia.

As the result of extensive studies of the pneumococcus infection of rabbits, Goodner and Stillman (548) pointed out that, in addition to the element of specific immunity usually considered as associated with antibodies, either cellular or circulating, another factor also appears of importance. This second factor concerns the capacity of the animal body to react in such a way as to facilitate the utilization of its specific elements of immunity and apparently conditions the functioning of such elements.

Additional evidence in regard to the importance of cellular factors in natural resistance was obtained by Webster and Clow (1392), who found during a study of the intranasal virulence of pneumococci for the mouse, an animal which presumably lacks natural circulating antibody, that to obtain results reproducible to within 10 per cent it was essential to use standard inbred strains of mice. Observations of similar import were also obtained by Rake (1058, 1059) in the mouse.

The role of the blood clearing mechanism in natural immunity to the pneumococcus is probably of considerable importance in many instances (see also pages 162–164).

In animals, natural immunity may vary with the species tested as previously pointed out (see pages 137–143). Evidence indicating or suggesting that other variables, such as genetic factors, age, and sex, may have a bearing on the demonstrable natural immunity of animals or man has been mentioned and is considered again below (see pages 185–203).

MECHANISM OF ACQUIRED IMMUNITY

Acquired immunity is discussed separately from natural immunity in the hope of clarifying some of the complexities of the problem of immunity to the pneumococcus. Immunity of an actively acquired nature may be developed as a consequence of infection or immunization. Accompanying the production of such active resistance, humoral antibodies demonstrable and measurable by their various actions frequently appear in the blood, and alterations occur in the reactivity of various groups of body cells to the pneumococcus and its derivatives. Extensive efforts have been made to determine the respective roles of humoral antibodies and of cellular factors in acquired immunity. General reviews of the literature embracing observations on immunity to the pneumococcus may be found in the discussions of Wadsworth (1361, 1362), Wright (1448), and White, with Robinson and Barnes (1417).

In view of the complexity of the pneumococcus as an antigen, it is not surprising that the nature of the antibodies evoked by immunization or infection is varied (see pages 133–134). However, as the relation of many of these antibodies to the presence or absence of acquired resistance appears negligible (see pages 127–131), chief attention will be directed to the role of type-specific antibodies in acquired immunity. Under suitable circumstances the passive transfer of antibodies having type-specific action will render a susceptible individual resistant or supplement the immunity of an individual of the resistant type. It appears probable that actively or passively acquired immunity to the pneumococcus is largely dependent upon an integrated system of cellular reactions conditioned by the presence in the blood and tissue fluids of specific antibacterial substances of a sensitizing nature.

Evidence of Altered Reactivity in Acquired Immunity

As the result of infection or artificial immunization, certain changes occur indicative of a bodily state of altered reactivity to the pneumococcus and its specific derivative, the capsular polysaccharide. Antipneumococcal immune substances commonly appear in the blood, the effectiveness of the mechanism for removing pneumococci from the circulation is enhanced, the ability to localize and resist infection with this organism is developed, and alterations of skin sensitivity occur. The antibodies and the state of altered reactivity produced are effective primarily against the specific type of pneumococcus in question, though certain minor exceptions to this generalization have been encountered, as previously noted (see pages 135–136). Each of the above changes may be considered briefly in turn.

APPEARANCE OF HUMORAL ANTIBODY. The artificial immunization of various animals was early shown to evoke the production of circulating antibodies. Protective substance was found by the Klemperers (724), Washbourn (1388), and Römer (1107) in the serum of immunized rabbits, and others demonstrated agglutinins (99, 932, 1360) and precipitins (932, 1360) in such serum. Protective substance was likewise found in immune horse serum (1389). Though these observations were made prior to Neufeld's first report on pneumococcus types (936) in 1909, some of the above investigators noted that the action of the antibodies engendered appeared effective only against the strain of pneumococcus used to incite their production.

Subsequently, specific antibodies were found in the blood or serum of various immunized animals as follows:

Agglutinins:
  Rabbit (1362, 785, 308, 628, 570, 532, 173, 1241, 1245, 540, 595)
  Horse (308, 33, 532, 414, 540)
Precipitins:
  Rabbit (1362, 33, 570, 623, 656, 625)
  Horse (363, 33, 617, 618, 619, 414, 623, 656, 625)
Opsonins:
  Rabbit (936, 1254, 1362, 785, 1448)
  Donkey (936)
  Horse (936, 937, 33, 414, 1383)
Protective substance:
  Mouse (939, 888)
  Rat (1126, 1137, 1136)
  Rabbit (936, 1363, 308, 570, 1090, 68, 532, 1241, 1245, 540, 595)
  Guinea pig (841)
  Donkey (936)
  Horse (936, 937, 308, 33, 407, 1090, 532, 414, 540)
Growth-retarding or bactericidal substance:
  Rabbit (628, 170, 1090, 1448)
  Chicken (174)
  Horse (362, 170, 407, 1090, 1379, 414)
Substances which aid in the *in vivo* immobilization of the organism:
  Horse (1077)

In similar fashion, specific humoral antibody has been identified in the blood or serum of man following immunization with pneumococcus vaccine (785, 228, 71, 72, 461, 1135, 1138, 433) or with the specific capsular polysaccharide or substances probably very similar to it (485, 459, 461, 1469, 478, 424, 433, 425). In several instances antibody determinations were made before and at various intervals after immunization.

Humoral antibody also frequently develops as a consequence of pneumococcus infection in animals, as has been demonstrated in mice (99), rabbits (99, 1363, 1097, 531, 532), cats (1097, 1290, 1291), dogs (169, 1290, 1291, 286, 285), and monkeys (231, 232). In addition, circulating antibodies commonly appear in the blood of man at about the time of spontaneous recovery from pneumococcus infections including pneumonia. While there may be doubt as to the specificity of action of the antibodies demonstrated under such circumstances in some of the older studies of infection in man, later investigations carried out with typed pneumococci have shown that the important actions of antibodies appearing as a result of infection are almost wholly type-specific in nature.

The Klemperers (725), Bezançon and Griffon (99), Römer (1106), Neufeld (932), and Wadsworth (1360) were among the first to investigate successfully antibody production during pneumococcus infections and pneumonia in man; and they and others identified agglutinins (99, 932, 1360, 1285, 1114), precipitins (1360), phagocytic-stimulating substances or opsonins (1285, 1115), and protective (1106) and curative (725) substances in the blood or serum of such patients.

Following the differentiation of pneumococci into types, many other observers demonstrated the appearance of specific humoral antipneumococcal immune substances in patients with similar infections; and the following were found:

Specific agglutinins (784, 257, 754, 118, 280, 1194, 815, 1321, 1312, 459, 577, 1429, 468, 469, 1087, 1010, 339, 340)
Precipitins (118)
Phagocytic-stimulating substances or opsonins (1254, 388, 278, 280, 5, 1194, 1087)
Growth-retarding or bactericidal substances (362, 912, 1194, 1379, 1275, 1087)
Protective substances (936, 937, 356, 278, 784, 61, 60, 635, 1194, 815, 1321, 1275, 820, 459, 577, 1429, 468, 469)

VARIATION IN ANTIBODY RESPONSE. The antibody response following immunization or infection varies with the type of pneumococcus and somewhat with age, being less marked in the young than in robust adults (see pages 186–192). Observations relating to the varied antigenic capacity of pneumococci of different types were made in several of the investigations cited above. In addition, specific comment concerning this matter may be found in the discussions of several workers relative to the amounts of antibody demonstrable after the immunization of animals with certain of nearly all the recognized types of pneumococci (308, 293, 992, 318, 1132, 1133, 320, 1245) and in reports dealing with the amounts of specific antibody demonstrable after infection in monkeys (232) and man (577, 1429, 468, 469).

In brief, the antibody response to immunization or infection with pneumococci of Type I or II is generally far better than the response to Type III. The response to pneumococci of Types V, VII, and VIII is also fairly good and is again better than the response to Type III.

INCREASED EFFICIENCY OF BLOOD-CLEARING MECHANISM. It has long been known that the intravenous injection into normal animals of suspensions of inanimate particulate matter, such as carbon particles or some of the common dyes, is followed by the rapid removal or clearing of these substances from the blood stream and their accumulation in certain phagocytic cells. The cells predominantly involved in this clearing process are the histiocytes or macrophages of the reticulo-endothelial system. The more active of these are the sessile histiocytes of the lymph glands, liver, spleen, and bone marrow and the wandering histiocytes in general (25, 1317). The functional activity of various groups of these cells may be different, and differences may occur in the activity of these groups in different animals. In some instances the polymorphonuclear leucocytes may also phagocytize particulate matter in the blood.

The special mechanism which operates to clear the circulation of bacterial cells of approximately the same size as the particles mentioned above appears essentially similar to this, and several studies have been made of the fate of pneumococci injected into the blood stream of either normal or immune animals or both (1363, 722, 1432, 169, 125, 1309, 1448, 1310, 377). Observations of a similar nature have also been carried out in some instances following the inhalation (1239) or intranasal instillation of pneumococci (1059). The cells of the reticulo-endothelial system of the liver, spleen, and kidney actively phagocytize bacteria and appear particularly involved in clearing organisms from the blood. The lung capillaries may also retain bacterial aggregates and thus assist in ridding the circulation of organisms (169, 1448). In addition, the polymorphonuclear leucocytes are especially active in phagocytizing bacteria, and these cells with their ingested organisms may, in turn, be engulfed by cells of the reticulo-endothelial system. Phagocytosis alone, however, does not necessarily ensure the destruction of the ingested organisms, and for the successful intracellular digestion of the latter the action of some additional factor, presumably of the nature of sensitizing antibody, seems required.

In the normal animal, periodic cultures of the blood following the sudden entrance into the circulation of a considerable number of pneumococci reveal that within a few minutes or hours all or nearly all the organisms disappear from the blood stream. In most cases following this there is a gradual reappearance or increase in the number of organisms in the blood, the reaction varying in degree and persistence with the virulence of the pneumococcus used and the resistance of the host. Bull (169) attributed the initial decrease in the number of circulating organisms to the action of *in vivo* agglutinins, but in a careful study Wright (1448) was unable to confirm this. This discrepancy of findings may possibly be related to differences in the native resistance of the animals used in their experiments, for Bull's observations were carried out on the dog, a naturally resistant animal, while Wright employed the rabbit, which is susceptible.

With strains of low virulence for the host, organisms usually do not reappear after their initial disappearance. If, however, strains of moderate or considerable virulence are administered to susceptible animals, such as the rabbit, the organisms apparently multiply faster than they can be removed from the circulation, their number increases, and, finally overwhelmed, the host succumbs to the infection (722, 1432, 1448). In animals of a more resistant nature, however, such as the dog, the initial clearing of the blood followed by the secondary increase in bacterial count occurs in similar fashion, but frequently after several days of bacteriemia acquired antibodies appear and the blood is sterilized (169). Bull (169) noted that following the successful clearing of virulent pneumococci from the blood, some organisms may become localized in foci inaccessible to the effects of the blood-clearing mechanism and in a few days produce a serious or fatal infection. Among others, an important place of refuge is offered by the lymphatics, the clearing mechanism of which appears very inferior to that of the blood and into which pneumococci rapidly migrate from the blood stream, as Drinker, Enders, Shaffer, and Leigh (377) have shown. The continued multiplication of organisms in the lymph with their subsequent outpouring into the general circulation offers a means of reinfecting the blood stream.

The effect of immunization is to increase markedly the efficiency of the vastly important natural mechanism for clearing organisms from the blood. In actively immunized animals this effect is type-specific and may begin to appear as early as five hours after the injection of the immunizing vaccine (Wright, 1448). Studies of the blood-clearing mechanism in rabbits reveal that it acts before any significant temperature rise occurs in the animal (1448), and is effective even when the total leucocyte count of the blood is markedly decreased by a previous injection of benzol (1432, 1448), or when the reticulo-endothelial system is blockaded by the injection of inanimate particulate matter (1448). It seems apparent that the mechanism responsible for clearing organisms from the blood is a complex one and involves a number of phenomena associated with bacterial adhesion and phagocytosis by integrated systems of cells and that it is probably not controlled by the operation of any single factor alone.

Topley (1317) has summarized the differences in the behavior of actively immunized and normal animals in respect to this mechanism by pointing out that the immunized animal behaves toward a virulent organism in the same way that a normal animal behaves toward a strain of the same organism having little or no virulence. The initial rapid removal of organisms from the circulation, so commonly encountered when ordinary cultures are used for producing infection, may be absent if virulent pneumococci in an active phase of growth are used (1448).

DEVELOPMENT OF ABILITY TO IMMOBILIZE ORGANISMS AND LOCALIZE INFECTION. Active immunization has been shown to give rise to changes within the body of animals (rabbit, 1077, and mouse, 218) which assist in immobilizing immediately pneumococci injected into their tissues. The organisms apparently clump and adhere to the cells at the site of injection, a phenomenon which either does not take place or occurs to only a limited degree in animals that have not been immunized. Rich (1077) regards the immobilizing action as dependent upon an immune substance contained in the body fluids of immunized animals. It is doubtless in many instances a great help in localizing infection; and the results of several studies in animals have clearly shown that active immunity develops parallel with the ability to localize infection. This has been observed following the active immunization of animals, such as the mouse (1243, 1244, 218) and the rabbit (1361, 922, 1258), and after recovery from infection in the dog (286).

In connection with the ability to localize infection, it was pointed out as early as 1904 (Wadsworth, 1361) that the resistance of the host must be balanced against the virulence of the organism. It was demonstrated that, following the intratracheal injection of living virulent pneumococci into rabbits, septicaemia developed in those that were normal, while in those possessing a low grade of resistance induced by active immunization a bronchopneumonic type of lesion usually occurred, and in still others, in which a higher initial resistance had been induced before infection, localization was more marked, and the resulting lesion was of the lobar variety.

PREVENTION OF SUBSEQUENT INFECTION AND ALTERATION OF COURSE. Observations relating to the production of immunity and to the effect of the acquired resistance in either lessening the severity of subsequent infections or preventing them altogether have been made during the course of numerous experimental studies on animals. In some instances investigations were carried out for precisely this purpose, while in others the findings were incidental to studies of different sorts, such as attempts to define the nature of the most suitable antigen for use in inducing active immunity or to measure the immune response to pneumococci or the specific capsular polysaccharide or allied substances administered by various routes. In any event, it is clear from the results obtained that the immunity of animals to pneumococcus infection may be markedly enhanced by subjecting them either to various immunizing procedures or to pneumococcus infection. In large measure the resistance produced is specific for the type of pneumococcus serving as antigen or source of the antigenic material.

Evidence of increased resistance to subsequent infection was obtained following the active immunization:

Of mice (1012, 1238, 1243, 440, 1011, 1160, 1369, 422, 1470, 41, 424, 218, 433)
Of rats (1126, 1127, 1128, 1130, 1131, 1132, 1135)
Of rabbits (1361, 936, 1362, 1363, 628, 922, 531, 532, 173, 737, 1245, 739, 740, 424)
Of guinea pigs (841)
Of dogs (727)
Of monkeys (125, 231, 240, 241, 242, 243, 1260, 738)

In addition to this, recovery from a frank pneumococcus infection has been found to be followed by a period of increased active resistance to subsequent infection in rabbits (532, 1097), cats (1097), dogs (1230, 286, 285), and monkeys (232). Arguing from analogy, it has seemed reasonable to expect that man's immunity to pneumococcus infection might also increase following infection of a spontaneous nature or immunization by various experimental means, and there is evidence suggesting that such may be the case (see pages 728–737, and 446–478).

ALTERATIONS IN SKIN SENSITIVITY. The antigens used for testing skin sensitivity have frequently been different in different studies, as already mentioned, and in consequence the results obtained are difficult to correlate. Various studies have been carried out on patients during and after pneumonia (103, 635, 1311, 742, 743, 459, 12) and on actively immunized animals (486, 700, 12, 595). The observations made may be considered from several points of view.

In testing skin sensitivity of patients with pneumonia, culture filtrates and extracts of pneumococci (635) have been used; also the whole organisms (742) and the specific capsular polysaccharide of various types (459, 12). Evidence was found suggesting that sensitivity to these materials on the part of patients in the acute stages of pneumonia was lower than that of normal individuals. This depression of skin sensitivity at such a time may be due to the general inhibition of specific cellular activities or to the development of circulating antibodies (635) incident to the production of a relatively solid immunity (743).

In actively immunized animals the intradermal injection of the specific capsular polysaccharide of pneumococci of homologous type usually, but not always (486, 12, 595), gives rise to a cutaneous reaction, and circulating antibody specific for the homologous type has always been found in animals showing such reactions. It seems clear, however, that sometimes humoral antibody may be present though skin sensitivity is absent. Nevertheless, the occurrence of a reaction to the intradermal injection of the specific capsular polysaccharide may probably be regarded as evidence that the host possesses some active immunity. The skin may be sensitive to the so-called nucleoprotein of the pneumococcus without any obvious correlation between sensitivity and the presence of circulating precipitins for that substance (486, 700, 595). In rabbits vaccinated with either S or R strains of pneumococci, skin sensitivity to nucleoprotein was found to occur independently of the presence of type-specific humoral antibody and skin sensitivity to the specific capsular polysaccharide.

As previously noted, cutaneous reactions to the specific capsular polysaccharide may be obtained in normal man in the presence or absence of circulating specific antibody (see pages 126–127). In pneumonia patients, however, the observations of Tillett and Francis (1311) and Finland and Sutliff (459, 460) reveal that sensitivity to these substances is found only at or shortly after crisis and in the presence of humoral antibody of homologous type. Such sensitivity may not develop in all cases even though circulating specific antibody is present. Skin sensitivity to pneumococcus nucleoprotein also develops at about the time of crisis in man with pneumonia (1311). In this instance circulating precipitins for the nucleoprotein were found in the blood, but, as in actively immunized animals, their concentration did not seem to affect the reaction.

The observation by Finland and Sutliff (460) that skin sensitivity to soluble specific substance persists longer after recovery in patients not receiving specific serum therapy than in those who receive such treatment suggests that such reactions may be indicative of the presence of a state of active immunity, the development of which is interfered with in patients receiving serum treatment.

It seems probable from the observations of the workers cited above that cutaneous reactivity to specific capsular polysaccharide in either animals or man may be regarded as evidence of the existence of some immunity to pneumococci of homologous type.

CELLULAR CHANGES. Observations on the type of cell involved in the reaction with the organism within the body have been made by many investigators. Though complete information is lacking, it seems probable that polymorphonuclear leucocytes, and perhaps to some extent large mononuclear leucocytes, are primarily concerned in the ingestion and destruction of organisms in naturally immune individuals. In the presence of acquired immunity, however, a large variety of cells may be active in disposing of pneumococci; and in recent years the role of the large monocyte, which is regarded as a histiocyte or macrophage, has been especially emphasized (1448, 1097, 1258, 1018, 1087, 218, 286, 285, 546, 547, 1095). Mention has been made of cells of this nature above and in the earlier discussion of the cellular changes associated with resolution in pneumonia (see pages 98–101). It appears clear that phagocytes other than the circulating leucocytes may be importantly concerned in the disposal of pneumococci, and Winternitz and Kline (1432) and Wright (1448) showed that the blood-clearing power of immunized rabbits was about the same in controls as in those whose circulating leucocytes had been largely destroyed by previous injections of benzol.

That the cells of the reticulo-endothelial system are probably intimately concerned in the mechanism of resistance has already been pointed out. Direct evidence suggesting their relation to actively acquired resistance was obtained by Neufeld and Meyer (939) and by Meyer (888), who were usually unable to induce a state of active immunity in mice which had been previously subjected to splenectomy and a blockading of their reticulo-endothelial system by intravenous injections of ferric saccharate. Meyer also found that by subjecting actively immunized mice to similar procedures it was frequently possible to "break" the immunity which had developed. The evidence is not all so clear-cut, however, for Wright (1448) found that blocking the reticulo-endothelial system of actively immunized rabbits had little or no effect on reducing the efficacy of their blood-clearing mechanism. In addition, as Meyer was easily able to induce passive immunity in splenectomized and "blockaded" mice, he regarded the effect of these procedures as probably due to an inhibition of antibody formation rather than to a decrease of the phagocytic activity of the cells of the reticulo-endothelial system.

Relation of Humoral Antibody to Acquired Immunity

The fact that specific antibodies having demonstrable antipneumococcal effects commonly appear in the blood in association with the development of immunity as a result of either immunization or infection strongly suggests that a probable relation exists between the presence of such substances and acquired immunity. The nature of the actions of these specific immune substances is varied, as is indicated above and in the sections dealing with circulating antibody (pages 115–125); and agglutinins, precipitins, opsonins (or tropins), and bactericidins, as well as substances having protective, curative, neutralizing, and immobilizing properties and the power to cause significant alterations in the biology of virulent pneumococci grown in contact with them, have been demonstrated under such circumstances. Moreover, the relation of specific humoral antibody of acquired origin to active immunity is such that its presence is usually indicative of the presence of immunity, though in individual instances some exceptions to this may be encountered (see pages 127–131).

PASSIVE IMMUNITY. *Protective power.* The fact that the passive transfer of specific humoral antibodies to a susceptible individual will render him temporarily resistant suggests that such substances may be importantly concerned in actively acquired immunity. Most significant in this respect is the demonstration that passively transferred antibodies have specific protective and curative properties. Many aspects of the protective action of immune serum have already been discussed and need not be repeated in detail (see page 120). It is clear that under suitable conditions the serum of an immunized animal affords protection of considerable degree against otherwise fatal doses of pneumococci of homologous type. Successful results depend largely upon the use of an optimum amount of serum and number of organisms; and in general, if an insufficient amount of serum is used or too many organisms are present, little or no protection is obtained.

Curative power. Investigations have also been made of the power of immune serum to cure an established infection in animals. Serum of this nature has been demonstrated to have curative value for mice (532, 1018, 909, 880), rabbits (724, 981, 1363, 168, 531, 532, 1151, 1152, 536, 377), guinea pigs (942), and dogs (1363), infected in various ways, and to assist in or to bring about the recovery of monkeys with pneumonia (233, 244). Such investigations have been carried out chiefly with the serum of immunized rabbits or horses.

The intravenous administration of specific immune serum to animals (rabbits) infected with pneumococci of homologous type causes an immediate agglutination of any circulating organisms with the resultant removal of the clumps by the liver, spleen, lungs, and possibly other organs (Bull, 168). In addition to increasing the extent of *in vivo* phagocytosis (170, 1018), the capacity of the mechanism for clearing the blood of organisms is markedly enhanced and the blood stream is rapidly sterilized (1432, 170, 233, 244, 1448, 531, 532, 1018, 536, 377). Little direct effect may be noted, however, upon organisms which have gained admission to the lymph vessels, as the lymphatic system apparently lacks the cellular elements so important in the blood-clearing mechanism (377).

Early treatment and an adequate amount of antibody are of great importance and will lessen the severity and shorten the course of the infection, as shown in animals infected by various routes (531, 532, 1018, 536, 377) as well as in monkeys with pneumonia (233, 244). While relatively small doses of antibody will suffice to bring about recovery in the early stages of infection, the amount required for this purpose increases very rapidly with the lapse of time, and a point is soon reached where no amount of immune serum will effect recovery (531, 532, 1018, 377). Petrie and Morgan's (1018) observations are of interest in respect to the importance of the time element here, for it was noted that the dose of immune serum adequate to cure mice twelve hours after intraperitoneal infection had to be increased about one hundredfold to be effective if given three hours later.

So far as the present discussion is concerned, it may be observed that in the use of immune serum for therapeutic purposes attention must be paid to the severity and extent of the infection present and the time after infection when such treatment is undertaken, as well as to the amount of antibody given. The curative power of specific immune serums for man with pneumococcus pneumonia has been demonstrated by many investigators. This matter is mentioned below (page 175) and is discussed in some detail in the chapters on Serum Treatment (page 805) and Results of Serum Treatment (page 880).

Passive immunity and skin tests. Skin tests have been carried out in a number of instances with specific capsular polysaccharide to determine the relation of cutaneous reactivity to the acquisition of passive immunity of homologous type. Studies of this nature have been made by Tillett and Francis (1311), Francis and Tillett (486), Finland and Sutliff (460), Alston and Lowdon (12), Francis (477), and Tilghman and Finland (1307).

The first observations were made by Tillett and Francis (1311) in patients with pneumococcus Type I pneumonia treated with Type I antipneumococcic serum. Subsequently, additional studies were made of both Type I and Type II cases receiving specific serum (460, 477) and of Type II and Type III cases treated with convalescent serum obtained from patients recovering from pneumonia of homologous type (460). In a few instances skin sensitivity was observed following the administration of antipneumococcic serum to normal animals (486, 12) and to normal man (460, 12, 1307).

In patients with pneumococcus pneumonia treated with specific antipneumococcic serum, skin sensitivity to the specific capsular polysaccharide of homologous type commonly appears at about the time of recovery (1311, 460, 477). Patients reacting in this way generally show specific circulating antibody, though in two instances Finland and Sutliff (460) obtained a positive skin reaction in the apparent absence of either agglutinin or protective substance in the serum. However, not all patients who have specific circulating antibody show a positive skin reaction; and this, in conjunction with the fact that apparently nearly every patient (though perhaps not every one [460]) treated with specific antipneumococcic horse serum who develops such skin sensitivity recovers, suggests that a positive skin reaction occurs only when both active tissue immunity and specific circulating antibody are present. The tests are sometimes positive in the presence of complications such as empyema.

Negative tests may be encountered in patients who recover (460, 477); and Finland and Sutliff (460) have obtained some evidence suggesting that the failure of skin sensitivity to develop may depend in part upon the dosage of immune serum given, upon certain characteristics peculiar to some lots of specific antiserum, or upon differences in the responsiveness of individual patients. In general, however, negative tests are usually encountered in patients whose illness ends fatally.

While Francis and Tillett (486) in passively immunized rabbits, and Finland and Sutliff (460) in a passively immunized human being, were able to "produce" skin sensitivity to the specific capsular polysaccharide by the administration of immune serum of homologous type, Alston and Lowdon (12) were unable to duplicate this finding in either animals or man. In addition, Finland and Sutliff noted that it was possible to produce a positive intradermal reaction to the specific substance a few minutes after the intravenous administration of specific serum to patients with lobar pneumonia.

In one instance human serum containing specific antibodies obtained from a patient showing skin sensitivity to the capsular polysaccharide of homologous type and convalescent from a Type II pneumonia was administered to another patient having Type II pneumonia. Skin reactivity to the Type II specific substance had been negative in this patient previously but became positive within one hour after the administration of this serum, and specific humoral antibody was demonstrable at that time. This condition was of short duration, however, for within two days both skin sensitivity and circulating antibody were absent, and subsequently the patient died.

A general consideration of the findings of the above investigators makes it probable that the occurrence of skin sensitivity to the specific capsular polysaccharide in passively immunized individuals indicates some resistance against pneumococci of homologous type and that at least a part of such immunity is derived from the antibody in the immune serum.

ANTIBODY ACTION. The Klemperers (724, 725) and others (1363, 290, 306) regarded some or all of the actions of antipneumococcic serum as antitoxic (see also pages 124–125). Römer (1106) attributed its effects to a purely bactericidal action. The observations of Pane (981), Neufeld and Rimpau (940, 941), Neufeld and Händel (936, 937, 938), and others (722, 362, 33, 170) made it clear, however, that antipneumococcic serum is primarily antibacterial in action.

The diversity of action of specific antibodies against the pneumococcus has already been mentioned; and as essentially all the actions of these antibodies may be specifically inhibited by the addition to test preparations of the specific polysaccharide derived from the capsule of pneumococci of homologous type, it appears that the demonstrable antibodies effective in pneumococcus immunity are those reactive with the surface antigen of the organism (see pages 131–132).

So far as known, the action of antibody on the pneumococcus is apparently the same whether derived from animals or man and whether functioning in natural (170) or actively or passively acquired immunity (937, 1432, 170, 939). Bactericidal tests reveal that the blood of susceptible animals can be rendered resistant to pneumococci of one type by the addition to it of the serum of animals immunized with virulent pneumococci of the same type (1090, 174). Little is known of the relative importance of the various actions of antibody in immunity, but it is likely that precipitins and perhaps neutralizing substances are of greater importance within the body, where pneumococcus growth products may be present in considerable amounts, than the results of tests *in vitro* would suggest. Agglutinins also presumably render important services within the body. However, as antibody sensitizes the organism and promotes not only phagocytosis but also intracellular digestion, and as this is the best authenticated explanation of the method by which the blood elements are able to kill the pneumococcus, it appears likely that opsonic action in its entirety may constitute the most important property of antibody, as Robertson, Woo, Cheer, and King (1097) have suggested.

SPECIFIC ANTIBODY OF THE RABBIT AND THE HORSE. There are several demonstrable differences between the properties of humoral antibody derived from the horse and from the rabbit. Some of these differences were observed by Zinsser and Parker (1465), Avery and Tillett (52), Francis and Tillett (486), Heidelberger and Kendall (623), and others (880, 625, 540, 656, 544), and have been summarized by Horsfall and his associates (656, 657).

Visible differences exist in the character of the precipitate formed when specific capsular polysaccharide is added to immune rabbit and to immune horse serum of corresponding type. Moreover, products related to the specific capsular substance form precipitates in immune horse serum but not in the corresponding rabbit serum (623, 625). Antipneumococcic rabbit serum will passively sensitize guinea pigs (52, 486, 880) and mice (880) so that when they are subsequently injected with soluble specific substance of homologous type, anaphylaxis results. Immune horse serum has no such effect in these animals. Although the role played by complement in the protective action of immune serum in animals is not clear it may be noted that immune rabbit serum was shown by Zinsser and Parker (1465) to fix complement in the presence of a substance probably closely related to specific capsular polysaccharide, while immune horse serum failed to do so. With organisms of homologous type, immune rabbit serum produces a satisfactory *Quellung* reaction (see pages 625–629), while immune horse serum usually does not. In protection tests in mice, immune horse serum shows a distinct prozone reaction not observed with the use of immune rabbit serum (540). The addition of nine volumes of distilled water will precipitate the antibody from immune horse serum but not from immune rabbit serum (656). The extraction of the phospholipins from immune rabbit or horse serum reduces or removes the agglutinating and precipitating properties of these serums (656). These properties can be restored to the extracted immune horse serum by the addition of lecithin and to the extracted rabbit serum by the addition of cephalin.

Such differences in the immunologic action and in the properties of the immune antibody of the horse and the rabbit may exist even though the curative value of the serums (for mice) are identical (880) and even though they are of equal antibody titer (540). Using Type I antipneumococcic serums, Goodner, Horsfall, and Bauer (544) demonstrated that the antibodies of immune rabbit serum are of smaller size than those of immune horse serum. Mention may be made of the fact that most of the differences in the antibody of the rabbit as compared with that of the horse have been shown using Type I serums.

The observations by Mehlman and Seegal (880) that immune rabbit serum was successful in passively sensitizing mice and guinea pigs, while horse serum was not, and that both of these serums passively sensitized dogs so that anaphylaxis was produced by the injection of the specific capsular polysaccharide of the corresponding type, suggest that the ability to confer passive sensitivity depends both on the nature of the antibody contained in the serums and on the species of the recipient.

Relation of Humoral Antibody to Course and Outcome of Infection

As is apparent from the discussion in the foregoing sections, there is impressive evidence that acquired immunity may be closely related to the presence and actions of specific humoral antibody. There is, however, evidence that other factors may also be significantly concerned in the mechanism.

It has already been pointed out that actively acquired immunity of considerable degree may be present in the absence of specific humoral antibody demonstrable by the methods usually employed for its recognition (see pages 129–131 and 136). Immunity to infection of varying degrees has been frequently observed following immunization or recovery from infection. This has been shown to be the case in rabbits, rats, dogs, and monkeys. The factors responsible for the observed active resistance in such instances are presumably those of a cellular nature. Additional evidence that cellular factors play an important part in acquired immunity is available as mentioned below.

ACTIVELY ACQUIRED ANTIBODY. There are many reports available in the literature relating to the occurrence of specific humoral antibody in the blood of animals or man suffering from pneumococcus infections including pneumonia. A number of these have already been cited in the foregoing sections. Since the differentiation of pneumococci into types, numerous investigators have attempted to correlate the time of appearance of humoral antibody with the time of recovery from pneumococcus infection. It has been observed in rabbits (531), cats (1097, 1291), and dogs (1291) that the appearance in the blood of specific humoral antibody regarded as of acquired origin usually marks the onset of recovery from infection. Many investigators, such as Neufeld and Händel (936, 937), Eggers (388), Dochez (356), and others (784, 257, 362, 754, 118, 280, 5, 61, 1194, 815, 1321, 820, 459, 577, 1429, 469), have studied antibody production in man during pneumococcus pneumonia and have noted that tests for humoral antibody having specific antipneumococcal actions, at first negative, usually become positive at about the time of recovery (see pages 729–735).

Without going into detail, it may be said that the bulk of the available evidence is highly suggestive that an intimate relationship exists between the appearance of specific circulating antibody and the recovery of patients from pneumonia, for most patients who develop such antibody recover and most of those who fail to do so die. Occasional and significant exceptions to this generalization have been found, however, which apparently make it impossible to assume that recovery from pneumococcus infections and pneumonia can be attributed solely to the elaboration and appearance in the blood of substances having demonstrable specific antipneumococcal actions. This is better understood when it is realized that specific circulating antibody may not be found in all instances among individuals who recover from such infections (936, 1254, 278, 61, 1097, 820, 1429, 468, 286, 285) and that in other instances antibody may appear in the blood early in the course of the disease and yet recovery be delayed until several days later (356, 60, 635, 1321, 1275, 820, 577, 1087) or that at times antibody may not be demonstrable until several days after recovery has taken place (356, 278, 815, 1087, 339). Various studies have shown that, though the presence of specific circulating antibody of actively acquired origin may assist in restraining the spread of the infection, extension may nevertheless occur in its presence (1087, 339) or fail to occur in its absence (1087). While bacteriemia is usually overcome by the appearance in the blood of acquired antibody (118, 61, 60, 1087), it may nevertheless develop or persist in the presence of such immune substances

(61, 1275, 820), and at other times it may fail to appear even though no antibody is demonstrable (1087). The presence of antibody of acquired origin does not necessarily prevent the development of focal infections such as empyema (1194, 1275, 459, 339).

A consideration of these facts, in addition to the demonstration by many workers that occasionally patients may die even though specific antibody is demonstrable in their blood (784, 118, 280, 60, 1275, 459, 1429, 468, 1087), justifies the conclusion either that the body brings into play more than one mechanism for localizing the infection and eventually bringing about a successful recovery or that the elaboration of circulating antipneumococcal immune substances represents but one phase of a specific reaction against the organism, as Robertson, Graeser, Coggeshall, and Harrison (1087) have pointed out.

PASSIVELY ACQUIRED ANTIBODY. The relation of passively acquired specific humoral antibody to the course and outcome of pneumococcus infections including pneumonia is apparently very similar to that existing between actively acquired antibody and recovery, and the available evidence strongly suggests that factors other than the presence of passively transferred antibody may frequently be of great importance in successfully terminating such infections.

It was pointed out above in the discussion of the passive transfer of immunity to the pneumococcus (page 168) that the injection of specific antipneumococcal immune substances into animals or man with pneumococcus infections including pneumonia may markedly affect the subsequent course and outcome of the disease. For details of many of the results of the specific serum treatment of patients with pneumococcus pneumonia the chapter on the Results of Serum Treatment (page 880) should be consulted.

Antibody of a kind that is ordinarily encountered only about the time of recovery usually becomes demonstrable in the blood of infected individuals as soon as specific antiserum has been injected intravenously. This has been observed in animals (168, 532) and man (33, 295, 297, 61, 60, 245, 1263, 815, 1275, 820, 1088). Though such injected antibody usually tends to decrease or disappear from the blood, presumably through its combination with the organism and its specific derivative, the capsular polysaccharide (295, 33, 992, 1088), it apparently enhances to a marked degree the capacity of the blood-clearing mechanism to remove any organisms in the circulation (as in infected animals). As a result, the blood is rapidly sterilized (306, 292, 293, 33,

297, 794, 61, 60, 245, 991, 299, 1269, 183, 1088) and reinvasion prevented (306, 33, 297, 1269). It is possible that this is the most important effect of the use of antiserum in pneumonia, and the effectiveness of this action of specific antibody is far greater in the early stages of pneumonia than it is after the third or fourth day of illness.

The injection into patients early in their illness of adequate amounts of antibody specific for the type of pneumococcus with which they are infected usually also has other related results. In addition to causing clinical improvement of the patients treated, it generally prevents the infection from spreading (292, 293, 33, 297, 1269, 24, 1088, 1272), usually shortens the duration of the acute phases of the pneumonia (292, 297, 60, 245, 176, 442, 1269, 24, 463, 930, 557, 1088, 1272, 184, 339, 447), and commonly reduces the case fatality rate (see pages 880–918). It may also possibly reduce the incidence of complications such as empyema (592, 557, 193, 446).

The facts described in the preceding paragraphs indicate that the relation of passively administered antibody to recovery is very intimate in many cases. It is clear, however, that the effectiveness of injected immune substances is largely limited to cases whose serum treatment is begun prior to the fourth day of illness. In addition, occasional exceptions have been reported to each of the commonly observed beneficial results of serum treatment. Thus, specific instances have been encountered, even early in the disease in some cases, where, despite the administration of a presumably adequate amount of antiserum, the usual effects have been absent: bacteriemia has persisted or developed (60, 183, 1088), extension of the pulmonary lesion has occurred (793, 1088, 1272), and the course of the illness has been little shortened if at all (793, 1450, 710). That complications have not been produced or prevented in many instances (297, 793, 245, 442, 238, 24, 1450) is perhaps beside the point at the moment. It has also been noted that in some instances, in spite of the early appearance of antibody in the blood after serum treatment, recovery may not occur until some days later (815, 1088) and, further and importantly, that a few patients may die even though they have considerable demonstrable circulating antibody in their blood at the time (Lord and Persons, 820; Robertson, Graeser, Coggeshall, and Sia, 1088). These observations, together with a review of the analyses of a number of series of patients who have died despite the fact that they received serum treatment (1365, 299, 238, 463, 779, 1272, 1088, 1051), which reveals that apparently there is a small percentage of cases, possibly in the neighborhood of 2 or 3 per cent, in which passive therapy alone in presumably adequate amounts is not effective in bringing about recovery, indicate that other factors may be importantly concerned in recovery from pneumonia (see pages 918–920).

Robertson, Graeser, Coggeshall, and Sia (1088) have commented extensively on this matter and have noted that the effect of antibody on the course of the disease is largely dependent upon the stage of the illness when the treatment is begun. Their findings may be regarded as representative of a summary of the available literature: for it was observed that in the early stages of pneumonia, before consolidation became maximum, the antibodies administered in specific antiserum appeared capable of affecting the pneumococcus in the lesion so as to bring about a rapid cessation of the disease process, while after this period the chief effect of injected immune substances was to confine the organism to the pulmonary lesion and to prevent the latter from spreading while the disease was being terminated by the still "unknown process of natural recovery."

Host Factors and Physiologic Variables

In view of the above testimony, it appears clear that certain factors inherent in the host may play an important part in the mechanism of acquired immunity. Judging from the rather limited observations available, these factors, though as yet rather ill defined, appear numerous, complex, and closely interrelated.

Genetic factors may be importantly concerned in resistance to the pneumococcus, as was pointed out in the discussion of natural immunity (see pages 137–153). Recognition of this fact has led to the use of standard inbred strains of rabbits (537) and mice (540, 546, 547) in investigations attempting to evaluate the role of cellular factors in protection tests (see also page 186). The use of animals of inbred strains in such studies permits more accurate determinations than does the use of ordinary animals of mixed stock. Extremely little is known of the possible relation of genetic factors to the acquired immunity of man.

The physiologic reactivity of the host, which is apparently related to age and maturation, also has a bearing on host resistance (see also pages 186–192). Though specific circulating antibodies for the homologous type commonly appear in the blood of man following infection or immunization with pneumococci of a given type, as earlier mentioned, antibody of this nature appears less regularly and, when demonstrable, is usually of a lower titer in infants and young children than in adults (1321). In young rabbits the cellular response to infection has been shown to be less extensive and intense than in the adult (494). Lauche (766) considers the inability of the very young to react vigorously to infection to account for the rarity of pneumonia in the lobar form in infants.

A number of physiologic variables affect acquired immunity as was noted by Stillman and Goodner (1245) in their study of the outcome of infection in actively immunized rabbits. The titer of the circulating antibody present at the time of infection was determined to have little relation to the latent but conditioned powers of the host to produce specific resistance factors quickly or to renew them after the stimulus of infection. As the degree and duration of active humoral immunity did not always parallel the observed active immunity to subsequent infection, investigations of other factors which might be concerned in such immunity were carried out by Goodner and his associates (536, 537, 546, 547) during the infection of passively immunized rabbits and mice. Among other variables studied were the outcome of infection in relation to the bacteriemia present and to the dose of infecting organisms injected, the count of circulating leucocytes as well as their estimated total number in the body, and age and weight in relation to the time of specific treatment or the amount of the immune serum administered. Though of considerable importance, no constant relation was noted between the presence and degree of bacteriemia and the ultimate outcome, and likewise only a very general correlation was found between the presence of a low leucocyte count at the time of infection and the resultant fatality rate. Body weight appeared important, however, and heavy animals seemed to be physiologically capable of utilizing more effectively the protective antibody of immune serum than did lighter ones. Studies of the cells involved in the host response to infection supported the general conception that the outcome is directly related to the cellular status at the time of infection; that is, a high content of circulating leucocytes in the blood and a generally robust physical condition in a mature animal were indicative of a satisfactory cellular status.

Goodner (537) has discussed the relationships to immunity of certain factors which he designated as the intrinsic and extrinsic factors. Body weight, which may be an expression of age, and the total leucocyte count of the blood were regarded as intrinsic factors, and the amount of antibody administered and the number of infecting pneumococci injected as extrinsic factors. These four variables appeared to determine the outcome in rabbits of protection tests carried out by injecting both the antibody and the organisms intravenously. While the relationship between the two extrinsic factors—the amount of antibody used and the number of organisms injected—appeared direct, the two intrinsic factors were not directly related to one another, and an increase in the total leucocyte count did not appear to compensate for a lack of weight, nor did an excess of weight appear to compensate for a lack of leucocytes. Nevertheless, all the factors were interrelated, the relation between the intrinsic factors being accomplished through the medium of the extrinsic factors.

Increasing the amount of immune serum used appeared to compensate for a lack of body weight but probably not for a lack of leucocytes. Thus the factors of body weight and amount of antibody appeared mutually compensatory, and the necessary amount of antibody was likewise directly related to the number of organisms used, which in turn was directly related to the leucocyte count. The general conclusion was that physiologically mature individuals who, as evidenced by their possessing a greater number of circulating leucocytes, are in a condition of high cellular reactivity have the advantage over others in utilizing the antibodies at hand. It may again be mentioned at this point that in normal mice the experimental mobilization of leucocytes (chiefly polymorphonuclears) prior to infection did not alone give evidence of an increased resistance (1253, 1159, 546). In the presence of injected specific antibody, however, a higher recovery rate from infection was obtained in rabbits (537) and mice (546, 547) whose leucocytes had been previously mobilized by various procedures than in controls receiving similar amounts of immune serum. The higher recovery rate in this instance seemed related to the increased number of polymorphonuclear leucocytes appearing under such conditions. Though considerable phagocytosis may occur in the absence of sensitizing antibody, the latter appeared necessary for rendering the organisms susceptible to digestion by the intracellular enzymes of the leucocytes.

It was revealed in a study of protection tests in mice by Goodner and Miller (546, 547) that monocytes formed the first line of defense in the peritoneal cavity. Age as well as weight seemed associated with a satisfactory degree of physiologic reactivity. A direct parallelism was noted between the type of cell initially present in the peritoneal cavity of the normal mouse and the effectiveness of the protective system. With a given number of leucocytes, better protection was obtained in small than in large mice, which presumably was due to the fact that monocytes formed a much higher proportion of the cells initially present in the peritoneal cavity of small mice than in large mice. The dominating relation between the factors studied in determining the outcome appeared to be between the number of monocytes initially present and the number of organisms injected. It was also noted, however, that the activity of the phagocytic cells might be greatly inhibited by excessive amounts of either immune serum or free specific capsular polysaccharide.

Local Lung Resistance

In some instances the cells in the lung may show an altered reactivity suggesting the presence of an area or areas of immunity which may be local and possibly not shared by the rest of the body. Numerous observations relating to this matter have been reported (1243, 1258, 1244, 1083, 470, 1087, 286, 285, 1095). Stillman and Branch (1243) immunized mice by subjecting them to the inhalation of dead pneumococci and, following the subsequent exposure of these animals to the inhalation of live pneumococci of homologous type, obtained some pulmonary localization of the resulting infection. These investigators also noted that previous studies of the same sort in mice had shown that immunization by the foregoing procedure produced little if any general immunity as determined by their reaction to intraperitoneal infection. In consequence, the occurrence of pulmonary localization in these mice, which were regarded as having no general immunity, was considered as possibly due to the presence of some local immunity in the lung. In a subsequent study their views were changed, however, for Stillman and Branch (1244) partially immunized mice both actively and passively by giving various agents by other than the pulmonary route and, after intoxicating them with alcohol, subjected them to the inhalation of live pneumococci of the corresponding type. The finding that pulmonary localization occurred among the animals immunized in this fashion but not among the controls made it probable that such localization occurred as a consequence of their possession of a general immunity of low grade.

Stuppy, Cannon, and Falk (1258) immunized rabbits by subjecting them to the inhalation of killed pneumococci, after which they were infected by the intrabronchial insufflation of living pneumococci of homologous type. A proliferative and exudative reaction was produced in the lungs in which the macrophage was the predominant cell in the inflammatory exudate. A similar though less marked reaction occurred after infection by the intrabronchial insufflation of pneumococci of heterologous types. The immunizing procedure was considered to have stimulated the phagocytic tissues to increased functional activity and to have aided in the mobilization of macrophages in the lung. Though the reaction was predominantly cellular, the participation of humoral antibodies could not be excluded.

At necropsies performed following death from pneumococcus pneumonia on patients not having demonstrable specific circulating antibody, Robertson and his associates (1087) found areas of local clearing or regional recovery in the lung. Pneumococci were rarely found in such areas, while in other regions close by and which were well consolidated they were present in considerable numbers. The suggestion was made that these areas of local lung recovery might represent examples of actively acquired antipneumococcal immunity of local tissue cells. Robertson and his co-workers (1083), Coggeshall and Robertson (286), and Coggeshall (285) also investigated this matter in dogs with experimentally produced pneumonia. It was observed that though specific humoral antibody appeared irregularly in the blood of dogs following recovery from repeated attacks of lobar pneumonia, perhaps the most significant and only definite evidence of increased resistance in such animals was found in the changes characterized by the "macrophage reaction" of the fixed tissue cells in the lungs. This reaction consisted of a swelling of the fixed tissue cells and a subsequent liberation of macrophages into the alveolar exudate. The macrophage reaction occurred regularly at the time of recovery from the initial attack, always accompanied resolution, and was associated with a local disappearance of the invading organism. In secondary attacks this reaction appeared while the inflammation was still extending; and as such attacks were more limited and of briefer duration, it was suggested that the reaction plays a role in controlling the infection. In short, the occurrence of the macrophage reaction was regarded as significant evidence of an increased resistance. In a later study Robertson and Uhley (1095) noted that though recovery from pneumonia may depend upon the presence of specific antibody together with a local cellular reaction in the lung, as yet they had been unable to find in either animals or man a constant relationship between the presence of circulating immune substance and the development of the macrophage reaction.

The findings of Finland and Winkler (470) are of interest in connection with the possible role of local lung resistance in some cases of pneumonia. These investigators studied fifty-seven recurrences of pneumonia in man and, after a careful analysis of the material presented, were unable to find any evidence that the recurrent lesions were affected by a local resistance in the lung due to a previous attack. It may be mentioned, however, that the average interval between attacks was twenty-eight months for those infected with pneumococci of the same type and was about four years for all cases. These intervals were considerably longer than those occurring between the experimentally induced repeated attacks of pneumonia in dogs studied by Coggeshall and Robertson (286) and Coggeshall (285), who reported that the elapsed time between attacks was usually a matter of only a few days or weeks.

RELATION OF HYPERSENSITIVENESS AND ALLERGY TO IMMUNITY

The extremely complex problems of anaphylaxis, hypersensitiveness, and allergy in relation to the pneumococcus and the possible bearing these states have on immunity to this organism have been rather widely investigated. The results of many studies have demonstrated that by various procedures a hypersensitive state can be induced in animals with living or dead pneumococci or with autolyzed cultures, extracts, or derivatives of these organisms. The response obtained from the injection of such substances into suitably sensitized animals is conditioned by many factors, but under the proper circumstances intradermal injection results in the appearance of skin reactions of various sorts (1465, 843, 1463, 1174, 1188, 700, 783, 1077, 1078, 595), intrabronchial administration may cause the appearance of pulmonary exudation (1174, 1258, 783, 286, 285), and injection into the body by other parenteral routes may give rise to various responses including acute anaphylaxis (1117, 279, 841, 783, 218). The uterine musculature of guinea pigs sensitized with pneumococci, when exposed to contact with solutions of this organism (1464), gave contractions typical of those produced by protein sensitization. The hypersensitive state is presumably dependent upon the presence of specific antibodies which have been withdrawn from the blood and fixed on or in the cells of the body (1317). Various aspects of the problem of allergy to the pneumococcus and its derivatives have been discussed in considerable detail by White, with Robinson and Barnes (1417).

In animals the relation between hypersensitiveness and allergy to the pneumococcus or its derivatives and resistance to this organism has been variously studied (1117, 279, 841, 843, 116, 700, 1077, 1078, 206, 218, 595, 286, 285). It has been demonstrated that the cells of animals immunized against the pneumococcus may acquire hypersensitivity or altered reactivity to this organism or its derivatives (279, 841, 843, 1077, 1078, 218, 595). However, altered reactivity or allergy to the pneumococcus may be produced in susceptible animals with but little (279) if any (843, 595) simultaneous increase in their resistance to this organism. The desensitization of such allergic animals may likewise be without effect in altering their susceptibility (843). In other instances the allergic state may be nearly or apparently wholly absent even in the presence of acquired immunity of high degree (841, 286, 285); or by suitable desensitizing procedures the allergic condition of immunized animals may be abolished without causing any measurable or significant decrease in their acquired immunity, as was clearly shown by Rich (1077) and Rich, Jennings, and Downing (1078).

In view of the observations made in the studies cited above, it seems likely that the relation between the condition of hypersensitiveness or allergy to the pneumococcus and that of acquired immunity may be very intimate; and while at times both allergy and immunity may be present in the same individual, in other instances either condition may be present in the absence of the other. It also appears likely, as Topley (1317) has stated, that

> . . . so far as our present knowledge goes it seems very probable that all the phenomena of anaphylaxis, of hypersensitiveness, and of immunity of the type dependent on the development of specific antibodies, result from the working of a single underlying mechanism, the character of the total reaction being determined in each particular case by a variety of secondary factors.

Rich (1077) and Rich, Jennings, and Downing (1078) studied the progress of pneumococcus infection in normal rabbits and in immune allergic and immune non-allergic rabbits. Marked resistance to infection was observed in the immune animals, and the operation of this immunity appeared entirely independent of the presence or absence of the allergic state. The amount of inflammation incited by infection of the immune animals was much greater in those in an allergic state than in those in which the latter condition had been abolished by previous desensitization or in others which had been passively immunized and were non-allergic. It was apparent that the exaggerated inflammatory reaction which occurred in the allergic state was not a necessary part of the immunity mechanism, and that immunity to infection could be clearly separated from allergic hypersensitivity. In fact, immunity seemed to supplement the protective power of the normal inflammatory mechanism, in that less rather than more inflammation was required to overcome the infection. As a result, and as others have suggested, the exuberant inflammatory response so commonly found in the presence of an allergic state may serve no essential purpose and may lead to an unnecessary destruction of the tissues involved in the reaction. In cases of acquired immunity without allergy, the situation seemed comparable to that in cases of natural immunity in that bacteria were effectively destroyed with a minimum of inflammatory response and tissue damage.

Observations similar in significance to those of Rich and his associates, who worked with rabbits, were made by Catron (218) in mice. From these studies it appeared clear that while a hyperergic or allergic response might frequently coexist with the operation of the mechanism of acquired immunity, the hypersensitive response was not essential to the successful functioning of the immune mechanism.

The possibility that a state of hypersensitiveness may play an important role in the production of pneumonia in the lobar form in man is discussed later (see pages 240–245). The development of a skin reaction following the intradermal injection of the specific capsular polysaccharide of the pneumococcus may probably be regarded, as was shown earlier, as evidence that the individual possesses some immunity to pneumococci of the homologous type (see pages 165–167 and 170–171).

Using rabbits as test animals, Harley (595) studied two types of allergic skin reactions to pneumococci and their products. The first of these was allergy to the specific capsular polysaccharide. This condition was induced by the intravenous injection of a vaccine composed of S forms of pneumococci; it was type-specific and was closely related to the presence in the blood of both specific circulating antibodies and the power of the serum of such animals to render guinea pigs anaphylactic when injected with the specific capsular polysaccharide of homologous type. The second type of reaction was non-type-specific, was independent of both humoral type-specific and anti-protein antibodies, and was induced by intracutaneous injections of vaccines composed of virulent or avirulent pneumococci alike.

Certain aspects of the possible relationship of pneumococcal allergy to immunity in man were investigated and discussed by Kramár and Gyüre (742, 743). Using several vaccines each containing pneumococci of a different type, skin tests were made on numerous healthy children and at various times during and after infection on a number of patients with pneumonia due to a variety of organisms including pneumococci of known type. It was concluded that allergy to the pneumococcus was a very labile condition, a view which Loeschcke (798) earlier propounded, and a condition which varied considerably with the individual and with age. Healthy human beings were classified into three groups depending upon their immune state toward the pneumococcus as shown by the diagrammatic representation below.

I		II		III
Anergic phase = *without protection*	→ ←	*Allergic phase =* *labile immunity*	→ ←	*Fastness =* *stable immunity*
Skin test negative. Newborn infants. Number decreases with age during nursing period. Senility (?).		Skin test positive. Number increases with age among nurslings. Majority of children and adults.		Skin test negative. Minority of children and adults. Persons artificially immunized.

While repeated minor pneumococcus infections, as well as recovery from frank infections of a clinical nature due to this organism, were considered as influencing an individual's condition in the direction of a state of immunity or "fastness," his condition might be influenced in the opposite direction, or toward the anergic phase in which no protection is present, by factors such as colds, exhaustion, fatigue, massive infection, and other diseases, and possibly by the advent of old age.

FACTORS AFFECTING VARIATIONS IN IMMUNITY

Numerous factors appear to have a bearing on the immunity of the individual to the pneumococcus. While many of these factors are still obscure, the nature and role of some are understood in varying degrees. Immunity appears to be dependent upon the functioning of integrated systems of cellular reactions conditioned by the presence of antipneumococcal immune substances. In many instances immunity is of a specific nature which presumably results from the interaction of cellular processes with specific antibodies of the kind frequently demonstrable in the blood. As body weight, the cellular activity of the host, one index of which is the total leucocyte count, and the extent, duration, and severity of the infection may be importantly related to the outcome in the presence of pneumococcus infection, as was pointed out above (pages 177–180), these factors may be regarded as having a significant relation to immunity. Several other factors which tend either to increase or decrease the quality and quantity of the demonstrable specific circulating antibody or specific resistance, or both, are considered in a broad way below.

Animal Species

Man in general, as well as some species of the lower animals, possesses considerable immunity to the pneumococcus (see pages 137–158). Such resistance, however, varies a great deal among individuals within the species.

Genetic Factors

It seemed probable from the work of Irwin and Hughes (679) with inbred strains of rats that immunity to infection might be importantly influenced by genetic factors. The natural resistance of mice and rabbits, various strains of which are commonly used in experimental studies with the pneumococcus, has been found to vary markedly. The results obtained by Webster and Clow (1392) and Rake (1058, 1059) with mice and by Goodner (537) with rabbits have demonstrated that the use of standard inbred strains of these animals largely eliminates a possible source of variation or error which might otherwise occur due to wide differences in the immunity of the test animals. Inbred strains of mice have also been used by other workers (540, 546, 547). As compared with ordinary strains of mice, the immunity of inbred strains appeared related to factors inherent in the tissues of the internal organs or in the body fluids (1059).

Whether or not genetic factors may influence the immunity of various groups of man to the pneumococcus is unknown. The problem of man's resistance is so complex that as yet statements concerning the influence of hereditary factors must be largely speculative. Certain findings relating to possible variations in the general immunity of members of different races are noted in the chapter on Epidemiology (page 258), and particularly in the section of that chapter dealing with the influence of race on the morbidity and mortality from pneumonia (see page 312). In respect to the relation of eye color and disease of the upper respiratory tract, Gafafer (505) observed 343 adults over a period of eight months and found no significant difference in the frequency or severity of attacks of the common cold in persons with blue or brown eyes.

Age

Immunity varies considerably with age. In normal animals, as the result of direct infection experiments or of tests of their blood or serum for specific circulating antipneumococcal antibodies, evidence has been obtained that the immunity of young chickens (171), rabbits (508, 1439, 1091, 1085, 494), and rats (1131, 1137) is less than that demonstrable in adults of the species (see also page 177). Resistance appears to decrease in old age, and in experimental lobar pneumonia in the dog, a naturally resistant animal, the prognosis was found to be poorest in the oldest animals (1292).

The immunologic mechanism responsible for the production of skin sensitivity following the injection of autolyzed cultures or bile solutions of pneumococci was observed by Zinsser and Grinnell (1463) to function more rapidly in adults than in young guinea pigs. With antigens other than pneumococci, Baumgartner (81, 82) found in immunized rabbits that adults produce a better quality and quantity of antibody than young animals. Some evidence was also obtained that aged rabbits were less able to produce antibody than were animals in the prime of life. In addition, and importantly, serums of the same antibody titer obtained from individuals of different ages appeared to have qualitative characteristics which were independent of titer and which allowed serums of the same titer to react differently, for it was found that some of the actions of antibody were more pronounced when the antibody was derived from the serum of robust adults than from the serum of young or very old rabbits.

The results of determinations for circulating antibody having various antipneumococcal actions (205, 577, 1270, 121, 462) and of intradermal tests for skin sensitivity to the specific capsular polysaccharide of some types of pneumococci (1270, 12) strongly suggest that the natural immunity of man likewise varies considerably with age. A consideration of the variations by age both of the case fatality rate of patients with pneumonia (see pages 703–710) and of the mortality rates from this disease (see pages 299–307) also gives presumptive evidence that the general characteristic of immunity to the pneumococcus varies markedly with age. On the basis of the available evidence, both direct and indirect, it may be stated that man's natural immunity to this organism, discounting whatever endowment he may have at birth, is low in infancy, progressively increases during early childhood, and is relatively high from late childhood through middle adult life, following which it appears to decrease. The term immunity is, of course, descriptive of only a relative and labile state, and marked individual variations may be encountered in persons of various ages.

It appears reasonable to assume that usually the presence in the blood of immune substances having specific antipneumococcal powers is indicative of the presence of a variable degree of immunity in the individual. Gundel (577) was unable to find either protective substance or agglutinins for pneumococci of Type I or II in the serum of a few newborn infants tested. However, the findings of Burhans and Gerstenberger (205), who demonstrated protective substance for Types I, II, and III in the serum of 40 per cent of parturient mothers and 30 per cent of their newborn infants, and those of Sutliff and Finland (1270), who found the incidence of whole blood pneumococcidal power for Types I, II, and III to be about the same in infants under ten days of age as in their mothers, indicate that a considerable proportion of infants probably have some immunity at birth. This is presumably derived from the mother by way of the placenta and after birth through the breast milk (766).

The reports of Sutliff and Finland (1270) and of Finland and Sutliff (462), who studied the incidence and amount of whole blood pneumococcidal power for pneumococci of several types in persons of various ages having no history of pneumonia, are of special interest. The observations indicate the probable variations of immunity with age.

Figure 1 is taken from the study of Sutliff and Finland (1270), who investigated the pneumococcidal power of the blood of 112 persons of various ages and of the mothers of 22 infants under ten days old for pneumococci of Types I, II, and III. The number of organisms killed by 0.5 cc. of defibrinated blood varied with the individual from about 10 to approximately 1,000,000; the specimens from by far the largest proportion of persons killed 10,000 organisms or less. There was but little difference between the three types of pneumococci or between the persons in different age groups in respect to the number of organisms disposed of, and only individuals 0.5 cc. of whose blood killed 30 or more pneumococci were regarded as having pneumococcidal power.

Bactericidal power was frequently present among the newborn and in infants under ten days old. In those a little older, in the group three to five weeks of age, and in others from two to fifteen months old, pneumococcidal power was absent or rare; while in children from two to eleven years old it was again about as frequent as among the newborn. The incidence of killing power for all three types was highest in young adults and tended to decrease considerably among persons in the older age groups. In all age groups variations were encountered in the incidence of pneumococcidal power for the different types, and killing power might be present for any one or two of the types in the absence of this power for the other types or type.

Tests for Type I, II, and III protective substance were also carried out on the serum of many of these individuals. While such substance was occasionally encountered in the serum of some persons, none was found in the serum of fifteen infants aged three weeks to fifteen months who were studied; and, except for this, no definite age distribution was noted. In addition, only a few of 142 individuals of various ages had type-specific agglutinins in their serum, and not any were found in infants from three weeks to fifteen months of age.

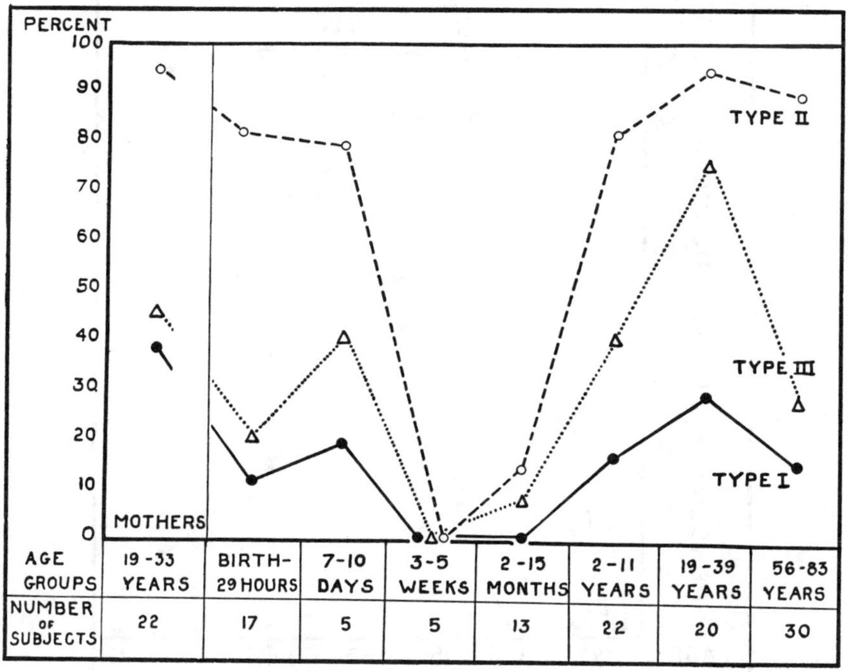

From Sutliff and Finland (1270)

Figure 1. Percentage of persons in different age groups whose blood was bactericidal for Type I, II, and III pneumococci

In a later report Finland and Sutliff (462) extended their study to include observations on the incidence of specific antibodies for the eight types, Types I, II, III, V, VIa, VIb, VIII, and IX. Bactericidal tests were carried out with the blood of 72 normal persons and hospital patients having no recent infection or history of pneumonia. In this group six were infants from two weeks to seven months of age, ten were children from one to nine years, and the remainder were adults, of which thirty-three were from sixteen to thirty-eight years of age, fifteen were from forty to fifty-eight years, and eight were over sixty-four years of age. In some instances tests with Type II, III, or VIa were omitted. The incidence of pneumococcidal power for 100 or more organisms of the various types in such individuals was shown graphically, as illustrated in Figure 2, which is taken from Finland and Sutliff's report.

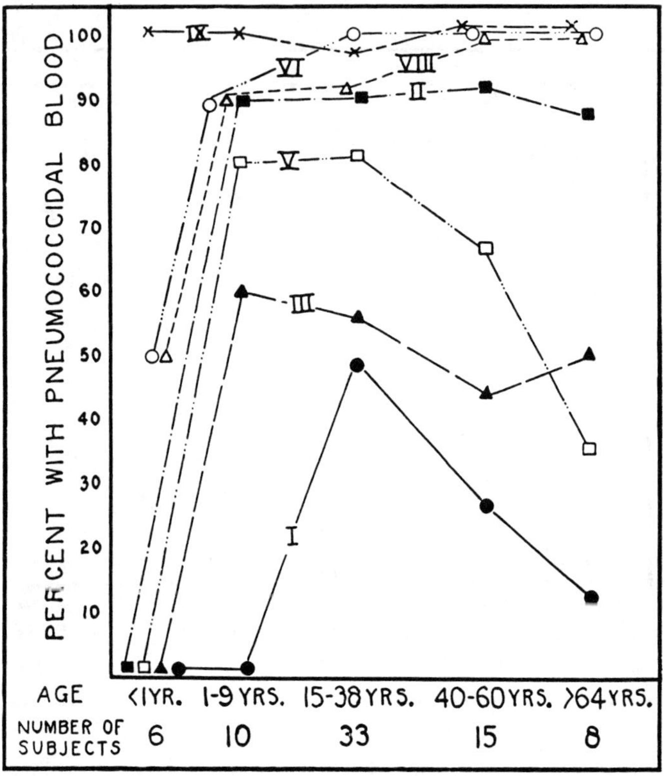

From Finland and Sutliff (462)

Figure 2. Percentage of persons in different age groups whose blood was bactericidal for various types of pneumococci

With minor variations, the general trend of the incidence of pneumococcidal power against the various types was uniform in indicating that such power is rare or absent in infants and common in children and in adults up to the age of about forty years, after which some decrease is often observed. As in the study of bactericidal power for Types I, II, and III shown in Figure 1, the relative incidence of such killing power for each of these three types was the same in all age groups.

The percentage incidence of killing power for the types investigated in persons in the various age groups is shown in Table 39. The results with Types VIa and VIb were essentially similar, and only the latter are shown.

TABLE 39. PERCENTAGE INCIDENCE OF BACTERICIDAL POWER IN THE BLOOD OF 72 NORMAL PERSONS IN DIFFERENT AGE GROUPS, BY PNEUMOCOCCUS TYPE

AGE GROUP	PER CENT INCIDENCE OF KILLING POWER BY TYPE						
	I	II	III	V	VIB	VIII	IX
2 weeks–1 year	–	–	–	–	50.0	50.0	100.0
1–9 years	–	90.0	60.0	80.0	88.9	90.0	100.0
16–38 years	48.5	90.3	56.0	81.2	100.0	93.9	97.0
40–60 years	26.7	91.7	44.4	66.7	100.0	100.0	100.0
Over 64 years	12.5	87.5	50.0	37.5	100.0	100.0	100.0

From Finland and Sutliff (462)

Though the number of individuals tested against any type in the different age groups was small and varied from six to thirty-three persons, the findings are doubtless of importance in indicating immunity variations with age.

Tests for protective substance against 100 or more lethal doses of Types II, III, V, VIb, and VIII or varying numbers of these types were carried out on the serum of 53 persons, all of whom were included in the studies of bactericidal power mentioned above (see Table 40). Infants under one year of

TABLE 40. PERCENTAGE INCIDENCE OF MOUSE PROTECTIVE SUBSTANCE IN THE SERUM OF 53 NORMAL PERSONS IN VARIOUS AGE GROUPS, BY PNEUMOCOCCUS TYPE

AGE GROUP IN YEARS	PER CENT INCIDENCE OF PROTECTIVE SUBSTANCE BY TYPE				
	II	III	V	VIB	VIII
1–9	–	–	–	25.0	–
16–38	21.7	18.8	15.4	40.9	30.4
40–60	–	30.0	8.3	61.5	7.7
Over 64	12.5	25.0	–	25.0	–

From Finland and Sutliff (462)

age were not included in the study of protective substance. From two to twenty-six persons were tested in each age group against the various types.

Protective substance against the types studied was rare in the serum of children, relatively frequent in the serum of adults, and somewhat less common in persons in the older ages.

Studies were also made of agglutinins in the serum of twenty-two young and middle-aged adults for the eight types mentioned above in relation to the pneumococcidal tests. Agglutinins were rarely found and were present in low dilution in three instances for Type VIa and for Type VIII pneumococci. Gundel (577) had previously reported a few observations on the occurrence of Type I and II protective substance and agglutinins in children and in adults and had noted that, while such antibodies were frequently found in adults, they were absent in children.

Sutliff and Finland (1270) studied the incidence in persons from birth to eighty-three years of age of skin reactions to the acetic-acid-precipitable proteins of four strains of pneumococci and to the autolysates of three strains of these organisms. The incidence of positive reactions among a group of more than forty persons tested with these materials increased with age. Skin tests were also made in persons of similar ages with the specific capsular polysaccharides of pneumococci of Types I, II, and III. In this instance, however, no significant alterations in the incidence of positive reactions with age were observed. A general erythematous reaction obscured the findings in infants. Alston and Lowdon's (12) findings with respect to skin sensitivity to the Type II capsular polysaccharide in normal persons from birth to forty years of age were different, and the percentage of those giving positive reactions was reported as markedly increasing with age. The incidence of positive reactions among fifteen persons from birth to one and one-half years of age was zero, while among 94 persons from one and one-half to twelve years old it was 50 per cent, and in 172 individuals from twelve to forty years old the proportion of reactors was 76 per cent.

Sex

Except for some indirect evidence relating to man, little is known of the possible variations of immunity to the pneumococcus with sex. Judging from the occasionally reported higher case fatality rates for lobar pneumonia in women than in men (see page 712), it might be presumed that women were less resistant to pneumonia than men. Since such a conclusion is based upon the fatality rates of hospitalized cases, its validity must be doubted, as Greenwood and Candy (567) have pointed out.

For determining sex differences in immunity in general to acute pulmonary infections, it is possibly more accurate to study mortality rates, as Doull, Harmon, and Fisher (373) have done. It seems likely as a result of their study of the death rates over several years for pneumonia and influenza together in most of the states in the registration area of the United States (see pages 310–312 and 328–329) that, in comparison with females of similar age, males are subject to two periods of excess mortality from pneumonia. The first period of excess male pneumonia mortality extends from birth to about puberty and does not vary with the degree of urbanization of the states studied; while the second and most marked period of excess pneumonia mortality in males is found in the groups aged twenty to sixty-nine years, and the rates in this large section of the male population vary definitely with the environment, being highest in urban and lowest in rural* states. This latter variation is presumably related to the greater opportunities for exposure to unfavorable conditions and infections prevalent in urban communities.

If the observations made have been correctly interpreted, they indicate that from infancy to early puberty males are inherently more susceptible to "pneumonia" than are females. This view is in accord with the finding of Van Volkenburgh and Frost (1348), who studied the incidence over two winters of minor respiratory infections in a group of families totalling 484 persons and reported that during the first ten years of life the males studied experienced a higher attack than females.

Infecting Organism: Virulence and Type

Immunity in general varies inversely with the virulence of the infecting organism, as has been well shown by animal experiments with the pneumococcus (487, 1285, 508, 1422, 1392). In spite of considerable immunity of natural or acquired origin, infection with pneumococci of high virulence may produce disease of great severity which frequently ends in death, while strains of low virulence may cause little or no apparent lesion. Even animals of great susceptibility, such as the normal rabbit, may prove resistant to pneumococci of little virulence, as mentioned earlier (see page 128).

Gaskell's (508) observations are of interest in respect to the relation of virulence to the type of lesion resulting from experimental infection. By maintaining the infecting dose of pneumococci above a certain minimum, and by controlling the virulence of the culture used he was able to a large

* States with a large proportion of their population engaged in agriculture such as Iowa, Kansas, and Oklahoma.

extent to control the type of pulmonary lesion induced by the intrabronchial infection of normal rabbits. Type I pneumococci of low virulence produced a patch of central pneumonia, strains of higher virulence produced a more widespread patchy lesion, and a further increase in virulence resulted in lesions of a lobar variety. With strains of the highest virulence massive blood invasion occurred, the localizing reaction in the lung seemed inhibited, and the animals died rapidly of septicaemia.

The degree of specific immunity resulting from the infection or artificial immunization of animals with pneumococci of maximum virulence is higher than when strains having little or no virulence are used (1361, 936, 1254, 1363, 308, 125, 231, 69, 1129, 1240, 486, 1260). Variations also occur in the antibody response to infection or immunization with pneumococci of different types, as previously described (page 161).

Fundamentally, the virulence of the infecting organism is of greater importance in relation to immunity than serologic type. Nevertheless, there is a general relationship between pneumococci of some types and virulence. For example, strains of freshly isolated Type I or II pneumococci, organisms which so commonly cause lobar pneumonia and a large number of deaths in man, are usually highly virulent for ordinary laboratory animals. In addition, the natural immunity of animals may vary against virulent pneumococci of different types (see pages 137–143), and animals of a given species may be more resistant against some types than others. In some instances immunity may be different against different strains of the same type (1439, 1392).

It would seem from studies of the specific humoral antibody of man in relation to natural immunity and from a consideration of the marked differences in the frequency with which pneumococci of the various types cause pneumonia (see pages 42–89), as well as of the differences in the resulting case fatality rates (see pages 663–667), that the immunity of man also varies against pneumococci of different types, and, further, that it probably varies against different strains of differing virulence within a single type.

Passage of Time

The immunity engendered by the immunization of animals or that resulting from their infection decreases with the passage of time (1388, 1128, 532, 1448, 1241, 422, 1470, 739). Stillman and Goodner (1245) have reported specific instances of this in rabbits immunized with pneumococci of Types I, II, and III whose level of specific circulating antibody and active resistance to infection with the homologous organism were followed for periods of a year or more. While some slight variations were encountered in the reactions of individual animals, the variations in the resulting antibody titer and active immunity of the group to infection were marked between the three types. The immunity of animals immunized with pneumococci of Type I was high at first, gradually and irregularly decreased during the succeeding months, and after the seventh month dropped to a low level. The titer of protective substance roughly paralleled the degree of resistance during this period, while the agglutinin titer was high for only a month or two. With Type II, active immunity was somewhat lower than for Type I but persisted moderately high for nine months. Most animals showed protective substance but rarely agglutinins. With Type III, however, no humoral antibodies were present, and active immunity was high for only a month and then decreased sharply and remained generally low.

The susceptibility of normal animals also varies with the passage of time; and with guinea pigs made carriers of pneumococci, Neufeld and Etinger-Tulczynska (935) observed differences in the immunity of the same animal to serious infection at different times.

It is apparent, too, that the general immunity of man changes with age as has already been pointed out (see page 187). The demonstrable immunity of man resulting from immunization (461, 1469, 988, 433) or pneumococcus infection (see pages 737–739) decreases over a period of a few to several months. In some instances the incidence of pneumonia among large groups of men in military organizations (246, 434) or engaged in industrial operations, such as mining or construction work, has been found to be high in the early period of their enrollment and to progressively decrease for several months following this (874, 549, 1008, 788; see also pages 329–332). Such decreases in the attack rate of pneumonia with the passage of time presumably result from the development of an increasing resistance.

In some instances the immunity of a relatively isolated population may apparently decrease over a period of years, as is suggested by Strøm's (1252) study of an outbreak of Type I pneumonia in a small isolated orphanage, for the attack rate was highest and the infection most severe among inmates who had lived there the longest.

In addition to the above evidence that man's immunity to the pneumococcus varies with the passage of time, direct antibody determinations were made on a few normal persons at various intervals by Ward (1379) and on more than fifty normal adults over periods of a few to many months by

Graeser and Harrison (551). The former study embraced observations on the pneumococcidal power of the blood for Types I, II, and III, and the latter for Types I and II. Though no significant alteration was found in the titer of the killing power present among the majority of individuals who had bactericidal power, a few showed gradual changes in the direction of an increase or a decrease in pneumococcidal power against some, but not necessarily all, of the types studied.

It is probable that the specific immunity of man may vary from time to time and may be different against pneumococci of various types at different times, just as it may be different against various types at the same time.

Immunization

Animals of several species and large numbers of humans have been subjected to immunizing procedures of one sort or another. Vaccines composed of pneumococci killed by various means, or of solutions of them, or of autolyzed cultures, culture filtrates, and extracts or derivatives of pneumococci have been used for this purpose. Barach (69) has reviewed much of the literature. Mention is made in the chapter on Measures for the Prevention of Pneumonia (page 395) of some of the details concerning the general circumstances surrounding the preparation and use of a number of the above agents. For a further discussion of these matters, see White, with Robinson and Barnes (1417).

VACCINES. The artificial immunization of animals with pneumococcus vaccines gives rise to the appearance of humoral antibody or immunity to infection or both. Usually the response following the use of suitable vaccines is of a specific nature (see pages 133–136).

The Klemperers (724) were the first to demonstrate antibody production following the immunization of animals (rabbits). Using animals such as the rabbit, guinea pig, chicken, cow, ass, or horse, similar observations were made by several other early investigators (1389, 981, 99, 932, 1360, 748, 1254, 1362, 1363). Their findings were amply confirmed, and to a considerable degree extended, by later studies in the mouse (939, 888), rabbit (785, 308, 628, 170, 570, 174, 68, 69, 1240, 486, 1241, 1245, 77, 595), rat (1126, 1127, 1137), guinea pig (841), chicken (750), dog (1127), horse (308, 532, 533), and monkey (240). Attention has already been called to the actions of the humoral antibody produced in many such instances (see pages 159–161). At times to ensure the production of antibody of high titer, the immunization of animals first with killed and later with living virulent pneumococci in small doses has been recommended (1389, 932, 308). In addition to finding that specific circulating antibodies which contribute to the immune state may appear following immunization with pneumococcus vaccines, it has also been shown that variable degrees of specific immunity may be acquired. This has been demonstrated in the mouse (1012, 1238, 1243, 888, 68, 69, 532, 434), rabbit (722, 1432, 922, 1448, 531, 532, 1258, 737, 434, 1078, 1077, 1245, 739), rat (1126, 1127, 1128, 1129, 1131, 1135, 1136), guinea pig (841), dog (727), and monkey (125, 240, 241, 242, 243, 738). In a few instances living organisms were used for immunizing purposes, and this resulted in the appearance of humoral antibody or immunity to infection or both (1388, 1361, 1363, 231, 841, 1260).

Following the observation of Wright and Douglas (1442, 1443, 1444) that the immunization of man with staphylococcus vaccine gave rise to the appearance of circulating antibody and an improvement in immunity specific for that organism, efforts were made to immunize man against the pneumococcus. Most investigations of the latter nature dealing with the use of pneumococcus vaccines were carried out in the direct attempt to reduce the incidence rates of pneumonia among men employed in certain industrial undertakings, such as mining on a large scale, and among troops in various military organizations, though in a few instances efforts were confined either to institutional or to other ordinary civilian groups (see pages 446–478).

The initial work among miners, begun under Wright's direction, was reported by Maynard (874) in 1913. Subsequently, Wright and his associates (1447) and other investigators reported similar studies (785, 786, 1376, 1008, 970, 973, 1219, 510, 788, 1007, 971). The use of pneumococcus vaccines for the immunization of soldiers was carried out by Cecil and Austin (228) and others (246, 140, 382, 859, 719), and for the immunization of institutional and other civilian groups by Rosenow and Sturdivant (1119) and several additional workers (1359, 693, 831, 988, 1249, 71, 72, 461, 1135, 1138, 731, 433, 1207). Though circulating antibody specific for the pneumococci used in the vaccine has been demonstrated to appear in the blood of man in several instances following immunization (785, 228, 71, 72, 461, 1135, 1138, 433), the evidence that a reduction in the incidence of pneumonia occurred among the persons vaccinated, while highly suggestive in some studies, was not conclusive in others.

It is probable that the failure of prophylactic vaccination to reduce the incidence of pneumonia in many instances was due to the fact that in some of the investigations cited above little attention was apparently paid to the details of the preparation of the vaccine used. As was indicated earlier in this chapter, it is now recognized that virulent pneumococci prepared for use in vaccines should be devitalized at the peak of their biologic activities with as little disarrangement of cellular integrity and of the relationships of the capsular substance and the nucleoprotein material of the cell body as is possible. Other matters, such as the route of administration, spacing of injections, total dosage, and types of pneumococci included in the vaccine, have also to be considered (see pages 408–440).

OTHER PREPARATIONS. In animals immunization with culture filtrates or solutions of pneumococci in bile or bile salts may be followed either by the appearance of specific circulating antibody (724, 1363, 69) or by an increase in specific immunity to infection (68, 69, 1129, 1131, 1132, 737, 1136), and administration of these substances to man may be followed by the appearance of specific circulating antibody (71, 1138). In animals immunized with autolyzed cultures prepared by special procedures, circulating antibody, presumably of a species-specific nature, appeared accompanying the development of some immunity either to infection (1118) or to the toxic action of anaerobically prepared autolysates or both (998, 114). Finland and Sutliff (461) reported that the single injection of an ordinary autolysate of pneumococci of Type I, II, or III into eleven persons was in most cases followed by the appearance of or increase in the pneumococcidal power of the blood for all three types, while protective substances and agglutinins appeared for the homologous type only.

Animals and man may also develop specific humoral antibody or specific immunity to infection or both as the result of immunization with certain extracts or derivatives of pneumococci, such as the specific capsular polysaccharide or substances which appear either identical with or closely related to it. The antigenicity of such substances has been demonstrated in mice (1012, 440, 1011, 1160, 1369, 422, 1470, 41, 395, 424), rats (1130, 1132, 1133, 1134), rabbits (424), horses (424), and man (485, 459, 461, 1469, 478, 424, 433, 425). The injection into animals of other fractions or extracts of pneumococci does not give rise to the appearance of specific antibody or resistance (1012, 1370, 1313).

Finland and Sutliff (461) observed some interesting differences in the antibody response of twenty-nine adults receiving intradermal injections of the specific capsular polysaccharide of pneumococci of Type I, II, or III. In persons whose blood showed no pneumococcidal power at the start, the administration of the specific substance was frequently followed by the appearance of such bactericidal power for the homologous type (only) with or without protective substances or agglutinins for the same type. Among other individuals, however, whose blood showed some killing power for various types prior to the intradermal injection of the specific substance, the response was somewhat different. In this group the injection was frequently followed by a decrease in the titer or a complete loss of the pneumococcidal power for both the homologous and heterologous types, accompanied by the appearance of protective substances or agglutinins or both for the homologous type only.

Presence of Infection or Other Disease

The presence of various infections and of other diseases may have a significant influence upon the resistance of the host. It has long been recognized that the occurrence of a mixed or secondary infection complicating the course of pneumococcus pneumonia seriously affects the prognosis, presumably by lessening the general immunity of the host. Secondary infections, especially with streptococci, are occasionally responsible for the death of patients with pneumococcus pneumonia who have received specific antipneumococcic serum treatment (see pages 918–920). The prognosis in dogs with experimental pneumococcus lobar pneumonia may be unfavorably affected by the occurrence of an intercurrent attack of snuffles (1292). Lesions produced by the intradermal injection of live pneumococci and *H. influenzae* into rabbits may progress more rapidly than if either organism is used alone (534), and the same appears true following the intranasal infection of mice with *H. influenzae* and influenza virus (664).

The common occurrence of pneumococcus pneumonia subsequent to outbreaks of infections such as the common cold, influenza, measles, scarlet fever, and the like suggests that these conditions may also depress the resistance of the host. Clear proof that a lessening of the total immunity, both circulating and cellular, occurs in such instances is, however, lacking. In fact, much of the data available tend to suggest that, rather than a lowering of host resistance in many such instances, more particularly in the presence of virus infections, there may occur an increase in the biologic activities of the organism present in the upper respiratory tract.

The only direct information at hand relative to possible variations of immunity as a consequence of infections such as those mentioned is apparently that obtained by Graeser and Harrison (551), who made observations on the bactericidal power of the blood for pneumococci of Types I and II in fourteen persons experiencing colds and in twelve with an influenza-like infection. Significant alterations in the incidence or degree of the killing power for these types were not found to occur as the result of such infections. In addition, Francis (480, 481), in a study of mice infected with a strain of influenza virus together with pneumococci, was unable to detect that the virus infection induced a transformation of degraded forms of pneumococci into actively pathogenic types. However, Shibley, Hanger, and Dochez (1181) and Dochez with these and other workers (369, 1182, 370, 1183, 366, 367, 359) have reported evidence suggesting that, in the presence of infections such as the infectious type of the common cold, organisms normally resident in the upper respiratory passages may become activated, with the result that their numbers and virulence are increased and pulmonary infection is frequently produced. These observations, together with those of other workers which presumably indicate that lobar pneumonia due to pneumococci of a given type may develop in individuals who possess considerable circulating antibody specific for that type, as earlier mentioned (see pages 127–129), give support to the view that under some conditions pneumonia may be brought about in consequence of the presence and activities in the upper respiratory tract of organisms of high virulence. Nevertheless, the changes necessary for the production of pulmonary infection may be as varied as they are complex (see pages 232–257), and it is clear that the presence in the upper respiratory tract of organisms of high virulence is not alone sufficient to cause pneumonia.

As elsewhere mentioned, there is some evidence suggesting that individuals who carry pneumococci in their nose or throat, more particularly those who are persistent carriers of these organisms, may be regarded as undergoing pneumococcus infection (see pages 155–157, and 373–378). Studies carried on over a considerable period of time by Gundel (577) in adults and by Gundel and Okura (580) in children failed to demonstrate the appearance of circulating antibodies specific for the types carried. Bull and McKee (172), however, observed the production of specific antibody in rabbits, and Neufeld and Etinger-Tulczynska frequently (933) but not always (934) observed the development of specific immunity to infection in mice, among those in which the carrier state was artificially induced; and Finland and Tilghman (465) occasionally found humoral antibody specific for the types carried among several normal persons studied. In man, carriers of pneumococci appear extremely common among individuals suffering from minor upper respiratory infections such as the common cold (see pages 342–378), and in several instances Winkler and Finland (1429) and Finland and

Winkler (468, 469) demonstrated in the blood of persons experiencing such infections the presence of circulating antibody specific for the type of pneumococcus carried. These observations presumably indicate that carriers of pneumococci may develop some immunity against the organism carried.

Variations of immunity also appear to occur in the presence of certain other conditions. It is probable that individuals suffering from some abnormal conditions and diseased states other than those immediately associated with acute infection may have a lowered resistance, for the general physical condition of patients with pneumonia may be an important factor in determining the outcome in many instances (see pages 699–702). Variations in general immunity are presumably reflected in variations in the incidence and mortality rates of pneumonia, and such rates appear influenced by numerous factors, as is pointed out in the chapter on Epidemiology (page 258).

Miscellaneous Factors

The evidence available suggests that immunity of a local or general nature or both may be depressed by exposure to certain unfavorable conditions, such as marked temperature variations, wetting, chilling, and trauma, or by the intimate contact of the pulmonary tissues with foreign substances. The most significant available data concerning the probable importance of the role played by these conditions are those relating to the morbidity and mortality rates of pneumonia in man (see pages 299–342).

The importance of temperature variations, wetting, and chilling in relation to resistance generally is also suggested by observations made in the course of the experimental infection of limited numbers of animals (918, 728, 940, 1259, 1292, 483, 954, 926). Though inconclusive, it appears from the pertinent evidence that experimental pulmonary infection may be successfully induced and may terminate fatally more often in animals who are subjected to intermittent heating and chilling and at times to wetting as well, than in controls not exposed to these conditions (918, 728, 1259, 954). In addition, McDowell (835) exposed rats to various temperature and humidity combinations before and after intraperitoneal infection. With high temperatures (83° F.), humidity appeared a significant factor, and immunity appeared optimum in such instances with a medium relative humidity ranging between 44 and 72 per cent. With medium temperatures (65°–71° F.), the relative humidity appeared of little importance. Animals acclimated to a medium temperature showed a lowered resistance when changed to a high temperature (83° F.) subsequent to pneumococcus infection.

While investigating experimental lobar pneumonia in dogs, Terrell, Robertson, and Coggeshall (1292) observed that the administration of morphine was followed by a considerable depression of body temperature for a period of several hours and that it was almost essential that such a phenomenon take place if a satisfactory lesion was to be produced. Doses of culture which regularly caused disease in morphinized dogs had little effect on dogs not receiving morphine. As the administration of morphine also caused some lowering of the pulse and respiration rates, the absolute significance of the lowering of body temperature alone in respect to the development of an extensive pulmonary lesion could not be determined. Francis and Terrell (483) obtained essentially comparable results in a study of experimental lobar pneumonia in monkeys. In this instance the animals with the most marked reduction in temperature following the use of morphine and ether became the sickest. In man following operative procedures, a decrease in body temperature is not uncommon, and at times post-operative pulmonary complications may develop (see pages 515–524).

Nedzel's (926) interesting experiments with dogs, in which thermocouples were planted in various places in the body following which the animals were exposed to high temperatures (hot water bottles) or chilling (ice bags), showed that the application of cold to the skin resulted in a drop in temperature of the skin and within the abdominal aorta and of the mucous membranes of the trachea at various levels. The reverse changes occurred following the application of heat to the skin. In both instances the most pronounced internal temperature variations were found in the mucous membranes of the upper trachea, while changes of temperature were less marked in the lower trachea and were least in the primary bronchi. Such changes occurred in an irregular wave-like manner and were attributed to alterations in the flow of blood through the tissues concerned due to reflex stimulation of the vasoconstrictor and vasodilator nerves.

The exposure of man to chilling due to drafts was shown experimentally by Winslow and Greenburg (1430) to produce a drop in skin temperature accompanied by drying and ischaemia of the nasal mucous membrane. In many persons, and especially in those having abnormalities of the nose, such as a deviated septum, exposure of the skin of the face or body to light rays from a dull red or dark source of heat produced congestion of the nasal mucous membrane with a narrowing of the airway (642, 1431).

Trauma to the pulmonary tissue of a local nature, such as that caused by the intrabronchial injection of sterile bouillon, killed broth cultures of pneumococci, starch, or other solutions of foreign matter, may under suitable circumstances lower the resistance locally and assist in the production of pulmonary lesions (1438, 146, 766, 1084, 483, 285). The inhalation of bromine (728) or of other irritating gases of the kind commonly used in present-day warfare frequently has a somewhat similar effect (see pages 340–342).

Alcohol appears to have a definitely unfavorable effect upon the general immunity of infected animals and to allow the frequent development of serious or even fatal infections not seen in controls (728, 1238, 1243, 534). Goodner (534) noted that a depression of general resistance occurred in intradermally infected rabbits which were placed in an abnormal position on their backs for several hours after infection, as septicaemia rather than localization of the infection occurred. In animals, avitaminosis (935, 564) and pregnancy (935) have also been reported to lead to a depression of general immunity.

In many respects the influence of season on general immunity appears striking, for in temperate zones pneumonia is most frequent during the winter months (see pages 289–295) and the fatality rates of cases occurring in the colder months appear higher than the rates of cases occurring at other times (see pages 679–681). Experimentally it has not been possible, however, to produce clear evidence of variation of host resistance in different seasons as the standards by which such alterations may be accurately measured are usually also subject to seasonal influences. In this connection the findings of Terrell, Robertson, and Coggeshall (1292) in dogs and of Francis and Terrell (483) in monkeys are of interest. In both studies it was observed that the susceptibility of the animals appeared generally greater in winter than in summer, as a serious pulmonary infection could usually be brought about by smaller doses of pneumococci in the former than in the latter period. Even though considerable individual variation was encountered with different animals, these findings likewise suggest that host resistance may be lower in winter than in summer. From a study of the marked seasonal variations shown in the incidence of pneumococcus carriers among various groups of normal people, Webster and Hughes (1393) also believe that the immunity of man is considerably influenced by seasonal changes and is lower in winter than in summer (see page 378).

Though the factors listed in the foregoing discussion appear to be a formidable group, it hardly seems that the list can yet be complete, and it is clear that fundamentally very little is known of the role in immunity of any of the factors above considered. It is desirable that additional observations be made.

CHAPTER FIVE

EXPERIMENTAL PNEUMOCOCCUS INFECTIONS AND PATHOGENESIS OF LOBAR PNEUMONIA

Experimental Pneumococcus Infections in Animals 204
Subcutaneous and Intradermal Infection 205
Intravenous Infection 212
Intraperitoneal Infection 213
Subarachnoid Infection 213
Intranasal Instillation of Pneumococcus Cultures 214
Exposure to Inhalation of Sprayed Cultures 217
Intratracheal Infection 218
Intrabronchial Infection 224
Infection by Other Routes 231
Summary 231
Pathogenesis of Pneumococcus Lobar Pneumonia 232
General Factors in Pathogenesis 233
Relation of Minor Respiratory Infections to Occurrence of Pneumonia 235
Allergy and Lobar Pneumonia 240
Route of Infection: Air, Blood, Lymph 245
Site and Nature of Initial Lesion 247
Atelectasis and Pathogenesis 250
Spread of Lesion 253
Summary 256

EXPERIMENTAL PNEUMOCOCCUS INFECTIONS IN ANIMALS

The experimental infection of animals with pneumococci given by various routes has been studied by numerous workers. Attention has already been called to the results obtained in many such instances, and frequent reference is made to pertinent experimental findings in the subsequent discussions in this chapter and in several other chapters. As a consequence of this thorough documentation of the text, it is unnecessary to present a detailed elaboration of the results obtained by the experimental infection of animals. However, where the special significance of certain observations has not been recorded elsewhere in the book, reference will be made to them here.

A general review of the data at hand reveals that, except in a few instances, as noted below, observers paid little or no attention to the fact that the native resistance of animals to the pneumococcus varies with the species and the breed. It is quite possible that certain discrepancies in the results of experiments may be attributed to failure to note this variation. Much of the older literature on the experimental infection of animals has been reviewed by Wadsworth (1361), and subsequent surveys have been made by other investigators (556, 1417).

Infections of an experimental nature have been incited in animals for various purposes, such as for determining the pathogenicity and virulence of pneumococci, estimating degrees of resistance, and investigating the mechanics of immunity, as well as for studying the pathogenesis and pathology of pneumococcus pneumonia. To avoid needless discussion, many of the reports at hand have been condensed and presented in tabular form. Table 41, in which the experiments are listed chronologically by animal and by route of infection, may prove of use for reference (pages 206–211).

It is apparent that the mouse, rabbit, monkey, and dog have been most widely used in experimental work with the pneumococcus. In relation to the pathogenesis of pneumonia, some interest attaches to the route by which organisms are administered. In nearly all the studies cited in the following discussion, the pneumococci used for the infection of animals were of moderate or high virulence, though occasional exceptions will be noted.

Subcutaneous and Intradermal Infection

The subcutaneous injection of pneumococci into normal animals, while giving rise to but little local reaction and practically no pulmonary lesion, rather commonly leads to a fatal septicaemia (1002, 1227, 1284, 1361, 122, 1377, 571, 218). Essentially similar to this, so far as the lack of pulmonary lesions and the frequency of occurrence of invasion of the blood are concerned, are the results obtained from the intradermal injection of normal rabbits with strains of Type I or II or with certain strains of Type III pneumococci virulent for this animal, and doubtless the response to the administration by this route of virulent pneumococci of other types would be somewhat the same. The local lesion, however, is usually pronounced, as Goodner (531, 532) and others have shown, and generally appears eight to twelve hours after infection followed by an abrupt rise in temperature. Bacteriemia may precede or follow the development of the visible lesion and is commonly progressive, in most instances leading to death within sixty to seventy hours. At times spontaneous recovery may occur accompanied by the appearance of specific humoral antibodies.

TABLE 41. AUTHORS AND REFERENCE NUMBERS OF ARTICLES DEALING WITH THE EXPERIMENTAL PNEUMOCOCCUS INFECTION OF VARIOUS ANIMALS, BY ROUTE OF INFECTION AND BY EXPERIMENTAL ANIMAL

ROUTE OF INFECTION	MOUSE	RABBIT	GUINEA PIG	MONKEY	CAT	DOG	RAT	PIGEON
Subcutaneous infection								
Pasteur, 1881	–	1002	–	–	–	–	–	–
Sternberg, 1881	–	1227	–	–	–	–	–	–
Tchistovitch, 1890	1284	1284	–	–	–	1284	–	–
Wadsworth, 1904	–	1361	–	–	–	–	–	–
Blake & Cecil, 1920	–	–	–	122	–	–	–	–
Wámoscher, 1926	1377	–	–	–	–	–	–	–
Griffith, 1928	571	–	–	–	–	–	–	–
Catron, 1935	218	–	–	–	–	–	–	–
Cooper, Gross, & Mellon, 1937	317	–	–	–	–	–	–	–
Intradermal infection								
Goodner, 1928	–	531	–	–	–	–	–	–
Goodner, 1928	–	532	–	–	–	–	–	–
Tillett, 1928	–	1310	–	–	–	–	–	–
Watson & Cooper, 1930	–	1390	–	–	–	–	–	–
Sabin, 1931	–	1150	–	–	–	–	–	–
Rhoads & Goodner, 1931	–	1076	–	–	–	–	–	–
Goodner, 1931	–	534	–	–	–	–	–	–
Blackman, Brown, & Rake, 1931	–	115	–	–	–	–	–	–
Goodner, Dubos, & Avery, 1932	–	539	–	–	–	–	–	–
Curphey & Baruch, 1932	–	336	–	–	–	–	–	–
Goodner & Dubos, 1932	–	538	–	–	–	–	–	–
Blake, 1932	–	–	121	–	–	–	–	–
Powell, Jamieson, Bailey, & Hyde, 1933	–	1047	–	–	–	–	–	–
Sabin, 1933	–	1152	–	–	–	–	–	–
Goodner, 1933	–	535	–	–	–	–	–	–
Goodner & Stillman, 1933	–	548	–	–	–	–	–	–
Gelari & Sabin, 1933	–	512	–	–	–	–	–	–
Rich, 1933	–	1077	–	–	–	–	–	–
Rich, Jennings, & Downing, 1933	–	1078	–	–	–	–	–	–
Goodner, 1934	–	536	–	–	–	–	–	–
Kolmer & Rule, 1934	–	740	–	–	–	–	–	–

TABLE 41 (*cont.*)

ROUTE OF INFECTION	MOUSE	RABBIT	GUINEA PIG	MONKEY	CAT	DOG	RAT	PIGEON
Intradermal infection (cont.)								
Kolmer & Rule, 1934	–	741	–	–	–	–	–	–
Kreidler, 1937	–	745	–	–	–	–	–	–
Intravenous infection								
Wadsworth, 1904	–	1361	–	–	–	–	–	–
Wadsworth, 1912	–	1363	–	–	–	1363	–	–
Cole, 1912	–	289	–	–	–	–	–	–
Kitagawa, 1914	–	722	–	–	–	–	–	–
Kyes, 1916	–	–	–	–	–	–	–	749
Bull, 1916	–	–	–	–	–	169	–	–
Blake & Cecil, 1920	–	–	–	122	–	–	–	–
Blake & Cecil, 1920	–	–	–	125	–	–	–	–
Schöbl & Sellards, 1926	–	–	–	1162	–	–	–	–
Wright, 1927	–	1448	–	–	–	–	–	–
Tillett, 1927	–	1309	–	–	–	–	–	–
Tillett, 1928	–	1310	–	–	–	–	–	–
Bull & McKee, 1929	–	173	–	–	–	–	–	–
Julianelle & Rhoads, 1932	–	702	–	–	–	–	–	–
Goodner, 1934	–	537	–	–	–	–	–	–
Fried, 1934	–	496	–	–	–	–	–	–
Nishikawa, 1935	–	954	–	–	–	–	–	–
Drinker, Enders, Shaffer, & Leigh, 1935	–	377	–	–	–	–	–	–
Rake, 1936	1059	–	–	–	–	–	–	–
Intraperitoneal infection								
Strouse, 1909	1253	–	–	–	–	–	–	1253
Neufeld & Händel, 1909	936	–	–	–	–	–	–	–
Neufeld & Händel, 1910	937	–	–	–	–	–	–	–
Morgenroth & Levy, 1911	910	–	–	–	–	–	–	–
Ungermann & Kandiba, 1912	1330	–	–	–	–	–	–	–
Dochez, 1912	356	–	–	–	–	–	–	–
Dochez & Gillespie, 1913	364	–	–	–	–	–	–	–
Clough, 1913	278	–	–	–	–	–	–	–
Avery, Chickering, Cole, & Dochez, 1917	33	–	–	–	–	–	–	–

TABLE 41 (*cont.*)

ROUTE OF INFECTION	MOUSE	RABBIT	GUINEA PIG	MONKEY	CAT	DOG	RAT	PIGEON
Intraperitoneal infection (*cont.*)								
Moore & Chesney, 1917	903	–	–	–	–	–	–	–
McDowell, 1923	–	–	–	–	–	–	835	–
Felton, 1924	407	–	–	–	–	–	–	–
Hirano, 1925	646	–	–	–	–	–	–	–
Felton & Bailey, 1926	426	–	–	–	–	–	–	–
Woo, 1926	–	1439	–	–	–	–	–	–
Rosenau, Felton, & Atwater, 1926	1111	–	–	–	–	–	–	–
Powell, Atwater, & Felton, 1926	1048	–	–	–	–	–	–	–
Jacobson, 1927	682	–	–	–	–	–	–	–
Griffith, 1928	571	–	–	–	–	–	–	–
Dawson, 1928	344	–	–	–	–	–	–	–
Whittle, 1928	1422	–	–	–	–	–	–	–
Goodner, 1928	532	–	–	–	–	–	–	–
Felton, 1928	412	–	–	–	–	–	–	–
Tillett, 1928	–	1310	–	–	–	–	–	–
Felton, 1930	414	–	–	–	–	–	–	–
Felton, 1930	415	–	–	–	–	–	–	–
Felton, 1930	416	–	–	–	–	–	–	–
Sabin, 1931	1150	–	–	–	–	–	–	–
Webster & Hughes, 1931	1393	–	–	–	–	–	–	–
Gundel & Wasu, 1931	584	–	–	–	–	–	–	–
Avery & Dubos, 1931	39	–	–	–	–	–	–	–
Shultz, 1932	1187	–	–	–	–	–	–	–
Gundel & Schwarz, 1932	582	–	–	–	–	–	–	–
Petrie & Morgan, 1932	1018	–	–	–	–	–	–	–
McDaniels, 1932	–	–	–	–	–	–	834	–
Schattenberg & Harris, 1932	1159	–	–	–	–	–	–	–
Felton, 1932	420	–	–	–	–	–	–	–
Felton, 1932	421	–	–	–	–	–	–	–
Cruickshank, 1933	331	–	–	–	–	–	–	–
Hartley, Parish, Petrie, & Smith, 1933	601	–	–	–	–	–	–	–
Morgan & Petrie, 1933	909	–	–	–	–	–	–	–
Webster & Clow, 1933	1392	–	–	–	–	–	–	–
Gundel & Seitz, 1933	583	–	–	–	–	–	–	–
Rosenthal, 1934	1122	–	–	–	–	–	–	–

TABLE 41 (*cont.*)

ROUTE OF INFECTION	MOUSE	RABBIT	GUINEA PIG	MONKEY	CAT	DOG	RAT	PIGEON
Intraperitoneal infection (*cont.*)								
Ross, 1934	–	–	–	–	–	–	1137	–
Maclachlan, Permar, Johnston, & Kenney, 1934	848	–	–	–	–	–	–	–
Hartley & Smith, 1935	602	–	–	–	–	–	–	–
Goodner & Horsfall, 1935	540	–	–	–	–	–	–	–
Goodner & Miller, 1935	546	–	–	–	–	–	–	–
Goodner & Miller, 1935	547	–	–	–	–	–	–	–
Schmidt, 1937	1161	–	–	–	–	–	–	–
Rosenthal, 1937	1123	–	–	–	–	–	–	–
Cooper, Gross, & Mellon, 1937	317	–	–	–	–	–	–	–
Felton & Stahl, 1937	432	–	–	–	–	–	–	–
Subarachnoid infection								
Stewart, 1927	–	1229	–	–	–	–	–	–
Stewart, 1927	–	–	–	–	–	1230	–	–
Stewart, 1928	–	–	–	–	–	1231	–	–
Stewart, 1928	–	–	–	–	–	1232	–	–
Kolmer, 1931	–	–	–	–	–	736	–	–
Intranasal instillation of organisms								
Bull & McKee, 1928	–	172	–	–	–	–	–	–
Bull & McKee, 1929	–	173	–	–	–	–	–	–
Neufeld & Etinger-Tulczynska, 1931	933	933	933	–	–	–	–	–
Neufeld & Etinger-Tulczynska, 1932	934	–	934	–	–	–	–	–
Greene, 1933	–	564	–	–	–	–	–	–
Webster & Clow, 1933	1392	–	–	–	–	–	–	–
Hoyle, 1935	664	–	–	–	–	–	–	–
Rake, 1936	1058	–	–	–	–	–	–	–
Rake, 1936	1059	–	–	–	–	–	–	–
Inhalation of sprayed cultures								
Blake & Cecil, 1920	–	–	–	122	–	–	–	–
Stillman, 1924	1237	–	–	–	–	–	–	–
Stillman, 1924	1238	–	–	–	–	–	–	–
Stillman & Branch, 1924	1243	–	–	–	–	–	–	–
Branch & Stillman, 1924	146	–	–	–	–	–	–	–

TABLE 41 (*cont.*)

ROUTE OF INFECTION	MOUSE	RABBIT	GUINEA PIG	MONKEY	CAT	DOG	RAT	PIGEON
Inhalation of sprayed cultures (cont.)								
Stillman, 1930	–	1239	–	–	–	–	–	–
Stillman, 1930	–	1240	–	–	–	–	–	–
Stillman & Branch, 1931	1244	–	–	–	–	–	–	–
Intratracheal infection								
Tchistovitch, 1890	1284	1284	–	–	–	1284	–	–
Wadsworth, 1904	–	1361	–	–	–	–	–	–
Newburgh, Means, & Porter, 1916	–	–	–	–	949	949	–	–
Kline, 1917	–	–	–	–	–	726	–	–
Wadsworth, 1918	–	–	–	–	–	1364	–	–
Winternitz, Smith, & Robinson, 1920	–	1433	–	–	–	–	–	–
Blake & Cecil, 1920	–	–	–	122	–	–	–	–
Blake & Cecil, 1920	–	–	–	123	–	–	–	–
Blake & Cecil, 1920	–	–	–	125	–	–	–	–
Cecil & Blake, 1920	–	–	–	231	–	–	–	–
Cecil & Blake, 1920	–	–	–	232	–	–	–	–
Cecil & Blake, 1920	–	–	–	233	–	–	–	–
Cecil & Steffen, 1921	–	–	–	240	–	–	–	–
Cecil & Steffen, 1922	–	–	–	241	–	–	–	–
Cecil & Steffen, 1923	–	–	–	242	–	–	–	–
Permar, 1923	–	1013	–	–	–	–	–	–
Permar, 1923		1014	–	–	–	–	–	–
Leake, Vickers, & Brown, 1924	–	–	–	–	–	772	–	–
Cecil & Steffen, 1925	–	–	–	243	–	–	–	–
Cecil & Steffen, 1925	–	–	–	244	–	–	–	–
Schöbl & Sellards, 1926	–	–	–	1162	–	–	–	–
Nakajima, 1926	–	922	–	–	–	–	–	–
Parker, 1929	–	–	998	–	–	–	–	–
Kramár & Gyüre, 1930	744	744	–	–	–	–	–	–
Stuppy, Falk, & Jacobson, 1931	–	–	–	1260	–	–	–	–
Francis & Terrell, 1934	–	–	–	483	–	–	–	–
Francis, Terrell, Dubos, & Avery, 1934	–	–	–	484	–	–	–	–
Fried, 1934	–	496	–	–	–	–	–	–
Intrabronchial infection								
Lamar & Meltzer, 1912	–	–	–	–	–	757	–	–
Wadsworth, 1912	–	–	–	–	–	1363	–	–

TABLE 41 (*cont.*)

ROUTE OF INFECTION	MOUSE	RABBIT	GUINEA PIG	MONKEY	CAT	DOG	RAT	PIGEON
Intrabronchial infection (cont.)								
Wollstein & Meltzer, 1913	–	–	–	–	–	1437	–	–
Kline & Meltzer, 1914	–	–	–	–	–	727	–	–
Kline & Winternitz, 1915	–	728	–	–	–	–	–	–
Gaskell, 1925	–	508	–	–	–	–	–	–
Christie, Ehrich, & Binger, 1928	–	–	–	–	–	269	–	–
Coryllos, 1929	–	–	–	–	–	322	–	–
Henderson, Haggard, Coryllos, & Birnbaum, 1930	–	–	–	–	–	632	–	–
Terrell, 1930	–	–	–	–	–	1290	–	–
Terrell, 1930	–	–	–	–	–	1291	–	–
Stuppy & Falk, 1931	–	1259	–	–	–	–	–	–
Kolmer & Rule, 1932	–	737	–	–	–	–	–	–
Terrell, Robertson, & Coggeshall, 1933	–	–	–	–	–	1292	–	–
Robertson, Coggeshall, & Terrell, 1933	–	–	–	–	–	1083	–	–
Robertson, Coggeshall, & Terrell, 1933	–	–	–	–	–	1084	–	–
Lieberman & Leopold, 1934	–	–	–	–	–	782	–	–
Francis & Terrell, 1934	–	–	–	483	–	–	–	–
Francis, Terrell, Dubos, & Avery, 1934	–	–	–	484	–	–	–	–
Coggeshall & Robertson, 1935	–	–	–	–	–	286	–	–
Coggeshall, 1935	–	–	–	–	–	285	–	–
Gross & Cooper, 1937	–	–	–	–	–	–	572	–
Intrapleural or intra-pulmonary infection								
Friedländer, 1883	–	–	–	–	–	501	–	–
Wadsworth, 1904	–	1361	–	–	–	–	–	–
Neufeld & Ungermann, 1912	–	–	942	–	–	–	–	–
Robertson, Woo, Cheer, & King, 1928	–	1097	–	–	1097	–	–	–
Terrell, 1930	–	–	–	–	1290	1290	–	–
Terrell, 1930	–	–	–	–	1291	1291	–	–
Infection of anterior eye chamber								
Tchistovitch, 1890	1284	1284	–	–	–	1284	–	–

After infection of the skin over the abdomen, the local lesion consists of a discolored swollen edematous area which frequently spreads so as to cover an area many centimeters in diameter. Much edema is present in the early lesion (1076), and by various procedures the spread of the lesion may be controlled by controlling the direction of the spread of the edema fluid. In this respect the effect of gravity on the edema fluid is important (534). The presence of other organisms in addition to pneumococci (534) or of autolysates prepared from an S or R culture of pneumococci of homologous or heterologous type (535) accelerates the development of the lesion and increases the severity of the infection.

Intradermal infections of decreasing severity were produced in the presence of increasing levels of natural (121) or of specific active or passive immunity (531, 532, 1310, 1390, 1152, 548, 512, 536, 740, 218, 336, 1077, 1078). The therapeutic value of various preparations other than specific immune serums was tested in intradermally infected rabbits. The preparations used were so-called antitoxic serum (1150), solutions of a specific enzyme (539, 538), heterophile antibody serum (1047), gold salts (512), and ethylhydrocupreine hydrochloride (optochin) and quinine (741), as well as sulfanilamide (745). The ability of pneumococci to give rise to nephritis in infected rabbits (115) was also tested.

Intravenous Infection

Many animals have been infected intravenously for the purpose of studying the factors important in the mechanism of natural immunity (1363, 722, 749, 169, 496, 377), active immunity (1363, 722, 125, 1309, 1448, 1310, 173, 702), or passive immunity (537, 377). Efforts to produce pneumonia by the intravenous injection of living virulent pneumococci into normal rabbits (1361, 954) and monkeys (*Macacus syrichtus,* 122, 1162, and *Cebus capucinus,* 122) were not successful.

Rake (1059), however, has reported the successful production of pneumonia in controlled breeds of normal mice following intravenous infection with carefully selected strains of pneumococci of Type I, II, III, or XIX of high intranasal or intraperitoneal virulence. It was necessary to use organisms of such virulence and breeds of mice of such resistance that the infected animals would live two days or longer after infection, and under these circumstances definite pneumonia was produced in twelve of eighty-seven mice infected intravenously and lesser pulmonary lesions occurred in most of the others. The interstitial reaction was marked. The early lesion consisted in a collection of fluid, monocytes, and polymorphonuclear leucocytes in the interstitial tissues of the alveolar septums. In advanced lesions the alveolar walls were many times their original thickness due to the infiltration of fluid and cells, and frequently an exudate of fluid and cells was present in the alveoli. In no instance did the number of leucocytes within the alveoli become so great that the exudate was predominantly cellular. This deficiency may have been due to the fact that the survival time was short and never exceeded four days. In any event, it was reported that the lesions produced resembled in no way the spontaneous pulmonary lesions occasionally found in mice. It seems, in consequence, that Rake, in 1936, demonstrated that pneumonia may be produced by the intravenous infection of normal mice not previously prepared by any immunizing procedure. This appears to be the first demonstration of the production of pneumonia by intravenous infection. In some instances lesions were also found in the spleen, liver, and kidney, and these varied somewhat with the serologic type of organism used, while the pneumonia produced did not show such variations.

Intraperitoneal Infection

In the presence of insufficient immunity the intraperitoneal infection of animals leads to a rapidly spreading peritonitis with the development of a variable, but usually progressive, septicaemia and other evidence of infection, resulting in death. Intraperitoneal infections have been largely used in the study of natural immunity (1253, 835, 1159, 1018, 1392, 1137), of active immunity (1310, 834), and of passive immunity (936, 937, 1330, 356, 364, 278, 407, 532, 412, 1310, 415, 416, 1018, 601, 909, 602, 540, 546, 547; see also pages 120–121). Such infections have also been incited for the purpose of estimating the virulence of pneumococci (936, 33, 426, 1439, 1111, 1048, 1422, 682, 571, 344, 584, 1393, 1187, 582, 420, 421, 646, 1392, 331) and for determining the therapeutic value of preparations other than specific immune serums (910, 903, 414, 39, 1150, 583, 848, 1122, 1161, 1123, 317).

Subarachnoid Infection

Experimental infections of the subarachnoid space have apparently been but little investigated. Stewart made a limited study of Type I infections of this nature in normal and actively and passively immunized rabbits (1229) and in normal dogs or in those which had recovered from a previous experimental meningitis (1230, 1231). Kolmer (736) also produced Type I meningitis in a few normal dogs. The therapeutic value of specific immune serum was tested in infected animals of both species, and at times ethylhydrocupreine hydrochloride (optochin) was added to the serum given to dogs. Stewart carried out similar investigations in normal dogs infected with pneumococci of Type II (1232).

Septicaemia rather than meningitis occurred in normal rabbits, while in those possessing some immunity slight localization occurred and meningitis was produced. In normal dogs localization was fairly good, though bacteriemia was frequent. The course of the infection in dogs that had recovered from an earlier meningeal infection was largely atypical, suggesting that some active resistance had been acquired. Type II infections gave rise to a more extensive outpouring of fibrin and cells than Type I infections and led to the rapid early production of subarachnoid blocks which appeared to reduce the possibilities of effective treatment.

Intranasal Instillation of Pneumococcus Cultures

The intranasal instillation of pneumococci in normal mice (933, 934, 664), rabbits (172, 173, 933, 564), and guinea pigs (933, 934) of unselected breeds has little effect on some animals, while in others a carrier state of many days' or weeks' duration may be induced (172, 933, 934) with the not uncommon occurrence of a bacteriemia, at times leading to a progressive systemic infection and death (172, 933, 934). By controlling the virulence of the organism used, Hoyle (664) was able to obtain bronchopneumonia following the intranasal infection of normal unselected mice under ether anesthesia.

In actively immunized rabbits, Bull and McKee (172) reported that the carrier state induced by intranasal infection lasted only twenty-four hours or less. Neufeld and Etinger-Tulczynska (933, 934) found the proportion of mice, rabbits, and guinea pigs which became carriers was not altered by a state of active or passive immunity, though in all groups the presence of such resistance did decrease the incidence of bacteriemia and serious infections. Some actively immunized mice exposed to contact with animals carrying pneumococci of Type I developed lesions of a bronchopneumonic type (934).

The detailed observations of Webster and Clow (1392) and of Rake (1058, 1059), who studied the results of the intranasal infection of selected inbred and other strains of normal mice with carefully chosen strains of pneumococci, are doubtless of even greater significance. Under circumstances in which the resistance of the animal was properly balanced against the virulence of the organism, the intranasal instillation of 0.03 cc. of a 1:100 dilution of an eighteen-hour broth culture of pneumococci containing approximately 150,000 organisms frequently gave rise to varying conditions, including pneumonia which at times was of the lobar form.

Webster and Clow (1392) observed that individual mice exhibited marked differences in their behavior toward the pneumococcus, as some were completely refractory while others became carriers of the organism for a few days or weeks and still others developed various forms of deep-seated infection often resulting in death. The incubation period of the serious infections was usually two days, with death occurring in from three to seven days after inoculation. The lesions incited were septicaemia, pneumonia, pleurisy, empyema, pericarditis, and cervical lymphadenitis. This report appears to be the first in the literature in which it was demonstrated that pneumonia could be produced by the intranasal infection of normal unprepared mice.

At least fifty strains of pneumococci of eleven types freshly isolated from man were used in Webster and Clow's study. Determinations were made of the comparative intranasal and intraperitoneal virulence of the strains used and of their ability to set up a carrier state or produce a fatal infection in contacts. Some strains showed individual characteristics with respect to their intranasal virulence and their ability to persist in survivors and spread to contacts. It was stated:

> The tests brought out a parallelism between degree of intranasal virulence and tendency to persist in survivors and spread to contacts to the extent that strains which spread to contacts were invariably of high intranasal virulence and strains which set up the carrier state in survivors were generally of moderate or high intranasal virulence.

It was also observed that in 50 per cent of the strains the degree of intranasal virulence did not parallel the degree of intraperitoneal virulence.

High intranasal virulence was accompanied by either high or moderate intraperitoneal virulence, and low intranasal virulence by low, moderate, or high intraperitoneal virulence. Most of the Type III strains used were of relatively high intranasal and intraperitoneal virulence, while the Type II strains were mostly of low intranasal but of high or moderate intraperitoneal virulence, and the Type I strains were of low intranasal but of either high or low intraperitoneal virulence. Most strains of other types were low in both intranasal and intraperitoneal virulence. Intranasal passage invariably led to a sudden drop in intranasal virulence from the level characteristic for the strain to zero without altering the intraperitoneal virulence of the strain or changing its usual form of smooth colony formation or its agglutinative properties. Intraperitoneal passage at times enhanced intraperitoneal virulence but did not alter intranasal virulence.

Rake's (1058, 1059) investigations dealt chiefly with the pathology and development of the lesions incited by the intranasal infection of inbred and unselected mice of various breeds. Lesions with quantitative differences could be produced in different breeds of mice by intranasal infection with pneumococci of the same type. Among the members of a single standard group of mice that died, the lesions produced were predictable and were closely similar for pneumococci of a given type even though the intranasal virulence of the strains differed, but the lesions varied with the type of the organism used. For example, so far as the lung lesions were concerned, pneumococci of Type I produced diffuse changes without special localization while those of Type II gave an ample alveolar exudate often with lobar distribution, and with Type III the most prominent feature was a localization of the lesion in the interstitial tissues of the alveolar septums. In the latter instance the exudate was gelatinous and was often accompanied by the appearance of a lobular pneumonia with an exudative pleurisy as well as by marked lesions of the lymphatic system including necrosis of the cervical and hilar lymph nodes and follicles of the spleen. The kidneys showed the most marked lesions of the other organs; and Type I infections frequently gave rise to acute diffuse nephritis, Type II to a predominantly tubular nephritis, and Type III to no special kidney lesion.

In some instances within one minute after the intranasal infection of mice with a strain of pneumococci of Type III, organisms of this type were obtained by culture from the trachea, heart, and lungs (Rake 1059). Of more than one hundred mice infected by the nasal route, positive blood cultures were obtained from the tail blood in 32.9 per cent during the first ten minutes after infection. The evidence seemed clear that organisms were present throughout the extent of the respiratory tract almost immediately after infection and that they promptly appeared in the blood. While it was uncertain at what region the invasion of the blood occurred, it seemed probable that organisms might enter the blood at one or more points in the respiratory tract. As points of entry, the mucous membrane of the nose (933) or the walls of the alveoli or both (1059) have been suggested.

Exposure to Inhalation of Sprayed Cultures

Blake and Cecil (122) sprayed the nose and throat of a few monkeys with a culture of Type I pneumococci. Though the animals remained well, all became carriers of these organisms for at least a month.

Stillman, either alone or with Branch, has observed the effects of subjecting normal or immunized mice (1237, 1238, 1243, 146, 1244) and normal rabbits (1239, 1240) to the inhalation of sprayed cultures of pneumococci of different types and varying virulence. In normal mice the inspired organisms were found on culture in the trachea and deep in the lungs shortly after exposure to the organisms in spray form (146). In most instances pneumococci disappeared from the lungs within three hours, and at the end of some time no bacteriemia was found (1237). The disposal of the organisms from the lung was delayed for as long as twenty-four hours in mice intoxicated by the intraperitoneal injection of a standard dose of alcohol, and positive blood cultures were found in 16 per cent of such animals. Death from septicaemia occurred in 3 per cent of the normal mice and in over 40 per cent of the intoxicated mice.

Repeated exposures to the inhalation of pneumococci in spray form induced a progressively increasing active immunity which was most marked in animals that had been intoxicated with alcohol at the times of exposure (1238). Normal mice dying after the inhalation of pneumococci usually showed a terminal septicaemia without any pulmonary localization of the infection, while in immunized mice septicaemia was less frequent and pulmonary localization was common. In some instances pneumonia of the lobar form was produced (1243).

The pathology of the lung lesions resulting from the inhalation of pneumococci by immunized mice while intoxicated with alcohol was studied by Branch and Stillman (146). In general, the lesions found assumed one of two forms, and either an exudative pleurisy and congestion of the alveolar capillaries was present or an exudative pneumonia which at times assumed the lobar form was found. Where the infection was localized, the earliest lesion was an interstitial inflammation or cellulitis, and much congestion and edema was present in the adjacent tissue. The lymphatics became involved secondarily and appeared to play but a minor role in the spread of the disease. In addition, the findings suggested that for the development of pneumonia having a lobar distribution it was necessary, even when virulent organisms were present deep within the respiratory tract, to break the normal defense barriers of the lung at some point by pulmonary injury. In this instance intoxication with alcohol appeared to be the damaging factor, though the precise nature of the action of alcohol in producing this damaging effect was not determined. Branch and Stillman's conception that pulmonary injury may be necessary for the production of lobar pneumonia has received considerable attention and has been widely quoted.

Pneumococci were also found deep in the lungs of normal rabbits shortly after inhalation (1239). Septicaemia often developed after such exposure to organisms of high virulence but was infrequent after the use of organisms of lower virulence. Specific humoral antibodies appeared more commonly in animals which successfully withstood the inhalation of virulent organisms than in those which had inhaled pneumococci of lower virulence (1240).

Intratracheal Infection

Intratracheal infection with pneumococci has been carried out for various purposes in the following cases:

Normal animals of susceptible species (1284, 1361, 1433, 1013, 922, 998, 744, 496)
Normal animals of more or less resistant species (1284, 949, 726, 1364, 122, 123, 125, 231, 232, 233, 240, 241, 242, 772, 243, 244, 1162, 1260, 483, 484)

Studies were also made of the response to infection by the intratracheal route:

In normal animals
- Mice (1284, 744)
- Rabbits (1284, 1361, 1433, 1013, 1014, 922, 744, 496)
- Dogs (1284, 726, 1364)
- Monkeys (122, 123, 240, 1162, 1260, 483)

In actively immunized animals
- Rabbits (1361, 922)
- Monkeys (125, 231, 232, 240, 241, 242, 243, 1260)

In guinea pigs passively immunized with an anti-autolysate serum (998)

In some instances, infection was incited for the purpose of determining the curative value of specific serums (233, 244) or of a specific enzyme preparation (484), or for other purposes (949, 726, 1364, 772).

In normal susceptible animals, such as the rabbit, intratracheal infection with pneumococci of high virulence was shown to lead to a rapidly developing septicaemia and death with but little pulmonary lesion (1361, 1013, 922). When strains of somewhat lower virulence were used, the pulmonary response was more definite, and at times pneumonia in the bronchopneumonic form was produced (1013, 922). However, by a proper balancing of the virulence of the infecting organism against the resistance of actively immunized rabbits, Wadsworth (1361) obtained pneumonia in the lobar form. The results of his study, carried out in 1904, were of special significance as Wadsworth was apparently the first worker ever to produce lobar pneumonia by experimental means. Nakajima (922) later repeated this study and obtained similar results.

The intratracheal injection of pneumococci into normal animals which possess considerable natural resistance to this organism commonly results in the development of pneumonia which is frequently of the lobar form, as was demonstrated in cats by Newburgh, Means, and Porter (949), in dogs by Tchistovitch (1284) and others (949, 726, 1364, 772), and in monkeys by Blake and Cecil (122, 123) and additional workers (233, 240, 244, 1162, 483). Blake and Cecil (122) infected thirty-seven normal monkeys and in thirty-two instances obtained lobar pneumonia which clinically was identical with lobar pneumonia in man. The case fatality rate was high. These investigators also noted that the contact of a normal monkey with another monkey having an induced Type I infection resulted in the development of a fatal Type I lobar pneumonia in the contact. In a few instances Stuppy, Falk, and Jacobson (1260) failed to obtain pneumonia in monkeys after the intratracheal inoculation of pneumococci of varying virulence.

Careful detailed studies were made of the pathology of the pneumonia produced by the intratracheal infection of normal rabbits (Permar, 1013) and monkeys (Blake and Cecil, 123, Schöbl and Sellards, 1162). In each instance the infecting dose of pneumococci was administered in 1 cc. of liquid.

The first investigation of this nature, in 1920, was that of Blake and Cecil (123), who performed necropsies on forty monkeys (*Macacus syrichtus* and *Cebus capucinus*) with experimentally produced pneumonia, chiefly of the lobar form. Most of the animals had been infected with pneumococci of Type I, but only a few were examined within the first twenty-four hours of infection. The general pathologic picture produced was stated to be identical with that of pneumococcus lobar pneumonia in man. At a number of places the epithelium of the large bronchi was damaged, and pneumococci were seen penetrating the bronchial walls at these points. Early lesions showed a thickening of the vascular adventitia and walls of the bronchi near the lung root, caused largely by edema, which was especially prominent around the blood vessels, and infiltration of polymorphonuclear leucocytes. A few large mononuclear cells and lymphocytes, as well as fibrin, were always present. The walls of the bronchi, interlobular septums, and arteries and veins were involved, and the perivascular, peribronchial, and septal lymphatics were distended and frequently contained large numbers of leucocytes. This early involvement of the interstitial framework of the lung and of the lymphatics was accompanied by an intense capillary engorgement and leucocytic infiltration of the alveolar walls and appeared to precede exudation into the alveoli. The pneumonia produced was regarded as primarily an interstitial infection of the lung. The infection spread rapidly, presumably from the grosser framework of the lungs into the alveolar walls through the interstitial tissues by way of the perivascular, peribronchial, and septal tissue and lymphatics, with the subsequent appearance of organisms and exudate in the alveoli. The lesion progressed through the stages of engorgement, and then red and gray hepatization, to resolution.

Exudation into the alveoli appeared first in the parenchymal tissue about the hilum and later involved the distal portions of the lung, leading to a rather uniform consolidation. Red hepatization was notable for the comparative absence of red blood cells in the fibrinous exudate, the red color being due largely to the marked engorgement of the alveolar capillaries. Interstitial lesions were less conspicuous from here on. After further progression of the process, typical gray hepatization was found, the alveoli being packed with polymorphonuclear leucocytes, a few large mononuclear cells, lymphocytes, and red blood cells in a network of fibrin threads. Alveolar walls were thin but well preserved. The epithelium of the bronchioles and bronchi was comparatively intact. Necrosis was not encountered. Areas first involved were the ones first to show gray hepatization. Resolution was accompanied by an active proliferation and desquamation of the alveolar epithelium. A variable degree of organization of the exudate was always found. The hilum lymph nodes were large and succulent and full of leucocytes.

Permar (1013) later studied the development of pneumonia following the intratracheal infection of normal rabbits with pneumococci of Type I. Preliminary studies with colored fluids showed that, after introducing such substances into the trachea, the fluid spread rapidly over the tracheal surface and down the subdivisions of the bronchial tree to reach the atria and alveoli. The direction of the spread of the fluid was importantly influenced by gravity. Following the use of living pneumococci, bronchopneumonia either well marked or of slight extent was produced in nineteen of twenty-seven rabbits. Early lesions were patchy and consisted of the rapid and nearly simultaneous development of inflammation of the trachea and bronchial tree and its terminal branches, including the communicating atrial and alveolar structures. The severity of the reaction increased toward the terminal bronchioles and was greatest in these and in the bud-like alveoli arising from them and in the alveolar ducts, atria, and alveoli. The reaction in the atria and alveoli consisted primarily of engorgement of the capillaries and the rapid accumulation of polymorphonuclear leucocytes in their walls, which was followed by the appearance in the air spaces of a serofibrinous exudate composed largely of polymorphonuclear leucocytes and endothelial cells accompanied by a variable amount of hemorrhage.

Shortly after this, the interstitial tissues, including all lymphatic networks and nodes, were seen to be involved, and this was followed by a more rapid spread of the lesion. In this instance, then, extension of the process through infection of the interstitial tissues and lymphatics appeared to be a secondary phenomenon. The process began as a bronchopneumonia and spread by peripheral extension, which led to a coalescing condition. In the course of this invasion of other tissues acute lymphangitis occurred, giving rise to acute interstitial pneumonia. Septicaemia was commonly found at necropsy, and the suggestion was made that it may have originated from direct infection of the blood due to ulceration of the vessel walls in the thin tissue surrounding the smaller air passages or to organisms entering the circulation by way of the lymphatic system. The interstitial involvement in rabbits appeared more intense than that usually seen in human pneumonia; otherwise the development of the lesions was regarded as essentially identical.

Subsequent to the previously described observations of Blake and Cecil (123), whose work on pneumonia in monkeys was carried out in a temperate climate (Washington, D.C.), Schöbl and Sellards (1162), working in the tropics (Philippine Islands), likewise studied the pathology of experimental pneumonia in monkeys (*Macacus syrichtus,* also known as *Pithecus philippinensis*). It was not possible to determine the effect of the climatic factor in altering the resistance of the test animals and the pathology of the lesions incited. It was reported, however, that, though the Type I pneumococci used were of the same degree of mouse virulence as the Type I strain used by Blake and Cecil (123), it was necessary in order to produce a fatal infection to give relatively larger doses of culture to monkeys in the tropics.

The results obtained were quite variable, but pneumonia occurred in ten of nineteen monkeys infected. It was again noted that gravity appeared to have an important effect on the direction of the spread of the intratracheally injected suspension of organisms. Superficially, the lesions produced resembled lobar pneumonia, but further examination revealed the absence over the most or the whole of a lobe of definite red or gray hepatization, and after draining off the large amount of edema fluid present the lesions appeared to resemble a confluent bronchopneumonia.

Consolidation began and was most intense about the hilum. The primary infection involved the tracheo-bronchial system, and inflammation was more pronounced in the neighborhood of the terminal bronchioli than in the larger proximal air passages. From this location the process extended directly to the alveolar passages, air sacs, and corresponding alveoli. The alveolar exudate was chiefly composed of polymorphonuclear leucocytes and a few large mononuclear and red blood cells. Some small areas of gray hepatization showed considerable fibrin. Toward the periphery of the lesion much edema fluid containing a few leucocytes was present and the blood vessels were engorged. In general the lesion closely resembled that reported by Permar (1013) in rabbits. Destructive lesions were found in the walls of the air passages in the terminal respiratory bronchioli. The infection probably extended directly and secondarily through these ulcerations into the perivascular lymphatics that surround the blood vessels which are close to the surface of the air passages at this point. The whole process of experimental pneumonia in monkeys appeared as a bronchopneumonia with a secondary interstitial inflammation. The striking feature, in contrast to human lobar pneumonia, was the extensive perivascular and interstitial inflammation seen in pneumonia in monkeys. The frequently encountered bacteriemia was regarded as a product of the secondary peribronchial lymphangitis.

There are certain significant points of similarity in the findings in the above three studies, in spite of the differences in the arrangement of the respiratory passages and subdivisions of the bronchi of the two animal species and also presumably in their native resistance. In each instance pneumonia was produced by the injection of living pneumococci. The initial process was observed to be an inflammatory reaction, beginning about the lower trachea and larger bronchi, which rapidly spread to the finer portions of the bronchial tree. In each instance involvement of the interstitial tissues was noted. The chief difference from the standpoint of the mode of origin of the disease in these studies was that, while Blake and Cecil (123) regarded the spread of the lesion with a perivascular lymphangitis, consequent interstitial pneumonia, and subsequent invasion of the alveoli to be part of the primary process, Permar (1013) and Schöbl and Sellards (1162) regarded the lymphangitis and acute interstitial reaction as secondary phenomena.

In view of the observations of Winternitz, Smith, and Robinson (1433), who questioned whether pulmonary lesions following intratracheal infection resulted from the activity of organisms placed in the lumen of the trachea or from the extension of an unrecognized infection of the tracheal submucosa, mention must be made of the technic usually used to inject organisms intratracheally. In practically every study cited in this section on intratracheal infection, the dose of infecting organisms was administered in one of two ways. One method consisted in the use of a needle and syringe, the needle being inserted through the skin of the neck and into the lumen of the trachea, where the dose of organisms was deposited, after which the needle was withdrawn. By the other method organisms were injected into the upper trachea through a small tube passed through the mouth and larynx. The former procedure was used by many workers including Blake and Cecil (122, 123), whose results are mentioned above, while the latter technic was employed by other investigators such as Permar (1013), whose findings are also cited in some detail.

Winternitz, Smith, and Robinson (1433) carried out the experimental infection of normal rabbits by injecting the organisms into the trachea with a syringe and needle. Various lesions including lobular pneumonia were produced. The tissues of the neck and trachea in the region through which the needle was inserted were subjected to careful examination. Infection along the path of the needle was regularly found, which was accompanied by lesions of the tracheal submucosa and also of the peritracheal and subcutaneous tissues. A leucocytic exudate was present, and a descending infection was noted around and within the lymphatics with which the trachea is richly supplied. This infection could be followed from the trachea into the larger bronchi near the hilum, where it involved the peribronchial and perivascular tissues and portions of the adjacent lung. The findings indicated that the lung infection resulted, not from organisms introduced intratracheally, but from infection of the loose tissue of the submucosa of the trachea, and that possibly the infection was carried by the lymphatics.

Winternitz and his associates carried out additional experiments with the catheter method of implanting organisms in the upper trachea by passing the catheter through the mouth and larynx. The results obtained were essentially identical to those just mentioned, and a small area of damage to the tracheal epithelium, which was presumably the result of trauma from the catheter, was always found just below the larynx. Infection was present in the submucosa of the trachea from this point downward and could be followed in this tissue to the larger bronchi.

These findings presumably constitute a serious challenge to the accuracy of the view that pulmonary infection frequently results from organisms injected intratracheally. Nevertheless, Blake and Cecil (122), who carried out an extensive series of experiments in monkeys, stated: "In no instance at autopsy has there been any evidence of local injury or infection in the trachea or in the tissue surrounding it."

Intrabronchial Infection

The results obtained following the intrabronchial pneumococcus infection of normal rabbits (728, 508, 1259), rats (572), dogs (757, 1363, 1437, 269, 322, 632, 1290, 1291, 1292, 1083, 1084, 782), and monkeys (483, 484), and of rabbits (737) and dogs (727, 286, 285) possessing some acquired resistance have likewise been variously studied. While many of these infections were induced for the purpose of studying the nature of the lesion incited by intrabronchial infection, others were carried out in an effort to determine the therapeutic properties of various general methods of treatment (269, 632, 782, 572), or the curative value of a specific enzyme preparation (484), or for other purposes (728, 1259, 1290, 1291).

The methods used to implant organisms in the bronchi have varied somewhat. Wadsworth (1363), Wollstein and Meltzer (1437), Kline and Winternitz (728), and others (727, 269, 1259, 1290, 1291, 737) have used the technic of Lamar and Meltzer (757), who injected organisms through a small tube passed down to a bronchus through the mouth and larynx. The procedure used by Gaskell (508) was similar except that the tube was passed into a bronchus through an opening in the trachea. A very satisfactory technic was developed and extensively used by Terrell, Robertson, and Coggeshall and their associates (1292, 1083, 1084, 286, 285). This involved injecting the organisms through a radiopaque ureteral catheter passed through the mouth and larynx, the position of the catheter being determined under the fluoroscope. This technic was also employed by Francis and Terrell and their coworkers (483, 484). In some instances Coryllos (322) and others (632, 782) have injected organisms through a bronchoscope.

Kline and Winternitz (728) infected normal rabbits by injecting pneumococci through a small catheter and reported that, when the culture was injected intrabronchially in this fashion using little force, pneumonia occasionally developed; while if the injection was made with considerable force, lobar pneumonia occurred. Such findings suggest that trauma to the pulmonary tissue may assist in the production of lobar pneumonia. These investigators also observed that, though pneumonia in the lobar form resulted from the forcible injection of organisms deep into a terminal bronchus, pulmonary lesions with bronchopneumonia were produced only irregularly if the culture was placed in the upper trachea just beyond the larynx. They also noted that foreign material was aspirated and pneumonia occurred in normal rabbits after both vagus nerves were cut even though no pneumococci were administered to these animals. These findings suggested that some sort of a protective mechanism was present in the upper respiratory tract which under normal conditions functioned to prevent infection from gaining access to the lower trachea and bronchi. Gaskell's (508) observations on experimental pneumonia in the normal rabbit are also in accord with this view, for it was observed that with a dose of Type I pneumococci of a particular size and virulence, little or no pulmonary lesion resulted when the organisms were placed in the upper trachea, while their intrabronchial instillation resulted in a definite pneumonia.

Gaskell (508) further reported that a significant relationship obtained between the virulence of the test culture and the type of pulmonary response produced in normal rabbits. With Type I pneumococci of low virulence, a small localized central pneumonia was produced. With the successive use of test cultures of progressively increasing virulence, a patchy, then coalescing lobular pneumonia, and finally lobar pneumonia was obtained. Further increases in virulence led to a rapidly fatal septicaemia with but little pulmonary response. In such instances the adjacent serous membranes were frequently involved. In the pneumonias produced, no damage was observed to the walls and lining epithelium of the bronchi or bronchioles in the early stages, and their involvement occurred later.

Variations in the nature of the inflammatory reaction were observed to occur and appeared dependent upon the virulence of the culture. With organisms of low virulence, little inflammatory reaction developed. As organisms of increasing virulence were used, the intensity of the response increased, as did the size but not the number of the individual foci of infection, and polymorphonuclear leucocytes appeared in increasing numbers. With organisms of sufficient virulence to produce a lobular lesion, the inflammatory reaction began to involve the perivascular lymphatics, and peribronchial lesions appeared. With organisms of sufficient virulence to cause lobar pneumonia, areas in all stages of development were seen within twenty-four to forty-eight hours after infection. Alveoli the farthest away from the initial lesion were the last to be involved. These first filled with a serous exudate, and later leucocytes appeared. At this point the perivascular reaction was often great, and the lymphatic reaction around the bronchi marked. Organisms were easily identified in the initially involved alveoli within twenty-four hours but later became scarce, their disappearance coinciding with the period of maximum perivascular reaction in the more severe lobular and lobar lesions. The frequently encountered bacteriemia was regarded as the result of the passage into the blood of leucocytes containing ingested but viable organisms.

Following the infection of rabbits by blowing pneumococci into their bronchi with an atomizer, Stuppy and Falk (1259) frequently obtained bronchopneumonia accompanied by a septicaemia. In a few instances interstitial lesions were produced.

The intrabronchial infection of normal animals of species which naturally possess considerable resistance to the pneumococcus usually results in the production of lobar pneumonia, as was shown by Lamar and Meltzer (757) and several additional workers (1363, 1437, 269, 322, 632, 1290, 1291, 1292, 1083, 1084, 782) in the dog, and by Francis and Terrell (483) in the monkey (*Macacus cynomolgos*).

Several studies have been made of the course and detailed pathology of the lesions incited by the intrabronchial infection of animals. Attention has already been called to Gaskell's (508) findings in the rabbit, which are given above. The most elaborate studies of this nature in the dog appear to have been carried out by Lamar and Meltzer (757), Wollstein and Meltzer (1437), Terrell, Robertson, and Coggeshall (1292), Robertson, Coggeshall, and Terrell (1083, 1084), and Coggeshall and Robertson (286). In the last instance observations were made on the pulmonary pathology of dogs experiencing repeated attacks of lobar pneumonia.

Lamar and Meltzer (757) produced lobar pneumonia similar to that occurring in man in forty-two of forty-eight infected dogs. The infecting dose varied in size but was large and usually consisted of 5 to 10 cc. of culture. Animals receiving very large doses generally died rapidly with a septicaemia and septic complications in addition to their lobar lesion. None of the animals was sacrificed earlier than seven hours after infection. Consolidation developed rapidly and was demonstrable within seven to twenty-four hours.

The involvement usually included the whole of one or more lobes. The lymph glands draining the affected region were enlarged and contained organisms. The exudate in the consolidated area consisted chiefly of a serous fluid containing numerous polymorphonuclear leucocytes and a few red blood cells. Organisms and edema fluid were present in the largest amounts at the periphery of the lesion. Fibrin appeared by the end of the second day, as did large mononuclear cells, and the latter showed evidence of phagocytosis. Transition from red to gray hepatization was not found. Spontaneous recovery usually began by the third or fourth day, and resolution was nearly always complete by the end of two weeks. In a few instances, especially in the presence of an accidental mixed infection, some organization of the exudate occurred.

A lobar pneumonia of lesser severity, without blood invasion and with a rapidly resolving exudate poor in fibrin, was produced by Wollstein and Meltzer (1437) in eighteen dogs by the intrabronchial insufflation of 10 to 30 cc. doses of cultures of pneumococci of low virulence.

The most detailed observations on the course and pathology of experimental lobar pneumonia in dogs were made by Terrell, Robertson, and Coggeshall (1292) and Robertson, Coggeshall, and Terrell (1083, 1084). Pneumococci of Type I or II were suspended in starch broth and implanted through a fine catheter by way of a bronchus far out in the lung periphery. The infection in more than one hundred dogs used assumed one of two general types and gave rise either to a localized pulmonary lesion in the form of lobar pneumonia with ensuing recovery or death or to a generalized infection developing at the outset or in the course of a localized infection, with or without lobar consolidation, and ending fatally. Severe and prolonged infection was produced with doses of 0.0001 to 0.00001 cc. of young virulent cultures given in a volume of 1 cc. of the starch suspension fluid. Death occurred in practically all dogs receiving over 0.1 cc. of culture. The course of the experimental pneumonia was generally short, averaging four or five days, and recovery was usually abrupt, simulating crisis.

Of fifty-eight dogs brought to necropsy, careful studies were made in thirty-nine, of which twenty showed lobar pneumonia (1083). In animals with localized lesions various stages of consolidation were found in different lobes of the lungs. Both red and gray hepatization was found, though the latter was much less common than in man as the pneumonia in dogs appeared to evolve more rapidly. Resolution was frequently encountered and was characterized by the appearance of the "macrophage reaction" consisting of a swelling and subsequent detachment of the cells of the alveolar walls, which then acted as phagocytes. Small areas of organization were not infrequent. Organisms were commonest near the spreading edge of the lesion and were present both in the alveoli and to a lesser extent in the interstitial tissues, where they were largely extracellular. Areas most intensely consolidated showed the fewest organisms, and in the older stages of red hepatization the numerous organisms present were practically all intracellular and apparently undergoing digestion. Bacteriemia was transient, moderate, or absent in animals showing the most intense consolidation and a well-marked alveolar cellular exudate.

In dogs with generalized lesions resulting in a fulminating infection with early death, two or more lobes were always involved, and the exudate was less uniform and contained more red blood cells. The lung structure was less well preserved, and more edema was present. In other animals in which a generalized infection developed after initial localization had occurred and in those dying with a marked bacteriemia, the lesions produced were varied. These dogs presented the picture of a combined lobar and lobular pneumonia with some interstitial pneumonitis and had frequent septic complications, such as empyema. In such instances the pulmonary exudate showed many extracellular organisms.

In dogs with typical lobar pneumonia the consolidation involved whole lobes and was intense, resulting in a firm, airless, liver-like lesion, but was less firm and less granular than the lobar consolidations of man. In the previous section (Intratracheal Infection) it was noted that both rabbits and monkeys exhibit considerable interstitial inflammation in the course of pneumonia. Such lesions were infrequent in the pneumonia of dogs. As compared with consolidation in man, the pneumonic lesions in the dog showed more marked peripheral and peribronchial edema, and the consolidation was usually less evenly distributed over the involved lobe or lobes. Dog lungs are more elastic and less fibrous than human lungs.

The pathogenesis of lobar pneumonia in the dog was carefully studied by Robertson, Coggeshall, and Terrell (1084), who performed necropsies on nineteen dogs killed at intervals of from one to twenty-four hours following infection. It is of interest to note that in two dogs killed *one hour* after inoculation definite changes were found which were discernible both by roentgenograms and by histologic examination of the involved tissue. The infiltration, consisting of starch, red blood cells, and edema fluid, was chiefly intra-alveolar and was most marked around the main bronchus and its branches. Alveolar hemorrhage was common. The most striking change in the blood vessels of the area was the frequent occurrence of an extensive perivascular edema. Pneumococci were present, not only in the lesion, but also in the walls of alveoli in areas of the normal lung some distance away. The visible lesion at this one-hour period was from 1.5 to 2.5 centimeters in diameter. Many alveoli contained fluid and small amounts of fibrin. The epithelium of the bronchi in the involved area showed signs of injury, and some cellular exudate was present in the bronchial lumina. The three-hour lesions showed a progression in the size and intensity of the reaction, and examination of the cut surface of the lung revealed a slightly depressed zone about one centimeter wide surrounding the involved area. In this zone alveoli were of varying size and many were partially or completely collapsed. Organisms were again present in the walls of apparently normal alveoli far from the lesion; they appeared in the alveolar spaces only after the exudation of edema fluid and were less frequent in the areas infiltrated with polymorphonuclear leucocytes, where the beginning of phagocytosis was seen, than in more distant areas.

Up to the six-hour period the development of the lesion was apparently similar regardless of the size of the infecting dose of organisms used. At this time, however, a difference became apparent, and in animals infected with the larger doses a more pronounced zone of edema surrounding the lesion was found. The alveolar exudate at this period contained a considerable number of polymorphonuclear leucocytes. At twelve hours the lesion was larger, darker, firmer, and more uniform, and organisms were less abundant in the walls of apparently normal alveoli in the zone beyond the edema than previously. The periphery of the consolidated area, however, showed organisms in great numbers within the alveoli filled with edema fluid. Advancing inward toward the main lesion, polymorphonuclear leucocytes and red blood cells began to appear in the alveoli. In the oldest part of the lesion organisms were rare, and nearly all were within leucocytes. By twenty-four hours dogs having well-advanced consolidation showed hepatization nearly complete and the alveoli evenly filled, largely with leucocytes. In some instances the beginning of the macrophage reaction was apparent at this time. In other dogs at this period showing a less regular and intense but a more extensive lesion, numerous lacunae of relatively normal tissue were seen within the consolidated area. In these animals red blood cells formed a large part of the cellular exudate, the macrophage reaction was absent, and organisms were widely spread throughout the whole lesion.

It seemed probable that the starch mixture in which the organisms were suspended at the time of injection played a role in the development of the pulmonary lesions, for immediately after the injection of the pneumococcus-starch mixture into a terminal bronchus a series of reactions indicative of local injury appeared. These consisted of an engorgement of the blood vessels, capillary hemorrhage into the alveoli, destruction of the architecture of the tissue in some places, exudation of fluid both into the alveolar spaces and into the perivascular and peribronchial tissue, and the mobilization of polymorphonuclear leucocytes. The injection of starch alone produced a reaction similar to this, but after six hours it did not progress; while if organisms were present, the progression was continuous. Attention was repeatedly called to the considerable amount of edema which appeared in the lesions of the infected dogs. The edema became extensive at about six hours, after which time the spread of the lesions was accelerated. It seemed probable that the early spread of the infection was principally by way of the lymphatics and capillaries, though the interstitial reaction was less than that found by other workers in monkeys or rabbits. It was not clear, however, how organisms were spread after the first few hours of infection, but their distribution suggested that they were carried by the edema fluid. Pneumococci were constantly seen in blood vessels in the parenchyma of the lung early in the infection, and this appeared to account for the frequently demonstrable bacteriemia at that time.

Various workers have noted the frequent occurrence of some atelectasis in dogs with experimentally induced lobar pneumonia (322, 632, 1292, 1084, 782). In these instances some displacement of the mediastinum and diaphragm toward the affected lobe was found. A similar phenomenon was observed to occur during resolution (1084).

Coggeshall and Robertson (286) studied the course and lesions produced in twenty-five dogs each undergoing from two to eleven attacks of lobar pneumonia induced at intervals of three days to nineteen months. One attack usually gave rise to some acquired immunity, and recurrent attacks were usually more mild, even when a larger number of infecting organisms were used, and bacteriemia was less common. Some differences were found in the pathology of the lesion produced by a recurrent attack as compared with that resulting from a primary attack. In the former instance, at the end of six hours the reinfected dogs showed larger and firmer lesions with a more extensive outpouring of edema fluid. Secondary lesions initiated in a previously affected lobe evolved more rapidly than primary lesions during the first twelve to sixteen hours. Secondary infections started in a new lobe, however, resembled primary infections with a non-fatal dose but differed from the latter in that the cellular response was more intense and even, hemorrhages were less frequent, and organisms were fewer in number and a larger proportion was intracellular.

Francis and Terrell (483) studied the production and course of pneumococcus pneumonia in the Java monkey (*M. cynomolgos*). Using the method of Terrell, Robertson, and Coggeshall (1292), intrabronchial infection was carried out with a starch suspension of Type III pneumococci virulent for rabbits. Doses of 0.25 to 0.5 cc. were usually given. Investigation showed that the addition of the starch mixture to the culture was not necessary, for typical lesions could be produced by injecting the organisms alone. Localized pulmonary lesions were found in sixty-eight animals, and the pneumonia closely resembled pneumococcus lobar pneumonia in man. Bacteriemia was common, occurring in 70 per cent of the animals, and frequently was extensive, accompanied by a high fatality rate (see page 793). In the absence of bacteriemia the average duration of the pneumonia was four to five days. Most animals that survived had one or two lobes involved, and recovery was usually by crisis.

Infection by Other Routes

The injection of pneumococci through the chest wall directly into the lung resulted in a septicaemia without pneumonia in rabbits (1361) and in the production of lobar pneumonia in one instance in dogs (501). In addition, intrapulmonary infection was carried out in guinea pigs for the purpose of studying the protective and curative value of specific immune serum (942). In some instances in the course of studies on immunity, rabbits and cats (1097) and cats and dogs (1290, 1291) have been infected by the intrapleural injection of pneumococcus cultures. Diffuse lesions with much sepsis resulted in rabbits, while in cats and dogs the lesions were usually more localized unless an overwhelming infection was produced by the injection of an extra large dose of organisms. The infection of the anterior eye chamber of mice, rabbits, and dogs gave rise to but little cellular response, and the aqueous humor of these animals provided an excellent medium for pneumococcus growth (1284).

Summary

The significance of many of the observations cited in relation to the experimental pneumococcus infection of animals appears essentially similar in that, where the virulence of the organism is not too great or the resistance of the host too low, infection with the pneumococcus usually evokes the production of a marked inflammatory response and the outpouring of edema fluid and a cellular exudate containing varying amounts of fibrin. On occasion, pulmonary lesions including lobar pneumonia may be produced in normal as well as in immunized animals of either susceptible or resistant species. Nevertheless, the presence of some immunity appears essential in every instance for the production of pneumonia in the lobar form. The development of lobar pneumonia in the experimentally infected normal dog, an animal possessing considerable natural resistance to the pneumococcus, may be cited as an example of this nature.

The findings also make it probable that under suitable circumstances the contact of the lungs of animals with the pneumococcus may give rise to lobar pneumonia without the preceding or accompanying activity of any other agent, such as a bacterial organism or virus. In many instances where pneumococci are present deep in the respiratory tract, damage to the normal defensive barriers of the lung, which may result from alcoholic intoxication or the direct contact of the pulmonary tissue with foreign substances, may play some role in assisting in the development of pneumonia in the lobar form.

As compared with the frequency with which pulmonary lesions occur when organisms are planted deep in the respiratory tract, the relatively infrequent occurrence of such lesions among animals carrying pneumococci in their nose and throat and the usual failure to produce pneumonia by implanting organisms in the upper trachea suggest that the upper respiratory tract and especially the larynx provide a barrier beyond which it is necessary for pneumococci to pass before pneumonia occurs.

The evidence at hand also suggests, and with increasing clearness, that the pneumococcus by itself is capable of rapidly penetrating epithelial tissues such as those which line the respiratory tract.

PATHOGENESIS OF PNEUMOCOCCUS LOBAR PNEUMONIA

The information available concerning the pathogenesis of pneumococcus lobar pneumonia is for the most part limited to observations made in experimental animals, and there is but little direct evidence relating to the spontaneous development of these infections in man. In many instances, however, it is probable that the factors influencing the production of pneumonia in animals are also concerned to some extent with the development of the disease in man. The production of pneumonia in animals is mentioned in the foregoing sections on experimental infection.

It is well recognized that pneumococci are commonly carried in the mouths of normal people and that in temperate climates they are most frequently found in such individuals in the colder months of the year when pneumonia is most frequent (see pages 342–385). Before considering the route and point of the initial infection and the means by which the lesion spreads, mention may be made of certain general factors which appear related in varying degrees to the development of this disease. The question of resistance and virulence is, of course, of importance. In many instances the production of lobar pneumonia appears facilitated by the presence of an acute minor upper respiratory infection in the host, and at times a condition of bacterial allergy or hypersensitivity to the pneumococcus may likewise assist in the process.

General Factors in Pathogenesis

Among the general factors of importance in the development of pneumonia, those concerned with the immunity of the host and with the virulence of the pneumococcus in question must be of great significance. The nature of many of the factors which affect host resistance has already been pointed out (see pages 185–203). It was seen that, in addition to several factors inherent in the host which appeared concerned in the operation of immunity (the species of the animal, factors of a genetic nature, age, and sex), resistance was shown to be related to the virulence and to some extent to the type of the infecting pneumococcus, and to vary with the passage of time or following immunization and possibly in the presence of infections and other diseases. Exposure to conditions lowering body temperature and to marked variations in temperature, chilling, wetting, trauma to the lung tissue, and the like appeared to favor the development of serious infection and, in consequence, have been interpreted as having a depressing effect upon either local or general resistance.

Studies of the virulence of pneumococci isolated from patients with pneumococcus infections, including pneumonia, have been made by several investigators, among which the observations of Whittle (1422, 1421), Gundel and Wasu (584), and Gundel and Schwarz (582) may be mentioned. It would appear from the findings of these workers that pneumococcus pneumonia in the lobar form is the result of infection with organisms of high virulence. Indeed, Whittle concluded that there is a certain specific minimal virulence below which pneumococci appear unable to infect the healthy human lung. Pneumococci of Types I and II, as well as those of some of the higher types isolated from patients with pneumococcus infections, were found to be of high virulence.

It was earlier shown that man in general appears to possess considerable immunity to the pneumococcus (see pages 143–150 and 187–192). A consideration of the available evidence strongly suggests that clinical syndromes characterizing lobar pneumonia are expressions of partial immunity, as Topley (1317) has mentioned. This being so, and as the natural resistance of man appears greatest in persons in the latter part of childhood and in early and middle adult life, it should not be surprising that, judging from the available reports, it is such individuals who develop perhaps a majority of the cases of lobar pneumonia which occur (see pages 299–307). The possession of resistance assists in the production of a localized lesion, as mentioned in the previous chapter. Pneumonia developing in the extremely young or old, whose resistance is naturally low, is more commonly diffuse and assumes a bronchopneumonic form.

As elsewhere noted, it appears probable from the limited data available that pneumococcus pneumonia may occur in individuals possessing humoral antibodies specific for the type causing the infection (see pages 127–129). It is perhaps somewhat of a paradox that pneumonia may develop in the lungs of individuals whose blood contains considerable specific circulating antibody, as Robertson and his associates (1094, 1084) have pointed out. Under the conditions initially present in the lung, however, the antipneumococcal effect of such antibodies presumably depends upon opsonization, phagocytosis, and intracellular digestion of the organism, as no strictly growth-inhibiting substance is present in the serum. As maximum opsonization seems dependent upon a quantitative relationship between the concentration of opsonins in the serum and the number of organisms at hand, it is probable that, if the number of organisms present exceeds a certain value, little opsonization occurs. In addition, an interval of time is necessary for the full action of the antibodies to be felt, and it is likely that organisms continue to multiply and spread in this interval. Robertson, Coggeshall, and Terrell (1084) also found evidence in studying the pathogenesis of experimental lobar pneumonia in dogs that a second factor is involved after the leucocytes arrive in the alveoli and before phagocytosis begins. In many respects it appeared likely that the first leucocytes to arrive did not find the organisms adequately prepared for phagocytosis, but later, when additional numbers of polymorphonuclear leucocytes were present and presumably more fluid containing opsonins as well, phagocytosis was general. Meanwhile organisms were spreading and a similar train of events was occurring at the periphery of the lesion.

The occurrence of marked variations in temperature, wetting, chilling, and similar unfavorable conditions appears to decrease host resistance, as already mentioned. The means by which this is accomplished is unknown. It is possible that these unfavorable conditions have an injurious effect upon the normal protective mechanism of the upper respiratory tract and permit the ready passage of organisms into the lower respiratory tract. Whether any accompanying alteration occurs in the functional capacity of the normal mechanism for removing organisms from the respiratory tract is unknown. Factors acting to traumatize the normal defensive mechanism of the lung parenchyma appear to alter the protective barriers of that tissue presumably by damaging the cellular mechanism which normally disposes of organisms deep in the lung.

The development of pneumonia has been regarded by numerous investigators as probably the outcome, not of an increase in the virulence of the pneumococcus concerned, but rather of a lessening in host resistance (1111, 1048, 298, 584, 300, 320, 582, 1068), and it seems clear that the latter is subject to considerable fluctuation. While it is, of course, probable that pneumonia might result from the entrance into the lower respiratory tract of a sufficient number of organisms of high virulence without the occurrence of any preceding or simultaneous decrease in the immunity of the host, it seems more in accord with the evidence at hand to consider that in the usual instance a local lowering of resistance or impairment of the natural defense mechanism occurs which permits virulent organisms to gain the lower respiratory tract and to set up an infection in the face of considerable general immunity.

Relation of Minor Respiratory Infections to Occurrence of Pneumonia

It has long been thought that an intimate relationship may exist between the presence of an acute minor respiratory infection and the occurrence of lobar pneumonia. This belief has arisen due to the many instances in which patients with pneumonia give a history of conditions such as coryza, rhinitis, pharyngitis, and laryngitis, with or without cough or other associated symptoms, either at the time of the onset of their more serious illness or within a week or two prior to it.

Minor upper respiratory infections previous to the onset of pneumonia have been found to be of common occurrence among patients with lobar pneumonia of the white race, and possibly of the yellow race as well (918, 1025, 1450). The incidence of such infections in various series of cases was reported as 40 per cent by Cole (297), 46.8 per cent by Cecil, Baldwin, and Larsen (230), 50 per cent by Finland and Sutliff (464), 60 per cent by Cole (302), 64 per cent by Loeschcke (798), 70 per cent by Dochez (359), 76 per cent by Lord and Heffron (813, 814), and 80 per cent by Bullowa (190). Cole (301) has stated that when patients were especially questioned concerning this matter, almost every one gave a history of some sort of previous upper respiratory infection. The evidence suggests, however, that in some patients lobar pneumonia may occur in the absence of any known predisposing cause of this nature.

In Africa, among persons of the black race with lobar pneumonia, Maynard (874) and Garnham and deSmidt (507) found that, as compared with Europeans, African natives seldom had an upper respiratory infection prior to the onset of pneumonia. The latter workers pointed out that, whereas minor infections of the respiratory tract were frequent in Europeans and Asiatics in tropical Africa, the resistance of the natives in the same locality (Kenya) was so low that instead of developing an infection of a similar nature they at once developed pneumonia. In respect to their general lack of resistance, African natives appear similar to young infants of the white race. In New York City, Kneeland and Dawes (732) observed a group of Hebrew infants and children and found that the youngest infants, aged eight to fourteen months, were very susceptible to respiratory diseases and pneumonia, while among individuals over eighteen months of age serious disease was less common and colds were more common.

In any event, the high incidence of colds and other acute minor respiratory disturbances prior to the onset of lobar pneumonia among white patients has given rise to the frequently expressed belief that the pneumococcus may be a secondary invader which causes serious pulmonary infection only after some preceding damage has been done by a primary agent, such as a virus, which was responsible for the initial minor infection. While this may be true in a large number of instances, it is fairly certain that the nature of the lesions incited and of the more serious symptoms, as well as the outcome of the disease, at least in cases due to infection with pneumococci of the more invasive types, such as Type I or II (300) or one of several of the higher types as well, are directly related to the character of these organisms.

Certain aspects of the relation of the common cold to the development of pneumonia are discussed below. The frequency with which pneumonia often follows influenza suggests that the filterable virus, which was shown by Smith, Andrewes, and Laidlaw (1214) and Francis (479) to cause at least one form of influenza, might commonly be the inciting factor in many cases of pneumococcus pneumonia. Francis and Magill (482), however, were unable to demonstrate the development of humoral neutralizing antibodies for influenza virus in a few patients recovering from pneumococcus pneumonia. As such antibodies had been found in patients recovering from influenza (1214, 479), the failure of such substances to appear following recovery from pneumonia presumably indicates, at least in the cases studied, that the influenza virus was not the inciting factor of the pneumonia. No information is at hand of antibody studies of a similar nature for the virus of the common contagious cold.

As above noted, the relation of minor acute infections of the respiratory tract to the onset of pneumonia appears very intimate in many cases. Though the precise nature of this relationship remains largely unknown, the findings of numerous investigations have suggested means whereby the occurrence of colds assists in bringing about pneumonia.

In recent years several studies of a clinical and epidemiologic nature have been made of minor upper respiratory infections including the common cold (1320, 849, 732, 1348, 358, 367, 311, 731, 1208). Continuous observations on a total of more than 18,000 persons over periods of many months have revealed that attacks of minor upper respiratory infections usually exhibit definite variations in their incidence, the curves for which show a double (1320, 849, 732, 367, 311, 731) or possibly a triple (358) peak. In general, these peaks occurred in the fall, midwinter, and spring months. The fall and spring peaks are usually low and the infections mild, while the midwinter peak in December or January is high, at which time the infections are most serious and are followed by the most severe secondary complications, such as pneumonia (see also pages 289–295). The curve for the carrier rate of pneumococci in the population at large also shows considerable seasonal variation and in the main appears very similar to the curve for these minor respiratory infections (see pages 378–385).

The general incidence of colds is highest in children (1320, 311), especially in those under five years of age (1348), and decreases with advancing age. It is evident, as the investigators cited below have pointed out, that the "common cold" implies more than a simple coryza and that the systemic reaction is more marked than is commonly believed. Townsend and Sydenstricker (1320) found that fever occurred in one-fifth of nearly 5,000 attacks, and Van Volkenburgh and Frost (1348) noted that almost one-quarter of the persons having 1,388 attacks were confined to bed at some period and that about the same proportion had fever. In the latter investigation nine-tenths of the patients had coryza, two-thirds had a cough, and approximately one-third suffered from a sore throat. The mean duration of the symptoms in all attacks was 15.9 days. In Collins and Gover's (311) study of nearly 3,000 persons over a period of thirty-three months the proportion of attacks accompanied by fever was highest in infants and children, while the incidence of attacks without fever was highest among adults twenty to forty years of age. These workers also reported that the proportion of attacks with fever annually increased as winter progressed.

The above studies of Townsend and Sydenstricker (1320) and Van Volkenburgh and Frost (1348) of minor acute respiratory infections reveal that normal persons experience from two to three attacks of such conditions each year. A point of epidemiologic interest may be mentioned here and an estimate made to ascertain the approximate frequency with which such attacks may be followed by lobar pneumonia. The 1935 population of Massachusetts was more than 4,350,000, and with two attacks of respiratory infection per person per year the total number of attacks would equal about 8,700,000. Using the data presented in Table 48 (page 292) and counting four cases for each death, it may be estimated that there are in the neighborhood of eight thousand cases of lobar pneumonia in Massachusetts each year. If all cases of lobar pneumonia were preceded by minor respiratory infections, then the total of over eight million such minor infections gave rise to about eight thousand cases of lobar pneumonia, indicating that about one in every one thousand attacks of minor respiratory infections may be followed by pneumonia in the lobar form. The inclusion of cases of bronchopneumonia in such an estimate might reduce this proportion to one in every five hundred to seven hundred. Such figures are, of course, simply gross estimates.

During the course of a common cold the number of pathogenic organisms, and especially pneumococci, in the upper respiratory tract usually exhibits a sudden and marked increase (see pages 374–377). Dochez, Shibley, and Mills (370) and their associates (1183, 366) have demonstrated this phenomenon in the chimpanzee, an animal whose basic flora of the upper respiratory tract was found similar to that of man; and Shibley, Hanger, and Dochez (1181), Smillie and Caldwell (1209), Webster and Hughes (1393), and others (1391, 732, 367, 359) have shown the same conditions in man in both children and adults.

Dochez, Shibley, and Mills (369) and their co-workers (370, 1183, 359, 366, 358) have found that at least one form of the common contagious cold is due to a filterable virus. These investigators suggested that the sudden increase in the number of pathogenic organisms in the upper respiratory tract which occurred during the course of a cold seemed due to the capacity of the virus to incite into biologic activity dangerous organisms, such as pneumococci, hemolytic streptococci, and *H. influenzae*. In this respect the observations of Dochez, Mills, and Kneeland (366) were of the greatest interest. Experimental colds were incited in two chimpanzees from whose nasopharyngeal cultures an R form of *H. influenzae* had been previously grown. Within forty-eight hours subsequent cultures showed the appearance of S forms of *H. influenzae,* which disappeared within three days in one ape but persisted for as long as six days in the other. The findings confirmed previous observations by these workers and indicated that one important effect of the cold virus was to incite activity on the part of potential pathogens present in the nasopharynx at the time of infection. Such organisms might then function as secondary invaders and extend and develop the injury inflicted by the primary agent and perhaps also increase the distribution of the secondary invaders in the community at large (Dochez, 358).

Smillie and Caldwell (1209) observed a number of persons with acute colds, several of whom became chilled and developed pneumonia. In the usual case in the latter instance the colds developed into pneumonia between the fourth and seventh days. Dochez, Mills, and Kneeland (367) studied the course of events during a wave of respiratory infections among a group of infants. It appeared that two agents were probably involved. The first was the initiating agent which gave rise to a mild disturbance, such as the common cold. The second agent also appeared operative in some instances but not in all. It was one or another of the pathogenic organisms which were empowered by the initiating agent to invade the host and give rise to the more severe secondary manifestations.

It may again be noted, however, that the exact means by which this secondary invasion occurs remains unknown.

Though the cold virus may activate some organisms and in the ape bring about a transformation of R to S forms, as Dochez, Mills, and Kneeland (366) have noted, Francis (480, 481), using the influenza virus and mice, was unable to produce a similar change in pneumococci.

Of course, pneumonia following influenza may develop for reasons other than the occurrence of any activation of organisms normally present in the upper respiratory tract. It also seems likely that in many instances pneumonia may develop in the absence of any immediately preceding upper respiratory infection. In animals such as the mouse, dog, or monkey, suitable experimental infection with virulent pneumococci commonly results in the production of pneumonia which is often of the lobar variety, as shown in the preceding section. It is highly unlikely that such uniform results could have been obtained in animals if a previous upper respiratory infection with a virus were essential to the production of such lesions. Robertson's (1082) observations on the accidental infection of a laboratory worker are also of interest in this respect. This person developed a Type I lobar pneumonia a few hours after washing out a jar that had been thoroughly sprayed with a virulent culture of Type I pneumococci. Recovery occurred following specific serum treatment. A few months later this same individual was accidentally exposed to pneumococci of Type II in spray form. The organisms, suspended in liquid gelatin, were being injected into a dog and some of the injection mass squirted out around the hilt of the needle. Type II lobar pneumonia occurred in this worker forty hours later, and again recovery followed the use of specific serum.

While it appears that pneumococcus lobar pneumonia in man commonly occurs during the course of or subsequent to minor upper respiratory infections, especially those presumably due to a virus, it is not clear that a virus infection is an essential prerequisite for the development of pneumonia in every instance, or indeed possibly in any instance.

Allergy and Lobar Pneumonia

In 1911, following the production of allergic reactions in guinea pigs immunized with derivatives of pneumococci, Rosenow (1117) advanced the suggestion that a state of hypersensitivity or allergy might be concerned in the production of lobar pneumonia. In several respects certain features of pneumococcus lobar pneumonia, such as the usual abrupt onset with the fairly rapid development of the massive lobar lesion, suggest, to the extent that it resembles a response to an antigen against which a condition of altered reactivity is present, that the onset of this disease represents a phenomenon of an allergic nature. There are numerous data at hand which contribute impressively to the view that a condition of allergy or hypersensitivity to the pneumococcus, or at least a state of altered cellular reactivity to this organism, does play a part in the development of lobar pneumonia. Though the matter cannot yet be definitely settled, the evidence favoring this view appears to be more significant than that opposed to it.

Reimann (1066) and Cole (300) have reviewed much of this material in considerable detail.

Contact with the pneumococcus appears frequently to give rise to evidence of demonstrable immunity, as shown by the appearance of specific circulating antipneumococcal immune substances in the blood of many individuals following minor or major infections with this organism. As the mechanism of the development of allergy seems intimately related to or identical with that controlling the production of demonstrable immunity (see pages 182–185), it seems likely that natural conditions which favor the production of an increased resistance, such as increasing age (up to middle or late adult life) and minor infections of the upper respiratory tract, such as the common cold, during the course of which pneumococci become numerous in the nose and throat, may frequently lead to a state of sensitivity to this organism. This sensitivity, of course, may and probably does vary in intensity and duration in different individuals, as Kramár and Gyüre (743) have suggested. A majority of normal adults appear to show skin sensitivity to pneumococci or their derivatives, and in patients with pneumonia this is diminished or absent and develops during or after convalescence (see pages 149–150 and 165–167). Functional capacities for both allergy and immunity to the pneumococcus may be relatively undeveloped in the very young and less effective in their operation in the very old than in individuals in other age groups (see pages 186–192). If such variation with age is shown to be true, and if a condition of sensitivity facilitates the production of pneumonia in the lobar form, a partial explanation is at hand for the infrequent occurrence of this form of pulmonary infection in newborn and young infants and its uncommon occurrence in the very old.

There is some evidence resulting from experimental studies which in all probability indicates that a condition of allergy, at least in the lower animals, has a significant relation to the extent of the pulmonary lesion incited by contact of the lung with the homologous antigen. Sharp and Blake (1174) sensitized rabbits with repeated injections of killed Type II pneumococci or with sterile autolysates of these organisms. Subsequently the animals were skin tested with the same autolysate and within twenty-four hours given intratracheal injections of this material. A day later they were sacrificed for necropsy studies. Acute exudative inflammation of the lungs frequently developed in animals that had been sensitized. A fairly close correlation was found between the degree of skin sensitivity present and the extent of the pulmonary lesion developed. In rabbits which gave negative or slightly positive reactions to the skin tests, little or no pulmonary inflammation occurred, while those with increasingly marked reactions developed pulmonary inflammations of increasing extent. Almost identical results with lobar lesions were obtained by Lindau (783) in sensitized guinea pigs. In this instance pneumococci of Type I were used, and it was noted that the skin sensitivity produced was species-specific in nature. In neither of the above studies were the autolysates toxic for the lungs of normal animals.

Following the repeated insufflation of killed pneumococci into the nose and throat of rabbits, Stuppy, Cannon, and Falk (1258) injected living pneumococci intrabronchially. The character of the pulmonary lesions produced gave evidence of the existence of an altered reactivity of the cells of the lung. Julianelle and Rhoads (702) immunized rabbits with pneumococcus protein or egg albumin. In either instance the subsequent intratracheal injection of the corresponding antigen produced a pulmonary exudate resembling that found in pneumonia, and the reactions appeared related to the presence of circulating antibody in the blood. Fried (495, 496) sensitized rabbits with horse serum. The later intratracheal injection of this material frequently gave rise to pulmonary inflammations which were extensive in some instances and resembled the lesions of lobar pneumonia.

Using a different procedure as well as a different and more resistant species of animal, Coggeshall (285) obtained results in dogs somewhat at variance with those demonstrated by the above investigators in rabbits or guinea pigs. The skin sensitivity to autolysates of pneumococci of homologous type was determined in dogs which had successfully recovered from experimental pneumococcus lobar pneumonia. None of the animals showed a positive skin reaction. The injection of such autolysates into the lungs of dogs which had recovered from pneumonia produced small lesions in some which were demonstrable by roentgenograms. Exudative lesions simulating a partly coalescing lobular pneumonia were found at necropsy, resembling the early reaction characteristic of the evolution of a recurrent infection in this animal. A similar, though less marked, reaction was found in a passively immunized dog, while a normal dog showed little if any evidence of an identical response. Nevertheless, considerable irregularity was noted in the response obtained in recovered and normal dogs, and three normal dogs also developed pulmonary lesions of similar appearance demonstrable by roentgenograms. In recovered dogs, no discernible relation was found between the severity of the preceding pneumonia and the presence or extent of the subsequent lesion induced by the autolysate injections, and dogs receiving repeated injections of autolysate reacted in the same manner on each occasion. Evidence was obtained, however, as Coggeshall and Robertson (286) likewise noted, that the tissue cells of the lungs of dogs which had been subjected to a previous pneumococcus infection reacted more rapidly to the presence of pneumococci or their products than did the cells of the lungs of normal dogs. For practical purposes it would seem immaterial whether or not this accelerated functional capacity may be classified as allergy, the important point being that a state of altered cellular reactivity was present.

The contentions of Lauche (766) are of special interest in respect to the possible role of allergy in the production of lobar pneumonia in man. Attention was called to the rarity of lobar pneumonia in the newborn and in very young infants. The existence of this peculiarity was regarded as due to the inability of infants to produce a vigorous reaction to pneumococcus infection as a consequence of their general lack of immunity, for what little immunity is present at birth is rapidly lost. During the first few days of life, however, when some immunity, and possibly some sensitivity, is present, lobar pneumonia may occur. Nine examples of such infections, with necropsies, were reported, and in each instance both the mothers and their newborn infants had lobar pneumonia. It was considered that for the production of pneumonia in the lobar form a definite relation must exist between the infected host and the invading organism. This must be of such a nature that the organism is permitted to settle and initiate infection and then, when its accumulated toxic products have reached a threshold value, the sensitized body is stimulated to produce a sudden extensive and powerful reaction which tends to render the organism harmless.

Lauche also pointed out that the available evidence appeared to show that such a sensitized state developed in consequence of a partial immunization against the pneumococcus, or rather a particular type of pneumococcus, which presumably resulted from the occurrence of previous infections with the organism. This state of partial immunization was considered to represent in a certain sense a hypersensitiveness to the pneumococcus which is similar in many respects to the allergic sensitivity which may be produced with various antigens. As the very young have not yet had sufficient opportunity to become sensitized to the pneumococcus, lobar pneumonia is infrequent in that group. With increasing age and consequently a longer period of opportunity for contact and infection with the pneumococcus, a proportional increase in the incidence of pneumonia in the lobar form is encountered. The peculiarities of the age incidence of this form of pulmonary infection Lauche regarded as understandable if lobar pneumonia is considered as a hyperergic response due to an infection in an allergic sensitized body having a partial immunity to the infecting type of pneumococcus.

Certain clinical differences between lobar pneumonia in the child and in the adult led Trask, O'Donovan, Moore, and Beebe (1321) likewise to suggest that the adult has some special reactivity to the pneumococcus which is different from that of the child and which may be the result of the acquisition of some sensitivity to the pneumococcus. Loeschcke (798), after a detailed study of the pathology of lobar pneumonia in man, also subscribed to the view that pneumococcus lobar pneumonia represents an allergic reaction of the lung following previous sensitization with this organism. This investigator further pointed out that if, when once acquired, the sensitized state were permanent, probably all the pneumonias in adults would be of the lobar form; and as this, of course, is not so, the probability is that the allergic state is labile and transient. As is necessary in many instances prior to the production of anaphylactic shock, the sensitization leading to lobar pneumonia was believed to occur a relatively short time before the pneumonia occurred. Minor upper respiratory infections, which so often precede the onset of pneumonia, were considered to be significantly concerned in the development of this sensitization. Gundel and Wasu (584) also regarded lobar pneumonia as a hyperergic reaction to the pneumococcus.

That the human lung may respond to stimulation by antigens presumably other than pneumococci with the production of allergic manifestations and a condition simulating pneumonia, upon which a secondary infection may or may not be superimposed, was shown by Waldbott and Snell (1373) and Miller, Piness, Feingold, and Friedman (891) in their studies of children having a constitutional allergic background.

The fact that pneumonia in the lobar form may be produced by the experimental infection of some normal animals does not necessarily indicate that lobar lesions may be developed in the absence of "sensitivity" to the pneumococcus. As Schöbl and Sellards (1162) found pneumococci in the mouths of a few normal monkeys, and Blake and Cecil (124) reported the occurrence of spontaneous pneumococcus lobar pneumonia in monkeys, it seems clear that such animals may normally experience some contact with this organism. Pneumococci are occasionally encountered in normal animals of other species as well (556, 1417). With the exception of one study, in none of the relevant investigations cited in the foregoing section dealing with experimental infections is mention made of sensitivity tests prior to infection. In this single instance, however, Francis and Terrell (483) failed to find evidence of any previous sensitization in the Java monkeys tested, yet the experimental infection of these animals gave rise to lesions resembling those present in lobar pneumonia in man (see page 231). Monkeys, of course, are presumably endowed with some degree of natural resistance, and this in itself doubtless aided in the production of the localized lesion.

In view of the above discussion, it seems possible that a condition of allergy or hypersensitivity to the pneumococcus may assist in the production of lobar pneumonia in many instances. While the essential feature for the production of this form of pneumonia would appear to be the presence in the host of a condition of altered cellular reactivity usually considered as indicative of some degree of immunity, the relation between allergy and immunity in this connection becomes more understandable if the difference between the anaphylactic and the immune state is considered to be a matter of the degree rather than of the kind of reactivity present, as Topley (1317) has pointed out. If, however, the allergic and the immune states are considered as entirely separate conditions, the possible relation of allergy to the development of lobar pneumonia becomes less clear.

Route of Infection: Air, Blood, Lymph

There is much conjecture and almost no direct evidence available as to the exact means by which pneumococci that give rise to spontaneous lobar pneumonia gain entrance to the lung. Under ordinary circumstances the infection must be borne to the lung by the air, blood, or lymph, as has been noted many times (297, 556, 766, 1317, 331, 765). A consideration of numerous factors influencing the production of this disease suggests that the infection is air-borne and that lobar pneumonia is bronchiogenic in origin.

Many years ago Rosenow (1114) suggested that pneumonia was a general infection with a secondary localization of the organisms in the lungs. This observation resulted from the finding that blood cultures were positive in many cases before physical signs of consolidation could be detected. As it is now known that lesions can commonly be demonstrated by roentgenograms in early cases when physical signs are still lacking, this observation seems of little significance. Apparently the only instance on record of the successful production of pneumonia by intravenous infection was that reported by Rake (1059) in mice. In this instance it was necessary, however, to balance carefully the resistance of the test animals against the virulence of the pneumococci used. Lauche (766), who regards lobar pneumonia as an allergic phenomenon, has stated that it is possible that a blood-borne infection might give rise to this disease and that the route of infection makes little essential difference so long as an allergic state is present within the lung. In addition, under experimental conditions it is likely, as Winternitz, Smith, and Robinson (1433) have shown, that pneumonia may be incited as a result of infection of the tissues and apparently the lymphatics in and around the trachea. However, neither Rake nor Winternitz and his associates obtained lobar pneumonia in their investigations here mentioned, and it seems clear from the observations cited in the previous section on experimental infections (page 204) that only when organisms are administered by way of the respiratory tract does lobar pneumonia result.

Various investigators (556, 331), including Lauche (766) and Loeschcke (798), strongly incline to the view that in the usual instance lobar pneumonia in man is the result of an air-borne infection.

Under normal conditions most organisms suspended in the inhaled air appear to be filtered out and held at or near the nasal orifices (1305). Many of those going further adhere to the film of mucus covering the nasal mucosa and are subsequently discharged or swallowed. Nasal mucus, while apparently not bactericidal, has growth-inhibiting properties, as Thomson and Hewlett (1305) have demonstrated. These investigators also reported that samples of air obtained from the nasopharynx seldom show organisms even though many are present in the inhaled air. The normal protective mechanism of the upper respiratory tract, concerning which little is known, presumably assists in the removal or destruction of organisms which come into contact with the mucous membranes in the region of the larynx. Once past the vocal cords, organisms may be dealt with mechanically following their adherence to the mucous membranes and be driven upwards by the ciliated epithelium. The physiology of respiration is such that the amount of "dead air" in the trachea and bronchial tree would probably preclude the chance of bacteria being drawn extremely deep into the bronchial tree at a single ordinary inspiration. This being so, it is likely that considerable opportunity is offered organisms to touch and adhere to the walls of the trachea and larger bronchi. Organisms gaining the deeper reaches of the bronchial tree are presumably removed and destroyed by phagocytic cells. Whether any other mechanism normally assists in this process is unknown.

Despite the usual filtering effect exerted by the passage of air through the somewhat devious channels of the upper respiratory tract, tending to remove foreign matter from the inspired air, particulate matter does reach the parenchyma of the lung, as is shown by the frequency with which anthracosis is encountered at necropsy. It would also seem clear that, where a sufficient concentration of organisms is present in finely divided droplets or droplet nuclei (1409, 1410) in the inspired air, they may gain the lower respiratory tract, and, as Stillman (1237, 1239) and Branch and Stillman (146) have shown in animals, they may be found at the periphery of the lung within a few minutes. As earlier indicated, numerous conditions appear to damage or interfere with the operation of the mechanism which normally acts to dispose of bacteria reaching the finer divisions of the bronchial tree. It seems likely that the assumption must be made, as Robertson and his associates (1094) have noted, that, as the result of some local change of this nature, the growth of pneumococci in the lung is protected from any destructive action of the blood elements. It is possible that a reaction of an allergic nature may assist in this process. After growth has been established and multiplication of the organisms has begun, their metabolic products accumulate in the surrounding area and, by producing an increasing injury to the tissue, cause the deposition of fibrin in the adjacent blood and lymph vessels, which further tends to shield the organisms from the action of any antipneumococcal immune substances contained in the blood.

There is considerable guess work in the above discussion concerning the route followed by an air-borne infection; but the route is even harder to trace when the infection develops as a consequence of the activation of pneumococci normally carried in the upper respiratory tract by a virus, such as that causing the common contagious cold. Smillie and Caldwell (1209) observed the development of pneumonia among a few individuals with an acute cold, in whose upper respiratory tract pneumococci had become prevalent. Though in most instances in persons with colds the organisms tended to disappear from the nasopharynx within a week or so, pneumonia occasionally developed in individuals who were exposed to chilling during that interval. The development of pneumonia within a few hours after chilling suggested that the entry of organisms into the lower respiratory tract had been rapid, but the route by which this infection occurred remains unknown.

Site and Nature of Initial Lesion

In animals, the site of the initial pulmonary lesion following the experimental injection of pneumococci into the trachea or bronchial tree is significantly influenced by variations in the technic and route of infection and consequently by the location of the area in which organisms first come in contact with the tissues of the respiratory tract. Where pneumococci are injected intratracheally, the pulmonary lesion commonly begins near the hilum, as was demonstrated in rabbits by Winternitz, Smith, and Robinson (1433) and in monkeys by Blake and Cecil (123) and Schöbl and Sellards (1162). In some instances, however, the initial involvement was of the median portion of the affected lobe, as was observed by Permar (1013) in rabbits and Francis and Terrell (483) in monkeys. In the latter instance the lesions exhibited a centrifugal spread. On the other hand, following the injection of organisms intrabronchially, the initial lesion begins in the immediately adjacent tissue, as was shown in rabbits by Gaskell (508); and in instances where the infecting organisms are planted in a terminal bronchus well out in the periphery of the lung, the initial lesion begins in that region, as was demonstrated by Robertson, Coggeshall, and Terrell (1084) in dogs and by Francis and Terrell (483) in monkeys.

In mice where pneumonia has resulted from the inhalation of pneumococci, Branch and Stillman (146) reported that the lesion might be either near to or distant from the hilum.

Little definite evidence is at hand indicating the site of the initial lesion in man, and the opportunity to study early lesions at necropsy is seldom encountered. As the result of his pathologic studies, Lauche (766) believes that pneumococci gain the trachea and at its bifurcation puncture the mucous membrane and enter the lymphatics at that point. The observations of Joannides and Steinman (685), however, suggest that the initial lesion is in the alveoli. Loeschcke (798) also considers that the initial lesion occurs in the alveoli, where inhaled pneumococci exert an irritating effect upon the cells of the alveolar epithelium, and that the beginning reaction is nearly always at the periphery of the lobe at or just under the pleura. Among fifty cases studied, the primary focus of infection was nearly always in dorsal dependent portions of the bronchial tree. In general, lesions usually began in areas embracing horizontal branches of the bronchi in the most dependent parts of the lobes; and the lower lobes, especially on the right, were most frequently the seat of the initial process. This peculiarity of distribution was regarded as due to the anatomic position of the main bronchi, which were more favorably situated to receive the deposition of aspirated material in some locations than in others.

Information relative to roentgenographic evidence of the site of the initial process in man is given in a following section on the spread of the lesion (see page 253).

So far as the nature of the initial lesion is concerned, the observations made in the course of the experimental infection of animals are of some interest, though it seems almost certain that a much larger number of organisms have been administered under such circumstances than ever ordinarily reach the human lung under normal conditions. In animals, as previously mentioned, the early lesions following infection by way of the respiratory tract frequently show some injury to the epithelium of the larger or smaller bronchi, and in many instances organisms have been found in the interstitial tissues and walls of the alveoli both within and at some distance from the lesion. Edema of increasing extent and some leucocytic infiltration of the involved area appeared.

Blake and Cecil (123) considered the inflammatory reaction in the interstitial tissues and walls of the bronchi with an accompanying lymphangitis as a part of the initial process in monkeys. Exudation into the alveoli was believed to occur secondarily. Robertson, Coggeshall, and Terrell (1084) found the very early lesion in dogs to be similar to this, though the interstitial reaction was less marked; and one hour after infection organisms were seen migrating in all directions away from the primary focus. Branch and Stillman (146) reported that the earliest lesion in mice was also an interstitial inflammation which involved the tissues around the bronchioli, atria, and alveoli and spread in the interstitial tissues around the blood vessels and bronchi and in the alveolar walls, but that both involvement of the lymphatics and exudation into the alveoli were probably secondary phenomena. Rake's (1058) findings in mice were almost identical to those of Branch and Stillman. In rabbits, Permar (1013) stated that the initial reaction involved the walls of the air passages, especially the smaller ones, which showed a degeneration and desquamation of their epithelial linings and a congestion of the subepithelial blood vessels. The striking early reaction was in the walls of the bronchioles, alveolar ducts, atria, and alveoli (indicating the presence of some early interstitial inflammation), following which exudation into the alveoli appeared with a subsequent involvement of the lymphatics and the development of an acute interstitial reaction. Schöbl and Sellards' (1162) findings in monkeys were nearly identical to those reported by Permar in the rabbit, and the acute interstitial inflammation with lymphangitis was considered a secondary reaction.

In the six studies cited above, involvement of the interstitial tissues and lymphatics was regarded as a part of the primary process by Blake and Cecil (123) and Robertson and his associates (1084), while Branch and Stillman (146), Rake (1058), Permar (1013), and Schöbl and Sellards (1162) viewed it as a secondary phenomenon.

In man, Lauche (766) considered the early lesion to be a penetration of the bronchial mucosa by the organisms, as noted above, following which they accumulated in the regional lymphatics, inciting an inflammatory reaction which induced a retrogressing flow of lymph back over the lobe, leading to an involvement of the alveoli. In this connection Miller's (893, 894, 895) extensive and detailed studies of the anatomy of the mammalian lung are of interest, for they indicate that the flow of lymph in the lymph vessels which accompany the pulmonary blood vessels and bronchi is presumably toward the hilum under ordinary circumstances. As such deep lymphatics have but few valves, it might be possible that the direction of their flow may be reversed in some areas and, by virtue of their anastomoses with the superficial lymphatics of the pleura, drain toward the periphery of the lung. This might assist in the rapid development of a pleurisy such as so commonly causes pain early in the course of human pneumonia. In dogs with experimental pneumonia, Robertson and his associates (1084) observed fibrin deposits on the pleura over the consolidated area within twelve hours of the time of infection.

Returning again to the early lesions in man, the observations of Joannides and Steinman (685) suggested that the initial lesion was in the alveoli; and, as a result of the irritation incited by the organisms, a considerable amount of fluid exuded into the alveoli. Loeschcke (798) also stated that the initial presence of pneumococci in the alveoli called forth a voluminous outpouring of edema fluid, with the subsequent appearance of leucocytes and fibrin. The entrance of organisms into the interstitial tissues and lymphatics was regarded as a secondary process.

Atelectasis and Pathogenesis

In recent years, due largely to the studies of Coryllos and his associates (322, 323, 632), the possible relation of atelectasis to the inception of pneumococcus lobar pneumonia has received considerable attention.

In dogs with experimental lobar pneumonia, Coryllos (322) observed that roentgenograms frequently showed considerable atelectasis and an increased density of the lung on the affected side with an elevation of the diaphragm and displacement of the heart and mediastinum toward the involved side. It was as a consequence of these findings and from a consideration of certain features of pneumococcus pneumonia in man, such as the common lobar distribution of the lesion, the frequency with which symptoms of an acute upper respiratory infection may precede the onset of the illness, and the sudden onset shown by many cases, that this investigator was led to suggest that atelectasis played an important role in the development of pneumococcus lobar pneumonia. His opinion was that a pneumococcus bronchitis occurred and that the thick tenacious exudate produced by this infection led to the occlusion of a bronchus, which resulted in the collapse of a lobe or parts of a lobe in which the infection spread and pneumonia developed. He regarded lobar atelectasis and lobar pneumonia as due to the same process, namely, the occlusion of a bronchus by retained exudate.

Certain observations made by other workers during the course of experimentally produced pneumonia in animals are of interest in relation to this point. The roentgenographic study of dogs showed that many exhibited evidence suggesting the presence of considerable collapse of the involved portions of the lung, as Henderson and his associates (632) noted. Robertson, Coggeshall, and Terrell (1083, 1084) pointed out that, in dogs having a slowly spreading and well-localized pulmonary lesion, little or no shift of the mediastinum occurred; but in other animals, in which the lesion was generalized and rapidly spreading, marked displacement of the heart toward the affected side was commonly encountered. It was noted that the fully consolidated lobe was of the same size as the normal lobe or slightly smaller and that a slight displacement of the heart and diaphragm in such instances was probably due to a fixation of lung size and a lack of aeration in addition to an increased elastic tension in the involved lung. Lieberman and Leopold (782) also observed that many dogs with experimental pneumonia showed a marked displacement of the heart and mediastinum toward the affected side accompanied by an elevation of the diaphragm on that side.

In monkeys at necropsy small areas containing collapsed alveoli were found by Blake and Cecil (123), and some collapsed bronchioli were reported by Schöbl and Sellards (1162). Lesions very similar to those noted by Blake and Cecil, showing varying degrees of alveolar collapse in the narrow zone surrounding the infected area but without involvement of the bronchi, were reported in dogs by Robertson, Coggeshall, and Terrell (1084). Mucous plugs were found only late in pneumonia in these animals.

In patients with pneumonia Cole (297) never found displacement of the heart or mediastinum in the absence of pleural fluid, though the diaphragm on the affected side was usually high. Coryllos (322) bronchoscoped nine patients with lobar pneumonia and found some exudate about the mouth of the bronchus of the affected lobe in all instances. This was removed and air blown into the bronchus with but little effect on the patient. Coryllos and Birnbaum (323) considered that, while some collapse of the lung was present in lobar pneumonia, mediastinal displacement was not marked as the exudate within the lung presumably prohibited much collapse. Henderson, Haggard, Coryllos, and Birnbaum (632) stated that atelectasis was especially likely to occur in post-operative patients and to give rise to post-operative pneumonia. Henderson (630) and Ross (1125) also favored this view. King (718), however, after an extensive study of post-operative pulmonary complications, which was carried out with unusual care, was led to the conclusion that pneumonia did not necessarily or even frequently develop in a collapsed area (see page 519).

Lord (808) mentions finding atelectasis of variable but usually slight degree in the roentgenograms of twenty-three of forty-seven patients with lobar pneumonia. He (811) also presented a comprehensive discussion of pulmonary collapse and its relationship to various pathologic states in man and noted that lung collapse of minor extent is frequent in both lobar pneumonia and bronchopneumonia but that massive collapse is rare in these diseases. In a series of 558 cases of pneumonia personally examined, Lord found evidence of massive collapse in only 14 or 2.5 per cent. In nine instances the patients had lobar pneumonia and in five bronchopneumonia. This investigator likewise reviewed the work of Coryllos and his associates and pointed out that their observations on the common occurrence of massive collapse in dogs undergoing an experimentally induced pneumonia probably cannot be applied to man, as relatively large doses of culture (10–15 cc.) were used in producing the experimental lesions and it is highly unlikely that such large doses are involved in the production of pneumonia in man. Other objections to the view that massive collapse is regularly concerned in the pathogenesis of lobar pneumonia were cited. It was pointed out that the finding of exudate in the bronchus of the involved lobe is not sufficient evidence of the lack of ingress or egress of air nor is mixture with mucus sufficient reason to believe that bloody sputum in pneumonia originates in the bronchus. Furthermore, and importantly, the physical signs in pneumonia are ordinarily those of consolidation with the large bronchi open and not those of collapse with a closed bronchus.

Graeser, Wu, and Robertson (552) took serial roentgenograms of the lungs of forty patients with lobar pneumonia, twenty of which were examined within the first forty-eight hours of illness. No collapse was found in any of the early cases. Nevertheless, some elevation of the diaphragm was commonly encountered at some stage of the disease, while in a few instances the motion of the diaphragm on the affected side appeared increased. Displacement of the mediastinum was seldom observed. As a result of their observations, these investigators concluded that atelectasis was not common in the pneumonia of adults. In children and dogs, whose mediastinum is more mobile, evidence of a mediastinal displacement was much more frequently encountered. As compared with human lungs, dog lungs are more elastic and less fibrous (1083). Davies, Hodgson, and Whitby (341) studied about 1,500 roentgenograms of 119 patients with pneumococcus pneumonia, only nine of whom were examined within the first forty-eight hours of illness. It was reported that, either coincident with or possibly preceding the development of the pulmonary consolidation, some elevation of the diaphragm on the affected side, and at times on the normal side as well, and a narrowing of the intercostal spaces over the involved lobe occurred. Such changes were commonly found. A shift of the mediastinum was rare, however, and appeared to occur only when the process developed with great rapidity. This latter finding is somewhat analogous with that reported by Robertson and his associates in dogs (1084), as mentioned earlier.

A consideration of the findings of the above investigators reveals that, while the role of atelectasis in the pathogenesis of pneumococcus lobar pneumonia is not clear, it seems probable that it is of relatively little importance in man in the usual case. It is possible in occasional instances, however, that atelectasis may be a factor in the development of pneumonia.

Spread of Lesion

Two general methods have been described by which the early lesion in pneumonia spreads. The infection may extend through the interstitial tissues and particularly the lymphatics of the lungs, or the organisms may be passively carried in edema fluid in response to the action of gravity and intrapulmonary pressure variations. It is likely in many instances that a combination of these methods is responsible for the extension of the lesion.

In mice, Branch and Stillman (146) described the spread of the process as occurring in an irregular fashion in the alveolar septums or interstitial tissues around the blood vessels and bronchi. Involvement of the lymphatics was considered to play a minor role in the process, which spread just as readily from the hilum outward as from the periphery in. Rake's (1058) findings in mice were essentially similar to these. In rabbits, Permar (1013) observed that, after the development of the initial lesion, the interstitial tissues and lymphatics became involved, following which the spread of infection through the lung progressed more rapidly. The lymphangitis was regarded as a secondary process and of extreme importance in the extension of the lesion. In monkeys, Blake and Cecil (123) considered that the spread of pneumococci in the lung was by way of the perivascular, peribronchial, and septal tissue and lymphatics. Schöbl and Sellards' (1162) observations of this animal were similar in this respect. In dogs, Robertson, Coggeshall, and Terrell (1084) found the lesion to extend in a regular manner. Though inflammation of the interalveolar septums was not conspicuous, the peribronchial and perivascular edema was marked. During the first few hours the organisms appeared to spread through the lung parenchyma in the lymphatics and capillaries, but after about six hours pneumococci were most numerous lying free in the edema fluid which filled the alveoli about the periphery of the lesion. It seemed probable that in this later period the organisms might be carried by the fluid through the small air passages into adjacent lobules. In this instance the possibility existed that the interstitial process, as well as the edema fluid, was importantly concerned in the spread of the infection.

Both Lauche (766) and Loeschcke (798) have regarded lobar pneumonia in man as an allergic manifestation occurring in a sensitized individual as already mentioned. The former considered that pneumococci, after gaining the lymphatics in the region of the hilum, multiplied and accumulated there in sufficient numbers to evoke considerable inflammatory reaction in the area, with a resultant blocking of the lymph channels, following which the infection spread throughout the entire lobe in the reversed flow of lymph. Organisms were presumed to enter the alveoli from the alveolar walls and there set up a hyperergic reaction. Loeschcke, however, disagreed with this conception of the spread of the lesion. His view was that the presence of air-borne organisms in the alveoli of the allergic sensitized lung caused an outpouring of edema fluid in which the bacteria multiply and accumulate, and that this fluid with its contained organisms spreads more or less quickly throughout the lobe. This process was accompanied by a rapid passage of organisms into the regional lymphatics. Pneumococci were always found in the alveolar edema fluid before being observed within the lymphatics. Before extensive coagulation of the exudate occurred, the edema fluid was considered to spread through the lobe by passing through the alveolar pores of Cohn into near-by acini, the process being aided by the negative pressure within the remainder of the lung. While the spread of infected edema fluid was largely stopped by the interlobar septums, penetration beyond these through various fenestrations and tissue bridges in these barriers was frequently found. Breathing and coughing assisted this process of spread, and attention was called to the possibility of violent coughing causing metastases in distant parts of the lung. Robertson and his co-workers (1084) pointed out the similarity of these findings with their own in their description of the spread of the infection in dogs with lobar pneumonia.

Loeschcke also carried out some interesting experiments in individuals having a radiopaque liquid in their bronchi, who were examined under the fluoroscope. Small columns of fluid were seen in the small bronchi, which oscillated during breathing and frequently spilled over and were aspirated into new areas in this manner. The liquid was seen to spread to entirely new bronchial areas with forced breathing and, on coughing, even to new lobes of the lung. Loeschcke considered that the mechanism of the spread of the infected edema fluid in pneumonia was essentially similar to this and in studying a group of twenty cases in which a metastasis of the lesion had occurred, noted that in nearly all instances the fluid had spread into more dorsal regions, which in the supine patient were in the most dependent position.

At this point it is well to consider other available evidence relating to the spread of pneumococcus infections by fluid exudates. The importance of gravity in controlling the direction of the spread of liquids injected into the bronchial tree was pointed out by Permar (1013), Schöbl and Sellards (1162), and Fried (496). Rhoads and Goodner (1076) found the earliest reaction in intradermally infected rabbits to be an extensive outpouring of edema fluid which contained many pneumococci. The spread of this fluid, and consequently the direction of the spread of the lesion, was chiefly affected by gravity. Goodner (534) confirmed these observations and reported that, due to the presence in the edema fluid of increased amounts of antithrombin, the fluid did not clot. The direction of the flow of the edema fluid was influenced by gravity to follow the line of least resistance rather than to follow the blood or lymph vessels. Robertson and his associates (1083, 1084) have emphasized the probable importance of the carriage of organisms by edema fluid in the spread of pneumonia in dogs; and in animals receiving the largest doses of infecting organisms, the lesions were generally the most extensive, the fatality rate was the highest, and the outpouring of edema fluid was the most marked. The presence in such fluids of the specific capsular polysaccharide of the infecting pneumococci, as well as of products of the autolysis of these organisms, may inhibit the action of any antibodies present and assist in making an already extensive injury more severe (see pages 131–132).

As the exudation of fluid into the alveolar spaces in pneumonia is always most pronounced about the periphery of the lesion, where pneumococci are the most numerous, these findings clearly suggest means by which the spread of the process may be facilitated, at least in the early stages of the lesion before extensive coagulation of the exudate occurs; and in man this period may apparently extend over an interval of several hours to a day or more.

Roentgenographic studies have been made in an effort to determine the probable location of the initial process in man and the usual direction of its spread. Sante (1158) reported that the lesion in children begins at the periphery of the lung and extends toward the hilum, while in adults it begins at the hilum and extends outward. There is fairly general agreement, at least so far as the usual case in adults is concerned, that the lesion begins in the neighborhood of the hilum and extends toward the periphery (297, 1329, 552, 341). This possibly may be interpreted to indicate that the initial pneumococcus invasion occurs in the region of the hilum. Nevertheless, it seems clear, as Graeser, Wu, and Robertson (552) and Davies, Hodgson, and Whitby (341) have demonstrated, that in occasional instances the process may begin elsewhere, such as at the periphery, and extend inwards. The latter workers reported that this somewhat unusual course of events occurred chiefly in cases due to pneumococci of Type III or one of the higher types. Ude (1329) and Davies and his associates (341) noted the appearance of soft linear shadows or thickened striae in early lesions or in overexposed films of later lesions which radiated from the hilum in the affected region. The arrangement of such shadows suggested that they represented an inflammatory engorgement of the vascular and lymphatic tissues surrounding the bronchi. Ude pointed out that lateral films of so-called hilum lesions frequently showed a triangular or cone-shaped area of consolidation, the base of which was usually at the periphery and the apex toward the hilum.

Summary

The available evidence suggests that for the development of pneumococcus lobar pneumonia a certain combination of circumstances must be present. It seems likely that (a) pneumococci of some virulence must have reached the lower respiratory tract; and that (b) against the organism some degree of resistance or enhanced cellular reactivity must be present, and this perhaps may or may not be confined to the lung of the host; it is also possible that (c) the action of the normal protective mechanism of the lung must be inhibited or damaged by some unfavorable condition which permits organisms to penetrate the parenchyma of the lung or protects them until their presence has incited sufficient local damage to allow the infection to get a foothold. These conditions closely resemble those described by Branch and Stillman (146) as controlling the production of lobar pneumonia in mice.

In so far as the conditions themselves are concerned, the first and second of those mentioned above appear to need little comment. In respect to the third condition, it may be noted, as was pointed out in various places in this and in the preceding chapter, that in animals damage to the pulmonary tissue may be necessary for the production of lobar pneumonia. Possibly the situation is somewhat similar in man, the injury being brought about by exposure to various unfavorable conditions such as not infrequently antedate the spontaneous development of lobar pneumonia in patients.

The problem is extremely involved, however, and it is not clear how any of the above conditions is affected by those factors generally regarded as predisposing individuals to pneumonia. As an illustration of this, consideration may be given the occurrence of acute minor respiratory infections, for, together, such conditions appear to constitute the single most commonly encountered predisposing factor in patients with lobar pneumonia. Whether the unfavorable action of an infection of this nature results from its influence on a single one of the above conditions or whether it affects one or both of the others as well, and possibly in different degrees, remains essentially unknown. To be sure, there is suggestive evidence that in occasional instances infections such as the common cold in some way facilitate the entrance of organisms into the lower respiratory tract and that possibly the degree of general host resistance or cellular reactivity remains unchanged or is somewhat increased at this time, yet it is not clear that the action of the normal protective mechanism of the lung is damaged as a consequence of a cold, and some additional factor may be necessary at such times to produce this injury. Till more information is available, explanations such as this must rest far more upon assumption than upon fact.

CHAPTER SIX

EPIDEMIOLOGY

Unreliability of Reports and Statistics 258
Geographic Prevalence 260
Frequency of Pneumonia and Pneumonia Death Rates 264
Trend of Pneumonia Death Rates 284
Climatic and Seasonal Distribution and Influence of Meteorological Factors 288
Accessory Factors Influencing Incidence of Pneumonia 299
Age 299
Sex 307
Race 312
Social Condition 316
Personal Condition 333
Exposure to Wet and Cold (Chilling) and Temperature Variations .. 336
Previous Respiratory Infections 339
Trauma and Aspiration of Noxious Substances 340
Transmission and Spread of Pneumococcus Lobar Pneumonia 342
Pneumococcus Carriers 342
Healthy Carriers not Having Contact with Pneumonia Patients 343
Healthy Carriers Having Contact with Pneumonia Patients 351
Total Number of Healthy Carriers in the Community 362
Secondary Carriers Produced by Contact with Carriers 365
Convalescent Carriers 366
Duration of Carrier State 367
Virulence Studies 372
Factors Affecting the Carrier State 373
Seasonal Prevalence of Pneumococci 378
Epidemics and Multiple Cases in Families 386
General Considerations of Epidemiology 390

UNRELIABILITY OF REPORTS AND STATISTICS

At the outset of any general discussion of the epidemiology of pneumonia it is well to appreciate that the absolute frequency of occurrence of this disease is unknown.* Statistics from official health organizations are available from many communities of the world, giving information on the total number of deaths from various causes including pneumonia. Such figures, however, do not reveal the actual number of cases which have occurred. In fact, in many instances, especially in Africa (770) and throughout the tropics in

* The preliminary returns from a recent governmental survey of 2,602,000 persons in 83 widely separated cities and towns and 24 rural counties in the United States over a twelve-

general (510), where deaths are frequently incompletely reported, official figures are not a reasonably accurate indication of even the number of deaths that have occurred.

Acute infections of the respiratory tract cause more disability (311) and a higher mortality at present than any other group of diseases (297, 200). In spite of inadequate reporting it is believed that under ordinary conditions the majority of fatal cases of acute lung disease are due to lobar pneumonia. In the United States, as in other countries, it is impossible to obtain morbidity figures indicating the exact prevalence of this disease, for neither pneumonia nor any one of its varieties has been made reportable by most states. In a few states, such as Massachusetts and New York, lobar pneumonia has been made notifiable; but in view of the number of cases and deaths reported in these states each year, it is probable that little over one-half (if that many) of the cases that occur are ever reported.

In temperate regions the epidemiology of lobar pneumonia with its definite seasonal variation appears to differ considerably from that of bronchopneumonia which is frequently erratic and lacks this periodicity (661, 837, 331). Clinical differentiation of the two diseases may be difficult or at times impossible, but in the main it is usually relatively easy to distinguish between them. Marked changes in the clinical diagnoses of diseases of the respiratory group have occurred during the past half-century. In the United States today there are fewer deaths attributed to undefined or unspecified pneumonia, bronchitis, and capillary bronchitis than there were fifty years ago. In consequence, in computing separate rates for the various forms of pneumonia, cognizance must be taken of this trend of diagnostic change; and to avoid unescapable pitfalls of error in computing rates over a long period of years, it is usually necessary to group all forms of pneumonia together.

There is no uniform method used throughout the world for reporting deaths from pneumonia. In some countries deaths are reported under the heading of "Pneumonia," while in others figures are given for "Bronchopneumonia Only" or "Lobar Pneumonia Only" and "Pneumonia, Type Unspecified," or various combinations of these terms may be used; while in a few places (notably some sections of India, 510) deaths from pneumonia are included under the general heading of "Respiratory Diseases."

The usual unreliability of both vital and hospital statistics for determining the morbidity of pneumonia has been lamented by various investigators (647, 510, 837, 1213). Because adequate morbidity figures are lacking, it will

month period in 1935–1936 reveal figures indicating that the annual incidence of pneumonia (all forms) was 558 cases per 100,000 population (1343).

be noted that much of the general discussion in the following sections is concerned with the number of deaths and the death rates from all forms or specific varieties of pneumonia. Observing due caution regarding the apparent accuracy and significance of such figures, certain points of interest will be mentioned. Among others, the *Epidemiological Reports of the Health Section of the Secretariat* of the League of Nations (768, 769), the United States mortality statistics (1335), and the mortality statistics for the State of Massachusetts (867) are of special value, but they too leave much to be desired.

GEOGRAPHIC PREVALENCE

Pneumonia is a ubiquitous, endemic, and at times epidemic disease. It has been reported from practically every country of the world from the arctics to the tropics. Though usually regarded as most prevalent in temperate zones, information is now at hand, as will be seen below, indicating its great prevalence in many of the warmer regions and true tropical areas of the world.

Among the older writers Hirsch (647) and Wells (1399, 1401) have both commented upon the world-wide prevalence of this disease and list hundreds of references supporting their observations. Their reports were made in 1886 and 1889. Judging from recent statistics, the situation with regard to the wide distribution of pneumonia has not changed, and it continues to be reported from all sections of the world. The following is a list of the countries, along with a selected group of available reports, which clearly indicate the world-wide distribution of this disease.

Countries from which pneumonia of various forms has been reported within recent years and a list of selected reports

North and Central America

CANADA
- *Canada Year Book* (213)
- League of Nations reports (771, 769)
- Mills (897)
- Howard (661)
- MacCordick (830)
- Brown (157)

UNITED STATES OF AMERICA
- Wells (1405)
- United States mortality statistics (1335)

North and Central America

UNITED STATES OF AMERICA (*cont.*)
- Tomanek and Wilson (1315)
- Wilson (1425)
- Massachusetts mortality statistics (867)
- Massachusetts Department of Public Health reports (865)
- League of Nations reports (769)
- Cecil (226)
- Anderson and Heffron (17)
- Heffron (613)
- Heffron and Robinson (615)

North and Central America (cont.)

HAWAIIAN ISLANDS
United States mortality statistics (1335)

MEXICO
Goodman (530)
League of Nations reports (769)
Hoffman (650)
Health department report (887)

PUERTO RICO
Suárez (1261)
United States mortality statistics (1335)

VIRGIN ISLANDS
United States mortality statistics (1335)

JAMAICA
Gifford, cited by Gautier (510)

GUATEMALA
League of Nations reports (769)

SALVADOR
Official statistical report (1157)
League of Nations reports (769)

HONDURAS
Phelps (1019)
Gautier (510)

SEVERAL CENTRAL AMERICAN AND NORTHERN SOUTH AMERICAN COUNTRIES
United Fruit Company reports (1331, 1332, 1333)

PANAMA REPUBLIC
Gautier (510)

PANAMA CANAL ZONE
Gorgas (549)
Clark (273)
Health department reports (979, 980)
League of Nations reports (769)

South America

BRITISH GUIANA
Gautier (510)

TRINIDAD AND TOBAGO
Report of Medical Inspector (1323)

VENEZUELA
League of Nations reports (769)

COLOMBIA
Egbert (387)
Official statistical reports (312)
League of Nations reports (769)

ECUADOR
Health department report (384)
Crespo, cited by Gautier (510)
League of Nations reports (769)
Ecuador statistical bulletin (385)

CHILE
Gonzalez (528)
Official statistical reports (262, 261)
League of Nations reports (769)

PARAGUAY
League of Nations reports (769)

ARGENTINA
Buenos Aires letter (1037)
Bachmann and Miravent (53a)
League of Nations reports (769)

URUGUAY
League of Nations reports (769)

BRAZIL
Austregesilo (29)
Health department report (80)
League of Nations reports (769)

Greenland
Cole (297)

Europe

ENGLAND AND WALES
Reports of Registrar General (559, 560)

Europe

ENGLAND AND WALES (*cont.*)

Griffith (571)
Glynn and Digby (520)
Canada Year Book (213)
League of Nations reports (771, 769)
Hay (606)
Langley (763)
Macnalty (852)
Davies, Hodgson, and Whitby (339, 340, 341)

SCOTLAND

Grant (553)
McLachlan (844)
Alston and Stewart (13)
Cruickshank (331)
Macgregor (837)
Blacklock and Guthrie (112)
Christie (267)
Therapeutic Trials Committee of Medical Research Council (557)
League of Nations reports (769)

NORTH IRELAND

League of Nations reports (769)

IRISH FREE STATE

Moore (902)
League of Nations reports (769)

NORWAY AND SWEDEN

Thjötta and Hanneborg (1294)
Strøm (1252)
Lindau (783)
League of Nations reports (769)

DENMARK

Christensen (265)
League of Nations reports (769)

THE NETHERLANDS AND BELGIUM

League of Nations reports (769)

FRANCE

Menetrier (882)

Europe

FRANCE (*cont.*)

Cotoni, Truche, and Raphael (324)
Feinblatt (406)
Canada Year Book (213)
League of Nations reports (771, 769)

SPAIN AND PORTUGAL

League of Nations reports (769)

ITALY

Pontano (1044)
Marginesu and Corda (860)
Levi (775)
League of Nations reports (769)

SWITZERLAND

Herzog (636)
League of Nations reports (769)

LUXEMBURG

League of Nations reports (769)

GERMANY

Canada Year Book (213)
League of Nations reports (771, 769)
Hallermann and Kähler (589)
Gundel and Linden (579)
Gundel and Schwarz (582)
Becker (84)

FINLAND

League of Nations reports (769)

ESTONIA, LATVIA, AND LITHUANIA

League of Nations reports (769)

SOVIET UNION (Russia)

League of Nations reports (769)
Viktorow, Semzowa, and Oettinger (1353)

POLAND

League of Nations reports (769)
Przesmycki, Kolago, and associates (1053)

Europe (cont.)

CZECHOSLOVAKIA

League of Nations reports (769)

AUSTRIA, HUNGARY, ROUMANIA, AND BULGARIA

League of Nations reports (769)

GREECE

Official statistical report (562)
League of Nations reports (769)

TURKEY

League of Nations reports (769)
Official statistical report (1327)

Africa

EGYPT

Official statistical report (389)
League of Nations reports (769)
Gohar and Abboud (526)

ANGLO-EGYPTIAN SUDAN

Whitehead (1419)
Gautier (510)

TUNISIA, ALGERIA, AND MOROCCO

League of Nations reports (769)

SENEGAL

Gautier (510)

FRENCH EQUATORIAL AFRICA

Vaucel and Salaün (1349)
Gautier (510)

BELGIAN CONGO

Walravens (1376)
Pearson and Mouchet (1008)
Gautier (510)

NORTHERN RHODESIA

Ordman (971)

UNION OF SOUTH AFRICA

Maynard (874)
Lister (784, 786)
Ordman (970)
Orenstein (973)
Lister and Ordman (788)

Africa (cont.)

MOZAMBIQUE (Portuguese East Africa)

Gautier (510)

TANGANYIKA TERRITORY

Lejeune (773)

KENYA

Garnham and deSmidt (507)
Gautier (510)

BRITISH SOMALILAND AND MAURITIUS

Gautier (510)

Asia

SYRIA AND PALESTINE

League of Nations reports (769)

PERSIA

Gilmour (517)

INDIA

Malone (857, 859)
Rogers (1103)
Cunningham and associates (334)
Health department reports (674, 673)
League of Nations reports (769)
Gautier (510)
Napier and Dharmendra (924)
Bhatnagar and Singh (100)

CEYLON

Gautier (510)
Health department report (247)

SIAM

Official statistical report (1196)

MALAY PENINSULA

Official statistical report (1200)
Macaulay (823)
McSwan (853)
Winchester (1428)
League of Nations reports (769)
Gautier (510)

Asia (*cont.*)

CHINA

Wu and Chiu (1450)
Health department reports (652, 653, 1173)

JAPAN

Ishida (680)
League of Nations reports (769)
Hirano (646)

PHILIPPINE ISLANDS

Cruz (332)
Vitug and Hizon (1357)
Official health reports (1020, 1021, 1022)
Monserrat (900)

Asia

PHILIPPINE ISLANDS (*cont.*)

League of Nations reports (769)
Albert and Abad (7)

DUTCH EAST INDIES

Gautier (510)
Kirchner (720)

Australia and New Zealand

Tebbutt (1287)
Penfold (1009)
Patterson (1003a)
Patterson and Williams (1003b)
Webster (1394)
Williams (1423)
League of Nations reports (769)

FREQUENCY OF PNEUMONIA AND PNEUMONIA DEATH RATES

In an extensive review of data on all forms of pneumonia Howard (661) found that from 2 to 6 per cent of all hospital admissions the world over were due to this disease and that it accounted for from 4 to 9 per cent of all deaths each year. These figures may be regarded as averages for communities in which pneumonia is fairly prevalent. In certain places in tropical and subtropical regions, however, the proportion of all deaths due to pneumonia may be very high, and figures of 16 to 49 per cent have been reported (1333, 874).

For the ten years of 1920 to 1929 inclusive, the mortality statistics for the United States registration area (1335) show that all forms of pneumonia accounted for 8.3 per cent or 1,006,869 of a total of 12,150,370 deaths. This is shown in Table 42 along with figures of a similar nature for Canada, England and Wales, France, and Germany. Though deaths from pneumonia are recorded in different ways in different countries and the figures in Table 42 for the countries mentioned above may not be strictly comparable to those of the United States, they nevertheless give an idea of the apparent relative importance of the disease in the countries listed. Of the total of over twenty-one million deaths from all causes, 7.4 per cent, or more than a million and a half, were due to pneumonia.

In the United States during the ten-year period mentioned above, pneumonia of all forms killed between 78,000 and 120,000 persons annually (see Table 43). Assuming that there are approximately four cases for each death,

TABLE 42. DEATHS FROM ALL CAUSES AND FROM PNEUMONIA, ALL FORMS. NUMBER AND PERCENTAGE, UNITED STATES, CANADA, ENGLAND AND WALES, FRANCE, AND GERMANY, FOR VARYING PERIODS, 1920–1929

	PERIOD	ALL CAUSES	PNEUMONIA OF ALL FORMS *Number*	*Per cent*
United States (1335)	1920–1929	12,150,370	1,006,869	8.3
Canada (213)	1924–1928	417,090	30,904	7.4
England and Wales (771)	1924–1928	2,344,681	176,555	7.5
France (771)	1925–1928	2,770,153	71,076	2.6*
Germany (771)	1924–1928	3,734,665	289,546	7.8
Total		21,416,959	1,574,950	7.4

* Judging from the death rates for pneumonia given in various League of Nations reports (768, 769) for several of the large cities of France, the proportion of 2.6 per cent of all deaths attributed to pneumonia seems too low. It is more probable that the correct proportion is about similar to that shown in the table for Germany.

TABLE 43. DEATHS FROM ALL CAUSES AND FROM PNEUMONIA, ALL FORMS, AND NUMBER AND PERCENTAGE OF DEATHS FROM LOBAR PNEUMONIA AND BRONCHOPNEUMONIA, UNITED STATES REGISTRATION AREA, 1920–1929

YEAR	ALL CAUSES	PNEUMONIA ALL FORMS*	LOBAR PNEUMONIA ALONE† *Number*	*Per cent*	BRONCHO-PNEUMONIA‡ *Number*	*Per cent*
1920	1,142,558	120,108	64,001	5.6	47,746	4.2
1921	1,032,009	78,263	37,871	3.7	34,889	3.4
1922	1,101,863	95,164	47,031	4.3	42,130	3.8
1923	1,193,017	105,680	52,480	4.4	46,221	3.9
1924	1,173,990	97,403	50,676	4.3	40,631	3.5
1925	1,219,019	96,432	51,407	4.2	39,820	3.3
1926	1,285,927	107,797	56,699	4.4	46,148	3.6
1927	1,236,949	87,230	46,694	3.8	36,574	3.0
1928	1,378,675	112,195	61,059	4.4	45,261	3.3
1929	1,386,363	106,597	57,547	4.2	43,690	3.2
Total	12,150,370	1,006,869	525,465	4.3	423,110	3.5

* Deaths from undefined pneumonia (numbering 58,294) included.
† Deaths from undefined pneumonia not included.
‡ Deaths from undefined pneumonia not included; capillary bronchitis included.

it may be estimated, as others have done (230, 17), that there are from 313,000 to 480,000 cases of pneumonia in this country each year. In England and Wales, where the case fatality rate of pneumonia appears to be somewhat lower than it is in this country (see pages 658–672), Hay (606) figured five cases for each death and estimated that there were 185,000 cases of pneumonia of all forms there in 1925. In similar fashion it may be estimated that in 1934 some 143,115 cases gave rise to the 28,623 deaths from pneumonia (852) which occurred there.

The number of deaths from all causes and the proportion due to pneumonia of various forms in the United States registration area for the ten years of 1920 to 1929 inclusive are shown in Table 43.

Of the total 12,150,370 deaths from all causes, lobar pneumonia alone (excluding undefined pneumonia, which is usually presumed to be lobar pneumonia) accounted for 4.3 per cent and bronchopneumonia (including capillary bronchitis) for 3.5 per cent of the deaths during the period in question. Of the 1,006,869 deaths from pneumonia of all forms during the ten years, 52 per cent were due to lobar pneumonia (excluding undefined pneumonia). In England and Wales the proportion of pneumonia deaths due to lobar pneumonia and undefined pneumonia together is very similar to this and was reported as 49.8 per cent in 1920 (661) and 49 per cent in 1934 (852).

The mortality statistics of the United States show that the rate for deaths from pneumonia of all forms averaged 88 per 100,000 population during the ten years of 1924 to 1933 inclusive (1335). In 1929 the disease was third among the commonest causes of death and was exceeded only by heart disease and cancer, in that order. According to Howard (661), the figure for deaths from all forms of pneumonia in Canada in 1926 was 90 per 100,000 population and the disease was also third among the commonest causes of death. In the United States in 1929, deaths from lobar pneumonia alone amounted to 49.5 per 100,000 population, and the disease was eighth among the commonest causes of death and was exceeded by heart disease, cancer, chronic nephritis, cerebral hemorrhage, accidental death, tuberculosis (all forms), and influenza, in that order.

The mortality statistics of Massachusetts (867) show that for the ten years of 1920 to 1929 inclusive, pneumonia of all forms has oscillated between the second and the fourth most important cause of death and has always been exceeded by heart disease and at times by cancer and cerebral hemorrhage. During the same period lobar pneumonia together with undefined pneumonia varied from seventh to ninth in frequency as the commonest cause of death. Deaths per 100,000 population for all forms of pneumonia for this same decade varied from 163 to 95 in this state, while the rate for lobar pneumonia and undefined pneumonia together varied from 74 to 46. In New York State, Cecil (226) has reported that pneumonia of all forms together with influenza was third among the commonest causes of death in 1933.

When the rank of pneumonia of all forms as a cause of death in Massachusetts is studied for individuals in different age groups, considerable variation is found (see Table 44). In general, pneumonia is a more important

TABLE 44. RANK OF PNEUMONIA, ALL FORMS, IN NUMERICALLY MOST IMPORTANT CAUSES OF DEATH, BY AGE GROUP, MASSACHUSETTS, 1906, 1916, AND 1926

AGE GROUP IN YEARS	RANK OF PNEUMONIA OF ALL FORMS *1906*	*1916*	*1926*	AGE GROUP IN YEARS	RANK OF PNEUMONIA OF ALL FORMS *1906*	*1916*	*1926*
Under 1	4	3	2	30–39	2	3	3
1–4	1	1	1	40–49	3	4	4
5–9	4	5	3	50–59	3	3	5
10–14	4	6	4	60–69	4	4	5
15–19	4	4	4	70 and over	3	4	6
20–29	3	5	5	Average	3	2	3

cause of deaths in infants and young children up to the age of five years than at other periods of life. The increasing importance of pneumonia as a cause of death in infants under one year of age, as shown by its change of rank from 1906 when it was fourth among the commonest causes of death to second place in 1926, may possibly be attributed to decreasing death rates among this group from other causes. In the age group seventy years and over, pneumonia was the third most important cause of death in 1906 and the sixth in 1926. This change in rank may be due to many factors, as, for example, increasing accuracy of diagnosis of diseases of the older age groups.

Just as life is continually changing, so both morbidity and mortality rates, being a product of life, are never stationary. The rates for pneumonia and its various forms vary continually and may be different in different places at the same time and vary considerably from year to year in the same place.

Individuals between the ages of twenty and sixty-five years may be regarded as constituting the most productive portion of the population. In the United States during the eight years of 1922 to 1929 inclusive approximately 36 per cent of the deaths from all forms of pneumonia occurred in persons between these ages; and during the ten years of 1920 to 1929 inclusive lobar pneumonia alone annually caused an average of over 52,000 deaths, of which 27,000 or more than 50 per cent were in patients within this age group. Assuming that these deaths represented but one-quarter of the cases which occurred in members of this group, it will be appreciated that a tremendous toll of sickness and death was taken among persons who were of the greatest economic importance to their communities.

During the past few decades pneumonia has become of tremendous economic importance among the natives, but not among the white population, in various tropical and subtropical regions. A review of numerous reports lends support to Gautier's (510) idea that the problem of the disease in these areas is chiefly limited to estates, plantations, mines, military groups, prisons, and so forth, where natives live and work in rather close contact under conditions which for them may be largely artificial.

In some regions either within the tropics, such as India (1103) and Central Africa (1008), or in which natives from the tropics were formerly employed, as in the gold and diamond mines of South Africa (874, 788), pneumonia has been recognized for thirty years or more as an important and perhaps the most important cause of death. The problem in those regions can hardly be regarded as a new one. In recent years, however, extensive areas in Central America and in tropical regions of Africa and the Far East have been opened up for exploitation, and reports are available from all these places attesting to the great prevalence of pneumonia.

It is common to find it stated in the literature dealing with this matter that pneumonia of all forms or lobar pneumonia alone is responsible for more deaths than any other disease. Statements of this nature may be found in the reports of the Tropical Division of the United Fruit Company, which operates largely in Central America and northern South America (1331, 1019, 1333, 1261). Official reports from Panama indicate that lobar pneumonia and bronchopneumonia are either first or second among the commonest causes of death (979, 980). Pneumonia mortality figures of from 200 to 1,500 per 100,000, with an average of 300 to 500, are common among the native gold and diamond miners in South Africa (874, 970, 788), and in central Africa both pneumonia and pneumococcus infections in general are extremely frequent (507, 1008, 1349, 773).* Pneumonia is also an important cause of

* Many foreign reports give death rates based on units of one thousand or 10,000 population. To simplify the text and make the figures readily comparable, all rates cited, unless otherwise mentioned, have been translated into units of 100,000 population.

death among the natives employed on the tea estates in India (924) and on the rubber plantations of the Malay Peninsula (823, 1428, 1036). Attempts to explain the great prevalence of pneumonia among natives in tropical regions have been made by various investigators, but much of the evidence presented is conflicting. The influence of several factors, such as climate, season, and race, on the prevalence of pneumonia is discussed in subsequent sections of this chapter.

North America

Judging from mortality statistics from various sources, pneumonia of all forms is more frequent in some cities and states in this country than in others. In other parts of the world the disease also appears specially prevalent in certain localities. In 1934 the Metropolitan Life Insurance Company of New York (886) called attention to the fact that, if the United States and Canada were considered as a whole and all areas with approximately similar rates for deaths from pneumonia were studied, certain regions, largely confined to two sections of the continent, appeared to show the highest pneumonia mortality rates. These two regions were designated as the "pneumonia belts."

One of these began in the northeastern portion of Canada in the region of Labrador and the Province of Quebec and, with a broad sweep and some minor variations, continued southward down along the Atlantic coastal states to include Georgia. This belt also extended inland in the region of the southern and central states to include Tennessee and Missouri. The second area of high pneumonia rates was in the mountain region of the west and included the four states of Colorado, New Mexico, Arizona, and Nevada. Several of the highest pneumonia death rates in the United States were found in these four western states.

As the figures used by the Metropolitan Life Insurance Company in this report covered only the two years of 1932 and 1933 and their source was not stated, it seemed advisable to attempt a similar compilation of data for the United States using the registration area mortality statistics for the ten years of 1924 to 1933 inclusive (1335). In the accompanying illustration (Map 3) the states having the highest death rates from pneumonia of all forms are represented by solid black and by crosshatching. The average rates per 100,000 in all states shown in solid black were above 88 for the ten-year period, which figure was the average for the entire country during that interval. Rates were not obtainable from a few states for all ten years, but what-

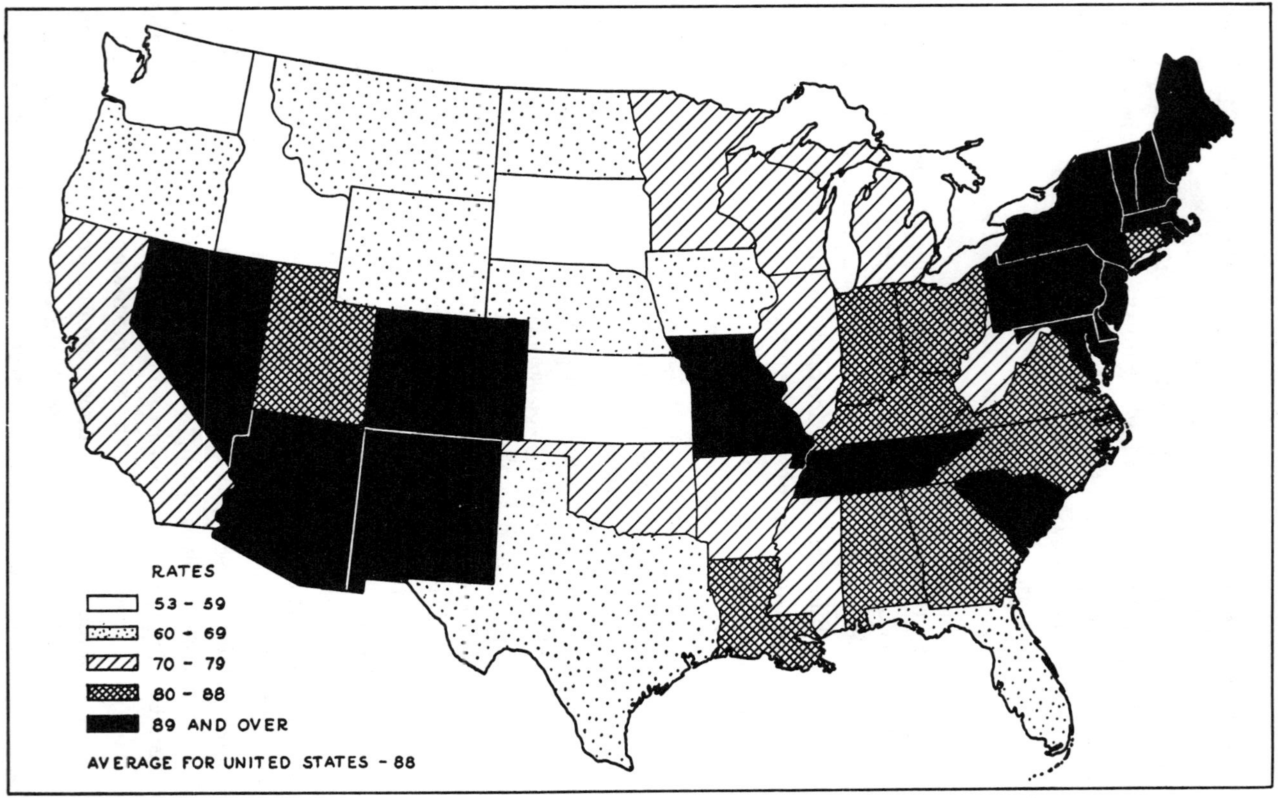

Map 3. Deaths per 100,000 population from pneumonia of all forms in the United States registration area, 1924–1933

ever data were available were used. This will be noted in the table (Table 45) accompanying Map 3, which lists all the states and the District of Columbia separately, giving the average death rates for bronchopneumonia (including capillary bronchitis), for lobar pneumonia (including undefined pneumonia), and for all forms of pneumonia.

The situation revealed by Map 3 clearly shows the two general areas of the country having the highest death rates from pneumonia and confirms the above-mentioned observations of the Metropolitan Life Insurance Company.* The first area is in the east and extends from Maine to Florida along the coast, and from Pennsylvania south extends westward to the Mississippi River to include all but West Virginia, Illinois, and Mississippi. Adjacent to this area on the west are included the states of Missouri and Louisiana. Maryland on the east, with a rate of 124, showed the highest rate in the United States (the rate for the District of Columbia was 121). Other states in the eastern area showed such high rates as 108 for Pennsylvania, 107 for Delaware, 106 for New York, 102 for Rhode Island, and 100 for Massachusetts. These six states have the highest rates in the eastern group and in 1930 held more than twenty-nine million persons or about 24 per cent of the total population of this country. Vermont with a rate of 94 and New Hampshire with 93 were next in order in the eastern group. Maine and South Carolina both had rates of 89. To the west and north of the latter, Tennessee showed a rate of 91 and Missouri of 99.

The second area, that in the far west, embraces the four states of Nevada (rate 122, the second highest in the United States), Arizona (rate 114), New Mexico (rate 113), and Colorado (rate 106). Utah with a rate of 81 may perhaps be included in this group.

No satisfactory explanation of the regional distribution of these high pneumonia death rates is at hand. Neither cold weather nor latitude can explain the findings, for the rate of Maine in the north with its cold climate is lower than that of Missouri and is the same as that of South Carolina in the south. Also, reports concerning pneumonia rates in Canada (769, 886) and those found for Montana and North and South Dakota in this country show that these northern regions which have long severe winters have low pneumonia death rates.

The high proportion of Negroes in the population of some of the southern states may be partly responsible for the high rates in states like South Carolina and Georgia. This alone, however, can hardly be the whole explanation; otherwise the rates of the neighboring states of Florida (rate 65)

* Findings very similar to these are shown in the *Report of Advisory Committee on Prevention of Pneumonia Mortality* of the United States Public Health Service (1343).

TABLE 45. AVERAGE FIGURES FOR DEATHS PER 100,000 POPULATION FROM BRONCHO-PNEUMONIA, LOBAR PNEUMONIA, AND PNEUMONIA ALL FORMS, UNITED STATES (CONTINENTAL) REGISTRATION AREA AND EACH STATE, FOR VARYING PERIODS, 1924–1933

	NUMBER OF YEARS INCLUDED IN RATE	DEATHS PER 100,000 POPULATION		
		*Broncho-pneumonia**	*Lobar pneumonia†*	*Pneumonia all forms*
U.S. Registration Area (continental)	10	37	51	88
Alabama	9	27	56	83
Arizona	8	53	61	114
Arkansas	7	23	48	71
California	10	39	40	79
Colorado	10	45	62	106
Connecticut	10	34	51	85
Delaware	10	47	60	107
District of Columbia	10	56	65	121
Florida	10	24	42	65
Georgia	7	28	59	86
Idaho	10	24	35	59
Illinois	10	32	46	78
Indiana	9	35	50	84
Iowa	10	28	40	68
Kansas	10	26	31	56
Kentucky	10	35	52	87
Louisiana	10	37	50	87
Maine	10	41	48	89
Maryland	10	61	63	124
Massachusetts	10	53	47	100
Michigan	10	34	45	79
Minnesota	10	34	38	72
Mississippi	10	20	55	75
Missouri	10	41	58	99
Montana	10	25	44	69
Nebraska	10	24	37	61
Nevada	4	43	79	122
New Hampshire	10	42	50	93

* Includes capillary bronchitis. † Includes undefined pneumonia.

TABLE 45 (*cont.*)

	NUMBER OF YEARS INCLUDED IN RATE	DEATHS PER 100,000 POPULATION *Broncho-pneumonia**	*Lobar pneumonia*†	*Pneumonia all forms*
New Jersey	10	35	57	92
New Mexico	5	53	60	113
New York	10	44	62	106
North Carolina	9	33	54	86
North Dakota	10	32	31	63
Ohio	10	38	44	82
Oklahoma	6	30	44	74
Oregon	10	29	36	65
Pennsylvania	10	43	65	108
Rhode Island	10	36	66	102
South Carolina	10	23	66	89
South Dakota	4	21	32	53
Tennessee	10	36	55	91
Texas	1	27	38	65
Utah	9	37	44	81
Vermont	10	39	55	94
Virginia	9	35	50	85
Washington	10	24	35	59
West Virginia	9	35	40	76
Wisconsin	10	32	41	73
Wyoming	10	25	38	63

* Includes capillary bronchitis. † Includes undefined pneumonia.

and Mississippi (rate 75), which have a Negro population as large as or larger than those states, might likewise be expected to be high (see Map 4).

Map 4 is taken from the United States census report of 1930 (1337) and shows the proportion of Negroes in the population of the various states. It offers an interesting contrast to Map 3, for it is clear that the heaviest concentration of the Negro population is in the southern states of this country, especially from Virginia and Tennessee south and extending westward to Texas. In general, these states have lower pneumonia death rates than many others farther north or to the west which have a much smaller proportion of Negroes in their population.

The larger part of the states in the west with high pneumonia death rates (Colorado, New Mexico, Arizona, Nevada, and possibly Utah) are included in the physical area of the Colorado Plateau; and, according to Goode's Atlas (529), this area is within the district (which also includes a portion of Wyoming and southern Idaho) having the highest mean rate of evaporation and the lowest average annual precipitation of any in the country. Further discussion of the relation of climate to pneumonia is given later (see page 288).

It is interesting that these western states with high rates for pneumonia are favored locations for patients with tuberculosis and for hospitals caring for this disease. Nevertheless, pneumonia is not common among patients with tuberculosis, though many patients with tuberculosis may previously have had pneumonia (918), and these states have high death rates for both tuberculosis and pneumonia. The New England states, however, with their high pneumonia death rates have low rates from tuberculosis. But, as was pointed out in the Metropolitan Life Insurance bulletin (886), many of the states with the highest pneumonia rates also have high tuberculosis death rates.

The relatively large proportion of native American Indians and of Mexicans in the populations of Arizona and New Mexico may also play some part in accounting for the excessive pneumonia rates shown by these states (886).

RATES AND AGE GROUPS. The data presented in Map 3 refer to rates for pneumonia of all forms in persons of all ages. Similar maps were prepared to show the death rates of pneumonia of all forms of persons in various age groups during the three years of 1924, 1927, and 1930. These, however, appeared to show nothing significant other than that many of the states which on Map 3 show low rates were among those with the highest rates for individuals seventy-five years of age and over; and several of the states with generally high rates, more especially in the eastern group, were usually among those having relatively low rates for these older persons. Along the Pacific coast California fell into the group of states with the highest pneumonia death rates in the country for persons in the age groups from birth to two years and from three to nine years. The rates for the states of Oregon and Washington were nearly always among the lowest even for the very young and the very old (for specific rates by age groups by states, see page 302).

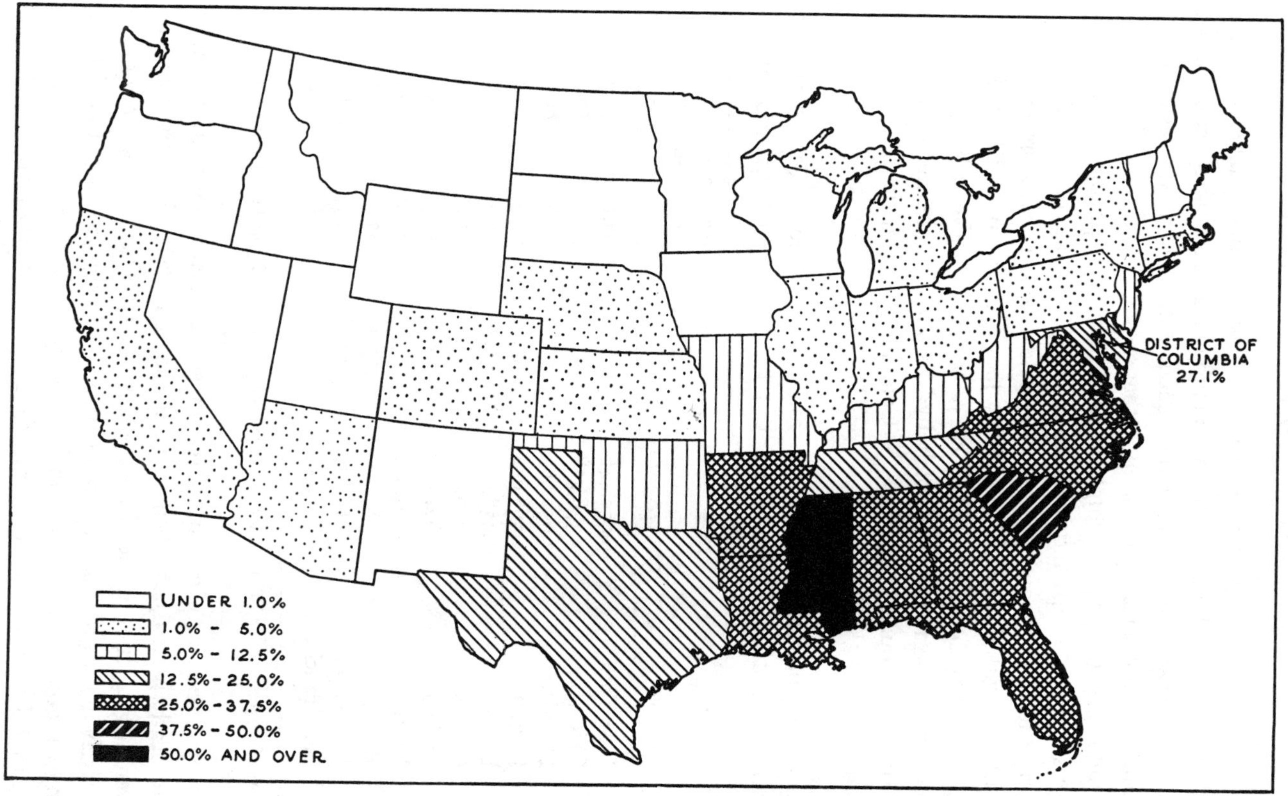

Map 4. Percentage of Negroes in the population of various states in 1930 (1337)

LOBAR PNEUMONIA AND BRONCHOPNEUMONIA. Two additional maps were prepared using the death rates for lobar pneumonia and bronchopneumonia as given in Table 45. The distribution of states with the highest rates for lobar pneumonia was essentially the same as that shown in Map 3 for all forms of pneumonia. States with the highest rates for bronchopneumonia roughly comprised three groups and included many, but not all, of the states with high rates for pneumonia of all forms and no others. The first group was in the east and, with the exception of New Jersey, Connecticut, Rhode Island, and Vermont, included all states north of Virginia and West Virginia. The second group was represented solely by Missouri, and the third group was made up of the four western states of Colorado, New Mexico, Arizona, and Nevada.

TABLE 46. DEATHS PER 100,000 POPULATION FROM PNEUMONIA, ALL FORMS, FOR THE ELEVEN LARGEST CITIES IN THE UNITED STATES, 1931, 1932, AND 1933

CITY	POPULATION*	DEATHS PER 100,000 PNEUMONIA OF ALL FORMS†		
		1931	*1932*	*1933*
New York	6,930,446	118.7	97.1	93.4
Chicago	3,376,438	75.0	65.1	63.9
Philadelphia	1,950,961	110.9	83.8	86.3
Detroit	1,568,662	65.5	67.9	51.7
Los Angeles	1,238,048	59.7	63.7	57.4
Cleveland	900,429	104.1	99.2	72.7
St. Louis	821,960	144.7	113.7	105.1
Baltimore	804,874	159.7	122.2	118.8
Boston	781,188	131.4	143.4	144.9
Pittsburgh	669,817	243.3	172.8	101.0
San Francisco	634,394	77.4	77.6	82.8

* As of 1930. † Rates are determined for the estimated population of each year.

RATES OF LARGEST CITIES OF THE UNITED STATES. Considerable variation is shown in the deaths per 100,000 population from pneumonia of all forms among the eleven largest cities in the United States (1335). These cities, arranged respectively in the order of the size of their populations, are listed in Table 46 along with their rates for 1931, 1932, and 1933.

In 1933 the rates varied from 51.7 for Detroit to 144.9 for Boston. Similar variations were present in 1931 and 1932. The size of the city does not correlate always with a high pneumonia rate, for Detroit with over twice the population of Boston, had a rate only about one-third as high in 1933. Other examples of this nature might be cited.

CITIES OF THE UNITED STATES WITH THE HIGHEST RATES. The United States mortality statistics report for 1932 (1335) gives the deaths per 100,000 population from pneumonia of all forms for several of the cities having a population of 100,000 or over in 1930. The cities with the ten highest rates in 1932 were as follows: Pittsburgh (rate 172), Boston (rate 143), Denver (rate 135), Washington, D.C. (rate 134), San Antonio (rate 130), Atlanta (rate 129), Kansas City, Missouri (rate 128), Memphis (rate 125), Nashville (rate 124), and Baltimore, Scranton, and Utica (rate 122 in each). Next in order were Minneapolis, Trenton, Cambridge, Camden, Cincinnati, Wilmington (Delaware), and more than a dozen others with rates of 100 or over. Though Pittsburgh heads the list with the highest rate in 1932, it appears from Table 46 that its rate decreased considerably by 1933 and it no longer held that position. During the past decade or two Pittsburgh had rates two or three times as high as any other city in the country, as others have pointed out (1314, 200, 1352, 162), but apparently this is no longer true.

It appears from the above-mentioned list of the pneumonia death rates for cities of 100,000 population or over that of the thirty-one cities having rates of 100 or over in 1932, all but six (Des Moines; El Paso; Kansas City, Kansas; Minneapolis; Omaha; and San Antonio) are within states shown on Map 3 as having the highest rates in the country. Minneapolis appears to be the only one of these six cities that is not close to other areas with high rates. Possibly San Antonio may be classed with Minneapolis in this respect, but it is close to Mexico; and though rates are not available for most of that country, they are very high for Mexico City, as will be seen below.

Countries Other than North America

A comparison of the death rates for pneumonia has been made for countries of the world other than the United States. Granted that it is difficult, if not impossible, to obtain accurate data from many countries, some use can be made of the available material. When extraordinarily high death rates for pneumonia are consistently reported from any community over a period of several years, they cannot be lightly disregarded.

The number of deaths and the death rates for pneumonia (chiefly for "pneumonia and bronchopneumonia" together) from many large cities throughout the world are given in the League of Nations epidemiologic re-

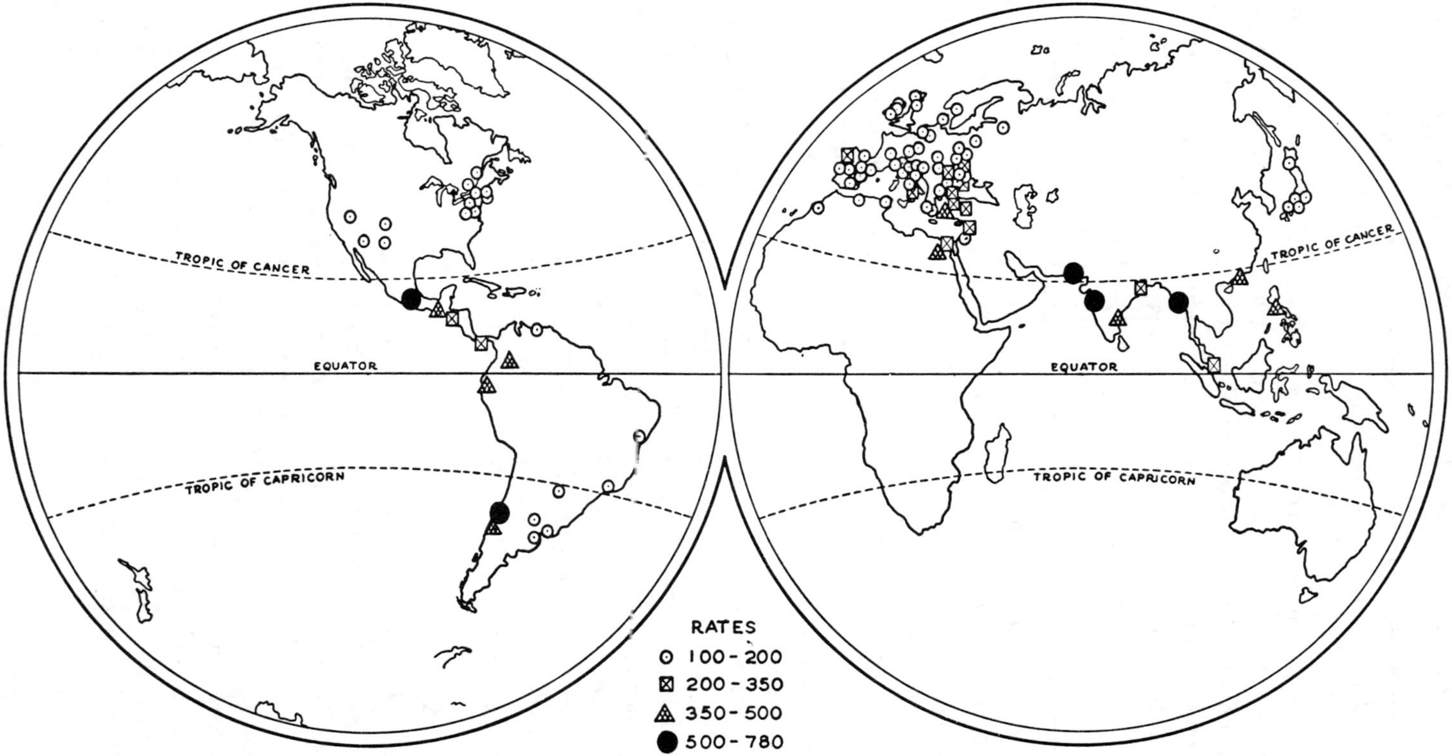

Map 5. Pneumonia (all forms) deaths per 100,000 population for certain cities throughout the world and of states in the United States having the highest death rates from this disease

ports (768, 769). Figures from this source have been used as a basis for the material presented in Map 5. Most communities having low figures for pneumonia deaths per 100,000 population over two, three, or more years were not further investigated. In many instances, however, extremely high rates obtained, and in all of these the League of Nations figures were sought for the past ten years. Such figures from Guatemala City, Guatemala, and Izmir (Smyrna), Turkey, were available for a period of only two years. Figures were obtained for from four to seven years for several cities with the highest rates in Central America and South America; for three years from Karachi, India; and for from five to ten years for the several other cities in India and elsewhere among those with the highest rates. In addition, wherever possible other outside sources giving figures for the same or different years were consulted to check rates that appeared excessive.

Nearly all the material available for comparing pneumonia death rates throughout the world is concerned with the rates for individual cities rather than for countries. At times, however, figures are given for several large cities in a single country, and this is more significant than rates for a single city. Nevertheless, it has been well known for years that probably the morbidity rate and certainly the mortality rate of pneumonia is usually higher in urban areas than in rural ones and is higher in the large cities than in the smaller ones (1403, 297, 200, 961, 674, 1335, 373, 852). The only report encountered which appeared at variance with this rule concerned death rates for pneumonia in Greece (562) where, over the period of 1921 to 1930 inclusive, the rates were always lower for persons in towns than for those in the country.

Table 47 accompanying Map 5 lists the various cities from which League of Nations reports (769) are available according to their death rates for one, two, or three of the years 1932–1933, 1933–1934, and 1934–1935. In several instances the reports are for the calendar years of 1932, 1933, and 1934, and at times, for investigative purposes, rates were studied for several other years. In some cities with high rates, such as Santiago and Valparaiso, Chile, no figures are available since 1930–1931. The number of years for which observations were at hand and the source of figures used to check these rates are indicated.

Because of the difficulty in obtaining necessary data, checking of the League of Nations figures was done only irregularly. When figures were checked, exact agreement was rare; but it was usual to find that if the League of Nations figures were very high, those from an outside source were

TABLE 47. DEATHS PER 100,000 POPULATION FROM PNEUMONIA ("PNEUMONIA" AND "BRONCHOPNEUMONIA" TOGETHER), FOR CERTAIN LARGE CITIES IN COUNTRIES OTHER THAN THE UNITED STATES, FOR VARYING PERIODS, 1924–1933 (LEAGUE OF NATIONS, 769, OR OTHER SOURCES, OR BOTH)

DEATH RATE	COUNTRY	CITY	NUMBER OF YEARS INCLUDED IN RATE	SOURCE OF DATA OTHER THAN REPORTS NO. 159, 166, 173, AND 179 LEAGUE OF NATIONS (769)
500 to 780	Chile	Valparaiso	4	League of Nations rep. (768) Official statistical rep. (262)
	India	Bombay	10	League of Nations rep. (768) Official health rep. (674)
		Karachi	5*	Official health rep. (674)
		Rangoon	10	League of Nations rep. (768) Official health rep. (674)
	Mexico	Mexico City	4†	Official health rep. (887)
350 to 500	Chile	Santiago	4	League of Nations rep. (768) Official statistical rep. (262)
	China	Hongkong‡	4	Official health rep. (652, 653)
	Colombia	Bogota	8	League of Nations rep. (768)
	Ecuador	Guayaquil	5†	Official health rep. (384)
	Egypt	Cairo	9	Official statistical rep. (389) League of Nations rep. (768)
	Guatemala	Guatemala City	2	
	India	Madras	9	League of Nations rep. (768)
	Philippine Islands	Manila	6†	Official health rep. (1021, 1020, and 1022)
	Turkey	Izmir (Smyrna)	3†	Official statistical rep. (1327)
200 to 350	Bulgaria	Plovdiv	2	
	Egypt	Alexandria	9	Official statistical rep. (389) League of Nations rep. (768)
	Greece	Salonica	7	League of Nations rep. (768)
	India	Calcutta	8	League of Nations rep. (768) Official health rep. (674)
	Italy	Naples	2	
	Panama	Panama City	6†	Official health rep. (979, 980)
	Portugal	Oporto	2	
	Roumania	Chisinau	2	

* Data for two years obtained from sources other than League of Nations, as indicated.
† Data for one year obtained from source other than League of Nations, as indicated.
‡ No League of Nations data available for Hongkong.

TABLE 47 (*cont.*)

DEATH RATE	COUNTRY	CITY	NUMBER OF YEARS INCLUDED IN RATE	SOURCE OF DATA OTHER THAN REPORTS NO. 159, 166, 173, AND 179 LEAGUE OF NATIONS (769)
200	Roumania (*cont.*)	Jassy	2	
to	Salvador	San Salvador	7	League of Nations rep. (768)
350	Straits Settlements	Singapore	11†	Official health rep. (1200) League of Nations rep. (768)
	Syria	Beyrouth	2	
	Turkey	Angora	6	
		Istanbul	5	Official statistical rep. (1327)
100	(North America)			
to	Canada	Ottawa	3	
200		Quebec	2	
	(South America)			
	Argentina	Buenos Aires	2	
		Santa Fé	2	
	Brazil	Rio de Janeiro	2	
		Salvador (Bahia)	2	Official health rep. (80)
	Paraguay	Asuncion	7	League of Nations rep. (768)
	Uruguay	Montevideo	2	
	Venezuela	Caracas	4	
	(Europe)			
	Belgium	Ghent	2	
		Liège	3	
	Bulgaria	97 Bulgarian towns	2	
		Sofia	2	
	Czechoslovakia	All of Czechoslovakia	2	
	Denmark	Copenhagen	3	
	France	Lyons	3	
		Marseilles	2	
		Nancy	3	
	Greece	Athens	6	League of Nations rep. (768)
		Piraeus	4	
	Hungary	Budapest	3	
	Ireland (North)	9 towns of North Ireland	3	
		Belfast	3	
	Irish Free State	Dublin	3	

† Data for one year obtained from source other than League of Nations, as indicated.

TABLE 47 (*cont.*)

DEATH RATE	COUNTRY	CITY	NUMBER OF YEARS INCLUDED IN RATE	SOURCE OF DATA OTHER THAN REPORTS NO. 159, 166, 173, AND 179 LEAGUE OF NATIONS (769)
100	(Europe) *cont.*			
to	Italy	Bologna	2	
200		Genoa	2	
		Milan	2	
		Rome	2	
		Trieste	3	
		Turin	2	
		Venice	2	
	Lithuania	Kowno	2	
	Luxemburg	Luxemburg	1	
	Norway	Oslo	3	
	Poland	Lodoz	2	
		Lwow	1	
		Warsaw	2	
	Portugal	Lisbon	2	
	Roumania	Bucharest	2	
		Cernauti	2	
		Galatz	2	
	Scotland	16 Scottish towns	2	
		Glasgow	2	
	Soviet Union	Leningrad	2	
	Spain	Barcelona	2	
		Bilbao	2	
		Granada	2	
		Madrid	2	
		Valencia	2	
		All of Spain	2	
	(Africa)			
	Algeria	Algiers	2	
	Morocco	Casablanca	2	
	Tunisia	Tunis	2	
	(Asia)			
	Japan	Hakodaté	2	
		Kobe	3	
		Kyoto	3	
		Osaka	3	
		Yokohama	2	
	Palestine	Jerusalem	3	

likewise high. Also, where the League figures indicated moderate or low rates, other figures were much the same. Because of this general correspondence in statistics from various sources, it seems probable that the situation revealed by Map 5 has in it certain fundamental elements of truth. In several instances rates overlapped from one group into another. In these cases the cities were classed in the group in which the larger proportion of their rates fell. In a few instances rates are given for whole countries or for a number of towns within a country. All the data for the city of Hongkong came from sources other than the League of Nations reports.

As pointed out above, nearly all the cities in the United States with the highest rates are in states shown on Map 3 as having the highest rates. To make the contrast of rates more marked on Map 5, the six states along the eastern seaboard of this country having the highest rates and the four western states with high rates, as previously described, have been included. It is obvious that their rates pale into insignificance by comparison with certain individual cities in other parts of the world in which the rates are much higher.

Detail is difficult to present in Map 5, but it hardly seems necessary, for it is apparent that the highest rates in cities have been reported from areas near or along the west coast of Mexico, Central America, and South America; from that portion of Asia and Africa bordering the eastern end of the Mediterranean Sea; and from India, southern China, and the Philippine Islands. It is a fact of no little interest that all of these cities lie either within or very close to the tropics, though the altitude of some is more than a mile.

These cities with excessive rates fall roughly into three geographic groups. The first of these, in Mexico, Central America, and South America, includes the six cities of Mexico City, Mexico (rate 400 to 600); Guatemala City, Guatemala (rate 260 to 460); Bogota, Colombia (rate 300 to 660); Guayaquil, Ecuador (rate 300 to 500); and Valparaiso (rate 500 to 700) and Santiago (rate 260 to 500 or over), Chile. The altitude above sea level is 7,500 feet at Mexico City, 4,850 feet at Guatemala City, 8,563 feet at Bogota, and 1,840 feet at Santiago. Both Guayaquil and Valparaiso are seaports, though part of the latter city is built on hills up to 1,700 feet high. The second or Mediterranean group is composed of Izmir (Smyrna), Turkey (rate 270 to 400), and Cairo, Egypt (rate 330 to 500). The former is a seaport and the latter is at an altitude of only a few hundred feet. The third or Asiatic group comprises: in India, the cities of Karachi (rate 540 to 780 or over), Bombay (rate 560 to 685), Madras (rate 300 to 680), and Rangoon (rate 400 to 630); in southern China, Hongkong (rate 370 to 560); and in the Philippines, Manila (rate 470 to 550), all of which are essentially at sea level. Reports of rates for a single year between 1930 and 1932 are available from other sources for three additional cities of India and range from approximately 500 for Bangalore City (673) and 395 for Delhi (674) to 282 for Colombo, Ceylon (247).

The rates of over eighty cities are spotted on Map 5. There are in addition over fifty other cities in which the rates are available from League of Nations sources. The rates for these latter cities were nearly always relatively low and were under 100 per 100,000 population. Included in this group with such low rates are some of the largest cities of the world, such as London, Berlin, Paris, Stockholm, Vienna, Amsterdam, and Montreal. In general, death rates for pneumonia appear low in cities along the northeastern coast of South America, in England, throughout much of France and most of Germany, Switzerland, and Belgium, and all of the Netherlands. Rates are also low for seven large cities in Australia and New Zealand.

TREND OF PNEUMONIA DEATH RATES

The trend of pneumonia mortality per 100,000 population in this country has been carefully studied over a number of years. Hospital statistics are of little value and may be misleading for this purpose. The following observations relative to the United States have been based on the mortality statistics of either the United States registration area or of Massachusetts.

In this country studies of the rates for pneumonia in the ten original registration states of 1900 were carried out for the years from 1900 through 1920 by Tomanek and Wilson (1315) and by Wilson (1425). This group of states was chosen for investigation because of its reasonably uniform population over a fairly long period. Though vagaries of classification and reporting may affect the figures to some extent, it has been possible to determine, and probably with a fair degree of accuracy, the trend of the rates for pneumonia and to determine whether the disease is becoming either more or less common. The excessive rates produced as a result of the influenza pandemic of 1918 were either discarded or adjusted.

The first report was by Tomanek and Wilson (1315) who stated:

> The general inference . . . is that the mortality as reported for all respiratory diseases, for lobar and undefined pneumonia, and for bronchitis is decreasing with a statistically significant trend, whereas bronchopneumonia is increasing and pneumonia of all forms is holding steady.

In conclusion, however, they further stated:

. . . all that we think it safe at present to infer is that pneumonia is neither increasing or decreasing, (and) that the human organism is reasonably in equilibrium with its environment with respect to this disease.

Further study of the data led Wilson (1425) to state:

The chief facts are that in the 10 original registration states mortality from: (1) Pneumonia (all forms) with a mean death rate of 152 per 100,000 has been running practically constant in the period 1900–1920; (2) Lobar and undefined pneumonia with a mean death rate of 105 has been decreasing about 2 units (2 per cent) per annum, or from 136 to 85; (3) Bronchopneumonia with a mean rate of 47 has been increasing 1.7 units (4 per cent) per annum, or from 30 to 64; (4) Bronchitis with a mean rate of 27 has been decreasing 1.3 units (5 per cent) or from 40 to 13; and (5) Respiratory diseases with a mean rate of 196 have been decreasing about 2.5 units (1 per cent) per annum or from around 220 to 170.

Tomanek and Wilson (1315) reported that in the ten original registration states from 1900 through 1920 the mean rate of pneumonia of all forms was 152.5 and the trend was -0.4 ± 0.3. An extension of this investigation was kindly carried out by Miss Angeline D. Hamblen.* The result shows that the mean death rate for pneumonia of all forms for these ten states for the more recent period of 1920 through 1932 was 104 with a downward trend of 3.72 ± 0.6. Combining these figures and including those for 1918, the mean rate for pneumonia of all forms for the ten states from 1900 through 1932 was 139 with a downward trend of 2.39 ± 0.7, indicating that annually a slight but definite decrease has occurred over the thirty-three-year period.

Lombard and Doering (800) studied the deaths per 100,000 population in the total "respiratory group" of diseases, which included pneumonia of all forms, bronchitis, and influenza, for Massachusetts alone. Their observations covered the years between 1842 and 1925. As several changes in the classification of the respiratory diseases occurred during the long period studied, it was obvious that the most accurate determination would be arrived at by studying the group as a whole rather than by attempting to follow the trends of separate diseases. The results of this investigation showed that, though the rate for the respiratory group of diseases had increased during the period from 1842 to 1892–1894, it had slowly decreased since the latter date.

In the course of an epidemiologic investigation (871, 615), carried out

* Principal statistical clerk of the Massachusetts Department of Public Health.

during the Massachusetts Pneumonia Study (869), data were obtained directly from the death certificates of more than 60,000 persons reported as dying of any form of respiratory disease, whether primary or secondary, during the eight years of 1892, 1902, 1912, 1921, 1922, 1928, 1929, and 1930. This material was analyzed statistically by Doctor Herbert L. Lombard.* The figure for deaths per 100,000 population for all respiratory diseases in Massachusetts was found to have been 353 in 1892 and, following an irregular course, to have decreased to 191.4 by 1930. This study, carried out with material collected directly from death certificates, confirms the above-mentioned observations of Lombard and Doering with regard to the general trend of the rates for all respiratory diseases in this state.

So far as the death rates of various forms of pneumonia in Massachusetts are concerned, Huber's (665) extensive study covering the years of 1849 to 1922 revealed findings much the same as those of Tomanek and Wilson and of Wilson, cited above, for the ten original registration states. The death rate for pneumonia of all forms was found to have shown little change during the past thirty years. Likewise, while the death rates for lobar pneumonia and undefined pneumonia and bronchitis were decreasing, the rate for bronchopneumonia was increasing. The tremendous increase in all respiratory disease deaths which occurred during the influenza pandemic of 1918 upset calculations considerably and made difficult the discernment of recent trends of these diseases. In 1925, however, after obtaining data for a few more years and making what appeared to be due allowances for changes in classification within the group of "diseases of the respiratory system," Kelley and Hamblen (706) stated:

> . . . we feel that the figures since 1918 are significant and that the death rate for pneumonia in Massachusetts is really decreasing.

Miss Hamblen has recently investigated this matter further and, including the figures for 1918, has found that from 1900 through 1934 the mean rate for pneumonia of all forms in Massachusetts was 152 with a trend of -2.88 ± 0.7, indicating a decrease of over two units per year. Though the decrease may have been slightly more rapid in Massachusetts, the mean rate of 152 from 1900 through 1934 is definitely higher than that of 139 previously mentioned for the ten original registration states from 1900 through 1932.

Wilson (1425) reported the results of a study of the rates for all respira-

* Director of the Division of Adult Hygiene of the Massachusetts Department of Public Health.

tory diseases in Michigan over the period of 1900 to 1920. All respiratory diseases with a mean rate of 146 showed a trend of -0.5 ± 0.6. The mean rate for pneumonia of all forms of 102 was low; and, though it showed little variation in its general trend, it tended to increase somewhat in the latter part of the period. The rate of 28.5 for bronchopneumonia, while low, had shown a slight upward trend of 1.5 ± 0.2. Lobar pneumonia and undefined pneumonia together also had a low rate (73.6), and this had been practically stationary over the period studied.

Figures for deaths per 100,000 population from pneumonia of all forms have been obtained for England and Wales for the fifty-seven-year period from 1875 to 1931 inclusive from the Registrar-General's reports (559). From 1875 to 1900 inclusive the rate gradually increased from in the neighborhood of 100 to around 125. Since 1901, however, the rate has shown a more or less steady and slow decline. The mean rate for the thirty-one-year period of 1901 through 1931 (including the 1918 rate) was 110.4 and exhibited a downward trend of 1.53 ± 0.3, indicating a decrease of a little more than one unit per year. It would appear then that, though the mean rate over a considerable period of years has been lower in England and Wales (rate 110) than in the ten original registration states in this country (rate 139), the annual decrease has been more rapid in the latter (—2.39) region than in the former (—1.53).

Except for information based on studies of pneumonia death rates over a considerable number of years for certain regions of the United States and for England and Wales, little information with regard to trends in the death rates for pneumonia is available. The course of death rates in native miners on the Witwatersrand, South Africa, over a period of two or more decades has been described by Ordman (970), Orenstein (973), and Lister and Ordman (788). Data from that region are difficult to interpret, for numerous efforts have been made there to lower the high morbidity and mortality rates for pneumonia by the vaccination of miners against various organisms (see page 448). This procedure was apparently moderately successful in the early years of its use, but of late, and especially since 1926, morbidity rates for pneumonia have again increased markedly. The observations of Lister and Ordman (788) suggest that this is due to a fundamental change in the nature of the infection now prevalent there and that steps can be and are being taken to correct the situation.

Mortality rates are available for several cities of India over a period of approximately twenty years (674), but show no uniform trend.

CLIMATIC AND SEASONAL DISTRIBUTION AND INFLUENCE OF METEOROLOGICAL FACTORS

Climatic Distribution

Climate has no great influence on the distribution of pneumonia. It was shown in the foregoing sections that the disease has been reported from practically all parts of the world. While it is very prevalent in some cities in certain of the warmer regions of the earth, it should be pointed out that the high pneumonia mortality rates in some cases, as for example in Bombay, Calcutta, and Karachi in India, are probably incident to the local conditions within those cities, rather than to climate, for the rates for neighboring outlying districts are markedly lower (674). Similar conditions probably explain the contrast between mortality rates in various mines, plantations, estates, prisons, and cities in tropical regions and the mortality rates in the region adjacent.

In some communities which geographically lie within the temperate zones, such as Valparaiso and Santiago, Chile (see Map 5, page 278), high rates are present throughout the whole country, in cities and rural districts as well (262). In the United States (see Map 3, page 270), nearly all of which also has a temperate climate, marked variations in rates are found in different sections of the country. And while these variations are not clearly related to any one set of climatic conditions, they are apparently related to the kind of community involved (see below). In England and Wales, likewise in the temperate zone, the mortality rate for pneumonia appears to vary and in general to increase from the south to the north (852).

When we compare the rates for the United States and for England with the rates for certain localities in other countries, particularly in warm areas, we find that the relation is much affected by the social conditions in the localities compared. For instance, while the mean rates for the United States and for England and Wales are much lower than for the cities of Bombay, Karachi, and Calcutta, they are considerably higher than for the regions adjacent to these cities. And the rates for rural areas and small cities (under 10,000 population) in the United States (1335) in 1920 (rate 107), 1931 (rate 68), and 1932 (rate 67) are also higher (though the difference is not so great) than the rates for rural regions in the vicinity of the Indian cities (674): Bombay and Karachi, 1930 (rate 59); Calcutta, 1930 (rate 44).

Lister (786) and Ordman (970) have called attention to the fact that in Johannesburg, South Africa, the pneumonia incidence and mortality rates vary a great deal in the different mines on the Rand and that the area of the gold fields is too small (about sixty by five miles) to account for these differences by climate. In fact, from the point of view of their mortality rates, Lister and Ordman (788) have divided some thirty-two mines into "bad" mines (mortality rate 5 per 1,000 or more per year) and "good" mines (rate less than 5 per 1,000 per year). Most of the "bad" mines were found to lie west of Germiston.

Seasonal Distribution

THE TROPICS. Gautier (510) has reviewed some of the literature dealing with the seasonal distribution of pneumonia in the tropics. When his findings are combined with other observations, it appears that in tropical regions reporting of pneumonia has shown a seasonal distribution in certain areas coincident with the dry or cold season or both, and to a lesser extent with the hot or the wet season, while in others no seasonal distribution has been found. Lack of precise figures, however, prevents accurate illustration of seasonal variation in most instances. In tropical Africa, pneumonia was found to be more prevalent on the Ivory Coast and in the Cameroons during the cold season, especially during the harmattan (510); on the Gold Coast its prevalence was attributed to the rainy season; and in Gabon, to the dry season (510). In Northern Rhodesia it was most prevalent just before the rainy season began (Ordman, 971); and in Katanga, Belgian Congo (1008) and in Dar-es-Salaam (Tanganyika Territory) it was most frequent during the hot period just prior to the rains; and in Nairobi (Kenya), during the dry season (510).

In India, especially in the North-West Province, pneumonia was most prevalent during the dry cold period in winter and was least prevalent during the warm wet summer season (859, 1103). In Sumatra the disease was most prevalent during or just after the heavy rains, while in Java no seasonal incidence was noted, and in the Celebes it was commonest when west winds prevailed (510). In South Borneo a high incidence of pneumonia coincided with a change of the monsoon, and in the Bismarck Archipelago with the onset and end of the rainy season (510). In the Carolines the beginning of the cold northeast monsoon marked the period of greatest frequency of pneumonia (510), as it did in the Philippines (332, 1357); and in the latter place this was just prior to the rains.

In Mexico City pneumonia appeared most prevalent just before the rains (530); while in Puerto Rico (1261), Honduras (1019, 1333), Panama, and British Guiana (510) the influence of season, temperature, and rainfall seemed negligible. With respect to Honduras, Phelps (1019) reported that in Puerto Castillo there is very little variation of temperature the year around, but often a considerable variation in the usually heavy rainfall there.

THE TEMPERATE ZONES. In countries in the north temperate zone pneumonia of all forms, but more especially lobar pneumonia, usually shows a pronounced seasonal distribution, approximately 60 to 70 per cent of the cases occurring during the winter and spring (647, 1402, 918). This has been shown for various communities within the United States (1168, 26, 1202, 563, 297, 1209, 951, 1206), and for Canada (661), Great Britain (837, 331, 267, 852), Germany (563, 84), and northern China (1450). In southern Australia in the south temperate zone pneumonia is usually most prevalent in the late fall and winter (1003a). Among the native gold miners on the Rand, Johannesburg, South Africa, pneumonia is most prevalent during the cold dry months of the winter and spring (874, 970, 788). The Rand is high (altitude more than 5,000 feet) and fairly dry, and has a high evaporation rate and a mild temperate climate.

In 1889 Wells (1402) reported that of a total of over 600,000 collected cases of pneumonia 70 per cent had occurred during the winter or spring. Greenberg (563) tabulated the deaths of over 88,000 individuals dying of lobar pneumonia in New York City during the period of 1901 through 1915 and found these showed a marked seasonal distribution. The distribution of these deaths by quarters of the years studied was as follows: first quarter, 38.1 per cent; second quarter, 25.8 per cent; third quarter, 10.9 per cent; and fourth quarter, 25.3 per cent. The maximum number of deaths occurred in March and the minimum in August.

Figures very similar to these have been found for 20,544 deaths occurring from lobar pneumonia (excluding undefined pneumonia) in Massachusetts during the ten-year period from 1921 to 1930 inclusive (867). In addition to this, lobar pneumonia is, as previously mentioned, a reportable disease in Massachusetts. During the ten years from 1921 to 1930 inclusive there were 47,947 cases of lobar pneumonia reported in this state (865). It is doubtful whether more than half the current number of cases are ever reported and it appears probable that the bulk of those reported were cared for by physicians who are in the habit of reporting. Despite the difficulty presented by incomplete reporting, the seasonal distribution of the cases which have been reported is interesting.

Figure 3 is a graphic representation of the incidence by months of reported cases of lobar pneumonia and deaths from this disease in Massachusetts during the ten years from 1921 to 1930 inclusive. In this figure, made on logarithmic paper, the twelve-month period begins with the first day of August and ends with the last day of July. By this method it is possible to show the full swing of the curves throughout the winter without a break.

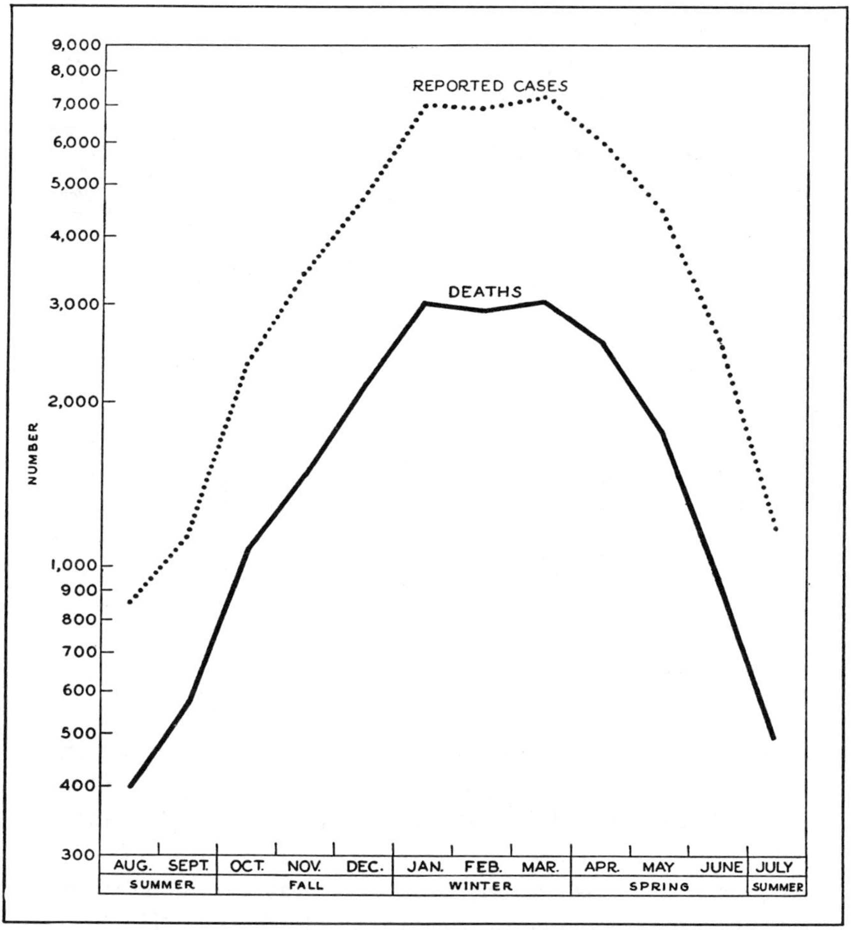

Figure 3. Distribution by months of 47,947 reported cases and 20,544 reported deaths from lobar pneumonia in Massachusetts during the ten-year period, 1921–1930

The two curves are very similar in general appearance; and the wider spread between them during the peak months of January through March would suggest that either a larger proportion of the cases that occur are reported then or that the case fatality rate is lower during that period. However, in view of the possible error in the reporting of cases, this matter cannot be settled with these figures. A larger number of the reported cases and deaths occurred during the six winter and spring months of December through May than in any other period of the years studied. While more

TABLE 48. LOBAR PNEUMONIA, REPORTED CASES AND DEATHS, BY MONTHS AND BY QUARTERS, MASSACHUSETTS, 1921–1930

MONTH	REPORTED CASES TOTAL	REPORTED CASES BY QUARTERS *Number*	REPORTED CASES BY QUARTERS *Per cent*	REPORTED DEATHS TOTAL	REPORTED DEATHS BY QUARTERS *Number*	REPORTED DEATHS BY QUARTERS *Per cent*
January	7,046			3,061		
February	6,913	21,197	44.2	2,949	9,040	44.0
March	7,238			3,030		
April	5,981			2,565		
May	4,440	12,988	27.1	1,793	5,313	25.9
June	2,567			955		
July	1,172			491		
August	858	3,166	6.6	395	1,452	7.1
September	1,136			566		
October	2,366			1,081		
November	3,417	10,596	22.1	1,483	4,739	23.1
December	4,813			2,175		
Total	47,947			20,544		

cases were reported in March, the largest number of deaths occurred in January (see also Table 48). Fewer cases and deaths were reported during the summer months of July, August, and September than at any other period.

The proportion of cases reported by quarters was very similar to the proportion of deaths reported by quarters (see Table 48). In both instances the first quarter of the years studied showed the highest figure and the second quarter was next, while the third or summer quarter was always the lowest. The proportion of reported cases during the first quarter was 44.2 per cent and of reported deaths 44 per cent. In the second quarter the figure for cases was 27.1 per cent and for deaths 25.9 per cent, while in the third quarter cases reported made up only 6.6 per cent of the total and deaths 7.1 per cent.

Of the total number of cases and deaths reported by months, the largest number of cases was reported in March and the largest number of deaths in January; while the smallest number of both cases and deaths was reported in August.

An examination of the working data used in the preparation of Table 48 reveals several minor points of interest. The number of reported cases and deaths varied in each of the years studied. The smallest number of cases reported in any year during the decade investigated was 4,080 in 1921, and the largest number was 5,544 in 1925. The smallest number of deaths reported was 1,749, in 1921; and the largest number was 2,315, in 1926. The maximum number of cases or deaths was not always reported in the same month each year. During the ten-year period the largest number of cases was reported in January three times, February once, March four times, and once each in April and May; while the smallest number occurred in August in nine years and in September in one. Among the reported deaths the largest number occurred in January three times, February once, March three times, April twice, and May once; while the smallest number occurred in July in one year and in August in the other nine.

From the foregoing it is clear that all forms of pneumonia, and especially lobar pneumonia, show a marked seasonal variation in the temperate zone; a variation which appears much less pronounced, or even absent, in certain areas within the tropics. In connection with this variation in the temperate zone and the possible relation of minor respiratory infections to pneumonia (see pages 235–240), the observations of Townsend and Sydenstricker (1320) of the United States Public Health Service are of interest. During 1924 they conducted an epidemiologic study of minor respiratory diseases (a few of which terminated in pneumonia) among more than 12,000 university students and in 775 families (chiefly of physicians) having a total population of 2,498 persons. These individuals were scattered over the whole country, but the largest proportion of the families lived along the Atlantic seaboard, more in large than in small cities and towns. Detailed information concerning the occurrence of respiratory disease in these persons was obtained by questionnaire. The data were regarded by Townsend and Sydenstricker as more representative of existing conditions than any others previously published.

During the year of 1924 there were several thousand attacks of minor respiratory infections (colds, bronchitis, sore throat, influenza, and so forth) among the total of more than 14,000 persons. Curves were prepared for students, families, and persons in the age group of fifteen to thirty-four years to show the incidence of these infections by months. Such curves revealed for the first time a double peak of incidence of these infections. Beginning at a low level in July, the curves were seen to mount rapidly to a high peak in September, followed by a drop in October, then by another rise in November, followed by a short drop in December, with a subsequent rise to the highest point in January. Following this, there was a gradual decrease to July. The two outstanding peaks occurred in September and in January. The authors believe the small secondary decline in December to be peculiar to the single year investigated and that it probably does not always occur.

The finding of a double peak in the curve of incidence of minor respiratory infections is of interest. In Figure 3 (page 291) showing the curves for reported cases and deaths from lobar pneumonia in Massachusetts, there is, in addition to the marked peak from January through March, the suggestion of a slight prominence of the curves during the period from September to October. In view of observations to be described below, this may be interpreted as an indication that the fall outbreak of respiratory infections is less frequently followed by pneumonia than is the winter outbreak. Also, it has long been recognized that pneumococci are more prevalent during the cold months of the year (see pages 378–385). In addition, in a study of pneumococcus carriers extending over a full year, Smillie (1206) found that the monthly incidence curve also showed a double peak and was nearly identical with the curve for minor respiratory infections reported by Townsend and Sydenstricker.

The study of McLean (849) is likewise of some interest in this connection. Though his report concerns only 153 infants and children, they were followed for the first five years of life. He too found that the curve for minor respiratory infections showed a double peak. The first peak, occurring in October, was for minor infections; and the second peak, occurring in December, was for the most severe infections of this nature.

Findings of essentially similar significance were reported by Kneeland and Dawes (732), Dochez, Mills, and Kneeland (367), Kneeland (731), and Collins and Gover (311). Dochez (358) finds that the peaks of incidence of the common cold in temperate climates tend to assume a cyclic character and in general to be three in number, one occurring in early fall, the second in midwinter, and the third in the spring. Kneeland and Dawes (732) conducted a study of the bacterial flora of the upper respiratory tract of infants. At the time of the outbreak of autumn colds the carrier rate of pathogenic organisms was low, no marked alteration of the basic flora of the upper respiratory tract occurred, and the colds were mostly mild. The colds, however, appeared to prepare the respiratory tract for other bacteria, for subsequently the proportion of infants carrying pathogenic organisms began to rise and by midwinter reached 80 per cent. This coincided with the winter wave of respiratory disease, and illnesses during this period were markedly more severe than those in the autumn.

Collins and Gover (311) studied the seasonal incidence of so-called minor respiratory infections in groups of families similar to those investigated by Townsend and Sydenstricker. These families, totalling nearly 3,000 people, contained some children and a large proportion of older individuals and were followed for nearly three years. Cases were classified by respiratory conditions such as colds and bronchitis, and by general symptoms such as fever, muscle aches or headaches, and chilliness. The curves for general incidence usually showed the double peak mentioned above. Further, the percentage of individuals with fever was low during the usual autumn outbreak and rose steadily during the winter. It appears then that the early fall outbreak was chiefly of a mild nature, while the midwinter one was much more severe. In general, children were more likely to show fever with an attack of minor respiratory infection than adults, and the proportion of individuals without fever was high in the adult group but low among the young and old. Likewise, fever occurred least often in infections largely limited to the nose, more often in those with symptoms of chest involvement, and most commonly in those with symptoms of throat lesions.

The seasonal incidence of pneumonia in a steel mill in this country, the employees of which have suffered much from this disease, was studied by Brundage and his associates (163, 162). No unusual distribution of cases by season was found, and the excess of pneumonia among steel workers appeared as great at one time of the year as at another.

Influence of Meteorological Factors on Prevalence

Numerous attempts have been made to correlate meteorological factors, such as temperature, rainfall and humidity, air, wind, ordinary dust, and barometric pressure, with the seasonal prevalence of pneumonia, and especially of lobar pneumonia (647, 1402, 918, 563, 297, 1103, 837). Though each of these factors, usually in combinations of two or more together, has been implicated at one time or another as affecting the occurrence of pneumonia, it now seems clear that wind direction and velocity and barometric pressure have no apparent relation to the prevalence of this disease.

The recent observations of Wells (1409) bearing on the problem of air and air-borne infection, and of Wells and Stone (1410) are of great importance. Under controlled conditions, by which temperature and humidity were kept constant, saline and broth cultures of various organisms were injected through an atomizer into a large enclosed tank. Studies were made of the size of droplets in relation to their time of fall. Minute droplets less than 0.1 mm. in diameter were found to settle slowly and to evaporate almost immediately, leaving any contained material, such as bacteria, suspended in the air as residue or droplet nuclei. Droplets of larger size rapidly fall to the ground before evaporation is complete. Droplets of saliva of various sizes may be expelled by persons talking, coughing, and sneezing; and while the larger ones rapidly fall to the ground, the smaller ones evaporate quickly, and each one may leave as many as 10,000 organisms suspended in the air as droplet nuclei. These may drift in the air for long periods or, if they settle, are easily lifted as dust by light air currents.

Cultures of organisms, including Type I pneumococci, representing inhabitants of the normal upper respiratory tract, and others including *B. coli* of the gastrointestinal group were atomized into the test tank. By means of an air centrifuge, samples of the tank air were obtained every few hours for culture. With the exception of the influenza bacillus, which usually died within one hour, organisms of the respiratory group remained viable and suspended in the quiet air of the tank for as long as three days; while those of the gastrointestinal group usually died before the end of the first day. To explain why the respiratory group of organisms has greater viability in air it was suggested that these organisms may be specially adapted to this form of transmission. It appeared that droplet nuclei settle so slowly that the time the organism may remain a source of danger and the distance it may travel depend more on the viability of the organisms in the air than upon the settling rate.

This work clearly points out the difference between the epidemiologic characteristics of droplet and droplet nuclei infection, for the former is essentially localized and concentrated while the latter is dispersed and dilute. Though it remains impossible to evaluate the role of droplet nuclei infection in the spread of pneumonia, these observations make it clear that the long-talked-of possibility of an air-borne infection has such significance that it cannot be lightly dismissed.

Though pneumococci may be found in the dust of rooms, and particularly those recently inhabited by patients with lobar pneumonia, as Stillman has shown (1235), the importance of this in relation to the spread of pneumonia is unknown. There is no clear relation of ordinary dust in the amounts encountered under ordinary circumstances to the incidence of pneumonia. It has been found, however, that exposure to heavy concentrations of soil dust, such as occurred in the so-called "dust bowl" area in the western part of this country in 1935, may be followed by increased morbidity and mortality rates for acute respiratory infections, including pneumonia. This matter was studied by Brown, Gottlieb, and Laybourn (155). The dust bowl area included the adjacent portions of the five states of Kansas, Colorado, New Mexico, Texas, and Oklahoma. Samples of dust obtained during several of the extraordinarily severe periodic dust storms which occurred in that area in the spring of 1935 were subjected to chemical and bacteriologic investigation. Previous workers had shown that the physiologic harmfulness of dust depends partly on its quartz (silica) content and that the diameter of the dangerous quartz particles usually ranges between 0.5 and 5.0 microns and is nearly always less than 10 microns.

An examination of the dust from the storms in question showed a range in particle size of from 2 to 770 microns, apparently most of the particles being above 10 microns in diameter. The silica content varied from 66.9 to 92.9 per cent in several samples examined. Further, though no evidence was found that the dust carried any pathogenic organisms, it was exceedingly irritating to the mucous membranes of the respiratory tract.

The two factors of temperature and humidity merit special consideration, for they appear to have an important influence, at least in certain instances, on the prevalence of pneumonia. Over fifty years ago Hirsch (647) observed that the incidence of pneumonia was markedly influenced by weather changes such as occur in winter and spring, especially sudden changes in temperature and extensive fluctuations in the proportion of moisture in the air. He also reported that in countries having the most sudden and severe temperature changes in winter, the incidence of the disease is correspondingly high at that time. Greenberg's (563) and Rogers' (1103) later observations led them to essentially the same conclusions, and both regarded marked temperature variations and a low humidity as being conducive to a high pneumonia rate. In addition, Greenberg found that, though variations in temperature alone failed to explain the seasonal distribution of pneumonia in the region around New York, he was forced to conclude that temperature variations per se were the most important controlling factors.

On study, this problem becomes very involved. Cole (297) and others have pointed out that exposure to cold or sudden temperature changes may irritate the mucous membrane of the throat and larynx and have suggested that crowding, with freer transmission of bacteria from person to person, may be a factor influencing the incidence of pneumonia during cold weather.

It is obvious from the situation revealed in a previous section that the cities of the world having the highest death rates from pneumonia do not all have the same climatic conditions. Even among those cities closest to this country, located in Mexico, Guatemala, Colombia, Ecuador, and Chile, there are certain differences which must be considered, for four of the cities are at considerable altitudes while the remaining two are at sea level. The cities with the highest rates elsewhere in the world, those in the Mediterranean and Asiatic groups, are close to sea level. Marked similarities of climate between these cities or groups of them are not apparent at this time. It may be said, however, that Mexico City, Guatemala City, and Bogota, Colombia, are all located at high altitudes, as are the four western states in this country which have a dry climate and exhibit some of the highest death rates of any of the states in the Union. On the other hand, other states with high rates are chiefly in the east where the altitude is lower and the climate very different from that of the western states.

In 1925 efforts were made by Rogers (1103) to determine the influence of various climatological conditions, such as rainfall, absolute humidity, temperature variations, and wind direction, on the incidence of pneumonia in India. The absolute humidity, which is the actual amount of vapor in the atmosphere expressed by weight in grains per cubic foot, was regarded as of greater significance than the relative humidity. For the purpose of this investigation Rogers used records of the jail population of more than a million and a half persons in India covering the period from 1896 to 1910 and compared his findings with somewhat similar observations made on the Indian Army. His study showed clearly that in the southeastern warm wet part of the country, which has an equitable climate, the morbidity rates for pneumonia were relatively low (rate 400 to 900 per 100,000 population). In districts in the northwest, however, where the daily temperature variations were more marked, the winter temperatures and the absolute humidity lower, and the climate dry and relatively cold, the rates were from five to more than ten times as high as in other areas, and in one cold area (South Indus Valley) reached the extreme figure of 5,020 per 100,000 population.

It appears that in certain instances the prevalence of pneumonia may be affected by low temperatures, especially marked variations in temperature in the lower ranges, and, possibly, a low humidity. So far as can be determined at present, this is true for many of the countries in the temperate zones, for some on the edge of the tropics, and for certain localities within the tropics which, because of their high altitude and dry climate, experience certain phenomena, such as sudden chilling, usually thought peculiar to regions in temperate zones.

While meteorological factors are presumably of importance in the regions mentioned, it is not clear that they explain the extraordinary amount of pneumonia which has been encountered in many sections of the tropics. As we have said above in discussing climate, it appears that the crowding together of groups of natives who are unusually susceptible to pneumococcus infections in general may have a determining effect. However that may be, it does not seem possible, even in warm countries, to ignore meteorological factors in considering the prevalence of pneumonia.

ACCESSORY FACTORS INFLUENCING INCIDENCE OF PNEUMONIA

Age

While pneumonia may occur at any period of life, it is probable that the incidence of pneumonia (of all forms) is highest in the young and in the old. In a foregoing chapter it was shown that some immunity to the pneumococcus (see pages 143–150) was possessed by the population at large and that this resistance appeared to vary with age, to be lowest at the extremes of age, and highest in the latter part of childhood and in the period of early and middle adult life. Though the part immunity plays in decreasing the incidence of pneumonia has not been clearly demonstrated (see page 154), it seems reasonable to expect that pneumonia would be most frequent during those periods of life when the general resistance is lowest. Conclusive proof of this is not available, however, for inadequacies in the reporting of pneumonia make it impossible to determine the exact incidence of the disease in persons in various age groups. Direct evidence concerning this matter comes chiefly from reports from hospitals and allied institutions, which at best can give little more than an index of the relative frequency of pneumonia in any age group.

Evidence of the relation of age to incidence is available in Massachusetts, but only with respect to lobar pneumonia, which is the only form of pneumonia reportable in this state. Figures have been obtained (866) showing that, during the ten-year period from 1921 through 1930, 47,947 cases of lobar pneumonia were reported to the State Department of Public Health. Of this number the ages were stated for 44,712 cases, a number which probably represents but little over half the cases that occurred during that decade.

The curve for the incidence of lobar pneumonia per 100,000 population in

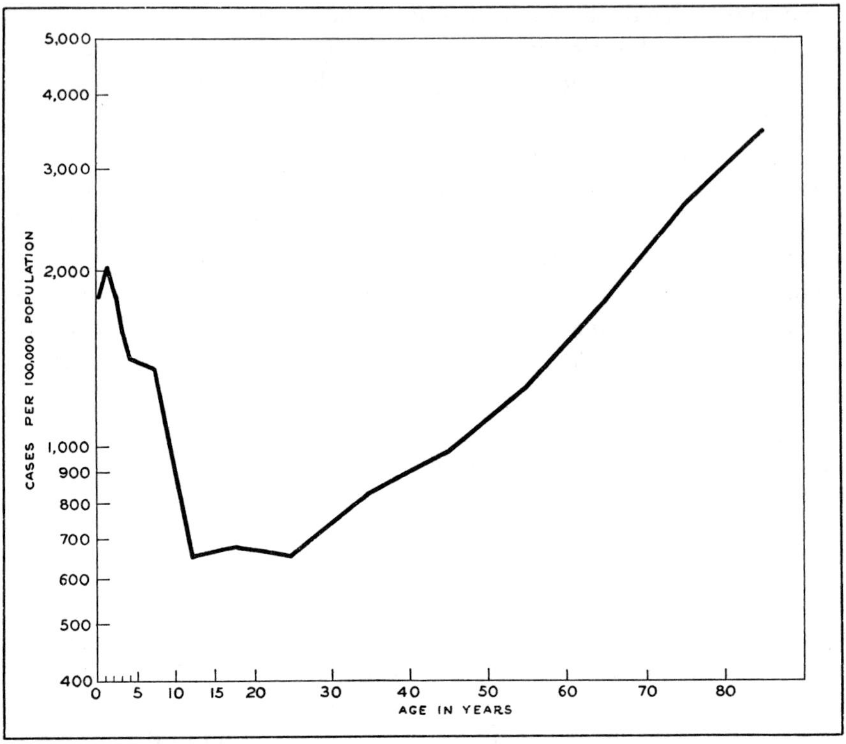

Figure 4. Reported cases of lobar pneumonia per 100,000 population, Massachusetts, 1921–1930, by age group*

this state by age groups (see Figure 4) indicates the greater frequency of the disease among the young and the old than among individuals in other age groups. The lowest rates are found for persons between the ages of ten and fifty years (644 to 977); while the rates for those in other age groups, especially in the group seventy years of age and over, are much higher (1,245 to 3,488).

* The rates are based on the estimated population in each age group for 1925 and are as follows:

AGE GROUP IN YEARS	RATE	AGE GROUP IN YEARS	RATE
Under 1	1,796	20–29	651
1–	2,017	30–39	835
2–	1,800	40–49	977
3–	1,569	50–59	1,245
4–	1,412	60–69	1,768
5–9	1,353	70–79	2,603
10–14	644	80 and over	3,488
15–19	672		

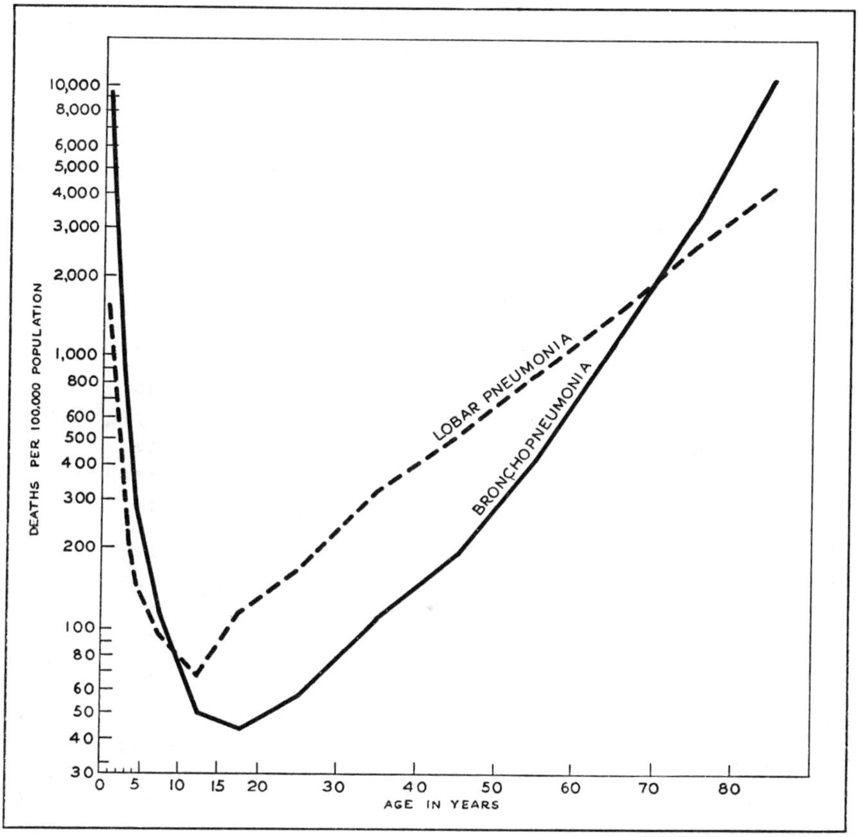

Figure 5. Deaths from lobar pneumonia and bronchopneumonia per 100,000 population, Massachusetts, 1921–1930, by age group*

Indirect evidence as to the great frequency of pneumonia among the young and the old is furnished by observations of the rates for deaths per 100,000 population for pneumonia of all forms. Using data from the United States mortality statistics (1335), such rates have been calculated for all the states and the District of Columbia in the continental registration area of this country for the year 1930 (Table 49).

It is apparent from these figures that the death rates for pneumonia of all forms are highest in the young and in the old and higher in the old than in the young. The lowest death rates are in the group 10 to 19 years of age. It is also clear that the death rates from pneumonia in the different age

* Rates are based on the estimated population of each age group in 1925.

TABLE 49. DEATHS PER 100,000 POPULATION FROM PNEUMONIA, ALL FORMS, BY AGE GROUP AND BY STATE, UNITED STATES (CONTINENTAL) REGISTRATION AREA, 1930

PLACE	ALL AGES	AGE IN YEARS 0–2	3–9	10–19	20–54	55–74	75 years and over
Alabama	85	363	22	24	60	214	730
Arizona	132	1,020	58	27	55	267	860
Arkansas	74	275	22	16	50	194	826
California	74	476	24	13	35	144	665
Colorado	118	725	26	20	50	255	1,209
Connecticut	81	350	19	11	43	211	825
Delaware	107	715	27	9	59	178	650
District of Columbia	122	637	36	16	79	230	625
Florida	61	298	15	17	41	121	517
Georgia	87	410	27	29	62	180	760
Idaho	83	405	26	19	39	223	823
Illinois	68	367	20	10	38	147	639
Indiana	80	376	22	14	38	148	780
Iowa	78	308	16	9	32	159	993
Kansas	55	254	17	12	20	105	647
Kentucky	92	405	27	16	49	215	895
Louisiana	89	550	28	21	56	194	648
Maine	91	370	17	17	34	181	805
Maryland	115	592	28	17	70	240	968
Massachusetts	92	446	25	10	44	208	855
Michigan	70	400	22	12	36	141	613
Minnesota	77	296	20	12	35	188	985
Mississippi	73	322	25	22	52	148	543
Missouri	92	390	24	16	46	205	905
Montana	80	304	25	18	51	200	820
Nebraska	66	289	18	12	27	136	865
Nevada	113	238[a]	38[b]	14	90	214	800
New Hampshire	84	322	20	11	27	174	810
New Jersey	77	478	29	12	44	172	590
New Mexico	128	474[a]	45[b]	23	66	232	799
New York	95	464	25	14	55	233	783
North Carolina	85	400	24	23	59	193	707
North Dakota	56	345	12	10	23	109	896

[a] Age group 0–5 years. [b] Age group 5–10 years.

TABLE 49 (*cont.*)

PLACE	ALL AGES	0–2	AGE IN YEARS 3–9	10–19	20–54	55–74	75 years and over
Ohio	76	377	21	11	37	160	796
Oklahoma	65	406	20	15	32	165	831
Oregon	65	211	13	13	35	160	660
Pennsylvania	96	523	25	12	56	211	735
Rhode Island	94	495	14	9	44	247	850
South Carolina	95	496	29	26	57	185	724
South Dakota	60	201[a]	13[b]	13	23	122	817
Tennessee	91	460	27	18	52	215	995
Texas[c]	–	–	–	–	–	–	–
Utah	89	520	24	22	40	172	791
Vermont	93	344	21	12	38	204	738
Virginia	95	380	30	19	65	210	835
Washington	64	300	17	12	32	137	750
West Virginia	85	457	23	14	38	210	945
Wisconsin	72	356	17	12	19	107	745
Wyoming	73	495	9	7	35	202	751

[a] Age group 0–5 years. [b] Age group 5–10 years.
[c] No data available for the whole state of Texas in 1930.

groups vary in the different states and that among the states showing the highest rates in each age group are Arizona, Colorado, and Maryland.

Additional information of a similar nature is available for Massachusetts (867). The deaths per 100,000 population for both lobar pneumonia and bronchopneumonia have been calculated by age groups for the ten-year period 1921 through 1930. The curve of these rates is shown in Figure 5. There were 20,544 deaths from lobar pneumonia and 26,130 deaths from bronchopneumonia (including one instance in which the age was unknown) in this state during that period.

The curves clearly show that the death rates of both lobar pneumonia and bronchopneumonia are extremely high in the young and in the old, and that at the extremes of life the rates were highest for bronchopneumonia (see also Table 50). The difference between the rates in the various age groups was most marked in infants and children up to the age of three years, when the rates for bronchopneumonia were from six to three times higher than the rates for lobar pneumonia, and in the group eighty years of age and over, when the rate of the former type of pneumonia was over twice that of the latter.

It is likewise apparent that the rates for bronchopneumonia exceeded those for lobar pneumonia in all the groups up to the age of ten to fourteen years. Between the ages of ten and seventy years the rates were higher for lobar pneumonia; and, everything considered, this may possibly be an indication that lobar pneumonia is more frequent than bronchopneumonia during that period of life.

It is well recognized that the case fatality rates of both lobar pneumonia and bronchopneumonia are high during the first year or two of life; and, assuming them to be approximately the same during that period, it is possible to gain some idea of the relative frequency of these two forms of pneumonia in early life. From the number of deaths due to lobar pneumonia and bronchopneumonia reported in Massachusetts during the ten-year period mentioned above, it appears that pneumonia of the lobar form is less frequent during the first few years of life, especially during the first and second year, than bronchopneumonia (see Table 50). In addition, if the case fatality rates of all forms of pneumonia are about the same after the age of seventy years, and there is reason to believe that they are, bronchopneumonia again appears more common than lobar pneumonia. This is especially marked in the group eighty years of age and over.

It is to be remembered that the figures used as the basis of these statements (see Table 50) represent the reported number of deaths from lobar pneumonia or bronchopneumonia as shown by data taken from death certificates and that there is doubtless some error in the accuracy of the diagnoses given on those certificates. It is not clear, however, that the margin of error is sufficiently great to alter the general significance of the findings.

There were 8,100 deaths from bronchopneumonia and 1,328 from lobar pneumonia in the group under one year of age, and 2,628 and 722 deaths respectively in the group between the ages of one and two years. After the age of two years differences in the number of deaths from these two forms of pneumonia are probably less significant, for it is known that at about that period the case fatality rate of pneumonia of the lobar form decreases markedly while that of bronchopneumonia shows little if any change. In the group 70–79 years old there were 3,554 deaths from bronchopneumonia and 2,781 from lobar pneumonia, and in those 80 years of age and over the number of deaths was 3,214 and 1,323 respectively.

Reports from clinics and hospitals dealing with the occurrence of pneumonia in persons in various age groups are common. Many of these have been mentioned previously in connection with the type incidence of pneumococci in both lobar pneumonia and bronchopneumonia in adults and in infants and children (see pages 57–89). Additional studies have been made by many other investigators, some of which will be mentioned later (1318, 874, 333, 885, 112, 7, 1212).

TABLE 50. DEATHS AND DEATHS PER 100,000 POPULATION FROM LOBAR PNEUMONIA AND BRONCHOPNEUMONIA, BY AGE GROUP, MASSACHUSETTS, 1921–1930*

AGE GROUP IN YEARS	LOBAR PNEUMONIA Deaths	LOBAR PNEUMONIA *Deaths per 100,000 population*	BRONCHOPNEUMONIA Deaths	BRONCHOPNEUMONIA *Deaths per 100,000 population*
Under 1	1,328	1,544	8,100	9,417
1	722	847	2,628	3,080
2	285	351	747	919
3	160	203	390	495
4	123	148	228	275
5–9	357	95	433	115
10–14	250	69	179	50
15–19	384	115	145	43
20–29	1,103	165	382	57
30–39	2,040	322	694	109
40–49	2,760	517	996	187
50–59	3,335	853	1,675	428
60–69	3,593	1,482	2,764	1,140
70–79	2,781	2,552	3,554	3,261
80 and over	1,323	4,292	3,214	10,428
Total	20,544		26,129	

* Rates are based on the estimated population of each age group in 1925.

Though uncommon, cases of so-called congenital lobar pneumonia have been described (766). Bronchopneumonia has also been found in the newborn and in infants dying within a few days of birth (1386, 1121). The evidence presented in numerous clinical reports is in accord with the supposition made above that the incidence of pneumonia (especially bronchopneumonia) is higher in infants and in very young children than in older children. Among cases of lobar pneumonia, for example, Cunningham (333) found that about 6 per cent of 1,488 cases in infants and children were in those under one year of age, over 55 per cent in those from one to five years of age, and the remainder or about 39 per cent in patients from five to thirteen years of age. This series was made up of cases treated at a single hospital between 1870 and 1915. Due to the operation of several factors, ideas have changed somewhat since that time concerning the frequency of lobar pneumonia in infants and children; and Grulee and Mulherin (574) reported that over a ten-year period ending in 1932, 25 per cent of 116 cases were in patients under one year of age, 57 per cent in those from one to five years of age, and the remainder or 18 per cent in others six to twelve years of age. It is apparent in both of these series that the largest proportion of the cases occurred among the younger children.

Reports from clinics and hospitals of the age distribution of large series of cases of primary bronchopneumonia are not available. However, many large series of cases of lobar pneumonia, which include patients of all ages, have been analyzed in this manner. The largest group of these comprises 32,681 cases collected by Musser and Norris (918). They found that 22,800 or 69.8 per cent of the cases were in patients between the ages of ten and fifty years (see Table 51). Ashton and Landis (26) found 61.4 per cent of 994 cases, and Shattuck and Lawrence (1176) 68.2 per cent of 2,882 cases, in patients between the ages of ten and fifty years. Others have likewise found that from 60 to 70 per cent or more of their cases of lobar pneumonia occurred in patients between these ages (1403, 254, 1357, 1103, 230, 830, 1450). Of the 44,712 reported cases of lobar pneumonia in Massachusetts in which the age was known (866), 43.5 per cent or 19,435 cases were in persons between the ages of ten and fifty years (see Table 51).

All the clinical reports cited above refer to the age distribution of patients seeking hospital care. The Massachusetts group, however, includes all reported cases regardless of where they were cared for; and, with the reservation that such cases are incompletely reported, the Massachusetts figures may be regarded as significant. When these variables are taken into consideration, it may be said that somewhere between 43 and 70 per cent of the cases of lobar pneumonia are in patients between the ages of ten and fifty years. As far as known, this would appear to hold true for persons living in temperate climates. During an epidemiologic study of respiratory disease deaths in Massachusetts (871, 615) it was observed that, when pneumonia deaths were subdivided according to the ages of the patients, the greatest number of deaths in hospitals was found to center in the group 20 to 40 years of age. This is perhaps an indication that patients with pneumonia tend to seek hospital care more frequently at that time of life and may to some extent explain the high proportion of cases in hospital series in the young and middle-aged adult groups. It is possible that, in some instances in tropical and subtropical regions, especially where highly susceptible natives are concerned, a much higher proportion of the cases occur in patients between the ages of ten and fifty years (874, 1103, 1008, 510). It is usually not possible to determine this with any degree of accuracy, however, for in most such instances the figures available come from industrial organizations where only selected natives of an estimated age of about eighteen to forty years are employed.

TABLE 51. LOBAR PNEUMONIA CASES. NUMBER AND PERCENTAGE BY AGE GROUP. MUSSER AND NORRIS (918) AND AS REPORTED TO THE MASSACHUSETTS STATE DEPARTMENT OF PUBLIC HEALTH, 1921–1930

MUSSER AND NORRIS SERIES				MASSACHUSETTS SERIES			
AGE GROUP IN YEARS	CASES Number	CASES Per cent		AGE GROUP IN YEARS	CASES Number	CASES Per cent	
0–5	1,249	3.8		Under 1	1,545	3.5	
5–10	3,132	9.6		1	1,720	3.8	
10–20	5,107	15.6	69.8 per cent	2	1,463	3.3	
20–30	8,041	24.6		3	1,235	2.8	
30–40	5,665	17.3		4	1,171	2.6	
40–50	3,987	12.2		5–9	5,078	11.4	
50–60	2,558	7.8		10–14	2,319	5.2	43.5 per cent
60–70	1,754	5.4		15–19	2,246	5.0	
Over 70	1,094	3.3		20–29	4,365	9.8	
Age not stated	94	0.3		30–39	5,291	11.8	
				40–49	5,214	11.7	
				50–59	4,869	10.9	
				60–69	4,284	9.6	
				70–79	2,837	6.3	
				80 and over	1,075	2.4	
Total	32,681				44,712		

That about one-half or more of all cases of lobar pneumonia in temperate regions occur in young and middle-aged adults is of interest from the standpoint of the immunity shown by the population at large, for it is at this period of life when resistance to the pneumococcus appears most pronounced. Variations in the frequency with which pneumococci of the various types cause pneumonia in infants and children and in adults were discussed earlier (see pages 74–89 and 42–74).

Sex

Pneumonia, and especially lobar pneumonia, is always regarded as more frequent in males than in females. Due to the lack of figures giving the true incidence of pneumonia in any considerable part of the population, this cannot be proved, but information of various kinds is available from numerous sources which lends great weight to the assumption.

Granted certain inadequacies in reporting, the proportion of males and females among the reported cases of lobar pneumonia in Massachusetts may still be offered as suggestive evidence of the greater frequency of this disease among males. During the ten years of 1921 through 1930, 47,947 cases of lobar pneumonia were reported to the State Department of Public Health by Massachusetts physicians (866). Of this number the sex was known in 47,364 cases. In each of the ten years more reported cases occurred in males than in females. Of the total 47,364 cases in which the sex was known, 27,464 or 58 per cent were in males and 19,900 or 42 per cent in females. Of the total group there were 44,684 cases in which both the age and sex were known, and of these, 25,981 were in males and 18,703 were in females. The incidence rates, if they can properly be called that, for these cases in males and females have been calculated by age groups (see Figure 6).

The curves show that the rates were always higher in males than in females. The lowest rates in males were for the group between ten and forty years of age, and in females for the group between ten and sixty years of age. The highest rates in both groups were in the young and the old, and this was especially pronounced in patients seventy years of age and over.

There are many reports in the literature based on data from clinics and hospitals which show the sex incidence of large series of cases of "pneumonia" or of lobar pneumonia. Such series are made up of cases in hospitals for patients of all ages or for adults only, and all contain approximately three times as many males as females. This higher proportion of males among cases treated in hospitals than among all cases reported by physicians in Massachusetts lends support to Cole's (297) belief that males with pneumonia seek hospital care more frequently than females.

The question of the proportion of patients with respiratory disease who are hospitalized has been little studied. In the course of an epidemiologic investigation (871, 615) carried out during the Massachusetts Pneumonia Study, the proportion of patients dying in hospitals of this state of all forms of respiratory disease during eight different years from 1892 through 1930 was determined. In the former year only 11.2 per cent of the deaths from respiratory disease occurred in hospitals, while in the latter year this proportion had gradually increased to 43.1 per cent. Throughout the period covered, a larger proportion of the deaths from respiratory disease in hospitals occurred in males than in females. In 1930, 48.1 per cent of all hospital deaths from respiratory disease occurred in males and 37.6 per cent of all such deaths in females. Further, the hospitalization of respiratory diseases occurred to a greater extent in the larger cities than in the small towns and more rural areas of the state. As this study embraced more than 60,000 deaths

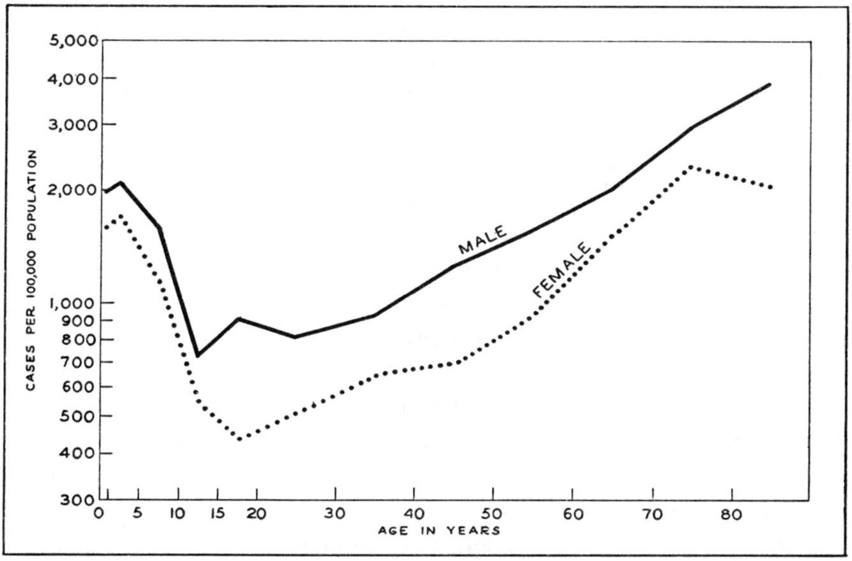

Figure 6. Reported cases per 100,000 population of lobar pneumonia in males (25,981) and in females (18,703), Massachusetts, 1921–1930, by age group*

from respiratory disease, these findings are regarded as significant, at least for Massachusetts. The extent of hospitalization per 100 deaths was determined for lobar pneumonia and bronchopneumonia. The findings show that for 1929 and 1930 the average hospitalization rate for lobar pneumonia was 50.4 for males and 40.6 for females, and for bronchopneumonia was 52.5 for males and 42.7 for females. All things considered, it seems likely that the

* The rates are based on the estimated population of each age group for 1925 and are as follows:

AGE GROUP IN YEARS	RATE *Male*	*Female*	AGE GROUP IN YEARS	RATE *Male*	*Female*
Under 1	1,983	1,586	30–39	922	648
1–4	2,076	1,681	40–49	1,255	698
5–9	1,540	1,152	50–59	1,556	939
10–14	732	547	60–69	2,009	1,524
15–19	904	438	70–79	2,958	2,344
20–29	803	514	80 and over	3,866	2,004

proportion of males with respiratory disease, and especially pneumonia, who enter hospitals is larger than the proportion of females.

Among cases of "pneumonia" Wells (1403) reported that 72.2 per cent of over 27,000 collected cases were in males, as were 75.2 per cent of 949 cases in adults reported by Sears and Larrabee (1168). Among patients of all ages with lobar pneumonia Musser and Norris (918) reported that 73.4 per cent or 8,881 of 12,098 collected cases were in males, as were 76.4 per cent of 991 cases studied by Ashton and Landis (26) and 85.1 per cent of 242 cases observed by Wu and Chiu (1450). In infants and children with lobar pneumonia Grulee and Mulherin (574) found 60 per cent of 116 cases were in males. Among adults with lobar pneumonia Musser and Norris found 69.7 per cent or 25,950 of 35,798 collected cases in males, and figures of similar significance have been reported for numerous smaller series of cases in adults (708, 254, 1357, 951, 830, 1385).

As long ago as 1889 Wells (1403) remarked that statements concerning the apparent excess of male morbidity of pneumonia are always accompanied by the simple and plausible explanation that the habits and occupation of the male lead to greater exposure and hence to an excess of opportunities of contracting this disease as compared with females. He also pointed out that this was only partially true, for in childhood and infancy, when no habit influence of this nature exists, males have more pneumonia than females. Observations of a somewhat similar nature have been made by Cole (297).

In recent years little attention seems to have been paid to this matter until the excellent study of Doull, Harmon, and Fisher (373) appeared in 1934. Studying the sex ratio of pneumonia mortality for states in the registration area of this country and its possible relation to occupation, they have advanced our knowledge of this matter considerably. Lacking satisfactory incidence figures, these workers used death rates for pneumonia of all forms and influenza and analyzed the rates of various states for several different years by age and sex, being careful to exclude years when influenza was prevalent. They found that there were two periods of life when the pneumonia mortality rate in males exceeds that in females.

The first period of excess male mortality from pneumonia began in infancy and, steadily and progressively diminishing, extended through childhood to disappear at about the time of puberty (age 10–14 years). At puberty the rates for both sexes were about similar. The second period of excess male mortality began in adolescence (age 15–19 years) to continue over a period of many years, and was much more conspicuous than the excess in childhood. In old age (70 years and over) the male excess pneumonia mortality was finally replaced by an excess mortality in females.

Efforts were made to correlate the two periods of excess male mortality with the degree of urbanization or lack of it shown by the various states. The excess male mortality of infancy and childhood appeared unrelated to the degree of urbanization. So far as the data allowed, the facts suggested that males at this time of life have a greater inherent susceptibility to pneumonia than females. At puberty, however, the resistance of the sexes was apparently similar.

The beginning of higher rates for males in adolescence did not appear to vary with the degree of urbanization, but the group between twenty and sixty-nine years of age, comprising the period of active adult life, showed that the sex ratio "varies definitely with the environment, the male excess being highest in urban states and lowest in rural." The higher male rates in adults were determined by factors different from those governing the higher male rates in childhood. Either the male must have a relatively greater exposure in urban districts than in rural, a belief which did not seem acceptable, or some environmental factor must be operative in urban areas which lowers the resistance of the male. Doull and his associates incline to the latter view and attribute the bulk of the excess adult male mortality to the effect of unfavorable factors associated with certain industries. The relation of pneumonia to occupation is discussed below (page 318).

The period of the greatest excess male mortality from pneumonia was found during the fifth decade of life. From the age of seventy years on, the female death rate was usually higher than the male, and this excess of female mortality did not appear affected by the degree of urbanization. The suggestion was made that this excess mortality in elderly females is due to the fact that the surviving male population, having been subjected for a long period to higher death rates for pneumonia, is more resistant than the surviving female population.

During the epidemiologic investigation (871) carried out in the course of the Massachusetts Pneumonia Study, the distribution of patients dying of all forms of respiratory disease in this state was determined by age and by sex over a period of eight different years. Males were found to have significantly higher death rates in the group under one year of age and between the ages of thirty and sixty years. This may be regarded as partial confirmation of the observations of Doull and his co-workers. Had the figures for the three years 1892, 1922, and 1929, when influenza was prevalent in Massachusetts, been omitted from this study, it is possible that a more complete agreement would have been obtained.

Race

Many years ago Hirsch (647) reported that the Negro was peculiarly subject to pneumonia when residing in a cold climate, and especially when moved from a warm or tropical climate to a colder one. While there is ample evidence that this is true (874, 892, 1295, 1335), it is now equally clear that under certain conditions even in warm climates Negroes show a pronounced susceptibility to pneumonia and to pneumococcus infections in general. Gorgas (549) has shown the high incidence of pneumonia among native laborers (chiefly Negro) employed in the construction of the Panama Canal. Other reports indicate the great prevalence of pneumonia among native laborers elsewhere in Central America (1331, 1019, 1332, 1333, 1261, 510). Further, it has been noted that necropsies on such patients rarely show pneumonia alone but very often pneumonia with septic complications. Natives employed in various enterprises in tropical Africa likewise experience extremely high morbidity and mortality rates for pneumonia and pneumococcus infections (507, 1008, 1349, 773, 510, 971). The incidence of pneumonia among natives in tropical Africa living under "natural" conditions has not been determined, yet it appears from the observations of Maynard (874) that the disease may not be rare, even under those circumstances. In fact, Livingstone (790) from his experience as a medical missionary in South Africa stated that in 1852 pneumonia was one of the commonest diseases of the natives of what presumably is now Bechuanaland.

The susceptibility to pneumonia of natives from tropical regions of Africa has been shown to vary with the district from which they came (Maynard, 874). Pearson and Mouchet (1008) pointed out that certain tribes or races of natives appear more resistant to pneumonia than others and, in addition, that "new" races are almost always more susceptible than others who have been accustomed to compound life for several years. Apparently most of the workers observed by these latter investigators were unmarried natives whom they divided into three groups: (a) those "voluntarily" applying for work, (b) those brought to the compounds by recruiting organizations, often from considerable distances, from a race which has supplied recruits for several years, and (c) those similarly recruited but who are members of a tribe which for the first time in its history is supplying men to the compounds. Natives in this last class were found to constitute the most susceptible form of labor and suffered much from pneumonia. They also observed that when natives of "new" susceptible tribes or races mixed in compounds with others of more resistant groups accustomed to compound life, the incidence of pneumonia tended to rise in the latter groups as well. Pearson and Mouchet also supplied interesting evidence of what appeared to be the result of the spontaneous immunization of various racial or tribal groups of natives in consequence of the degree of habituation to life in the compounds shown by each group. Local natives, accustomed to the conditions of climate, food, and compound life, had a rate for pneumonia deaths of 12.36 per 1,000; natives of another district, from a group having a shorter record of contact with compound life, had a rate of 18.45; while natives of three other groups introduced comparatively recently into the compounds had a rate of over 40.

The great frequency of pneumonia among African Negroes employed in the gold and diamond mines in the vicinity of Johannesburg, Pretoria, and Kimberley, in the more temperate regions of southern Africa, has been the subject of much investigation and even governmental legislation (874, 785, 786, 973, 970, 788, 1007). Natives from tropical areas, especially those coming from north of 22° South Latitude, suffered more from pneumonia than did others from the more temperate regions. This difference of susceptibility has been regarded as a racial characteristic. However, nearly all the supply of mine labor is drawn from regions throughout South Africa which, according to the League of Nations reports (770), are peopled by natives of a single ethnological group, the Bantu race; and Lister and Ordman (788) suggest that the susceptibility shown by groups of natives from various parts of South Africa is best termed a "territorial" rather than a racial susceptibility. This also appears applicable to natives throughout most of South Africa, including the Rhodesias and Belgian Congo as well.

From the above and other reports (768, 769), it is likewise apparent that, as compared with white people living and working in the same districts, Negroes have very high morbidity and mortality rates for pneumonia. This has been regarded as proof of a difference in susceptibility between these races. Inasmuch as nearly all the studies mentioned above note that the immunity of even the most susceptible natives appears to increase markedly after the lapse of a few months' time in their new environment, it seems probable that the unusual severity of pneumonia among these natives is due not so much to a fundamental difference in race as to the fact that such natives have had little previous exposure to pneumococci and, consequently, have but little initial effective resistance against these organisms. If this be so, one of the dubious fruits of our civilization is the responsibility for introducing large susceptible populations to the highly invasive pneumococcus. Nevertheless, it is probable that no such simple explanation will account for the susceptibility shown by all Negroes under all circumstances. It is clear, however, that the problem of environmental change is in many instances closely associated with high pneumonia incidence rates (see pages 329–333).

Whether the apparent differences between the reported susceptibility of other races is closely associated with a lack of previous exposure to pneumococci is less clear. In China, Wu and Chiu (1450) regard the susceptibility of the Chinese as about similar to that of Europeans, and in Singapore, Winchester (1428) found that Tamils had nearly three and one-half times as much pneumonia as did Chinese. These observations are based upon the proportional number of lobar pneumonias encountered among more than 41,000 hospital admissions in the first instance and among more than 19,900 admissions in the second. Because the source of these data are hospital statistics, they must be received with caution for such figures are notoriously subject to hidden influences which may greatly affect their significance. It seems likely, however, that Tamils are quite susceptible, and this may be a part of the reason for the high morbidity and mortality rates shown by certain groups of the population in India (1103, 924). Gautier (510) studied such rates for the Indian armies over a period of eight years and found that the native Indian troops had about three times more pneumonia and five times more deaths per thousand from this disease than the white troops there.

In the United States, so far as differences in the susceptibility of the white population as compared with the colored population (which includes Negroes) or with the Negro population alone are concerned, recourse must be had to the death rates for each of these groups, as morbidity figures are not available. According to the United States census report (1337), the population of this country in 1930 was composed of several racial groups: white 88.7 per cent, Negro 9.7 per cent, and other colored races 1.6 per cent.

The following death rates have been taken from the United States mortality statistics for 1932 (1335) and are based upon the estimated population for each group as of July 1, 1932. The figure for deaths per 100,000 from pneumonia of all forms for the total population of the continental United States registration area (including the District of Columbia) in 1932 was 76.8. The calculated rate for the white population in this area was 71.5 as compared with the rate of 121.3 shown by all colored races and a rate of 111.0 shown by Negroes alone. The higher rate for the total colored as compared with the Negro population appears due to the inclusion in the former group of races such as the American Indian with a rate of 153.5 and the Chinese with a rate of about 140.

The United States mortality statistics for 1932 give the estimated populations and death rates for pneumonia of all forms for both the white and colored populations of fourteen states in this country (see Table 52). It is apparent from the percentages mentioned above that nearly all the colored population is made up of Negroes, and the proportion of these in various states in this country was earlier shown on Map 4 (see page 275).

TABLE 52. POPULATION AND DEATHS PER 100,000 POPULATION FROM PNEUMONIA, ALL FORMS, BY COLOR, IN FOURTEEN STATES OF THE UNITED STATES, 1932

STATE	WHITE Population	WHITE Pneumonia death rate	COLORED Population	COLORED Pneumonia death rate
Alabama	1,731,000	59.3	951,000	80.2
Arkansas	1,386,000	67.2	481,000	75.5
California	5,268,000	61.8	679,000	134.3
Florida	1,083,000	44.0	445,000	80.9
Georgia	1,855,000	64.6	1,055,000	115.8
Kentucky	2,413,000	74.5	225,000	164.0
Louisiana	1,345,000	62.4	793,000	100.9
Maryland	1,372,000	81.6	281,000	198.6
Mississippi	1,014,000	46.8	1,022,000	62.1
North Carolina	2,289,000	65.7	955,000	109.1
Oklahoma	2,161,000	60.3	279,000	92.8
South Carolina	959,000	69.7	786,000	107.3
Tennessee	2,169,000	72.9	481,000	138.9
Virginia	1,789,000	63.6	646,000	131.1

It is shown in Table 52 that the pneumonia death rates were, without exception, higher for the colored than for the white populations in the states listed. In four states, California, Kentucky, Maryland, and Virginia, the rates were more than twice as high in the colored as in the white population. The highest rate for both the white and the colored population occurred in Maryland (rates 81.6 and 198.6 respectively); and, as elsewhere noted, Maryland had the highest average rate in the United States during the ten years of 1924 through 1933 (see page 271).

The mortality statistics report for the United States in 1932 (1335) lists the deaths per 100,000 population from pneumonia of all forms for a number of the cities in this country having a population of 100,000 or over in 1930. In this tabulation pneumonia death rates of 200 or over were found only in the colored population. Among the cities listed, there were ten in which the death rates for pneumonia in this group were 200 or over. These were as follows: Atlanta, Baltimore, Chattanooga, Dallas, Fort Worth, Kansas City (Missouri), Louisville, St. Louis, Washington (D.C.), and Wilmington (Delaware). In each of these cities death rates for pneumonia of all forms in the colored population were from more than two to nearly five times (Dallas: rates, colored 251.1, white 58.8) as high as in the white. All of these cities are located in states in the southern section of this country, and most of them in states in that area having the highest average rates (see Map 3, page 270). The high rates of Negroes in southern states have been commented upon by others (1209, 438, 1385).

It is unfortunate that no satisfactory morbidity figures are available for Negroes in this country. It must also be remembered that no relatively great mass migration of Negro labor occurs in the United States such as takes place each year in connection with the employment of new hands at certain of the mines in various parts of Africa. Though the figures for pneumonia deaths per 100,000 population for the Negro in this country are relatively high, they appear extremely low in comparison with such rates as 1,200 to 5,700 which have been reported from tropical Africa (1008, 971) and 800 to 5,100 from South Africa (874, 788, 1007).

In consequence of the facts revealed by these reports, it is obvious that many of the colored races, and especially the Negro, appear far more susceptible to pneumonia than the white race.

Social Condition

OVERCROWDING. Marked overcrowding, usually intimately associated with a low economic status, undoubtedly favors the direct transmission of pneumococci and tends to increase the incidence of pneumonia. Observations supporting this view have been reported by many investigators (647, 549, 296, 297, 1008, 682, 298, 961, 1187, 510, 1007). However, the influence of crowding is not always apparent (1206, 1210). Where overcrowding exists, bacteria are probably spread in the particles of saliva and spray of persons coughing and sneezing, and organisms suspended in droplet nuclei in the air and contained in dust may be passed to many persons (1235, 297, 1409, 1410, 1408).

Blake and Cecil (124) observed an epidemic of thirty-two cases of spontaneous lobar pneumonia in a shipment of overcrowded monkeys. Outbreaks of pneumonia have occurred in the crowded quarters of ships, barracks, and prisons (647, 1399, 1031, 510; see also pages 386–390). As a result of correcting an overcrowded condition, Gorgas (549) reported a dramatic lessening of the incidence and mortality rates for pneumonia among natives employed in the construction of the Panama Canal (see Table 53). These workers were chiefly Negroes from Jamaica and Barbados. In the early years of the project, when forty to fifty thousand workers a year were employed, pneumonia morbidity and mortality rates were high. During this period the natives were housed in crowded barracks, each accommodating eighty-four men, each man having approximately thirty square feet of floor space. A uniform diet, consisting of food of a nature different from that to which most of the men were accustomed, was supplied.

TABLE 53. PNEUMONIA DEATHS PER 1,000 POPULATION FOR NEGROES EMPLOYED IN THE CONSTRUCTION OF THE PANAMA CANAL, 1906–1912

YEAR	PNEUMONIA DEATH RATE
1906	18.74
1907	10.61
1908	2.6
1909	1.66
1910	1.66
1911	2.24
1912	1.3

From Gorgas (549)

In 1908 the barracks were closed, and the natives allowed to bring in their families and live in separate scattered huts along the banks of the Canal. Concurrent with this, a change was made in the food supplied; and the men were issued raw food of a nature to which they were accustomed, which might be prepared by their wives.

It is apparent from the data in Table 53 that a sharp decrease in the mortality rate occurred during 1908, when the figure dropped from 10.61 per thousand in 1907 to 2.6. It is highly improbable that the alteration in diet alone could have brought about this result. The usual term of employment at the Canal was one year, and in many instances, at the conclusion of this period, workers would return home and later come back to work again. In this fashion the proportion of the native population there which probably had acquired some immunity to the pneumococcus was gradually increased. The possible benefits derived from this situation appear to have arrived too late to explain the marked lowering of both the morbidity and mortality rates which occurred at the time the barracks were closed.

The investigations of Pearson and Mouchet (1008) relative to native miners employed in the Belgian Congo in tropical Africa have shown that the death rates, not only for pneumonia, but for all diseases as well, are considerably lower in compounds housing only two or three hundred natives than they are in others having five to ten times this number of inhabitants.

At the mines in South Africa, where natives are lodged in barracks rather than in huts concentrated in compounds, Peall (1007) found evidence that infection causing multiple cases of pneumonia occurred in overcrowded barrack rooms rather than as a result of transmission from one gang of miners to another while at work.

As pneumonia rates are so high in Negroes, it is not surprising that most of the direct evidence concerning the effects of overcrowding is based upon observations concerning them.

OCCUPATION. For many years it has been believed that individuals employed in certain occupations, such as day laborers, sailors, and others engaged in heavy manual labor out of doors, tend to have a relatively high incidence of pneumonia (918, 1168, 256, 230, 1450). Such conclusions have been based upon the analyses of series of hospital cases, however, and until recent years no accurate information has been available in regard to the influence of occupation upon the occurrence of pneumonia.

In 1920 the Industrial Fatigue and Research Board of Great Britain (558), using the sickness records of more than 20,000 men employed in the iron and steel industry during the six years of 1913 through 1918, obtained data on the incidence of various groups of diseases. Respiratory diseases (other than asthma and pulmonary tuberculosis) comprised one of the groups studied. Of the six occupational classes considered, steel melters, teemers, and pit men were found to head the list with an average per person of 23 per cent more time lost from all sickness than all the workers; and puddlers with an excess of 20 per cent were next. While the excess of sickness from respiratory diseases among men in the first group was only 10 per cent, it was 35 per cent among puddlers. Both groups had considerable "rheumatism." Among tin plate men the excess of sickness from respiratory diseases amounted to only 5 per cent. Men in all three groups work under conditions exposing them to trying variations in temperature. Puddlers, with the highest excess rate for respiratory diseases, alternate periods of about twenty minutes of intense labor with periods of rest without shelter; while melters' heavy work comes in bursts followed by long rest periods, during which they retire to shelters and occasionally change shirts. Tin plate men, with the lowest excess rates for respiratory diseases, work steadily and seldom rest sufficiently long (usually four minutes by actual observation) to become chilled. Information of this nature gives definite evidence that the incidence rates, at least for respiratory diseases as a group, may be considerably higher among men engaged in certain occupations than among those engaged in other occupations within the same industry.

Mortality rates for all causes and for individual causes among all men and among those in various age groups engaged in 178 different occupations in England and Wales from 1921 through 1923 were given in the Registrar-General's report (560). This report shows that in males the mortality from all respiratory diseases is more closely associated with social status than is the mortality from other diseases. This was true whether or not pulmonary tuberculosis was included. In general, the highest rates, and especially for pneumonia alone, were found among persons in the lower classes (see Tables 54 and 55). Among occupied males the highest mortality rates for all respiratory diseases were found in tin and copper miners; cutlery grinders; kiln and oven men engaged in manufacturing china; cotton strippers and grinders; potters, metal grinders, cotton blow room operatives, stevedores, and costermongers.

Subsequently observations of similar significance were reported by Whitney (1420) for occupied males in the United States. Her data were based on figures obtained from the United States Census Bureau for 1930.

Table 54 lists the comparative mortality figures for males between the ages of twenty and sixty-five years in certain classes and those engaged in specific occupations having the highest mortality from pneumonia of all the 178 occupational groups shown in the Registrar-General's report (560).

The highest mortality rates for pneumonia alone among men in specific occupational groups were found in brass foundry furnacemen and laborers, cutlery grinders, stevedores, cotton blow room operatives, iron foundry furnacemen and laborers, cotton card and frame (not spinning frame) tenders, puddlers, metal glazers and polishers, "other" dock laborers, and costermongers, in the order named. This may also be seen in Table 55. Men in three of these occupations, namely, brass and iron foundry workers and puddlers, are exposed to marked variations in temperature, and brass foundrymen have the additional hazard of exposure to zinc oxide fumes. Cutlery grinders, stevedores, cotton blow room operatives and carders, metal glazers and polishers, and dock laborers are exposed to considerable dust. The dust

TABLE 54. STANDARDIZED MORTALITY (COMPARATIVE MORTALITY FIGURES)* FOR ALL CAUSES AND FOR CERTAIN SELECTED CAUSES OF DEATH IN MALES AGED 20 TO 65 YEARS IN ENGLAND AND WALES, 1921–1923, BY CLASS AND OCCUPATIONAL GROUP

OCCUPATIONAL GROUP NUMBER	GROUP	ALL CAUSES	DISEASES OF RESPIRATORY SYSTEM (97–107)†	BRONCHITIS (99)	PNEUMONIA ALL FORMS (100, 101)
–	All males	1,013	151.3	49.0	85.2
–	All occupied and retired civilian males	1,000	151.7	49.6	85.1
–	Social class I (upper and middle) (Civilians only)	812	96.2	12.7	70.5
–	Social class II (intermediate) (Civilians only)	942	115.1	27.2	71.6
–	Social class III (skilled workers) (Civilians only)	951	139.2	46.5	76.2
–	Social class IV (intermediate) (Civilians only)	1,007	168.2	59.4	91.1
–	Social class V (unskilled workers) (Civilians only)	1,258	236.5	87.4	127.8
	Occupation				
20	Earthenware, china, etc., kiln and oven men	1,830	445.3	242.8	141.2
24	Certain skilled glass workers (not blowers or finishers)	1,417	299.7	123.9	146.6
27	Persons engaged in smelting, rolling, converting of iron or steel‡	1,025	219.2	63.9	128.7
27A	Puddlers (included in above group)	1,250	319.1	133.2	173.4
28	Metal moulders	1,137	252.6	85.5	145.4
29	Iron foundry furnacemen and laborers	1,116	298.3	90.3	193.2
30	Brass foundry furnacemen and laborers	1,530	320.1	98.7	212.1
40A	Cutlery grinders	3,295	699.5	361.2	207.6

From Table C in the Registrar-General's report (560).

* Standardized death rates based on a population so chosen as to yield exactly 1,000 deaths at the death rates for different ages prevailing among all occupied and retired civilian males in 1921–1923.

† Numbers in parentheses are disease title numbers from the International List of Causes of Death, third revision, Paris, 1920. Diseases of respiratory system do not include influenza or pulmonary tuberculosis.

‡ This group is included for comparative purposes.

TABLE 54 (*cont.*)

OCCUPATIONAL GROUP NUMBER	GROUP	ALL CAUSES	DISEASES OF RESPIRATORY SYSTEM (97–107)†	BRONCHITIS (99)	PNEUMONIA ALL FORMS (100, 101)
	Occupation (cont.)				
41	Metal glazers, polishers, buffers, and moppers	1,443	285.8	97.3	172.4
51	Cotton blow room operatives—skilled	1,516	368.9	149.8	193.9
53	Cotton card and frame (not spinning frame) tenders	1,601	314.2	81.7	185.6
103	Shipyard laborers (unskilled)	1,351	303.6	121.8	166.2
118	Stevedores	1,619	354.4	101.8	207.1
119	Coal boat loaders and dischargers	1,231	290.2	98.3	166.7
120	Other dock laborers	1,532	322.0	124.3	170.6
122	Porters	1,497	280.4	107.9	152.3
127	Costermongers, hawkers, and street sellers	1,660	331.6	133.4	168.4
153	Barmen	1,955	288.8	99.0	162.9
164	General and undefined laborers	1,438	264.3	96.5	143.4

† Numbers in parentheses are disease title numbers from the International List of Causes of Death, third revision, Paris, 1920. Diseases of respiratory system do not include influenza or pulmonary tuberculosis.

to which cutlery grinders are exposed has a high silica content, and to a lesser extent the same type of exposure is suffered by metal glazers and polishers. Stevedores, cotton workers, and dock laborers are exposed to dust of other kinds. Costermongers appear exposed to weather variations alone. Tin and copper miners (not included in Table 54) exposed to dust (high silica content) had high mortality rates for chronic interstitial pneumonia but not for acute pneumonia.

Table 55 gives comparative mortality figures for males between the ages of twenty and sixty-five years in certain classes and those engaged in specific occupations associated with the highest mortality from pneumonia, along with the mean annual figure for deaths per 100,000 for these groups by ages. Table 55 also gives the mean annual death rate for certain age groups. The highest pneumonia mortality rate among younger men occurred in coal boat loaders and dischargers (rate 333 for age group 16–19 years), while the

TABLE 55. STANDARDIZED MORTALITY (COMPARATIVE MORTALITY FIGURES)* AND DEATH RATES PER 100,000 FOR PNEUMONIA, ALL FORMS, BY AGE GROUPS, FOR CERTAIN CLASSES OF MALES AND FOR SPECIFIC OCCUPATIONAL GROUPS HAVING THE HIGHEST PNEUMONIA MORTALITY RATES

OCCUPATIONAL GROUP NUMBER	GROUP	COMPARATIVE MORTALITY FIGURE*	MEAN ANNUAL DEATH RATE PER 100,000 AT AGES† 16–19	20–24	25–34	35–44	45–54	55–64	65–69
–	All males	1,001	23	29	41	72	103	168	264
–	All occupied and retired civilian males	1,000	21	28	40	72	103	170	276
–	Social class I (upper and middle) (Civilians only)	828	8	16	26	63	93	144	232
–	Social class II (intermediate) (Civilians only)	841	16	20	33	62	87	145	244
–	Social class III (skilled workers) (Civilians only)	895	20	27	37	63	91	153	258
–	Social class IV (intermediate) (Civilians only)	1,071	22	31	45	80	109	174	275
–	Social class V (unskilled workers) (Civilians only)	1,502	24	41	61	111	154	251	368
	Occupation								
20	Earthenware, china, etc., kiln and oven men	1,659	–	–	25	188	169	286	324
24	Certain skilled glass workers (not blowers or finishers)	1,723	–	95	64	79	109	444	296
27	Persons engaged in smelting, rolling or converting iron or steel‡	1,512	14	57	68	121	123	258	311

From the Registrar-General's report (560)

* Comparative mortality figures for pneumonia among males between the ages of 20 and 65 years. The rate for all occupied and retired civilian males is taken as 1,000. Taken from Table D in the report cited.

† Taken from Abstracts in the report cited. ‡ This group is included for comparative purposes.

TABLE 55 (*cont.*)

OCCUPATIONAL GROUP NUMBER	GROUP	COMPARATIVE MORTALITY FIGURE	MEAN ANNUAL DEATH RATE PER 100,000 AT AGES 16–19	20–24	25–34	35–44	45–54	55–64	65–69
	Occupation (cont.)								
27A	Puddlers (included in above group)	2,038	–	114	70	73	248	386	543
28	Metal moulders	1,709	55	33	67	134	155	321	323
29	Iron foundry furnacemen and laborers	2,270	57	103	116	158	217	336	359
30	Brass foundry furnacemen and laborers	2,492	68	–	107	338	223	246	–
40A	Cutlery grinders	2,439	–	93	99	57	490	231	833
41	Metal glazers, polishers, etc.	2,026	68	77	26	183	277	254	253
51	Cotton blow room operatives—skilled	2,278	–	177	100	104	161	482	–
53	Cotton card and frame (not spinning frame) tenders	2,181	–	–	38	227	121	560	469
103	Shipyard laborers (unskilled)	1,953	91	87	92	223	149	206	469
118	Stevedores	2,434	–	98	69	247	130	496	176
119	Coal boat loaders and dischargers	1,959	333	149	82	129	204	251	351
120	Other dock laborers	2,005	31	62	71	155	199	345	470
122	Porters	1,790	39	17	90	143	171	299	449
127	Costermongers, etc.	1,979	53	42	78	163	217	295	438
153	Barmen	1,914	14	21	86	205	137	313	311
164	General and undefined laborers	1,685	34	45	65	120	173	297	414

highest rates among individuals of older ages occurred among cutlery grinders (rate 833 for age group 65–69 years).

Though the above observations on the pneumonia rates in different classes of males in England and Wales, and in the United States among male workers in specific occupational groups, relate entirely to mortality, they nevertheless serve to focus attention on the pneumonia problem associated with certain occupations.

In the United States the excellent studies of Russell, of Brundage, and of Thompson and their associates of the United States Public Health Service (1929–1933) have thrown considerable light upon the relation of some occupations to the incidence as well as to the mortality of the respiratory diseases, including pneumonia (1143, 163, 162, 1301, 161). These reports concerned the health of workers in dusty trades, each dealing with a different kind of dust, as follows: (a) calcium dust (cement plant); (b) silica dust (granite industry); (c) metal dust (silver polishing); (d) carbon dust (coal industry); (e) vegetable dust (cotton-milling industry); and (f) municipal dust (street sweeping).

Russell and his co-workers (1143) studied the health of workers in the granite industry. The employees in this industry were found to have a higher incidence of pneumonia than others employed in hard rock gold mining (American mines—high silica content in dust), cement making, hard coal mining, cotton milling, silver polishing, and the combined general industrial groups whose sick-benefit associations send sickness reports to the United States Public Health Service. The incidence rate for pneumonia in men in the granite industry was exceeded only by the rates for workers in the iron and steel industry and for soft coal miners. Further, granite industry workers showed a higher mortality rate for respiratory diseases, especially tuberculosis, than all other occupied males in the registration area in the years (1908–1909) used for analysis. Omitting tuberculosis, granite workers also showed a higher mortality rate for all other respiratory diseases, and especially pneumonia, than the all-other-occupied-male group. Individuals exposed to the heaviest concentration of dust showed more lost time and a higher mortality rate for respiratory diseases than those exposed to smaller concentrations of dust. This was most pronounced among the group of pneumatic tool workers in general and cutters in particular. Nearly all men exposed to the most intense concentrations of granite dust developed silicosis after a period of years. Such dust has a high percentage of quartz (free silica) content.

Extending these studies, Thompson and his associates (1301) made a similar type of analysis of the data concerning men exposed to dust in coal mining, textile and silverware manufacturing, and street cleaning. It was again observed that dust with the highest quartz content was the most damaging. The highest total dust exposure was found in coal mines, granite quarries, and cement plants; but the highest percentage of quartz was found in granite dust. Relatively high rates for respiratory diseases (about twice those found in men in other industries) were also found in hard coal miners and cement plant workers. In other instances soft coal miners, textile, silverware, and street-cleaning employees showed an incidence rate only slightly above that shown by male industrial workers generally.

In connection with the above study, Brundage (161) analyzed the mortality rates from various causes shown by hard coal miners in and about Wilkes-Barre, Pennsylvania, over a period of nine or more years, and similar data were obtained for soft coal miners in the states of Indiana, Illinois, Missouri, and Wyoming. In general, miners of both sorts, but more particularly hard coal miners, appeared to have higher mortality rates for respiratory disease, and especially for pneumonia and influenza, than other adult male non-miners of the same communities. The excess pneumonia mortality of hard coal miners was shown chiefly by the older men (over forty-five years of age) and was prominent both during and in the interval between epidemics of influenza. The highest differential mortality in soft coal miners in epidemic periods was also in the older men, but in inter-epidemic periods of so-called "normal times" it was most apparent in the group from sixteen to forty years of age.

The study of Brundage and his associates (163, 162) of the morbidity and mortality of pneumonia among iron and steel workers revealed probably the most significant findings in the relation of this disease to occupation. Data were obtained from a number of companies in the iron and steel industry, and an extensive investigation was carried out using the sickness records of one large steel company (unnamed) in Pennsylvania.

For many years the reports of several industrial sick-benefit associations to the United States Public Health Service had consistently shown a higher case incidence of pneumonia among employees in the iron and steel industry than among workers engaged in other industries as a whole. Figures for pneumonia incidence per thousand men showed considerable variation in different steel companies, and rates varying from 2.2 to 13.7 were recorded. It was found, however, that the incidence rate of pneumonia among workers in the steel industry in general was 69 per cent above the rate for workers in public utilities and 52 per cent higher than that for all other reporting industries as a group for the years 1922 through 1928. The average incidence of pneumonia among general industrial workers was shown to be from 2.5 to 3 per thousand per year, while the figure for workers in the steel industry was found to be 4.4 per thousand. Further, employees in the steel industry showed high rates, not only for pneumonia, but for most other diseases of the organs of respiration as well.

Detailed analyses of the rates for individuals employed in specific occupations within the steel company investigated showed that certain occupations appeared unusually hazardous so far as the incidence of pneumonia was concerned. Rates were computed for general laborers obliged to work out of doors during inclement weather, and for men subjected to great heat with wide variations in temperature but not particularly exposed to any other kind of industrial health hazard. It was determined that the frequency of pneumonia in these two groups was 13.6 and 12.6 cases per thousand per year respectively as compared with a rate of 3.9 in other workers in the same mill exposed to none of the above conditions. The suggestion was made that the unusually high incidence rate shown by general laborers, whose chief industrial exposure appeared to be out-of-door work in all kinds of weather, resulted from the opportunities for chilling afforded by periods of irregular physical activity during inclement weather. Intermittent exposure to intense direct heat offered a similar hazard and may well account for the high rates in the other group subjected to marked temperature variations.

As compared with the pneumonia incidence rate of employees in "all other departments" of the steel company studied (3.8 cases per thousand per year), the rates in the following departments were over twice as high: blast furnace, general labor for mills, coke ovens, open hearth, rod and wire mills, shops (steel car, plumbing, boiler, roll, and disc shops), and coal mines. The excess of pneumonia in these departments over that of "all other departments" amounted to 268 per cent, 184 per cent, 182 per cent, 124 per cent, 95 per cent, 55 per cent, and 37 per cent respectively. The highest pneumonia incidence rate was found in the blast furnace department. The distribution of cases was uneven, however, and most were concentrated in a few occupations within this department. Nearly all occurred either in the general laborers or in men in occupations associated with stacks and stoves (casting), especially among the first and second helpers. The former group was exposed to all kinds of weather conditions, and the latter did heavy work with exposure to heat with wide temperature changes and to gases and smoke.

Occupations which intermittently exposed workers to extremely high temperatures in the blast furnaces, coke plants, open hearth steel-making department, and open hearth rolling mills were found to be associated with high pneumonia incidence rates. Equally high rates were found among chippers, who performed somewhat sedentary but fatiguing work under damp and drafty conditions. In general, employees of the steel company in question not doing out-of-door work in all kinds of weather or exposed to heat with wide temperature changes, dust, gas, or smoke, or performing strenuous labor showed an annual incidence of pneumonia of 3.9 per thousand, while for other employees exposed to one or more of these conditions the figure was 12.1 per thousand. No significant data were obtained on the relation of pneumonia incidence to race, alcoholism, dust, or exposure to gases.

In relation to the high incidence of pneumonia found among employees in the steel industry as a whole, it was pointed out that the average figures for pneumonia deaths per 100,000 population between 1910 and 1920 were extraordinarily high for cities having a large steel industry, such as East Youngstown, Braddock, Pittsburgh, Carnegie, Johnstown, Gary, Pueblo, and Duquesne. In such cities having a large proportion of their population engaged in the steel industry, it appeared possible that the high mortality rates of these municipalities were directly related to the increased hazard encountered by the employees in their occupation. Additional evidence of this nature was obtained by the study of the pneumonia death rates of the population of the city (unnamed) in which the above-mentioned steel company was located. The figure for deaths per 100,000 from pneumonia for females in the general population of that city was 56 and for males in the general population 107, while males employed in the steel works there showed a rate of 124 and those employed in certain departments of the steel works (blast furnaces, coke ovens, open hearth, coal mines, and general labor departments) showed a rate of 241.

Mention has already been made of the apparent lowering of the pneumonia mortality rate of Pittsburgh in the past few years (see pages 276–277). Doubtless the marked reduction in the rate of operations and output of steel experienced by the whole industry, which resulted from the general economic depression in recent years, has had some influence in this connection. The same, of course, would probably hold true of various other cities having a large proportion of their population engaged in the steel industry.

During the course of the above investigations, made by members of the United States Public Health Service, an independent study of the incidence of "pneumonia" from 1925 through 1930 among the employees of a large coal, iron, and railroad company was carried out by Kibbey (714). The incidence per thousand men per year in the various departments was found to be 11.3 for underground iron ore miners, 5.6 for surface workers (includes all surface workers and, in addition, clerks, superintendents, nurses, physicians, and so forth), 4.6 for coal miners (includes all men working underground), and 4.3 for "all dependents" (workers' families). It is apparent that the rate of 11.3 for underground iron ore miners was the highest and was nearly double that of any other group. The high pneumonia incidence rate among men in this single department was believed due to sudden and marked temperature changes to which they were exposed on regaining the surface after their day's work (see pages 337–338). Apparently a considerable proportion of the employees of this company were Negroes, but incidence figures by race were not given.

As earlier mentioned in this chapter in the discussion of the relation of sex to the occurrence of pneumonia, Doull, Harmon, and Fisher (373) studied the possible relation of occupation to the observed variations in the sex ratio of the mortality from pneumonia. These workers demonstrated that the excess male mortality from pneumonia in adults in different states in the United States varied definitely with the degree of urbanization shown by those states. Those most highly industrialized appeared to have the highest excess adult male pneumonia mortality. Doull and his associates regarded it as most probable that this was due to some environmental factor which was most potent in lowering the resistance of males in urban states. They further pointed out that, if it be assumed that this variation in the sex ratio of mortality with urbanization is chiefly due to unfavorable industrial conditions, then such conditions must either be more universal than is generally believed or else men in a relatively small number of occupations must have extraordinarily high pneumonia death rates. A study was made of the rates of several highly industrialized states where about one-half the males gainfully employed were engaged in the extraction of minerals and in manufacturing and mechanical occupations. It appeared that to account for the sex ratio of pneumonia mortality in these states the employees in such occupations would have to have death rates approximately three times as high as other males and females; and even taking into account the findings in the above-mentioned reports of the Registrar-General (560) and of Brundage and his associates (163, 162), this seemed improbable. In consequence, it appeared that either the list of "harmful" occupations has to be enlarged so as to include others not now recognized as such, or that only a part of the excess pneumonia mortality in adult males in industrial states can be attributed to occupation.

The foregoing observations in this section relate primarily to the relation of occupation and pneumonia in white populations. Relatively little information is at hand concerning this problem in colored populations. In connection with studies of the prevalence of pneumonia among natives employed in the gold mines in South Africa, Lister and Ordman (788) determined that the incidence of pneumonia and other acute respiratory diseases was higher in men working underground than in those doing surface work. The incidence of pneumonia in the former group of workers did not appear affected by the depth underground at which the work was done. Incidence rates were highest in such workers among laborers in one occupational group, that of loaders. Exposure to considerable variations of temperature, with opportunities for chilling, was offered by underground working conditions and upon the return of miners to the surface. In the copper mines of Northern Rhodesia (tropical Africa) findings of similar significance were obtained by Ordman (971), and the pneumonia incidence and mortality rates in underground miners were found to be three times that of surface workers.

From the above discussion it is obvious that persons engaged in certain occupations, especially those requiring fatiguing physical labor out of doors in all kinds of weather; and those who perform certain occupations associated with the smelting, rolling, or converting of brass, iron, or steel, who experience intermittent exposure to intense heat; and those exposed to some forms of dust may have higher pneumonia morbidity or mortality rates, or both, than others not so employed. This also appears true of underground miners who may be exposed to considerable changes of temperature in the course of their work and upon their return to the surface. It is the factors accessory to the occupation rather than the execution of the precise occupation itself, then, which appear of so much importance in this respect.

ENVIRONMENTAL CHANGE AND ALTITUDE. The broad problem of environmental change in relation to the occurrence of pneumonia involves a consideration of several factors. Considerable data are at hand suggesting that the reported high incidence of pneumonia which in certain instances has followed environmental change is the result of the increased opportunities for infection this affords, presumably by bringing persons into contact with organisms against which they may have but little resistance. The initial immunity of the population in question appears to be of prime importance. Race, differences between the old and the new environment, and general climatic conditions may also be involved.

Excellent material for the study of this problem has been furnished by observations on large groups of Negroes who, for the purposes of supplying labor in some enterprises, such as the mining of copper, gold, and diamonds in Africa and the construction of the Panama Canal, have been transported, by various means, distances of several hundred miles or more. The term of employment in such enterprises has usually been short. At the gold mines on the Witwatersrand (commonly referred to as the Rand), South Africa, for example, natives usually enlist for a six-month period of work, and few remain there more than twelve months. In former years some 200,000 natives were employed in the mines, but of late the number has been increased to nearly 250,000, and now, as before, the annual labor turnover is nearly 100 per cent (788). The periods of enlistment, and consequently discharge from the mines, are staggered, and during many months of the year there is a constant stream of natives coming to and returning from the mines. It is clear, then, that the continued operation of this single group of mines involves the mass migration of nearly a quarter of a million native laborers each year.

Maynard (874) made a study of pneumonia among several thousand natives transported from various districts in Africa to the gold mines on the Rand. These natives were chiefly from the low regions of Portuguese East Africa (north of 22° South Latitude), the tropical climate of which was considerably different from the high, dry, and mild temperate climate of the Rand. Natives from the above region were referred to as "tropical" natives and following their arrival on the Rand were kept in observation compounds for an average of three weeks before being allowed to do any underground work. The attack rates and mortality rates from pneumonia (nearly all lobar pneumonia) were highest forty-eight hours after the arrival of such natives at the observation compound and from then on steadily decreased for several months. It is of interest that though the attack rate decreased with a lapse of time, little or no change was observed in the case fatality rate, which suggests that the factors governing resistance to this infection are somewhat different from those involved in the mechanism concerned in recovery after infection has developed. Table 56 shows the pneumonia attack rate experienced by 45,291 tropical natives during their first nineteen days on the Rand.

TABLE 56. PNEUMONIA CASES IN 45,291 TROPICAL NATIVES OBSERVED ON THE RAND, SOUTH AFRICA. NUMBER AND PERCENTAGE ATTACKED BY DAY AFTER ARRIVAL AT MINES

DAY AFTER ARRIVAL	NUMBER ATTACKED	PER CENT ATTACK RATE
0–4	526	1.16
5–9	389	0.86
10–14	314	0.69
15–19	275	0.61

From Maynard (874)

The highest attack rates occurred in newly arrived natives, and this phenomenon was not affected by seasonal changes. Between the time of arrival and the end of the nineteenth day the attack rates decreased from 1.16 per cent to 0.61 per cent. The pneumonia attack rates for 8,123 of these tropical natives were followed for a period of over five months. During that interval work in the mines was begun, but the attack rates steadily declined, as is shown in Table 57.

During the interval between the first and the fifth month after arrival on the Rand the attack rate decreased from 3.89 per cent to 1.22 per cent.

In addition to Maynard's report, Gorgas (549) found that among the native laborers employed in the construction of the Panama Canal, most cases of pneumonia occurred in newly arrived natives rather than in those who had been at the Canal some time. In this instance the new natives had four and one-half times as much pneumonia as those who had been there for some months. Observations of the same import were made by Pearson and Mouchet (1008) on native miners in the Belgian Congo. Climatic differences between the old and the new environment of natives were much less in this instance, as well as in that reported by Gorgas, in comparison to the differences experienced by tropical natives in their sojourn on the Rand. Reports from other sources have likewise shown that changing the environment of Negroes has been accompanied by high pneumonia incidence rates, followed by a gradual decline over a period of several weeks or longer (140, 324, 510). It is almost a foregone conclusion that in each of the above instances Negroes have been removed from their usual sphere of life, which in the tropics ordinarily is one of relative isolation, and plunged into the midst of a crowded existence. Concurrent with this abrupt change, under ordinary conditions, the maximum incidence of pneumonia occurred.

TABLE 57. PNEUMONIA CASES IN 8,123 TROPICAL NATIVES OBSERVED ON THE RAND, SOUTH AFRICA. NUMBER AND PERCENTAGE ATTACKED BY MONTH AFTER ARRIVAL AT MINES

MONTH AFTER ARRIVAL	NUMBER ATTACKED	PER CENT ATTACK RATE
0	312	3.89
1	203	2.58
2	155	2.00
3	139	1.83
4	125	1.68
5	89	1.22

From Maynard (874)

Certain other information is at hand concerning the relation of environmental change to the occurrence of pneumonia. Maynard (874) remarks that Grundler found that recruits in the German army had a much higher incidence of pneumonia than did seasoned troops. Similar findings were reported for American soldiers at Camp Wheeler, Georgia, by Cecil and Vaughan (246). In addition, soldiers moved from the south into northern camps during the World War suffered very high morbidity rates for respiratory diseases in general, as Cole (297) has noted.

The direct relation of altitude alone to the incidence of pneumonia is not clear. Cole (297) has regarded altitude as of little importance in this matter. It was earlier pointed out that, though certain states and cities in this country and some cities in other countries located at high altitudes have very high pneumonia death rates, other communities in the same or different countries located practically at sea level have experienced rates as high or higher (see pages 269–284). It is apparent, however, that a high altitude, in conjunction with a low annual rate of precipitation and a high rate of evaporation, contributes to frequent rapid and extensive variations in temperature, which in turn might tend to increase the incidence of pneumonia. It is said that there is great fear of pneumonia in some mining camps located at very high altitudes (10,000 to 15,000 feet). Information is lacking as to whether this feeling has resulted from experience with a high morbidity rate or, as is perhaps readily understandable, with a high case fatality rate in such regions.

Personal Condition

ALCOHOL. Though both acute and chronic alcoholism appear to heighten susceptibility to pneumonia, actual proof of this is lacking. The assumption that alcoholism predisposes to pneumonia rests largely on the observations of several investigators who have obtained a history of alcoholism from varying proportions (5 to 19 per cent) of patients with lobar pneumonia (918, 256, 1176). Findings of similar significance have been reported from other sources (230, 760, 464). For example, Cole (297) states that among 488 cases of lobar pneumonia treated at the Johns Hopkins Hospital an alcoholic history was obtained in 144 or 30 per cent of the cases; and of these, 30 had been on sprees shortly before admission. Further, among 537 cases at the Hospital of the Rockefeller Institute for Medical Research, 102 or 18.9 per cent were classed as heavy drinkers and 153 or 28.5 per cent as moderate drinkers.

From his study of pneumonia among Negro laborers in Panama, Gorgas (549) states, but presents no figures in support of his belief, that the use of alcohol tends to increase the risk of pneumonia. If the human consumption of alcohol actually tends to increase the incidence of pneumonia, the precise nature of the mechanism involved is unknown. A lowering of local or general resistance is to be considered.

The observations of Stillman (1237, 1238) and of Stillman and Branch (1243) on the effect of alcoholic intoxication upon the fate of pneumococci inhaled by mice under experimental conditions are of much interest in this respect. Mice were subjected to the inhalation of pneumococci by spraying broth cultures within a closed chamber. It was determined by the direct culturing of portions of their lungs that under ordinary conditions pneumococci are disposed of and disappear from their lungs within about four hours. In other mice first stupefied by the intraperitoneal injection of a standard dose of alcohol and then subjected to the inhalation of a similar intensity of sprayed culture, the findings were different. In this instance pneumococci were found to persist in the lungs for about twenty-four hours. Alcoholic intoxication, then, appeared to slow the normal mechanism of disposal of the inspired organisms. While only 3 per cent of normal mice died of septicaemia following the inhalation of pneumococci, some 40 per cent of the intoxicated group died of this. Results very similar to these were also obtained using cultures of hemolytic streptococci and influenza bacilli. It was concluded that in some unknown way alcoholic intoxication alters the natural defense mechanism so as to depress the resistance of the host.

The extent to which these findings can be applied to the problem in man is not clear. An impairment of the normal mechanism for disposing of organisms deep in the respiratory tree may be a factor in the causation of pneumonia in certain cases of acute alcoholism where, due to certain conditions, such as a lessening of the cough reflex, infected material may be aspirated. In addition, unusual exposures to wet and cold probably also play a part in the predisposition of many alcoholics to respiratory infections, including pneumonia.

DIET. Individuals living on grossly inadequate diets (often found in confirmed alcoholics), and particularly those with scurvy or rickets, are regarded as especially susceptible to pneumonia (549, 1025, 1109, 1008, 788). Due to the presence of numerous complicating factors, it appears impossible, however, to obtain a clear concept of the relation of diet alone to susceptibility. As earlier mentioned, Gorgas (549) reported an abrupt and marked decrease in the incidence of pneumonia among Negro laborers at the Panama Canal following a relief of their overcrowded condition and an improvement in their diet (see page 317). He stated that a part of this decrease may possibly have been due to the change in diet. Better evidence of the importance of diet in relation to the occurrence of this disease has been supplied by Maynard (874), Pearson and Mouchet (1008), and Lister and Ordman (788). These observers found that many of the Negroes who seek employment in the mines of Africa do so only after a period of several months of partial starvation at home, and thus arrive at the mines in an undernourished condition. Maynard and Pearson and Mouchet note that among such natives the incidence of all forms of illness, including pneumonia, is high and is much higher than among other groups of natives who are in better condition at the time of their arrival at the mines. Winchester (1428) regards Tamils as more susceptible to pneumonia than the Chinese and attributes the low incidence of the disease in the latter to the fact that the diet of the Chinese is better balanced, while that of the Tamils consists largely of carbohydrate (rice) with but little protein and fat.

Shibley and Spies (1185) studied the effect of Vitamin A on the common cold and found that feeding extra Vitamin A to adults had no influence on the incidence or severity of the colds experienced by these individuals, but the colds that occurred in this group were consistently of shorter duration than those which occurred among control groups. This finding is in accord with the conclusions of Clausen (274), who made an extensive review of the literature in relation to the influence of nutrition on resistance. He observed that, in general, susceptibility to infection was usually not markedly affected by diet, but that resistance to infection after it is established may be greatly reduced by deficiencies in diet. This appeared true of deficiencies of Vitamins A and C and possibly of Vitamin B complex. No evidence was found that a lack of Vitamin D lowered resistance. In addition, however, Clausen stated that the existence of a partial deficiency of vitamins may lead to a loss of resistance to infection, though proof of this is lacking.

TABLE 58. PNEUMOCOCCUS LOBAR PNEUMONIA. NUMBER AND PERCENTAGE OF CASES WITH SYSTEMIC DISEASE, BY TYPE

	TOTAL CASES	CASES WITH SYSTEMIC DISEASE	
		Number	*Per cent*
Type I	298	61	20.4
Type II	203	67	33.0
Type III	131	83	63.3
Group IV	370	116	31.3
Total	1,002	327	32.6

From Cecil *et al.* (230)

FATIGUE AND OTHER FACTORS. In persons subject to debilitating influences, such as marked fatigue (558, 162, 961), or to acute infections, such as influenza, measles, scarlet fever, typhoid fever, tic fever, or dysentery, the incidence of pneumonia may be high (918, 807, 297, 1008). The presence of chronic disease, such as chronic non-tubercular infections of the respiratory tract (464), or of systemic diseases, such as degenerative vascular disease, valvular heart disease, nephritis, or malignant disease, may likewise increase susceptibility to pneumonia (918, 256, 807, 230, 245, 961, 120, 464).

Cecil and his associates (230, 245), Blake (120), and Finland and Sutliff (464) have found that pneumococcus Type III infections are especially liable to occur among patients with chronic disease. In Cecil, Baldwin, and Larsen's (230) series of 131 Type III cases of lobar pneumonia, 83 patients or 63.3 per cent had systemic disease of some sort (see Table 58); and in Blake's

(120) series of 119 cases, 79 patients or 66 per cent had one or more chronic diseases.

It is apparent in Table 58 that systemic disease was present in about one-fifth of the Type I cases, one-third of the Type II cases, and two-thirds of the Type III cases. Finland and Sutliff (464) found a high proportion of chronic disease among patients with Type VIII pneumonia. The incidence of chronic disease presumably increases with the age of the group considered, and it is among the older group that most investigators have found the largest proportion of Type III and Type VIII cases (see pages 60–67).

Exposure to Wet and Cold (Chilling) and Temperature Variations

Exposure to wet and cold and to extensive variations in temperature, with the associated opportunities for chilling, has long been regarded as extremely important in relation to the prevalence of pneumonia (647, 1361, 918, 297). It is almost certain that this view is correct, though the matter is difficult of proof. As pointed out in several of the earlier sections of this chapter, many observations have been made in recent years which lend important support to this view (see pages 289–295 and 295–299). In the discussion of pathogenesis in the preceding chapter (pages 233–235) it was shown that exposure to wet or cold or both, or to other conditions tending to lower body temperature, occupies a prominent place among the factors which appear to depress host resistance and thus, under certain circumstances, permits pulmonary infection to become established. As there noted, direct observations in support of this view have been cited by numerous investigators (918, 728, 1209, 1259, 1430, 1292, 483, 954, 926).

Among patients with lobar pneumonia Musser and Norris (918) found that more than 17 per cent of 4,244 collected cases, and Chatard (254) that more than 19 per cent of 658 cases gave a history of exposure to bad weather before onset. Findings of like significance have been reported by numerous other investigators. For the purpose at hand such information is of far less value, however, than that derived from other sources, as described below.

In Rogers' (1103) interesting study of pneumonia in India, data were obtained on 14,266 cases, most of which were believed to be cases of lobar pneumonia. His experience of twenty years in medical work in India would appear to make his observations of special value. It was clearly shown that the yearly incidence per thousand increased steadily from the region of Burma, Assam, and the lower portion of Madras in the east and south to that of the Indus Valley in the northwest. The rates in the former regions were from 4.2 to 7.6, while in the latter they were from 25.8 to 50.2. The area with the lowest rates had the warmest, most even climate, while the northwest portion was the coldest and showed the most extensive seasonal and daily temperature variations. During the two coldest months of the year (December and January there) the incidence rates in this northwest area were up to 100 per cent in excess of the rates for all India. The same area with the highest rates had the lowest absolute humidity as compared with other divisions of the country, while in areas with the lowest rates the reverse was true.

It was suggested that the extremely high incidence of pneumonia in northwestern India was due to the repeated chilling of the natives, who bathe in the river in the cold early morning clad only in loin cloths which are allowed to dry on them. Chilling is caused by the rapid evaporation of water due to the dry air and cold winds.

Smillie and Caldwell's (1209) observations in regard to a direct effect of cold weather are of interest. In a small isolated community in Alabama they found that a period of cold weather was followed by an epidemic of colds which tended to spread throughout the families in the neighborhood. Two or three days after the onset of the colds pneumococci overgrew all other organisms in the nose and throat of those affected and were found in almost pure culture for about a week. These organisms were most prevalent in the nose and throat from the fourth to the eighth day after the onset of the cold, and during that period individuals who were exposed to low temperatures or chilling tended to develop pneumonia. Pneumonia did not develop in those suffering exposure alone; but it frequently developed in individuals with an acute cold who were exposed to chilling.

In the section on occupation above, it was seen that high pneumonia incidence and also mortality rates appeared common among individuals whose occupations involved conditions exposing them to wet, cold, chilling, and extensive temperature variations (see page 318). Among the industrial groups in the coal, iron, and railroad company studied by Kibbey (714), the highest pneumonia incidence was found among underground iron ore miners (11.3 per thousand) and was nearly twice as high as the rate shown by underground coal miners or surface workers and their dependents. The higher rate in ore miners was believed due to the fact that these workers were perspiring and hot when they came up from the mines and in many instances had to walk a half mile or so in the open air to the bath-houses, which were kept too warm (80° F.). After changing clothes there, they again walked in the open air about a mile to the car line. These walks offered two good chances for chilling, especially at certain seasons of the year. It was believed that these facts, rather than the presence of pneumoconiosis in ore miners, more nearly accounted for the prevalence of pneumonia in that group. In favor of this view was the finding that, even with a higher incidence rate, ore miners had a lower case fatality rate than other workers without pneumoconiosis. Though nearly 100 per cent of the coal miners had anthracosis, their pneumonia incidence rate was low, as was their case fatality rate. The observation that the group having one of the lowest pneumonia incidence rates (surface workers) had the highest case fatality rate is in accord with the demonstration of Rogers (1103) that individuals in areas of India having the lowest incidence rates had the highest case fatality rates.

In their studies of pneumonia incidence among gold miners on the Rand, Ordman (970) and Lister and Ordman (788) have commented upon the importance of underground working conditions and the wide temperature changes to which native miners are subjected on entering and leaving the mines. This was especially true during the fairly cold weather of winter, when the temperature often dropped abruptly in the late afternoon, producing a definite chilling effect. In some mines improvements in ventilation were introduced, and covered roadways or tunnels were built through which miners had to travel before reaching the open air. It was suggested that the issue of a heavy coat or jacket to every miner to wear when entering or leaving the mines would also lessen the menace of chilling.

The importance of exposure to wet and cold and to temperature variations among men employed in the iron and steel industry was clearly pointed out by Brundage and his associates (163, 162). It was noted that among the occupational groups studied, the highest pneumonia incidence was 13.6 per thousand and was found among men whose occupation involved only exposure to inclement weather; while the next highest rate was 12.6, and this was found in those exposed to heat with wide changes in temperature but having no other industrial health hazard.

A review of all the departments of the company investigated showed that men in the blast furnace department had the highest incidence rates. Within this department the rates were highest for individuals in a few occupations, as previously described, and nearly all cases occurred among general laborers or men in occupations associated with stacks and stoves (casting), especially the first and second helpers. The stove keepers and helpers had exposure to heat with extreme variations in temperature, to gases and smoke, and to some extent to dust and inclement weather; and this group had thirteen times as many cases as would be expected from the control group. Hot blast men and stove cleaners, also employed in this department, had as much gas, dust, smoke, and out-of-door work in all kinds of weather as the other groups but, together with the blowers, experienced less severe exposure to heat with wide temperature variations and had only four times the number of cases as expected from the control group. It was concluded that the performance of strenuous work under intermittent exposure to high temperatures seemed to intensify the pneumonia hazard. The highest incidence rates were found in men intermittently exposed to high temperatures, in those doing unsheltered work in the open, and in those performing sedentary but fatiguing work in a damp and drafty environment. The one unfavorable factor common to all these occupations seemed to be a sudden cooling or chilling of the body.

In view of these observations it appears that either or both sudden or prolonged exposure to extensive variations in temperature must be regarded as one of the most important predisposing factors of pneumonia.

Previous Respiratory Infections

The relation of minor respiratory infections to the occurrence of lobar pneumonia has already been discussed (see pages 235–240 and 289–295). Considered together, infections of this nature appear to be the commonest recognized predisposing factor in lobar pneumonia in white patients. Minor infections of the upper respiratory tract are usually followed, not only by an increase in the number of pneumococci carried by an individual, but also by an increased incidence of pneumococcus carriers in the community (see also pages 374–377) and by an increase in the occurrence of pneumonia.

The common cold is one of the most frequent of the minor upper respiratory infections. Though world-wide in distribution (1205, 359, 1208), it is probably most prevalent in temperate zones where the temperature and climatic conditions are most variable (Dochez, 359). Influenza also has a world-wide distribution (1304). Pulmonary lesions may develop subsequent to an attack of either the common cold or influenza. Colds appear more likely to be followed by lobar pneumonia than by bronchopneumonia, while after influenza the latter form of pneumonia is more common.

The problem of true mixed infections and of consecutive or superinfections was discussed earlier (see pages 11–16).

It has long been recognized that no other acute infectious disease of such severity is so likely to recur in the same patient as pneumonia (Wells, 1403,

Osler, 976, Cecil, 224, Norris and Landis, 961). Judging by the available reports, from 4 (830) to 41 per cent (807) of patients with pneumonia give a history of having had one or more previous attacks of this disease. The matter is considered in some detail elsewhere (see pages 533–535).

Trauma and Aspiration of Noxious Substances

TRAUMA. Trauma to the chest may be followed by pneumonia (1361, 26, 297, 807, 961). Under these circumstances the pneumonia usually does not begin until one or two days after the injury; and, as Lord (807) has stated, it differs chiefly from ordinary pneumonia in the hemorrhagic character of the sputum. Either lobar pneumonia or bronchopneumonia may occur, and the prognosis may be made more serious by the presence of shock.

According to Lord (807), Litten divided cases of post-traumatic pneumonia into those with "traumatic pneumonia" in which there was direct injury to the lung, and those with "contusion pneumonia" in which the lung was injured in consequence of concussion. Lord remarks that "Actual injury to the pulmonary substance probably occurs in both forms, but in the latter may take place without obvious lesion of the chest wall." The pneumonia may affect the injured side or the side opposite. In such cases autoinfection by the pneumococcus or other organism present in the upper respiratory tract at that time would be favored.

Among 991 cases of lobar pneumonia studied by Ashton and Landis (26) trauma may have been an important predisposing factor in 7 (0.7 per cent). Cole (297) states that, in general, a history of preceding chest injury may be obtained in from one to 4 per cent of all cases of lobar pneumonia. Nevertheless, none of the 770 cases studied by him gave such a history.

ASPIRATION OF NOXIOUS SUBSTANCES. The inhalation of noxious substances in solid, liquid, or gaseous form may give rise to a pneumonia which is less often of the lobar than of the bronchopneumonic variety. The inhalation of some dusts, particularly those containing a high content of silica, leads to a high incidence of respiratory diseases, including pneumonia (1143, 1301, 155; see pages 295–297 and 318–329). The findings of Haythorn and Meller (607) suggest that anthracosis, even in the more severe grades, is not a significant factor in influencing the occurrence of pneumonia. The inhalation of an alkaline dust of high silica content may lead to acute silicosis (253).

It is not clear how inhaled dust may act to give rise to pneumonia. Limited bacteriologic studies of ordinary dust were made by Stillman (1235), who found pneumococci in the dust of eighteen of sixty-two rooms examined in which no case of pneumonia had been cared for. Dust from other rooms, in which cases of Type I or II pneumococcus lobar pneumonia had been cared for, showed pneumococci present in 40 per cent of 183 specimens examined. Of 74 strains of pneumococci isolated, 25 or 33.8 per cent were Type I, 23 or 31 per cent were Type II, 2 or 2.7 per cent were Type III, and the remaining 24 or 32.4 per cent were of other types. Together, Types I and II accounted for 64.8 per cent of the strains found. Brown, Gottlieb, and Laybourn (155) studied the bacteriologic content of soil dust obtained during the tremendous dust storms which occurred in the region of western Kansas in 1935. No pathogenic organisms were found in such dust, but it proved exceedingly irritating to the mucous membranes of the respiratory tract.

From the United States Army report on the medical aspects of gas warfare, which summarizes the experience of more than 70,000 men admitted to hospitals for gas poisoning during the War, it is clear that the irritating effect on the lung of chlorine, bromine, phosgene, and some other gases is often pronounced (1344). Edema and necrosis of the lining of much of the respiratory tract occurred. Pneumonia, seldom of the lobar form, was by far the commonest cause of death in cases ending fatally. An analysis of the necropsy findings of 546 gassed men revealed that the cause of death in 440 (80.6 per cent) was tracheobronchitis and pneumonia (14 others had lobar pneumonia). The next most common cause of death was gas asphyxiation, which occurred in 33.

In infants pneumonia may occur as a result of the aspiration of amniotic fluid (1386, 1121) and in other persons may follow immersion in water (807). The aspiration of oily substances, which occasionally occurs in children or debilitated individuals, leads to a foreign body reaction within the lung with an outpouring of large mononuclear phagocytic cells (1024, 1055). Such lesions, referred to as "lipoid pneumonias," are occasionally lengthy in course and may have an acute pneumonia superimposed upon them. Repeated roentgenograms may be necessary to differentiate this lesion from that of pulmonary tuberculosis.

The result of careful experimental work in animals suggests that the inhalation or direct injection of substances irritating to the lung has the effect of injuring a portion of the tissue and locally reducing its resistance to infection (728, 146, 1084, 1013, 508; see also pages 231–235). The matter is extremely complicated, however, and results either at variance with this view or so interpreted have been reported (1162, 1013, 483). Nevertheless, it is possible that in man a decrease in resistance, either local or general, or both local and general, may result in some instances from the inhalation of irritant dusts, chemicals, fumes, gases, and liquids, and thus provide suitable conditions for the occurrence of pulmonary infection. In such instances infection would probably result from organisms already in the upper respiratory tract.

TRANSMISSION AND SPREAD OF PNEUMOCOCCUS LOBAR PNEUMONIA

Pneumococcus Carriers

Sternberg (1227) in 1881 was probably the first to show that pneumococci may be present in the mouths of healthy persons. Subsequently this was also demonstrated by Washbourn (1388). By 1905 it was clear that pneumococci could be obtained from the mouths of from 45 to 60 per cent of all normal persons (1405, 994, 803, 166, 648). As the following discussion will show, this has been confirmed many times since then. The repeated examination of groups of individuals over a period of many months indicates that nearly all normal persons carry pneumococci in their mouths for variable periods each year (648, 1048, 1393, 578, 267, 133).

Though, as seen above, early investigators did establish that pneumococci were carried by approximately one-half of all normal persons, little real headway was made in solving the epidemiologic problems presented by pneumococcus pneumonia until the discovery of pneumococcus types in 1909–1912. The separation of pneumococci into Types I, II, and III, and later into the higher types, has been of the utmost importance in assisting in this work. The fact that the great majority of all pneumococci encountered can now be classified is of invaluable aid in following the spread of such organisms among individuals in the community.

Many epidemiologic studies of pneumonia have been made since the advent of pneumococcus typing. Among the most important of these the reports of the following investigators may be mentioned: Dochez and Avery (360, 361); Stillman (1234, 1235); Rosenau, Felton, and Atwater (1111); Powell, Atwater, and Felton (1048); Jacobson (682); Smillie and Caldwell (1209); Gundel and Linden (579); Webster and Hughes (1393); Shultz (1187); Cruickshank (331); Smillie (1206); Smillie and Leeder (1210); Viktorow, Semzowa, and Oettinger (1353); Christie (267); Bliss, McClaskey, and Long (133); Bunim and Trask (201); and Smillie (1207).

Saliva or washings or swabs from the throat and in some instances cultures from the nose or nasopharynx of several thousand healthy persons, some of whom were in intimate contact with patients with pneumococcus pneumonia, have been examined to determine the presence of pneumococci. A combination of cultural methods, together with the injection of some of the material into white mice with the subsequent typing of any pneumococci obtained, has proved most satisfactory for this purpose. In some instances similar examinations have been carried out on patients convalescent from pneumococcus pneumonia.

Studies of this nature have revealed that carriers of pneumococci may be divided into three broad classes: (a) healthy persons having no known contact with pneumonia patients, (b) healthy persons with such contact, and (c) patients convalescent from pneumonia. As will be noted later, there are numerous accessory factors which appear to influence the carrier state of various of these groups of individuals, such as the type of pneumococcus concerned, the season of the year, and the presence of upper respiratory disease in the individual or his immediate contacts.

In the following pages, healthy persons not in contact with patients with pneumonia will be referred to as "non-contacts," and healthy persons having such contact will be designated "contacts."

HEALTHY CARRIERS NOT HAVING CONTACT WITH PNEUMONIA PATIENTS. Dochez and Avery (360) and Stillman (1234, 1235) were probably the first to call attention to the fact that, whereas pneumococci of Types I and II were responsible for more than one-half of all cases of pneumococcus lobar pneumonia, these two types were seldom found in the mouths of normal persons not in contact with patients with pneumonia. This observation has been amply confirmed by subsequent investigations.

The carrier rate of pneumococci of Types I, II, III, and of Group IV has been studied by numerous investigators and data for several hundred non-contact infants and children have been assembled in Table 59. Of the 531 individuals examined, only 188 or 35.4 per cent were found to carry these organisms. Also, only 4 or 0.8 per cent of the 531 carried Type I; 8 or 1.5 per cent, Type II; and 6 or 1.1 per cent, Type III; while a much larger group of 170 or 32 per cent carried pneumococci of Group IV. Further comment concerning the incidence of the types found among these carriers is reserved till later.

The pneumococcus carrier rate of a larger group of non-contact individuals made up chiefly, but not entirely, of adults and based on the studies of several workers is presented in Table 60. In several instances the total number of pneumococcus strains found was larger than the number of pneumococcus carriers, for at times more than one type was obtained from a given carrier.

TABLE 59. NON-CONTACT INFANTS AND CHILDREN. NUMBER AND PERCENTAGE OF CARRIERS OF PNEUMOCOCCI AND DISTRIBUTION OF STRAINS FOUND BY TYPE; PERCENTAGE INCIDENCE OF TYPES IN TOTAL NON-CONTACT GROUP

SOURCE	PERSONS EXAMINED			STRAINS FOUND				
		CARRIERS FOUND						
	TOTAL	*Number*	*Per cent*	TOTAL	TYPE I	TYPE II	TYPE III	GROUP IV
					Number			
Wollstein, 1923 (1435)	33	12	36.4	12	–	–	–	12
Plummer, Raia, and Shultz, 1930 (1029)	43	27	62.8	27	–	–	2	25
Raia, Plummer, and Shultz, 1931 (1057)	53	28	52.8	28	1	3	2	22
Ishida, Nagai, and Saito, 1931 (681)	244	60	24.6	60	1	5	2	52*
Blacklock and Guthrie, 1933 (112)	158	61	38.6	61	2	–	–	59
Total	531	188	35.4	188	4	8	6	170
					Percentage incidence in total non-contact group			
					0.8	1.5	1.1	32.0

* Includes 8 with "rough" pneumococci.

Of the 1,801 persons examined, 812 or 45.1 per cent were found carrying pneumococci. Type I was found in only 8 or 0.4 per cent and Type II in 14 or 0.8 per cent of the 1,801 persons, while Type III was more frequent and was recovered from 189 or 10.5 per cent. Pneumococci of Group IV were commonest and were found in 628 or 34.9 per cent of the whole group.

For various reasons three series of considerable size have been omitted from Table 60. The first of these is that of Sailer, Hall, Wilson, and McCoy (1155), who found only 111 or 16 per cent of 700 soldiers carrying pneumococci. This figure appears unusually low, for pneumonia was prevalent among the troops at the time the study was carried out. Mice were not used for the isolation of pneumococci from the cultures taken in this instance.

Among the 111 carriers found, 6 carried Type I; 15, Type II; 5, Type III; and 85, strains of Group IV. The second series is that of 950 persons examined by Jacobson (682), who found pneumococci of Types I, II, and III in 7 or 0.7 per cent, 5 or 0.5 per cent, and 82 or 8.6 per cent respectively of the

TABLE 60. NON-CONTACTS. NUMBER AND PERCENTAGE OF CARRIERS AND DISTRIBUTION OF STRAINS FOUND BY TYPE; PERCENTAGE INCIDENCE OF TYPES IN TOTAL NON-CONTACT GROUP

SOURCE	PERSONS EXAMINED			STRAINS FOUND				
	TOTAL	CARRIERS FOUND *Number*	CARRIERS FOUND *Per cent*	TOTAL	TYPE I *Number*	TYPE II *Number*	TYPE III *Number*	GROUP IV *Number*
Stillman, 1916 (1234)	398	172	43.2	188	4[a]	4	44	136[b]
Stillman, 1917 (1235)	297	116	39.1	121	1	–	34	86[c]
Sydenstricker and Sutton, 1917 (1282)	50	19	38.0	19	–	1	1	17[d]
Rosenau, Felton, and Atwater, 1926 (1111)	180	85	47.2	91	2	4[e]	9	76
Strøm, 1932 (1252)	50	30	60.0	30	–	–	14	16
Smillie, 1933 (1206)	493	212	43.0	212	1	3	67	141
Viktorow, Semzowa, and Oettinger, 1934 (1353)	308	168	54.5	168	–	2	20	146
Napier and Dharmendra, 1935 (924)	25	10	40.0	10	–	–	–	10[f]
Total	1,801	812	45.1	839	8	14	189	628
					Percentage incidence in total non-contact group			
					0.4	0.8	10.5	34.9

[a] Includes 3 obtained from persons in contact with Type I pneumonia.
[b] Includes 26 atypical Type II strains. [c] Includes 22 atypical Type II strains.
[d] Includes 1 atypical Type II strain.
[e] Strains of atypical Type II are included as they are not given separately.
[f] Includes 3 strains of two types observed locally in India.

group. He, however, gave no data on the incidence of Group IV in his series. The third series omitted is that reported by Christensen (264), who examined 1,474 non-contacts (all but 23 were soldiers) and found only 230 or 15.6 per cent of the group carrying pneumococci. Type I was found in 1 or 0.06 per cent, Type II in 3 or 0.2 per cent, Type III in 21 or 1.4 per cent, and Group IV in 205 or 13.9 per cent. Both the carrier rate for all pneumococci and the incidence of the various types individually are so low in this series as to raise doubts as to the adequacy of the determinations. No mice were used in the isolation of pneumococci in this instance, and Christensen remarked that had this been done the proportion of carriers found might have been larger.

In comparing the carrier rate of Types I, II, III, and of Group IV in infants and children (Table 59) with that of the larger group composed chiefly of adults (Table 60), it appears that pneumococci were found in 35.4 per cent of infants and children and in 45.1 per cent of the adults. The most striking difference between the two groups is in the carrier rate of Type III. While pneumococci of this type were found in only 1.1 per cent of the infants and children, they were recovered from 10.5 per cent of the older group.

The groups in Tables 59 and 60 have been combined to obtain a composite view of the usual frequency with which pneumococci are carried by healthy non-contact persons (see Table 61).

TABLE 61. NON-CONTACTS (TABLES 59 AND 60 COMBINED). NUMBER AND PERCENTAGE OF CARRIERS AND DISTRIBUTION OF STRAINS FOUND BY TYPE; PERCENTAGE INCIDENCE OF TYPES IN TOTAL NON-CONTACT GROUP

SOURCE	PERSONS EXAMINED			STRAINS FOUND				
	TOTAL	CARRIERS FOUND *Number*	CARRIERS FOUND *Per cent*	TOTAL	TYPE I *Number*	TYPE II *Number*	TYPE III *Number*	GROUP IV *Number*
Infants and children (Table 59)	531	188	35.4	188	4	8	6	170
Older group (Table 60)	1,801	812	45.1	839	8	14	189	628
Total	2,332	1,000	42.9	1,027	12	22	195	798
				Percentage incidence in total non-contact group	0.5	0.9	8.4	34.2

One thousand or 42.9 per cent of the 2,332 persons studied were carrying pneumococci, and from this group 1,027 strains were recovered. Pneumococci of Type I (carried by 0.5 per cent of persons in whom pneumococci were found) and Type II (0.9 per cent) were seldom found, while those of Type III were more common (8.4 per cent). Strains of Group IV were the commonest and were carried by approximately one-third (34.2 per cent) of the entire group.

Information is available on another group of healthy non-contact individuals (mostly children) who have been studied in a somewhat different way. Over a period of many months this group was subjected to examinations repeated at intervals of about one to four weeks (see Table 62); 2,422 examinations being made on 287 persons. Pneumococci were obtained in 66 per cent of the examinations, which yielded 1,598 strains.

TABLE 62. EXAMINATIONS OF 287 NON-CONTACTS. DISTRIBUTION OF STRAINS FOUND BY TYPE AND PERCENTAGE INCIDENCE OF TYPES IN TOTAL EXAMINATIONS MADE*

SERIES	EXAMINATIONS MADE	STRAINS FOUND TOTAL	TYPE I	TYPE II	TYPE III	GROUP IV
		Number				
Powell, Atwater, and Felton (1048), 1926 (93 adults)	418	299	13	20†	32	234
Gundel and Linden (579), 1931 (84 children)	890	565	17	28	89	431
Gundel (578), 1933 (110 children)	1,114	734	9	5	75	645
Total	2,422	1,598	39	53	196	1,310
		Percentage incidence in total examinations made				
		66.0	1.6	2.2	8.1	54.1

* The reports of Webster and Hughes (1393), who carried out over 3,000 examinations on 105 non-contacts, and of Bliss, McClaskey, and Long (133), who made 1,016 examinations of 20 such individuals, have not been included in Table 62, as neither of these reports presents the results obtained in sufficient detail for the purpose. Also omitted were Hirano's (646) findings in an unknown number of non-contacts in Japan. Pneumococci of 49 strains were obtained in this study: 5, or 10.2 per cent Type I; 4, or 8.2 per cent Type II; one, or 2 per cent Types I and II (agglutination occurred in serums for both types); 5, or 10.2 per cent Type III; and 34, or 69.4 per cent Group IV. Hirano also carried out 1,121 other examinations for the presence of pneumococci in patients with influenza and found pneumococci in 448 instances.

† Atypical Type II's are included as they are not given separately.

Pneumococci of Type I were found in 39 or 1.6 per cent of the 2,422 examinations made, and Type II in 53 or 2.2 per cent, Type III in 196 or 8.1 per cent, and Group IV in 1,310 or 54.1 per cent. This group shows a somewhat higher incidence of pneumococci in general (66 per cent) than either the group of infants and children (35.4 per cent) listed in Table 59 or the older group (45.1 per cent) in Table 60, and a considerably higher incidence of

Type III than the infant and children group (8.1 per cent versus 1.1 per cent, Table 59), as well as a somewhat higher incidence of Group IV than the older group (54.1 per cent versus 34.9 per cent, Table 60). The reports of Gundel and Linden in Table 62 comprise the bulk of the examinations listed in that table and were made on children in Germany. In connection with the relatively high incidence of Type III found in this group, it is of interest to note that it was earlier pointed out (Table 5, page 45) that pneumococci of this type appear especially prevalent among cases of lobar pneumonia in the region of Germany.

It is important to examine the proportion of the various types found among the strains isolated from healthy non-contact individuals. For this purpose the 188 strains obtained from infants and children, as listed in Table 59, may be added to the combined group of 1,299 strains isolated by Gundel and Linden, as seen in Table 62. Together these total 1,487 strains, and the proportion of the various types in this group may be compared with that obtained from the older group of non-contacts. The latter comprises the 839 strains as listed in Table 60 and the 299 strains isolated by Powell and his associates from adults, shown in Table 62, totalling 1,138 strains (Table 63).

Of the total 2,625 strains, only 51 or 1.9 per cent were Type I and 75 or 2.9 per cent were Type II, while 391 or 14.9 per cent were Type III, and the remaining 2,108 or 80.3 per cent were Group IV. The total number of strains isolated is fairly large, and it seems likely that these figures represent the approximate proportion of the various types found among the pneumococci carried by healthy non-contacts. Several years ago it was observed that non-contact carriers seldom give a history which might possibly explain the source of the pneumococci they are carrying (1234, 1111, 1048).

Certain differences are found in the incidence of the various types among the strains carried by the younger and by the older group. The incidence of Type I and of Type II among the pneumococci carried by both the younger and the older group of non-contacts is essentially similar and is low. Type III, however, shows the most marked difference and is less frequently found among the strains carried by the younger group (11.4 per cent) than by the older group (19.4 per cent). Pneumococci of Group IV make up the largest proportion of all the strains carried by both groups but are somewhat more common among young persons (83.8 per cent) than older ones (75.7 per cent).

On a few occasions determinations of the incidence of the types of pneumococci carried by non-contacts have been extended to include varying numbers of the higher types. Among 734 strains isolated from non-contact school children and typed from I through XXXII, Gundel (578) in Germany found that Types XVIII (109 strains), VI (103 strains), IV (77 strains), III (75 strains), and X (71 strains) were the commonest. Other studies were carried out in this country. Smillie (1206) determined the incidence of Types I through XIX among 281 strains recovered from non-contacts in the population at large. Apparently the individuals from which these strains came were largely adults. In his series the types most frequently encountered were Types III (67 strains), XVIII (34 strains), VI (21 strains),

TABLE 63. NON-CONTACT CARRIERS. NUMBER AND PERCENTAGE DISTRIBUTION OF PNEUMOCOCCUS STRAINS FOUND BY TYPE

		STRAINS FOUND							
		TYPE I		TYPE II		TYPE III		GROUP IV	
SOURCE	TOTAL	*Number*	*Per cent*	*Number*	*Per cent*	*Number*	*Per cent*	*Number*	*Per cent*
Infants and children (Tables 59 and 62)	1,487	30	2.0	41	2.8	170	11.4	1,246	83.8
Older group (Tables 60 and 62)	1,138	21	1.8	34	3.0	221	19.4	862	75.7
Total	2,625	51	1.9	75	2.9	391	14.9	2,108	80.3

XV (10 strains), and X (9 strains). Among the strains isolated from 103 non-contact carriers in an institution for the feeble-minded which were examined for all thirty-two types, Smillie and Leeder (1210) found Types III, VII, X, and XVIII most frequently, but no single type predominated. Bliss, McClaskey, and Long (133) carried out typing for all thirty-two types on the pneumococci obtained from 350 positive cultures from adults. Strains of Type VI were most frequently encountered, while those of Type XI were next most common. From these studies it appears that each of four types was mentioned in three different reports as among the commonest in non-contacts. These were Types III, VI, X, and XVIII.

When the incidence of the various types of pneumococci found among the strains carried by healthy non-contacts is compared with that found among cases of pneumococcus lobar pneumonia, striking differences are revealed. In Table 64 the incidence of the various types found among strains isolated from non-contact infants and children (Table 63) has been compared with their incidence among cases of pneumococcus lobar pneumonia in a similar younger group (Table 24, page 81). A further comparison has been made in Table 64 of the types found in the older group of non-contacts (Table 63) and those found in patients (Table 5, page 46).

In non-contact infants and children, Type I accounted for only 2 per cent of the strains carried whereas it was responsible for more than ten times this proportion or 22.4 per cent of the cases of pneumonia in the same age group. A less marked, though still considerable, difference was observed between the incidence of Type II in non-contacts (2.8 per cent) and in cases (8.1 per cent). Type III, however, was found more often in non-contact carriers (11.4 per cent) than in cases (5.5 per cent), and pneumococci of Group IV were also somewhat more common in carriers (83.8 per cent) than in cases (64 per cent); though in the latter instance the difference is less marked than between the incidence of these strains in carriers and cases in the older groups. Types I and II, then, were commonest among the cases, but Type III and Group IV were most frequent among the carriers.

TABLE 64. NON-CONTACTS (INFANTS AND CHILDREN AND OLDER GROUP), PERCENTAGE DISTRIBUTION OF STRAINS FOUND; AND PNEUMOCOCCUS LOBAR PNEUMONIA CASES (INFANTS AND CHILDREN AND OLDER GROUP), PERCENTAGE DISTRIBUTION BY TYPE

SOURCE	TYPE I	TYPE II	TYPE III	GROUP IV
Infants and children				
1,487 strains from non-contacts (Table 63)	2.0	2.8	11.4	83.8
826 cases of pneumococcus lobar pneumonia (Table 24)	22.4	8.1	5.5	64.0
Older persons				
1,138 strains from non-contacts (Table 63)	1.8	3.0	19.4	75.7
16,813 cases of pneumococcus lobar pneumonia (Table 5)	32.6	19.6	10.8	36.9

Among persons in the older groups, Type I accounted for only 1.8 per cent of the strains obtained from non-contact carriers, while it was found in about eighteen times this proportion or 32.6 per cent of the cases. Type II also showed a marked difference in incidence in the two groups and accounted for but 3 per cent of the strains from carriers, as compared with nearly seven times this proportion or 19.6 per cent of those from cases. Strains of both

Type III and Group IV made up a much larger proportion of the pneumococci obtained from non-contact carriers than from cases. The incidence of Type III in the carrier group was 19.4 per cent and was but 10.8 per cent among the cases, and the incidence of Group IV strains in these series was 75.7 per cent and 36.9 per cent respectively.

In both the younger and the older groups, pneumococci of Types I and II together accounted for a much smaller proportion of the strains obtained from carriers than from cases, while with strains of Type III and Group IV the reverse was true, and they made up a larger proportion of the pneumococci obtained from carriers than from cases. Such differences were most marked among individuals in the older groups. Further, Types I and II together accounted for 4.8 per cent of the strains isolated from non-contacts, while among cases these types were responsible for 30.5 per cent of the series in the younger group and for 52.2 per cent of those in the older group. When Type III and Group IV pneumococci are considered, the situation is quite different; for together in non-contacts they made up 95.2 per cent of the strains obtained from the younger group and 95.1 per cent of those from the older group, while in cases they were found in 69.5 per cent in the younger group and in 47.7 per cent in the older group.

These differences in the incidence of pneumococci in the above groups clearly suggest that a marked difference exists between the epidemiology of pneumococcus Type I or II pneumonia and that of pneumonia due to Type III or strains of Group IV, considering the latter as a single entity. This was recognized as early as 1915 (360, 361), and, in consequence, in most epidemiologic studies special attention has been paid to pneumococci of Type I and Type II. The emphasis which has been placed upon these two types is reflected somewhat in the following discussion.

HEALTHY CARRIERS HAVING CONTACT WITH PNEUMONIA PATIENTS. Healthy persons in contact with patients having pneumonia due to pneumococci more often carry these organisms than other individuals not having such contact. The carrier rate of pneumococci and of Types I, II, and III, and of Group IV has been reported in the literature for a considerable group of contacts. The data have been assembled and presented in Table 65. At times more than one strain was obtained from some carriers. As most of the persons examined were family contacts, the group includes both children and adults. Of the 1,782 contacts examined, 977 or 54.8 per cent were found carrying pneumococci of 1,018 strains. Of the 1,782 contacts 3.3 per cent harbored

Type I; 2.7 per cent, Type II; 10 per cent, Type III; and 41 per cent, strains of Group IV.

In Table 66 a comparison is made of the incidence of pneumococcus carriers in the non-contact groups (Table 61) and the contact groups (Table 65) and of the proportion of the various types found among the strains obtained from non-contacts (Table 63) and contacts. A larger proportion of persons in contact with patients with pneumococcus pneumonia were found carrying pneumococci (54.8 per cent) than were found among others not exposed to such contact (42.9 per cent). Further, in each instance pneumococci of Types I, II, III, and Group IV were more commonly carried by contacts than by non-contacts. Significant differences between the carrier rate in these two groups of healthy persons also appeared in relation to the incidence of the first two types found among the strains isolated, for Type I

TABLE 65. CONTACTS. NUMBER AND PERCENTAGE OF CARRIERS AND DISTRIBUTION OF STRAINS FOUND BY TYPE; PERCENTAGE INCIDENCE OF TYPES IN TOTAL CONTACT GROUP

SOURCE	PERSONS EXAMINED			STRAINS FOUND				
		CARRIERS FOUND			TYPE I	TYPE II	TYPE III	GROUP IV
	TOTAL	*Number*	*Per cent*	TOTAL	*Number*			
Stillman, 1917 (1235)	645	334	51.8	365	33	22	51	259*
Rosenau, Felton, and Atwater, 1926 (1111)	270	117	43.3	124	10	6†	22	86
Smillie and Caldwell, 1929 (1209)	73	49	67.1	49	2	3	1	43
Plummer, Raia, and Shultz, 1930 (1029)	46	30	65.2	30	1	–	2	27
Shultz, 1932 (1187)	86	41	47.7	41	–	–	5	36
Smillie, 1933 (1206)	582	347	59.6	347	11	18	87	231
Bunim and Trask, 1935 (201)	80	59	73.8	62	2	–	11	49
Total	1,782	977	54.8	1,018	59	49	179	731
					Percentage incidence in total contact group			
					3.3	2.7	10.0	41.0

* Includes 52 atypical Type II strains.
† Strains of atypical Type II are included as they are not listed separately.

accounted for 5.8 per cent of those in contacts and only 1.9 per cent of those in non-contacts, and Type II for 4.8 per cent in contacts as compared with 2.8 per cent in non-contacts. The incidence of the carrier rate of strains of Type III and of Group IV did not appear to show any marked difference between the two groups, though in each instance the proportion was somewhat higher in the contacts.

TABLE 66. NON-CONTACTS AND CONTACTS. PERCENTAGE OF CARRIERS AND PERCENTAGE INCIDENCE OF TYPES IN GROUP EXAMINED; STRAINS FOUND AND PERCENTAGE DISTRIBUTION BY TYPE

	Persons examined					
			PERCENTAGE INCIDENCE OF TYPES IN TOTAL GROUP			
SOURCE	TOTAL	PER CENT CARRIERS	*Type I*	*Type II*	*Type III*	*Group IV*
Non-contacts (Table 61)	2,332	42.9	0.5	0.9	8.4	34.2
Contacts (Table 65)	1,782	54.8	3.3	2.7	10.0	41.0

	Strains found				
		PERCENTAGE DISTRIBUTION BY TYPE			
	TOTAL	*Type I*	*Type II*	*Type III*	*Group IV*
Non-contacts (Table 63)	2,625	1.9	2.8	14.9	80.3
Contacts (Table 65)	1,018	5.8	4.8	17.5	71.8

More important than the analysis of the strains found in contacts in general is the analysis of the strains isolated from the contacts of patients with pneumonia due to specific types of pneumococci. Contacts, and especially the family contacts, of patients with pneumonia due to certain types of pneumococci frequently become carriers of the types to which they are exposed, as will be seen later. Dochez and Avery (361) and Stillman (1234, 1235) early recognized that, though carriers of Type I or Type II pneumococci were seldom encountered in the general population, carriers of these types were frequently found among the contacts of patients having pneumonia due to these types. With Type III, however, these and other investigators (1111) pointed out that strains of this type were found only slightly more often in contacts with Type III cases than in non-contacts. In addition to this, pneumococci of Types I and II appeared of greater epidemiologic significance than those of Type III, for they passed from the sick to the well more rapidly than did Type III and were responsible for a much larger proportion of the cases of lobar pneumonia than Type III. These findings have been confirmed many times.

It is only within recent years that efforts have been made to carry out typing for many of the higher types, to establish what proportion of cases were due to these types and whether such types were more frequent in contacts than in non-contacts, and thus to determine their epidemiologic significance. In regard to this latter point the observations of Smillie (1206) are of special value. The data available are still insufficient, however, to permit comparing the proportion of each of the thirty-two recognized types found in contacts with that in non-contacts.

In his investigation of the types carried by over a thousand family contacts and non-contacts, Smillie (1206) carried out typing for Types I through XIX. He observed that strains of some types were far more prevalent in the family contacts of cases due to those types than in non-contacts. Table 67 lists Smillie's findings.

TABLE 67. FAMILY CONTACTS WITH CASES OF PNEUMONIA DUE TO PNEUMOCOCCI OF SPECIFIC TYPE. NUMBER AND PERCENTAGE CARRYING PNEUMOCOCCI OF HOMOLOGOUS TYPE AND NUMBER AND PERCENTAGE OF CARRIERS OF THESE TYPES IN THE GENERAL POPULATION

TYPE TO WHICH EXPOSED	NUMBER OF CONTACTS EXPOSED	CONTACTS CARRYING HOMOLOGOUS TYPE		CARRIERS OF PNEUMOCOCCI IN THE GENERAL POPULATION	
		Number	*Per cent*	*Number*	*Per cent*
I	186	10	5.4	1	0.2
II	126	14	11.1	3	0.7
III	61	13	21.3	67	13.6
V	32	5	15.6	2	0.4
VI	6	1	16.7	21	4.3
VII	31	1	3.2	5	1.0
VIII	31	7	20.1	3	0.6
IX	15	4	31.0	7	1.4
XIV	2	1	50.0	5	1.0
XVIII	23	4	17.4	34	6.9
All others	81	–	–	345	–
Total	594			493	

From Smillie (1206)

Smillie pointed out that the number of contacts with cases of pneumonia due to pneumococci of Types VI, IX, and XIV was too few to permit conclusions to be drawn from the available data and, further, that the incidence of homologous strains in the contacts of patients having pneumonia due to Types VII, XVIII, and possibly Type III as well, "is not significantly greater than the general prevalence of these strains in the population at large." The data for Types I and II, however, were significant; Type I was twenty times more prevalent among contacts with Type I cases than in the population at large, and Type II was more than ten times more prevalent among individuals having exposure to this type. In addition, Types V and VIII also tended to show a much greater prevalence among contacts exposed to such types than among the general population.

Pneumococci of Types I and II, and possibly Types V and VIII, then, tend to pass more frequently from the sick to the well than from normal person to normal person, or at least to be found more frequently among contacts with cases due to these types than among other persons. In Smillie's study the data for Type VII and possibly Type III gave no evidence of the occurrence of such a phenomenon. Though these observations were made on groups containing some children, they are of particular interest in view of the fact, earlier pointed out, that pneumococci of Types I, II, III, V, VII, and VIII are responsible for about seventy-five per cent of the cases of lobar pneumonia in adults (pages 51–54). This point alone is sufficient to cause all strains of these types to be regarded with suspicion. All the available data suggest that of these six types only Type III accounts for a larger proportion of the strains isolated from healthy carriers (contacts or non-contacts) than from cases and that, in consequence, pneumonia due to this organism may be regarded as an autogenous infection. Assuming this to be true, most infections with pneumococci of the other types listed above may be regarded as of exogenous origin, the organisms being acquired either by direct contact with an active case or by association with a healthy or convalescent carrier of one of these types.

As already mentioned, the incidence of homologous types among the family contacts of cases of pneumonia due to such types has been determined by several investigators in addition to Smillie. The reported results are given in Table 68. A summary of the findings presented in this table may be seen in Table 69.

Of the total 1,701 family contacts examined, 204 or 11.4 per cent were found carrying pneumococci of the type homologous with that to which

TABLE 68. FAMILY CONTACTS WITH CASES OF PNEUMONIA DUE TO PNEUMOCOCCI OF SPECIFIC TYPE. NUMBER AND PERCENTAGE CARRYING PNEUMOCOCCI OF HOMOLOGOUS TYPE (DATA COLLECTED FROM LITERATURE)

TYPE TO WHICH EXPOSED	SOURCE	PNEUMONIA CASES	CONTACTS EXAMINED		
			TOTAL	CARRYING HOMOLOGOUS TYPE *Number*	*Per cent*
Type I	Stillman, 1916 (1234)	24	44	2	4.5
	Stillman, 1917 (1235)	28	107	16	15.0
	Avery, Chickering, Cole, and Dochez, 1917 (33)	–	160	21	13.1
	Rosenau, Felton, and Atwater, 1926 (1111)	23	216	8	3.7
	Jacobson, 1927 (682)	16	36	6	17.0
	Smillie and Caldwell, 1929 (1209)	–	17	2	11.8
	Shultz, 1932 (1187)	6	21	5	23.8
	Smillie, 1933 (1206)	48	186	10	5.4
	Smillie and Leeder, 1934 (1210)	17	62	15	24.2
	Bunim and Trask, 1935 (201)	3	21	2	9.5
	Total		870	87	10.0
Type II	Stillman, 1916 (1234)	17	40	3	7.5
	Stillman, 1917 (1235)	24	77	5	6.0
	Avery, Chickering, Cole, and Dochez, 1917 (33)	–	149	18	12.1
	Jacobson, 1927 (682)	7	29	14	48.0
	Smillie and Caldwell, 1929 (1209)	–	7	3	42.9
	Shultz, 1932 (1187)	4	16	–	–
	Smillie, 1933 (1206)	34	126	14	11.1
	Smillie and Leeder, 1934 (1210)	10	37	6	16.2
	Total		481	63	13.1
Type III	Rosenau, Felton, and Atwater, 1926	5	54	6	11.2
	Shultz, 1932	2	7	2	28.5
	Smillie, 1933	16	61	13	21.3
	Bunim and Trask, 1935	2	11	3	27.2
	Total		133	24	18.0

TABLE 68 (*cont.*)

TYPE TO WHICH EXPOSED	SOURCE	PNEUMONIA CASES	CONTACTS EXAMINED TOTAL	CARRYING HOMOLOGOUS TYPE *Number*	*Per cent*
Type IV	Shultz	1	5	–	–
Type V	Shultz	2	7	1	14.2
	Smillie	8	32	5	15.6
	Total		39	6	15.4
Type VI	Shultz	3	14	1	7.1
	Smillie	3	6	1	16.7
	Bunim and Trask	3	23	–	–
	Total		43	2	4.7
Type VII	Shultz	2	11	2	18.1
	Smillie	8	31	1	3.2
	Total		42	3	7.1
Type VIII	Smillie	12	31	7	20.1
	Bunim and Trask	1	3	3	100.0
	Total		34	10	29.4
Type IX	Shultz	1	5	–	–
	Smillie	2	15	4	31.0
	Total		20	4	20.0
Type XI	Bunim and Trask	1	5	–	–
Type XIV	Smillie	1	2	1	50.0
	Bunim and Trask	1	4	–	–
	Total		6	1	16.7
Type XVIII	Smillie	7	23	4	17.4

they were exposed. Of the types to which the largest number of contacts were exposed, Types I, II, III, V, and VIII produced the largest proportion of carriers of the homologous type. This proportion was 10, 13.1, 18, 15.4, and 29.4 per cent respectively for these types.

Though carriers of Type I or II pneumococci are frequently found among the contacts of cases due to these types, not all cases produce such carriers. Dochez and Avery (361) determined that carriers of Type I pneumococci were found in association with 37.5 per cent of eight Type I cases. The reports of Stillman (1234, 1235); Rosenau, Felton, and Atwater (1111); and Jacobson (682) show that 25.3 per cent or 23 of their combined 91 Type I cases gave rise to carriers of the homologous type. Carriers of Type II pneumococci were found in association with 41.7 per cent of 24 cases observed by Dochez and Avery (361), and the combined reports of Stillman (1234, 1235) and Jacobson (682) show that 27 per cent or 13 of their 48 Type II cases gave rise to carriers of pneumococci of this type.

TABLE 69. FAMILY CONTACTS WITH CASES OF PNEUMONIA DUE TO PNEUMOCOCCI OF SPECIFIC TYPE. NUMBER AND PERCENTAGE CARRYING PNEUMOCOCCI OF HOMOLOGOUS TYPE (SUMMARY OF TABLE 68)

TYPE TO WHICH EXPOSED	NUMBER OF CONTACTS EXAMINED	CONTACTS CARRYING HOMOLOGOUS TYPE	
		Number	*Per cent*
I	870	87	10.0
II	481	63	13.1
III	133	24	18.0
IV	5	–	–
V	39	6	15.4
VI	43	2	4.7
VII	42	3	7.1
VIII	34	10	29.4
IX	20	4	20.0
XI	5	–	–
XIV	6	1	16.7
XVIII	23	4	17.4
Total	1,701	204	11.4

In connection with observations on contacts, Stillman (1235) and Rosenau, Felton, and Atwater (1111) determined the prevalence of carriers of the homologous types among the family contacts in various households. Among 51 households harboring patients with Type I pneumonia, family contacts carrying the homologous type were encountered in 16 or 31.4 per cent. Among 24 households with Type II pneumonia, 5 or 21 per cent yielded contacts carrying the same type. Thus, in addition to finding that 10 per cent of the family contacts with Type I cases and 13 per cent of those in contact with Type II cases are carriers of these types, it has been shown that carriers of the homologous types are found in association with approximately one-quarter of the Type I and Type II cases and in about the same proportion of households harboring such cases.

In addition to the reports cited above concerning the incidence of pneumococci in family contacts, several investigators have studied the incidence of these organisms in the hospital contacts of pneumonia patients (682, 1187, 331, 1210, 1353, 267). Data have been obtained on either patient contacts or hospital staff contacts or both. The results of investigations of this nature carried out in this country are somewhat different from the results obtained in Europe, as will be noted below.

In the United States, Jacobson (682) and Shultz (1187) together examined 87 hospital attendants (physicians, nurses, and orderlies) working on pneumonia wards and found the number and percentage carrying pneumococci of Types I, II, and III and of Group IV to be about the same as that found in the general population. Smillie and Leeder (1210) determined the incidence of Types I and II among 94 hospital patient contacts of 31 Type I and Type II cases and 71 hospital staff contacts of 6 cases of these types (see Table 70). Pneumococci of these types were found in only 2.1 per cent of the cultures from patient contacts and 2.8 per cent of those from attendant contacts and were thus but slightly more frequent than their combined

TABLE 70. CONTACTS WITH TYPE I OR TYPE II LOBAR PNEUMONIA CASES (HOSPITAL PATIENTS, HOSPITAL STAFF, AND FAMILY). NUMBER OF CASES, CONTACTS, AND CONTACT DAYS, AND NUMBER AND PERCENTAGE OF NASOPHARYNGEAL CULTURES YIELDING PNEUMOCOCCI OF HOMOLOGOUS TYPE

				CULTURES			
	CASES	CONTACTS	CONTACT DAYS	NEGATIVE	POSITIVE AND NOT HOMOLOGOUS	POSITIVE AND HOMOLOGOUS	
	Number	*Number*	*Number*	*Number*	*Number*	*Number*	*Per cent*
Hospital patient	31	94	707	63	75	2	2.1
Hospital staff	6	71	610	42	27	2	2.8
Family contacts	27	99	287	22	56	21	21.2

From Smillie and Leeder (1210)

prevalence of 1.4 per cent found in non-contacts, as shown in Table 61. These workers did find, however, that a very much larger proportion of the family contacts with such cases carried strains of these two types, as will be seen later.

In Europe, Viktorow, Semzowa, and Oettinger (1353) in Moscow made the interesting observation that pneumococci as a group were carried by 54.6 per cent of 308 non-contacts, 60.3 per cent of 186 hospital staff contacts, and 72.7 per cent of 77 family contacts of patients with pneumonia. The distribution of the types found among the hospital staff contacts was essentially similar to that observed in the population at large except that Type I was encountered six times among the 112 carriers.

As compared with the American studies, the most marked difference in the incidence of pneumococci in hospital contacts was reported from Great Britain. Among 139 cultures from nurses in contact with cases of Type I or II pneumonia, Cruickshank (331) found 25 or 18 per cent showed pneumococci of these types, while in 88 nurses not having such contact these types were never found. Further, among 156 patient contacts on pneumonia wards Types I and II were found in 26 or 16.6 per cent. Such positive cultures were obtained either at the first, or more frequently at the second or third examination. Christie (267), also in Great Britain, studied the pneumococcus carrier rate of 100 healthy nurses over a period of several months. At one point, when pneumonia was prevalent in the community, the incidence of Types I and II in this group was as high as 10 per cent and during the rest of the period remained between 1 and 5 per cent.

Over the period of a year Christie also followed the prevalence of pneumococci of various types in the throats of 60 nurses working on pneumonia wards and compared this with the incidence of types obtained from a group of 75 nurses working on other wards. Pneumococci of Type I were found in 13.3 per cent and of Type II in 21.7 per cent of the pneumonia ward nurses, while none of the nurses on the other wards showed Type I and only 2.7 per cent showed Type II.

It appears from these findings that in Great Britain at least pneumococci of Types I and II may pass more frequently to the contacts of hospitalized patients having pneumonia due to these types than in this country. The considerable differences between the carrier rates of pneumococci of Types I and II in hospital patient and attendant contacts in these two countries suggest that differences exist in the epidemiology of pneumonia due to these organisms in these places. Other evidence at hand indicates that some difference also exists between pneumonia due to these organisms in the two countries. It has already been shown (pages 42–48) that Types I and II cause a larger proportion of the cases of lobar pneumonia in Great Britain than in this country, and it will be seen later (pages 664–669) that the fatality rate of cases due to these two types is lower there than in the United States. These variations all appear to reflect differences in host response to the organisms in question. Further, Webster and Hughes (1393) in this country have found evidence in experimental animals that those types, such as Types I and II, which are associated with serious disease spread relatively infrequently among normal animals, while other types less often producing serious lesions tend to survive and spread relatively easily among normal animals. Whether or not Types I and II may actually be regarded as less often producing severe disease in Great Britain than other types or other organisms, and consequently tend to spread more widely among normal contacts there, is unknown. If this were so, the carrier rate of these two types in the general population might also be expected to be higher there than in the United States; and, as far as known, no considerable series of non-contacts have been examined there to determine this.

As earlier mentioned, family contacts have been studied by several workers (361, 1234, 1235, 1111, 682, 1209, 1187, 1206, 1210, 1353, 201). The findings of Jacobson (682), Smillie and Caldwell (1209), Shultz (1187), and Smillie (1206) suggested the desirability of giving special attention to this very important group of individuals. Considering the United States, it was gradually becoming apparent that of all the contacts of patients with pneumonia those *in the immediate family* of such patients appeared especially likely to be found carrying pneumococci of the homologous type. The study of Smillie and Leeder (1210) clearly illustrates this and has served to focus attention on the matter (Table 70). As shown in their study, among the groups of contacts exposed to pneumococcus Type I and Type II cases, only 2.1 per cent and 2.8 per cent of the hospital patient and staff contacts respectively were carriers of these types, as compared with 21.2 per cent among the family contacts. Observations of a similar nature were subsequently reported by Viktorow, Semzowa, and Oettinger (1353). Among their group of 77 family contacts with Type I and II cases, 25 per cent (8.9 per cent Type I and 16.1 per cent Type II) were found carrying strains of these types, while 112 hospital staff contacts showed only 5.4 per cent of such carriers.

This extraordinary difference in the carrier rates of the three groups of individuals in Table 70 is further emphasized by the fact that although the hospital groups were in contact with patients many more days than the family groups, relatively few of them became carriers of the types to which they were exposed.

Smillie and Leeder have pointed out that of 62 family contacts exposed to 17 Type I cases for a total of 153 days, 15 or 24.2 per cent carried pneumococci of this type as compared with one or 1.6 per cent of homologous type carriers among 61 hospital patient contacts of 20 Type I cases exposed for 426 days. The findings for contacts of Type II cases were much similar. Among 37 family contacts having 134 days' exposure to 10 Type II cases, 6 or 16.2 per cent proved carriers of the homologous type as compared with one or 3.0 per cent among 33 hospital patient contacts with 11 Type II cases having 281 contact days. Likewise, 610 days of exposure of 71 hospital staff contacts of five Type I and one Type II cases yielded only 2 or 2.8 per cent of carriers of these types.

One of the most significant observations made by these investigators was that a study of family contacts showed that the proportion of carriers of the homologous types found among those exposed to pneumococci of Type I or II was about as great in those examined on the first day of their exposure as after a week of exposure. Thus, the number of contact days following the onset of lobar pneumonia did not appear to affect the carrier rate of family contacts. This observation, together with the recognized low rate of spread of Type I or II in hospital contacts, suggested that some factor other than contact alone determined whether pneumococci of these types produced carriers among those exposed. Much evidence, direct and indirect, has been obtained concerning the nature of this additional factor, which appears to be the presence of upper respiratory infection in the contacts, as will be seen later.

TOTAL NUMBER OF HEALTHY CARRIERS IN THE COMMUNITY. In the foregoing discussion the proportion of both healthy non-contacts and healthy contacts carrying pneumococci of various types was pointed out, and a comparison was made between the carrier rates of these two groups. The normal population of the community, of course, includes the members of both these groups. For the purpose of determining the relative incidence of the pneumococcus and various of its types in the community, the findings in the total group of non-contacts (Table 61) and contacts (Table 65) have been combined in Table 71. Data presented by Dochez and Avery (361) on a combined group of contacts and non-contacts, which have not been listed above, have been included with the table.

There are two points it is well to appreciate in connection with the interpretation of the data summarized in Table 71 (and Table 72 too). First, as the proportion of contacts in the general population is ordinarily insignificant in comparison with the numbers of non-contacts and no allowance is made for this difference in Table 71 (or Table 72), the higher carrier rate of the contact group included tends to make the carrier rate of the total group somewhat too high. Second, most, but not all, of the studies made of

TABLE 71. NON-CONTACTS AND CONTACTS. NUMBER AND PERCENTAGE OF CARRIERS AND DISTRIBUTION OF STRAINS FOUND BY TYPE; PERCENTAGE INCIDENCE OF TYPES IN TOTAL GROUP EXAMINED

SOURCE	PERSONS EXAMINED TOTAL	CARRIERS FOUND *Number*	CARRIERS FOUND *Per cent*	STRAINS FOUND TOTAL	TYPE I *Number*	TYPE II *Number*	TYPE III *Number*	GROUP IV
Non-contacts (Table 61)	2,332	1,000	42.9	1,027	12	22	195	798
Contacts (Table 65)	1,782	977	54.8	1,018	59	49	179	731
Contacts and non-contacts (Dochez and Avery, 361)	113	66	58.4	66	3	8	–	55
Total	4,227	2,043	48.3	2,111	74	79	374	1,584
					Percentage incidence in total group examined			
					1.8	1.9	8.8	37.5

the pneumococcus carrier rate in both contacts and non-contacts have been limited to observations carried out during the colder seasons of various years, and, as will be seen later, it is at such times that pneumococci in general appear the most prevalent. Thus the carrier rates shown by the grand total of the 4,227 persons listed in Table 71 would under ordinary circumstances appear to indicate the maximum rates for carriers in the community.

Among a grand total of 4,227 healthy individuals examined, 2,043 or 48.3 per cent were carrying pneumococci. Strains of Type I were encountered in 74 or 1.8 per cent of the 4,227 persons examined, strains of Type II in 79 or 1.9 per cent, of Type III in 374 or 8.8 per cent, and of Group IV in 1,584 or 37.5 per cent.

Pneumococci may be obtained, then, from nearly one-half (48.3 per cent) of the population of the community. Among the population at large, most of the carriers harbor strains of Group IV (37.5 per cent); and though strains of Type III are less often found (8.8 per cent), they are nearly three times as common as strains of Types I and II together (3.7 per cent).

The proportion of pneumococci of various types among the strains isolated from this total group of "community carriers" is shown in Table 72. This table includes the total number of strains isolated from non-contacts (Table 63) and contacts (Table 66) and the combined group reported by Dochez and Avery (361) mentioned above.

TABLE 72. NON-CONTACT AND CONTACT CARRIERS. NUMBER AND PERCENTAGE DISTRIBUTION OF STRAINS FOUND BY TYPE

SOURCE	TOTAL STRAINS FOUND	TYPE I		TYPE II		TYPE III		GROUP IV	
		Number	*Per cent*	*Number*	*Per cent*	*Number*	*Per cent*	*Number*	*Per cent*
Non-contacts (Table 63)	2,625	51	1.9	75	2.8	391	14.9	2,108	80.3
Contacts (Table 65)	1,018	59	5.8	49	4.8	179	17.5	731	71.8
Contacts and non-contacts (Dochez and Avery, 361)	66	3	4.5	8	12.1	–	–	55	83.3
Total	3,709	113	3.0	132	3.6	570	15.4	2,894	78.0

Of the total of 3,709 strains of pneumococci isolated from healthy persons, only 3.0 per cent were Type I and 3.6 per cent Type II; while 15.4 per cent were Type III, and members of Group IV made up by far the largest proportion (78 per cent).

At this point the number of healthy carriers of pneumococci in the state of Massachusetts may be estimated. If the figures used for the proportion of carriers in the population are taken from Table 61, which gives the incidence of these among non-contacts only, and such individuals comprise the bulk of the population, the number of estimated carriers is much lower than if the proportions used for calculation are taken from Table 71 or 72, which include both contacts and non-contacts. In any event, even using the minimum proportions (Table 61), the number of estimated carriers of pneumococci in Massachusetts alone is in the vicinity of 1,800,000 (42.9 per cent of the 1935 population of 4,350,910). This huge group includes over 21,000 carriers of Type I, 39,000 carriers of Type II, 365,000 carriers of Type III, and 1,488,000 carriers of Group IV strains. The maximum estimated number of Type I carriers is 78,000 and of Type II carriers 82,000. Even the minimum estimates are rather appalling in revealing the size of the carrier groups in the population of this single state and indicate that there is an enormous reservoir of these organisms in the community. These figures may possibly hold true for only the colder seasons of the year, yet it would appear clear that any attempt to control the prevalence of pneumonia by simply isolating current cases, whose number is insignificant in proportion to the size of the carrier group, must under ordinary circumstances hold but little promise.

SECONDARY CARRIERS PRODUCED BY CONTACT WITH CARRIERS. The production of a secondary group of carriers by the contact of normal persons with healthy carriers of pneumococci offers another means of spreading these organisms throughout the community. Rosenau, Felton, and Atwater (1111) studied this matter in some detail. They found that of 33 persons exposed to contact with 3 healthy carriers of pneumococci of Type I, only one or 3 per cent became a carrier of this type. This proportion of Type I carriers is nearly double that found in the community in general (1.8 per cent), as shown in Table 71. Of 65 persons exposed to 8 carriers of Type II strains, none became carriers of this type; and of 122 persons exposed to 17 carriers of Type III strains, 8 or 6.6 per cent apparently became carriers of the homologous type. This latter figure is somewhat lower than the proportion (8.8 per cent) of carriers of this type found in the population at large, as shown in Table 71.

In comparing the above figures for the proportion of secondary carriers produced by contact with healthy carriers with the proportion of carriers of these types found among non-contacts in their study, it appeared that Type I carriers produced about three times the number of carriers of this type as were found in non-contacts, and Type III carriers produced approximately the same proportion of carriers of this type as were found in non-contacts. As is described later, Webster and Hughes (1393) also reported a few instances in which a secondary group of carriers were produced by the contact of normal persons with carriers.

Though the number of observations concerning this matter is small, it seems clear that carriers may produce secondary carriers of the homologous types in occasional instances. Though this may not occur with great frequency, as Rosenau, Felton, and Atwater (1111) and Smillie and Leeder (1210) have found, this means of spreading pneumococci cannot be disregarded. As may be seen below in the discussion of the factors affecting the carrier state, the presence of some pathologic condition of the upper respiratory tract may facilitate the production of secondary carriers.

Cases give rise to a much larger proportion of carriers among their contacts than do carriers and, in consequence, have been regarded as the most important means of transmitting pneumococci from person to person. Among a total of 78 normal persons having no contact with cases but exposed to contact with carriers of Types I, II, and III, as reported by Rosenau and his associates (1111), only one or 1.3 per cent became a carrier. This proportion may be compared with the finding of 174 or 11.7 per cent of carriers of the homologous types found among 1,484 contacts with cases due to pneumococci of these three types, as shown in Table 69. The spread of organisms by healthy carriers is generally considered a very important means of transmitting infection, and this conclusion appears inescapable though but few specific instances in which infection of a clinical nature apparently resulted from such transmission have been reported (956, 1395, 1412, 331, 1207).

CONVALESCENT CARRIERS. Patients convalescent from pneumococcus pneumonia may continue to carry strains of the infecting organism in their nasopharynx for days, weeks, or months. This has been observed repeatedly both in children and in adults, as will be seen below (360, 361, 1234, 682, 1187, 1252, 331, 1210). In consequence, convalescent carriers are regarded as a potential source of infection to persons in contact with them and doubtless aid importantly in spreading pneumococci throughout the community (see also page 369).

In general, after the acute phases of pneumonia are over, the infecting organism, which tends to persist for a variable period in the upper respiratory tract, is gradually lost; and pneumococci of some type or types commonly carried by normal individuals or some other organism may appear in its place. At times what appear to be unclassified pneumococci seem to supplant the infecting agent. Shultz (1187) attempted to ascertain whether such organisms were true immunologic unclassified strains or whether they represented degraded forms of the type which formerly was present and caused the infection. According to the method advocated by Griffith and others, representatives of these strains were injected into mice in the attempt to increase their virulence and possible specificity. In four instances after such treatment pneumococci were obtained which appeared identical with the types originally responsible for the infection. Additional study is needed to determine the significance of this observation. Similar efforts were made by Webster and Hughes (1393) to develop the specificity of atypical strains of pneumococci obtained from healthy carriers. In this instance, however, no evidence of alteration of specificity or virulence change was obtained.

DURATION OF CARRIER STATE. *Non-contacts.* The results of the repeated examination of various groups of healthy individuals are uniform in indicating that some persons may be classified as true chronic carriers of pneumococci (1234, 1048, 1393, 582, 1391, 578, 267, 133). In certain instances pneumococci of a single type have been repeatedly obtained from the same individual for periods ranging from three months to more than three years. Among 39 persons examined at approximately seven-day intervals for from seven months to three and one-half years, Webster and Hughes (1393) found that 8 or 20.5 per cent could be classified as chronic carriers. These investigators have divided normal individuals into four classes: (a) non-carriers, who are nearly always free of pneumococci; (b) transient or intermittent carriers, who may carry different types at different times; (c) periodic carriers, who may carry strains of a single type for many weeks alternating with free intervals between such periods; and finally, (d) chronic carriers, who, as above mentioned, may carry a single type for long periods.

As an example of the tendency of some persons to remain free from carrying pneumococci while others assume the carrier state, these investigators noted that even persons working and living together exhibited differences in their disposition to become carriers of various sorts. These differences were regularly observed and were not regarded as due to chance of exposure alone; for of seventeen persons exposed over a period of several months to a carrier of Type III, eleven remained entirely free from this organism, while cultures were occasionally positive in four, and one individual carried strains of this type for three months. Among seven other persons exposed to a carrier of Type XIII, one remained free from the organism; in two, cultures were positive once; while three others carried this type for from seven to fifteen months.

Bliss, McClaskey, and Long (133) also investigated this matter and arrived at conclusions which, though differing from those of Webster and Hughes in some respects, were essentially similar in regard to their general significance. Bliss and her associates would divide normal individuals into two broad classes: (a) chronic carriers, and (b) non-carriers, and believe that no intermediate group exists. Their group of chronic carriers would correspond to a combination of the groups of periodic and chronic carriers of Webster and Hughes, as described above. The inclusion of the periodic carriers in the group of chronic carriers seemed reasonable, for such individuals tended to carry the same type over long periods and to show apparent interruptions of the carrier state at some examinations at which no pneumococci or strains of a different type were found. These interruptions were not regarded as real, however, as strains of the original type subsequently reappeared in the cultures, and it seemed improbable that such individuals could be continually reinfected with the same type. In consequence, this phenomenon was regarded as due to the presence of two or more types in these persons, and the failure to find the same type at each examination was regarded as probably due to variations in the numbers of organisms present in the culture or to variations in the mouse virulence of the strain. Bliss and her co-workers confirmed the observations of Gundel and Okura (580) who, by their blocking experiments in which sputum was injected into mice along with antiserum for the dominant type present, had shown the simultaneous presence of two, three, or more types in many instances in a group of healthy persons examined; and who in some instances obtained strains of two types from normal individuals. The fact that healthy individuals may occasionally carry pneumococci of more than one type was previously observed by others, as was indicated earlier (see pages 344–350).

Bliss and her co-workers would class as non-carriers individuals showing no recurrence of a given type in serial cultures. Among a group of twenty persons examined repeatedly over a period of two academic years, none of those regarded as non-carriers showed over 10 per cent of positive cultures, while among the chronic carriers only one had less than this proportion.

In the course of epidemiologic studies of pneumonia Powell, Atwater, and Felton (1048) found that, though the carrier state of normal persons having no more contact with pneumonia than that suffered by the population at large was usually less than thirty days for Type I, II, or III, one individual was observed to carry strains of Type I for at least ninety days and another, strains of Type III for 120 days.

Contacts. The duration of the carrier state of pneumococci of the type homologous with that to which they are exposed among normal persons in contact with patients with pneumococcus pneumonia has been studied by several investigators (361, 1234, 1235, 682, 1252, 331, 1210, 267, 1353). The duration of this state among a group composed chiefly of family contacts was found by Dochez and Avery (361) to be about twenty-three days. In a group of a similar nature Stillman (1235) found the average carrying period to be twenty-five days for strains of Type I and forty-three days for Type II. Subsequently, however, Jacobson (682) reported the instance of a contact in a family in which three cases of Type II pneumonia occurred who carried this organism for at least 141 days, after which period no further examinations were made. In addition, Smillie and Leeder (1210) determined that some of the family contacts of Type I or II cases may continue to harbor these organisms for periods of several weeks to months.

Among a group of boys in an orphanage whose contact with each other was in some respects similar to that shown by many family contacts, Strøm (1252) determined the carrier rate of Type I pneumococci at the time of an outbreak of pneumonia due to this organism. Ten boys were found carrying Type I, and at a subsequent examination seventy-three days later this type was again recovered from four of these individuals.

Cruickshank (331) and Christie (267) have found that the duration of the carrier state of Type I or II among hospital staff (nurse) contacts is usually short. The former, however, observed one instance in which this condition was "persistent." Though many hospital patient contacts were only transient carriers of these types, others became persistent carriers of them.

The data at hand suggest that not only are a larger proportion of family contacts, as compared with hospital staff or patient contacts, carriers of the type homologous with that to which they are exposed, as previously pointed out, but also as compared with other contacts this carrier condition is usually of longer duration among family contacts.

Convalescent patients. The length of time the organism persists in the nasopharynx of convalescent patients varies somewhat with the different types of pneumococci. In children Shultz (1187) found that, as measured from the time of onset of the pneumonia, the duration of the carrier period for pneumococci of Type I varied from 3 to 145 days with an average of 50 days. While strains of Type II were always lost by 21 days, those of Type III persisted longer and were carried from 15 to 152 days, averaging 64 days. Types I and III, then, showed the longest carrying period, and this was in marked contrast to the duration of the carrier state of pneumococci of many of the higher types studied, for in this instance the carrier period was shorter (2 to 30 days) and averaged 10 days.

In adults the duration of the carrier state for pneumococci of Type I, II, or III was found by Dochez and Avery (360, 361) and by Stillman (1234) to vary from 7 to 108 days and to average about two to three weeks. Though Jacobson's (682) findings were much similar to this, he observed that strains of Type I or II may persist for as long as five months in some instances. The observations of Strøm (1252) on convalescent carriers of Type I and of Cruickshank (331) on similar carriers of Type I or II are in general accord with these findings. The latter investigator, however, has presented certain data which clearly illustrate that, following recovery from pneumococcus Type I or II lobar pneumonia, a considerable proportion of individuals may continue to carry strains of these types for several weeks and in some instances apparently for many months (see Tables 73 and 74).

TABLE 73. TWO HUNDRED FIFTY PATIENTS CONVALESCENT FROM TYPE I OR TYPE II LOBAR PNEUMONIA. NUMBER EXAMINED AND NUMBER AND PERCENTAGE SHOWING HOMOLOGOUS TYPE IN THEIR SPUTUM, BY DAY AFTER CRISIS

DAYS AFTER CRISIS	NUMBER OF CASES	PATIENTS SHOWING TYPE I OR II IN THEIR SPUTUM	
		Number	*Per cent*
0–4	184	114	60.8
8	122	58	47.5
12	89	39	43.8
16	52	26	50.0
20	43	18	41.8
24	26	9	36.6
25–42	29	18	62.0

From Cruickshank (331)

While waiting for patients to be discharged from the hospital, Cruickshank (331), in conjunction with Montgomery in Great Britain, examined the sputum at intervals of four to seven days of 250 patients recovering from Type I or II pneumonia. The proportion of carriers of these types decreased from 60.8 per cent within four days after crisis to 36.6 per cent at the end of about three weeks. Among a group of 29 patients who because of the presence of complications, such as delayed resolution and empyema, were detained in the hospital for a period of from 25 to 42 days, 18 or 62 per cent remained carriers of Type I or II.

Another group of patients convalescent from Type I or II pneumonia was examined at intervals of two months following their discharge from the hospital. Some of these patients had been out of the hospital for six months before the first follow-up examinations were made. In all, 122 patients were examined for periods varying from two to twenty-six months (see Table 74).

TABLE 74. ONE HUNDRED TWENTY-TWO PERSONS RECOVERED FROM TYPE I OR TYPE II LOBAR PNEUMONIA. NUMBER EXAMINED AND NUMBER AND PERCENTAGE CARRYING HOMOLOGOUS TYPE, BY MONTH AFTER RECOVERY

MONTHS AFTER RECOVERY	NUMBER OF CASES	PERSONS CARRYING TYPE I OR II	
		Number	*Per cent*
2–4	52	19	38.4
6	49	11	22.4
8	59	10	16.9
10	55	7	12.7
12	35	7	20.0
14	25	4	16.0
18	11	2	–
26	16	2*	–

From Cruickshank (331)

* One positive at 21 and one at 25 months.

The results of this study are extraordinary in indicating that some 38 per cent of these patients apparently still carried Type I or II when examined two to four months after recovery, and even at the end of fourteen months 16 per cent were found to be carriers of these types. In two instances individuals showed these types as long as twenty-one months, or nearly two years, after recovery. Because of the lack of data on the incidence of carriers of these types in the general population in Great Britain, as previously mentioned, the exact significance of these findings is not clear. Despite this, it would appear obvious that following recovery from Type I or II pneumonia some individuals may continue to carry these organisms for periods of many months. It is possible that the duration of the carrier state of these types is somewhat longer in Great Britain than in this country. Nevertheless, Smillie and Leeder (1210) in Boston cultured at various intervals a few patients who had recovered from Type I or II pneumonia and obtained strains of these types from such individuals for periods of a few months up to nearly a year later. In some instances, as positive findings were not obtained at every examination, either the carrier condition was periodic or the organism was missed at the time of culture.

While it is probable that every individual carrying pneumococci must be regarded as potentially dangerous to the community, it would seem that persons harboring such organisms for the longest periods are of the greatest importance in this respect. From this point of view true chronic carriers of pneumococci, whether they be non-contacts, contacts (particularly the family contacts), or convalescent patients appear to deserve the most attention.

VIRULENCE STUDIES. A number of observations have been reported which deal with the virulence of strains of pneumococci isolated from non-contact, contact, and convalescent carriers and from patients with pneumonia (1111, 1048, 682, 584, 582, 1187, 1252, 331, 1353). In all of these studies conclusions have been based chiefly upon the observed virulence for white mice of the strains tested. This method of determining virulence is open to numerous possible variations, as earlier mentioned (see page 27).

Rosenau, Felton, and Atwater (1111) felt that the virulence of strains of Types I and III isolated from the contacts of cases due to those types might be slightly higher than that of strains of the same types obtained from persons not exposed to such contact. In addition, the strains of Group IV isolated appeared of generally lower virulence than the strains of Type I, II, or III. In a continuation of this study in which determinations were made of the virulence of strains obtained from healthy carriers, Powell, Atwater, and Felton (1048) confirmed this latter point but were unable to find any other significant difference in the virulence of the strains isolated.

Though Jacobson (682) reported that the virulence of different strains within the same type may vary widely, his findings, and those of Shultz (1187), Strøm (1252), and Viktorow and his co-workers (1353), led these investigators to regard the virulence of strains of some types obtained from carriers as lower than that of other strains of these types isolated from patients with pneumonia. The findings of Gundel and Wasu (584), of Gundel and Schwarz (582), and of Cruickshank (331) were different from this and in general resembled those of Powell and his collaborators described above. Gundel and his associates found the virulence of pneumococci of a given type to be essentially the same whether the strains were obtained from persons who were sick or well, and Cruickshank observed no special difference between the virulence of strains of a given type isolated from acutely ill or convalescent patients and those obtained from contacts or non-contacts.

In view of these variations of the results of testing the virulence of strains of a given type isolated from different sources and of the technic used (mouse inoculation), which is not very satisfactory for this purpose, no conclusion would appear justified from these reports. Other indirect information, however, suggests that there is no essential difference between the virulence of strains of a given type whether obtained from cases or carriers.

FACTORS AFFECTING THE CARRIER STATE. The carrier state is importantly affected by the type of pneumococcus considered. As shown in Table 63, strains of Type I or II are seldom obtained from healthy non-contacts, while strains of Type III are much more frequent, and those of Group IV constitute about 80 per cent of all the strains carried by such persons. Additional examples of this nature might be cited from the foregoing tables among both the non-contacts and the contacts.

Age appears to affect the carrier state to some extent. Within a few days (581) to a few months (730, 681) after birth pneumococci appear in the respiratory tract of infants, but children under two or three years of age less often carry pneumococci than children over this age (681, 112, 1353). As shown in Tables 59 and 60, about 35 per cent of non-contact infants and children are carriers of pneumococci as compared with 45 per cent of adults.

Rosenau, Felton, and Atwater (1111) studied the relation of the types found and the proportion of individuals carrying pneumococci among 180 non-contacts and 270 contacts of various ages and were unable to discover any significant variations with age. They also determined that age appeared of little importance in relation to the groups of carriers producing secondary carriers. Viktorow and his associates (1353) reported the incidence of carriers among persons of various ages to be highest in the group 10–20 years of age. These reports are somewhat at variance with that of Gundel and Linden (579) who, as a result of repeatedly examining various groups of non-contact persons, regarded children as especially prone to carry pneumococci. From the examination of a group of children in families in which pneumonia was present, Bunim and Trask (201) arrived at the same conclusion. In this instance it was found that of 41 contacts under eleven years of age, only 10 per cent showed no pneumococci, while among 39 older contacts 43 per cent were without these organisms. However, a much larger proportion of the younger than of the older persons in this study exhibited symptoms of a minor respiratory infection, so that the influence of age alone is not clear in this series.

Sex may be of no great importance in relation to the carrier state in non-contacts (1048), and about the same proportion of strains of the various types is found in males as in females, though Gundel (578) found Types X and XVIII carried somewhat more frequently by boys than by girls. Gundel and Okura (580) found boys more often carry strains of two or three types than girls, though this finding was regarded as a coincidence.

Data on the influence of race on the carrier state are too scanty to serve as the basis for any conclusion (682, 681, 1407, 510, 924).

Season of the year markedly affects the proportion of pneumococcus carriers found, as will be noted in the following section (see page 378).

Social status has no clear relation to the proportion of individuals carrying pneumococci or to the types carried. About the same proportion of carriers, having an approximately similar distribution of the types searched for, was found among various groups of students, laboratory workers, nurses, dispensary patients, and inmates of a tuberculosis sanatorium (1282, 1048, 682, 1393). Social status and the presence or absence of overcrowding are usually intimately related. Jacobson (682) reported an instance of a single family in which there were three Type II cases having eleven contacts, and seven of these carried this type. One child in the family had measles. This extraordinary group existed in four dark, filthy rooms ten feet below the sidewalk level. From the limited data available in his study Smillie (1206) obtained no evidence that pneumococci were harbored more frequently by individuals living under overcrowded conditions than by others in less crowded quarters. He also found no evidence that persons with pneumonia living under crowded conditions tended to infect their contacts any more frequently than others living under more favorable circumstances.

Smillie and Leeder (1210) introduced a healthy carrier of Type I pneumococci into the crowded living quarters of a group of feebleminded individuals in an institution, and over a ten-day period no evidence was found that the organism had spread to any of the contacts. It was noted that the ten-day period may have been too short to obtain the evidence sought and, further, inasmuch as the experiment was made in the summer, that the seasonal factor may have had a bearing on this point. In one instance cited, these investigators found no evidence of spread of pneumococci of Type II from a hospital patient to his patient contacts in a small ward, though infection did spread from a Type I case to several hospital staff contacts. Viktorow and his co-workers (1353) have followed the spread of pneumococci of Type I from a patient to his ward contacts.

One of the most important factors affecting the carrier state is the presence or absence of minor respiratory infections in otherwise healthy individuals. Among such infections the common contagious cold is especially important though itself due, as Dochez and his associates have shown, to a filterable virus (898, 369, 1182, 370, 359, 812). It has been demonstrated that usually there is a marked increase in the number of pathogenic organisms, and especially pneumococci, in the upper respiratory tract during the common cold both in animals (chimpanzees: 370, 1183, 366) and in man (1181, 1209, 1393, 1391, 367, 359), though possibly this may not occur in the latter in all instances (1210). Individuals having frequent colds usually (730, 1391), but not always (133), show the highest carrier rate for pneumococci, and in some instances during the later stages of a cold these organisms have been found in pure culture for a period of several days.

The division of healthy carriers into various groups, as suggested by Webster and Hughes (1393) and Bliss, McClaskey, and Long (133) has already been mentioned. The former workers obtained evidence that a carrier is really an infected individual in the sense that the organism is growing in the nasopharyngeal tissues. Evidence was obtained which suggested that pneumococci of Type III and some strains of the higher types, especially Type XIII, were actually spreading from person to person. No evidence was found, however, that strains of Type I or II spread with such facility among normal persons. A strain of Type I of high mouse virulence obtained from a carrier was planted in the nose and the throat of a healthy non-carrier. Cultures from the nose three hours later showed this organism still present, but subsequent cultures from both the nose and the throat were all negative. Five of eight chronic carriers studied by them had sinus or tonsil infections and experienced frequent attacks of coryza, sore throats, and the like each winter; while five non-carriers observed for periods of seven months to three years were free of upper respiratory infections. Extending this investigation, Webster and Clow (1391) studied the association of pneumococci, influenza bacilli, and hemolytic streptococci in persons of various ages with the occurrence of coryza and sinusitis. The results of this work led to the classification of normal individuals into three groups. It was observed that: (a) those who showed few or none of these organisms present in nasopharyngeal cultures were almost free of all types of respiratory infections and sinusitis; (b) those who occasionally showed some of these organisms present had occasional colds and minor respiratory infections; and (c) persons who were chronic carriers of these organisms had frequent respiratory infections and often suffered from chronic sinusitis. It would appear from the foregoing that chronic carriers were more subject to minor respiratory infections than non-carriers. Bliss, McClaskey, and Long (133), who also studied this matter, were unable to confirm this finding, however; and in their investigation of twenty persons extending over two academic years, no special difference was found between the number of these infections in carriers and non-carriers; and the duration of colds was the same in both groups. As all three of these studies, detailed as they are, embrace observations on a relatively small total group of persons, additional studies are needed to settle this matter.

Cruickshank's (331) report is of interest in respect to the observations of Webster and his collaborators (1393, 1391) on the frequent finding of pathologic conditions present in the upper respiratory tract of normal persons who are chronic carriers of pneumococci. The former studied convalescent patients who became chronic carriers of the infecting pneumococcus and found that the majority of these had some pathologic condition of the upper respiratory tract or had chronic bronchitis, while in non-carriers such conditions were much less frequent. An unhealthy condition of the mucous membrane of the upper respiratory tract may be a definite factor affecting the carrier state.

In Table 59 it was seen that approximately 35 per cent of healthy infants and children carry pneumococci. In contrast to this, Wollstein (1435) found pneumococci in 87.5 per cent of children with bronchitis, and Plummer and his associates (1029, 1057) found 81.4 per cent of children with upper respiratory infections carried these organisms. The latter reported that among children observed in their first study pneumococci were no more frequent in contacts (65 per cent) than in non-contacts (63 per cent) but were most often found in a group of contacts who also had respiratory infections (83 per cent). In a group of individuals of various ages Smillie and Caldwell (1209) found pneumococci present in 82 per cent of 34 persons having an acute cold at the time of examination, as compared with 53 per cent of 28 others who had just recovered from a cold and 54 per cent of 11 individuals having no history of a recent cold. In addition, it has already been shown that persons exposed to contact with patients having pneumonia usually carry pneumococci more frequently, and especially of the types to which they are exposed, than others not having such contact (see pages 351–362). And further, persons residing in camps or institutions in which pneumonia is prevalent may carry pneumococci, especially of the prevalent types, more often than others not having such exposure (1235, 1282, 1252, 267, 1207).

It was earlier remarked that Smillie and his associates (1209, 1206, 1210) suggested that some factor other than contact alone appears to determine whether or not contacts become carriers of the homologous type of pneumococcus to which they are exposed. It seemed possible that this factor was the presence of the common cold. Most significant in this respect was the finding by Smillie and Leeder (1210) that of the various classes of contacts of patients with pneumonia the family contacts are especially liable to harbor strains of the homologous type; and among 25 such contacts with Type I or Type II cases who carried these types, 19 or 76 per cent had colds at the time they were cultured. Details were presented showing the occurrence of colds among the family contacts of two cases of Type II and one of Type I pneumonia. In the first instance six contacts were examined, and two of the four carrying Type II had acute colds. In the second, of ten contacts examined six carried Type I, and nine of the ten had acute colds when cultured.

Bunim and Trask (201) obtained results of a similar nature in the course of an examination of eighty family contacts with children having pneumonia due to pneumococci of various types. They also observed that the age of the contacts appeared to be an important factor in combination with the presence of upper respiratory infections. Some 46 per cent of the contacts under eleven years old had symptoms of upper respiratory infection, while such symptoms were found in only 20 per cent of persons over this age. Also, in the older group of contacts pneumococci were found just as frequently in those without as in those with respiratory infections, but in the younger group only 5 per cent having infections of this nature were free of pneumococci as compared with 13 per cent of those without such infections. It was further found that in thirteen of fourteen families studied, one or more members besides the patient gave a history of respiratory infection, and in six families upper respiratory infection was epidemic. When pneumonia occurred in a child, it was common to find that other members of the family suffered from some sort of respiratory infection.

Bunim and Trask likewise note that the increase in the incidence of carriers of pneumococci in family contacts with colds was related to an increased incidence of both homologous and heterologous types. The fact that individuals exposed to respiratory infections show a generally higher pneumococcus carrier rate than others not having such exposure has already been mentioned.

A consideration of the data at hand makes it highly probable that the presence or absence of respiratory infection is one of the most significant factors influencing the carrier state.

Relatively little is known of the complex problem of the relation of the carrier state to immunity. Neufeld and Etinger-Tulczynska (933, 934, 935) observed that the instillation of pneumococci into the nose of experimental animals resulted in many instances in their becoming carriers of these organisms for several weeks. In animals this carrier state was produced and persisted even though a high degree of immunity for the homologous type had been developed in some by active or passive procedures. No apparent loss of virulence occurred in the organism carried. Whether or not the carrier state developed seemed to depend upon the individual disposition of the animal.

An investigation of the relation of the carrier state to the presence or absence of humoral antibody in patients convalescent from pneumococcus pneumonia was reported by Cruickshank (331). Early in convalescence, type-specific protective antibody was usually demonstrable in carriers and in non-carriers alike and tended to disappear equally in both groups. Such studies were presumably confined to individuals "early" in convalescence. Judging by the results of this and the above investigations, apparently no evidence was obtained suggesting the existence of any particular relation between the presence of immunity and the presence or absence of the carrier state.

The observations of Webster and Hughes (1393) on healthy human carriers suggest that a person carrying pneumococci is really an infected individual in the sense that these organisms are growing in the nasopharyngeal tissues, as previously mentioned. They further regard the presence or absence of the carrier state as being dependent upon the amount of immunity of the host to a given type and consider this resistance to be a variable property which decreases in the winter and increases during the warmer months of the year. After additional study Webster and Clow (1391) suggested that the dosage of pneumococci in the community is controlled by the resistance of carriers and of contacts.

It is apparent from these somewhat dissimilar observations that additional information is needed to determine the relation of antipneumococcal immunity in the host to the presence or absence of the carrier state. It is possible that the factors governing the carrier state in convalescent patients, at least for a short period following recovery from pneumonia, may be somewhat different from those concerned in the regulation of this state in healthy individuals.

Seasonal Prevalence of Pneumococci

The seasonal prevalence of pneumococci and of various types of this organism isolated either from patients with pneumonia or from pneumococcus carriers or both has been commented upon by numerous workers (803, 956, 264, 1048, 682, 1393, 239, 616, 732, 837, 1206, 367, 464, 267, 1353, 201, 734).

The fact that respiratory infections, and especially lobar pneumonia, ordinarily have a definite seasonal variation in many parts of the world has already been pointed out (see pages 289–295). The curve of the incidence of respiratory infections appears to have at least two peaks each year, one in early fall (September) and the other in midwinter (January). A third peak occurring in midspring has been described (358). The fall outbreak is made up largely of infections of a mild nature, while the midwinter wave is composed of much more severe infections, as illustrated by the high proportion of the cases of lobar pneumonia which occur in midwinter and early spring. The midspring outbreak is often associated with less severe lesions than the midwinter outbreak.

The curve for the percentage of carriers of pneumococci among the combined groups of contacts and non-contacts in the population is similar to the curve of respiratory infections and tends to have a double peak with the highest points occurring in the fall and in midwinter to early spring. This was pointed out by Smillie (1206), whose data on the carrier incidence among persons of various ages covered the period of a full year. In retrospect, the findings of Powell, Atwater, and Felton (1048) on the distribution of carriers over a period of seven months (September through March) among a group of healthy adults having no more contact with cases of pneumonia than the population at large seem to show the same thing. The curves illustrated in both these reports appear identical in their significance in this respect.

In Smillie's report the curve shown was for the incidence of pneumococci of all types considered as a group. It was also found that wherever the number of strains of the various types encountered was large enough to be considered significant, a similar seasonal distribution was observed. Strains of Types III, VI, and XVIII, for example, were found throughout the year but were far more prevalent in the spring months. No one type appeared limited to one season nor appeared suddenly and then disappeared. The report of Powell and his associates gave separate curves for Types I, II, and III and for Group IV, all of which appeared essentially similar in their trends.

Presumably the groups of persons included in the above two studies were chiefly adults. In infants somewhat different findings have been reported. Kneeland and Dawes (732) studied the carrier rate of several pathogenic organisms, including pneumococci, among approximately three hundred inmates of an infants' home over two winter periods. While a double peak of respiratory infections was observed, it was found that accompanying the fall outbreaks of these disturbances there was little change in the carrier rate of the organisms studied, though by midwinter the rate was extremely high (80 per cent).

Despite this variation in the carrier rate as shown by infants, it may be said that the above and other studies show that pneumococci in general exhibit a definite seasonal prevalence, being most commonly found in the colder months of the year (803, 1393, 616, 367, 267). The findings of Jacobson (682) on the incidence of carriers of Types I, II, and III and of Viktorow and his collaborators (1353) on carriers of Types I and II are likewise in accord with this view.

In Webster and Hughes' (1393) study of carriers among normal persons it was found that chronic carriers of pneumococci frequently suffered attacks of upper respiratory infection each winter, as mentioned previously. During such attacks pneumococci increased in the nose and throat of these individuals, often to the point of being the only organism in cultures. The incidence of these organisms in healthy persons underwent seasonal variations similar to the incidence of respiratory infections in the same individuals, and the incidence of a given type in each chronic carrier was subjected to the same sort of variation. It was also observed that the number of carriers and the quantity of organisms carried by the group of chronic carriers likewise exhibited seasonal variations similar to the incidence of coryza, sore throat, and other respiratory diseases. As already seen, these variations were regarded as dependent upon host resistance to a given type, which was believed to vary and to be lower during the colder months of the year than during warm weather.

Smillie (1206) has summarized his findings on the proportion of contacts and non-contacts found carrying pneumococci in various seasons, as shown in Table 75. In both groups examined pneumococci were much less prevalent in the summer than in the winter; and, as might be expected, the proportion of carriers was lower among non-contacts than among contacts in all seasons, though no significant difference between the seasonal variation of the types found in these groups was apparent.

In connection with the seasonal variation shown by the prevalence of pneumococci in healthy carriers, it is of interest to note the distribution of certain types isolated from the sputum of patients with pneumonia and some other respiratory infections during the course of the Massachusetts Pneumonia Study (869) as compared with the proportion of reported cases and deaths from lobar pneumonia in Massachusetts by quarters of the year, as earlier listed in Table 48 (page 292).

TABLE 75. NON-CONTACTS AND CONTACTS. NUMBER EXAMINED AND PERCENTAGE CARRYING PNEUMOCOCCI, BY SEASON OF THE YEAR

PERSONS EXAMINED	AUTUMN		WINTER		SPRING		SUMMER	
	Number of persons	*Per cent positive*	*Number of persons*	*Per cent positive*	*Number of persons*	*Per cent positive*	*Number of persons*	*Per cent positive*
Contacts	130	57	218	56	212	67	22	36
Non-contacts	62	48	184	48	194	45	53	15

From Smillie (1206)

As Types I, II, III, V, VII, and VIII have proved to be the commonest in the region of Massachusetts as well as in some other places (see page 52), the number and proportion of strains of these types obtained from specimens sent for bacteriologic diagnosis to the Massachusetts State Bacteriologic Laboratory in Boston have been determined over a period of thirty-six consecutive months. Most, but not all, of such specimens came from patients with some variety of pneumonia (see Table 76).

Though strains of Types I and II were found in all months of the three years studied, they were most frequently encountered during the winter and spring months of December through April. Of the 480 strains of these types isolated, the proportion obtained in January (16.3 per cent) and in March (15.3 per cent) was larger than in other months of the year. An examination of the percentage incidence of these types by months for each of the three years included in Table 76 (percentages not given in table for each year separately) shows that during two winters the largest proportion of Type I and II strains was found in January, while during the other it was found in December. Though the proportion of these types found in each of the months showed some variation from year to year, this was most marked during the summer and fall months of August through November. Their incidence was low during these months but at times no lower than during June or July. Despite these variations there was nevertheless considerable uniformity in the general incidence of these types in a given month for each of the different years.

TABLE 76. PNEUMOCOCCI OF TYPES I AND II AND OF TYPES III, V, VII, AND VIII ISOLATED FROM THE SPUTUM OF PATIENTS WITH PNEUMONIA OR SOME OTHER RESPIRATORY INFECTION. NUMBER AND PERCENTAGE DISTRIBUTION BY MONTHS, DURING THREE YEARS (MASSACHUSETTS STATE BACTERIOLOGIC LABORATORY, BOSTON)

YEAR	TOTAL NUMBER	*Aug.*	*Sept.*	*Oct.*	*Nov.*	*Dec.*	*Jan.*	*Feb.*	*Mar.*	*April*	*May*	*June*	*July*
							TYPES I AND II						
1932–33	140	1	8	9	8	9	24	19	23	16	12	8	3
1933–34	183	1	2	5	26	29	27	20	24	20	17	10	2
1934–35	157	4	2	10	13	13	27	11	26	22	18	6	5
Total	480	6	12	24	47	51	78	50	73	58	47	24	10
Per cent		1.3	2.5	5.0	9.8	10.4	16.3	10.4	15.3	12.1	9.8	5.0	2.1
							TYPES III, V, VII, AND VIII						
1932–33	196	4	5	12	7	11	52	19	26	33	18	4	5
1933–34	272	6	3	17	24	43	55	38	33	16	20	11	6
1934–35	257	1	3	30	14	24	51	35	30	23	32	9	8
Total	725	11	11	59	45	78	158	92	89	72	70	24	16
Per cent		1.5	1.5	8.1	6.2	10.8	21.5	12.7	12.3	9.9	9.7	3.3	2.2

Though strains of Types III, V, VII, and VIII were also encountered in all months, they were likewise commonest in the winter and spring. The largest proportion of the 725 strains of these types found was encountered in January (21.5 per cent) and in February (12.7 per cent). In each of the three years the largest proportion was found in January. The proportion of these types in a given month also showed some variation from year to year, which again was most pronounced during the months of August through November or possibly December, when their incidence was generally low but frequently no lower than in June or July. As with Types I and II, the proportion found in the same month in each of the years was in general fairly similar. It may be said, however, that for all the types considered the least variations in incidence were found during the months of late winter and of spring, and for Types I and II from January through May nearly the same proportion was found in each of these months in one year as in another, and this was true of the other types for the shorter period of January through March.

The incidence of each of these six types is shown separately in Figure 7. In each instance the number of strains of a given type found during the same month in the three different years has been added together.

Type I appears to show the widest general spread throughout the year and to have a peak in January and in March. The curve for Type III is somewhat similar and shows an even higher peak in January. The curve for Type VIII is much similar to this only at a lower level, while at a still lower level the Type VII curve resembles that of Type I. Though somewhat different from the other types, the curve for Type II is much similar to that for Type V, and both show their highest peaks in March. Types V, VII, and VIII all show sub-peaks in October. Though the highest incidence of strains of Types I, III, VII, and VIII occurred in January and of Types II and V in March, these data only cover a period of three "normal" pneumonia years; and it seems probable that at times individual types may show a distribution different from this.

In Table 77 the data have been combined to show the proportion of carriers of pneumococci found by season (compiled from Table 75) as compared with the proportion of Types I and II and of Types III, V, VII, and VIII isolated from the sputum of patients with respiratory infection by season (Table 76), and with the distribution by season of reported cases and deaths from lobar pneumonia in Massachusetts (Table 48, page 292).

The proportion of pneumococcus carriers in the population appears to

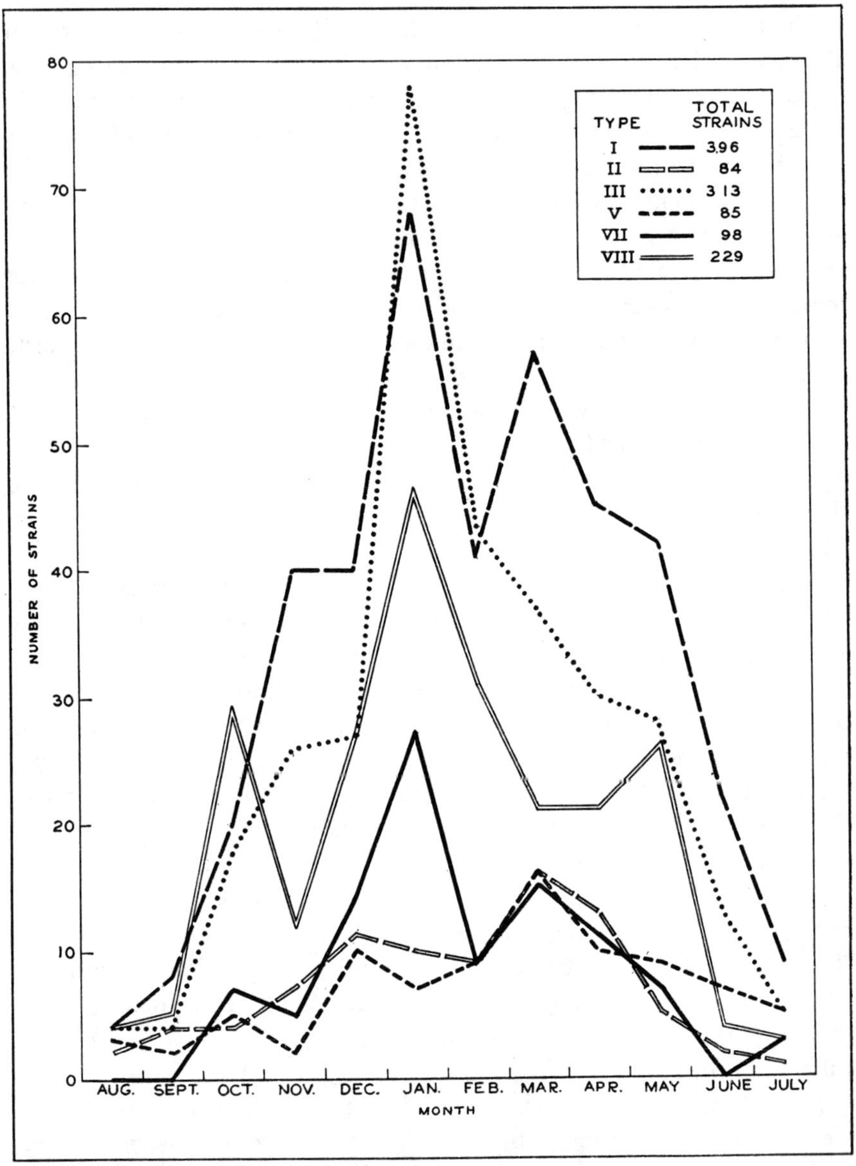

Figure 7. Monthly incidence of pneumococci of Types I, II, III, V, VII, and VIII isolated from the sputum of patients with pneumonia and some other respiratory infections over a period of three years

show considerable, though less, variation in the different seasons than the proportion of the types isolated from patients with respiratory infection or the proportion of reported cases or deaths from lobar pneumonia. The seasonal differences in the proportion of the types obtained from patients with respiratory infection and of the reported cases and deaths from lobar pneumonia are remarkably similar. The considerable variations shown in Table 77 may be regarded as evidence not only of seasonal variations in the prevalence of pneumococci, but presumably also of seasonal variations either in the virulence of these organisms or in the resistance of man to them.

TABLE 77. CARRIERS, CONTACTS AND NON-CONTACTS; STRAINS OF FIVE TYPES OF PNEUMOCOCCI FROM PATIENTS WITH RESPIRATORY INFECTION; AND REPORTED LOBAR PNEUMONIA CASES AND DEATHS IN MASSACHUSETTS. PERCENTAGE DISTRIBUTION BY SEASON

SEASON OF YEAR	PNEUMOCOCCUS CARRIERS*		STRAINS FROM PATIENTS WITH RESPIRATORY INFECTION†		REPORTED LOBAR PNEUMONIA CASES AND DEATHS‡	
	Contacts	*Non-contacts*	*Types I and II together*	*Types III, V, VII, and VIII together*	*Cases*	*Deaths*
Autumn	21.4	14.1	25.2	25.1	22.1	23.1
Winter	35.3	41.3	41.9	46.8	44.2	44.0
Spring	41.0	40.8	26.9	22.9	27.1	25.9
Summer	2.3	3.8	5.9	5.2	6.6	7.1

* Compiled from Table 75. † From Table 76. ‡ From Table 48.

Studies of the virulence of strains of pneumococci obtained from healthy carriers led Powell, Atwater, and Felton (1048) to suggest that virulence may vary in different seasons and be different for each type of pneumococcus. As the result of investigations of the spread of pneumococcus and other infections in experimental animals and of pneumococci isolated from human carriers, Webster and Hughes (1393) suggested that the prevalence of the carrier state and of pneumococcus infections is determined by variations and differences in the resistance of the host to a relatively stable and unchanging organism. The matter is not yet settled, however; and, as mentioned in these studies, much additional evidence is needed before it can be definitely determined whether such variations can be attributed to seasonal alterations of virulence or of host resistance or both.

Epidemics and Multiple Cases in Families

Pneumonia is endemic nearly everywhere and upon occasion may assume epidemic characteristics. Hirsch (647) lists a number of epidemics extending back to the sixteenth century, and Wells' (1399) classic compilation of similar events contains more than two hundred examples beginning with outbreaks reported in 1440. For various reasons it seems logical, as Wells mentions, to assume that some of the epidemics these investigators cited may have been outbreaks of some other disease, such as pneumonic plague.

Though secondary pneumonia, chiefly of the bronchopneumonic form, tends to be pandemic on occasions in the course of pandemics of influenza, it is highly improbable that any such extensive outbreaks of lobar pneumonia have ever occurred. An examination of the reports of many epidemics of pneumonia supports this view. "Pneumonia" or lobar pneumonia may at times be unusually prevalent in certain regions or even over considerable portions of whole countries, at which times the opinion is frequently expressed that a "big pneumonia year" is in progress. It is the localized outbreaks of this disease, however, which are usually most striking and in consequence comprise the bulk of the literature on epidemics of pneumonia.

In addition to Hirsch (647) and Wells (1399) other writers have considered the matter of pneumonia epidemics (297, 807, 661, 510, 331). Many examples of outbreaks localized to camps, barracks, prisons, asylums, and similar institutions have been reported (918, 874, 387, 1235, 952, 1282, 892, 985, 1289, 969, 773, 1008, 1294, 1165, 961, 510, 1252, 1207). In some instances epidemics have occurred on ships or in certain houses (1399, 918, 807, 1031, 661, 141, 510).

While many of the foregoing instances concern epidemics among individuals of the white race, an unusual prevalence of pneumonia is by no means confined to this race, as was apparent earlier in this chapter. Natives of Alaska (1399), Puerto Rico (985), Jamaica, Barbados, and Central America (549), and the Philippines (1031) have suffered from pneumonia in epidemic form, as have Negroes in Africa (647, 874, 773, 1008) and in this country (1289).

During the past decade or more special attention has been paid to identifying the etiologic agent responsible for epidemics of pneumonia. Several epidemics apparently due chiefly to pneumococci of Type I have been reported. In an outbreak of pneumonia in an institution for boys (New York) Stillman (1235) found three of six cases due to this organism. The examination of 56 other boys in this institution showed six or 10 per cent to be carriers of Type I. Likewise, four of six cases occurring among the inmates of an asylum were due to pneumococci of Type I, strains of which were recovered from 2 per cent of 148 other inmates examined. During an outbreak of pneumonia occurring in an army camp (Texas) during the War, Nichols (952) recovered Type I from 56 per cent and Type II from 22 per cent of 150 cases. In an isolated community of laborers (Maryland) Sydenstricker and Sutton (1282) observed 27 cases of pneumonia, 15 of which were due to Type I and one to Type II. Six per cent of 100 other men in this community were carriers of Type I, and six per cent were carrying Type II. Park and Chickering (985) reported an outbreak of pneumonia among laborers in an army camp (South Carolina). Of 51 cases studied, 22 were due to Type I. In another epidemic in an army camp (New York) Tenney and Rivenburgh (1289) found 68 of 135 cases caused by pneumococci of this type. Strom (1252) reported an outbreak in a boys' orphanage in Norway. Twelve cases of pneumonia and two of otitis media occurred. Among the twelve cases of pneumonia, six were typed during the acute illness and five proved due to Type I. The examination of thirty other boys during the height of the epidemic showed ten or 33.3 per cent were carriers of this type; and a subsequent examination of sixty-five boys, made nearly three months later, showed eleven or 16.9 per cent still carrying this organism.

An epidemic of Type II pneumonia with 17 cases occurring in a hospital for the insane (Massachusetts) was investigated by Smillie (1207). Of 267 inmates without pneumonia and from whom 450 cultures were obtained, 30 were proved to be carriers of Type II. In a few the carrier state was demonstrated to persist for periods up to a year or more. An epidemic believed due to pneumococci of Type V was reported by Schroder and Cooper (1165). This occurred in an institution in New York City housing more than 700 children. Of this number a considerable proportion became ill, and 132 cases were studied closely. Of those seriously afflicted 38, or 31 per cent, had pneumonia. Of the 9 cases typed 7 showed pneumococci of Type V. Other examples much similar to those cited above may be found in the literature.

At times pneumonia may appear in epidemic form among animals. Blake and Cecil (124) observed an epidemic of lobar pneumonia in a consignment of monkeys received by them. Among the 32 cases which occurred, 28 were found due to one or the other of two separate strains of pneumococci of Group IV.

Though outbreaks of pneumonia in families have not been found with great frequency (1025, 1048, 616), they nevertheless occur. Where suitable studies have been carried out among the members of such families in which two or more cases have occurred either simultaneously or within a short period, it has been found that these family outbreaks are nearly always due to pneumococci of a single type (821, 682, 1210, 1068, 201). Also, and as might be expected in view of the high proportion of the family contacts of cases found carrying pneumococci of the homologous type, as mentioned above (see pages 353–362), healthy carriers of the type causing the pneumonia are often found among the members of such families. Among the eleven contacts of three Type II cases occurring in one family, Jacobson (682) found seven carrying strains of this type. Examples of a similar nature have been reported by Smillie and Leeder (1210) and by Bunim and Trask (201).

With respect to the recognition of instances of family outbreaks of pneumonia due to pneumococci of a single type, the experience of the Massachusetts Pneumonia Study (869) is of interest. During the course of that investigation, carried out over a five-year period, arrangements were made for the examination of sputum and other material and for pneumococcus typing in sixty-six laboratories throughout the state. The number of specimens obtained from patients with respiratory disease and sent to such laboratories for examination steadily increased throughout the period of the study. As a result of this widespread application of bacteriologic diagnosis, it became apparent that the number of family outbreaks of pneumonia and other infections due to a single type was by no means so small as had previously been believed. Though the number of such instances thus far recorded in a given year in the whole state is not large and may perhaps be in the neighborhood of a dozen or so, still it is sufficient to indicate what must be occurring elsewhere with the same regularity. Of course, occurrences of this nature can only be recognized on a large scale when facilities for bacteriologic diagnosis are generally available. Specific examples of regional and of family outbreaks of pneumonia and other infections due to pneumococci of a single type, particularly to those of Type I, will be noted in a report to be published by members of the Massachusetts State Department of Public Health.*

Numerous possibilities might be mentioned to account for the occurrence of epidemics or of a series of cases occurring in a single family. Exposure to wet and cold, overcrowding, poor ventilation, inadequate diet, the pres-

* A report on this topic has now been published; Gilman, B. B., and Anderson, G. W., *A Community Outbreak of Type I Pneumococcus Infection,* Am. J. Hyg., 28:345, Nov. 1938.

ence of other diseases, including minor respiratory infections, in the group considered, and climatic variations are some of the factors which have been cited as of importance.

The problem of epidemic disease has been extensively studied by Gill (516). Though his specific data were concerned with epidemics of malaria, influenza, and plague, he formulated a theory which he regarded as sufficiently broad to explain epidemics of all diseases which may occur in this form. He stated that the origin of epidemics is controlled by four factors, which are (a) the reservoir of the parasite, (b) the parasite, (c) the immunity, and (d) the transmission factor. Quantitative changes in these factors resulting in a temporary upset in the equilibrium between infection and resistance were believed to explain all epidemic manifestations of disease. The transmission factor was stated to comprise atmospheric conditions favoring the passing of infection from host to host and in its broadest sense to embrace the influence of atmospheric states on the specific parasite while both in and outside of the body of the host.

With respect to the problem of pneumonia it may be noted that the high proportion of pneumococcus carriers in the population at large provides a more than ample reservoir of the parasite. Some seasonal variation in the prevalence of pneumococci has been demonstrated; and during periods when the organism is most prevalent, pneumonia is most prevalent. The factor of immunity is extremely complex, but man as a species may be regarded as possessing a considerable but probably constantly varying resistance to the pneumococcus. The direct influence of climatic and meteorological factors on the organism is less clear; for in some instances it may die within a few hours when outside of the body and yet at other times remain alive for a day or more suspended in the air. However, in the colder seasons of the year there is much crowding of the population for the sake of obtaining warmth and shelter, and the transmission of organisms from person to person at such times must be fairly direct.

Gill's explanation of the genesis of epidemics takes into account the severe outbreaks of disease occasionally seen when a susceptible population first comes into contact with an organism with which it previously had no contact and against which it consequently had no immunity. Localized epidemics of this nature he refers to as "artificial epidemics," which appears to be an apt designation when the broader aspects of the problem are recognized.

The multiplicity of factors involved in the production of this disease would seem to account for the feeble tendency to focal concentration of pneumonia cases in spite of the widespread distribution of pneumococci.

GENERAL CONSIDERATIONS OF EPIDEMIOLOGY

Pneumococcus pneumonia is not a single disease, for it may be caused by any one of many types of pneumococci, each of which has specific immunologic characteristics. The pneumococcus is a rather strict obligate parasite which lives and multiplies chiefly in man and not in his environment, as Rosenau, Felton, and Atwater (1111) have pointed out. In consequence, man is the chief source and reservoir of the organism, strains of which have been encountered in nearly all parts of the world and are presumably present wherever people may be found.

A large proportion of the healthy population carry pneumococci in their nose and throat at some time each year. The evidence at hand makes it probable that carriers are the most important means of spreading pneumococci throughout the community. Non-contact, contact, and convalescent carriers assist in the widespread dissemination of these organisms. Of the greatest importance in this respect are individuals who carry a single type for periods of weeks or months. The incidence of the carrier state is especially high in persons having minor acute respiratory infections, particularly if they are in contact with patients with pneumococcus pneumonia at the time, and is considerably affected by seasonal variations, being highest in individuals in temperate zones during the colder months of the year.

Most pneumococci carried by normal persons are strains of types other than Type I or Type II. The occurrence of strains of Type III in 15.4 per cent of such individuals carrying pneumococci (Table 72, page 364) reveals that the incidence of this type may be somewhat more frequent in healthy persons than in those with lobar pneumonia (incidence 10.8 per cent, Table 5, page 46) and much the same as in patients with bronchopneumonia (incidence 16 per cent, Table 19, page 71) due to pneumococci.

Non-contact carriers greatly outnumber the contact or convalescent carriers in the community. As shown in Table 61 (page 346), pneumococci of Type I or II may not be frequently encountered in healthy non-contact carriers and strains of Type I may be found in only 0.5 per cent of normal persons and strains of Type II in but 0.9 per cent. However, if these incidence figures are applied to the United States, the population of which was more than 122,000,000 in 1930, it appears that there may be in the neighborhood of 610,000 carriers of Type I and 1,098,000 carriers of Type II pneumococci in this country. It is thus apparent that the number of carriers of these types far exceeds the number of cases of pneumonia due to them in any year, for it was estimated that there were about 480,000 or less cases of pneumonia of all forms in the United States each year (see page 266); of this number of cases approximately three-quarters may be ascribed to pneumococci of the various types, and possibly around 127,000 such cases are due to strains of Type I or II (613). A consideration of figures such as these suggests that the reservoir of carriers of these types in the healthy population is sufficient to account for the number and widespread distribution of infections caused by them.

The high incidence of Type I and II infections in patients with lobar pneumonia (see Table 5, page 46), as contrasted with the low carrier incidence of pneumococci of these types in the general population, has led to the view that Type I or II pneumonia is an infection of exogenous origin, the organisms being acquired by contact with a patient having a homologous type pneumonia or with a healthy or convalescent carrier of these types (361, 33, 297, 298, 584, 300, 1206, 331, 1210, 1353, 1068). The limited data at hand suggest that the situation with respect to certain other pneumococci, such as Types V, VII, and VIII, may be somewhat analogous, for these types also tend to be found more frequently in cases than in carriers. As pneumococci of types other than those mentioned above are found about as frequently among the strains carried by normal persons as among those isolated from patients with lobar pneumonia, it seems likely that pneumonia due to any one of these types is the result of a chance infection with organisms commonly carried in the mouth and, in consequence, may be regarded as of "autogenous" origin. It appears, then, that pneumococci of Types I and II especially, and possibly to a lesser degree those of Types V, VII, and VIII as well, are endowed with an unusual invasive power largely lacking in strains of other types. Exceptions to this generalization may be encountered at times, especially among infants and children in whom the incidence of the various types in pneumonia is somewhat different from that found in adults (see pages 79–84 and 342–378).

The high proportion of carriers of the homologous type found among persons in contact with cases of pneumococcus lobar pneumonia, a situation which is largely limited to the family contacts of such cases, has been interpreted to indicate that cases commonly infect their contacts. Although it seems clear that at times cases may infect their contacts, there is an accumulating body of evidence, similar to that presented by Smillie and Leeder (1210), which suggests that in the usual instance the sequence of events is somewhat different from this. The majority of patients with lobar pneumonia give a history of having had an acute minor respiratory infection prior to the onset of their pneumonia; and, among others, Smillie and Caldwell (1209), Shultz (1187), Smillie (1206), Smillie and Leeder (1210), and Bunim and Trask (201) have found that the investigation of the families of patients with pneumococcus pneumonia frequently reveals that minor respiratory infections are common or epidemic in the family. It appears that a given type of pneumococcus may invade a family or group of individuals in close contact and spread in that group, especially in the presence of outbreaks of minor respiratory infections, until a high proportion of the individuals become carriers of the type in question. If under such circumstances some factor or combination of factors which tends to depress host resistance becomes operative, one or more individuals in the group may come down with pneumonia due to the organism carried. Suitable culturing of the immediate contacts of the patient at this time will, of course, reveal the presence of numerous carriers of pneumococci of homologous type.

In addition to the spread of infection among normal persons by their contact with healthy and convalescent carriers and with patients with pneumococcus pneumonia, such carriers and cases, when in contact with other cases (969, 445), may at times be the source of organisms which give rise to mixed or successive infections in the same patient.

Pneumococci are spread chiefly through the secretions and discharges of the mouth and respiratory tract and usually by direct contact with persons carrying these organisms or with patients having pneumonia. In most instances pneumococci are probably directly acquired by droplet infection, the droplets emanating from persons talking, laughing, coughing, sneezing, and spitting. At times indirect infection through food or drink, by hand-to-mouth contamination, or by contact with articles, such as eating or drinking utensils or toys, which have recently been mouthed may also occur (Rosenau, 1110). In addition, pneumococci may be present in dried sputum (1440) and in dust (1235) and may be suspended in the air as droplet nuclei which are readily carried and spread by air currents (Wells, 1409). Suspended in the air, these organisms may remain alive for a day or more (1410). Wells (1408) has demonstrated that the air in crowded rooms contains many organisms and that during the act of sneezing thousands of droplets are expelled into the atmosphere, each of which may carry with it its quota of bacteria.

It is apparent, of course, that the mere presence in the upper respiratory tract of pneumococci of any type is not alone sufficient to bring about pulmonary infection, and it is likewise clear that the production of pneumonia is a complex matter. Alterations in the virulence of the organism carried are presumably not alone sufficient to account for the development of the disease, and there is evidence that many strains of pneumococci carried by healthy people possess considerable virulence. While it seems likely that pneumococci of considerable virulence are essential to the production of pneumonia in the lobar form, the evidence at hand also suggests that in the presence of such organisms the disease occurs in the usual instance as the result of a temporary lowering of host resistance. Many investigators have called attention to this matter and have stressed the importance of various factors which depress host resistance and facilitate the production of lobar pneumonia. Those most often mentioned are: acute minor respiratory infections or other infectious diseases; exposure to temperature variations, chilling, wetting, and fatigue; and conditions which may damage the lung tissue or favor the aspiration of organisms (1008, 1111, 682, 1048, 298, 1209, 119, 320, 444, 1068; see also pages 199–203 and 232–235).

Following the demonstration by Griffith (570, 571) and others that there are variants of the pneumococcus, and also that under experimental conditions pneumococci of one type may be transformed into those of another type, the question was at once raised whether under adverse environmental conditions in the host rough pneumococci or those of a type possessing little virulence might be transformed into strains of a virulent type and thus give rise to infection (1187, 837, 331, 267). Thus far, however, there is no direct evidence that any such biologic alteration occurs under ordinary conditions in the pneumococci carried by normal persons (1393, 1392). The suggestion that pneumococci might change their type and virulence under some circumstances and thus possibly facilitate the development of infection may be attractive in some of its aspects. It would perhaps appear to explain the occurrence of cases of pneumonia due to pneumococci such as those of Type I or II in relatively isolated individuals who presumably had had no contact with a known carrier of the homologous type. Of great interest in this connection is Smillie's (1207) illuminating study of an outbreak of Type II pneumococcus pneumonia which occurred in a hospital for insane patients. Cases developed in patients residing in several buildings of the institution. Smillie found that:

> The incidence of each case, if considered separately and without the carrier study, would have been most mysterious. Everything became quite clear, however, when the carrier studies were made, since each case could be linked closely to a carrier.

The number of carriers of pneumococci of Type II exceeded the number of cases which actually developed. The existence of this widespread carrier condition for the type of pneumococcus in question appeared to account for the distribution of the cases that developed, without the necessity of invoking a consideration of the theoretically possible occurrence of a transmutation of type. As Cruickshank (331) and Smillie (1207) have mentioned, a marked similarity exists between the epidemiology of pneumococcus pneumonia and that of meningococcus meningitis.

Man in general possesses considerable immunity to the pneumococcus. This resistance appears to be in most individuals both type-specific and species-specific. Blake (921) considers that the immunity effective in controlling pneumonia morbidity is a broad species-specific antipneumococcal immunity. According to other observations of Blake (119), and to evidence available from additional sources, the factors controlling the prevalence of pneumonia under ordinary conditions seem to be: (a) the nature of the infective organism, (b) the opportunities for acquiring the infection, (c) the nature of the predisposing factors to which the individual is exposed, and (d) the host and his resistance. In temperate zones lobar pneumonia exhibits a marked seasonal variation. This presumably results from the fact that pneumococci are most prevalent in the general population during the colder months of the year. At this time the opportunities for direct person-to-person infection are most marked because of crowding and the frequent occurrence of minor respiratory infections, with a consequent increase in coughing and spitting, and possibly also because of an increase in the biologic activities of the organism present. Also, doubtless many predisposing factors are of more widespread importance during cold weather than at other times, and at such periods host resistance may be generally lower than during the warmer months of the year.

CHAPTER SEVEN

MEASURES FOR THE PREVENTION OF PNEUMONIA

General Measures of Prevention 395
Personal Hygiene 396
Community Hygiene 398
Patients with Pneumonia: Care and Isolation 401
Carriers of Pneumococci: Isolation and Treatment 403
Immunization Against Pneumonia and Minor Respiratory Infections 406
Active Immunization Against the Pneumococcus 408
Character of the Immunizing Agent 410
Route of Administration 415
Dosage: Vaccines and Similar Preparations 418
Dosage: Specific Capsular Polysaccharides and Allied Agents 429
Type of Pneumococcus and Immune Response 432
Time of Appearance of Immune Response 434
Duration of Immune Response 437
Results of Immunization of Animals Against Experimental Pneumococcus Pneumonia 440
Results of Immunization of Animals Against Contact Infection 446
Results of Immunization of Man Against Pneumococcus Pneumonia ... 446
Active Immunization 446
South African Studies 448
Other Studies of Prophylactic Vaccination 463
Discussion of Studies of Prophylactic Vaccination 475
Reactions to Immunizing Agents and Contraindications to Their Use 478
Passive Immunization 483

GENERAL MEASURES OF PREVENTION

RESPIRATORY diseases as a group have proved notoriously difficult to control or prevent, a situation which has presumably resulted from the varied nature of the factors which, as pointed out at the end of the preceding chapter, govern the prevalence of such infections. The prevalence of pneumonia appears related to (a) the invasive power of the organism, (b) the opportunities for acquiring infection, (c) the predisposing conditions to which the individual is exposed, and (d) the host and his resistance.

Despite the lack of any generally accepted measures of prevention for pneumonia, evidence is at hand for parts of this country and for England

and Wales, indicating that the mortality rates, and probably the incidence rates as well, have shown a significant decrease during the past quarter of a century (see pages 284–287). Numerous circumstances, including improvements in general hygiene, have presumably contributed to this decrease. Nevertheless, the pneumonia mortality rates are still far higher than need be. The material presented in several sections of the foregoing chapter and in the chapter on Aspects of Immunity (page 113) suggests means which might be taken to reduce still further the incidence and mortality rates for pneumonia. There is, however, great need of additional careful and extended epidemiologic investigations of pneumonia and other respiratory diseases, not only in this country, but in other regions as well.

Although numerous general measures of prevention are cited, the following discussion includes recommendations directed primarily at the prevention of pneumonia caused by pneumococci. Doubtless the adoption of many of the measures suggested would have a desirable effect. However, as was pointed out by Shattuck (1177) in 1841, the number and the involved nature of the factors controlling the occurrence of pneumonia make it extraordinarily difficult to determine the relative value of any measure or combination of measures suggested.

Personal Hygiene

PRECAUTIONS AGAINST SPREADING DISCHARGES OF THE RESPIRATORY TRACT. Pneumococci are commonly present in the secretions and discharges of the mouth and respiratory tract and it is probable that the chief means of spreading infection with these organisms is by contact with droplets from such sources. It is advisable to adopt measures tending to reduce the risk of droplet infection. The mouth and nose should be covered when coughing or sneezing. Wells (1408) has demonstrated that the use of a handkerchief in the latter instance largely smothers the spray of organisms disbursed while sneezing. Promiscuous spitting should be prohibited. Pneumococci may be present in the air and dust and be spread by air currents, kissing, soiling the hands with sputum containing these organisms, and contact with contaminated things, such as handkerchiefs, clothing, bed linen, furniture, rugs, and similar articles.

AVOIDANCE OF CONTACT WITH PERSONS HAVING RESPIRATORY INFECTION. As patients with pneumonia and their contacts, and persons with lesser acute respiratory infections as well, more often have pneumococci in their upper respiratory tracts than other individuals, contact with them should be avoided whenever possible. Further, contact with individuals having any general infectious disease should also be avoided, and it is likewise advisable not to mingle in crowds if it can be helped.

It is well to recognize that the invasive power of pneumococci differs somewhat with the various types. Pneumococci of Types I and II, and possibly those of Types V, VII, and VIII as well, which appear responsible for 70 per cent of the cases of pneumococcus lobar pneumonia, must be considered as possessing unusual invasive powers as elsewhere mentioned (see pages 390–394). In consequence, contact with patients known to be infected with organisms of one of these types or with persons carrying them should be avoided whenever possible.

Among white patients in temperate zones an acute minor respiratory infection is probably the commonest single recognized predisposing factor in lobar pneumonia. Certain phenomena appear to be associated with the occurrence of the minor respiratory infections. Their appearance is followed by an increase in the frequency with which pneumococci are encountered in the upper respiratory tract, especially in persons in contact with patients having pneumonia due to these organisms, and leads to an increase in the biologic activity and the number of pneumococci in the nasopharynx of the individual afflicted. Such respiratory disturbances in persons in contact with patients having pneumococcus pneumonia may be an important factor in determining whether or not the individual becomes a carrier of organisms of the type to which he is exposed (1210). Furthermore, outbreaks of minor respiratory infections are usually followed by an increased incidence of pneumonia, particularly in the colder months of the year.

Thus, as there apparently is a close association between the prevalence of minor respiratory disturbances and the prevalence of pneumonia, the avoidance of the former would doubtless lead to a decrease in the occurrence of the latter. It is not clear at the present time, however, that any reliable method of avoiding or preventing minor respiratory infections other than by positive and absolute isolation is known. For practical purposes such isolation can hardly be considered to exist. It is hoped that future work may reveal some method of preventing these lesser respiratory disturbances. In the interim, individuals having such infections should be especially cautious of their own activities during their affliction, particularly during the first week of it, and avoid conditions tending to chill their body surface, all excesses, and unusual exposure. It is at such times in particular that patients with pneumonia or with any infectious disease and their known contacts, as well as crowds, should be avoided. It would doubtless be advisable in large industrial organizations, mines, mills, institutions, military organizations, and similar groups to separate or isolate from other members of the group individuals with minor respiratory infections, at least during the early and acute stages of such infections. Observations relative to the importance of the control of the minor respiratory disturbances in respect to the prevention of pneumonia have been made by several investigators (222, 301, 226, 1208).

AVOIDANCE OF MARKED TEMPERATURE CHANGES, WETTING, CHILLING, AND THE ASPIRATION OF FOREIGN SUBSTANCES. Exposure to marked variations in temperature, particularly if sudden or prolonged, to wetting or to chilling, predisposes to high rates for pneumonia incidence or mortality, or both, as mentioned in the foregoing chapter, and is to be avoided whenever possible. Likewise, it is desirable to prevent the inhalation of irritating dusts, especially siliceous dusts, fumes and similar noxious substances which were also seen in the previous chapter to lead to high pneumonia rates.

Certain procedures of use in the prevention of post-operative pulmonary complications, including pneumonia, are described in Chapter X (pages 523–524).

AVOIDANCE OF EXCESS. The avoidance of alcoholism, exhaustion, excessive worry, loss of sleep, and inadequate diets, all of which presumably favor the occurrence of pneumonia, is to be recommended.

In temperate zones host resistance may be depressed during the colder months of the year. At such periods individuals should be especially watchful of their general physical condition and, so far as possible, avoid situations which tend to afford opportunities for infection to be acquired.

Community Hygiene

OVERCROWDING. The overcrowding of living, working, or recreational quarters should be prevented, for under such conditions pneumococci may be rapidly passed from person to person. The factor of overcrowding would appear of special significance in temperate zones during the colder months of the year.

OCCUPATIONAL HAZARDS. As already mentioned it was shown in the previous chapter that conditions such as exposure to marked variations in temperature, wetting, chilling, and irritating dusts, particularly siliceous dusts, as well as the performance of strenuous fatiguing labor out of doors in inclement weather, commonly lead to an increased incidence or mortality rate, or both, from pneumonia. Individuals performing certain occupations appeared to suffer an unusual exposure to conditions of this nature (see pages 318–329). Brundage and his co-workers (163) have reported specific recommendations for overcoming many of the exposure factors which operate among some workers in the iron and steel industry. Among other things it was advised that blowers and cool air ventilation be supplied, that high temperature work be mechanized in many instances, and that shelters be provided for out-of-door laborers. Doubtless workers in many occupational groups would experience an improved health record were these and similar suggestions adopted. Further, wherever needed, arrangements should be made to prevent the aspiration of such foreign substances as irritating gases and fumes (see pages 340–342).

SPECIALLY SUSCEPTIBLE POPULATIONS. Certain groups of individuals, such as the native inhabitants of most tropical regions, and in some instances, as in South Africa, of the more temperate areas as well, may be considered as especially susceptible to pneumonia (see pages 268–269, 312–316, and 329–332). This susceptibility is particularly obvious in Negroes. In addition, the experience in several army camps in this country during the last war also showed the great susceptibility of individuals moved from rural districts into crowded camps and from the southern and warmer parts of the United States into camps in northern states.

Thus, persons from isolated, rural, or warm regions when massed together and subjected for military or other purposes to more or less crowded living and working conditions may be considered, so far as pneumonia is concerned, as constituting a susceptible population. Measures to prevent the occurrence and spread of all respiratory diseases, including pneumonia, are specially needed among such groups. Not only should attention be given those points mentioned above, which may apply to the groups under consideration and be useful in preventing such diseases, but certain extra precautions appear definitely indicated.

As in nearly all instances the attack rates and mortality rates from pneumonia are highest among the newest arrivals in the group, most attention should be paid to such individuals. Various investigators have commented on the general measures to be used in army camps. Among others, Cole (296) has considered this matter and Opie, Blake, Small, and Rivers (969) have discussed it at some length. Care should be taken not to overcrowd troop trains and barracks for recruits. Overexhaustion and undue exposure during the first few months of training should be avoided. Promiscuous spitting should be forbidden and handkerchiefs supplied. Facilities should be provided for the prompt care of pathologic conditions of the mouth and upper respiratory tract. Individuals with respiratory infections should be isolated at once. During the first few weeks in camp, mass meetings and the crowding of quarters provided for recreational purposes should be forbidden.

Cole (296) has pointed out the advisability of maintaining two kinds of hospitals in army camps, each of which should have a separate staff. All infectious and contagious diseases may be cared for in one hospital and all other conditions in the other. Within the infectious disease hospital, patients with pneumonia should be kept isolated in separate cubicles (296, 591). This, however, may not prove sufficient, and Opie, Blake, Small, and Rivers (969) regard separate rooms as a necessity. In addition, patients with uncomplicated diseases, such as measles, whooping cough, or influenza, should be kept entirely isolated from persons with pneumococcus infections, who, in turn, should be separated from those with scarlet fever or other streptococcus infections. Attendants carrying hemolytic streptococci in their upper respiratory tract should be excluded from the hospital (969), as presumably should all individuals who might come in contact with patients and who are carrying pneumococci of the more invasive types, such as Type I, II, V, VII, or VIII. Aseptic nursing technic should be used and the wearing of gowns and masks made compulsory for all attendants. Concurrent bacteriologic examination of sputum, throat cultures, blood, and necropsy material from patients with pneumonia should be carried out to determine the nature of the etiologic agent and to evaluate the success of the measures used to prevent the spread of the infecting organisms. Opie, Blake, Small, and Rivers (969) have pointed out that, with an adequate expenditure, the deaths of "thousands of recruits within one month" of entering service might be avoided.

Many of the above measures might be applied with distinct success and considerable profit among groups of individuals gathered together for other than military purposes. Overcrowding must be prevented and close contact in living and recreational rooms avoided. Attention should be given the matter of avoiding chilling while going to or from work or at work and during rest and sleep. Provision should be made to ensure the intake of an adequate diet, and, at mines, work underground should be prohibited during the first few weeks of employment. Special attention should be paid individuals in poor general physical condition. Persons with minor respiratory infections should be isolated from their fellows and not permitted to work until the condition subsides. It would seem highly desirable in the group under discussion to enforce, so far as possible, the strict isolation of all patients with pneumonia, as Gautier (510) has suggested.

In all the groups mentioned in this section, as in other groups made up of individuals employed in occupations associated with high pneumonia incidence and mortality rates, the possibility of using immunizing procedures to increase host resistance is to be considered. This matter is discussed in some detail below (pages 446–478). In especially susceptible groups, where the incidence of pneumonia may be highest within a few days of arrival at the place where residence is to be established, immunizing procedures would presumably yield the best results if undertaken about two weeks in advance of the contemplated change of residence. In many instances it would probably be advisable to repeat the immunizing process at the end of about two months.

Patients with Pneumonia

CARE. Patients with pneumonia, especially in the early days of their illness when the sputum usually contains considerable numbers of the infecting organism, must presumably be regarded as a focus of infection to be avoided. In consequence, most patients when hospitalized are placed in isolation or semi-isolation (see also Isolation, below) and are cared for by attendants observing the usual precautions against infection.

The sputum of patients with pneumonia should be collected in paper receptacles or on paper handkerchiefs or pieces of cloth and at once burned. If metal sputum cups are used, they should be boiled. Concurrent sterilization by boiling should be carried out on all linen, cloth handkerchiefs, dishes, and other articles used by the patient. If sputum comes in contact with the bed, floor, walls, or similar objects, it should be wiped up with disinfectant before it dries. The walls and floors of rooms previously used by patients should be given a thorough wet cleaning before any attempt is made to sweep or stir up dust in any similar manner. Recommendations similar to these have been advanced by several workers (1405, 1440, 33, 296, 297, 298, 301, 852).

Whenever possible, suitable treatment of cases of pneumococcus pneumonia with immune serum specific for the type of pneumococcus causing the infection usually shortens the course of the acute illness when undertaken early, and may possibly also shorten the period during which the patient is actively disseminating considerable numbers of organisms in his immediate surroundings and thus at times shorten the interval during which he may be a menace to his contacts.

ISOLATION. The strict isolation of patients with pneumonia, especially if they are found to be infected with pneumococci of Type I or II, has been advocated by several investigators (33, 296, 591, 297, 969, 1352, 298, 510, 301, 445, 852, 447). For many years Cole (297, 298, 301) has advised the isolation of all cases, and the few visitors who are allowed to see pneumonia patients at the Hospital of the Rockefeller Institute for Medical Research and all the professional attendants of such patients wear masks and gowns. Though he recognized the difficulty of determining the value of such procedures, Cole has suggested that they be followed elsewhere. Cruickshank (331) reported that over a period of several years the isolation of patients with lobar pneumonia had become increasingly common in Glasgow but that results did not seem to justify the practice.

The mortality rates for pneumonia (all forms) in Pittsburgh, Pennsylvania, were formerly the highest of any city in the United States (see pages 276–277). In 1924 a regulation was adopted by which all cases of pneumonia were isolated, as reported by Vaux (1352), and when a case was cared for at home the house was placarded, the patient was isolated in the home, and visitors were prohibited. So long as the isolation was satisfactory, the movements of the family were not restricted. In Pittsburgh this form of modified quarantine has presumably been continued. Subsequent to the adoption of this regulation Pittsburgh's previously large number of pneumonia deaths and high mortality rates from this disease showed an irregular but apparently progressive decrease. How far quarantine and isolation of cases were responsible for the decrease in rates, it is impossible to estimate because of the varied nature of the diseases under consideration and because of accessory factors which may be importantly concerned in this matter, as elsewhere mentioned (see pages 327–328).

As about one-half or more of all persons in the general population may carry pneumococci in their nose or throat at some time each year, it is obvious that these organisms are practically universal in their distribution and are present in the mouths of millions of individuals, only a comparatively few of whom develop pneumonia. At any given time, the number of healthy carriers of pneumococci *of any type* appears to greatly exceed the number of current cases of pneumonia due to representatives of that type. This would appear as true for pneumococci of Type I or II, strains of which are the least frequently encountered among normal persons, as for those of Type III and of the higher types, which are more commonly found in the mouths of normal individuals. Because of this enormous reservoir of organisms in the general population, it seems unlikely that isolation or quarantine, or both, of patients with pneumonia could ever be very effective in controlling the spread of infection under ordinary circumstances (1048, 331).

Smillie and Leeder's (1210) finding of about ten times the proportion of carriers of the homologous type among the family contacts of patients with Type I or II pneumonia as among the hospital contacts of such cases (see pages 359–361) suggests that attention should be directed to the care and isolation of patients treated at home. However, as indicated at the end of the foregoing chapter, this high proportion of homologous type carriers among the family contacts may be the result of the previous spread of pneumococci within the family group. It would appear of considerable importance that this matter be further investigated, for if, as the evidence now suggests, numerous members of the family were already carrying strains of the type in question at the time the patient became ill, it would seem of little use under such circumstances to insist upon the isolation of the case in the hope of preventing the dissemination of the infecting organism to the family contacts of the patient. Despite the difficulties attendant upon the evaluation of procedures such as the isolation or quarantine of patients with pneumonia in reducing the spread of the disease, it may be said that the isolation of patients from all individuals suffering from an acute respiratory infection such as a common cold and from all children should be insisted upon. Persons in the latter groups appear to carry pneumococci and allied pathogenic organisms more frequently than other "normal" individuals and to acquire such organisms easily from patients with pneumonia (see pages 351–362 and 373–377). The isolation of patients from such individuals affords protection from cross infection both to the patient and to the contact.

Carriers of Pneumococci: Isolation and Treatment

As indicated in the previous chapter, it is likely that carriers of pneumococci are far more important in spreading these organisms in the community at large than are cases. Some but not much attention has been paid to carriers, and an effort has been made in only a few instances to isolate pneumococcus carriers and to try by various procedures, such as the local application of medication to the nose and throat, to overcome the carrier condition. Such an undertaking was suggested by Avery, Chickering, Cole, and Dochez (33) and was put into practice for more than one hundred carriers by Sailer, Hall, Wilson, and McCoy (1155), as mentioned below. It was pointed out by the former investigators, however, that the use of local applications to the nose and mouth might be of no avail in curing the carrier condition of convalescent patients, for such individuals may harbor pneumococci in the deeper parts of the respiratory tract.

Gundel and Wasu (584) reported that all carriers of pneumococci of Type I or II must be regarded as suspicious and have recommended that such individuals be isolated and treated to cure the carrier condition or instructed how to avoid spreading the organisms carried. Smillie (1207) isolated all recognized carriers of pneumococci of Type II encountered in an institution during an outbreak of Type II lobar pneumonia. Eventually the inmates were immunized against this type and the epidemic stopped. As carried out, the procedure of isolating the known carriers was regarded as of "questionable" value. It is readily conceivable that, in the future, occasions may arise when groups of individuals carrying pneumococci of a single type may be isolated during attempts to stop outbreaks of infection due to pneumococci of the same type. As little is known of successful methods of treating such carriers in order to eradicate the carrier condition, additional investigations along this line are indicated.

Before considering the measures that have been used in the attempt to cure the carrier condition in man, certain findings relative to the carrier state induced in animals by the intranasal instillation of living pneumococci may be reviewed. Two studies of this nature were reported by Neufeld and Etinger-Tulczynska (933, 934). In their first study it was observed that many mice infected intranasally with Type I or Type II pneumococci became carriers of the corresponding type and that some of these carriers developed a generalized fatal infection. The subcutaneous injection or nasal douching with "optochin" (see pages 778–782) prior to the instillation of pneumococci into the nose did not alter the proportion of animals that became carriers or the subsequent death rate.

In the second investigation mentioned, both guinea pigs and mice were infected intranasally with pneumococci of Type I. Their subsequent injection with potent immune serum of homologous type did not appear to clear up the carrier state. When the specific serum was applied locally as a douche to the nasal passages of similarly infected animals the initial smears showed many extracellular organisms in the nasal secretions, while those made three hours after the use of the serum revealed the presence of active phagocytosis, and at this time most of the organisms were intracellular. Nevertheless, the carrier condition was not completely eradicated by this treatment. In a few guinea-pig carriers, the parenteral administration of 5 cc. of specific immune serum on the second and third days after infection, in combination with nasal irrigations twice a day with the same serum, resulted in a cure of the carrier condition after one or two days. Results of similar significance were obtained in mice. In both mice and guinea pigs the use of normal horse serum for a similar purpose was without effect. In addition to these experiments, the nasal passages of mice carrying pneumococci of Type I were irrigated with certain chemicals to determine whether these substances could cure the carrier state. The daily intranasal instillation of optochin base in oil, of optochin hydrochloride, or of a 5 per cent solution of trypaflavin for periods of several days had little effect on the carrier condition. One-half of one per cent solutions of similar preparations of optochin or of solutions of hydrogen peroxide instilled into the nose twice daily for a week or more also failed to clear up the spontaneous carrier state of guinea pigs carrying pneumococci of Type XIX.

Apparently few attempts have been made to overcome the carrier state in man by means of sprays and applications to the nose and throat. Sailer and his associates (1155) treated in this way 111 men in an army camp who were carriers of pneumococci of Type I, II, or III, or Group IV. The carriers were isolated in the hospital and divided into separate groups containing sixteen men, each group being subdivided into squads of four men each. The same treatment was given the men in each squad in a given group, but the intensity of treatment and frequency of its administration were varied. Periodic cultures were taken of the nose and throat to determine the efficacy of the measures used. Eleven preparations, such as Dichloramin-T dissolved in eucalyptol or in chlorcosane, phenol in oil or glycerin, quinine sulphate, tincture of iodine in oil, and the like, were used. The first-named preparation was given by intranasal spray for fifteen seconds in each nostril and was sprayed in the throat for thirty seconds. Phenol in oil was administered intranasally by dropping the solution into the nose. (This proved the most effective means of avoiding the occurrence of middle ear infections with this material.)

In general, two treatments a day gave the best results. An oily solution of phenol or iodine was the most effective preparation though results were also good with Dichloramin-T dissolved in eucalyptol. In a number of instances pneumococci were reported to have disappeared from the nasopharyngeal cultures of the carriers within a week after the institution of such treatment. In view of the circumstances surrounding the experiment and the somewhat unsatisfactory technic used to detect pneumococci in the cultures, the observations may be considered of interest but not necessarily reproducible on another occasion.

Neufeld and Etinger-Tulczynska (934) failed to cure the carrier state in eight infants, each of whom over a period of several days received an intranasal instillation twice a day of a few drops of a 5 per cent solution of optochin base in oil.

The animal experiments reported above suggest that it is possible to cure the carrier state by combining local and general therapeutic measures. It would be of interest to determine how far the local treatment of human carriers was successful when combined with immunizing procedures of an active or passive nature. Because of the large number of persons involved, it would appear futile to advocate the treatment of all carriers of pneumococci in the hope of eradicating their carrier condition. However, in localized outbreaks of pneumonia, when pneumococci of a single type are involved, some effort to control carriers might be made while other procedures for combating the outbreak were being instituted.

Individuals suffering from nasal obstruction, tonsillitis, sinusitis, and allied conditions may carry pneumococci more frequently than other persons not experiencing such difficulties. The correction of pathologic conditions of this nature would presumably assist in clearing up or forestalling the development of a carrier condition (see pages 375–376).

Immunization Against Pneumonia and Minor Respiratory Infections

In various localities numerous efforts have been made to increase the resistance of man by active immunization against the pneumococcus and in this way to effect a decrease in the incidence of pneumonia due to this organism, as is discussed in some detail later (pages 446–482). Such measures have also been used in an attempt to decrease the incidence of minor acute respiratory infections, including the common cold, in the immunized group. In the latter instance, following the use of vaccines containing pneumococci, and at times other organisms as well, a suggestive (Maynard, 874) or definite (Peall, 1007) reduction in the incidence of such minor disturbances was obtained among vaccinated Negroes in Africa. Success was also reported by Duckwall (382) among American army troops in this country. However, among various groups of white civilians in this country, Von Sholly and Park (1359), Park (988), and Jordan and Sharp (693), and, in England, Ferguson, Davey, and Topley (436) found immunization to be of little or no value in reducing the incidence of minor respiratory infections; and Brown (160) in the United States failed to obtain a reduction in the incidence of the common cold following such a procedure.

Stoltenberg (1249) gave immunizing injections of a mixed autogenous vaccine to a group of 487 infants and children in Norway in an effort to reduce the incidence of respiratory infections among such individuals who had been hospitalized for various reasons (see also pages 472–473). The patients immunized received three subcutaneous injections of varying doses of vaccine at intervals of four to six days. The study extended over a period of nearly four years. As suitable controls were lacking, the incidence of various respiratory infections in the vaccinated group was compared with the incidence of such disturbances in 496 patients of similar ages who had been cared for in the same hospital during a period of about three years prior to the introduction of the immunizing procedure. The incidence of all respiratory and allied infections, which included bronchitis, pneumonia, otitis media, and the like, was 47.9 per cent in the control group as compared with 20.1 per cent in the vaccinated group. The findings suggested that immunization was responsible for the lowered incidence of such infections in the vaccinated children. Results were most marked in infants under one year of age, as the immunized individuals in that group had only one-fifth as many respiratory infections as the controls of similar age. The mean duration of all infections was nearly the same in both the immunized and the control groups regardless of age. It should be noted that Stoltenberg's study embraced observations on the incidence of many of the more serious infections of the respiratory tract and was not limited to those of lesser severity such as the common cold.

Kneeland (731) carried out a somewhat similar investigation in a group of twenty-three children in an infants' home in New York City. These infants were given two courses of subcutaneous injections of increasing doses of a mixed vaccine containing pneumococci of Type I and selected strains of streptococci and influenza bacilli. The first course consisted of nine weekly injections begun in October, and the second of seven injections was begun in February. The study period extended from October through May.

The number of colds was the same in both the vaccinated and the control groups, but there was a significant reduction in the severity of the more serious secondary forms of respiratory infection among the immunized. The findings suggested that the protection afforded by vaccination against secondary invaders during colds was due to the immunity engendered, the duration of which was about two months. Observations of similar significance covering a two-year period were reported from a children's home in New York City by Wallfield (1375). Eight semi-weekly subcutaneous injections of increasing doses of a mixed stock vaccine were given nineteen infants and children under six years of age the first year, and thirty-four received such vaccine the second year. In each year a single course of injections was given beginning in October. The incidence of colds was influenced little if at all among the vaccinated, but the severity of the secondary infections which occurred was reduced.

The above observations suggest that adequate immunizing procedures might be of value in reducing the incidence or severity of the more serious secondary complications which so frequently follow minor respiratory infections. Additional studies are necessary, however, to extend these findings and to define the nature of the most satisfactory vaccine for use and the optimum dosage and time of administration. It is possible that the constitution of the vaccine yielding satisfactory results in infants and children would need alteration and the elimination or addition of some other organisms to prove effective in adults. If success follows such investigations and a suitable vaccine or other immunizing agent of known antigenicity can be obtained, it would seem advisable to consider the periodic administration of immunizing agents to selected individuals or groups of individuals in whom, under ordinary circumstances, acute minor respiratory infections are frequent and are commonly followed by the occurrence of severe secondary complications.

ACTIVE IMMUNIZATION AGAINST THE PNEUMOCOCCUS

Much evidence that immunizing procedures may be of value in the prophylaxis of pneumonia was presented in the chapter on Aspects of Immunity (page 113). The resistance of many of the higher animals to infection with pneumococci of a given type has often been markedly increased by their artificial immunization with a suitable antigen containing or prepared from pneumococci of the homologous type, as shown by the appearance in their blood of circulating antibodies specific for pneumococci of the same type (see pages 127–129, 158–168, and 196–199). The resistance or antibody, or both, engendered by vaccination is largely, but not always wholly, type-specific in nature (see pages 133–136).*

As the mechanism of acquired immunity in man appears to function in a manner analogous to that in many animals, it has seemed reasonable to hope that the immunization of man would also lead to an increase in resistance and so to a decrease in the incidence of pneumonia. While immunity does not develop to the same degree in all individuals following immunization, and in some cases no resistance may become demonstrable, there is evidence to suggest that on the whole the immunologic mechanism in man is more responsive than in animals. While both commonly respond to the administration of a suitable immunizing agent with the production of immunity of a type-specific nature, a response for some heterologous type or types appears to develop much more frequently in man than in animals. Moreover, the duration of the immune response following immunization may possibly last longer in man than in animals.

Prior to discussing the results obtained from the use of immunizing procedures in an effort to prevent pneumococcus pneumonia in animals and man, certain aspects of the problem of increasing immunity to the pneumococcus by vaccination and the more obvious factors which influence the level of the active immunity or antibody evoked need discussion. For this purpose consideration must be given to observations which were carried out chiefly but not entirely on experimental animals. Certain studies in man in which data were obtained on the development of circulating antibodies will be included in the review. In the following section attention will be directed primarily to the use of immunizing agents made from or containing pneumococci of known type. The results of numerous extensive experiments are of importance in clearly indicating the great need for attention to detail in the conduct of immunizing programs. Many references will be given to pertinent studies, which with some exceptions will be considered in a general way. The literature has been reviewed by Barach (69) and White, with Robinson and Barnes (1417), and the latter workers have prepared an extensive survey of matters relating to immunization.

In this discussion, the development of humoral antibody or of resistance to infection will frequently be considered to indicate the acquisition of immunity. Comment will be confined chiefly to the production of immunity

* The somewhat peculiar non-specific variety of immunity produced by the immunization of rabbits with large doses of the whole cells of smooth or rough strains of pneumococci, as determined by Tillett (1309, 1310) and Julianelle (699), is considered elsewhere (see page 136).

of a type-specific nature. It is apparent that numerous factors concerned with the procedures used have a bearing on the successful outcome of efforts made to actively immunize against the pneumococcus. Consideration will be given to the character of the immunizing agent, the route of injection, the doses and schedule of injections used, and the types of pneumococci represented in the antigen. Variations in one or more of these factors may have a significant relation to the degree, time of appearance, and duration of the immunity induced and, in consequence, have a bearing on the active immunization of man for the prevention of pneumonia.

It should be noted at this point that during the past twenty-five years or so one or more of several kinds of tests have been applied to measure the quality of the active resistance (or antibody) evoked by immunization. These tests have not all been carried out under comparable conditions. Many of the reports available state that the immunity produced in animals was sufficient to protect against a determined number of minimum fatal doses of live pneumococci of the homologous type. It is now apparent that the virulence of the live organisms used for such tests may vary markedly with the passage of time and be different in different laboratories, or even within the same laboratory at different times. In addition the inherent resistance of the usual stock strains of animals used in protection tests may and does vary widely. It is only within recent years that suitable protection tests for antibody determinations have been carried out in parallel, one group of animals receiving the serum of unknown titer under test and the other a standard serum of known potency, in order that the potency of the test serum might be determined in terms of a standard. As a consequence of the situation here briefly outlined, caution must be exercised in attempting to compare too closely the results of many investigations dealing with the efficacy of immunizing procedures.

Character of the Immunizing Agent

Numerous agents, such as suspensions of pneumococci killed in various ways, or autolysates, solutions, or culture filtrates of pneumococci, or solutions of chemical components of these organisms, such as the specific capsular polysaccharide or substances presumably closely allied to this material, have been employed for immunizing purposes. The immune response is importantly affected by the immunizing agent used. The response, when pneumococcal vaccine is administered, is usually greater the more closely the organism used approaches the natural state of the intact, living, vigorous, fully specific, virulent cell, as mentioned in the chapter on Aspects of Immunity, where it was also pointed out that the antigenic properties of intact pneumococcus cells are different from those exhibited by many preparations of disrupted cells, the former being superior to the latter as immunizing agents for the production of specific immunity, as Avery and his associates (43, 46, 51, 44) have clearly shown (see pages 133–134).

Though the matter is chiefly of academic interest from the standpoint of prophylactic vaccination, live virulent organisms used for immunizing purposes evoke the most pronounced immune response (1388, 1389, 932, 1361, 1363, 308, 231, 1238, 1243, 841, 1240, 1260). Where killed pneumococci are employed, experience has shown that vaccines containing many autolyzed organisms should be avoided, as should those prepared from feebly growing cultures of dubious specificity and little virulence. In the usual instance, the higher the virulence of the culture used as a source of the vaccine, the better is the immune response, as Neufeld (932) and others have demonstrated (1361, 936, 33, 231, 240, 1243, 69, 1129).

Efforts have been made to determine the comparative value of vaccines made from cultures grown on various kinds of media (874, 1447, 785, 786, 125, 788), but the results have appeared largely inconclusive. In the usual instance virulent pneumococci freshly isolated from a human case of pneumonia have been found most satisfactory. Such organisms grown in beef heart infusion broth with the addition of a small amount of dextrose and acid sodium phosphate or some similar buffer presumably make a suitable antigen (1207). The use of a large inoculum to ensure rapid growth would also appear of importance. The fraction of a per cent of phenol, tricresol, formaldehyde, or some other chemical is usually added to the vaccine as a preservative. Lister and Ordman (788) consider the factors primarily concerned in the preparation of an efficient vaccine are:

> . . . (a) the medium used for the isolation of the organism, (b) the number and frequency of subcultures made of the organism before it was killed, (c) the mode of killing of the organism, e.g., by heat, antiseptics, etc., (d) the preservative used in making up the final vaccine, (e) the length of time and mode of storage of the vaccine before it is used prophylactically.

Suspensions of pneumococci may lose their antigenicity during a period of two months even if stored in the refrigerator (433), and each batch of vaccine prepared should be tested for antigenicity before being released for use (125, 222, 434).

While it is apparent that under suitable conditions intact-cell or whole-cell vaccine will make a reasonably adequate antigen, it is now also obvious that some immunity will be produced following the administration of various soluble derivatives of the pneumococcus. Whether cell-free solutions or certain preparations of autolysates of pneumococci or filtrates, either of cultures or of suspensions of shaken organisms, are used, the specific immunity that results is presumably due primarily to the specific capsular polysaccharide or allied substance contained in such mixtures, which has been shown to be antigenic in both animals and man.

SUSPENSIONS OF KILLED PNEUMOCOCCI. Pneumococci killed by various means and suspended in saline, glucose, broth, or some similar vehicle have been more widely used for immunizing purposes than any other pneumococcus antigen. In animals, following the administration of an antigen of this nature, a variable degree of immunity was shown to develop:

In mice (1012, 1238, 1243, 68, 69, 434, 433)
In rabbits (932, 936, 1363, 785, 628, 1448, 68, 69, 532, 173, 698, 699, 1258, 1241, 737, 1078, 1077, 1245, 739, 77)
In guinea pigs (841)
In rats (1129, 1131, 1135, 1136, 1137)
In donkeys (936)
In horses (936, 33)
In monkeys (125, 240, 738)

In man, the use of such antigens was considered to have produced immunity:

Either because specific humoral antibody became demonstrable (785, 228, 71, 72, 1135, 1138, 433)
Or because the incidence of pneumonia in the immunized group apparently decreased or was lower than that experienced in groups chosen as controls (874, 1447, 785, 786, 228, 382, 140, 1359, 988, 1249, 731, 788, 1007, 971, 1207)

In most instances the pneumococci in the vaccines used have been killed by heating the culture or a suspension of the organisms at 55° to 60° C. for an hour or more (936, 1447, 785, 308, 33, 228, 628, 125, 240, 1012, 1238, 1243, 68, 69, 173, 698, 699, 1258, 71, 1241, 1131, 737, 434, 1078, 1077, 1245, 77, 788). Heat-killed vaccines were used almost exclusively in the early investigations of the resistance induced by immunization with this organism and are still widely employed for this and similar purposes. In addition, and especially in recent years, attention has been paid to the use of vaccines containing pneumococci killed by the action of dilute carbolic acid, hydrochloric acid, formaldehyde, or other chemicals (785, 786, 308, 1129, 1131, 737, 434, 738, 739, 1135, 1136, 1138, 77, 433, 1207). In either instance pneumococci from young vigorously growing cultures (usually seven to nine hours old) which are killed at about the time of their maximum rate of multiplication and before significant autolysis appears have proved the most satisfactory.

Comparisons of the antigenicity of various vaccines and allied immunizing agents have been made by numerous workers. In several instances the results obtained are difficult to correlate with the conclusions reached or with the findings of other studies, for the different preparations used were not given by the same routes. In general, however, it seems that a suitable intact-cell vaccine usually evokes an immune response which is frequently better or appears somewhat earlier than that obtained by solutions of the whole organisms or by culture filtrates or similar agents (785, 1238, 68, 69, 699, 71, 737). Nevertheless, in several instances when intact, killed pneumococci, desiccated mechanically disrupted organisms, or bile-salt solutions of the organisms were used as antigens under more or less identical conditions, the response to the various agents administered was reported to be about the same with each antigen (Ross, 1129, 1135, 1136, 1138).

Vaccines containing acid-killed pneumococci may be inferior to those containing organisms killed by other chemicals (738, 739). While formalin-killed vaccines may be somewhat better than heat-killed (434), there is good evidence that in animals the amount of antibody developed as a consequence of the injection of these antigens is about the same in both cases but that the immune response may appear earlier after the use of heat-killed vaccines (Barnes and White, 77). In man, acetone-killed vaccines may be more efficient than heat-killed vaccines (Felton, Sutliff, and Steele, 433). The problem of the most suitable method of killing pneumococci for use in vaccines is involved and seems by no means to be settled as yet.

The immunity induced by the vaccination of animals with suspensions of pneumococci is largely (936, 938, 785, 33, 1448, 69, 1258, 77) but not always wholly type-specific in nature (628, 1243, 173, 699). Using vaccines containing acetone-killed pneumococci of Type I or II, Felton, Sutliff, and Steele (433) obtained in animals an antibody response for the homologous type only, while in man some heterologous type antibody also became demonstrable.

In a few instances pneumococcus lipovaccines have been used for immunizing purposes. The dried organisms were suspended in olive or cottonseed oil to which at times a small amount of lanolin was added (246). The immunization of animals with vaccines of this nature gave rise to a low grade of immunity (628, 125), and the immunization of man probably lessened the incidence of pneumonia among the immunized, as reported in some studies (246, 1119), though this effect was not always observed (831). Cecil (221, 222) reviewed this work and concluded that the results obtained with pneumococcus lipovaccines were far inferior to those secured by the use of vaccines containing organisms suspended in saline.

AUTOLYSATES, CULTURE FILTRATES, AND SOLUTIONS OF PNEUMOCOCCI. The administration of certain autolysates, filtrates of cultures or shaken suspensions of pneumococci, or solutions of these organisms prepared by dissolving pneumococci with bile salts has given rise to the appearance of a variable but usually not marked degree of immunity in animals (724, 1363, 308, 1118, 1012, 68, 69, 1129, 1131, 1132, 737, 1135, 1136) and to the occasional development of humoral antibody in man (71, 461, 1138). In the latter instance Ross (1138) reported that the level of the demonstrable protective antibody which developed was about the same as that appearing in the blood of humans convalescent from pneumococcus lobar pneumonia, which is usually rather low, being in the neighborhood of protection against 5,000 minimum lethal doses or less in most instances. An immune response is less regularly evoked by autolysates, culture filtrates, or solutions of pneumococci than by whole-cell vaccine, and, if it appears, is usually of a lower grade and slower in development.

SPECIFIC CAPSULAR POLYSACCHARIDES AND ALLIED AGENTS. The antigenicity of chemical derivatives of the pneumococcus, such as the specific capsular polysaccharide or substances presumed to be closely allied, has already been mentioned (see pages 133–134). Because of their potential importance as immunizing agents, great interest has been aroused in such substances. Once prepared, they are relatively stable and much easier to handle on a large scale than are most other immunizing agents.

Schiemann and Casper (1160) immunized mice, either with derivatives of pneumococci of Type I, II, or III, which they regarded as probably identical with the specific capsular polysaccharide of these organisms, or with intact-cell vaccines of these types. In the case of Type III only, the antigen produced a more pronounced specific immune response than the vaccine of this type. Evidence somewhat similar to this was reported by Felton (422) whose study of mice receiving a single injection of the preparations under test suggested that Type I and II antigens induced a higher level of immunity than did whole-cell vaccine of these types. After the administration of specific capsular polysaccharides or more or less closely related preparations, immunity for the homologous type, and in some instances for some heterologous types in addition, may become demonstrable in animals (1470) or man (461, 433, 425). In the course of antibody studies in human beings following their injection with either vaccines or antigens prepared from pneumococci of Type I or II, Felton, Sutliff, and Steele (433) observed that the antigens employed produced a much greater heterologous antibody response than vaccine.

Despite the theoretical implications of the above findings, conclusive evidence is as yet lacking that chemical derivatives of the pneumococcus are superior to properly prepared vaccines for immunizing purposes. In fact the reverse seems to be true, at least in so far as the use of such agents for the production of specific antipneumococcic serum of high antibody titer is concerned.

For practical purposes the use of specific derivatives of pneumococci as immunizing agents is, of course, still in the experimental stage. The technical difficulties of preparing suitable antigens of this nature are at times considerable. In large doses these derivatives of the pneumococcus appear to inhibit rather than to stimulate the development of immunity (see pages 131–132). For immunizing purposes the best results have been obtained with small doses. During the past few years the immunization of man on a large scale with substances of this nature made available by Felton (425) has been undertaken in various localities in this country in an effort to ascertain the value of such derivatives for the prevention of pneumonia. His preliminary figures (425) suggest that the incidence of pneumonia was reduced among the immunized groups (see page 474).

Route of Administration

The immune response elicited by pneumococcus immunizing agents may be importantly affected by the route by which these preparations are given (724). Parenteral injection has been the means most often employed. The results obtained by giving suspensions of pneumococci and related preparations by various routes will be considered first, following which the response to pneumococcus specific capsular polysaccharide or some allied substance will be dealt with.

When pneumococcus vaccines, solutions of these organisms, or culture filtrates are used, the response to injection by the intradermal, subcutaneous, or intramuscular route is of lower grade than the response to injection by the intraperitoneal or particularly the intravenous route. Reports of studies of immunization by different routes are listed below:

Intradermal (698, 699, 71, 461, 1077, 595)
Subcutaneous (785, 228, 240, 71, 1241, 72, 738, 739, 740)
Intramuscular (1241, 72)
Intraperitoneal (841, 68, 1258, 1241)
Intravenous (936, 785, 308, 33, 240, 698, 699, 1241, 71, 1077, 77, 595)

In most of the reports cited, observations were limited to experimental studies of animals. In the few instances where the results of studies of man were given, it appears that the antibody response was greater following vaccination by the intravenous route (Lister, 785, Barach, 71) than by the intradermal (Barach, 71), subcutaneous (Lister, 785, Cecil and Austin, 228, Barach, 71, 72), or intramuscular (Barach, 72) route. The level of the antibody appearing under these various conditions is discussed in the following section on dosage (page 418). Barach's (71) observations on a group of human beings given injections of the filtrates either of cultures or suspensions of shaken pneumococci or of vaccine are of interest. Each of the preparations was tested intravenously, and at times intradermally or subcutaneously as well. Among twenty-three individuals given vaccine intravenously, homologous type protective substance appeared in the blood of twenty or 87 per cent, as it did in the blood of 89 per cent or in eight of nine persons receiving intravenous injections of filtrates. However, after the intradermal injection of vaccine such antibody appeared in only ten or 42 per cent of twenty-four persons inoculated, and in two individuals given vaccine subcutaneously no protective substance became demonstrable.

Routes other than those mentioned above have also been used to administer vaccines for immunizing purposes. The intratracheal injection of vaccine into monkeys (241, 243) gave rise to about as favorable an immune response as the intravenous injection of identical preparations, while little if any immunity was produced in similar animals by merely spraying the vaccine into their throats. Considerable immunity developed in mice and rabbits subjected to the inhalation of sprayed vaccines or to the intranasal instillation of suspensions of killed pneumococci (1238, 1243, 1258, 933). The injection of vaccine into the buccal submucosa of rabbits also gave rise to resistance (1258).

During the past decade or more, attempts have been made to produce immunity to the pneumococcus by the oral administration of vaccines, culture filtrates, or solutions of these organisms. In animals the immunizing agent has been administered in the food or by stomach tube, while in man it has usually been dried and given between meals in capsules or suspended in water. Oral immunization, with the consequent appearance of some immunity, was demonstrated by Ross, who fed rats and dogs the tissues of other animals dead from pneumococcus infection (1126, 1127). This investigator obtained similar results in rats fed with dead or living pneumococci, solutions of these organisms, or culture filtrates (1127, 1129, 1131, 1135, 1136, 1137). Ross (1135, 1138) also demonstrated that humoral antibody production followed the oral administration of vaccines to man. In most instances the level of the antibody which developed was about the same as that usually found in the serum of patients convalescent from pneumococcus pneumonia. Findings essentially similar to those reported by Ross were obtained by Kolmer and Rule in rabbits (737, 739, 740) and in a few monkeys (738). The quality of the immunity obtained was compared with that resulting from the subcutaneous vaccination of similar animals. Even after the use of larger doses of vaccine, the resistance evoked by oral immunization was usually of lower grade and shorter duration than that produced by subcutaneous vaccination. Thus far, oral immunization has proved rather unreliable and of limited value. Nevertheless, the above observations may be of importance and open up new fields of endeavor which at present appear in need of further investigation.

So far as the quality of the immune response elicited is concerned, the intravenous administration of vaccines would appear to be the technic of choice, and the intravenous route has proved the most suitable means of immunizing animals for the production of specific diagnostic and therapeutic serums of high antibody titer. For the purpose of vaccinating large numbers of humans in an effort to prevent pneumonia, however, this method of administering immunizing agents is cumbersome and time consuming and, in consequence, the subcutaneous route has been most often used. For human use, the relative ease with which various preparations may be given orally may prove a factor of prime importance in later investigations.

Some information is at hand relating to the immune response obtained as a result of the administration by several routes of pneumococcus specific capsular polysaccharide or of what appear to be closely related chemical fractions of these organisms. The intraperitoneal injection of such preparations has produced definite immunity in the mouse (1160, 422, 1470, 41, 395), as has subcutaneous injection (1012, 1011, 1470) or intravenous injection (422, 1470) into this animal, the time of appearance and the degree of immunity developed being about the same regardless of the route of injection employed (Felton, 422, Zozaya and Clark, 1470). The oral administration of several preparations of the specific capsular polysaccharides was shown by Ross (1130, 1132, 1133, 1134) to lead to the subsequent development of some active immunity in rats but not in mice. The level of the immunity developing in rats fed with such agents appeared slightly less than that produced by feeding intact-cell vaccine or solutions of pneumococci..

In man, the intradermal injection of specific capsular polysaccharides or presumably related compounds is usually followed by the appearance of some humoral antibody (485, 459, 461, 1469, 478). Though previously absent, protective substances against from 10 to 10,000 or more otherwise fatal doses may appear, as may pneumococcidal power of sufficient degree to allow 0.5 cc. of blood to kill from 1,000 to 10,000 or more pneumococci of homologous type (Finland and Sutliff, 461, Zozaya and Clark, 1469, Francis, 478). As the intradermal injection of the specific capsular polysaccharide in man evokes the production of humoral antibodies which are almost wholly type-specific in nature, the results obtained by its use seem to differ somewhat from those obtained by the injection into the skin of whole-cell vaccine, which less frequently gives rise to the appearance of type-specific immune substances. Felton, Sutliff, and Steele (433) vaccinated a group of normal individuals subcutaneously with various chemical fractions of the pneumococcus which apparently owed their antigenicity to the characteristics responsible for this action in the specific capsular polysaccharide of these organisms. In most instances vaccination resulted in the appearance of protective substance or in a tenfold increase in the level of this antibody in the blood of these persons. Similar antigens given in like fashion were demonstrated by Felton (425) to give rise to the appearance of humoral protective substance in the blood of 97 per cent of 180 inoculated men within one month after the injection. Protective substance varying in amount from "one protective unit per c.c. of serum to 0.01 unit" appeared in the blood of these men.

Dosage: Vaccines and Similar Preparations

In the more exact sense, little attention was apparently paid in some of the early studies of animals to the dosage and schedule of injections of the immunizing agent. Nevertheless, the Klemperers (724) and Washbourn (1389) used repeated injections and in 1909 Neufeld and Händel (936) clearly stated that the most satisfactory procedure was to give repeated, gradually increasing doses of vaccine at frequent intervals over periods of several weeks or months.

Unless otherwise stated, the results discussed below relate to the immunity developed against pneumococci of the homologous type. In most cases the preparations used were made from cultures or contained pneumococci of Type I or II, though at times pneumococci of some other type or types were represented in the antigen.

In general, it seems likely that so long as the optimum amount of the preparation is used, dosage has less importance in respect to the effect on the time of appearance of immunity than on the level and duration of the resistance incited. The optimum amount of an immunizing agent may vary with animals of different species and between individuals within the species and from man to man.

VACCINES AND SIMILAR PREPARATIONS IN ANIMALS. The effect of varying the dosage of vaccines and preparations of a similar nature has been rather widely studied. Though small doses of such agents may suffice to immunize small animals, larger doses are usually required in the larger animals. In a general way, following the administration by any route at intervals of one to several days of gradually increasing doses of vaccines or related preparations made from or containing pneumococci of considerable virulence, the highest and most durable immunity is produced in those animals receiving the largest total dose of the antigen used. The findings of numerous investigators involving the use of mice (1238, 1243, 69, 434), rabbits (785, 308, 33, 1258, 1241, 434, 739, 77), rats (1126, 1127, 1135, 1136), horses (308, 33), and monkeys (125, 231, 240) support such a conclusion. Nevertheless, if the individual doses given are too large, little or no immunity becomes demonstrable. Furthermore, in specific instances the route of injection is of considerable importance, as mentioned above. In consequence it seems desirable to compare, so far as possible with the data available, the quality of the immunity induced when varying doses of antigens are administered by similar routes.

Intravenous route. Repeated intravenous injections of suspensions of killed pneumococci were given by Lister (785), Cole and Moore (308), and several other workers (33, 240, 69, 1241, 1245, 77). In addition, studies were made of the effects of single intravenous injections of several agents of this nature by Cole and Moore (308) and Barach (69), and of single injections of vaccine by Stillman (1241).

Lister (785) gave rabbits an injection of vaccine every seven days for three weeks. Specific antibody production was demonstrated (agglutinins and opsonins); and, with preparations containing pneumococci of a single "group" (see page 22) or type, the immune response was better following doses of 400 million organisms each than following doses of 100 million organisms. Essentially similar results were obtained following the injection according to the same schedule of divided doses of vaccine containing pneumococci of five groups or types, the amount given individual animals totaling 2,000, 3,000, or 6,000 million organisms. Antibodies developed for each of the types included in the vaccine, and the response was greatest in the animals receiving the largest doses. Very large doses, however, totaling 30,000 million organisms each, failed to evoke the production of demonstrable antibodies. With three injections at seven-day intervals of doses of about 400 million pneumococci each, sufficient immunity developed to protect rabbits from infection with live pneumococci of homologous type to the extent of eight times the usual fatal dose, the latter being taken as 100 million organisms.

In a more extensive study of this nature Cole and Moore (308) investigated the most satisfactory immunizing schedule in rabbits for the production of immune serum of high antibody titer. Several groups of animals were used, each series receiving intravenous injections according to a different schedule. It was demonstrated that, if injections were given at intervals of seven or eight days, considerable difficulty was encountered in producing much immunity, and, in fact, if large doses were given at such intervals, antibody production appeared depressed. A satisfactory response was obtained when the first doses were small, each for example containing about the same number of organisms as are contained in from 2 to 5 cc. of the original broth culture, and subsequent doses of increasing size were given at weekly intervals till the individual doses contained the number of organisms in from 1 to 2 liters of broth culture. The original twelve to fifteen hour broth cultures from which the vaccine was prepared contained about 200 to 300 million pneumococci per cubic centimeter. Much better results were obtained, however, when the rabbits received several series of daily injections of a small dose of vaccine for seven days, with a week's rest between each series. In this instance the individual doses were much smaller and varied in size from the number of organisms contained in from 1 to 2 cc. of the original culture. Specific agglutinins became demonstrable in dilutions as high as 1:400 and protective substance against approximately 100,000 minimum fatal doses. Where the daily immunizing injections were continued for fourteen days before allowing a rest period, the results were less satisfactory. Cole and Moore (308) continued their work and immunized horses for the production of therapeutic antipneumococcic serum. Repeated intravenous injections were given, first of gradually increasing doses of killed organisms at daily intervals with rest periods between each group of seven or eight injections, and later of increasing doses of live organisms injected according to a similar schedule. Antibody in relatively high titer was produced as a result of these procedures.

Barach (69) also obtained a good antibody response from the intravenous injection of rabbits with several doses of vaccine at daily intervals, the total amount averaging 2 to 5 billion organisms per animal. Stillman's (1241) findings in the rabbit were much the same, and he noted that the titer of the protective substance which appeared in the blood was as high after administering a single dose of 1 cc. of vaccine as after fifteen doses of the same size, though protective substance persisted longer when the larger doses were used. Stillman and Goodner (1245) likewise produced a good immune response in rabbits given three injections of vaccine at four-day intervals. Each injection contained the number of pneumococci present in 30 cc. of the original culture.

Barnes and White (77) recently reinvestigated the immunization of rabbits by intravenous injections of vaccine. Doses of different size were given at varying intervals. The results obtained were graded according to determinations of the titer of the antibody produced. Three series of three injections at one-day intervals with a week's rest between each series were found preferable to three series of five injections at daily intervals with weekly rest periods between each course. The doses used varied from 0.1 to 4.0 cc. of vaccine, which was standardized by the Gates apparatus at 1.5. The number of organisms in 1 cc. of vaccine was equivalent to that in about 2 to 3 cc. of the original broth culture. It was found best to give doses of gradually increasing size till fairly large doses (3 to 4 cc. of vaccine) were used, and then give doses of about the same size as "holding" doses, rather than to give small, then large, doses, and then drop back to small and subsequently increase again to large doses. With the former technic, serums of high antibody content were produced. The titer of the protective substance in these serums was determined in units and measured from 1,800 to more than 2,000 units per cubic centimeter. Such titers were possibly equivalent to many million minimum fatal doses. While it was observed that those rabbits receiving the largest total doses of vaccine had the highest titer of protective substance in their serum, it was nevertheless definitely noted that the optimum dosage for immunizing purposes was still not clear.

With various extracts and solutions of pneumococci given intravenously to rabbits in repeated doses, Cole and Moore (308) were able to obtain only a low grade of immunity. They also pointed out that frequent small doses of such antigens given at intervals of a few days to a week were much more effective than were larger doses at longer intervals. Barach (69) gave single intravenous injections of similar preparations to rabbits and obtained some antibody in each instance.

Cecil and Steffen (240) produced good active immunity in monkeys (*Macacus rhesus*) with four intravenous injections of vaccine given at intervals of seven days. The doses used contained 300, 400, 800, and 1,200 million pneumococci.

Subcutaneous route. Varying amounts of vaccine have been administered subcutaneously to rabbits (785, 1241, 434, 739) and monkeys (125, 231, 240, 242, 738). In the former animal, Lister (785) employed three doses at seven-day intervals, the total amounts given ranging from 3,000 to 9,000 million organisms. The antibody response to the largest doses was considered as good as that obtained from the injection of smaller doses intravenously. Stillman (1241) made the unusual observation in rabbits vaccinated subcutaneously that the protective antibody which appeared persisted longer and was of higher titer when two or three doses were given than when fifteen doses were given. This finding appeared anomalous, however, for, using other routes to inject vaccine, protective substance persisted longest in animals receiving the largest number of doses. A fair active resistance was produced in rabbits injected with doses of 100 to 500 million or more pneumococci given three or more times (434, 739).

In monkeys, as Blake and Cecil (125) showed, doses of vaccine containing avirulent pneumococci totaling 16 billion organisms given subcutaneously failed to protect these animals from a subsequent experimental infection. Nevertheless, with larger doses of a suitable vaccine containing virulent pneumococci, Cecil and Steffen (240) obtained good active resistance in such animals (*M. rhesus, M. syrichtus,* and *C. capucinus*). In this instance three subcutaneous injections were usually made, and individual doses of 20, 40, and 60 billion organisms were given at seven-day intervals, the total dose amounting to 120 billion pneumococci. In another study Cecil and Steffen (242) demonstrated the presence of resistance in monkeys vaccinated in similar fashion, the total doses ranging from 120 to 200 billion organisms. Though less conclusive, results somewhat similar to these were also obtained in monkeys by Kolmer and Rule (738). Amounts of vaccine equivalent to 20 million organisms per kilogram of body weight were injected every five days for six doses.

Intraperitoneal route. Varying doses of vaccines and related preparations have been injected intraperitoneally into mice (68, 69, 434) and rabbits (1241). Mice receiving single doses of such agents equivalent to 200 million pneumococci successfully resisted subsequent infection with 10,000 minimum fatal doses of live culture (Barach, 68). In a similar investigation Barach (69) used both single and repeated daily injections in mice, the total dose administered averaging from 200 to 400 million organisms, and with the larger doses obtained protection against as many as 100,000 minimum infecting doses. In a few mice given three injections of vaccine at three- to five-day intervals, Ferguson (434) obtained protection against 10,000 lethal doses with amounts of vaccine equivalent to three million organisms. With doses of vaccine of increasing size, the immunity produced tended to increase; and, with quantities of vaccine totaling twelve million pneumococci, protection was obtained against 100,000 minimum infecting doses. Stillman (1241) demonstrated the development of an antibody response in rabbits vaccinated intraperitoneally which, when from six to fifteen 1 cc. doses were used, approached the quality of the immune response obtained by the intravenous injection of like doses.

Oral route. The effect of giving varying doses of vaccines and similar agents orally has been investigated in rats by Ross (1126, 1127, 1129, 1136, 1137) and in rabbits (737, 739) and monkeys (738) by Kolmer and Rule. Ross (1126) observed that rats fed for several days 7 grams a day of the tissues of animals dead of pneumococcus infection developed sufficient immunity to withstand intraperitoneal infection with 1,000 minimum lethal doses of live culture. Several daily feedings of the live pneumococci contained in 50 cc. of a twenty-four-hour broth culture likewise produced considerable resistance. Continuing observations of this nature, Ross (1127) observed the effect of varying the dose of the live organisms fed to rats. Doses of 2 cc. of live culture fed daily for from nine to twenty-one days produced only slight immunity, and the resistance resulting from the use of 10 to 18 cc. of culture daily was but little better. However, when the organisms from 50 cc. of live culture were fed daily, a fairly good immune response was obtained. When heat-killed pneumococci were fed in doses of about comparable size, the immunity incited was much less marked. The use of 5 cc. of the filtrate of a twenty-four-hour culture daily for several days yielded little result.

The oral administration to rats of doses of heat-killed vaccines, dried mechanically disrupted pneumococcus cells, and bile-salt solutions of these organisms was also studied by Ross (1129). Doses prepared from the original culture or containing the number of organisms found in from 3 cc. to 50 cc. of the original culture and given daily on three to seventeen successive days, produced immunity to from 1,000 to 10,000 minimum fatal doses. The results of experiments in which rats were given single feedings of the bile-salt dissolved solution of pneumococci in still smaller doses revealed that it was necessary to administer an amount of solution representing the number of organisms contained in between 1 and 5 cc. of the original culture to obtain evidence of resistance and that the level of immunity thus produced (immunity to as many as 10,000 minimum fatal doses) was greater than that resulting from feeding an amount of solution representing the organisms contained in 50 cc. of the culture (immunity to 1 to 100 minimum fatal doses). In this instance, then, the immunity evoked by one administration of such a solution of pneumococci was greater after a small than after a large dose, and in this respect the results obtained are somewhat analogous to those reported following the use of solutions of the specific capsular polysaccharide or some similar agent, as discussed below. The level of the immunity produced by a single small dose of a suspension of acid-killed degraded pneumococci was about the same as that resulting from the use of solutions of virulent pneumococci representing an equivalent number of organisms. Findings of similar significance were also obtained by Ross in subsequent investigations (1136, 1137).

Suspensions containing pneumococci from 10 cc. of culture or solutions of pneumococci representing the cells in 5 cc. of culture were administered orally to rabbits on seven successive days (Kolmer and Rule, 737); resistance to subsequent infection developed. These workers also demonstrated (739) that, with a single oral dose of vaccine containing about 1,000 million pneumococci per kilogram of body weight, rabbits developed considerable immunity but that immunity of a higher degree was obtained by the use of a minimum of five doses of this size given at daily intervals. Seven such doses gave even better results. Kolmer and Rule (738) gave monkeys oral doses of 1 cc. of vaccine every five days for six doses, and obtained evidence of the development of a slight amount of immunity to later infection.

Other routes. The findings resulting from the administration of varying doses of vaccine by several other less often utilized routes all tend to support the general view that, with doses of the size customarily used, those animals receiving the largest total doses ordinarily develop the highest immunity (1238, 1243, 241, 243, 1258, 933, 1241).

VACCINES AND SIMILAR PREPARATIONS IN MAN. Though pneumococcus vaccines and similar preparations have been administered to many thousand human beings, the number of reports on the level of the immune substances appearing in the serum following such procedures is decidedly limited. Many of the observations of this nature were made during the course of large-scale efforts to prevent pneumonia in man by prophylactic vaccination. From the data available it appears that, as in animals, the degree of the demonstrable immunity produced in man following vaccination varies much with the individual, for some persons develop a considerable antibody response after receiving only small doses of an immunizing agent, while in others even huge doses fail to produce this reaction.

In the course of immunizing several thousand men against pneumonia in 1911, Wright, Morgan, Colebrook, and Dodgson (1447) undertook to study the antibody response in human beings who received varying doses of killed pneumococci, but because of various difficulties, this phase of their work was soon terminated. Nevertheless, it was reported that with the limited information available the injection of a total dose of about 200 to 300 million pneumococci suspended in saline solution appeared to stimulate the production of some humoral antibody. This investigation was carried out largely, if not wholly, on African natives and was concluded before the discovery of pneumococcus types. Subsequently, several other studies were made.

Lister (785), who also worked in Africa, studied the development of type-specific humoral agglutinins and opsonins in nine men vaccinated intravenously and fourteen vaccinated subcutaneously. Previous tests had revealed the absence of such antibodies from the blood of these individuals. The vaccines used contained equal numbers of pneumococci of five types or groups (designated by Lister as Groups A, C, D, F, and G; see also Appendix B, page 946) and were standardized so that each cubic centimeter held a total of approximately 10,000 million organisms. Weekly doses were given for three weeks in each instance. The intravenous injections were made with heat-killed pneumococci which had been grown on blood agar plates and suspended in saline solution. Some individuals vaccinated intravenously received doses containing from 2,000 to 4,000 or 8,000 million organisms in each dose, while others received successive doses of increasing size which varied from 2,500 to 10,000 million pneumococci per dose at the start to the large final doses of 10,000 to 40,000 million organisms each. With the smaller doses no humoral antibodies became demonstrable until after the third and last injection, but with the larger doses these substances appeared after the first dose and were found in increasing concentration after the second and third doses.

The first five men Lister vaccinated subcutaneously were given injections of the same heat-killed vaccine mentioned above, the doses varying in size from 2,000 to 12,000 million organisms per dose. As antibodies were produced irregularly and in low titer, a second vaccine was made. This was prepared from broth cultures and consisted of a saline suspension of the same five groups of pneumococci listed above, but carbolic acid (0.25 per cent) rather than heat was used to kill the organisms. Nine men received subcutaneous injections of this preparation at weekly intervals for three weeks. Three individuals receiving doses each totaling 10,000, 20,000, or 30,000 million organisms per injection developed an antibody response which was regarded as fairly satisfactory, and this was most marked in persons receiving the largest doses. The remainder of the group received doses of increasing size, the three individual doses ranging from approximately 20,000 to 30,000 million pneumococci at the start to 20,000 to 40,000 million at the end. The antibody response to these doses was about comparable to that produced by the three men who also received subcutaneous doses of the acid-killed vaccine. Lister remarked that in man there was little difference whether the vaccine used was given subcutaneously or intravenously provided a suitable dosage was given for the method used. It seemed likely that to obtain a similar antibody response subcutaneous vaccination required larger doses than intravenous vaccination. It was considered, in any instance, that more than one dose must be given. The procedure recommended was to give three subcutaneous injections at seven-day intervals, each dose consisting of 6,000 million organisms of each group or type of pneumococcus against which immunity was desired. Later, however, this plan was altered and experience suggested that somewhat smaller doses might suffice (786).

Observations similar to those just cited were made by Cecil and Austin (228) who gave subcutaneous injections of a heat-killed saline suspension of pneumococci of Types I, II, and III to forty-two men. In the beginning, eight men received a single injection of 24,000 million organisms (8,000 million of each of the three types). Due to the occurrence of some rather severe reactions in a few individuals in this group, the remainder of the group were given four or five smaller doses at intervals of three to seven days, the total number of pneumococci in each dose varying from about 1,000 to 12,000 million per injection. In the blood of many, but not all, of the vaccinated men, agglutinins appeared in low titer and protective substance against from 100 to about 10,000 minimum lethal doses became demonstrable. It was concluded that the immune response as measured by antibody determinations depended upon the total dose of organisms used and was but little influenced by the number of individual doses into which the total dose was divided. As a rule, individuals receiving the largest total amounts of vaccine developed the greatest immune response. Weekly doses of the order of 1,000, 2,000, 4,000, and 4,000 million organisms of each type of pneumococcus contained in the vaccine were regarded as satisfactory.

In another report Cecil and Vaughan (246) cite the observations of Whitmore on the development of protective substance in one man given a single dose of lipovaccine containing about 10 billion pneumococci of each of the types, I, II, and III, or a total of 30 billion organisms. Tests for Type I antibody demonstrated that protective substance for approximately 10 to 100 lethal doses appeared in the serum of this individual.

Barach (71) investigated the antibody response of thirty-seven human beings following the single or repeated injection of various agents prepared from cultures of pneumococci of Type I, II, or III. Culture filtrates or filtrates of suspensions of shaken organisms were injected intravenously in doses totaling from 1 to 7 cc., as were doses of saline-suspended heat-killed vaccine totaling from 1 to 5 billion organisms. The latter preparation was also given intradermally in several instances in doses totaling from 1 to 3 billion organisms, and two persons received subcutaneous doses of it totaling 5 billion or 9 billion organisms. The individuals used for these tests were patients with pneumococcus pneumonia or some other disease. The immunizing agent given to the pneumonia patients was made from cultures or contained pneumococci of a type believed different from that responsible for the pneumonia in the patient. Most of the patients vaccinated intravenously developed antibody for the homologous type or types. When vaccine was given in this fashion, protective substance against as many as 10,000 to 100,000 minimum lethal doses became demonstrable; when filtrates were administered by the same route, antibody appeared less often in this concentration. Patients to whom doses of vaccine were given intradermally rarely developed such a marked antibody response, and no antibody appeared in the blood of two persons vaccinated subcutaneously.

In a subsequent study Barach (72) immunized several healthy blood donors against pneumococci of Types I, II, and III with the end in view of using their blood to transfuse patients with pneumonia due to one of these organisms. Injections of heat-killed saline vaccine or of filtrates of cultures or suspensions of shaken pneumococci were given subcutaneously or intramuscularly in doses containing, or ranging from, the equivalent of one to twenty-five billion pneumococci once or twice a week for several weeks to a year. When all the doses were taken together, the number of pneumococci administered was as large as 80 billion Type I, 170 billion Type II, and 170 billion Type III, but in some instances the numbers were smaller. The concentration of the humoral antibody produced by such procedures was disappointing in that, at most, it appeared to protect against but 100,000 minimum infecting doses, and even this level was only irregularly attained.

Felton, Sutliff, and Steele (433) prepared a vaccine containing acetone-killed vacuum-desiccated pneumococci of Type I or II. A single dose of two milligrams of the dried agent, equivalent to about 200 million organisms, was suspended in saline and injected subcutaneously into about twenty persons. The majority of this group had protective substance in their serum against approximately ten lethal doses of live culture of homologous type prior to the vaccine injections, and nearly all showed a ten to one hundred-fold or occasionally greater increase in the titer of their specific protective antibody. The uniformity and degree of the response elicited was marked and seemed better following the use of a single dose of such vaccine than most previous workers had obtained with repeated doses ten or more times as large of vaccines prepared in other ways. Persons receiving Type I vaccine occasionally also showed an increase in the titer of their protective substance for Type II and vice versa.

The observations of Ross (1138) on the oral immunization of man are of great interest. One or more of four different immunizing agents were given to a group of sixty-three persons. The preparations administered were made from cultures of pneumococci of Type I, II, or III. A suspension of acid-killed organisms in water was used, as was a similarly prepared vaccine in which the organisms were dried. Two different solutions of pneumococci were likewise employed, the first of which was a Berkfeld filtrate of a bile-salt solution of these organisms diluted in water, while the second consisted of a similarly prepared agent which had been dried and powdered. The dry preparations were put into capsules or emulsified in water just before ingestion. In practically every instance a single dose was given each day for from two to ten days, and occasionally, if no protective substance developed following this procedure, a second set of feedings was given. In many cases, however, no antibody developed even after a second set of feedings. Some individuals received preparations containing pneumococci of a single type, while many persons were given agents representing organisms of two or three types.

In comparison with the dosage of organisms usually administered to man parenterally, the doses given by mouth could almost be classed as heroic. From five to ten feedings or more were given in some instances of preparations each containing the equivalent of the number of pneumococci in from 1,200 to 2,400 or even 3,600 cc. of the original broth culture, which in this instance presumably contained about 100 million organisms per cubic centimeter. In consequence, total doses of the order of 150 to 1,000 billion or more pneumococci were ingested by some individuals. While the technic used in this instance for the demonstration of humoral protective substance could have been improved, Ross reported that evidence was obtained that antibody of this nature either developed or increased in titer in about two-thirds of the vaccinated persons. This reaction did not seem to be accompanied by the appearance of agglutinins. The response was largely type-specific, though at times some heterologous type antibody also appeared. In the usual case the titer of the protective substance, when it appeared or increased, was sufficient to protect mice against about 5,000 minimum lethal doses, though the quality of the response obtained varied considerably from person to person.

The demonstrable results were about similar with each of the antigens used. As a practical procedure, Ross considered that feeding the pneumococci from 1,200 cc. of the culture of each type on each of six to ten successive days might prove satisfactory. This investigator also suggested that, if specially prepared cultures could be obtained, smaller doses, possibly in the neighborhood of from 2.5 to 12 per cent of this size, might suffice to immunize man. Proof of this contention is lacking.

Dosage: Specific Capsular Polysaccharides and Allied Agents

In animals the dose of the specific capsular polysaccharide or allied preparation has a significant bearing on the level of the immunity incited. Comparative tests have been made of the adequacy of the immune response elicited by the administration of varying amounts of these agents. The findings of Perlzweig and Steffen (1012), Schiemann and Casper (1160), and others (1470, 41, 395, 424) have clearly indicated that the best results are obtained with single or repeated very small doses and that large doses almost invariably produce no demonstrable immunity. Less is known of the range of effective dosage of these substances in man.

With the limited data available, the influence in the case of either animals or man of administering varying amounts of the specific capsular polysaccharide or presumably similar agents by various routes on the quality of the immune response produced is not clear. It has been shown, however, that possibly a small dose (0.25 mgm.) injected intravenously into mice may give rise to as much immunity as a dose twice as large given intraperitoneally (422).

SPECIFIC CAPSULAR POLYSACCHARIDES AND ALLIED AGENTS IN ANIMALS. Small doses of SSS and such preparations have been administered by various routes to animals of several species, as earlier mentioned. The exact dosage required to produce in mice immunity against from 100 to 100,000 or more minimum lethal doses of the infecting organism of homologous type was less clear in some of the initial observations (1012, 440) than in several of the later studies. Schiemann and Casper (1160) found a total of 0.03 mgm. caused the development of this degree of immunity whereas the use of larger doses produced toxicity but no immunity. Felton (422) gave a single injection of from 0.25 to 0.5 mgm. and obtained resistance to from 100 to 1,000 minimum infecting doses. This degree of immunity was reported to be many times higher than that resulting from the administration of a single dose of vaccine regardless of the size of the dose of the latter agent. Zozaya and Clark (1470) obtained no immunity after the injection of specific capsular polysaccharide in dilutions of 1:10,000, yet this material in a dilution of 1:150,000 produced specific resistance against 10,000 minimum infecting doses. Findings of like significance were also reported by the latter workers following the administration of varying dilutions of these soluble derivatives adsorbed on carbon or collodion particles.

After an injection of the specific capsular polysaccharide every three days for three doses, the total dose given amounting to only 0.00075 mgm., Avery and Goebel (41) obtained specific immunity in mice. Humoral antibody failed to develop in rabbits, however, to which considerably larger doses were given. In the latter instance injections were given on six consecutive days, followed by a week's rest, after which the whole course was repeated twice more. Some of the rabbits received a total dose of 0.18 mgm. while others received a total of 1.8 or 18.0 mgm. Enders and Wu (395) found the optimum dose in mice to be 0.0005 mgm. and noted that the resistance evoked was of a lower level when a dose ten times this size was used and that little if any immunity was produced by a still larger dose. Felton (424) also showed the importance of using small doses in the immunization of mice. Dilutions of 1:100,000 failed to immunize while dilutions ranging from 1:1 million to 1:20 or 50 million produced immunity. He likewise determined that small doses produced active immunity but no demonstrable antibody in rabbits. The injection of 1 or 2 mgm. into horses gave rise to demonstrable antibody, but the latter decreased and disappeared as the dose was increased.

The oral immunization of rats was carried out by Ross (1130, 1132, 1133), who fed solutions of the specific capsular polysaccharide to these animals in doses up to 6 mgm. Following the ingestion of a single dose of 0.5 mgm. of such a substance, specific immunity against from 100 to 1,000 minimum infecting doses of pneumococci occasionally appeared. By feeding rats doses of similar size on each of two or three successive days, resistance of the same or of a somewhat higher order was produced with greater regularity. In mice, however, the oral administration of total doses ranging from 0.002 to 0.3 mgm. failed to produce any immunity.

SPECIFIC POLYSACCHARIDES AND ALLIED AGENTS IN MAN. Francis and Tillett (485), Finland and Sutliff (459, 461), and other workers (1469, 478) have shown that amounts of pneumococcus specific capsular polysaccharide as small as 0.01 mgm. injected intradermally into man frequently give rise to the development of specific humoral antibody. In many instances doses of this size were given repeatedly at intervals of one to several days with similar results, but the titer of the antibody produced was apparently little if at all higher than that evoked by a single injection. Francis and Tillett (485) reported that the largest amount of such a substance which gave rise to demonstrable antibody was a total of 0.05 mgm. and that no antibody appeared in the blood of individuals who received still larger amounts. So far as the production of humoral antibody is concerned, there is evidence that, while one to four injections of 0.01 mgm. each at intervals of from one to seven days may be considered a relatively satisfactory dosage schedule with this agent, additional observations are needed to define the most suitable technic for use in man.

Felton (424) and Felton, Sutliff, and Steele (433) investigated the antigenic properties of several fractions of the pneumococcus cell which either contained pneumococcus specific capsular polysaccharide or were presumably more or less akin to that substance. A single subcutaneous injection of the preparations used was given to at least twenty persons, the individual doses ranging from 1 to 10 mgm. A dose of 2 mgm. was found to produce about the same concentration of serum antibodies as that found in the serum of patients convalescent from pneumonia.

In all, then, doses ranging from a total of 0.01 to 10 milligrams of the various agents under discussion have been injected intradermally or subcutaneously into man, but the optimum dose for human beings has not yet been determined for any one of the antigens studied (485, 459, 461, 1469, 478, 424, 433, 425).

Type of Pneumococcus and Immune Response

It has long been known that the antigenic properties of pneumococci of various types are not identical and that some types give rise to a much more adequate immune response than others, as earlier pointed out (see pages 161–162). This has been amply demonstrated by the results obtained from the injection into animals of pneumococcus vaccines of various sorts by various routes: parenterally (785, 240, 242, 69, 1258, 434, 1245, 738) or orally (737, 738, 1136, 1137). The investigations cited have embraced the use of rabbits (785, 69, 1258, 737, 434, 1245), mice (69, 434), rats (1136, 1137), and monkeys (240, 242, 738). Similar observations have been made following the administration to man of vaccines parenterally (785, 228, 71, 72) and orally (1138). It hardly seems surprising, therefore, that the administration by several routes of derivatives of pneumococci, such as the specific capsular polysaccharide and allied agents, to animals (mice 1012, 1470 and rats 1132, 1133), and possibly also to man (459, 433), has apparently been followed by a similar variation in the immune response.

In general, the demonstrable immune response to Type I antigens is the most pronounced and is somewhat better than the response produced by corresponding preparations of Type II, which in turn is usually far superior to the response induced by like antigens containing or prepared from pneumococci of Type III. Occasional exceptions to this generalization have been reported, however. Among rats fed the specific capsular polysaccharides of pneumococci of Type I, II, or III, less specific resistance developed in animals receiving the Type II preparation than in those fed either the Type I or Type III preparation (Ross, 1132, 1133). The antibody response in rats to the oral administration of various vaccines prepared from pneumococci of Type I, II, III, IV, V, or VI also suggested that the Type II preparations were less antigenic than those representing Type I or Type III (Ross, 1136, 1137). While the response to the other types was even less marked than the response to the Type II vaccine, it was more pronounced with the Type IV preparation than it was with that of Type V and was least definite in the case of Type VI.

Barach (72) made a study of the antibodies appearing in the blood of a few human beings undergoing a prolonged course of immunization with several filtrates of cultures or shaken organisms, and vaccines prepared from or containing pneumococci of Type I, II, or III. In some instances after receiving such preparations once or twice a week for from six weeks to a year in presumably adequate doses, antibody became demonstrable for one or two of the types represented in the antigen but not for the other or others. For example, one individual received Type I, II, and III vaccines regularly for a year, at the end of which time his serum contained no protective antibody against pneumococci of Type I; yet such substances were present against 10,000 minimum lethal doses of Type II and against 1,000 such doses of Type III. Another person who also received similar amounts of the same immunizing agents for a year showed protective substance against 10 minimum lethal doses of pneumococci of Type III and no antibody for Type I or II. In the serum of still another individual who had been immunized in much the same fashion, protective substance was present chiefly for Type II, while the serum of two additional similarly vaccinated persons showed no antibody for this type. These observations are illustrative of the well-recognized fact that a comparable demonstrable response fails to develop in all individuals in a group each simultaneously receiving approximately equal amounts of the same antigen. In view of such a circumstance, it appears that the immune response to vaccination with antigens representing pneumococci of various types may at times be fundamentally altered by characteristics of an unknown nature resident within the individual host (see pages 177–180).

In the usual instance, qualitative determinations of the active immunity induced by the administration of Type I, II, or III vaccines to animals have revealed that the response is most pronounced with Type I, while that with

Type II is somewhat less marked, and that for Type III generally the least (240, 242, 69, 1258, 737, 434, 1245, 738). The situation is essentially comparable with respect to the titer of the demonstrable humoral antibodies appearing as a consequence of such immunization. In the rabbit, Stillman and Goodner (1245) observed that agglutinins in low titer (1:10) were regularly produced for Type I, were seldom developed for Type II, and rarely if ever appeared for Type III. The findings of these investigators also largely agreed with those of Barach (69) in that protective substance may appear against as many as 100,000 minimum lethal doses of Type I, against about 10,000 such doses of Type II, while it is usually absent or present in only very low titer (about 100 minimum lethal doses or less) against Type III.

Findings similar to these have been reported with respect to human beings immunized with vaccines containing pneumococci of Types I, II, and III. Cecil and Austin (228) demonstrated that agglutinins developed in titers of 1:3 to 1:10 for Type I or II, though such antibodies were seldom found for Type III. These workers also noted the frequent appearance of protective substance against from 100 to 10,000 minimum lethal doses of Type I or II, while antibody of this nature was seldom found for Type III and, when present, was in much lower titer. Results of like significance were reported by Barach (71). In addition, after the oral administration of various vaccines or solutions of pneumococci containing or representing strains of Types I, II, and III, Ross (1138) failed to find agglutinins, as elsewhere noted, but reported that protective substance appeared or increased in titer in the blood of 74 per cent of fifty-three persons fed Type I preparations and of about 60 per cent of thirty persons fed Type II antigens, and approximately the same proportion of sixty persons fed Type III antigens. In the latter instance, however, the response was slighter and more irregular than the response to the other two types. Mention may also be made of the fact that, even though two sets of feedings were given to many of the persons under test, antibody did not appear in about 25 per cent of the individuals fed Type I preparations or in approximately 40 per cent of those fed Type II or Type III preparations.

Time of Appearance of Immune Response

A number of reports are available which give information as to the time between administration of the antigen and appearance of the immune response in rabbits (724, 785, 1118, 1448, 69, 531, 532, 1258, 1245), mice (68, 69), rats (1129, 1135), monkeys (240), and man (785, 228, 71, 1138) by the administration of one or more doses of pneumococcus vaccines or of solutions, filtrates, or autolysates of cultures of these organisms. In many instances, however, the tests were not repeated often enough to determine the precise time of appearance of the immune response. A limited amount of data of a similar nature is available concerning the use of chemical derivatives of the pneumococcus in mice (422, 1470, 395) and man (485, 461, 433, 425). Presumably consideration should be given to the species of the animal and the character of the antigen, as well as to the size of the dose and the route of its administration. For want of adequate information, only a rather general discussion of the effect of such factors on the time of appearance of the immune response is possible.

Immunity as determined by the presence of humoral antibodies or by active resistance to infection commonly becomes demonstrable in animals within three to fourteen days after the administration of one or more doses of vaccines or of the filtrates of either cultures or suspensions of shaken organisms, or of solutions of pneumococci (724, 785, 1118, 1448, 68, 69, 531, 532, 1129, 1135). In several cases where especially detailed observations were made, immunity of considerable degree was frequently present within three to six days after the use of a single dose of any one of several antigens, and occasionally evidence of immunity was noted as early as the first day (1448, 68, 69, 531, 532, 1129, 1135). In general, immunity develops earliest after the use of an intact-cell vaccine, and evidence of it may be obtained at times within one to three days. After the use of filtrates either of cultures or shaken pneumococci or of solutions of these organisms usually (1448, 68, 69), but not always (1129, 1135), immunity appears after a longer interval, measuring four or more days.

Of great theoretical importance were Wright's (1448) findings in a study of rabbits immunized by the parenteral injection of Type I vaccine. Evidence was obtained that the capacity of the blood-clearing mechanism to remove pneumococci of homologous type from the blood stream was increased by this process and that this altered state of reactivity began to appear as early as *five hours* after the vaccine injection. Wright's study is presumably the first in the literature to report evidence of such an early development of immunity after immunization. Ross (1129) reported what he considered evidence of the early development of a slight degree of active immunity to infection in two rats fed bile-salt solutions of pneumococci. Within twenty-four hours resistance was present against ten minimum lethal doses of the infecting organism.

After becoming demonstrable following the administration of a single dose of vaccine or some similar preparation, immunity rapidly increases in degree until a peak is reached by the fifth to the seventh day, following which it decreases over an interval of about ten or more days. The results appear the same regardless of whether the antigens used are administered parenterally (1448, 68, 69) or orally (1129, 1135).

The limited data available suggest that the sequence of events differs little if at all in man. Lister (785) reported that humoral antibody did not become demonstrable in man following three moderate-sized weekly intravenous injections of vaccine until several days after the last injection. With larger doses, however, antibody appeared a few days after the initial dose, increased in titer after each of two subsequent doses, and was possibly still higher at the end of six weeks after the last dose. Antibody likewise became demonstrable seven days after the last of three large subcutaneous doses at weekly intervals. Cecil and Austin (228) also found that antibody had developed in man following the last of three or four rather large weekly subcutaneous injections of vaccine. Barach (71) showed the average interval between administration of the antigen and appearance of humoral antibody in human beings receiving a single injection of vaccine intravenously or intradermally to be 4.4 and 4.5 days respectively. In other individuals receiving the cell-free filtrates of shaken pneumococci intravenously, the average interval was slightly longer, or 5.6 days. The vaccines used contained pneumococci of Type I, II, or III and the filtrates were of shaken suspensions of strains of Type I or II. The time of antibody appearance seemed to be little if at all influenced by the type of pneumococcus represented in the antigen. Ross (1138) demonstrated the appearance of antibody in man two or three days after giving six feedings on successive days of either pneumococcus vaccines or bile-salt solutions of these organisms or both.

The following reports are concerned with the time when immunity appeared in mice following their injection with a small dose of the specific capsular polysaccharide or some allied pneumococcus derivative. After the use of such preparations, the elapsed interval before resistance becomes demonstrable appears about the same as that mentioned above in instances where vaccine is administered to animals. For example, Felton (422) reported immunity to be present within forty-eight to seventy-two hours following the injection of one of the agents under discussion. In addition, Zozaya and Clark (1470) found demonstrable immunity within four days, and Enders and Wu (395) obtained evidence that a slight amount of immunity might develop as early as twenty-four hours after the injection of 0.005 mgm. of an antigen of this nature. After its appearance, the immunity usually increased to a considerable extent up to the fourth to seventh day, following which the maximum level reached was maintained with but little variation for two or three weeks.

In man after one or more intradermal injections of the specific capsular polysaccharide, Francis and Tillett (485) and Finland and Sutliff (461) observed that humoral antibody frequently became demonstrable within six to ten days, though at times its appearance might be delayed several days longer. Using antigens of a presumably similar nature, Felton, Sutliff, and Steele (433) found that two weeks after the subcutaneous injection of a single 2 mgm. dose antibody had appeared or increased in the blood of nearly all the persons receiving the injections.

The foregoing observations suggest that, as a rule, following the use of any of the above mentioned antigens, immunity becomes demonstrable at an earlier period in animals than in man. This may be more apparent than real however, as many of the tests for immunity which can be applied satisfactorily to animals cannot be used for man. Among the lower animals on which suitable observations are available, the interval necessary for the development of immunity in general appears to vary to only a minor degree with the species of the animal used. However, the rapidity with which the immune response appears after vaccination may at times be affected to some extent by the character of the antigen employed and the route by which it is injected. In some instances, even when within the usual range of dosage, the amount of the immunizing agent administered may also influence the speed with which the immune response develops.

Duration of Immune Response

The duration of the immune response elicited by the administration of pneumococcus vaccines prepared in various ways or of bile-salt solutions of these organisms has been studied to some extent in rabbits (1448, 532, 1241, 1245, 739), rats (1128, 1129, 1135), and man (785, 1135, 1138, 433). Information of a similar nature is also available concerning the results obtained from the injection of chemical derivatives of the pneumococcus into mice (422, 1470, 395) and man (485, 459, 461, 1469, 433, 425). The following studies are of particular interest:

Studies of animals by

Ross (1128, 1135), Wright (1448), Stillman (1241), Felton (422), Zozaya and Clark (1470), Stillman and Goodner (1245), Enders and Wu (395).

Studies of man by

Lister (785), Finland and Sutliff (459, 461), Zozaya and Clark (1469), Ross (1138), Felton and his associates (433, 425).

As determined by antibody studies in man and by studies of acquired immunity to infection as well in animals, the duration of the demonstrable immune response to a comparable amount of the same antigen may, in any instance, be longer in man than in animals, as Lister (785) has pointed out. Considerable individual variation may be encountered in this respect, however. Time, of course, is an important element in affecting the level of the measurable resistance following vaccination (see pages 194–196).

Animals receiving vaccines or solutions of pneumococci frequently show an immune response for periods of two to four months (1128, 532, 739, 1135) or for even as long as nine or ten months (1448, 1241, 1245). Following the use of similar preparations the antibody response in man can frequently be demonstrated to persist for from three to fourteen months and in a few instances for over twenty months (785, 1135, 1138, 433). Following the injection of specific capsular polysaccharide or some allied agent, the immune response obtained may persist for from four to seven weeks in some animals (422, 1470, 395) and for periods of several days to three months or more in man (485, 459, 461, 1469, 433, 425). Such findings suggest that the immune response to the administration of vaccines may persist longer than the response following the use of chemical derivatives of the pneumococcus. Additional observations are necessary to confirm this supposition. In orally immunized rats the response elicited may remain demonstrable slightly longer when living rather than dead pneumococci or solutions of these organisms are fed (Ross, 1135).

Numerous factors other than the responsiveness of the individual concerned have an important bearing on the observed duration of the immune state produced by immunizing procedures. For example, the test used must be considered, as is clearly illustrated by Wright's (1448) findings in rabbits given pneumococcus Type I vaccine. The agglutinins which appeared were usually no longer demonstrable after the third week, and evidence of the presence of opsonins seldom persisted for over a month, yet precipitins were occasionally found for as long as three months while the capacity of the blood-clearing mechanism to remove pneumococci of homologous type from the circulation appeared enhanced for as long as ten months. The antibody studies of Stillman (1241) and a combination of such studies along with determinations of active resistance by Stillman and Goodner (1245) in the rabbit are of identical significance in this respect. Agglutinins, if they appear, usually disappear after an interval of some days, while protective substance may persist for several and even for many months and active immunity to infection may be present even longer.

In animals, as might be expected, the immune response to immunization usually persists the longest in those receiving the largest total dose of vaccine (1129, 1241, 1135), though this difference may be less marked when doses of relatively small size are used (532, 1135). In the usual instance the specific resistance to infection or antibody produced by the administration of immunizing agents either parenterally by various routes (1241) or orally (1129, 1135) remains demonstrable but a week or two after a small total dose but may persist for many weeks or months following the administration of more doses of the same size or of a number of larger doses. No observations on the possible relation of dosage to the duration of the antibody response in man are at hand.

The route of immunization also has a bearing on the duration of the immune response. Stillman (1241) gave Type I vaccine by various routes to a considerable number of rabbits. The results obtained in animals receiving comparable dosage (approximately fifteen doses of 1 cc. each) showed that after intravenous vaccination agglutinins might persist for periods up to one hundred days, while protective substance was frequently found for as long as four hundred days, and in one animal it persisted for eight hundred and eighty days. Following intraperitoneal vaccination, agglutinins disappeared earlier, usually within ten to forty days, while protective substance remained demonstrable for periods as long as three hundred to six hundred days. When the vaccine was injected intramuscularly, agglutinins never lasted longer than forty days and protective substance also disappeared earlier and usually was not demonstrable after one hundred days. After subcutaneous vaccination no agglutinins appeared and protective substance persisted for only a few days. In general, then, the duration of the antibody response was longer in animals vaccinated intravenously or intraperitoneally than in those vaccinated intramuscularly or subcutaneously.

In rats (1128, 1135) and rabbits (739) immunized by the oral administration of vaccines, the active immunity to infection induced was highest the first month or so and by the end of two to six months had disappeared. The oral immunization of man (1135, 1138) with similar preparations gave rise to antibody which was commonly demonstrable for six or seven months and at times may have persisted for about twenty-two months. In this instance, however, relatively huge doses were used for immunizing purposes.

The persistence of the immune response following vaccination likewise varies with the type of pneumococcus contained in the vaccine (1245, 1138). Specific immunity may be demonstrable for many months after the suitable administration of Type I vaccines, and for nearly as long after the use of

Type II preparations, while the response to Type III usually disappears in the course of a few weeks or less.

It is well recognized, of course, as above pointed out (see page 410), that the quality of the immunity evoked by immunizing procedures may be vitally affected by the nature of the antigen used. Few attempts have been made, however, to compare the duration of the immunity resulting from the administration by similar routes of what are believed to represent comparable amounts of antigens having different characteristics. Some evidence of this nature has been presented by Ross (1135, 1136), who administered vaccines killed by acid or heat or mechanically disrupted pneumococci or bile-salt solutions of them to both rats and man. The results obtained were about the same with each of the antigens used. Felton, Sutliff, and Steele (433) obtained some data of a similar nature on the duration of the antibody response in human beings receiving either a single subcutaneous 2 mgm. dose of a dried acetone-killed vaccine or a dose of 2 mgm. of any one of the several chemical derivatives of the pneumococcus studied. While not definite, the findings suggested that after a single dose of the amount used the immune response persisted longer in a larger proportion of the group receiving a chemical fraction of the pneumococcus than of the group receiving the whole-cell vaccine.

RESULTS OF IMMUNIZATION OF ANIMALS AGAINST EXPERIMENTAL PNEUMOCOCCUS PNEUMONIA

Active Immunization

The course of events subsequent to the intratracheal or intrabronchial infection of animals actively immunized in various ways has been studied by several investigators (727, 125, 231, 240, 241, 242, 243, 1258, 737, 434, 738, 739). Studies of this nature have been made in dogs (727), monkeys (125, 231, 240, 241, 242, 243, 738), and rabbits (1258, 737, 434, 739). With the exception of the observations in dogs (727) and one of the studies in rabbits (1258), the reports cited deal with attempts to prevent experimental pneumococcus pneumonia by active immunizing procedures. Vaccines containing presumably intact pneumococci killed in various ways have generally been used for immunizing purposes, though in one study in monkeys small doses of living virulent or avirulent pneumococci (Cecil and Blake, 231) were given subcutaneously, and in another instance in rabbits bile-salt solutions of these organisms as well as vaccines were administered orally (Kolmer and Rule, 737).

In the usual instance vaccines prepared from virulent cultures have produced a more satisfactory immune response than those containing avirulent pneumococci (125, 231, 240). In monkeys immunizing agents have been given subcutaneously (125, 231, 240, 242, 738), intravenously (240), intratracheally (241, 243), by throat spray (241, 243), or orally (738) in varying doses, and in rabbits subcutaneous (434, 739) or oral (737, 739) administration has been employed. In general, active immunity of a rather high order may be obtained from the use of three or four intravenous or intratracheal injections of a suitable vaccine. Subcutaneous inoculation appears less effective unless much larger doses are used, and the limited data available suggest that still larger doses are required when the immunizing agent is given orally. In fact, the value of oral immunization for the prevention of pneumonia in animals has not been clearly demonstrated. Very large doses repeatedly sprayed into the throats of monkeys gave rise to but slight evidence of an enhanced resistance.

Inasmuch as many of the studies above mentioned merit more than passing consideration, the findings obtained in each are briefly presented. The work of Blake and Cecil (125), Cecil and Blake (231), and Cecil and Steffen (240, 241, 242, 243) in monkeys, reported between 1920 and 1925, appears of the greatest importance in respect to the prevention of pneumonia in animals by active immunization. Although many of the vaccinated animals developed sufficient immunity to protect them from pneumonia of homologous type, specific antibody only irregularly became demonstrable in their blood (see also pages 129–131). Three types of monkeys were used in these experiments (*Macacus rhesus, Macacus syrichtus,* and *Cebus capucinus*), and adequate immunization was shown to protect even the Philippine monkey (*M. syrichtus*), which was regarded as the most susceptible, from a subsequent experimentally induced pneumonia.

In 1914, Kline and Meltzer (727) observed that in many instances after intrabronchial infection the lungs of immunized dogs became sterile within a period of twenty-eight to forty-five hours. This rapid disappearance of organisms from the lung was not seen in control animals. Findings of like significance were later obtained in the course of various studies by Cecil and Steffen (240, 241, 242, 243) in monkeys and by Stuppy, Cannon, and Falk (1258) in rabbits.

In most of the reports at hand the procedures followed in attempting to determine the value of immunization as a method of protecting monkeys against experimentally induced pneumonia have been quite similar. The process consists of stimulating the development of immunity by administering three or more doses of the antigens under test at intervals of five to seven days, the total dose varying somewhat depending upon the route of administration, the type of pneumococcus contained in the vaccine, and the group of animals used. From two to four weeks after the last dose of vaccine, each inoculated monkey, as well as one or more controls, is given a single intratracheal injection of living pneumococci of homologous type (0.1 to 0.001 cc. of an eighteen-hour broth culture). Rather large doses are commonly used for this purpose, though the number of live organisms injected may vary from 400 to 2 million or more. Observations are then made on the subsequent condition of the animals and the clinical course of the infection if any develops. At times the animals are sacrificed a few days after infection for careful pathologic and bacteriologic study. Importantly, such investigations in monkeys have shown that animals in the immunized and infected group usually have normal sterile lungs when killed six or seven days after infection, while pulmonary lesions, commonly in the form of lobar pneumonia and from which the infecting organisms can be isolated, are found in the similarly infected but non-immunized controls.

Blake and Cecil (125) immunized monkeys with a weekly subcutaneous injection for three or four weeks of a vaccine containing an old degraded avirulent heat-killed strain of Type I pneumococci. A lipovaccine, as well as a saline vaccine, was used. The doses in each instance were about comparable and totaled approximately 16 billion organisms in several animals, while in others smaller amounts were given. The immunity induced by these procedures was not sufficient to prevent the development of pneumonia following the intratracheal injection of live pneumococci of this type two or three weeks later. Vaccination did, however, cause a modification in the severity of the experimentally produced pneumonia, for, as compared with the controls, the disease was milder and the fatality rate lower among animals in the immunized group. It was likewise observed that three small doses of vaccine produced less protection than a single large dose.

Cecil and Blake (231) also immunized monkeys by the subcutaneous injection of living pneumococci of Type I. In this instance either virulent or avirulent degraded organisms were used. A small dose of the live virulent organisms numbering about 400,000 pneumococci was found to stimulate a degree of active immunity sufficient to protect the animals from pneumonia due to infection with the homologous type. Resistance of approximately this same degree could be obtained from vaccination with the avirulent strain of pneumococci if doses about twice as large were used.

Subsequently, other studies were carried out in monkeys by Cecil and Steffen (240, 241, 242, 243) using vaccines containing virulent pneumococci killed by heat. The relative value of subcutaneous and intravenous immunization with a vaccine containing pneumococci of Type I was studied (240). Three large doses, consisting of 20, 40, and 60 billion organisms, totaling 120 billion, were given subcutaneously, and in some instances four smaller doses of 300, 400, 800, and 1,600 million organisms, or 3.1 billion, were given intravenously. Good protection against experimentally induced Type I pneumococcus pneumonia was obtained in each instance. About the same level of resistance was developed by animals receiving the three large subcutaneous doses as by those given the four much smaller doses intravenously. As the subcutaneous dose totaled approximately forty times that of the intravenous dose, the superiority of the intravenous route of immunization appeared marked. Attention was also called to the finding that, as compared with Blake and Cecil's (125) previous failure to obtain protection in monkeys given subcutaneous doses of an avirulent Type I vaccine totaling 16 billion organisms, the use of vaccine containing virulent pneumococci in an amount nearly ten times this size stimulated the production of sufficient immunity to give almost uniform protection against pneumonia of homologous type.

In a similar study Cecil and Steffen (242) investigated the immunizing value of vaccines containing killed pneumococci of Type II or III, or a single strain of Group IV. The usual three subcutaneous doses at weekly intervals were given and the animals tested two weeks later by the intratracheal injection of living pneumococci of the homologous strain. All the animals receiving a total dose amounting to 190 billion organisms of Type II and those given 120 billion pneumococci of the strain of Group IV were protected, as were about one-half of those which had received from 120 to 200 billion pneumococci of Type III. It may be noted that, as in the preceding study, the doses used are relatively enormous for small animals such as the monkey and are very large even for man.

In several instances Cecil and Steffen (241, 243) also immunized monkeys by the intratracheal injection of vaccine. The antigen was delivered with a syringe and needle through the tissues of the neck directly into the trachea. An interval of five to seven days was allowed between each of the three doses given. With the Type I vaccine a total dose of 120 billion organisms gave protection against intratracheal infection with 0.001 cc. of an eighteen-hour broth culture of the same type. With a total vaccine dose of about one-tenth the above amount, adequate protection was obtained against an infecting dose of a similar culture one-tenth (0.0001 cc.) as large. In comparison with some of the previous findings of these workers in monkeys, the evidence suggested that a comparable degree of immunity could be produced by intratracheal vaccination with doses only one-tenth the size of those used subcutaneously.

Among the animals inoculated against Type II or Type III, protection was obtained from pneumonia due to infection with the homologous type after the intratracheal injection of vaccine doses totaling 210 billion Type II or 200 billion Type III pneumococci. Encouraged by the results of intratracheal vaccination, efforts were made to immunize other monkeys by spraying Type I vaccine into the nose and throat with an atomizer. The doses used were very large and varied from 20 billion pneumococci given daily for nineteen to twenty-four days to 40 billion organisms given every three or four days for five weeks. In no instance were these animals protected against a later experimental pneumonia due to this type though, judging by the milder course of the infection experienced by some of them, it seemed probable that a slight degree of resistance had occasionally developed. The inadequacy of this method of immunization was attributed to the apparent failure of the sprayed organisms to pass the larynx and reach the deeper portions of the bronchial tree, for the animals allowed little or none of the atomized liquid to reach the larynx, as was later demonstrated with India ink.

Kolmer and Rule (738) administered vaccine containing pneumococci of Types I, II, and III to a few monkeys (*M. rhesus*) subcutaneously and orally. The doses were similar in each instance and consisted of 20 million organisms of each of the three types per kilogram of body weight given every five days for six doses. Two weeks later intratracheal infection was carried out with strains of Type I or II. While the results obtained were not definite, the findings suggested that with the same doses of vaccine a higher immunity resulted from subcutaneous than from oral immunization and that the resistance incited was better for Type I than for Type II. The total dose of organisms in the vaccine used in this study apparently amounted to only a few hundred million pneumococci of each type. This amount is approximately from one hundred to one thousand times smaller than the total dose used by Cecil and Steffen in those instances in which they were successful in immunizing monkeys against pneumonia by vaccination with killed pneumococci, as noted above.

Studies of the efficacy of active immunization for the prevention of experimental pneumonia in rabbits (737, 434, 739) are less extensive and less conclusive than many of the observations cited above in monkeys. In most cases the work was confined to a study of the bacteriemia occurring as a consequence of the later intratracheal or intrabronchial infection or of the resulting fatality rate.

Both oral and subcutaneous vaccination were practiced with preparations representing or containing pneumococci of Type I, II, or III. The vaccines were administered daily for five to seven days or at intervals of four to seven days for two or three doses. The subcutaneous doses varied from a total of 300 million to a billion or more of the pneumococci of each type contained in the vaccine, while the number of organisms given orally was nearly five times this amount. Such procedures generally appeared to limit the bacteriemia and to permit recovery from infecting doses which were fatal to controls. The results obtained were always best after subcutaneous vaccination and with the preparations containing pneumococci of Type I.

In summary, the evidence seems clear that monkeys may be successfully immunized against an experimentally induced pneumonia due to pneumococci of Type I, II, or III. Also apparent is the fact that adequate protection with killed pneumococci has resulted only when large doses of vaccine were used. Effective protection was obtained with total doses of approximately 3 billion organisms given intravenously or with 120 to 200 billion given subcutaneously or intratracheally. In a few instances where the size of the infecting dose was reduced to about one-tenth that ordinarily used, satisfactory protection from Type I pneumonia was obtained with a total dose of vaccine containing around 12 billion organisms given intratracheally. Mouse protective antibody seldom appeared in the blood, and the limited data available suggest to some extent that the active resistance developed was largely type-specific in nature.

Passive Immunization with Specific Antipneumococcic Serum

Attention has already been called to the value of passively transferred immune substances for the prevention and cure of many pneumococcus infections (see pages 120–121 and 168–171). There is, nevertheless, relatively little information available as to the value of specific antipneumococcic serum in the prevention of pneumococcus pneumonia of homologous type. Cecil (222) reported having demonstrated in some unpublished experiments that monkeys receiving injections of antipneumococcic serum were immune and failed to develop experimental pneumonia of homologous type when infected the following day. Monkeys were also immune when the serum and organisms of the homologous type were injected simultaneously. Parker's (998) observations on guinea pigs passively immunized with an anti-autolysate pneumococcus serum and subjected to a later intratracheal infection with a mixture of a toxic autolysate preparation and living pneumococci were presumably of similar significance. The value of passive immunization against Type I or II for the prevention of severe or fatal infections in mice, rabbits, and guinea pigs carrying pneumococci of these types was demonstrated by Neufeld and Etinger-Tulczynska (933, 934).

RESULTS OF IMMUNIZATION OF ANIMALS AGAINST CONTACT INFECTION

Whether artificially acquired immunity to the pneumococcus is a safeguard against contact infection has been little studied in animals. This matter in its broadest aspects would appear to be of fundamental importance in relation to the problem of controlling the incidence of pneumonia in man by prophylactic vaccination. In the course of Blake and Cecil's (125) earlier mentioned unsuccessful attempt to fully immunize monkeys with a saline solution or a lipovaccine containing avirulent degraded pneumococci of Type I, one of the animals after vaccination was placed in the same cage with another undergoing an experimentally induced Type I pneumonia. Contact infection apparently occurred, for within a few days the vaccinated monkey also came down with pneumonia due to this organism. Neufeld and Etinger-Tulczynska (934) reported a few observations relating to the spread of Type I pneumococci from four guinea pigs, in which the carrier state of this organism had been induced, to fifteen actively or passively immunized mice placed in contact with them. Over half the immunized and exposed mice became carriers of Type I pneumococci within a period of a week. None of these animals died, however, which possibly was in some contrast to the previously observed fatality rate of 20 to 30 per cent among normal mice carrying pneumococci of the same type. In this instance the possession of immunity may have prevented the development of serious infection in these animals which so frequently accompanies the carrier state of similar organisms.

RESULTS OF IMMUNIZATION OF MAN AGAINST PNEUMOCOCCUS PNEUMONIA

Active Immunization

It is unfortunate that, although a million or more men have been subjected to prophylactic vaccination against pneumonia, there is no unanimity of opinion as to the usefulness of such a procedure. Although numerous investigations of this matter have been made, many observers consider that much of the evidence thus far reported is incomplete and the results obtained inconclusive. This is probably not surprising in view of the fact that vaccination against pneumonia has been carried out under such widely varying circumstances that each study should be considered by itself. Nevertheless, there appears, in general, to be more evidence in favor of the value of immunization than against it. Much more work remains to be done, however, before the true possibilities and limitations of prophylactic vaccination become clear. The available data on the subject present a more or less confusing picture. An effort will be made to point out in the following sections some of the reasons for this confusion.

From the foregoing discussion in this chapter and elsewhere, it is obvious that many complicated factors must be considered when undertaking programs for the immunization of man in the hope of preventing pneumonia and when estimating the degree of success attained. Since presumably little is to be gained by presenting a detailed analysis of all the pertinent reports available, only brief summaries will be given. Attention has already been called in this and in the preceding chapter to efforts that have been made to reduce the frequency of pneumonia in certain groups by active immunization. Investigations of this kind have been carried out in many parts of the world, but prophylactic vaccination has been used longer and far more extensively among miners and other native workers employed in the gold and diamond mines in the Union of South Africa, particularly in the neighborhood of Johannesburg, than among other groups elsewhere (see Table 78). In addition to miners, however, soldiers and members of various civilian groups, including some persons residing in institutions, have been similarly vaccinated, as previously mentioned in the chapter on Aspects of Immunity (see pages 196–199).

Attempts to prevent pneumonia in man by active immunization against the pneumococcus were begun in South Africa in 1911 under the direction of Wright and were reported first by Maynard (874) in 1913, and later in 1914 by Wright, Morgan, Colebrook, and Dodgson (1447). Much of this work, as well as the bulk of the many later studies made in Africa, was carried out under the auspices of the South African Institute for Medical Research. As there is a certain homogeneity about these studies, they will be considered first, and subsequently many other investigations carried out elsewhere will be reviewed. The list of the reports at hand, as shown in Table 78, has been arranged to follow this order. Several reports, chiefly containing discussions of the studies listed in this table, are referred to in the text.

As shown in Table 78, vaccination against pneumonia has been carried out in Africa, the United States, Europe, and India. Although the number of vaccinated individuals listed is only about 400,000, it is clear from the detailed review of the vaccination experiments on the Witwatersrand Goldfields by Lister and Ordman (788) that during several of the years since 1918 nearly all the annual labor complement of 200,000 or more men there were immunized each year. In all but the last of the studies mentioned in Table 78 the antigen used consisted of a vaccine containing pneumococci, usually of several types, and in some cases of other organisms as well which had been killed in various ways, though chiefly by the application of heat. In these instances, one or more doses (usually three) of the vaccines used were administered subcutaneously, as mentioned below. Such doses were commonly injected into the subcutaneous tissues of the pectoral region or near the insertion of the deltoid. Local or general systemic reactions of a mild type were occasionally encountered, as will be seen later (see page 478). In the last study in Table 78, reported by Felton (425), a single dose of a chemical derivative of pneumococci of Type I and Type II was administered.

SOUTH AFRICAN STUDIES. Attention has been previously called to the magnitude of the pneumonia problem among native laborers in Africa (see pages 268–269, 312–316, and 329–332). The susceptibility of these workers to pneumonia appears greatest among individuals newly arrived at the mines and varies considerably among natives of different tribal or territorial groups coming from different regions. East Coast natives and those from the low-lying tropical districts suffer the highest incidence and mortality rates from this disease. As a rule, among natives employed in mines, those working underground have higher pneumonia incidence and mortality rates than surface workers. Under ordinary circumstances the population of the native laborers employed at the mines and works in the Transvaal is large, numbering from 200,000 to 250,000 men, and is constantly changing. The average length of stay at the gold mines is only about eight months and is even shorter than this at the diamond mines. Almost all the pneumonia in African natives has been in the form of lobar pneumonia, though this situation may have changed somewhat in recent years, as elsewhere mentioned. In former years bacteriologic studies indicated that practically all the cases of lobar pneumonia were due to pneumococci. In the following attempt to

TABLE 78. ACTIVE IMMUNIZATION OF MAN AGAINST PNEUMONIA. REPORTS FROM VARIOUS COUNTRIES, WITH APPROXIMATE NUMBER AND KIND OF PERSONS VACCINATED BY YEAR REPORTED

YEAR REPORTED	REPORTED BY	COUNTRY	PERSONS VACCINATED *Kind*	PERSONS VACCINATED *Approximate number*
1913	Maynard (874)	South Africa	Native miners	23,000
1914	Wright, Morgan, Colebrook, and Dodgson (1447)	South Africa	Native miners	31,000
1917	Lister (786)	South Africa	Native miners	33,000
1932	Rep. South African Inst. Med. Research (1219)	South Africa	Native miners	40,000
1935	Lister and Ordman (788)	South Africa	Native miners	many thousands
1935	Peall (1007)	South Africa	Native miners	68,000
1935	Ordman (971)	Northern Rhodesia, Africa	Native miners	4,000
1918	Cecil and Austin (228)	U.S.A.	Soldiers	12,500
1919	Cecil and Vaughan (246)	U.S.A.	Soldiers	13,400
1919	Rosenow and Sturdivant (1119)	U.S.A.	Civilians	93,400
1920	Borrel (140)	Native African troops in France	Soldiers	2,300
1920	Duckwall (382)	U.S.A.	Soldiers	1,300
1921	Von Sholly and Park (1359)	U.S.A.	Civilians	1,500
1921	Walravens (1376)	Belgian Congo, Africa	Native miners	probably several thousands
1921	Jordan and Sharp (693)	U.S.A.	Civilians	2,800
1922	McCoy, Hasseltine, Wadsworth and Kirkbride (831)	U.S.A.	Civilians	17,700
1923	Pearson and Mouchet (1008)	Belgian Congo, Africa	Native miners	unknown
1925	Cecil (222)	U.S.A.	Soldiers	4,000
1925	Cecil (222)	American troops in France	Soldiers	45,800
1925	Malone (859)	India	Native soldiers	3,000
1932	Stoltenberg (1249)	Norway	Infants and children	500
1932	Kneeland (731)	U.S.A.	Infants	23
1936	Smillie (1207)	U.S.A.	Institutionalized war veterans	600
1937	Felton (425)	U.S.A.	Men in C.C.C. camps	47,000

evaluate on the basis of reported studies vaccination as a means of preventing pneumonia, consideration will often be given to factors mentioned above (such as environment of the host and character of the disease) and to other factors, such as diet and housing, all of which may have contributed to produce spontaneous alterations in the pneumonia morbidity and mortality rates.

Prior to the general recognition of pneumococcus types, Maynard (874) and Wright and his associates (1447) reported immunizing several thousand native African miners with a pneumococcus vaccine. Three individual studies were mentioned by Maynard. The first of these concerned a considerable number of men who received two subcutaneous injections at intervals of seven to twelve days of either a vaccine prepared in London and shipped to South Africa or a vaccine prepared locally. Individual doses varied in size and contained from 40 to 60 million organisms at first, while a few months later doses of 200 to 300 million organisms were used. As the records of the vaccinated and the control miners became mixed up, this study was discarded.

The second experiment was referred to as the "8,000 experiment" in which four of every five of more than 8,000 well "tropical" natives entering the mining companies' compounds at Johannesburg in August 1912 were vaccinated. The unvaccinated men in the same group were kept as controls. All natives were under observation for six months. Those immunized received one or two subcutaneous injections of from 250 to 2,500 million pneumococci, and in a few instances even larger doses were used. Over a six-month period the figure for pneumonia attacks per thousand men was 19.5 for the inoculated and 26.4 for the controls. Vaccination seemed of benefit, though the effect only appeared to last about two months. Nevertheless, not only did the incidence of pneumonia appear decreased in the immunized men during the first two months, but the results obtained suggested that the attack rates of respiratory diseases other than pneumonia were also decreased in the vaccinated group. The fatality rate of individuals coming down with pneumonia, however, did not appear lowered as a consequence of their previous vaccination.

The third study described by Maynard (874) was carried out at two different mines. Among several thousand men employed, three of every four tropical East Coast and Basute natives were vaccinated, leaving the fourth as a control. A single subcutaneous dose of 1,000 million pneumococci was given to more than 15,000 men with little effect. The inconclusive results obtained were attributed to a lack of careful observation of the natives at some of the mines and to the fact that the men were of mixed tribal or territorial groups who had been working at the mines for varying lengths of time. It was known of course, as already mentioned, that each of the latter factors was important in influencing the incidence of pneumonia among the native laborers there. The combined returns for four months among the vaccinated and control groups are given in Table 79.

TABLE 79. REPORTED PNEUMONIA ATTACK RATE PER 1,000 AMONG VACCINATED AND CONTROL AFRICAN NATIVES, BY MONTHS

	VACCINATED NATIVES		CONTROL NATIVES	
MONTH AFTER VACCINATION	*Number*	*Hospital admissions with pneumonia per 1,000 per month*	*Number*	*Hospital admissions with pneumonia per 1,000 per month*
First	15,701	5.3	5,212	5.6
Second	14,938	3.7	4,916	3.3
Third	13,922	2.8	4,599	4.8
Fourth	13,018	2.9	4,320	1.4

From Maynard (874)

Several studies of a similar nature, some of which were discarded for various reasons, were reported by Wright and his co-workers (1447). Between October 1911 and April 1912, vaccination was carried out on 5,963 natives and 5,671 others were kept as controls. The immunized were given two separate doses of vaccine at intervals of eight to ten days. The average total number of pneumococci injected was about 300 million, and, though the dosage varied somewhat, it never exceeded a total of 600 million organisms. During the next two months the pneumonia attack rate experienced by the vaccinated group was reported to have been much lower than that of the controls.

In the latter part of 1912 another group of natives was inoculated with varying doses of vaccine. It was concluded that doses ranging from a total of 250 to 1,000 million pneumococci had a marked effect in decreasing the incidence of pneumonia and in lowering the fatality rate of such cases as occurred among the inoculated. With a dose of 500 million organisms, the incidence rate was apparently reduced by 25 to 50 per cent and the death rate by 40 to 50 per cent. These effects were considered to last for about three months after vaccination. The observation was also made that in instances where natives received doses of over 1,000 million organisms (from 2,500 to 12,500 million organisms were given) there seemed temporarily to be a slight increase in the incidence rate of pneumonia. Wright and his associates also reported giving vaccine doses containing from 200 million to 1,000 million organisms to a large number of native diamond miners. This investigation was carried on at the Premier Diamond Mine during the full year of 1912, and the reported results are shown in Table 80.

TABLE 80. NUMBER OF MEN AND NUMBER AND PERCENTAGE OF CASES AND DEATHS FROM PNEUMONIA AMONG INOCULATED AND UNINOCULATED NATIVE MINERS AT THE PREMIER DIAMOND MINE, 1912

	Results for average whole native population at mines				
	DAILY AVERAGE NUMBER OF NATIVES	PNEUMONIA CASES		PNEUMONIA DEATHS	
		Number	*Per cent*	*Number*	*Per cent*
Inoculated	9,909	508	5.13	154	1.55
Uninoculated	4,502	467	10.33	145	3.21
	Results for natives beginning work during 1912				
	NUMBER OF NATIVES WHO JOINED MINE	PNEUMONIA CASES		PNEUMONIA DEATHS	
		Number	*Per cent*	*Number*	*Per cent*
Inoculated	17,431	376	2.16	120	0.7
Uninoculated	6,771	348	5.14	120	1.77

From Wright *et al.* (1447)

During the whole period, the average daily number of vaccinated men at the mine was approximately ten thousand, while the controls numbered nearly half as many. The pneumonia attack rate amounted to 5.13 per cent in the vaccinated group and was 10.33 per cent, or more than twice as high, among the controls. Similar results were obtained among new laborers beginning work at the mine during the same year, for pneumonia occurred in 2.16 per cent of the 17,431 vaccinated men as compared with 5.14 per cent of the 6,771 controls. The proportion of the individuals in both the total group and the group of natives entering service at the mine that year who died of pneumonia was about twice as high among the controls as among the vaccinated.

Subsequent to the above studies the discovery of pneumococcus types was announced and efforts were made to carry out the bacteriologic diagnosis of natives with lobar pneumonia. Lister (785) in 1916, using his own classification of pneumococcus types (see page 22), reported the incidence of the types found in 96 cases which were examined between 1913 and 1915, and late in 1917 he (786) reported similar figures for 148 cases typed from 1913 through part of 1917. From these apparently limited studies, it was concluded that from 63 to 76 per cent of all cases of lobar pneumonia in native miners were due to pneumococci of Group A, B, or C.* As a consequence of this observation and of other findings relating to the antigenicity of pneumococcus vaccine (see pages 425–428), it was recommended that three subcutaneous injections at weekly intervals of a vaccine containing 6,000 million pneumococci of each of the above three groups or types be used for immunizing purposes. For various reasons, including the fact that by 1917 it was apparent that four other groups of pneumococci (Groups E, H, J, and K) were also frequently found in the pneumonias in natives at some mines, it was recommended that strains of these organisms might well be included in the vaccine prepared for future work.

Rather than follow the previous practice of vaccinating a part of the men at a mine and reserving the remainder for controls, Lister (785, 786) advanced reasons why it seemed preferable to vaccinate all or almost all the men at a given mine and determine whether or not the incidence and death rates of pneumonia in the whole group might thus be reduced. He concluded that at a mine with part of the labor force vaccinated, the unvaccinated members reaped a benefit which could not be computed statistically. This benefit was considered to derive from the belief that vaccination, by causing a reduction in the number of current cases of pneumonia, breaks the epidemiologic chain by which pneumococci are spread from case to carrier or person to person. While proof of such a contention is lacking, there is much in the epidemiology of this disease to recommend this point of view, the validity of which has apparently never been seriously challenged.

To return again, further consideration must be given Lister's (786) results reported in 1917. Observations were made in respect to the results obtained by the prophylactic vaccination of newly arrived miners in three different mines, each of which had a bad pneumonia record. Broth cultures of

* In terms of the current classification of pneumococci generally used, Lister's Group A corresponds to one of the higher types; his Group B, Type II, and his Group C, Type I, as elsewhere noted; see Appendix B, page 946.

pneumococci were centrifuged and the organisms suspended in saline (0.85 per cent) and killed by the addition of 1.5 per cent of a proprietary agent named "Medical Bacterol" which apparently was a product related to or containing cresol.

The first study was carried out at the Premier Diamond Mine, an open surface mine which had been closed in 1914 at the beginning of the war but had been reopened a short time previous to the study. By the third quarter of 1916 from forty to fifty-five cases of pneumonia were occurring there each month and the disease was epidemic. Prophylactic immunization had been undertaken with a vaccine containing about equal proportions of pneumococci of the three groups, A, B, and C, in an effort to stop the outbreak. All resident miners were given two subcutaneous doses at seven-day intervals, the total dose received by each man amounting to 8,000 million organisms. This procedure apparently brought the epidemic under control. The experiment was continued for twelve months. During this period only newly arriving miners were vaccinated, and heavier doses were used than previously. These workers were given three subcutaneous doses of a vaccine containing the above same three groups of pneumococci at intervals of seven days, totaling 21,000 million organisms per man. In all, over 10,000 new miners were vaccinated. The mean population of native laborers at the mine during the whole year was 5,621 men, yet there occurred only seven cases of lobar pneumonia with one death among individuals receiving three doses of vaccine.

The second study was carried out at the large Crown Mines, where some 14,000 or more natives were employed. In 1915, because of the high pneumonia incidence of 41 per thousand, all miners were given a single dose of a polyvalent vaccine containing 2,000 million pneumococci. Several months later revaccination was carried out, and, subsequently, all were reinoculated every three or four months. A concurrent reduction occurred in the pneumonia attack and death rates. Following this, a separate study was undertaken, and over a nine-month period the regular three-group vaccine (Groups A, B, and C), containing a total of 7,000 million pneumococci per dose, was given three times at weekly intervals to all newly arriving miners. In all, more than 10,000 natives were vaccinated. During the study period a still further decrease occurred in the pneumonia incidence, which dropped from 24.8 to 13.8 per thousand, and the figure for deaths declined from 4 to 2.9 per thousand. These decreases were also accompanied by some lowering of the case fatality rate among individuals in the inoculated group who developed pneumonia.

In the eighty-two cases that occurred among the vaccinated miners, none was due to pneumococci of Group A, B, or C, the three groups contained in the vaccine. As Lister estimated that without vaccination probably about 120 cases due to these organisms would have occurred, he concluded that the results secured were clearly due to the vaccine used and constituted proof of the efficacy of this method of vaccination against lobar pneumonia. The figures cited are impressive and, if they do not clearly indicate, they certainly strongly suggest that prophylactic vaccination was effective in lowering the incidence and death rates from pneumonia. However, the failure to carry out or to report bacteriologic studies of cases occurring at this mine in the period just prior to the beginning of the above study makes it somewhat dangerous to draw sweeping conclusions as to the failure of Group A, B, or C cases to appear in the vaccinated men. All in all, Lister considered this particular study to be one of the most significant ones he had made.

The third experiment reported in 1917 by Lister (786) was that conducted among native diamond miners at the DeBeers Mines in Kimberley. Formerly employing about 13,000 natives, only about 7,400 miners were working at the mines at the time the study was carried out, but, as previously, pneumonia was very common there. According to Lister, pneumococci of Groups A, B, and C were about as prevalent in cases of pneumonia at the diamond mines as they were in cases at the gold mines on the Rand, though no bacteriologic data were shown to illustrate this point. Pneumococci of Group H were also frequently encountered in cases at the diamond mines, and in consequence organisms of this group were added to the vaccine used. The latter, then, contained pneumococci of Groups A, B, C, and H and totaled 8,000 million organisms (per cubic centimeter) per dose. Over a period of six months all of 6,466 new arrivals at the mines received a subcutaneous dose as above on each of three occasions at intervals of seven days. The average length of service at the mines was five months, and by the end of the study nearly 800 men had left employment there. In addition, as only the newly arrived miners were vaccinated, it was not until toward the end of the study period that the proportion of the immunized to the uninoculated natives became high. Despite these difficulties, the evidence obtained suggested that both the number of cases and number of deaths from pneumonia were somewhat reduced.

At this point it may be noted that one real obstacle to a more enthusiastic reception by distant workers of the reports of Lister and others from South Africa is the lack of bacteriologic evidence that the groups or types of pneumococci most prevalent there in lobar pneumonia were included in the vaccine used. In Lister's (786) 1917 report he stated that from 63 to 76 per cent of all cases of lobar pneumonia in native miners were due to pneumococci of Group A, B, or C, as already mentioned. This highly important conclusion was, however, apparently supported solely by the bacteriologic findings in 96 cases examined from 1913 to 1915 (785) and the findings in 148 cases (786) studied over the five years of 1913 through 1917. It would appear that the size of the group so examined is far too small to be necessarily a fair sample of all the cases occurring in the gold mines on the Rand. This seems a safe assumption, for Lister (786) remarked that the number of native miners on the Rand averaged about 200,000 per year and that over the three-year period of 1913 through 1915 the mean yearly death rate of lobar pneumonia for all native laborers at the mines and works in the Transvaal was 6.16 per thousand. Assuming there was little significant change in this rate during the next two years as well, there were presumably 1,232 deaths a year from this disease. With an average of four times this number of cases there may have been approximately 4,900 cases yearly. Over a five-year period, then, nearly 25,000 cases may have occurred, yet bacteriologic findings were given in only about 250 or one per cent of these cases. Although there may be some margin of error in the above mathematics, such figures will serve to call attention to the point made. Moreover, the bacteriologic findings in pneumonia in miners may vary from mine to mine, as Ordman (970) has reported, a fact which serves further to emphasize the need of more extensive bacteriologic investigations. Presumably the difficulties in carrying out studies of this nature have been great. It may also be noted that lack of similar data has seriously handicapped the drawing of suitable conclusions in many other studies of prophylactic vaccination against pneumonia.

As a result of the apparent success of Lister's work, as described above, arrangements were made by 1918 to inoculate all new native miners with three doses of pneumococcus vaccine at weekly intervals. While this procedure was not uniformly carried out in all mines on the Rand, yet for the next six years a large majority of newly arriving natives apparently received at least one or two doses of vaccine. The preparation used had a wider antigenic coverage than the vaccine previously administered, for it contained 1,000 million of the pneumococci of each of eight different groups or types (970). As to the success of this wholesale vaccination, Lister and Ordman (788) stated, "The results were generally admitted to be satisfactory and the whole six-year period was characterized by a far lower mortality from lobar pneumonia than that of any similar period in the history of the gold mines."

It was considered that the control of the pneumonia problem was well in hand.

In the latter part of 1926 and in 1927, a situation arose, however, which indicated that the eight-group pneumococcus vaccine in use was no longer controlling the ravages of pneumonia as it formerly had, for both the incidence and the mortality rates from pneumonia began gradually to rise. The bacteriologic examination of cases occurring around that time revealed that organisms other than the pneumococcus were causing a considerable proportion of the cases. Whereas in former years it was believed that nearly all cases were due to pneumococci and that approximately 70 per cent were caused by Group A, B, or C, as earlier mentioned, these groups were found less often in 1927, and in 95 cases examined in that year they were present in but 42 per cent of the cases (Lister, 787). This and other evidence of like nature (Ordman, 970, Lister and Ordman, 788, Peall, 1007) suggested that pure pneumococcus pneumonia was becoming scarce on the Rand and that cases due to the streptococcus, influenza bacillus, staphylococcus, Friedländer's bacillus, and other organisms were increasing in number. In several instances mixed infections in which two or more organisms were obtained from the lungs by lung puncture or at necropsy were also encountered. Such cases had seldom been found in earlier years. In brief, the limited bacteriologic evidence available suggested that a significant and rather abrupt change had occurred in the variety of the organisms causing pneumonia. This alteration appeared to be accompanied by changes in the clinical and pathologic nature of the cases, for the massive lesions of lobar pneumonia were found less frequently and the consolidated areas appeared wetter and showed more congestion than formerly. In addition, cases of atypical pneumonia or bronchopneumonia increased in number to a considerable degree. While in former years most cases of pneumonia were primary, a large proportion of all current cases were of a secondary nature.

This general change in the character of the cases occurring on the Rand and in other neighboring areas in the Union of South Africa was attributed to the invasion of a virus of some sort which was considered to be responsible for the initial infection in many cases. There was not complete agreement, however, that any such important change as outlined had occurred (973, 788). While clinically the evidence for such a change may have been considerable, though this was strongly challenged by Orenstein (973), certainly the bacteriologic data cited are so limited that generalizations concerning a changing etiology would appear hazardous. However, what bacteriologic evidence was presented (787, 970, 1219, 788, 1007) appears to support the conclusion drawn. In addition, from statements made by Lister and Ordman (788), it seems probable that the results of most of the bacteriologic and necropsy examinations made at many of the mines on the Rand have never been published.

In any event, the changing etiology of pneumonia in South Africa was regarded as the reason for the failure of the eight-group pneumococcus vaccine in use to continue to control the morbidity and mortality rates from this disease. In consequence, it was decided to prepare a mixed vaccine which was to contain pneumococci of several groups or types and strains of some of the miscellaneous organisms found in current cases as well. Such a preparation was aptly termed a "community autogenous vaccine" and has been used to a variable extent since 1930 (1007). In 1935 Lister and Ordman (788) stated:

The vaccine used in pneumonia prophylaxis on the mines of the Witwatersrand contains 11,000 million organisms per c.c. and has at present the following constitution:—

Pneumococcus	A	1,000	million	per	c.c.
"	B	2,000	"	"	"
"	C	1,000	"	"	"
"	E	1,000	"	"	"
"	K	1,000	"	"	"
"	R	1,000	"	"	"
"	S	1,000	"	"	"
"	T	1,000	"	"	"
Streptococcus pyogenes		500	"	"	"
Streptococcus salivarius		200	"	"	"
B. influenzae (Pfeiffer)		500	"	"	"
M. catarrhalis		200	"	"	"
Staphylococcus aureus (haem.)		500	"	"	"
Bacillus of Friedländer		100	"	"	"

. . . The dosage of the constituents of the vaccine, other than the pneumococcus, is empirical and is subject to any alteration that future experience may dictate.

In preparing the vaccine, the pneumococci are grown from seven to nine hours and the other organisms for longer periods. Broth is used for culturing the pneumococci and the streptococci, while the remaining organisms are grown on solid media. The broth cultures are centrifuged and the organisms taken up in physiologic saline, and the same vehicle is used to suspend the organisms grown on solid media. The bacteria in these suspensions are killed by heating in a water bath for one hour at 60° C., after which phenol is added so that the final concentration of this preservative is 0.5 per cent.

At some of the mines natives newly arriving for work receive three subcutaneous doses of 1 cc. each of the above vaccine. The doses are given at seven-day intervals. During the first two years the new vaccine was in use, the results obtained in about 40,000 natives suggested it was of value (1219). Later observations covering a period of nearly five years (788, 1007) were of similar significance. As an example of the direct bacteriologic evidence available as to the usefulness of such a vaccine, the data in the accompanying table (Table 81), as given by Lister and Ordman (788) may be cited.

As seen in Table 81, the proportion of cases showing no pneumococci was higher in the vaccinated community (31.2 per cent) than in the uninocu-

TABLE 81. PERCENTAGE DISTRIBUTION OF GROUPS OF PNEUMOCOCCI IN THE LUNG AND LUNG-JUICE SPECIMENS FROM CASES OF PNEUMONIA IN NATIVES IN INOCULATED AND UNINOCULATED COMMUNITIES, BY PNEUMOCOCCUS GROUP, 1930–1934

PNEUMOCOCCUS GROUP FOUND	INOCULATED COMMUNITY (224 SPECIMENS)	UNINOCULATED COMMUNITY (86 SPECIMENS)
A*	–	1.2
B*	4.0	27.9
C*	8.0	16.3
E*	11.6	3.5
K*	4.5	9.3
N	0.5	–
R*	4.9	3.5
S*	5.8	5.7
T*	0.5	1.2
V	0.9	–
Z	1.3	–
"Unclassified"	26.8	19.8
No pneumococcus	31.2	11.6
Pneumococcus groups represented in vaccine	39.3	68.6

From Lister and Ordman (788)

NOTE: The specific types to which many of these groups of pneumococci correspond are listed in Appendix B, page 946.

* Groups represented in the vaccine.

lated community (11.6 per cent). In addition, pneumococci of the groups represented in the vaccine given were isolated from a much smaller proportion of the cases from the vaccinated area (39.3 per cent) than from the other area (68.6 per cent). The most striking difference in the incidence of pneumococci of the different groups in these cases was in the incidence of strains of Group B, which were found in only 4 per cent of the cases in the immunized group but were present in 27.9 per cent of the cases in the unvaccinated group.

Peall (1007) reported using the "community autogenous vaccine" over a period of three and one-half years in 68,828 natives at one of the mines in the Transvaal, the Randfontein Estates Gold Mine. This mine employed from 18,000 to 21,000 men and in 1929 had a mortality from pneumonia and influenza of 8.3 per thousand per year. In the early part of 1930 both the incidence and the mortality rates increased sharply. The vaccination of all new recruits was begun in July 1930 using the customary three doses of 1 cc. each. The results obtained were striking and were attributed to the vaccine used. The incidence rates for pneumonia decreased markedly and soon dropped considerably below such rates for all other gold mines on the Rand, as shown in Table 82. Apparently immunizing programs were carried out in few if any of the other gold mines during the period covered. While the figures for pneumonia morbidity for all other gold mines on the Rand decreased between 1930 and 1933 from 37 to 21 per thousand, the rates at the Randfontein Estates Mine dropped from 45 to 9. The mortality rates for pneumonia and influenza decreased in similar fashion, and in 1933 the figure per thousand per year was 1.1 for the Randfontein Estates Mine, which was 57 per cent below the average rate of 2.6 for all other gold mines. Peall (1007) concluded:

> That, following the prophylactic inoculation of all recruits at the Randfontein Estates G. M. Co. with a Community Autogenous Vaccine, the morbidity and mortality rates from pneumonia were greatly reduced in comparison with the previous pneumonia incidence on the mine and with the incidence on all other gold mines of the Witwatersrand during the experimental period.

In many instances the miners employed worked for the usual period of a few months and then left the mines and later returned for another period of work. Some evidence was obtained that those men who at their first enlistment had been vaccinated and, after working and later leaving the mines, had subsequently returned for work again were less susceptible to pneumonia than others with a similar history but who had not been previously vaccinated. This suggested that a certain residual of the immunity induced by immunization had persisted for many months. In addition to these findings, Peall reported that the results obtained from vaccination also suggested that the incidence rates of influenza and other respiratory diseases as well were lowered by the use of the mixed vaccine.

TABLE 82. PNEUMONIA MORBIDITY PER 1,000 PER YEAR FOR THE RANDFONTEIN ESTATES GOLD MINE AND ALL OTHER GOLD MINES ON THE RAND, BY YEAR, 1928–1933

YEAR	ALL OTHER GOLD MINES ON RAND *Pneumonia cases*	*Rate per 1,000*	RANDFONTEIN ESTATES MINE *Pneumonia cases*	*Rate per 1,000*
1928	6,791	37.79	574	32.71
1929	5,223	30.56	924	54.02
1930	6,720	37.72	838	45.59*
1931	5,824	31.48	504	26.43
1932	4,606	23.90	250	12.96
1933	4,394	21.27	212	9.85†

From Peall (1007)

* Vaccination begun the latter part of this year.
† 53 per cent below average of all other mines.

In 1931, before the reported value of the "community autogenous vaccine" had been recognized, Orenstein (973) in Johannesburg, who had a wide experience with native miners on the Rand, reviewed all of the previous work on the vaccine prophylaxis of pneumonia in that region. He concluded that in almost every instance such efforts had accomplished little. A study of this report serves to indicate the need for caution in attempting to appraise with accuracy the results of immunizing programs.

It is clear that there is not complete agreement among the physicians in South Africa as to the value of prophylactic vaccination against pneumonia. The possibility exists that too much has been expected of such procedures. The pneumococcus vaccine used for several years may have been fairly successful in reducing the incidence of pneumonia due to the types of pneumococci included in the vaccine. In recent years, however, such beneficial results were no longer obtained and the incidence of pneumonia again increased. Most of this increase was attributed to the occurrence of cases due to organisms not included in the vaccine, and, in consequence, the composition of the vaccine was changed, as previously mentioned. A consideration at this distance of the apparent general situation in South Africa suggests that the character and severity of the predisposing factors which contribute to a high pneumonia morbidity, such as overcrowding, exposure to wet, cold, marked temperature variations, and the like, and to which the susceptible African native is exposed in varying degree, are sufficiently numerous and intense to result in a continued high general incidence of pneumonia. The reports available likewise suggest that, if the development of pneumonia due to organisms included in the vaccine is blocked by previous immunization, acute pulmonary infection may occur with some allied organism. Under such circumstances it is possible that prophylactic vaccination can never effect a long continuing decrease in the incidence of pneumonia in the groups under consideration unless some alteration is also made in the nature of the predisposing factors to which these groups are exposed.

A study similar to that of Lister and Ordman (788) and that of Peall (1007) was carried out by Ordman (971) at the Roan Antelope Copper Mine in Northern Rhodesia. The average monthly native population at this mine was around 2,000 to 4,000 men, most of whom were of the "tropical" variety which at the mines along the Rand in South Africa had proved so susceptible to pneumonia that their importation for work in the gold fields had been prohibited by law since 1913. Between 1926 and 1931 the pneumonia incidence figures were about 50 to 80 per thousand and the mortality figures in the vicinity of 18 to 20 per thousand. A group of forty-two cases of pneumonia of various kinds was examined bacteriologically in an effort to determine the identity of the organisms causing pneumonia in this community. Pneumococci were found only twice, and in both cases these were members of Group B. Certain other organisms, but particularly strains of *Streptococcus pyogenes,* were frequently encountered. With this work as a background a vaccine was made up containing representatives of the organisms most often isolated from the lesions of patients with pneumonia. Each cubic centimeter of the vaccine contained the following number of organisms in millions: pneumococcus Group B 4,000, *Streptococcus pyogenes* 2,000, *Streptococcus salivarius* 1,000, *Micrococcus catarrhalis* 500, and *Staphylococcus aureus haemolyticus* 500, totaling 8,000 million organisms. The usual three subcutaneous doses of 1 cc. each were given at seven-day intervals.

The inoculation of newly arrived natives was begun in October in 1931, and the present study embraced observations made on the whole population of the mine over the subsequent period of two years. A comparison of the mortality rates for pneumonia of all forms among natives at this mine for the two years prior to beginning vaccination and the two following years showed that the figure of 13.96 per thousand in the former period had been reduced to 2.41 in the latter period. Such a striking effect indicated a reduction in the mortality rate of 82.7 per cent. This marked result was obtained even though the proportion of men working underground was more than doubled during the experiment and reached 59 per cent by 1933. In addition, and contrary to previous experience at this mine, after beginning vaccination there were periods of several consecutive months in which no deaths from pneumonia occurred. While housing, diet, general hygiene, and other matters which might have affected the pneumonia rates were studied, no suitable explanation of the lowered rates was found other than that this effect resulted from prophylactic inoculation. However, there was a concurrent marked reduction in the mortality rates from all diseases as well as pneumonia during the vaccination period, and presumably a part of this reduction in each case may have been due to factors other than vaccination (see Table 83).

As shown in Table 83, the death rates from all diseases as well as pneumonia decreased during the inoculation period. In addition to this, the proportion of the total mortality experience which was attributed to pneumonia decreased from about 50 to 80 per cent to about 35 per cent.

The above studies have been presented in some detail, for, despite the fact that African natives of considerable susceptibility were dealt with, they constitute much of the most suggestive evidence available as to the possible efficacy of prophylactic vaccination against pneumonia.

OTHER STUDIES OF PROPHYLACTIC VACCINATION. The first extensive investigation of prophylactic vaccination against pneumonia outside of Africa was made in American soldiers (mostly white) in 1918 at Camp Upton, New York, by Cecil and Austin (228). The vaccine used contained pneumococci of Types I, II, and III and consisted of a saline suspension of heat-killed organisms obtained from centrifuged twelve to fourteen hour broth cultures with 0.3 per cent of tricresol added. The antigenicity of varying doses of this preparation was first determined by inoculating human volunteers, as earlier described (see pages 425–427). As the result of such tests the decision was made to use moderate total doses of the order of 6,000 to 9,000 million pneumococci of each of Types I and II and 4,500 to 6,000 million of Type III to be given in three or four small subcutaneous doses at weekly intervals. The volume of the doses was adjusted to 0.5 cc. in each instance.

Approximately 40 per cent of the strength of the camp, or 12,519 men, were vaccinated on this basis, though in several instances only one or two doses were administered. A bacteriologic survey of the pneumonias in camp

TABLE 83. AVERAGE POPULATION AND MORTALITY RATES FROM ALL DISEASES AND PNEUMONIA OF ALL FORMS PRIOR TO AND DURING THE INOCULATION PERIOD AT THE ROAN ANTELOPE MINE, BY VARIOUS PERIODS, 1926–1933

YEAR (OCTOBER TO SEPTEMBER)	AVERAGE NATIVE POPULATION	MORTALITY RATE PER 1,000 PER YEAR		PER CENT OF ALL DEATHS DUE TO PNEUMONIA
		All diseases	*Pneumonia (all forms)*	
Prior to inoculation period				
1926–27	975	49.23	35.90	72.9
1927–28	1,664	28.25	23.44	83.0
1928–29	2,792	29.37	18.27	62.2
1929–30	3,661	27.31	14.48	53.0
1930–31	4,849	24.33	14.64	60.2
Inoculation period				
1931–32	2,800	7.50	2.86	38.1
1932–33	2,663	6.38	2.25	35.3

From Ordman (971)

prior to the vaccination period revealed that among the first cases examined, which numbered nearly one hundred, 70 per cent were due to pneumococci, of which about one-half were strains of Type I, II, or III. The period of investigation after beginning the inoculations lasted ten weeks. During that interval no case of Type I, II, or III pneumonia developed in persons in the inoculated group who had received two or more doses of vaccine; while among the control group, which numbered more than 19,400 men, there were twenty-six cases due to pneumococci of these types. (One Type I case occurred among the vaccinated men, and this case appeared twenty-four hours after the first dose of vaccine was given.)

The vaccinated group, however, was apparently composed of seasoned troops, as was about three-quarters of the control group, and individuals of this type are less susceptible to pneumonia than are raw recruits such as those who made up the remainder of the controls. Even after making allowances for this factor, the results obtained favored the use of vaccination; for, together, the number of pneumonias due to all organisms totaled but 17 in the vaccinated group as compared with 110 cases in the seasoned troop controls. There were, in addition, 63 cases among the control recruits, making a grand total of 173 cases for the controls. Computed on the basis of an annual number per thousand, the pneumonia death rate was 12.8 in the control troops and only 0.83 in the vaccinated.

Evidence was obtained that vaccination reduced the incidence and mortality rates for all pneumonias (especially pneumococcus and streptococcus cases) in general and the rates for cases due to those types of pneumococci included in the vaccine in particular. As the troops were moved from camp at the end of ten weeks, the duration of these effects could not be determined.

In a later study, also carried out in 1918 on American soldiers and conducted at Camp Wheeler, Georgia, Cecil and Vaughan (246) attempted to lessen the work of immunizing a large body of men by using a single subcutaneous dose (1 cc.) of a lipovaccine. This preparation contained 10,000 million pneumococci of each of the types I, II, and III. Pneumonia was rife in the camp, and most all cases were primary pneumococcus lobar pneumonia, of which about 43 per cent were due to one or another of the above three types. The general conditions at this camp differed considerably from those which existed at the time the above study was made at Camp Upton. Most of the men were raw recruits from rural regions, about one-sixth of them were Negroes, and early in the study an influenza epidemic struck the camp which greatly reduced the resistance of the vaccinated and control groups alike. In addition, the camp population was rapidly changing and increased from about 9,000 men in mid-September to nearly 16,000 by the middle of November. Approximately two weeks later demobilization of the troops was begun, and within the next three weeks the population had decreased to 4,000. The period of investigation relative to the value of inoculation extended from September 21 through December 20. Influenza appeared about October first, and within two weeks the attack rate was high. A great many cases of secondary pneumonia occurred, but the incidence rates were about twice as high in the control as in the immunized group.

Vaccination was begun in mid-September, and approximately 75 per cent of the old seasoned troops then in camp were inoculated. Most of the incoming recruits were vaccinated within twenty-four hours of arrival. By early November 13,460 men or about 80 per cent of the troops in camp had been vaccinated, and the remainder or 3,415 men served as controls. In the four preceding months Types I, II, and III together had caused 43.2 per cent of all the cases of pneumococcus pneumonia which had occurred there, while during the interval of about three months when influenza was prevalent (which corresponded closely with the vaccination period) these types were less common and were found in only 11.5 per cent of all pneumococcus cases.

In the large group of vaccinated men during the study period, pneumonia due to Type I, II, or III occurred thirty-two times, while in the 20 per cent of the troops that were unvaccinated it occurred forty-two times. The situation was very similar in respect to the incidence of cases due to all other pneumococci as well, for there were 298 such cases in the vaccinated men and 256 such cases in the controls. Together, cases due to all organisms numbered 363 in the inoculated troops and 327 in the uninoculated.

The total fatality rates for all cases in the groups under comparison were essentially the same and amounted to 21.7 per cent for the inoculated and 22.3 per cent for the uninoculated. A difference in such rates was observed, however, in the recruits and seasoned troops depending upon whether the pneumonia was primary or secondary. For recruits with primary pneumonia the case fatality rate was 11.5 per cent for the vaccinated and 33.3 per cent, or nearly three times as high, for the controls; whereas for secondary cases the rates were about the same in each group (around 25 per cent). The situation was very similar for the seasoned troops in the various groups.

Other data indicated that the incidence rates for pneumonia were always higher among the Negro than among the white troops in comparable groups (see Table 84). Further, the incidence rates for any particular group, whether white or Negro, recruits or seasoned men, were considerably lower for the vaccinated members of the group than for the unvaccinated. This difference, however, was most marked in the case of the seasoned white troops where the incidence of pneumonia per thousand for the controls (rate 40.0) was nearly eight times that for the vaccinated men (rate 5.2). Nevertheless, results of considerable significance were likewise obtained among the vaccinated seasoned Negro troops as well. Also of importance was the fact that the pneumonia incidence rates were only about one-half as high for all vaccinated recruits (rate 58.2) as for all unvaccinated recruits (rate 115.2).

TABLE 84. NUMBER OF MEN AND CASES OF PNEUMONIA AND INCIDENCE FIGURES PER 1,000 IN VACCINATED AND CONTROL WHITE AND NEGRO RECRUITS AND SEASONED TROOPS DURING A STUDY PERIOD OF THREE MONTHS AT CAMP WHEELER

	NUMBER OF MEN	NUMBER OF CASES OF PNEUMONIA	PNEUMONIA INCIDENCE RATES PER 1,000 MEN LISTED
Recruits			
White			
Vaccinated	3,832	148	38.7
Unvaccinated	919	59	64.0
Negro			
Vaccinated	1,113	140	125.0
Unvaccinated	157	65	413.0
Total vaccinated	4,945	288	58.2
Total unvaccinated	1,076	124	115.2
Seasoned men			
White			
Vaccinated	6,570	34	5.2
Unvaccinated	1,919	77	40.0
Negro			
Vaccinated	1,828	27	14.8
Unvaccinated	383	30	78.4
Total vaccinated	8,398	61	7.2
Total unvaccinated	2,302	107	46.4

From Cecil and Vaughan (246)

Although many of the rates cited in this study were based upon relatively small groups of men, their trend was the same in practically every instance. It was concluded that, even though the rapidly changing population at this camp, combined with an epidemic of influenza, produced less striking results than had been obtained at Camp Upton, as already noted, the results were distinctly encouraging. The suggestion was made that prophylactic inoculation be further applied both in civil and in military life.

Cecil (222) subsequently reported that during the winter of 1918–1919 pneumococcus vaccine was extensively used in the United States Army, both for men in this country and for those abroad, and cited a memorandum from the Surgeon General's Office in Washington, D.C., to this effect.

Though lacking in detail, one instance in particular seems of interest. This concerned the results obtained following the vaccination of 45,849 troops in the American Expeditionary Forces, 49,463 others serving as a control series. The pneumonia incidence per 100,000 was 83.5 in the vaccinated group and 168 in the unvaccinated group. The pneumonia deaths per 100,000 in these same groups were 10.8 and 22.5 respectively.

In an attempt to prevent influenza and pneumonia among civilians, Rosenow and Sturdivant (1119) distributed a mixed lipovaccine to a large number of physicians to use for their patients. This vaccine was made up of 30 per cent pneumococci of Types I, II, and III, 40 per cent pneumococci of Group IV and green streptococci, 20 per cent hemolytic streptococci, and 10 per cent *Staphylococcus aureus*. Three subcutaneous inoculations were given at weekly intervals, the individual doses containing 2.5, 5.0, and 7.5 billion organisms respectively.

Data were studied relative to 93,476 persons who received the three doses as above; and while the records obtained were stated to have been far from satisfactory, it was reported that over a six-week observation period the average incidence of influenza and pneumonia in this group was about one-third that experienced by a control group of considerably larger size and that the average mortality rate for the inoculated individuals was about one-fifth that of the uninoculated. Bacteriologic study of the cases was apparently not made.

Borrel (140) vaccinated a group of native African troops sent to France during the war. The vaccine contained three strains of pneumococci and totaled 6,000 million organisms per cubic centimeter. In his first experiment two injections of this preparation (0.5 and 1.0 cc.) were given a week apart. The reported results are shown in Table 85. The pneumonia incidence and mortality rates in the men in two different battalions studied were always lower in the vaccinated than in the control groups.

Subsequently, Borrel increased the number of pneumococci in the vaccine to 8,000 million per cubic centimeter and inoculated another group of African troops. In this instance three doses were given (0.5, 1.0, and 2.0 cc.) which totaled 28,000 million pneumococci. The results obtained were considered not very satisfactory, though the incidence and mortality rates were lower for the vaccinated than for the control group. For 2,393 individuals vaccinated the morbidity figure was 65 per thousand, while for 919 controls it was 95. The mortality figures per thousand in these groups were 19 and 28 respectively.

In this and in several of the following investigations, apparently no study was made of the bacteriology of cases occurring before or during the vaccination period. Under such circumstances it is impossible, of course, to determine the effectiveness of any vaccine in preventing the occurrence of pneumonia due to the organisms contained in the preparation used.

The enthusiastic report of Duckwall (382) describes another investigation somewhat similar to the one above. He used a saline suspension of pneumococci of Types I, II, and III containing 1,000 million organisms per cubic centimeter and reported giving 1,002 American soldiers three inoculations of this vaccine (0.5, 1.0, and 1.0 cc.) at intervals of seven to ten days. More than 300 other men received either one or two doses of the same preparation, and 5,820 men served as controls. The hospital admission figure for pneumonia per thousand per year over the four-month study period was 14.9 for the group receiving three injections of vaccine as compared with the higher rate of 54.0 for the controls. This latter rate was also higher than the rates for men who received but one or two injections of vaccine. The hospital admission rates for influenza, tonsillitis, bronchitis, coryza, and pharyngitis were all proportionally lower for the vaccinated than for the unvaccinated group. The figure for pneumonia deaths per thousand per year was 2.99 for the troops receiving three inoculations and 8.76 in the controls. Duckwall concluded that the vaccine protected against pneumonia and the common respiratory diseases in the proportion of about five to one.

TABLE 85. PNEUMONIA MORBIDITY AND MORTALITY FIGURES PER 1,000 IN VACCINATED AND UNVACCINATED NATIVE AFRICAN TROOPS IN FRANCE

	MORBIDITY PER 1,000	MORTALITY PER 1,000
95th Battalion		
Vaccinated troops	36	–
Control troops	130	33
96th Battalion		
Vaccinated troops	73	7
Control troops	85	18

From Borrel (140)

In another effort to prevent respiratory infections including pneumonia, Von Sholly and Park (1359) inoculated 1,536 civilian office workers, of whom 1,293 received three subcutaneous injections at weekly intervals of one of two vaccines. These preparations contained pneumococci of several types as well as streptococci and one or two other organisms frequently found in respiratory infections. Approximately 3,000 additional office workers were used as controls over the six-month observation period. While little evidence was obtained that the use of these vaccines reduced the incidence of respiratory diseases in general, the results were suggestive of a favorable effect on the incidence of pneumonia. Only one case of pneumonia occurred in the inoculated group as compared with eleven cases among the controls. On a percentage basis, pneumonia was about five times as frequent in the control group (0.36 per cent) as in the vaccinated group (0.075 per cent).

In the Katanga, Belgian Congo, where African natives are extensively employed in the mining of copper, Walravens (1376) and Pearson and Mouchet (1008) have reported making various efforts to vaccinate native laborers. The vaccine used contained strains of pneumococci obtained from Lister in South Africa, and in some instances strains locally prevalent were also included. The exact number of men inoculated and the results obtained were not reported in either instance. Pearson and Mouchet's investigation was interrupted by an epidemic of influenza and vaccination was discontinued.

Jordan and Sharp (693) in the United States inoculated a group of civilian adults and children who, for the most part, were living in institutions. The study extended over a period of about seven months and embraced observations on 3,193 controls and 2,873 individuals who had received three vaccine injections. A mixed vaccine was used in subcutaneous doses at weekly intervals. The initial dose contained the following number of organisms in millions: pneumococcus Type I, 1,000; Type II, 1,000; Type III, 500; influenza bacillus, 500; hemolytic streptococcus, 500; and *Streptococcus viridans,* 500; totaling 4,000 million. The second and third doses were double this size. The incidence of pneumonia, being 5.9 per cent (7 cases) among the vaccinated individuals and 7.9 per cent (12 cases) among the controls, was much the same in both groups. As no bacteriologic studies were made, it is impossible to tell what the prevailing organisms were in cases there either before or during the vaccination period.

A similar type of study was carried out in several institutions in New York State by McCoy, Hasseltine, Wadsworth, and Kirkbride (831). A single 1 cc. dose of a lipovaccine containing approximately 10 billion pneumococci of each of the types I, II, and III was given to 17,752 inmates of institutions, while 18,595 others in the same hospitals were left as controls. Over a period of approximately two winters there were in these groups respectively 253 and 340 cases of pneumonia, most of which were in the form of terminal bronchopneumonia. Bacteriologic examination was carried out for about one-half of these cases.

Of special interest were the findings for cases in the control group and in another group of 103 cases occurring in patients admitted to the hospitals too late for inoculation. Together these two groups, which were examined bacteriologically, totaled 289 cases. In contrast to the usual high incidence of Type I and Type II cases in lobar pneumonia in ordinary civilian life, there were in this total group, which consisted chiefly of cases of atypical pneumonia, only nine (3.1 per cent) Type I and six (2.1 per cent) Type II cases. Type III accounted for 49 cases and pneumococci of Group IV for 86, while the remaining 139 cases were due to streptococci or other organisms. Such findings suggested that the organisms prevalent in pneumonia in these institutions were to a large extent different from those included in the vaccine administered. Of the 122 cases in the vaccinated group that were studied bacteriologically, Types I, II, and III caused one, two, and sixteen cases respectively. Considering the nature and composition of the vaccine used in this experiment, it is not surprising that but little evidence was obtained as to its favorable effect for the vaccinated group.

Encouraged by studies of prophylactic vaccination against pneumonia made elsewhere, Malone (859) and King (719) in 1925 reported their efforts to vaccinate native troops along the North-West Frontier Province of India. Pneumonia was a frequent and serious illness among the troops in that region. After considerable work, however, no evidence was obtained that the vaccine used was of any help in solving the pneumonia problem in that area. The explanation of this failure may have lain in the unhappy method by which the vaccine was produced. As pneumococci of Types I and II were the organisms most frequently found among seventy-eight cases of pneumonia examined, a vaccine was prepared containing equal numbers of these organisms and totaling 5,000 million pneumococci per cubic centimeter. In the preparation of this material broth cultures of the organisms were grown for periods as long as two or three days before the growth was harvested by centrifuging. It is well recognized now that cultures of such age contain chiefly the débris of autolyzed pneumococci which is of little use in stimulating an effective immune response.

In any event, the first effort made to immunize several thousand men was discarded as troop movements precluded observing them for any length of time. During the winter of 1922–1923 a second attempt was made and two subcutaneous injections of the above vaccine of 1 cc. each were given a week apart to 2,996 men while 5,227 others served as controls. During the next few months there were twenty-eight cases of either lobar pneumonia or bronchopneumonia in the former group and fifty-six in the latter group. This represented a case rate per thousand of 9.3 for the vaccinated and 10.7 for the unvaccinated troops, from which it was rightly concluded that the preparation used had failed to influence the incidence of pneumonia.

Stoltenberg's (1249) apparent success in reducing the incidence of respiratory infections including pneumonia in a group of 487 hospitalized infants and children in Norway has already been alluded to (see page 407). Three injections of a mixed autogenous vaccine were given. During the latter part of this study, which covered a period of nearly four years, each cubic centimeter of the vaccine contained the following number of recently isolated organisms in millions: pneumococci of Types I, II, and III, 200; Pfeiffer's bacilli, 300; Friedländer's bacilli, 50; staphylococci, 200; *M. catarrhalis,* 100; and streptococci, 150. The doses administered were varied according to the age and the response of the patient. The first dose of this preparation consisted of a total of from 75 to 250 million organisms, while the second dose contained from 100 to 500 million and the third dose from 250 to 1,000 million organisms. "Pneumonia" or bronchopneumonia was about one-half as frequent (11 cases) among the 487 vaccinated children as among the 496 children used as controls (21 cases). A proportional reduction also occurred in the attack rates of the lesser respiratory infections among individuals in the vaccinated group.

In a study of like nature carried out in New York City, Kneeland (731) reported obtaining results essentially similar to those of Stoltenberg. A mixed vaccine was used consisting of selected strains of pneumococci of Type I (40 per cent), *H. influenzae* (30 per cent), and streptococci (30 per cent). Two courses of weekly subcutaneous injections of increasing doses were given to twenty-three infants while a like number of others were retained as controls. The first course, begun in October, was of nine injections, the initial dose totaling 45 million organisms and the final dose 750 million. The second course, begun in February, was of seven injections of larger size, the initial dose totaling 190 million organisms and the final dose 1,000 million. Over a study period of approximately eight months two cases of pneumonia occurred among individuals in the inoculated group and five in the controls. In addition to this apparently favorable result, there was a marked lessening of the severity but not in the number of many of the lesser respiratory infections among the vaccinated. The findings suggested that it was necessary to administer a considerable amount of vaccine before any effect was obtained and that the duration of the resistance induced was about two months.

In 1936 Smillie (1207) reported a study of great interest. Prophylactic vaccination of the patients and attendants in a hospital for the insane was carried out in an effort to stop an outbreak of pneumococcus Type II pneumonia which was current there. The vaccine used was prepared from a strain of Type II pneumococcus freshly isolated from a patient in the institution who had pneumonia due to this organism. Unusual care was taken in preparing the vaccine to prevent autolysis of the organisms. Young broth cultures were centrifuged and the sediment was suspended in saline solution to which 0.2 per cent of formalin was added to kill and preserve the organisms. "Smears from the finished vaccine showed heavy capsulation." Three subcutaneous injections of the vaccine, which contained 750 million Type II pneumococci per cubic centimeter, were administered to 590 patients and 40 attendants who lived or worked in and around the wards in which pneumonia due to this organism had occurred. Weekly doses of 0.5, 1.0, and 1.0 cc., totaling 1,875 million organisms, were given.

Prior to the vaccination period seventeen cases of Type II lobar pneumonia had occurred in this institution over an interval of about a year and they apparently were becoming more frequent. Nasopharyngeal cultures were made in 267 patients and attendants, and 30 carriers of Type II pneumococci were found. Although the vaccination period began January 5, 1936, no case of pneumonia developed after January 1, 1936.

Under the circumstances the question at once arises whether the epidemic stopped as a result of vaccinating the exposed population or whether it terminated for some other and unknown reason. While no definite answer is available, the evidence obtained strongly suggested that the immunizing procedures used were responsible for ending the outbreak. Even though a number of persons in the vaccinated population continued to carry pneumococci of Type II for the next few months, no new carriers of this organism or cases of pneumonia developed. Smillie stated:

The results secured seem to be of significance, but the series of vaccinated persons is too small to warrant an unqualified conclusion that a serious recrudescence of widespread infection was prevented by the specific measures that were employed.

It is hard to be more conclusive than this in evaluating the procedures used because too little is known of the natural history of an outbreak of an infection of this nature. As a result, one cannot be sure what the usual course of events might be. Although a number of small epidemics of pneumonia have been studied, careful bacteriologic observations have been carried out in only a few such instances (see pages 386–390). In consequence there exists a crying need for more information relating to the usual "life cycle" of epidemics of this nature. An understanding of the usual course of such outbreaks will aid in determining the value of immunizing procedures for their control. This matter is particularly important in the present age with its various huge institutions for the care of sick and handicapped persons who not infrequently become involved in an outbreak of pneumococcus infection of considerable severity.

If efforts similar to those of Smillie, just described, prove successful in stopping epidemics of pneumococcus infections, a definite advance in the control of suffering, loss of life, and economic waste will have been made.

As earlier noted, efforts are now being made to prevent pneumonia by immunization with chemical derivatives of pneumococci of Type I and Type II. A brief preliminary report of such an attempt was made by Felton (425). Three experiments were carried out on young men (average age about twenty-three years) enrolled in the Civilian Conservation Corps camps in this country. Work begun in December 1933 is still under way. In the initial experiment 3,000 men were immunized by a single injection (presumably given subcutaneously) of 2 mgm. each of a Type I and Type II soluble antigen. This preparation is apparently similar or closely related to the specific capsular polysaccharide of these organisms. A group of 9,000 other men in the same or similar camps constituted a control for the study. Specific antibody formation was demonstrated in a number of the immunized men. Over a period of about four months there were 8 cases of pneumonia with 2 deaths in the control group of 9,000 men and no cases in the inoculated group of 3,000 men.

In a second experiment 14,000 men were inoculated and a similar number used as controls. In this instance dosage of 1 mgm. of the Type I and Type II antigen was used rather than the 2 mgm. amount previously employed. The occurrence of reactions after the larger dose made this reduction in the amount injected advisable. Over an observation period of about six months during the winter and spring of 1934–1935 there were 13 cases of pneumonia with no deaths in the group of 14,000 inoculated men and 23 cases with 2 deaths in the 14,000 men in the control group. In a third experiment mentioned, 30,000 men were being inoculated but the work was not yet finished.

No statement was made in this initial report as to the nature of the organisms responsible for the cases of pneumonia which developed.

DISCUSSION OF STUDIES OF PROPHYLACTIC VACCINATION. The following discussion relates primarily to the findings in studies employing vaccines. Little is known as yet of the use of chemical derivatives of pneumococci for the prevention of pneumonia.

The general impression gained from the reported results of prophylactic vaccination against pneumonia is that many of the efforts achieved a considerable degree of success. However, such a conclusion cannot be accepted without definite reservations. In many instances the groups studied were so small that the difference of a very few cases of pneumonia in either the vaccinated or the unvaccinated series could have influenced the figures to a significant degree. In addition, the factors which govern the occurrence of pneumonia appear so complex and so varied in nature that frequently reasonable doubt may exist as to the similarity of the conditions, such as environment, work, diet, hygiene, and the like, to which the immunized and control groups were exposed. Furthermore, the natural resistance of the individuals comprising the study groups was possibly not always comparable.

In the light of present-day knowledge, certain general criticisms of a bacteriologic and immunologic nature may also be leveled at many of the above studies. Frequently too little attention was paid to the character of the organisms selected for inclusion in the vaccine administered to the immunized groups. In preparing the vaccine sufficient care was often not taken in growing the organisms, and at times cultures which had been incubated for one or two days or more were used. As a rule, little was known of the physical state of the cells in the finished product, and frequently the antigenicity of the vaccine was unknown, though there were a few conspicuous exceptions (1447, 785, 228) in this respect (see pages 425–428). In several instances there was little or no evidence that the bacteria included in the vaccine represented the organisms most often encountered in current cases of pneumonia in the same locality. The successful determination of this latter point involves a considerable amount of initial and continued bacteriologic study, without which under ordinary circumstances either no benefits or only those of a limited or transient character would appear obtainable.

Despite difficulties of this nature, it seems important that the general conclusion of almost all the investigators is similar and that success in varying degree was obtained by prophylactic vaccination. Clearly two things must be given consideration in deciding upon the value of immunizing procedures in the control of pneumonia. The first is whether or not the total incidence of pneumonia may be reduced by the use of a vaccine or related preparation of limited antigenic coverage. Although some of the evidence at hand suggests such a reduction in incidence may occur, there are reasons why this would appear to remain a highly debatable point. The second matter is whether or not a preparation containing pneumococci of a few specific types or derivatives of these organisms will to a large extent, when used in suitable doses, prevent the occurrence of pneumonia due to these same organisms. Although conclusive proof may be lacking, there is evidence of a nature difficult to refute that such a result can be obtained in many individuals (but probably not all), at least for a period of a few months. Additional carefully conducted investigations of the problem under discussion are needed.

Studies of immunity in man make it probable that at a given time the constituent members of a group possess a widely varying individual resistance to the pneumococcus; that whatever effective resistance can be produced by the usual immunizing procedures does not last much longer than two to four months; and that, in a given locality under ordinary circumstances, the incidence of various organisms and the many different types of pneumococci in lobar pneumonia, and probably in other forms of pneumonia as well, is rarely if ever the same over an interval of some months (see pages 57–60). The operation of these variable factors serves to complicate and render more difficult large-scale attempts to prevent pneumonia by prophylactic measures. This is particularly true when the limited use of the same vaccine is continued over some period of time. It seems unreasonable to expect that a single course of injections of a vaccine containing pneumococci of the same few types, even when an ideal preparation is used with great care, can ever produce a lasting reduction in the general incidence of pneumonia. Presumably the best effects might be obtained by the administration of two or more courses of injections at intervals of about two months of a vaccine the composition of which is changed frequently to suit the immediate need shown to exist by the bacteriologic examination of current cases of pneumonia. Ordman (970) has reported success with a procedure very similar to this.

In the past the usual total dose of organisms in the vaccine used for the prevention of pneumonia in man has seldom amounted to more than 24 billion organisms and commonly was less. Such doses seem small in comparison with the size of the inoculations given monkeys (usually 120 to 200 billion organisms) to protect them from an experimentally induced pneumonia, as discussed earlier (page 442). It is doubtful, however, that the large doses used in these animals could be used subcutaneously in man without causing frequent severe reactions, as Cecil and Steffen (240) have mentioned. In fact such large doses may not be necessary, for the natural resistance of man to the pneumococcus may be higher than that of the monkey (see pages 139–148), and the dose of organisms which gives rise to spontaneous infection in man is probably smaller than the intratracheal dose customarily used to produce experimental pneumonia in immunized monkeys.

Where immunizing procedures have been carried out in animals other than monkeys, the best results have usually been obtained by the daily administration of vaccine for several successive days. This is followed by a rest period and subsequently the course of injections with a period of rest is repeated one or more times. No information is at hand relating to the parenteral vaccination of man along these lines. In nearly every instance in the foregoing studies of prophylactic vaccination in human beings, the vaccine doses have been given at weekly intervals. It would seem advisable that attention be paid to the possibility of shortening the interval between doses in man.

The evidence available suggests that, to evoke a satisfactory immune response in man with pneumococcus vaccine, repeated injections must be given of several billion organisms of each of the types against which immunity is desired. The not infrequent occurrence of systemic reactions when very large individual doses are given, however, definitely limits the size of the doses which may be used. This in turn limits the number of types of pneumococci against which a presumably effective resistance can be obtained. This limitation, in conjunction with the varied etiology of pneumonia in the population at large and the short duration of the resistance resulting from immunization, makes any present scheme to vaccinate the whole of large civilian populations distinctly impracticable.

At times certain population groups may doubtless be considered to present a special problem. Among the more obvious examples of this nature are occurrences of localized epidemics of pneumonia due to pneumococci of a single type or situations where in a more or less controlled population over a short period of time cases due to any one of a few organisms are numerous, such as among African natives during their first few months of work at some mines. Recruits in military organizations probably also fit into this category. In such instances it is possible that adequate inoculation with a suitable vaccine may serve to stop epidemics or to check the occurrence of pneumonia during the important first few months when new work is being carried on in a new environment (see also pages 399–401).

The value of prophylactic vaccination for the prevention of pneumonia among individuals employed in particular occupations, such as those involving exposure to marked variations in temperature, intermittent wetting, chilling, and the like, which appear associated with high pneumonia morbidity or mortality rates, needs special consideration and study. Persons who at frequent intervals are subject to severe respiratory infections including pneumonia may be aided by one or two series of prophylactic inoculations each winter, as Cecil has mentioned (221, 222).

REACTIONS TO IMMUNIZING AGENTS AND CONTRAINDICATIONS TO THEIR USE. *Reactions to vaccines.* The occurrence of reactions following the parenteral administration of pneumococcus vaccine or mixed vaccine has been noted by many observers (785, 228, 246, 1359, 221, 859, 222, 71, 731, 788). In many respects these reactions closely resemble those produced by typhoid vaccine and may take the form of a local irritation or a general systemic reaction. In no instance has a reaction of great severity been reported.

The local type of reaction may occur after the subcutaneous administration of vaccine. This is manifested by the development of an area of tenderness and induration about five to ten centimeters in diameter at the site of the injection. If the vaccine injections are made under the skin of the upper arm, the area of reaction is usually oval in shape. At times the axillary glands may become swollen and tender. Within three or four days the tenderness and induration about the involved area usually disappear. A response of this nature is not uncommon, and Von Sholly and Park (1359) reported that, of 1,293 persons receiving three injections of mixed vaccine at weekly intervals, 63 per cent had a mild local reaction of this type to the first dose. Similar reactions occurred in 63 per cent after the second dose and in 60 per cent after the third dose. Another 10 to 20 per cent of the vaccinated individuals had a little larger or more intense reaction of this kind.

In some instances Cecil and Austin (228) found that an additional complication of a local nature may occur. This consists of a slowly developing, small, painful, tender nodule involving the subcutaneous tissues at the point of inoculation. The nodules are frequently two or three centimeters in diameter and come to fluctuation by the sixth or seventh day. Such infiltrations are sterile, shortly become cold and painless, and resolve spontaneously. Though of no great importance, the lesions are bothersome and may develop after any dose of vaccine, while in a few instances they may follow each dose. Among more than 12,500 men inoculated, most of whom received three or four doses of a saline-suspended pneumococcus vaccine, Cecil and Austin (228) found that small infiltrations of this variety developed in 152 or in one of every 82 men (about 1.2 per cent). Reactions of this type occur much more frequently after the use of a saline vaccine than after the use of a lipovaccine; for, among more than 13,000 men given a single subcutaneous injection of a lipovaccine, Cecil and Vaughan (246) observed only five such reactions (0.04 per cent).

General, systemic, or constitutional reactions of a degree sufficient to impair an individual's working ability or to require hospitalization after the use of vaccine subcutaneously are not very common. At times these reactions do not appear till twenty-four hours after the vaccine is given. Cecil and Austin (228) have described them as simulating an attack of influenza. General malaise, chilly sensations, a rise in temperature of one or two degrees, headaches, and muscle pains may occur. In a few instances symptoms appear which are referable to the respiratory tract, such as coryza, sore throat, cough, and pain in the chest (228, 1359). Among more than 12,500 soldiers in an army camp vaccinated by Cecil and Austin (228), general reactions of this nature developed in only 25 or one in every 500 men (0.2 per cent). These individuals were confined to their quarters or to the hospital for a few days before returning to their usual duties. Most of the men vaccinated in this experiment received three or four doses of a saline vaccine. In the study made by Cecil and Vaughan (246) in which a single injection of lipovaccine was given to some 13,000 troops, all reactions were infrequent and the general reactions were usually mild. Only 0.7 per cent of the men had to be admitted to the hospital. Nearly all of the hospital admissions were among recruits, and only 3 of more than 8,000 seasoned men were temporarily incapacitated by these reactions.

Von Sholly and Park (1359) observed mild general reactions consisting of headaches, dizziness, nausea, or malaise in from 19 to 27 per cent of more than 1,200 civilian office workers after each of three injections of mixed vaccine. After each dose about 3 per cent of the inoculated group showed more intense general reactions. These individuals had chills or chilly sensations, fever, general pains, or mild prostration. In all, approximately 26 per cent of the whole group inoculated had general reactions of some kind. Such a high proportion of general reactions is unusual and doubtless may be attributed partly to the fact that practically all general symptoms occurring after vaccination were counted in this instance as a reaction.

In African natives mild local reactions are "common" but the more incapacitating general reactions are apparently seldom encountered (874, 1447, 785, 786, 788). Possibly the low incidence of the latter type of reaction is more apparent than real, as not infrequently an illness must be of considerable severity before native laborers will seek medical care. Among nearly 3,000 native troops in India receiving two doses of vaccine, Malone (859) stated that less than 2 per cent of the men reported sick from reactions.

In a study of twenty-three infants who received two courses consisting first of nine and later of seven weekly injections of a mixed vaccine, Kneeland (731) reported that some local redness and induration occurred after the larger doses used but that no general reactions were observed.

Neither the frequency nor the severity of the reactions following the subcutaneous injection of vaccine is sufficient to impair the possible usefulness of prophylactic vaccination against pneumonia. A number of factors appear to influence the reactions following vaccination. Different individuals show wide variations in their tendency to develop such reactions. The character of the vaccine used is important, and some preparations are more irritating or more likely to produce reactions than are others. The dosage of the organisms used is also important. As a rule, reactions are much less frequent after small than after large individual doses, but of course the larger doses produce the most satisfactory immune response. The route by which vaccine is administered also appears to be a factor in this matter, for subcutaneous inoculation seems to give rise to the general type of reaction less frequently than does intravenous vaccination. This point is not definite, however, for apparently few persons have ever received pneumococcus vaccine intravenously. Although Lister (785) reported that only a very slight general reaction occurred in a few African natives vaccinated intravenously with large individual doses containing as many as 20,000 to 40,000 million pneumococci, the vaccine he used must have been unusually bland as repeated intravenous doses of 20,000 million organisms in rabbits or subcutaneous doses of from 30,000 to 60,000 million in guinea pigs produced no evidence of toxicity.

With respect to the occurrence of the small sterile subcutaneous infiltrations described by Cecil and Austin (228) as mentioned above, these investigators obtained evidence suggesting that such lesions were more frequent among individuals of the white race than among those of the black race. In a total of more than 12,500 men inoculated, these lesions developed in 152 or about 1.2 per cent, while among 1,500 Negroes included in this group apparently only one man had such a reaction. The suggestion was made that a response of this nature may be related to the basic natural resistance of the individual vaccinated.

Reactions to specific derivatives of pneumococci. Little information is available relating to the effect of specific derivatives of pneumococci in the prevention of pneumococcus pneumonia in man. Since the potential importance of these materials is great, it seems advisable to describe the character of the reactions produced by such agents, as reported by Felton, Sutliff, and Steele (433).

The antigens used were prepared by treating pneumococci of Types I and II with acid or alkali in various ways (424) or by digestion with pancreatin or trypsin, and in some instances various preparations of the specific capsular polysaccharides were also used. In all, seven different agents were prepared from pneumococci of Type I, and a similar group of antigens from Type II. These materials were administered subcutaneously in small doses to a number of individuals, as described previously (see pages 414–415) and the response was noted.

Felton, Sutliff, and Steele (433), who carried out this investigation, stated:

No untoward or severe reaction was obtained by using as much as 10 mgs. in a single injection. Daily observations in twenty subjects injected with amounts ranging from 1 mg. to 10 mgs. each, showed local swelling and slight tenderness, or, in nine instances local swelling, slight tenderness and erythema which lessened considerably after 48 hours. The temperature was elevated to 99° in four subjects, malaise appeared in two, and in one elderly person a chill occurred. In subsequent experience among forty ambulant persons receiving 2 mgs. of various fractions or dried vaccines only one complained of malaise and eight showed swollen, red local reactions after 48 hours.

These observations suggest that the more or less immediate response of various individuals to the injection of small doses of certain specific derivatives of pneumococci is not unlike that elicited by the use of vaccines. In Felton's (425) later report of the administration of derivatives of pneumococci to 3,000 men, the 2 mgm. dose used occasionally caused reactions which were stated to be severe. Details as to the character of the response obtained were not given. Subsequently the dose was decreased to 1 mgm. and apparently this was more satisfactory for it was used in two different experiments embracing the inoculation of 44,000 men.

Contraindications to immunizing procedures. Relatively little information is available relating to circumstances under which immunizing procedures are contraindicated. From the observations of Wright and Douglas (1444), Cecil and Austin (228), Cecil (221, 222), and Stoltenberg (1249) on the use of vaccines in persons having infections at the time, it would appear advisable to exclude from the group to be inoculated all individuals with acute infections or with pulmonary tuberculosis. This is especially important for individuals with an acute infection of the respiratory tract, for vaccine injections tend to increase the severity of the illness (228, 1249). An increase in the severity of the infection is presumably related to the so-called "negative phase" which Wright and Douglas described (1444) as a state of temporarily reduced resistance lasting in the neighborhood of twenty-four hours or more following an injection of a vaccine containing organisms of the kind already active in infecting the host. Such an effect may be due to the presence in the vaccine of substances antagonistic to the immunity of the inoculated individual (see pages 131–132). In animals it has been demonstrated that the injection of a considerable dose of an antigen for which specific antibodies of either natural or acquired origin are present results in a temporary decrease in the level of those antibodies in the circulating blood (1317). This phase in turn is usually followed by a rise in antibody titer above the previous level.

In addition to individuals with infections there are also other classes of people with whom precautions must be taken. Cecil (221, 222) considers it unwise to give large doses of vaccine to patients with chronic cardiac or renal disease or to invalids or pregnant women. He would, in addition, exclude women from vaccination while menstruating.

There is no definite or strongly suggestive evidence, despite the possible theoretical dangers of such a procedure, that inoculation with vaccine predisposes the individual to pneumonia. To be sure, Wright and his associates (1447) suggested that the use of a dose of pneumococci totaling from 2,500 to 12,500 million organisms in African natives may possibly have temporarily increased the incidence of pneumonia in these individuals, as earlier mentioned. The evidence presented to support this view was very slight indeed, however, and the subsequent use of still larger doses in thousands of such natives has apparently failed to confirm this suggestion.

Passive Immunization

Cecil (222) has mentioned that the passive immunization of man by the injection of specific antipneumococcic serum might in certain instances be useful in preventing pneumonia. Conceivably situations might arise when passive immunization would be of value, as for instance with an acute bronchitis due to or associated with a carrier state of pneumococci of a type for which a potent immune serum was available. No evidence is at hand that antiserum has been administered under these circumstances for the purpose of preventing pneumonia.

CHAPTER EIGHT

SYMPTOMS OF LOBAR PNEUMONIA

General Description of the Disease 485
- Incubation Period 486
- Mode of Onset 487

Predominant Symptoms at Onset 487
- Chill 488
- Pain 488
- Cough and Respiratory Distress 490
- Fever 490
- Other Symptoms at Onset 490

Symptoms During Course 491
- Fever 491
- The Circulatory System 492
  - The Heart and Pulse 492
  - Cardiac Irregularities 494
  - Blood Pressure 496
  - Cyanosis 496
- The Blood 497
  - White Blood Cells 497
  - Red Blood Cells 498
  - Coagulation Time of the Blood and Platelets 499
  - Oxygen and Carbon Dioxide Content of the Blood 499
- Metabolic Changes and Acidosis 500
- The Respiratory System 500
  - Respiration Rate 500
  - Cough and Sputum 501
- The Gastrointestinal System 502
  - Jaundice 502
- The Urinary System 503
- The Central Nervous System 504
- The Skin 505

THERE is little that is new in relation to the symptoms or clinical aspects of lobar pneumonia; and, as there are numerous admirable clinical discussions of the disease available in the medical literature, no attempt will be made to review this matter exhaustively. In addition to the discussions of pneumonia in various textbooks of medicine, the more extensive articles by Cole (297), Lord (807), and Howard (661) are especially to be recommended.

The symptoms of lobar pneumonia are both local and general and have been well known for centuries (644). Local symptoms are referable to changes occurring in the lung and neighboring tissues as a consequence of the infection, while the general symptoms are similar to those of many infections. In spite of numerous repeated efforts to ascribe the general symptoms of pneumococcus lobar pneumonia to the action of some toxic substance, which either is elaborated by the infecting organism or arises from its disintegration within the body, the true cause remains unknown. Cole (292, 300) has discussed this matter in considerable detail. Although some derivatives of pneumococci which have been studied are toxic for animals, evidence is lacking that the general symptoms of pneumonia in man can be directly attributed to the presence of these substances in the body. Cole (300) has suggested that perhaps the symptoms of pneumonia arise from cellular injuries produced as a result of the metabolic activities of the organisms present, the injuries being brought about without the actual injurious substance being detectable or possibly without the formation of specific chemical substances.

In the following presentation of the symptomatology of lobar pneumonia, attention will be called, so far as possible with the data available, to the relative frequency of the various symptoms in cases of lobar pneumonia in general and in cases due to pneumococci of a particular type. Although pneumococci of the various types may at times cause pneumonia in various forms, significant evidence is gradually accumulating indicating that Types I, II, V, VII, and VIII are especially prone to give rise to lobar pneumonia, while pneumococci of the remaining types are usually most often encountered in pneumonia of other forms and in other infections (see pages 42–57).

GENERAL DESCRIPTION OF THE DISEASE

In most instances the onset is abrupt, the five cardinal symptoms being pain in the side, chill, fever, cough, and the expectoration of rusty or blood-tinged sputum. Pain, chill, and cough usually appear first and may occur simultaneously. The pain is commonly distressing and limits respiratory movements. At first dry, the cough generally becomes productive within a few to twenty-four hours. The chill lasts for half an hour or more and is associated with or followed by a rise in temperature. At times the chill is repeated. The temperature is usually elevated to 102° to 104° F. within a few hours. The pulse and respiratory rates also increase at the beginning of the disease.

Frequently at the time of onset the patient is found lying on the affected side, the alae nasi dilating with inspiration, and a short audible grunt heard with expiration. The face is commonly flushed and the lips cyanotic. In many instances the patient has an expression of distress which suggests the diagnosis.

The extent of the pulmonary process and the severity of the symptoms are quite variable, some patients becoming desperately ill with only a small area of consolidation while others may be far more comfortable and less seriously sick with lesions of the same or of larger size. Examination of the chest usually reveals numerous physical signs, as described in Chapter IX (page 506). In some instances the cough is not distressing and the sputum is slight in amount or absent. Pain may be absent and the respiratory and pulse rates as well as the temperature but little elevated. Hardy or uninformed persons may continue their usual activities even though very ill until their collapse brings them much-needed medical attention (807, 1331, 1008). In any instance predictions as to the outcome are unsafe, for at times the condition of the patient may change rapidly and within a few hours an apparently mild case may turn into one of great severity. Nevertheless, changes for the worse usually develop gradually and are associated with an increasing severity of many of the symptoms and frequently an extension of the pulmonary process. The general severity of the symptoms is usually a better guide to the condition of the patient than the apparent extent of the pulmonary involvement. As a rule, approximately three-quarters of the patients recover.

Incubation Period

While the exact incubation period of lobar pneumonia is unknown, it seems likely it is relatively short, possibly in the neighborhood of a few to about forty-eight hours. The disease may begin within a few hours after wetting or chilling. The report of Robertson (1082) in respect to the incubation period is of considerable interest. He observed an instance of two accidental laboratory infections in a Philippine laboratory assistant. This individual came down with pneumococcus Type I lobar pneumonia a few hours after exposure to cultures of the organism in spray form, and, after recovering, five months later developed a Type II lobar pneumonia forty hours after a similar exposure to a Type II culture. Other evidence that the incubation period is relatively short was reported by Pearson and Mouchet (1008) in discussing the health of native laborers in tropical Africa. These investigators found that cases of pneumonia almost invariably occurred among such individuals within a few hours following their transportation overnight in an open railroad car.

In experimental animals infected intratracheally or intrabronchially, evidence of a developing lesion may be obtained within one to a few hours; and in those subjected to the intranasal instillation of pneumococcus cultures or to the inhalation of sprayed cultures, serious lesions frequently develop within one to two days, as earlier mentioned (see pages 214–231). Presumably the number and character of the organisms concerned, the condition of the host, and the severity of the predisposing factors to which he is exposed all have a bearing on the length of the incubation period.

Mode of Onset

In a large majority of patients the beginning of the disease is sudden. Onset is usually dated from the chill or pain in the side, and many patients can tell practically to the hour when their illness began. Persons going to bed well may awake during the night feeling restless and cold and have a sudden shaking chill or pain in the chest. In other individuals, following an indefinite period of malaise, coryza, cough, and other respiratory symptoms, such symptoms all suddenly become worse. This is accompanied by a chill, which is followed by a rapid rise of the temperature to 102° to 104° F. within a few hours. In such cases also the time of onset may usually be accurately determined. In some cases, however, the onset is insidious and the exact time the process began is impossible to determine. Patients having lobar pneumonia following a coryza or mild respiratory infection occasionally exhibit this type of onset.

Among 949 cases of "pneumonia" studied by Sears and Larrabee (1168), the onset was sudden in 660 (nearly 70 per cent) and insidious in 126 (13 per cent). The manner in which the disease began in the remaining 163 cases was not stated. Wu and Chiu (1450) reported that among 234 typed cases of pneumococcus lobar pneumonia the onset was sudden in 82 per cent and gradual in 17 per cent and that the mode of onset did not appear related to the type of pneumococcus concerned. Among other typed cases, Sutliff and Finland (1272) found the onset to be sudden in 95 per cent of 239 Type I cases, and Finland and Sutliff (464) reported that the onset was abrupt in 72 per cent of about 150 Type III cases and in 81 per cent of 66 or more Type VIII cases.

PREDOMINANT SYMPTOMS AT ONSET

The chief symptoms at onset are chill, pain in the chest, and cough. At times certain other symptoms may also appear, as is mentioned below. The chill may appear first and be followed shortly by pain and cough, or the chill, pain, and cough may occur coincidentally. There may, however, be considerable variation in the symptoms at the time of onset.

Chill

Chill occurs in one-half or more of all cases. Of 949 "pneumonias" studied by Sears and Larrabee (1168) and 991 cases of lobar pneumonia analyzed by Ashton and Landis (26) approximately 50 per cent had a chill. Among 9,851 cases collected by Musser and Norris (918) 58 per cent had a chill, 12 per cent had repeated chills, while in 30 per cent only a feeling of chilliness was present. Nearly identical observations have been reported in other series of cases as well (Cole, 297, Lord, 807). The chill is usually ushered in with a feeling of coldness associated with general malaise and restlessness.

While always exceeding 55 per cent, the incidence of chills in typed cases of pneumococcus lobar pneumonia has tended to vary somewhat with the series of cases reported and with the type of pneumococcus causing the infection. In a total of 409 cases Richardson (1080) reported that a shaking chill occurred in 73 per cent of 117 Type I cases, 67 per cent of 87 Type II cases, 62 per cent of 34 Type III cases, and 87 per cent of 171 Group IV cases. In an analytical study of the symptoms shown by 1,000 patients Cecil, Baldwin, and Larsen (230) found that chill occurred most frequently in cases of Type I infection (70 per cent) and least frequently in cases due to Group IV pneumococci (55 per cent). Chill occurred in more than 55 per cent of 234 cases analyzed by Wu and Chiu (1450) and was about as common in cases due to pneumococci of one type as in those due to another type. These cases were classified as being due to pneumococci of Type I, II, III, or Group IV. In 239 Type I cases investigated by Sutliff and Finland (1272), chill occurred in 79 per cent, and it was also common among the Type III and Type VIII cases observed by Finland and Sutliff (464).

Chill is often absent in the young and the old, in alcoholics, and when pneumonia complicates acute or chronic disease (807).

Pain

Pain is one of the most common initial symptoms and is due to invasion of the pleura. It may precede or accompany chill. The character of the pain varies in different patients from a diffuse soreness or "stitch in the side" in some to an acute sharp stabbing pain in others and is aggravated by exertion, deep breathing, or cough. It is often severe enough to make the patient cry out, double up, or wake from sleep. In children or persons with apical or central pneumonia or in delirious patients, pain may be less prominent or absent. The pain is usually localized to the chest, but in some patients may be referred to the neck, abdomen, or flank on the affected side. In rare instances it may be felt on the opposite side or both sides (807, 1450). When severe, pain contributes to the dyspnea. As the disease progresses pain usually decreases or disappears.

More than 68 per cent of the 991 cases studied by Ashton and Landis (26) had pain, as did more than 75 per cent of 770 cases investigated by Cole (297). In the latter series pain was noted as the first symptom in 107 cases.

Some data are available on the incidence of pain in typed cases of pneumococcus lobar pneumonia. In Richardson's (1080) series of 409 cases pain was present in 81 per cent of 117 Type I cases, 87 per cent of 87 Type II cases, 75 per cent of 34 Type III cases, and 91 per cent of 171 Group IV cases. In this instance then, pain was least frequent in Type III cases and most frequent in Group IV cases. Among 1,000 patients investigated by Cecil, Baldwin, and Larsen (230), pain in the side occurred in more than 80 per cent of the cases due to Type I, II, or III. These three types apparently accounted for about two-thirds of the cases in the series. In the remaining cases, due to pneumococci of Group IV, pain was less common and was present in about 60 per cent.

In a total of 234 typed cases studied by Wu and Chiu (1450), pain occurred in 147 or 60 per cent. It was present in 55 per cent of the Type I cases, 64 per cent of the Type II cases, about 43 per cent of the Type III cases, and in almost 68 per cent of the Group IV cases, and was thus, as in Richardson's series, the least common in Type III and the most common in Group IV cases. Sutliff and Finland (1272) examined 239 Type I cases and reported that pain was present in 79 per cent. It seems clear from the above figures that the incidence of pain in cases due to pneumococci of various types may vary considerably and that no marked correlation exists between the occurrence of this symptom and the type of the invading pneumococcus.

The mechanism by which the pleurisy in lobar pneumonia causes pain was demonstrated by Capps (214) in his excellent monograph, *A Clinical Study of Pain*. The visceral pleura is not endowed with pain sense, while the parietal pleura is. Capps states that lesions occurring in the region of the parietal thoracic pleura give rise to pain immediately overlying the lesion. Further, if the *outer* rim of diaphragmatic pleura be irritated by pleurisy, the pain will be referred through the last six intercostal nerves to the lower thorax, lumbar region, or abdomen. The more intense the irritation, the greater is the tendency of the pain to spread down over the lower abdomen. If, however, the initial pleurisy irritates the *central* portion of the diaphragmatic pleura, that part which covers the dome of the diaphragm, the pain will be referred through the phrenic nerve to the neck on the corresponding side. In that region the pain will usually be localized rather sharply and a point of maximum tenderness will develop which has a remarkable tendency to appear in the skin overlying the anterior edge of the trapezius muscle. The segmental distribution of the fourth cervical nerve embraces the skin area in this region.

With respect to diaphragmatic pleurisy, Capps states: "In our experience, between five and ten per cent of lobar pneumonia patients give such evidence of diaphragm involvement." Pain felt in either the abdomen or neck under such circumstances is true referred pain and in the abdomen often produces a sensitive area with a point of maximum tenderness and muscular rigidity which may lead to unnecessary surgical procedures in some patients with early pneumonia (see also pages 653–654).

Cough and Respiratory Distress

While cough usually is one of the important early symptoms, its absence at the time of onset is not uncommon. When the disease begins abruptly, cough frequently does not appear at once and several hours may elapse before it becomes prominent (297). Although the cough may be dry and painful in the first few hours, it rapidly becomes productive and the expectoration is generally rusty and tenacious within twenty-four hours (808). Respiratory distress or difficult or rapid breathing are among the less common symptoms at onset. In the event that respiratory symptoms were present prior to the pneumonia, they all usually become intensified after the onset.

Fever

Ordinarily the temperature rise begins abruptly and in nearly all cases reaches a peak within twelve to twenty-four hours following the chill (961). Temperatures of 102° to 104° F. or more are the rule.

Other Symptoms at Onset

Cole (297) observed that vomiting may frequently occur as one of the early symptoms of pneumonia in adults and it was present in 27 per cent of his series of 770 cases. Cunningham (333) reported the occurrence of vomiting in 60 per cent of 1,500 cases in children, and Adams and Berger (4) found it present in nearly the same proportion (58 per cent) of 145 cases in children. Vomiting may occur once or twice with or preceding the chill, or, less commonly, a tendency to nausea and vomiting may persist throughout the duration of the disease.

In adults, acute maniacal symptoms (976) or convulsions may rarely usher in an attack of pneumonia (297). In children, convulsions and lesser disturbances, such as rigidity of the neck or tenderness of it on motion, or strabismus, may occur (976); such symptoms were found in 8 per cent of 1,500 cases by Cunningham (333). Adams and Berger (4) state that 4.8 per cent of 145 cases in children had symptoms suggesting the presence of meningitis and were admitted to the hospital with that diagnosis (see also page 654).

Headache may occur. Diarrhea develops at times in adults, but as an early symptom is much more common in children. Great weakness, fainting, vertigo, or epistaxis may also occur at onset but are rare.

SYMPTOMS DURING COURSE

After the onset the symptomatology of the disease is fairly characteristic and patients, unless delirious, are usually quiet. Moving patients frequently causes them pain, and generally their one desire is to remain undisturbed and be left alone.

Fever

Fever appears to be the one symptom constantly present in lobar pneumonia (297, 807, 230, 1450). During the acute stages the fever is usually fairly high and ranges over 102° F. More than two-thirds of Cole's (297) 770 cases had maximum temperatures between 104° and 106° F. The temperature was usually fairly constant or showed only slight variations. Nevertheless, cases with a morning remission of temperature of from one to two degrees or more are common (Lord, 807).

Uncomplicated cases showing very wide temperature variations during the acute stages of the disease may occur but are not common. An occasional severe case may be seen in which a low temperature is maintained throughout the course. Cases with a constantly low temperature appear to be rare, however, even in the aged, but low temperatures are much more common in the aged and debilitated than in the young and vigorous. Among 770 cases studied by Cole (297), there were but 15 in whom the temperature never exceeded 102° F. Under ordinary circumstances mouth temperatures are unreliable and rectal temperatures should be taken at four-hour intervals.

In 70 per cent of 1,987 cases collected by Musser and Norris (918), the fever ended between the fifth and the tenth day. Of the total group only 4, or 0.2 per cent, had fever of two days' duration and 32, or 1.6 per cent, had fever of three days' duration. Although cases of such short duration are occasionally seen, the disease may run a protracted course of two weeks or more. Rapid elevation of temperature with the exacerbation of other symptoms usually means extension of the pulmonary process or the development of some complication.

Cruickshank (331) determined that the duration of the fever was a day or so shorter in patients under thirty-five years of age than in older individuals. This investigator also reported the duration of fever in 100 cases each of Type I and Type II lobar pneumonia and in 60 cases attributed to pneumococci of Group IV as 7.6, 7.7, and 7.5 days respectively. The Type I cases showed a sustained temperature, usually about 102° F., throughout the course, whereas in Type II infections the temperature generally fell to a much lower level after reaching a high point at the time of onset. In a smaller series of cases (40 cases) due to pneumococci of various types, Graeser, Wu, and Robertson (552), however, were unable to detect any correlation between the course of the temperature and the type of pneumococcus causing the infection.

The Circulatory System

Symptoms referable to the circulatory system are prominent and easily detectable in pneumonia, yet from the evidence available it appears that the circulatory system plays no more than a minor role in the outcome of the usual case.

THE HEART AND PULSE. The condition of the heart should be carefully determined at the time of the first visit to the patient. It is important to note and record its size by percussion and the point farthest down and out toward the left at which the apex impulse can be palpated for comparison with subsequent findings, should the question of cardiac displacement or variations arise from effusions, whether pleural or pericardial.

Although dilatation of the heart during pneumonia is not often demonstrated, Levy (777) showed some dilatation in 61.9 per cent of 21 cases of lobar pneumonia by roentgen-ray measurements. Dilatation may have been slightly less frequent in a few patients receiving digitalis. Davies, Hodgson, and Whitby (341), however, found only 3 of 119 patients showed cardiac enlargement by roentgen-ray examination and consider it a rare occurrence in pneumonia.

Large consolidations of the left lung, atelectasis, or effusions may displace the heart. The right border of the heart may be obscured by consolidation of the middle lobe. Coryllos (322) states that especially in the early stages of pneumonia displacement of the mediastinum and of the diaphragm to the affected side is more frequent than is generally believed and can be found if carefully looked for. Displacement of the heart in such cases may be ascribed to atelectasis. Lord (811) reports that he, Holmes, and King found roentgenographic evidence of varying and usually slight lung collapse in 23 of 47 patients with lobar pneumonia. Massive lung collapse is infrequent. Among 558 cases of pneumonia examined by Lord (811) a complicating lung collapse involving a sufficiently large area to lead to clinically demonstrable cardiac displacement was found in 14, or 2.5 per cent. Nine of the patients had lobar pneumonia and five bronchopneumonia.

Systolic murmurs, apparently functional in origin, may appear during the course of the acute disease and disappear in convalescence. Diastolic murmurs appearing during the course are much less common and almost invariably indicate a complicating acute, or pre-existent chronic endocarditis.

The pulmonic second sound may be accentuated due to back pressure caused by the consolidation obstructing the pulmonary circulation, and the daily lessening of its intensity may indicate a failing heart. Lord (807) states: "A shortening of the first sound and approach to the second in quality (embryocardia), increased rapidity and weakness of the pulse, cyanosis, aggravated dyspnea, with or without nervous symptoms may come on gradually or suddenly." Cardiac weakness before the third day is unusual. Such weakness may occur at the time of crisis or, uncommonly, after crisis. Patients with considerable cardiovascular embarrassment often have cyanotic, cold, clammy extremities.

In 1915 Newburgh and Porter (950) demonstrated that the contractions of the hearts of normal dogs were much impaired when perfused with the blood of dogs having pneumonia. However, they also showed that the hearts of dogs which have died from pneumonia contract normally when fed normal dog blood and concluded that the heart muscle is not functionally impaired in this disease. It is now generally conceded that the effects of pneumonia on the heart muscle in the usual case are not so marked as was previously believed (807, 796, 1418, 1384). The relation of the heart to death in pneumonia is discussed elsewhere (see pages 544–546).

In most cases the pulse remains full and in good force throughout the disease. DeGraff, Travell, and Yager (349) studied 7,480 electrocardiographic tracings taken on 975 patients with lobar pneumonia. In 80.5 per cent of the series nine tracings were taken in each case. Although nearly one-half of the patients received varying amounts of digitalis, ample data were obtained for a study of the heart rate in patients treated without this drug. The findings indicate that in pneumonia the heart rate varies within very narrow limits and remains within these narrow limits from day to day during the acute course of the disease, even in the presence of marked fluctuations in temperature. During the febrile period, 27 per cent of the cases showed a variation in rate of less than 10 beats per minute and 66 per cent showed a maximum variation of less than 21 beats per minute.

In some instances an increase in the pulse rate occurs in the presence of a concurrent rise in temperature. The normal ratio of pulse to respiration of 1:4 is usually upset and may be reduced to 1:3, 1:2, or even 1:1 (807). Among 770 cases studied by Cole (297), 459 had a maximum pulse rate between 110 and 140. A rate of more than 140 is usually an unfavorable sign (see pages 720–722). Rapid rates are often encountered in children, women, and people of small stature.

Dicrotic pulse is seldom noted but was reported by Chatard (254) as occurring in about 8 per cent of 658 cases. The pulse may get smaller and less forceful as the disease progresses.

Bradycardia may occur during the illness and DeGraff, Travell, and Yager (349) found 11 per cent of more than 900 cases had a heart rate of from 70 to 89 per minute during the febrile period, even though many patients had a high temperature at the time. Bradycardia may also occur during the first few days after crisis (807; see also page 547).

CARDIAC IRREGULARITIES. The incidence of various minor and major cardiac irregularities varies from 10 to 20 per cent or more as determined in three large series of cases (254, 297, 349). The majority of these irregularities, however, were due to auricular or ventricular extrasystoles and were probably not of significance. In the series of 975 patients on whom DeGraff, Travell, and Yager (349) took 7,480 electrocardiograms, approximately one-quarter of all cases showed transitory electrocardiographic changes at some time during the course of the disease. Abnormalities of rhythm were found in 10 per cent, disturbances of conduction in 10 per cent, and in 2.4 per cent inversions of the T wave other than in Lead 3 were encountered.

In these 975 patients, 562 were treated without digitalis and 413 received varying doses of the drug. As the incidence of abnormal basic rhythms was small and was about the same in each group, the findings were given for the two groups together. Auricular fibrillation or flutter occurred in 35 cases, or 3.6 per cent. In a series of 612 cases observed by Cole (297), these conditions were found in 3.7 per cent.

The findings of DeGraff and his associates with respect to the incidence of various forms of abnormal basic rhythm in the 975 cases they investigated are shown in Table 86. Auricular fibrillation occurred in 27 (2.8 per cent),

TABLE 86. INCIDENCE OF ABNORMAL BASIC RHYTHMS IN 975 CASES OF LOBAR PNEUMONIA AS DETERMINED BY ELECTROCARDIOGRAPHIC STUDY*

TYPE OF ARRHYTHMIA	CASES	
	Number	*Per cent*
Auricular fibrillation	27	2.8
Auricular flutter	10†	1.0
Paroxysmal tachycardia	6	0.6
Wandering pacemaker	8	0.8
Total	51	5.2

* Varying doses of digitalis were given 413 of the patients.

† Two of the cases of auricular flutter also showed fibrillation and are included in both groups.

auricular flutter in 10 (one per cent), paroxysmal tachycardia in 6 (0.6 per cent), and wandering pacemaker in 8 (0.8 per cent). Cases with abnormalities of the basic rhythm were about five times as frequent in patients over 40 years of age as in younger patients.

A survey of 1,456 cases by Cohn and Lewis (288) at the Hospital of the Rockefeller Institute for Medical Research showed that auricular fibrillation occurred in 37 cases, or 2.5 per cent. Many of the patients received digitalis in varying dosage and this series presumably includes the group of 612 cases reported by Cole (297) and referred to above. Again the incidence of cases with abnormal rates was shown to vary with age and in Cohn and Lewis' series the incidence of auricular fibrillation was only 0.7 per cent in patients under forty years of age, as compared with 6.6 per cent in older patients.

In DeGraff, Travell, and Yager's (349) group of 562 patients receiving no digitalis, certain abnormalities of conduction were noted in electrocardiograms. Prolongation of the auriculo-ventricular conduction time was present in 9.2 per cent of the cases, dropped beats in 0.5 per cent, and complete dissociation in none. Some evidence of block, first appearing during the febrile period, was found in 22 per cent of the cases.

BLOOD PRESSURE. There is little uniformity among the results of reported studies of the blood pressure in pneumonia, and apparently the findings are of little significance (297, 807, 1450) and vary from case to case.

A fall in systolic blood pressure associated with a persistently rapid pulse may be of serious significance, however. Studies of the circulation in pneumonia, such as those of Perry (1015), indicate that a tendency toward a rise in pulse pressure exists and that circulatory failure in lobar pneumonia is commonly due to a failure of the circulation at the periphery as a consequence of a vasomotor paralysis seriously affecting the peripheral vessels. The nature of this paralysis is largely unknown but appears related to the degree of toxemia present (see pages 545–546).

CYANOSIS. Cyanosis of some grade is an almost constant symptom of the more severely ill patient. Cole (297) points out that Peabody made the suggestion that a portion of the cyanosis present might be due to the formation of methemoglobin by the action of the pneumococcus on the blood hemoglobin. Stadie (1223) demonstrated that this was probably not the case, as any methemoglobin formed was rapidly removed from the circulation. Certain extracts of unwashed pneumococci do have the power, however, of converting hemoglobin into methemoglobin, as Neill and Avery (927) and Morgan and Neill (908) have shown.

Haldane (587), Stadie (1223), and others have clearly demonstrated that cyanosis is directly related and frequently proportional to the degree of oxygen unsaturation of the arterial blood. Incomplete oxygen saturation of the blood in the lungs seems largely due to the operation of such factors as the presence of edema in and about the alveolar walls, clogging of the alveolar spaces with exudate, mechanical interference with the circulation through the consolidated areas, and incomplete aeration of a large portion of the lungs due to restricted shallow and rapid breathing (see also pages 759–762). The degree of cyanosis present may not always be wholly dependent upon the nature and extent of the pulmonary lesion and may be related to the severity of the infection.

When present, cyanosis is usually greatly increased by effort. At times cyanosis only becomes clinically demonstrable when the patient is asleep. It is most easily detected on the ears, lips, or under the nails. In unfavorable cases a gray pallor may supersede the cyanosis.

The Blood

Several changes in the content of the blood occur during pneumonia. Those relating to bodily changes in metabolism are discussed below (see page 500). The appearance of pneumococci in the blood is described in the chapters on Complications (page 548) and Prognosis (page 655). Certain other changes are noted here.

Two important substances commonly appear in the blood during the course of the illness. One is the soluble specific substance derived from the capsule of the infecting pneumococcus and having the power of nullifying the actions of specific antibody (see pages 131–132). The other is spontaneously produced antibody, the appearance or lack of which seems intimately related, respectively, to recovery or to death (see pages 173–175 and 728–735).

The possibility of lobar pneumonia arising as a secondary manifestation of a pneumococcus septicaemia is discussed elsewhere (see pages 245–246).

WHITE BLOOD CELLS. Leucocytosis occurs in a large proportion of all cases and usually begins at the time of the chill or within a few hours after it, to continue throughout the disease. Leucocyte counts, either high or low, are generally maintained at a nearly constant level during the acute illness. The total white blood count in the peripheral circulation is commonly between 10,000 and 40,000 cells per cubic millimeter. Cole (297) found only 6 per cent of 463 cases with a white blood count under 10,000, and only 8 per cent with a count over 40,000. These figures are practically identical with those reported by Chatard (255), who analyzed 582 cases, and with those of Lord (807), who analyzed 500 cases. Adams and Berger's (4) findings in 145 cases in children two to fifteen years old were the same. The average count in Chatard's cases was 24,000. He pointed out that of all the acute febrile diseases lobar pneumonia gave rise to the highest white blood counts. These were usually between 15,000 and 40,000, and in most uncomplicated cases between 20,000 and 30,000. The highest count recorded by Chatard was 105,000.

The leucocyte response in patients over thirty years of age, and especially in those over fifty, may be less vigorous than the response in younger patients, as Chatard observed.

Although a general relationship may obtain between the severity of the disease and degree of lung involvement, and the height of the white blood count in that the highest counts tend to occur in patients with the most severe and extensive lesions, there are many exceptions to this, as noted by the above investigators. Graeser, Wu, and Robertson (552) were also unable to find any definite correlation between the two factors.

A possible relationship between the type of pneumococcus causing the infection and the leucocyte count in patients not given specific serum therapy has been sought by various observers without any striking degree of success (552). Counts averaging about 19,000 to 22,000 at the height of the fever have been reported in Type I cases (277, 1080, 331, 339), while in Type II cases the average counts were slightly lower and ranged from about 15,000 to 18,000 (1080, 331, 340), and in Type III cases the averages were quite variable and were in the neighborhood of 10,000 to 30,000 (277, 1080, 331, 464, 340). Richardson (1080) reported an average count of 18,000 in 171 Group IV cases, and Finland and Sutliff (464) reported that the counts in Type VIII cases were much the same as in Type III cases. The number of cases in each of the above series referred to is so small it is probable that the findings given are of little significance.

Differential white blood counts have been done in a great many cases and the findings extensively studied. They show, in general, the presence of a polymorphonuclear neutrophile leucocytosis of 80 to 90 per cent (255, 807, 890). The presence of young forms of leucocytes is the rule (713, 890, 1074) and attempts have been made to use the percentage increase of such forms found as a prognostic guide. As Middleton and Gibbon (890) point out, however, no final conclusions can be drawn from such efforts except that the failure of leucocytosis to develop is an unfavorable sign and the occurrence of leucopenia ominous. There is universal agreement with this conclusion (see also pages 723–725).

A monocytosis of moderate degree and usually of short duration frequently appears at or about the time of recovery, as Hickling (639) and Reznikoff (1074) have shown.

Following crisis or lysis the number of leucocytes does not decrease at once with the drop in temperature, but usually falls slowly and in favorable cases may reach normal within seven to ten days (807). If complications or delayed resolution occur, leucocytosis may persist for a longer period.

RED BLOOD CELLS. Experimental evidence has shown extracts of pneumococci to possess some hemolytic power (306, 292, 50, 701, 1069, 328). As the course of the usual case of pneumonia is short, however, little or no marked anemia occurs (297, 976) but mild secondary anemia may occasionally be seen for a week or so after defervescence (807). Bullowa (190) considers anemia may result in some instances from pneumococcus Type V or Type VI infections, particularly during pregnancy.

COAGULATION TIME OF THE BLOOD AND PLATELETS. The coagulation time of the blood is prolonged during the acute illness and returns to normal after convalescence (Dochez, 357). This change is attributed to the presence in the blood of an increased amount of anti-thrombin (357, 534). There is also a concurrent decrease in the number of platelets present. As compared with a demonstrated average platelet count of about 250,000 per cubic millimeter in normal man, Reimann (1062) found the number of platelets in the blood in lobar pneumonia to be around 125,000 to 243,000. Several hours after the termination of the fever in favorable cases, the number of platelets increased and during the subsequent six to nine days rose to considerably above normal. The highest count recorded in 13 cases studied was 748,000.

In mice the injection of pneumococcus extracts was followed by a marked and abrupt fall in the number of platelets in the blood. Where recovery occurred the platelet count rose to normal within four to nine days and continued to increase for several days more before dropping back to normal (Reimann and Julianelle, 1069).

OXYGEN AND CARBON DIOXIDE CONTENT OF THE BLOOD. Normally the oxygen saturation of the hemoglobin of arterial blood is 95 per cent and of venous blood about 70 per cent (1449). During pneumonia, although there is no special decrease in the total amount of circulating hemoglobin, the oxygen saturation of the hemoglobin is commonly less than the normal values given above (587, 1223, 876, 1449). Cyanosis results from the unsaturation of the available hemoglobin and is a product of the infection, especially as it relates to factors impeding the proper aeration of the blood in its passage through the lungs, as already described.

The carbon dioxide content of the blood normally (1449) varies from about 45 to 56 volumes per cent (45 to 56 cc. of the gas per 100 cc. of blood). A slight reduction in the carbon dioxide content of the blood may be present in pneumonia (Peabody, 1006) and determinations of 40 to 50 volumes per cent in the venous blood are common. Peabody found one case in which the carbon dioxide content was 29 per cent, an unusually low figure for pneumonia. The carbon dioxide content bears little relation to the severity of the disease but tends to be lower in the more severe cases or in the terminal stages of pneumonia. In general the content of this gas in the blood parallels the output of ammonia in the urine (see also pages 759–762).

Metabolic Changes and Acidosis

Although the general metabolic changes occurring in pneumonia appear to be of only minor importance, few of them are understood. It has been known for many years that the excretion of chlorides in the urine decreases and may stop until defervescence, when excretion again begins, often in increased amounts (1006, 807, 830, 565). The reasons for this are little understood. The excretion of phosphorus in the urine is apparently variable (565).

During pneumonia potassium concentration in the blood may increase (1262, 565). The calcium, chloride, and sodium concentrations decrease, as does the total base bound by protein (1262, 565). While the albumin of the blood decreases the globulin content increases, so that the content of total protein remains little changed (1262). The magnesium content of the blood (1262) and the blood sugar level are about normal (830). Haldane (587) demonstrated an increased alkali tolerance during pneumonia and considered this to be due chiefly to a retention of alkali on the part of the body as a compensatory mechanism to facilitate the ease with which oxygen diffused from the blood into the tissues. This was well described by Means and Barach (876), who showed further that the hydrogen-ion concentration of the blood in pneumonia usually remains normal.

Gastric acidity is low until after crisis, when it returns to normal (1262). Other metabolic changes, including an increased excretion of ammonia as found by Peabody (1006), and of sulphur, creatinin, and creatin, are discussed by Lord (807).

The slight acidosis present as reported by Palmer in 1917 (978) is due partially to the presence of an unknown acid which can be demonstrated in the blood and urine and is not betahydroxybutyric acid so common in diabetes and some other metabolic diseases. The acid is apparently excreted as rapidly as it is formed (876). There is general agreement that the acidosis which exists in pneumonia is slight and of little significance. That resulting from an increased retention of carbon dioxide causing a carbonic acid acidosis is mild indeed, as Means and Barach (876) demonstrated.

The Respiratory System

RESPIRATION RATE. An increase in the respiratory rate is a practically constant feature of pneumonia. In typical cases the respiratory movements are restricted and short. Respiratory rates of 25 to 40 per minute are found in the milder cases. In the more severe cases rates of 50 to 60 or even 70 or more per minute may occur.

The respiratory distress in pneumonia is quite different from that seen in cardiac disease. Orthopnea is rare and patients seldom request to be propped up in bed.

The sensitivity of the respiratory centers in the central nervous system may be decreased in pneumonia. In dogs and cats with experimental pneumonia Newburgh, Means, and Porter (949, 948) demonstrated a marked reduction in the sensitivity of the respiratory centers to increased concentrations of carbon dioxide in the blood. Animals with the most severe infections were the least sensitive in their respiratory reactions. These changes were found in animals with pneumonia but were absent in others having only septicaemia. The depression of the activity of the respiratory centers in the above animals with pneumonia was apparently due to the influence of afferent stimuli conveyed from the chest by the vagus nerves, for section of these nerves was followed by the prompt return of activity of the respiratory centers to normal.

COUGH AND SPUTUM. Cough is almost always present (26, 1080, 807) and is often the most distressing symptom in typical cases, especially when the sputum is tenacious and difficult to raise (297). It may be less prominent or absent in the aged, debilitated, or delirious, or in patients with upper lobe lesions. Lord (807) remarks that von Jürgensen states with justice, "Cough is rarely of use, always troublesome and sometimes dangerous."

The sputum is quite typical of the disease in about one-half to three-quarters of the cases (807, 1450) and is rusty, tenacious, glairy, and more or less transparent. Rusty or "prune-juice" sputum usually appears during the first or second day but may be absent until later in the illness. The reddish brick-dust appearance is due to the mixture of red blood cells and hemoglobin with the sputum. Ordinary mucopurulent or thin saliva-like sputum containing purulent masses with or without a rusty appearance or streaks of unchanged blood may be present. In jaundiced patients the sputum may be greenish (297). Frankly bloody sputum or true hemoptysis may occur in pneumonia but tuberculosis should be suspected when these are encountered.

Sutliff and Finland (1272) found bloody sputum present in 75 per cent of 239 cases of Type I lobar pneumonia in adults. During the early years of the Massachusetts Pneumonia Study (869) the character of the sputum was noted in 685 cases of lobar pneumonia in adults. Bloody or blood-tinged sputum was present in approximately 75 per cent of the cases. Nearly all of the cases were due to pneumococci of Type I, II, or III, or Group IV and the proportion of cases having blood in the sputum was about the same in each of these groups. Greenish sputum was encountered in nearly 10 per cent of all cases.

Most of the exudate is absorbed rather than coughed up (918) and the amount of sputum usually averages from one to two ounces daily. In the cases mentioned above that were investigated during the Massachusetts Pneumonia Study, the amount of sputum raised was essentially the same whatever the type of the infecting pneumococcus.

Fibrinous bronchial casts may be found but are rare. Uncommonly no sputum will be expectorated during the course of the illness. Children and aged patients are likely to swallow sputum, as are those greatly debilitated, stuporous, or delirious. During resolution the sputum becomes more fluid, less tenacious, and not infrequently more purulent (297, 275, 1450).

The Gastrointestinal System

The tongue is usually white and furred, and in toxic cases dry. The appetite is lost and nausea may be present. Constipation is more common than diarrhea. Meteorism is a distressing symptom and may be dangerous (see pages 756–758). Vomiting is not common and is more frequent in children (4) than in adults. Vomiting from irritation of the pharynx by tenacious sputum may, however, be troublesome (807). Nausea, vomiting, constipation, or diarrhea may occur in about one-third of the cases (1168, 1450). Hiccough is not common.

JAUNDICE. Cole (297) reported jaundice as occurring in some 5 to 10 per cent of all cases. It was present in 11.5 per cent of 658 cases investigated by Chatard (254) and in about 10 per cent of 242 cases studied by Wu and Chiu (1450).

Jaundice may arise from one cause or several, such as an increased production of bile pigments by the spleen and perhaps some other organs due to blood destruction, the inability of the liver cells to remove such pigment from the blood, or a blocking of the bile ducts of the liver due to inflammation, neoplasm, or other abnormal condition. Infection of the bile ducts, gall bladder, or liver, or hypostatic congestion, or the "toxic" effects of pneumonia, about which little is known, may serve either to block the drainage of bile or to depress the function of the liver cells. Although the complete explanation of its occurrence may be uncertain, Keefer (705) states that jaundice can usually be explained on the basis of depressed liver function together with an increase in the production of bilirubin. As the function of the liver cells appears impaired during the acute illness, the usual amount of bile pigment is not withdrawn from the blood. The accumulation of pigment in the blood stream gives rise to subclinical or clinically recognizable jaundice.

Certain patients, more especially those with marked cyanosis, may show an increase in their red blood cell counts. The cyanosis results from anoxemia as earlier pointed out, and the polycythemia of such patients may result from a physiologic effort to combat this. Keefer notes that jaundice during pneumonia may become more intense as the illness subsides. Whether or not a part of the jaundice in pneumonia is due to destruction of an excess number of red blood cells as patients begin to improve is unknown. The relation of jaundice to the severity of the attack of pneumonia is uncertain and may not be significant (see page 727).

The spleen may be enlarged.

The Urinary System

Albuminuria, usually transient in nature, is a frequent finding in pneumonia. Its presence has been noted in from about one-quarter to more than three-quarters of the cases in various series (1168, 26, 254, 297, 830). In infants and children albuminuria may be less frequent, and Cunningham (333) discovered it in only 40 per cent of 897 cases.

Approximately one-quarter of all cases show casts during the height of the disease. Both albumin and casts tend to disappear from the urine following defervescence. In spite of the great frequency with which signs of kidney damage appear, permanent renal damage is rare (see pages 608–610).

As elsewhere described, soluble specific substance (SSS) may appear in the urine during the course of pneumococcus pneumonia (see page 25). Thus Dochez and Avery (363) found it present as early as twelve hours after the initial chill, and Avery and his associates (33) demonstrated its presence in the urine at some stage of the disease in 65 per cent of 111 cases due to pneumococci of Type I, II, or III. Studies of a similar nature have been made by other investigators (1054, 754, 118, 297, 1321, 1010). Quigley (1054) tested the urine of 82 patients with Type I, II, or III lobar pneumonia two or three times a day during the acute illness and obtained a precipitin reaction for SSS in 81 per cent of the cases. In many instances the strength of the reaction increased for three or four days and persisted for from two to nineteen days, following which it gradually disappeared. No regularity of appearance, persistence, or disappearance of the reaction was discernible and apparently it was not particularly influenced by crisis. Blake (118) found that some patients who never excreted SSS in the urine during the acute illness may excrete it in small amounts for a week or two after crisis.

The available evidence indicates that SSS is found most frequently and in the most significant amounts in the urine of patients with severe infections and that its presence in the urine may, in consequence, be of prognostic importance (see page 693). The presence of SSS in the urine may at times also be of value in determining the type of pneumococcus responsible for the infection (see pages 637–639). In convalescence the urinary excretion of specific capsular polysaccharide may persist for twenty-one to fifty-eight days (363, 1054).

The Central Nervous System

All grades of central nervous system symptoms may be seen. Anxiety, restlessness, and disorientation are found in a majority of cases. Headache is common. Meningismus, while not frequent in adults, is fairly common in children.

Sears and Larrabee (1168) and Chatard (254, 255) find delirium present in about one-quarter of all cases. Cole (297), whose observations are similar, adds that the low muttering delirium such as seen in typhoid fever is seldom present. Patients should never be left alone, as delirium may develop suddenly and unexpectedly and they may injure themselves or others.

It is frequently stated that severe delirium is most likely to be present with apical pneumonia (807, 976, 661). Clear evidence of this is not available. Among cases of "pneumonia" in adults studied by Sears and Larrabee (1168) delirium occurred in about the same proportion (24.6 per cent) of 138 cases with upper lobe lesions as was found (28.1 per cent) in 427 cases with lesions confined to the lower lobes.

Delirium is usually severe and about twice as frequent in alcoholic patients as in others, and in such persons the onset of pneumonia may be marked by the onset of typical symptoms of delirium tremens. Among the patients with "pneumonia" analyzed by Sears and Larrabee (1168), 256 were alcoholics and delirium occurred in 126, or 49.6 per cent, while it was found in only 108, or 24 per cent, of 441 non-alcoholics.

Osler (976) remarks that hemiplegia may occur as a result of thrombosis, embolism, abscess, or edema. Transient aphasia with or without hemiplegia may occur. Inequality of the pupils may be present.

The Skin

The skin is usually hot and dry during the acute stages and may show a diffuse erythema or furunculosis (807) and rarely purpura (955, 83) or gangrene (661).

Herpes, occurring in from 5 to 40 per cent or more of cases, has a higher incidence in pneumonia than in any other disease (297, 4, 807, 976) and may in consequence be of diagnostic importance. The eruption usually appears by the second or third day of illness but may occur at any time. Although the lesions are commonest on the lips and nose, they may occur on the ears, chin, cheeks, tongue, genitals, or anus. They are not generally found on the trunk or extremities.

CHAPTER NINE

PHYSICAL SIGNS IN LOBAR PNEUMONIA

Inspection 507
Palpation 507
Mensuration 507
Percussion 508
Auscultation 508

THE physical signs in the chest in lobar pneumonia vary to a considerable extent depending upon the nature, size, and location of the underlying lesion or lesions. Loeschcke (798) regards an outpouring of edema fluid containing organisms to represent the earliest lesion, as described in the section on pathogenesis (page 250). He considers it very unlikely that a clinical diagnosis can be made on the basis of physical signs at this period in the development of the process.

The usual demonstrable manifestations in the early case were described more than a century ago by Laënnec (755) as consisting of a small area of crepitous rales which sound equal in size and hardly wet. Dulness is absent at this stage.

Lord (807) presents an excellent discussion of the physical signs in lobar pneumonia, in the course of which he says:

Within twenty-four hours of the onset, physical signs are usually limited to slight dulness and fine consonating rales with long breath or cough. Harsh inspiration, broncho-vesicular breathing and slight changes in voice, whisper and tactile fremitus may be demonstrable, but are often lacking. Diminished breathing may be the only sign. In some cases at this early period the lungs are negative. Usually by the second or third day the pulmonary findings are outspoken. Inspection shows restricted motion of the affected side, over which there is dulness, bronchial breathing, increased voice, whisper and tactile fremitus. In the absence of diffuse bronchitis, fine consonating rales can usually be heard over the involved region during the early period of the disease, but may disappear while it is at its height. In typical cases the extent of the involvement gradually increases until involvement of the greater part or the whole of one lobe may be determined. In atypical cases the evidence on physical examination may be uncertain for a time or remain so throughout the disease. In from five to ten days the temperature usually falls by crisis or lysis, and with defervescence signs of resolution may be heard in the affected lung. The fine consonating rales, redux crepitus, of the period of invasion return and the percussion note becomes more resonant.

The characteristic physical signs which may be demonstrated over a fully consolidated lobe are: (a) dulness to percussion, (b) bronchial or tubular breathing, (c) crackling rales, (d) increased voice and whisper, and (e) increased tactile fremitus. After crisis has occurred these signs usually persist a few days to a week or more. Rarely, such signs may persist for weeks or months. Patients who enjoy complete recovery seldom show abnormal physical signs after a few weeks.

Inspection

The patient usually presents a fairly typical picture of an acutely ill person having some grade of cyanosis, rapid, somewhat restricted, labored breathing, herpes, and cough. Unilateral flushing of the face, which may or may not be on the side of the involvement, is occasionally seen.

The chest on the affected side generally shows restricted motion, which is largely voluntary and dependent upon the amount of pleurisy and pain present. Decreased excursion of the diaphragmatic shadow may also be noted on the involved side.

Palpation

Variation in the expansion of the two sides of the chest may be better felt than seen. Occasionally coarse rales and friction rubs may be palpated. A perceptible increase in the temperature of the skin overlying the lesion may be found.

Tactile fremitus is generally increased over the involved area and usually becomes more marked with progress of the infiltration, providing the pleura is not much thickened, in which case it may be diminished. Lord (807) points out that if the bronchi are filled with secretion, tactile fremitus may be diminished or absent and that the removal of this material by cough may be followed by the reappearance of fremitus. Owing to the high pitch of the voice in women and children, attempts to elicit changes in tactile fremitus in such individuals may be of little aid. Patients with central pneumonia may show no alterations in fremitus.

Mensuration

The involved side of the chest may be somewhat smaller than the unaffected side.

Percussion

The importance of percussion as a means of demonstrating physical signs in the chest was first emphasized by Auenbrugger (28) in 1762. Both light and heavy percussion should be used (807). Light percussion will demonstrate dulness due to superficial pulmonary infiltration, and heavy percussion, dulness due to deep infiltration.

All parts of the chest, including the apex of the axilla, should be percussed. When an area of sufficient size is involved percussion during the stage of engorgement usually reveals dulness which at times has the tympanitic quality referred to as Skoda's resonance. The cause of this tympanitic quality, while not evident, may be due to the nearness of exudate or consolidation to air-containing tissues or organs and is perhaps most commonly observed in apical lesions. In the presence of consolidation of considerable size in the lower lobe a zone of relative resonance may be detected in the paravertebral region on the affected side. This is probably due to spinal resonance from the normal lung of the opposite side and is known as the Sonorous Triangle of Lord.

Dulness may be absent in the early stages. During the stage of red hepatization the degree of dulness varies and although the note may be flat, the total absence of resonance and the sense of resistance to the finger as found in large effusions are lacking. The area of dulness varies and may be limited to a part or the whole of one or more lobes. Dulness to percussion may give more accurate evidence of the extent of the lesion than the occurrence of abnormal breath sounds or of rales (552).

In central pneumonias often only slight dulness may be demonstrable over the site of the involvement, while in other instances dulness is absent throughout the course of the disease. Compensatory emphysema or hyperresonance over the involved region or of the nearby lung may mask the underlying infiltration.

Auscultation

All parts of the lung should be examined with a stethoscope as the signs on auscultation vary considerably with the location of the lesion and with the individual. One of the first signs of pneumonia is usually a suppression of breath sounds. A slight blowing quality is frequently present in the early stages which later becomes harsher and more intense, resembling tubular breathing. Likewise during the early period, an intensification of whispered voice is important for diagnosis (297, 828). Fine consonating moist rales of the crepitant variety are commonly heard toward the end of inspiration or forced inspiration at this stage as a succession of minute crackles. They are attributed to a disturbance by the incoming air of the sticky exudate in the finest branches of the bronchi.

The breath sounds over an area of definite consolidation are usually bronchial or tubular, and as Lord (807) remarks, "In no other disease does bronchial breathing reach such a degree of intensity as in croupous pneumonia, due to the propagation of laryngeal and tracheal sounds through the solid lung." Thickened pleura or plugged bronchi, such as occur in massive pneumonia, will alter breath sounds and tactile fremitus as well, so that either may be diminished or absent. Relief of the bronchial obstruction by cough will be followed by the reappearance of bronchial breathing.

Persistent rales at one place during repeated examinations may in rare instances be the only auscultatory sign obtained. Crepitant rales in pneumonia may be distinguished by their clear-cut, sharp, distinct, or resonating (consonating) quality from the non-consonating rales arising in the bronchi in cases in which there is no consolidation of the surrounding tissue (Lord, 807). This distinction is at times difficult to make, but is of value as a means of distinguishing between consolidation and simple bronchitis, edema, and hypostatic congestion. During the height of the disease crepitant rales disappear, to reappear during resolution (*redux crepitus*), as described by Laënnec (755).

Over the consolidated area the spoken voice is usually loud and high pitched (bronchophony), probably due to a direct conduction of sound through the solid tissue. Following the spoken voice there is usually a short interval of bronchial expiration. Bronchophony is usually more marked in men than in women or children, due to the deeper pitch of the voice, and may be absent in massive pneumonia. Egophony, the peculiar bleating or nasal quality of the voice, is heard at times.

CHAPTER TEN

CLINICAL VARIETIES OF PNEUMONIA AND ASSOCIATION WITH OTHER CONDITIONS

Clinical Varieties of Pneumonia 510
Apical Pneumonia 510
Abortive Pneumonia 511
Central Pneumonia 512
Double Pneumonia 512
Massive Pneumonia 512
Migratory Pneumonia 513
Terminal or Secondary Pneumonia 513
Pneumonia in Childhood and Old Age 513
Post-operative Pulmonary Complications and Pneumonia 515
Origin and Nature 515
Factors Influencing Occurrence 519
Incidence 520
Prognosis 521
Bacteriology 522
Prevention and Treatment 523
Inhalation or Anesthesia Pneumonia 524
Association with Other Conditions 524
Collapse of Lung 525
Tuberculosis 525
Other Diseases 525

CLINICAL VARIETIES OF PNEUMONIA

NUMEROUS factors appear to influence the nature of the lesion produced in lobar pneumonia (see pages 232–245). The location and extent of the involved areas are variable and at times several areas may be involved simultaneously or in succession. In addition some clinical and other differences exist between the usual case in adults and that in children or in aged patients and in individuals in whom pneumonia occurs as a secondary or terminal event.

Apical Pneumonia

Among others, Osler (976) reports that stupor, delirium, hyperpyrexia, and signs of meningeal irritation may be more common with lesions involving the upper lobes than with those confined to other lobes. Confirmation of this observation is lacking (807). As elsewhere indicated, involvement of the upper lobes may occur in from about 10 to 14 per cent of cases and appears approximately twice as frequent on the right as on the left (see pages 107–109). The findings of Fabyan (399) in 195 cases of lobar pneumonia at necropsy and of Berry (96) in 400 cases similarly examined suggest that the prognosis with apical lesions, particularly on the right, is more serious than that resulting from the occurrence of lesions in other lobes.

Abortive Pneumonia

Lobar pneumonia of very brief duration occurs but is rare. Cases of one day's duration have been reported. As earlier noted, in a series of 1,987 collected cases Musser and Norris (918) found only 4 of two days' duration (0.2 per cent) and 32 of three days' duration (1.6 per cent). In a group of 200 cases studied by Lord (807, 808) one case of two and another of three days' duration were observed. Osler (976) states that abortive pneumonia of two or three days' duration is especially likely to occur in institutions in which pneumonia is prevalent.

The probability exists that in any case the duration of the illness is significantly influenced by such factors as the dosage and virulence of the infecting organism and the immunity of the host. In this connection, Gaskell's (508) findings in a study of the experimental production of pneumonia in rabbits are of interest. Using pneumococci of controlled virulence it was observed that a certain minimal effective dose of organisms must reach the lung in order to produce typical pneumonia. When pneumococci in smaller dose or of less virulence were used, the organisms were rapidly dealt with and pneumonia of an abortive type resulted.

The observations of Cecil (223) and of Robertson, Graeser, Coggeshall, and Harrison (1087) in man also relate to the matter under discussion. One case of abortive lobar pneumonia was reported by the former worker and two cases by the latter investigators; in each instance humoral antibodies were demonstrable in significant amounts as early as the first day of their illness. It is likely that these antibodies were present at the time of onset (see pages 127–129 and 233–234). In one of the cases reported by Robertson and his associates all the classical symptoms of lobar pneumonia were present but lasted less than eighteen hours. No evidence of consolidation could be found by roentgen-ray or by physical examination, although the sputum contained virulent pneumococci of Type II. The findings suggest that in some instances at least, individuals possessing a relatively high immunity at the time of onset may experience an abortive form of pneumonia.

Central Pneumonia

As already mentioned, consolidation in the usual case in adults apparently begins at the lung root and extends slowly toward the periphery (see pages 253–256). In occasional cases, and perhaps in children especially, the initial lesion may be at the periphery. In cases of central pneumonia the lesion is confined to the central portion of one or more lobes and physical signs may be absent for several days or throughout the entire illness. In these cases other manifestations, such as the acute onset with chill, fever, rusty sputum, rapid respiration, leucocytosis, and roentgenographic findings, will assist in making the diagnosis (808). The presence in the sputum or blood of one of the more invasive types of pneumococci, such as Type I, II, V, VII, or VIII, is suggestive. In some instances the diagnosis may be in doubt until crisis occurs. Howard (661) states that many of these cases were described in the older literature under the terms "latent" or "larval" pneumonia.

Double Pneumonia

Double pneumonia usually refers to involvement of one or more lobes on both sides of the chest. Involvement of the two lower lobes may be found during life in approximately 10 per cent of all cases (694) and was reported by Cecil, Baldwin, and Larsen (230) in 16.3 per cent of 1,896 cases of lobar pneumonia due to pneumococci of Type I, II, or III, or Group IV (for findings at necropsy, see pages 109–111). The course is similar to that of ordinary pneumonia but the prognosis is somewhat less favorable (see pages 696–698).

Massive Pneumonia

In massive pneumonia, which is rare, the bronchi of the involved region are filled with fibrinous exudate (Lord, 807, Howard, 661). These cases are likely to show such physical signs as flatness to percussion and diminished or absent respiration, voice sounds, whisper, and tactile fremitus. If the lesion is confined to the lower part or the whole of one lung, pleurisy with effusion may be simulated. Coughing may expel fibrinous plugs from the bronchi and allow demonstration of the physical signs of consolidation. In ordinary instances lack of displacement of the heart away from the lesion is an indication that an effusion is not present but an exploratory puncture may be necessary to settle the diagnosis.

Migratory Pneumonia

Pneumonia of the migratory type is seen in a small number of cases. Its occurrence usually indicates a lack of resistance on the part of the patient as a result of which the infection spreads from lobe to lobe, resolution occurring in one place while infiltration progresses in another. In this manner all lobes of one or both lungs may be successively involved, and, in rare instances, a lobe previously attacked may become reinfected (see pages 532–533). A prolonged and severe illness is likely to result, and complications not infrequently develop (661).

In view of Loeschcke's (798) observations on the role of uncontrolled cough in disseminating infected edema fluid throughout many areas of the lungs, it is perhaps surprising that more clinical evidence of lesions of the wandering or migratory type is not available (see pages 254–256). That a great many pneumonias belong in this group is shown by the frequency with which extension from one to another neighboring lobe is found at necropsy (874, 807, 808, 798; see also pages 110–111).

Terminal or Secondary Pneumonia

Occasionally lobar pneumonia and more frequently bronchopneumonia may be the terminal event in such chronic diseases as arteriosclerosis, chronic heart or kidney disease, cancer, diabetes, cerebral hemorrhage, fractures, cirrhosis of the liver, and the like (256, 297, 807, 230, 464, 470). The initial chill, pain in the side, and raising of sputum are often lacking. There may be little or no increase in temperature and the disease may remain unsuspected. Prognosis is poor.

Among 658 cases of lobar pneumonia studied by Chatard (256), there were 35 cases, or 5.3 per cent, in which the disease could be called terminal, as these patients all had some chronic disease as well. In 24 of the 35 cases the lobar distribution of the pneumonia was confirmed at necropsy. As compared with the high incidence of pneumococci of Type I or II, or Group IV in most series of cases of lobar pneumonia, infection with Type III is particularly prone to occur in such patients, as was pointed out earlier (see pages 335–336). When secondary pneumonia occurs in the bronchopneumonic form it is usually due to pneumococci of one of the less common types or to other organisms.

Pneumonia in Childhood and Old Age

The natural immunity of man to the pneumococcus appears low in infancy, progressively increases during childhood, and is relatively high from late childhood through middle adult life, after which it shows a general decrease, as previously mentioned (see pages 156–157 and 187–192). The possession of some resistance assists in the production of a localized lesion such as occurs in lobar pneumonia (see pages 256–257). Although pneumonia developing in the extremely young or old frequently results in scattered lesions of the bronchopneumonic form, lobar pneumonia may be found among individuals in these age groups.

There is no agreement as to the frequency of occurrence of lobar pneumonia in infants and children, and some pathologists incline to the belief that a true lobar lesion is rare in young children (885, 112). Many clinicians, however, consider that lobar pneumonia is a common form of pneumonia among infants and children (1318, 333, 574, 7), but because children usually recover, the diagnosis in their case is seldom confirmed by necropsy. In fact, Smith (1212), from his observations at Bellevue Hospital, New York City, states that the most frequent variety of pneumonia he has encountered is one closely resembling the lobar form in adults. He considers this the most common variety of pneumonia at all ages and remarks that in patients over three years of age it is almost the only type seen. In addition, according to Bullowa (190), most of the primary pneumonias of children are of the lobar variety.

Numerous investigators state that pneumonia in infants is usually bronchopneumonia, while in children after the age of two or three years lobar pneumonia is commonest (333, 1025, 899, 766, 1321, 710). Pneumonia in newborn and stillborn infants, commonly associated with trauma or hemorrhage at birth, is usually an aspiration pneumonia and patchy in distribution (Warwick, 1386, Rosenthal, 1121). Lobar pneumonia may occur, however, in the first few days of life and was found at necropsy within one or two days of birth in nine cases studied by Lauche (766). In each instance the mother also had the disease at the time of delivery.

Lobar pneumonia in infants and children may differ in several respects from that in adults. The initial chill is less common and symptoms referable to the central nervous system, such as convulsions or delirium, may occur instead. Gastrointestinal disturbances, especially vomiting and diarrhea, are more likely to be prominent features. Abdominal pain is not uncommon. Cough is usually present but not distressing. Children under about five to eight years old rarely expectorate and usually swallow their sputum (1318, 808). The temperature is frequently at a higher level and the pulse rate proportionally more rapid than in adults. As the physical signs of consolidation may not appear until late in the illness, the diagnosis may be in doubt for several days. An acute onset with fever, cough, rapid respiration, expiratory grunt, and leucocytosis may be the only definite indications (808). The leucocytosis is generally higher than in adults. Roentgen-ray examination is of importance in determining the nature of the illness.

The case fatality rate may be in the neighborhood of 20 per cent or more in infants, but is considerably lower in older children (see Prognosis: Age, pages 703–707). Lyon (821), Trask, O'Donovan, Moore, and Beebe (1321), and Bullowa (187) point out that the incidence of bacteriemia in pneumococcus pneumonia in infants and children is much lower, possibly about one-third of that seen in adults. It may even be less common, however (see pages 555–557). Associated with the generally lower fatality rate both the incidence and the degree of blood invasion are less in cases in children than in adults. The appearance of type-specific humoral antibodies during the course of the illness is likewise less common in the younger patients (1321). The explanation of these differences is obscure, although a lack of physiologic maturation may be assumed the cause of some of them (see pages 186–192). Complications such as empyema and otitis media are more common in children than in adults and delayed resolution may be less common.

The frequency with which various organisms, including pneumococci of many types, are found in the pneumonias of infants and children, has already been discussed (see pages 74–89). In cases of pneumococcus lobar pneumonia Types XIV, I, VI, V, and VII in approximately that order were the types most commonly encountered. Type XIV is especially prominent in cases in infants and Type I in the older children.

The pneumonias of old age are chiefly of the bronchopneumonic variety. Uncommonly, however, true lobar pneumonia may occur. Frequently insidious in nature, the condition is similar to the terminal pneumonia discussed in the foregoing section and may be unsuspected during life. A general lack of resistance may be assumed to account for the more frequent development of bronchopneumonia in elderly individuals and for the high case fatality rate of pneumonia in any form.

Post-operative Pulmonary Complications and Pneumonia

ORIGIN AND NATURE. As a post-operative pulmonary complication true lobar pneumonia is uncommon (1414, 297, 807, 1228, 154, 1272, 464) and most such disturbances are the result of other forms of infection, such as bronchitis, pneumonitis, or bronchopneumonia. Lobar or lobular atelectasis may also occur and be accompanied by an underlying infection in some portion of the bronchial tree. The infection, in all probability, usually arises from organisms present in the mouth and throat at the time of operation.

As the factors instrumental in producing post-operative pneumonia appear largely inseparable from those concerned in the development of other related pulmonary abnormalities after operation, the following discussion will not be limited to pneumonia alone. Many of the factors of importance in giving rise to such conditions, as described by Whipple (1414) and tabulated by Cole (297), are outlined below.

(1) Lowering of local resistance due to:
  (a) Irritation—from ether or gas
  (b) Congestion—from partial asphyxia or defective respiratory excursion, lowered blood pressure, or prolonged recumbent position
  (c) Inhibition of respiratory movements—from binders, dressings, muscle splinting, from pain or peritonitis
(2) Lowering of general resistance due to:
  (a) Shock of operation or hemorrhage
  (b) Infection or other pathologic condition responsible for necessity to operate
  (c) Exposure in hospital before, during, or after operation
(3) Access to the lungs of bacteria in the mouth and throat due to abolition of laryngeal and bronchial reflexes

In most instances, presumably, it is a combination of factors such as these which operates to cause post-operative pulmonary complications. The role of many of these factors in such conditions has been reviewed by numerous workers (1414, 270, 1422, 1167, 914, 259, 632, 630, 405, 154, 1156, 716, 717, 811, 89, 282, 718, 1276).

Following abdominal operations Whipple (1414) finds considerable restriction in respiratory movements due to muscle splinting from pain. Accompanying this there is a marked reduction in vital capacity as shown by Churchill and McNeill (270). Respiration becomes more rapid and shallow, accompanied by a reduction in total lung volume. In experimental animals a reduction in lung volume follows immediately upon producing distention of the stomach, intestine, or peritoneal cavity, as Beecher, Bradshaw, and Lindskog (89) have demonstrated. After laparotomy the lung assumes the position normally found at the time of expiration, which Henderson (630) terms the acapnial position. He likewise considers that vascular stasis, perhaps resulting from a general decrease in muscle tonus, which also affects the diaphragm, may occur. The ensuing impairment of respiration produces a condition of hypoventilation, as mentioned by Muller, Overholt, and Pendergrass (914) and Coburn (282) and allows the collection of secretion in the bronchi, as pointed out by Churchill and McNeill (270) and others (1422, 632, 154, 1156, 716, 717, 1276). Facilitated by an impairment of the mechanism for removing the secretions from the bronchial tree, atelectasis or pneumonia may result (1414, 630, 811, 405). The role of nervous reflex activity in the etiology of these conditions is not apparent but seems small (1167, 632).

The failure of Ward (1379) to find any reduction in the pneumococcidal powers of the blood of patients following operation, even though pneumonia developed in one case, led him to suggest that a lowering of local resistance was probably of more importance in the production of post-operative pneumonia than a lowering of general resistance. The reports of workers such as Whittle (1422), Brown and Debenham (154), and King (716, 717) further indicate that abolition of the normal laryngeal and bronchial reflexes, in addition to a lowering of local resistance, with a resultant bronchitis and its sequel of pulmonary infection with or without atelectasis, is of the utmost importance in causing such complications. Whipple (1414) and King (716) find, however, that patients whose general resistance is low, such as those in the terminal stages of cancer, have a very high incidence of post-operative pulmonary complications.

A careful investigation of post-operative pulmonary complications was made by King (716, 717) over a two-year period in Boston at the Massachusetts General Hospital. His study was confined to the type of pulmonary disturbance occurring in the first three or four days after operation. These complications were almost always accompanied by fever, leucocytosis, cough, and purulent sputum. Cases of bronchitis, pulmonary embolism, tuberculosis, empyema, and so forth were excluded. The type of complication investigated is variously termed in the literature as bronchopneumonia, "pneumonitis" (1414), or collapse (atelectasis). The report covered some 7,000 operations, following 426 of which such pulmonary complications developed.

Three types of pulmonary complication were found:

(a) There were a few cases of bronchopneumonia and these were of the greatest importance, as most deaths occurred in this group. Stewart (1228) also found this true in a much larger series reviewed by him;

(b) There were a few cases of typical massive collapse diagnosed clinically and by roentgenograms, produced by the occlusion of a large bronchus by exudate and clearing quickly when the plug was expelled by cough;

(c) Intermediate between the above two forms was a large group of cases difficult to classify for the lesion was not pneumonia in the "medical" sense, as it ran a much shorter course with less toxemia.

This last form of lesion was responsible for a very large percentage of the complications in this series and, as Whipple (1414) earlier mentioned, is the type of post-operative pulmonary complication commonly encountered. King summarizes the explanations advanced by various observers:

(a) Whipple ably described the lesion and named it "pneumonitis"—meaning a pneumonia in which the alveolar exudate is caused by a relatively avirulent pnemococcus and is lacking in fibrin, in consequence of which the exudate is quickly absorbed.

(b) Cutler regarded it as an embolic pneumonia—a contention difficult of proof.

(c) Coryllos believed it due to pulmonary collapse and stated that the steps in the development of post-operative pneumonia are: bronchitis, obstruction of a bronchus by infected exudate, atelectasis due to the obstruction, and pneumonia developing in the collapsed area.

King considers the differential diagnosis lies between a low-grade bronchopneumonia, better termed a pneumonitis, and lobar or lobular atelectasis. He notes that the diagnosis of atelectasis has become much more general in recent years. At the Massachusetts General Hospital in 1928 less than one-third of the total post-operative pulmonary complications were diagnosed as atelectasis, while in 1931 two-thirds of the cases were so recorded.

The exact physical signs found must be noted with care and their correct interpretation is important for diagnosis. Lord has repeatedly shown that obstruction of a bronchus from any cause will produce (a) dulness, (b) absent or diminished breathing without bronchial breathing, (c) absent or diminished voice without egophony, (d) diminished whisper, and (e) diminished tactile fremitus. If in a given instance the bronchial obstruction is removed and the collapse persists, the signs change and are those of consolidation in which bronchial breathing is prominent. In consequence bronchial breathing may indicate *either* pneumonic consolidation (infection) *or* a collapsed area with an open bronchus.

With respect to the cause of post-operative pulmonary complications, King (716) states:

We believe, therefore, that a purulent bronchitis develops in a large percentage of postoperative cases; that in some cases the infection is limited to the bronchi; and that in the intermediate group of pulmonary complications, now under discussion, there is an accompanying "pneumonitis," combined at times with atelectasis due to occlusion of the bronchi by exudate. We have found no evidence that atelectasis necessarily precedes pneumonitis and have been able to prove atelectasis in only 47 per cent of our series of cases.

He adds:

In most instances a sharp distinction cannot be drawn between pneumonitis and collapse in this intermediate group, the underlying lesion in all cases being *purulent bronchitis*. (Italics supplied.)

FACTORS INFLUENCING OCCURRENCE. *Sex and type of operation*. King found that the sex of the patient and the type of the operation were the two most important predisposing factors in his series and showed that males have at least twice as many pulmonary complications as females, and that such complications are more than *twelve* times as frequent after laparotomy and hernia operations as after operations in the non-abdominal group.

Post-operative pulmonary complications after non-abdominal operations occurred most frequently following thyroid operations. Their average incidence was 7.5 per cent after 130 operations in 1930 and 6.9 per cent after 102 operations in 1931.

Sepsis and perforation. Patients, and especially male patients, operated upon because of the presence of sepsis or perforation of a viscus showed an extraordinarily high percentage of pulmonary complications. This was found to be due largely to the generally unfavorable pre-operative condition of the patient. Appendectomy with drainage, for example, was complicated by pneumonia almost four times as often as simple appendectomy (see below).

Pre-operative respiratory infections. Only 14 per cent of the total 426 patients with post-operative pulmonary complications had acute or chronic pre-operative respiratory infections.

Anesthesia. Of patients on whom laparotomies or hernial operations were performed, 12.7 per cent developed pulmonary complications after having inhalation anesthesia, 16.6 per cent after spinal anesthesia, and 18.4 per cent after local anesthesia. The explanation of the higher rates for spinal and local anesthesia apparently lies in the fact that anesthesia in these forms was used either on patients extremely ill from infection or on those in the terminal stages of malignancy and requiring palliative operations. In a group of 35 patients having operations of the same kind who were given Avertin anesthesia, three, or 8.6 per cent, developed pulmonary sequelae.

King's finding that pulmonary complications occurred more often after the use of spinal than after inhalation anesthesia is similar in significance to the earlier observation of Brown and Debenham (154). The latter reported the occurrence of such complications in 1.3 per cent or 6 of 474 cases after inhalation anesthesia and 7.4 per cent or 25 of 338 cases after subarachnoid anesthesia. These investigators also pointed out that operations performed under spinal anesthesia were on the average 50 per cent longer than those under a general anesthetic. After spinal anesthesia, the depth and force of the respiratory movements were definitely inhibited for a considerable period and the patients tended to remain quiet for some hours. Moreover, possibly the secretions of the bronchial tree underwent an increase in viscosity and tenacity.

INCIDENCE. Lord (807) states that post-operative pneumonia follows laparotomy in from 1 to 4 per cent of the cases. In investigations made with great care, the incidence is usually higher, as doubtless many of the lesser complications are included in the tabulations. The incidence alone of post-operative massive atelectasis was reported by Scott and Cutler (1167) as 0.6 per cent in one series of 2,000 patients, and as 0.2 per cent in a second series of 1,000 cases. In Brown and Debenham's (154) series totaling 812 patients, 31 or 3.8 per cent suffered some sort of post-operative pulmonary complication. In 1932 Stewart (1228) reviewed much of the literature dealing with the incidence of these complications. In a collected series of 144,336 operations a post-operative pulmonary complication was reported as occurring in 2,801 or 1.9 per cent.

In King's series, discussed above, pneumonia, pneumonitis, or collapse developed after 6 per cent of all operations, after 14 per cent of laparotomies or hernial operations, and after 7.2 per cent of thyroid operations. The incidence after a simple appendectomy was 6 per cent, as contrasted with 22.5 per cent in patients having appendectomy with drainage. Among males the incidence of these complications was 46.8 per cent after operations on the stomach and duodenum, 35.6 per cent after gall-bladder operations, and 26.2 per cent after intestinal operations. The rates in these three groups were so high that King coined the expression "bad risk" group to identify patients needing operations on the organs mentioned. Among females in the "bad risk" group the rates were about one-half as high. Following gastrostomies and palliative operations for intestinal obstruction on patients of both sexes, 22.2 per cent experienced pulmonary complications, and after gastric and duodenal suture the incidence was 61.8 per cent! Of 34 patients operated upon, 21 developed pulmonary complications. The explanation of the very high rates in this series was not clear.

The general incidence of post-operative pulmonary complications was listed by King (718) as shown in the accompanying summary:

	Number	*Per cent having post-operative pulmonary complications*
Laparotomies and hernial operations	3,037	13
Other operations	4,028	1
Total	7,065	6

The findings in males and females, after limiting the field to abdominal operations, are as follows:

	Per cent of post-operative pulmonary complications	
Operation	*Male*	*Female*
Stomach and duodenum	47	17
Gall bladder	36	14
Intestine	26	13
Appendix	14	6
Hernia	9	4
Gynecological operations	–	6
Miscellaneous abdominal operations	11	5

As a rule when considering abdominal operations, the closer the operative field approaches the diaphragm the higher is the incidence of pulmonary complications (154, 716, 717, 718).

Seasonal variation in incidence. King (716) found much less seasonal variation in the incidence of the post-operative pulmonary complications in his series than has been reported by others (1414, 807). His series, however, did not include any patients with urogenital diseases, many of whom are old and in whom a marked seasonal incidence of pulmonary complications following operation is often found. Nevertheless, further elaboration of this point is needed.

PROGNOSIS. King (716) found that although pulmonary complications followed 6 per cent of all operations, the complication itself was regarded as primarily responsible or as the major cause of death in 0.5 per cent of the total number of operations performed, and in 1.2 per cent of the laparotomy and hernial operations. Lord (807) considered the matter from a different angle and stated that post-operative pneumonia is responsible for about one-quarter of all deaths after operation under general anesthesia.

BACTERIOLOGY. No extensive bacteriologic investigations of post-operative pulmonary complications have yet appeared in the literature. A few investigators, however, have made studies of limited scope (1414, 1422, 259, 716, 1272, 464, 1276). Whipple (1414), Whittle (1422), Chickering (259), and King (716) are in agreement in stating that whenever pneumococci are isolated from cases of post-operative pulmonary complications they are largely of the less virulent types. Nevertheless, cases of pneumonia due to the more invasive types, such as Type I, II, or III, may occur post-operatively (1414, 1272, 464, 1276).

Whipple (1414) in 1918 reported finding pneumococci of Group IV in the sputum of patients with post-operative pulmonary complications. Examination of the sputum of 97 patients revealed the presence of these organisms in 42 per cent of the cases, both before and after operation. In several instances agglutinins specific for the strain of pneumococcus isolated from the sputum appeared in the blood within seven to fourteen days after the onset of the complication. King (716) carried out bacteriologic investigation of the sputum of forty-four patients with pulmonary complications and found typical pneumococci in thirty instances. Strains of Type III were present in ten specimens and strains of Group IV in the other twenty. The remaining fourteen specimens contained too few pneumococci to type.

Sutliff and Finland (1272) observed several cases of pneumococcus Type I lobar pneumonia which occurred a few hours either after operation on the nose or throat or after a normal delivery. The attendant circumstances suggested that direct infection from the upper respiratory tract had taken place. Observations of similar significance were made by Finland and Sutliff (464) in studying a number of Type III and Type VIII pneumonias. In these instances only a few of the cases secondary to operation were of the lobar variety and bronchopneumonia was the commoner.

Sutliff and Steele (1276) made a bacteriologic investigation of the oral flora of 16 patients about to undergo abdominal operation. After operation more than two-thirds of the patients showed evidence of some comparatively severe pulmonary complication. Further bacteriologic investigation was carried out in all instances. A correlation appeared between the presence of pathogenic organisms, especially pneumococci and streptococci in the throat before operation or in throat or sputum after operation, and the occurrence of some pulmonary complication. The findings revealed that patients not carrying pneumococci at the time of operation showed minimal post-operative pulmonary changes. A group of 6 patients showed pneumococci or *Beta*-hemolytic streptococci constantly or intermittently but without relation to pulmonary complications. Instances of bronchitis, atelectasis, bronchopneumonia, and infarct occurred in this group. In another group of 7 patients organisms of similar varieties or a Friedländer's bacillus were present either before or after operation, or both before and after. In a few of these cases pneumococci of a type different from that previously found or streptococci previously absent appeared in the sputum after operation. The source of these organisms was not discovered. Patients in this third group suffered the most severe pulmonary complications, five having bronchopneumonia. One patient with Type III bronchopneumonia died.

The pulmonary signs appearing after operation in the patients studied were regarded as being caused by the organisms mentioned. The severity of the pulmonary lesion incited was considered proportional to the virulence of such bacteria. Whipple's (1414) conclusions many years ago were similar. An extension of observations of this nature is desirable.

PREVENTION AND TREATMENT. Specific recommendations for the prevention and treatment of post-operative pulmonary complications have been considered by several investigators (1414, 1167, 632, 630, 631, 1156, 717, 811, 405, 282, 718, 447). Many of the measures useful in the prevention of pneumonia in general have already been discussed (see pages 395–483), and procedures of aid in the treatment of pneumonia are described later (see pages 741–804 and 805–879). The general principles of the prevention and treatment of post-operative pulmonary complications may be outlined here.

Whenever possible, operation should be avoided in the presence of respiratory infections. The warmer months of the year should be chosen for operations when it is possible to plan for them. Care should be taken at all times, before, during, and after operation, to avoid undue exposure of the patient. Overheating, chilling, or exposure to sudden or prolonged temperature changes should be avoided. After operation efforts should be made to prevent restriction of the movement of the lungs and to facilitate bronchial drainage. Tight chest swathes should be avoided. The relief of pain by judicious medication may assist in obtaining better respiratory movements. Attention should be given to the prevention of intercurrent infections. Frequent changes in posture, occasional deep breathing, and the application of measures to relieve or prevent tympanites are of value. Attention to oral hygiene both before and after operation may be of assistance.

King (717), in a study of several carefully controlled series of cases treated in various ways, has well described his efforts to prevent the development of post-operative pulmonary complications in patients after abdominal and hernial operations. Post-operative inhalations of from 5 to 25 per cent of carbon dioxide in air or oxygen were administered in varying amounts at various intervals to many of the patients in the treated groups without any striking reduction in the total incidence of pulmonary disturbances. There may, however, have been some decrease in the occurrence of the more severe complications in these groups. No case of massive atelectasis occurred in the treated patients. Nevertheless, King considered that equally good results can be obtained by the routine use of frequent changes of posture alone.

Frequent change of position may give immediate and striking relief if the symptoms present are due to the retention of tenacious material in the bronchi. In all instances specimens of sputum should be sent to the laboratory for bacteriologic diagnosis. Should pneumococci be present of a type for which a therapeutically effective specific antiserum is available and serious symptoms develop, the advisability of treating the patient with this agent should be considered (see pages 805–879). In suitable cases excellent results have been obtained by the antiserum treatment of patients with post-operative pneumonia. The response to serum resembles that of patients with lobar pneumonia treated in like manner.

Inhalation or Anesthesia Pneumonia

The designation inhalation, anesthesia, or ether pneumonia is old and is based on the erroneous assumption that irritation by the vapor of a volatile anesthetic such as ether is the cause (1414). The relation of several anesthetics to the incidence of post-operative pulmonary complications is discussed in the foregoing section on anesthesia (page 519).

ASSOCIATION WITH OTHER CONDITIONS

Uncommonly, lobar pneumonia may be associated with other conditions or diseases.

Collapse of Lung

The occurrence of atelectasis in pneumonia was discussed in Chapter V (see page 250) and in the preceding section on post-operative pneumonia (page 517) in this chapter.

Although not common, obstruction atelectasis may complicate lobar pneumonia, especially in the young. Lord (808) considers it due to bronchial plugging by retained tenacious secretion with absorption of the air in the part of the lung supplied by the occluded passage. Maintaining one position for a long time favors its development. Massive collapse is seldom encountered. Collapse of sufficient degree to lead to clinically demonstrable cardiac displacement was found by Lord (811) in only 2.5 per cent (14 cases) of 558 cases of pneumonia examined personally. Lobar pneumonia was present in 9 of the cases and bronchopneumonia in 5.

Tuberculosis

Pneumococcus lobar pneumonia may occur in patients with active pulmonary tuberculosis but is rare (Lord, 807, Cecil, Baldwin, and Larsen, 230).

Other Diseases

Lobar pneumonia has long been known to occur occasionally in association with such other diseases as smallpox, scarlet fever, typhoid or paratyphoid fever, diabetes, heart disease, renal disease (256), malaria, and insanity (807). In typhoid fever the pulmonary lesion produced may be caused by either the pneumococcus or the typhoid bacillus (976, 807). The pneumonia may begin at the onset of typhoid fever, or at the height of the latter illness, making diagnosis difficult, or at times in convalescence from it (Lord, 807). Pneumococcus lobar pneumonia may complicate paratyphoid infections (182). Among 530 cases of diabetes reviewed by Lord (807), pneumonia occurred as a complication in 6 (one per cent) and all died.

CHAPTER ELEVEN

SPECIAL FEATURES IN THE COURSE OF THE DISEASE

Duration of the Disease 526
  Crisis and Lysis 527
  Prolongation of Illness 531
Relapse 532
Recurrence 533
Resolution and Delayed Resolution 540
  Resolution 540
  Delayed Resolution 542
Termination in Fibrosis 543
Death 544
Convalescence 546
Persistence of Carrier State 547

Most of the symptoms occurring in the course of the usual case of lobar pneumonia are described in Chapter VIII (page 484). Although there may be great variability in the symptoms encountered, a large majority of cases pursue a rather typical course for five to ten days. A marked and fairly uniform increase in temperature, rapid pulse and respiration, considerable cough and sputum, a varying amount of pleuritic pain, usually notable and continued dyspnea, and some cyanosis are generally present. Patients usually look very ill and have the appearance of being "toxic." In addition to these general features of the disease, one or more of certain special features of importance are also observed in such cases.

DURATION OF THE DISEASE

In approximately 70 per cent of cases the disease may be expected to end in from five to ten days (918, 874, 807, 961, 1450, 464, 288, 186). Cases that last one, two, or three days are uncommon and have already been described (see pages 511–512). Occasionally the acute disease lasts two or three weeks or more. In cases due to a type of pneumococcus for which an effective specific antiserum is available, appropriate serum treatment, particularly when given early, will materially shorten the course of the acute illness, as described later (see pages 880–887).

In the United States, in various European countries, and in China the duration of the acute course averages from 5.8 to 7.9 days (Musser and

Norris, 918, Cohn and Lewis, 288, Wu and Chiu, 1450). In African natives, however, Maynard (874) believes the average course to be 5.3 days and thus possibly somewhat shorter, while in Indian (Tamil), Malayan, and Chinese laborers in the Malay Peninsula, McSwan (853) considers the average duration to be from nine to twelve days and thus definitely longer. As the findings of these two investigators are based on a combined series of less than 600 cases, these determinations are possibly of little significance. In Cohn and Lewis' (288) series of 1,456 cases of lobar pneumonia at the Hospital of the Rockefeller Institute for Medical Research, New York City, the average duration for all cases was 7.89 days. The etiology was unknown in 70 of the cases and in the remainder, the causative agent was pneumococci of Type I, II, or III, or Group IV. Most of the Type I and a few of the Type II cases received specific serum therapy. In the total series, the average duration in recovered cases, excluding seven which lasted more than twenty days, was 7.9 days.

In a series totaling 692 patients who spontaneously recovered from pneumonia due to pneumococci of Type I, II, or III or Group IV, Cecil, Baldwin, and Larsen (230) measured the average length of illness in cases due to these various organisms. It was found to be 8.8 days, 8.6 days, 9.1 days, and 8.7 days respectively, thus showing little variation in each group. In a similar study of 168 cases due to pneumococci of Type I, II, or III or Group IV, Wu and Chiu (1450) were also unable to show any marked correlation between the variety of pneumococcus causing the infection and the duration of the illness.

The duration of the illness was studied by Finland and Sutliff (464) in cases of pneumococcus Type III and Type VIII pneumonia (including both lobar pneumonia and bronchopneumonia) and by Bullowa (186) in Type VIII cases of similar nature. The former workers observed that 73 per cent of the Type III cases terminated before the end of the tenth day and that 70 per cent of the Type VIII cases terminated before the end of the ninth day. About 10 per cent of the cases due to each of the types lasted more than fifteen days. In Bullowa's series of Type VIII cases most ended on or before the eighth day.

Crisis and Lysis

The phenomena which characterize crisis probably constitute the most remarkable obvious feature of this or any other disease. A desperately ill patient may, in the course of a few hours, be changed into an exhausted patient on the road to recovery. Accompanying this change there is a coincidental drop in the temperature to or below normal, and a marked subjective sense of relief with a disappearance of the toxemia. Examination of the chest, however, may reveal little or no apparent alteration in the signs of consolidation. This unusual occurrence, as Zinsser (1461) has said, suggests that a sudden neutralization of a toxin has taken place. As yet, however, the existence of a toxin in pneumonia remains undemonstrated.

To a large extent, the recovery of patients treated without specific antiserum is to be attributed to the spontaneous development of sufficient immunity to overcome the infection. In most cases the spread of the local inflammation ends with the beginning of crisis. The effectiveness of immune substances in bringing about crisis and in stopping the spread of infection is clearly evident in suitable cases receiving specific serum treatment (see pages 880–888).

Rosenow (1117) has suggested that crisis may be anaphylactic in nature and represents a reaction to an acquired sensitivity to the infecting organism. Thomas and Parker (1298), by the use of repeated lung punctures in seventy-three patients, determined that in some favorable cases the number of organisms present within the consolidated area may diminish to a great extent before crisis occurs. They regard the death of the organisms as unrelated to the occurrence of crisis and state that the detoxifying effect so noticeable at crisis may be the result of the action of local chemical factors within the lung (see page 734).

A return of the temperature to about normal or under for a period of twelve to twenty-four hours may be termed crisis (807, 961). Crisis, nevertheless, is a variable and a somewhat relative phenomenon and evades precise definition. Cole (297) states that the fall of an elevated temperature to normal or under within an interval of thirty-six hours may be deemed crisis. He advocates evaluating the clinical picture as a whole and considering as crisis the drop in temperature, pulse, and respiration, with a coincident change in the general condition of the patient for the better. Few of the reported series of cases in which this matter is dealt with, however, have been analyzed in this fashion.

Lord (807) notes that defervescence most commonly occurs in the late evening hours and that signs of resolution usually appear just before, at, or after it. A disappearance of restlessness, delirium, flushing of the face, and anxiety usually foretells the beginning of crisis. Patients are generally exhausted and soon pass off into a sleep, at first broken, which gradually deepens and may last twelve hours or more. During this interval a rapid drop of temperature occurs accompanied by a profuse sweat. The pulse and respiration rates drop and the cough becomes looser.

Crisis is more frequent in children than in adults and more often occurs in adults in the prime of life than in aged patients (918, 1003, 808, 1450, 464). It may be infrequent in lobar pneumonia in infants and children under three years of age, however, for in Albert and Abad's (7) series of 254 cases it was seldom found. In 1,500 cases in infants and children under thirteen years of age, Cunningham (333) observed a fall in temperature, pulse, and respiration by crisis in 72 per cent. Among adults as age increases the proportion of cases with crisis decreases, and the proportion ending by lysis or in death increases, as Patterson (1003a) has found. The proportion of his cases in various age groups ending in crisis or lysis is shown in Table 87. Although the number of cases in his series is not large (521 cases), the results illustrate that with increasing age a decreasing proportion of cases end by crisis.

TABLE 87. LOBAR PNEUMONIA. NUMBER AND PERCENTAGE OF CASES ENDING BY CRISIS OR LYSIS, BY AGE GROUP

AGE GROUP	TOTAL CASES	CASES ENDING BY CRISIS		CASES ENDING BY LYSIS	
		Number	*Per cent*	*Number*	*Per cent*
10–19	72	59	82.0	13	18.0
20–29	126	68	54.0	47	37.3
30–39	132	71	53.8	43	32.6
40–49	86	29	33.7	30	35.0
50–59	54	15	28.5	18	33.3
60–69	41	3	7.3	13	31.7
70–79	10	1	10.0	1	10.0
Total	521	246	47.2	165	31.7

Crisis is more common in vigorous adults than in persons debilitated by acute or chronic disease, and is more common in patients in whom the disease runs a short course than in others (808).

Uncommonly crisis may occur as early as the second or as late as the nineteenth day (1168) but is usually found between the fifth or sixth and the ninth day (1168, 26, 918, 1003, 230, 1357, 1385, 464). Sears and Larrabee (1168) find crisis to be rare after the tenth day. Maynard (874) reports the average time of crisis to be about four and one-half days in his series of 975 recovered cases in African Negroes. This was somewhat shorter than the average time of crisis in the European series he used for comparison.

The exact incidence of crisis in adult cases varies considerably with the criteria used to define it. It has been reported in from 15 to 58 per cent of all cases (1168, 918, 830, 297, 1003, 230, 1450). Musser and Norris (918) state it was present in 53.1 per cent of 10,159 collected cases, while Cole (297) reports true crisis occurred in but 15 per cent of his series of several hundred cases. Among recovered cases only, the incidence is much the same and is reported in from 35 to 49 per cent (874, 1357).

The incidence of crisis and lysis in 744 cases due to pneumococci of Type I, II, or III or Group IV was reported by Cecil, Baldwin, and Larsen (230), as shown in Table 88. No specific treatment was given these cases. Crisis occurred in 56.6 per cent of 285 Type I cases, in 50 per cent of 122 Type II cases, and was found less frequently in Type III cases (39.3 per cent of 89 cases) and in Group IV cases (45.5 per cent of 248 cases).

TABLE 88. PNEUMOCOCCUS LOBAR PNEUMONIA. NUMBER OF CASES AND NUMBER AND PERCENTAGE OF CASES NOT RECEIVING SPECIFIC SERUM THERAPY ENDING BY CRISIS OR LYSIS, AND BY TYPE

	TOTAL CASES	CASES ENDING BY CRISIS		CASES ENDING BY LYSIS	
		Number	*Per cent*	*Number*	*Per cent*
Type I	285	146	56.6	112	39.3
Type II	122	61	50.0	61	50.0
Type III	89	35	39.3	54	60.7
Group IV	248	113	45.5	135	54.4
Total	744	355	49.6	362	48.7

Among 168 cases due to pneumococci of various types studied by Wu and Chiu (1450), crisis was likewise most commonly observed in Type I and Type II cases. These workers attempted to correlate the onset of the illness, whether sudden or gradual, with the mode of termination of the disease. Their findings suggest that Type II and Type III cases having an abrupt onset are most likely to end by crisis, while Type I and Group IV cases failed to show any such correlation. These results are of interest, although the number of cases in each group was too small of course to yield significant findings.

Among recovered cases of lobar pneumonia Finland and Sutliff (464) report that crisis occurred in 33 per cent of Type III infections and in 27 per cent of Type VIII infections. In recovered cases of bronchopneumonia, however, the occurrence of crisis with either type was less frequent.

Occasionally toward the end of the disease the temperature may fall rapidly, to be followed by its abrupt rise, and a day or so later the permanent temperature drop may take place. Such an occurrence is spoken of as a modified or atypical crisis or pseudo-crisis, and may be present in about 15 per cent of cases (874, 297). Cole (297) is convinced from personal experience and inquiry among physicians that the most common ending of lobar pneumonia is by lysis or modified crisis. Defervescence taking place over an interval of twenty-four to thirty-six hours is referred to by Lord (807) as protracted crisis and that requiring over thirty-six hours as lysis.

Lysis is commonest in the debilitated, in patients with other acute or chronic disease, and in those with complications (Musser and Norris, 918). Lord (807) finds complications are nearly four times as frequent in cases ending by lysis than by crisis.

Lysis has been reported as occurring in from 25 to 70 per cent of cases (874, 297, 230, 1357, 830). In Musser and Norris' (918) series of 8,667 collected cases, 24.9 per cent ended by lysis. More cases among the aged than among the young end by lysis. A suggestion of this is seen in the results presented in Table 87. Cecil, Baldwin, and Larsen (230) observed lysis in nearly half of their series of 744 cases, due to pneumococci of Types I, II, III, and Group IV (Table 88). It was commoner in Type III and Group IV cases than in Type I or Type II. Wu and Chiu (1450) found that 41.7 per cent of 168 typed cases of pneumococcus lobar pneumonia terminated by lysis.

The usual time of lysis is about the sixth to the tenth (1003, 1357) day of illness, but in some instances may be delayed until the twelfth day or longer (1168). It is distinctly uncommon before the fourth day (1357). The more prolonged the attack, the more likely it is to end by lysis. The average duration of the illness in uncomplicated cases ending by lysis was reported by Warr and Alperin (1385) as twenty-one days.

Prolongation of Illness

At times the course of the illness may be unusually prolonged. There may be a re-elevation of temperature with a return of various symptoms after the apparent termination of the disease, or a prolongation of the initial attack.

In a review of more than 600 cases of lobar pneumonia at the Johns Hopkins Hospital, McCrae (832) found a number of conditions might cause a re-elevation of temperature after defervescence. The commonest of these were empyema, delayed resolution, and tuberculosis, coexisting with pneumonia or with a tuberculous pneumonia wrongly diagnosed. Other complications, such as endocarditis, pericarditis, thrombosis, meningitis, or a migratory pneumonia with gradual extension of the pulmonary process were also the cause in some cases. Conditions such as these may likewise occasionally be responsible for the continuance of fever after the time of its expected decline, as Lord (808) has noted. In addition, a mixed infection (see pages 11–16) or relapse may account for a prolongation of the illness.

RELAPSE

In rare instances, a few days after the subsidence of the original attack a fresh invasion of the same or of a different lobe occurs (918, 1299, 961, 765). Loeschcke (798), in a study of the pathology of pneumonia, investigated some sections of lungs showing the presence of a new infection superimposed on an incompletely resolved area. He considered that reinfection of a lobe is possible at the stage when the lobe begins to "breathe" again—namely, at about the time of beginning resolution.

The occurrence of relapse was reported in 0.06 per cent or 36 of 5,966 cases collected by Norris (961), and Lord (807) states that Wagner found relapse in 0.18 per cent or in 2 of 1,100 cases. Of 1,500 cases of lobar pneumonia in infants and children, Cunningham (333) found reinfection had developed in 1.8 per cent.

The generally low incidence of relapse is doubtless due to the effect of the humoral and cellular immunity of the host in restraining the activities of organisms present in the lung or upper respiratory tract. This, however, may be only part of the explanation and the absence of some preceding injury to the lung tissue, such as that which in mice results from their intoxication with alcohol, may be a factor, as Branch and Stillman (146) have mentioned (see pages 217–218). During the course of experimental pneumococcus infections in cats and rabbits, or after recovery, Robertson, Woo, Cheer, and King (1097) observed that secondary infections with streptococci or Gram-negative bacilli were more or less common. Terrell, Robertson, and Coggeshall (1292) found that in dogs undergoing an experimental pneumococcus lobar pneumonia the occurrence of snuffles was followed by a generalization of the pneumonia, which promptly ended fatally. It was noted that, in contrast to the usual finding of a pure culture of pneumococci in the lungs, these animals generally showed a mixed bacterial flora in the involved areas at necropsy.

In man relapse may indicate a general lack of resistance and have serious consequences. In pneumococcus pneumonia the reinfection may be due either to pneumococci of the type causing the original invasion or to those of a different type or to some other organism. Hemolytic streptococci or staphylococci appear to be the commonest offenders in the latter instance, as was pointed out in the discussion of mixed infections (page 11). Langley (765) views relapse as a less serious matter. He states that it occurs within seven days of the previous crisis, is rarely or never fatal, and runs a brief course, usually lasting but three days.

After an apparently successful recovery following treatment with the appropriate antipneumococcic serum, relapse may develop and be due to pneumococci of the same type. This presumably is most likely to occur in cases to whom insufficient serum dosage had been given, as Cecil (224) has pointed out. In adequately treated cases, however, relapse is more often due to a pneumococcus of some other type or to some other organism. Thomas (1299) reports relapse in several serum treated Type I cases in which pneumococci of this type were replaced in the sputum by those of a different type. Parsons and Myers (1000), Sutliff and Finland (1271), and Finland (446) have clearly demonstrated that in cases of serum treated pneumococcus pneumonia relapse is followed by a rapidly fatal termination. In a number of cases the pneumococcus originally present had disappeared and cultures of the lung and blood at necropsy revealed the presence of some other organism which was responsible for the fatal outcome. In several instances the secondary infection was caused by *Beta*-hemolytic streptococci. Intense toxemia, marked bacteriemia, and death within two or three days are not uncommon in cases of this nature. An attack of this kind coming on after recovery in a serum treated case of pneumococcus pneumonia may be responsible for the apparent failure of specific serum therapy (see pages 918–920).

The distinction between a relapse and a recurrence is at times an arbitrary one, as the interval between attacks is variable.

RECURRENCE

Recurrence is more commonly seen in pneumonia than in any other acute infectious disease (Osler, 976, Cecil, 224, Norris and Landis, 961). The incidence in various series of patients with a history of one or more previous attacks of pneumonia varies greatly in different reports. Musser and Norris (918) found 13.6 per cent or 1,615 of 11,081 collected cases had such a history. The incidence of recurrence was 22 per cent in Cole's (297) series of 607 cases, 12.7 per cent in Patterson's (1003a) series of 521 cases, 16.4 per cent in Warr and Alperin's (1385) series of 2,039 cases, and 16.5 per cent in Finland and Winkler's (470) series of 1,000 consecutive typed cases of pneumococcus pneumonia at the Boston City Hospital. The latter investigators also pointed out that among 1,000 patients on the medical wards of the hospital for afflictions other than pneumonia, 14 per cent gave a history of one or more attacks of pneumonia. Lord (807), in three small series collected from the literature, found the incidence of recurrence to vary from 26 to 41 per cent.

Patients should be carefully questioned with regard to previous attacks before their statements concerning the matter are accepted. Possibly it was because this precaution was not taken that recurrence was reported in only 6.5 per cent of 4,000 cases investigated by Shattuck and Lawrence (1176) and in but 4 per cent of 525 cases studied by MacCordick (830).

In a study of pneumonia in native miners on the Rand, Johannesburg, South Africa, Maynard (874) found that among 1,129 men who had recovered from the disease, 80 had a second attack within thirty days from the time their temperature dropped to normal. The figure for attacks in this group was 70 per thousand, as contrasted with a figure of 40 per thousand for miners contracting a first attack of pneumonia within thirty days of their arrival at the mines. In another group of natives studied over a period of a full year, the figure for first attacks was 3.8 per thousand, as compared with 7.5 per thousand for attacks among men in the recovered-case group.

Instances have been reported in which as many as ten (1003a) to twenty-eight attacks (874, 297) have occurred in the same patient. Among the cases cited by Cole (297) there were 30 with a history of more than one previous attack of pneumonia. Of these, 18 had two previous attacks, 9 had three, 2 had four, and one had eighteen. Also in Cole's series, there were 107 patients who had only one previous attack and in 9 of these it had occurred within one year. In 38 the initial attack had occurred from one to five years before, in 19 five to ten years before, in 25 from ten to twenty years before, and in 16 more than twenty years before. Among the 57 typed cases of pneumococcus pneumonia reported by Finland and Winkler (470) the shortest interval between attacks was four weeks and the longest nearly twelve years.

Cecil (222, 223) remarks that recurrent attacks are nearly always due to a type of pneumococcus different from the one causing the initial infection. However, he mentions several instances in which Type III or Group IV infections (224) have been repeated in the same patient. In such instances the interval between attacks is usually over a year. In 607 cases studied by Cole (297) only one patient had two attacks of Type I pneumonia. These occurred at an interval of eight months. No repeated attacks with Type II pneumococci were found in his series. Thomas (1296) also reports a Type I case in a twenty-nine-year-old male Negro, whose infection with the same organism was repeated thirty-one days later. Specific serum treatment was given in both attacks, with recovery. One of Thomas' patients had a Type II pneumonia in May and a Type I the following October. A patient observed by Robertson (1082) had a Type I pneumonia which was followed five months later by an attack due to Type II. Serum treatment was also used on each occasion, with recovery. An occurrence of Type II pneumonia repeated after a year's interval was reported by Cruickshank (331). This patient had been a chronic carrier of pneumococci of Type II in the interval between attacks. One of Cole's patients, twenty-four years of age, had 18 attacks of pneumonia, the last 7 of which were typed. Pneumococci were found on each of these latter occasions and were identified, following the chronological order of the attacks, as strains of Type I, Type III, Group IV, Type III, Type III, Type III, and Type II atypical.

The most adequate and detailed clinical and bacteriologic study of recurrences in pneumonia yet to appear is that by Finland and Winkler (470), which embraces data on 57 cases from which serologically identified pneumococci were obtained during each of two or more attacks. This series includes cases of lobar pneumonia and those having bronchopneumonia or atypical involvements. The findings with respect to the question of the incidence of the various types in recurrences appear of significance and are as shown in Table 89.

TABLE 89. RECURRENT CASES OF PNEUMOCOCCUS PNEUMONIA. NUMBER AND PERCENTAGE DISTRIBUTION OF 57 CASES BY TYPE RECOVERED DURING THE EARLY ATTACK AND DURING THE RECURRENCE

FIRST ATTACK			RECURRENCE			
Type	*Number*	*Per cent*	*Type I*	*Type II*	*Type III*	*Others**
I	20^{8}	33	4^{2}	5^{2}	3	8^{4}
II	12^{5}	20	5^{2}	2^{2}	1	4^{1}
III	6	10	3	1	1	1
Others*	22^{2}	37	7^{2}	2	1	12
Total	60	100	19	10	6	25
Per cent			32	17	10	42

NOTE: Superior figures represent the number of cases treated with specific serum during earlier attack.

* Type II atypical included.

As these workers state:

When due allowance is made for the small numbers concerned, the distribution of cases among the various types during the early attacks and during the recurrences is very similar to that found in any large series of cases of pneumococcus pneumonias. There was obviously no correlation between the types obtained during the different attacks. For example, the 20 cases with Type I pneumococci during the first attack had about the usual distribution of types during the succeeding pneumonia and, conversely, the 19 patients having Type I pneumococci in the latter attack were similarly distributed among the different types during the first attack. The same was true for the other types.

In some instances organisms other than pneumococci were also isolated from these cases.

The average interval between attacks due to the same type of pneumococcus in a given patient in Finland and Winkler's (470) series was twenty-eight months, while the interval between attacks for all cases was approximately four years. Of 19 cases recurring within one year, 4 were due to pneumococci of the same type.

Data on the character of the pulmonary lesion, duration of disease, and mode of termination in the initial and recurrent attacks in 57 cases (Table 90) were also presented by Finland and Winkler (470). In 72 per cent of the cases, the pulmonary lesion was lobar in distribution during each observed attack. Six patients had three such attacks and one patient had four. In all but four of the remaining cases, scattered patchy lesions were observed only during the recurrence. Recurrences differed from the initial attacks with respect to the kind of lesion produced, in that bilateral involvement was twice as frequent and the disease was chiefly of the bronchopneumonic variety. Successive attacks in each individual were quite similar with respect to the duration and mode of termination of the infections.

In 45 per cent of the recovered cases the duration of the acute disease was essentially the same in the first and subsequent attacks, and in 69 per cent of the cases the mode of termination of the disease, by either crisis or lysis, was also the same in the initial invasion and in the recurrence. Blood cultures were made in 47 of the cases in the first attack and were positive in 9, or 19 per cent. In the second attack, 6, or 12 per cent of 52 cases, had positive blood cultures. The incidence of bacteriemia was regarded as lower in these cases than that ordinarily found in pneumococcus pneumonia, which was considered to be about 30 per cent.

Wells (1403) in 1889 stated that recurrence most often occurred when the

TABLE 90. COMPARISON OF EARLY ATTACKS AND RECURRENCES BY VARIETY OF LESION IN 57 CASES AND DURATION OF DISEASE AND MODE OF TERMINATION IN RECOVERED CASES

FIRST ATTACK	RECURRENCE	NUMBER OF CASES
	All Cases	
Pulmonary lesion		
Lobar	Lobar	41 (72%)
Lobar	Atypical	12
Atypical	Lobar	2
Atypical	Atypical	2
	Recovered Cases	
Duration of acute disease		
Same (±1 day) in both attacks		23 (45%)
Recurrence 2 or more days longer		11
Recurrence 2 or more days shorter		17
FIRST ATTACK	RECURRENCE	NUMBER OF CASES
Mode of termination		
Crisis	Crisis	25 } (69%)
Lysis	Lysis	12 }
Crisis	Lysis	8
Lysis	Crisis	7
Crisis	Empyema	1
Empyema	Lysis	1

initial lesion was in the left lung. He remarked that the same lung is apt to be infected repeatedly though not necessarily in the same part. In Finland and Winkler's (470) series, however, no consistent relation obtained between the site of the initial involvement and that of the reinfection.

In 1921 Thomas (1296) reported that there was no evidence of the persistence of passive immunity in serum treated cases beyond about four weeks. He also suggested that the action of specific serum in aborting pneumonia may lessen the antigenic value of the attack. Finland and Winkler's (470) findings are in accordance with these observations and in a serum treated Type II case the homologous type antibodies disappeared from the blood within two weeks. And further, in a Type I case with spontaneous recovery, a high titer of antibody for this type persisted in the blood for several months.

Although specific serum therapy in the first attack had little obvious effect on the character of the recurrence, early recurrence with the same type was more frequent among serum treated cases.

The explanation of the apparent tendency for pneumonia to occur more often in patients once having had it than in patients who never had it (1403) is unknown. Various current theories used to explain this situation were summarized by Finland and Winkler (470). Maynard (874) remarks that either a first attack predisposes to a second, or second attacks occur in persons peculiarly susceptible to pneumonia. The duration of the demonstrable immunity acquired as a consequence of the infection in cases with spontaneous recovery appears rather short and probably does not exceed six to twelve months in the usual instance (see pages 737–739). It is possible some second attacks occur in patients of unusual general susceptibility (331, 470). Finland and Winkler (470) conclude that no marked change in the local or type-specific susceptibility occurs after one or more attacks.

The available evidence relating to this question obtained by the production of repeated attacks of pneumonia in monkeys is inconclusive (Cecil and Blake, 232). That relating to dogs, however, may be more definite, as Coggeshall and Robertson (286) have so ably demonstrated. In 25 dogs, 78 attacks of pneumonia were produced at intervals of three days to nineteen months. As the intervals between the induced attacks were usually only a matter of a few weeks or months, it is possible that it is invalid to make a direct comparison of the results obtained with the usual findings in man. Humoral antibody appeared only with great irregularity in the dog and seemed unrelated to the course of the illness. By and large, recurrent attacks in this animal were milder than primary attacks, and when the same lobe was involved in the recurrence, the lesions tended to evolve more rapidly in the early stages of the infection. This was accompanied by the early appearance of the macrophage reaction, which was regarded as possible evidence that the animal possessed an increased resistance (see pages 181–182). In addition, one of the most striking features observed was a difference in the occurrence of bacteriemia in the first and succeeding attacks, for while it was frequent in the former it was rare and only of slight extent in the latter instances. This may be of significance and similar in import to the findings of Finland and Winkler (470) in man, as described above, although the number of observations in either group is too small to be certain.

In discussing the role of allergy to the pneumococcus in affecting the occurrence of lobar pneumonia, Reimann (1066) ventures the suggestion that possibly recurrences are found in patients who are in a continual hypersensitive state or are unusually hypersensitive to this organism (see also pages 240–245).

The case fatality rates among two groups of African Negroes studied by Maynard (874) were 32 and 39 per cent in natives having first attacks of pneumonia, as contrasted with fatality rates of 22 and 33 per cent for second attacks. Although these figures suggest the presence of a lower rate in cases with recurrences, Maynard realized that for the second attacks the numbers of cases (60 and 80) were too small to yield significant conclusions. Findings similar to these were reported by Warr and Alperin (1385). In their series the fatality rate of 1,704 patients in an initial attack was 28.3 per cent, as compared with a rate of 22.6 per cent for 335 patients with a history of one or more previous attacks. Possibly Finland and Winkler's (470) cases reveal a similar situation, for the fatality rate in their group of 57 cases with recurrence was lower than that usually found in the general run of cases in the same hospital and was 19.0 per cent (11 deaths). They also remark that the 57 cases suffered a total of 122 attacks. The fatality rate in 26 attacks among patients receiving specific serum therapy was zero and in 96 others not given such treatment it was but 11.5 per cent. Findings such as these suggest that the case fatality rate in succeeding attacks may be lower than in first attacks.

On the other hand, Cohn and Lewis (288) consider that the number of previous attacks a patient has undergone does not influence the prognosis. Indeed, Shattuck and Lawrence (1176) report that the fatality rate may even be higher in succeeding than in first attacks. Of 42 of their patients with a history of preceding pneumonia 33 per cent died. This was a higher fatality rate than that of their whole series of 4,000 cases, of whom 25 per cent died.

It may be said in summary that the evidence at hand suggests that the attack rate of pneumonia is higher in patients who have once had the disease than in individuals who have not. The type incidence, location of the lesion, mode of termination by either crisis or lysis, and duration of the infection appear little influenced by the occurrence of the previous attacks. Although the infecting organism from one attack may persist in the respiratory tract and perhaps give rise to a second attack later, it seems highly unlikely that this is the usual course of events. The incidence of bacteriemia and the case fatality rate may be lower in recurrences than in initial attacks, due to the acquisition of some immunity, probably of a cellular nature. Thus an immunologic paradox is arrived at in which persons with some sort of increased resistance appear more likely to get pneumonia than do others. Possibly this situation may be correlated with the observation made earlier that the possession of some immunity favors the development of lobar pneumonia (see pages 256–257). There are, however, difficulties in the ready acceptance of such a conclusion at this time.

RESOLUTION AND DELAYED RESOLUTION

Resolution

As already indicated, evidence of the beginning of resolution may occasionally be detected at the time of crisis. Resolution, however, does not appear directly related to the occurrence of crisis, as Cole (297) and Graeser, Wu, and Robertson (552) have noted. It may precede, occur with, or, as is more common, follow crisis. The bulk of the exudate is slowly and rather irregularly absorbed, as described in the chapter on the Pathology of Lobar Pneumonia (see page 97). The physical signs of consolidation gradually diminish. Alteration of the voice or breath sounds is more likely to persist during resolution than is dulness, and not infrequently increased whisper is the last sign to disappear (552). In children the lung clears rapidly, while the process is slower in robust adults (297) and may be still slower in aged patients (341). In most instances resolution appears complete within a week or two. On roentgen-ray examination the shadow of the involved area gradually becomes less dense and uniform and takes on a mottled appearance. Usually it is a matter of a few weeks to a month or more before essentially every trace of the lesion disappears from roentgenograms.

By roentgenographic observations in 40 patients with pneumococcus lobar pneumonia of known type, Graeser and his associates (552) found the rate of resolution to be irregular and that the process may extend over a period of three or four to more than seventy days. Although no uniformity in the rate was noted, the process was often complete within fourteen to twenty-one days. Slight accentuation of the bronchovascular markings, however, usually persisted in the involved areas. A similar type of study was made by Davies, Hodgson, and Whitby (341) of 119 cases of typed pneumococcus lobar pneumonia. On the average, resolution was complete in all cases by the twentieth day. Type I cases required from ten to fifty days, or twenty days on the average, to complete resolution and no traces of the lesions remained. In Type II infections, however, some evidence of the attack persisted, as shown by a slight increase in the density and extent of the pulmonary striae. In Group IV cases an average of thirty days was required for restitution of the lung to normal.

Davies and his collaborators (341) report that consolidations which form rapidly often resolve rapidly. Cole (297) considered that the areas first involved were the last to clear. Graeser and his co-workers (552) investigated the matter and found that this sequence occurred in some cases, but that usually resolution appeared first in the older lesion. At times the process might occur simultaneously throughout the involved areas. In addition, it was noted that resolution may occur in one area while the disease is spreading to involve new portions of the lung in another. However, these workers, as well as Davies, Hodgson, and Whitby (341), are unanimous in their conclusion that generally densities about the hilum are the slowest to subside. The latter investigators also pointed out that at the time resolution begins, and not before, a globular swelling of the hilar glands takes place on both the affected and the normal sides. Enlarged hilar glands were commonly found associated with rapid resolution, but the presence of calcified glands was often a portent of a delay of the process.

Graeser, Wu, and Robertson (552) observed roentgenograms in resolution which perfectly simulated single or multiple lung abscesses or widespread tuberculosis. Repeated films were necessary to rule out these conditions. The occurrence late in the acute illness or in the early part of convalescence of a pulmonary lesion, designated by Kessel (712) and Gleich (518) as an aputrid pulmonary necrosis, is mentioned in the chapter on Complications (page 606). The condition is described as a symptom-free abscess of the lung, not in communication with a bronchus and so not exposed to mixed infection, which heals rapidly. During life the differential diagnosis of such a complication from the normal alterations in the appearance of the lung occurring in resolution must be difficult.

That subtle changes may persist in the lung for some time after resolution appears complete is suggested by the interesting finding of Graeser (550). He was able to demonstrate the presence of specific capsular polysaccharide in the lungs of dogs following experimental pneumococcus pneumonia as long as two months after the inflammatory exudate had disappeared. Control observations on the lungs of normal dogs were negative.

Hickling (639) finds a monocytosis present at the time of resolution and considers the monocyte intimately related to resolution. Reznikoff (1074) also notes the usual occurrence of a monocytosis at about the time of beginning resolution in pneumonia. In addition, however, he observed its presence at the time of recovery from some other infectious diseases as well. As elsewhere described, any relation the monocyte may have to resolution is not clear (see pages 98–100).

The factors responsible for recovery in pneumonia are chiefly those of an immunologic nature. The process of resolution, however, seems largely of a chemical nature and occasionally after recovery resolution may be delayed for days or weeks (see below) or at times may never occur (see page 543). Davies, Hodgson, and Whitby (339, 340) demonstrated the appearance of agglutinins in the blood of Type I, II, and III cases during recovery and consider the presence of these antibodies an indication of the occurrence of resolution. This is highly unlikely.

Large mononuclear cells of various descriptions are commonly found in resolving areas. Some of these may come from the blood. In addition, the cells of the alveolar walls enlarge and are extruded into the exudate, where they function as phagocytes and become the predominant cells of the thinning exudate in late resolution. This process was described by Robertson and his associates (1083, 286, 1095), who termed it the "macrophage reaction," as already seen (see pages 99–101). It may represent a type of immune response on the part of the pulmonary tissue cells (1087, 1095).

Delayed Resolution

Clinically, resolution is practically complete in the usual case within about two weeks after crisis or lysis, though some reduction in vital capacity may be demonstrable for one or two weeks longer and remnants of the lesion may be seen in roentgenograms for an even longer period, as mentioned above. Uncommonly, however, the gross process of the liquefaction, absorption, and removal of the exudate may be delayed. The leucocyte count may remain elevated for some weeks under these circumstances (918). Local physical signs of a variable amount of consolidation may persist and some general manifestations such as fever, increased pulse and respiration, cough, weakness, or other symptoms may be present (833). Roentgen-ray examination is essential in diagnosis, which may be difficult, and conditions such as empyema, tuberculosis, relapse, organizing pneumonia ending in fibrosis, or lung abscess must be excluded. Except for the prolongation of the illness, delayed resolution alone is usually not serious.

Delayed resolution was present in 4.1 per cent or 105 of 2,548 cases collected by Musser and Norris (918), and McCrae (833) found it in 3.7 per cent or 30 of 805 cases studied at the Johns Hopkins Hospital. Similar observations were reported by Chatard (254). A study of the possible factors influencing the occurrence of delayed resolution was made by McCrae (833). He determined in a series of 30 cases that there was considerable yearly variation in the incidence of the condition, a variation parallel to that for the occurrence of pericarditis in the total series of 805 cases of lobar pneumonia investigated. Age did not appear to influence the occurrence of delayed resolution. Cunningham's (333) finding of this condition in 4.1 per cent of 1,500 cases in infants and children also suggests that youth may be of little consequence in influencing its occurrence. Factors such as sex or alcoholism seemed to have little, if any, effect on the incidence in McCrae's (833) series, and delayed resolution was no more common after upper lobe lesions than after infections in other lobes. Race, however, appeared of importance, and the incidence was much higher among Negroes than among white patients. McSwan's (853) observations on natives in the Malay Peninsula were possibly of similar significance, for he observed that in such individuals resolution was often protracted for a month or more, following which the consolidation would suddenly resolve over a period of three or four days. Davies, Hodgson, and Whitby (341) pointed out that in general consolidations which form slowly frequently end in delayed resolution.

In McCrae's series resolution was delayed at times for as long as fifty days. He remarks that predictions cannot be made as to the absolute restoration of the lung to normal, for permanent changes may occur and appear rapidly (see below).

The cause of delayed resolution is not clear, but it probably results from an upset of the ferment–anti-ferment balance within the consolidated lesion, as already mentioned (see page 100).

TERMINATION IN FIBROSIS

In rare instances, resolution fails to occur and the remaining exudate becomes organized, as was earlier described (see page 101). Chatard (254) found 4 cases (0.6 per cent) of unresolved pneumonia among 658 cases of lobar pneumonia. According to Lord (807) Fränkel investigated 1,000 cases of croupous pneumonia at necropsy and found an organizing or indurative pneumonia in only 7. In Lord's (807) series of 210 cases of lobar pneumonia at necropsy at the Massachusetts General Hospital, 16 or 7.6 per cent had a similar lesion. He observes that a delay of resolution beyond three weeks may, in general, be regarded as evidence of developing pulmonary induration and that the condition is commoner after bronchopneumonia.

Hart (599) concluded from a roentgenographic study of the post-pneumonic lung that along with the fibrosis of an organizing pneumonia a chronic non-tubercular infection or suppuration of the lung with the formation of an abscess cavity may develop. Bronchial dilatation, bronchiectasis, and bronchiectatic abscesses may appear. Areas of massive fibrosis resulting from the healing of abscesses or a diffuse fibrosis throughout the involved area may occur. Consolidations which form slowly may at times terminate in fibrosis (341). Anthracosis may be a factor in influencing the occurrence of organizing lesions (607; see also page 101).

DEATH

The day of illness on which death took place was studied by Sears and Larrabee (1168) in 283 patients dying of "pneumonia." Death occurred before the fourteenth day in 78 per cent, before the eleventh day in 64 per cent, and before the seventh day in 22 per cent. In Musser and Norris' (918) series of 2,613 collected deaths from lobar pneumonia, the sixth to the eighth day was the commonest time of exitus. The bulk of the deaths in Menetrier's (882) group of 400 lobar pneumonias and bronchopneumonias investigated at necropsy occurred between the third and the tenth day. Cohn and Lewis (288) analyzed a series of 1,456 cases of lobar pneumonia at the Hospital of the Rockefeller Institute for Medical Research. Most of the cases were due to pneumococci of known type and most of the Type I cases and a few of the Type II cases received specific serum therapy. The average duration of the illness of the 287 patients who died, excluding 11 in which the disease lasted more than twenty days, was 7.88 days. Death may occur as early as the second or be delayed until the twentieth (288) to thirty-eighth day (882). Death rates in pneumonia are considered in the chapter on Epidemiology (page 258) and case fatality rates chiefly in the chapters on Prognosis (page 655), and Results of Serum Treatment (page 880).

As death approaches, the temperature seldom falls and usually rises. It may, however, drop to normal or subnormal (807). The degree of the toxemia present is generally independent of the height of the temperature and the extent of the lung involvement (807). The heart beats faster and weaker, the pulse becoming very rapid and often almost imperceptible before respiration ceases. In some cases the pulse and heart beat remain good almost up to the minute of death (297). Respirations become more superficial and ineffectual. Cough disappears, sputum is retained, the extremities become cold, and cyanosis is replaced by an ashen pallor. Death usually comes insidiously (918). Thrombosis of the heart or lung may cause death abruptly, but the terminal stages generally occupy several hours.

Extensive bacteriemia or septicaemia is commonly present in fatal cases (223, 153, 187; see also page 561) and in such instances pulmonary edema is not infrequent (187). Death may occur, however, in the absence of bacteriemia, and in three instances with necropsy studied by Sutton and Sevier (1277) massive lung lesions, but no septic complications, were present in two. The cause of death in the third patient, in which the only discoverable lesion was an involvement confined to two lobes, was attributed to "toxemia." Robertson, Graeser, Coggeshall, and Sia (1088) have considered the matter of death in pneumonia with small lesions and no complications in the absence of an infected blood stream. They point out that little pertinent information is available but report some unpublished observations of Sutliff and of Finland relating to the occurrence of death in Type I and Type II cases not receiving specific serum treatment. Sutliff had 19 patients with Type I pneumonia who died with only a single lobe involved. Six showed sterile blood cultures during life and 3 died without complications. Finland had 24 fatal Type II cases in which the pneumonic process was confined to one lobe, and 5 died without detectable bacteriemia. No information as to the presence of complications was given in Finland's data. The occurrence of death with small localized lesions and sterile blood cultures following serum treatment is uncommon (see also pages 918–920).

Signs of cardiac failure are frequently prominent at the time of death. Cohn and Lewis (288) observe that the proximity of death does not determine the onset of auricular fibrillation, for in their cases having this condition it ceased in 10 of 18 patients before death occurred.

Among 200 consecutive necropsies on patients dying of lobar pneumonia or bronchopneumonia, Brooks (153) states that definite evidence of a preexisting cardiac disorder was present in 116, and that in 77 instances death was apparently due to cardiac failure. Possibly the findings in this series of cases cannot be regarded as typical. In any event, the bulk of the evidence available indicates that the signs of cardiac failure seen shortly before death in pneumonia are largely secondary effects resulting from vasomotor paralysis (223). Perry (1015) has found evidence of such paralysis in the peripheral vessels in pneumonia, a condition which was most marked at the time of crisis or death. Warfield (1384) considers that the toxicity resulting from the infection increases vascular permeability and leads to vascular stasis, a decrease in blood volume, and a decrease in the amount of blood returned to the heart. To compensate for these changes, the heart decreases in size and increases its rate of contractions. A progressive increase in the heart rate leads to anoxemia of the cardiac muscle, which is augmented by the anoxemia usually present in severe cases. This results in dilatation of the heart which occurs shortly before death. The finding of dilatation of the heart at necropsy has already been mentioned (see page 112).

The vasomotor paralysis, as earlier noted, leads to circulatory failure, which is fundamentally a failure of the circulation at the periphery (see page 496). The condition which results is similar to that seen in shock. In discussing the relation of the heart to pneumonia, White (1418) states, "Although at postmortem examination the heart muscle cells may show some changes like cloudy swelling, such a finding does not mean heart disease." He further observes that "the weakness and collapse due to pneumonia are not the result of cardiac failure, but are the result of the infection."

Newburgh, Means, and Porter (949, 948) studied the cause of death in dogs and cats with experimentally induced pneumonia. Their investigations showed that death is due to failure of the respiratory center and not to cardiac deficiencies. Cole (297), Lord (807), and Locke (796) have expressed similar views regarding the cause of death in patients dying of pneumonia.

CONVALESCENCE

Following defervescence, many patients exhibit a subnormal temperature for several days, while others may have a slight evening rise in the temperature for the first few days. In the absence of complications the pulse and respiration are usually within normal limits. The mind becomes clearer, the patient begins to take an interest in his surroundings, and his appetite and strength gradually return.

Individuals vary greatly but, in general, it may be said that should the patient's strength permit, he may be allowed to sit up in bed about a week after the termination of the disease. The lungs are usually clear within approximately two weeks and if the general condition of the patient is good he may gradually be permitted to get up. In any instance, where the progress of convalescence is not satisfactory or resolution is delayed, roentgenograms of the chest may be taken at intervals for follow-up purposes (599). Patients should not be allowed to return to their former occupations for at least six weeks after defervescence, and preferably eight weeks or longer should be allowed for convalescence.

Sudden death may occur in patients who appear to be convalescing in the usual manner. Lord (807) describes two instances of this nature which occurred on the second and the eighth day after recovery. Pulmonary thrombosis was present in one patient at necropsy and pulmonary embolism in the other. In some patients cerebral symptoms may occur after crisis and persist during and after convalescence as a toxic psychosis in which the outlook is usually favorable (976, 807).

Perry (1015) has produced evidence indicating that the decreased tonicity of the peripheral blood vessels, which is most obvious immediately before crisis or death, requires three or four weeks or more to disappear in convalescence. Other evidence that abnormalities of the cardiovascular system may occur in the recovery period was obtained by DeGraff, Travell, and Yager (349) in studying serial electrocardiograms in 562 patients with lobar pneumonia treated without digitalis. Exceedingly slow heart rates due to sinus bradycardia were not uncommon after the temperature reached normal. In convalescence, heart rates of less than 60 per minute were found in approximately one-third (32 per cent) of the patients in this series who recovered. In the total group of 562 cases, nearly 10 per cent had prolongation of the auriculo-ventricular conduction time or dropped beats. Of these, 22 per cent showed some evidence of block first appearing during the course of the disease but in 78 per cent, prolongation of the P-R intervals first became demonstrable in convalescence. More than one-half of the patients developed an increased P-R interval during the first three days of convalescence and in about one-half of these the conduction time returned to normal in the interval while the patients were still under observation. In many instances abnormalities of rhythm or disturbances of conduction, and less often inversions of the T wave other than in Lead 3, first became demonstrable in the post-febrile period.

PERSISTENCE OF CARRIER STATE

Persons convalescent from pneumococcus pneumonia carry the infecting organism in their nose or throat for periods of several days to many months. Various factors, including the type of pneumococcus concerned, appear to influence the duration of the carrier state. Observations relating to convalescent carriers and the duration of the carrier period are discussed in the chapter on Epidemiology (see pages 366 and 369).

CHAPTER TWELVE

COMPLICATIONS: INCIDENCE AND TREATMENT

Complications Primarily of Bacterial Origin 548
Bacteriemia 549
Pneumococcus Lobar Pneumonia and Pneumococcus Pneumonia: Type I cases; Type II cases; Type III cases; Group IV cases; Type I, II, III, and Group IV cases: comparison; Type V cases; Type VII cases; Type VIII cases; Type XIV cases ... 551
Pneumococcus Pneumonia: Type I–XXXII cases 555
Factors Influencing Incidence 555
Relation to Certain Complications 560
Septicaemia 561
Treatment 562
Summary 563
Pleurisy with Effusion 564
Empyema 566
Otitis Media and Mastoiditis 585
Pericarditis 586
Endocarditis 589
Meningitis 592
Arthritis 598
Parotitis 600
Peritonitis 601
Abscesses, Cellulitis, Mediastinitis, and Furunculosis 603
Lung Abscess and Gangrene 604
Croupous Gastritis, Colitis, and Similar Conditions 607
Rhinitis, Tonsillitis, and Laryngitis 607
Conjunctivitis 607
Miscellaneous Complications 608

COMPLICATIONS PRIMARILY OF BACTERIAL ORIGIN

It is remarkable in pneumococcus pneumonia that septic complications are not more frequent for pneumococci can be isolated from the circulating blood of a considerable proportion of all patients. In most cases the organisms are swept from the circulation by an efficient mechanism for clearing the blood (see pages 162–164), and the general immunity of man to the pneumococcus must be considerable in the usual instance to prevent the development of septic complications. Such conditions are likely to develop, however, in places where the organism can spread directly from the lung or in such places as are especially susceptible to some form of pyogenic infection. The closed body cavities, lined with epithelial tissues such as the pleura, pericardium, meninges, and peritoneum, are particularly liable to these secondary focal infections (297). The ability of the pneumococcus to penetrate epithelial tissues with considerable ease was commented on earlier (see page 232).

Various factors appear to influence the occurrence of complications in pneumonia. The patient's immunity and general physical condition are important, and also the nature of the infecting organism and matters such as age, year, season, and frequently the presence or absence of bacteriemia.

In pneumococcus cases febrile complications appear especially likely to develop with Type V infections, those that develop with Type I infections being next in frequency, according to Sutliff and Finland (1271, 1272). Including empyema, as mentioned later, febrile complications occurred in 28 per cent of the Type V cases and in 18.1 per cent of the Type I cases in their series. It seems probable from the additional evidence cited below that Type II infections are particularly likely to give rise to bacteriemia, endocarditis, or meningitis. It is possible that in many such reported instances the infecting pneumococcus was a Type V rather than a Type II as stated, for until recently the differentiation between Type II and related strains of this organism, such as Type V, was not always practicable.

In general, the occurrence of complications lessens the chances of recovery (see pages 695–696).

Bacteriemia

Although as a complication bacteriemia is not usually thought of in the same sense as some of the other septic conditions which may follow pneumonia, such as empyema, yet the evidence suggests that in many respects the factors which govern the development of bacteriemia may also be prominent in influencing the occurrence of many of these related conditions as well.

The term "bacteriemia" as used here indicates merely the presence of bacteria in the blood stream. The results of studies in animals reveal that their experimental inoculation by various routes with living pneumococci is accompanied by the appearance of these organisms in the blood within a few minutes to hours in a large percentage of all instances, as previously mentioned (see pages 204–231).

In man with lobar pneumonia, positive blood cultures have been obtained in a varying proportion of cases. Prochaska in 1910, as cited by Lord (807), demonstrated pneumococci in the blood of 100 per cent of 50 cases. Rosenow

(1114) in 1905 found bacteriemia present in 91 per cent of 175 cases, and in 1915 Mathers (872) reported its occurrence in 75.7 per cent of 128 cases. These incidence figures are much higher than those obtained in recent years using ordinary culture methods. The explanation of the high proportion of bacteriemic cases in the series cited is not clear, although it may lie in the fact that in the cases studied blood cultures were repeated at frequent intervals. Avery, Chickering, Cole, and Dochez (33) found that bacteriemia could be demonstrated in 30.3 per cent of 448 cases cultured once or twice, while

TABLE 91. PNEUMOCOCCUS LOBAR PNEUMONIA. NUMBER OF CASES AND NUMBER AND PERCENTAGE WITH POSITIVE BLOOD CULTURES

REPORTED BY	NUMBER OF CASES CULTURED	CASES WITH POSITIVE CULTURES *Number*	*Per cent*
Alexander, 1917 (9)	93	21	22.6
Cole, 1920 (297)	728	202	27.8
Bloomfield, 1923 (136)	198	69	35.0
Cecil, Baldwin, and Larsen, 1926 (230)	326	89	27.3
Kessel and Hyman, 1927 (713)	56	15	26.8
Bullowa, Rosenblüth, Park, and Cooper, 1928 (195)	500	112	22.2
Koch, 1932 (733)	130	42	32.4
Sutliff, 1932 (1267)	280	62	22.1
Wu and Chiu, 1933 (1450)	218	47	21.6
Cruickshank, 1933 (331)	329	84	25.5
Total	2,858	743	26.0

in 37 in which blood cultures were made at frequent intervals the cultures were positive in 50 per cent of the cases.

Employing the customary blood culture technic, using 5 to 10 cc. of blood in broth and occasionally 1 cc. for each of one or more agar pour plates, bacteriemia was demonstrated in from 15 (1357) to 32 (1385) per cent of the cases in several series of lobar pneumonias in which the causative organism of the pneumonia was largely or wholly unknown. Cultures were made by Vitug and Hizon (1357) in 423 such cases, by MacCordick (830) in 187 cases, by Warr and Alperin (1385) in 281 cases, and by Hamilton (592) in 37 cases. Together these workers examined the blood of 928 cases and found bacteriemia in 198, or 21.3 per cent.

Of greater interest, however, are the findings of numerous other investigators who determined the incidence of bacteriemia in cases due to pneumococci of known type.

PNEUMOCOCCUS LOBAR PNEUMONIA AND PNEUMOCOCCUS PNEUMONIA. In pneumococcus lobar pneumonia in general, bacteriemia has been found in from 21.1 to 35 per cent of the 2,858 cases, listed in Table 91. All or almost all of these cases were in adults. Of the total series bacteriemia was present in 743, or 26 per cent. The occurrence of bacteriemia in children is discussed later (page 557).

TABLE 92. TYPE I LOBAR PNEUMONIA. NUMBER OF CASES AND NUMBER AND PERCENTAGE WITH POSITIVE BLOOD CULTURES

REPORTED BY	NUMBER OF CASES CULTURED	CASES WITH POSITIVE CULTURES	
		Number	*Per cent*
Bullowa, Rosenblüth, Park, and Cooper, 1928 (195)	149	50	35.0
Cole, 1929 (299)	431	138	32.0
Cecil and Plummer, 1930 (238)	470	90	19.2
Blake, 1931 (120)	194	71	36.6
Sutliff, 1932 (1267)	51	22	43.0
Wu and Chiu, 1933 (1450)	91	20	22.0
Cruickshank, 1933 (331)	114	37	32.4
Massachusetts Pneumonia Series, 1937 (869)	532	139	26.1
Total	2,032	567	28.0

In adults with pneumococcus pneumonia (lobar pneumonia and bronchopneumonia together) the incidence of bacteriemia appears much the same as the above figure. It was present in 24.8 per cent of 1,719 cases studied by Bullowa and Wilcox (198) and in 33.4 per cent of 296 cases examined by Kohl and Reitzel (734). Combining these two series, bacteriemia was found in 26.1 per cent, or 526 of 2,015 cases investigated.

Type I cases. A number of studies have been made to determine the incidence of bacteriemia in cases of pneumococcus Type I lobar pneumonia. The results shown in Table 92 indicate that bacteriemia may be present in from 19.2 to as many as 43 per cent of such cases. In the combined total of 2,032 Type I cases, bacteriemia was found in 567, or 28 per cent.

In Type I pneumococcus pneumonia (lobar pneumonia and bronchopneumonia together) bacteriemia occurred in 27.4 per cent of 468 cases (see Table 97, page 556) reported by Bullowa and Wilcox (198) and in 48.7 per cent of 119 cases studied by Kohl and Reitzel (734). The latter figure is unusually high for Type I infections. Nearly all the Type I cases were in adults.

Type II cases. The available reports indicating the incidence of bacteriemia in patients with Type II lobar pneumonia are summarized in Table 93. The reported incidence has varied from 15 to 46.4 per cent. In the total group of 732 cases, bacteriemia was demonstrated in 320, or 43.7 per cent.

TABLE 93. TYPE II LOBAR PNEUMONIA. NUMBER OF CASES AND NUMBER AND PERCENTAGE WITH POSITIVE BLOOD CULTURES

REPORTED BY	NUMBER OF CASES CULTURED	CASES WITH POSITIVE CULTURES *Number*	*Per cent*
Bullowa, Rosenblüth, Park, and Cooper, 1928 (195)	95	30	31.0
Blake, 1931 (120)	79	32	40.5
Cecil and Plummer, 1932 (239)	202	164	46.4
Wu and Chiu, 1933 (1450)	40	6	15.0
Cruickshank, 1933 (331)	136	34	25.0
Massachusetts Pneumonia Series, 1937 (869)	180	54	30.0
Total	732	320	43.7

The occurrence of bacteriemia in cases of pneumococcus Type II pneumonia (lobar pneumonia and bronchopneumonia together) was studied by Bullowa and Wilcox (198) and by Kohl and Reitzel (734). The former workers found it in 38.7 per cent of 194 cases (see Table 97, page 556) and the latter in 31.3 per cent of 32 cases. Practically all cases were in adults.

Type III cases. Investigation of cases of Type III lobar pneumonia reveals the occurrence of bacteriemia in from 18.1 to 25 per cent in the larger series. The tabulated findings in several series are shown in Table 94. Among a group of 255 collected cases bacteriemia was demonstrated in 56, or 22 per cent.

In cases of Type III pneumococcus pneumonia in general (lobar pneumonia and bronchopneumonia together) the incidence of bacteriemia seems somewhat higher. It was demonstrated by Finland and Sutliff (464) in 35

TABLE 94. TYPE III LOBAR PNEUMONIA. NUMBER OF CASES AND NUMBER AND PERCENTAGE WITH POSITIVE BLOOD CULTURES

REPORTED BY	NUMBER OF CASES CULTURED	CASES WITH POSITIVE CULTURES	
		Number	*Per cent*
Cecil, Baldwin, and Larsen, 1926 (230) ...	36	10	27.7
Bullowa, Rosenblüth, Park, and Cooper, 1928 (195)	66	17	25.0
Blake, 1931 (120)	116	21	18.1
Wu and Chiu, 1933 (1450)	14	1	7.1
Cruickshank, 1933 (331)	8	4	50.0
Massachusetts Pneumonia Study, 1935 (869)	15	3	20.0
Total	255	56	22.0

TABLE 95. GROUP IV LOBAR PNEUMONIA. NUMBER OF CASES AND NUMBER AND PERCENTAGE WITH POSITIVE BLOOD CULTURES

Cecil, Baldwin, and Larsen, 1926 (230) ...	90	15	16.6
Bullowa, Rosenblüth, Park, and Cooper, 1928 (195)	190	15	7.8
Wu and Chiu, 1933 (1450)	73	20	27.4
Cruickshank, 1933 (331)	71	9	12.6
Massachusetts Pneumonia Study, 1935 (869)	73	9	12.3
Total	497	68	13.7

per cent of 131 cases, by Bullowa and Wilcox (198) in 29.7 per cent of 182 cases (see Table 97, page 556), and by Kohl and Reitzel (734) in 33.3 per cent of 27 cases. The higher incidence in these cases is presumably due to the greater frequency of the condition in the atypical forms of pneumonia. The cases in the above series were wholly or almost wholly in adults.

Group IV cases. Several series of cases of lobar pneumonia attributed to pneumococci of Group IV have been examined and the occurrence of positive blood cultures noted, as seen in Table 95. Bacteriemia was found in from 7.8 to 27.4 per cent of the cases in various series. In the total of 497 cases examined only 68, or 13.7 per cent, had positive blood cultures.

In 875 cases of pneumonia (lobar pneumonia and bronchopneumonia together) due to pneumococci of one or another of the types, Type IV through Type XXXII, Bullowa and Wilcox (198) found bacteriemia in 150, or 17.1

per cent (see Table 97, page 556). As in the above series cited, essentially all cases were in adults.

Type I, II, III, and Group IV cases: comparison. In Table 96 is shown a summary of the findings in Tables 92–95. It is seen that in a total of 3,516 cases of pneumococcus lobar pneumonia bacteriemia occurred in 1,011, or 28.8 per cent (see also Table 91, page 550). Among cases due to pneumococci of Type I, II, or III, bacteriemia was found least often in Type III cases (22 per cent), somewhat more frequently in Type I cases (28 per cent), and most frequently in Type II cases (43.7 per cent). In cases attributed to pneumococci of Group IV, bacteriemia was found less frequently (13.7 per cent)

TABLE 96. PNEUMOCOCCUS LOBAR PNEUMONIA. NUMBER OF CASES AND NUMBER AND PERCENTAGE WITH POSITIVE BLOOD CULTURES, BY TYPE

PNEUMOCOCCUS	NUMBER OF CASES CULTURED	CASES WITH POSITIVE CULTURES Number	Per cent
Type I (from Table 92)	2,032	567	28.0
Type II (from Table 93)	732	320	43.7
Type III (from Table 94)	255	56	22.0
Group IV (from Table 95)	497	68	13.7
Total	3,516	1,011	28.8

than in those due to Type I, II, or III. The latter finding is probably of little importance in view of the observations below, as already mentioned, relating to the occurrence of bacteriemia in cases due to various of the individual higher types.

Type V cases. Of 17 cases of Type V lobar pneumonia included in the Massachusetts Pneumonia Series (869) 4, or 29.4 per cent, had positive blood cultures.

Among 147 patients with pneumococcus Type V pneumonia (lobar pneumonia and bronchopneumonia together) Bullowa and Wilcox (198) found bacteriemia in 42, or 28.6 per cent (see Table 97, page 556). Nearly all the Type V cases were in adults.

Type VII cases. The incidence of bacteriemia in cases of Type VII pneumococcus pneumonia (lobar pneumonia and bronchopneumonia together) was determined by Bullowa and Wilcox (198) and by Kohl and Reitzel (734). The former found this condition in 11 per cent, or 15 of 136 cases (see

Table 97), and the latter in 14.2 per cent, or 2 of 14 cases. In Type VII cases then, bacteriemia is rather infrequent. All or practically all of the Type VII cases studied in these series were in adults.

Type VIII cases. In cases of Type VIII pneumococcus pneumonia (lobar pneumonia and bronchopneumonia together) the incidence of bacteriemia was higher than in Type VII cases. Finland and Sutliff (464) recorded its presence in 31 per cent, or 21 of 68 cases examined, and Bullowa and Wilcox (198) observed it in 21 per cent, or 25 of 119 cases (see Table 97). Nearly all cases were in adults.

Type XIV cases. In adults with pneumococcus Type XIV pneumonia (lobar pneumonia and bronchopneumonia together) Bullowa (187) found bacteriemia in 30 per cent, or 13 of 43 patients (see also Table 97).

PNEUMOCOCCUS PNEUMONIA: TYPE I–XXXII CASES. Bullowa and Wilcox (198) have reported the incidence of bacteriemia in a series of 1,719 cases of pneumococcus pneumonia (lobar pneumonia and bronchopneumonia together) at the Harlem Hospital, New York City, collected over the years of 1928–1933, as shown in Table 97. All or nearly all of these cases were apparently in adults. Bacteriemia was present in 24.8 per cent, or 427 of the 1,719 cases due to pneumococci of one or another of all the thirty-two recognized types.

The incidence varied considerably in cases due to the various types. The proportion of Type I, II, III, V, VII, and VIII cases in this series that had bacteriemia has been stated in the preceding sections dealing with this matter by types. In Type XIV cases the incidence was 30.2 per cent.

Bacteriemia was demonstrated in 16.1 per cent, or 19 of 118 Type IV cases. The number of cases due to each of the remaining types is so small that though the figures are of interest, they are not of great significance. The absence of bacteriemia in cases attributed to Types XI, XVI, XXII, XXVII, XXVIII, XXX, XXXI, and XXXII should be noted.

FACTORS INFLUENCING INCIDENCE. It is obvious from the foregoing discussion that the incidence of bacteriemia may vary considerably depending upon the particular type of pneumococcus invading the host. Furthermore, as may be seen in Table 97, bacteriemia was not demonstrated in cases due to any one of eight types, possibly because the series of cases due to those types (Types XI, XVI, XXII, XXVII, XXVIII, XXX, XXXI, and XXXII) was so small and organisms of these types seldom invade the blood, or perhaps because pneumococci of the types in question were not actually the cause of

TABLE 97. PNEUMOCOCCUS PNEUMONIA (LOBAR PNEUMONIA AND BRONCHO-PNEUMONIA TOGETHER). NUMBER OF CASES AND NUMBER AND PERCENTAGE WITH POSITIVE BLOOD CULTURES, BY TYPE

PNEUMOCOCCUS TYPE	NUMBER OF CASES CULTURED	CASES WITH POSITIVE CULTURES *Number*	*Per cent*
I	468	128	27.4
II	194	75	38.7
III	182	54	29.7
IV*	118	19	16.1
V	147	42	28.6
VI	33	8	24.2
VII	136	15	11.0
VIII	119	25	21.0
IX	49	6	12.2
X	13	1	7.8
XI	14	–	–
XII	17	6	35.3
XIII	21	1	4.8
XIV	43	13	30.2
XV	7	2	28.6
XVI	9	–	–
XVII	11	1	9.2
XVIII	36	10	27.8
XIX	19	8	42.1
XX	21	4	19.0
XXI	7	2	28.6
XXII	11	–	–
XXIII	7	3	42.8
XXIV	8	1	12.5
XXV	8	2	25.0
XXVII	3	–	–
XXVIII	6	–	–
XXIX	10	1	10.0
XXX	2	–	–
XXXI	3	–	–
XXXII	3	–	–
Total*	1,719	427	24.8

From Bullowa and Wilcox (198)

* Pneumococci of the types IV through XXXII caused 875 of the cases and bacteriemia was demonstrated in 150, or 17.1 per cent of these cases.

the illness. Other than the type of pneumococcus, many additional factors, some of which are known, also appear to cause variations in the frequency with which bacteriemia is found.

Age seems of great importance in this respect. Infants and children generally have a lower incidence of bacteriemia than adults, as was found by Wollstein and Benson (1436) and later pointed out by Lyon (821) and others (1321, 1057, 710, 187). And, as will be seen below, young adults have a lower incidence of bacteriemia than do more elderly patients.

Among a combined total of 54 cases of lobar pneumonia in infants and children studied by Wollstein and Benson (1436) and by Lyon (821), bacteriemia was found in only 6, or 11.1 per cent. It was also present in 27.2 per cent, or 3 of 11 cases of bronchopneumonia in patients of similar age, reported by the latter investigator.

In cases of pneumococcus pneumonia of various forms in infants and children Raia, Plummer, and Shultz (1057) report the occurrence of bacteriemia in only 4.9 per cent, or 16 of 329 cases. In a series of similar cases studied by Kereszturi and Hauptmann (710) it was found in 6 per cent, or 4 of 65 cases. Combining these two series there is a total of 394 cases and bacteriemia was demonstrated in only 20, or 5.1 per cent. These observations suggest that the proportion of cases of pneumococcus pneumonia in children which show positive blood cultures is only about one-fifth the proportion of cases in adults with pneumococcus lobar pneumonia, as seen in Table 91 (page 550), or with pneumococcus pneumonia in general, as seen in Table 97.

Among adults as age advances, the outlook for successful recovery from pneumonia becomes progressively poorer (see pages 707–710). This is doubtless due to the occurrence of a generalized decrease in resistance to the pneumococcus with an increase in age. It might be expected then that older patients with a decreased immunity would show a higher incidence of bacteriemia. Evidence of this was sought at various times among the cases treated during the Massachusetts Pneumonia Study and Continuing Program (869). As early as 1934 the findings were suggestive of such a phenomenon but the number of cases on which the observations were based was considered too small to be significant. Subsequently, however, an additional number of cases became available for tabulation and the findings appear of greater value.

Table 98 lists by age group the Type I cases of lobar pneumonia from whom satisfactory blood cultures were obtained in the Massachusetts Pneumonia Series (869) from 1931 through June 30, 1937. These cases received varying amounts of specific immune serum during the course of their illness but the great majority of them had only one blood culture and this was made prior to or at the time of the first serum injection.

TABLE 98. TYPE I LOBAR PNEUMONIA. NUMBER OF CASES AND NUMBER AND PERCENTAGE WITH POSITIVE BLOOD CULTURES, BY DECADE OF LIFE

AGE GROUP	NUMBER OF CASES CULTURED	CASES WITH POSITIVE CULTURES	
		Number	*Per cent*
0–9	4	1	25.0
10–19	71	12	16.9
20–29	123	28	22.8
30–39	137	31	22.6
40–49	110	38	34.5
50–59	47	11	23.4
60–69	32	12	37.5
70 years and over	12	7	58.3
Total	536	140	26.1

Cases from the Massachusetts Pneumonia Series

Positive blood cultures were found in 26.1 per cent, or 140 of 536 cases cultured. Among individuals ten or more years of age the incidence of bacteriemia is seen to advance from 16.9 per cent in 71 cases ten through nineteen years of age to 58.3 per cent in 12 persons seventy years of age and over.

The available evidence suggests that the effect of age on the occurrence of bacteriemia is similar for each of the types. Some evidence of this nature is at hand relating to the occurrence of this condition in cases included in the Massachusetts Pneumonia Series, as shown in Table 99. Varying amounts of specific antiserum were used in the treatment of these cases but in most instances as above, only a single blood culture was made and this was done prior to or at the time of the initial injection of serum. In Type I cases the incidence of positive blood cultures was 24.7 per cent in patients ten through forty-nine years of age, in contrast to the 33 per cent incidence found in patients fifty years of age and over. In Type II cases the proportion with bacteriemia was 28.1 per cent in the younger group and 36.6 per cent in the older. The findings in Type V cases were similar in that 16.6 per cent of the younger and 40 per cent of the older patients experienced bacteriemia, but the total number of Type V cases cultured (17 cases) is too small to be more than of interest.

The occurrence of bacteriemia among cases of pneumococcus pneumonia due to any one of each of several of the more common types, such as Types I, II, III, IV, V, VI, VII, VIII, IX, XIV, and XVIII, was demonstrated by Bullowa and Wilcox (198) to vary from year to year. In Type I cases, for example, over a period of five consecutive years the incidence of bacteriemia varied from around 16 per cent in some years to more than 30 per cent in others.

TABLE 99. TYPE I, TYPE II, AND TYPE V LOBAR PNEUMONIA. NUMBER OF CASES AND NUMBER AND PERCENTAGE WITH POSITIVE BLOOD CULTURES, BY AGE GROUP

	10–49 years of age			*50 years of age and over*		
	NUMBER OF CASES CULTURED	CASES WITH POSITIVE CULTURES		NUMBER OF CASES CULTURED	CASES WITH POSITIVE CULTURES	
		Number	*Per cent*		*Number*	*Per cent*
Type I	441	109	24.7	91	30	33.0
Type II	139	39	28.1	41	15	36.6
Type V	12	2	16.6	5	2	40.0

Cases from the Massachusetts Pneumonia Series

As may be seen in the chapter on Prognosis (page 679), the case fatality rate in pneumonia appears to vary considerably with the season of the year and higher rates are present during the colder months. Other evidence also suggests that a seasonal variation of host resistance occurs both in animals and in man (see pages 201–203) and it seems not unreasonable in consequence to suggest that in the future when suitably analyzed series of cases are available, the incidence of bacteriemia may also be found to exhibit some seasonal variation.

Possibly the site of the pulmonary lesion may influence the occurrence of bacteriemia, though such a circumstance would be difficult to comprehend. In any event, Vitug and Hizon (1357) observed that in lobar pneumonia the incidence of bacteriemia was 11 per cent in patients with right sided involvements, 15.6 per cent in patients with left sided involvements, and 30.5 per cent when the lesions were bilateral. The occurrence of a higher incidence of bacteriemia in patients with bilateral as compared with unilateral lesions is, of course, probably to be expected.

Possibly also the duration of the illness may influence the frequency with which bacteriemia is found. In commenting on this matter Blake (120) stated that although invasion of the blood in Type I or Type II cases is usually heavy and occurs early in the disease, the invasion with Type III infections is usually slight and most often occurs late in the illness. Cruickshank (331) took blood cultures from a series of 330 patients with pneumococcus lobar pneumonia, and found bacteriemia in 33 per cent of cases having blood cultures on the first day of illness, in 28 per cent cultured on the second day, in 42 per cent cultured on the third day, in 22 per cent cultured on the fourth day, and in 15 per cent cultured on the fifth day.

In the presence of mixed infections bacteriemia is frequent and was found by Bullowa and Wilcox (198) in 47.1 per cent of a small group of pneumonias in this category.

In pneumococcus lobar pneumonia early hospitalization alone does not appear to influence the proportion of cases developing bacteriemia (195).

RELATION TO CERTAIN COMPLICATIONS. In pneumococcus lobar pneumonia certain septic complications appear more common in patients experiencing bacteriemia than in others whose blood cultures are sterile. Evidence of this is shown by the findings in some of the Type I cases in the Massachusetts Pneumonia Series (869), as seen in Table 100. Varying amounts of specific antiserum were administered to these patients. The proportion of cases having negative blood cultures that developed empyema was 7.4 per cent, as contrasted with an incidence of this complication of 18.8 per cent in patients with bacteriemia. Empyema was then more than twice as common in cases having bacteriemia. The situation was even more striking with respect to the occurrence of pericarditis or endocarditis in the two groups. These complications developed in only 0.3 per cent of cases with negative blood cultures, in comparison to their occurrence in 4 per cent of cases having bacteriemia.

The presence of bacteriemia is of great prognostic importance and the fatality rate of cases having this condition is several times that of others with negative blood cultures, as is mentioned elsewhere (see pages 681–693). Prognosis is poorest in cases with the heaviest blood invasion. Koch (733) determined that blood cultures from cases in the first three days of illness show decreasing bacterial counts and that after the third day the counts were usually the same or tended to increase. A few to 2,000 or more organisms per cubic centimeter may be found in the blood during life or at death (297, 807), and as many as 180,000 pneumococci per cubic centimeter have been found at the time of death (1277). Blake (120) studied 122 cases of Type III lobar pneumonia and found that bacteriemia was usually light in such cases, for only 9 cases showed more than 10 colonies per cubic centimeter of blood. Finland and Sutliff (464) found that colony counts of the blood in bacteriemic cases of Type III pneumococcus pneumonia usually show under 20 colonies per cubic centimeter. In a few cases, however, counts of over 1,000 colonies were present. In Type VIII cases most of the bacteriemic patients had counts of about 10 colonies, although a few had as many as 2,000 colonies per cubic centimeter.

TABLE 100. TYPE I LOBAR PNEUMONIA. NUMBER OF CASES AND NUMBER AND PERCENTAGE WITH OR WITHOUT BACTERIEMIA EXPERIENCING CERTAIN COMPLICATIONS

	With negative blood cultures			*With positive blood cultures*		
		CASES DEVELOPING COMPLICATION			CASES DEVELOPING COMPLICATION	
COMPLICATION	NUMBER OF CASES	*Number*	*Per cent*	NUMBER OF CASES	*Number*	*Per cent*
Empyema	340	25	7.4	112	21	18.8
Pericarditis or endocarditis	340	1	0.3	112	5	4.0

Cases from the Massachusetts Pneumonia Series

SEPTICAEMIA. The term "septicaemia" is frequently used to indicate the occurrence of active growth and multiplication of organisms in the blood stream. It is difficult if not impossible to obtain suitable data relating to such a situation in pneumococcus pneumonia, for ordinarily it is impossible to be sure, in a given case, that a condition of this nature prevails. It is well recognized, however, that in fatal cases blood cultures taken just before or at the time of death usually show a higher percentage of positive results than those taken early in the course of the disease (793, 61, 60, 195). This does not necessarily mean in every instance that the organisms are multiplying in the blood stream, but often that they are probably more or less constantly being poured into the blood from the infected lesion, and in conjunction with a failure of the vital mechanism for clearing the blood of organisms, their numbers increase. If the number entering the blood could be controlled, there is ample evidence that the blood would tend to sterilize itself as is usual following the adequate treatment of suitable cases with specific antiserum (see pages 885–886).

The findings of various investigators clearly indicate the high proportion of positive blood cultures obtained in fatal cases of pneumococcus lobar pneumonia. Cecil, Baldwin, and Larsen (230) report that bacteriemia was demonstrated in only 7.2 per cent, or 15 of 207 patients that recovered, while it was found in 62.1 per cent, or 74 of 119 fatal cases. The observations of Bullowa, Rosenblüth, Park, and Cooper (195), as seen in Table 101, are similar. Of 378 recovered patients from whom blood cultures were taken, the results were positive in only 45, or 11.9 per cent, while positive cultures were found in 54.9 per cent, or 67 of 122 fatal cases cultured. In general, then, positive cultures are about five to eight times more frequent in cases ending in death than in recovery.

TABLE 101. PNEUMOCOCCUS LOBAR PNEUMONIA. NUMBER OF CASES AND NUMBER AND PERCENTAGE OF POSITIVE BLOOD CULTURES IN PATIENTS RECOVERING OR DYING FROM PNEUMONIA, BY TYPE

	Recovered cases			*Fatal cases*		
	NUMBER OF CASES CULTURED	CASES WITH POSITIVE CULTURES *Number*	CASES WITH POSITIVE CULTURES *Per cent*	NUMBER OF CASES CULTURED	CASES WITH POSITIVE CULTURES *Number*	CASES WITH POSITIVE CULTURES *Per cent*
Type I	106	21	19.0	43	29	67.0
Type II	63	12	19.0	32	18	56.0
Type III	42	4	9.0	24	13	54.0
Group IV	167	8	4.0	23	7	30.0
Total	378	45	11.9	122	67	54.9

From Bullowa *et al.* (195)

Lord (807) reported the results of examining the blood of 152 cases of pneumococcus lobar pneumonia at necropsy, at the Massachusetts General Hospital. Positive blood cultures were obtained in 27 per cent (42 cases). Had similar cultures been taken at the time of death and before the delay incident to the postmortem examination, doubtless the proportion of cases with positive cultures would have been higher.

TREATMENT. As pointed out in Chapter IV (see pages 168, 174–177), the appearance in the blood of actively or passively acquired antibody specific for the type of pneumococcus responsible for the infection commonly brings about a sterilization of the blood stream and prevents the reappearance of bacteriemia. Uncommonly, however, bacteriemia may persist or develop in the blood of patients having considerable humoral antibody for the homologous type. Nevertheless, the adequate use of a potent therapeutic serum specific for the type causing the infection will, in cases due to any one of several of the types, ordinarily sterilize the blood stream, prevent the reappearance of bacteriemia, and bring about a marked reduction in the otherwise expected high case fatality rate, as is shown elsewhere (see pages 885–886 and 912–916). Such effects are especially prominent in well-treated Type I cases. While the results appear similar in significance in Type II cases, the findings thus far are less conclusive. Doubtless satisfactory results may be obtained with many of the types above Type III as well. With Type III, however, the results with horse antiserum therapy have been disappointing. The intradermal or subcutaneous injection of pneumococcus vaccine has been tried in such cases with little, if any, certain benefit (see pages 795–804). The use of drugs such as ethylhydrocupreine (optochin) might prove of aid in some cases, although the hazard of incurring a temporary or permanent impairment of vision makes the administration of this particular drug generally inadvisable. Sulfanilamide or one of its allied compounds may be of more value (see page 783).

SUMMARY. In pneumococcus lobar pneumonia in adults bacteriemia has been found in 28 per cent of Type I cases, in 43.7 per cent of Type II cases, in 22 per cent of Type III cases, and in 29.4 per cent of Type V cases, and among these types is thus commonest in Type II infections. In cases of this disease in adults attributed to pneumococci of Group IV (Types IV–XXXII together), bacteriemia is found in 13.7 per cent.

Much the same as these figures are those relating to the incidence of bacteriemia in cases of pneumococcus pneumonia (lobar pneumonia and bronchopneumonia together) due to these same types, as may be seen in Table 97 (page 556).

The highest percentage of positive blood cultures is found in cases ending fatally. The occurrence of bacteriemia is also influenced by factors such as the type of pneumococcus concerned, age, year, day of illness, and the presence of mixed infections. Possibly variations in incidence also occur in different seasons of the year and with pulmonary lesions located in various regions of the lungs. The presence of bacteriemia seems to influence the incidence of complications such as empyema and endocarditis and pericarditis.

Pleurisy with Effusion

Pleurisy occurs in nearly every case of lobar pneumonia. Chatard (254) reported its occurrence in more than 51 per cent of 658 cases and remarked that it was so common its presence was frequently not recorded. Blake and Cecil (123) observed the production of pleurisy in monkeys following an experimental pneumococcus Type I lobar pneumonia. At necropsy all of 40 animals showed gross or microscopic evidence of a fibrinous pleurisy with leucocytes present in the exudate. Lesions such as this lead to the accumulation of fluid in the pleural cavity. Observations of a similar nature were made in rabbits by Gaskell (508), who, by producing pulmonary lesions with pneumococci of differing virulence, was able to control the kind of lesion developed. With organisms of high virulence the infection was not confined to a lobe of the lung but spread directly to the pleural surface, causing an acute pleurisy which was usually bilateral.

As was mentioned earlier, in pneumonia in man the bacteria probably reach the pleura through the lymphatics of the lung (see page 248). The resultant exudate is usually fibrinous and, as Cole (297) remarks, in the majority of instances phagocytosis rapidly occurs, preventing the growth of organisms and severe injury to the pleura. In a few cases, however, bacterial growth does occur and a purulent exudate forms. Early in the disease the exudate is thin and contains few leucocytes. As the fluid increases in amount, the number of leucocytes rapidly increases, until it becomes thick and purulent. The kind of organism present, and certain other factors as well, appear to affect the occurrence of empyema to a considerable extent, as is mentioned below.

In practically every case of pneumonia there is some increased formation of fluid on the affected side, although the amount is small in most cases. The fluid is usually sterile and until pus is demonstrated cannot be termed an empyema. Scott and Finland (1166) have studied the various kinds of cells likely to be encountered in pleural effusions and have reviewed much of the literature dealing with this matter.

The condition of the pleura at necropsy following lobar pneumonia has been reported by several workers. Fabyan (399) studied 195 cases at postmortem in which the condition of the pleura was noted in 164, or 84.1 per cent. Fibrinous pleurisy was present in 155, or 94.6 per cent. The nature of the fluid present was noted in a number of the cases. The exudate was serous in 30 cases, thick in 29, purulent in 9, and hemorrhagic in 6. Maynard (874) found pleural effusions in 40.4 per cent of 556 cases in African Negroes at necropsy and cites Musser and Norris as finding similar conditions in 41.5 per cent of 974 collected necropsies. In Lord's (807) series of 154 necropsies, a varying but usually small amount of fluid was present in 55, or 35 per cent of the cases. The fluid was clear or cloudy in 40, purulent in 9, and hemorrhagic in 6 cases.

Berry's (96) observations in 400 postmortems are also of interest. The pleura was affected on the left side in 48, on the right side in 97, and bilateral involvement was found in 228. His related observations are shown in the accompanying summary:

Abnormalities of the pleura and pleural cavities found at necropsy in lobar pneumonia

CONDITION	UNILATERAL LESION	BILATERAL LESION
Fibrinous exudate	121	40
Fibrous exudate	126	71
Fibrinous and fibrous exudate	65	9
Serofibrinous exudate	18	2
Hydrothorax	5	3
Hemothorax	2	–
Total	337	125

Doubtless many instances of pleurisy with effusion are missed clinically and commonly the amount of fluid present is so small as to render its detection of no particular importance. Cole (297) has reported the occurrence of pleurisy with effusion in 3.8 per cent, or 28 of 770 typed cases of pneumococcus lobar pneumonia, and states that Musser and Norris found the condition diagnosed clinically in 6.26 per cent of 25,511 cases of lobar pneumonia in general. Among 525 similar cases MacCordick (830) observed it in 14, or 2.6 per cent. Cecil and Plummer (238) reported finding sterile effusions in 2.3 per cent, or 26 of 1,131 cases of Type I lobar pneumonia and in 1.5 per cent, or 15 of 991 Type II cases (239).

The diagnosis of pleural effusion rests on the demonstration of evidence of fluid by physical signs, roentgenograms, and the withdrawal of some of the fluid by aspiration. The character of any fluid obtained should be determined (see pages 643–644). The physical signs encountered in the presence of fluid and matters pertaining to the diagnosis of this condition are discussed under the appropriate sections in the following discussion of empyema. In some of Cole's (297) cases referred to above, the accumulated fluid was removed by repeated chest taps and in a few instances amounted to 2,200 cc. per patient. He considers that when extensive the early and repeated aspirations of sterile fluids may occasionally prevent the development of empyema.

Empyema

Empyema is the commonest complication of lobar pneumonia and should be suspected in every case in which the temperature continues or becomes re-elevated after defervescence. The onset is insidious, rendering early detection difficult. The development of empyema may be regarded as an indication that the host possesses some immunity in that the infection is being localized.

Finland (443) demonstrated the appearance of specific circulating antibodies in the blood of patients recovering from pneumococcus pneumonia and found that these antibodies may be present in practically the same concentration in the pleural fluids of such patients, providing the fluids are sterile. Pneumococci growing in pleural exudates give off their specific capsular polysaccharide into the surrounding fluid, as Cole (295) has shown. The inhibiting effect of this substance on immune bodies is such that if present in sufficient amount the antibodies are prevented from affecting the invading pneumococci (see pages 131–132). The fate of specific capsular polysaccharide in the body is uncertain but at least a part of it is excreted in the urine, and in patients with pneumococcus Type I, II, or III empyema soluble specific substance may be detected in the urine in some instances as late as the fiftieth day (363).

GENERAL INCIDENCE. Maynard (874) found empyema in 2.8 per cent, or 19 of 688 cases of lobar pneumonia in African Negroes at necropsy. In Berry's (96) series of 400 cases at necropsy at the Boston City Hospital, the complication was present in 14.7 per cent, or 59. A much higher proportion of cases with empyema was found at postmortem examination in patients dying during the last influenza pandemic. Feinblatt (406) examined 139 cases of lobar pneumonia under these circumstances and empyema* was present in 38.1 per cent, or 53. The common occurrence of pericarditis in association with empyema in cases of lobar pneumonia and bronchopneumonia at necropsy was clearly described by Stone (1250).

Some data are also at hand indicating the incidence of empyema at post-

* In such cases streptococci rather than pneumococci are usually the cause of the empyema.

mortem in cases due to pneumococci of certain types. Cecil and Plummer (239) report that of 52 cases of Type I lobar pneumonia at necropsy, empyema was present in 14, or 27 per cent, and in 79 Type II cases it was found in 9, or 11 per cent.

The expected frequency with which empyema complicates the clinical course of lobar pneumonia in general varies somewhat in different reported series of cases. Howard (661) has combined many of the larger series and finds that among 24,730 cases collected from the literature, 739 or approximately 3 per cent had empyema. In Table 102 are presented several additional series not included in Howard's tabulation and totaling 9,133 cases. Empyema occurred in 292, or 3.2 per cent. Nearly all these cases were in adults. Under exceptional conditions, such as in the presence of pneumonia associated with epidemics of influenza or measles, the proportion of cases developing empyema may rise to as high as 21 (1251) to 45 per cent (892), as was noted during the War, and the influenza epidemic of 1917–1919. Most such outbreaks result from streptococcus pneumonia. Cases of this nature commonly exhibit a high incidence of other complications as well, such as meningitis, pericarditis, septicaemia, and the like, occurring in conjunction with the empyema (638). It is of interest that McCrae (832) reports that few cases of empyema were seen during the great influenza epidemic of 1889–1892.

TABLE 102. LOBAR PNEUMONIA. NUMBER OF CASES AND NUMBER AND PERCENTAGE OF CASES DEVELOPING EMPYEMA

REPORTED BY	NUMBER OF CASES	CASES WITH EMPYEMA *Number*	*Per cent*
Shattuck and Lawrence, 1918 (1176)	4,000	120	3.0
Locke, Thomas, and O'Hara, 1920 (797)	447	23	5.1
Patterson, 1922 (1003a)	521	45	8.6
Locke, 1923 (793)	71	5	7.0
Lord, 1925 (807)	500	19	3.8
Vitug and Hizon, 1928 (1357)	1,030	16	1.6
MacCordick, 1931 (830)	525	12	2.3
Warr and Alperin, 1933 (1385)	2,039	52	2.6
Total	9,133	292	3.2

Although Pisek and Pease (1025) found empyema in only 41, or 4.1 per cent of 1,000 cases of lobar pneumonia and bronchopneumonia in infants and children under six years of age, the condition is ordinarily much more common in infants and children than in adults (see below, page 571). Raia, Plummer and Shultz (1057) observed empyema in 7.2 per cent, or 24 of 329 cases of lobar pneumonia and bronchopneumonia in infants and children under twelve years of age. In 131 similar cases reported by Kereszturi and Hauptmann (710) it occurred in 11 per cent. These figures are in contrast to the 3.2 per cent incidence for adults, shown in Table 102.

INCIDENCE IN PNEUMOCOCCUS CASES. The occurrence of empyema in several series of cases of pneumococcus lobar pneumonia is illustrated by the figures in Table 103. Nearly all cases were in adults. Of the total of 3,709 cases, empyema developed in 182, or 4.9 per cent.

TABLE 103. PNEUMOCOCCUS LOBAR PNEUMONIA. NUMBER OF CASES AND NUMBER AND PERCENTAGE OF CASES DEVELOPING EMPYEMA

REPORTED BY	NUMBER OF CASES	CASES WITH EMPYEMA	
		Number	*Per cent*
Cole, 1920 (297)	770	41	5.3
Cecil, Baldwin, and Larsen, 1926 (230)	1,913	99	5.2
Kessel and Hyman, 1927 (713)	56	3	5.4
Wu and Chiu, 1933 (1450)	242	23	9.5
Cruickshank, 1933 (331)	728	16	2.2
Total	3,709	182	4.9

The occurrence of this condition in clinical series of typed cases of pneumococcus lobar pneumonia is illustrated in Table 104. Practically all cases were in adults. The total number of collected Type I, II, III, and Group IV cases in Table 104 is 5,393 and empyema occurred in 286, or 5.3 per cent. In the 2,528 Type I cases this complication was found in 161, or 6.4 per cent. An unusually high incidence of empyema in cases of Type I lobar pneumonia was reported by Sutliff and Finland (1272). The condition was found in 12.6 per cent, or 30 of 239 cases in their series. As most of these cases are included in the Massachusetts Pneumonia Series (869), they are not listed in Table 104.

As shown in Table 104, empyema was present in 4 per cent, or 63 of 1,570 Type II cases; in 4.4 per cent, or 17 of 386 Type III cases; and in 5 per cent,

TABLE 104. PNEUMOCOCCUS LOBAR PNEUMONIA. NUMBER OF CASES AND NUMBER AND PERCENTAGE OF CASES DEVELOPING EMPYEMA, BY TYPE

REPORTED BY	NUMBER OF CASES	CASES WITH EMPYEMA *Number*	*Per cent*
Type I			
Cecil and Plummer, 1930 (238)	1,131	73	6.5
Wu and Chiu, 1933 (1450)	99	4	4.0
Cruickshank, 1933 (331)	255	10	3.9
Massachusetts Pneumonia Series, 1937 (869)	1,043	74	7.1
Total	2,528	161	6.4
Type II			
Cecil and Plummer, 1932 (239)	991	38	3.8
Wu and Chiu, 1933 (1450)	45	7	15.6
Cruickshank, 1933 (331)	253	3	1.2
Massachusetts Pneumonia Series, 1937 (869)	281	15	5.3
Total	1,570	63	4.0
Type III			
Cecil, Baldwin, and Larsen, 1926 (230)	268	10	3.7
Blake, 1931 (120)	104	5	4.8
Wu and Chiu, 1933 (1450)	14	2	14.3
Total	386	17	4.4
Group IV			
Cecil, Baldwin, and Larsen, 1926 (230)	633	32	5.1
Wu and Chiu, 1933 (1450)	84	10	11.9
Cruickshank, 1933 (331)	192	3	1.6
Total	909	45	5.0
Grand total	5,393	286	5.3

or 45, of 909 cases attributed to pneumococci of Group IV. Empyema was thus more frequent in pneumonia due to Type I (6.4 per cent) than in pneumonia due to pneumococci of Type II, Type III, or Group IV.

In recent years data have appeared relating to the occurrence of empyema in cases of pneumococcus pneumonia due to some of the higher types. Sutliff and Finland (1271) reported the incidence of purulent complications in 910 cases of lobar pneumonia and bronchopneumonia due to one or another of the types of pneumococci from Type I to Type XX inclusive. Among these cases pneumococci of Type V caused empyema in 7 of 47 cases, or 14 per cent, and gave rise to this condition in a higher proportion of cases than did any of the other types. Type I infections gave rise to empyema in 32, or 12 per cent, of 273 cases, and in consequence this type was relegated to second place as a cause of the complication. In cases of lobar pneumonia in the Massachusetts Pneumonia Series (869), however, empyema was observed in only 5.9 per cent, or 1 of 17 Type V cases, while among 1,043 Type I cases it was found 74 times, or in 7.1 per cent. None of Sutliff and Finland's (1271) Type V cases mentioned above are included in the Massachusetts series but many of their Type I cases are.

In the preceding section on bacteriemia it was observed that empyema tended to occur most frequently in bacteriemic cases and that bacteriemia is apparently more frequent in Type II infections than in those due to other types. The expectation might be, then, that empyema would be commoner in Type II cases, an assumption not borne out by the observations listed in Table 104. The explanation of this discrepancy will have to await further studies. Possibly the fact that specific antiserum was used in the treatment of many of the cases in Table 104 is the answer.

Of the Type I and Type II cases in Table 104, probably a majority received varying amounts of specific antipneumococcic horse serum for the treatment of their pneumonia. It is likely that in such instances the action of the antibody of the serum tends to assist in localizing the infective process. This might result, as Cole (33, 299) has suggested, in an increased incidence of suppurative complications (see page 887) and permit the localization of infections which otherwise would lead to death. In recent years with the more general use of serum therapy in pneumonia has come the recognition that to obtain the most satisfactory results, cases must be treated as early as possible after the onset of the illness. In consequence, serum therapy is now commonly used in early cases and in such instances evidence is accumulating which suggests that the incidence of septic complications such as empyema may be reduced by this form of therapy (see page 888). Possibly similar effects may be obtained by the specific serum treatment of children with pneumococcus pneumonia (930).

FACTORS AFFECTING INCIDENCE. Among others, Locke (795) has shown that about one-half of all empyemas that occur follow lobar pneumonia. The nature of the infecting organism is important and the incidence is generally higher in pneumonias due to streptococci than to pneumococci, and in the latter instance appears higher in cases due to some types than to others, as seen above. The occurrence of bacteriemia may also affect the incidence of empyema, as already noted. Observations by Webster (1394) suggest that just as yearly variations occur in the incidence of the many types of pneumococci and other organisms in causing pneumonia, so variations occur in the frequency with which these organisms give rise to empyema. Further, variations in the occurrence of empyema in different years were demonstrated by several investigators (892, 1251, 1394), as Heuer (638) has remarked.

Patterson (1003a), in a study of 521 cases of lobar pneumonia, finds a definite seasonal variation in the occurrence of this complication, as seen in Table 105. Empyema was found in only 8 per cent of the cases occurring in

TABLE 105. LOBAR PNEUMONIA. NUMBER OF CASES AND NUMBER AND PERCENTAGE OF CASES WITH EMPYEMA, BY SEASON

SEASON	NUMBER OF CASES	CASES WITH EMPYEMA	
		Number	*Per cent*
Spring	101	11	11.0
Summer	115	9	8.0
Autumn	138	8	6.0
Winter	167	16	10.0

From Patterson (1003a)

the summer, and in only 6 per cent in the autumn. In winter, however, 10 per cent of the cases had empyema, as did 11 per cent in the spring. The groups on which these observations are based are too small to render Patterson's findings significant and additional data are needed.

In infants and children with pneumococcus Type I pneumonia, Lyon (821) found empyema in 37.8 per cent, or 12 of 32 cases, and Cecil and Plummer (238) reported its presence in 16.7 per cent, or 5 of 30 similar cases. Of 7 cases of Type II bronchopneumonia in infants and children, Wollstein (1435) observed empyema in 43 per cent. Among 54 similar cases in the series due to pneumococci of Group IV, this complication was present in 5.5 per cent. Blacklock and Guthrie (112) studied a series of 66 pneumococcus empyemas in infants and children and found that 30, or 45.5 per cent, were due to pneumococci of Type I. Only one case was due to Type II, and the remainder were caused by Group IV pneumococci. Studies such as these have called attention to the especially common occurrence of Type I empyema in infants and children having Type I infections. Blacklock and Guthrie (112) also demonstrated that among children, as age increases, the proportion of empyemas due to pneumococci of Type I increases.

It is apparent from the findings discussed above and elsewhere that the incidence of empyema is affected by age and is higher in infants and children than in adults. Possibly among adults the proportion of cases developing this condition may be higher in older than in younger patients, as Patterson's (1003a) findings suggest (Table 106). Nevertheless, Patterson's

TABLE 106. LOBAR PNEUMONIA. NUMBER OF CASES AND NUMBER AND PERCENTAGE OF CASES DEVELOPING EMPYEMA, BY AGE GROUP

AGE GROUP	NUMBER OF CASES		CASES WITH EMPYEMA *Number*		*Per cent*	
10–19	72	330	7	24	9.7	7.3
20–29	126		11		8.7	
30–39	132		6		4.6	
40–49	86	191	10	21	11.6	11.0
50–59	54		5		9.3	
60–69	41		5		12.4	
70–79	10		1		10.0	
Total	521		45		8.6	

From Patterson (1003a)

series of cases is probably too small to settle this matter. Of the cases of pneumonia in Table 106, there were 330 in patients in the age group of ten to thirty-nine years, and 24, or 7.3 per cent, had empyema; while among the 191 cases over forty years of age the complication was more frequent and was found in 21, or 11 per cent.

In an intensive study at the Johns Hopkins Hospital of the occurrence of empyema after lobar pneumonia, McCrae (832) found the complication in 29 of 809 cases. He concluded it was more common in males than in females and more common in Negroes than in individuals of the white race. The predisposition of males to develop this condition may have been more apparent than real, for although there were about four times as many empyemas in males as in females in his series, there is usually nearly this same proportion of males to females in all large series of cases of lobar pneumonia. So far as the influence of race is concerned in affecting the incidence of empyema, Miller and Lusk (892), in a series of pneumococcus lobar pneumonias totaling about 100 cases each in Negroes and in whites, found the incidence of this condition to be 8.6 per cent in Negroes and 13 per cent in whites. In cases of streptococcus pneumonia in similar groups, these same workers found the incidence of empyema to be 20 per cent in Negroes and 45 per cent in whites. If empyema is considered evidence of an immunologic reaction assisting in the localization of the infection, Miller and Lusk's observations are readily understandable, for as a rule resistance in certain of its phases appears lower in Negroes than in whites. Maynard's (874) findings in Africa, as earlier mentioned, and those of Vitug and Hizon (1357) in the Philippines, are also of interest in this matter. The former studied 688 cases of lobar pneumonia in Negroes at necropsy and found empyema in only 19, or 2.8 per cent; and the latter workers in 1,030 cases in patients, probably largely of the yellow race, at the Philippine General Hospital, Manila, observed this condition in only 16, or 1.6 per cent.

McCrae (832) is of the opinion that empyema is more likely to develop after severe than after mild cases of pneumonia. Evidence supporting this view has been presented by Heuer (638).

KIND OF LESION. In empyemas as a group, the kinds of lesions produced are, in the approximate order of the frequency with which they occur: massive or general, interlobar, sacculated, bilocular, bilateral, and necessitatus, as Harloe (596) has shown. Among 351 cases of empyema in patients of all ages the distribution of cases by the variety of lesion as given by this investigator was as follows:

Kind of lesion	*Occurrence in per cent*
Massive or general	76.9
Sacculated or interlobar	18.6
Bilocular	2.3
Bilateral	2.3

There were also two cases of massive empyema necessitatus in his series.

In 285 cases developing in conjunction with pneumonia, Locke (795) found that 70 per cent were encapsulated and that the majority of these were located in the lower and posterior portions of the pleural cavity. Bilateral empyema was uncommon, as others have also shown (96, 383, 1225, 596). It may be more frequent in children than in adults, but from the collected cases of Steinke (1225) there appears little difference in the incidence of bilateral empyema among such patients. Including his own cases, Steinke has collected reports of 54 cases. His figures suggest, as noted above, that about 1 to 2 per cent of all empyemas may be bilateral. This is particularly true among cases examined at necropsy.

Although contralateral empyema may rarely occur, in a series of 29 cases of empyema studied by McCrae (832) empyema always occurred on the same side as that involved in the pneumonia and in every instance in his series the pneumonic lesion was in a lower lobe. Dunham (383), in a series of 3,889 empyemas occurring in army camps during the War, found the right side involved slightly more often than the left. This is probably the natural outcome of the inherent tendency for pneumonia to occur more often on the right than on the left side (see pages 107–111). Empyema, however, occurs about as often after pneumonia on the left side as on the right side.

Under ordinary circumstances the great majority of all empyemas are caused by pneumococci, hemolytic streptococci being next in frequency (795). Staphylococci and other organisms are less often found. An important difference exists in the usual type of exudate appearing in cases of pneumococcus and streptococcus empyema. In nearly every instance where pneumococci invade the pleural cavity and grow rapidly, the fluid which appears thickens and soon changes to greenish-yellow pus containing large amounts of fibrin. Such a plastic exudate probably contributes to the stabilization of the mediastinum. In streptococcus cases the exudate is ordinarily thin, serous, bloody, or slightly purulent, has but little fibrin, and probably does little to aid in immobilizing the mediastinum. Likewise, the pathology found in cases of pneumococcus empyema is usually very different from that found in streptococcus cases. Simple empyema, usually pneumococcal in origin, may be considered an intrapleural abscess of varying size and location. Empyema of streptococcus origin, however, is not usually simple and frequently coexists with other purulent complications, as previously noted.

As a rule in streptococcus pneumonia, empyema due to this organism appears early in the course of the illness while the patient is still acutely ill with the pneumonia. The fluid frequently accumulates rapidly in such cases, necessitating early drainage. On the other hand, empyema of pneumococcus origin generally does not appear until late in the pneumonia, or as is more common, until after crisis or lysis. In such cases the accumulation of fluid is slow and the need for immediate drainage not imperative. It will be obvious, then, that these two types of cases present problems with important differences, as is generally recognized.

Pericarditis occasionally occurs in conjunction with empyema, as already indicated. McCrae (832) noted this association and Stone (1250), in reviewing 300 necropsies of patients dead from either lobar pneumonia or bronchopneumonia, had the unusual experience of finding that a high proportion of cases with empyema also had pericarditis. Apparently streptococci (hemolytic) were the cause of about 72 per cent of all the pneumonias in this series and the cause of about 75 per cent of the cases with pericarditis. Of 48 cases of empyema which were operated on and later ended in death, extensive pericarditis, usually purulent, was found in 15, or 31.2 per cent. Among 100 patients with empyema dying without operation, the proportion with pericarditis was even higher, and it was present in 46 per cent of the cases.

SYMPTOMS. In cases in which empyema develops following the acute stages of pneumococcus lobar pneumonia, the temperature, pulse, and respirations either do not fall at the time of the expected defervescence, or within a few days following their fall they again begin to rise. The commonest symptom is persistence of fever, which may vary from approximately normal to over 103° F. In some cases, the temperature remains persistently elevated and in others the septic type of "picket-fence" temperature is seen. The pulse and respiratory rates are usually elevated. Cough, chills, sweats, and rapid emaciation, accompanied by a sallow and unhealthy color, are common. Some patients are comfortable, while others suffer great distress from dyspnea and, uncommonly, pain. Vital capacity is usually decreased and the decrease is progressive and often marked.

In streptococcus cases the symptoms are generally much more severe (638). Severe toxemia is often present with a rapid pulse, urgent respiration, and an appearance of being desperately ill. The symptoms may seem all out of proportion to what might be expected from a simple empyema. Should death occur, and it often does early in such cases, necropsy frequently reveals, in addition to the empyema, some other serious septic condition, such as pericarditis, peritonitis, meningitis, or septicaemia.

PHYSICAL SIGNS. Inspection is generally not important but diminished motion of the affected side of the chest may be seen. Palpation frequently reveals a diminished but not necessarily absent tactile fremitus. This change may be impossible to detect if the amount of fluid is small. The percussion note becomes duller and at times sounds flat or wooden, and there is a sense of solid resistance to the finger. At the end of the acute stage of the pneumonia in patients who shortly develop empyema, a decrease in dulness over the consolidated area is frequently followed by a return of dulness as the empyema appears. Diminished and bronchial breathing, diminished voice, egophony, and increased whisper are usually found over free fluid. Neither bronchial breathing nor egophony may be heard unless the accumulation of fluid is large. Rales once loud tend to become faint.

DIAGNOSIS. A daily examination of the chest should be made throughout the acute illness and convalescence in all patients with pneumonia. The presence of a friction rub over the affected area may indicate a dry pleurisy but does not exclude the possibility of free or encapsulated fluid elsewhere. If any suspicion of fluid arises, a needle should be inserted to ascertain its nature. With effusions of some size, displacement of the heart away from the fluid may be demonstrated. The heart is rarely displaced toward the effusion should a massive collapse occur on the affected side (808). At times, displacement of the trachia toward the unaffected side may be determined by palpation in the region of the suprasternal notch.

The small amounts of fluid which so often accompany pneumonia are usually serofibrinous and sterile but may contain varying amounts of blood and occasionally dead organisms (808). Large effusions occurring with or after pneumonia are usually purulent. The occurrence of such effusions in children under five years of age generally means an empyema. Nearly all patients with empyema show a marked leucocytosis and counts of 10,000 to 30,000 are to be expected (832, 255, 807). This finding may be of diagnostic aid, particularly in patients late in convalescence, although where serum was used in the treatment of the pneumonia, serum sickness may develop in late convalescence and also cause a leucocytosis.

Roentgen-ray examinations, and especially when made on several consecutive days, are often of great diagnostic aid. The use of a portable roentgen-ray apparatus is of great assistance when patients are too ill to be moved from bed, and films taken in this manner are usually satisfactory. If possible, films should be taken with the patient upright or, if the patient is too ill for this, an anterioposterior film with the patient lying on one side should be included in the series. Otherwise the presence or absence of air, as well as fluid, in the pleural sac will be missed. With the patient in the upright position, the presence of free pleural fluid is suggested by obliteration of the costophrenic angle and a homogeneous increase of density at the base of the lung, reaching its highest level at the axillary region unless pneumothorax is present, when it assumes a hydrostatic level. A profile view is also desirable for the purpose of detecting an encapsulated effusion in the interlobar fissure. Encapsulated effusions may occur at any place but are most commonly basal or in the region of the interlobar septums and are of even density with sharply defined margins. The detection of an encapsulated effusion from physical signs alone may be difficult. The finding of a small area of dulness with diminished breathing, voice, and tactile fremitus may be suggestive. For the early diagnosis of empyema in general, Davies, Hodgson, and Whitby (341) find roentgenograms of less value than physical signs.

The only certain diagnostic procedure available is the chest tap. By this method alone can one ascertain whether a fluid is infected and the nature of the organism present. Exploratory puncture is best done under local anesthesia with a needle of sufficiently large bore to aspirate fluid or somewhat thick pus, should it be encountered. Any unusual thickness of the pleura causing resistance to the needle may be noted at the time of the tap. In performing a chest tap for free effusions, the site of choice is in the seventh intercostal space in the region of the angle of the scapula; this site being in a dependent region is the one most likely to yield fluid if it is free within the chest. The site of puncture for encapsulated fluids should be over the area of the effusion, which is best determined by roentgen-ray examination. Specimens of all fluid obtained, no matter how small the amount, should be saved and submitted for examination (see pages 643–644). Fluid obtained from diagnostic or therapeutic chest taps should be examined by Gram-stained smear and both aerobic and anaerobic cultures should be made. It is desirable from the standpoint of successful treatment to establish the identity of the infecting organism. A high proportion of polymorphonuclear leucocytes in such fluids suggests the presence of infection, and when bacteria are present approximately all the cells found are of this variety (808, 1166).

PROGNOSIS. Heuer (638), in his excellent discussion of empyema, has shown with startling clearness that in comparing the results of treatment in empyema, it is of the utmost importance not only to classify cases as to their etiology, but also to ascertain whether such cases are simple or complicated. Simple cases usually recover and are those in which empyema occurs alone in conjunction with the residual pneumonia. Most of the mortality associated with empyema occurs in cases complicated by the presence of some other septic process, such as septicaemia, meningitis, pericarditis, or lung abscess (638, 596).

It should be remembered that although empyema is the commonest complication of lobar pneumonia, its frequency, severity, and mortality vary in different years as McCrae has shown (832). This has also been emphasized by Heuer (638), who states:

> . . . respiratory infections vary in type and in virulence in different localities and in the same locality in different years; that the pathologic conditions to which they give rise, may be a simple empyema or an empyema associated with other serious conditions; that the mortality in empyema varies in different age groups, in different types of infection, in different localities and in different years; and that these variations in the mortality are dependent in greater degree upon the incidence of pathologic conditions other than empyema than upon the empyema itself, or the kind of operation performed.

In McCrae's (832) series of 29 cases and in the 99 cases reported by Cecil, Baldwin, and Larsen (230), the great majority of empyemas were first recognized during the second to fourth week following the onset of pneumonia (see Table 107). The onset of frank empyema early in the acute course of pneumonia is of serious prognostic significance (230, 1145). This is illustrated by the findings of Cecil and his associates (230) in cases developing in the course of or following pneumococcus lobar pneumonia, as shown in Table 107. The highest fatality rate was found in patients in whom empyema appeared during the first week of the pneumonia. Of 11 cases in this group death occurred in 10, or 90 per cent. Among 27 cases first recognized from the seventh to the fourteenth day after the onset of the pneumonia, 51.8 per cent died, while of 61 cases in which empyema developed on and after the fourteenth day, only 22.9 per cent died. The average fatality rate of the total 99 cases was 38.3 per cent and was somewhat higher than that found in the series of more than 1,000 cases of lobar pneumonia studied by these investigators.

Heuer (638), in a review of the necropsy findings in 583 cases of empyema, reports that death from absorption from a simple empyema is uncommon. He further found that most fatal cases show purulent complications in addition to the empyema, which may have been adequately drained. It also appeared from the clinical and pathologic findings in his cases that such purulent complications are probably the result of the original respiratory infection and are not due simply to the presence of the empyema.

In general, the fatality rate from acute pneumococcus empyema is approximately 10 per cent, and that of streptococcus empyema about 20 per cent. As mentioned above, the fatality rates vary markedly with the presence of complications in addition to the empyema. Muller (913) and Heuer (638), among others, find the case fatality rate of simple uncomplicated empyema to be in the neighborhood of 1 to 7 per cent, while that of cases complicated by other purulent conditions varies from 35 to 45 per cent, or more. Age, too, is an important factor. Fatality rates are high in the very young and in the old.

TABLE 107. PNEUMOCOCCUS EMPYEMA. NUMBER OF CASES AND NUMBER AND PERCENTAGE OF DEATHS, BY DAY AFTER THE ONSET OF PNEUMOCOCCUS LOBAR PNEUMONIA THE CONDITION DEVELOPED

TIME OF DEVELOPMENT OF EMPYEMA RELATIVE TO ONSET OF PNEUMONIA	NUMBER OF CASES	DEATHS	
		Number	*Per cent*
Before seventh day	11	10	90.0
Seventh to fourteenth day	27	14	51.8
On and after fourteenth day	61	14	22.9
Total	99	38	38.3

From Cecil *et al.* (230)

Harloe's (596) findings with respect to the fatality rate of cases in various age groups are of interest. His data include observations on a total of 351 cases, as shown in Table 108. The fatality rate was zero in children eight through fourteen years of age, was low in children four through eight years old and in young adults, and was higher in the still younger children and in adults in the older age groups. In the group of 233 cases in infants and children there were 22, or 9.9 per cent of deaths. This fatality rate is very similar to that of 7.8 per cent reported by Mason (863) for 103 cases in infants and children.

In Harloe's series as shown in Table 108, there were 70 patients in the first two years of life, of whom 12, or 19.1 per cent, died. In Mason's series there were 31 patients under three years of age, of whom 7, or 22.5 per cent, died. McEnery and Brennermann (836), in a series of 94 cases in infants and children, found that the fatality rate of 67 patients with pneumococcus infections was 7.5 per cent. Of 9 staphylococcus cases 44.4 per cent died, of 7 cases due

TABLE 108. EMPYEMA. NUMBER OF CASES AND NUMBER AND PERCENTAGE OF DEATHS, BY AGE GROUP

AGE GROUP	NUMBER OF CASES	DEATHS *Number*	DEATHS *Per cent*
	Children		
1 year or less	20	6	30.0
1–2	50	6	12.0
2–4	69	7	10.2
4–6	53	2	3.8
6–8	26	1	3.9
8–10	7	–	–
10–12	8	–	–
Total	233	22	9.9
	Adults		
12–14	5	–	–
14–20	27	2	7.4
20–30	34	1	2.9
30–40	24	4	16.6
40–50	19	2	10.1
50–60	4	1	25.0
60–70	4	1	25.0
70–80	1	–	–
Total	118	11	9.3

From Harloe (596)

to hemolytic streptococci 28 per cent died, of 3 with streptococcus viridans infections 33 per cent died, and of 8 due to other organisms none died. Staphylococcus infections caused only one-tenth of the cases, but were responsible for about one-third of the deaths in the whole series and for most of the deaths in the first year of life among infants with empyema. Children with Type I pneumonia and a bacteriemia are especially likely to develop empyema with eventual recovery (1321).

Death occurred in 9.3 per cent, or 11, of 118 of the cases in adults, shown in Table 108. In Cole's (297) 41 cases of empyema occurring after pneumococcus lobar pneumonia 7, or 17.1 per cent, died. All or nearly all of these cases were in adults. Cecil, Baldwin, and Larsen's (230) experience with 99 similar cases due to pneumococci of known type is given in Table 109. The fatality rate of Type I cases was 36.3 per cent, of Type II cases 38.4 per cent, of Type III cases 33.3 per cent, and of Group IV cases 43.7 per cent. In the total 99 cases there were 38 deaths, or 38.3 per cent. As these cases were in adults, this rate seems rather high. This series, however, was made up of cases entering the Bellevue Hospital, New York City, a large charity hospital, and many patients in the group may be expected to be in very poor physical condition at the time of their admission to the hospital. Cecil and Plummer (238) subsequently reported a fatality rate of 51.7 per cent for 29 cases of pneumococcus Type I empyema occurring after lobar pneumonia due to this organism.

TABLE 109. PNEUMOCOCCUS EMPYEMA. NUMBER OF CASES AND NUMBER AND PERCENTAGE OF DEATHS, BY TYPE

	NUMBER OF CASES	DEATHS	
		Number	*Per cent*
Type I	44	16	36.3
Type II	13	5	38.4
Type III	10	3	33.3
Group IV	32	14	43.7
Total	99	38	38.3

From Cecil *et al.* (230)

The occurrence of empyema in association with severe outbreaks of pneumonia, such as took place in many of the army camps in this country during the War, was usually followed by very high case fatality rates. In Dunham's (383) collected series of 3,889 cases of empyema occurring under such circumstances and due to various organisms, 1,260, or 32.4 per cent, died. Death from pneumococcus infections occurred in from 34.2 per cent (1251) to as high as 57 per cent (892) of white patients and in about 70 per cent of Negro patients (892). Death from streptococcus infections occurred in 58 to 65 per cent (892, 1251) of white patients, and in 44 to 56 per cent (219, 892) of Negro patients. Cole (298) reports the fatality rate of streptococcus cases as 43 per cent.

Bilateral cases are likely to be very severe, with a fatality rate in the neighborhood of 25 (596) to 75 per cent (1225).

Stone, Phillips, and Bliss (1251) found a seasonal variation in the fatality rate with empyema, the highest rate occurring at the end of winter (March).

In review, the prognosis in empyema is seen to vary considerably and to be affected by such factors as age, race, the nature of the organism present, the occurrence of additional septic complications in the patient at the time, the time after onset of the pneumonia the condition develops, whether the lesion is unilateral or bilateral, and the season of the year. The occurrence of infections such as measles and influenza preceding the onset is likewise important, as is the mode of treatment used.

TREATMENT. In every case of empyema, whether in a child or an adult, surgical advice should be sought, for operative intervention is usually necessary before recovery can occur. In nearly all instances patients should not be operated on for empyema until the pleural exudate has been examined bacteriologically and the presence of living pyogenic organisms demonstrated.

In streptococcus cases, thin bloody exudate may collect rapidly in such large amounts early in the disease that early and repeated aspirations are essential for the continuance of life. With respect to the treatment of such cases, the experience at the time of the War during the influenza epidemic of 1917–1919 is interesting (297, 638). Cases of streptococcus empyema occurring in the first part of this epidemic were treated by rib resection with open drainage. Fatality rates as high as 40 to 60 per cent were usual. Later in the epidemic the methods of treatment were changed. Repeated aspirations were resorted to first to tide patients over the acute stages of their pulmonary disease, and, if necessary, drainage by surgical measures was carried out later. Accompanying this change in handling cases, there occurred a marked drop in their fatality rate which decreased to about 15 per cent and later to 10 per cent. It was assumed that this decrease was due entirely to a change in the methods of treatment. Subsequent experience, however, with the latter method of treatment and a careful review of the War cases of empyema make this extremely unlikely, as Heuer (638) has shown. He finds that probably the decrease in the fatality rate from streptococcus empyema observed in the latter part of the influenza epidemic was due largely to a decrease in the general severity of the pulmonary infections which occurred at the time. Early in the epidemic when the fatality rate from empyema was high, the incidence of other septic complications, such as septicaemia, pericarditis, peritonitis, and mediastinitis in these cases was also very high, while later in the epidemic empyema was less often complicated by other purulent conditions, and the fatality rate of the cases in that period was much lower.

In pneumococcus empyema early and frequent aspirations are usually not necessary, as the pus accumulates slowly and seldom appears in large quantities until relatively late in the disease or during convalescence. Thoracic surgeons usually advise waiting for the empyema to "ripen" before initiating surgical procedures. This interval gives time for the formation of adhesions which assist in stabilizing the mediastinum, and lessens the likelihood of producing an undesirable open pneumothorax at the time of operation.

The methods of treatment which have been widely used for empyema are (a) repeated aspirations with or without some subsequent procedure, (b) closed aspiration drainage by the insertion of a tube between the ribs, and (c) intercostal incision or rib resection with open drainage. No single method of treatment is universally accepted. Neither Muller (913) nor Heuer (638) advises open drainage, and the latter states that he uses rib resection only in order to allow the introduction of a larger tube. Both observers have stressed the fact that in cases of simple (uncomplicated) empyema the fatality rate is likely to be low, while in cases complicated by other purulent conditions it is likely to be high, as already mentioned. This appears true regardless of the method of treatment. Practically, the proper use of one good method appears better than the random use of several. Although occasional cases of empyema in adults have been cured by repeated aspirations alone, such a procedure should never be relied upon and surgical opinion on the treatment of these cases should be requested.

In few cases of pneumococcus empyema is there any great need of hurry to operate. A large majority of so-called "chronic" empyemas have been improperly or inadequately drained. At times tuberculosis may be the cause.

Muller (913) states: "Always in babies, usually in children, frequently in adults, one or more aspirations are done, especially if there is cyanosis, displacement of the heart or dyspnea." The treatment of empyema in children is discussed below.

After the acute stages of the pneumonia are over, aspiration may be followed by tube drainage between the ribs if the pus is thin, and especially if the empyema is massive. If much fluid is present, small amounts are removed at first and increasing amounts later. When the cavity is sufficiently emptied, or if only a small amount of exudate is present, the outer end of the tube may be inserted into a bottle partly filled with water, and placed at a level lower than that of the chest, to obtain siphon drainage. In a few days irrigations with Dakin's solution may be useful if no bronchial fistula exists and if much fibrin is present; otherwise saline solution may prove best. Satisfactory results have been obtained without the use of irrigations and many surgeons prefer not to use them. The irrigation of empyema cavities with other kinds of solutions and disinfectants has been tried with but slight success. If the clinical course of the patient is not satisfactory, a rib resection may be done within two weeks and a larger tube inserted. This was necessary in 60 per cent of 99 cases reported by Muller (913). While Harloe (596) advises the use of the closed negative pressure operation employing a trochar thoracotomy with tube drainage, Mason (863) regards the rib resection method with open drainage after repeated aspirations as preferable.

The post-operative and convalescent care of empyema patients includes the use of a high caloric diet, heliotherapy, and other general supportive measures. Blood transfusions may be of value at times. The use of blow bottles and breathing exercises to assist in re-expanding the lung play an important part in the aftercare of these cases.

In adults the treatment of pneumococcus empyema by washing out the cavity with antipneumococcic horse serum has been tried repeatedly with no obvious success. The intravenous administration of such serums has likewise proved of no avail. This failure to cure empyema by the use of antipneumococcic horse serum is perhaps not unexpected. Sutliff and Rhoades (1275) have shown that many patients with complications already have spontaneously produced specific antibodies in their blood and it is unlikely that the injection of additional antibodies would have any particular effect on the empyema. As earlier mentioned, Cole (295) has shown that as pneumococci grow in pleural exudates they give off their specific capsular polysaccharide (SSS) into the surrounding fluid. This substance accumulates in the exudate in such large amounts that, as Cole remarks, one cannot expect to treat an empyema with antiserum locally or by intravenous injection unless the exudate surrounding the organisms is drained off as the SSS present inhibits the actions of the immune substances of the serum. As it is usually impossible to drain off all the exudate, which is constantly forming, the treatment of empyema with immune horse serums is now seldom attempted. In treating empyema due to hemolytic streptococci, however, Amos and Craven (14) were encouraged by the results, in a few cases, of the intravenous and intrathoracic injection of antistreptococcus serum.

Following the drainage of empyema in the usual manner, little or no disfigurement of the thorax occurs. Rarely, marked scoliosis with mediastinal displacement may result. Such cases are encountered much less commonly now than formerly. Bronchiectasis and fibroid changes in the lung have been reported (832).

Many of the septic complications of empyema have already been noted. Tuberculosis may also be found as a complication. Perforation into a bronchus may occur. In unrecognized or untreated cases spontaneous perforation through the chest wall may occur, as described long ago by Hippocrates (645).

TREATMENT OF EMPYEMA IN CHILDREN. Muller (913) states that opening the chest of children during pneumonia seems especially harmful. Surgical drainage should be carried out only after the acute phases of the pneumonia have subsided, the principles of therapy being much the same as in adult cases. Repeated aspirations can usually be relied upon to tide patients over to an opportune time for operation. At operation, closed drainage through a tube, without rib resection, seems the method of choice, although if necessary rib resection may be done to accommodate a larger tube. Mason (863) feels that irrigations should not be used unless especially indicated.

Various chemicals have frequently been employed in the treatment of empyema in children. Solutions of mercurochrome, as well as ethylhydrocupreine (optochin), have been used to irrigate the pleural cavity (1322). In some instances the pus has been removed and replaced by the injection of air, a procedure McEnery and Brennermann (836) do not think advisable. Considerable discussion is centered about the proper treatment for cases in children and some investigators hold that repeated aspirations alone without operation are all that is required. McEnery and Brennermann report that 72 per cent of 94 cases of empyema were cured by repeated aspirations. Among their cases, however, if a patient did not do well with simple aspirations, operation was resorted to at once. These workers feel that the best results are obtained by letting empyemas "ripen," if possible, for many days before operation.

Otitis Media and Mastoiditis

Acute inflammation of the accessory nasal sinuses or middle ear may precede pneumonia or occur during or after it. The condition may be overlooked during the course of pneumonia until some untoward occurrence such as the development of meningitis leads to its discovery. Lesions of this nature are commoner in children than in adults.

Among 400 cases of lobar pneumonia at necropsy, Berry (96) found acute sinusitis in 2, acute otitis media in 27 (6.8 per cent), and acute mastoiditis in 9 (2.3 per cent). These cases were almost wholly in adults.

As a clinically recognized complication during pneumonia Cunningham (333) found purulent otitis media in 13.1 per cent of 1,500 cases of lobar pneumonia in infants and children. Raia, Plummer, and Shultz (1057) recorded its occurrence in 329 cases of lobar pneumonia and bronchopneumonia in patients of similar age. Acute purulent otitis media was found in 12.5 per cent, or 41, of the cases. In all but 13 instances it was due to pneumococci of some one of the higher types. Observations much similar to these were made by Blacklock and Guthrie (112), who examined the ears of 497 infants and children with pneumonia. Purulent otitis media was the commonest complication found and was present in 183, or 36.8 per cent. In 33 cases of pneumococcus otitis media, typing revealed that the pneumococci in 31 were of Group IV, while Type I and Type II were found in one case each.

During lobar pneumonia in adults purulent otitis media was found in 9 (1.4 per cent) of 658 cases by Chatard (254), in 44 (2.2 per cent) of 2,039 cases by Warr and Alperin (1385), and in 3 (1.2 per cent) of 242 cases by Wu and Chiu (1450). In the latter instance the cases were of known type and pneumococci of Type I were found in otitis media in one case and of Type II in two cases. When the customary treatment of this complication is undertaken the occurrence of otitis media in pneumonia does not appear to alter the prognosis.

Many of the types common in lobar pneumonia may be found in middle ear or mastoid infections in general (1271), and Finland and Sutliff (464) report that pneumococci of Type III especially, and less often those of Type VIII, are found in such infections.

Pericarditis

Pericarditis is an occasional and a serious complication of pneumonia. Many cases escape detection clinically and are found only at postmortem examination. In some instances the complication does not begin until a few hours before death.

The incidence of this condition in necropsied cases has been reported by various workers. In lobar pneumonia Musser and Norris (918) found it in 12.6 per cent of 2,128 collected necropsies. The findings of additional investigators are as follows:

Cases of lobar pneumonia at necropsy. Incidence of pericarditis

OBSERVER	TOTAL	WITH PERICARDITIS *Number*	*Per cent*
Fabyan (399)	195	34	17.4
Maynard (874; African Negroes)	688	67	9.7
Berry (96)	400	42	10.5
Feinblatt (406)	139	28	20.1
Cruz (332; Filipinos)	400	13	3.3

In cases of lobar pneumonia and bronchopneumonia together at necropsy Stone (1250) found pericarditis in 24 per cent of 300 cases, and Menetrier (882) in 5.5 per cent of 400 cases. At necropsy, then, pericarditis has been found in about 4 to 24 per cent of cases. Feinblatt's series and Stone's series, however, are made up of patients dying of pneumonia in army camps during the War. The unusually severe pneumonias prevalent then doubtless contributed to the high incidence of pericarditis found and in Stone's series streptococci were the cause of about 75 per cent of the cases of pericarditis.

In cases of pneumococcus Type I lobar pneumonia at necropsy Cecil and Plummer (239) found suppurative pericarditis in 3.8 per cent of 52 cases, and in 79 Type II cases it was found in 2.5 per cent.

Among 1,500 infants and children with lobar pneumonia, Cunningham (333) observed pericarditis in only three cases. The frequency may be somewhat greater in adults. In a collected series of 40,773 cases Musser and Norris (918) found it in 1.2 per cent. The reports of additional workers are as follows:

Cases of lobar pneumonia. Incidence of pericarditis

OBSERVER	TOTAL	WITH PERICARDITIS	
		Number	*Per cent*
Chatard (254)	658	35	5.3
Cole (297)	770	17	2.2
MacCordick (830)	525	4	0.8
Warr and Alperin (1385)	2,039	16	0.8
Wu and Chiu (1450)	242	2	0.8

In 19 of Chatard's 35 cases cited above the complication was not found until necropsy. In Cole's series empyema was the commonest complication found and pericarditis the second most common.

Cecil, Baldwin, and Larsen (230) reported the incidence of pericarditis in 1,913 typed cases of pneumococcus lobar pneumonia, as seen in Table 110. In the whole series of 1,913 cases it was found in 10, or 0.5 per cent. The incidence in Type I cases was 0.6 per cent, in Type II cases 0.8 per cent, in Type III cases 0.4 per cent, and in Group IV cases 0.3 per cent. Subsequently Cecil and Plummer (238) reported the occurrence of this complication in 0.6 per cent of 1,131 Type I cases. The same authors (239) also later reported finding pericarditis in 0.3 per cent of 991 Type II cases. These latter series apparently include the Type I and Type II cases in Table 110.

Fabyan (399) listed the type of lesion encountered in his series of 34 cases of pericarditis. It was fibrinous in 23 cases and serous in 11. In Stone's (1250) group of 72 cases 19.4 per cent, or 14, showed acute serofibrinous pericarditis; 61.1 per cent, or 44, had acute purulent pericarditis; and in 19.4 per cent, or 14, a subacute fibrinoplastic and purulent condition (shaggy heart) was present. At times an associated endocarditis (882) or empyema may be found. In Stone's series mentioned above, empyema was present in 87.5 per cent, or 63, of his 72 cases. McCrae (833) noted a close relation between the occurrence of pericarditis and delayed resolution, as was earlier stated (see page 543). The amount of fluid in the pericardial sac may vary from a few cubic centimeters to a liter or more. In Berry's (96) series of 400 lobar pneumonias at necropsy the pericardium was involved in varying degrees in nearly one-third of the cases.

TABLE 110. PNEUMOCOCCUS LOBAR PNEUMONIA. NUMBER OF CASES AND NUMBER AND PERCENTAGE OF CASES WITH PERICARDITIS, BY TYPE

	NUMBER OF CASES	CASES WITH PERICARDITIS	
		Number	*Per cent*
Type I	644	4	0.6
Type II	368	3	0.8
Type III	268	1	0.4
Group IV	633	2	0.3
Total	1,913	10	0.5

From Cecil *et al.* (230)

The question of the mode of origin of pericarditis in pneumonia has been discussed in the literature for years (833, 1250, 297, 807, 332). Acute fibrinous pericarditis and fibrino-purulent pericarditis have been observed in monkeys (123) and rabbits (508) undergoing an experimentally induced pneumococcus pneumonia where the lesion seemed to occur as a result of the direct extension of the infection.

At necropsy in man Stone (1250) and Cruz (332) found pericarditis slightly more often in cases of pneumonia involving the left lung. Fabyan (399) observed it more frequently in cases with right-sided involvements. Both Fabyan and Stone, however, find the condition considerably more frequent in the presence of bilateral pulmonary involvements. In Stone's (1250) series of 72 cases of pericarditis found at necropsy the complication was associated with pneumonia in the right lung in 25 per cent of the instances, with pneumonia in the left lung in 29 per cent, and with bilateral involvements in 46 per cent. In addition it usually occurred in the presence of empyema, as already mentioned, and was twice as common when the empyema involved the left pleural cavity as when it involved the right or was bilateral. Nevertheless, Stone concluded that the evidence was insufficient to decide whether pericarditis was more frequent after pneumonia on the left than on the right side.

Diagnosis is often difficult. At the daily examination of the heart all changes in size of the area of cardiac dulness should be noted. With effusions of some size the area of cardiac dulness is enlarged both to the right and to the left and distention of the neck veins may appear. Roentgenograms are of considerable aid in diagnosis. Stone (1250) regarded as the clinical sign of utmost importance a to-and-fro friction sound not transmitted beyond a limited area, usually first heard over the base of the heart in the fourth or fifth intercostal space near the sternum, and practically synchronous with the heart beat. At times the rub could be detected by palpation. Occasionally pleural rubs may obscure a pericardial rub. Stone considers paracentesis of the pericardial sac a most important diagnostic and prognostic procedure.

The prognosis with pericarditis is poor. Case fatality rates of from 75 to 100 per cent have been reported (254, 297, 830, 1324, 1385).

When the diagnosis of exudate in the pericardial sac is made, and especially if fluid is present in sufficiently large amounts to embarrass the heart, the fluid should be aspirated. Withdrawal of the fluid should be continued even though what appears to be thin blood is encountered, for at times a hemopericardium occurs.

When pericarditis is accompanied by purulent effusion due to pneumococci, surgical drainage should be considered. Special conditions surrounding each case determine whether or not operation should be performed. Truesdale's (1324) findings suggest that the most satisfactory results are obtained when the pericardium is drained by an incision through its extreme lateral and most dependent point. Such drainage offers practically the only hope of recovery, as the use of type-specific horse antiserum for the treatment of pneumococcus cases has proved of little value. In Stone's (1250) series, due chiefly to streptococci, in which nearly all cases were complicated by the presence of other serious conditions such as empyema, the patients were so gravely ill that incision and drainage of the pericardium were not attempted.

Endocarditis

Endocarditis is a rare and nearly always fatal complication of pneumonia. The literature dealing with this condition was reviewed by Preble (1050) and by Thomas and O'Hara (1297).

At necropsy after lobar pneumonia Musser and Norris (918) found endocarditis in 5.8 per cent of 2,693 collected cases. The complication was found in other series as follows:

Cases of lobar pneumonia at necropsy. Incidence of endocarditis

OBSERVER	TOTAL	WITH ENDOCARDITIS *Number*	*Per cent*
Fabyan (399)	195	12	6.1
Berry (96)	400	14	3.5
Feinblatt (406)	139	1	0.7
Lord (810)	337	14	4.2
Brooks (153)	200	14	7.0

Other reports giving figures much similar to these have appeared (1050, 882). Cecil and Plummer (239) found endocarditis in 5.8 per cent of 52 cases of pneumococcus Type I lobar pneumonia at necropsy and in 11.4 per cent of 79 Type II cases, and pointed out that the condition appears considerably more common in Type II than in Type I cases.

During life endocarditis occurred with or after lobar pneumonia in 0.3 per cent of 1,500 cases in infants and children studied by Cunningham (333). The condition seems somewhat more frequent in adults. Musser and Norris (918) report that endocarditis was recognized in 0.44 per cent of 32,349 collected cases. The findings in additional series of cases are as follows:

Cases of lobar pneumonia. Incidence of endocarditis

OBSERVER	TOTAL	WITH ENDOCARDITIS *Number*	*Per cent*
Chatard (254)	658	13	1.9
Vitug and Hizon (1357; Filipinos)	1,030	7	0.7
Rosenblüth and Block (1112)	150	5	3.3
Warr and Alperin (1385)	2,039	4	0.2

Endocarditis is commonly considered to occur in about 5 per cent of fatal cases and in about one per cent of all cases.

Cecil and Plummer (239) found endocarditis in 0.4 per cent, or 4, of 1,131 cases of pneumococcus Type I lobar pneumonia and in 1.2 per cent, or 12, of 991 Type II cases. Many of these Type I and Type II cases received specific serum treatment. Endocarditis is rare in Type III cases (230, 120). Among 633 Group IV cases reported by Cecil, Baldwin, and Larsen (230) this complication was found in 0.6 per cent.

Preble (1050) considers the condition about twice as frequent in females as in males. In a series of 23 cases of pneumococcus endocarditis reviewed by Lord (810), however, the sex distribution was about equal. Approximately two-thirds of all cases developing in pneumonia occur in patients from forty to seventy years of age (1050, 810). Preble observed that nearly one-half of 50 necropsied cases showed evidence of a previous chronic endocarditis. Not all pneumonia patients with an existing chronic valvular lesion develop acute endocarditis, however.

Pneumococcus endocarditis makes up about one-quarter of all cases of bacterial endocarditis and lobar pneumonia is the commonest predisposing cause. If the complication develops in association with an attack of pneumonia the chances are nearly four to one that it will be of the ulcerative or malignant type, but the proliferative variety may occur. The vegetations vary in size from minute to large masses, are grayish or yellowish in color, and are usually soft and friable but may be dense and firm (1050, 810). Infarcts are frequent and occur in about one-half of the cases (1050, 1297).

Necropsy studies reveal that although the pneumococcus, as with other organisms causing endocarditis, is most likely to attack the left side of the heart, it attacks the aortic valve twice as commonly as other organisms and attacks the right heart more frequently and the tricuspid valve twenty times as often as other organisms (1050). Any one or more of the valves may be affected and the lesion may involve the adjacent endocardium as well.

Irregular fever, chills, sweats, anemia, and leucocytosis are common symptoms. The duration of the fever in 132 cases studied by Preble (1050) varied from seven to one hundred eighty days with an average of thirty. The pulse is usually increased and subjective symptoms are ordinarily few. Joint pains, arthritis, and clubbing of the fingers may occur. A few cases show purpuric spots and the spleen is often enlarged and frequently contains infarcts. Infarcts in the lungs may produce alterations of the respiratory rhythm with or without dyspnea and hemoptysis, and in the kidneys may lead to pain and hematuria. An associated meningitis is found in approximately one-half of the cases.

Examination of the heart may reveal nothing of importance. When they develop under observation (810) harsh, loud, or musical systolic murmurs may be regarded as significant, and diastolic murmurs of the utmost diagnostic importance. Bacteriemia, often severe, is commonly present. The occurrence of bacteriemia after defervescence regardless of the apparent progress of convalescence is suspicious.

After the subsidence of the fever in pneumonia, its re-elevation which cannot be otherwise explained, the occurrence or persistence of bacteriemia, the appearance of infarcts, purpuric spots, arthritic pains, clubbing of the fingers, and the development of diastolic or of loud harsh systolic murmurs, all tend to indicate the presence of endocarditis. It is doubtful whether a true case of pneumococcus origin has ever recovered, but Preble (1050) reports recovery in 4 of 132 cases. Lord (810) has emphasized the importance, in making the diagnosis of pneumococcus endocarditis at necropsy, of insisting upon the demonstration of the organisms in the endocardial lesion proper.

The only specific therapeutic agent available is antipneumococcic serum. Past experience with the treatment of pneumococcus endocarditis with this agent has apparently failed to produce a recognized cure in any case. If such therapy is to be used in patients previously treated with serum during the acute stages of their pneumonia, particular caution must be exercised with respect to sensitivity to horse serum (see pages 836–842). Patients may already have spontaneously produced antibody in their blood (810) and the injection of additional immune substances appears of little or no use. In pneumonia, if serum treatment is begun early in suitable cases, there is ample evidence that such therapy will prevent or cure bacteriemia in most instances (see pages 885–886). By reducing the frequency of bacteriemia it is possible that the development of endocarditis may be avoided in some instances, although proof of this contention is as yet lacking. The use of quinine or its derivatives or of sulfanilamide or related preparations (see pages 775–782 and 783–790) and vaccines (see pages 795–804) may be worthy of trial, though probably little can be expected of them.

Meningitis

In patients with lobar pneumonia acute meningitis was found at postmortem in 3.5 per cent of 4,833 cases collected by Musser and Norris (918). The findings in reports from other sources are as follows:

Cases of lobar pneumonia at necropsy. Incidence of meningitis

OBSERVER	TOTAL	WITH MENINGITIS *Number*	*Per cent*
Fabyan (399)	195	8	4.1
Maynard (874; African Negroes)	688	72	10.5
Berry (96)	277	14	5.1
Feinblatt (406)	139	1	0.7
Lord (807)	154	4	2.5

In Menetrier's (882) series of 400 necropsies on cases of lobar pneumonia and bronchopneumonia together it was present in 2.5 per cent, or 10. In addition to the cases of meningitis observed by Fabyan in his series, 2 cases of pachymeningitis and one of congestion of the choroid plexus were found. Similarly, in Berry's series hemorrhage of the brain was present in 4 and brain abscess in one.

Among patients with pneumococcus lobar pneumonia at necropsy Cecil and Plummer (239) found meningitis in 11.5 per cent of 52 cases with Type I infections and in 12.7 per cent of 79 with Type II infections.

Clinically, meningitis was found in lobar pneumonia in 0.4 per cent of 49,028 collected cases by Musser and Norris (918). In other series the complication was found as follows:

Cases of lobar pneumonia. Incidence of meningitis

OBSERVER	TOTAL	WITH MENINGITIS	
		Number	*Per cent*
Chatard (254)	658	13	1.9
Cole (297)	770	8	1.1
Lord (807)	500	2	0.4
Vitug and Hizon (1357; Filipinos)	1,030	20	1.9
MacCordick (830)	525	3	0.5
Warr and Alperin (1385)	2,039	35	1.7

Pneumococcus meningitis may occur with considerable frequency in Negroes of low resistance (773).

The occurrence of this complication in cases of lobar pneumonia due to pneumococci of known type was reported by Cecil and his associates (230, 238, 239) as shown in Table 111. Many of the Type I and Type II cases received specific serum treatment. In the total 3,023 cases due to pneumococci, meningitis occurred in 56, or 1.8 per cent. It was present in 1.8 per cent of the Type I cases, in 2.4 per cent of the Type II cases, in 1.1 per cent of the Type III cases, and in 1.4 per cent of the Group IV cases. The incidence was highest in Type II cases. In Wu and Chiu's (1450) series of 242 typed cases, meningitis was found in 5, or 2.1 per cent. In 99 Type I cases the complication was present in 3 (3 per cent) and the remaining 2 cases occurred among 84 patients with Group IV infections (2.4 per cent). None of 45 Type II or of 14 Type III cases developed meningitis. In cases in children, which are uncommon, pneumococci of Group IV are commoner than are those of Type I, II, or III (112).

Meningitis may appear at any time during the disease or in convalescence, but usually begins during the height of the illness (297, 807). The symptoms are similar to those of meningitis caused by other pyogenic organisms. Direct extension from an infected middle ear, mastoid, or nasal sinus is not unusual. Preble (1050) found approximately 30 per cent of meningitis cases associated with acute endocarditis. Menetrier (882) also noted a similar association of these two conditions.

TABLE III. PNEUMOCOCCUS LOBAR PNEUMONIA. NUMBER OF CASES AND NUMBER AND PERCENTAGE OF CASES WITH MENINGITIS, BY TYPE

REPORTED BY	NUMBER OF CASES	CASES WITH MENINGITIS *Number*	*Per cent*
Type I			
Cecil and Plummer, 1930 (238)	1,131	20	1.8
Type II			
Cecil and Plummer, 1932 (239)	991	24	2.4
Type III			
Cecil, Baldwin, and Larsen, 1926 (230)	268	3	1.1
Group IV			
Cecil, Baldwin, and Larsen, 1926 (230)	633	9	1.4
Total	3,023	56	1.8

Lindau's (783) observations, in experimental animals, on the relation between allergic sensitivity to the pneumococcus and the severity of the symptoms incited by the injection into the basal cistern of sterile autolysates of these organisms are of interest. Guinea pigs were sensitized by the repeated parenteral injection of autolysates or vaccines made from pneumococci of Type I. Subsequently skin sensitivity to these preparations was demonstrated in many animals, following which sterile autolysates of the organisms were injected into the cistern of a number of the allergic and non-allergic animals. At necropsy the next day the resulting lesions were studied. In the sensitized animals that had shown a positive skin test, a pronounced inflammatory infiltration of the meninges was present with many leucocytes, macrophages, and some edema. Reactions of this kind were not found in animals whose skin test previously had shown them to be non-allergic. Also, and more importantly, 4 of 16 animals in the allergic group died within six to ten hours, showing a pronounced meningeal reaction, while among 24 guinea pigs in the non-allergic series no deaths occurred.

What part sensitivity of an allergic nature may play in the production of meningitis in man or in the rapid development of the lesion once it has begun is unknown. The possible relation of allergy to the inception of lobar pneumonia was mentioned earlier (see pages 240–245).

The diagnosis of meningitis can be made by lumbar puncture and examination of the spinal fluid. Cloudy fluid under increased pressure is usually obtained, showing a decrease in sugar content and a marked increase in protein and in cellular constituents. A high proportion of polymorphonuclear leucocytes are usually found. The presence of organisms such as pneumococci can be demonstrated microscopically and by culture. Any pneumococci found should be typed as specific serum is commonly used for treatment in suitable cases. Typing can often be carried out rapidly by the use of the Neufeld or of a simple precipitin method (see page 644).

The prognosis in pneumococcus meningitis is poor, the case fatality rate usually being in the neighborhood of 95 to 100 per cent. Globus and Kasanin (519), Harkavy (594), and many others have called attention to the alleged cases of pneumococcus meningitis with recovery which are frequently reported in the literature and to the lack of sufficient laboratory data in these cases on which to base a diagnosis.

Reviews of the literature in relation to prognosis and therapy have been made by Ratnoff and Litvak (1061), Carbonell and Cook (216), Globus and Kasanin (519), and others (527). These reports show that the condition is fatal in most instances, but that occasional cases of recovery are reported without any special treatment, or with varying forms of treatment.

Carbonell and Cook (216) report recovery in one case following the administration of ethylhydrocupreine and Huntoon's antibody solution. Globus and Kasanin (519) report recovery in a case with a Group IV pneumococcus infection following repeated lumbar and cisternal punctures and the subcutaneous use of a staphylococcus vaccine. Harkavy (594) reports the recovery of a Type I case following intraspinal and intravenous injections of concentrated antipneumococcic serum. Both lumbar and cisternal punctures were used in conjunction with the serum treatment. Kolmer (736) reports the recovery of a patient following repeated bilateral intracarotid injections at eight-hour intervals of concentrated antipneumococcic serum reinforced with 1 cc. of a sterile 1:100 solution of ethylhydrocupreine hydrochloride to each 20 cc. of serum used. This mixture was given both by lumbar and by cisternal puncture as well as by injection into the carotid arteries.

Recovery occurred in a case asserted by Reveno and McLaughlin (1072) to have been due to pneumococci of Type I and Type II. A total of 120,000 units of concentrated bivalent antiserum was used in divided doses over a seven-day period. Both lumbar and cisternal punctures were employed. This patient had a right-sided facial paralysis on the fourth day and paralysis of the right abducens nerve on the second day. The former cleared up rapidly and the latter slowly, over a period of two months.

Litchfield (789) and Gray (555) report 11 cases of pneumococcus meningitis with 5 recoveries following the use of Kyes' immune chicken serum (see pages 809–812). Intraspinal injections of from 5 to 20 cc. of this serum were given one to three times daily and intravenous injections of 5 to 10 cc. were given once or twice daily. The bacteriologic diagnosis of some of these cases was not clearly established. To these 11 cases may be added 16 others collected by Kyes (751), who states that of the total 27 cases, recovery occurred in approximately 50 per cent. This is an amazing record and the properties of this serum bear further investigation.

The experimental production of pneumococcus meningitis in animals has been undertaken to a limited extent, as was mentioned earlier (see page 213). Stewart produced the disease in rabbits (1229) and dogs (1230, 1231, 1232), and Kolmer in dogs (736). Rabbits were discarded as they usually died of septicaemia rather than meningitis. Stewart investigated methods of treating Type I or Type II meningitis in dogs. The most successful treatment combined lavage of the accessible subarachnoid space with intraspinal instillation of mixtures of specific antiserum and ethylhydrocupreine. The lavage was accomplished by passing sterile saline solution from the lumbar region to and out of the cisternal region by means of appropriately placed needles. Evidence was obtained which suggested that the serum thus administered penetrated fairly well around the base of the brain. Early treatment produced the best results. Involvement of the lateral ventricles of the brain did not appear until late in the illness. Recovery occurred in some of the dogs with Type I infections but in none with Type II infections.

Stewart (1230) also found evidence that dogs after recovery from meningitis possess some resistance to reinfection of the subarachnoid space. This immunity seemed chiefly of a cellular nature, for antibodies (agglutinins) were rarely found in the spinal fluid. He also reported that some differences may exist between the pathology of Type I meningitis and that of Type II.

In Type II cases an especially marked and heavy exudation of fibrin occurred early in the illness with a resulting tendency to the early development of subarachnoid blocks.

Kolmer (736) used Type I pneumococci or hemolytic streptococci in the production of meningitis in dogs. In animals with pneumococcus Type I infections, treatment with specific immune serum reinforced with ethylhydrocupreine, when carried out before the third day, resulted in a considerable number of recoveries. All animals treated after three days died. Usually treatment was begun within about twenty-four hours of infection and consisted in (a) cisternal drainage, (b) the injection into each common carotid artery of 0.5 cc. per kilogram of body weight of a mixture of immune serum or Huntoon's antibody solution and a 1:100 solution of ethylhydrocupreine hydrochloride (1 cc. of a 1:100 solution added to each 20 cc. of serum), followed by (c) the intracisternal injection of 0.5 cc. of the mixture. These treatments were repeated at intervals of about every eight hours.

As already indicated, the usual therapeutic procedure, other than the simple drainage of spinal fluid is the lavage of the subarachnoid space (a) with saline solution alone or (b) in conjunction with the injection either of a specific serum, if one is available for the type of pneumococcus concerned, or of a solution of chemicals.* At times the serum and drug are used in combination and injected into the veins or into the common carotid arteries, while additional amounts are given by ventricular, cisternal, or lumbar puncture as well, at intervals of six to eight hours. Lumbar and cisternal drainage should follow the injections into the blood stream and precede the injections into the ventricle or subarachnoid space. The earlier that treatment can be instituted, the greater will be the chance of recovery.

Repeated drainages by both lumbar and cisternal punctures are in themselves often useful for obtaining symptomatic relief in early cases, and in favorable cases are doubtless of great value in assisting recovery. Such procedures aid in removing large amounts of the accumulated plastic exudate and organisms. Stewart (1230) finds that lumbar-cisternal lavage with sterile saline solution removes great quantities of organisms which are easier to dislodge than the leucocytes, which adhere to the exudate more firmly.

* See also Finland, M., Brown, J. W., and Rauh, A. E., *Treatment of pneumococcic meningitis: A study of ten cases treated with sulfanilamide alone or in various combinations with specific antipneumococcic serum and complement, including six recoveries,* New England J. Med., 218:1033, June 23, 1938, which was published subsequent to the preparation of this section. These workers report obtaining strikingly good results in the treatment of pneumococcus meningitis.

In the absence of intraspinal block Kubie and Retan (747) suggest using forced spinal drainage. Intravenous injections of a liter or less of a hypotonic saline solution, usually about 0.45 per cent concentration, which is just above the point where hemolysis of red blood cells occurs, may be given. Following this the patient is placed on a Bradford frame and a lumbar puncture performed. Drainage through the lumbar needle can then be carried out constantly over a period of several hours. The solution injected accelerates the formation of spinal fluid and thus by increasing its flow through the needle may assist in washing out accumulated products of the infection from the subarachnoid space.

Arthritis

Purulent arthritis due to pneumococcus infection is a rare and grave complication of pneumonia. Its occurrence usually denotes a serious generalized infection. It was found by Fabyan (399) in one of 195 cases of lobar pneumonia at necropsy.

In reviewing the records of patients with lobar pneumonia Chatard (254) found purulent arthritis in 0.4 per cent of 658 cases. Howard (660) noted the occurrence of arthritis in 0.1 per cent of 4,256 cases of pneumonia collected from the European literature in 1910. Bulkley (167) reviewed the literature in 1914 and in a collected series of 12,364 cases of pneumonia (chiefly from European sources) pneumococcus arthritis was found in 17, or 0.1 per cent. It may be pointed out that although the etiologic agent responsible for most of the pneumonias in this collected series was probably never determined, the figure for the incidence of arthritis relates only to cases recognized as due to the pneumococcus. In consequence, the incidence of this condition in cases of pneumococcus pneumonia is doubtless higher than that given by Bulkley, a possibility that is corroborated by the figures in Table 112.

Warr and Alperin (1385) found arthritis in 0.2 per cent, or 4, of 2,039 cases of lobar pneumonia in general and it was present in 0.2 per cent, or 2, of 770 pneumococcus cases reported by Cole (297).

The reported incidence of septic arthritis among typed cases of pneumococcus lobar pneumonia was determined by Cecil and his co-workers (230, 238, 239) as shown in Table 112. Arthritis was found in 0.6 per cent, or 18, of the total 3,023 typed cases. It was commonest in Type I cases and was present in 0.9 per cent. The incidence of this condition in Type II cases was 0.5 per cent, in Type III cases 0.4 per cent, and in Group IV cases 0.3 per cent.

Septic arthritis may occur at any age and is commoner in children than in adults (660, 1145, 112), but the secondary form after pneumonia is probably more frequent in adults (167). It may be more frequent in men than in women (660, 167). Pneumococcus arthritis may appear with considerable frequency in Negroes of low resistance (773). From 70 to 90 per cent of all cases of this condition follow either lobar pneumonia or bronchopneumonia (660, 167). There may be single or multiple joint involvement and in about 60 to 75 per cent of the cases the involvement is single (660, 167). Any joint may be attacked, or several may be involved at once or in succession. Nevertheless, it is usually confined to a single joint and most often occurs in a large joint such as the elbow, knee, or shoulder (167, 1112, 1145).

TABLE 112. PNEUMOCOCCUS LOBAR PNEUMONIA. NUMBER OF CASES AND NUMBER AND PERCENTAGE OF CASES WITH SEPTIC ARTHRITIS, BY TYPE

REPORTED BY	NUMBER OF CASES	CASES WITH ARTHRITIS	
		Number	*Per cent*
Type I			
Cecil and Plummer, 1930 (238)	1,131	10	0.9
Type II			
Cecil and Plummer, 1932 (239)	991	5	0.5
Type III			
Cecil, Baldwin, and Larsen, 1926 (230)	268	1	0.4
Group IV			
Cecil, Baldwin, and Larsen, 1926 (230)	633	2	0.3
Total	3,023	18	0.6

In Bulkley's (167) collected series of 173 cases of pneumococcus arthritis, the condition followed pneumonia in 73. It appeared from the first to the twentieth day after the onset of the pneumonia and on the average usually began on the eleventh day. At times, however, it may not develop until as late as the ninth week. The temperature is variable but in severe cases is high. Chills and sweats may be frequent. Endocarditis, pericarditis, empyema, or meningitis not infrequently accompanies joint involvement. The general picture is usually one of severe toxemia with considerable prostration. Bacteriemia may be present.

The involved joint is nearly always hot and swollen. Discoloration of the overlying skin may not be present and pain is variable but is likely to be exquisite on pressure or motion of the joint. The diagnosis rests on aspiration of the joint and the demonstration of the organism in the exudate removed.

In serum treated cases, arthralgia due to serum sickness must be considered in the differential diagnosis. The joint involvement of serum sickness is commonly confined to the smaller joints, is frequently accompanied by urticaria and, of course, clears up spontaneously within a few days without impairment of function.

The prognosis with septic arthritis is not good. Howard (660) states that the fatality rate of such cases is approximately 60 per cent. The findings of Chatard (254), Bulkley (167), Cole (297), and Warr and Alperin (1385) are in general agreement with this.

The usual treatment when only one or a few joints are involved is incision and drainage. If a heavy infection is present through and through drainage and irrigation of the joint with saline solution, followed by tight closure of the joint and immobilization with subsequent aspiration if necessary, frequently give satisfactory results (1112, 1145, 765). Repeated aspirations may suffice with light infections, as Lejeune (773) has observed.

In the older literature ankylosis was considered to occur rather frequently after pneumococcus arthritis (167), but subsequent findings show that ankylosis is likely to be rare (1145). However, cartilage and ligaments within the joint may be destroyed. Pus may escape from the joint capsule and burrow between neighboring structures in untreated cases.

In convalescence, physiotherapy and massage of the adjacent muscles and, a few weeks after operation, passive motion of the joint followed by muscle exercises later are useful. Provided treatment is undertaken early, complete return of joint function is to be expected.

Parotitis

Parotitis is an associated condition rather than a true complication of pneumonia. In 400 cases of lobar pneumonia at necropsy Berry (96) observed it twice. Clinically, Chatard (254) found it in 4 of 658 cases, Cole (297) in 2 of 770 cases, and Warr and Alperin (1385) in one of 2,039 cases.

Cecil and Plummer (239) and Wu and Chiu (1450) reported the occurrence of parotitis in a few of many patients with lobar pneumonia due to pneumococci of known type. It was present in 5 of 1,131 Type I cases and in 2 of 991 Type II cases examined by the former workers. In Wu and Chiu's series of 242 cases due to various types it occurred once in a patient with a Group IV infection.

The involvement is usually unilateral and may be caused by the pneumococcus or some other organism. Occasionally pus can be expressed from Stenson's duct (807). Spontaneous recovery may occur but operative intervention and drainage of the lesion may be necessary.

Peritonitis

Musser and Norris (918) found peritonitis in 2.1 per cent of 971 necropsied patients after lobar pneumonia. It was also found after lobar pneumonia by Fabyan (399) in 2 per cent of 195 necropsies; by Berry (96) in 4 per cent of 400 necropsies; by Feinblatt (406) in 4.3 per cent of 139 necropsies; and by Lord (807) in 3.2 per cent of 154 necropsies. The above series consisted almost wholly of adults and in them the condition was uncommon. In infants and children secondary peritonitis after pneumonia is also uncommon and in 497 necropsies on such patients Blacklock and Guthrie (112) found only 2.4 per cent, or 12, with this complication.

Rolleston (1105) reported finding peritonitis in 0.2 per cent or 11 of 4,454 collected cases of "pneumonia" and Rischbieth (1081) found it in only 0.02 per cent, or one of 6,000 similar collected cases. The condition was described as occurring in 0.3 per cent of 8,132 cases of lobar pneumonia collected by Musser and Norris (918) and was present in 0.2 per cent of 2,039 cases in Warr and Alperin's (1385) series.

Cecil, Baldwin, and Larsen (230) have reported finding this complication in 0.16 per cent, or 3 of 1,913 cases of lobar pneumonia due to pneumococci of known type, as seen in Table 113. It occurred in 0.16 per cent of the Type I cases, in none of the Type II cases, in 0.37 per cent of the Type III cases, and in 0.16 per cent of the Group IV cases.

Secondary peritonitis is distinctly rare in adults but may be found somewhat more often in children (1105, 1081, 112). Peritonitis may of course be either primary or secondary in persons of any age. Pneumococcus cases are rare under any circumstance. Blacklock and Guthrie (112) in a study of primary pneumococcus peritonitis found it in only 1.2 per cent, or 24 of 2,000 consecutive necropsies on infants and children. Most cases reported are of a primary nature and most have occurred in young girls. In Blacklock and Guthrie's (112) 12 secondary cases, 10 were in infants under two years of age. The primary cases reported by these workers and by M'Cartney

(827) were mostly in girls between the ages of three to seven years. Struthers' (1255) findings in a few cases were similar.

All of M'Cartney's 10 primary cases were in young girls and were due to pneumococci of Type I or II. All had a bacteriemia and all showed pneumococci of the corresponding type in their vaginal secretions. This investigator demonstrated that primary cases nearly always occur in young girls, usually of the underprivileged, poorer classes, and are most common during the summer months. Such children frequently suffer from vulvovaginitis and pneumococci homologous in type with that causing the peritonitis can often

TABLE 113. PNEUMOCOCCUS LOBAR PNEUMONIA. NUMBER OF CASES AND NUMBER AND PERCENTAGE OF CASES WITH PERITONITIS, BY TYPE

	NUMBER OF CASES	CASES WITH PERITONITIS *Number*	*Per cent*
Type I	644	1	0.16
Type II	368	–	–
Type III	268	1	0.37
Group IV	633	1	0.16
Total	1,913	3	0.16

From Cecil *et al.* (230)

be isolated from their vaginal secretions. Using a female monkey M'Cartney demonstrated the portal of entry of the pneumococcus in such cases is by way of the vagina, cervix, uterus, and Fallopian tubes into the peritoneal cavity. The pathway of primary infection in young boys is not clear (112).

Including 15 cases of their own, Blacklock and Guthrie's (112) series of collected cases of primary pneumococcus peritonitis totals 72. Pneumococci of Type I were found in 53 cases and of Type II in 9 cases, making 86 per cent due to these two types. The occurrence of virulent organisms of this nature in such primary infections has been noted by others (1422, 584).

In pneumonia the diagnosis of peritonitis is made difficult by the fact that some patients may have abdominal pain from other causes, and spasm and tenderness may be present in the absence of peritonitis (4, 807, 214). Gibson (514) states that in severe forms of ordinary peritonitis the total leucocyte count is relatively low, but the percentage of polymorphonuclear leucocytes is high, while in pneumococcus cases both the total count and the proportion of polymorphonuclear neutrophile leucocytes is high. He regards this finding as of importance in differentiating pneumococcus peritonitis from appendicial and other non-pneumococcic forms of peritonitis.

A variable amount of exudate may be present. The lesion may be diffuse or localized and at times gathers and points toward the navel with the occasional spontaneous rupture and discharge of pus. Pelvic abscess may occur.

The literature contains considerable discussion as to the advisability of carrying out laparotomy in suspected cases of pneumococcus peritonitis for the sake of establishing a diagnosis or for therapeutic purposes (1145, 112, 967, 1060). While it is doubtful if any final decision can be arrived at, it is probable that operation or at least paracentesis of the abdominal cavity will have to be carried out to establish the diagnosis.

The case fatality rate even after providing adequate peritoneal drainage is reported to be in the neighborhood of 60 per cent (661, 827), but may be considerably lower in some primary cases in children (1145). With a circumscribed lesion recovery may occur following operative procedures. Any pneumococci obtained from peritoneal exudate should be typed (see page 644). If a suitable serum is available for the type found, ample amounts should be injected intravenously, taking due precautions to avoid treating sensitive patients and especially patients to whom serum was administered previously (see pages 836–842). Rappaport and Brescia (1060) gave 510,000 units of Type I serum in divided doses intravenously over a period of four days to a young girl with primary pneumococcus Type I peritonitis with recovery. Blacklock and Guthrie (112) also reported good results from serum therapy under such circumstances providing large doses were used.

Abscesses, Cellulitis, Mediastinitis, and Furunculosis

Abscesses, occurring in various locations and in various tissues including the skin, may be found in pneumonia but are not common (918, 399, 96, 297, 1385, 112, 869). In cases of pneumococcus pneumonia, pneumococci of the same type as that causing the pulmonary lesion are usually found in the abscess. At times other organisms may be encountered. Abscess of the lung is discussed in the following section.

Abscesses due to primary pneumococcus infection in the absence of pneumonia may occur in some instances but are uncommon. Moore and Brown (901) report obtaining pneumococci from a perinephritic abscess in one instance. This patient also had a pneumococcus bacteriemia. These investigators likewise made the unusual observation that cultures of the urine of 329 individuals suffering from urogenital infections were positive in 96 cases (approximately 30 per cent) for pneumococci. In each of 27 instances where the organisms were typed they were found to be representatives of Type XIV. In a few instances organisms of this type were also obtained from the blood of the patients examined and in some cases humoral agglutinins for the homologous type were found. Observations in control patients were negative. Confirmation of these extraordinary findings is as yet lacking.

Cellulitis is usually rare although Cecil and Plummer (239) report finding 32 cases among 1,131 patients with pneumococcus Type I lobar pneumonia and 17 among 991 patients with Type II lobar pneumonia. In pneumococcus pneumonia the condition is usually due to other organisms. The treatment of abscess and cellulitis is similar to that generally used for these conditions.

The occurrence of mediastinitis is ordinarily an indication of lowered resistance and is an ominous sign. Mediastinitis was found at necropsy after lobar pneumonia in 2 per cent of 195 cases examined by Fabyan (399); in 2.8 per cent of 400 cases reported by Berry (96); and in 1.4 per cent of 139 cases reported by Feinblatt (406). In 956 cases of lobar pneumonia investigated during the Massachusetts Pneumonia Study (869) mediastinitis occurred in 0.1 per cent, or in one patient. This patient, oddly enough, was a professional sword swallower. He had a Type I pneumonia which became generalized, leading to many complications and death.

Diagnosis may be very difficult and roentgenograms are often of aid. If accessible localized abscesses form they should be drained. At times great difficulty in swallowing is present.

Furunculosis is chiefly an associated condition rather than a true complication in pneumonia. It may be found in emaciated and weakened patients following a long period of illness as occurs in some cases in the presence of complications such as empyema. Cole (297) considers it an unfavorable sign and in one of his patients death occurred as a result of furunculosis.

Lung Abscess and Gangrene

True lung abscess or gangrene following pneumococcus lobar pneumonia is rare, but occurs sometimes following pneumonia due to other organisms. Loss of microscopic amounts of tissue occurring as an accident of resolution is not uncommon. Lesions of this sort are usually easily repaired in recovery but may be observed in various instances at necropsy, and larger lesions may occasionally be observed in roentgenograms taken during life.

In fatal cases of lobar pneumonia, lung abscess or gangrene was found at postmortem in 5.2 per cent, or 100 of 1,914 collected cases by Musser and Norris (918); in 4.6 per cent, or 9 of 195 cases by Fabyan (399); in 4.8 per cent, or 19 of 400 cases by Berry (96); in 0.7 per cent, or one of 139 cases by Feinblatt (406); and in 10 per cent, or 5 of 50 cases by Loeschcke (798). McSwan (853) reports having found these conditions occasionally at necropsy, and Lord (807) states that including both microscopic and gross lesions these complications were present in 27 per cent, or 14 of 51 cases examined at postmortem.

As with most other complications in pneumonia, the proportion of cases which show gangrene and lung abscess at necropsy is usually higher than the proportion of total cases which show these conditions. In typed cases of pneumococcus lobar pneumonia at necropsy Cecil and Plummer (239) observed lung abscesses in 5.8 per cent, or 3 of 52 Type I cases, and in 7.6 per cent, or 6 of 79 Type II cases. In about half the instances the abscesses were multiple and minute. In studying cases of pneumococcus Type III and Type VIII lobar pneumonia and bronchopneumonia at necropsy Finland and Sutliff (464) found that Type III cases, especially with lobar pneumonia, rather frequently showed microscopic or gross evidence of lung destruction and abscess formation.

Musser and Norris (918) report the occurrence of gangrene in 0.49 per cent of 27,761 collected cases of lobar pneumonia. Chatard (254) observed lung abscess in 1.4 per cent, or 9, of 658 cases; Cole (297) in only one of 770 cases; Lord (807) in 0.4 per cent, or 2, of 500 cases; MacCordick (830) in one of 525 cases; and Warr and Alperin (1385) in 0.4 per cent, or 9, of 2,039 cases.

The occurrence of lung abscess among typed cases of pneumococcus lobar pneumonia was reported by Cecil and Plummer (239) and by Wu and Chiu (1450). The former investigators observed it in 4 (0.4 per cent) of 1,131 Type I cases and in 5 (0.5 per cent) of 991 Type II cases, and the latter workers found it but once among 242 Type I, II, III, and Group IV cases, and this occurred in one of their 99 Type I cases (one per cent).

In most of the reports cited it is not possible to determine the exact nature of the lesions referred to as lung abscess or gangrene although they sometimes appear clearly due to accidents of resolution. It is probable that there is little or no relation between lobar pneumonia and the occurrence of true putrid lung abscess or gangrene, and the latter may be regarded as independent of the accidents of resolution and due to the aspiration of putrefactive organisms into the deeper parts of the respiratory tract. This view is suggested by the rarity with which these conditions follow lobar pneumonia, the foulness of the sputum which cannot be ascribed to pneumococcus infection alone, the probable importance of an anaerobic group of organisms as inciting agents, and the rarity with which, on careful analysis, the evolution and grouping of the initial symptoms in abscess and gangrene are consistent with lobar pneumonia. With true putrid lung abscess or gangrene the sputum eventually becomes abundant and foul. With gangrene of the lung, prune-juice or chocolate colored sputum is likely to be present. Constitutional symptoms of great severity are usual. Roentgenograms and examinations of the sputum are of assistance in making the diagnosis. Mixed infections are the rule in such conditions. At times operative intervention may assist recovery but the case fatality rate is generally high (254, 807, 1385).

Loss of pulmonary substance occurring as an accident of resolution may be considered separately. Such lesions were probably present in the necropsied cases above mentioned which were reported by Lord (807), Loeschcke (798), Cecil and Plummer (239), and Finland and Sutliff (464) and may have been present in most of the additional cases in the above series. Lesions of this nature may result from necrosis of tissue due to an impaired circulation in the area or perhaps from the effect of direct cellular injury by the organisms present, a mechanism which seems to be operative in staphylococcus cases (see pages 10–11). In the latter instance the rupture of small abscesses just beneath the pleura is instrumental in producing empyema. Evidence is lacking that empyema in pneumococcus cases has a similar cause. Possibly some post-pneumonic lung lesions with a loss of pulmonary tissue result from an excess of enzyme within the consolidated area or from a deficit of anti-enzyme in the region (Lord, 806; see also pages 97–100).

During resolution roentgen-ray films may reveal a condition typical of the usual appearance of lung abscess, as was mentioned earlier (see page 541), but which disappears in the course of a few weeks without showing other manifestations. The observations of Kessel (712) are of interest in this connection. He has described a lesion occurring in the lung in resolution which he refers to as an aputrid pulmonary necrosis. He reviewed the literature and found that the condition had previously been described pathologically but never clinically, and reported 8 cases with clinical and roentgen-ray findings. Necropsies were performed on 3 of these patients.

According to Kessel, the essential points for diagnosis are that roentgenograms taken in the latter part of an acute pneumonia or in early convalescence may show an appearance typical of lung abscess with a fluid level within the consolidated area. The sputum, however, never becomes foul or profuse, clubbing of the fingers never occurs, and spontaneous and complete recovery follows within two or three weeks. Kessel considers the lesion to result from thrombosis of an artery about which necrosis and abscess formation develop. As there is no communication with a bronchus, secondary infection does not occur and healing may take place rapidly. Abscesses of this nature are symptom free and are usually found only by roentgen-ray examination.

Gleich (518) reported a case which appeared to be of this type occurring in a child with recovery in two weeks. Among the serum treated cases of lobar pneumonia in the Massachusetts Pneumonia Series (869) a similar condition was seen in roentgenograms in an adult following a Type II pneumonia. Roentgenologists considered it a typical lung abscess. The patient never had symptoms referable to abscess formation and the lesion entirely disappeared over a period of about three weeks.

In addition, whether lung abscesses, such as those described by Graeser, Wu, and Robertson (552) and possibly also by Davies, Hodgson, and Whitby (341), which are revealed during resolution by roentgenogram and which rapidly clear up, are due to the presence of the type of lesion described by Kessel or to changes of a different nature cannot be determined with the data available.

Croupous Gastritis, Colitis, and Similar Conditions

Pneumococcus gastritis and colitis with the formation of fibrinous membranes have been observed but are rare (976, 807). Ulcerative glossitis, gangrenous stomatitis, multiple gastric ulcers, acute duodenitis, acute enteritis, hemorrhagic colitis, and intestinal ulcers have also been observed in a few cases of lobar pneumonia (399, 1385).

Rhinitis, Tonsillitis, and Laryngitis

Conditions such as rhinitis, tonsillitis, or laryngitis may accompany the onset of pneumonia or, as is much less common, occur during the course of the disease (see also pages 111–112). When they appear during the course of the illness, they are commoner in children than in adults. Cunningham (333) found rhinitis in 11 per cent of 1,500 cases of lobar pneumonia in infants and children and acute exudative tonsillitis in 3 per cent. Laryngitis with aphonia is a rare complication (661).

Conjunctivitis

Lord (807) observed conjunctivitis in 3 of 500 adults with lobar pneumonia and notes that corneal ulcers, panophthalmitis, and infiltrations of the retina may occur. Cunningham (333) found conjunctivitis in 5 per cent of 1,500 cases in infants and children.

MISCELLANEOUS COMPLICATIONS

Myocarditis

Although myocarditis is frequently present in patients dying of lobar pneumonia (399, 96, 1357, 153), myocardial changes during the illness are generally insignificant and, as already mentioned, pneumonia does not cause heart disease (see pages 492–494 and 544–546).

Nephritis

True acute nephritis is an uncommon complication of lobar pneumonia. Evidence of mild renal irritation can be obtained in a large percentage of all cases, as was earlier pointed out (see pages 503–504). The finding of pneumococci in the urine of patients with urinary tract infection is mentioned elsewhere (see page 603).

Acute nephritis at necropsy has been observed by many workers and its reported incidence varies considerably, doubtless primarily because of the varied criteria used to characterize the condition (1168). Musser and Norris (918) report finding nephritis in 19 per cent of 7,020 collected necropsies. Fabyan (399) found it in 4.1 per cent, or 8, of 195 cases at necropsy. In Berry's (96) series of 400 cases similarly examined "toxic" damage of the kidney was present in 157 but acute nephritis was found in only 4 (one per cent). Feinblatt (406) found "toxic nephrosis" in 10.7 per cent of 139 cases at necropsy and acute diffuse glomerular nephritis in one, or 0.7 per cent. In 42 fatal cases of lobar pneumonia studied at necropsy by Neale (925) cloudy swelling of the kidney was present in 17, or 40.5 per cent, and acute inflammation in 3, or 7.1 per cent. In a series of 400 cases of lobar pneumonia and bronchopneumonia at necropsy Menetrier (882) found nephritis in 4 (one per cent), congestion of the kidneys in 19 cases, and a recent infarct of the kidney in 4 cases.

Blackman and Rake (116) studied sections of 95 kidneys selected from among 4,000 necropsies on patients dying from pneumococcus lobar pneumonia or from some complication of it. In a series of young infants acute nephritis was found in 9.5 per cent and in none was it recognized before death. In older children and adults a few or a moderate number of scattered lesions were present in the glomeruli and tubular epithelium in 76.8 per cent but none had gross acute nephritis. From their studies and related observations Blackman and Rake concluded that the kidneys of young children appeared especially susceptible to injury during pneumococcus infection.

Experimental observations and necropsy studies of animals injected with autolysates of pneumococci prepared by the method of Parker (997) have revealed that these mixtures contain a substance highly toxic for the kidney (115, 114, 1398). In addition, Rake (1058) found in unselected mice infected by the intranasal instillation of pneumococcus cultures that strains of Type I gave rise to a diffuse pneumonia which was frequently associated with an acute glomerular nephritis. With Type II, a confluent pneumonia resulted and at times a tubular nephritis occurred, while Type III produced pneumonia in other forms but without special changes in the kidney.

In lobar pneumonia in man Musser and Norris (918) found acute nephritis in 1.2 per cent of 30,042 collected cases. Cole (297) reported that 0.6 per cent, or 5 of 770 cases gave evidence of acute kidney inflammation. A similar condition was noted by Neale (925) in 3.4 per cent, or 10 of 287 cases. Vitug and Hizon (1357) found acute nephritis in 2.5 per cent, or 26, of 1,030 cases in the Philippines. It was present in 1.2 per cent, or 3, of 250 cases examined by Rosenblüth and Block (1112) and in 0.7 per cent, or 7, of 1,004 cases reviewed by Seegal (1169).

In Cunningham's (333) series of 897 cases of lobar pneumonia in infants and children, evidence of marked renal irritation was found in 3 per cent and acute nephritis with edema and hematuria in 0.7 per cent.

The nephritis occurring as a complication of lobar pneumonia is always acute, generally glomerular, and rarely if ever leads to a chronic nephritis. It is also known as a larval nephrosis. Blackman (114) has shown in rabbits that there is an essential similarity between nephritis and nephrosis, for each could be produced with the same bacterial toxin (solutions of autolyzed pneumococci) when used in different quantities. The larger doses gave rise to the glomerular lesions and with smaller doses the tubular lesions and many other changes of nephrosis resulted. In the latter instance, using repeated small injections of the autolysate, it was observed that as immunity to this material developed the toxin appeared less and less damaging to the tissues and albuminuria decreased, as did the level of the blood cholesterol. Immunity of this nature disappeared after some months.

In pneumonia acute nephritis may appear between the fourth to the twenty-first day after the onset of the illness (925, 1112, 1169). The urine usually shows a large amount of albumin, some red blood cells, white blood cells, and granular and tubular casts. Hematuria may be a dominant feature. Retention of blood non-protein nitrogen occurs along with a variable loss in the power of the kidneys to concentrate urine. The urinary excretion of substances such as dyes or urea is usually impaired.

Abnormalities of kidney function may persist along with a rise in blood pressure and then gradually subside within a few to several months (297, 807, 1112). The prognosis is generally good. In children the course is usually shorter.

Phlebitis, Thrombosis, and Embolism

Phlebitis with peripheral venous thrombosis is uncommon. Steiner (1224), in a review of the literature up to 1910, collected 51 cases, to which he added 3 of his own. Numerous other cases have subsequently been reported. Occasionally pneumococci may be cultured from the clot.

At necropsy, Fabyan (399) found pulmonary thrombosis in 5 of 195 cases of lobar pneumonia and pulmonary infarcts in 6. In 400 cases at necropsy reported by Berry (96) pulmonary infarct was present in 6 and 3 showed thrombi in their hearts. In Feinblatt's (406) group of 139 necropsies pulmonary infarct was found only once. In 400 cases of lobar pneumonia and bronchopneumonia investigated at postmortem by Menetrier (882), arterial pneumococcus thrombosis was observed in 25, pulmonary thrombosis without infarct in 10 (and with infarct in 9 others), cerebral thrombosis in 5, and thrombosis in an extremity in 2.

The general incidence of phlebitis and thrombosis in cases of lobar pneumonia varies between 0.5 and 1 per cent (1224, 230, 239). Phlebitis may occur during the acute illness, but is much more common during convalescence, probably developing as a consequence of the generally weakened state of the patient. Judging from Steiner's (1224) findings, the condition is commonest in middle-aged patients and may be more frequent in males than in females. Any vessel may be affected but most frequently the veins of the legs, and especially the left femoral vein, are involved.

Local swelling and redness are likely to be present with edema and tenderness. Chilly sensations may occur and a sense of weight or stiffness may be found if the lesion is in an extremity. Death occurred in 14 of the 54 cases (26 per cent) analyzed by Steiner (1224) and in 8 was due to pulmonary embolism.

The most satisfactory treatment is bed rest and immobilization of the affected part for several weeks. In favorable cases patients should probably not be allowed to walk for at least forty days after the lesion is recognized.

Sudden death due to pulmonary embolism may rarely occur during the acute illness (807) or during convalescence (297, 807). Numerous examples of pulmonary infarcts and embolism have been reported, as is mentioned above. Embolism of the smaller arteries, while less common, has been reported (807).

Peripheral Neuritis

Neuritis may occur either during the acute disease or during convalescence, but is very uncommon. As Howard (661) states, "It may be ocular, facial, palatal, laryngeal or peripheral in distribution." The condition is regarded as "toxic" in origin (976, 807). The brachial plexus may be involved. Musser and Norris (918) observe that most young patients recover and most of the old ones die.

Wilson and Hadden (1426) and Young (1456) report neuritis and multiple neuritis as infrequent complications of serum treatment and regard them as manifestations of anaphylactic phenomena. In view of the dearth of knowledge relating to the exact etiology of neuritis and the fact that it also occurs in cases not treated with serum, caution should be exercised in accepting this view.

Tympanites and Acute Dilatation of the Stomach

Tympanites, which may be associated with obstinate constipation, is not uncommon. Its presence is attributed to the paralyzing effects on the musculature of the bowel of "toxins" produced during the infection. Marked tympanites embarrasses respiration and heart action and may endanger the life of an acutely ill patient. The treatment of this condition is discussed elsewhere (see pages 756–758).

Acute dilatation of the stomach is a rare complication. Fussell (504) reports collecting 6 cases from the literature, to which he added 5 of his own. Six of the 11 patients died. In 8 cases dilatation of the stomach occurred before crisis. Vomiting, abdominal pain, distention, constipation, visible gastric peristalsis, and collapse suggest the diagnosis. Suitable palpation may elicit splashing sounds in the stomach. The abdominal distention is often relatively sudden in onset. Nothing should be given by mouth and the stomach tube should be passed at once in almost every instance, even if the patient's condition is poor. Evacuation of the stomach contents, especially if massive and foul, may bring almost immediate relief.

Pneumothorax

Lord (807) states that lobar pneumonia may be regarded as the cause of pneumothorax only in so far as it leads to complications such as lung abscess or empyema to which the condition may be secondary. Perforation of an empyema into a bronchus or of an area of abscess or gangrene into the pleura may establish free air communication between the outside and the pleural cavity leading to a pyopneumothorax (807, 661).

CHAPTER THIRTEEN

DIAGNOSIS

General Diagnostic Features 612
Bacteriologic Study 614
  Routine Procedures 614
  Importance of Etiologic Diagnosis 615
  Relation of Clinical Aspects to Type of Infecting Pneumococcus 616
  Collection of Specimens for Pneumococcus Typing 617
  Bacteriologic Examination of Sputum 620
  Methods of Pneumococcus Type Determination 620
    Neufeld Method 625
    Krumwiede Method 629
    Sabin Method 630
    Tube Agglutination and Precipitin Methods 633
    Avery Cultural Method 635
    Urine Precipitin Test 637
    Other Typing Methods 639
  Examination of Blood Cultures 641
  Examination of Throat Cultures 642
  Examination of Pleural Fluids 643
  Examination of Material Removed by Lung Puncture 644
  Examination of Pus 644
  Examination of Spinal Fluids 644
The Leucocyte Count 645
Roentgen-ray Examination 645

GENERAL DIAGNOSTIC FEATURES

It is not always possible to separate the pneumonias clinically into lobar pneumonia and bronchopneumonia, and at times it may be difficult or impossible to do so even at necropsy. Indeed, such differentiation loses much of its former significance in view of the importance of the pneumococcus as the infecting agent in both. Although other organisms commonly give rise to pneumonia of the atypical or bronchopneumonic form, about one-half or more of the cases, as well as most cases of lobar pneumonia, are caused by pneumococci. In pneumonia in any form it is of great importance that the infecting organism be identified.

The diagnosis of lobar pneumonia is commonly regarded as one of the easiest to make with accuracy. In 1912 Cabot (207) reviewed 3,000 general necropsies at the Massachusetts General Hospital and found lobar pneumonia successfully diagnosed in 74 per cent of the cases and bronchopneumonia in 33 per cent. In 1934 a similar type of investigation was made by Swartout (1280) in 1,805 necropsied cases at the New Haven Hospital. This revealed an apparent increase in the accuracy of diagnosis in recent years, for lobar pneumonia was reported as successfully diagnosed in 99 per cent of the cases and bronchopneumonia in 87 per cent. It seems doubtful, however, if such a high proportion of correct diagnoses are obtained in the general run of all cases.

For the accurate diagnosis of lobar pneumonia, dependence must be placed chiefly upon the history, physical signs, and roentgenographic and bacteriologic findings. Nevertheless, a large proportion of lobar pneumonia cases are typical and in many of these a probable diagnosis can be made from the history alone. The history of abrupt onset with chill, rapid temperature rise, pain in the side, cough with rusty sputum, and dyspnea, and on examination, rapid, shallow respiration, dulness and crepitant rales, bronchial breathing, increase of voice, whisper, and tactile fremitus over a localized area of the chest are characteristic features of the disease. Herpes may be present. A leucocytosis and the presence of pneumococci, especially of one of the types commonly found in lobar pneumonia, give confirmatory evidence.

Pulmonary consolidation can be demonstrated either by physical signs or by roentgenograms. Graeser, Wu, and Robertson (552) searched for a correlation between physical signs and roentgen-ray findings in 40 patients with pneumococcus lobar pneumonia. As a rule, up to the period of the maximum consolidation (see page 96), roentgenograms were more accurate than physical signs in revealing the extent and character of the lesion. In all but one of 14 cases examined within five to thirty hours of the onset, though physical signs were absent or minimal at the time of the initial examination, evidence of lobar pneumonia was found by roentgenograms. These observations point to the superiority of roentgenograms as compared with physical signs as a diagnostic aid in early cases. The physical signs present early usually gave no indication of the extent of the lesion as shown by roentgen-ray films, an observation concurred in by Davies, Hodgson, and Whitby (341). Films taken soon after the onset of symptoms were of assistance in substantiating a presumptive diagnosis and facilitated early specific serum therapy in appropriate cases (see also page 645).

Pneumonias caused by organisms other than pneumococci occasionally show special features, such as the salmon pink "anchovy sauce" sputum noted by Chickering and Park (260) in staphylococcus cases (see pages 9–11). Streptococcus or influenzal pneumonias are usually atypical in onset and have diffuse lesions. Friedländer's bacillus pneumonia is usually severe, but marked physical signs may be absent. Differential diagnosis in pneumonia must rest on bacteriologic studies and the nature of the etiologic organism should be determined.

BACTERIOLOGIC STUDY

Routine Procedures

The bacteriologic study of patients with pneumonia involves the routine examination of the sputum and blood. In some instances cultures from the throat and specimens of urine, pleural or peritoneal fluid or exudate, spinal fluid, material removed by lung puncture, and pus are also examined. At times cultures from various sources such as infected joints or abscesses, or from the blood and lungs or other tissues at necropsy are likewise studied. In short, any source from which the infecting organism or substances revealing its identity might be obtained may be investigated. Such examinations afford the only certain means of determining the nature of the infecting organism without immunologic study.

Adequate facilities for the bacteriologic examination of sputum and other material obtained from patients having or suspected of having pneumonia should be generally available at all times. The laboratories supplying this service should be manned by suitably trained technicians under competent supervision.

Plummer (1027) in 1932 summarized the usual routine procedures carried out in the bacteriologic study of patients with pneumonia at the Bellevue Hospital, New York City, as follows:

1. As soon after admission as the diagnosis of pulmonary disease is made, a sputum specimen is obtained. If the patient is not expectorating, a throat swab is procured. The specimens obtained from patients with pneumonia, or suspected of pneumonia, are sent to the laboratory for examination and typing. Sputum procured from patients with chronic pulmonary disease is examined and studied microscopically by the Ziehl-Neelsen and dark-field methods.

2. At the same time that the sputum or swab is obtained, cultures are made from the blood of all patients with pneumonia, or suspected pneumonia.

3. When the first sputum obtained from pneumonia patients has not shown a predominance of Type I or Type II pneumococcus, a second specimen is pro-

cured in order to confirm the initial findings. If sputum specimens of tuberculous patients give negative findings, other specimens are obtained, at regular intervals, for microscopic study.

4. When initial blood cultures taken on pneumonia patients are positive, they are repeated daily until the procedure is no longer indicated; when negative, they are repeated every second day until the toxemia subsides.

5. Spinal fluids, chest fluids, joint fluids, and pus obtained from infected foci are obtained whenever possible and sent to the laboratory for bacteriologic study.

6. Exudate is occasionally obtained by lung puncture and then only when the sputum or swab gives ambiguous or unsatisfactory results.

Importance of Etiologic Diagnosis

The importance of carrying out the etiologic diagnosis of respiratory diseases including pneumonia has been stressed by many investigators beginning with Neufeld and Händel (936, 938). Cole (290, 293, 297, 298, 301, 302) has repeatedly emphasized the significance of such determinations, as have many other workers (260, 230, 987, 119, 582, 1027, 1067, 183, 813, 814). The course of respiratory diseases and usually the prognosis in cases of lung infection vary greatly with the organism responsible for the infection. Progress in the specific treatment and cure of pneumonia, as well as in the proper pursuit of epidemiologic studies leading to the adoption of rational measures for the prevention and control of the disease, is dependent upon determining the nature of the infecting organism in each case.

Infections due to pneumococci, streptococci, staphylococci, influenza bacilli, tubercle bacilli, and other organisms can be identified by bacteriologic means. Pulmonary infection with hemolytic streptococci leads to pathologic changes which differ considerably from those resulting from infection with the influenza bacillus and these in turn are different from the lesions incited by the pneumococcus, staphylococcus, or another organism. In consequence, if it is known at onset that pneumonia is of influenzal origin, one is better prepared to interpret persisting signs of infection with bronchitis and often destructive bronchiectasis and other lesions, as Blake (119) has pointed out. Likewise, if it is known that the infection is caused by the hemolytic streptococcus, careful watch can be kept for the early development of empyema which may require treatment while the patient is still acutely ill with pneumonia. When the staphylococcus is the cause, care must be taken in making a prognosis, as recovery is rare.

When the infection is due to pneumococci, it is important to identify the type causing the infection, for the type of pneumococcus has an important bearing on the occurrence of certain complications, is usually significantly related to the prognosis, and may be a type for which a suitable specific antiserum is available, permitting the immediate administration of serum with a resulting prompt recovery. Serum treatment seems the only means at present available of favorably modifying the case fatality rate in pneumococcus pneumonia. The serums used are type-specific in action and unless typing is carried out there is no means of knowing whether serum for Type I, Type II, or for some other type should be given. Typing should be carried out for as many of the known types as possible, and in every case for those types for which specific therapeutic antiserums of accredited value are available. Pneumonias due to infection with Type I, Type II, Type III, and many, if not all, of the higher types of pneumococcus, are specific infections, each giving rise to an immunologic response on the part of the patient which is largely type-specific in nature (see pages 49–51). This fact is of the utmost significance with respect to the use of specific immune serum for treatment.

Relation of Clinical Aspects to Type of Infecting Pneumococcus

While certain clinical aspects of pneumonia may furnish suggestive evidence as to the infecting organism, it is impossible to determine the identity of the etiologic agent by other than laboratory means. Nevertheless, the grouping of the initial symptoms in a typical explosive onset, though common to all types of acute pneumococcus pneumonia, is generally observed most often in cases due to pneumococci of Type I or Type II (Lord, 808; see also page 487).

The data available, although limited with respect to some of the types of pneumococci, suggest that representatives of most of the types may give rise to any of the various forms of pneumonia (1271, 198) and that the form of pneumonia caused by a certain type varies with the individual host. Nevertheless, pneumococci of some types, particularly of Type I or Type II and possibly also those of Type V, VII, or VIII, are more likely to be found in cases of lobar pneumonia than in cases of pulmonary lesions of other forms. In consequence, the expectation is that in typical cases of lobar pneumonia, the incidence of these types will be high. In atypical cases, such as may occur after operation, in the very young or in elderly patients, or as a complication of some chronic illness, the infection is likely to be due to one of the other types or to some organism other than the pneumococcus.

The age (557) and sex of the patient also appear of importance for most Type I and Type II cases occur in young male adults, as was previously described (see pages 60–67). Type III cases, in most instances, are commonest in patients with some chronic illness, especially females over fifty years of age (see also pages 335–336). The scanty evidence available relating to several of the other individual types suggests that most cases due to such organisms are in patients under fifty-nine years of age.

There are, however, no special distinguishing clinical features in cases due to any particular type of pneumococcus. For example, the general clinical features of Type III and Type VIII cases (464) or of Type XIV cases (187) are much the same and are similar to those seen in Type I or II pneumonias.

Collection of Specimens for Pneumococcus Typing

Under ordinary circumstances typing may be carried out on pneumococci obtained from any source. Occasionally strains found in the sputum or lung at about the time of crisis or those found in broth cultures shortly before undergoing autolysis may fail to type (24, 1153, 1298, 188). For the usual diagnostic purposes in pneumonia, sputum is most satisfactory. The character of the sputum generally reflects the changes occurring in the lung. Suitable specimens come from the deep air passages and are relatively free from saliva and nasal secretions. These generally contain some blood and tend to be thick and sticky. Usually, thin watery specimens are not satisfactory. Various workers have commented on the necessity of obtaining satisfactory specimens for typing purposes (32, 117, 33, 297, 807, 1264).

Though relatively small amounts of sputum may suffice at times, whenever possible at least one or two teaspoonfuls should be obtained. Lord and Heffron (814) state:

> The specimen should be collected in a clean, wide-mouthed bottle or cardboard sputum box and sent at once to the laboratory. Sputum receptacles should be clean, but not necessarily sterile. Inasmuch as the determination of type may depend on the presence of living organisms, no antiseptic should be added. Though the patient may have difficulty in raising sputum, a specimen can almost always be obtained if its importance is explained and the physician is sufficiently insistent. If pleural pain with cough is troublesome, morphia may be given. A hot drink may promote the expectoration. Irritation of the pharynx with a swab may induce retching and a sample may then be secured.

The very young and the old are likely to swallow sputum. In children, gastric aspiration has been used at times to obtain swallowed specimens. If sputum is not procurable, typing may be carried out on pneumococci obtained from swabs of the pharynx or larynx and from various cultures, including blood cultures. In some instances also urine or sputum can be tested for precipitins, or material removed by lung puncture or infected spinal or pleural fluids may be examined.

Gastric aspiration is apparently frequently employed by Wittes and Bullowa (1434) to obtain material for pneumococcus typing from infants and children with pneumonia. A small tube is passed down into the stomach, intermittent suction applied with a syringe, and the suction maintained while the tube is withdrawn. Any mucus or other material in the tube is then flushed into a test tube with 10 cc. of saline solution and portions of this are used for typing by the Neufeld method (page 625) or one or more of the other methods described below. Gastric aspirations are ordinarily carried out the first thing in the morning when the patient is fasting and are considered by Wittes and Bullowa to be more successful as a means of obtaining material for typing than pharyngeal or laryngeal swabs and, in certain patients with atypical lesions, to give a higher proportion of positive results than lung puncture.

Throat cultures are made by swabbing the posterior nasopharynx with a sterile swab which is at once placed in a tube containing 3 to 4 cc. of Avery broth (page 636) or plain or blood broth and sent to the laboratory. Laryngeal cultures can be made with the use of a laryngoscope and are treated similarly.

Blood cultures are taken aseptically by removing about 7 to 12 cc. of blood from some convenient vein. All but 2 cc. are at once inoculated into from 50 to 100 cc. of broth. The remaining 2 cc. are divided equally between two agar pour plates. As soon as completed the cultures are at once sent to the laboratory for incubation. A beef infusion dextrose (0.1 to 0.3 per cent) broth having a pH of 7.8 is satisfactory for pneumococcus cultures. Details of the preparation of such a broth are given by White, with Robinson and Barnes (1417).

It is of special importance that the blood be cultured in all cases treated with specific immune serum (see pages 855–858). The usual cotton-stoppered flasks are satisfactory for taking blood cultures on patients in hospitals. Blood culture medium for obtaining cultures in patients treated at home may be easily transported without contamination if placed in a four or a six-ounce wide-mouthed bottle with a cork or rubber stopper. Several thicknesses of sterile gauze on each side of a layer of absorbent cotton are folded over the top of the stopper. The stopper covered with gauze is inserted loosely into the mouth of the bottle and the whole outfit sterilized. After sterilization the stopper is tightened and the gauze fastened in place with string. The gauze covering prevents subsequent contamination of the stopper, neck, and rim of the container. In making a culture the string is untied and the stopper grasped through the gauze and removed. Blood is then inoculated directly into the medium in the bottle, the stopper with its gauze cover replaced, the string retied, and the whole sent to the laboratory. Outfits of this description (see Figure 11, page 854) were successfully used in the Massachusetts Pneumonia Study and Continuing Program (869). Outfits of similar nature should be generally available to physicians for use in patients outside of hospitals.

Where pneumococci are sought in pathologic exudates such as empyema fluids or pus, specimens of these materials may be sent to the laboratory in sterile containers. At least 10 cc. and preferably more should be sent for examination, for at times difficulty is encountered in identifying the infecting organisms in substances of this nature. Infected spinal fluids for examination should also be sent to the laboratory in about the same volume. Cultures may be made of any of these substances as described later (see pages 643 and 644).

In collecting urine for precipitin type determination, a fresh specimen of about six ounces is obtained in a clean glass vessel and sent to the laboratory. No preservative should be used.

In some instances typing may be done on pneumococci obtained by lung puncture or lung suction (1298, 797, 112, 710, 526, 188). A long sterile needle of fine bore is attached to a sterile 10 cc. or 20 cc. syringe containing a few cubic centimeters of sterile broth. Bullowa (190) advises the use of a flexible stainless steel needle four inches long (22 gauge, 35° bevel) with a medium point. Under novocaine anesthesia the needle is inserted through the prepared skin overlying the consolidated area and then, maintaining suction with the syringe and while the patient holds his breath for a moment, the needle is rapidly pushed into the lung and pulled out again. The contents of the syringe are then washed into a tube for culture and any pneumococci found are typed by one or more of the methods described below. Most investigators are hesitant to use this method of obtaining material for typing. Bullowa (190), however, reports performing more than 2,500 lung punctures. Air embolism occurred four times, persistent hemiplegia twice, some hemoptysis twenty-five times, and death within two minutes of the puncture once. He considers that accidents occur less frequently after this operation than after thoracic aspiration for pus or a therapeutic pneumothorax.

Bullowa believes that the value of lung puncture offsets its hazards, particularly in cases where doubt exists as to the nature of the organism responsible for the infection. In infants and children Blacklock and Guthrie (112) find lung puncture of little use in the etiologic diagnosis of cases of bronchopneumonia. Nemir (930) and Kereszturi and Hauptmann (710) regard the throat swab simpler to use in pneumonia in infants and children, and about as satisfactory.

Bacteriologic Examination of Sputum

In examining sputum, the color, consistency, amount, odor, and any unusual characteristics of the specimen are observed and recorded. A Gram-stained smear is made and examined routinely to determine the number and presence of organisms. Other smears are prepared and stained with an acid-fast stain, such as the Ziehl-Neelsen, and examined for tubercle bacilli.

Steps are then taken to determine the type of any pneumococci present by the methods described below, and if desirable, loopfuls of the specimen may be streaked on to blood-agar plates for incubation and subsequent observation and examination of the organisms in the colonies which appear. Organisms isolated in this fashion may be tested for bile solubility for their identification as pneumococci by washing up colonies in saline solution and setting up a test similar to that described later in the discussion of the tube agglutination method of typing (page 634).

Methods of Pneumococcus Type Determination

Several bacteriologic methods are available for determining the type of pneumococcus causing an infection. As already mentioned, these include procedures for identifying the type of pneumococcus obtained from sputum or other materials and the testing by a precipitin reaction of fluids to determine the presence or absence of a soluble substance which is probably pneumococcus specific capsular polysaccharide.

The relative merits of the various methods of typing may be mentioned. For general diagnostic purposes in pneumonia the Neufeld method (932, 933) is the most satisfactory. It is simple, rapid, and in the hands of suitably trained individuals probably as accurate as any single method of typing known (24, 1153, 86, 321, 188). No laboratory animals are needed to carry out this test. Added advantages are that the individual organisms are seen and but little diagnostic serum is required. The latter is an important item when examination is made for all the known types. If pneumococci are very scarce in the specimen examined, the chance of their being overlooked is always great, but with the Neufeld method they are less likely to be overlooked under such circumstances than with other methods. This seems especially true with pneumococci such as Type I or Type II which at times may be few in number when sputum is obtained early in pneumonia and when other types or organisms, probably contaminants from the mouth, may be numerous. Uncommonly, strains of pneumococci are encountered, more particularly among the higher types, which either fail to develop the *Quellung* reaction of Neufeld or show only slight evidence of it in the presence of rabbit diagnostic serum of the homologous type.

The Krumwiede (746) and Sabin (1146) methods of typing are also relatively rapid and are accurate (616, 239). Because many specimens of sputum fail to coagulate on heating or when they do coagulate fail to yield a clear fluid, and because relatively large amounts of both sputum and diagnostic serum are needed, the use of the Krumwiede test is limited. It may, however, be of aid in some instances when few or no pneumococci can be seen in the sputum on direct examination. Mice are not used in the Krumwiede test but must be used with the Sabin method. At times the Sabin technic may yield positive results in the typing of those few strains of pneumococci which fail to show a positive reaction by the Neufeld method.

The precipitin method of typing from the urine (33) may likewise be classed as a relatively rapid method. Its disadvantage, however, is that usually the urine of patients with pneumococcus pneumonia does not yield a positive reaction sufficiently early in the illness to be of much assistance in making a prompt bacteriologic diagnosis, which is so important from the standpoint of instituting specific serum therapy at the earliest possible moment. Nevertheless, in some instances, a positive test may be obtained at an early period and in the absence of suitable results with any other typing method. No laboratory animals are needed in the performance of this test, but the amounts of diagnostic serum required are relatively large.

The tube agglutination method of typing, with or without the associated precipitin method, was for many years the standard method of type determination and continues to be valuable for this purpose and for checking the results obtained by the more rapid methods, particularly when the latter methods fail (117, 33, 616, 86). The tube agglutination method is usually much slower than any of the procedures mentioned above and, while accurate, involves the use of laboratory animals, such as albino mice, and relatively large amounts of diagnostic serum.

A cultural method of typing described by Avery (32) in 1918 and occasionally called the "artificial mouse" method has been used to a limited extent. As with the tube agglutination method, this method ordinarily involves a delay of several hours before sufficient organisms are obtained to be tested.

A few additional methods of typing, thus far relatively little used, have been described, as mentioned below (see page 639). The Rosenthal and Sternberg (1120) method is a precipitin test which may be applied directly to sputum or pathologic exudates, is rapid, and does not require animal inoculation. The Calder (209) technic may be combined with the Avery cultural method or require the use of mice and is much slower.

As indicated above, one or another of several methods or combinations of methods are of assistance in carrying out typing with sputum, urine, pathologic exudate, pus, and cultures of various descriptions, without involving the use of animals. The Neufeld, Krumwiede, urine precipitin, Rosenthal and Sternberg, and Avery cultural methods are of value for this purpose. In addition, organisms obtained by culture and without the use of animals may be typed by the Sabin, tube agglutination, or Calder technic.

The experience of the State Bacteriologic Laboratory of the Massachusetts Department of Public Health in carrying out typing for all the recognized types without the use of animals is of interest. Records kindly supplied by Miss Edith A. Beckler, director of the laboratory, show that during 1936 a total of 1,075 specimens of sputum alone were submitted to the laboratory for typing. Of this number 489 (45.6 per cent) were typed directly by applying the Neufeld technic to the sputum and for the remaining 586 specimens it was necessary to resort to the Avery cultural method in order to determine the presence or absence of pneumococci and to establish the type of any of these organisms found. For many of the latter specimens, however, which showed pneumococci, the original testing of the specimen by the Neufeld method was not carried out for all types because of a press of work. Had this been done, the findings suggest that considerably more than one-half of the total 1,075 specimens examined could have been typed immediately by the use of the Neufeld method alone. Even so, approximately 92 per cent of all the specimens containing pneumococci of Type I, II, V, VII, or VIII were identified at the first examination with the Neufeld technic.

Where laboratory animals are needed in carrying out the typing of pneumococci, white mice are universally used. In the absence of mice young rabbits have been employed with considerable success in a few instances (Faber,

398). Intraperitoneal injections of about three times as much inoculum were given as are used for mice. Young albino rats have also been employed with apparent satisfaction (Garnham and deSmidt, 507).

The peritoneal fluid of the albino mouse acts to a certain extent as a selective medium in which to grow pneumococci. Pneumococci present in the sputum or similar material injected intraperitoneally multiply rapidly. Exudate obtained from the resulting peritonitis usually contains pneumococci in considerable numbers and these may be typed by the Neufeld, Sabin, tube agglutination, or other appropriate technic, as described below. The use of mice, however, involves the loss of many valuable hours, and in some instances contaminating organisms may outgrow the pneumococci and the latter be lost. Pure cultures of pneumococci can be obtained from the heart's blood more frequently than from the peritoneal exudate.

In the past, before typing was carried out to any extent for the higher types, the Krumwiede, Sabin, and tube agglutination methods were shown to be more than 95 per cent accurate (1264, 616). When the results of the latter two procedures were negative for Types I, II, and III and pneumococci were present, they were assumed to be representatives of Group IV. Sutliff (1264) and Bullowa (176) determined that there is an error of approximately 15 per cent in diagnosing Group IV infections in this manner, for about that proportion of cases when typed a second time were found to have Type I, II, or III infections. From many of these cases, the initial specimens of sputum examined were considered unsatisfactory. The above discrepancy in results may doubtless be attributed to the scarcity of the infecting organisms in the sputum early in the illness and to the contamination of the sputum with pneumococci normally inhabiting the mouth. The use of the Neufeld method of typing would seem more suitable under such circumstances for even though organisms are few in number they can, with the application of some diligence, usually be observed directly. In every instance, however, when pneumococci of some type other than Type I or Type II are found in the sputum or throat cultures of patients with pneumonia, it is advisable to repeat the typing on a second specimen obtained a few hours later.

The finding of pneumococci of Type I or Type II in the sputum is practically conclusive evidence that the infection is due to the type found, as these organisms are seldom obtained from the mouths of normal persons (see pages 342–367). Pneumococci of the other types, however, may be found in the mouths of many normal individuals, though some types, such as Types V, VII, and VIII, are commoner in patients with pneumonia than in healthy people.

In recent years, with the wider application of the Neufeld and other methods of typing to the bacteriologic diagnosis of pneumonia, observations such as those of Sutliff and Finland (1271) and of Bullowa (188) have shown the general reliability of sputum typing. Bullowa (188) found that examination of the sputum gave the correct type in 93.7 per cent of cases. As a rule the Neufeld method of typing alone will reveal the type of pneumococcus present in the sputum in a very high proportion of instances (Beckler and MacLeod, 86; Cooper and Walter, 321) and in the great majority of cases the organism found is the type responsible for the infection (Bullowa, 188).

Finland (445) has pointed out that in general the frequency with which multiple strains of bacteria are isolated from the patient is directly proportionate to the diversity of the methods employed in searching for the etiologic agent. Nevertheless, when one of the types commonly causing lobar pneumonia is found in the sputum of a patient with a typical lobar pneumonia, it is strong presumptive evidence that the type found is responsible for the infection. If uncertainty exists as to the significance of the organism found, the typing should be repeated on a second specimen. And further, a blood culture should be made in all cases, regardless of the results of sputum typing. Such cultures will be positive in about 25 to 30 per cent of cases of pneumococcus pneumonia, and identification of the organism in the blood will give significant evidence as to the nature of the infecting agent in essentially all of these cases. In addition, the demonstration of a bacteriemia is important for prognosis, and in pneumococcus cases treated with specific immune serum it is a clear indication that much more than the usual amounts of serum should be administered (see pages 855–858).

In addition to the equipment needed for carrying out pneumococcus typing, diagnostic serums must be available. Satisfactory serums for this purpose can be obtained from state or municipal laboratories in many communities and from several of the commercial firms supplying biologic materials. White (1415) states that standard monovalent diagnostic antiserums for Type I and for Type II, prepared in the League of Nations Center in the Staatens Seruminstitut, Copenhagen, Denmark (Dr. Th. Madsen, Director), may be had upon application to that laboratory.*

* The production of satisfactory antiserums for diagnostic purposes is described by White, with Robinson and Barnes (1417).

In some instances difficulty may be encountered in separating the immunologically related strains of pneumococci of Type II from Type V or of Type III from Type VIII (469, 464, 188). Attention to the titer of the diagnostic serum used will overcome this difficulty and usually the differentiation can be made by the Neufeld method more easily than by any other method of typing.

Schematic representations of the commoner methods of typing are shown in Figures 8, 9, and 10 (pages 627, 631, and 638). These figures were prepared for use in the Massachusetts Pneumonia Study (869). Copies of them have been distributed to pathologists, bacteriologists, technicians, and medical students and to physicians in general practice.

NEUFELD METHOD. First described by Neufeld (932) in 1902, the method of typing now bearing his name was redescribed by this investigator in association with Etinger-Tulczynska (933) in 1931 and since then has gained practically universal acceptance. It is perhaps the most rapid of all typing methods, requiring only five to thirty minutes to perform in the usual instance, and is simple and accurate. For these reasons it has proved of great value in general investigations of pneumonia and has made possible the earlier administration of therapeutic serum to suitable cases (22, 799, 23, 24, 1153, 995, 86, 321, 446, 188, 813, 869, 814). This latter advantage is well illustrated by Beckler and MacLeod's (86) findings during the Massachusetts Pneumonia Study (869), for by using the Neufeld method of typing it was possible to give an immediate report on 94.6 per cent of the specimens containing pneumococci of Type I, II, or III in which pneumococci could be seen in the sputum.

Pneumococci obtained from sources such as sputum, pleural or other pathologic exudates, cultures, or spinal fluids can be rapidly typed by this method. Whereas typing by other procedures is ordinarily done with diagnostic antipneumococcic horse serum, rabbit diagnostic serum is required to obtain the best results with the Neufeld method (933, 86, 557, 321).

To type pneumococci in sputum, a small loopful is transferred to a glass slide or cover slip and mixed directly with the undiluted type-specific rabbit antiserum. The mixture is examined microscopically after the addition of a small amount of Loeffler's alkaline methylene blue stain. Variations in the intensity of the color of these solutions may make it desirable to add a small amount of the dry stain to the standard solution of Loeffler's alkaline methylene blue if the final mixture looks too pale. A positive reaction is denoted by an apparent swelling of the capsules of the pneumococci without any obvious change in size of the organism within. Neufeld termed this the *Quellung* effect. It occurs only when pneumococci come in contact with suitable antiserum of the homologous type (see Figure 8).

The swollen appearance of the capsule may result from the deposition of antibody on it or within it. In any event the enlarged zone immediately surrounding the organism does not take stain and has a typical ground-glass appearance, while the enclosed cell body is stained and not enlarged.

The test is easy to set up but to a person unused to the method it may be difficult to read until a number of known positives have been examined. The wet preparations are examined under the oil immersion lens and constant attention to the lighting apparatus (mirror, diaphragm, and so on) and to the focus is required.

Technic. If the specimen is to be tested against all thirty-two types, nine loopfuls of the sputum are placed about one inch apart on a 9 by 2 inch plain glass slide (86). Type I antiserum is added to the first drop, and to save time combinations of previously prepared pooled monovalent antiserums are added to the other drops, flaming the loop between each transfer, as follows:

*Pool**	*Types included*
A	Types II, IV, V, and VII
B	Types III and VIII
C	Types IX, XI, XIII, and XV†
D	Types VIa, VIb‡, XVII, and XVIII
E	Types XII, XIV, XVI, and XXVIII
F	Types X, XIX, XX, and XXI
G	Types XXII, XXIII, XXIV, and XXV
H	Types XXVII, XXIX, XXXI, and XXXII

* Pooled typing serums obtained from commercial sources usually include different combinations of types from those here listed (see also page 924).

† Type XXX is now usually classified with Type XV.

‡ Type VIb was formerly Type XXVI (320).

To the second drop two loopfuls of the combined serum of pool A (Types II, IV, V, and VII) are added, and to the third two loopfuls of the serum of pool B, and so on. Two loopfuls of stain are added to each mixture and after thorough mixing the preparations are immediately covered with a number 1 cover slip to prevent drying.

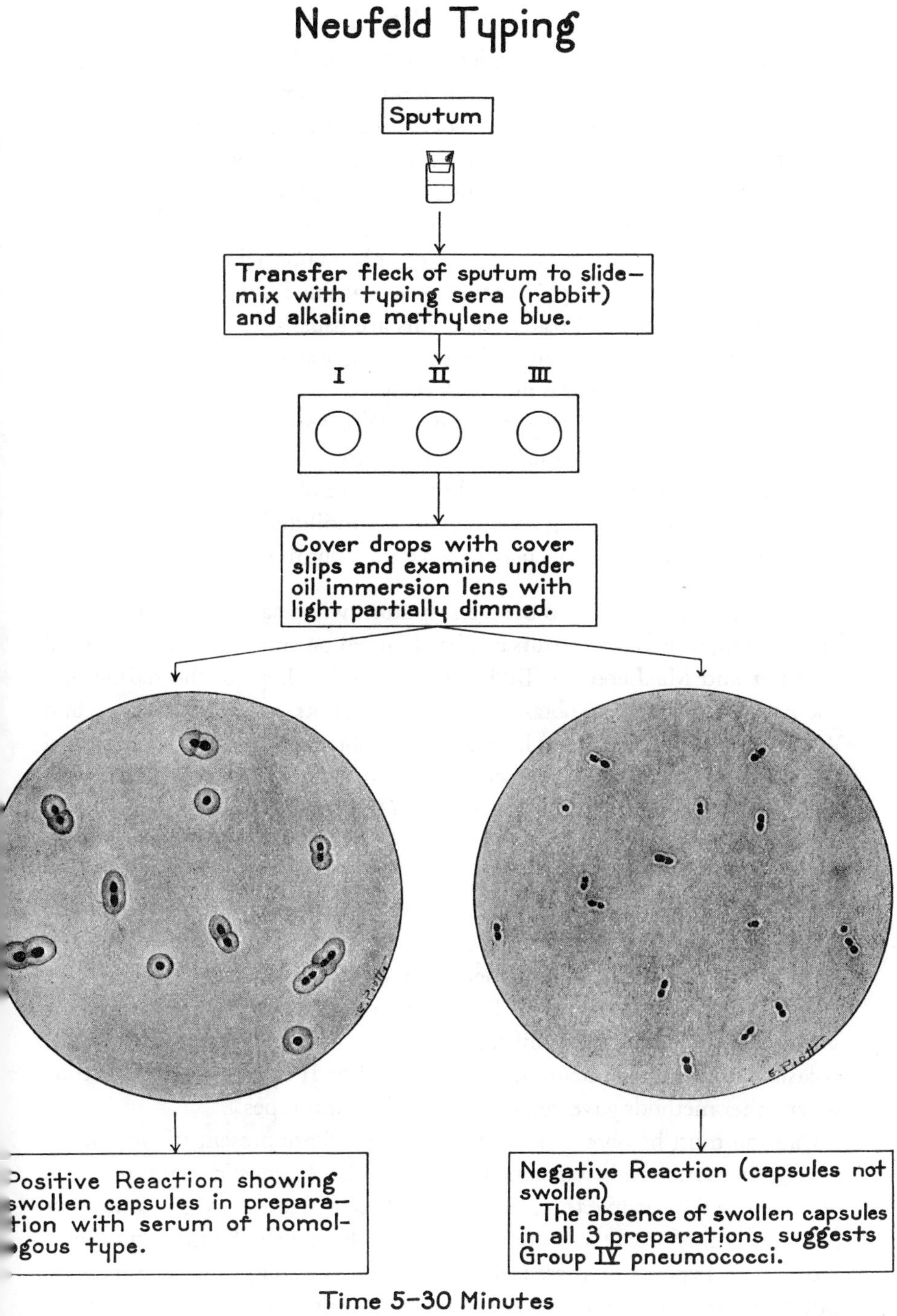

Courtesy of Massachusetts Department of Public Health

Figure 8. The Neufeld or *Quellung* method of type determination

The examination is made under the oil immersion lens with a strong light partially dimmed (diaphragm about three-fourths closed). Pneumococci are stained a deep blue color and occur in pairs or short chains. In mixtures of pneumococci and antiserum of homologous type the swollen, definitely outlined capsules present an unstained, pale greenish-gray and characteristic ground-glass appearance. By contrast, pneumococci ordinarily show no capsules or only a faint halo of light. If no reaction is evident, the preparation is re-examined after an interval of about thirty minutes. Positive reactions are usually apparent immediately, though at times when the sputum is especially viscid, the reaction may take a few minutes to develop.

A positive test in the drop mixed with Type I antiserum indicates the presence of Type I pneumococci. If the reaction is present in one of the other drops, as in the drop mixed with serum of pool A for example, the test is repeated, using two loopfuls of undiluted monovalent antiserum of each type in this pool to separate loopfuls of sputum.

Although it is desirable to use fresh sputum when carrying out typing by this method, satisfactory results can be obtained on sputum many hours old (Beckler and MacLeod, 86; Bullowa, 188) and if kept in the refrigerator good results have been obtained after two weeks or more (Cooper and Walter, 321). Positive results have also been obtained on dead pneumococci (Neufeld, 932) and on pneumococci in sputums inadvertently mixed with solutions of formalin, tricresol, or phenol (Bullowa, 188).

On rare occasions an error may be made in carrying out typing by this method. During the Massachusetts Pneumonia Study and Continuing Program (869) such errors consisted chiefly of reporting as Type III, pneumococci which later proved to be Type VIII; but also, when very few pneumococci were present in the specimen, they were sometimes not seen at the original examination, although Type I, II, or III was subsequently found by some other method. Also significant, however, as earlier mentioned, was the occasional finding of pneumococci of Type I or II by the Neufeld method when other methods gave negative results for these types.

Caution must be observed when pneumococci are present in large numbers as there may be insufficient antibody in the diagnostic serum to give a positive reaction. While this may occur in the presence of large numbers of pneumococci of any type, it appears particularly likely to happen with pneumococci of Type III. In these instances diluting the sputum with saline solution and repeating the test will usually give the desired result. The presence of pneumococci of Type III in the initial preparation examined may be suspected if precipitated material (probably SSS) having a characteristic stringy mucoid appearance is seen in the mixture. At times with pneumococci of Type V a positive reaction may be slow in developing or the swollen capsules in preparations showing a positive reaction may be difficult to detect and the outline of the capsule less distinct than with other types. As Cooper and Walter (321) state, with any type the characteristic appearance of the capsule when swollen is a more dependable indication of a positive reaction than a mere increase in size.

KRUMWIEDE METHOD. When the reaction to the test is positive, the Krumwiede (746) method of typing sputum usually yields a result within fifteen to thirty minutes. Thin watery sputums are generally unsatisfactory for testing by this method. Specimens giving the appearance of having been raised from deep within the lung coagulate more or less firmly when heated at 100° C. The liquid which escapes from the coagulum frequently contains a soluble agent, presumably specific capsular polysaccharide, which can be detected by layering it over diagnostic serum of the corresponding type (see Figure 9).

Technic. In performing the test, about 2 to 10 cc. of the sputum is poured into a centrifuge tube and placed in boiling water for ten to twenty minutes until a more or less firm coagulum results, which is broken up with a platinum loop or a glass rod. If only a small amount of fluid is present, about 0.5 cc. of isotonic (0.9 per cent) saline may be added to the tube. About 0.2 cc. of fluid is needed in the test for each type. Overdilution with saline solution should be avoided. The tube is replaced in the boiling water again for a few minutes to extract the soluble agent from the coagulum. The contents are stirred several times to assist the process. The tube is removed and the clear fluid in it decanted. If necessary, the tube may be centrifuged to throw down the broken clot. If the fluid resulting from these procedures is too cloudy it cannot be used for the test.

When testing the fluid for Types I, II, and III, 0.2 cc. of each of the undiluted specific antiserums for these types is placed in separate agglutination tubes. Horse diagnostic serum is usually employed for the test. An equal amount of the clear fluid obtained from the sputum is slowly added to each tube, running it down the side to form a layer over the serum. The tubes are then placed in a water bath at 50°–55° C. or in the incubator at 37.5° C. and observed at intervals of a few minutes, for an hour.

A positive reaction is indicated by the appearance of a definite contact ring at the line of juncture of the two fluids in one of the tubes. The occurrence of such a reaction in the tube containing the Type I antiserum indicates that the sputum came from a patient with a Type I infection. Negative tests are of no significance in indicating the type of infection present and the failure of the reaction to develop may be due simply to a lack of sufficient precipitable substance in the sputum.

Sabin method. In 1929 Sabin (1146, 1147) introduced a microscopic slide agglutination method of typing which proved very useful (1148, 177, 196, 616). As mice are needed, the time required before the test can be made is about three to five hours, but more time may be necessary. Drops of peritoneal exudate, obtained from previously inoculated mice, are smeared on a slide, typing serum and stain added, and the preparation observed under the microscope for evidence of agglutination which indicates a positive reaction (see Figure 9). As the mouse is not killed, peritoneal fluid may be obtained for testing at intervals of an hour or so if necessary. The procedure requires considerably less time and less diagnostic serum than the tube agglutination test and has the added advantage that the organisms are seen under the microscope.

Technic. In carrying out either the Sabin or tube agglutination methods of typing with materials such as sputum, a mouse is inoculated according to the following procedure.

When sputum is used, a bean-sized kernel is washed in three or four changes of sterile isotonic (0.9 per cent) saline solution to remove surface contamination. The sputum is then ground in a sterile mortar. If necessary, 1 or 2 cc. of saline may be added, and 0.5 to 1 cc. of the emulsion is injected intraperitoneally into a white mouse.

Three to five hours later a part of the abdomen of the mouse is cleaned with alcohol and the peritoneal cavity punctured through this area with a sterile needle attached to a sterile hypodermic syringe or with a sterile capillary pipette. Clear, turbid exudate or no exudate may be obtained. To procure the turbid exudate needed, manipulation of the syringe or pipette may be necessary. The material obtained is placed in a small tube from which drops may be transferred with a loop to a slide.

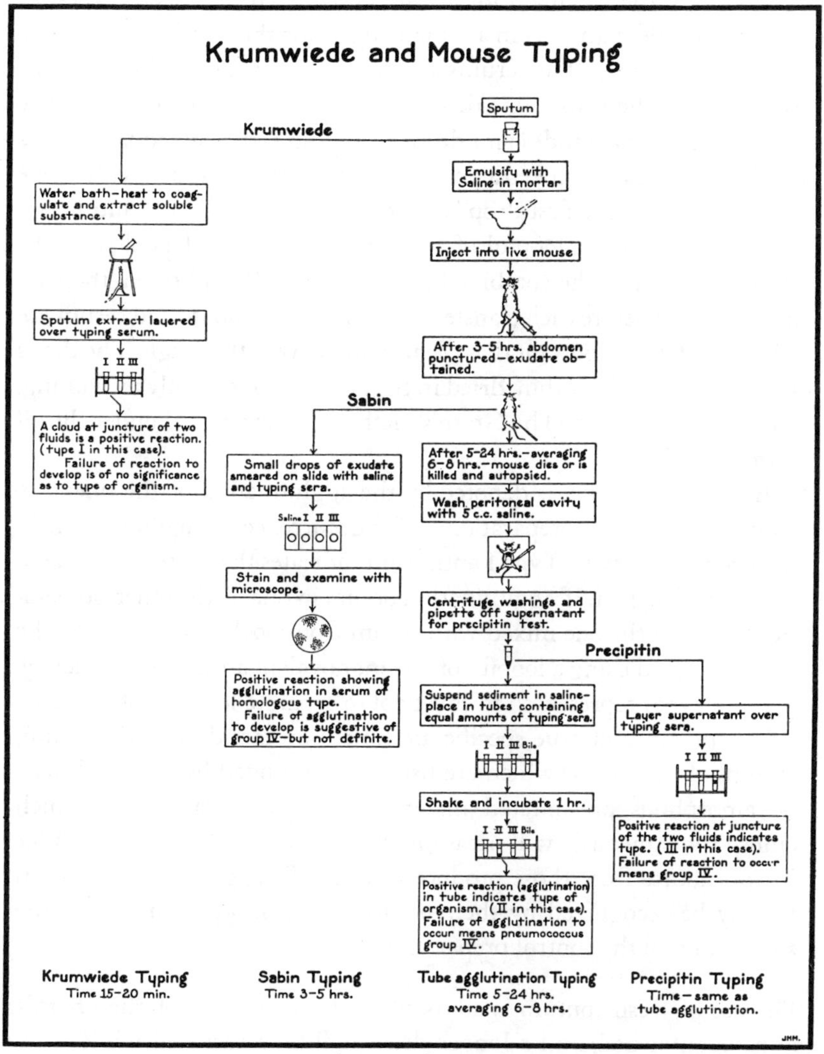

Courtesy of Massachusetts Department of Public Health

Figure 9. The Krumwiede, Sabin, tube agglutination, and precipitin methods of type determination

In testing the specimen for all the known types, pools of type-specific monovalent antiserum are made up as for the Neufeld method of typing (page 626). The serums are diluted according to directions accompanying the vials. Nine drops of peritoneal exudate of equal size are placed on glass slides and drops of typing serum of equal size are added. If desirable, an extra drop of exudate can be mixed with saline as a control. To the first drop is added a loopful of Type I antiserum, to the second drop a loopful of the combined serum of pool A, to the third a loopful of the combined serum of pool B, and so on, the loop being flamed before each transfer. The drops of exudate and serum are stirred and it is important that the mixing be very thorough. The drops are then smeared out thin, dried in the air, and fixed gently by flaming. The smears are stained by Gram's method and examined under the oil immersion lens.

A positive reaction is denoted by the agglutination of the pneumococci in one of the preparations. The occurrence of agglutination in the drop mixed with Type I antiserum indicates the presence of pneumococci of Type I. If agglutination occurs in one of the other preparations, such as the one mixed with serum from pool A for example, the test is repeated using a loopful of the monovalent antiserum of each of the four types represented in this pool to separate loopfuls of exudate.

The presence of true specific agglutination is indicated by finding clumps of organisms which are usually surrounded by a stained mass of amorphous precipitated material. Groups of organisms which clump spontaneously will occasionally be seen. These, however, differ in appearance from those produced by specific agglutination and can usually be recognized by their occurrence in more than one of the smears and in the control preparation.

The use of fresh sputum is advisable; otherwise some of the organisms may have autolyzed, and a longer delay will be occasioned while waiting for growth. It may be necessary to repeat the test at intervals of an hour or so if too few organisms are present to obtain satisfactory results.

In the case of pneumococci of Type III, Sabin (1147) finds that sufficient organisms for a microscopic slide agglutination test may be present as early as two hours after mouse inoculation. The appearance of the specific reaction with Type III differs somewhat from that obtained with other types. This is attributed primarily to the larger size of the capsule of the organism.

The clumps appear larger and the organisms farther apart or in mucoid strings. Mouse peritoneal exudate containing Type III pneumococci is nearly always mucoid and stringy.

TUBE AGGLUTINATION AND PRECIPITIN METHODS. Mice are required in performing the tube agglutination method of typing and the same mouse used for the Sabin method may also be used in this test (see Figure 9). Usually macroscopic tube agglutination can be carried out from five to twenty-four hours after mouse inoculation. It can be done at any time before, should the mouse die, but the average time required is about six to eight hours. So long a delay is a distinct handicap in early diagnosis and specific treatment, yet at times, when the sputum contains few pneumococci, type determination may not be possible until after such an interval is allowed for growth of the organisms.

Technic. The technic of mouse inoculation is the same as that used in preparation for the Sabin test (see page 630). Following inoculation the mouse should be killed (chloroformed) and necropsied as soon as it becomes very sick or when Gram-stained smears of its peritoneal exudate obtained by capillary pipette puncture show numerous organisms per high-power field. If allowed to live until death occurs, contaminating organisms may overgrow any pneumococci present.

To obtain the exudate necessary for the test, the mouse is necropsied and the peritoneal cavity opened aseptically. One-half of a blood-agar plate is streaked with peritoneal exudate and, if this has not been done previously, a smear is made for staining by Gram's method. The peritoneal cavity is rinsed with 4 or 5 cc. of sterile saline solution and the washings collected in a centrifuge tube. The heart is exposed aseptically and a loopful of heart's blood is streaked on the other half of the blood-agar plate for subsequent incubation if desirable, as described below.

The tube containing the washings is centrifuged four or five minutes at low speed to throw down the leucocytes and other cells present, which are discarded. The supernatant is decanted into a second tube and centrifuged at high speed for twenty to thirty minutes to throw down the organisms, following which the supernatant fluid is drawn off or decanted and saved for the precipitin test. The sediment is reserved for the agglutination test.

A. Agglutination test. The sediment is diluted with saline solution to the density of a moderately heavy suspension of organisms (about similar to the density of an eighteen-hour broth culture). In carrying out the test for Types I, II, and III, 0.2 cc. of the suspension of organisms is added to agglutination tubes, each containing 0.2 cc. of Type I, II, or III diagnostic antiserum, both diluted and undiluted, according to the directions accompanying the vials of typing serum. Horse diagnostic serum is generally used. To a similar tube is added 0.4 cc. of the suspension of organisms and 0.1 cc. of sterile ox bile. The tubes are placed in a rack and shaken thoroughly and removed to a water bath at 50°–55° C. or the incubator at 37.5° C. They are observed and the findings recorded at the end of fifteen minutes', thirty minutes', and one hour's incubation. If the reaction is not definite incubation is continued for two hours.

A positive reaction is indicated by the appearance of gross agglutination in one of the tubes containing diagnostic serum. The occurrence of agglutination in a tube containing Type I serum indicates the presence of pneumococci of Type I. Atypical Type II pneumococci may agglutinate in the presence of Type II serum. This difficulty may usually be overcome by using the dilutions recommended in the directions accompanying the vial of Type II diagnostic serum. Such atypical Type II pneumococci are frequently representatives of Type V and may be tested against serum of that type if any is at hand.

If specific agglutination fails to appear in any tube and the bile clears, the results indicate the presence of pneumococci of some other type. Additional tests can be carried out in similar fashion for any number of the remaining types, providing the appropriate diagnostic serums and sufficient exudate are available.

B. Precipitin test. The precipitin test requires only a few minutes after the exudate is obtained. It is useful for confirming the results of type determinations by other methods, and is of special value where the mouse peritoneal exudate contains many contaminating organisms, which may interfere with a specific agglutination test (117). A positive reaction is presumably due to the presence of pneumococcus specific capsular polysaccharide in the exudate, which precipitates when in contact with antiserum of the homologous type (see Figure 9).

The clear supernatant fluid from the second centrifuging, as described above, is used. In testing for Types I, II, and III, 0.2 cc. of undiluted diagnostic antiserum is added to each of three small tubes. Horse diagnostic serum is ordinarily used. Type I antiserum is added to the first tube and 0.2 cc. of the clear supernatant fluid is layered over it. To the second tube, Type II serum and supernatant fluid are added and to the third, Type III serum and supernatant fluid.

A positive reaction is denoted by the appearance, either immediately or within a few minutes, of a cloudy ring at the juncture of the serum and the supernatant in one of the tubes, the other tubes remaining clear. Incubation is usually not necessary. The occurrence of a positive reaction in the tube containing the Type I antiserum is indicative of the presence of Type I specific substance. If the reaction develops in the tube with Type II or Type III serum, the presence of those types, respectively, is indicated. The test can be carried out in similar fashion for any of the higher types, providing diagnostic serums for those types and sufficient supernatant fluid are available.

C. Cultures from mouse. As mentioned above, one-half of a blood-agar plate is streaked with peritoneal exudate and the other half with the heart's blood of the inoculated mouse. If advisable or desirable to check the type determined by the tube agglutination or precipitin test, the blood-agar plate is incubated at 37.5° C. Colonies can then be fished from the plate for subculturing, typing, and storage, if required. In the latter instance, subcultures made in blood broth or on a blood-agar slant, incubated four to six hours at 37.5° C. and stored in the refrigerator, will prove satisfactory (see also page 21).

For checking the results of previous type determinations by the use of blood-agar plate cultures, a few drops of saline solution are poured on to the surface of a freshly incubated plate and the colonies washed up in it. Typing may be carried out on the organisms in the resultant suspension by applying the Neufeld, Sabin, or tube agglutination technic. When such checking is carried out with organisms stored in blood broth, fresh subcultures are made and incubated. Typing may be done by the Neufeld, Sabin, or tube agglutination technic.

AVERY CULTURAL METHOD. The Avery cultural method (32, 87) is valuable for carrying out typing without the use of mice. The method was evolved by Avery (32) during the War, when mice were almost unobtainable. It proved of considerable aid at the time (219, 829, 1351, 1295, 1350, 985) and has been employed intermittently since then (86).

Avery's (32) original method called for the inoculation of sputum into glucose blood (rabbit) broth, incubation, removal of the pneumococci by centrifuging, and either typing them by the macroscopic tube agglutination method or dissolving them in bile and setting up a precipitin test with the bile solution and diagnostic serums. The addition of glucose or dextrose and rabbit blood to the medium accelerates the initial growth of pneumococci. Many modifications of the above method have been used. The procedures described below have proved satisfactory.

Technic. A selected bean-sized kernel of sputum is washed in three or four changes of sterile saline and ground in a sterile mortar with 0.5 to 1 cc. of broth; 0.5 cc. of the mixture is then inoculated into a centrifuge tube containing 4 cc. of special medium. The special medium used is a beef infusion broth, pH 7.8, containing 0.3 per cent dextrose and from 2 to 5 per cent of sterile defibrinated rabbit, horse, or sheep blood. Rabbit blood is probably preferable. Medium of this composition is frequently referred to as Avery broth. The tube is shaken, and incubated three to six hours at 37.5° C. A subculture is made from this by streaking a loopful of the broth on to a blood-agar plate, from which a pure culture may later be obtained for confirmation of the type found.

Various tests may now be applied to the contents of the tube. If organisms are numerous, loopfuls of the culture may be mixed directly with diagnostic antiserum and typing carried out as described above under the Neufeld method (page 625). If few organisms are present, it may be necessary to use the sediment of a centrifuged specimen.

When contaminating organisms are not so plentiful as to mask the reaction, typing can be done by either the microscopic or macroscopic agglutination method. The tests may be performed directly with the culture or the tube may be centrifuged two minutes at low speed to throw down the blood cells, the supernatant fluid transferred to a second tube which is centrifuged at high speed to throw down the organisms, and the tests made on a suspension of the bacterial sediment. In carrying out microscopic agglutination, small drops of the suspension of organisms are mixed on a slide with diagnostic antiserums, dried, stained, and examined, as described under the Sabin test above (page 630). For macroscopic agglutination the bacterial suspension is mixed with typing serums in small tubes, as mentioned under the agglutination technic above (page 633).

Precipitin tests can also be made with supernatant fluid from a second centrifuging of the bacterial suspension, as described above under the precipitin test (page 634). If many contaminating organisms are present, a second type of precipitin test may be of value. After the culture is centrifuged at low speed to throw down the blood cells, the supernatant fluid is drawn off or decanted into another centrifuge tube containing 1 cc. of sterile ox bile and incubated twenty minutes at 37.5° C. to dissolve the pneumococci. Contaminating organisms may then be removed by centrifuging and the supernatant bile solution used for the test by layering 0.2 cc. amounts over equal volumes of diagnostic serums.

False precipitin reactions may occasionally occur and it is advisable to check positive findings of this method by carrying out the typing of any pneumococci present by some other means. Broth subcultures of the plate previously inoculated can be used as the source of organisms.

Urine precipitin test. When it is being tested for specific substance, the urine is layered over diagnostic serum in small tubes (see Figure 10) and observed for the appearance of a precipitin reaction at the juncture of the two fluids (363, 33, 1010). A positive test indicates the presence in the urine of pneumococcus specific capsular polysaccharide given off during the growth of the organism in the body. In most instances, the reaction is negative early in the disease, thus restricting the usefulness of the test. At times, however, the test will be positive as early as the first or second day and will thus allow an immediate type determination. The urine test is also useful in confirming the results of typing carried out by other methods.

The test is simple, requiring only a few minutes to set up, and may be repeated as often as indicated. It is of value in some cases in the absence of results by other typing methods. If the initial test is unsatisfactory the urine may be concentrated (33, 1010) and the test repeated. Negative tests are of no diagnostic importance. Positive tests of increasing intensity are of prognostic significance (see page 693).

Technic. To test unconcentrated urine, a specimen is cleared of débris by centrifuging at high speed for a few minutes and the supernatant fluid layered in 0.2 cc. amounts over equal volumes of undiluted diagnostic antiserums in agglutination tubes, the serum of each type being placed in a separate tube. A positive reaction is denoted by the appearance of a precipitate at the line of juncture of the urine and antiserum. The intensity of the reaction may vary from an almost im-

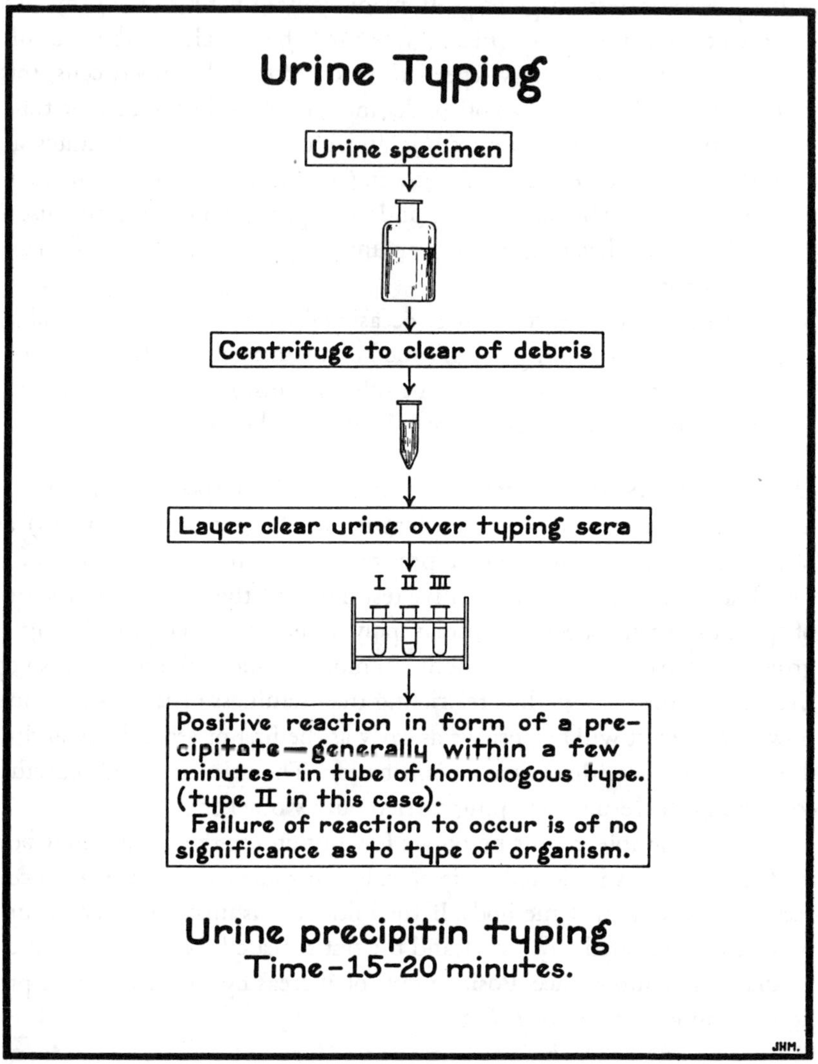

Courtesy of Massachusetts Department of Public Health

Figure 10. The urine precipitin method of type determination

perceptible cloud to a heavy flocculent precipitate, and may appear at once or within an hour's incubation at 37.5° C. The tubes should be observed frequently. Bacterial growth may obscure the test if the incubation is prolonged.

To concentrate urine for the test, 2 or 3 drops of glacial acetic acid are added to about 25 cc. of urine, preferably from a twenty-four-hour specimen, and boiled down to about 5 cc. over a free flame, after which it is filtered through paper to remove any precipitate. The filtrate is added to 8 to 10 volumes of 95 per cent alcohol, centrifuged to collect the precipitate which forms, and dried rapidly to remove the excess alcohol. The residue is extracted with 2 or 3 cc. of saline solution which redissolves the specific substance and the solution cleared by centrifuging. The test is set up as described above, using the cleared supernatant fluid in place of urine.

The above procedures were outlined by Dochez and Avery (363) and by Avery, Chickering, Cole, and Dochez (33) in their studies of the urine test. Subsequently the matter was further investigated by Pepper (1010) who devised two new methods of concentrating urine and reported that a theoretical loss of about 50 per cent of the precipitable substance occurred when either of his methods was employed. Pepper's methods, however, permitted obtaining a fivefold to tenfold concentration of the precipitable substance in the urine.

The first of Pepper's methods was an ultrafiltration procedure using collodion sacks in which to dialyze the urine. The specific substance is retained in the sack. Thirty cubic centimeters of urine may be reduced to 3 cc. in eight to fifteen hours by using a negative pressure of about 100 mm. of mercury and a precipitin test set up with the solution remaining in the dialyzing bag. In the second method, 30 cc. of cleared urine are evaporated to dryness at 70° C.; the residue dissolved in water and cleared by filtering. The tests are set up in the usual manner, using the clear filtrates.

OTHER TYPING METHODS. As early as 1910 attempts were made by Neufeld and Händel (938) to devise a rapid method of identifying certain varieties of pneumococci. Mice were inoculated intraperitoneally with sputum and three hours later with 1 cc. of antipneumococcic serum. Necropsy was performed after a further interval of about an hour. The phagocytic cells of the peritoneum and the liver and other organs were examined for ingested pneumococci which, if found, indicated that the pneumococcus in the sputum was homologous in type with that of the serum injected. The results were equivocal and the method was little used.

In recent years, numerous efforts, some of which will be mentioned here, have been made to reduce the time required for carrying out typing (784). Using Sabin's technic for the abdominal puncture of mice inoculated with sputum four hours earlier, Armstrong (22) applied the Neufeld method of typing to pneumococci obtained from peritoneal exudate. Logan and Smeall (799) also used this procedure and considered it easier and superior to other rapid methods. Subsequently, however, these workers altered their technic and carried out the Neufeld method directly on the sputum.

A relatively simple precipitin method of typing directly from the sputum was devised by Rosenthal and Sternberg (1120).

Technic. From 1 to 3 cc. of sputum are placed in a small test tube. About an equal amount of a borax-boracic acid mixture (borax 15 gm., boracic acid 15 gm., and water 100 cc.) is added to this, drop by drop, and stirred with a glass rod until a homogeneous mixture results. The amount of the borax-boracic acid solution required varies somewhat with the character of the sputum. Following this, 0.25 to 0.5 cc. of 3 per cent hydrogen peroxide is added and the mixture stirred again. After centrifuging at high speed for two or three minutes, the mixture separates into three layers. Solid material collects at the bottom and a foamy pellicle forms at the top. The zone of fluid between these two layers may be clear or of varying degrees of cloudiness. This middle layer is poured through the foam at the top into a small tube and centrifuged at high speed for five minutes. The bottom of a Petri dish is then covered with wet cotton to supply moisture, and on this are placed two wooden applicator sticks about two inches apart to serve as supports for a slide. In examining for Types I, II, and III a slide is marked off into three divisions labeled I, II, and III and a drop of the appropriate diagnostic antiserum is placed on each of the corresponding sections. To each drop, a drop of the clear supernatant fluid from the second centrifuging is added with a glass rod. The slide is placed on the supporting sticks in the Petri dish, and the dish covered and set in the incubator at 37.5° C. At ten-minute intervals the drops are examined under the microscope (low power) for flocculation. The reaction may occur almost at once or within ten to sixty minutes.

The occurrence of a positive reaction is denoted by the appearance of masses of flaky precipitated material in one of the preparations. The absence of flocculation in any of the drops is of no significance, as the failure of the reaction to develop may be due only to a lack of sufficient soluble precipitin (presumably specific capsular polysaccharide) in the sputum. A positive reaction, however, is of definite significance (86). Empyema fluids may also be typed by this method. No mice and only relatively small amounts of diagnostic serum are needed.

Calder (209) has described an agglutination method of typing employing organisms obtained from the peritoneal exudate of mice previously inoculated with sputum or those obtained by the use of the Avery method.

Technic. In either instance, after centrifuging at low speed to remove the various blood and body cells, the supernatant fluid is again centrifuged in a second tube and at high speed, to throw down the organisms. Blood cultures may be treated in similar fashion. Drops of the sediment of organisms are transferred to individual cover slips lightly stained with gentian violet. Diagnostic serum is then added, a drop of each type to each cover slip, and mixed with the organisms. The cover slips are inverted over the trough of a hollow-ground glass slide, rimmed with vaseline, and placed in a small shaking machine suspended by springs. The machine is operated by the motor of an electric buzzer. Five minutes' shaking is usually sufficient to give readable results and the preparations are examined under the microscope for agglutination.

Calder reports good results with this method and as incubation is unnecessary it is apparently more rapid than the tube agglutination method. The procedure may be carried out without mice and is economical of serum.

Examination of Blood Cultures

Broth blood cultures are observed after about eight to twelve hours' incubation at 37.5° C. If bacterial growth is not evident, incubation is continued and the culture observed at intervals for at least seventy-two hours, and preferably for seven days (33). In positive broth blood cultures the supernatant fluid ordinarily shows a diffuse turbidity and on agitation the mixture appears brownish-red to chocolate in color. Usually a sufficient number of organisms is present, as shown by a Gram-stained smear of the culture, so that the Neufeld technic may be applied directly to loopfuls of the culture and typing carried out immediately without centrifuging. If pneumococci are few in number, it is advisable to remove 10 cc. of the medium to an appropriate tube with a sterile pipette and centrifuge at low speed to remove the blood cells. The supernatant fluid is poured into a second tube and centrifuged at high speed to throw down the organisms. If desired, the clear supernatant fluid may be saved and used for a precipitin typing as described above (page 634). A saline suspension is made of the remaining sediment of organisms which may be typed by the Neufeld (page 625), Sabin microscopic agglutination (page 630), tube agglutination (page 633), or Calder method.

Blood-agar pour plates are incubated twelve to eighteen hours at 37.5° C. and examined for the number of colonies per plate. Any pneumococci present may be typed by subculturing them into broth and using the organisms so obtained; or a small amount of saline may be added to the plate and used to make a suspension of the organisms which can be immediately typed by the Neufeld or Sabin microscopic agglutination method.

Examination of Throat Cultures

The swab used in culturing the posterior nasopharynx or larynx is at once placed in a tube containing 3 to 4 cc. of Avery broth (page 636) or if this is not available, blood broth or plain broth. Vinograd, Nemir, and Park (1354) point out that valuable time may be saved by removing the particles of sputum by whirling the stick rapidly back and forth in the broth, centrifuging the suspension at high speed, and applying the Neufeld technic (page 625) to the sediment. If this procedure is not used, the culture is incubated three to five hours at 37.5° C. Loopfuls are transferred to a slide and any pneumococci present typed by the Neufeld technic. If the type cannot be determined by this method, about 1 cc. of the culture is injected into the peritoneal cavity of a mouse and typing subsequently carried out by the Neufeld, Sabin (page 630), or tube agglutination method (page 633).

The reliability of throat swabs as a means of identifying the etiologic agent in pneumococcus pneumonia has been investigated somewhat extensively. Kelly and Gussin (709) found the method satisfactory and successful results have been reported in from 73 (188) to 88 per cent of cases (1029, 1057, 112, 930, 710, 1354). It is always advisable, however, when typing is done from throat cultures, to confirm the findings by repeating the procedure on a second specimen obtained some hours later. Throat or laryngeal cultures are most often used to obtain organisms for typing from infants and children with pneumonia. In Kereszturi and Hauptmann's (710) series, it required from six hours to two days with an average of one and four-tenths days to type children by the use of throat cultures. In 75 per cent of their cases results were successful with a single culture and in the remainder additional cultures were necessary.

At times more than one organism may be obtained from a throat culture and repeated throat cultures, blood cultures, and urine precipitin tests may be needed to determine the infecting organism (see also pages 11–16). In infants and children there is an added disadvantage with respect to the latter two tests, however, for in such individuals positive blood cultures are less frequently found and the urine less often contains specific precipitable substance than in adults.

Examination of Pleural Fluids

The gross character of pleural fluids, whether serous, serofibrinous, hemorrhagic, or purulent should be recorded (808). If sufficient amount is available, the specific gravity is taken. As a rule the specific gravity of transudates is relatively low (1.010 to 1.015) and that of exudates higher (1.018 or above). Direct microscopic examination of the fluids by the Neufeld method (page 625) should be made at once. If the type cannot be determined in this fashion, cultures of the fluids should be made immediately and before they have stood for several hours at room temperature. Such cultures are best made on blood-agar plates or in Avery (page 636) or blood broth (page 618) by adding to the media a few drops of the fluid from the syringe used for the thoracic puncture. Cultures incubated anaerobically will occasionally yield a growth of pneumococci when aerobic cultures fail to do so. Thin smears of the fluid should be examined for organisms by Gram stain, for tubercle bacilli by an acid-fast stain, and for blood cells by Wright's stain (1166).

Immediate microscopic examination should be made of serofibrinous fluids as spontaneous coagulation is likely to occur and enmesh any cells present, remove them from the fluid, and render the results of subsequent examinations faulty. If the examination cannot be made at once, coagulation may be prevented by adding to the fluid an equal volume of one per cent sodium citrate in 0.85 per cent saline solution. Both red and white blood cell counts are desirable on bloody fluids. Lord (808) states that the finding by differential white counts of a predominance of polymorphonuclear neutrophile leucocytes in serofibrinous fluids may, in general, be regarded as an indication of a severe infection. An excess of lymphocytes in exudative fluids may indicate a less intense inflammation.

Purulent exudates should be cultured in the usual way, as described above. Smears should be examined for organisms. Any pneumococci found should be typed. Should no organisms be found in smear or culture, the empyema may be tuberculous and a guinea pig should be inoculated under the skin with a small amount of the fluid.

The precipitin test (page 634) affords a simple and rapid means of determining the type of pneumococcus present if the supernatant fluid of a centrifuged specimen is clear (117, 33). The supernatant fluid is layered over diagnostic antiserum and observed at intervals for a positive reaction. The Rosenthal and Sternberg technic (page 640) may also be of use as a precipitin method of typing purulent exudates. The results of the determination of types by these methods may be checked later by typing the organisms obtained from cultures or mouse inoculation by the Neufeld (page 625), Sabin slide agglutination (page 630), or tube agglutination technic (page 633).

If pneumococci can be seen easily in smears, they may be typed by placing loopfuls of the exudate on a slide and adding diagnostic antiserums as described above under the Neufeld technic. The Sabin microscopic slide technic may also be used if organisms are plentiful. Pneumococci obtained from the cultures made may likewise be typed by these methods or by the tube agglutination method. If desirable, and if no organisms are seen in smears, it is advisable to centrifuge a portion of the material at high speed for thirty minutes, suspend the sediment in saline, and inoculate a mouse (page 630) or an Avery culture (page 635) with it. Typing can be subsequently carried out on any pneumococci obtained by these procedures.

Examination of Material Removed by Lung Puncture

Cultures of material removed by lung puncture are examined in much the same manner as throat cultures (see page 642). It is usually necessary, however, to incubate cultures of this nature for several hours before pneumococci become sufficiently numerous to proceed with typing.

Examination of Pus

Pus is examined in the same manner as are purulent exudates mentioned above. Cultures of any pathologic exudates may be accorded treatment similar to that used in the examination of blood cultures (page 641).

Examination of Spinal Fluids

Gram-stained smears of the spinal fluid should be examined for the presence of pneumococci. If the fluid is heavily infected a Neufeld test (page 625) is set up at once. A precipitin test may be made for confirmation using a technic similar to that already described (page 634). If many pneumococci are present, drops of the fluid may be transferred to a slide and typing also carried out by the Sabin microscopic technic (page 630).

In all cases, however, when spinal fluids are to be tested, cultures should be made in the usual manner (117). As satisfactory cultures of spinal fluid are often difficult to obtain, they should be made in duplicate or triplicate. Likewise, some of the fluid should be streaked on a blood-agar plate or cultured on a Loeffler's blood-serum slant, and a few cubic centimeters incubated in a sterile tube separately. Occasionally cultures made in the latter fashion are positive when all others fail to show growth. Following incubation of the cultures, any pneumococci which grow out may be typed by the same technic as is used for blood cultures (page 641).

If desirable, in addition to making the cultures indicated above, some of the fluid may be inoculated into a mouse. A portion of the specimen is centrifuged at high speed for about thirty minutes to throw down the organisms present, the sediment taken up in 1 cc. of sterile saline solution and injected into the peritoneal cavity of a mouse. Pneumococci present in the peritoneal exudate subsequently obtained may be typed by the Neufeld, Sabin slide, or tube agglutination technic.

THE LEUCOCYTE COUNT

The demonstration of a leucocytosis in patients with an acute onset of illness with chill, pain, cough with or without bloody expectoration, and temperature is of aid in the diagnosis of pneumonia, even in the absence of definite physical signs of consolidation. A leucocytosis of 10,000 to 40,000 is usually found and is commonly present at the time of onset or shortly after, as already pointed out (see pages 497–498). The counts are likely to be higher in young patients than in older ones. About 80 to 90 per cent of the cells are usually polymorphonuclear.

The demonstration of a leucocytosis in patients having an atypical onset of their illness, such as children with meningismus or gastrointestinal upsets, or patients with delirium tremens, or the aged, should lead to the closest scrutiny of the chest by physical examination and roentgenograms. Late in the disease the persistence of an elevated leucocyte count or a re-elevation of the count usually indicates delayed resolution or the presence of a septic complication. In cases treated with an alien serum it may mark the occurrence of serum sickness.

ROENTGEN-RAY EXAMINATION

Roentgen-ray examination is of great value in confirming the results of physical examination and for the demonstration of central or multiple lung lesions not otherwise to be found. In adults consolidation usually begins at the hilum and extends toward the periphery, though in occasional cases and perhaps in children especially, the initial lesion may be at the periphery, as already mentioned (see pages 253–256).

In lobar pneumonia the increased density shown in roentgenograms is usually somewhat uneven and mottled with ill-defined margins, but may be homogeneous and sharply defined. As a rule, the diaphragm is high on the affected side. In addition, fluoroscopy usually shows a diminished excursion of the diaphragm on that side. By taking a roentgenogram a permanent record of conditions within the chest is obtained, which may be of great value later in the illness should the question of extension, effusion, or other intrathoracic complication arise. Davies, Hodgson, and Whitby (341) in a roentgenographic study of 119 cases of lobar pneumonia, state that although exceptions were found, densely consolidated lesions were usually associated with the most severe symptoms and hazy opacities were likely to be found in the milder cases.

Ude's (1329) observations on the matter of central pneumonias as shown by roentgenographic findings in 120 cases of lobar pneumonia are of interest. Fifty of the cases were examined early and many of these showed cone-shaped densities on the films. He finds that on a flat anteroposterior or posteroanterior plate such densities appear as central or hilum pneumonias. By taking lateral views, however, these hilar lesions were shown not to be true hilum pneumonias but were triangular or cone-shaped areas of consolidation with the base toward the periphery and the apex at the hilum occurring in the posterior part of the lower portion of an upper or the upper portion of a lower lobe. Ude regards these lesions as representing an early "posteromedial" pneumonia.

In a roentgenographic study of 40 cases of pneumococcus lobar pneumonia Graeser, Wu, and Robertson (552) find that the early appearance of density in roentgen-ray films is not characteristic of the disease except when considered together with the history of the patient. Nevertheless, the rapid development of such density, when its probable age is known, and its visual localization from a single focus in any lobe serve to differentiate the lesion from that due to most any other acute pulmonary infection.

As earlier mentioned, roentgenograms are superior to physical signs for detecting early lesions and for disclosing the extent of the process, while consolidation is developing (see pages 612–614). Almost without exception films taken by the end of twenty-four to forty-eight hours show abnormal densities (552, 341) and if the lesion is not apparent by the end of this period the diagnosis should be questioned (552). Graeser and his associates (552) report one case of Type I lobar pneumonia of nineteen hours' duration which failed to show definite roentgenographic evidence of the lesion at that time. This patient later had the signs and symptoms of an advanced case, yet repeated films showed only a slight haziness in the involved region. In most cases, however, after the lesions are maximum, physical signs and roentgenographic findings correlate well.

In their studies of lobar pneumonia Graeser, Wu, and Robertson (552) and Davies, Hodgson, and Whitby (341) report having detected that pneumococcus Type I and Type II cases tend to show the most uniform type of lobar distribution and have the most dense opacities while Type III and Group IV cases seemed to present the greatest variation in the character and spread of the lesion. The findings of the latter workers also suggested that the lesions in Type III and Group IV cases were more likely to be peripheral than central. Great individual variation may be found, however.

Davies and his associates (341) were also impressed with the frequency with which cases with lesions in more than one lobe were encountered. In 16 of 37 Type I cases (43.2 per cent) abnormalities were observed in roentgenograms in an adjacent lobe of the lung or in the opposite lung, although physical signs of these additional lesions were present in only 3 cases. When the lesion involved other lobes, only a part of the additional lobe was affected. Many lesions of this nature have been observed at necropsy (see pages 111–112) and their formation may often be due to the spread of infected edema fluid by cough and gravity as Loeschcke (798) suggests (see pages 255–256).

In addition to aiding in determining the presence, location, size, and density of the pulmonary lesions in pneumonia, roentgenograms are also of value in differentiating consolidation from conditions such as collapse of the lung and pleural effusions, as discussed in Chapter XIV. Films taken during the course of pneumonia may be of value in diagnosing conditions such as delayed resolution (page 542), termination in fibrosis (page 543), or certain complications (page 548). At times they will also show evidence of resolution when neither the physical signs nor the temperature indicates approaching crisis.

CHAPTER FOURTEEN

DIFFERENTIAL DIAGNOSIS

Bronchopneumonia 648
Pulmonary Infarct 650
Acute Tuberculous Pneumonia 650
Obstruction Atelectasis 651
Pleurisy with Effusion 652
Pulmonary Lesions Associated with Rheumatic Fever 652
Abdominal Pain at Onset of Lobar Pneumonia 653
Meningismus at Onset of Lobar Pneumonia 654

Patients with atypical onsets may present difficult diagnostic problems and lobar pneumonia may be confused with conditions such as bronchopneumonia, pulmonary infarct, or pleural effusion. Less commonly, acute tuberculous pneumonia or pulmonary collapse from various causes may also offer some difficulty. As previously mentioned, variation from the typical picture in lobar pneumonia is not uncommon in children in whom the disease may simulate meningitis or appendicitis (see pages 513–515). In the aged, in debilitated persons, or in those with chronic disease, the clinical course of bronchopneumonia and lobar pneumonia may be very similar. Under such circumstances terminal lobar pneumonia may be overlooked and central pneumonia may be in doubt for several days (807).

BRONCHOPNEUMONIA

Less importance attaches to the differentiation of lobar pneumonia from bronchopneumonia now than formerly. Most cases of the former and perhaps a majority of the cases of the latter are due to pneumococci and if the type responsible for the infection is one for which an effective specific antiserum is available, serum treatment may be inaugurated at once in suitable cases.

In bronchopneumonia in general, pneumococci of Type I and Type II are much less often encountered than in lobar pneumonia (see pages 67–74). In primary bronchopneumonia, it seems probable that the distribution of the remaining types is not markedly different from that in lobar pneumonia. Other organisms, especially streptococci, are frequently the cause of bronchopneumonia in the primary form and perhaps usually of the disease in the secondary form. Cases in infants and children under about three or four years of age are usually primary, while in older individuals they are as a rule secondary to an associated infection, particularly of the respiratory tract, or to some other condition.

Finland and Sutliff (464) studied a group of 225 Type III and 105 Type VIII pneumococcus pneumonias in adults. With lobar pneumonia due to these types the onset was abrupt in 72 and 81 per cent of the cases respectively, while with bronchopneumonia it was abrupt in only 40 and 33 per cent of the cases. The commonest initial symptoms in their cases of bronchopneumonia were fever, cough, and dyspnea, but no single symptom occurred at onset in more than one-quarter of the cases. Chill, pain, and rusty sputum were found in 73 and 85 per cent of the cases of lobar pneumonia due to Type III and Type VIII, respectively, but were present in only 25 and 35 per cent of the cases of bronchopneumonia due to those types. Approximately one-fifth of the Type III cases and one-third of the Type VIII cases were bronchopneumonic in form. Thus bronchopneumonia was commoner with Type VIII than with Type III infections.

The clinical differentiation of bronchopneumonia from lobar pneumonia is usually not difficult. The onset is commonly insidious and the involvement patchy, and the illness generally occurs as a secondary complication of other diseases. The temperature is nearly always irregular. The only physical signs may be widely scattered moist rales. At times multiple small areas of consolidation may be demonstrated. Recovery is usually by lysis, resolution slow, and relapse not uncommon.

On the other hand, the differentiation of a confluent bronchopneumonia from lobar pneumonia may be impossible since the physical signs are essentially identical. Frequently in children, and at times in adults, atelectasis may be observed in the course of a bronchopneumonia but, as Lord (807) points out, the signs are more likely to suggest pleural effusion or massive pneumonia than lobar pneumonia. The signs are caused by collapse of the lung, due to occlusion by tenacious secretion of a bronchus supplying the affected area, and may be made to alter or disappear following expulsion of the secretion by cough.

In bronchopneumonia, in contrast to lobar pneumonia, roentgen-ray examination shows a patchy character of the areas of increased density. Multiple foci are more often present and the involved regions are more widely separated. Confluent lesions usually cannot be differentiated from lobar pneumonia.

PULMONARY INFARCT

Pulmonary infarction may give rise to a symptom complex which is for a time nearly or wholly indistinguishable from lobar pneumonia. Lord (807, 808) has considered the matter and points out that infarction should be first thought of when there is sudden onset of pulmonary symptoms in patients who have chronic heart disease or cardiac decompensation; uterine sepsis (with or without relation to childbirth); operation for abdominal sepsis; or otitis media or mastoid disease complicated by sinus thrombosis; or in patients who have suffered injuries to the veins of the extremities, especially when thrombosis is present.

Marked dyspnea and cyanosis may appear suddenly when there is occlusion of a large branch of the pulmonary artery. Pain in the side and cough with bloody sputum are common. Attention to the order in which the symptoms appear will assist in making diagnosis (807). Bloody sputum may appear within a few hours of onset or be delayed two or three days. The blood may be in the form of streaks or thoroughly mixed with the sputum. The examination of washed sputum particles may show no bacteria microscopically or by culture. Chill less often occurs at the onset than in lobar pneumonia. In the latter disease the temperature rises almost at once with the beginning of symptoms, while in infarct the rise is more gradual, the temperature generally reaching a maximum, seldom of more than 103° F., only after a day or two.

The physical signs are commonly indistinguishable from those of lobar pneumonia. Pleurisy, with or without hemorrhagic effusion, may be present, as well as a moderate leucocytosis. In favorable cases the temperature falls by lysis and the signs slowly disappear.

Parsons and Myers (1000) note that the occurrence of severe secondary streptococcus infections complicating recovery from pneumococcus lobar pneumonia may give rise to a clinical picture suggestive of pulmonary infarct. In such cases a streptococcus bacteriemia can usually be demonstrated.

ACUTE TUBERCULOUS PNEUMONIA

Though of rare occurrence, an acute tuberculous pneumonia may sometimes be encountered, and when it occurs, it usually simulates acute pneumococcus pneumonia. The patient is likely to have a family history of tuberculosis or a history of contact with tuberculous patients, of hemoptysis or, occasionally, of a primary pleurisy or adenitis, and may show cervical scars.

At times such patients will give a history of slowly failing health, cough with sputum, and an evening temperature with night sweats for some weeks prior to their acute illness.

Although the initial symptom complex may be typical (808), chill and pain are less common than in pneumococcus cases (814). Rusty sputum may occur but greenish sputum is more common. The occurrence of hemoptysis as an initial symptom is suspicious. Pallor rather than cyanosis may be present and the temperature intermittent or remittent; polymorphonuclear leucocytosis may be absent.

Physical and roentgen-ray examination may reveal signs of apical disease or a diffuse mottling above the anterior portion of the third rib, in addition to signs of consolidation elsewhere. The etiologic diagnosis may be in doubt several days and frequently repeated examinations of the sputum for tubercle bacilli must be made before the diagnosis can be established. Lesions in the upper lobes are more often found than in pneumococcus cases.

OBSTRUCTION ATELECTASIS

Collapse of one or more lobes of the lungs during pneumonia (see page 525) occurs very seldom. In otherwise healthy patients, collapse of one of the lower lobes may be mistaken for pneumonia. It may be associated with conditions which produce an excess of bronchial secretion, such as acute bronchitis, or with hypertrophy of the heart or large pericardial effusions (961). Foreign body or neoplasm may also be responsible. The condition may come on with great suddenness and cause some dyspnea, pain, and viscid expectoration of about a day's duration. Examination of the chest may show retraction of the affected side, slight dulness, diminished or absent breathing, and the absence of vocal fremitus and rales. The apex of the heart is commonly displaced toward the affected side.

Roentgenograms are of aid in diagnosis. Collapse of an entire lower lobe may be recognized by the presence of a homogeneous shadow in the cardiophrenic angle with a sharply defined outer border, slanting down and outward to the diaphragm. Should collapse of the middle lobe be present, a similar homogeneous shadow will be observed in the right lower lung field, with a sharply limited, nearly horizontal upper margin and a vertical outer border. Further, in unilateral atelectasis, examination shows elevation of the diaphragm, narrowing of the intercostal spaces, and increased downward inclination of the ribs on the affected side, with displacement of the heart and mediastinum toward the lesion.

PLEURISY WITH EFFUSION

The distinction between pleural effusion and lobar pneumonia may at times be difficult to make, particularly in complicated cases. In primary cases of serofibrinous pleuritis, Lord (807) states that the onset is more often gradual than sudden, and chilliness rather than chill is common. In the more unusual case the onset is abrupt, with chill, fever, and pain, but seldom with any bloody sputum.

In outspoken cases of lobar pneumonia the breath sounds are bronchial, with increased voice, whisper, and tactile fremitus over the involved area, while with typical pleural effusions the breath sounds though bronchial are diminished, with diminished or absent voice, whisper, and tactile fremitus. Norris and Landis (961) remark, however, that occasionally the signs peculiar to one of these conditions may occur in the other. When there are large effusions, diminished motion on the affected side, displacement of the heart and trachea away from the affected side, and the usual physical signs of fluid are characteristic features (see page 575). The greatest difficulty arises in distinguishing between small effusions and pneumonia. With small effusions visceral displacement may not be present. Grocco's paravertebral triangle of dulness may be demonstrated on the side opposite the accumulation of fluid and there is relatively less resonance on the affected side in the paravertebral region than when pneumonia is present, as Lord (807) has shown. Roentgen-ray examination may aid in differentiating between the two conditions. In all doubtful cases a chest tap should be performed. Compression of the lung at the back, over a free effusion in the base of the pleural sac, gives rise to signs of consolidation which may be detected above the area having signs of fluid.

PULMONARY LESIONS ASSOCIATED WITH RHEUMATIC FEVER

In some instances patients with acute rheumatic fever may have pulmonary symptoms. The terms "rheumatic pneumonia" or "rheumatic lung" have been used to describe these cases. The condition, though apparently first described by British investigators, has presumably been known in this country for many years (165).

In patients with acute rheumatic fever, pulmonary signs and symptoms are not uncommonly encountered (776, 662). Though the nature of the pathologic lesion in the lung in such patients seems uncertain (Mallory, 856), it has been studied by Naish (921) who reports clinical data on six cases together with necropsy findings.

All of Naish's patients, aged seven to thirty-three years, had symptoms of acute rheumatic fever or rheumatic heart disease and in most of the six cases a clinical diagnosis of pneumonia was also made. The onset of pulmonary symptoms was atypical. Each patient had pain in the chest, several had dyspnea, and some had cough with a little sputum and fever, besides the obvious signs of acute rheumatic fever or cardiac lesion. Left lower lobe lesions were commonest at onset, but initial lesions in other lobes were described. The "pneumonias" were progressive, lasting several days to several weeks with increasing signs of consolidation. The temperature in these patients could be controlled by salicylates. Cyanosis was not marked until late, but was then intense. In some cases the lesions were observed to spread from a small area till they involved both lungs extensively within four days. Patients affected in this manner were apparently gradually suffocated.

At necropsy bronchopneumonia was found to coexist with the rheumatic lesion in one patient and the remainder showed lung lesions which Naish (921) states were unlike anything previously described. The pulmonary process resembled a pneumonia caused by fibrosis and the lung felt like India rubber, was tough, non-friable, and fairly dry. Large areas were frequently involved. Microscopically the lesions had the histologic structure of Aschoff bodies and appeared due to a tremendous thickening of the alveolar walls. In many places buds from the alveolar walls had completely occluded the alveolar cavities, the predominant cell being the large endothelial cell which apparently originated from the walls of the alveolar capillaries. Multinucleate cells were occasionally seen.

Naish believes that cases of this nature occur more often than are recognized and do not always end in death. One of his patients suffered a typical attack of this kind, after which all the symptoms and signs cleared up. A year or so later this same patient suffered a second attack, which was fatal.

ABDOMINAL PAIN AT ONSET OF LOBAR PNEUMONIA

Lobar pneumonia may occasionally begin with abdominal pain, as earlier mentioned, which leads to diagnosis of some acute abdominal surgical condition (see pages 488–490). Such pain may be accompanied by tenderness and some muscle spasm in the abdomen and is due to sensations referred from the chest through the last six intercostal nerves (214).

Abdominal pain at the onset of lobar pneumonia is more frequent in children than in adults. In children up to thirteen years of age Cunningham (333) found abdominal pain in 15 per cent of 1,500 cases of lobar pneumonia. Townsend (1318) and Grulee and Mulherin (574) also reported the frequent occurrence of abdominal pain in children at the onset of pneumonia. In Adams and Berger's (4) series of 145 hospitalized cases of lobar pneumonia in children, the admission diagnosis for 25 (17.6 per cent) was appendicitis. Twenty-three per cent of the 145 cases had abdominal signs of some kind. Tenderness, usually superficial, was most frequent and spasm was less often found. In differentiating lobar pneumonia from appendicitis these investigators note that the white blood count is of value for it is nearly always more than 15,000 with the former condition and under that level with the latter. They also point out that a history of vomiting, abdominal pain, and diarrhea is found with equal frequency with either condition in children but that patients with pneumonia usually look much sicker than those with appendicitis and have physical signs of pulmonary disease. Roentgen-ray examination is of aid in demonstrating lung lesions in doubtful cases.

In adults, abdominal pain at onset was noted in 10 of 770 cases (1.3 per cent) of lobar pneumonia observed by Cole (297) and in 12 of 200 cases (6 per cent) studied by Lord (807). Chatard (254) and MacCordick (830) have also reported the occasional occurrence of abdominal pain in adults at the time of onset of pneumonia in the lobar form.

MENINGISMUS AT ONSET OF LOBAR PNEUMONIA

Uncommonly in adults and somewhat frequently in children the onset of lobar pneumonia may be marked by symptoms simulating those of meningitis. As seen in Chapter VIII (page 491), symptoms of this nature may be encountered in from 5 to 8 per cent of cases in infants and children early in the illness. Such symptoms are due to meningeal irritation and usually subside at the time of crisis or shortly after.

Severe headache, fever, irritability, incontinence, increased peripheral reflexes in the arms and legs, and inability to extend the lower leg with the thigh flexed (Kernig's sign), delirium or coma may occur in such realistic fashion that the disease is considered meningitis. The pupils and eye grounds are invariably normal and localized or convulsive movements or paralyses are lacking. In a large majority of instances lumbar puncture shows the spinal fluid to be under increased pressure and to rise normally with jugular compression. The fluid is clear, shows no increase in cell count, and is sterile on culture. The globulin and sugar content are normal. Repeated examinations of the lungs at daily intervals will usually permit establishing a diagnosis of pneumonia. Roentgenograms are of great assistance.

CHAPTER FIFTEEN

PROGNOSIS

General Case Fatality Rates 656
Pneumonia and Lobar Pneumonia 658
Bronchopneumonia 663
Effect of Various Factors on Prognosis 663
Type of Pneumococcus 663
Type I cases; Type II cases; Type III cases; Group IV cases; Type V cases; Type VII cases; Type VIII cases; Type XIV cases .. 664
Pneumococcus Pneumonia 674
Pneumonia Due to Organisms Other than Pneumococci 677
Year and Season 677
Bacteriemia 681
Type I cases; Type II cases; Type III cases; Group IV cases; Total Type I, II, III, and Group IV cases 683
Pneumococcus Pneumonia 687
Pneumonia Due to Organisms Other than Pneumococci 689
Additional Aspects of the Relation of Bacteriemia to Prognosis .. 689
Infants and Children with Bacteriemia 693
Soluble Specific Substance in Urine 693
Complications and Previous Attacks of Pneumonia 695
Extent of Pulmonary Involvement 696
Chain-Forming Pneumococci 698
Factors Affecting the Individual 699
General Physical Condition 699
Age as Factor in Prognosis 703
Race as Factor in Prognosis 710
Sex as Factor in Prognosis 712
Pregnancy as Factor in Prognosis 713
Occupation and Social and Environmental Conditions 713
Alcoholism as Factor in Prognosis 718
Prognostic Significance of Certain Signs and Symptoms 719
Temperature Height 719
Pulse Rate 720
Blood Pressure 722
Leucocyte Count 723
Respiration Rate 725
Cyanosis 726
Miscellaneous Signs and Symptoms 726

Pneumonia in any form must always be regarded as serious. The factors governing the outcome in any instance are numerous, many are closely interrelated, and the nature of some of them is known, as will be pointed out. Basically, prognosis is dependent upon the virulence and pathogenic properties of the infecting organism and the resistance of the host. In a general way, there is a relationship between virulence and some types of pneumococci which can frequently be demonstrated in laboratory animals, as previously mentioned (see pages 193–194). In addition, since the natural resistance of both animals (page 137) and man (page 143) varies with pneumococci of different types, the prognosis of pneumonia may also vary with the type of pneumococcus causing the infection.

Man has a relatively high resistance to the pneumococcus. This immunity is dependent on many factors and may vary with the individual and even in the same individual, as shown in the chapter on Aspects of Immunity (see pages 185–203). In pneumonia the extent, severity, and duration of the disease have an important bearing on outcome, as do individual characteristics such as the patient's general physical condition, age, and the like, as discussed below. It is also likely that the intensity and duration of exposure to various factors predisposing to pneumonia, such as chilling, wetting, marked variations in temperature, or the intimate contact of the pulmonary tissues with some foreign substances, may affect the outcome to a variable degree.

In addition to the many general factors affecting prognosis, there are certain specific features of prognostic importance which may be noted by observing the response of a patient to his infection, as mentioned later.

The prognosis in many cases of pneumonia may be significantly altered by the early application of suitable therapeutic measures. The discussion in this chapter is restricted to cases not treated with specific serum, unless otherwise noted.

GENERAL CASE FATALITY RATES

The cases for which fatality rates are given in this section exclude for the most part patients treated with serum, men in military groups, and infants and children. When individuals from these groups are included, mention of the fact is made. In cases due to a type of pneumococcus for which a clinically effective immune serum is available, prompt and adequate treatment will usually bring about a marked lowering of the fatality rate; the fatality rates for cases treated with specific serum are given in Chapter XIX (page 880). Rates for men in military groups and for infants and children are discussed

TABLE 114. LOBAR PNEUMONIA. NUMBER OF CASES AND NUMBER AND PERCENTAGE OF DEATHS IN THE UNITED STATES AND CANADA

SOURCE	HOSPITAL	REFERENCE NUMBER	NUMBER OF CASES	DEATHS *Number*	DEATHS *Per cent*
Townsend and Coolidge, 1889	Massachusetts General	1319	1,000	250	25.0
Ashton and Landis, 1905	Philadelphia General (Penn.)	26	991	533	53.0
Chatard, 1910	Johns Hopkins (Md.)	254	658	200	30.3
Shattuck and Lawrence, 1918	Massachusetts General	1176	2,882	788	27.3
Locke, Thomas, and O'Hara, 1920	Boston City (Mass.)	797	1,795	621	34.6
Kelly, 1926	Cook County (Chicago, Ill.)	708	6,531	2,351	36.0
Cecil, Baldwin, and Larsen, 1927	Bellevue (New York City)	230	1,107	342	30.8
Park, Bullowa, and Rosenblüth, 1928	Harlem (New York City)	991	830	266	32.0
Finland, 1930	Boston City (Mass.)	442	213	70	32.9
MacCordick, 1931	Montreal General (Canada)	830	525*	132	25.1
Nichol, 1931	Jackson Memorial (Miami, Fla.)	951	152	41	27.1
Blake, 1931	New Haven General (Conn.)	120	606*	185	30.5
Warr and Alperin, 1933	Memphis General (Tenn.)	1385	574*	140	24.2
Sutliff and Finland, 1933	Boston City (Mass.)	1271	770†	286	37.1
Massachusetts Pneumonia Study, 1937	Several (Mass.)	615	705‡	155	22.0
Benjamin, Blankenhorn, Ruegsegger, and Senior, 1937	Cincinnati General (Ohio)	94	201*	55	27.3
	Total		19,540	6,415	32.8

* Possibly specific serum was used in the treatment of a few of these cases.

† This series includes cases due to pneumococci of the types from I through XX. Of 268 Type I cases included, specific serum was used in the treatment of 97, and similar treatment was given 46 of the 142 Type II cases in the series.

‡ Of the total 705 cases in the Massachusetts group, 338 were treated at home, with 70 deaths or 20.7 per cent.

in sections of this chapter where matters pertaining to these particular groups are considered.

Pneumonia and Lobar Pneumonia

Probably the largest series of collected cases of "pneumonia" ever reported was that presented by Wells (1404) in 1904. He gathered from the world literature, largely between the years of 1800 and 1900, approximately 500 series of cases, and found that among a total of 465,400 cases there were 94,826 deaths, yielding a case fatality rate of 20.4 per cent. At least 90,000 of these cases, however, were in patients in military groups which had very low fatality rates. Examples of low rates in similar groups are cited below (see page 699). When these 90,000 cases are excluded from the larger series, the fatality rate rises to approximately 24 per cent for more than 375,000 cases.

Sears and Larrabee (1168), in a series of 949 cases of "pneumonia" at the Boston City Hospital, found that 341 or 35.9 per cent died, and in Glasgow, Smith (1213) reported that 21.8 per cent, or 2,727, of 12,517 cases of lobar pneumonia and bronchopneumonia together died. The case fatality rate was thus apparently lower in the series from Glasgow than in the series from the United States, a matter which will shortly be elaborated.

Data relating to the fatality rate of reported cases of lobar pneumonia alone, whether or not the etiologic agent responsible for the infection was identified, may be seen in Tables 114 and 115. Table 114 gives data collected from the American and Canadian literature. Of a total of 19,540 cases, 6,415, or 32.8 per cent, died. The fatality rates in the individual series included varied from 22 per cent (615) to 53 per cent (26) but were usually in the neighborhood of 30 per cent. A large majority of these cases occurred subsequent to 1918, although the cases in Townsend and Coolidge's (1319) series extend as far back as 1821, and in Ashton and Landis' (26) series, as far back as 1897.

Table 115 presents data from other countries. Of a total of 31,220 cases, death occurred in 7,466, a rate of 23.9 per cent. The addition of the cases in Table 114 to those in Table 115 gives a grand total of 50,760 cases of lobar pneumonia with 13,881 deaths, a rate of 27.3 per cent.

Attention may be focused for a moment on Table 115 and the 11,182 cases which occurred in Great Britain and Sweden with 1,944 deaths, a rate of 17.4 per cent. The fatality rate of these cases is only a little more than one-half the rate, 32.8 per cent, for lobar pneumonia in the United States and

TABLE 115. LOBAR PNEUMONIA. NUMBER OF CASES AND NUMBER AND PERCENTAGE OF DEATHS IN COUNTRIES OTHER THAN THE UNITED STATES AND CANADA

SOURCE	NUMBER OF CASES	DEATHS	
		Number	*Per cent*
Great Britain			
Greenwood and Candy, 1911 (567)	5,116	997	19.5
Macgregor, 1933 (837)	1,077	158	14.7
Langley, 1933 (765)	189	44	23.3
Guys Hospital Reports, 1933 (1145) ...	154	24	16.0
Davies, Hodgson, and Whitby, 1935 (339)	859	163	19.0
Sweden			
Huss, 1855, cited by Greenwood and Candy (567)	2,710	375	13.8
Lindau, 1933 (783)	1,077	183	17.0
Total	11,182	1,944	17.4
Tropical Regions			
Goodman (Mexico), 1905 (530)	101	40	39.8
Maynard (Africa), 1913 (874)	1,809	709	39.2
Pearson and Mouchet (Africa), 1923 (1008)	800	124	15.5
Rogers (India), 1925 (1103)	14,266*	3,709	26.0
United Fruit Company (Central America), 1927 (1331)	771	242	31.4
McSwann (Malay), 1927 (853)	200	63	31.5
Vitug and Hizon (Philippines), 1928 (1357)	1,030	243	23.5
Winchester (Singapore), 1929 (1428) ..	540	280	51.9
Total	19,517	5,410	27.7
Other countries			
Patterson (Australia), 1922 (1003a)	521	112	21.5
Grand total	31,220	7,466	23.9

* A few cases of bronchopneumonia are apparently included in this series.

Canada (Table 114) and is considerably lower than that, 27.7 per cent, for the same disease in the tropics (Table 115).

Observations relating to the apparently lower case fatality rate for lobar pneumonia in certain sections of Europe, notably in Great Britain and the

Scandinavian countries, have been made by numerous investigators. Christensen (264) reported a fatality rate of about 12 per cent for 110 cases in Denmark. His cases, however, may have been in soldiers and not in civilians. Thjötta and Hanneborg (1294) state that the case fatality rate in Norway was only about 13 to 18 per cent between the years 1865 and 1917, and Lindau (783) reports that fatality rates are lower in Norway and Sweden and in several other European countries than in the United States.

Findings of similar significance have been reported for Great Britain (1109, 1145) as emphasized by Macgregor (837), Cruickshank (331), and Davies, Hodgson, and Whitby (339). Further, Wu and Chiu (1450) consider that the fatality rate of cases in Peiping, China, is lower than that found in the United States.

Judging from the reports from tropical and semi-tropical areas of the world, shown in Table 115, and from additional observations in Central America (549, 1019), Puerto Rico (1261), and Africa (973), the case fatality rate for lobar pneumonia is about the same in those regions as it is in the United States and Canada. In fact, from the excellent summary of matters relating to pneumonia in the tropics made by Gautier (510) in 1932, it is possible that the rates may be even somewhat higher in the warmer areas of the earth (see Table 116). Gautier collected a total of 48,137 cases of "tropical pneumonia" (lobar pneumonia and bronchopneumonia together) from a number of hospitals in the tropics. These cases had a weighted average fatality rate of 37.9 per cent, as shown in Table 116.

Practically all the cases referred to above in this chapter were cared for in hospitals and the fatality rate in such cases is probably higher than for cases not hospitalized, as is mentioned below (see page 715). It is clear from the results shown in Tables 114, 115, and 116 that the fatality rates may vary markedly in different hospitals.

The fatality rates may also vary in different places in the same country or in different groups in the same place (see also pages 677–681 and 714–718). Rogers (1103), in an extensive study of pneumonia in India (see page 298), found that the disease was much more frequent in the relatively dry, cold parts of the country than in the warm and moist regions. His figures, which are based on 14,266 cases, nearly all of lobar pneumonia (see Table 115), also show that case fatality rates were lowest in areas having the highest attack rates and *vice versa*. In areas with the highest incidence rates, fatality rates were in the neighborhood of 23 to 26 per cent, while in regions having the

TABLE 116. TROPICAL PNEUMONIA (LOBAR PNEUMONIA AND BRONCHOPNEUMONIA TOGETHER). NUMBER OF CASES AND PERCENTAGE OF DEATHS IN CENTRAL AND SOUTH AMERICA, AFRICA, AND ASIA

COUNTRY AND HOSPITAL	PERIOD	NUMBER OF CASES	DEATHS *Per cent*
America			
British Guiana			
Public Hospital, Georgetown	1910–1913	1,265	40.5
Honduras			
Hospital Puerto Castillo	1921–1929	672	39.1
Central America			
United Fruit Company's Hospital	1920–1925	3,367	38.6
	1926–1929	1,463	31.8
Panama Republic			
Santo Thomas Hospital, Panama	1920–1923	427	47.5
Africa			
French Congo			
General Hospital, Brazzaville	1927	588	33.4
Pointe Noire Hospital	1927	494	40.0
Senegal			
Native Hospital, Dakar	1926–1928	193	25.4
Belgian Congo			
Native Hospital, Katanga	1923–1924	778	21.6
Sudan			
Native Hospital	1928	447	28.2
British Somaliland			
Berbera Hospital	1925–1928	216	13.9
Kenya			
Hospitals	1920–1928	10,435	22.4
Portuguese East Africa			
Hospitals	1925–1927	665	22.4
Mauritius			
Hospitals	1920–1925	922	40.6
	1927–1928	545	31.2
Asia			
Ceylon			
Hospitals	1928	4,433	26.1
India			
Sambunath Hospital, Calcutta	1928	43	58.0

TABLE 116 (*cont.*)

COUNTRY AND HOSPITAL	PERIOD	NUMBER OF CASES	DEATHS *Per cent*
Asia (cont.)			
Straits Settlements			
General Hospital, Singapore	1926–1928	540	51.8
	1929	264	45.4
Tan Tock Seng Hospital, Singapore ..	1925–1927	1,048	53.7
District Hospital, Penang	1922–1924	319	58.3
Federated Malay States			
Hospitals	1925–1929	13,482	47.5
Netherlands East Indies			
Central Civilian Hospital, Batavia	1919–1921	1,572	49.1
Central Civilian Hospital, Sourabaya ..	1919–1921	953	47.8
Central Civilian Hospital, Batavia	1923	219	38.4
Central Civilian Hospital, Sourabaya ..	1923	218	33.5
Central Civilian Hospital, Semarang ..	1923	305	70.2
Central Civilian Hospital, Batavia	1922	742	50.0
Sourabaya and Semarang, 171 hospitals	1924	1,164	30.3
Central Municipal Hospital, Batavia ..	1911–1915	358	37.5
Total		48,137	37.9*

From Gautier (510)

* Weighted average

lowest incidence, fatality rates of 30 to 39 per cent obtained. As all the cases in this study occurred in the jail population of India and embraced but few very young or very old individuals, it is possible that the groups investigated tended to be uniform with regard to personal factors, such as age, sex, and physical condition.

Kibbey's (714) findings in a group of mine workers and their dependents in Alabama gave results somewhat similar to Rogers' observations. Kibbey's study was based on 2,603 cases of "pneumonia" occurring over a six-year period and it was noted that although the incidence of pneumonia was lowest in wage earners working above ground, this group had the highest case fatality rate. The various groups studied were not large, however, and neither were the differences in their case fatality rates. The fatality rate of 560 cases occurring in surface workers was 29.6 per cent (166 deaths), as compared with a rate of 23 per cent (62 deaths) among 270 cases in underground coal and ore miners.

Bronchopneumonia

As far as can be determined from the data available, the fatality rate in bronchopneumonia is as high as that in lobar pneumonia or higher. Lord (807) reports that among 339 cases of bronchopneumonia at the Massachusetts General Hospital, death occurred in 89, a rate of 26 per cent. In Cole's (298) series of 211 cases at the Hospital of the Rockefeller Institute for Medical Research, which were due to various organisms 68, or 32.2 per cent, died. Finland (449), at the Boston City Hospital, finds a fatality rate of 55 per cent among 619 cases of pneumococcus bronchopneumonia. Two Type VII patients in this series received serum treatment and one died. No specific treatment was given the remaining 617 cases (see Table 126, page 675).

Among 137 cases of "influenzal" bronchopneumonia observed by Locke, Thomas, and O'Hara (797) at the Boston City Hospital, the fatality rate was 38 per cent. These cases occurred during the last influenza pandemic. In a similar series of 916 patients with influenzal bronchopneumonia in Copenhagen, Denmark, Bie (102) found a fatality rate of 23 per cent (209 deaths).

Stone, Phillips, and Bliss (1251), during the War, reported the occurrence of 181 cases of "measles pneumonia" (atypical or bronchopneumonia) with 83 deaths, a rate of 45.8 per cent, in the troops at Camp Riley, Kansas (see also pages 3–17).

EFFECT OF VARIOUS FACTORS ON PROGNOSIS

Type of Pneumococcus

Under ordinary circumstances in pneumonia due to pneumococci a general relationship exists between the prognosis and the type of infecting pneumococcus. Some types are nearly always associated with higher case fatality rates than others. Doubtless the inherent invasive capacity of certain types, as well as their ability to produce varying amounts of specific capsular polysaccharide during growth, significantly influences the chances of recovery. It has long been known that pneumococci of Type I produce relatively small amounts of the specific capsular polysaccharide in their growth, while strains of Type II usually produce larger amounts, and those of Type III the largest (617, 618, 619). As these substances have the ability specifically to inhibit the action of antipneumococcal antibodies (see pages 131–132), it is not surprising that the fatality rates in pneumonia due to each of these three types progressively increase from Type I to Type III. Cruickshank (331) has stressed this relationship. As yet little is known of the relationship between prognosis with infections due to other types and the relative abilities of pneumococci of these types to produce their specific capsular carbohydrate.

TYPE I CASES. Data are available relating to the outcome of a large group of cases of pneumococcus Type I lobar pneumonia treated in the United States and Canada (Table 117) and in various other sections of the globe (Table 118).

TABLE 117. TYPE I LOBAR PNEUMONIA. NUMBER OF CASES AND NUMBER AND PERCENTAGE OF DEATHS IN THE UNITED STATES AND CANADA

SOURCE	PERIOD OF INVESTIGATION	NUMBER OF CASES	DEATHS *Number*	DEATHS *Per cent*
Cole (291)	1912	34	8	23.5
Richardson (1080)	1913–1914	39	12	30.8
Mathers (872)	1914–1915	50	13	26.0
Frissell and Famulener (503)	1915	9	1	11.1
Clough (277)	1915–1916	19	7	36.8
Alexander (9)	1913–1917	14	6	42.9
Hartman and Lacy (604)	1917	36	12	33.3
Quigley (1054)	1917–1918	33	13	39.4
Jones (691)	1918	26	1	3.9
Locke, Thomas, and O'Hara (797)	1919–1920	57	15	26.3
Thomas (1299)	1917–1921	10	–	–
Locke (793)	1919–1922	71	12	16.9
Wadsworth (1365)	1915–1923	344	65	18.9
Park, Bullowa, and Rosenblüth (991)	1926–1928	105	33	31.4
Cecil and Plummer (238)	1920–1929	405	109	26.9
Finland (442)	1924–1929	70	22	31.4
Baldwin (59)	1926–1930	20	5	25.0
Lord (809)	1917–1931	93	23	24.7
Howard and Fullerton (663)	1929–1931	7	–	–
Buchanan and Ashley (164)	1934	15	3	20.0
Massachusetts Pneumonia Study (615)	1931–1935	190	50	26.3
Finland (449)	1930–1936	365	157	43.0
Benjamin, Blankenhorn, Ruegsegger, and Senior (94)	1935–1937	83	22	26.5
Total		2,095	589	28.1
Additional Type I cases				
Kohl and Reitzel (734)	1932–1935	119*	52	43.7
Bullowa (190)	1928–1936	100*	30	30.0
Grand total		2,314	671	29.0

* Pneumococcus pneumonia (lobar pneumonia and bronchopneumonia together).

TABLE 118. TYPE I LOBAR PNEUMONIA. NUMBER OF CASES AND NUMBER AND PERCENTAGE OF DEATHS IN COUNTRIES OTHER THAN THE UNITED STATES AND CANADA

SOURCE	NUMBER OF CASES	DEATHS	
		Number	*Per cent*
Great Britain			
Ferguson and Lovell, 1928 (437)	50	13	26.0
Alston and Stewart, 1930 (13)	53	12	22.6
Leys, 1933 (779)	15	3	20.0
Therapeutic Trials Committee of Medical Research Council, 1934 (557)	301*	45	15.0
Langley, 1935 (763)	158	33	20.9
Irish Free State			
Moore, 1923 (902)	36	6	16.7
Denmark			
Christensen, 1925 (265)	42	9	21.4
Total	655	121	18.5
Other countries			
Marginesu and Corda (Italy), 1923 (860)	16	4	25.0
Wu and Chiu (China), 1933 (1450)	54	7	13.0
Levi (Italy), 1933 (775)	25	5	20.0
Bhatnagar and Singh (India), 1935 (100)	24	12	50.0
Total	119	28	23.5
Grand total	774	149	19.3

* Only patients twenty to sixty years of age were included in this series, and all patients dying within twenty-four hours of admission to hospitals were omitted.

As seen in Table 117, of a total of 2,095 cases in the United States and Canada 589, or 28.1 per cent, died. When the additional cases in the table are included, the total number of cases is 2,314, of which 671, or 29 per cent, died.* Probably no considerable error is entailed by including these additional series, which are of Type I pneumococcus lobar pneumonia and bronchopneumonia, for in such series due to Type I (and to Type II as well) almost all cases are of the lobar form, as Sutliff and Finland (1272) have dem-

* Early compilation of data on a smaller total number of cases showed a fatality rate of 25 per cent.

onstrated. As the number of cases in the grand total is fairly large and has been collected from the literature over a period extending back as far as 1912, it seems probable that the fatality rate found is fairly representative for Type I infections in this part of the world.

Table 118 gives a number of series of cases of Type I lobar pneumonia collected from the foreign literature. Inasmuch as the figures in earlier tables in this chapter indicated a probable lower fatality rate for cases of lobar pneumonia in Great Britain and the Scandinavian countries than in this country, the series in Table 118 are tabulated so as to reveal a similar relation between the fatality rates in Great Britain and Scandinavia and other countries if it exists. The grand total of all the Type I cases in Table 118 is 774, of which 149, or 19.3 per cent, died. This finding suggests that the fatality rate of Type I cases is somewhat lower in other parts of the world than in this country. Among 655 cases occurring in the British Isles and in Denmark, 121, or 18.5 per cent, died, a fatality rate which again is considerably lower than the rate of 29 per cent for Type I cases in the United States and Canada. The inclusion in the British series of the 301 selected cases reported by the Therapeutic Trials Committee of the Medical Research Council (557), which had a rate of 15 per cent, probably makes the rate in the total British group somewhat lower than the actual rate in that country. Combining the cases in Tables 117 and 118 we have a total of 3,088 Type I cases almost wholly of lobar pneumonia, of which 820, or 26.6 per cent, died.

As a rule, Type I lobar pneumonia is a moderately severe illness. Atypical pneumonia or bronchopneumonia due to pneumococci of Type I may be more serious, and Finland (449), at the Boston City Hospital, has reported a fatality rate of 89 per cent for 28 cases of this nature (see Table 126, page 675).

TYPE II CASES. More Type II than Type I cases die, as is revealed by a tabulation of reports from the United States and Canada (Table 119) and from other countries (Table 120). In Table 119 the fatality rate for 1,592 cases of Type II lobar pneumonia is 36.6 per cent. Combining this series with the other Type II cases in the table, there is a grand total of 1,753 cases with 651 deaths, a rate of 37.1 per cent.* In all series containing 25 or more cases, the fatality rates are rather uniformly high. Type II pneumonia is usually a severe disease.

In Table 120 are listed the Type II cases from other countries. These total

* Early compilation of data on a smaller series of Type II cases revealed a fatality rate of 41 per cent.

TABLE 119. TYPE II LOBAR PNEUMONIA. NUMBER OF CASES AND NUMBER AND PERCENTAGE OF DEATHS IN THE UNITED STATES AND CANADA

SOURCE	PERIOD OF INVESTIGATION	NUMBER OF CASES	DEATHS *Number*	DEATHS *Per cent*
Richardson (1080)	1913–1914	28	7	25.0
Mathers (872)	1914–1915	25	7	25.0
Frissell and Famulener (503)	1915	7	4	57.1
Clough (277)	1915–1916	3	–	–
Alexander (9)	1913–1917	22	9	40.9
Hartman and Lacy (604)	1917	29*	10	34.5
Hart (600)	1917–1918	30	13	43.3
Quigley (1054)	1917–1918	36	13	36.1
Jones (691)	1918	19	1	5.3
Locke, Thomas, and O'Hara (797)	1919–1920	66	21	31.8
Thomas (1299)	1917–1921	26	9	34.6
Park, Bullowa, and Rosenblüth (991)	1926–1928	61	18	29.5
Finland (442)	1924–1929	32	11	34.4
Baldwin (59)	1926–1930	29	15	51.7
Cecil and Plummer (239)	1920–1931	441	215	48.8
Blake (120)	1921–1931	79	32	40.5
Howard and Fullerton (663)	1929–1931	12	1	8.3
Cohn and Lewis (288)	1911–1932	388†	98	25.3
Buchanan and Ashley (164)	1934	17	5	29.4
Massachusetts Pneumonia Study (615)	1931–1935	51	11	21.6
Finland (449)	1930–1936	165	73	44.2
Benjamin, Blankenhorn, Ruegsegger, and Senior (94)	1935–1937	26	9	34.6
Total		1,592	582	36.6
Additional Type II cases				
Kohl and Reitzel (734)	1932–1935	32‡	9	28.1
Bullowa (190)	1928–1936	129‡	60	46.5
Grand total		1,753	651	37.1

* Three cases were atypical Type II.
† Specific serum was used in the treatment of a few of these cases.
‡ Pneumococcus pneumonia (lobar pneumonia and bronchopneumonia together).

627, with a fatality rate of 29 per cent, suggesting that the fatality rate with Type II infections is somewhat lower in the countries listed than in the United States and Canada. The possibility of Type II cases having a lower fatality rate in Great Britain than in this country was mentioned by previous

TABLE 120. TYPE II LOBAR PNEUMONIA. NUMBER OF CASES AND NUMBER AND PERCENTAGE OF DEATHS IN COUNTRIES OTHER THAN THE UNITED STATES AND CANADA

SOURCE	NUMBER OF CASES	DEATHS Number	DEATHS Per cent
Great Britain			
Ferguson and Lovell, 1928 (437)	5	1	20.0
Alston and Stewart, 1930 (13)	75	23	30.7
Leys, 1933 (779)	23	6	26.1
Therapeutic Trials Committee of Medical Research Council, 1934 (557)	305*	82	26.9
Langley, 1935 (763)	67	33	49.3
Irish Free State			
Moore, 1923 (902)	25	8	32.0
Denmark			
Christensen, 1925 (265)	41	4	19.0
Total	541	157	29.0
Other countries			
Marginesu and Corda (Italy), 1923 (860)	5	–	–
Wu and Chiu (China), 1933 (1450)	42	8	19.0
Levi (Italy), 1933 (775)	21	5	23.8
Bhatnagar and Singh (India), 1935 (100)	18	12	66.7
Total	86	25	29.1
Grand total	627	182	29.0

* Only patients twenty to sixty years of age were included in this series, and all patients dying within twenty-four hours of admission to hospitals were omitted.

investigators (557). The fatality rate of 29 per cent for 541 cases in the British Isles and Denmark is essentially the same as that of 29.1 per cent for 86 cases from other foreign countries. The number of cases in the latter group is of course small. Combining the cases in Tables 119 and 120 there is a grand total of 2,380 Type II cases, among which death occurred in 833, or 35 per cent.

Among 15 cases of atypical pneumonia or bronchopneumonia due to pneumococci of Type II, Finland (449), at the City Hospital in Boston, had 12, or 80 per cent of deaths (see Table 126, page 675).

As mentioned in Chapter II (pages 42–47) and as shown in Tables 5 and

6 (pages 43 and 48), the incidence in pneumococcus lobar pneumonia of cases due to Type I and Type II appears definitely higher in Europe, particularly in Great Britain and the Scandinavian countries, than in the United States and Canada. Further, as shown in Tables 117–120, the fatality rates of cases due to either of these two types are lower in the European countries mentioned than in this country. The question arises whether or not the lower fatality rate in the older civilizations of Europe could be the product of a longer exposure to the types in question, with the result that the infections these organisms produce are more frequent but less fatal. The possible effect of resistance upon the production of lobar pneumonia was mentioned earlier (see pages 232–235). It would seem that either host resistance is generally higher in Europe and that the immune response to infection is more prompt and vigorous than in this country, as is also suggested by the occurrence of a lower fatality rate in bacteriemic cases in Great Britain (331, 557), or that the organisms are less invasive there. Judging from the somewhat limited data available relative to the incidence of bacteriemia in Type I and II cases in Europe (331, 557), which may be about the same as that in the United States, and from the great frequency with which these organisms cause pneumonia abroad, there seems little reason to believe that any marked difference exists in the invasiveness of these types in the two places. Much additional study is needed, however, to clarify the matter.

TYPE III CASES. In Table 121 are summarized the available figures relating to the fatality rate of cases of Type III lobar pneumonia. The fatality rate of 1,109 cases occurring in the United States and Canada is 46 per cent (510 deaths) and that of 105 cases occurring in other countries is 39 per cent (41 deaths), the rate being somewhat higher for cases in the United States and Canada group. In all there is a grand total of 1,214 cases of Type III lobar pneumonia, of which 551, or 45.4 per cent, died. Type III cases then have a higher average fatality rate than the combined total of either the Type I cases (26.6 per cent) or the Type II cases (35 per cent), mentioned in the sections above.

The explanation of the high fatality rate in Type III cases lies, in part, with the tendency of pneumococci of this type to attack individuals over fifty or sixty years of age (see pages 60–64) and especially if some chronic illness has already lowered their resistance (see pages 335–336). The fatality rate of Type III cases in young adults is much lower than in elderly patients (464).

Information is also at hand relating to the fatality rate of cases of Type

TABLE 121. TYPE III LOBAR PNEUMONIA. NUMBER OF CASES AND NUMBER AND PERCENTAGE OF DEATHS IN VARIOUS COUNTRIES

SOURCE	NUMBER OF CASES	DEATHS *Number*	DEATHS *Per cent*
United States and Canada			
Quigley, 1918 (1054)	13	1	7.8
Locke, Thomas, and O'Hara, 1920 (797)	45	21	46.7
Cecil, Baldwin, and Larsen, 1927 (230)	161	67	41.6
Park, Bullowa, and Rosenblüth, 1928 (991)	92	27	29.3
Finland, 1930 (442)	17	7	41.2
Bigelow, 1931 (104)	9	4	44.4
Blake, 1931 (120)	122	54	44.3
Howard and Fullerton, 1932 (663)	16	5	31.3
Buchanan and Ashley, 1935 (164)	14	5	35.7
Cohn and Lewis, 1935 (288)	181	75	41.4
Massachusetts Pneumonia Study, 1937 (615)	104	40	38.5
Finland, 1937 (449)	335	204	61.0
Total	1,109	510	46.0
Other countries			
Marginesu and Corda (Italy), 1923 (860)	6	2	33.3
Moore (Ireland), 1923 (902)	7	–	–
Macgregor (Great Britain), 1933 (837)	42	18	42.9
Wu and Chiu (China), 1933 (1450)	14	4	28.6
Levi (Italy), 1933 (775)	16	9	56.3
Davies, Hodgson, and Whitby (Great Britain), 1935 (340)	20	8	40.0
Total	105	41	39.0
Grand total	1,214	551	45.4

III pneumococcus pneumonia (lobar pneumonia and bronchopneumonia together). Finland (449) reported a fatality rate of 60.6 per cent for 434 cases with 263 deaths, and Bullowa (190) 39.6 per cent for 273 cases with 108 deaths. Together these two sizable series total 707 cases with 371 deaths, a rate of 52.5 per cent (see Tables 126 and 127, pages 675 and 676). Finland's series includes his 335 cases with 204 deaths listed in Table 121. The proportion of deaths in Finland's series is extraordinarily high (60.6 per cent) but is probably largely influenced by the fact that most of the patients admitted

TABLE 122. GROUP IV LOBAR PNEUMONIA. NUMBER OF CASES AND NUMBER AND PERCENTAGE OF DEATHS IN VARIOUS COUNTRIES

SOURCE	NUMBER OF CASES	DEATHS Number	DEATHS Per cent
United States and Canada			
Locke, Thomas, and O'Hara, 1920 (797)	77	29	37.7
Cecil, Baldwin, and Larsen, 1927 (230)	373	109	29.2
Park, Bullowa, and Rosenblüth, 1928 (991)	324	83	25.6
Finland, 1930 (442)	94	30	31.9
Blake, 1931 (120)	211	54	25.6
Buchanan and Ashley, 1935 (164)	38	10	26.3
Cohn and Lewis, 1935 (288)	326	47	14.4
Massachusetts Pneumonia Study, 1937 (615)	321	48	15.0
Total	1,764	410	23.2
Other countries			
Marginesu and Corda (Italy), 1923 (860)	17	4	23.5
Moore (Ireland), 1923 (902)	42	6	14.3
Ferguson and Lovell (Great Britain), 1928 (437)	61	15	24.6
Macgregor (Great Britain), 1933 (837)	237	20	8.4
Wu and Chiu (China), 1933 (1450)	76	17	22.4
Levi (Italy), 1933 (775)	23	4	17.4
Davies, Hodgson, and Whitby (Great Britain), 1935 (340)	49	7	14.3
Total	505	73	14.5
Grand total	2,269	483	21.3

to the Boston City Hospital are from the lowest social classes. This obviously is not the sole explanation, for Bullowa's patients at the Harlem Hospital, New York City, come from about the same level in the social scale. Finland's patients, however, tend to be somewhat older on the average than Bullowa's, as elsewhere mentioned (see pages 63–64). In addition, it is possible that Bullowa's cases are more representative of the general situation in the community and it is likely that in comparison with the cases treated at the Boston City Hospital, those cared for at the Harlem Hospital represent a higher proportion of all cases occurring in the immediate vicinity of the institution. As a consequence of this situation, Finland's cases may be considered representative of about the most severe and unfavorable type of case encountered and typical of the cases entering many large charity hospitals in the country, which draw their patients from the whole city in which they are located rather than from one special section of it. Possibly other factors also are concerned in the explanation of the differences in the fatality rates of cases in these two institutions.

TABLE 123. TYPE V PNEUMOCOCCUS PNEUMONIA. NUMBER OF CASES AND NUMBER AND PERCENTAGE OF DEATHS IN THE UNITED STATES*

SOURCE	NUMBER OF CASES	DEATHS *Number*	DEATHS *Per cent*
Finland and Tilghman, 1936 (466)	197	90	45.7
Massachusetts Pneumonia Study, 1937 (615)	44†	11	25.0
Benjamin, Blankenhorn, Ruegsegger, and Senior, 1937 (94)	36†	11	30.6
Bullowa, 1937 (190)	166	31	18.7
Rosenblüth and Block, 1937 (1113)	29	11	37.9
Total	472	154	32.6

* Thirty-nine cases with 14 deaths (35.9 per cent) reported by Cooper, Rosenstein, Walter, and Peizer (320) are omitted from the table as it is probable that many of these cases are included in Bullowa's (190) series as shown, and that others are in the series of Rosenblüth and Block (1113)

† Cases of lobar pneumonia.

GROUP IV CASES. The fatality rates in numerous series of cases of Group IV lobar pneumonia have been reported from various places in the world. A number of series are tabulated in Table 122. Of the cases reported from the United States and Canada, death occurred in 23.2 per cent, or 410, of 1,764 cases, as compared with 14.5 per cent, or 73, of 505 cases reported from other countries. In the grand total of all these cases the fatality rate is 21.3 per cent for 2,269 cases (483 deaths).

The fatality rates in cases due to many of the individual higher types included in Group IV are mentioned below (see also Tables 126 and 127, pages 675 and 676).

TYPE V CASES. The fatality rate of reported cases of Type V pneumonia is shown in Table 123. All cases included are from American sources. As indicated in the table, the cases in two of the series are of Type V lobar pneumonia, while those in the remaining three series are of Type V pneumonia (lobar pneumonia and bronchopneumonia together). Together there are 472 cases and death occurred in 154 or 32.6 per cent. Pneumococci of Type V are immunologically related to those of Type II and, as the accompanying figures indicate, not infrequently give rise to severe infections.

TYPE VII CASES. Table 124 lists five series of Type VII cases collected from the American literature. In two series as indicated the cases are of lobar pneumonia, while in the remainder they are of pneumonia (lobar pneumonia and bronchopneumonia together). In all there are 383 cases with 94 deaths, a rate of 24.5 per cent, and the fatality rate is lower in these cases than in those due to Type V, mentioned above.

TABLE 124. TYPE VII PNEUMOCOCCUS PNEUMONIA. NUMBER OF CASES AND NUMBER AND PERCENTAGE OF DEATHS IN THE UNITED STATES*

SOURCE	NUMBER OF CASES	DEATHS	
		Number	*Per cent*
Kohl and Reitzel, 1936 (734)	14	3	21.4
Finland, Ruegsegger, Dowling, and Tilghman, 1937 (456)	130	50	38.5
Massachusetts Pneumonia Study, 1937 (615)	41†	2	4.9
Benjamin, Blankenhorn, Ruegsegger, and Senior, 1937 (94)	25†	6	24.0
Bullowa, 1937 (190)	173	33	19.1
Total	383	94	24.5

* Thirty-six cases with 10 deaths (27.8 per cent) reported by Cooper, Rosenstein, Walter, and Peizer (320) are omitted from the table as it is probable that many if not all of these cases are included in Bullowa's (190) series here listed.

† Cases of lobar pneumonia.

TYPE VIII CASES. The available Type VIII cases are mostly of pneumococcus Type VIII pneumonia (lobar pneumonia and bronchopneumonia together) and are all from American sources, as shown in Table 125. Among a total of 520 cases 119, or 22.9 per cent, died. The 227 cases of Finland (449) and the 197 cases of Bullowa (190) are the two largest series among those shown. The fatality rates in these two series are markedly different, for the rate in the former series is 34.8 per cent, as compared with 12.7 per cent in the latter.

TABLE 125. TYPE VIII PNEUMOCOCCUS PNEUMONIA. NUMBER OF CASES AND NUMBER AND PERCENTAGE OF DEATHS IN THE UNITED STATES*

SOURCE	NUMBER OF CASES	DEATHS Number	DEATHS Per cent
Kohl and Reitzel, 1936 (734)	8	4	50.0
Massachusetts Pneumonia Study, 1937 (615)	66†	8	12.1
Finland, 1937 (449)	227	79	34.8
Benjamin, Blankenhorn, Ruegsegger, and Senior, 1937 (94)	22†	3	13.6
Bullowa, 1937 (190)	197	25	12.7
Total	520	119	22.9

* Twenty-seven cases with 7 deaths (25.9 per cent) reported by Cooper, Rosenstein, Walter, and Peizer (320) are omitted from the table as it is probable that many if not all of these cases are included in Bullowa's (190) series here shown.

† Cases of lobar pneumonia.

Here again, as with the Type III cases mentioned earlier, the kind of patient these observations are based on is possibly largely responsible for the differences observed, and the patients in Finland's group were probably older than those in Bullowa's series, as suggested by the findings mentioned elsewhere (see pages 63–64). The Type VIII pneumococcus is immunologically related to Type III, but usually gives rise to a less serious illness than the latter.

TYPE XIV CASES. In adults Type XIV infections are likely to be serious. In the Massachusetts Pneumonia Study (615) death occurred in 3 of 14 patients having Type XIV lobar pneumonia. Finland (449) has reported a fatality rate of 42.7 per cent in 75 Type XIV cases (32 deaths) of pneumococcus pneumonia (lobar pneumonia and bronchopneumonia together) in adults, and Bullowa (190) a rate of 31.9 per cent among 91 similar cases‡ (29 deaths). Combining these three series, there is a total of 180 cases with 64 deaths, a rate of 35.6 per cent. (For cases in infants and children see pages 704–707.)

PNEUMOCOCCUS PNEUMONIA. Finland (449) has summarized his findings relating to the fatality rates in cases of lobar pneumonia or of atypical pneu-

‡ It is probable that 5 cases with 2 deaths earlier reported by Cooper, Rosenstein, Walter, and Peizer (320) are included in Bullowa's (190) series above mentioned.

monia (bronchopneumonia) due to one or another of nearly all the individual types of pneumococci from Type I through Type XX, as shown in Table 126. The table also includes cases due to all other types. The cases included were studied at the Boston City Hospital over a period extending from the middle of 1930 through June 30, 1936. The severity of the pneumonias in that hospital is attested by a fatality rate of 41 per cent for a total of 1,759 cases of pneumococcus lobar pneumonia, and the rate was even higher than this among the 617 cases of pneumonia of atypical forms.

TABLE 126. PNEUMOCOCCUS PNEUMONIA IN ADULTS. NUMBER OF CASES AND PERCENTAGE OF DEATHS IN PATIENTS WITH LOBAR PNEUMONIA AND ATYPICAL PNEUMONIA (BRONCHOPNEUMONIA), BY TYPE

PNEUMOCOCCUS TYPE	LOBAR PNEUMONIA NUMBER OF CASES	LOBAR PNEUMONIA DEATHS *Per cent*	ATYPICAL PNEUMONIA (BRONCHOPNEUMONIA) NUMBER OF CASES	ATYPICAL PNEUMONIA (BRONCHOPNEUMONIA) DEATHS *Per cent*
I	365	43	28	89
II	165	44	15	80
III	335	61	99	59
IV	46	39	18	67
V	167	42	30	67
VI	28	39	30	50
VII	100	33	30	57
VIII	159	24	68	60
IX	30	30	12	50
X	37	32	40	50
XI	29	24	18	44
XII	38	29	8	63
XIV	51	39	24	50
XVII	19	26	20	40
XVIII	38	29	32	66
XIX	19	26	12	8
XX	36	17	35	46
All others*	99	26	98	42
Total	1,759†	41	617‡	

From Finland (449)

* Includes some cases of unknown type.

† Early compilation of data on the fatality rate of cases of lobar pneumonia due to pneumococci of the higher types was based on a combined total of 493 cases reported by several investigators with 139 deaths or 28.2 per cent.

‡ Two Type VII cases are omitted, as they received serum treatment.

Bullowa (190) has also reported a large series of cases studied at the Harlem Hospital, New York City, over the period from July 1, 1928 through June 30, 1936 (see Table 127). These cases were of pneumococcus pneumo-

TABLE 127. PNEUMOCOCCUS PNEUMONIA IN ADULTS. NUMBER OF CASES (LOBAR PNEUMONIA AND BRONCHOPNEUMONIA TOGETHER) AND NUMBER AND PERCENTAGE OF DEATHS, BY TYPE

PNEUMOCOCCUS TYPE	NUMBER OF CASES	DEATHS	
		Number	*Per cent*
I	100	30	30.0
II	129	60	46.5
III	273	108	39.6
IV	151	30	19.9
V	166	31	18.7
VI	43	8	18.6
VII	173	33	19.1
VIII	197	25	12.7
IX	67	18	26.9
X	16	3	18.8
XI	21	4	19.0
XII	46	11	23.9
XIII	28	6	21.4
XIV	91	29	31.9
XV	15	5	33.3
XVI	23	5	21.8
XVII	25	8	32.0
XVIII	58	14	24.2
XIX	45	14	31.2
XX	38	8	21.0
XXI	19	2	10.5
XXII	25	2	8.0
XXIII	19	5	26.3
XXIV	12	2	16.7
XXV	11	1	9.1
XXVII	6	–	–
XXVIII	9	1	11.1
XXIX	13	2	15.4
XXX	4	–	–
XXXI	6	2	33.3
XXXII	7	–	–
Unclassified	257	54	20.4
Total	2,093	521	24.9

From Bullowa (190)

nia (lobar pneumonia and bronchopneumonia together) and wherever possible were classified as to the type causing the infection. Among his series of 2,093 cases listed in Table 127, the fatality rate was 24.9 per cent (521 deaths), which is only about one-half as high as the fatality rate of Finland's cases shown in Table 126.

It is clear from the findings recorded in Tables 123–127 that pneumonia due to pneumococci of any one of many of the higher types may cause death in a considerable proportion of the cases.

Pneumonia Due to Organisms Other than Pneumococci

Bullowa (190) reported a series of 756 cases of pneumonia (lobar pneumonia and bronchopneumonia together) due to organisms other than pneumococci, among which 249, or 33 per cent died. The fatality rate of 99 cases due to *Beta*-hemolytic streptococci included in this series was 39.4 per cent (39 deaths). A rate of 82 per cent was found in 39 cases (32 deaths) due to Friedländer's bacillus, and of 43.9 per cent for 73 cases (32 deaths) with multiple infections. Additional information relating to the fatality rates of pneumonia due to organisms other than pneumococci is presented elsewhere (see pages 3–17).

Year and Season

It has long been recognized that the general fatality rate of pneumonia and of lobar pneumonia varies each year and that at times the variations may be marked (1319, 1176, 1008, 807, 708, 713, 1357, 1385, 331). The explanation of such variations remains largely unknown but may be due to changes either in the virulence of the infecting organism or to alterations in host resistance. Thus far attempts to measure alterations of virulence in different years have been unsuccessful. Cruickshank (331) observes that variations in fatality rates in different years may arise from differences in the type distribution of the cases occurring in the various years quite apart from any change in the virulence of a given type (see also pages 57–60). Doubtless this is involved in the problem, but marked differences in the fatality rates of cases due to a single type may occur in successive years (see Table 128).

In a series of 1,000 cases of lobar pneumonia at the Massachusetts General Hospital occurring between 1821 and 1889, Townsend and Coolidge (1319) reported a gradual rise in the fatality rate over the period investigated, the rate rising from 10 per cent for cases in the first decade studied to 28 per cent for cases in the last decade. Due to the difficulties encountered in the diagnosis of some of the early cases in this series, too much reliance cannot be placed upon the finding of an apparently low fatality rate in the early part of the period. This investigation was later extended by Shattuck and Lawrence (1176) to embrace cases occurring at the same hospital up to 1917, thus permitting a review of lobar pneumonia in a single institution over a span of nearly a century (95 years). The total number of cases investigated was about 4,000. They confirmed Townsend and Coolidge's findings and also stated that when considered by decades there was no evidence that the fatality rates had changed perceptibly since 1881.

TABLE 128. PNEUMOCOCCUS LOBAR PNEUMONIA. TOTAL NUMBER OF CASES AND TOTAL NUMBER OF DEATHS AND PERCENTAGE OF DEATHS IN TYPE I, II, III, AND GROUP IV CASES, BY YEAR*

YEAR	NUMBER OF CASES	DEATHS NUMBER	TYPE I *Per cent*	TYPE II *Per cent*	TYPE III *Per cent*	GROUP IV *Per cent*	AVERAGE YEARLY *Per cent*
1920–1921	377	93	20.4	29.4	35.2	22.4	24.6
1921–1922	534	138	17.1	39.3	43.3	18.9	25.8
1922–1923	319	89	11.9	39.8	40.0	25.1	27.9
1923–1924	275	96	20.0	50.9	45.4	34.0	34.9
1924–1925	408	128	21.9	41.4	53.1	30.4	31.3
Total	1,913	544					28.4

From Cecil *et al.* (230)

* Many cases received specific serum treatment.

A very similar study was made by Greenwood and Candy (567) in 1911 in London at the London Hospital. The records were searched back as far as 1784, but the most reliable data pertained to cases treated there during the last fifty years, and during that interval there were 5,116 cases with 997 deaths, a rate of 19.5 per cent. Their findings indicated that no particular change in the fatality rate had occurred over the fifty-year period.

Except as modified by the use of specific therapy in recent years, there seems no evidence that the fatality rate of pneumonia treated by other means has changed for a century or more and it is doubtful if it has changed much for a still longer period. Yearly variations in the fatality rate, however, almost invariably occur.

In 800 cases of lobar pneumonia in African natives, studied over a three-year period, Pearson and Mouchet (1008) found the fatality rate varied from 12.8 to 21.6 per cent in different years. Lord (807) studied a series of 2,025 cases occurring at the Massachusetts General Hospital between 1897 and

1913 and found that 507, or 25 per cent, died. The lowest fatality rate in any year was 15.3 per cent (20 of 130 cases died) and the highest was 31.6 per cent (38 of 120 cases died). Lord also mentioned that in a series of 500 cases the largest number of consecutive recoveries was 16. In 1926 Kelly (708) investigated 6,531 cases of lobar pneumonia which occurred at the Cook County Hospital in Chicago over a period of seven and a half years, and found the fatality rate to vary from 26.6 per cent to 41.4 per cent in different years. Among a series of 1,030 cases occurring over a nine-year period in the Philippines, Vitug and Hizon (1357) report that the fatality rate varied from 15 to 35 per cent in different years.

Cecil, Baldwin, and Larsen (230) studied variations of the fatality rates of 1,913 cases of pneumococcus lobar pneumonia, of which 544, or 28.4 per cent, died over a five-year period at the Bellevue Hospital, New York City (Table 128). Many of the cases received varying amounts of specific serum in treatment. As seen in Table 128 the fatality rate of Type I cases varied in different years from a low of 11.9 per cent to a high of 21.9 per cent. The minimum and maximum rates for Type II cases were 29.4 and 50.9 per cent, for Type III cases 35.2 and 53.1 per cent, and for Group IV cases 18.9 and 34 per cent. The proportional variation was least marked with Type III cases. A yearly variation in the fatality rate for all the cases was also apparent. Findings of like significance were reported for Type I and Type II cases by Park, Bullowa, and Rosenblüth (991), for Type I cases by Cecil and Plummer (238), and for Type I and Type II cases in Great Britain by several workers (557).

In addition to apparently unpredictable yearly differences in the fatality rates in lobar pneumonia, seasonal variations of the rates also occur. In 1889 Wells (1402) reported that from his findings in a collected series of more than 600,000 deaths from "pneumonia" there was some evidence that death was most frequent in the winter and spring months. Evidence indicating a similar phenomenon has been accumulated from subsequent reports.

Patterson (1003a) studied a series of 521 cases of lobar pneumonia over a two and one-half year period in Australia, and found the fatality rate of 115 cases occurring in summer to be 20 per cent (23 deaths) and of 138 cases in the autumn to be 16.7 per cent (23 deaths), while in cases occurring in the winter the rate was 24.6 per cent for 167 cases (41 deaths) and in the spring 25 per cent for 101 cases (25 deaths). Observations much similar to these were made in 2,629 cases (of which 825, or 31.7 per cent, died) by Cecil, Baldwin, and Larsen (230). The fatality rate of 1,195 of their cases with 421 deaths was 35.2 per cent in the late winter and early spring (January, February, and March), as compared with a rate of 27.2 per cent for 253 cases (69 deaths) in the summer (July, August, and September). It is probable that many of the cases in the series of Cecil and his associates received specific serum therapy.

Results very similar, though less striking, have been reported in 1,030 cases from the Philippines by Vitug and Hizon (1357), and findings about as definite as those of Cecil and his collaborators were obtained by Macgregor (837) in 1,077 cases in Glasgow. Kelly (708), in Chicago, in a series of 6,531 cases occurring over a period of seven and one-half years, also reports that some seasonal variation in the fatality rate was present in his series. This variation, however, was different from that mentioned above, for the highest rate (41.8 per cent) occurred in the fall (October), and the lowest rate (32.4 per cent) was in early summer (June). No additional data are given by Kelly concerning this matter.

Also of interest in connection with the problem of seasonal variation of fatality rates were the findings obtained during the Massachusetts Pneumonia Study and Continuing Program in a series of 1,043 Type I and 281 Type II cases treated with specific immune serum from January 1, 1931 through June 30, 1937 (see Table 129). The Type I results were reported by Lord and Heffron (814). Of 299 Type I cases treated during the months of April through September (late spring and summer) 28, or 9.4 per cent, died. Of 217 Type I cases occurring from October through December (early fall and winter) 26, or 12 per cent, died, and during January through March (late winter and early spring) there were 527 cases of which 91, or 17.3 per cent, died. The fatality rate increased, then, from the warmer to the colder period of the year and was highest in the winter months, being nearly double that for the summer months. The results appeared somewhat similar for the serum treated Type II cases but the groups are too small to be of significance. With Type II, however, the highest rate obtained in the spring months of April through June, rather than in the late winter and early spring, as with Type I (see also pages 381–385).

The explanation of these differences is not clear. Perhaps the greater prevalence of colds and other acute respiratory tract infections, the more rapid transfer and larger dosage of organisms through crowding, and a decreased host resistance during the winter months are responsible. Evidence that host resistance is depressed in winter was discussed previously (see pages 201–203), and the facts that about 70 per cent of the cases and the same proportion of all deaths from this disease occur in the first six months of each year in Massachusetts, as elsewhere mentioned (see pages 290–293), seem also to point in the same direction.

Bacteriemia

The frequency with which organisms are found in the blood in pneumonia was mentioned in the discussion of complications (pages 549–563), where

TABLE 129. PNEUMOCOCCUS LOBAR PNEUMONIA. NUMBER OF TYPE I AND TYPE II CASES AND NUMBER AND PERCENTAGE OF DEATHS, BY QUARTERS OF THE YEAR

PERIOD IN WHICH CASES OCCURRED	NUMBER OF CASES	DEATHS Number	DEATHS Per cent
		Type I cases	
April 1—June 30	256	25	9.8
July 1—September 30	43	3	7.0
October 1—December 31	217	26	12.0
January 1—March 31	527	91	17.3
Total	1,043		
		Type II cases	
April 1—June 30	58	14	24.1
July 1—September 30	13	2	15.4
October 1—December 31	79	17	21.5
January 1—March 31	131	30	22.9
Total	281		

Cases from the Massachusetts Pneumonia Series. All received varying amounts of specific antipneumococcic serum.

it was noted that Rosenow (1114) examined 175 cases of lobar pneumonia and obtained positive blood cultures from nearly all cases. As bacteriemia was so common in his series, he concluded its presence was without value in estimating the outlook in any case. Subsequent findings, however, make it clear that the occurrence of bacteriemia in the usual instance is of great prognostic importance. In fact, Cole (299) considers the presence or absence of invasion of the blood in pneumococcus cases the most important prognostic feature. The effect of bacteriemia in influencing the prognosis in children with pneumonia is considered separately below (see page 693).

Many series of cases are available, giving information as to the fatality rate in cases without or with bacteriemia. The fatality rate of cases with bacteriemia is several times higher than that of cases with sterile blood cultures. Combining the series of lobar pneumonias reported by MacCordick (830) and by Warr and Alperin (1385), which include a number of cases of unknown etiology, the fatality rate of 345 cases without bacteriemia was 21.2 per cent (73 deaths), as compared with a rate of 54.5 per cent for 123 cases

TABLE 130. PNEUMOCOCCUS LOBAR PNEUMONIA. NUMBER OF CASES AND NUMBER AND PERCENTAGE OF DEATHS IN CASES WITHOUT AND WITH BACTERIEMIA

SOURCE	WITHOUT BACTERIEMIA			WITH BACTERIEMIA		
	NUMBER OF CASES	DEATHS *Number*	DEATHS *Per cent*	NUMBER OF CASES	DEATHS *Number*	DEATHS *Per cent*
Alexander, 1917 (9)	72	14	19.4	21	15	71.4
Bloomfield, 1923 (136)* ..	187	34	18.2	70	39	55.7
Baldwin and Rhoades, 1925 (61)*	70	7	10.0	37	29	78.4
Cecil, Baldwin, and Larsen, 1927 (230)*	240	45	18.8	89	74	83.1
Bullowa, Rosenblüth, Park, and Cooper, 1928 (195)	205	28	13.7	49	40	81.6
Koch, 1932 (733)	nr	nr	nr	45	34	75.6
Sutliff, 1932 (1267)	218	59	27.1	62	42	67.7
Wu and Chiu, 1933 (1450)*	164	15	9.1	44	33	75.0
Cohn and Lewis, 1935 (288)†	1,002	84	8.4	399	198	49.6
Total	2,158	286	13.3	816	504	61.8

nr = no record.

* Serum was used in the treatment of some of these cases.

† There are 501 Type I cases in this series, most of which received specific serum treatment, as did a few of the 388 Type II cases included. The etiology was unknown in 70 of the cases.

with bacteriemia (67 deaths). The fatality rate with bacteriemia was thus between two and three times as high as without it.

Of greater value are the findings in other series in which the etiology of the cases was known. The findings in a number of such series composed almost wholly of pneumococcus lobar pneumonia are shown in Table 130.

The fatality rate in 2,158 cases without bacteriemia in Table 130 is 13.3 per cent (286 deaths) in contrast to the rate of 61.8 per cent for 816 cases (504 deaths) among patients having bacteriemia. Even though some of the cases in these series received specific serum treatment, as indicated in the table, the importance of bacteriemia is striking and death occurred from four to five times as often in cases with invasion of the blood stream as in others without it. In each individual series in Table 130 the fatality rate with bacteriemia is uniformly high, as compared with the rate in the corresponding series in cases without this condition.

The findings in cases of pneumococcus pneumonia in general (lobar pneumonia and bronchopneumonia together), without and with bacteriemia, are given in Table 136 (page 688).

TYPE I CASES. In Table 131 are listed a number of series giving the fatality rate of cases of Type I lobar pneumonia in the absence or presence of bacteriemia

TABLE 131. TYPE I LOBAR PNEUMONIA. NUMBER OF CASES AND NUMBER AND PERCENTAGE OF DEATHS IN CASES WITHOUT AND WITH BACTERIEMIA

SOURCE	WITHOUT BACTERIEMIA			WITH BACTERIEMIA		
	NUMBER OF CASES	DEATHS *Number*	DEATHS *Per cent*	NUMBER OF CASES	DEATHS *Number*	DEATHS *Per cent*
Baldwin and Rhoades, 1925 (61)*	28	3	10.7	11	6	54.5
Bullowa, Rosenblüth, Park, and Cooper, 1928 (195)	48	8	16.7	22	18	81.8
Cecil and Plummer, 1930 (238)	80	18	22.5	45	30	66.7
Chickering, 1930 (258)	nr	nr	nr	30	10	33.3
Sutliff, 1932 (1267)	29	4	13.8	22	17	77.3
Bullowa, 1933 (183)	nr	nr	nr	10	8	80.0
Wu and Chiu, 1933 (1450)*	71	2	2.8	20	10	50.0
Cruickshank, 1933 (331)	nr	nr	nr	37	5	13.5
Warr and Alperin, 1933 (1385)	nr	nr	nr	31	14	45.2
Therapeutic Trials Committee of Medical Research Council, 1934 (557)†	72	11	15.3	23	4	17.4
Finland, 1936 (448)	129	24	18.6	100	81	81.0
Total	457	70	15.3	351	204	58.1

nr = no record.

* Probably some cases received specific antiserum.

† Only patients twenty to sixty years of age were included in this series, and all patients dying within twenty-four hours of admission to hospitals were omitted.

TABLE 132. TYPE II LOBAR PNEUMONIA. NUMBER OF CASES AND NUMBER AND PERCENTAGE OF DEATHS IN CASES WITHOUT AND WITH BACTERIEMIA

SOURCE	WITHOUT BACTERIEMIA			WITH BACTERIEMIA		
	NUMBER OF CASES	DEATHS *Number*	DEATHS *Per cent*	NUMBER OF CASES	DEATHS *Number*	DEATHS *Per cent*
Avery, Chickering, Cole, and Dochez, 1917 (33)*	99	9	9.1	49	36	73.5
Baldwin and Rhoades, 1925 (61)*	8	1	12.5	14	13	92.9
Bullowa, Rosenblüth, Park, and Cooper, 1928 (195)	32	7	21.9	17	13	76.5
Chickering, 1930 (258) ..	10	3	30.0	11	10	90.9
Cecil and Plummer, 1932 (239)	71	6	8.5	64	56	87.5
Wu and Chiu, 1933 (1450)*	32	5	15.6	6	2	33.3
Cruickshank, 1933 (331)..	nr	nr	nr	34	18	52.9
Warr and Alperin, 1933 (1385)	nr	nr	nr	10	9	90.0
Bullowa, 1933 (183)	nr	nr	nr	35	27	77.1
Therapeutic Trials Committee of Medical Research Council, 1934 (557)† ..	73	8	11.0	22	11	50.0
Finland and Dowling, 1936 (452)	39	10	25.6	53	38	71.7
Total	364	49	13.5	315	233	74.0

nr = no record.

* Probably some cases received specific serum treatment.

† Only patients twenty to sixty years of age were included in this series, and all patients dying within twenty-four hours of admission to hospitals were omitted.

emia. The rate without this complication was 15.3 per cent in 457 cases (70 deaths), as compared with 58.1 per cent in 351 cases (204 deaths) in patients with bacteriemia, and was thus nearly four times as high in the latter group. Considerable variation is seen between the rates in each individual series in both groups. With respect to comments made earlier in this chapter in discussing the prognosis of pneumonia by type and to the probable occurrence of lower fatality rates in some European countries than in this country, it is of interest to note that the lowest fatality rates with bacteriemia seen in Table 131 are in the cases from Great Britain reported by Cruickshank (331; rate 13.5 per cent) and by the Therapeutic Trials Committee of the Medical

Research Council (557; rate 17.4 per cent). As the latter series includes only cases selected as indicated in the table, perhaps the rate noted is lower than actually occurs there in the usual run of Type I cases.

TYPE II CASES. Among 364 cases of Type II lobar pneumonia with sterile blood cultures 49, or 13.5 per cent, of the patients died, as compared with 74 per cent, or 233, of 315 patients with positive blood cultures, as seen in Table 132. The death rate in Type II cases is more than five times as high with bacteriemia as without it.

Here again the cases with bacteriemia with the lowest fatality rates were from foreign countries. In Wu and Chiu's (1450) series from China, and in the British series of Cruickshank (331) and of the Therapeutic Trials Committee of the Medical Research Council (557), the fatality rates with bacteriemia did not exceed 52.9 per cent, yet in the remainder of the series, which are of American origin, the rates were always above 71 per cent.

TYPE III CASES. The fatality rate of cases of Type III lobar pneumonia with bacteriemia is extraordinarily high. As seen in Table 133, 86.1 per cent, or 62

TABLE 133. TYPE III LOBAR PNEUMONIA. NUMBER OF CASES AND NUMBER AND PERCENTAGE OF DEATHS IN CASES WITHOUT AND WITH BACTERIEMIA

SOURCE	WITHOUT BACTERIEMIA			WITH BACTERIEMIA		
	NUMBER OF CASES	DEATHS *Number*	DEATHS *Per cent*	NUMBER OF CASES	DEATHS *Number*	DEATHS *Per cent*
Avery, Chickering, Cole, and Dochez, 1917 (33)	39	11	28.2	16	16	100.0
Baldwin and Rhoades, 1925 (61)	7	1	14.4	4	3	75.0
Cecil, Baldwin, and Larsen, 1927 (230)	26	11	42.3	10	8	80.0
Bullowa, Rosenblüth, Park, and Cooper, 1928 (195)	23	4	17.4	7	6	85.7
Wu and Chiu, 1933 (1450)	13	4	30.8	nr	nr	nr
Cruickshank, 1933 (331) ..	nr	nr	nr	4	4	100.0
Warr and Alperin, 1933 (1385)	nr	nr	nr	10	4	40.0
Bullowa, 1935 (186)	nr	nr	nr	21	21	100.0
Total	108	31	28.7	72	62	86.1

nr = no record.

of 72 cases with this condition, died, while in 108 cases without it 31, or 28.7 per cent, died. In each instance, however, the groups of cases are small. As the incidence of bacteriemia in cases of Type III lobar pneumonia is lower than in cases due to almost any other if not all of the commoner types, its demonstration in Type III cases may serve as an indication that the patient possesses an unusually feeble resistance. This view is supported by the observations of workers such as Cole (297), Blake (120), Finland and Sutliff (464), Finland and Winkler (468), and Bullowa (186), who have reported that bacteriemia in Type III cases is nearly always fatal.

GROUP IV CASES. The fatality rate of cases of Group IV lobar pneumonia without and with bacteriemia is seen in Table 134. Among 331 patients with

TABLE 134. GROUP IV LOBAR PNEUMONIA. NUMBER OF CASES AND NUMBER AND PERCENTAGE OF DEATHS IN CASES WITHOUT AND WITH BACTERIEMIA

SOURCE	WITHOUT BACTERIEMIA			WITH BACTERIEMIA		
	NUMBER OF CASES	DEATHS *Number*	DEATHS *Per cent*	NUMBER OF CASES	DEATHS *Number*	DEATHS *Per cent*
Avery, Chickering, Cole, and Dochez, 1917 (33)	79	3	3.8	21	11	52.4
Baldwin and Rhoades, 1925 (61)	27	2	7.4	8	7	87.5
Cecil, Baldwin, and Larsen, 1927 (230)	75	12	16.0	15	14	93.3
Bullowa, Rosenblüth, Park, and Cooper, 1928 (195)	102	9	8.8	3	3	100.0
Wu and Chiu, 1933 (1450)	48	4	8.3	18	11	61.1
Warr and Alperin, 1933 (1385)	nr	nr	nr	16	7	43.8
Cruickshank, 1933 (331)	nr	nr	nr	9	1	11.1
Total	331	30	9.1	90	54	60.0

nr = no record.

negative blood cultures 30, or 9.1 per cent, died, while death occurred in 60 per cent, or 54, of 90 patients whose blood cultures were positive. The number of cases in the latter group in particular is small. The proportion of the patients with bacteriemia who died varied considerably and was 11.1 per cent in Cruickshank's (331) series (from Great Britain) and was as high as 93 (230) to 100 per cent (195) in some of the other series (American cases).

TOTAL TYPE I, II, III, AND GROUP IV CASES. For ease of comparison the total series of cases with and without bacteriemia shown in Tables 131–134 may be combined, as seen in Table 135. In all there are 1,260 non-bacteriemic cases with 180, or 14.3 per cent of deaths, and 828 cases with bacteriemia with 553, or 66.8 per cent of deaths. The fatality rate of the bacteriemic cases was nearly five times that of the non-bacteriemic cases.

TABLE 135. PNEUMOCOCCUS LOBAR PNEUMONIA. NUMBER OF CASES AND NUMBER AND PERCENTAGE OF DEATHS IN CASES WITHOUT AND WITH BACTERIEMIA, BY TYPE

	WITHOUT BACTERIEMIA			WITH BACTERIEMIA		
	NUMBER OF CASES	DEATHS *Number*	DEATHS *Per cent*	NUMBER OF CASES	DEATHS *Number*	DEATHS *Per cent*
Type I (from Table 131)	457	70	15.3	351	204	58.1
Type II (from Table 132)	364	49	13.5	315	233	74.0
Type III (from Table 133)	108	31	28.7	72	62	86.1
Group IV (from Table 134)	331	30	9.1	90	54	60.0
Total	1,260	180	14.3	828	553	66.8

With respect to the cases without bacteriemia, the fatality rate was highest in Type III cases (28.7 per cent) and lowest in Group IV cases (9.1 per cent). In cases with bacteriemia the highest fatality rate was also in Type III cases (86.1 per cent), the rate in Type II cases being somewhat lower (74 per cent), and the lowest rates being in Group IV and Type I cases (60 and 58.1 per cent respectively). In pneumococcus lobar pneumonia the demonstration of bacteriemia must be considered important evidence that a serious deficiency exists in the resistance of the host to the invading organism.

PNEUMOCOCCUS PNEUMONIA. Some information is at hand relating to the fatality rates with and without bacteriemia of cases of pneumonia (lobar pneumonia and bronchopneumonia together) due to one or another of almost all the recognized types of pneumococci. Combining the series of Type V cases reported by Bullowa and Wilcox (199), Finland and Tilghman (466), and Rosenblüth and Block (1113), 236 cases showed negative blood cultures and death occurred in 33, or 14 per cent. Among their cases with bacteriemia, however, death occurred in 73.3 per cent, or 88, of 120 cases and in consequence was about five times as frequent in such cases (see also Table 136).

TABLE 136. PNEUMOCOCCUS PNEUMONIA (LOBAR PNEUMONIA AND BRONCHO-PNEUMONIA TOGETHER) IN ADULTS. NUMBER OF CASES AND NUMBER AND PERCENTAGE OF DEATHS WITHOUT AND WITH BACTERIEMIA, BY TYPE*

PNEUMOCOCCUS TYPE	WITHOUT BACTERIEMIA			WITH BACTERIEMIA		
	NUMBER OF CASES	DEATHS		NUMBER OF CASES	DEATHS	
		Number	*Per cent*		*Number*	*Per cent*
I	76	11	14.5	24	19	79.3
II	69	13	18.8	60	47	78.5
III	198	36	18.2	75	72	96.1
IV	124	9	7.3	27	21	77.8
V	127	8	6.3	39	23	59.0
VI	37	5	13.5	6	3	50.0
VII	151	16	10.6	22	17	77.4
VIII	161	10	6.2	36	15	41.7
IX	58	11	19.0	9	7	77.7
X	15	2	13.3	1	1	100.0
XI	20	3	15.0	1	1	100.0
XII	33	2	6.1	13	9	69.3
XIII	27	5	18.5	1	1	100.0
XIV	63	8	12.7	28	21	75.0
XV	13	4	30.8	2	1	50.0
XVI	22	4	18.2	1	1	100.0
XVII	23	7	30.4	2	1	50.0
XVIII	48	7	14.6	10	7	70.0
XIX	33	4	12.1	12	10	83.3
XX	31	3	9.7	7	5	71.5
XXI	17	1	5.9	2	1	50.0
XXII	23	1	4.4	2	1	50.0
XXIII	15	3	20.0	4	2	50.0
XXIV	9	1	11.1	3	1	33.3
XXV	8	–	–	3	1	33.3
XXVII	6	–	–	–	–	–
XXVIII	9	1	11.1	–	–	–
XXIX	12	1	8.5	1	1	100.0
XXX	4	–	–	–	–	–
XXXI	6	2	33.3	–	–	–
XXXII	6	–	–	1	–	–
Unclassified	241	45	18.1	16	9	56.3
Total	1,685	223	13.2	408	298	73.0

From Bullowa (190)

* Cases treated without specific serum therapy.

In the Type VII cases investigated by Finland, Ruegsegger, Dowling, and Tilghman (456), the fatality rate in 80 cases without bacteriemia was 26 per cent (21 deaths) and 90 per cent in 30 cases (27 deaths) with bacteriemia (see also Table 136).

Among cases of Type VIII pneumonia Finland and Sutliff (464) report that 21 per cent of 47 cases without bacteriemia died, while death occurred in 43 per cent of 21 cases having bacteriemia. The fatality rates in Bullowa's (184) cases are somewhat lower, and of 70 cases with negative blood cultures 9, or 12.8 per cent, died, as did 33.3 per cent, or 5, of 15 cases with positive blood cultures (see also Table 136).

In a series of Type XIV cases (in adults) examined by Bullowa (187) 9, or 69.2 per cent, of 13 patients with bacteriemia died, and of 30 cases without bacteriemia 23 per cent died (see also Table 136).

In addition to these cases of pneumococcus pneumonia (lobar pneumonia and bronchopneumonia together) a large series divided by type was reported by Bullowa (190), as seen in Table 136, which includes the above cases reported by Bullowa and his associate, already mentioned. The cases in Table 136 were cared for at the Harlem Hospital, New York City, during the period of July 1, 1928–June 30, 1936. In all there are 1,685 cases without bacteriemia with 223 deaths, a rate of 13.2 per cent, and 408 cases with bacteriemia with 298 deaths, a rate of 73 per cent.

The cases with bacteriemia in this table are of interest. Among the various types where the number of cases is greater than 20, the fatality rate is highest in Type III infections (96.1 per cent in 75 cases) and lowest in Type VIII infections (41.7 per cent in 36 cases). Among the non-bacteriemic cases where the number due to each type is greater than 20, the fatality rate is highest in Type XVII infections (30.4 per cent in 23 cases) and lowest in Type XXII infections (4.4 per cent in 23 cases).

PNEUMONIA DUE TO ORGANISMS OTHER THAN PNEUMOCOCCI. In a series of 643 cases of pneumonia (lobar pneumonia and bronchopneumonia together) due to various organisms other than pneumococci and without bacteriemia, Bullowa (190) found that 146, or 22.7 per cent, died, as compared with 91.3 per cent, or 103 of 113 similar cases with bacteriemia. The serious prognostic significance of bacteriemia in such cases was also mentioned earlier (see pages 3–16).

ADDITIONAL ASPECTS OF THE RELATION OF BACTERIEMIA TO PROGNOSIS. The relatively low fatality rate in pneumonia in the absence of bacteriemia, in contrast to the high proportion of deaths which occurs when this condition is present, strongly suggests that so long as invasion of the blood does not exist, the patient is rarely in danger (223). Apparently death may occur, however, even in the absence of bacteriemia, as was previously mentioned (see page 545), but usually at the time of death bacteriemia may be demonstrated (see page 561).

The presence of organisms in the blood, even if few in number, is usually an indication that collapse of the defensive mechanism of the body has begun and that in a sense, and in the absence of the use of specific treatment, the patient is doomed, as Bloomfield (136) has stated. Numerous aspects of bacteriemia and its relation to the efficiency of the blood-clearing mechanism

TABLE 137. PNEUMOCOCCUS LOBAR PNEUMONIA. NUMBER OF CASES AND NUMBER AND PERCENTAGE OF DEATHS WITHOUT AND WITH BACTERIEMIA, AND BY PERIOD IN WHICH BACTERIEMIA DEVELOPED*

BLOOD CULTURE AND PERIOD	NUMBER OF CASES	DEATHS	
		Number	*Per cent*
Negative within first 3 days	55	9	16.3
Positive within first 3 days	11	7	63.6
Positive after first 3 days	27	23	85.1

* Specific serum may have been used in the treatment of a few of these cases.

and other matters have been investigated in laboratory animals (169, 1237, 1243, 508, 1239, 834, 206, 483, 484, 286, 1328, 1083, 536), as elsewhere pointed out (see pages 162–164).

In man, the time during the illness when bacteriemia develops has an important relation to prognosis. Although serious at any time, positive blood cultures early in the disease usually mean less than the appearance of bacteriemia at a later period. Bloomfield (136) stated that a negative blood culture early in the illness means only that the issue is still an open one. He likewise mentioned that if the blood continues sterile until the sixth or seventh day there is much less likelihood that bacteriemia will develop and the prognosis in such cases is generally good. Baldwin and Rhoades' (61) observations relating to the significance of the time of development of bacteriemia are of importance and are shown in Table 137. As seen in that table, the fatality rate in 55 cases of pneumococcus lobar pneumonia having sterile blood cultures within the first three days of illness was 16.3 per cent, and among 11 cases with positive blood cultures in the first three days the fatality rate was 63.6 per cent. In comparison to this latter figure, however, death occurred in 85.1 per cent of 27 cases in which bacteriemia developed after the third day of illness.

The degree of persistence of bacteriemia in pneumonia is also an important factor in prognosis. Cohn and Lewis' (288) study of more than 1,200 cases of lobar pneumonia, nearly all of which were due to pneumococci of some type, illustrates this point very well. Their group includes several hundred Type I cases treated with specific antiserum and a few Type II cases similarly treated. The fatality rate of 1,002 cases with negative cultures was

TABLE 138. PNEUMOCOCCUS LOBAR PNEUMONIA. FATALITY RATE OF NON-BACTERIEMIC CASES AND OF BACTERIEMIC CASES, BY NUMBER OF ORGANISMS PRESENT PER CUBIC CENTIMETER OF BLOOD

BLOOD CULTURE FINDINGS	FATALITY RATE
Negative cultures	11.1
Positive cultures	
Colonies of organisms per cubic centimeter of blood	
1–2	31.3
2–5	40.0
5–10	40.0
10–20	33.3
20–50	85.7
50–100	100.0
100–500	80.0
Over 500	100.0

8.4 per cent (84 deaths, see Table 130, page 682). Among 253 cases which showed positive blood cultures only once, 101, or 40 per cent, died, as compared with a rate of 66.4 per cent among 146 cases (97 deaths) having positive blood cultures two or more times. In contrast to the fatality rate of cases without bacteriemia (8.4 per cent), the rate for cases having this condition was more than four times as high, and in cases with persistent bacteriemia the rate was about eight times as high.

As a rule, with bacteriemia, patients having the largest number of organisms in the blood have the highest fatality rate, as Avery, Chickering, Cole, and Dochez (33) and others (297, 661, 733) have reported. Cole's (297) findings in this connection in Type II and Group IV cases of lobar pneumonia are of interest and are shown in Table 138. No Type I cases were included in Cole's tabulation, as nearly all of his cases of this type received specific serum treatment. His Type III cases were also omitted, as all but two of several having bacteriemia died. The exact number of bacteriemic cases on which the observations in Table 138 are based was not stated, but presumably it was not less than 50.

In the absence of bacteriemia the fatality rate was 11.1 per cent, while in cases with from 1 to 20 colonies of organisms per cubic centimeter of blood the fatality rate varied from 31.3 to 40 per cent. In cases with more than 20 colonies per cubic centimeter of blood the prognosis was poorest and death occurred in from 80 to 100 per cent of the cases under those circumstances.

Koch (733) investigated a number of patients having pneumococcus lobar pneumonia and bacteriemia and reported that among 12 patients whose bacterial counts per cubic centimeter of blood gradually decreased, only 2 died, while among 20 patients showing stationary or increasing colony counts, all died. No patient with more than 30 colonies per cubic centimeter survived.

With respect to the omission by Cole (297) of Type III cases from the data shown in Table 138 because nearly all died, it is of interest to note that Blake (120) pointed out that in cases of this type bacteriemia is not so frequent or so heavy, as is mentioned elsewhere (see page 560), or so often encountered among fatal cases as it is among cases due to Type I or II. Similar findings were reported by Finland and Sutliff (464).

In 1917 Sutton and Sevier (1277) reported that in general the incidence of bacteriemia in cases of pneumococcus lobar pneumonia due to a particular type is about the same as the usual fatality rate of the cases due to that type. In consequence the incidence of bacteriemia in such cases is a rough index of the respective fatality rate for a given type. Among others, Baldwin and Rhoades (61), Baldwin and Cecil (60), Park, Bullowa, and Rosenblüth (991), and Cecil and Plummer (239) confirmed this observation for a few of the types, as did Bullowa (188) for cases of pneumococcus pneumonia due to one or another of many of the higher types. At least one notable exception to this generalization exists and that is with Type III, for as shown in Table 94 (page 553) the incidence of bacteriemia with this type is but 22 per cent, yet the usual fatality rate of such cases is approximately 45 per cent (see Table 121, page 670). In contrast to these variations the situation with Type I and to a less extent with Type II is different. With the former type the incidence of bacteriemia is 28 per cent (Table 92, page 551) and the usual fatality rate about 27 per cent (page 666), and with the latter type the corresponding figures are 43.7 per cent (Table 93, page 552) and 35 per cent (page 668).

INFANTS AND CHILDREN WITH BACTERIEMIA. In pneumonia in infants and children bacteriemia is less often found than in adults, as was earlier pointed out (see page 557), and in the usual case is of less serious prognostic significance, as was mentioned by Lyon (821) and Trask, O'Donovan, Moore, and Beebe (1321). Findings of similar significance were reported by Bullowa (187) for cases of Type XIV pneumococcus pneumonia in infants and children. Bacteriemia may, however, be of serious import, particularly in infants, as Bullowa's (190) findings reveal, for of 25 patients under two years of age, with pneumonia (lobar pneumonia and bronchopneumonia together) due to pneumococci of various types, who had positive blood cultures, 22, or 88 per cent died, while of 14 older children with bacteriemia only 6, or 42.8 per cent, died. The demonstration of bacteriemia in infants and children who are seriously ill with pneumonia is likewise a bad token, and in small groups of cases (6 to 15 in each series) fatality rates of from 50 to 80 per cent were observed under such circumstances by Plummer and his associates (1029, 1057) and by Nemir and her co-workers (931).

Soluble Specific Substance in Urine

Avery, Chickering, Cole, and Dochez (33) demonstrated that the presence of soluble specific substance (SSS) in the urine in pneumococcus pneumonia is of prognostic significance. The frequency with which this substance is found in the urine was discussed in another chapter (see pages 503–504). Tests for its detection were also described elsewhere (see pages 637–639). The intensity of the reaction in the urine bears a fairly close relationship to the severity of the infection in Type I, II, and III cases (33, 118, 1054, 297, 807, 224, 1010). Pepper's (1010) frequent failure to find soluble specific substance in the urine of 9 cases due to pneumococci of various of the higher types led him to suggest that this substance does not appear in the urine so regularly in cases of this nature and that in such instances its appearance is of different prognostic significance than in Type I, II, or III cases. Additional study of this matter is desirable.

The observations of Quigley (1054) and of Cole (297) relating to the occurrence of soluble specific substance in the urine in cases of lobar pneumonia due to pneumococci of Types I, II, and III, together with the fatality rate of such cases, are given in Table 139. As all patients with Type I infections in Cole's series were treated with specific antiserum, the fatality rate of these cases was omitted from his report.

As seen in Table 139, with Type I, II, or III infections the demonstration of a specific precipitin reaction in the urine indicates a severe infection and the fatality rate of patients whose urine shows such reaction is higher than the rate in cases in which the reaction is absent. Mild cases usually fail to show a positive reaction. Cole (297) has pointed out that when the urine reaction is intense and becomes more so every day, the prognosis is very poor.

It is clear from the findings in Table 139 that SSS was not found in the urine of all patients with Type I, II, or III pneumonia. Pepper (1010), however, reports that by concentrating the urine in such cases a positive reaction can be obtained in nearly every case.

TABLE 139. PNEUMOCOCCUS LOBAR PNEUMONIA. NUMBER OF CASES TESTED FOR PRESENCE OF SOLUBLE SPECIFIC SUBSTANCE IN THE URINE, NUMBER WITH POSITIVE OR NEGATIVE REACTIONS, AND NUMBER AND PERCENTAGE OF DEATHS IN EACH GROUP, BY TYPE

	TOTAL NUMBER OF CASES	POSITIVE REACTION IN URINE			NEGATIVE REACTION IN URINE		
		NUMBER OF CASES	DEATHS		NUMBER OF CASES	DEATHS	
			Number	*Per cent*		*Number*	*Per cent*
		Cases reported by Quigley (1054)					
Type I	33	24	10	41.7	9	3	33.3
Type II	36	32	12	37.5	4	1	25.0
Type III	13	11	1	9.1	2	–	–
		Cases reported by Cole (297)					
Type I	35	20	nr	nr	15	nr	nr
Type II	28	20	10	50.0	8	–	–
Type III	17	12	7	58.0	5	1	20.0

nr = no record. No information is given concerning the number of deaths in Type I cases in Cole's series, as the patients were treated with specific antiserum.

Blake (118) studied the daily urinary excretion of soluble specific substance in lobar pneumonia. His series comprised twelve Type I and four Type II cases and two cases due to pneumococci of the higher types. Blood cultures and blood agglutinin and precipitin tests were likewise made at daily intervals. His cases appeared to fall into one of three groups, as follows: (a) patients with mild infections who recovered and had negative blood cultures and no detectable SSS in the blood or urine during the course of the illness; (b) patients with clinically severe infections but with recovery who showed an early bacteriemia with considerable SSS in the urine but none detectable in the blood; (c) patients who died and had bacteriemia with increasing amounts of SSS in both the urine and the blood.

Blake was unable to find any demonstrable relationship between the excretion of SSS in the urine and the presence or absence of blood agglutinins and reported, as did Pepper (1010), that SSS may continue to be excreted in the presence of humoral agglutinins. In Blake's (118) cases, however, the blood precipitins were closely related to the excretion of SSS in the urine, and all patients having SSS in the urine during their illness failed to show humoral precipitins except in two cases, in which both were present in small amounts.

Trask, O'Donovan, Moore, and Beebe (1321) tested the urine of several children with pneumococcus pneumonia for evidence of SSS and found it in a few instances, as did Kereszturi and Hauptmann (710). In cases investigated by the former workers the amount in the urine increased in two of six patients with Type I pneumonia coincidental with recovery. In the remaining cases of the series the amount in the urine remained stationary during the acute disease and until several days after recovery. Blake (118) earlier pointed out that in adult patients with SSS in the urine the amount excreted usually decreases at the time of recovery, and about a week later increases. Some patients who did not excrete SSS during the course of their pneumonia showed SSS in the urine about a week or two after recovery.

Complications and Previous Attacks of Pneumonia

The presence of complications increases the fatality rate in pneumonia, as earlier mentioned (see page 549). This is the case with empyema, especially if other septic conditions are also present, as frequently happens in cases due to streptococci. Fatality rates approaching 100 per cent occur with pericarditis, endocarditis, or meningitis, and rates in the neighborhood of 50 to 60 per cent prevail with septic arthritis or peritonitis. With mediastinitis also the outlook is not good.

Shattuck and Lawrence (1176) found that the fatality rate of 688 cases of lobar pneumonia with complications was 43.4 per cent (299 deaths), as compared with a rate of 21.6 per cent for 2,469 cases without complications (534 deaths). The proportion of deaths in their series was thus about doubled in the presence of complications. In pneumonia a variety of infections or diseases may depress host resistance so as to make the prognosis very poor indeed (see also pages 199–201), and the presence of systemic disease is an unfavorable factor, as mentioned below (page 701).

Cohn and Lewis (288) have emphasized the effect of complications and allied factors upon the fatality rate in lobar pneumonia. They list eight factors such as septic complications, cardiovascular affections, multiple lobe involvements, bacteriemia, alcoholism, occupation, and the like, and note that in the presence of only one of these conditions, if it is of relatively little importance, such as the type of work the patient does, the fatality rate may be only about 10 per cent or less; but as the number of unfavorable factors present in a given case increases, the fatality rate rapidly increases. In the presence of only one of the more serious conditions, however, such as certain septic complications, rates of 100 per cent may obtain.

The effect of previous attacks of pneumonia on the prognosis in a succeeding attack cannot be stated with certainty. It was previously pointed out, however, that possibly the fatality rate of second and subsequent attacks may be less than with primary attacks (see page 539).

Extent of Pulmonary Involvement

The extent of pulmonary involvement is importantly related to prognosis. Although death may occur when only a small area is involved (see pages 544–545), the outlook is poorest when the disease extends from lobe to lobe, and it is probable in such instances that the patient has little resistance, as Cole (297) has mentioned. Maynard's (874) necropsy findings in African natives dying of pneumonia, and observations of experimentally induced pneumonia in dogs (1083) and monkeys (483), support this view.

The frequency with which various lobes are involved in pneumonia was discussed earlier (see pages 107–111). As the number of lobes involved increases, the fatality rate increases, as many investigators have shown (1168, 255, 96, 230, 1357, 830, 1385, 288), the rate being highest in the presence of the most extensive lesions even in the absence of bacteriemia (1267). Fatality rates of from 8.5 to 32 per cent have been reported with single lobed lesions (1168, 255, 230, 1357, 288), as compared with rates of 24 to 36 per cent with two lobed lesions (1168, 230, 288; see also Table 140).

Cohn and Lewis (288) reported the fatality rate of more than 1,400 cases of lobar pneumonia treated at the Hospital of the Rockefeller Institute for Medical Research by the number of lobes involved. Several hundred of the pneumococcus Type I cases and a few of the Type II cases included in this series received specific serum therapy. Of 801 cases with one lobe involved 68, or 8.5 per cent, died. Of 428 cases with two lobes involved 105, or 24.5 per cent, died; with three lobes involved 70 of 172, or 40.7 per cent, died; with four lobes involved 30 of 44, or 68.2 per cent, died, and with five lobes involved all of 11 cases died.

In a series of 1,030 cases of lobar pneumonia in the Philippines, Vitug and

Hizon (1357) found the fatality rate lowest with lesions confined to the right base, and death occurred in 11 per cent, or 39, of 351 cases with such involvement. Cases with lesions in the left base had a fatality rate of 16.7 per cent or somewhat higher.

TABLE 140. PNEUMOCOCCUS LOBAR PNEUMONIA. NUMBER OF CASES AND NUMBER AND PERCENTAGE OF DEATHS IN CASES WITH ONE OR MORE LOBES INVOLVED, BY TYPE*

	NUMBER OF CASES	DEATHS Number	DEATHS Per cent	NUMBER OF CASES	DEATHS Number	DEATHS Per cent
	Single lobe			*Two lobes*		
Type I	375	51	13.6	174	43	24.7
Type II	214	70	32.7	110	48	43.6
Type III	156	55	35.3	97	46	47.4
Group IV	413	67	16.2	174	65	37.4
Total	1,158	243	21.0	555	202	36.4
	Three lobes			*Four lobes*		
Type I	77	21	27.3	6	4	66.7
Type II	33	16	48.5	8	5	62.5
Type III	12	8	66.7	3	1	33.3
Group IV	32	18	56.3	19	9	47.4
Total	154	63	40.9	36	19	52.8

From Cecil *et al.* (230)

* Specific serum was used in the treatment of many of these cases.

In a series of 582 cases, Chatard (255), at the Johns Hopkins Hospital, reported that the fatality rate of cases with involvement on the right side was about 26 per cent, while in those with lesions on the left side the rate was 20 per cent or somewhat lower. In Vitug and Hizon's (1357) experience the reverse was true, and patients with lesions in the right lung had a slightly lower fatality rate (18 per cent) than those with left sided lesions (20.6 per cent).

The fatality rate is high in cases with double pneumonia where involvement occurs on both the right and the left side, and rates varying from 39 to 80 per cent have been found under such circumstances (1168, 255, 830). Warr and Alperin (1385) reported that when lesions are on both the right and the left, the rate is higher than when two lobes of the same lung are attacked. In patients having recurrent attacks of pneumococcus pneumonia, Finland and Winkler (470) observed that bilateral involvement is about twice as common as in primary attacks, yet the fatality rate in such instances may not be increased.

Fabyan (399) and Berry (96) have both remarked on the frequency with which upper lobe lesions, especially on the right side, are found in cases at necropsy. Their observations suggest that the prognosis with such lesions may be poorer than with other single lobed lesions. Among patients with single lobed lesions in Vitug and Hizon's (1357) series of 1,030 cases of lobar pneumonia, those with apical involvements had the highest fatality rate of all, the rate being 19 per cent for lesions of the right apex and 22 per cent for lesions of the left apex. Sears and Larrabee (1168), however, in a series of 949 "pneumonias," found little difference between the fatality rate of apical and other single lobed lesions, and Cole (297) also was unable to confirm the finding that apical lesions are more serious than other lesions involving a single lobe.

The only report at hand giving the fatality rate with single or multiple lobe involvements in cases of pneumococcus lobar pneumonia by type is that of Cecil, Baldwin, and Larsen (230), whose findings in nearly 2,000 cases are presented in Table 140. Specific serum was used in the treatment of many of these cases. Among 1,158 cases with single lobed lesions the fatality rate was 21 per cent, in 555 cases with two lobes involved it was 36.4 per cent, in 154 cases with three lobes involved it was 40.9 per cent, and in 36 cases with four lobes involved it was 52.8 per cent. Where the number of cases is large enough to judge, similar increases in the fatality rates with an increasing number of lobes involved occurred in cases due to each of the types, Types I, II, and III, and to pneumococci of Group IV.

Chain-Forming Pneumococci

Bullowa and Wilcox (197, 186) report that certain strains of pneumococci recovered from sputum, blood cultures, or material removed by lung puncture, when grown in broth, exhibit a tendency to grow in long chains and that possibly this tendency may be correlated with the severity of the patient's illness. The presence of chain-forming pneumococci appeared to indicate a less severe infection. In the experience of these investigators about 4 per cent, or 49, of 1,152 cases of pneumococcus pneumonia yielded organisms which grew in chains. Occurrences of this nature were most frequent in Type V cases, although they were also rather common in Type VIII (186) cases. Such pneumococci did not appear especially virulent for mice.

Factors Affecting the Individual

Although often difficult or impossible to assess in a given case, numerous factors affecting the individual may affect his resistance and influence prognosis.

GENERAL PHYSICAL CONDITION. The prognosis in patients in good physical condition at the time of onset of their illness is much better than in patients who, because of enfeeblement due to previous or co-existent disease or to the operation of other untoward influences, are in less vigorous health. The importance of previous good health in favorably influencing the outlook with pneumonia is probably nowhere more strikingly illustrated than among men chosen for physical fitness to serve in various military organizations throughout the world. Müller (915) reports that among soldiers in the Prussian army between the years of 1878 and 1898 there were more than 85,000 cases of "pneumonia" and that the fatality rate of these cases varied from 3.1 to 4.3 per cent. These rates are extraordinarily low, yet similar findings have been reported from numerous sources.

In Wells' (1404) collected series of 465,400 cases of pneumonia earlier mentioned in this chapter a number of series of cases from military sources were included, among which the following, being some of the largest, may be cited:

SOURCE	CASES *Number*	DEATHS *Number*	DEATHS *Per cent*
British Army, 1854	12,271	413	3.5
British Navy, 1896	3,099	136	4.0
German Army, 1880	42,467	1,524	3.6
German Army, 1896–1901	19,169	735	3.8
Italian Army, 1890–1899	12,442	1,874	15.6

The low fatality rate in most of the groups listed is perhaps not so amazing on second thought, for in the vast majority of instances the men having pneumonia were presumably young adults in excellent health and the resistance of such individuals is high.

Additional figures of like significance are at hand. Musser and Norris (918) reported that between 1868 and 1902 there were 6,838 cases of lobar pneumonia among men in the United States Army and that the fatality rate in this group was 10.75 per cent. Further, the reports of the Surgeon General of the United States Army (1345) for the ten years of 1926 to 1935 inclusive, show that lobar pneumonia occurred in 2,059 men, of whom 277, or 13.5 per cent, died. Reports dealing with the health of the British Army (561) reveal findings very similar. From 1922 to 1931 inclusive, among warrant officers, non-commissioned officers, and army men in the United Kingdom there were 2,715 cases of pneumonia of all forms with 275 deaths, a rate of 10.1 per cent. In men of similar rank in the whole regular British Army at home and abroad (excluding the native troops in various countries) from 1922 to 1931 inclusive, there were a total of 6,335 cases of pneumonia of all forms with 646 deaths, a rate of 10.2 per cent. In this same period, in commissioned officers there were 218 cases with 40, or 18.3 per cent, of deaths. The higher fatality rate for the officers as compared with the men is probably due in large measure to the fact that the officers are older on the average than the men. Excluding native troops, the British Army in India during the years of 1922–1931 had 2,155 cases of pneumonia of all forms in warrant officers, non-commissioned officers, and men, with 239 deaths, a rate of 11.1 per cent, and in a like interval in Egypt and in the nearby territory the fatality rate was 6.1 per cent for 505 cases (31 deaths).

The evidence is clear that under ordinary circumstances the fatality rate of young healthy men is very low, even though no special form of therapy is used (see also pages 330–332 and 333–336). During times of war, when respiratory and other infections may be epidemic among soldiers, higher fatality rates are usual. Wells (1404) reported a fatality rate of 26 per cent for United States Army troops during the period of the Civil War (1860–1865). Of 77,335 cases 20,116 ended in death. Relatively high fatality rates were also seen during the Great War, and Stone, Phillips, and Bliss (1231) found that 23 per cent, or 154, of 668 men with lobar pneumonia died. Thomas (1295) reported a fatality rate for lobar pneumonia of 22 per cent for 127 cases in white soldiers (28 deaths) and of 27 per cent for 37 cases of bronchopneumonia (10 deaths) among similar individuals.

Efforts were made in many army camps in this country during the Great War to carry out pneumococcus typing and to treat Type I cases with specific antiserum, as is mentioned elsewhere (see pages 890–892). During that period data were obtained on a small number of cases of Type I pneumonia, all or nearly all of the lobar form, in which no serum was used, as is shown in Table 141. In a collected series of 93 cases, death occurred in 18, a rate of 19.4 per cent. Thomas (1299) has reviewed these cases and states that Miller and Lusk (892) had an additional 63 Type I cases with 2 deaths, which might be added to those given in Table 141, bringing the total number of cases up to 156 with 20 deaths, a rate of 12.8 per cent. This latter figure, as well as the 19.4 per cent rate in Table 141, is considerably lower than the fatality rate of 29 per cent found in Type I cases in civilian patients in the United States and Canada, as shown in Table 117 (page 664).

In contrast with the usually low fatality rate of pneumonia in men in military organizations who are young and robust, the fatality rate for older and debilitated patients, and especially for those with chronic systemic diseases, is much higher. The frequent occurrence of Type III infections among

TABLE 141. TYPE I LOBAR PNEUMONIA IN AMERICAN ARMY CAMPS. SOURCE, NUMBER OF CASES, AND NUMBER AND PERCENTAGE OF DEATHS, IN THE UNITED STATES, 1917–1924*

SOURCE	CAMP	NUMBER OF CASES	DEATHS	
			Number	*Per cent*
Nichols (952)	Mobilization (Texas), 1917	18	7	38.9
McClelland (829)	Beauregard (La.), 1918	2	–	–
Cecil (219)	Upton (N.Y.), 1918	9	2	22.2
Stone, Phillips, and Bliss (1251)	Fort Riley (Kansas), 1918	5	1	20.0
Leopold (774)	Dix (N.J.), 1918	10	1	10.0
Thomas (1295)	Meade (Md.), 1918	7	–	–
Greenway, Boettiger, and Colwell (566)	Bowie (Texas), 1919	17	–	–
Park and Chickering (985)	Jackson (S.C.), 1919	2	–	–
Tenney and Rivenburgh (1289)	Upton (N.Y.), 1919	5	–	–
Wadsworth (1365)	Several, 1924	18	7	38.9
Total		93	18	19.4

* All or nearly all of these cases were apparently lobar pneumonia.

such individuals was mentioned previously (see pages 335–336). Cecil, Baldwin, and Larsen (230) have analyzed 1,002 cases of lobar pneumonia due to pneumococci of Types I, II, III, and Group IV, to show the proportion of deaths among patients with or without some chronic systemic disease, as illustrated by the figures in Table 142. Many of the cases received specific serum treatment.

Among 327 cases in Table 142 having systemic disease, death occurred in 155, or 47.4 per cent, while in 675 cases without such conditions the fatality rate was only about one-half as high, as only 161, or 23.9 per cent, died.

Among the cases with systemic disease the fatality rate was highest (66.3 per cent) with Type III infections and lowest (33.6 per cent) with Group IV. In cases without systemic disease the highest rate was in Type II cases (36.8 per cent) and the lowest rate in Type III (8.3 per cent).

The fatality rate for all the cases in Table 142 was 31.5 per cent, and Cecil and his associates (230) reported that the fatality rate of cases with acute alcoholism was 55.8 per cent, with auricular fibrillation 60 per cent, with chronic myocarditis 78.2 per cent, with any form of chronic valvular heart disease 45.8 per cent, with emphysema 40.5 per cent, and with syphilis 39.9 per cent.

TABLE 142. PNEUMOCOCCUS LOBAR PNEUMONIA. NUMBER OF CASES AND NUMBER AND PERCENTAGE OF DEATHS IN CASES WITH OR WITHOUT SYSTEMIC DISEASE, BY TYPE*

	WITH SYSTEMIC DISEASE			WITHOUT SYSTEMIC DISEASE		
	NUMBER OF CASES	DEATHS *Number*	DEATHS *Per cent*	NUMBER OF CASES	DEATHS *Number*	DEATHS *Per cent*
Type I	61	23	37.7	237	37	15.6
Type II	67	38	56.7	136	50	36.8
Type III	83	55	66.3	48	4	8.3
Group IV	116	39	33.6	254	70	27.6
Total	327	155	47.4	675	161	23.9

From Cecil *et al.* (230)

* Specific serum was used in the treatment of many of these cases.

Brooks (153) studied 200 necropsies of patients dying of lobar pneumonia or bronchopneumonia and found evidence of chronic cardiac disease in more than one-half (116 cases) of the patients. He concluded that as a rule cardiac patients are a bad risk in pneumonia. The matter was further studied by Cohn and Lewis (288) in a clinical investigation of 1,456 cases of lobar pneumonia, many of which received specific serum treatment. Their findings indicated that, in general, cases with cardiovascular complications in the second, third, and fourth decades of life had higher fatality rates than other patients of similar age without such conditions. From the fifth decade on in their series the fatality rates were about the same, whether or not some cardiovascular lesion was present. In consequence, the presence of lesions of this nature appears of greater prognostic significance in patients under than over fifty years of age.

AGE AS FACTOR IN PROGNOSIS. Age is one of the most important factors in prognosis. The fatality rate is extremely high in very young and very old patients in whom resistance is low, while patients of intermediate age usually have a higher immunity with a resulting lower fatality rate (see also pages 186–192).

Cases in infants and children. With pneumonia in any form the fatality rate is high during the first two or three years of life, and usually from 20 to 35 per cent or more of infants with pneumonia die (333, 1025, 1436, 821, 1435, 930, 7, 931, 190). The form of the pulmonary lesion seems of little importance in affecting the prognosis in infants (see also pages 513–515).

TABLE 143. LOBAR PNEUMONIA IN INFANTS AND CHILDREN. NUMBER OF CASES AND NUMBER AND PERCENTAGE OF DEATHS, BY AGE GROUP

AGE GROUP IN YEARS	NUMBER OF CASES	DEATHS	
		Number	*Per cent*
0–1	29	6	20.7
1–2	91	12	13.2
2–3	147	6	4.1
3–4	123	6	4.9
4–5	75	4	5.3
5–6	77	1	1.3
6–13	313	2	0.6
Total	855	37	4.3

From Cunningham (333)

Cunningham (333), in a series of 855 cases of lobar pneumonia (see Table 143) in infants and children, had 29 cases in patients under one year of age with 6 deaths, a rate of 20.7 per cent, and in infants one to two years of age the fatality rate of 91 cases with 12 deaths was 13.2 per cent. Higher rates in cases of lobar pneumonia in infants were reported by Pisek and Pease (1025), for 40.2 per cent of 75 cases in patients under one year of age died, as did 34 per cent of 97 patients from one to two years of age. Albert and Abad (7), in the Philippines, reported a fatality rate of 23.5 per cent for 412 cases of lobar pneumonia (97 deaths) in patients under two years of age, and in individuals of similar age a rate of 20.7 per cent for 1,937 cases of bronchopneumonia (400 deaths). Among 1,000 cases of lobar pneumonia and bronchopneumonia together in infants and children under six years of age, Pisek and Pease (1025) found a fatality rate of 34.3 per cent. Neither in Cunningham's nor in Albert and Abad's series was any mention made of the etiologic agents responsible for the cases.

After the age of two or three years the fatality rate of bronchopneumonia tends to decrease somewhat but still continues high, while the rate for pneumonia in the lobar form decreases markedly (1318, 333, 1025, 930, 710). The effect of advancing age upon the fatality rate in cases of lobar pneumonia in infants and children is shown by the figures in Table 143, which were compiled from Cunningham's (333) findings. The fatality rate decreased from 20.7 per cent for 29 patients in the first year of life to the very low rate of 0.6 per cent for 313 cases in patients 6 to 13 years of age. In a series of 227 cases of lobar pneumonia in patients under six years old reported by Pisek and Pease (1025), the fatality rate decreased from 40.2 per cent for 75 cases under one year of age to 34 per cent for cases under two years of age, and for cases in the succeeding years was 12.9, 16, zero, and 0.7 per cent.

The total fatality rate of infants and children of various ages with lobar pneumonia is low, as illustrated by the collected cases tabulated in Table 144. In this table there are 2,923 cases, of which only 128, or 4.4 per cent, died. The fatality rates of the individual series included in the table varied from a low of 2.5 per cent among 1,138 cases collected by Townsend (1318) to a high of 12.7 per cent for 79 cases studied by Mitchell (899).

A few cases of lobar pneumonia in infants and children due to pneumococci of known type have been reported (1436, 1025, 899, 821, 793, 1321, 931). Of the Type I cases available Mitchell (899) had 9, and Lyon (821) 14 with no deaths, and Locke (793) 63 cases with 7 deaths, and Trask, O'Donovan, Moore, and Beebe (1321) 36 cases with 2 deaths, making a total of 122 Type I cases with 9 deaths, a rate of 7.4 per cent. In Mitchell's (899) series the fatality rate was 20 per cent in 10 Type II cases (2 deaths), 33.3 per cent in 3 Type III cases (1 death), and 12.3 per cent in 57 Group IV cases (7 deaths). Among 30 Group IV cases reported by Trask and his co-workers (1321) 3, or 10 per cent, died.

A few cases of bronchopneumonia in infants and children due to pneumococci of known type have also been investigated (1436, 1025, 821, 1435, 931). Among 28 cases due to pneumococci of Type I, II, III, or Group IV in Wollstein and Benson's (1436) series, approximately 43 per cent died. The number of deaths in 20 similar cases investigated by Pisek and Pease (1025) was not stated, while in Lyon's (821) cases one of 3 Type I cases died, one Type II case died, both of two Type III cases lived, and 17 per cent of 13 Group IV cases died. In Wollstein's (1435) series all of 3 Type I cases lived, while the fatality rate was 55 per cent for 7 Type II cases (4 died) and 26 per cent for 54 Group IV cases (14 died).

Considering pneumonia of various forms due to various organisms in infants and children together, Raia, Plummer, and Shultz (1057) report a fatality rate of 17 per cent for 329 cases (56 deaths). In this series 308 cases with 16.6 per cent, or 51 deaths were due to pneumococcus infections. Including

TABLE 144. LOBAR PNEUMONIA IN INFANTS AND CHILDREN. NUMBER OF CASES AND NUMBER AND PERCENTAGE OF DEATHS

SOURCE	NUMBER OF CASES	DEATHS	
		Number	*Per cent*
Townsend, 1889 (1318)	1,138*	28	2.5
Cunningham, 1916 (333)	855	37	4.3
Mitchell, 1917 (899)	79	10	12.7
Webster, 1924 (1394)	626†	39	6.2
Locke, 1923 (793)	129	8	6.2
Trask, O'Donovan, Moore, and Beebe, 1930 (1321)	96	6	6.3
Total	2,923	128	4.4

* Collected cases. † All cases in children two to fourteen years of age.

the total series (329 cases) of Raia and her associates (1057), which were investigated at the Bellevue Hospital, New York City, Nemir, Andrews, and Vinograd (931) subsequently reported that over a period of seven consecutive winters at the same hospital there was a grand total of 1,362 cases of pneumonia in infants and children with 18.3 per cent of deaths. Of this number of cases, 1,033 were observed by the latter workers alone and in their series there were 186 deaths (18 per cent), of which only 19 occurred in patients over two years of age. In addition, most of the deaths were associated with pneumonia of the bronchopneumonic (atypical) form, and the fatality rate of such cases was 50.2 per cent, as compared with a rate of only 5.5 per cent for other patients having pneumonia in the lobar form.

Several series of pneumococcus pneumonias (lobar pneumonia and bronchopneumonia together) of some size have been reported, as seen in Table 145. Of 1,348 collected cases in the table, 233 or 17.3 per cent died. The fatality rates in the different series varied from 11.7 per cent (190) to 40.7 per cent, the latter figure being for Blacklock and Guthrie's (112) cases from Glasgow. These workers attributed the high proportion of deaths in their series to the fact that their patients came from the lowest social classes. It may also be mentioned that of their 140 cases 112 were in children under three years of age.

TABLE 145. PNEUMOCOCCUS PNEUMONIA (LOBAR PNEUMONIA AND BRONCHOPNEUMONIA TOGETHER) IN INFANTS AND CHILDREN. NUMBER OF CASES AND NUMBER AND PERCENTAGE OF DEATHS

SOURCE	NUMBER OF CASES	DEATHS *Number*	DEATHS *Per cent*
Trask, O'Donovan, Moore, and Beebe (1321)	182	41	22.5
Raia, Plummer, and Shultz (1057)	308	51	16.6
Blacklock and Guthrie (112)	140	57	40.7
Bullowa (190)	718	84	11.7
Total	1,348	233	17.3

The fatality rate of pneumonia (lobar pneumonia and bronchopneumonia together) due to pneumococci of some of the commoner types in infants and children of various ages, as given by Nemir, Andrews, and Vinograd, is shown in Table 146. Among 26 Type I cases in infants under two years of age, the fatality rate was 26.9 per cent (7 died), while of 116 older children with Type I pneumonia death occurred in only 1.7 per cent (2 died). The situation is much the same with the other six types listed (Types III, V, VI, VII, XIV, and XIX), the rates being very much higher in the younger than in the older children. In infants under two years old the highest fatality rate is in the Type XIX cases (34.8 per cent) and the lowest in Type V cases (14.4 per cent). The rate for Type XIV cases is 16.8 per cent in the younger group and 2 per cent in the older group. Among children two to twelve years of age the highest fatality rate is in Type V cases (5.3 per cent) and the lowest in Type VII and Type XIX cases, among which there were no deaths.

As elsewhere mentioned, Type XIV is one of the commonest types encountered in the pneumonias of infants and children (see pages 74–89). To the total 175 cases with 22 deaths due to pneumonia with this type, as seen in Table 146, may be added the 20 cases with 2 deaths previously reported by Raia, Plummer, and Shultz (1057) and the 116 cases with 14 deaths subsequently reported by Bullowa (190), yielding a grand total of 311 cases of Type XIV pneumococcus pneumonia in infants and children of all ages with 38 deaths, a rate of 12.2 per cent.

TABLE 146. PNEUMOCOCCUS PNEUMONIA (LOBAR PNEUMONIA AND BRONCHO-PNEUMONIA TOGETHER) IN INFANTS AND CHILDREN. NUMBER OF CASES AND NUMBER AND PERCENTAGE OF DEATHS IN PATIENTS OF DIFFERENT AGES, BY TYPE

PNEUMOCOCCUS TYPE	UNDER 2 YEARS OF AGE			2 TO 12 YEARS OF AGE		
	NUMBER OF CASES	DEATHS *Number*	DEATHS *Per cent*	NUMBER OF CASES	DEATHS *Number*	DEATHS *Per cent*
I	26	7	26.9	116	2	1.7
III	15	4	26.7	22	1	4.5
V	7	1	14.4	38	2	5.3
VI	68	20	29.4	47	1	2.1
VII	12	2	16.7	20	–	–
XIV	125	21	16.8	50	1	2.0
XIX	46	16	34.8	10	–	–

From Nemir *et al.* (931)

In pneumonia of various forms in infants and children due to organisms other than pneumococci, Raia, Plummer, and Shultz (1057) find that death occurred in 5, or 23.8 per cent, of 21 cases. In Nemir, Andrews, and Vinograd's (931) series, streptococci and staphylococci together caused death in 76 per cent, or 57, of 75 cases in infants under two years of age, as compared with 8.2 per cent, or 5, of 61 cases in children two to twelve years of age. In Bullowa's (190) series similarly divided by age and due to various organisms other than pneumococci, death occurred in 25.7 per cent, or 104, of 405 cases in infants under two years of age, and in but 5.6 per cent, or 22, of 377 cases in children over this age.

Cases in adults. The low fatality rate with lobar pneumonia seen in the latter part of childhood continues into adult life up to the age of approximately twenty years, the rates during this period being about 10 per cent or less. In a series of 142 pneumococcus cases in patients five to fifteen years of age, some of which received specific serum therapy, Macgregor (837) in Great Britain reported a fatality rate of only 1.4 per cent (2 deaths). Among 66 cases of "pneumonia" of unknown etiology in patients fifteen to nineteen years old, Sears and Larrabee (1168) found that 7, or 10.6 per cent, died.

In patients ten to nineteen years of age with lobar pneumonia Shattuck and Lawrence (1176) found that 10 per cent of 329 cases died (see Table 147). This figure is somewhat higher than that of 6.5 per cent reported by Cohn and Lewis (288) for 186 cases in the same age group with 12 deaths. A number of the cases in the latter series, however, received specific serum treatment. Nevertheless, it is usual in adults to find the lowest fatality rates in patients under twenty years of age (1319, 1168, 567, 1176, 297, 230, 1357, 837, 288). After this age the proportion of cases dying increases approximately 10 per cent with each decade of life.

TABLE 147. LOBAR PNEUMONIA. NUMBER OF CASES AND NUMBER AND PERCENTAGE OF DEATHS, BY AGE GROUP

AGE GROUP IN YEARS	NUMBER OF CASES	DEATHS	
		Number	*Per cent*
Under 10	476	66	13.9
10–19	329	33	10.0
20–29	626	115	18.4
30–39	580	169	29.1
40–49	431	154	35.7
50–59	292	145	49.7
60–69	100	72	72.0
70 and over	48	34	70.8
Total	2,882	788	27.3

From Shattuck and Lawrence (1176)

The influence of advancing age on prognosis was well shown in Shattuck and Lawrence's (1176) investigation of 2,882 cases of lobar pneumonia admitted to the Massachusetts General Hospital between 1889 and 1917. Death occurred in 788, or 27.3 per cent of all the cases. The cases and deaths were divided by decades according to the age of the patient, as seen in Table 147. The proportion of 329 patients ten to nineteen years of age who died was 10 per cent, as above mentioned, and the proportion of fatalities steadily increased with age till it reached about 70 per cent for patients sixty years of age and over. Similar findings have been reported in other series (1319, 1168, 567, 1357). Among the pneumococcus cases reported by Cecil, Baldwin, and Larsen (230; see Table 149) and the cases of Cohn and Lewis (288; see Table 148) which were nearly all due to pneumococci, the fatality rates did not increase so rapidly with increasing age, possibly because many of the

TABLE 148. LOBAR PNEUMONIA. NUMBER OF CASES AND NUMBER AND PERCENTAGE OF DEATHS, BY DECADES OF LIFE*

DECADE OF LIFE	NUMBER OF CASES	DEATHS Number	DEATHS Per cent
1st	38	–	–
2nd	186	12	6.5
3rd	418	38	9.1
4th	361	66	18.3
5th	234	68	29.1
6th	138	61	44.2
7th	72	34	47.2
8th	8	7	87.5
9th	1	1	100.0
Total	1,456	287	19.7

From Cohn and Lewis (288)

* Nearly all cases were due to pneumococci. This series includes 501 Type I cases and nearly all were given specific serum treatment, as were a few of the 388 Type II cases included.

TABLE 149. PNEUMOCOCCUS LOBAR PNEUMONIA IN ADULTS. NUMBER OF CASES AND PERCENTAGE OF DEATHS IN TYPE I, II, III, AND GROUP IV CASES, BY AGE GROUP*

	NUMBER OF CASES	DEATHS Per cent	NUMBER OF CASES	DEATHS Per cent	NUMBER OF CASES	DEATHS Per cent
	Under 20 years		*20 to 30 years*		*30 to 40 years*	
Type I	59	8.4	187	16.0	179	17.8
Type II	16	18.7	89	17.9	91	38.4
Type III	8	12.5	33	15.1	62	29.0
Group IV	51	13.6	142	13.3	155	21.2
Total	134	11.1	451	15.5	487	24.2
	40 to 50 years		*50 to 60 years*		*60 to 70 years*	
Type I	110	21.0	60	26.6	32	31.2
Type II	84	53.5	60	45.0	22	63.6
Type III	63	44.4	43	69.7	54	59.2
Group IV	136	29.4	76	38.1	55	54.5
Total	393	34.8	239	42.7	163	52.7

From Cecil *et al.* (230)

* Specific serum was used in the treatment of many of these cases.

cases in those series were treated with specific serum. The rate increased from 6.5 per cent for patients in the second decade of life to 47.2 per cent for those in the seventh. The rates were still higher in the older groups, but the numbers of cases in the latter groups are too small to be significant.

Many of the cases in Table 148 were previously studied by Cole (297), who considered that the influence of age on the fatality rate was slight for adults under the age of 55 years. Evidence presented elsewhere, however, suggests that the factor of age may be of definite importance in patients by the time they reach their fortieth year, for the proportion of cases with bacteriemia is higher in the older than in the younger groups (see pages 557–559).

As alluded to above, Cecil, Baldwin, and Larsen (230) reported the fatality rates of adult patients with lobar pneumonia due to pneumococci of Types I, II, III, and Group IV by age, as shown in Table 149. The proportion of deaths in all cases in patients under twenty years of age was 11.1 per cent and the rate advanced in older patients to 52.7 per cent for those sixty years of age and over. The results were nearly the same with cases due to pneumococci of Type I, II, III, or Group IV in each age group, although with Type I the fatality rate advanced more slowly with increasing age, probably as many of the cases received specific serum therapy. Findings fundamentally similar to these though less detailed were presented by Sutliff and Finland (1272) and Finland and Sutliff (464) for cases of Types I, II, III, and VIII lobar pneumonia and bronchopneumonia (see also pages 909–911).

RACE AS FACTOR IN PROGNOSIS. It is unlikely with the available data that any reliable statement can be made relating to the relative resistance or lack of it shown by groups of individuals of different races, as determined by their respective case fatality rates. True, the incidence rates and the death rates for pneumonia per unit of population are usually much higher for the colored or for Negroes than for white persons, as earlier pointed out (see pages 312–316), yet there must remain considerable doubt whether race is a factor of definite significance in the prognosis in a given case. It may be in some instances, as earlier stated (page 338), that among individuals with high attack rates the fatality rate is low. However, as Negroes, especially in the tropics, so frequently show evidences of widespread infection at necropsy after pneumonia (see page 312), it is easy to conclude their resistance is markedly lower than that of individuals of the white race. Probably the most striking evidence that race affects prognosis is that mentioned above in this chapter in relation to the fatality rate of pneumonia and lobar pneumonia (page 658).

It was seen there that among a series of more than 19,000 cases of lobar pneumonia collected from the American and Canadian literature there was a fatality rate of 32.8 per cent and that among a series of more than 11,000 cases from Great Britain and Sweden the fatality rate was 17.4 per cent. Together these series total more than 30,000 cases, having a fatality rate of 27.2 per cent, and this rate is considerably lower than the rate of 37.9 per cent reported by Gautier (510) for more than 48,000 cases occurring in natives in tropical countries, most of which were in colored persons (see Table 116, page 662). His cases were of "pneumonia" and not of lobar pneumonia as in the other series. Suggestive but meager information has been reported from other tropical sources in a few isolated instances, which also tends to indicate that individuals of other races exhibit a poorer prognosis in pneumonia than do white persons (1008, 1428).

Nevertheless, no clear evidence is available in the United States that the fatality rate for Negroes is very different from that for white persons. Chatard (254) at the Johns Hopkins Hospital had 408 cases of lobar pneumonia in white patients and 250 in Negroes with a fatality rate of about 30 per cent in each group. Nichol (951) in Florida reported a fatality rate of 28.5 per cent for 91 cases in white patients (26 died) and of 24.5 per cent for 61 cases in colored patients (15 died), the rate being slightly higher in the white than in the colored patients.

Kibbey (714), in a study of "pneumonia" in mine workers and their dependents in Alabama, obtained some data suggesting that Negroes may have a poorer prognosis than white patients. Kibbey divided his patients into five groups depending on their status at the mines (coal and ore mines) and determined the fatality rates of cases occurring in the various groups by race. In all there were more than 2,600 cases of pneumonia and, with the exception of one group in which the fatality rate was slightly higher in white patients, the rates for Negroes were nearly double those for white persons in the other groups. Such data, however, are insufficient for the task at hand. Further, in Bullowa's series of 2,093 cases of pneumococcus pneumonia listed in Table 127 (page 676) the fatality rate was 24.9 per cent, as compared with a rate of 41 per cent for Finland's series of 1,759 cases of pneumococcus lobar pneumonia shown in Table 126 (page 675). Also, Finland's cases of bronchopneumonia had a still higher proportion of deaths. Approximately 85 per cent of Bullowa's patients are colored persons, mostly Negroes, while few of Finland's cases are in colored persons, yet the fatality rate was much higher in Finland's series than in Bullowa's.

During the War the fatality rate for Negroes with pneumonia was reported as higher than that for white patients in some army camps (892) and lower (1295) in others.

SEX AS FACTOR IN PROGNOSIS. It seems unlikely that suitable information has appeared in the literature to determine the effect, if any, of sex on prognosis. Males may have more pneumonia, particularly at certain times of life, than females, as was earlier mentioned (see pages 307–312). Judging from the collected cases of lobar pneumonia of Musser and Norris (918), the fatality rate is likely to be lower in males than in females. In their series there were 33,351 males with 19.3 per cent of deaths (6,449 died) and 12,927 females, of whom 26.5 per cent died (3,431 died). Subsequently Cohn and Lewis (288) reported the fatality rates of males and females with lobar pneumonia at the Hospital of the Rockefeller Institute for Medical Research. Many of the cases in this series received specific serum therapy. Of 1,863 cases in males 201, or 18.9 per cent, died, and in 393 cases in females 86, or 21.9 per cent, a slightly larger proportion, died.

Many factors need consideration, however, in studies of this nature and the series of cases cited above refer only to hospitalized cases, so that the true significance of sex in relation to prognosis is not known, for the proportion of all cases in either sex in any community is unknown. In fact, the figures may be weighted in favor of males, as more males than females with pneumonia are hospitalized, at least in Massachusetts (871, 615), and possibly the smaller number of females entering hospitals do so because they represent the more severe cases in their sex group. Such an occurrence would tend to cause a high fatality rate among the females hospitalized.

Greenwood and Candy (567) in London found the fatality rate of 1,315 females with lobar pneumonia to be 16.1 per cent (212 died), as compared with a rate of 20.7 per cent for 3,801 cases in males (785 died). After careful consideration of these and several thousand additional collected cases, they decided that the material was inadequate for reliable conclusions as to the effect of sex upon the case fatality rate in pneumonia.

In a study of Type I, II, III, and VIII cases of pneumonia (lobar pneumonia and bronchopneumonia together) Finland and Sutliff (464) found the fatality rate for Type I and Type II cases about the same in either sex. With both Type III and Type VIII, however, females had higher fatality rates than males and this was chiefly confined to the older females with Type III infections and to females under the age of sixty years with Type VIII infections.

PREGNANCY AS FACTOR IN PROGNOSIS. Although lobar pneumonia may be uncommon during pregnancy, and Musser and Norris (918) collected 13,611 cases of pregnancy and found pneumonia in only 120 or 0.8 per cent, when it occurs it is likely to run a severe course and lead to abortion in about one-half or more of the instances (918, 807, 350, 338). As pregnancy advances, the frequency of abortion and the maternal fatality rate increases. If abortion does not occur in the first few days of illness, the prognosis is better (918). Bacteriemia is not infrequent and may be heavy and persistent.

Bie (102) studied a group of 85 pregnant patients who had "influenzal" bronchopneumonia, and reported that the prognosis was poorest in the fifth to the ninth month of pregnancy. Of 65 cases in women at this stage of pregnancy 34, or 52 per cent, died. In the total series of 85 cases 38, or 45 per cent, died, as compared with 17 per cent, or 78, of 459 cases in non-pregnant women. In Bie's series, the fatality rate for pregnant women with single lobed lesions was 29 per cent and for pregnant women with bilateral involvements was 54 per cent. Death occurred in 66 per cent of the patients who aborted or delivered during the pneumonia and in 34 per cent of the women who did not. In his series about one-third of all pregnant patients aborted or delivered.

OCCUPATION AND SOCIAL AND ENVIRONMENTAL CONDITIONS. *Occupation.* Cole (297) has remarked that little evidence is available relating to the effect of occupation upon the prognosis in pneumonia. He and Howard (661), however, consider that possibly patients who have been performing heavy work have somewhat higher fatality rates than others not so occupied. Cohn and Lewis (288) analyzed more than a thousand cases of lobar pneumonia to determine how far being engaged in physical work of varying severity affected prognosis. Many of their cases received specific serum therapy. The fatality rate of 249 patients with a history of having done light work was 14.1 per cent (35 died). Among 664 who did work of medium intensity the fatality rate was 17.2 per cent (114 died), while among 603 others who did heavy work the rate was higher, 22.9 per cent (138 died). Factors other than having done heavy work were also present in some of the latter cases and after a careful review of the data, Cohn and Lewis concluded that alone the performance of heavy work in the past might be of no special importance in influencing the outlook in pneumonia.

In the chapter on Epidemiology it was pointed out that those occupations calling for exposure to certain unfavorable conditions, such as wetting and chilling, marked temperature variations, and the inhalation of some dusts or irritating fumes, appeared associated with high pneumonia attack rates (see pages 318–329). Some evidence is available that a number of such factors may operate to lower the resistance of the host, as elsewhere described (see pages 201–203). In Great Britain (560, 852) and in the United States (1143, 163, 162, 1301, 161, 1420) factors of this nature appear to influence resistance at least to the extent of contributing to high morbidity and mortality rates from pneumonia and possibly they also unfavorably affect the prognosis when pneumonia develops, although little direct evidence relating to this matter is at hand. Patterson's (1003a) findings (in Australia) are of interest in this respect. Among a total of 521 cases of lobar pneumonia in adults he reported that 112, or 21.5 per cent, died. Included in this series were 30 cases, of whom 11 or 36.8 per cent died, in patients giving a history of having been somewhat exposed to heat and cold during their work. The number of cases is small and the findings cited possibly misleading, for he considers as individuals exposed to heat and cold, cooks, laundresses, blacksmiths, and engine firemen. No mention was made of the possible effect of age on the fatality rate of the special group cited.

Social condition. A general relationship exists between economic or social status and prognosis and it has been noted many times in the study of hospitalized cases of pneumonia that hospitals admitting chiefly patients from the lower social levels have the highest fatality rates from this disease. Specific mention of this was made by several workers (26, 567, 297, 223, 1213, 238, 225, 112).

The general fatality rate of pneumonia in hospitals which admit patients in moderate or well-to-do circumstances may be in the neighborhood of 20 per cent; while in large municipal institutions where patients from the lower classes comprise most of the admissions, fatality rates of from 35 to 45 per cent or more are not unusual. Ashton and Landis (26) reported a fatality rate of 53 per cent for 991 cases of lobar pneumonia for patients of the latter variety at the Philadelphia General Hospital (see Table 114, page 657), and Finland (449), among 1,759 patients of the same class with lobar pneumonia, found the fatality rate to be 41 per cent, as earlier mentioned (see page 675). The possible reasons for the discrepancy between the high fatality rate in Finland's series and the lower rate in Bullowa's cases, shown in Table 127 (page 676), were discussed above (page 670). Differences in the fatality rates with pneumonia may be found at the same time in different hospitals in the same community depending upon the class of patient admitted (238).

Smith (1213) studied the relation of social or environmental factors to the outcome of pneumonia (lobar pneumonia and bronchopneumonia together) in infants and children under five years of age in Glasgow. A comparison was made of the fatality rates of cases in the private and in the charity wards of various hospitals. This showed that the proportion of children dying from pneumonia was from four to seven times higher among patients in poor circumstances than among those whose economic status was of a higher level. Blacklock and Guthrie (112) of Glasgow have commented on this study and attribute the high fatality rate of 40.7 per cent for 140 cases of pneumonia (57 deaths) in infants and children in their own series from that city to the fact that their patients were derived from the lowest social classes.

Not only may the general fatality rate of cases treated in some hospitals be lower than the rate for patients cared for in others, but differences in the rates may apparently be found when the outcome of cases treated in hospitals is compared with the outcome of those cared for at home. Little is known, however, of the fatality rate of home-treated cases, and from inquiry among a large number of physicians in private practice it is obvious that although the fatality rate may be low in cases treated at home, its usual level is unknown. Greenwood and Candy (567) have discussed this matter and cite a series of cases of lobar pneumonia in Great Britain gathered by the Collective Investigation Committee of the British Medical Association many years ago (before 1900). None of the cases were cared for in hospitals. Among a total of 1,039 cases 186, or 17.9 per cent, died. The fatality rate of 687 cases in males with 117 deaths was 17 per cent, and of 352 cases in females with 69 deaths was 19.6 per cent.

Although the proportion of deaths (17.9 per cent) appears low in the above series of home-treated cases, it is but little lower than the fatality rate of 19.5 per cent found in a series of 5,116 cases cared for at the London Hospital, as reported by Greenwood and Candy (567) and as shown in Table 115 (page 659). Both these series are of British origin and, as earlier mentioned, it is probable that the general fatality rate from pneumonia in Great Britain is lower than in the United States.

Cole (297) cautions against accepting a fatality rate in the neighborhood of 15 per cent for cases treated at home, as the number of cases in most series is too small to be representative. During the course of the Massachusetts Pneumonia Study (869) efforts were made to obtain information on a number of cases of lobar pneumonia treated in the patients' homes in various parts of the state. For a number of reasons the attempt was only partially successful and the series gathered is open to the suspicion that in some instances at least some selection of the cases was made. In any event, data were obtained on a group of 338 cases, of which 70, or 20.7 per cent, died (615; see footnote of Table 114, page 657). These cases are shown in Table 150.

Of the home-treated cases in this table, death occurred in 25 per cent of 84 Type I cases; in 16.7 per cent of 18 Type II cases; in 41.2 per cent of 51 Type III cases; and in 12.7 per cent of 157 cases due to pneumococci of all other types. The fatality rate of 22 cases from whom no pneumococci were obtained was 13.6 per cent, and of 6 cases due to organisms other than pneumococci was 33.3 per cent.

TABLE 150. LOBAR PNEUMONIA IN PATIENTS TREATED IN THEIR HOMES. NUMBER OF CASES AND NUMBER AND PERCENTAGE OF DEATHS, BY ORGANISM FOUND*

ORGANISM	NUMBER OF CASES	DEATHS	
		Number	*Per cent*
Pneumococcus			
Type I	84	21	25.0
Type II	18	3	16.7
Type III	51	21	41.2
Type IV	10	4	40.0
Type V	12	3	25.0
Type VII	20	2	10.0
Type VIII	33	1	3.0
All other types	82	10	12.2
No pneumococci found	22	3	13.6
Miscellaneous organisms	6	2	33.3
Total	338	70	20.7
All cases due to pneumococci of the higher types†	157	20	12.7

* Neither vaccine nor specific serum therapy was used in the treatment of these cases.
† All pneumococcus cases except those due to Types I, II, and III.

During the same period that the cases in Table 150 were collected, another series of 367 cases with 85 deaths, a rate of 23.2 per cent, which occurred in various hospitals, chiefly small ones, throughout Massachusetts and which were treated without specific serum therapy, was also collected (615). As neither this series nor the series of home-treated cases is very large and their fatality rates are very similar, no reliable conclusion can be drawn as to differences in the relation of deaths to cases in patients treated at home or in many of the hospitals of Massachusetts. The fatality rate of these two series together, however (705 cases with 155 deaths), is 22 per cent and this is much lower than the rate of 41 per cent for 1,759 cases treated at the Boston City Hospital at about the same time by Finland (449), as already mentioned. This and other information (615) suggests that cases treated in large hospitals have a higher fatality rate than those treated in small hospitals or at home. The following facts may perhaps explain why these differences exist. Patients entering large hospitals, particularly of the municipal variety, are usually from the lower social classes, their general physical condition is not good, and alcoholism is common among them (297), while these factors are less often encountered in patients cared for in small hospitals, especially of a private nature, or at home. Furthermore, hospitals as a group are likely to deal with the more severely ill cases which have been removed from the home because they failed to progress satisfactorily.

Environmental condition. The relation of environment alone to the prognosis in pneumonia is complex and difficult to determine. Changes in environment may be followed by high attack rates of pneumonia without appreciable change in the fatality rates of the resulting cases, according to Maynard (874), as pointed out previously (see pages 329–332). Pearson and Mouchet (1008), however, find that under similar circumstances following a change of environment the case fatality rate may be high among individuals in a group for a few weeks, following which it decreases.

The relation of altitude to prognosis has never been adequately investigated. It was shown in the chapter on Epidemiology (pages 274 and 283) that pneumonia attack rates may be high in some cities located at high altitudes and it might be presumed that the prognosis of cases occurring in a rarefied atmosphere would be more or less unfavorably affected. Cole (297), Lord (807), and Howard (661), however, point out that there is little evidence that this is so. Boothby (137) remarks that a less severe pneumonia will cause more serious anoxemia in patients at high altitudes than at sea level, and reports that in some mining villages located in the mountains it is common practice to send pneumonia patients down to lower levels as rapidly as possible. Such a practice is apparently in vogue in this and some other countries.

Goodman (530) studied 101 adults with lobar pneumonia in Mexico City, which has an altitude of about 7,500 feet. These cases were nearly all in American patients and had a fatality rate of 39.8 per cent. He attributes at least a part of this high rate to altitude. Nevertheless, Cole (297) mentions examining the records of several hundred cases of pneumonia occurring at a South American mining camp located at an elevation of 7,000 feet and among 440 cases of lobar pneumonia and 71 of bronchopneumonia the fatality rate was low, 16.2 per cent. Possibly these cases were in young adults, and youth may have been a factor in their favor.

ALCOHOLISM AS FACTOR IN PROGNOSIS. A history of alcoholism is an unfavorable factor in prognosis. Alcoholic intoxication may act to depress host resistance, as previously mentioned (see page 333), and the fatality rate of alcoholic patients with pneumonia, particularly in heavy drinkers, is much higher than in non-alcoholics (1168, 1176, 215, 297, 230, 288).

Shattuck and Lawrence (1176) studied the effect of alcoholism on prognosis in a series of cases of lobar pneumonia at the Massachusetts General Hospital. Of 526 cases in non-alcoholics 116, or 22.1 per cent, died, while among 214 chronic alcoholics 98, or 41.5 per cent, died. These findings suggest that the fatality rate may be about doubled in chronic alcoholics. Similar observations were made by Cohn and Lewis (288) in patients with lobar pneumonia at the Hospital of the Rockefeller Institute for Medical Research. Many of the cases in this series received specific serum treatment. The results of this study are shown in the accompanying summary:

Relation of alcoholism to prognosis

ALCOHOLIC HISTORY	CASES *Number*	DEATHS *Number*	DEATHS *Per cent*
Never drank	554	89	16.1
Mild drinker	301	57	18.9
Moderate drinker	106	41	38.7
Heavy drinker	42	20	47.6

The high proportion of deaths among patients with a history of moderate or heavy alcoholic addiction is clear.

In neither of the above series, however, is the factor of age stated, and as Cole (297) points out, age is important in attempting to draw conclusions from such data, as most abstainers are among the younger patients, which by itself would give a lower fatality rate in the non-drinkers.

Capps and Coleman (215) have considered this matter further and, over an eight-year period at the Cook County Hospital in Chicago, investigated 3,422 cases of lobar pneumonia in males eighteen years of age and over. The cases were divided into three groups according to their alcoholic history. Patients in the first group never drank or drank less than two glasses of beer daily, and had an average age of about thirty-five years. Of 884 cases in this group 198, or 22.5 per cent, died. The second group included patients who regularly drank two or more glasses of beer or one or two glasses of spirits daily, and the average age in this group was forty years. Among 1,095 cases in the second group 385, or 34.4 per cent, died. The third group was composed of patients who regularly drank considerable beer or spirits and were occasionally drunk, and had an average age of forty-three years. Of 1,443 cases in this group 720, or 49.9 per cent, died. In these three series, then, the fatality rates increased in proportion to the history of alcoholism from 22.5 per cent to 34.4 per cent to 49.9 per cent, without any marked accompanying change in the average age of the patients included; and the unfavorable effect of alcoholism, particularly when marked, upon prognosis was obvious. Additional detailed studies of the cases in the various groups by age also confirmed this observation and likewise made it clear that the highest fatality rates for alcoholics occurred among the oldest patients and, although fairly high, the rates were considerably lower for the younger patients.

PROGNOSTIC SIGNIFICANCE OF CERTAIN SIGNS AND SYMPTOMS

As no single sign or symptom is of outstanding prognostic importance in pneumonia, reliance must be placed upon the whole clinical picture.

Temperature Height

Although temperature range is of little help in estimating prognosis, cases with persistently low temperatures due to overwhelming infections are very serious. Among 86 cases of "pneumonia" investigated by Sears and Larrabee (1168) in which the temperature remained under 102° F., 38 or 44.1 per cent died, while in 297 cases with temperatures ranging from 102° to 104° F., 90 or 30.3 per cent died, and among 71 cases with temperatures between 104° and 106° F., only 12 or 16.9 per cent died.

Long-continued temperatures or very high temperatures alone are of little prognostic significance. Cole (297) studied the relation of the temperature height to prognosis in 768 cases of pneumococcus lobar pneumonia at the Hospital of the Rockefeller Institute for Medical Research. Many of Cole's cases received specific serum treatment and his findings are shown in Table 151. As seen in this table, the resulting fatality rate of cases with temperatures at different levels does not show any particular relation between the degree of the fever and the outlook. Those groups containing more than 100 cases each had maximum temperatures ranging from 103° to 106° F. and fatality rates varying from 15.6 to 27.2 per cent. The groups of cases with maximum temperatures below or above these levels also showed great variability of the fatality rate, but the groups are small. In nine cases with temperatures above 107° F., a chill reaction occurred during the course of their treatment with specific antiserum, which was regarded as the cause of the high temperature. Of these nine cases death occurred in one.

TABLE 151. PNEUMOCOCCUS LOBAR PNEUMONIA. NUMBER OF CASES AND NUMBER AND PERCENTAGE OF DEATHS IN CASES WITH MAXIMUM TEMPERATURES OF VARIOUS HEIGHTS*

MAXIMUM TEMPERATURE RANGE IN DEGREES FAHRENHEIT	NUMBER OF CASES	DEATHS	
		Number	*Per cent*
100–101	4	–	–
101–102	11	2	18.2
102–103	30	3	10.0
103–104	119	32	26.9
104–105	275	43	15.6
105–106	252	52	20.6
106–107	61	22	36.1
107–108	12	3	25.0
108 and over	4	3	75.0
Total	768		

From Cole (297)

* Many cases received specific serum treatment.

Pulse Rate

During the first few days of pneumonia the pulse rate generally gives no special information concerning prognosis. At a later period a gradually increasing rate is usually of serious consequence. Cases in which the maximum rate per minute is 120 or under have a better prognosis than others in which the rate exceeds this figure, as Sears and Larrabee (1168), Chatard (254), Cole (297), and other workers (1385, 349) have demonstrated. Women and children and persons of small stature may maintain a rapid pulse throughout their illness.

Cole (297) has presented an analysis of 768 cases of pneumococcus lobar pneumonia which reveals the fatality rate of cases having maximum pulse rates at various levels, as shown in Table 152. Many of Cole's cases received specific serum therapy. In this series, the fatality rate is seen to increase from about 5 per cent or less in patients whose maximum pulse rate did not exceed 120, to around 62 per cent in cases with maximum rates of 160 and over. Cole mentions, however, that these figures give a somewhat false impression, for in many instances the highest pulse rates were frequently found in fatal cases and occurred shortly before death.

TABLE 152. PNEUMOCOCCUS LOBAR PNEUMONIA. NUMBER OF CASES AND NUMBER AND PERCENTAGE OF DEATHS IN CASES WITH MAXIMUM PULSE RATES OF VARIOUS LEVELS*

MAXIMUM PULSE RATE PER MINUTE	NUMBER OF CASES	DEATHS	
		Number	*Per cent*
Under 100	28	–	–
100–110	89	1	1.1
110–120	114	6	5.3
120–130	206	24	11.7
130–140	139	28	20.1
140–150	108	55	50.9
150–160	41	19	46.3
160 and over	43	27	62.8
Total	768		

From Cole (297)

* Many cases received specific serum treatment.

DeGraff, Travell, and Yager (349), in a study of repeated electrocardiographic tracings in 975 patients with lobar pneumonia, reported findings much like those in Table 152. Many of these cases also received specific serum treatment and 562 were given varying amounts of digitalis as well. DeGraff and his associates observed, as previously mentioned (see page 494), that relatively little variation of the pulse rate occurred from day to day in these cases, even in the presence of marked swings of the temperature. Nearly two-thirds of the patients who subsequently recovered had ventricular rates under 110 per minute during the course of their illness and, conversely, in patients later dying, more than two-thirds had rates exceeding 110. The development of a high ventricular rate late in the illness was particularly serious.

The findings of DeGraff and his collaborators (349) with respect to the proportion of cases recovering who had heart rates at varying levels, as determined by electrocardiographic tracings, are shown in the accompanying summary:

Expectancy of life for rate groups

HEART RATES	NUMBER OF TRACINGS	CASES RECOVERED *Per cent*
70–89	177	90.4
90–100	551	78.1
109–129	495	56.6
130–149	155	31.6
150 and over	25	16.0

The occurrence of irregularity of the pulse in pneumonia may be of grave import, particularly when due to such abnormalities of the basic rhythm as are caused by auricular fibrillation or flutter (297, 349). Irregularities due to extra systoles are usually of little consequence. The occurrence of auricular or nodal premature contractions or both, alone or in conjunction with ventricular premature contractions, may be somewhat more serious (349).

In their electrocardiographic study of the heart in lobar pneumonia, DeGraff, Travell, and Yager (349) determined the fatality rate of a number of cases with abnormal basic rhythms, as seen in Table 153. These cases are from their series of 975 patients mentioned above (and elsewhere, see pages 494–496). Many received specific serum treatment, and nearly one-half of the whole group got digitalis in varying doses. Of the total 51 cases with abnormal basic rhythms shown in Table 153 death occurred in 32, or 62.8 per cent. DeGraff and his co-workers contrast this high fatality rate with that of 34.2 for the remaining 924 cases in the series they studied, in which such conditions were absent. The seriousness of abnormal basic cardiac rhythms was as evident in the cases reported by the above investigators in patients under forty years of age as in those over this age.

Blood Pressure

Blood pressure changes in pneumonia, unless extreme, are usually of little importance. The prognostic value of Gibson's rule concerning the relation of pulse pressure to pulse rate is of practically no significance in this disease (297, 661, 1015).

Rapid changes in blood pressure are more important than the absolute pressure. A rapid fall in systolic pressure, especially if accompanied by an increase in pulse rate, is a bad omen, and frequently indicates a serious circulatory disturbance arising from intoxication or progressive infection (297, 830, 1015).

TABLE 153. LOBAR PNEUMONIA. NUMBER OF CASES AND NUMBER AND PERCENTAGE OF DEATHS IN CASES WITH VARIOUS ABNORMAL BASIC CARDIAC RHYTHMS*

TYPE OF ARRHYTHMIA	NUMBER OF CASES	DEATHS	
		Number	*Per cent*
Auricular fibrillation	27	17	63.0
Auricular flutter	10†	7	70.0
Paroxysmal tachycardia	6	4	66.7
Wandering pacemaker	8	4	50.0
Total	51	32	62.8

From DeGraff *et al.* (349)

* Many of these cases received specific serum treatment and varying amounts of digitalis as well.

† Two cases of auricular flutter also showed fibrillation and are included in both groups.

Leucocyte Count

The leucocyte count is, in general, an unreliable prognostic guide in pneumonia in man (1114, 255, 297, 807, 194, 1073, 890, 552) and in pneumococcus infections in animals as well (122, 1097, 1292, 483). In man with pneumonia, counts of 15,000 to 40,000 are usual and as a rule the prognosis is best in patients with counts within these ranges. High fatality rates are found in the presence of leucopenia, and judging from a few cases reported by Chatard (255) and Osler (976) with total counts of more than 50,000, the prognosis may be poor with unusually high counts. In the latter instance, however, other factors may enter into the matter which also unfavorably affect prognosis. Nevertheless, the outlook is not always poor with high counts, as seen below.

Avery, Chickering, Cole, and Dochez (33) have reported the fatality rate of 463 cases of lobar pneumonia in adults according to the leucocyte count found during the illness, as shown in Table 154. Doubtless many of these cases received specific serum treatment. Of 29 cases with a leucocyte count under 10,000, 65.5 per cent died. The proportion dying with counts of 10,000 to 20,000 was 23.7 per cent; and with counts of 20,000 to 30,000, 18 per cent; and with counts of 30,000 to 40,000 death occurred in 14.4 per cent. The lowest fatality rate, which was 11 per cent, occurred in 9 cases with counts of more than 50,000. A decrease in the total leucocyte count occurring during the course of the illness may mark the invasion of a new lobe. Rosenow (1114) considered that cases with the lowest counts were the most likely to have bacteriemia. No additional evidence is at hand relating to this matter in man, but in animals with experimentally induced pneumococcus infections observations of a similar nature have been made in some instances (1114, 122, 531) but not in others (122, 1275).

TABLE 154. LOBAR PNEUMONIA IN ADULTS. NUMBER OF CASES AND PERCENTAGE OF DEATHS AMONG CASES WITH LEUCOCYTE COUNTS OF VARYING NUMBERS*

LEUCOCYTE COUNT	NUMBER OF CASES	DEATHS *Per cent*
Under 10,000	29	65.5
10,000–20,000	143	23.7
20,000–30,000	177	18.0
30,000–40,000	76	14.4
40,000–50,000	29	24.1
Above 50,000	9	11.0
Total	463	

From Avery *et al.* (33)

* Many of the cases in this series probably received specific serum therapy.

Leucocytes are importantly concerned in the destruction of the invading organisms in pneumonia and their phagocytic functions may be regarded as essential to recovery (see pages 117–120). In the usual instance the leucocytes apparently maintain their ability throughout the illness to destroy virulent pneumococci, as suggested by the findings of Robertson, Graeser, Coggeshall, and Harrison (1087).

At times in severe pneumonias degenerate forms of polymorphonuclear leucocytes may be present in large numbers in blood smears. The cells stain poorly, their nuclei are fragmented, and their cytoplasm presents a picture suggesting cloudy swelling (Avery, Chickering, Cole, and Dochez, 33). Their demonstration may be of some prognostic value (33, 194).

Numerous studies of the leucocyte response to infection as measured by an estimation of the number of young forms of polymorphonuclear leucocytes in stained smears of the blood have been made, the cells grouped into from two to five classes depending upon the conformation of their nuclear material, and the number in each class compared with the number found in the blood of healthy individuals. Such investigations have resulted in the development of the Arneth, Shilling, and other similar indices (1073, 404, 890, 1074).

A single determination of an Arneth, Shilling, or other index is of little value, but the results of several blood examinations of this nature made at intervals of a few hours may be of some prognostic aid. Nevertheless, investigation of the matter by Reznikoff (1073), Farley, Huston, and Reisinger (404), and Middleton and Gibbon (890) led them to the unanimous conclusion that in prognosis undue dependence cannot be placed upon such determinations.

Respiration Rate

The respiration rate and character of the breathing are important and give information concerning the severity of the infection and the probable outcome of the case (297, 661). Sears and Larrabee (1168) analyzed 949 cases of "pneumonia" so as to reveal the relation of the maximum respiratory rate per minute to the outcome, and similar analyses were made in 658 cases of lobar pneumonia by Chatard (254) and in 768 pneumococcus cases by Cole (297; see Table 155). In all three series the results are essentially similar and show that low fatality rates prevail in cases in which the maximum respiratory rate is under 40 per minute.

TABLE 155. PNEUMOCOCCUS LOBAR PNEUMONIA. NUMBER OF CASES AND NUMBER AND PERCENTAGE OF DEATHS IN PATIENTS WITH MAXIMUM RESPIRATORY RATES OF VARIOUS LEVELS*

MAXIMUM RESPIRATION RATE PER MINUTE	NUMBER OF CASES	DEATHS	
		Number	*Per cent*
Under 20	–	–	–
20–30	25	–	–
30–40	178	8	4.5
40–50	312	48	15.4
50–60	165	60	36.4
60 and over	88	44	50.0
Total	768		

From Cole (297)

* Many cases received specific serum treatment.

The findings in Cole's (297) series are shown in Table 155. Many of his cases received specific serum treatment. In patients with maximum respiratory rates under 40 per minute the fatality rate was about 4 per cent or less. With respiratory rates of 40 to 50 per minute, the proportion dying was 15.3 per cent, with rates of 50 to 60 per minute death occurred in 36.3 per cent of the cases, and of those with respirations of 60 and over, 50 per cent died.

Cole (297) further stated that the character of the respiration rather than the rate alone is of greater prognostic significance. Rapid shallow breathing is of serious consequence and in extreme cases each breath is a struggle, the secondary muscles of respiration, especially the neck muscles, being called into play.

Cyanosis

The degree of cyanosis present bears a relation to the severity of the infection and is of prognostic importance (1223, 106, 138). Cases showing marked cyanosis frequently have a high fatality rate, and in such instances a high degree of arterial blood oxygen unsaturation (20 per cent or more) is usually present (1223, 106). Patients with extensive spreading lesions are apt to have "wet" lungs and anoxemia with cyanosis of considerable degree (106).

The effect of oxygen want on the outcome of pneumonia has not been determined (297), and as Locke (796) states, the high fatality rate of patients with extensive cyanosis is not due to the anoxemia but to the underlying condition responsible for its development (see also pages 759–767).

Bullowa (190) has presented some figures indicating the occurrence of a higher fatality rate in patients with cyanosis than in those without it. His series is composed of cases of Type I pneumococcus pneumonia (lobar pneumonia and bronchopneumonia together) with or without bacteriemia or cyanosis who received specific serum treatment. Among the cases without bacteriemia there were 157 not having cyanosis and death occurred in 6, or 3.8 per cent, as compared with 9.8 per cent, or 16, of 164 cases with cyanosis. The findings were of much the same significance in the bacteriemic group and death occurred in 23 per cent, or 11, of 47 cases without cyanosis and in 50.5 per cent, or 46, of 91 cases with cyanosis.

Miscellaneous Signs and Symptoms

In addition to the signs and symptoms already mentioned, certain others may occasionally be of prognostic aid. The prognostic value of herpes seems doubtful, but Lord (807) notes it has been regarded as a favorable sign. Persistent tympanites may be dangerous. Bullowa (186) has called attention to the serious significance of diarrhea, pulmonary edema, and dehydration.

Sears and Larrabee (1168) and Patterson (1003a) have considered the prognostic value of the demonstration of albuminuria. The former workers analyzed 624 cases of "pneumonia" and found no albumin in the urine in 175 cases of which 32, or 18.3 per cent, died. Of 493 cases showing a trace or less in the urine 152, or 30.8 per cent, died. In other cases having increasing amounts in the urine, higher fatality rates obtained, and 15 of 16 cases (93.3 per cent) with more than a large trace present died. In a series of 403 lobar pneumonias studied by Patterson (1003a), the findings were very similar. His observations are shown in the summary below:

AMOUNT OF ALBUMIN IN URINE	CASES *Number*	DEATHS *Number*	*Per cent*
Absent	170	23	13.5
Trace	91	15	16.5
+	128	36	28.1
++	14	6	42.9
Total	403		

The relation of jaundice to the prognosis in pneumonia is not clear. Lord (807) and Howard (661) have considered the subject at some length. Lord states that the fatality rate in some reported series of cases is higher for patients with jaundice than for those without it, while in other series there is little difference between the rates for the two groups. In a series of 34 cases of lobar pneumonia with jaundice observed by Warr and Alperin (1385) death occurred in 44 per cent, which was nearly double the proportion of deaths these workers found for several hundred other cases without jaundice.

Delirium in pneumonia, especially when marked, is an unfavorable sign. Sears and Larrabee (1168), in a group of 949 "pneumonias," found delirium occurred most often in alcoholic patients and the fatality rate of alcoholics with delirium was greater (rate 62.7 per cent) than among non-alcoholics with delirium (rate 50 per cent). Among 149 cases of lobar pneumonia with delirium observed by Chatard (254), 45 per cent died, as compared with a fatality rate of 30.3 per cent for his whole series of 658 cases. In addition, in a series of 2,039 cases of lobar pneumonia investigated by Warr and Alperin (1385), 27 per cent died, and included in this group were 86 cases having delirium with a fatality rate of 74 per cent.

CHAPTER SIXTEEN

RECOVERY FACTORS AND DURATION OF IMMUNITY

Recovery Factors 728
Immunity Factors 728
Humoral Antibodies 729
Cellular Factors 735
Miscellaneous Factors 736
Summary 737
Duration of Immunity 737
Following Spontaneous Recovery 737
Following Specific Serum Treatment 739

RECOVERY FACTORS

THE changes occurring during the course of pneumococcus pneumonia are so numerous and complex that the nature of the factors responsible for the survival of all cases recovering spontaneously has thus far eluded detection. Man normally possesses considerable immunity against the pneumococcus and recovery from pneumonia appears largely due to the acquisition of an increased immunity developing as a consequence of the infection. Other factors may also be intimately concerned in the process. Relatively little is known of the mechanism of recovery in cases due to organisms other than pneumococci but presumably the process is essentially similar to that occurring in pneumococcus cases.

Immunity Factors

The immunologic changes occurring as a result of pneumococcus pneumonia in man have been investigated by testing the blood at various stages of the illness for the presence of antibodies having various actions and by performing skin tests with several substances in an effort to detect the occurrence of an altered state of cellular reactivity. Cultures of material removed by lung puncture at different times in the disease or of sputum have likewise been made and observed for the appearance of a change in the number or in the character of the infecting pneumococci. In some instances also the lungs of fatal cases have been examined at necropsy for evidence of areas of local recovery, as manifested by the presence of the macrophage reaction. A discussion of immunity to pneumococcus infections, including pneumonia, is given in Chapter IV (page 113). Certain aspects of the findings indicated there are reviewed here along with additional observations relating to the subject under discussion.

HUMORAL ANTIBODIES. In 1891 the Klemperers (725) demonstrated that the serum of patients convalescent from pneumonia possessed properties not present in the serum of normal persons and that its administration to laboratory animals with pneumococcus infections had curative effects. In addition, the investigations of Bezançon and Griffon (99), Römer (1106), Neufeld (932), and Wadsworth (1360) showed that antibodies appeared in the blood of many patients with pneumococcus pneumonia at about the time of recovery. Prior to the discovery of the existence of pneumococcus types these workers, as well as others, identified agglutinins (99, 932, 1360, 1285, 1114), precipitins (1360), phagocytic-stimulating substances or opsonins (1285, 1115), and protective substances (1106) in the blood or serum of patients. Subsequent to the discovery of types many additional studies of this matter were made and the appearance of specific humoral antipneumococcal immune substances having various actions was demonstrated in the blood of numerous patients with pneumococcus pneumonia. Agglutinins were found by Lister (784), Chickering (257), Lacy and Hartman (754), Blake (118), and others (280, 1194, 815, 1321, 485, 1312, 459, 577, 1429, 468, 469, 1087, 1010, 339, 340). Blake (118) also found precipitins under these circumstances, and phagocytic-stimulating substances or opsonins were found by Strouse (1254), Eggers (388), Clough (278), and additional workers (280, 5, 1194, 1087). In similar fashion growth-retarding or bactericidal substances were noted by Dochez and Avery (362), Müller (912), Sia, Robertson, and Woo (1194), and others (1379, 1275, 1087), while beginning with Neufeld and Händel (936, 937) and Dochez (356) protective substances were found by many workers (278, 784, 280, 61, 60, 635, 1194, 815, 1321, 1275, 485, 820, 459, 577, 1429, 468, 469). The growth-retarding substances studied by Dochez and Avery (362) inhibited the proteolytic and glycolytic activities of pneumococci and this effect was termed an "antiblastic" immune response.

The findings of the many investigators cited have shown that tests of the blood or serum for antibody are usually negative in the first three or four days of illness, following which a variable but increasing proportion of favorable cases show positive tests as crisis approaches. At about the time of crisis a majority of patients have demonstrable humoral antibody, although in some instances antibody does not appear until during convalescence, as Dochez (356), Clough (278), Lord and Nesche (815) and others have shown (1094, 820, 809, 1087, 468, 339, 340). In some cases antibody has not been found until sixteen days or more after recovery (Dochez, 356, Lord and Persons, 820) and in still others it has never been found.

The amount of antibody per cubic centimeter of blood which may become demonstrable in pneumonia or after recovery is small. Illustrative examples may be given. Protective substance is often found for from 10 to 1,000 pneumococci of the homologous type and may occasionally be present for 10,000 to a million or more (61, 60, 820, 809, 459, 1429, 468, 469). Finland and Winkler (469) found protective substance for 100 to a million or more organisms in many Type II cases, and in Type V cases protection was frequently present for 10,000 to a million or more pneumococci. In Type III cases the same investigators (468) found protection for 10 to 1,000 pneumococci in some cases and uncommonly for one million, and in Type VIII cases it was often present for 100 to 100,000 organisms and occasionally for a million. Likewise in cases due to any one of several of the higher types* Winkler and Finland (1429) commonly demonstrated protection for 1,000 to 100,000 pneumococci of the homologous type; in some patients it was absent, or present against only 10 organisms, and in others it was present against 10 million. In terms of units these amounts of protective substance are small and presumably represent less than one unit of antibody per cubic centimeter of blood in the usual case.

Agglutinins may be present in dilutions up to about 1:64 in many instances, as workers such as Finland and Sutliff (459) have shown. Agglutinins are frequently found in Type II cases in dilutions of 1:4 to 1:8 and occasionally in dilutions of 1:16, while in Type V cases they are common in dilutions up to 1:64 and may reach 1:256 (469). In Type III infections agglutinins may be demonstrated in dilutions of 1:4 to 1:8 in some cases and at times in dilutions of 1:64, and in Type VIII cases are commonly found in dilutions of 1:4 to 1:16 and occasionally in dilutions of 1:64.

Sutliff and Rhoades (1275) observed that the blood of patients with pneumococcus pneumonia had pneumococcidal power against from 10,000 to several million organisms. In acutely ill patients tested one to five days before crisis, one cubic centimeter of blood had pneumococcidal power for from none to 10,000 or more organisms, and in patients tested one to three days after crisis the blood had higher killing power and one cubic centimeter was pneumococcidal for from 100,000 to a million organisms. Robertson and

* The cases included in this investigation had pneumonia due to pneumococci of Type II, III, IV, V, VII, VIII, XII, XIV, XVII, XVIII, or XIX.

his associates (1087) measured the killing power of the serum of a number of patients* and gave the results in terms of the highest dilution of serum killing all of 500 to 1,000 pneumococci in test preparations. Killing power was frequently demonstrated in dilutions of 1:20 to 1:40 and occasionally in dilutions of 1:320 or over.

The antibody response to infection appears to vary much with the individual patient and with age. Humoral antibody may occur less often in the blood of children than of adults with pneumonia and least often in the youngest children (1321, 577, 1145). Further, the antibody response in pneumonia appears to differ somewhat depending upon the type of pneumococcus causing the infection, much as it does in man following immunizing procedures (see pages 432–434). The response to Type I and Type II infections is usually relatively good, and also the response to many of the higher types (1429, 468, 469), as already mentioned. With Type III cases, however, little or no antibody is often found (257, 577, 468). With the immunologically related types, Type II and Type V, some cross immunity may occur in the blood of patients recovering from infections due to either of these types, as Finland and Winkler (469) have demonstrated, and a Type II case may show some antibody for Type V and vice versa. The heterologous antibody production of these two types, however, is less often found and is of a lower grade than is the cross immunity resulting from a Type III or Type VIII infection (468). In either lobar pneumonia or bronchopneumonia the results are very similar.

The demonstrable type-specific humoral antibodies appearing in pneumococcus pneumonia are those reactive with the surface antigen of the organism (see pages 171–172), producing alterations in its capsule. The reaction sensitizes pneumococci and promotes both their phagocytosis and their intracellular digestion by the leucocytes and allied cells. The death of the organisms occurs as the result of this process, which apparently is the only recognized means by which the blood elements are able to kill pneumococci, as Robertson, Woo, Cheer, and King (1097) have pointed out. In the presence of an excess of pneumococcus specific capsular polysaccharide, however, the action of the antibody is inhibited and the development of immunity is definitely impaired and retarded, as earlier described (see pages 131–132). Indeed, when relatively large amounts of the specific soluble carbohydrate are present, as may occur in severe cases and particularly in Type

* The cases included in this investigation had pneumonia due to pneumococci of Type I, II, IIa, III, or Group IV.

III infections or with extensive bacteriemia, the immune mechanism may be largely blocked.

The exact relation of the appearance of specific circulating antibody to recovery from pneumonia is not clear. It may be said, however, that most patients who develop demonstrable specific humoral antibody survive and most of those who fail to do so die. The results are nevertheless variable and exceptions occur. Extension of the pulmonary process is usually restricted when antibody appears in the blood, but at times it may extend even when antibody is demonstrable (1087, 339) or fail to do so in its absence (1087). In similar fashion complications such as empyema may develop in the presence of specific circulating antibody or fail to occur in its absence (61, 60, 1194, 1275, 459) or, as Davies, Hodgson, and Whitby (339) report, antibody already present may disappear from the blood when a complication develops and reappear later when the condition has subsided.

There is considerable evidence that possibly the most important function of antibody is to prevent the appearance of bacteriemia, and when humoral antibody becomes demonstrable bacteriemia if present is usually overcome, as Blake (118), Baldwin and Rhoades (61), Baldwin and Cecil (60), and Robertson and his associates (1094, 1087) have shown. Robertson, Terrell, Graeser, and Cornwell (1094) observed in studying the pneumococcidal power of the blood of patients with pneumonia that when the killing power present was above a specified threshold level bacteriemia was absent but if it fell below this level or was absent bacteriemia might develop. Nevertheless, in some instances bacteriemia may develop or persist in the presence of considerable amounts of circulating antibodies having various actions (61, 1275, 820) and it does not always appear even in the absence of such immune substances (1087). Antibody may be present simultaneously with severe toxemia.

It is likewise clear that recovery may occur in pneumococcus pneumonia without specific circulating antipneumococcal immune substances ever becoming demonstrable, as Neufeld (932), Neufeld and Händel (936), Strouse (1254), Dochez (356), and numerous additional workers have shown (278, 61, 1097, 820, 1429, 468, 286, 285), and that in other instances antibody may appear in the blood relatively early in the illness, perhaps by the fourth or fifth day, yet recovery be delayed until several days later, as illustrated by the findings of Dochez (356), Baldwin and Cecil (60), Herrold and Traut (635), and similar investigators (1321, 1275, 820, 577, 1087). And although patients frequently die in the absence of the development of humoral antibody, they may occasionally die even when specific antibody is present, as Lister (784), Blake (118), Clough (280), Baldwin and Rhoades (61), and other workers have shown (60, 1275, 1321, 820, 459, 1429, 468, 1087). In many instances where death has occurred under such circumstances some complication or an unusually extensive lesion has been present. If organisms become isolated in places not easily accessible to humoral antibodies, the outcome may be fatal (see also page 163).

As Lord (809) has mentioned, the chief objections to accepting the production of humoral immunity as the sole explanation of recovery in pneumonia are the discrepancy between the small amount and inconstant presence of antibody during the disease and the decisive nature of crisis, and the occasional delay of the favorable termination of illness until the usual time in spite of the very early appearance of immune substances.

The problem of the role of specific acquired antibody in influencing the outcome of pneumonia was further reviewed by Robertson, Graeser, Coggeshall, and Harrison (1087). Their conclusion that either the body brings into play more than one mechanism for localizing the infection and bringing about recovery or that the elaboration of specific circulating antipneumococcal immune substances represents but one phase of a specific reaction to the organism, seems justified from the data at hand. Of course, the procedures ordinarily used to detect the presence of humoral antibody may not be suitable or sufficiently sensitive to permit its demonstration in all instances and some tests may be more sensitive than others, as previously noted (see pages 127 and 130–131). Further, possibly the antibody appearing in the blood is only an excess over that usually needed to combat the infection and in consequence could not be expected to be found in all cases.

In addition to the frequent appearance in the blood of type-specific antibodies, other antibodies having actions of a non-specific nature may often be demonstrated. Species-specific antibodies reacting with the protein component of pneumococci of any type may be found, as Tillett and Francis (1311, 1312) and Trask and his associates (1321) have shown. Humoral precipitins for C substance may appear within twenty-four hours of the onset and persist until a day or two after crisis, as Tillett and Francis (1312) have also observed. The role of neither of the above antibodies in pneumococcus infections is understood, however, and it is doubtful that antiprotein antibodies have any special significance (see pages 127–131 and 133–135). Heterophile antibody may occasionally be found in the blood before, during, and after pneumonia but there is no evidence that its presence has any influence on the course or outcome of pneumonia in man, as mentioned in Chapter IV (see pages 124–125), where it is likewise noted that any "antitoxins" appearing in the blood in this disease seem to play no demonstrable part in immunity to the pneumococcus or in recovery from pneumonia.

In favorable cases, in addition to the successful operation of the immune mechanism, other factors, some of which will be discussed later, may contribute to reducing the number of pneumococci in the lung during the late stages of pneumonia. One of these factors may be a change in the characteristics of the organism, since in the late stages of the disease smooth virulent S forms have been shown to become avirulent R forms. However, as this change is presumably due to contact of the organisms with immune substances, the matter is considered at this point.

Thomas and Parker (1298) reviewed some of the pertinent literature and remarked that the number of organisms in the lung seemed to decrease as crisis approached. Moreover, numerous lung punctures performed by these investigators on 73 patients with lobar pneumonia showed that cases yielding live organisms after the sixth day of illness had a fatality rate twice as high as those with negative punctures after the sixth day. At times the number of organisms found decreased markedly prior to crisis, but this did not occur in all cases recovering. The decrease in number in favorable cases may begin three or four days prior to crisis, according to these workers, who likewise state that crisis is unrelated to the death of the organisms and that the organisms may die twenty-four hours before crisis or not until twenty-four hours after. They consider that two somewhat independent mechanisms are involved in recovery and that a bactericidal process is necessary to gain control of the infection, following which a detoxifying mechanism neutralizes "toxic" products and relieves the acute symptoms. Somewhat in contrast with the findings of Thomas and Parker were the results of a subsequent investigation by Bullowa (188), who did not find any appreciable decrease in the number of organisms obtained by lung puncture at the seventh or eighth day in 218 cases of Type I pneumococcus pneumonia.

Shibley and Rogers (1184) reported carrying out lung punctures on 20 cases of lobar pneumonia during life or after death. Cultures of material removed by this procedure were positive in all but four cases and these were in the stage of crisis or lysis at the time. In fatal cases the R form of pneumococci was found in one of ten cultures made at postmortem, the S form in another, and both R and S forms in eight. Lung puncture in one case early in the illness yielded few pneumococci of the R form, while a second puncture at the time of crisis gave organisms largely of the R form.

Griffith (571), Paul and Lawrence (1005), and Sabin (1153) have all reported findings indicating that in many instances at the time of defervescence the biologic characteristics of the infecting pneumococcus may be altered, probably as a result of the action on the organism of immune substances. Pneumococci of the smooth virulent S form present in the sputum may gradually become changed at about the time of crisis into rough avirulent forms; as Griffith (571) states, they appear to escape death at the expense of losing their virulence and type-specific characteristics. Such changes do not appear uniformly, however, for virulent type-specific pneumococci of the kind responsible for the illness can be obtained from the mouths of many patients during and after convalescence, as earlier pointed out (see pages 366 and 369).

CELLULAR FACTORS. If recovery is to be attributed chiefly to the successful functioning of the immunologic mechanism, and it has been shown that the appearance of humoral antibody is doubtless due to the operation of such a mechanism, then cellular factors are of paramount importance. Direct tests for ascertaining the nature of the cellular status in pneumonia have been made with varying degrees of success by injecting one or more of a number of substances, such as specific capsular polysaccharide or pneumococcus nucleoprotein, into the skin of patients at various stages of their illness. Positive tests with pneumococcus capsular polysaccharide specific for the type causing the infection have often been found at crisis or shortly after, and in the presence of humoral antibody of the homologous type, as earlier described; and skin sensitivity to pneumococcus nucleoprotein may also develop at about the time of crisis (see pages 126 and 165–167). Tests with the former substance are positive only in the presence of active tissues and specific circulating antibodies.

In addition to the leucocytes, particularly those of the polymorphonuclear variety, which play such a significant role in phagocytizing and digesting pneumococci in pneumonia, other cells such as the histiocyte or macrophage also appear of importance. Robertson, Graeser, Coggeshall, and Harrison (1087) examined several patients not having demonstrable humoral antibody, and in these patients at necropsy found areas of local lung clearing or regional recovery in the lung, as mentioned in Chapter IV (see pages 180–

182). Pneumococci were nearly absent in these areas, while in neighboring consolidated regions they were numerous. It was suggested that the clearing might have resulted from the acquisition of immunity by the local tissue cells which brought about recovery in the region. The macrophage was the predominant cell in the reaction, and the appearance of the macrophage reaction was, on the basis of numerous studies, considered evidence of an increased resistance. Robertson and Uhley (1095) point out that, although recovery may depend upon the presence of circulating antibody in addition to the occurrence of a local cellular reaction in the lung, they were unable to find a constant relationship in either animals or man between the presence of humoral immune substances and the development of the macrophage reaction (see also page 99).

Miscellaneous Factors

Factors other than those related to the immunologic processes may be concerned in recovery from pneumonia. Doubtless some impairment of the circulation exists in the consolidated area (see page 95) and it is also probable that at least partly because of this the acidity of the area increases, pneumococci tend to be destroyed along with the leucocytes and other cells present, and the enzymes thus liberated initiate the digestion of the exudate, as elsewhere described (see pages 96–101). The occurrence of the macrophage reaction may assist in the destruction and removal of pneumococci. The possible role of enzymes in aiding the destruction of pneumococci was considered many years ago and still commands attention (292, 300), especially in view of the findings of Avery and Dubos (38) in 1930. These investigators isolated from a living organism an enzyme capable of specifically decomposing the capsular material of the Type III pneumococcus, thus rendering the latter readily susceptible to phagocytosis and intracellular digestion (380). The therapeutic use of this enzyme solution in mice (38, 39), rabbits (539, 538), and monkeys (484) with pneumococcus Type III infections has given promising results.

Additional evidence that non-specific factors may assist in recovery from pneumococcus infections was obtained by Gelari and Sabin (512), who treated intradermally infected rabbits with subeffective amounts of specific immune serum and gold salts. Test rabbits receiving either of these preparations alone had a very high fatality rate, but the majority of animals given both preparations recovered.

Summary

There are probably other factors involved in recovery from pneumonia but so far as present knowledge is concerned the outcome is chiefly influenced by the degree of natural resistance of the patient, his power to elaborate and utilize specific immune substances during the course of the illness, and his capacity to withstand the ill effects of the pneumococcus toxemia. Pneumococcus toxemia, complicated by the degenerative changes incidental to advancing age, is one of the most important factors in limiting the success of the natural forces of recovery and of the use of specific serum in treatment.

The effect of actively acquired specific humoral antibody upon the course and outcome of pneumococcus pneumonia is apparently very similar to that of passively acquired antibody in the form of specific antipneumococcic serum. The only means at present available of favorably modifying the outlook in pneumococcus pneumonia is by the early administration of adequate amounts of serum specific for the type responsible for the infection (see pages 805 and 880). The use of certain recently introduced chemicals, particularly when administered with specific antiserum, may subsequently be shown to yield even better results (see pages 783–790).

DURATION OF IMMUNITY

Considerable evidence is at hand concerning the duration of the immune response following recovery from pneumonia (257, 754, 118, 297, 1296, 912, 222, 1194, 223, 1097, 815, 1275, 459, 460, 995, 1088, 1429, 470, 286). The duration of the immunity arising as a consequence of immunization is in some respects analogous and is discussed elsewhere (see pages 437–440).

In comparison with the duration of the immunity produced by certain other diseases, that following pneumococcus pneumonia may be considered very short.

Following Spontaneous Recovery

After spontaneous recovery from pneumococcus pneumonia, the persistence of immunity varies somewhat with the different types of the infecting organism concerned, and humoral antibodies homologous in type with that causing the infection generally persist longer after infection with Type I or Type II or with some of the higher types than after infection with Type III (754, 297, 459, 1429). The percentage of cases with demonstrable antibody is high early in recovery, progressively decreases with the lapse of time, and after several weeks is very low. However, in some instances antibody may be detected for as long as a year or more (257, 754, 1194, 1275, 459, 1429, 470).

Chickering (257) observed that serum agglutinins in Type I, II, and Group IV cases persisted for weeks in a few instances, as did Lacy and Hartman (754). Lord and Nesche (815) were able to demonstrate that agglutinins and protective substance remained in the serum of many patients for days or weeks after recovery. Sia, Robertson, and Woo (1194) examined the serum of a number of patients for pneumococcidal power and reported that in one case it lasted only ten days, though in others it persisted in low titer for weeks or months. In a similar study Sutliff and Rhoades (1275) found that the blood of patients in the first week after crisis killed from 100,000 to one million organisms, while blood from patients in the second, third, and fourth week of recovery killed only 1,000 to 100,000 organisms.

Finland and Sutliff (459) demonstrated the frequent persistence of agglutinins in Type I, II, and III cases for periods up to twenty-three days, but they were rarely present when tested for from five to fourteen months after crisis. These same workers found that protective substance in Type I, II, and III cases was commonly present for at least twenty-three days and was occasionally demonstrable at five to fourteen months after crisis. In the same patients and at the same intervals they also carried out skin tests for reactivity to the specific capsular polysaccharide of the type homologous with that responsible for the infection. Skin sensitivity was usually present for shorter intervals than antibody. In each instance in this part of their study, the tests were made on groups of patients not previously tested. In the experience of Davies, Hodgson, and Whitby (339) with Type I cases, agglutinins always disappeared from the serum within ten to twelve days after recovery.

In cases due to one or another of several of the higher types, Winkler and Finland (1429) observed that agglutinins and protective substance frequently persisted for as long as one to slightly more than two months, and in some cases the results were still positive at the time of the last test.

Sia, Robertson, and Woo (1194) stated that tests of killing power in the blood of patients during pneumonia and after recovery suggested that patients having the most intense immune response seemed to carry demonstrable antibody the longest. The findings in various studies by Finland and his associates (459, 460, 1429) suggest that tests for protective substance are positive longer after recovery than are tests for other antibodies or for skin sensitivity (see page 127).

Cecil (222) points out that as pneumonia seldom recurs in the same patient in less than a year's time, it is likely that the immunity following an attack lasts for six to twelve months in most cases and also that probably there is a small but variable amount of cross immunity against types other than the one which caused the infection. Subsequently Finland and his co-workers (459, 469, 468, 1429) not infrequently found some antibody of heterologous type in the blood after pneumonia.

Finland and Winkler (470), in a study of patients with recurrent attacks of pneumonia, reported an observation which further suggested that the immunity engendered by the infection is not of very long duration, for the types responsible for the second or subsequent attacks had about the same distribution among the cases as the types causing the primary attacks (see pages 535–538). The average interval between attacks of pneumonia due to the same type of pneumococcus in a given patient was twenty-eight months. Among 19 cases recurring within one year 4 were due to pneumococci of the same type. These workers also observed one patient who had humoral antibody for the type causing his original pneumonia when he developed a second attack due to the same organism a year later. Another patient who had recovered from Type I pneumonia had a high titer of antibody in his blood for several months, but suffered a recurrent attack of Type I pneumonia three years later.

It is clear from the findings in animals that immunity of considerable degree may be present at times in the absence of demonstrable humoral antibody (see pages 129–131) and it seems likely that this is also true with man in many instances.

Following Specific Serum Treatment

Following specific serum treatment, the duration of the demonstrable immune response in man is shorter than after spontaneous recovery. Thomas (1296) pointed out that the use of serum apparently lessens the antigenic value of the attack. He likewise observed that after such treatment it was doubtful if immunity lasted longer than about four weeks, and reported an instance of a patient with Type I pneumonia who recovered following specific serum therapy and had a recurrence due to the same organism thirty-one days later.

Finland and Sutliff (460) studied the length of time that humoral antibody and skin sensitivity to SSS of homologous type were demonstrable in several patients recovering from Type I or Type II pneumonia who had been treated with specific immune serum. Positive skin tests were frequent up to the tenth to the twenty-second day after serum administration and in a few cases apparently the tests were still positive five to fourteen months later. The results with tests for agglutinins gave about the same results as skin tests in the early period after serum treatment, but tests made five to fourteen months later revealed that agglutinins were absent. Protective substance was present in many Type I and Type II cases in the early period but was not found at the later period. Finland and Sutliff pointed out that, in general, immune reactions were rarely demonstrable later than one month after recovery when patients have received serum treatment, whereas when recovery has been spontaneous such reactions may persist several months.

Robertson, Graeser, Coggeshall, and Sia (1088) studied the pneumococcidal power of patients' serum after specific serum treatment and found that although occasionally killing power disappeared within three or four days after serum administration was stopped, more commonly it gradually decreased over a period of several weeks.

Finland and Winkler (470) observed the complete disappearance of antibodies from the blood of a patient with Type II pneumonia within two weeks after serum treatment. Nine months later this patient had a recurrent pneumonia due to pneumococci of the same type. In a group of recurrent cases studied it was observed that although serum treatment in the first attack had little apparent effect on the character of the recurrent attack, early recurrence of an infection with the same type was more frequent among serum treated cases.

CHAPTER SEVENTEEN

GENERAL THERAPEUTIC MEASURES

General Management 742
Hospitalization 743
Home Care 743
Nursing Care 744
Diet and Fluid Intake 746
Care of the Bowels 747
Non-Specific Treatment 748
Treatment for Pain 748
Treatment for Cough 749
Cardiovascular Medication 749
Caffeine 753
Camphor 753
Strychnine 754
Alcohol 754
Epinephrine and Ephedrine 754
Sedatives 755
Treatment for Tympanites 756
Hydrotherapy 758
Treatment for Pulmonary Edema 758
Treatment for General Collapse 759
Special Treatment 759
Oxygen and Carbon Dioxide Treatment 759
Other Forms of Special Treatment 768
Chemotherapy 775
Quinine 775
Ethylhydrocupreine (Optochin) 778
Miscellaneous Chemicals 782
Sulfanilamide and Related Preparations 783
Vitamins and Enzymes 790
Vaccine Treatment 795

THE treatment of pneumonia has changed considerably during the past one hundred years or more. Townsend and Coolidge (1319), in a review of the methods used at the Massachusetts General Hospital from 1821 to 1889, called attention to the procedures in use at three different periods during that interval. Prior to 1850, patients were subjected to "heroic" measures, consisting of frequent bleeding, purging, and the administration of large amounts of numerous drugs. A gradual transition and moderation of therapeutic measures occurred between 1850 and 1860. From 1860 to 1889 the expectant form of treatment was in vogue and has continued to be of service in many cases. Townsend and Coolidge remark that the fatality rate of cases treated prior to 1850 was no higher than that of cases subsequently treated and that in view of the drastic nature of the treatment used in the early period this was rather surprising. A new era in the treatment of pneumonia, or at least in the treatment of many cases of pneumococcus pneumonia, was initiated by Neufeld and Händel (938) in 1910, who, as described elsewhere, first made use of specific serum therapy (see page 807). Recent discoveries in the field of chemistry offer hope of the introduction of a chemical compound which alone or in conjunction with antiserum will prove useful in the treatment of pneumonia. The general therapeutic measures other than serum therapy are considered in this chapter.

GENERAL MANAGEMENT

A number of matters must be given consideration in the general medical treatment of pneumonia. Efforts should be made to conserve the patient's strength, to relieve discomfort, to neutralize the effects of the disease upon the circulatory, respiratory, and other systems of the body, to destroy the infecting agent by specific measures wherever possible, and to give such attention as is necessary to the care of any complications that may arise. In all cases it is desirable to obtain the maximum of rest compatible with suitable nutrition, elimination, and whatever special care is indicated. Bed rest throughout the disease is essential and good nursing important. Further, care should be taken to prevent the spread of the infection to members of the patient's family and to his attendants, as earlier mentioned (see pages 401–403).

The general management of patients is frequently of great importance, particularly in severe cases where the outlook is dubious. Direct symptomatic treatment continues to be of value in spite of the use in many cases of specific antiserum or certain chemotherapeutic agents. The problem in pneumonia is fundamentally that of combating an acute infection, and a rational basis for symptomatic treatment should be sought in the pathologic physiology resulting from the infection (796). Medication of little or doubtful value should be avoided. Cole (297) has called attention to the seriousness of the promiscuous administration of drugs and remarks that unfortunately many patients have to fight not only the disease but varying degrees of drug poisoning as well.

Means and Barach (876, 875) have considered the marked functional changes resulting from pulmonary infection during pneumonia. Factors such as the increased metabolism due to fever, impaired blood flow through the lungs, and anoxemia give rise to an increased respiratory rate or hyperpnea. The efficiency of the respiratory system is markedly reduced, while at the same time the functional demands on it are far above normal. The impaired efficiency of the respiratory system is largely the result of consolidation, excessive bronchial secretion, and pain caused by the pulmonary lesion. Occasionally some edema of the uninvolved alveoli, possibly of cardiac origin, and pleural effusion may be contributing factors.

Hospitalization

Patients are usually first seen in their homes and a decision should be made within the first day or two of illness as to the advisability of hospitalization. Consideration must be given to the advantages and disadvantages offered by the home for the proper care and treatment of the patient and these should be weighed against the unavoidable excitement and expenditure of energy on the part of the patient consequent to his removal to a hospital. In the usual instance the chance of receiving adequate nursing care is better for patients in the hospital than in the home, but all details of treatment can be carried out in the home if adequate service can be provided. If patients are to be hospitalized, they should be taken to the hospital early in the illness and not left at home until acutely ill or in extremis. Delay in hospitalization has doubtless cost the life of many patients. The patient should be carried to the hospital on a stretcher and preferably by ambulance and should not be dressed or permitted to sit up during the trip.

Home Care

When the patient is cared for at home, a light airy room with ample ventilation is desirable, as fresh air in abundance is required. The room should be quiet and an open fireplace is an advantage for purposes of ventilation. The patient should be screened from drafts. The exposure of patients to very cold air, a procedure widely used several years ago, failed to produce beneficial effects (333, 796) and has been replaced by the more moderate practice of maintaining an adequate supply of cool but not cold air. A room temperature of about 60°–65° F. is usually suitable but it is well to be guided by the patient's desires and some patients may feel better and have less labored respirations in cold air. With other patients exposure to very cold air will incite cough. If possible the humidity of the room should be maintained at about 40 to 60 per cent, although a higher humidity may be of aid if cough is bothersome and the bronchial secretions tenacious. Freedom from worry about household or business affairs is important and visitors should be restricted to an absolute minimum. Neither attendants nor visitors suffering from any form of infection of the respiratory tract should be permitted to approach patients with pneumonia (see page 403).

Nursing Care

It is generally conceded that there are few diseases in which competent nursing care is more important than in pneumonia, for every effort should be made to conserve the patient's strength. The exact importance of nursing care, however, can probably never be determined. Several good discussions of the nursing care of pneumonia are available (297, 807, 1017, 1454) but that prepared by the Bureau of Pneumonia Control of the New York State Department of Health (945) is especially to be recommended.

The patient should be fed by the nurse with as little effort on his part as possible. Liquids and food should both be taken in the recumbent position, liquids being given preferably from a glass by means of a bent tube. The urinal or bed pan should be used from the beginning and under no circumstances should the patient be allowed out of bed to go to the bathroom. Surface bathing may be given once a day providing the room is previously warmed and it does not fatigue the patient. The unnecessary exposure of large areas of the body to room air during the bath should be avoided.

The patient's bed should be single and so placed as to be approachable from both sides. It should be sufficiently high, moreover, to facilitate attendance on the patient by the physician and nurse. A firm mattress covered with rubber and draw sheets should be used. As orthopnea is uncommon in pneumonia, most patients are more comfortable flat in bed. If the semi-sitting position proves desirable and the bed cannot be suitably manipulated, pillows may be supplied to assist in maintaining it. The bed clothing should be of sufficient warmth to protect the patient from cold but not heavy enough to produce respiratory embarrassment or sweating. A short woolen night shirt or pyjamas are desirable and whichever is used should be slit up the whole length of the front to facilitate examining the patient without the necessity of his assuming a sitting posture. The patient should be examined daily; turning him on his side will make it possible to examine his back while he is lying down. Turning the patient on the affected side is less likely to aggravate the cough. At times examination of the patient twice a day may be desirable but there is little excuse for more frequent examinations.

To avoid the danger of hypostasis and of massive pulmonary collapse from retained pulmonary secretions, the patient's position should be changed about every two hours (807). Watch should be kept for the development of pressure areas, particularly over bony promontories. The skin should be kept dry and after the back has been washed or rubbed, cold cream or an alcohol bathing solution and powder should be applied.

The temperature (rectal), pulse, and respiration should be noted and recorded at four-hour intervals. The character and amount of nourishment given and the fluid intake and output are likewise recorded. It is unwise to leave patients alone at any time, as the sudden appearance of unexpected delirium may lead them to injure themselves or others. Careful attention to the bed and pillows will assist in securing comfort for the patient without the expenditure of energy on his part. Sleep is to be coveted and it is seldom necessary or advisable to wake the patient for food or medicine.

Proper care of the mouth and nose is important. Dyspneic patients usually breathe through their mouths, which leads to a drying of the mucous membranes of the mouth and throat that is irritating if marked and makes respiration more difficult. It likewise interferes with giving food, for taste is nearly always impaired. The mouth and tongue may be swabbed every two hours with an alkaline solution, followed by the application of albolene to the tongue and cold cream to the lips. Lord (807) recommends a mouth wash consisting of 4 drams of boracic acid and 4 ounces each of lemon juice and glycerine for use in swabbing the mouth. The nose should be kept clean and sprayed with albolene every few hours as necessary.

The first specimens of sputum obtained from the patient should be sent to the laboratory for bacteriologic examination and the typing of any pneumococci found (see pages 620–637). All other sputum collected should be disinfected or burned. A suitable receptacle for sputum, such as a cardboard sputum cup, should be kept within easy reach of the patient. Extremely ill patients may find it difficult to expectorate into a special receptacle. Small pieces of gauze, linen, or cotton, or handkerchiefs of paper may be used to wipe sputum from the lips, following which they are placed in a paper receptacle and burned. Preparations such as carbolic acid or formaldehyde are useful for carrying out concurrent disinfection, but should not be kept in places accessible to the patient.

The nurse should be able to put on a suitable chest binder, apply stupes, and give enemas; she should also be capable of recognizing distention, approaching collapse, or the appearance of any unusual symptoms, which should be reported to the physician at once. If possible, she should be familiar with the usual methods of administering oxygen and where specific serum is used in treatment she may be called upon to recognize and treat certain untoward reactions and to give assurance if chills or vomiting occur or itching and joint pains from serum sickness develop.

Diet and Fluid Intake

As a rule the duration of the illness is so short that the diet is of relatively minor importance (297, 807, 606, 796, 1441). Bullowa (190), however, feels that the caloric intake in pneumonia is of great importance and advises the use of a relatively high-caloric, bland, low-residue diet. Doubtless such diets are advisable for grossly underfed patients and in instances where a high temperature may persist for several weeks, as with an empyema.

Anorexia is liable to be marked, particularly in the early stages of the illness. All food taken during the acute stages should be in the form of very soft solids or liquids. Milk, if well tolerated, is the simplest and perhaps the best food and, as Cole (297) remarks, it is not certain that milk gives rise to distention. Cole (302) has administered in some cases from 5 to 8 grams of sodium chloride daily in addition to that in the diet and notes that it may have been of aid in relieving distention and the symptoms of toxemia. Very large doses should be avoided, otherwise subcutaneous or pulmonary edema may occur. Salt given in capsules may cause some nausea and vomiting. Enteric coated pills may be tried. Occasionally a part of the extra salt may be mixed in salty foods or sprinkled on crackers and given in the diet.

If the patient refuses food it is probably best not to urge it upon him too much. Food may be offered at intervals of about two hours while the patient is awake.

The foods useful in pneumonia include milk and simple milk dishes such as matzoon, koumiss, zoolak, buttermilk, and eggnogs. Cream, butter, and starches in the form of gruels, macaroni, rice, toast, stale bread, cooked cereals, and baked or mashed potato, as well as eggs, custards, broths, beef juice, scraped beef, minced chicken, fruit juices, and cooked fruits are of value. Care should be taken to avoid feeding an excess of sugars or of fats, as the former may aggravate or incite tympanites and the latter give rise to diarrhea (796).

The maintenance of a relatively high fluid intake in the usual case is important. Patients should receive about three liters (3,000 cc.) of fluid every twenty-four hours during the acute stages of the illness. The apparently beneficial action of water at such a time is little understood. There is little if any reason to insist that eight or ten liters of fluid be given daily and it may often be dangerous to administer such large quantities, as the circulatory system is already under considerable strain. In the presence of pulmonary edema Bullowa (190) advises restricting fluids to a minimum.

Fluid in some form may be offered the patient every hour or two. Small bits of cracked ice may be given him to suck. In severe cases small amounts of fluid given at frequent intervals with a spoon may be of great value, while in very toxic patients or in those unable to swallow, fluids may be given subcutaneously, intravenously, or by slow rectal drip.

In addition to plain water, milk, buttermilk, bouillon, soups, barley water, fruit juices well diluted, black coffee and tea in moderate amounts, and simple carbonated waters and ginger ale will often be useful. Water containing glucose and flavored with lemon juice will furnish both calories and liquid and is usually acceptable. Maclachlan, Kastlin, and Lynch (846) advise dissolving 200 grams of dextrose (glucose) powder in 1,000 cc. of water and adding the juice of two or three lemons. If the administration of this mixture is prolonged over many days it may lead to nausea and vomiting.

Care of the Bowels

It has long been the custom, if the bowels have not moved at the onset, to administer a mild saline cathartic such as sodium phosphate (45 grains) in half a glass of warm water, a Seidlitz powder, or a saline cathartic water, as Lord (807) has described. Bullowa (190) considers this unnecessary and frequently inadvisable because of the water loss it entails.

Drastic catharsis should not be attempted. If the patient is dehydrated or dyspneic, cathartics are best avoided, otherwise one-half to one ounce of magnesium hydrate or one or two teaspoonfuls of the fluid extract of cascara may be used (190). During the course of the illness it is preferable, if necessary to keep the bowels open, to employ a daily saline or soapsuds enema. If vomiting or flatus is bothersome, the amount of nourishment may be restricted and albumin water alone be given. Every care should be taken to prevent tympanites (see page 756). In some instances lack of food rather than the peculiarities of any particular food may contribute to this condition.

With vomiting and abdominal distention of rather abrupt onset, the possibility of acute dilatation of the stomach should be kept in mind, as elsewhere described (see page 611).

NON-SPECIFIC TREATMENT

Innumerable preparations have been used in the general treatment of pneumonia, a number of which will be mentioned. The evidence relating to the value of several of these agents is conflicting, however, and it is well to appreciate that no final judgment can be rendered as to the usefulness of many of them. Cole (301) has remarked that he feels convinced that no great saving of lives results from the use of many of the non-specific preparations. This view is unquestionably correct. Considerable symptomatic relief may often be obtained, however, by judicious medication.

The evidence at hand suggests that the toxemia occurring in pneumococcus pneumonia has notable effects on smooth muscle. Circulatory insufficiency in this disease appears to be due usually to peripheral vasomotor paralysis with capillary stasis; acute gastric dilatation or tympanites, to the effect of toxemia on the musculature of the gastrointestinal tract; and the occurrence of abortion or delivery in pregnant patients, to the effect of toxemia on the uterine muscle.

Treatment for Pain

Pain in the chest is present in a large majority of cases of lobar pneumonia but in many, due to its mildness, is of little moment. Frequently, however, distressing and persistent pain may occur and may be of great importance because of its interference with respiration and to a lesser degree with cardiac functions and sleep. Counterirritants applied to the chest over the painful area, such as iodine, mustard, or cantharides plasters, and the use of wet or dry cupping and leeches have been tried but such procedures ordinarily do little except add to the patient's discomfort (297, 807, 796).

Perhaps the most satisfactory local method of controlling pleural pain is the use of a chest binder, preferably one that may be drawn tightly about the chest and strapped and buckled over the shoulder so it will fit properly. Such a binder may, however, interfere too much with breathing. Strapping the affected area with adhesive tape after shaving the skin may offer more advantages if a number of strips are used and are carried sufficiently well across the midline of the chest and the back. Adhesive strapping, however, stretches or slips. It cannot be tightened after being applied, it makes examination of the chest difficult, and it is frequently painful to remove. On the other hand, it has the obvious advantage that it can be restricted to a unilateral area which it is desired to immobilize. The application of dry heat or of an icebag to the painful area may be tried but is generally insufficient to give relief. Diathermy may be of some value in relieving such pain (110) but danger from burns or shocks limits its usefulness (190). Cole (297) finds that ordinary flaxseed poultices applied after the skin has been well oiled often give great relief.

Many instances are encountered in which the simpler methods do not suffice. At such times codeine is usually inadequate and it may be necessary to use morphine in doses of 1/8 to 1/6 grain or more. Care must be taken not to depress the respirations too much by the indiscriminate use of morphine. If the pulmonary lesion is extensive or "wet," the use of morphine is best combined with oxygen therapy (Davis, 343). The production of an artificial pneumothorax may be tried if lesser measures fail (606, 287, 1356) and pain is frequently relieved in a few minutes by this procedure, but it is not without its dangers (see page 771).

Treatment for Cough

Cough may be the source of much trouble. If it is harassing and unproductive, if it interferes with sleep or intensifies pain, or if it is fatiguing to the patient, one-quarter grain of codeine, one-twelfth grain of heroin, or one-eighth grain of morphine may be given. Usually codeine alone or in conjunction with some preparation such as phenobarbital sodium (sodium luminal) is considered safest and preferable (605, 1455, 447). Where bronchial secretions are abundant or with widespread lesions it is not advisable to use morphine (807, 106, 343). If sputum is raised with great difficulty potassium or sodium iodide or ammonium chloride given once or twice at four-hour intervals may be of assistance, but numerous physicians feel expectorants are of no value. Markedly increasing the humidity of the air in the room may aid (190).

Cardiovascular Medication

Symptoms referable to the cardiovascular system are often prominent, particularly in the later stages of pneumonia, as earlier mentioned (see pages 492–497 and 545–546), and their treatment may constitute a vital part of the general therapeutic program. Many serious cases show evidence either by physical signs or by roentgenograms of some dilatation of the heart, and dilatation of the right heart is not unusual at necropsy. Actual pathologic alterations of the myocardium are insignificant in pneumonia, however, and seemingly not sufficient to cause heart failure (1418). Dilatation of the peripheral capillary bed, both superficial and deep, which may be attributed to the paralyzing effect of the toxemia on the smaller blood vessels, doubtless is commonly the cause of the cardiovascular collapse seen in some cases of pneumonia (1015, 153, 1384). Such effects are probably present in some degree in most cases and, when severe, produce a condition similar to that seen in shock.

All means available should be used to support the heart and preserve good vascular tone. The relief of tympanites and regulation of the bowels nearly always act favorably on the cardiovascular system. Attention to the fluid and salt intake will assist, particularly in very toxic patients. Other things that ease the burden on the heart are reasonable control of a harassing cough, judicious use of sedatives for restlessness and excitability, and freeing the patient of anxiety. Hydrotherapy may be of considerable aid (796). Brooks (153) has called attention to the fact that there is little specific medication that is of use in combating the peripheral circulatory collapse in pneumonia but mentions that pituitrin or epinephrine may aid at times. The action of both drugs is relatively fleeting. Yens (1455) finds small repeated subcutaneous doses of epinephrine very useful. Warfield (1384) notes that digitalis fails to increase vascular tone at the periphery and believes strychnine in subcutaneous doses of 1/20 to 1/15 grain every two or three hours is the most satisfactory preparation for this purpose.

Digitalis and strophanthin. Many discussions and much advice are available relating to the use of digitalis in pneumonia (297, 777, 713, 991, 119, 637, 953, 1452, 796, 1385, 1441, 686, 288, 1384, 302). Digitalis may be of great value to a few patients and perhaps of some use to many others. Its action is the same whether or not fever is present, it does not increase blood pressure, and it may be life-saving in patients with auricular fibrillation or flutter. Levy (777) reported that his roentgenographic study of the size of the heart in pneumonia showed that possibly cardiac enlargement occurs less often in patients taking digitalis. His observations were limited to a few cases.

In times past the use of digitalis was frequently a matter of routine in all cases. The careful study of Niles and Wyckoff (953), and the similar report of Wyckoff, DuBois, and Woodruff (1452), however, have largely resulted in the discontinuance of this practice. These workers studied a group of 835 patients with pneumococcus lobar pneumonia over a two-year period at the Bellevue Hospital, New York City. The patients were divided into groups according to whether they had routinely received digitalis or specific antipneumococcic serum, or both or neither of these agents. The potency of the digitalis preparations used was carefully investigated. The findings reported showed that of 404 cases treated without digitalis 136, or 33.7 per cent, died, as compared with 41.4 per cent, or 140, of 338 cases receiving digitalis. The difference between the fatality rates of these groups of cases suggests that the fatality rate may be somewhat less in cases not routinely given this drug. Each of these groups was further subdivided according to the age, sex,

TABLE 156. PNEUMOCOCCUS LOBAR PNEUMONIA. NUMBER OF CASES AND NUMBER AND PERCENTAGE OF DEATHS IN PATIENTS TREATED WITHOUT OR WITH DIGITALIS, BY AGE GROUP*

AGE GROUP IN YEARS	TREATED WITHOUT DIGITALIS			TREATED WITH DIGITALIS		
	NUMBER OF CASES	DEATHS		NUMBER OF CASES	DEATHS	
		Number	*Per cent*		*Number*	*Per cent*
10–29	94	15	16.0	73	19	26.0
30–39	109	30	27.5	76	25	32.9
40–49	99	40	40.4	99	44	44.4
50 and over	102	51	50.0	90	52	57.8
Total	404	136	33.7	338	140	41.4

* Many cases received specific serum treatment.

type of pneumococcus, and the presence or absence of various complications. The figures relating to the difference in the fatality rates of patients in various age groups who were treated without or with digitalis, as reported by Niles and Wyckoff (953), are shown in Table 156. The age group showing the most marked difference between the fatality rate of cases treated without or with digitalis is that of 10 through 29 years. Of 94 cases in this group not given the drug 15, or 16 per cent, died, while 26 per cent, or 19, of 73 cases receiving it died. The differences were less marked in the other groups and the number of cases in all groups is too small and the possible number of complicating factors affecting the fatality rates appears too large to permit drawing final conclusions from such data. The fatality rates of the groups treated without or with digitalis and having bacteriemia were essentially the same. Of 54 cases with bacteriemia who did not receive this drug, 43, or 79.6 per cent, died, while of 53 cases treated with digitalis 42, or 79.2 per cent, died. From these findings, it was concluded that there was no justification for the continued routine use of digitalis in lobar pneumonia.

Subsequently the matter was even more exhaustively studied by Cohn and Lewis (288) in a series of 1,456 cases at the Hospital of the Rockefeller Institute for Medical Research. Of 448 cases treated without digitalis 47, or 10.5 per cent, died, while among 1,008 cases receiving the drug 240, or 23.8 per cent, died. Cohn and Lewis subdivided these series into many groups which were carefully analyzed. Their findings were such that they stated:

> Whether digitalis was given or was not, whether the size of the dose was small or, in our judgment, adequate, whether it was given early or late—all of these considerations appear to be of no deciding consequence.

The important factors in influencing the outcome were the severity of the disease and the resistance of the host, rather than the administration of digitalis. To be sure, Cohn and Lewis reported a somewhat higher fatality rate for cases treated with digitalis. This appeared to be because cases of a more severe nature more often received the drug than did others which were less severe and less frequently had complicating factors present, such as advanced age with pre-existing cardiovascular disease. The observations support the view that there is no apparent value in the routine use of digitalis nor does its routine administration appear to influence the outcome in the general run of cases. The problem is complex, however, and much larger series of cases are needed to arrive at a final judgment.

There are certain cases in which the use of digitalis is indicated. It is of value for patients with congestive heart failure or with auricular fibrillation or flutter. With sudden decompensation, Locke (796) advises giving dram doses of a standard tincture of digitalis every four hours for three doses and then 15 minims three times daily as needed to maintain the digitalis effects. Under ordinary conditions when digitalis is indicated it is best to use one of the standardized preparations of the dried leaves in the form of 1½ grain (0.1 gram) pills. Depending upon the patient's weight, two or three pills are usually given three times daily for two days and then one pill a day as a maintenance dose. The use of the standard tincture in doses of one dram every six to eight hours for three doses and then 15 minims two or three times daily as needed is usually satisfactory, but the dosage cannot be so accurately controlled as when pills are used. With either preparation the individual doses can be further divided so that the drug can be stopped at once if toxic symptoms appear.

When the condition of the patient is critical and immediate digitalization advisable, one of the standard solutions of digitalis may be given intravenously in doses equivalent to 0.3 to 0.4 grams of the leaves and repeated if necessary in two or three hours. In such cases, if digitalis has not previously been given, strophanthin may be administered intramuscularly or intravenously in doses of 1/160 to 1/120 of a grain dissolved in two drams of normal saline solution. Ouabain (crystalline strophanthin) may be used in the same manner in doses of 1/160 of a grain. In taking over the care of any patient the physician must learn whether or not digitalis has been given and, if it has, how much. If strophanthin is given a patient who has had digitalis within three weeks, immediate death may result. The action of strophanthin is only a little more prompt than that of digitalis if the latter is given intravenously (796) or in divided large doses by mouth (297) and there seems little need to use this potentially dangerous drug.

Caffeine

The action of caffeine on the heart and circulation is complex and not well understood. It may, however, somewhat increase the per minute output of blood by the heart. Prompt improvement of some degree in the quality of the pulse with an accompanying rise in blood pressure may follow its use but these changes are of brief duration (796). According to Warfield (1384) caffeine is of no value in the treatment of circulatory difficulties due to a failure of the circulation at the periphery. The most important action of this drug is as a stimulant to the central nervous system, particularly the respiratory center, resulting in an increase of both the rate and the depth of respiration. Caffeine may be useful in combating collapse in severe cases but should not be given to delirious or excited patients. The drug may be administered in the form of coffee by mouth or by rectum but in patients in acute need is best administered in the form of caffeine sodio-benzoate given hypodermically in doses of 3 to 7½ grains, repeated within fifteen to thirty minutes as necessary.

Camphor

The literature concerning the action and uses of camphor has been somewhat extensively reviewed by Haman (590) and Marvin and Soifer (862). Locke (796) notes that camphor has long been considered to possess almost unique powers as a cardiac stimulant in cases of cardiac failure occurring in infectious diseases, but that the drug has been used but little in recent years in this country.

In attempting to ascertain the value of camphor in oil as a cardiac stimulant for patients with advanced congestive heart failure, Marvin and Soifer (862) administered doses varying from 9 to 45 grains to a number of patients. No evidence was obtained that camphor in these doses had any action whatever on the heart rate, respiration, blood pressure, vital capacity, electrocardiogram, or general condition of the patient. Although the drug may have some temporary stimulating effect on the central nervous system (297) and favorable clinical impressions may be formed as a result of its use (590), evidence is lacking that it occupies a definite place in the treatment of pneumonia (796, 862, 302). "Coramin" may prove of more use for stimulating the respiratory center. Alpha-lobeline hydrochlorate 1/6 grain is likewise effective, but because of its greater toxicity the dosage must be carefully watched. Both these drugs may be of aid in an emergency.

Strychnine

Almost without exception clinicians frown upon the use of strychnine in pneumonia (297, 796, 606). Locke (796) suggests that its usefulness, if any, is confined to its administration in conjunction with digitalis. Warfield (1384), as above mentioned, however, considers subcutaneous doses of 1/20 to 1/15 grain every two or three hours for several doses as needed are of considerable aid in combating circulatory failure due to peripheral vasomotor paralysis resulting from toxemia.

Alcohol

Evidence is lacking that alcohol is of value in the treatment of pneumonia (297, 606, 1441, 302, 190). It is seldom routinely used, although to patients who are chronic alcoholics alcohol in some form is frequently given and in generous amounts. Bullowa (190), however, does not use alcohol under such circumstances. Locke (796) considers that alcoholic beverages such as whiskey, brandy, or champagne are valuable adjuncts in the care of patients with considerable toxemia, in the aged, and in those who take little food.

Epinephrine and Ephedrine

The primary effect of epinephrine (adrenalin) is that of a powerful vasomotor and cardiac stimulant, but its action is transitory. As an emergency measure in doses of 3 or 4 minims of a 1:1,000 dilution administered intravenously and repeated once or twice at intervals of a few minutes it may be of value in cases of acute cardiac collapse developing during pneumonia (796). In repeated small subcutaneous doses it may also be of assistance in certain cases of serious circulatory insufficiency (1455) or for a progressively decreasing blood pressure (302). Ephedrine may likewise be of some aid in the latter instances.

Sedatives

Sedatives have long been used in the treatment of pneumonia. Generally speaking, morphine is probably more useful in this disease than any other drug, particularly early in the illness and in the presence of marked pleural pain (297, 606, 343, 119, 302). Morphine has a depressing effect upon the respiratory center and appears to retard intestinal peristalsis to some extent. The action of dilaudid is similar to that of morphine but produces a more marked depression of the respiratory center (386).

Davis (343) reviewed much of the literature on the use of morphine and its effect on the respiration in pneumonia. He likewise carried out considerable clinical experimental work on a number of patients with pneumonia and demonstrated that occasionally in patients having marked pleural pain its relief after the administration of morphine was followed by an increase of pulmonary ventilation, which resulted in a rise in the percentage of oxygen saturation of the arterial blood. He remarked that for other patients the benefits which may result, such as the relief of pain, a reduction of the metabolic rate, and ability to sleep, undoubtedly outweigh the possible ill effects of a slight reduction in pulmonary ventilation and increase in anoxemia. Davis' findings indicate that the effect of morphine on the respiratory movements and on the oxygen content of the blood is slight in the usual case and is ordinarily not sufficient to contraindicate its use. He further showed, however, that in cases having extensive pulmonary involvement accompanied by profuse moisture in the lungs or in cases where a severe oxygen deficiency already exists, the use of morphine may lead to acute anoxemia. Morphine should not be used in such patients unless oxygen therapy (see page 759) is also given.

Cole (297) has pointed out that when patients are restless, coughing, and tossing, better and more prompt results follow the administration of morphine than of any other drug. The most satisfactory means of giving the drug is in repeated small doses of 1/8 to 1/6 grain subcutaneously. With unusually troublesome cough, codeine may be preferable, as mentioned elsewhere (see page 749).

In patients without marked pain who are suffering from sleeplessness, which may be most distressing, or from nervous excitement, restlessness, or delirium, chloral hydrate, bromides, or paraldehyde may be used. Chloral hydrate should not be given patients taking alcohol. The use of barbital and its derivatives was reported by Blake (119) to cause excitement in patients with pneumonia. Locke (796) states that the best sedative in the presence of either delirium or insomnia is hydrotherapy (see page 758). In such instances Bullowa (190) finds a warm wet pack at 100° F. of aid, as well as oxygen therapy when an oxygen chamber is available. An icebag applied to the head may assist in quieting some patients.

The control of delirium or marked excitement by morphine should not be attempted without some consideration, for at times the use of enough of the drug to be effective may markedly depress the respirations and produce serious gastrointestinal symptoms. Anorexia, nausea, and vomiting may occur and, more seriously, intestinal peristalsis may be greatly diminished, with the almost unavoidable appearance of tympanites and obstinate constipation, the treatment of which is very exhausting to an extremely sick patient (796). In certain instances, however, 1/6 grain of morphine combined with 1/150 grain of scopolamine, given subcutaneously, may be effective. With marked delirium physical restraint of the patient may be required.

Treatment for Tympanites

As earlier mentioned, care of the bowels and maintenance of an adequate fluid intake with ample food and salt in the diet are of aid in the control and prevention of abdominal distention. The fats and sugars of the diet should be carefully supervised if tympanites develops (796) and it is probably advisable to omit milk temporarily from the diet under such circumstances (297). Tympanites is attributed to the paralyzing effects of toxemia on the musculature of the intestines. Bullowa (190) intimates that tympanites is commonly associated with the presence of bacteriemia and states that it usually persists as long as the latter is present. The limitation of diaphragmatic movement and aggravation of respiratory and cardiac distress may be considerable with marked distention. Beecher, Bradshaw, and Lindskog (89) showed in dogs that distention of the intestine causes an immediate decrease in lung volume.

Patients should be carefully watched for signs of beginning distention. If tympanites develops, prompt and, if necessary, drastic measures for relief must be adopted. Hot fomentations and turpentine stupes usually afford sufficient relief. The combination of a turpentine stupe with an enema of some kind is preferable. The rectal tube alone may help to bring away gas but without the aid of some form of enema, it is generally insufficient to relieve distention. Bullowa (190) finds that distention is less frequent in patients receiving oxygen therapy and that within eighteen to twenty-four hours following the institution of such treatment distention may be improved.

Enemas of several types are useful in the treatment of tympanites. Perhaps the simplest and best is a soapsuds enema. One consisting of two ounces each of magnesium sulphate, glycerine, and water often facilitates the release of gas. Locke (796) regards the injection of one pint of a mixture of equal parts of warm milk and molasses as most effective. Bullowa (190) mentions the use of enemas containing ox gall, magnesium sulphate, or castor oil and considers them safer than cathartics.

Satisfactory methods of applying stupes have been discussed by Cole (297) and Peterson (1017). When ordering turpentine stupes, explicit directions must be given and followed up later to see that they have been carried out correctly. A suitable stupe may be given by spreading evenly over the abdomen, without rubbing it in, a mixture of one part of turpentine to three or four parts of cottonseed or olive oil. This may be applied with a small absorbent applicator and over it is placed two layers of dry gauze. The stupe cloths are made out of old blankets cut about one yard square. One of these is wrung as dry as possible from boiling water and then so folded within another dry blanket that, when placed on the abdomen, a layer of dry blanket and the gauze are between the wet blanket and the skin. Care must be taken to avoid burning the patient. A fresh stupe should be applied about every five minutes for from fifteen minutes to an hour. The process is then discontinued for an hour and repeated if necessary. To diminish the absorption of the turpentine and the chance of blistering the skin, the turpentine mixture should not be applied to the abdomen oftener than once a day. When applying the stupes, a tube should be inserted in the rectum to facilitate the passage of gas. After the stupes it is usually best to give an irritant enema consisting of one dram of turpentine to a quart of soap suds.

In the event that stupes do not produce the desired result, pituitrin in 0.5 to 1.0 cc. doses given hypodermically sometimes meets with prompt response, although on the whole the results are much less striking than in cases of post-operative abdominal distention. In desperate cases physostigmine salicylate (eserine), 1/60 grain, may be given subcutaneously and repeated in a few hours if needed. Emulsion of asafetida, three to five ounces, given as an enema may produce relief when all other methods fail.

Hydrotherapy

There is considerable difference of opinion concerning hydrotherapy in pneumonia. Cole (297), Howard (661), and Langley (765) do not advocate it, while Cecil (224), Locke (796), and Bullowa (190) consider it helpful. Lord (807) states that it may occasionally be of use but points out that there is no convincing evidence that it modifies or shortens the course of the disease in any way. He and others, however, have found that it may prove quieting to nervous and excited patients.

Locke (796) is the most enthusiastic advocate of hydrotherapy and has stated that it is almost as beneficial in pneumonia as it is in typhoid fever. He believes the exact form in which the water is applied is of small importance so long as the technic of the particular type of bath used is accurately followed. He mentions the use of a cold chest compress, the sheet bath, and the cold sponge, as well as the alcohol rub. With high fever and the persistence of toxemia, the bath or rub may be given every three or four hours. Locke states:

> The objective signs of favorable reaction of the baths are almost always definite. The cyanosis disappears, dyspnoea is relieved, cardiovascular tone is improved, fever lowered, respiration stimulated, elimination increased, delirium lessened and the patient is relaxed, often dropping off into a sound sleep.

Treatment for Pulmonary Edema

Bullowa (190) has discussed the treatment of pulmonary edema at some length. The condition is less common in well-nourished patients and in those receiving oxygen therapy and specific antiserum treatment. When pulmonary edema develops he advocates restricting the fluid intake to twenty-eight ounces a day and the intravenous injection of 100 cc. of a 50 per cent sucrose solution. Glucose (dextrose) solutions given intravenously (181) may produce only a temporary beneficial effect which is often followed by an aggravation of the condition. Bullowa also mentions the use in some cases of oxygen under a positive pressure of 10 cm. of water given by means of a Haldane face mask.

Treatment for General Collapse

General collapse may occur, particularly at about the time of crisis, at which time the patient's strength may be spent and he may die of exhaustion or linger a while between life and death. Careful watch of patients should be kept during that period and if collapse occurs, supportive measures used. Hot drinks, warm blankets, the application of hot water bottles or radiant heat, intravenous injections of saline or glucose solution, and cardiac stimulation may be necessary. Absolute quiet and the application of dry heat to the body should be provided first of all. Aromatic spirits of ammonia one dram, or one half to one ounce of brandy or whiskey may be given in an effort to cause reflex stimulation of the heart and medullary centers. The inhalation of ammonia or smelling salts may have a similar effect. Epinephrine (adrenalin solution) may be injected intramuscularly in doses of 15 minims of a 1:1,000 dilution, or if the collapse is sudden and acute, intravenous doses of 4 or 5 minims may be used. Caffeine sodiobenzoate in 7½ grain doses subcutaneously may aid. If needed, strophanthin in a dose of 1/120 grain may be injected into a muscle or vein if the patient has not previously had digitalis (796). Oxygen may be administered as anoxemia is nearly always present.

SPECIAL TREATMENT

Oxygen and Carbon Dioxide Treatment

Deficient oxygen saturation of the blood is of frequent occurrence during pneumonia. The nature of the "respiratory battle" occurring in this disease was clearly described by Means and Barach (876, 875). Before considering the matter further a few points of general importance may be reviewed.

GENERAL CONSIDERATIONS. Normally human arterial blood is about 95 per cent saturated with oxygen and that present is in one of two forms. A small part, about one-fiftieth, in human arterial blood is available in *free solution* and the remainder is combined with hemoglobin as the easily dissociated compound oxyhemoglobin. The readiness with which the tissues are supplied with oxygen depends primarily upon the pressure of the oxygen in free solution and as Haldane (587) states, *"Thus, it is the oxygen in free solution and not the total available oxygen in the blood that is of immediate importance."*

Under normal conditions, as the oxygen in free solution is taken up by the body cells, its diffusion pressure tends to fall, which decrease is at once made up by additional oxygen flowing out from the oxyhemoglobin of the red blood cells. In pneumonia the oxygen saturation of the hemoglobin of arterial blood is often less than normal and in these cases there is less oxygen available in the red blood cells to go into solution in the blood. The oxygen pressure of the blood, and consequently of the tissues, falls, causing in the latter the abnormal condition of "oxygen want."

A sample of air obtained at the end of a rapid maximal expiration is regarded as "alveolar" air and, under standard sea level conditions, normally contains on the average about 14 per cent of oxygen, 5.6 per cent of carbon dioxide, and 80 per cent of nitrogen, along with water vapor at body temperature (1449). The carbon dioxide is under an average tension of 40 mm. Hg and the tension of the oxygen is 100–105 mm. Hg. As elsewhere mentioned, the oxygen saturation of the hemoglobin of arterial blood is normally 95 per cent and that of the venous blood about 70 per cent. The tension of the oxygen and carbon dioxide in arterial blood is largely dependent upon the concentration of these gases in the alveolar air and is normally about the same.

Anoxemia denotes a lowered oxygen content of the blood. Haldane (587) has pointed out that the body has no means of storing oxygen and that "anoxemia not only stops the machine but wrecks the machinery." Anoxemia is of several forms and that existing when the *pressure* of oxygen in the arterial blood is lower than normal, as in pneumonia, is termed the anoxic type. Other varieties, such as that due to a decrease in the total amount of circulating hemoglobin or the stagnant type occurring with a sluggish circulation, are far less often encountered in pneumonia. For the purposes of this discussion the term anoxemia will be used to indicate anoxemia of the anoxic type.

Deficient oxygen saturation of the arterial blood in pneumonia may be attributed to several factors. The causes listed by Potts (1045) are as follows: (a) a failure of adequate pulmonary ventilation due to rapid, shallow breathing; (b) some intrinsic alveolar disturbance due to factors such as (i) the mechanical interference of alveolar exudate preventing air from giving up its oxygen to the blood, (ii) dysfunction of the alveolar membranes due to edema and faulty nutrition, and (iii) interference with the circulation in the alveolar walls by the formation of fibrin plugs within the capillaries; (c) intrinsic changes in the circulating blood due to changes in the behavior of the hemoglobin with the formation, for example, of methemoglobin; and (d) an intrinsic tissue disturbance. Binger (106) has pointed out that anoxemia is likely to be worse when patients have very "wet" lungs, a condition which is likely to accompany extensive spreading lesions. He further notes that the amount and character of the exudate present are more important factors in the production of anoxemia than is rapid shallow breathing. Oxygen diffuses slowly through thick exudate and rapidly through thin exudate.

In pneumonia as a result of conditions such as those mentioned, the blood takes up an insufficient amount of oxygen during its passage through the lungs, thus giving rise to anoxemia. The symptoms caused by this type of anoxemia are similar to those which prove so distressing to persons with mountain sickness, that is, cyanosis, rapid pulse, disturbed breathing, nausea, vomiting, fatigue, and delirium, leading to collapse. It would seem unwise, of course, to add these difficulties to others already present in severely ill patients, and as Boothby (137) remarks, such patients have neither the time nor the ability to compensate for acute anoxemia, and oxygen should be of benefit to them. Binger (106) observes that if anoxemia is a contributory cause of death in pneumonia, it is so by its action on the vital tissues, particularly the heart muscle and the medulla. It may be mentioned, however, that there is little evidence to show that anoxemia increases the risk of death from pneumonia in the usual instance.

In 1918 Hoover (655) pointed out that part of the blood flowing through the partially consolidated area will not be relieved of its carbon dioxide and on its return to the heart will mix with aerated blood from other portions of the lungs in sufficient quantity to cause cyanosis in the peripheral vessels. Additional observations indicate that as the consolidation increases, more and more blood will be shunted to uninvolved parts of the lungs, where it may rid itself of its carbon dioxide, and in consequence at such times and in the absence of an extensive lesion, cyanosis may decrease.

Although the degree of cyanosis present often parallels the extent of the anoxemia, this relationship is not always exact (137, 178). For practical purposes, however, the extent of the cyanosis may be considered as revealing the approximate degree of anoxemia of the blood and oxygen want present in the tissues. Cyanosis is usually first demonstrable under the nails and later may be seen in the mucous membranes and skin. Stadie (1223) and others (137) have found that when cyanosis can just be detected under the nails and on the lips, the oxygen unsaturation of the arterial blood equals approximately 10 per cent, when cyanosis is definite the blood is about 15 per cent unsaturated, and when it is marked it will be 20 to 30 per cent unsaturated.

In any illness accompanied by fever, the oxygen requirements of the tissues mount rapidly. Added to this in pneumonia is a marked reduction of vital capacity. An increase of the heart rate will partially compensate for the reduction of oxygen in the blood by sending the red blood cells about the body more rapidly. In spite of this the oxygen unsaturation often increases, the amount of available oxygen in the inhaled air remaining constant, and the respiratory rate increases, producing more rapid and shallower respirations with added fatigue (1045). The vicious circle so established can often be broken by increasing the oxygen concentration of the inspired air. Apparently, however, anoxemia cannot always be overcome by this procedure (655, 877).

CLINICAL USE AND RESULTS. Though Wells (1404) mentions giving oxygen inhalations for the treatment of pneumonia in 1904, the therapeutic administration of oxygen was but little used prior to the War (1914–1918), during the latter part of which Haldane (587) advised its administration to gassed soldiers. Since then its use has been extensively investigated. Among the more recent reports dealing with the therapeutic use of oxygen in pneumonia, those of Barach (70), Binger (106), Bullowa (178), Boothby (137), and Potts (1045) may be particularly recommended, and Bullowa (190) has considered the matter in great detail.

The indications for oxygen therapy in pneumonia were reviewed by Bullowa (190), who advises instituting such treatment when the depth of the breathing is increased considerably and the rate is 36 per minute or over, when the accessory muscles of respiration are being used, when the pulse is increased to 120 or more, and when cyanosis or dyspnea is present. He would likewise administer oxygen to patients with distention. Such therapy should also be given when the level of the oxygen saturation of arterial blood indicates the presence of anoxemia of appreciable extent.

Many methods for the administration of oxygen to patients with pneumonia have been tried. In addition to giving it by inhalation it has been injected subcutaneously and intravenously. Neither of the latter procedures is of value, as they do not provide sufficient oxygen. Reviews of the advantages and disadvantages of the commonly used methods of oxygen administration are given by Barach (67), Bullowa (178, 190), and Palmer (977). The usual means employed for giving oxygen by inhalation are (a) the tube and funnel, (b) nasal catheter, (c) nasal inhaler, (d) face mask, (e) rebreathing apparatus, (f) portable oxygen tent, and (g) oxygen chamber.

As the body has no facilities for storing oxygen, if its administration is indicated, it should be given continuously and not at short intervals (137,

1045, 190). It is preferably used early in the disease and, when given at all, should be used in sufficient concentration to be of benefit. Ordinary room air contains 21 per cent oxygen and any effective means of giving oxygen by inhalation must raise the concentration in the inspired air to 30 per cent or more.

The tube and funnel and face mask methods are of little use, for with these methods it is extremely difficult to increase the percentage of oxygen in the inspired air and consequently in the alveolar air and blood (67) and both methods require constant supervision. Some physicians find the nasal catheter method gives satisfactory results in the milder cases. With an oxygen flow of 2 liters per minute Barach (67) found an oxygen concentration of 30 per cent in the inspired air. In such instances where the oxygen is run from the tank through a wash bottle before being delivered to the catheter, Palmer (977) demonstrated that if the flow was slow enough to count the bubbles the patient was receiving only about one-quarter of a liter of oxygen per minute. For the desired effect he should receive from 2 to 6 liters per minute (74, 190). Certain details of administering oxygen by this and the other most useful methods are given below.

A nasal inhaler may be used. This is a metal tube ending in a curved fork with rubber tips or extensions on the paired arms which may be inserted into the nostrils. The type described by Bullowa (190) has a flat band attached near the intake end of the tube which may be fastened to the forehead with adhesive tape, the oxygen supply being fed in through a rubber tube from over the head. With an apparatus of this type an oxygen flow of 4 liters per minute increases the concentration of oxygen in the alveolar air from around 14 or 15 to 29 per cent, an increase of more than 90 per cent. A greater increase occurs with a more rapid flow.

Barach (67) found that a rebreathing apparatus with a nosepiece or a mouthpiece and a soda lime container to absorb the excess carbon dioxide in the expired air gave good results. Such an apparatus is readily portable but must be bothersome to the patient. Oxygen concentrations in the inspired air of 40 per cent were easily maintained with this apparatus and its efficiency was confirmed by determinations of the oxygen saturation of arterial blood.

Oxygen tents of various kinds have been devised. The tent is a hood of some description which covers the head and shoulders or in some cases additional parts of the body as well. In the front and usually in the sides also there are fireproof, flexible, transparent, non-breakable windows through which the patient can see and be observed. The oxygen and other gases present are cooled by being run over cracked ice or by some other method. Excess moisture usually condenses on the cooling apparatus. By means of a blower, convection currents, or by the pressure of the oxygen as it comes from the tank (237), a constant circulation of cooled air containing from 40 to 60 per cent of oxygen circulates through the tent. In most tents the exhaust air is drawn off and run through a soda lime container to remove excess carbon dioxide, recharged with oxygen, and used again. At times provision is made to run the air over activated charcoal for the removal of odors (190). Such an apparatus, while very satisfactory for hospital use, is relatively expensive, cumbersome, and difficult to transport outside, so that tents have been used but little in the treatment of patients at home. Completely equipped oxygen tents can now be rented as desired, however, from a number of the medical supply stores and chemical companies in many cities in this country. If necessary, patients may be kept in oxygen tents continuously for days and months.

Probably the simplest apparatus of this nature is the oxygen box described by Burgess and Burgess (204, 203), which consists of a small tent large enough to cover the head. It has transparent sections in the front, an ice container for cooling, and an open top. The sides extend about eighteen inches or more above the head. The oxygen run in near the bottom fills the box and is allowed to spill out of the top continuously. This method is not unduly wasteful of oxygen as all tents leak considerably and with a flow of 4.5 liters per minute a 50 per cent concentration of oxygen may be maintained at the level of the patient's nose. The Burgess box is economical but appears more suitable for infants and children than for adults (190).

A few large hospitals have constructed permanent oxygen chambers or rooms large enough to accommodate one or two beds with their patients and attendants. The oxygen and carbon dioxide content of the air can be kept closely regulated in these rooms, as may the temperature and humidity. Such chambers are of course very satisfactory but are expensive to build and maintain.

For the treatment of pneumonia, ordinary commercial oxygen is used and large tanks containing 220 cubic feet under a pressure of about 2,000 pounds per square inch are the most economical. Every oxygen tank used should have suitable gauges attached for recording the pressure within the tank and the flow of oxygen in liters per minute. Float gauges are desirable for showing the rate of flow. The high pressure within the tank is stepped down with a reducing valve. All oxygen regulators and gauges should be tested every few weeks to ensure their accuracy (185, 190). Tents should be inspected and tested periodically for leaks and after use scrubbed with soap and water and washed with or dipped into a 1:1,000 solution of bichloride of mercury or some similar disinfectant.

In general, for the administration of oxygen in the hospital or home, the nasal inhaler and the oxygen tent are the most satisfactory. The nasal catheter in times past has also been extensively employed. When a single or double catheter or a nasal inhaler is used, the oxygen flow from the tank should be about 4 liters a minute, though a faster flow may be required. Barach (67) was previously enthusiastic about the use of the nasal catheter but subsequently he altered his views somewhat and reports (73) that after considerable experience he finds the catheter method frequently inadequate, necessitating the use of a tent. In consequence he advises using a tent or oxygen chamber from the start if this form of therapy is needed. Bullowa (190) likewise does not favor the use of nasal catheters.

If the catheter is used, however, three or four holes should be cut or punched in the sides of the tube near the end to distribute the discharge pressure of the oxygen against the mucous membranes. The catheter is lubricated, the tip inserted in the nostril, and pushed along the floor of the nose until it is visible through the mouth against the posterior wall of the pharynx, after which it is withdrawn about one-half inch. The outer end may be fastened over the forehead or ear with adhesive tape. When this method is used the tube or tubes should be cleaned every four hours, the nose sprayed with albolene, and the tube or tubes replaced, preferably by a physician. The oxygen from the gauge on the tank should be led through a suitable apparatus containing water to humidify it; otherwise the mucous membranes may become excessively dry and irritated.

The nasal inhaler is simpler to use, easier to keep clean, produces less irritation, and is just about as efficient as the catheter. Bullowa (190) states that an oxygen flow up to 15 liters per minute is tolerated with the forked inhaler.

When tents are employed care must be taken to maintain the movement of air within the tent and to keep it at an even temperature, free of odors, and at a satisfactory relative humidity. It is desirable that a thermometer and a hygrometer be placed inside the tent where they are out of the way, not unduly affected by the incoming air, and easily visible. The oxygen concentration should be tested at least three times daily and should be maintained at from 40 to 60 per cent. Unless a simple gas analysis apparatus is attached no tent can be considered properly equipped. The continued use of oxygen concentrations higher than 60 per cent may have detrimental effects on the patient, causing pulmonary edema and aggravating the pulmonary lesion present (106). The carbon dioxide content must likewise not be allowed to rise too high and concentrations of 4 or 5 per cent or more will accelerate the respirations and unduly fatigue the patient. Due to the almost inevitable occurrence of air leaks about the patient and his bed clothes, and at times in the tent as well, and the rapidity with which carbon dioxide is removed from the air by passing it across soda lime, the content of this gas in the tent seldom increases to the point where it causes trouble. Bullowa (190) states, relating to the ideal conditions for tent operation:

We usually specify odorless operation, an effective temperature of 66 to 68° F., humidity of 50 per cent, air movement of less than 50 linear feet per minute, oxygen concentration of 50 per cent, and carbon dioxide of less than 1 per cent.

Great danger from *fire* exists whenever oxygen tents or chambers are used. Open flames and sparks must be avoided. Suitable notices to this effect should be attached to all tents and chambers and it is advisable to have proper fire extinguishers at hand.

Some tents lacking motors to circulate the air and force it through the cooling apparatus may be unsuitable in hot, humid weather. All tents, however, give the patient a shut-in feeling, and excited or delirious patients frequently will not tolerate them. The cost of the oxygen administered by the nasal catheter or inhaler method is commonly in the vicinity of three or four dollars a day. The cost of tent operation is approximately double this amount, including the charge for ice as a refrigerant and the soda lime, but may be more if much oxygen is lost through leaks.

The symptomatic relief following the adequate exhibition of oxygen is frequently so marked that the temptation is to forget that the method has but restricted powers to alter the fatality rate of the cases treated. The beneficial effects are most obvious with patients treated in tents or chambers where the oxygen concentration can be maintained at from 40 to 60 per cent as long as required. Soon after placing patients in a suitable tent or chamber they appear more comfortable, cyanosis lessens or disappears, and at times dyspnea is relieved. In many, a drop of pulse or respiration may be noted and in a few, a drop in temperature may occur. The pulse rate is more often slowed than the respiration but in severe cases the latter effect may be the most prominent (67). Occasionally the temperature may decrease two or more degrees after instituting oxygen treatment (138, 137). When the oxygen saturation of arterial hemoglobin is only 70 or 80 per cent, as not infrequently occurs in pneumonia, oxygen treatment may be of considerable benefit because it increases the amount of the gas in the blood by as much as 20 to 30 per cent, thus increasing the oxygen pressure in the tissues.

In patients who have received oxygen treatment for some time, care must be taken not to remove them from the tent or chamber too abruptly. Boothby and Haines (138) observed that the sudden withdrawal of high concentrations of oxygen may lead to acute anoxemia with serious consequences. Bullowa (190) has made similar observations and states that a rise in temperature of 1° to 1.5° F. and an increase in the pulse of 10 to 16 beats per minute are usually observed when patients are removed from an oxygen chamber. To avoid abrupt changes the oxygen concentration within the tent or chamber may be gradually lowered over a period of several hours prior to removing the patient, or oxygen may be given with a nasal inhaler after his removal. Barach (73) further points out that patients who have recovered from their acute infection may be removed rather suddenly from a tent or chamber without difficulty.

Aside from instances of mechanical obstruction of the airways, the most marked beneficial effects of oxygen treatment are seen in cases of postoperative bronchopneumonia or pulmonary edema rather than in patients with severe lobar pneumonia. This might be expected considering the differences in the nature of the pulmonary lesion present in each instance.

Attempts to show a reduction in the fatality rates of cases treated with oxygen have been largely disappointing (876, 875, 138, 70, 299, 106, 796, 137, 703) and the method cannot be regarded as having any particular curative value. Its value as a supportive measure is generally agreed upon and it is probable that in some instances the use of oxygen may prolong the life of the patient until his immune mechanism can achieve recovery. The opinion of Palmer (977), Locke (796), Boothby (137), Bullowa (178), and Potts (1045) is similar to that of Boothby and Haines (138), who state that,

> Oxygen treatment is of value only in relieving the patient of the added load and danger of anoxemia, and it must be continued until the cause of the anoxemia is relieved. There is no evidence that oxygen increases the patient's resistance to infection, but it does prevent the lowering of his resistance which occurs when he becomes anoxemic and, therefore, its administration should be initiated at the very first sign of cyanosis.

In addition to the usual forms of oxygen therapy mentioned above, certain special forms may be considered. Joannides (684) has treated dogs with experimentally induced pneumonia by the administration of compressed air and feels the procedure worthy of trial in man. This would appear to be a hazardous undertaking.

The advisability of combining carbon dioxide, in concentrations up to 5 to 10 per cent, with the oxygen used in the treatment of pneumonia has been discussed by Henderson, Haggard, Coryllos, and Birnbaum (632, 630, 631) and the matter reviewed by Boothby (137), Saklad (1156), and Bullowa (190). This combined form of therapy would rarely if ever appear to be desirable, as Finland (447) and Bullowa (190) mention.

Other Forms of Special Treatment

ALKALI AND GLUCOSE THERAPY. There is but little acidosis present in pneumonia, as previously mentioned (see page 500). Although alkali in the form of sodium bicarbonate has long been used in treatment (1114) and Means and his associates (876, 877) early studied the rationale of such a procedure and believed the occurrence of a carbonic acid acidosis to be of some importance, no obvious beneficial effects have resulted from alkali therapy (796, 686). It may be remarked that in a subsequent discussion of Brooks' (153) paper on the cause of death in pneumonia, Means reported that he no longer considers carbonic acid acidosis of importance in this disease.

Glucose has been administered by mouth, subcutaneously, intravenously, and by rectum for the treatment of pneumonia. In solutions it provides a simple means of giving calories as well as fluids, and Locke (796) considers the intravenous injection of a few hundred cubic centimeters of a 10 per cent solution of value in the treatment of markedly toxic patients. The use of similar injections in the treatment of pulmonary edema was mentioned earlier (see page 758).

Maclachlan, Kastlin, and Lynch (846) have emphasized the virtues of glucose therapy and regard it as especially valuable in the treatment of toxemia, particularly in the presence of bacteriemia. These workers administered at least 400 grams of dextrose (glucose) a day in water by mouth, or 200 grams daily in divided doses if given intravenously. Twenty-five per cent solutions were administered four to six times a day. Treatment of this nature is still used to some extent but it must be regarded as a supportive measure and one that has little influence on the outcome of the disease in nearly all cases, as Maclachlan and his associates (847) subsequently pointed out.

VENESECTION. Venesection has been used in the treatment of pneumonia since the time of Hippocrates (644). Opinions as to the usefulness of the procedure vary. Cole (297) and Lord (807) consider it of little value, while Locke (796), Hess (637), and others (1016, 606) believe it is frequently helpful. Its proponents consider it of value in those cases where pulmonary congestion or marked dilatation of the right heart develops, and that under such circumstances the removal of several hundred cubic centimeters of blood may afford striking relief.

Petersen and Levinson (1016) reviewed a number of reasons for the liberal use of venesection in pneumonia. The removal of blood doubtless removes a certain amount of presumably toxic material, as these investigators note, but it also removes any immune substances present and, if persisted in, is likely to create a serious condition and the circulatory insufficiency due to peripheral vascular dilatation already present in the usual case may be aggravated. In the absence of the usual medical indications for it venesection cannot be recommended.

ARTIFICIAL PNEUMOTHORAX. In the course of making lung punctures to obtain material for bacteriologic study, Rood (1108) in 1919, inadvertently produced an artificial pneumothorax in a few patients and as clinical improvement resulted he treated three patients by this method. As a consequence of his observations Rood suggested that pneumothorax be tested as a therapeutic measure in selected cases. Friedemann's (498) observations on seven cases treated in 1921 aroused little interest, but Coghlan's (287) report of the treatment of six cases in 1932 appeared striking and was followed by other similar studies (1356, 780, 905, 782, 90, 920, 643, 128, 193). Summaries of the literature were made by Lieberman and Leopold (782) and Behrend and Cowper (90), and also by Blake, Howard, and Hull (128), who made an exhaustive study of artificial pneumothorax therapy. In addition, some experimental work was carried out by Lieberman and Leopold (782) in dogs with pneumococcus pneumonia. The animal work gave encouraging results, although the findings are open to several interpretations.

The method used by Coghlan (287) in the treatment of patients with pneumonia was to inject 400 to 600 cc. of air into the pleural cavity on the affected side. He reported that following this procedure collapse of the lung occurred, and that cyanosis began to clear within fifteen to thirty minutes, pain stopped, a feeling of well-being appeared, and the patients developed a profuse sweat. In one patient the urinary output of chlorides increased 400 to 600 milligrams per cent and the white count dropped. In six cases given two or three injections of air each, the temperature fell sharply two or three hours after each injection, but rose gradually, as the air was absorbed, within eighteen to twenty-four hours. Five of the six patients recovered. None of the patients developed pleural effusion or empyema. The relief of pain by separating inflamed pleural surfaces is easy to understand but the mechanism of the other responses obtained was unknown and still remains so.

As mentioned by Blake, Howard, and Hull (128), artificial pneumothorax has been used in the treatment of at least 124 patients. The clinical effects most commonly observed following such therapy are a prompt relief of pleural pain, a variable relief of dyspnea, and often a striking decrease in toxicity. These changes are nearly always temporary, however, the symptoms returning as the air is absorbed and the lung re-expands. In addition, a critical fall of temperature which also is usually temporary may or may not occur.

The technic of treatment has undergone numerous changes and at first two or three injections of 300 to 600 cc. of air were given at intervals of six hours or more. This proved inadequate and later three to five injections at about four-hour intervals were given in an effort to maintain a mean positive intrapleural pressure of about 1 or 2 cm. of water. Subsequently this technic was altered and Blake and his associates (128) found it most satisfactory to give larger doses of air but to give them more slowly. The speed of introducing the air averaged about 10 to 15 cc. per minute and the doses ranged from about 1,800 to 2,400 cc. At this rate it must have taken around two hours each to give many of the doses used. These workers state that not more than four to eight hours should elapse between the first and the second and the second and the third doses, although some variation occurs depending upon the pressure first obtained, the amount of air given, and the nature of the clinical response.

The customary procedure of Blake and his collaborators was to examine the patient and take a roentgenogram to confirm the diagnosis of pneumonia and to be sure the lesion was unilateral. Before beginning treatment, morphine was administered and the patient was placed in a lateral position with the involved side uppermost. With a technic similar to that used for the production of artificial pneumothorax in pulmonary tuberculosis, air was allowed to flow into the chest under the negative pressure developed in inspiration until the intrapleural pressure nearly reached atmospheric pressure. Roentgenograms of the chest were made, after one or another of the initial doses, to determine the extent of the pulmonary collapse and the presence or absence of adhesions.

The results of pneumothorax treatment have shown that prompt improvement with recovery can be obtained at times in very early cases (within twenty-four hours of onset usually) providing that the lesion is unilateral, that no adhesions are present, that the patient suffers no unfavorable reaction, that bacteriemia is not present or does not develop, and that a sufficient volume of air is kept in the chest to maintain compression of the lung. The results in cases treated after about forty-eight hours or more of illness are negligible in most instances. Blake and his co-workers (128) found no evidence that therapy of this nature induced an earlier antibody response to the infection. These investigators stated:

> Artificial pneumothorax, when administered so as to induce and maintain complete collapse of the lung on the involved side, would appear to be a useful therapeutic procedure in the treatment of lobar pneumonia but only when used early in the disease, preferably within twenty-four hours after onset.

They also mention that "There is no evidence to support the view that it is of curative value later than seventy-two hours after onset."

The treatment of patients by artificial pneumothorax is not a simple procedure and, as generally stated, it should be carried out only by physicians who are familiar with pneumothorax technic. In addition to the handicap imposed by the necessity of instituting treatment very early and in cases with unilateral lesions, there are numerous other factors that preclude the widespread use of this method. Adhesive pleuritis, which is commonly present in pneumonia and which Fabyan (399) found in 57 per cent of 195 cases of lobar pneumonia at necropsy, prevents the development of satisfactory collapse in many instances. If, when adhesions are present, the introduction of air into the pleural sac is persisted in, the lung may be torn and air embolism or pyopneumothorax may occur (643). Bacteriemic cases do not respond well to pneumothorax treatment and such treatment is no insurance against the late development of bacteriemia (Bullowa and Mayer, 193). Selective collapse of the involved lobe is impossible and collapse of the normal parts may aggravate dyspnea. The lesion may spread to another lobe of the same lung or to one on the opposite side, and the incidence of empyema may be increased, as in Bullowa and Mayer's (193) series, where it occurred in 18.7 per cent of 16 cases. Other investigators, however, have not reported any unusual increase in the occurrence of empyema (287, 90, 128). Further, patients may be unduly fatigued by the necessary frequency and prolonged duration of the treatments used. Extreme displacement of the mediastinum may cause death.

Considerable enthusiasm was aroused for pneumothorax treatment a few years ago, but it has subsequently largely subsided. The procedure may be of use in a few selected, very early cases and for the relief of intractable pleural pain, as previously mentioned (see page 749).

DIATHERMY. A careful review of the physical and biologic factors involved in the use of diathermy for the treatment of pneumonia was made by Binger and Christie (107, 108, 109, 268, 110) and Christie, Ehrich, and Binger (269) in 1927 and 1928. Experiments in dogs demonstrated that normally the lungs are cooled by the circulation of blood through them and that treatment with diathermy did not cause more than a fraction of a degree (0.3°–0.4° C.) rise in the temperature of the normal lung unless the pulmonary circulation was first stopped. Diathermic currents of the strength usual in treatment were also applied to the thorax of dogs with an experimentally induced pneumonia. Thermocouples were inserted directly into the consolidated areas and after treatment their position was confirmed at necropsy. In such instances in comparison with the temperature in the normal lobes the final increase in temperature in the involved lobes amounted to slightly more than 1° C. (269).

A similar type of experiment was carried out in three patients with lobar pneumonia in which thermocouples were introduced into the lung and varying doses of diathermy were given over periods of thirty to sixty minutes (110). The temperature of the human lung failed to rise as a result of the treatment. Diathermy was of some assistance in alleviating pleural pain, however, but did not lessen cyanosis.

Reports are available in the literature of the use of diathermy in the general treatment of pneumonia (1441, 1233, 1413). None of the evidence yet cited, however, concerning the alleged benefits of this procedure in man is convincing. Stewart (1233) makes the statement unsupported by other data that the fatality rate of his series of nearly 1,000 cases treated by diathermy is 11.9 per cent. Apparently some or perhaps many of his cases were in men in the navy. The usual low fatality rate of pneumonia in individuals of this nature was pointed out in the chapter on Prognosis (see pages 699–700).

ROENTGEN THERAPY. Powell (1046) has reported using roentgen-ray therapy in the treatment of pneumonia due to pneumococci or other organisms.

From 250 to 350 roentgens of 0.3 angstrom unit of effective radiation (135 kilovolts with 3 mm. aluminum filter) were given anteriorly or posteriorly over the involved area. Symptomatic relief was reported to result occasionally from this procedure. Defervescence was stated to occur within twelve to thirty-six hours, accompanied by a decrease in the leucocyte count. If the white blood count or the temperature remained elevated a second treatment was given. Powell was enthusiastic about the results obtained. Over a period of four and one-half years he states this form of therapy was used in 104 cases of lobar pneumonia with 5 or 4.8 per cent of deaths. Results with the roentgen-ray treatment of bronchopneumonia were regarded as less striking.

The findings of this study are difficult if not impossible to interpret, as no control series treated by other means over the same interval was reported and significant matters, such as the nature of the infecting organism responsible for the cases treated or the age of the patients, were omitted. It would also be of interest to know the day of illness on which roentgen therapy was begun.

HEMOTHERAPY. Hemotherapy has been used in some instances in pneumonia. The use of convalescent serum in treatment is considered elsewhere (see pages 812–814).

Gautier (510) reports finding that 238 cases of pneumonia were treated with repeated small transfusions (50 cc.) of convalescent blood in the Belgian Congo with indefinite results. He further states that in Guatemala patients were given autohemotherapy and blood was withdrawn from the patient and injected directly into the consolidated region of his lung. Such methods of treatment are of no avail and the latter in particular is dangerous.

DEUTEROPROTEOSE THERAPY. Deuteroproteose, prepared from the fibrin of ox blood by digestion with hydrochloric acid and pepsin and subsequent precipitation with ammonium sulphate, was used several years ago by Brooks (149) in the treatment of a number of diseases and infections including pneumonia. In small doses in animals no toxic effects appeared and it was stated that a leucocytosis rapidly developed which lasted several hours (150, 152). Parenteral doses in the neighborhood of 3 cc. or more of a 10 per cent solution produced severe reactions with convulsions in albino rats (152).

Subsequently Brooks (151) reported treating with unusual success a large series of cases of pneumonia of all forms with deuteroproteose. It was noted that the preparation used contained several different protein compounds of unknown characteristics. A sterile 10 per cent aqueous solution of the deuteroproteose was usually given intramuscularly or intravenously without dilution. In cases of moderate severity in adults intramuscular doses of 2 or 3 cc. were given twice daily, in severe cases 3 or 4 cc. were used twice daily, and in desperate cases 4 or 5 cc. were generally administered twice daily. Similar injections were used twice a day until clinical improvement was marked and the temperature normal, after which the same or a smaller dose was injected once a day.

For children with pneumonia of moderate severity, doses of 0.02 or 0.03 cc. of the 10 per cent solution per pound of body weight were generally given twice daily. With more severe cases the individual doses were increased to 0.04–0.06 cc. per pound of body weight. Doses of the same or of smaller size were given once a day in convalescence.

Brooks (151) states that such treatment reduces the case fatality rate and lessens the severity and duration of the disease. No untoward reactions occurred in the treated cases. Brooks' (151) series of treated and control cases embraced patients of all ages and with pneumonia of all forms. He reports a fatality rate of 8 per cent for 287 cases of lobar pneumonia (25 deaths) in patients treated with deuteroproteose and of 39 per cent for 300 cases (118 deaths) not given such treatment. With bronchopneumonia the fatality rate was 9 per cent for 598 treated cases (54 deaths) and 35 per cent for 602 untreated cases (212 deaths). In all four of these groups of cases approximately 80 per cent or more were in infants and children and in adults under the age of forty years.

The apparently favorable action of the deuteroproteose used by Brooks should be further investigated. In spite of the absence of untoward reactions in the treated cases there is the question of possible danger in the parenteral injection of an alien protein. As mentioned later (see page 796), there is no evidence from analogy in favor of the effectiveness of a specific antigen in combating an existing infection and its value in pneumonia is uncertain. A non-specific antigen would theoretically seem even less likely to be effective. In view of the apparently favorable results in Brooks' series, however, further treated and control cases should be studied. The inciting agent should be determined.

In addition to the comparison of case fatality rates, such other evidence as the speed of development and degree of specific immunity in both groups is desirable. Inasmuch as Brooks (150) states that his hemoproteose induced a marked leucocytosis, determination of the white count in the treated and control groups would also be desirable. As seen in Chapter IV, however (see pages 117–119 and 178–179), although a minimum number of leucocytes is necessary for the successful destruction of pneumococci, there is no evidence (at least in experimental animals) that increasing the number of leucocytes by various means has any favorable effect, in the absence of injected specific antibodies, upon the outcome of pneumococcus infections.

CHEMOTHERAPY

No wholly satisfactory chemotherapeutic agent has yet been discovered for the treatment of pneumonia. Some preparations are loosely considered of value in the treatment of pneumococcus cases but in the main sufficient evidence has not yet been obtained to confirm or refute this view. In several instances new compounds are being tried. Cole (297) considers that the ideal therapeutic agent for pneumonia would be one which without harm to the patient destroyed the infecting organisms or inhibited their growth and neutralized their toxins. Most chemical preparations thus far tried for pneumococcus cases seem either to be without value or to expose the patient to unusual and often unwarranted dangers.

As Locke (796) pointed out, probably the clearest evidence that no drug possesses specific therapeutic properties in pneumonia is the large number of such compounds for which these actions are claimed. Nevertheless, the fact that certain preparations of the quinine group and related groups, in addition to other substances as well, have been shown to exert a variable degree of bactericidal or bacteriostatic effect on the pneumococcus, either *in vitro* or *in vivo* or both, is a finding of considerable significance. The continued preparation and investigation of the properties of new substances may ultimately lead to the production of a chemotherapeutic agent of real value for the treatment of pneumococcus pneumonia. The direct action of a number of chemicals on the pneumococcus has been reviewed by White, with Robinson and Barnes (1417).

Quinine

During the past quarter of a century quinine in various forms has been somewhat widely used in the treatment of pneumonia, particularly in Germany. Marked pneumococcidal powers are claimed for the drug, though Morgenroth and Levy (910), who early investigated the properties of quinine, found it to be of no value in overcoming pneumococcus infections in mice. Cole (297) notes that while the drug has a slight bactericidal action in the test tube, this effect is small when compared to ethylhydrocupreine (see page 778) and that *in vivo* no effects on the pneumococcus from quinine have been demonstrated. By protection tests in animals Felton (414) found antipneumococcic serum to be a million times more active than quinine and a hundred thousand times more effective than ethylhydrocupreine. If quinine exerts a beneficial effect in pneumonia, the mechanism of its action is unknown.

In 1927 Cahn-Bronner (208) in Germany reviewed the results of ten years' experience with the quinine treatment of lobar pneumonia. A group of 252 treated pneumococcus cases was studied. This investigator reported that though such treatment may not markedly affect any single symptom of pneumonia, it tends to cause a rapid defervescence, relieve toxic symptoms, and hasten crisis. Empyema was not prevented in the treated cases. He regards quinine as better than optochin for the treatment of pneumococcus lobar pneumonia and notes that the most marked effects are obtained when treatment is instituted within the first three days of illness. He further mentions that the drug is ineffective in sepsis or meningitis due to the pneumococcus and is of uncertain value in bronchopneumonia due to this organism.

Cahn-Bronner (208) tried various quinine preparations but preferred the daily intramuscular injection of 0.5 gram of quinine hydrochloride in solution for three or four doses. Subcutaneous, intradermal, or repeated intramuscular injections in the same spot produced considerable pain. In his series of 252 cases of pneumococcus lobar pneumonia, quinine treatment of 175 patients was begun during the first three days of illness. The total 252 treated cases had a fatality rate of 7 per cent, as compared with a rate of 20.5 per cent for 341 control cases. He also collected several series of cases from the literature and added these to his own. The fatality rate for the 977 quinine treated cases in the combined group was 9.6 per cent, in contrast to a 20 per cent rate for 2,275 cases used as controls.

It is difficult to reconcile the enthusiasm of some German workers (84) for quinine treatment with the general pessimism in regard to it prevailing on this continent. Possibly the cases occurring here are of a more serious nature, as is suggested to some extent by the findings mentioned earlier (see pages 658–669). Even in Germany, however, opinions differ as to the value of such treatment, for Hess (637), in reviewing the literature in that country in 1931, concluded that better results have been obtained with ethylhydrocupreine than with quinine. In North America, Cole (297, 302), Lord (807), Howard (661), and others do not favor the use of quinine. Warr and Alperin (1385), however, gave quinine in association with other drugs to a series of 163 cases and considered that it might have been of some aid.

Locke (796) noted that several additional quinine preparations have replaced the use of quinine sulphate by mouth, and reports that quinine-urethane (quinine hydrochloride 0.5 gram, and urethane 0.5 gram in 5 cc. of water) given intramuscularly twice daily is the one in most frequent use. Cahn-Bronner (208) finds the inclusion of urethane to be unnecessary and of no value. Kolmer (735) has advocated the use of a similar quinine-urethane mixture or, instead, 0.5 gram of ordinary quinine with urea hydrochloride dissolved in 2 or 3 cc. of hot sterile water. He recommends that intramuscular injections of either of these mixtures be given at once and repeated in twenty-four hours if the temperature has not fallen. Subsequently, if crisis does not occur within forty-eight hours Kolmer advises that a third injection of the same size be given. In the same patients at the same time this worker would likewise use ethylhydrocupreine hydrochloride in 2½ grain capsules by mouth every three hours until a total of 20 grains has been administered. Subsequently, however, Kolmer with Rule (741) found administration of quinine and urea hydrochloride by stomach tube and intramuscularly to rabbits with intradermal pneumococcus Type I infections to be without value.

As a consequence of these varied observations the conclusion appears inescapable that evidence of the value of quinine in the usual form in pneumonia is conflicting, inconclusive, and inadequate.

In addition to the above studies, other investigations have been made using new quinine preparations not previously tried. Gundel and Seitz (583) tested the *in vitro* and *in vivo* pneumococcidal power of a number of these and mention specifically hydroquinine, *alpha* and *beta* isoquinine, and ethylapoquinine. The last preparation they considered the best, although its toxicity for mice was considerable. In 1934 Maclachlan, Permar, Johnston, and Kenney (848) investigated thirty-five compounds of the quinine group and reported that only three had any appreciable pneumococcidal power. These were ethylapoquinine, hydroxyethylapoquinine, and hydroxyethylhydrocupreine. The first-named preparation apparently was the least toxic and had greater protective and curative power in mice than optochin. Only a few patients have thus far been treated with this agent and no decision as to its value can be made, although it seems likely that none of these preparations will prove suitable. Johnston (686) has reviewed some of these studies.

Ethylhydrocupreine (Optochin)

Ethylhydrocupreine and its related compounds are derivatives of quinine and their effects *in vitro* and *in vivo* on the pneumococcus have been variously studied and discussed (910, 1445, 1446, 881, 903, 293, 904, 297, 324, 62, 1061, 735, 216, 1322, 414, 1283, 796, 637, 934, 741, 302, 845). Ethylhydrocupreine is marketed under the proprietary name of "Optochin."

In 1911 Morgenroth and Levy (910) discovered that ethylhydrocupreine had a specific bactericidal effect on pneumococci in test-tube preparations, and that when given to infected mice brought about recovery in a high proportion of instances. The bactericidal power of this drug was also studied by Wright, Morgan, Colebrook, and Dodgson (1445), Moore and Chesney (903, 904), and Baldwin and Rhoades (62) among others. Moore and Chesney (903) found the specific germicidal action of this preparation to be greater than that of any other compound in the following series examined by them, namely quinine, hydroquinine (methylhydrocupreine), isopropylhydrocupreine, isobutylhydrocupreine, and isoamylhydrocupreine.

Ethylhydrocupreine was used in the treatment of pneumococcus pneumonia with varying results by Wright and his associates (1446), Mendel (881), Moore and Chesney (903, 904), Baldwin and Rhoades (62), Cross (330), Szenti (1283), Hess (637), and others. The drug has also been given for meningitis (1061, 216) and empyema (1322) due to pneumococci and has been suggested (735), and tried without success, for the cure of a pneumococcus carrier state in both animals and man (934). Its administration to intradermally infected rabbits failed to overcome the infection (741).

The dose and preparation of ethylhydrocupreine used in pneumonia have varied somewhat in different studies. Mendel (881) gave optochin base by mouth in conjunction with a milk diet. Doses of 0.3 gram in capsules were administered every five hours day and night so long as the temperature remained elevated. With each dose, 200 cc. of milk were given in order to slow down absorption, to lessen the concentration of free acid in the stomach, and thus, by increasing the time of conversion of the base into the acid salt, to prevent the toxic symptoms caused by too rapid absorption into the blood stream of a too strong concentration of the drug. Moore and Chesney

(903) gave ethylhydrocupreine hydrochloride according to various dosage schedules and observed that a general relationship held between the patient's weight and the amount of the drug administered orally on the one hand and the degree of the bactericidal power developed in his serum on the other. They state (904) that when an amount of the drug represented by 0.024–0.026 gram per kilogram of body weight is given by mouth every twenty-four hours moderate bactericidal power of the serum develops, as shown by *in vitro* tests. Daily dosage of this size may be used for several days. The most suitable dosage scheme was to divide the total amount of the drug so that the initial dose was relatively large and to follow this at intervals of not more than three hours by smaller, equal-sized doses. When an average-sized patient was to receive 1.5 grams in twenty-four hours, a first dose of 0.45 gram was given, and this was followed by successive doses of 0.15 gram each at regular intervals. In this fashion a total of 1.5 grams may be given every twenty-four hours. Doses totaling 9.9 grams were used in the course of several days. Subcutaneous injection of the drug produced irritation, and intramuscular injection appeared to slow its absorption. The hydrochloride is soluble in distilled water but only partly so in saline solution.

Baldwin and Rhoades (62) gave optochin base in 4 grain capsules five times each twenty-four hours until fifteen doses had been given, which was considered the full dose. They remark that optochin base, also available as the proprietary compound "Numoquin-base," was used in preference to the hydrochloride as it less often gives rise to toxic symptoms. Milk was also given with each dose and no solid food was allowed during the period of treatment. It was demonstrated that frequently but not always the serum of patients who received from 20 to 40 grains or more of the base had bactericidal power, approximately 2 cc. of serum killing from 300 to 500 pneumococci over a period of many hours. In the investigation carried out by Cross (330), dosage similar to that of Baldwin and Rhoades was given along with milk.

When given by mouth the hydrochloride of ethylhydrocupreine is absorbed much more readily than is the base (904). With dosage as used by Moore and Chesney (903, 904), bactericidal effects became demonstrable in the serum in about twelve hours. Such action was also demonstrated in pericardial exudate.

Toxic symptoms not infrequently occur after the administration of optochin, such as ringing or roaring in the ears or partial deafness of a temporary nature, and various degrees of dimming of the vision, which may or may not result in permanent blindness, as was first noted by Wright and his associates (1446) and confirmed in a great many cases later (903, 904, 62, 330). Moore and Chesney (903) collected from the literature 787 cases treated with optochin and 36, or 4.5 per cent, had either amaurosis or amblyopia, and in one case at least permanent and almost total blindness resulted. Possibly toxic symptoms occur less frequently after the use of the base than after hydrochloride (62).

In 75 cases treated by Moore and Chesney (904) some degree of amblyopia occurred in 9, or 12 per cent. Mild ringing in the ears is usually the first toxic symptom and may appear after administering from 4 to 42 grains of the drug, as Baldwin and Rhoades (62) found. Administration should be stopped at the first appearance of any of the toxic symptoms, or if they do not occur, after the full dosage has been given.

In the series of 787 optochin treated cases collected by Moore and Chesney (903) the fatality rate was 12.96 per cent. Nearly all of the cases were from European sources, which may have been part of the reason for the low proportion of deaths (see pages 658–669). In their own detailed study (903, 904) of the treatment of 75 cases of pneumococcus lobar pneumonia of known type with ethylhydrocupreine at the Hospital of the Rockefeller Institute for Medical Research, no lowering of the fatality rate occurred when the drug was used in full doses. The fatality rate of the whole group was 37.3 per cent (28 died). Eliminating unsuitable cases due to late or unsatisfactory treatment, there remained 51 cases, of whom 16, or 31.3 per cent, died. The reasons for the failure of the treatment as suggested by these workers were that (a) the action of the drug is confined to the general circulation and apparently it does not penetrate the local lesion or inhibit a spread of the process, (b) its action is slow, requiring several hours to kill organisms in the blood stream, and (c) during the treatment pneumococci in some instances become "fast" or resistant to the drug. The course of the illness was not shortened in any instance and no effect was noted suggesting that ethylhydrocupreine was of value in the prevention or cure of bacteriemia. At times vomiting may occur after the drug is given, rendering uncertain the dosage available for absorption. The margin of safety between the therapeutic and the toxic dose is extremely narrow and precluded obtaining better results with ethylhydrocupreine.

Baldwin and Rhoades (62) treated 27 cases of pneumococcus lobar pneumonia with much the same findings and concluded that the most that could be said was that the results were suggestive that some benefit had accrued to the patients treated. More enthusiastic over the results of such treatment were workers such as Mendel (881), who treated more than 50 cases, Cross (330), with 126 cases, Hess (637), with 127 cases, and Szenti (1283), with 44 cases in children. Details were frequently lacking from their reports. All except Cross' series were of German origin and low fatality rates in the treated and untreated cases were not infrequent in these groups. In Cross' series from Brooklyn, New York, however, the fatality rate was 26.1 per cent for 126 treated cases (33 died), as compared with 31 per cent for 100 cases used as controls (31 died). The latter also reported an unpublished series of 3,008 cases treated in the United States and collected by Kraus. Cross states that this series probably contains cases of "respiratory influenza and acute pulmonary congestion" as well as of pneumonia. These cases were treated with optochin base, and death occurred in 153, or 5.08 per cent. Due to the varied nature of the cases in this large series, the reported findings cannot be considered of significance.

White, with Robinson and Barnes (1417), in reviewing certain aspects of the action of cinchona compounds on the pneumococcus, notes that in several instances the combined administration of ethylhydrocupreine and specific immune serum to animals with pneumococcus infections has produced a synergistic effect. The action of the two agents together was many times that of the simple total of the two individually. The combined use of these preparations in man has been occasionally employed in the treatment of meningitis, as was mentioned earlier (see page 595). No reports are available relating to the effects on patients with pneumonia of treatment of this nature.

While the action of ethylhydrocupreine on pneumococci in the body is perhaps more pronounced than that of any other related drug which can be similarly used, its absorption is uncertain, its action is especially feeble on cultures of young pneumococci of high virulence (903, 904), and its proclivity to produce dimness of the vision and possibly permanent blindness would militate against advocating the routine use of this drug in the treatment of pneumonia. It is to be hoped that subsequent studies may reveal compounds of greater usefulness, as the findings of Matsuda (873) for ethylapocupreine and of Maclachlan (845) for hydroxyethylapocupreine suggest. The latter reports that essentially no toxic symptoms and no evidence of blindness were seen in about 200 cases of pneumonia treated with his preparation. The daily dose for adults consisted of 120 grains given by mouth in capsules over a period of several days. Total doses up to 800 grains or more in the course of a week were used in some cases. Intramuscular injection produced necrosis.

Miscellaneous Chemicals

In addition to quinine and the related preparations mentioned above, a host of miscellaneous drugs and chemicals have been used in the treatment of pneumonia at one time or another and although the value of none has been demonstrated, many workers appear more or less enthusiastic about their use. None of these miscellaneous preparations mentioned, however, can be recommended.

Creosote in various forms has long been used in pulmonary diseases, including pneumonia, and has been given by inhalation, rectal injection (918), and by intravenous injection (984).

Mercurochrome has had little if any beneficial effect (491, 735, 1019, 1331, 1332, 1333). In infants and children Freeman and Hoppe (491) administered a one per cent solution intravenously, the average dose being 0.005 gram per kilogram of body weight. Occasionally two or three doses of this size were given. In adults Phelps (1019) generally used one intravenous dose of 20 cc. of a one per cent solution, but a few patients were given two doses. He reports treating 144 cases of lobar pneumonia in and around Central America with this drug, with 33 deaths, or 22.9 per cent.

Potassium permanganate, 2 grains to 1.5 pints of warm water, has been given slowly as an enema (1331, 1164). The amounts used varied from 3 ounces to the full pint and a half, depending upon the age of the patient. The doses were usually repeated at two to four-hour intervals for the first twenty-four to thirty-six hours. At times additional enemas were given after the temperature reached normal and in adults these were combined with the oral administration of one-half grain of thyroid twice daily for two weeks. Enemas, as above described, were given by Schottstaedt (1164) in California to 64 patients with lobar pneumonia with 5, or 7.8 per cent of deaths. In several other cases he also administered 4 ounces of the permanganate solution by mouth every three hours.

Sodium salicylate was used by Couvy and Poppoff (325) either intravenously or by mouth. They report treating 140 cases of lobar pneumonia in African Negroes with this drug mixed in glucose solution, with a fatality rate of 5 per cent. No data were given as to the fatality rate of untreated cases in the same locality. Symptomatic improvement with a lessening of toxemia, the development of a sense of well being, and a rapid temperature drop were reported to have occurred. The latter may probably be attributed to the antipyretic effect of the drug. The maximum dose used was 11 grams in six days. Generally 30 cc. doses containing approximately 2 grams of the drug were injected intravenously twice daily until the temperature fell.

Colloidal silver solutions have been used (918), as have colloidal gold, sodium nucleinate, and iodine (510), as well as bile salts given subcutaneously (510) or intravenously (1459). Lamb (759) in Great Britain reported treating 11 cases of lobar pneumonia with 2 deaths with 2 cc. subcutaneous doses of "Nuclein," a proprietary preparation containing about 5 per cent nucleinic acid, but was not particularly enthusiastic about the results obtained. Intravenous injections of collosol iodine (presumably a colloidal preparation) were used by Murphy (916) in 90 cases with 9 deaths. Doses of 10 cc. were generally given once or twice daily until six to twelve doses had been injected.

Rosenthal (1122, 1123) investigated the action of formaldehyde sulphoxylate. The drug was without pneumococcidal effect *in vitro,* but in tests of its curative power, when given subcutaneously, brought about recovery in a high proportion of mice infected with pneumococci of Type I. It was without effect, however, on infections due to pneumococci of strains or types other than the Type I strain (NIH strain) of the National Institute of Health, Washington, D.C. (1123). The chemotherapeutic effect was related to the sulphoxylate portion of the molecule and was not dependent upon the formaldehyde.

Rosenthal (1123) likewise reported that the following substances have been found devoid of chemotherapeutic activity against the pneumococcus: *ortho-, meta-,* and *para*-aminobenzene sulphonic acids; *meta*-aminobenzene sulphonamide, *meta*-nitrobenzene sulphonamide, *p*-aminobenzene sulphinic acid, *p*-acetyl aminobenzene sulphonamide, *p*-aminobenzene sulphonyl chloride, and benzoylsulphimide.

Sulfanilamide and Related Preparations

Essentially all the miscellaneous preparations mentioned above that have been used clinically have been administered on an empirical basis and without experimental evidence as to their possible value. The situation regarding the administration of sulfanilamide and some of its related preparations in recent years is better. It should be noted in passing that probably the most outstanding advance ever made in the chemotherapeutics of bacterial infections was made with the introduction of sulfanilamide for the treatment of infections due to *Beta*-hemolytic streptococci and some other organisms. Its action on the pneumococcus, however, is less marked and striking than that of one of its related preparations (M. & B. 693), as noted below.

The usefulness of sulfanilamide and related compounds in combating infections due to organisms such as hemolytic streptococci, as first described by Domagk (372), led to the investigation of their possible value in pneumococcus infections. These substances are azo dyes or closely related preparations. Rosenthal (1123) investigated the curative power of some of the sulphonamide and related compounds in mice with pneumococcus infections. Prontosil (4-sulphonamide-2-4 diaminobenzol) and Prontosil soluble (4-sulphonamide-phenyl-2-azo-7-acetylamino-1-hydroxy-naphthalene-3, 6-sodium desulphonate) gave negative or only slight effects. However, sulphonamide (*p*-aminobenzenesulphonamide), later termed sulfanilamide and bearing the trade name of "Prontylin," gave fairly consistent chemotherapeutic results on seven strains of pneumococci of Types I, II, and III, and the life of infected mice was frequently prolonged and in some instances saved by its administration.

The infecting dose usually varied from 10 to 100 lethal doses and was injected intraperitoneally. Treatment was begun within an hour and all doses were given subcutaneously. Two daily injections of about 0.5–0.7 gram of sulphonamide (sulfanilamide) per kilogram of body weight suspended in olive oil were needed for five to eight days to obtain the best results.

Rosenthal (1124) also demonstrated that sulphonamide had *in vitro* effects on pneumococci and that although it was not antiseptic in the ordinary sense of the term, it was bactericidal and bacteriostatic to pneumococci in high dilutions (1 : 10,000–1 : 100,000).

Sulfanilamide is readily absorbed from the gastrointestinal tract in animals and man and may be demonstrated in the blood, urine, and spinal fluid. With the usual dose, it is possible to reach and maintain concentrations in the blood as high as 1 : 5,000 or 1 : 10,000 as Marshall, Emerson, and Cutting (861) have demonstrated. The drug is rapidly excreted in the urine and may be entirely eliminated within forty-eight to seventy-two hours, providing the kidneys are normal.

The manner in which sulfanilamide acts has been variously studied. Its bactericidal and bacteriostatic action *in vitro* has already been mentioned. It appears to assist in localizing the infection and in reducing the intensity of the bacteriemia in mice (1123) and rabbits (745) infected with pneumococci. Studies of its effect on the streptococcus also suggest that its chief action is to inhibit the growth and multiplication of the organisms, thus permitting the body to mobilize its defensive forces (1397, 132, 105, 975). It may, however, cause a depression of the leucocyte count even to the point of leucopenia or agranulocytosis (105).

In addition to the studies of mice by Rosenthal, mentioned above, the following reports of favorable results from the sulfanilamide treatment of animals infected with pneumococci have been published: of rabbits (745); of mice (1161, 317); and of rats (572). Kreidler (745) observed sterilization of the blood, clinical improvement with recession of the lesion, and frequent recovery when rabbits with an intradermal pneumococcus Type I infection were treated with sulfanilamide. A dose of 100 cc. of a one per cent solution of the drug was given by stomach tube twice daily for several days, the daily dose being approximately 2 grams. Treatment begun about six hours after infection gave better results than that begun later.

Schmidt's (1161) findings in mice with pneumococcus Type XIV peritonitis were similar. He used 0.5 cc. of a one per cent aqueous solution of sulfanilamide every four hours intraperitoneally. Treatment begun later than four hours after infection was of little or no value. Cooper, Gross, and Mellon (317) found that daily doses of 12.5 milligrams given by mouth usually cured mice with peritonitis resulting from infection with pneumococci of Type III. Curative power was demonstrated for 10 fatal doses (0.5 cc. of a 1:1,000,000 dilution of a twenty-hour broth culture).

Extending their study Gross and Cooper (572) produced Type III pneumonia in twenty-seven albino rats infected intrabronchially with a dilute twenty-four-hour culture suspended in mucin. Thirteen of the animals were given 125 milligrams of sulfanilamide by mouth immediately after infection and daily thereafter for about fifteen days. The fatality rate of the thirteen treated rats was 23.1 per cent, as compared with 85.7 per cent for fourteen untreated rats with Type III pneumonia.

Subsequently the drug was used in the treatment of a number of cases of Type III pneumococcus pneumonia in man (627, 190) and in a case of Type III meningitis (896). In pneumonia due to Type III, Heintzelman, Hadley, and Mellon (627) gave oral doses of 5 to 10 grains of sulfanilamide every two to four hours daily for five to seven days, or in some cases 30 to 50 grains were given daily for four or five days. Several of the treated cases also received a few intramuscular injections of prontosil. They report treating 9 cases with 2 deaths, or 22 per cent, which they compare with the 80 per cent fatality rate of 10 control cases. The results were considered favorable but difficult to assess, for certain unfavorable factors were present in the untreated cases that were absent in those receiving the drug.

Bullowa (190) used sulfanilamide as well as prontosil in a few cases with Type III pneumococcus pneumonia, some of which had bacteriemia. In three cases with a light bacteriemia recovery occurred. When bacteriemia occurs in Type III cases it is generally slight (see pages 560–561) but of unusually serious significance, as elsewhere mentioned (see pages 685–686).

Millett (896) reported treating a patient with Type III meningitis and septicaemia with prontosil soluble.* After drainage of the spinal fluid, 20 cc. of a 2.5 per cent solution were introduced intrathecally and a similar dose was given intramuscularly. Both doses were repeated several hours later but the patient died. Necropsy showed that the dye had diffused generally throughout the subarachnoid space with a minimum of irritation.

Toxic effects may result from the administration of sulfanilamide (1123, 1124) and in patients nausea, vomiting, dizziness, hyperpyrexia, and cyanosis have been described (105, 190). Fatal agranulocytosis has been reported. The cyanosis is associated with methemoglobinemia or sulfhemoglobinemia, which may last several weeks (1397). Bullowa (190) advises the daily observation of smears of the blood while the drug is being used for the appearance of abnormal forms of red and white blood cells as evidence of toxicity. The administration of large amounts of fluid will speed elimination of the drug if toxic symptoms develop.

The use of certain other amino compounds related to sulfanilamide has been reviewed by Whitby (1414a, 1414b). In his second paper he pointed out that sulfanilamide consists of a benzenesulphonamide with an amino group in the para position. He noted that more than a thousand allied compounds have been studied in various laboratories. Whitby (1414b) stated that the more important of these compounds can be divided approximately into three groups. His classification, omitting his reference numbers, is as follows:†

(1) Those in which substitution has been made in the amino group: sulphamido-chrysoidin; prontosil soluble, benzyl-aminobenzenesulphonamide (Proseptasine), and Soluseptasine.

* See also the footnote on page 597.

† The designation M. & B. 693 which occurs in the quotation is the proprietary name given by May & Baker, Ltd., to the pyridine compound mentioned. The proprietary name used by Merck & Co., Inc., is Dagenan.

(2) Those in which one hydrogen atom of the sulphonamido group has been substituted: Uleron; 2-(*p*-aminobenzenesulphonamido) pyridine (M. & B. 693); 4-4′ diaminobenzenesulphonanilide; 4-amino 4′-dimethylaminobenzenesulphonanilide; and 4-3′ diaminobenzenesulphonanilide.

(3) Compounds of sulphone type which are chemically unrelated to the sulphonamides: 4-4′ acetamidodiphenylsulphone; 4-4′ diamino diphenylsulphone.

Whitby (1414b) mentioned that drugs in the first of these groups had but little action on the pneumococcus, while the action of those in the second and third groups (including effects on certain other organisms, particularly the streptococcus) had been increased to include some effects on this organism. However, as the toxicity of drugs in the third group rendered them unsuitable for clinical trial, those preparations included in the second group alone deserved special mention; and of these 2-(*p*-aminobenzenesulphonamido) pyridine* (M. & B. 693) was by far the most effective.

Whitby (1414a) described 2-(*p*-aminobenzenesulphonamido) pyridine (M. & B. 693) as a white, crystalline, almost tasteless solid, soluble in water at ordinary room temperatures to the extent of about one part in 1,000. The drug was shown by Whitby (1414a, 1414b), among others, to have considerable activity against the pneumococcus as demonstrated by *in vitro* and *in vivo* tests. The protective effect of the drug given by stomach tube was determined in mice infected intraperitoneally with pneumococci of one of several types. Six doses of 30–40 mgm. each, given over a period of three or four days, gave protection against 10,000 lethal doses of Type I pneumococci. With six individual doses of 20–40 mgm. each, protection was likewise obtained against pneumococci of Type VII or VIII. Where strains of Type II, III, or V were used, protection was not complete, though fairly good. Whitby (1414b) stated that in mice the curative blood level for massive pneumococcal blood stream infections was 15–25 mgm. per 100 cc.

In animals the toxicity of this preparation was low, the average lethal dose in mice being 16.6 mgm. per gram of body weight and in rats 15.8 mgm. per gram of body weight. Its daily administration in one-gram doses for several days to cats and dogs had no effect on the blood, urine, or general health of the animals. Although the drug is relatively insoluble in water, it is more rapidly absorbed from the gastrointestinal tract than sulfanilamide,

* Since the preparation of material for this section, the Council on Pharmacy and Chemistry of the American Medical Association has formally named this product "sulfapyridine." (See J.A.M.A., 112:49, Jan. 7, 1939.)

but it is excreted in the urine somewhat more slowly than the latter (1414b). During excretion, the urine contains about equal proportions of the free drug and the conjugated acetylated form.

Evans and Gaisford (395a) in Great Britain reported treating 100 cases of lobar pneumonia in adults and 40 cases of bronchopneumonia in infants and children with M. & B. 693 with good results. The drug was made up in 0.5 gram tablets and given by mouth. For adults the routine method of treatment was to give 2 grams at once and one gram every four hours for several days. The total dosage used averaged about 25 grams, a few patients receiving somewhat more than this. Cyanosis appeared in some of the cases and methemoglobin was found in six cases. Sulphemoglobinemia was not found. The fatality rate of the 100 treated cases in adults was 8 per cent, while that of 100 cases used as controls was 27 per cent. These results suggest that the drug may have some value. It is unfortunate, however, that the etiology of most of the cases (both treated and controls) was not determined and that not enough detail was given concerning both the treated cases and the controls to be convincing. Determinations of the concentration of the drug in the blood or urine during treatment were apparently not made. The most marked clinical effect seen in the treated cases was a more prompt temperature drop than in the controls. It was stated that nausea did not follow administration of the drug, which seems unusual judging by experience with this preparation in several clinics in this country. In three cases the leucocyte count fell below 5,000, though all recovered. Agranulocytosis did not occur in any of the treated cases. In general it seems likely that the toxic effects of the compound may be similar to the toxic effects of sulfanilamide.

The dosage given the forty infants and children with bronchopneumonia treated by Evans and Gaisford (395a) was about one-quarter to one-half that used in adults. Older children received more than infants. Death occurred in two patients in this series and both had complicating factors.

Whitby's (1414b) comments on dosage of M. & B. 693 are of interest. He recommends a relatively high initial dose followed by a sufficient regular four-hourly dose to maintain the blood level at an adequate concentration. In pneumococcus pneumonia he uses 5 grams in the first twenty-four hours in lots of 2 grams, 2 grams, and one gram, four-hourly, followed by one gram at four-hour intervals, until a total of about 23 grams is given. With this dosage the concentration of the drug in the blood frequently reaches about 8 mgm. per 100 cc. in the first twelve hours and is maintained at that level during the course of treatment. Whitby states that the drug disappears from the blood within twenty-four hours of stopping treatment but that traces of it remain in the urine for about forty-eight hours.

The drug appears to exert a bacteriostatic action on the pneumococcus, retarding or inhibiting its multiplication and possibly affecting its capsule, and does not seem either to stimulate or to depress the immune mechanism of the host. Whitby (1414b) mentions that the immunity produced in animals cured of an infection by M. & B. 693 appears to be fundamentally the same "in *quantity, quality,* and *speed of production* as the immunity created by orthodox active immunization." Whether any direct bactericidal effect may be caused by the drug seems uncertain.

The findings in both *in vivo* and *in vitro* tests indicate that in the presence of an adequate concentration of M. & B. 693 about six or seven hours are required before the effects of the drug begin to be demonstrable as measured either by a slowing down of the multiplication rate of the organisms or by a decrease in the incidence or intensity of blood stream infection (1414a, 1414b). The possibility that some strains of pneumococci become "fast" or resistant to the drug is suggested by Whitby (1414b).

In conclusion it may be stated that there is but little reported evidence that sulfanilamide is of value in pneumococcus infections, and its effects on this organism appear slight; the evidence relating to the use of M. & B. 693, however, although still limited, seems more promising. Although the clinical use of these chemical compounds in pneumococcus infections must still be regarded as experimental, continued study of the mode of action of such preparations is desirable and may subsequently permit the manufacture of a more suitable chemotherapeutic agent. The available data suggest that possibly the use of some of these compounds in conjunction with specific antiserum would, in suitable cases of pneumococcus pneumonia, give a better therapeutic response than the use of either preparation alone. While this is by no means certain at this time, the matter may be settled in the not too distant future, for therapeutic tests of this nature are in progress in a number of places. Whitby's (1414b) comments on the matter are timely:

> A survey of our unpublished experiments confirms the now generally accepted hypothesis that these drugs are not specifically concerned with the immunity mechanism. Hence it would be most unwise to jettison all those devices for producing specific immunity which have been a stand-by for so many years.

In addition, it is desirable that study be made of the value of preparations such as sulfanilamide and M. & B. 693 for the treatment of pneumonia due to certain organisms other than pneumococci, particularly pneumonia caused by hemolytic streptococci.

Vitamins and Enzymes

VITAMINS. The complexity of the relationship of vitamins to resistance to bacterial diseases is generally recognized and the problem little understood. Greene (564) considers deficiency of vitamin A or D may be a factor in reducing the resistance of rabbits to pneumococcus infections. Clausen (274) has reviewed considerable of the literature and states that some evidence is available suggesting that a deficiency of vitamins A and C appears to lower resistance to infection. Possibly a lack of vitamin B complex may do the same but no such effect has been shown with certainty to result from a lack of vitamin D. Most of the observations made, however, were on animals which were frequently maintained on unusual and often grossly abnormal diets and in consequence the results secured appear practically impossible to interpret in so far as they might relate to the use of vitamins in the treatment of pneumonia in man.

Orenstein (974) states that in 1929 he treated 299 cases of lobar pneumonia and bronchopneumonia in African natives with a diet high in vitamin A with apparently favorable results. The patients were fed either beef liver or a concentrated vitamin A preparation. Subsequently this investigator studied a series of 764 cases of lobar pneumonia in African males. Vitamin A was used in the treatment of 375 of these, of which 38, or 10.1 per cent, died, while in 389 control cases 40, or 10.2 per cent, essentially the same proportion, died. The treated cases received from six to twelve capsules daily, each containing 2 minims of a vitamin A preparation said to contain one hundred and fifty times as much vitamin A as the same volume of good cod liver oil. The period of hospitalization, proportion of cases with complications, and related matters, were the same in both groups and it was concluded that large doses of vitamin A do not exert a favorable influence on the outcome of lobar pneumonia.

Fox (475) studied the vitamin A content of the livers of 70 African natives dying from either accidents or pneumonia and found an ample supply of the vitamin in individuals of both groups. He concluded that pneumonia is usually of such short duration that changes in the amount of available vitamin A within the body are of little if any importance.

As a general dietetic measure in pneumonia if the patient is emaciated

Bullowa (190) advises feeding vitamin B_2 in the form of autolyzed yeast or dried sprouting barley. He considers that the vitamin supply may become depleted during the course of a long-continued fever and states that the reserve of cevitamic acid is lowered in some cases and notes that fruit juices or green vegetables may be included in the diet as a precautionary measure.

ENZYMES. Of theoretical interest at the moment is the possibility that at some time in the future solutions of enzymes may become available for the treatment of pneumonia. This hope has arisen from the extraordinary findings of Avery and his associates (38, 380, 39, 539, 538, 484, 301, 379, 381).

Following the discovery of the specific capsular polysaccharides of pneumococci and the recognition that they are vital factors in the defensive mechanism of the organism, efforts were made to find some agent which would decompose these substances. Initial success along these lines was gained by Avery and Dubos (38) at the Hospital of the Rockefeller Institute for Medical Research in 1930, who state:

A systematic search for enzymes capable of hydrolyzing the polysaccharides found in the capsular material of pneumococci of the various types has been carried on in this laboratory for several years. A number of enzymes from animal and plant sources, known to be active in the hydrolysis of simpler carbohydrates, were tested, but none of them were found capable of attacking the polysaccharides of pneumococcus origin. In addition, cultures of various moulds, yeasts, soil actinomycetes and bacteria, many of which were known to decompose cellulose, were tested without success. Recently, however, a bacillus has been isolated from the organic matter of soil taken from the cranberry bogs of New Jersey, which is able to split the specific capsular polysaccharide of pneumococci of Type III. The micro-organism is a pleomorphic, Gram negative bacillus, motile and spore-bearing.

They also added:

From cultures of this bacillus it has been possible to extract a soluble principle which, in the absence of the living cell, decomposes this specific carbohydrate. The decomposition of the specific polysaccharide is indicated by the appearance of reducing sugars in the hydrolyzed mixtures and by the simultaneous disappearance of serological specificity. The rate of reaction and the total amount of specific substance decomposed appear to bear a quantitative relationship to the concentration of the active principle.

The active substance present in the sterile bacterial extracts is heat labile, being destroyed by exposure to a temperature of 60° to 65° C. It is extraordinarily specific in its action against the polysaccharide of pneumococci of Type III, since the capsular carbohydrates of the specific types of Friedländer's bacillus, and even those of pneumococci of Types I and II, are unaffected. The fact that the reacting substance is a product of living cells, that it is specific and heat labile and that its action seems to conform to the laws of enzymatic reactions strongly supports the view that the active principle is of the nature of a specific enzyme.

The specific enzyme was not bacteriolytic or bacteriostatic nor did it kill the pneumococci in contact with it, but it did denude them of their capsules. The organisms then lost their specific agglutinability. Their power of elaborating the capsular carbohydrate was not destroyed, however, as shown by the reappearance of this substance when the organisms were transferred to a medium devoid of the active hydrolyzing agent. In such instances specific agglutinability likewise reappeared. The enzyme, then, acts directly on the carbohydrate of the capsule without significantly affecting the organism.

The function of the enzyme in specifically decomposing the capsular polysaccharide of the Type III pneumococcus was shown not to be impaired or retarded by the presence of fresh animal serum (38, 380). The injection of this agent into the abdominal cavity of mice was demonstrated to have protective and curative effects against infections due to the intraperitoneal injection of pneumococci of Type III (38, 39). Its action *in vivo* was similar to that *in vitro* and the organisms were denuded of their capsules. Removal of the capsules permitted the prompt phagocytosis and subsequent destruction of the naked cells.

Encouraged by these observations, investigators have pursued this line of research further, and the specific enzyme in solution was shown by Goodner, Dubos, and Avery (539) and Goodner and Dubos (538) to have a marked curative action when given intravenously twenty-four hours after infection to rabbits with intradermal pneumococcus Type III infections. In the absence of such treatment the fatality rate was 95 per cent, whereas in animals treated with the enzyme only 5 per cent died. Where large doses of enzyme were used at the outset recovery occurred and subsequent tests of the animals showed that no immunity to the Type III pneumococcus had developed. When smaller therapeutic doses were used and recovery occurred, subsequent studies revealed that some immunity to this organism had developed. The minimal amounts of enzyme required to bring about survival bore a definite relationship to the severity of the infection as gauged by the number of pneumococci present in the circulating blood, and larger doses had to be used in those animals which showed the heaviest bacteriemia.

These studies were pushed further and in 1934 Francis, Terrell, Dubos, and Avery (484) tested the therapeutic action of the enzyme in monkeys (the Java species, *Macacus cynomolgos*) which developed pneumonia following their infection by the intratracheal or intrabronchial route with pneumococci of Type III. Preliminary studies by Francis and Terrell (483; see also pages 210 and 231) showed that these monkeys develop a lesion closely resembling lobar pneumonia in man, though in monkeys bacteriemia is

TABLE 157. PNEUMOCOCCUS TYPE III PNEUMONIA IN JAVA MONKEYS. NUMBER OF ANIMALS AND NUMBER AND PERCENTAGE OF DEATHS IN ANIMALS TREATED WITHOUT OR WITH ENZYME THERAPY, BY KIND OF LESION*

KIND OF LESION	TREATED WITHOUT ENZYME			TREATED WITH ENZYME		
	NUMBER OF ANIMALS	DEATHS *Number*	DEATHS *Per cent*	NUMBER OF ANIMALS	DEATHS *Number*	DEATHS *Per cent*
Pneumonia without septicaemia	20	–	–	8	–	–
Pneumonia with septicaemia (1–250)†	20	9	45.0	15	–	–
Pneumonia with septicaemia (250–2,000)†	12	9	75.0	9	1	11.1
Pneumonia with septicaemia (2,000 or more)†	16	16	100.0	8	7	87.5
Total	68	34	50.0	40	8	20.0

From Francis and Terrell (483)

* Classification made on the basis of the height of the septicaemia present during the first three days of illness.

† Numbers in parentheses refer to the number of organisms present per cubic centimeter of blood.

more frequent and intensive. Seventy per cent of the animals had bacteriemia and more than a third showed 250 or more organisms per cubic centimeter of blood. A comparison of the outcome in monkeys treated without or with the specific enzyme solution is shown in Table 157. Recovery occurred in all instances in the absence of septicaemia regardless of whether or not enzyme treatment was given. The best results obtained were in animals having a light to a fairly heavy septicaemia. When enzyme was not given, death occurred in 45 per cent, or 9, of 20 monkeys having from one to 250 organisms per cubic centimeter in their blood, and in 75 per cent, or 9, of 12 monkeys having from 250 to 2,000 organisms per unit of blood. Together these two groups total 32 animals with 18 deaths, or 56.2 per cent, which may be contrasted with a 4 per cent fatality rate (one death) for a total of 24 monkeys in the groups treated with enzyme. In the total group of 68 untreated animals in Table 157, 34 or 50 per cent died, and in the total group of 40 animals that received treatment, 8 or 20 per cent died. The fatality rate of the 48 untreated monkeys with septicaemia was 70.8 per cent (34 died), in contrast to 25 per cent for the 32 treated animals with septicaemia (8 died).

In all the treated animals intravenous injections of the enzyme solution were given within the first three days of illness. The enzyme administered appeared to stop the spread of the lesion and either to accelerate or to make possible the initiation of resolution. Sterilization of the blood was promoted, the temperature dropped, and the occurrence of complications was prevented or lessened.

Dubos (379) and Dubos and Bauer (381) have described methods of producing the enzyme in considerable amount and of concentrating it so as to yield a forty-two-fold concentration in volume by means of dialysis with collodion membranes of controlled pore size. These matters have been discussed in considerable detail by White, with Robinson and Barnes (1417).

Difficulties exist, however, in the use of this specific enzyme. Goodner, Dubos, and Avery (539), in their experiments on the treatment of infected rabbits with this agent, noted that intravenous injections often produced a reaction, the temperature rising two or three degrees for three or four hours, and the leucocyte count first falling and then rising again as the temperature dropped. Disturbances of a similar nature occurred in the monkeys with pneumonia treated with enzyme (484). It appeared impossible with existing information to produce enzyme of uniform activity and purity. Occasional lots produced febrile reactions and leucopenia. During treatment leucopenia seemed especially likely to occur in those animals already having a depressed white count.

The continuation of studies such as these is desirable in the hope that this preparation of specific enzyme or one of a similar nature may later prove applicable to the treatment of suitable infections in man.

Sickles and Shaw (1198) in 1933 announced that they had isolated three organisms somewhat different from the one studied by Avery and Dubos (38, 380) and had obtained from these organisms an enzyme which in sterile solutions was also capable of specifically decomposing the capsular polysaccharide of pneumococci of Type III. It likewise had a protective and therapeutic action in mice infected with pneumococci of this type. Sickles and Shaw (1198) also isolated an organism which specifically utilized the capsular substance of Type II pneumococci in its growth. They were unable, however, to separate the enzyme from the living organism in this instance. Their further studies (1199) on an organism capable of decomposing the specific capsular carbohydrate of Type I were similar and they were unable to separate the enzyme from the organism. In discussing the observations of Avery and his collaborators relative to the isolation of the enzyme specific for Type III pneumococcus capsular polysaccharide, Cole (301) in 1934 stated that these investigators had also separated from a newly isolated organism an enzyme which destroyed Type II capsular substance but which was less active than their original enzyme for Type III.

VACCINE TREATMENT

Theoretical Considerations

From time to time vaccines of various kinds have been used in the treatment of pneumonia in many places throughout the world. Beginning with Rosenow (1118) in the United States, studies of this nature were carried out in this country (1251, 760, 1278, 1279, 989, 761, 1164), in Africa (785, 1008, 507), in India (858), and in Great Britain (1453, 759). Considered chronologically according to the date of reporting the observations made, the first study at hand was that of Lister (785) in 1916, who was followed by Rosenow (1118) and numerous others (1251, 1008, 858, 760, 1453, 1278, 759, 1279, 989, 507, 761, 1164).

Numerous aspects of the use of vaccine and allied preparations in the production of active immunity to infection or demonstrable humoral antibody or both were considered in Chapter VII (pages 408–440). It may be seen there that the character of the antigen used, the size and spacing of the doses, and the route by which they are given have an important bearing on the immunity engendered. Many of the factors discussed in that chapter are applicable to the use of vaccines and other agents in the treatment of patients with pneumonia.

Practically all the reports relating to the treatment of pneumonia with vaccine are of a clinical nature, and detailed information so essential to establishing the value, if any, of this procedure is conspicuously lacking. The vaccine used generally contained a mixture of organisms or was of unknown composition. The antigenicity of the preparations was almost wholly unknown in every instance. Bacteriologic diagnosis was seldom carried out in the treated cases, so there was no means of knowing, even if the composition of the vaccine were known, whether the preparation used contained organisms similar to those infecting the patient. Whereas the immune response is nearly always better when vaccine is given intravenously, this route was used in only a few instances in the treatment of pneumonia, and antibody studies were seldom made.

It is perhaps well that smaller doses of vaccine are almost invariably used for therapeutic than for prophylactic purposes. For treatment individual doses of a few million to a billion or more killed organisms have ordinarily been used subcutaneously, intradermally, or intramuscularly at intervals of about six to eight hours.

Although it seems certain that the suitable immunization of animals, and perhaps even of man in some instances, will prevent the occurrence or abort the course of pneumonia under special circumstances, as elsewhere described (see pages 440–482), incontestable evidence that the use of vaccine will alter the course of a pneumococcus infection when administered *after the illness has begun* has never been produced. The so-called rationale of vaccine therapy is based on the assumption that the parenteral injection of devitalized organisms will accelerate the immune response. There is no reason to believe, however, that the administration of vaccine in pneumonia will elicit a more prompt or significant stimulation of the immune mechanism than the disease itself. Live organisms are a far better antigen than those killed and otherwise mutilated by various means, and in pneumonia large numbers of live organisms are in the lung and many gain access to the blood stream as well. Under such circumstances the body is flooded with antigenic substances. In fact, for immunizing purposes it would seem impossible to improve on an attack of pneumonia as a means of stimulating the development of immunity.

During pneumonia the pneumococcus is continually being split up into its component fractions, the specific capsular polysaccharide and the nonspecific cellular carbohydrate (C substance) and protein. Zinsser's (1462) view, outlined in 1929, that in order to obtain suitable active immunity in pneumonia, intact organisms must be used as neither the specific capsular substance nor the protein fraction of the organisms will produce the kind of antibodies needed, may now be modified to some extent, for it has been subsequently shown that the capsular carbohydrate is antigenic and gives rise to a type-specific immune response. Furthermore, some alteration of this view is necessary under any circumstances, for the implication is that antibodies are only uncommonly produced in pneumonia, while the reverse is the case, as mentioned in the chapter on Recovery Factors and Duration of Immunity (page 728).

As already indicated, evidence is lacking that vaccine treatment stimulates a more prompt immune response than would otherwise occur. In the usual instance in pneumonia, spontaneously produced humoral antibody rarely becomes demonstrable before the third or fourth day of the illness. There is no evidence that the injection of immunizing agents into normal man results in a still earlier appearance of the immune response, as seen in Chapter VII (pages 434–437). Nor is there any evidence, judging from Barach's (71) and Lambert's (761) findings in a number of cases of pneumonia receiving vaccine injections that immune substances of this nature appear earlier in cases given vaccine, for these investigators found that antibody was generally not demonstrable until the fourth or fifth day under such circumstances. In the section of Chapter VII referred to above, it may be seen that acquired resistance may begin to appear in animals as early as five hours after immunizing procedures are instituted. Possibly this may also be the case for man after suitable vaccination and, if so, acquired resistance probably also begins to appear as promptly after the onset of pneumonia. The early appearance of resistance in animals after immunization was discovered when tests were made of the ability of the blood-clearing mechanism to remove from the circulation live virulent pneumococci injected intravenously, tests that cannot be applied to man.

Barach (71), after injecting into patients with pneumonia a suitable vaccine containing pneumococci different from the type causing the disease, found that the antibody response yielded protective substance for from 10,000 to 100,000 minimum lethal doses of pneumococci of the same type as that contained in the vaccine (see pages 427–428). This titer is about the same as that of the protective substance usually appearing in patients not treated with vaccine who have recovered from the disease (see pages 729–731). Lambert (761), however, contends that following vaccine therapy possibly more antibody may be produced than occurs in cases not treated with vaccine. His findings suggest that protective substance of the order of more than one million minimum lethal doses may frequently be found at some period after vaccine therapy. The significance of this observation is unknown. He notes, however, as others earlier found, that in some patients no antibody ever becomes demonstrable and that at times death may occur even if antibody is present.

Clinical Use and Results

Pneumococcus vaccine was apparently first used as a therapeutic agent in pneumonia by Rosenow (1118) in Chicago, who states that in 1913 with Hektoen he treated 146 cases of lobar pneumonia with a partially autolyzed pneumococcus vaccine. Pneumococci, presumably of several types, were grown for twenty-four hours, suspended in saline solution, ether added, and the mixture shaken and incubated three to five days to facilitate autolysis. When approximately 95 per cent of the organisms had become Gram-negative the ether was vaporized off, a preservative added, and sterility tests made. These investigators considered that certain toxic substances were the cause of the primary negative phase following the injection of vaccine and that these could be eliminated by autolysis. Of the 146 cases treated with this agent 23 per cent died, as contrasted with 38 per cent of the alternate control cases.

At a later period Rosenow (1118) extended this work and treated many additional cases with a similar autolyzed vaccine. The etiologic diagnosis of nearly all these cases was apparently unknown. One cubic centimeter of this preparation containing the residue of approximately 20 billion pneumococci was given to adult patients each day so long as the temperature was elevated. In all, 200 patients were treated, with 14 deaths, or 7 per cent. Among these cases were 95 in which treatment was begun within the first two days of illness with 3 per cent of deaths, while the remaining 105 cases treated later in the illness had 11 per cent of deaths. The fatality rate of control cases was not recorded. The vaccine used did not appear appreciably to alter or shorten the course of the treated cases.

Stone, Phillips, and Bliss (1251) treated 70 cases of lobar pneumonia with Rosenow's autolyzed vaccine, with 9 or 12.8 per cent of deaths. These cases occurred in men in an army camp in this country and as their fatality rate was slightly lower than that of other cases not given vaccine, it was concluded that vaccine may be of some value. Daily doses of 1 or 2 cc. were given subcutaneously for four or five days. As far as known, the use of autolyzed vaccine has been discontinued. From observations made elsewhere it seems likely that such an agent would stimulate but little specific immunity (see pages 410–414).

Lister (785) in South Africa employed a vaccine containing pneumococci of five different groups or types which was given to seven patients, all of whom recovered. Each patient received three intravenous doses containing from 2,500 to 5,000 million organisms. All developed agglutinins and opsonins for each of the five types included in the vaccine. Although pneumonia is an outstanding medical problem in some localities in South Africa, as previously described, and prophylactic vaccination has been carried out on thousands upon thousands of native laborers there (see pages 448–463), no one since Lister has used vaccine for the treatment of current cases in that region, as Orenstein (973) has noted. Pearson and Mouchet (1008) in the Belgian Congo treated a few cases with vaccine with indifferent success and Garnham and deSmidt (507) in Kenya (Africa) had similar results. The latter prepared an autogenous vaccine from the saline washings of the peritoneal cavity of a mouse injected with the patient's sputum the day previously. The organisms were heat killed and carbolic acid added as a preservative. Subcutaneous doses of 0.3 to 1 cc. or more were given at daily intervals. The fatality rate of 38 treated cases of "pneumonia" was 15.8 per cent and was the same as that in 38 untreated cases. No evidence was obtained that the acute illness was shortened.

Malone (858) with a phenol-killed vaccine containing pneumococci of Types I, II, III, and Group IV treated 29 cases of "pneumonia" in India and considered that such therapy shortens the course of the illness if begun before the fourth day and lowers the fatality rate. Evidence supporting these statements was not given.

Lambert (760) at the Bellevue Hospital, New York City, carried out over the period 1922–1926 an extensive clinical study of adults with pneumonia (apparently both lobar pneumonia and bronchopneumonia together) whom he treated with a mixed stock vaccine. The vaccine was commercially prepared, sterilized without heat, and of such concentration that 1 cc. contained one billion organisms. The content of the preparation in millions of bacteria was as follows: influenza bacilli 200, forty strains of pneumococci of Types I, II, III, and Group IV 100, streptococci 100, *Micrococcus catarrhalis* 200, *Staphylococcus aureus* 200, and *Staphylococcus albus* 200.

Doses of 1 to 2 cc., usually 1.5 cc., were given intramuscularly every six hours as long as the temperature was over 99° F., after which the dose was repeated once or twice at twelve-hour intervals and was then given once daily for a day or two more. Lambert's cases treated over the four-year period mentioned were subsequently augmented by an additional series in adults similarly treated over a later four-year interval (761) and the whole large series considered together (Table 158).

Lambert considered that the administration of vaccine diminished the severity of the disease without shortening the course or affecting it in any marked way. Apparently bacteriologic diagnosis was carried out on but few of his cases, for no tabulation of the results by type was given in his 1933 summary (761). Some mention of this matter was made in his earlier report (760), however, and the fatality rate of cases treated with and without vaccine respectively was stated to be 8 per cent and 17 per cent for Type I cases, 16 per cent and 72.7 per cent for Type II cases, 12 per cent and 35 per cent for Type III cases, and 17 per cent and 27 per cent for Group IV infections. Nevertheless, in no instance was the number of treated or untreated cases in these different groups given.

TABLE 158. PNEUMONIA (LOBAR PNEUMONIA AND BRONCHOPNEUMONIA TOGETHER). NUMBER OF CASES AND NUMBER AND PERCENTAGE OF DEATHS IN CASES TREATED WITH OR WITHOUT VACCINE THERAPY, BY TIME OF BEGINNING TREATMENT

TIME OF BEGINNING TREATMENT	TREATED WITH VACCINE			TREATED WITHOUT VACCINE		
	NUMBER OF CASES	DEATHS *Number*	DEATHS *Per cent*	NUMBER OF CASES	DEATHS *Number*	DEATHS *Per cent*
Within 48 hours	97	9	9.3	97	39	41.2
Within 72 hours	107	17	15.8	115	45	39.1
After 72 hours	270	89	32.9	270	131	48.5
Total	474	115	24.3	482	215	44.6

From Lambert (761)

No untoward reactions occurred in his treated cases and Lambert was enthusiastic about this mode of therapy. Antibody studies were made in a number of the cases in his second series. His final figures make interesting reading, as seen in Table 158.

Among 97 cases in which treatment with vaccine was begun within the first forty-eight hours of illness, as seen in Table 158, death occurred in only 9, or 9.3 per cent, whereas in 97 untreated cases it occurred in 39, or 41.2 per cent. The difference in the fatality rates of the treated and untreated cases was nearly as marked in the groups treated before or after seventy-two hours of illness. In the total series there was a fatality rate of 24.3 per cent for 474 vaccine treated cases (115 died), as compared with a rate of 44.6 per cent for 482 cases used as controls (215 died).

The results of treatment with vaccine in this series seem striking. It appears impossible, however, to grasp the significance of these figures, as Park

(William H.) noted in discussing Lambert's (761) summary, presented by the latter before the Association of American Physicians.

In a study reported by Wynn (1453), a mixed stock vaccine was also used for treatment; the vaccine used in cases of bronchopneumonia contained equal numbers of pneumococci, streptococci, and influenza bacilli and that used for lobar pneumonia contained several "strains" of pneumococci. Individual doses of unstated number were given, each containing 100 million organisms. Wynn considered the results especially good when treatment was begun within the first three days of illness. Of 100 consecutive cases treated, only 13, or 13 per cent, died. This series includes 49 cases treated in the first three days of illness with only one death (2 per cent). These cases occurred in Great Britain and no statement was made as to their etiologic diagnosis or the fatality rate of untreated or control cases. Attention was called earlier to the usual finding of a low fatality rate in pneumonia in that country (see pages 658–669).

Another report from Great Britain is that of Lamb (759), who treated 24 cases of lobar pneumonia with a commercial mixed stock vaccine which presumably contained some strains of pneumococci. Subcutaneous doses of 100 to 200 million organisms were used for adults and doses containing one-half as many organisms for children. At times a total of four or five doses was given. Of the 24 cases treated, 8 (33.3 per cent), an unusually high proportion, died.

The remaining series at hand are of cases treated in the United States. Sutton (1278) at the Cook County Hospital in Chicago treated many cases of "pneumonia" (apparently lobar pneumonia, bronchopneumonia, and terminal cases together) with a mixed stock vaccine of identical composition to the one used by Lambert, as mentioned above. Over a period of about eighteen months all cases admitted to one ward of the hospital received vaccine treatment, while those admitted to a neighboring ward were kept as controls. The etiology of these cases was apparently not determined. On admission the cases to be treated were given a 1.5 cc. dose of the vaccine subcutaneously, which was repeated every six hours until the temperature was normal, after which a similar dose was given twice daily for two days.

In all, Sutton treated 128 cases, of which 49, or 39.2 per cent, died, as compared with 61.2 per cent, or 80, of 148 untreated cases. He likewise reports a number of cases previously treated in similar fashion by Tice. In the latter series death occurred in 25 per cent, or 13 of 52 treated cases and in 36.7 per cent, or 18 of 49 control cases. Sutton combined these two series and subdivided them further, as seen in Table 159. No untoward reactions occurred in any of the treated cases.

TABLE 159. PNEUMONIA (LOBAR PNEUMONIA, BRONCHOPNEUMONIA, AND TERMINAL PNEUMONIA). NUMBER OF CASES AND NUMBER AND PERCENTAGE OF DEATHS IN CASES TREATED WITH OR WITHOUT VACCINE, BY VARIOUS SPECIAL GROUPS

GROUP	TREATED WITH VACCINE			TREATED WITHOUT VACCINE		
	NUMBER OF CASES	DEATHS *Number*	DEATHS *Per cent*	NUMBER OF CASES	DEATHS *Number*	DEATHS *Per cent*
Treatment begun within 48 hours of onset	25	3	12.0	32	19	59.3
Treatment begun within 72 hours of onset	51	7	13.7	69	34	49.2
All cases except those dying within 24 hours of admission	160	45	28.1	173	73	42.1

From Sutton (1278)

Among the cases whose treatment was begun within the first forty-eight hours of illness, as seen in Table 159, death occurred in 12 per cent, or 3, of 25 cases receiving vaccine therapy, as compared with 19 deaths, 59.3 per cent, in 32 control cases. The findings were about as striking in cases whose treatment was begun within seventy-two hours of onset; only 13.7 per cent of the 51 treated cases died, as compared with 49.2 per cent of the 69 untreated cases. In the total group, omitting those dying within twenty-four hours of admission to the hospital, death occurred in 28.1 per cent of 160 treated cases, and in 42.1 per cent of 173 untreated cases.

In view of these results it is hardly surprising that Sutton was favorably impressed with vaccine therapy. Subsequently a study of a similar nature was reported by Sutton, Kendall, and Rosenblum (1279). In this instance, a commercially prepared vaccine of unstated composition containing organisms chemically killed (by the addition of "Merthiolate") was used in doses of 1 to 1.5 cc. every six hours until the temperature became normal, following which a dose of the same size was given twice daily for two days. The vaccine used was termed a "Natural Bacterial Antigen," for it was considered that the organisms contained in it more closely approximated their natural state than those in most stock vaccines. Each dose was divided into four equal parts and each part was given subcutaneously in a different area. Subsequent to this study, Sutton, in a personal communication, stated that intradermal injections of this nature were being used.

Apparently the etiologic diagnosis of the cases treated was almost wholly unknown. The figures reported refer to the results obtained in adults treated with or without vaccine after those cases dying within twenty-four hours of admission to the hospital were excluded. Among 129 cases receiving vaccine therapy, there were 29 deaths, or 22.5 per cent, while among 339 cases considered as controls there were 143 deaths, or 42.1 per cent. These results were regarded as good as those obtained by specific antiserum treatment in pneumonia. It is impossible, however, to compare these results with those obtained by serum treatment, for the etiology of the cases in the above series was unknown and many were probably due to organisms other than pneumococci.

In 1931 Park (989) attempted to determine whether or not vaccine is efficacious in pneumonia and treated a series of 30 cases of lobar pneumonia with a mixed vaccine and contrasted the results with those obtained in 30 control cases. He states, "If we had not known that the vaccine was given to one-half of them we never would have suspected from the course of the disease that any special form of treatment was given." He concluded that as far as could be told, vaccine had no effect on the disease.

Schottstaedt (1164) reports treating 42 cases of lobar pneumonia with a commercially prepared "antigen" of unknown composition. Doses of 1.5 cc. were given every six hours for six days and death occurred in 8, or 19 per cent, of the cases, as compared with 30 per cent of 90 cases used as controls.

It appears impossible from the above reports to evaluate the merit of vaccine in the treatment of pneumococcus pneumonia. In spite of its use in a considerable number of cases all told and an apparent reduction in the case fatality rates on comparison with controls, the evidence is not convincing. Lack of attention to the bacteriologic diagnosis, the somewhat indiscriminate grouping of lobar pneumonia and bronchopneumonia together, and uncertainty as to the quality and composition of the vaccine limit the value of the observations. Treatment of an existing infection by vaccination has not been proved to be of value in any other disease and there is, in consequence, no support from analogy for its use in pneumococcus pneumonia. Laboratory studies have failed to show that vaccination of the patient with pneumococcus pneumonia produces an immune response more quickly than the infection itself. In view of Lambert's (761) findings, mentioned earlier, that possibly patients given vaccine produce more antibody than others not so treated, however, further observations are desirable on the amount of humoral immune substances produced in vaccinated and unvaccinated patients with pneumococcus pneumonia.

It is reassuring to note that there is no evidence in the reported vaccine treated cases and controls that this method of treatment was harmful. There is some evidence in animal experiments, as pointed out in Chapter IV (see pages 131–132) that the injection of specific pneumococcus products increases susceptibility to pneumococcus infection. It would appear that if the use of very large doses of a vaccine of considerable antigenicity is pushed it might easily overcome whatever resistance the patient has and lead to disaster. The possible dangers of using a vaccine in the presence of an acute pneumococcus infection were regarded as sufficient to cause editorial comment in the form of a warning concerning the matter in the *Journal of the American Medical Association* (315) in 1933.

Numerous investigators such as Cole (297), Cecil (221), Lord (807), Bullowa (176, 190), Howard and Fullerton (663), Langley (765), Park and Williams (995), and Finland (444) consider the value of vaccine therapy unproved and that it probably is of no use in the treatment of pneumonia. From a careful consideration of the available evidence, no other conclusion would appear justified.

CHAPTER EIGHTEEN

SERUM TREATMENT

History of Serum Treatment 806
Treatment with Miscellaneous Serums 809
Immune Chicken Serum 809
Human Convalescent Serum 812
Huntoon's Antibody Solution 814
Heterophile Antipneumococcic Serum 820
Non-Specific Serum 821
Treatment with Specific Antipneumococcic Horse Serum 822
Preparation and Standardization of Immune Horse Serum 823
Preparation of Unconcentrated Antipneumococcic Serum 824
Preparation of Concentrated Antipneumococcic Serum 825
Standardization of Antipneumococcic Serum 826
Test for Chill-Producing Substances 830
Antibodies in Immune Serum and Probable Mode of Action 832
Selection of Cases for Serum Treatment 832
Contraindications to Serum Treatment 835
Precautions against Sensitivity to Horse Serum 836
History 837
Tests for Sensitivity 839
Eye Test 839
Skin Test 840
Interpretation of Reactions 840
Unreliability of Attempted Desensitization 841
General Considerations 841
Summary: Circumstances Under which Serum Treatment May be Hazardous 842
Route of Serum Injection 843
Dosage with Antipneumococcic Horse Serum 845
General Considerations 845
Type I Cases 846
Type II Cases 848
Type V Cases 850
Type VII, Type VIII, and Type XIV Cases 851
Dosage for Infants and Children 852
Plan of Treatment 853
Initial Dosage 855
Technic of Treatment 856

Dosage with Antipneumococcic Horse Serum (*cont.*)
Additional Dosage and Guides to Subsequent Treatment 858
Use of Unconcentrated Serum 862
Serum Reactions and Their Treatment 863
Allergic Reactions 864
Chill or Thermal Reactions 867
Serum Sickness or Serum Disease 869
Treatment with Immune Rabbit Serum 872
Methods of Preparation and Standardization 873
Clinical Use of Rabbit Antiserum 875
Precautions in the Use of Rabbit Antiserum 875
Administration of Antipneumococcic Rabbit Serum 876
Reactions and Their Treatment 878

FOLLOWING a brief outline of the history of the development of serum treatment in pneumonia, the use of several different kinds of serum will be considered. The results obtained from the injection of a number of these serums will be mentioned in the sections dealing with their administration. The results obtained from the use of specific antipneumococcic horse or rabbit serum, however, are discussed in the following chapter (page 880).

HISTORY OF SERUM TREATMENT

The development of specific immune serum against the pneumococcus has been a long, slow, and irregular process which is by no means completed. The important stages in its development were first the observation by Fränkel (488) in 1886 that rabbits recovered from an experimental pneumococcus infection were resistant to a subsequent inoculation with the same organism. This important finding was confirmed by Foà and Bordoni-Uffreduzzi (472, 473, 474). What may be considered the second stage was the demonstration by the Klemperers (723, 724, 725) that the young of actively immunized mother rabbits usually acquired protection and, furthermore, that the serum of actively immunized rabbits, when injected into the blood stream of normal rabbits, protected the latter from an otherwise fatal infection due to their inoculation with pneumococci twenty-four hours later. To these workers also must go the credit for demonstrating that serum obtained from patients convalescent from pneumonia had a curative effect on experimentally infected rabbits. The Klemperers (725) in 1891 then proceeded to treat six pneumonia patients with small subcutaneous doses of immune rabbit serum. As far as known, this was the first attempt made to administer immune serum for the treatment of pneumonia.

It was therefore established as early as the eighteen-nineties that pneumococci introduced parenterally into the animal body acted as antigens in that they induced immunity and that the serum of animals thus immunized possessed protective properties (see also pages 159–177). In the same decade Mosny (911), Emmerich (391), Denys (352), Pane (981), Mennes (884), Washbourn (1389), and Eyre and Washbourn (396) immunized various animals with pneumococci or derivatives of these organisms and attempted to standardize the serum and to administer it to patients with pneumonia. Stimulus was given these efforts by the fact that at about the same time diphtheria antitoxin began to yield successful results in the treatment of diphtheria. It is obvious that at that time, however, because of the meager knowledge existing concerning the pneumococcus, serum therapy for pneumonia was much of a hit-or-miss affair. By 1904 Anders (16) was able to collect from the literature 535 cases which had been treated with subcutaneous doses in the neighborhood of 20 cc. every six to twelve hours for many days, of the serum of immunized horses, rabbits, dogs, or turkeys with but indifferent success. Occasionally, however, the results obtained with the then new agent kept alive the belief that antipneumococcic serum possessed curative properties and in one way or another its production was intermittently continued in various places.

The discovery that all pneumococci were not alike and that they may be divided into a number of serologic types marked the next important step in the evolution of antipneumococcic serum (see pages 22–24). This permitted the preparation and use of specific serums and helped explain many of the past failures with serum treatment. Numerous observations of fundamental importance relating to this matter were made by Neufeld and Händel (936, 937, 938) in 1909 and 1910. They outlined suitable means of producing specific serums of high potency and developed measures for their standardization. They emphasized the necessity in pneumonia of the immediate intravenous administration of large doses of highly potent specific serum in order to obtain the highest possible concentration of immune substances in the blood within a very brief period. In addition, they reported treating three cases of lobar pneumonia with 10 to 30 cc. doses of immune horse serum in this fashion.

By 1913 Cole and his associates (306, 290) in this country at the Hospital of the Rockefeller Institute for Medical Research were so impressed with the findings of Neufeld and Händel and the results of their own observations that they undertook to determine the nature of the infecting organism present in their cases of lobar pneumonia and to treat those with pneumococcus Type I or II infections with specific immune horse serum (291, 292, 293, 294, 295, 33, 296). These efforts were largely responsible for the successful development of specific serum therapy and Cole's studies were continued (297, 298, 299, 300, 301, 302). The contribution of various workers at the above hospital to the study and treatment of pneumococcus pneumonia has been one of outstanding importance.

Treatment with immune horse serum was tried in a number of places in this country, but met with indifferent success at times, particularly during the War (see pages 890–891), apparently in many instances because the serums used had little or no potency. Further, it became apparent that it would be desirable if possible to eliminate from the serum much of the extraneous protein it contained. It seemed probable such an accomplishment would simplify the technical difficulties attendant upon the intravenous injection of large doses and that possibly the occurrence of serum reactions could be substantially reduced. Efforts in this direction were made by Avery (30) and by Gay and Chickering (511) in 1915 and by Huntoon and his associates in 1921 (669, 670, 671). Serum prepared by the method of the latter workers was used in the treatment of a number of cases (see page 814). More successful, however, was Felton (407) in 1924, and as seen below (page 825), immune horse serums concentrated largely by one or another of his methods are widely used today.

The introduction of concentrated serum must be regarded as an important stage in the development of this form of therapy, for it was a long step forward in making the procedure practicable. Good results from the use of concentrated immune horse serum in suitable cases were reported in 1928 by Cecil (223), Bullowa, Rosenblüth, Park, and Cooper (195), Park, Bullowa, and Rosenblüth (991), and Cecil and Sutliff (245), and shortly afterward other favorable reports appeared by Bullowa (176), Finland (442), Cecil and Plummer (238), Baldwin (59), Lord (809), and by Cecil and Plummer (239) again. The findings of these investigators were based almost wholly on cases treated in large hospitals. Their observations suggested that concentrated antipneumococcic horse serum might be successfully used by physicians in general practice for the treatment of cases in small hospitals and in the patient's home (Bigelow, 104). Confirmation of this supposition was obtained during the Massachusetts Pneumonia Study and Continuing Program (614, 17, 813, 615, 814) and by results in the New York Pneumonia Control Program (1102).

During the past ten years and more, while the preparation and use of horse serums concentrated by Felton's methods were being extended, several other methods of serum concentration were described (see page 825), but were never widely used. In addition, efforts were made to produce an improved therapeutic agent by developing an "antitoxic" serum (Parker, 998, Parker and McCoy, 999) but its use in animals (Sabin, 1150, Park, 989) and man (Cecil, 223) showed it of little if any merit (see also page 125). Jamieson and Powell (683) also prepared an antitoxic serum of a somewhat different nature but its administration to a few patients did not give encouraging results. Further, the therapeutic value of antipneumococcic serum containing heterophile antibody was likewise investigated without success, as mentioned below (page 820) and in several instances treatment with nonspecific serum has likewise failed to assist in bringing about recovery (see page 821).

Other serums also have been used at various times. In 1911 Kyes (748) demonstrated the presence of immune substances in the serum of chickens immunized against the pneumococcus. Serum of this nature was subsequently used in the treatment of pneumonia, as mentioned below. Human convalescent serum has been employed in the treatment of a number of cases (see page 812). Barnes and White (77) in 1934, in an experimental study of the immunizing value of pneumococci killed in various ways, found that serum of much higher specific antibody content could be obtained from rabbits than from horses. Horsfall, Goodner, MacLeod, and Harris (659, 658) and Bullowa (190, 189) subsequently reported favorable results in the treatment of a number of cases of pneumococcus pneumonia with specific immune rabbit serum. The available evidence suggests that antiserum produced in the rabbit may have certain advantages over that produced in the horse (see also pages 172–173).

TREATMENT WITH MISCELLANEOUS SERUMS

Immune Chicken Serum

The resistance of chickens to the pneumococcus was mentioned elsewhere (see page 142). In 1911 Kyes (748) demonstrated the presence of agglutinins and protective substance in the blood of chickens following their repeated intramuscular injection with large doses of live virulent pneumococci. Brahma cockerels were frequently used and in the preparation of immune serum for therapeutic purposes the immunizing injections of large doses of many strains of living pneumococci were given intraperitoneally (750, 752). Apparently the types of pneumococci included among the organisms injected were unknown, for their identity was not revealed. The injections were given every two weeks and after six or eight doses bleedings of 30 to 40 cc. were begun at two-week intervals, alternating with the injections of organisms.

In 1918 Kyes (750) reported treating a number of patients having lobar pneumonia at the Cook County Hospital, Chicago, with whole immune chicken serum. Intravenous doses of 2.5 cc. were given once or twice daily until the temperature fell to 100° F. From one to twelve doses per patient were used, with an average of three. The fatality rate of 115 cases so treated was 20.8 per cent (24 died), as compared with a rate of 45.3 per cent for 538 cases (244 died) used as controls. In that same year Stone, Phillips, and Bliss (1251) treated with a similar preparation 30 cases of lobar pneumonia in soldiers at Fort Riley, Kansas. They reported one death, or 3.3 per cent, which they contrasted with a 14.2 per cent fatality rate in cases not so treated.

The use of this serum was continued and McClellan (828) reported treating a number of cases of lobar pneumonia with it in soldiers at Camp Grant, Illinois, in 1917–1918. Doses of 2.5 cc. were given intravenously or intramuscularly once or twice daily during the acute stages. About two-thirds of the cases were diagnosed during the first or second day of illness, so presumably serum treatment was begun early in a large proportion of them. The results of treatment are shown in Table 160.

As shown in that table, 7.7 per cent, or 25, of a total of 322 cases died. This fatality rate is much the same as that of other cases in military groups not receiving any special form of treatment, as mentioned in the chapter on Prognosis (see pages 699–700), and is but little lower than the 10.7 per cent rate mentioned by Locke (793) for 6,964 cases of lobar pneumonia (747 died) in the whole American Army in 1918.

Continuing the work of McClellan at Camp Grant, Gray (555) treated 234 cases of influenzal bronchopneumonia with Kyes' immune chicken serum, with a fatality rate of 16.7 per cent, which he compares with the rate of 53.6 per cent for 1,684 cases not receiving serum. The treated cases occurred in 1918 during the course of the widespread influenza epidemic then prevalent. The very nature of this report, however, coupled with the author's admission that the latter series may not be suitable as control cases, renders the significance of these figures uncertain. Apparently little bacteriologic work was done on any of the cases, though they were said to have been caused by pneumococci. Gray also reported a fatality rate of 4.3 per cent for 118 cases of atypical pneumococcus pneumonia treated during the last months of 1918 and early in 1919 during the latter part of the influenza epidemic. It may be noted in connection with this matter that during the latter part of that epidemic, in 1918–1919, the fatality rate of the atypical forms of pneumonia was observed to undergo a marked spontaneous decline from its higher point early in 1918, as Lord (807) and Heuer (638), among others, have pointed out. Such being the case, the interpretation of Gray's findings is rendered even more difficult.

TABLE 160. LOBAR PNEUMONIA. NUMBER OF CASES AND NUMBER AND PERCENTAGE OF DEATHS IN CASES GIVEN KYES' IMMUNE CHICKEN SERUM, BY TYPE

	NUMBER OF CASES	DEATHS	
		Number	*Per cent*
Type I	43	4	9.3
Type II	56	8	14.2
Type III	13	–	–
Group IV	199	13	6.5
Untyped	11	–	–
Total	322	25	7.7

From McClellan (828)

All the serum used by Gray was given intravenously; larger doses were used than in the previous studies and generally 5 to 10 cc. were given twice daily. A few patients received 30 cc. daily and Gray states that those who recovered commonly received a total dose of 60 to 90 cc. With respect to the effect of this serum on the patient, he remarks, "No marked changes were regularly seen after serum administration that were not seen in individual cases not treated with serum."

Immune chicken serum has frequently caused severe chills with hyperpyrexia in a considerable proportion of the cases treated (1251, 828, 752) but in Gray's (555) experience only about 5 per cent of the cases had any appreciable chill after such treatment. Kyes and Carey (752, 753) report devising methods to free chicken serum from most of its chill-producing properties.

It seems doubtful if sufficient data are at hand to properly evaluate immune chicken serum as a therapeutic agent in pneumonia. Presumably it continues to be used to some extent, chiefly by physicians in and around Chicago. The treatment of meningitis with this preparation was mentioned earlier (see page 596). Until more is known of chicken serum and its sphere of usefulness, it would seem unwise to advocate its routine administration in pneumonia.

Human Convalescent Serum

Sporadic attempts have been made to treat pneumonia patients by the administration of large amounts of whole blood or serum obtained from patients convalescent from pneumonia (840, 797, 1226) or pneumococcus pneumonia of homologous type (88, 460) or from normal persons following their immunization with pneumococcus vaccine (72).

Stengel (1226) in 1921 discussed the use of convalescent serum in pneumonia and reviewed a considerable sampling of the literature. Gundel (576, 577) has also considered this matter and remarks that although the antibody titer of convalescent serum is lower than that of the serum of suitably immunized animals there are certain points in favor of its use in that anaphylactic reactions and serum sickness may be largely avoided. Although this is so, the potency of antiserum of human origin in comparison with the potency of satisfactory antiserum of animal origin is extraordinarily low (see also pages 729–734).

In 1919 McGuire and Redden (840) at the Naval Hospital in Chelsea, Massachusetts, reported treating 151 cases of post-influenzal bronchopneumonia with serum obtained from patients with the same disease. Their observations were made in the latter part of the widespread influenza epidemic of 1917–1919 and these workers reported, as had others already referred to, that the severity of the infection toward the end of the epidemic was much less than it had been earlier. For treatment intravenous doses of about 120 cc. each were given. Most cases received three or even fewer injections of this size and most were treated within the first four days of illness. No control series of cases was available. Only 6, or 4 per cent, of the total 151 patients died. The course of the illness seemed shortened by the treatment and in approximately one-half the cases the temperature was normal within forty-eight hours. Bacteriologic diagnosis was carried out on but few cases. No anaphylactic reactions or serum sickness occurred but a few patients had chills following treatment. Study of this report suggests that the findings may possibly be considered as representative of the use of convalescent serum in the treatment of influenza of mild form rather than of its use in the treatment of frank pneumonia alone. Most patients had leucocyte counts of 10,000 or under and the most striking results were obtained in these cases. The treated cases were all in men in the navy, and youth and good physical condition are favorable factors in this group, as earlier mentioned (see pages 699–700).

In 1920, Locke, Thomas, and O'Hara (797) at the Boston City Hospital reported treating 22 cases of influenzal bronchopneumonia with human serum from convalescent cases with no special results. Twelve cases of this nature with apparently more favorable results were given similar treatment by Stengel (1226).

Stengel (1226) likewise treated eight or ten cases of lobar pneumonia with serum from patients convalescent from pneumonia of the same form. In only one or two instances, however, was bacteriologic diagnosis carried out and specific human serum given. These patients received one intravenous dose of from 10 to 50 cc. of the serum and most of them recovered. Data such as these appear of no value in determining whether or not human convalescent serum is of use in the treatment of pneumonia.

In 1930 Beebe and Sutliff (88) reviewed some of the literature relating to treatment with convalescent serum. In the same article, they reported the treatment, within three or four days of the onset of illness, of two cases of Type II and one case of Type III lobar pneumonia with large amounts of specific convalescent serum obtained in the first week of recovery from patients convalescent from pneumonia due to pneumococci of homologous type. Intravenous doses totaling from 310 to 440 cc. per patient were administered over a period of forty-eight hours with no apparent beneficial effect. The Type III case and one of the Type II cases died. Chills with some increase in temperature accompanied treatment in both the fatal cases. Subsequently Finland and Sutliff (460) treated one Type II and two Type III cases with specific human convalescent serum in much the same fashion. All three cases died. The Type II case received 130 cc. of convalescent serum and the Type III cases were given 75 and 310 cc. respectively. The Type III case receiving the larger dose had a progressively increasing bacteriemia. Although negative before treatment was given, the skin test in the Type II case became positive to specific capsular polysaccharide of the homologous type one hour after receiving 130 cc. of the serum. In addition, humoral antibodies previously absent became demonstrable at this time. Two days later, however, the skin test was negative, circulating antibodies were not found, bacteriemia developed, and the patient shortly died.

Barach (72) immunized healthy blood donors by giving repeated intramuscular and subcutaneous injections of pneumococcus vaccine for several months (see page 428). Blood from these donors immunized with the appropriate type was used to transfuse two patients with Type II and six with Type III pneumococcus lobar pneumonia. Amounts of blood totaling from 1,000 to 1,600 cc. were given in two or three transfusions over an interval of twenty-four hours with no apparent effect.

As a consequence of these findings of somewhat limited extent, it appears that the results of treatment with convalescent serum or human immune blood are not satisfactory. These methods of treatment are of course cumbersome and difficult to carry out.

Huntoon's Antibody Solution

In 1915 Gay and Chickering (511) devised a method for concentrating the antibody of immune horse serum by means of specific precipitation which may be briefly described as follows. Pneumococci of a given type such as Type I were cultivated and then precipitated from the culture by the addition of alcohol or acetone. The precipitate was dried, ground, and extracted with saline and the nearly clear extract obtained mixed with antipneumococcic serum of homologous type. The resulting precipitate was collected, washed free of serum, and dissolved in saline solution. The final solution contained about as much protective substance as the original serum and was almost free of horse protein. Somewhat modifying this procedure Huntoon and his associates (669, 670, 671) in 1920 evolved what seemed to be a more successful means of separating the immune substances in antipneumococcic serum from its other constituents. The resulting product was termed Huntoon's Antibody Solution and was used intermittently for the treatment of pneumonia for several years (236, 314, 229, 244, 60, 713, 223, 238, 93). This means of concentrating serum was also investigated by Felton and Bailey (427).

Cecil and Larsen (236) studied the therapeutic properties of such an antibody solution containing immune substances for pneumococci of Types I, II, and III. Protective effects were obtained by administering the solution to mice prior to infection and curative effects were demonstrated in monkeys with pneumonia. The results were most satisfactory against Type I infections and were less marked with Type II and least marked with Type III infections. Cecil and Steffen (244) later reported their detailed observations on the cure of experimentally induced pneumococcus pneumonia in monkeys with Huntoon's antibody solution. With otherwise fatal Type I infections in these animals, intravenous injections in doses of 10 to 20 cc. one to three times daily begun seventy-two hours after the onset of the illness exercised a specific therapeutic effect, promptly freed the blood of pneumococci, and brought about recovery. The solution was also effective in the experimental Type II cases but less so than with Type I. In this instance larger doses were necessary, blood cultures remained positive longer, and treatment had to be instituted by the end of twenty-four hours to yield suitable results. No effect was observed in monkeys with pneumonia due to pneumococci of Type III or some strains of Group IV treated with the antibody solution. The subcutaneous injection of the solution in monkeys with Type I pneumonia was effective but required a longer time to produce results. Doses administered intratracheally were of no value. These findings were later reviewed by Baldwin and Cecil (60).

Several hundred patients with pneumonia due to various organisms have been treated with Huntoon's antibody solution containing antibodies for Types I, II, and III. The first investigation of this nature was that reported by Cecil and Larsen (236), who treated more than four hundred patients with lobar pneumonia at the Bellevue Hospital, New York City. The medical wards of the hospital were divided into two groups and all cases entering one group were treated with this preparation, while all those admitted to the other wards were used as controls. No selection of the cases was made at entry. The treated cases received 50 to 100 cc. of antibody solution intravenously one to three times daily as long as the temperature remained above 100° F. From three to six injections were ordinarily given and the average total dose per patient was 225 cc.

No immediate untoward reactions or serum sickness occurred but severe chill or thermal reactions developing twenty to forty minutes after the injections were the rule. The chill generally lasted fifteen to thirty minutes, accompanied by cyanosis and an increase of dyspnea, during which time the temperature became elevated. Temperatures of 106° to 109° F. were rather frequent and in one case a rectal temperature of 113.1° F. occurred. The hyperpyrexia lasted thirty to sixty minutes, after which sweating occurred and the temperature usually fell to normal or under, defervescence in some instances being permanent. Such reactions were considered as representative of a foreign protein reaction, usually followed each injection, and exhibited a tendency to decrease in severity with each reaction. Death occurred in three patients probably as a consequence of these reactions. Delirium, cyanosis, dyspnea, rapid weak pulse, sweating, pulmonary congestion, and coma ending in death were encountered.

Clinical improvement was not infrequent, especially in Type I cases. Several Type I cases having bacteriemia showed negative blood cultures after a single injection of the antibody solution. In Type II and Type III cases no effect on bacteriemia was noted.

The cases of lobar pneumonia treated by Cecil and Larsen (236), as well as the untreated cases used as controls, are shown in Table 161. In a total of 424 treated cases due to pneumococci of Type I, II, III, or Group IV, death occurred in 91, or 21.5 per cent, as compared with 28.3 per cent, or 116, of 410 untreated cases. The total fatality rate was thus somewhat lower in the treated cases.

TABLE 161. LOBAR PNEUMONIA. NUMBER OF CASES AND NUMBER AND PERCENTAGE OF DEATHS IN CASES TREATED WITH AND WITHOUT HUNTOON'S ANTIBODY SOLUTION, BY CAUSATIVE ORGANISM

ORGANISM	TREATED WITH ANTIBODY SOLUTION			TREATED WITHOUT ANTIBODY SOLUTION		
	NUMBER OF CASES	DEATHS *Number*	DEATHS *Per cent*	NUMBER OF CASES	DEATHS *Number*	DEATHS *Per cent*
Pneumococcus						
Type I	158	21	13.3	162	36	22.2
Type II	83	23	27.7	67	27	40.3
Type III	73	29	39.7	60	24	40.0
Group IV	110	18	16.4	121	29	24.0
Total	424	91	21.5	410	116	28.3
Streptococcus and others	48	24	50.0	35	12	34.3
Unclassified	36	14	38.9	47	20	42.6

From Cecil and Larsen (236)

Among the Type I cases in the two groups in Table 161 the fatality rate of 158 treated cases was 13.3 per cent, in contrast to the rate of 22.2 per cent for 162 untreated cases. The treated Type II cases had a fatality rate of 27.7 per cent, while it was 40.3 per cent in the untreated cases. The proportion of deaths in the Type III cases was 39.7 per cent in those treated and 40 per cent in the control cases, and in Group IV cases the corresponding figures were 16.4 per cent and 24 per cent.

The data suggested that Huntoon's antibody solution might have some effect in reducing the fatality rate in Type I, II, and Group IV cases. Among the cases due to organisms such as streptococci in Table 161, however, the fatality rate of 48 cases in the treated group was 50 per cent, as compared with 34.3 per cent for 35 untreated cases, and was thus higher in the treated group.

Conner (314) at the New York Hospital, New York City, likewise treated a number of cases with Huntoon's antibody solution. No series of control cases was observed. Daily intravenous doses of 50 cc. were used for males and 25 cc. for females. As in the above study, severe chill reactions followed essentially every injection given and in one instance death occurred as a result of the reaction. Clinical evidence of beneficial effects resulting from the treatment was very irregularly seen. The effect on the leucocyte count was also irregular and most cases showed little if any special change in the white count after treatment. The fatality rate of 23 Type I cases was 13 per cent (3 died), of 9 Type II cases 22.2 per cent (2 died), of 9 Type III cases 33.3 per cent (3 died), and of 49 Group IV cases 4.1 per cent (2 died). These results were interpreted to indicate that the treatment had some beneficial effect on Type I and probably on Type II and Group IV cases as well, and Conner was inclined to attribute these results to a non-specific action of the preparation administered.

The severity of the chill reactions generally produced by the antibody solution was such that Cecil and Baldwin (229) in 1924 made efforts to avoid them and to determine the curative power of the solution when administered to patients subcutaneously. Larger doses were used than previously, and ordinarily in the vicinity of 100 to 200 cc. were given as the initial injection, which was repeated in ten to twelve hours. If required, two more injections of about similar size were given the next day and another on the following day. The total dose per case averaged about 650 cc. No chill reactions occurred, although a few patients had chilly sensations or a rise in temperature of 1° to 2° F.

In all, Cecil and Baldwin (229) treated 91 Type I, II, III, and Group IV cases of lobar pneumonia with subcutaneous injections with a fatality rate of 34 per cent, as compared with a rate of 35 per cent in 100 control cases. Wherever treatment could be begun within the first forty-eight hours of illness, however, the treated cases had a considerably lower fatality rate than the untreated cases, the rate for 53 cases in the former group being 20 per cent and for 59 cases in the latter group 40 per cent.

The findings suggested that this form of treatment was of some value in Type I, II, and Group IV cases when given very early, but not in Type III cases. Nevertheless, the results were so irregular after subcutaneous treatment and so poor in comparison with the results of intravenous treatment that Cecil and Baldwin advocated a return to the latter method. Baldwin and Rhoades (61) found that antibody administered subcutaneously only irregularly became demonstrable in the blood and then only in low titer. At about the time the report of Cecil and Baldwin (229) was made in 1924, Felton's (407) method of concentrating immune horse serum appeared and the use of Huntoon's antibody solution was largely abandoned, as Cecil (223) and Cecil and Plummer (238) have described.

Nevertheless, other efforts were made to continue treatment with this preparation. Kessel and Hyman (713) at the Mt. Sinai Hospital, New York City, subsequently reported treating 56 cases of lobar pneumonia with Huntoon's antibody solution with 19 deaths, or 34 per cent. Although no control series was studied, this fatality rate appeared to be much the same as that usually encountered in the same hospital. Doses of 50 cc. intravenously were given at the start of treatment in each case and increased to 100 cc. every six hours later as needed. The treated cases averaged a total of 350 cc. per patient. Chill reactions were usual with some rise in temperature, which rarely exceeded 3° F. Death occurred in one patient as the result of a reaction following a single dose of 100 cc. These investigators concluded that good results occasionally occurred and these seemed due to the specific nature of the antibody solution and to be independent of the non-specific chill reaction, but that the results were not sufficiently striking to warrant the routine use of this agent in the treatment of lobar pneumonia in a general hospital.

In 1934 Belk and Sharpe (93) at the Bryn Mawr Hospital, Bryn Mawr, Pennsylvania, reported another study of the administration of Huntoon's antibody solution. The preparation they used was manufactured by a slightly different process than had been employed previously and they attributed the almost complete absence of chill reactions in their treated cases to this change.

These investigators treated 130 cases of lobar pneumonia in adults and children and compared the results with those obtained in 52 untreated cases which they stated were not strictly controls. Doses were usually given intravenously but in many instances intramuscular injections were given. For adults doses of 50 to 100 cc. three times daily were administered and in children 25 to 50 cc. were used. The average amount injected totaled more than 400 cc. in many adults and 193 cc. in children. No severe chill reactions occurred and apparently in the total group of several hundred injections given only five were followed by chill reactions.

The cases in the treated series were divided in various ways and Belk and Sharpe were enthusiastic about the results obtained. The nature of their report makes satisfactory comparison of the findings difficult. A compilation of their total results in adults is shown in Table 162. The fatality rate of 79 treated cases with 19 deaths was 24.1 per cent, while 36.4 per cent, or 12 of 33 untreated cases, died. Belk and Sharpe consider the difference in

TABLE 162. LOBAR PNEUMONIA IN ADULTS. NUMBER OF CASES AND NUMBER AND PERCENTAGE OF DEATHS IN CASES TREATED WITH AND WITHOUT HUNTOON'S ANTIBODY SOLUTION, BY TYPE

	TREATED WITH ANTIBODY SOLUTION			TREATED WITHOUT ANTIBODY SOLUTION		
	NUMBER	DEATHS		NUMBER	DEATHS	
	OF CASES	*Number*	*Per cent*	OF CASES	*Number*	*Per cent*
Type I	11	6	54.5	7	3	43.9
Type II	8	4	50.0	4	–	–
Type III	17	4	23.5	5	3	60.0
Group IV	32	5	15.6	6	2	33.3
Untyped	11	–	–	11	4	36.4
Total	79	19	24.1	33	12	36.4

From Belk and Sharpe (93)

these two fatality rates evidence of the value of this form of treatment. The findings are suggestive that the antibody solution aided some of the treated cases, but inasmuch as the low rate for the total treated group is due wholly to the lower rates for the Type III, Group IV, and untyped cases, and the number of cases in the individual series as well as in the total groups is so small, there appears to be little reason for sharing their belief that Huntoon's antibody solution is of great value.

Of 12 untreated cases of lobar pneumonia in infants and children Belk and Sharpe report that 7, or 37 per cent, died as compared with 6 per cent, or 3, of 48 treated cases. Most of the treatment in children was given intramuscularly.

A review of all the reports mentioned in this section suggests that Huntoon's antibody solution has at times shown some effect in Type I, II, and Group IV cases. To what extent this effect may be attributed to a non-specific action is unknown, but such an action may have played some part in producing the results obtained, as evidenced by the not infrequent lowering of the fatality rate in the Group IV cases. The benefits derived from treatment with this agent, however, appear so unpredictable and so irregularly obtainable and its propensity to produce severe or fatal thermal reactions so great that its general use in pneumonia cannot be advised.

Heterophile Antipneumococcic Serum

The claim has been made by Bailey and Shorb (55) and by Powell, Jamieson, Bailey, and Hyde (1047) that immune serum containing heterophile antibodies possesses advantages over immune serum containing only type-specific antibodies. Heterophile antigen was found to be present in some pneumococci and heterophile antibody was demonstrated not to be type-specific in its actions. It was considered that antibody of this nature played a part in bringing about recovery in pneumonia and in consequence that such antibody might be of value in the treatment of cases due to any and all types of pneumococci. Further observations by Finland, Ruegsegger, and Felton (457, 458), however, indicate that heterophile antibody probably is of no value in combating pneumococcus infections in man (276).

In the usual instance heterophile antibody serum is made by adding to bivalent Type I and II antipneumococcic horse serum a variable amount of rabbit serum containing heterophile antibodies. Some danger may be attached to the use of this serum, for although patients are generally tested for evidence of sensitivity to horse serum prior to its administration, the fact that they must also be tested for sensitivity to rabbit serum is frequently overlooked.

Thompson and Kelly (1300) reported treating 42 cases with heterophile antibody serum and believed it might be of some use. Similar observations were made by Rockwell and Tyler (1100), who treated 68 cases with 42.6 per cent of deaths, by Noble and Kibler (958), who treated 50 cases with 18 per cent of deaths, and by Callomon and Ungar (210), who treated 24 cases with 12.5 per cent of deaths. Many of these cases were of pneumococcus pneumonia but in perhaps one-half the instances no data were given as to the etiologic agent responsible for the illness and apparently it was unknown. In a majority of instances the use of heterophile antibody serum appears analogous to the use of non-specific serum therapy.

The Council on Pharmacy and Chemistry of the American Medical Association, acting on a review of the problem relating to the use of heterophile antibody serum submitted by Plummer (1028), concluded that it was unwise and unwarranted to recommend the general use of Type I and II antiserums containing heterophile antibodies. Evidence is lacking that heterophile antibody is of therapeutic value for the treatment of pneumonia in man.

Non-Specific Serum

Over a period of many years various substances of a non-specific nature such as preparations containing proteins have been used in the treatment of pneumonia. Their trial has usually resulted in no special benefit to the patient (1423). In monkeys (233) with an experimentally induced pneumococcus Type I pneumonia and in rabbits (532) with intradermal infections due to the same organism, the intravenous injection of normal horse serum or of typhoid vaccine did not in any way alter the progress of their infection, although in other animals similarly infected the administration of type-specific antiserum resulted in the prompt sterilization of the blood stream and their rapid recovery.

A temporary effect may be seen in some instances after non-specific serum therapy, the mechanism of which is little understood. Goodner (532) showed in rabbits with an intradermal pneumococcus infection that the use of non-specific therapy in the form of normal horse serum or typhoid vaccine frequently caused the *temporary* disappearance of bacteria from their blood. After an hour or so the organisms again reappeared in the blood of these animals. Further, in an occasional patient receiving non-specific serum treatment or antiserum containing no antibodies for the organism causing the infection, a drop in temperature of several degrees, which is generally temporary, may occur. A response of this nature was presumably the cause of the occasionally reported benefit in Group IV cases following their treatment with Huntoon's antibody solution containing antibodies for Types I, II, and III only, as mentioned above.

Sutliff, Finland, and Hunnicutt (1273) studied this matter in thirteen patients with pneumococcus Type I lobar pneumonia treated with a non-specific serum (antimeningococcic serum). It was demonstrated that following the injection of non-specific serum a temporary drop in temperature usually occurred, lasting from one to a few hours. In several instances patients given repeated doses of this serum continued to get worse, necessitating their treatment with type-specific antiserum to alter the progress of the infection. In these individuals, prompt and permanent sterilization of the blood stream and recovery occurred after instituting specific treatment. The findings indicated that in comparison with the results in cases given only specific serum, non-specific serum treatment was of no value in preventing the development of bacteriemia or in its treatment, nor did it prevent extension of the pulmonary lesion, as this was a frequent occurrence in these cases, and it did not appear to shorten the course of the illness.

Various investigators have remarked that if non-specific serum treatment were of real merit in reducing the fatality rate in pneumonia, then the Type III and Group IV cases, treated with serum containing antibodies for Types I and II only, should show a substantial reduction in their fatality rates. This, however, has not occurred, as Cecil (225) has shown. Certain data obtained during the course of the Massachusetts Pneumonia Study (869, 615) are of interest with respect to this matter. During the early part of that investigation 128 Group IV cases received varying amounts of Type I and II antiserum. Death occurred in 23, or 18 per cent, of these cases, as compared with 15 per cent, or 48, of 321 similar cases gathered at the same time which did not receive any serum (see also page 671).

In summary, it may be noted that the non-specific serum treatment of pneumonia is almost wholly without value and cannot be recommended.

TREATMENT WITH SPECIFIC ANTIPNEUMOCOCCIC HORSE SERUM

Data accumulated since 1910 indicate that the best therapeutic agent available for use in pneumonia is highly potent specific antipneumococcic serum of animal origin. The advantages of such preparations are many, as is apparent in considering the results obtained by their use (see pages 880–918) and the relative ease with which the concentrated products may be given. There are, however, certain unavoidable disadvantages in the use of alien serums. Their action is type-specific and therefore a single serum will not benefit all cases of pneumococcus pneumonia, relatively large doses must be used, the expense of the serum is considerable, and they may at times give rise to untoward reactions. Nevertheless, adequately used specific antipneumococcic serum appears to be the only known agent which can be shown to cause prompt and striking symptomatic improvement *regularly* and a marked reduction in the expected fatality rate in cases due to pneumococci of a type for which a clinically effective serum is available.

Although goats, sheep, asses, fowl, rabbits, and horses have all been employed for the production of antipneumococcic serum, for economic reasons it is the horse that has supplied the vast bulk of all serum thus far used in the treatment of patients. The rabbit, however, is gaining favor as the animal used in the production of serum against a number of types, particularly those less frequently encountered (see page 918). As evidence is accumulating that rabbit antiserum can be successfully employed, the clinical use of this product is discussed on page 872.

PREPARATION AND STANDARDIZATION OF IMMUNE HORSE SERUM*

Specific antipneumococcic horse serum has been rather widely used in the treatment of pneumococcus pneumonia, more particularly in this country. Whole immune serum has been used to a variable degree, but in recent years most of the serums prepared have been concentrated and their use is rapidly extending.

Horses may be immunized against a single type or against two or more types of pneumococci. Because the greatest demand has been for serums for Types I and II, it has been the custom of manufacturers to provide a bivalent serum for both, as well as monovalent serums for each type. The close immunologic correspondence between Types II and V is a reason for the production of serums containing antibodies for these two types and it is possible that similar relationships yet to be demonstrated between other types for which suitable antiserums may be obtained may result in still other combinations. The employment of two types in immunizing a horse does not detract seriously, if at all, from the ability of the animal to develop antibodies for both types to as high a level as though a culture of a single type were used as the immunizing antigen.

In the preparation of specific antiserum pure and authentic strains of pneumococci of high virulence for mice are grown in a suitable nutrient broth, harvested at the stage of optimal growth by centrifugal separation, suspended in isotonic saline solution, and then killed by formalin or by an exposure to a degree of heat sufficient to devitalize the cells but not high enough to rob them of their antigenic properties. The suspension is then standardized for pneumococcal content by appropriate physical or chemical methods, and the dose for every injection is accurately measured. In some instances in the past, living pneumococci were used in the latter part of the course of immunization but such a practice has been largely abandoned.

Gradually increasing amounts of the suspension of organisms are injected into the jugular vein of a healthy horse in repeated series, interrupted by rest periods between each series. From time to time test bleedings are taken and when the serum shows a high antibody content the animal is subjected to a

* Those interested will find an exhaustive account of the methods of serum production, concentration, and standardization in White, with Robinson and Barnes (1417).

schedule of serial injections of antigen and bleedings, separated by regular intervals to allow time for all the antigen to disappear from the blood, as well as to procure the blood as nearly as possible at the peak of antibody response (see also pages 419–422).

Under aseptic precautions the blood is taken from the jugular vein into suitable containers, the serum or plasma is allowed to separate from the clot or sedimented cells, and then drawn off. The serum or plasma thus obtained is held for concentration or, if the unconcentrated product is to be made, a chemical preservative is added to the serum, after which it is put through the usual filtration procedures to ensure the elimination of all formed blood elements and bacteria.

Banzhaf and Curphey (65) employed a method for immunizing purposes somewhat similar to that above and in addition administered repeated intramuscular doses of the infected pleural exudate of a horse to stimulate antibody production. Curphey and Baruch (335) reported findings which they believe suggested that the so-called "exudate" antiserum so produced was more potent than that otherwise obtained, but this method of immunization has never gained general acceptance.

Preparation of Unconcentrated Antipneumococcic Serum

In the days before reliable and economical methods had been devised for the concentration of antipneumococcic serum, the native serum as it came from the clot was the only product available for clinical use. After having a chemical preservative added to maintain sterility, it was passed through bacteria-proof filters and finally tested for sterility, potency, and harmlessness. Unconcentrated serums generally contain about 8 or 9 per cent of solids. The potency of whole immune serum varies somewhat with each lot depending upon such factors as the length of time the horses have been undergoing immunization, the intervals between their injections with antigen, and factors inherent in the individual horse.

For some time after concentrated serum appeared on the market, some physicians, among them Cole (299), still preferred serum in its natural state. The repeated intravenous injection of large amounts of whole serum is time consuming, requires the use of special apparatus, and is too complicated a procedure to be readily applicable outside of hospitals. These facts, coupled with the common occurrence of serum sickness of some severity following its use, were disadvantages which led to the abandonment of whole serum as soon as the quality of the concentrated product improved.

Preparation of Concentrated Antipneumococcic Serum

Several methods are used for the refinement of antipneumococcic serum, but all have as their purpose the concentration of specific antibodies in small bulk and the elimination of non-immune serum proteins and other constituents, some of which may give rise to shock, chills, or thermal reactions, and serum sickness.

One of the first preparations of concentrated serum was the pneumococcus antibody solution of Huntoon and his associates (669, 670, 671), who modified the specific absorption method of Gay and Chickering (511), as mentioned above (see page 814).

Avery (30), however, was the first to reveal the close relation between pneumococcal antibody and a globulin fraction of immune horse serum and to demonstrate that 38 to 42 per cent saturation of the serum with ammonium sulphate completely precipitated the antibodies. The principle once established, a variety of methods were devised and used for a time in concentrating antipneumococcic serum. Banzhaf (64) employed the same procedure as Avery, after first dialyzing the whole serum. Felton (407), whose extensive studies (408, 409, 427, 428, 410, 412, 413, 414, 416, 418, 417, 429, 419, 423) not only laid the foundation for this phase of serum production but gave us a reliable and usable product, first used acidulated water for the precipitation of the immune globulin. Later (413) he used sodium sulphate as the precipitant and then devised the alcohol method (418), which, with one modification or another, is now usually employed in manufacturing laboratories. Other methods of concentration were described by Banzhaf and Klein (66), Goodner (533), and Kirkbride, Hendry, and Murdick (721).

In brief, antibody solution made by Felton's alcohol method is prepared by adding ethyl alcohol to immune serum in the proportion of one to five, the two components of the mixture being previously chilled and the process being carried out at a temperature only slightly above the freezing point in order to avoid denaturation of the immune globulin. The resulting precipitate is filtered or centrifuged out of the mixture and washed in cold distilled water to remove the water-soluble protein. The so-called acid fraction (410, 411, 429) is then removed and the insoluble globulin containing the desired antibody is dissolved in the requisite volume of salt solution. The solution is freed from any bacteria or particulate matter acquired during the several steps of the process by filtration, then tested for potency and blandness, after which it is filled into final containers, again tested for sterility, and if satisfactory, the serum is ready for distribution. The final product should be clear, limpid fluid, free from sediment, containing 10 to 12 per cent of total solids and approximately 0.2 per cent phenol or a sufficient amount of any other chosen germicide to ensure sterility. Good concentrated horse serum is in the neighborhood of five to ten times as potent as the average whole immune serum. The potency of different lots varies to some extent depending upon the nature and potency of the unconcentrated serum used in its preparation and the method of concentration employed.

Standardization of Antipneumococcic Serum

Quantitative measurement of the potency of antipneumococcic serum is necessary in the estimate of proper dosage for treatment in pneumonia and as a guide to workers engaged in the production of such serums. Thus far determination of the mouse protective titer of the antiserum has proved the most practical method of testing. Uniform results in repeated tests are sometimes difficult to obtain, at least partly because strains of pneumococci may differ in virulence, in abundance of growth, and in neutralizing power, and because mice may have varying susceptibility to the infection, as elsewhere noted (see pages 120–121, 131, and 186). Details of the procedures used in standardization are well presented and discussed by White, with Robinson and Barnes (1417). The protection test, developed by Neufeld and Händel (936), modified by Avery, Chickering, Cole, and Dochez (33), and later further modified and used by the United States Hygienic Laboratory (now the National Institute of Health) has since been found unsuitable for testing the potency of antipneumococcic serums. In its final form a standard amount of serum (0.2 cc.) was used with a uniform amount of culture.* A second type of protection test as developed by Felton (407, 412, 415, 416, 432) and used by other workers, including those at the National Institute of Health, has been widely used (1018, 540, 721). In this test a constant amount of culture is used with varying doses of serum. Park and Cooper's (988) modification of the test is now probably the most commonly used procedure (1417).

A tentative unit has been agreed upon. As originally defined by Felton (407, 412), the unit is that amount of antibody which will protect at least 50 per cent of a series of inoculated standard white mice against 1,000,000 fatal doses of a standard pneumococcus culture of the same type. The matter of standardization is extraordinarily involved, however, and changes in the value of the unit from time to time have not simplified it.

* In the early days of the use of this test varying amounts of culture were used.

Further studies of the problem were also made by Felton (415, 416, 432) and to facilitate comparison of the potency of serums produced in various laboratories he (415) distributed a serum designated F146 to be used as a standard. On the basis of protection tests Felton assigned a value to this serum of 500 units of protective substance per cubic centimeter for both Type I and Type II. Subsequently, however, as mentioned by the Council on Pharmacy and Chemistry of the American Medical Association (18), this value was decreased to 200 units and the unit described as 1/200 of a cubic centimeter of the serum F146. This latter value was accepted by the League of Nations Permanent Commission on Biologic Standardization (767a) in 1935. Hartley and his colleagues (601) prepared serums which were standardized against F146, and portions of them were dried to ensure stability of potency. The above commission recommended that the definition of the unit as mentioned by Hartley and his associates be accepted. At present, then, as Hartley and Smith (602, 603) point out, one unit of Type I antibody is represented by 0.0886 mgm. of the dry standard preparation and the unit of Type II is represented by 0.0894 mgm. of its dry standard serum. They advocate the international adoption of these standards and universal adherence to them is of great importance in rendering experimental and clinical findings obtained in laboratories and hospitals throughout the world more readily and directly comparable.

For ascertaining the antibody content of any given lot of antipneumococcic serum a sample is tested simultaneously with a standard serum of known potency, usually supplied from some governmental source.* The determination is based upon the comparative protective effect of the two serums against a strain of pneumococcus of homologous type and of exalted and known virulence. With bivalent serums the potency is determined by separate protection tests against each type. The findings resulting from the tests are translated into units and the serum, in amounts of ten thousand units or multiples thereof, is filled into the vials or syringes bearing a label upon which are given the name of the manufacturer, the name of the product, the type, the total number of units,† a lot number, and the date beyond

* The National Institute of Health of the United States Public Health Service furnishes a standard bivalent serum of Types I and II and standard monovalent serums of Types V, VII, and VIII for the comparative titration of all antipneumococcic serums of these types manufactured under federal license. It is probable that in Great Britain similar standard serums, at least for Types I and II, may be obtained from the National Institute for Medical Research, and laboratories of any country desiring standard serums for the first two types may apply to the League of Nations Center at the Staatens Seruminstitut, Copenhagen, Denmark.

† Actually a somewhat larger number of units is contained in each vial than the number recorded on the label. This excess number of units is included to make up for the decrease in

which the potency may not be relied upon. Concentrated antipneumococcic serum is usually given an expiration date of about a year, but the sooner after its preparation it is used, the greater its potency should be, and perhaps also the less likely it will be to produce reactions. A flier or leaflet* giving directions for testing for sensitivity to horse protein and for using the serum is included with the serum in the final package.

It is desirable, so far as possible, to adopt standardized conditions under which the tests for potency are made, and the inclusion in the mouse protection test of a standard antiserum as a control is an advance in this direction. Stability in the standard antiserum is, however, essential, inasmuch as the measurement of the potency of the serum under test is determined in terms of the potency of the standard at the time the test is made. The reliability of the method may be increased by the use of dry standard control antiserums, as Hartley and his associates (601) have shown for Type I and Smith and his collaborators (1215) for Type II.

In the United States the official standard Type I and Type II antiserum (1339), P 11, is dispensed by the National Institute of Health for use as a control in potency tests of Type I and Type II antiserum. The potency of the control serum P 11 is 300 units per cubic centimeter for Type I and 150 units per cubic centimeter for Type II. This serum is furnished in the liquid state but a reserve supply has been dried and will be used if the supply of the liquid preparation is exhausted or if there is evidence of a loss of potency. The potency of the control serums for Types V, VII, and VIII as recently adopted is 500, 900, and 250 units per cubic centimeter, respectively.

It is advisable that a standard method of testing be adopted with respect to virulence and dosage of pneumococci and strains and number and length of the period of observation of the mice used. At present there is, in the United States, no official method. The method outlined by the American Drug Manufacturers' Association is frequently used, as noted by Lord and Heffron (814). In general the methods employed are based on the use of several doses of serum and a fixed dose of culture.

The biologic assay of the potency of antiserum is somewhat uncertain at best and it is to be hoped that subsequent investigations will reveal more suitable methods of testing. Numerous *in vitro* tests have been described

potency which occurs with the lapse of time before the expiration date is reached. Decrease of potency with a lapse of time may be ascribed to the occurrence of subtle alterations of the character of the proteins of the serum.

* The instructions given on the fliers enclosed with the antipneumococcic serum distributed by the State Antitoxin and Vaccine Laboratory in Massachusetts may be seen in Appendix A, pages 940–945.

and suggested for use but none has been generally accepted for determining the potency of horse antiserum* (1090, 174, 502, 1468, 1366, 601, 602; see also page 116).

Over a period of years there has been considerable experience with tests for the potency of Type I and Type II serums. Much more recent, however, has been the testing for potency of serums of other types, particularly Types V, VII, VIII, and XIV. In the past, the potency of serums of these types has shown marked variation and at times has been uncertain. Owing to the relative avirulence of certain of the higher types of pneumococci which are used for the tests, the standardization of serums for many of the higher types presents a special problem which is being studied in several places.

In this country all antipneumococcic serum that enters interstate commerce must be prepared according to federal regulations and meet all specifications as to identity, purity, and potency.† In Great Britain, the product comes under the British Therapeutic Substances Act and, therefore, must fulfill the stipulations of that law. The policy of the National Institute of Health governing the serums used in the United States is to permit the release for distribution of only those lots of Type I and Type II therapeutic horse serum which have a potency of more than 500 units per cubic centimeter for the unconcentrated preparations and a potency of more than 1,000 units for the concentrated. Good concentrated serums frequently contain two or more times this number of units for Type I but are commonly somewhat less potent for Type II than for Type I. No minimum potency has apparently yet been established, however, for the other types.

Specific serums for many of the higher types were introduced by Cooper and her associates (318, 320). Concentrated antipneumococcic horse serums are now available for Types I, II, V, VII, VIII, and XIV, while serums for other of the serologic types are being developed. In Massachusetts therapeutic horse antiserums prepared by the State Department of Public Health Antitoxin and Vaccine Laboratory are available for Type I, II, V, VII, and VIII infections. In New York State, the Division of Laboratories and Research, New York State Department of Health, distributes antiserums against pneumococci of these same types (947) and the manufacture of serums against some additional types is under way. Serums for many of these and at times for certain additional types as well are now also generally avail-

* The potency of rabbit antipneumococcic serum for types other than Types I, II, V, VII, and VIII is, however, determined at times by antibody-nitrogen tests, see pages 874–875.

† These regulations and specifications are altered from time to time as advancing knowledge and necessity dictate. Information concerning them may be obtained by inquiry of the Director, National Institute of Health, Washington, D.C.

able in many other states in the country and in several cities, such as New York City. In Massachusetts, New York State, New York City, and Michigan these serums are provided free to all needing them. Similar provision has been or is being made in a number of other localities in the United States (see page 930).

Favorable results with antiserums for Types I, II, and certain of the higher types make it desirable that specific serums be made available for trial against other higher types. In view of the low incidence and considerable and unpredictable yearly variation in frequency of the less common types, there is difficulty in providing the relatively small amounts of an expensive product for an uncertain demand. Possibly the introduction of rabbit antiserums will assist in helping solve this problem.

Test for Chill-Producing Substances

One of the undesirable and troublesome features of present-day antipneumococcic serum is the property exhibited by some lots to cause chills or thermal reactions when administered to patients intravenously. The intravenous injection of any one of a large number of substances is liable to give rise to a reaction of this nature (1417). Felton and Kauffmann (411, 410, 429) have studied the factors in serum assumed to give rise to chills following the use of concentrated antipneumococcic horse serum. Such factors as denaturation of the protein constituents of the serum, its physical state, the presence in it of a so-called acid fraction which may be precipitated out of solution by suitable means have been considered the usual cause. The material obtained by acid precipitation is a phosphorus-containing lipoid substance. At times, however, serums with the acid fraction removed may continue to produce chill reactions and the identity of the chill-producing factor must be regarded as unknown.

Several schemes have been tried for the identification of lots of serum that are likely to cause chill reactions. Bullowa, Rosenblüth, and Merkin (194) studied the circulating leucocytes of patients receiving injections of concentrated horse antiserum to see if any characteristic changes appeared in these cells which would allow them to identify chill-producing lots. Their efforts were unsuccessful.

Sabin and Wallace (1154) injected the serum intravenously into dogs. They considered it was possible in this way to determine whether or not a lot of serum was likely to give rise to chill reactions when used in man. If the temperature of the dog rose 1.5° F. or more after receiving the serum the reaction was considered positive regardless of whether or not a chill occurred. This method of testing serum has not been widely used.

The subsequent test designed by Barnes and Kramer (75), consisting in the intravenous injection of monkeys with varying amounts of the serum under examination, has been extensively employed in the preparation of suitable concentrated horse antiserums for use in the Massachusetts Pneumonia Study and Continuing Program (76, 615). It was demonstrated that serum known to produce chills or thermal reactions in patients gave rise to a more or less similar response in monkeys, typical reactions being characterized by a sudden elevation of the temperature, often of several degrees, and a shaking chill of some severity. Both the chill and the temperature rise are variable, as in man. The monkey test for the chill-producing properties of serum has been routinely used in Massachusetts in recent years and the results suggest that it has been of value in detecting those lots of serum likely to cause severe reactions in patients. Such lots are withheld from distribution and are reprocessed in an effort to render them bland.

It is apparent, however, that lots of serum causing no chills in monkeys may not prove completely chill-free when used in patients. Nevertheless, patients treated with such serums appear to have fewer chills than others and when these occur they have been comparatively mild. Barnes and Robinson (76) demonstrated a 50 per cent reduction in the incidence of chills in patients treated with serums causing no chills in monkeys. Inasmuch as this test is not always readily carried out or easily interpreted, it is the practice of many manufacturers to submit a few samples of each lot of serum prepared for clinical trial and only when the serum is found to be bland in its physiologic action is the remainder of the lot approved for distribution.

It may also be mentioned that most lots of concentrated horse antiserums prepared appear largely free of chill-producing properties and that with added experience the quality of the product has greatly improved. The tendency to produce chill reactions does not lie wholly within the serum itself, for the patient also is a factor. Some patients will have a chill reaction after the injection of serum which produces no such reaction in other patients.

It is desirable that additional studies of the matter of chill-producing substances be made, and that either methods of producing chill-free antiserum be devised or a simple reliable test for detecting lots of serum likely to give rise to chill reactions on intravenous administration be developed (615). A method designed to detect lots of immune rabbit serum likely to produce thermal reactions is considered below (see page 875).

Antibodies in Immune Serum and Probable Mode of Action

Following their suitable immunization with pneumococci, the serum of animals contains varying amounts of antibodies having numerous actions chiefly of a type-specific nature. Under such circumstances agglutinins, precipitins, opsonins, and bactericidins have been demonstrated, as well as substances having protective, curative, neutralizing, and immobilizing properties and the power to cause significant alterations in the biologic characteristics of virulent pneumococci grown in contact with them. These findings, as well as the role of specific antibodies in acquired immunity and the curative power of immune serum in both animals and man, are described in general throughout Chapter IV (page 113) and in particular in the sections of that chapter associated with the discussion of the passive transfer of immunity to the pneumococcus (pages 168–171). In the same chapter it may be seen that the action of specific antipneumococcic serum is primarily antibacterial. The demonstrable antibodies effective in pneumococcus immunity are those reactive with the surface antigen of the organism and their actions may be specifically inhibited by the presence of specific capsular polysaccharide of homologous type (see page 131). This latter substance is of great importance because it is able, even in high dilution, to combine with antibody of homologous type so as to render it ineffective and to impair and retard the development of immunity, thus opposing the defense mechanism of the patient (see also pages 729–735).

SELECTION OF CASES FOR SERUM TREATMENT

In using serum for the treatment of pneumococcus pneumonia, consideration must be given to the severity and extent of the infection present, the time after onset at which such treatment is begun, and the general condition of the patient. Descriptions of the clinical use of specific antipneumococcic serums in pneumonia have been published in convenient handbook form by Lord and Heffron (813, 814), from which much of the following discussion is taken.

The stage of illness at which treatment is instituted is of great significance. Experiments in animals, particularly those of Cecil and Blake (233) in monkeys, Goodner (531, 532) in rabbits, and Petrie and Morgan (1018) in mice, indicate that with pneumococcus Type I infections the earlier serum treatment is begun, the better the chances of recovery and the smaller the doses of serum required to check the invasion of the blood stream by the infecting organisms. In highly susceptible animals there is a time limit beyond which serum therapy is ineffective in saving the life of the animal (531, 532, 1018, 377). Petrie and Morgan (1018) found that the dose of immune serum adequate to cure mice twelve hours after infection had to be approximately *one hundred times larger* to bring about recovery if given *three hours later*.

In man as in experimental animals the fatality rate rises rapidly with the lapse of time between the onset of the illness and the beginning of specific treatment (see pages 894–897). This is because delay in beginning treatment gives time for bacteriemia to develop, for large amounts of specific capsular polysaccharide (SSS) to accumulate, for consolidation to become maximal, and for the disease to become so severe that the essential tissues of the body are damaged by toxemia and possibly anoxemia.

In the Pneumonia Study and Continuing Program in Massachusetts (869) the distribution of antipneumococcic serum by the State Department of Public Health was restricted to physicians who certified that the patient had not been ill longer than four days (ninety-six hours). Limitation of the use of antiserum to this period seemed justifiable at the time in the absence of definite evidence of benefit after this period and accomplished the double purpose of conserving an expensive product, the supply of which was limited, and of emphasizing the importance of early treatment. Evidence has accumulated, however, which indicates that no time limit can be set beyond which serum is ineffective and that in consequence patients should not be deprived of the benefit of specific treatment even though it is begun late in the course of the illness (see pages 896–897). As a result, the restriction by the Massachusetts Department of Public Health of the use of antiserums to patients who had not been ill longer than four days was removed in March 1937 (249).

In Massachusetts antipneumococcic horse serums are now available from the State Department of Public Health to physicians, provided that:

1. Sputum or other material from the patient is first typed and found to contain Type I, Type II, or other type of pneumococcus for which a specific serum is available;

2. As soon as the patient is discharged the physician agrees to send a record of the case to the State Department of Public Health on a form enclosed with the serum.

Pneumococcus pneumonia must always be regarded as serious. The importance of treating apparently mild cases is well recognized, for in such cases there may be a rapid or gradual transition from a condition of apparent safety to one of great gravity. In consequence, it is desirable to treat all cases at the earliest possible moment, for otherwise life may be unnecessarily lost.

Specific serums for many types of pneumococci are now available. Their value, however, varies somewhat with the different types. Specific serum is known to be effective against Type I and Type II pneumococcus pneumonia, but the results are more satisfactory against Type I than Type II. No favorable effects with specific horse antiserum have been obtained against Type III. There is as yet less information regarding the merits of antipneumococcic serum in the treatment of the higher types. As these types less commonly cause pneumonia than Types I and II, some time will be required for the accumulation of the needed evidence. Even so, sufficient data are already available to suggest that specific treatment for Types V and VII is of value. The results are promising for Types VIII and XIV as well, although the findings are less definite for the latter than for the former type (see pages 903–906).

As pneumococci of many types for which specific antiserums are available may cause pneumonia, it is necessary to carry out bacteriologic diagnosis and the typing of any pneumococci found (see pages 620–644) prior to beginning serum therapy, in order to know which is the proper serum to use. The importance of early therapy, together with the fact that more than 50 per cent of all cases of lobar pneumonia are caused by pneumococci of Types I and II (see Table 5, page 46), has naturally raised the question of the desirability of treating all cases of lobar pneumonia with bivalent Type I and II antiserum without waiting for typing to be carried out (991, 245, 258, 326, 104, 661, 611, 614, 813). To do so, however, is to subject nearly one-half of the patients to the possibility of untoward reactions from the alien serum and to needless expense (297, 446, 557, 340, 813, 814). With the development and widespread use of the rapid Neufeld method of typing it is usually possible to obtain a diagnosis of type within a few minutes after the sputum reaches the laboratory and the time element may be largely disregarded. Facilities for typing can and should be made easy of access and generally available through the laboratories of hospitals and departments of health. Now that antiserums are obtainable for a number of the higher types, which are not uncommon in bronchopneumonia as well as in lobar pneumonia, the distinction between lobar pneumonia and bronchopneumonia is immaterial from the point of view of specific treatment. It is essential, of course, to determine the type of infection in all cases to be treated.

Specific serum has been little used thus far in the treatment of pneumococcus pneumonia in children. It is usually difficult to obtain sputum for typing from children under twelve years of age (see also pages 617–618). Owing to the low fatality rate, the small size of the veins, the difficulty of making repeated intravenous injections, and the lack of any conclusive results thus far obtained, the specific treatment of children is generally not attempted. Nevertheless the findings of Nemir (930), Kereszturi and Hauptmann (710), Webster (1394), and Bullowa (190) suggest that in some instances satisfactory results may be obtained in infants and children. The most obvious beneficial results have followed the treatment of Type I or Type XIV cases in such patients. Pneumococci of these two types are especially common in the pneumonias of infants and children (see pages 74–89). Consideration of the results of specific serum treatment on the children's wards of the Bellevue Hospital, New York City, led Smith (1212) to conclude that such treatment will be more commonly used for children in the future. Although serum treatment may be difficult to carry out, there is no apparent reason why these patients should be denied the benefits of specific therapy; and in the presence of severe infections, and especially when bacteriemia is demonstrated, specific serum treatment would seem advisable (190, 814).

CONTRAINDICATIONS TO SERUM TREATMENT

Patients already in a desperate state of illness with such serious manifestations as ashy cyanosis, cold, clammy skin, rapid thready pulse, and low blood pressure, and those in stupor or coma should not be given serum therapy. Such patients are likely to die before adequate dosage can be given, and even a mild reaction from an alien serum may hasten the fatal termination (176, 444, 446, 1051, 813, 814). An illness of such severity is seldom encountered within the first few days. Age, regardless of its extremes, is not a contraindication to serum treatment, although it is advisable to proceed cautiously in elderly patients. Patients eighty years of age and over may be successfully treated under such circumstances.

Cecil and Sutliff (245) have successfully treated patients having cardiac decompensation and pneumonia with specific serum but advise the use of great caution on such occasions. Finland (444, 446) also recommends caution in the treatment of patients having an irregular pulse and a low blood pressure. In such cases smaller doses than usual should be employed and these given very slowly at longer intervals than usual.

It is important to exclude from treatment patients to whom, in consequence of a natural or acquired sensitiveness, the administration of serum may be dangerous. This precaution applies not only to the serum treatment of pneumonia, but also to the treatment of any disease in which the therapeutic serum is derived from an alien species. A more extensive discussion of this matter is given in the following section on precautions against sensitivity.

A summary listing circumstances under which the use of serum may be hazardous is shown on page 842.

PRECAUTIONS AGAINST SENSITIVITY TO HORSE SERUM

Certain precautions are necessary as a means of avoiding the administration of serum to sensitive patients. The precautions relating to the use of horse serum are considered here and those desirable in the use of rabbit serum are presented later (see page 875).

Undue apprehension regarding the hazard of the intravenous injection of horse serum has often needlessly deprived patients of the benefits of specific treatment. Though the intravenous injection of this alien serum is attended with more risk than administration by other routes, the danger is in fact small. As noted in the section on serum reactions below (see page 863), death has occurred in a few patients as a consequence of its use. Of the six deaths (0.3 per cent) occurring among 1,755 patients in the Massachusetts Pneumonia Series* (869, 814) three were attributed to allergic reactions and three to thermal reactions.† Death from reactions occurred in 8 (0.2 per cent) of 3,250 of Bullowa's (190) cases in adults and in 2 (1 per cent) of his 205 cases in children. Methods of guarding against thermal reactions are discussed elsewhere (see page 869). The precautions against the use of horse serum in sensitive patients are considered here.

Reactions of an allergic nature are unrelated to the curative properties of specific immune horse serum. They are due to the parenteral introduction of substances common to the horse and at times toxic for man. Separation of the antibodies from these substances does not seem possible with present knowledge, and reactions can be prevented only by excluding from treatment patients who are sensitive to horse serum. Methods for the recognition of sensitiveness fall short of perfection and untoward reactions are ap-

* The instructions distributed with the serum dispensed by the Antitoxin and Vaccine Laboratory of the Massachusetts Department of Public Health relating to the precautions advisable in the use of serums may be seen in Appendix A, page 940.

† It is not always possible to make a distinction between allergic and thermal reactions. For the sake of completeness these cases are mentioned here and are referred to in more detail in the section on reactions (see pages 865 and 868).

parently unavoidable in a small proportion of cases (986, 1372, 24, 1316, 557, 813, 814). It may be mentioned that numerous British workers (24, 557) and Toomey (1316) in this country are highly skeptical of the value of any of the ordinary tests for sensitiveness to serum. Where there is doubt regarding the advisability of using serum on account of possible sensitiveness, a consultation is desirable to share the responsibility. General discussions of sensitiveness and the relation of it to the use of serum have been presented by numerous workers (936, 802, 316, 1220, 986, 842, 1056, 1372, 1316, 1140, 403).

There are three known groups of patients to whom the administration of horse serum may be dangerous. Patients in these groups may be allergic to horse serum in varying degree. The first and most hazardous includes spontaneously sensitive individuals, usually those subject to asthma or hay fever. The second and less hazardous comprises those who have had a previous injection of horse serum. There is a third group of those whose history is apparently negative both for allergic diseases and the previous administration of horse serum, but who may have undiscovered sensitivity to the serum. The only means of detecting sensitiveness in this group before the intravenous injection of serum is by the use of the skin or eye test or both.

There are, therefore, two precautions which should invariably be taken before serum is given. First, the history of the patient in relation to allergic manifestations should be ascertained and second, he should be tested for sensitivity to horse serum by means of the eye or skin test or both.

History

Patients should be asked whether they have had asthma or hay fever. Special inquiry should be made concerning the occurrence of asthma or vasomotor rhinitis under exposure to emanations from horses. Clinical and experimental data indicate that sensitiveness to horse dander may be combined with sensitiveness to horse serum. An affirmative reply with respect to sensitiveness to emanations from horses places the patient in the class of those to whom the administration of horse serum is known to be dangerous, and it seems best to exclude such patients from specific treatment. Antipneumococcic serum has, nevertheless, been given in spite of a history of horse asthma. Alexander (8) successfully treated three patients with such a history, although considerable difficulty was encountered and asthma of menacing severity was induced by the injections.

With a history of asthma or hay fever unrelated to horses the contraindication is less clear. In the course of the Pneumonia Study and Continuing Program in Massachusetts, at least fifteen patients with a history of asthma and two with a history of hay fever were treated without unfavorable reactions. It has not been established that an increased hazard results from the injection of horse serum into patients with a family history of asthma or hay fever or a personal or family history of such other diseases of allergy as eczema, urticaria apart from serum sickness, and angioneurotic edema. There is a tendency for allergic conditions to run through various members of succeeding generations of a family (965). In view of the possibility of increased risk for patients in this group, it is desirable to observe special precautions. Both the skin and the eye test should be made and serum not given unless the tests are negative. Further, if serum is given, epinephrine (adrenalin solution) should first be injected (see page 841). The initial dose of serum should be smaller and injected more slowly than usual.

Inquiry should also be made concerning any previous administration of serums such as diphtheria, tetanus, or other antitoxin, antimeningococcic or antipneumococcic serum, or diphtheria toxin-antitoxin mixture. It is important to appreciate in this connection that diphtheria toxoid contains no horse serum. Diphtheria toxin-antitoxin mixture contains a small amount of horse serum, and in communities where this method of immunization is used, nearly a third of the children show skin sensitivity to horse serum. Park (986) and Mackenzie and Hanger (842) note, however, that such sensitivity is usually of a mild nature. Tuft (1325) finds that a positive skin test is more likely to be present in children with a family or personal history of asthma or hay fever. Care must be taken that the history obtained is reliable, and in the case of patients who are very ill, or of children, it may be necessary to question other members of the family. The distinction between serum and vaccine is often not understood. Previous vaccine treatments are not of importance with respect to sensitivity to serum.

Some importance attaches to the incubation period of sensitiveness following the administration of horse serum. A first injection of such serum ordinarily causes no immediate symptoms, and injections can be repeated for from seven to ten days without danger. After this interval which serves as an incubation period, sensitiveness to serum develops and serum disease may appear (see page 869). Repetition of intravenous injections after seven to ten days from the time of giving the first dose, or in the presence of serum disease, may be dangerous and should not be attempted. During serum disease the skin test is frequently negative, but usually becomes positive after its termination and may remain so for a variable number of years.

The previous administration of horse serum gives rise to sensitiveness which is greater in degree the larger the amount of the initial injections, but which is less dangerous than spontaneous sensitiveness in such allergic diseases as asthma and hay fever, and diminishes with the lapse of time. Sensitiveness to horse serum is, in general, of maximum intensity during the first two or three months, and repetition of the injection during this period is likely to be followed by severe immediate general reactions and even death (see pages 842 and 865). Should a second attack of pneumonia occur or meningitis, endocarditis, or peritonitis develop at this time, it is rarely safe to attempt the further administration of serum. Reinjections after this interval are usually followed by the accelerated development of serum disease, and when years have elapsed repetition may be followed by serum disease after the usual incubation period.

Tests for Sensitivity

As a second precaution, in addition to taking the history, all patients should first be tested for sensitivity by the eye (conjunctival) test. As an extra added precaution in certain cases, the skin (intradermal) test should also be used. In patients with a history of allergic diseases or a previous injection of serum, it is desirable to use both tests as an added precaution. Before either test is made, a 1:1,000 dilution of fresh epinephrine (adrenalin chloride solution), together with a serviceable hypodermic syringe and needle, must always be at hand, and before serum treatment is begun the syringe must be filled and ready for immediate use.

Tests for sensitivity are facilitated by having on hand normal horse serum diluted 1:10 with physiologic sodium chloride solution,* to be used in the eye test. It is desirable also to have on hand normal horse serum diluted 1:100 with physiologic sodium chloride solution* for the intracutaneous test. In addition, physiologic saline solution* should be available to be used as a control in the intradermal test.

Eye Test

In performing the eye test, both eyes should first be observed for any evidence of inflammation of the conjunctivae. A drop of diluted or undiluted normal horse serum is then placed in the conjunctival sac of one eye, leaving the other eye as a control. If normal horse serum is not available, some of the serum it is planned to inject may be used in the eye test. A positive reaction

* Provided to physicians by the State Department of Public Health in Massachusetts.

is indicated by the occurrence within thirty minutes of itching, watering, and diffuse reddening of the eye. If this does not occur the test is regarded as negative. Positive reactions are not common (444, 813, 814). When they occur they will usually subside within an hour or two. A drop or two of 1:1,000 epinephrine (adrenalin solution) in the conjunctival sac will control severe reactions. The test is likely to be unsatisfactory in young children, who may wash out the serum by crying.

Skin Test

In making the skin test, if only one syringe is used, a control injection of physiologic salt solution is first made into (not under) the skin of the anterior surface of one forearm in amount sufficient to cause a small white elevation. In a corresponding location on the other arm an equal amount of normal horse serum diluted 1 : 100 with physiologic salt solution is similarly injected. Dilute normal horse serum is used, as concentrated antipneumococcic serum causes positive intradermal tests in a large proportion of patients with (1269) or without pneumonia (804) and is unsuited for the determination of skin sensitivity. Before the injection is made some of the normal horse serum is ejected from the needle to remove any water or saline remaining in the needle. When the test is negative the elevations caused by the injections tend to disappear within a few minutes, but the elevation produced by the serum may subside less quickly than that produced by the saline solution. A positive test is indicated by the appearance within five to twenty minutes of a genuine urticarial wheal with surrounding erythema. Irregular finger-like extensions of the central wheal indicate higher and more dangerous degrees of sensitiveness. The reaction usually subsides within one to two hours.

The performance of the intradermal test is not wholly devoid of danger and in rare instances may be followed by severe general reactions and even death in spontaneously allergic subjects (316). As patients known to be subject to horse asthma or horse vasomotor rhinitis should not be treated with serum, they need not be tested.

Interpretation of Reactions

The evidence furnished by the history and these tests, though not infallible, is the best obtainable with present knowledge. The intradermal test is more sensitive than the eye test, and a mildly positive intradermal test may indicate a degree of sensitivity below the level of clinical importance (1220, 986,

1372, 272, 1140). In rare instances sensitive individuals may fail to react to either test. If the history and both tests are negative, or either of the tests if only one is used, serum may be given, but it is always desirable to have adrenalin ready for injection.

A positive reaction to the eye test is so nearly an absolute contraindication to intravenous serum therapy that serum cannot be given under any circumstances without great risk (1220, 986, 897, 842, 156, 1140, 446, 813, 814, 403). A strongly positive intradermal test is to be regarded as equally significant of danger. A negative eye test with a positive skin test and a history of asthma or hay fever is a contraindication to serum therapy. If the history is negative and reaction to either the eye or the skin test is doubtful and it is nevertheless decided to give serum, a subcutaneous injection of 5 to 15 minims of a 1:1,000 dilution of epinephrine (adrenalin chloride solution) should be given six minutes by the clock before the injection of serum. Atropine has been used under such conditions to block the occurrence of an allergic reaction (1423), and although Hill and Martin (641) consider it to give the best results, Bullowa (190) believes it of little or no value.

Unreliability of Attempted Desensitization

The attempt to "desensitize" sensitive patients is of uncertain value at best and should not be relied upon for the prevention of accidents (1372, 1316, 1140, 403). Waldbott (1372) has collected two deaths occurring after a so-called desensitizing procedure had been carried out and others may be found in the literature. It is desirable, however, to adopt the precautions suggested by animal experiments which may diminish the risk in patients with undiscovered sensitiveness.

General Considerations

Investigations by Besredka (97) show that in sensitized animals a full injection of serum may be tolerated after preliminary small or repeated doses and, among others, Friedberger and Mita (497) and Lewis (778) find that otherwise fatal doses can be given when diluted serum is given slowly. Intravenous injection should, in consequence, be given in divided doses and the initial dose should be small. All injections should be given slowly. Unconcentrated antipneumococcic serum should be diluted with an equal volume of physiologic salt solution. Concentrated serum cannot always be so diluted without the formation of a precipitate.

Neufeld and Händel (936) and Cole (297) have suggested that all patients to be treated should receive a small dose (0.5 to 1.0 cc.) of the specific antiserum subcutaneously for desensitizing purposes an hour or so prior to the first intravenous injection. Longcope (801), however, from his experience with the use of other kinds of serums, found that such a procedure was of little or no use in preventing immediate serum reactions.

SUMMARY: CIRCUMSTANCES UNDER WHICH SERUM TREATMENT MAY BE HAZARDOUS

In considering the administration of antipneumococcic horse serum, it should be appreciated that there are circumstances under which its use may be hazardous. Though these matters are discussed more fully above, principally in a preceding section (page 835), the circumstances under which caution is necessary are grouped in the following outline by the degree of risk involved.

Group I

Horse serum treatment entails more than the usual risk when given:

1. To those with a family or personal history of asthma or hay fever, eczema, urticaria, or angioneurotic edema (pages 837–838);
2. To those who have had a previous administration of horse serum such as diphtheria, tetanus, or other antitoxin, antimeningococcic or antipneumococcic serum or diphtheria toxin-antitoxin mixture (page 838);
3. To those giving a mildly positive reaction to an intradermal test (page 840).

Group II

Horse serum should NOT be given:

1. To those with a history of asthma or vasomotor rhinitis under exposure to emanations from horses (page 837);
2. To those giving a positive reaction to an eye test or a strongly positive reaction to an intradermal test (page 841);
3. To those in extremis (page 835);
4. To those who have received horse serum several days to several months previously. No strictly accurate limits can be placed on this period, but roughly it may be defined as about seven days to three months (pages 838–839).

Group III

Horse serum treatment should be discontinued when:

The patient has a severe, shock-like reaction, an asthmatic attack or urticaria (page 867), or alarming thermal reaction (page 869) following any injection.

ROUTE OF SERUM INJECTION

In nearly all instances the intravenous route is preferable for the administration of specific serum in pneumonia, as was pointed out in 1910 by Neufeld and Händel (937, 938). Such treatment permits the immediate widespread distribution of immune substances within the body, and the maximum beneficial effects are obtained (297, 244, 1075, 61, 245, 195, 813, 1307, 814).

Experiments in animals with various serums have shown that following intratracheal administration the alien serum is only slowly absorbed and does not appear in the blood for three or four hours or more (Jones, 687, 688, Cecil and Steffen, 244). In some instances antibody so administered may never appear in the blood (Rhoades, 1075). Absorption is somewhat more rapid after intraperitoneal injection, though from one-half hour (687, 688) to more than two hours (1075) may be required before the serum or antibodies become demonstrable in the blood. After subcutaneous injection absorption is slow and may require seven to twenty-four hours (Rhoades, 1075), seriously affecting the therapeutic value of specific antibodies, as Cecil and Steffen (244) demonstrated in monkeys with an experimentally induced pneumonia and given Huntoon's antibody solution. The intramuscular and intravenous administration of Type I antipneumococcic serum in rabbits having an intradermal Type I infection was studied by Curphey and Baruch (336). Providing bacteriemia was not marked the curative effects obtained were about the same with either technic. When bacteriemia was heavy, however, the intravenous route of serum administration gave the best results. These investigators considered the evidence sufficient to warrant a careful trial of intramuscular treatment in man.

In persons not having pneumonia Rhoades (1075) found that after the subcutaneous injection of from 250 to 400 cc. of Huntoon's antibody solution protective substance rarely appeared in the blood. In one instance it was present within two hours after serum administration and then only in very small amounts. In similar subjects she also demonstrated that when such a preparation was given by mouth or by rectum no antibody appeared in the blood. Cecil and Sutliff (245) gave an intravenous injection of either whole or concentrated immune serum to eight individuals not having pneumonia and demonstrated the appearance of protective substance in their blood within a period of thirty minutes.

Tilghman and Finland (1307) investigated the appearance of specific antibody in the blood after intravenous, intramuscular, or subcutaneous injection of 20,000 to 30,000 units of Type I or II concentrated antiserum in 21 subjects not having pneumonia or other respiratory infection. Tests for agglutinins and protective substances were made prior to the injections and after them at five-hour, ten-hour, and twenty-four-hour intervals, and at various additional intervals for nearly a month. Their findings indicate that the maximum circulating antibody titers were usually demonstrable at five hours after intravenous injection of antibody, at ten hours after intramuscular injection, and at twenty-four hours after subcutaneous injection. A greater concentration of antibody was attained in the blood more constantly, it appeared more rapidly, and persisted longer after intravenous injection than after intramuscular or subcutaneous injection. The concentration of protective substance in the blood after intravenous injection was usually one hundred or more times that attained after injection by other routes, though in an occasional subject titers nearly as high occurred after intramuscular injection.

The subcutaneous use of Huntoon's antibody solution in man with pneumonia was mentioned earlier (see page 817), and Cecil and Baldwin (229) found this route of administration to give only irregular and feeble therapeutic results. Bullowa and his co-workers (195) note that absorption is slow if concentrated antipneumococcic serum is given under the skin. The intramuscular injection of antiserums in man with pneumonia also delays absorption and reduces the therapeutic effect obtained (61, 195, 897, 1307, 814). Mills (897) considers that intramuscular injection reduces the potency of the serum given by one-half. Bullowa (176) states that although intramuscular injection may be suitable for some cases in adults seen very early in their illness, he always gives serum intravenously.

In infants and children with pneumonia both the intravenous and the intramuscular routes have been used. Nemir (930) usually gave the initial dose intravenously and many of the later ones intramuscularly. The practice of Kereszturi and Hauptmann (710) was very similar. In Type XIV cases in infants and children Bullowa (187) reports that nearly all doses were given intramuscularly. This investigator (190) recommends intramuscular administration in infants with pneumonia and notes that after the injection the site should be massaged. He further cautions, however, that if bacteriemia is present intravenous treatment is usually essential and it may be necessary to cut down on a vein in order to give it. Injection of the serum through a fontanelle should not be tried, as uncontrollable subdural hemorrhage may result. In children over three or four years of age intravenous treatment can usually be carried out without much difficulty.

DOSAGE WITH ANTIPNEUMOCOCCIC HORSE SERUM

General Considerations

So far as the effect on the disease is concerned, the results obtained by the adequate use of unconcentrated serum are identical with those resulting from the similar use of concentrated serum. In general, with either product patients should be treated as early in the course of the disease as possible and it is desirable to give the necessary amount of antibody within as short a time as is consistent with safety. Experience has shown that as a rule treatment carried out persistently whether by day or by night is more successful and requires less serum than treatment interrupted by relatively long intervals (many hours to a day or more). The number of units needed is likely to increase with the lapse of time between the onset of the disease and the inauguration of specific therapy. Other conditions, under which more than the usual amounts of antiserum are advisable, are listed on pages 856 and 858.

In estimating the required dosage, reliance must be placed chiefly on previous observations of the fatality rates in groups of cases which are large enough to make the figures significant and for which the dosage is recorded in standard units or units which it is possible to translate into standard units. Mouse protection tests require too long a time for completion to be of service as a guide to the treatment of any individual patient but may serve to indicate the variability of desirable dosage in different cases. Thus samples of blood taken not less than eight hours after serum treatment may show protection against a million lethal doses in each cubic centimeter of the patient's serum after the injection of as small an amount as 25,000 units of antibody in one case, and yet an equal amount of protection may be absent after the injection of 400,000 units in another (820, 814).

The required dosage, then, varies with a number of factors. In the earlier cases treated with whole immune horse serum, repeated doses of from 50 to 100 cc. each were given, the total amount used averaging from 147 cc. to over 400 cc. per patient (292, 33, 797, 297, 1299, 793, 176). Total doses in the neighborhood of a liter and a half were occasionally used. When first introduced, concentrated serum was used cautiously and doses of about 10,000 units or more three times daily were advised (992, 993). These amounts were soon increased and treated cases commonly received an average of from 50,000 to 500,000 units (195, 991, 245, 176, 442, 897, 238, 326, 990, 820, 1269, 225, 24, 463,

1001, 779, 995, 444, 1272, 446, 557, 447, 1051). The serums used for most if not all the cases treated in the older series were standardized in various ways and without uniformity. In consequence it is usually impossible to interpret the dosage used in the earlier cases in terms of the present-day standard unit and the findings in the earlier cases must be largely disregarded when attempting to arrive at an optimum dosage.

The dosage used in the treatment of the pneumonias in children is considered separately below (see page 852).

Type I Cases

In the Massachusetts Pneumonia Series* 956 cases of pneumococcus Type I lobar pneumonia were treated during the first four days of illness with concentrated horse antiserum of known potency, with 134 deaths (14 per cent). Analysis of these cases (Table 163) by years and by average total dose of serum in cubic centimeters and in standard units† shows fluctuation in the case fatality rate: low rates prevailed during the first three years (1931–1933) and higher rates during the last four years (1934–1937) without any very significant relation to dosage in units. In the series, among the first 459 cases (1931–1935), however, there were 50 deaths, a case fatality rate of 10.9 per cent. In this group each case received an average of 95,327 units in divided doses. Among the last 497 cases there were 84 deaths, or 16.9 per cent, and in this group each case received an average of 80,404 units.

Analysis of the 1936 and 1937 series by Robinson and Philbrook shows that the relatively high fatality rate of the 1937 series (20.5 per cent) as compared with the 1936 series (13.4 per cent), may be more apparent than real, owing to the small number of cases involved. It should also be noted that the 1937 cases include only those for the first half of the year, a period during which more serious infections occur, as elsewhere mentioned (see pages 680–681), and the higher fatality rate for these cases may also in part be seasonal.

The fatality rate in Type I cases given optimum specific treatment is unknown but would no doubt be lower than that of any reported series. In

* In these cases, as in all the Type I and II cases of the Massachusetts series analyzed in the following pages, none is included which during 1931–1935 received less than 16 cc. of serum or during 1936–1937 received less than this amount or less than 20,000 units. See Appendix A, page 938.

† The serums used in the treatment of these Type I cases, and of the Type II cases which follow, were tested either against the standard control serum P 11 or against another serum which was later titrated against a second serum, the potency of which was compared directly with P 11. In consequence, the dosages of the Type I and II Massachusetts cases referred to in the text and shown in Tables 163 and 164 are expressed in standard units (see page 827).

Cole's (302) 462 cases at the Hospital of the Rockefeller Institute for Medical Research, there were 48 deaths, or 10.4 per cent, in the series as a whole. The death rate was 8.2 per cent for cases treated within the first four days, as against 14 per cent in the Massachusetts series, suggesting that the latter received insufficient dosage. Comparison of the two series with respect to age factors cannot be made with the data at hand. Though the average dosage in units in Cole's series is not known, it is likely that it was much larger than in the Massachusetts cases. In his earlier reported series (299) of 371 cases,

TABLE 163. TYPE I LOBAR PNEUMONIA: CASES TREATED WITH SERUM OF KNOWN POTENCY DURING THE FIRST FOUR DAYS OF ILLNESS. DISTRIBUTION BY YEARS OF 956 CASES SHOWING NUMBER AND PERCENTAGE OF DEATHS, AVERAGE DOSE OF SERUM IN CUBIC CENTIMETERS, AND AVERAGE DOSE IN UNITS*

YEAR†	TOTAL CASES	DEATHS		AVERAGE TOTAL DOSE	
		Number	*Per cent*	*In cc.*	*In units‡*
1931	8	–	–	74.8	85,215
1932	78	5	6.4	76.2	61,818
1933	119	10	8.4	82.4	92,407
1934	122	17	13.9	68.1	118,582
1935	132	18	13.6	53.6§	96,881
1936	253	34	13.4	36.5‖	76,108
1937¶	244	50	20.5	36.7	84,858
Total	956	134	14.0	58.8**	87,569

* Cases were taken from the Massachusetts Pneumonia Series.
† Calendar year. ‡ Based on serum P 11 as the standard. § Based on 131 cases.
‖ Based on 252 cases. ¶ Through June 30. ** Based on 954 cases.

each patient received an average of 420 cc. of unconcentrated serum. In his later report (302) concentrated serum is recommended in doses of 15 to 30 cc., or 90,000 units, repeated every four hours until definite results are obtained.

Abernethy (1) treated 25 Type I cases at the Hospital of the Rockefeller Institute for Medical Research with concentrated antiserum of known potency, without a death. The skin test with capsular polysaccharide was used as a control of dosage and serum was administered until the test became positive. The average total dose per patient amounted to 83 cc., or 335,000 units, and it was estimated that 57 cc., or 203,000 units, were necessary for the average uncomplicated case. Nevertheless, no definite conclusion regarding optimum dosage can be based on so small a series.

Finland (448), at the Boston City Hospital, treated 219 cases of Type I pneumococcus pneumonia (lobar pneumonia and bronchopneumonia together) with serum of known potency.* The fatality rate of this group was 18 per cent (40 deaths) as compared with a rate of 39 per cent (113 deaths) for 289 similar cases not given serum. Many of the treated cases of lobar pneumonia in the series are included in the Massachusetts series above. The average total dose in Finland's treated cases was 94 cc., or 147,000 units. The amounts of serum given varied from 5 to 340 cc., or from 4,000 to 1,700,000 units.

It is important that further data on the optimum effective dosage for Type I cases be obtained. It is probable that severe cases due to any type will require a larger total dose of antiserum than mild cases. This fact should be borne in mind in outlining dosage recommendations for use in hospitals where unusually severe cases are encountered, as in the Boston City Hospital (see pages 666, 671, and 675), and in organized pneumonia programs covering cities, counties, and states. There should be sufficient flexibility in such recommendations to take care of both severe and mild cases.

At present in Massachusetts a total of AT LEAST 60,000 units† of antibody divided into three injections at two-hour intervals is recommended for Type I cases as the INITIAL amount. IN EVERY INSTANCE, HOWEVER, SUBSEQUENT ADDITIONAL DOSES SHOULD BE GIVEN AS THE INDIVIDUAL CASE REQUIRES (see page 858). The importance of following treatment through in this manner can hardly be overemphasized.

Type II Cases

In the Massachusetts series, 259 Type II cases were treated with antiserum of known potency during the first four days of illness, with 57 deaths (22 per cent). Analysis of the cases (Table 164) by years, and average dosage in cubic centimeters and in units per case, shows fluctuations in the case fatality rate, higher rates occurring during the first five years (1931–1935) and lower rates during the last two years (1936–1937). It should be noted that the cases for 1937 include only those treated in the first half of the year. Among the first 126 cases there were 31 deaths, a case fatality rate of 24.6 per cent. In this

* The strength of the serums used was stated in units standardized by tests against serum P II.

† This number of units can be obtained in a volume of about 20 to 50 cc. depending on the potency of the individual lot of serum.

group each case received an average of at least 59,700 units in divided doses. Among the last 133 cases there were 26 deaths, or 19.6 per cent, and in this group each case received an average of 123,996 units. The lower fatality rate in the more recent cases may be ascribed to an increase of dosage. As the fatality rate is still high, however, it would seem desirable to give still larger dosage in Type II cases.

TABLE 164. TYPE II LOBAR PNEUMONIA: CASES TREATED WITH SERUM OF KNOWN POTENCY DURING THE FIRST FOUR DAYS OF ILLNESS. DISTRIBUTION BY YEARS OF 259 CASES, SHOWING NUMBER AND PERCENTAGE OF DEATHS, AVERAGE DOSE OF SERUM IN CUBIC CENTIMETERS, AND AVERAGE DOSE IN UNITS

YEAR†	TOTAL CASES	DEATHS		AVERAGE TOTAL DOSE	
		Number	*Per cent*	*In cc.*	*In units‡*
1931	3	–	–	80.0	4,933
1932	14	5	35.7	143.0	26,224
1933	33	7	21.2	127.8	25,280
1934	28	8	28.6	108.1	55,857
1935	48	11	22.9	69.8	98,794
1936	69	13	18.8	80.2	108,720
1937§	64	13	20.3	70.4‖	140,466
Total	259	57	22.0	88.6¶	92,718

Cases were taken from the Massachusetts Pneumonia Series
† Calendar year. ‡ Based on serum P 11 as the standard.
§ Through June 30. ‖ Based on 60 cases. ¶ Based on 255 cases.

Finland and Dowling (452), at the Boston City Hospital, treated a group of cases of Type II pneumococcus pneumonia (lobar pneumonia and bronchopneumonia together) with serum of known potency* and compared the results obtained during 1929–1932 with those during 1932–1935. Many of the treated cases of lobar pneumonia are included in the Massachusetts series above. The fatality rate of 148 untreated cases in Finland and Dowling's series covering the whole period of investigation was 51 per cent (76 died). Of 48 treated cases in the early period of their study 11, or 23 per cent, died and these cases received an average of 169 cc., which was considered to rep-

* The dose in units given these cases was expressed in terms of the standard unit using P 11 as the standard test serum.

resent 453,000 units of antibody. Of 38 cases in the later period of the study 16, or 42 per cent, died and the average total dose used was 145 cc. or 136,000 units. The better results in the early treated cases were attributed to the much larger average dose used in that group (it was about three times the size of the later dose). The difficulties of estimating dosage in many of the early cases in terms of the present standard unit are considerable and the findings reported open to some discussion. Nevertheless, the more adequate treatment given those in the earlier period may be regarded as responsible for the more satisfactory results in this series. The number of cases in both treated series is, however, small.

Further information based on large series of Type II cases is desirable for the purpose of determining the optimum effective dosage.

At present in Massachusetts a total of AT LEAST 100,000 units* of antibody divided into three or more doses at two-hour intervals is recommended in Type II cases as the INITIAL amount. As WITH TYPE I, HOWEVER, IT IS IMPORTANT THAT SUBSEQUENT ADDITIONAL INJECTIONS BE GIVEN AS THE INDIVIDUAL CASE REQUIRES (see page 858). Failure to pursue treatment in the face of an obvious need for it may result in the loss of the patient.

Type V Cases

In the Massachusetts Pneumonia Series there were 17 Type V cases treated with serum of known potency within the first four days of illness, with one death (5.9 per cent). These cases received an average of 101,853 units per case. Of 26 Type V cases treated with antiserum within the first four days of illness by Finland and Tilghman (466) death occurred in 4, or 15 per cent. From their experience they recommend an initial dosage of 60,000 units in patients under thirty years of age, and 100,000 units in those over thirty and in patients during pregnancy and the puerperium. Additional doses of 60,000 to 100,000 units are advised as soon as bacteriemia is demonstrated. Eighty-six Type V cases were treated by Bullowa and Wilcox (199). Nineteen, of whom 11 died, were excluded from their analysis because of inadequate treatment. Of 67 remaining, 5, or 7.5 per cent, died. The dosage was increased during the period of the investigation from an average of 152,000 units to an average of 383,500 units for patients without bacteriemia. Larger amounts were given to bacteriemic patients.

At present in Massachusetts the same dosage is recommended for Type V

* This number of units can be obtained in a volume of about 40 to 100 cc. depending on the potency of the individual lot of serum.

as for Type II cases, namely, AT LEAST 100,000 units in divided doses as the INITIAL amount, with additional injections as the individual case may require (see page 858). The unit of Type V antibody has only recently been standardized, thus rendering all cited dosage recommendations in units tentative.

Type VII, Type VIII, and Type XIV Cases

There were no Type VII, VIII, or XIV cases in the Massachusetts series.* Finland, Tilghman, Ruegsegger, and Dowling (467) treated 30 cases of Type VII pneumococcus pneumonia (lobar pneumonia and bronchopneumonia together) with specific antiserum. In 23 cases, treatment was begun within ninety-six hours of the onset of the illness; in 4 cases early on the fifth day; and in the 3 remaining cases on or after the sixth day. Of the 30 cases, 3, or 10 per cent, died. Among the earlier cases the total initial dose was about 200,000 units given in three injections within a period of four hours. This was later reduced to between 60,000 and 100,000 units with additional dosage, when available, for bacteriemia and when the clinical response to the initial dose was not entirely satisfactory. Their experience suggested that doses of 80,000 to 100,000 units are adequate for most uncomplicated cases if the blood is sterile before treatment, and that twice that amount is probably required in cases with bacteriemia and possibly also in those whose pulmonary lesion has extended before treatment.

Benjamin, Blankenhorn, Ruegsegger, and Senior (94) treated 18 cases of Type VII lobar pneumonia within the first four days of illness with no deaths. These cases all received at least 60,000 to 80,000 units of antibody.

A number of cases of Type VIII pneumococcus pneumonia (lobar pneumonia and bronchopneumonia together) were treated by Bullowa (184, 186). Of 37 treated cases only 2, or 5.4 per cent, died. The average dose was in the neighborhood of 50,000 to 70,000 units per patient. Benjamin and his associates (94) treated 8 cases of Type VIII lobar pneumonia in the first four days of illness with no deaths. These patients all received at least 60,000 to 80,000 units of serum.

Bullowa (187) reports treating six cases of Type XIV pneumococcus pneumonia (lobar pneumonia and bronchopneumonia together) in adults, with 2 deaths, or 33 per cent. The total doses used in this series varied from

* Type VII and Type VIII serum was first dispensed by the Department of Public Health in Massachusetts in 1938. An initial dosage of at least 60,000 to 90,000 units is recommended in Type VII cases and of at least 100,000 units in Type VIII cases. See Appendix A, page 943. It is probable that serum for Type XIV cases will be dispensed at a later date.

15,000 to 235,000 units. More would probably have been given had additional serum been available in some instances.

In summary, it may be stated that in uncomplicated Type VII, VIII, and XIV cases an INITIAL dosage of AT LEAST 60,000 to 100,000 units may be used. As the standardization of serums for Types VII and VIII (as well as for Type V) mentioned earlier (page 828), is a recent development, and as no standard has yet been adopted for any other of the higher types, the present dosage recommendations for cases due to any of these types may be modified by later experience.

Favorable results in the use of specific antiserum against Types I, II, V, VII, and VIII justify the hope of successful treatment of many other types. Serum for experimental trial should be made available for these types as soon as possible. Meanwhile every effort should be made to collect large series of cases of pneumonia due to the higher types to serve as satisfactory controls of serum treated cases. Comparative studies of serum treated and control cases will be necessary before the merit of this extension of the method can be determined.

Dosage for Infants and Children

Relatively little information is available relating to the serum treatment of children and the dosage used. Some data, however, have been reported which have a bearing on this matter. Nemir (930) treated a number of cases of both lobar pneumonia and bronchopneumonia in infants and children having Type I, II, IV, V, VI, VII, XIV, XV, XVIII, XIX, or XXII infections. The number of cases due to each type was small. In a grand total of 81 such cases treated 8, or 9.8 per cent, died, while death occurred in 16.6 per cent, or 20, of 120 similar untreated cases. The dose of specific serum used was approximately 300 to 800 units per pound of body weight, varying in relation to the severity of the disease. The average dosage for twenty-four hours was generally from 6 to 9 cc. for an infant and from 15 to 25 cc. for a child. A total of three or four doses was frequently sufficient and never more than seven were given.

A study similar to this was made by Kereszturi and Hauptmann (710), who used specific serum for eight different types for cases of pneumococcus pneumonia. The results were indifferent, however, as the fatality rate of 32 treated cases was 9 per cent, as compared with a rate of 7 per cent for 28 control cases. Efforts were made to give approximately 1,000 units per pound of body weight per day to children over two years of age, and 2,000 units per pound of body weight per day to infants.

Bullowa (187) treated a number of infants and children with Type XIV pneumonia (lobar pneumonia and bronchopneumonia together). In 15 cases death occurred in one, or 7 per cent. Most patients received a total of from 10,000 to 50,000 units of antibody, though occasionally larger amounts were given.

Plan of Treatment

As concentrated antiserums are now generally used, the following discussion will be concerned chiefly with their administration. The technic of giving unconcentrated antiserum is described separately below (see page 862).

In adults, and wherever possible in children, all doses of antipneumococcic serum are given intravenously. The usual equipment needed for administering concentrated serum is listed as follows, and shown in the accompanying illustration (Figure 11).

Equipment for Testing Sensitiveness and Administration of Serum

For testing sensitiveness:

1. Before either test is made, a 1:1,000 dilution of fresh epinephrine (adrenalin chloride solution) and a serviceable hypodermic syringe and needle should be at hand;
2. For the eye test, antipneumococcic serum or diluted* or undiluted normal horse serum are required (page 839);
3. For the skin test, a 1:100 dilution of normal horse serum in physiologic saline,* physiologic saline* for the control, a tuberculin syringe and a fine needle (gauge 26) are needed (page 840).

For serum treatment:

1. Fresh epinephrine (adrenalin chloride solution) in 1:1,000 dilution in a syringe ready for administration in case of an allergic reaction;
2. Warm antipneumococcic serum;
3. A 2 cc. syringe for the first injection of serum and a 10 and 20 cc. syringe or two 20 cc. syringes with appropriate needles for subsequent injections of serum;
4. Physiologic saline solution for rinsing the syringes if they have been sterilized by boiling;
5. Alcohol and iodine for disinfecting the skin over the vein;
6. A tourniquet;
7. Material for taking a blood culture.

* These solutions are provided by the State Department of Public Health in Massachusetts and dispensed with the serum.

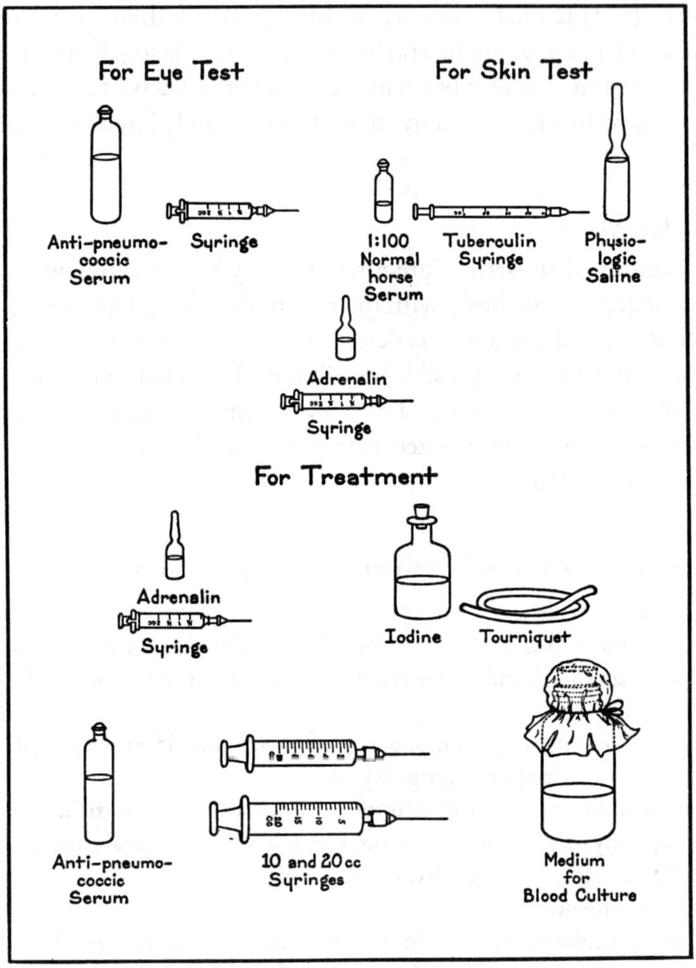

Figure 11. Equipment for testing sensitiveness and serum administration

In all cases experience has shown the advisability of beginning serum treatment cautiously. The required antiserum should never be given in one dose but always in divided doses. The initial dose is a test injection and should consist of only a small amount of serum given very slowly to guard against the possibility of a reaction in a patient with undiscovered sensitiveness. An interval of two hours is allowed to elapse between doses, as reactions, if they occur, are likely to take place within this period.

Blood culture medium should be a part of the equipment. The importance of obtaining a blood culture previous to the first injection of serum and as occasion may require during the course of treatment should be more generally appreciated. Extraordinarily high fatality rates obtain in bacteriemic cases not given serum (see pages 681–693) and in those inadequately treated.

FAILURE TO DETERMINE THE PRESENCE OF BACTERIEMIA IN SERUM TREATED CASES DEPRIVES THE PHYSICIAN OF ONE OF THE MOST IMPORTANT GUIDES FOR DOSAGE. Provision should be made to supply culture medium and facilities for the bacteriologic investigation of cultures. The desirability of making such provision on a large scale is suggested by the experience in Massachusetts, where blood cultures were taken in only 635, or 47.4 per cent, of 1,341 Type I, II, or V cases of lobar pneumonia. There is reason to believe that had such cultures been made in practically every case and the larger amounts of serum needed been given routinely to bacteriemic patients, the fatality rate of the treated cases would have been considerably lower than that actually obtained (see pages 912–916).

With the patient in a hospital and the laboratory at hand, culture medium in cotton-plugged flasks can be utilized. For use in the home, to avoid contamination in transit, fluid culture medium in bottles should be generally available at such typing stations as are approved for blood culture examination (see also page 618). This provision is now made in Massachusetts.

Before the administration of serum, care should be taken to see that it is of the proper type and to note the lot number and the potency recorded on the label of the vial. The serum should be warmed before injection by placing the vials in water at about body temperature. If the water is too hot, the serum will coagulate and be unfit for use. Concentrated antipneumococcic serum should not be diluted with water, as the resulting precipitate may incite a chill reaction. The syringes and needles should, therefore, be dry sterilized or sterilized by boiling and then either dried or rinsed with sterile saline solution. Some manufacturers provide serum in syringe vials ready for immediate use.

Initial Dosage

It is impossible to lay down any schedule of dosage which will apply to every case. It is important to remember that successful serum therapy is chiefly dependent on early and adequate specific treatment. Delay may entail the costly and time-consuming administration of extra doses of serum and the risk of losing the patient.

At present in Massachusetts* it is recommended, subject to the precautions previously outlined (pages 836–842), that patients with Type I pneumococcus pneumonia be given an INITIAL DOSAGE of at least 60,000 units, those with Type VII at least 60,000–90,000 units, and those with Type II, V, or VIII infections at least 100,000 units.

Until further evidence is available an INITIAL DOSAGE of at least 60,000 to 100,000 units in Type VII, VIII, and XIV cases is advised. Doubtless a similar recommendation would serve to initiate treatment in cases due to any other of the higher types as well.

In every case this initial dosage should be AT LEAST DOUBLED if

1. Treatment is begun after the third day of the disease;
2. The patient is over forty years of age;
3. The patient is pregnant or in the first week of the puerperium;
4. There is involvement of more than one lobe;
5. Pneumococcus bacteriemia is known to be present.

Recommendations very similar to these have been made by other workers (452, 448, 190).

It also seems likely, in view of the nearly doubled fatality rate of cases occurring in the late winter and early spring months, as compared with those occurring at other times (see pages 679–681), that the usual initial dosage employed should be at least doubled in treating cases occurring in the former period of the year.

Doses totaling 300,000 to 400,000 units or more may be necessary at times.† In pregnancy and immediately following delivery, in view of the high death rate from pneumococcus pneumonia, doses totaling about 400,000 to 500,000 units are often required.

Technic of Treatment

The injections are usually most easily made into a vein in the cubital space, but any vein may be used. The overlying skin is cleansed with alcohol and painted with tincture of iodine and a tourniquet applied to the upper arm.

The first blood culture is made at this time. The needle of an empty syringe is inserted into a vein and 5 to 10 cc. or more of blood withdrawn for

* In the New York State Pneumonia Control Program, the minimum dosage recommended for Type I cases is 100,000 units and for Type II, 160,000 units (235).

† The prozone phenomenon such as occurs with the use of large doses of horse antiserum in mouse protection tests (see page 121) has never been demonstrated to occur in man following the administration of large doses.

the culture (see also page 618). The tourniquet is released, the syringe disconnected, leaving the needle in the vein, and the blood is ejected into a flask containing 50 cc. or more of sterile bouillon. Agar pour-plate cultures may also be made at this time. Before any injection of serum it is well to be sure that the needle is securely in place in the vein by the withdrawal of a small amount of blood into the syringe. Serum which perchance escapes into the perivascular tissues during the injection is harmless.

The following suggestions are made with respect to the initial course of injections of concentrated serum:

The customary first dose is 2 cc. of the warmed serum. A small syringe is attached to the needle still in place in the vein and the injection begun. The serum should be injected with extreme slowness at a rate not to exceed one cubic centimeter per minute by the watch.

Following the first dose an interval of about two hours is allowed to elapse and a second dose consisting of the remainder of the first vial (about 8 to 13 cc. depending upon the volume of serum in the vial) is given during a period of five to ten minutes.

After a further delay of two hours, the contents of two vials are given.

The volume of serum and the number of units in the three vials thus far administered will depend on the amount in the vials and the potency of the serum. If the volume is 30 cc. and the potency 2,000 units per cubic centimeter, 60,000 units will have been given; or if each of the three vials used contained 20,000 units, 60,000 units will have been injected.

For the fourth and subsequent injections, if these are necessary, the contents of three or more vials may be given as the individual case may require.

In the course of treatment it seems best that no single injection exceed 50 cc. in volume.

Where commercially prepared serum in syringe vials is used it is customary to administer 10,000 units as the initial dose. While the volume of serum comprising this dose varies somewhat from lot to lot, it is often less than 5 cc. Following this dose after an interval of two hours, a second dose, consisting of 20,000 units (about 8 to 13 cc. depending on the potency of the serum), is given. After a further delay of two hours the contents of two 20,000 unit vials or of one vial of this size and one of the 10,000 unit size is given. In this fashion an initial dosage of 60,000 to 70,000 units is achieved. Subsequent doses in multiples of 10,000 units totaling from this amount up to 60,000 units or more may be injected for the fourth and additional doses if necessary. It is advisable that no single dose exceed 50 cc. in volume.

As therapeutic antipneumococcic serums are likely to vary in amount per vial and potency, the volume of the serum which must be given to obtain the desired dosage should be determined from information furnished by the manufacturer with respect to the particular lot in question.

A schematic presentation of the usual procedures undertaken in the course of initiating serum therapy is shown in Figure 12.

After initiating treatment the clinical response of the patient is observed. For several hours after the administration of the INITIAL DOSAGE of antiserum, no change is likely to be apparent, but within eight to twenty-four hours there may be a marked improvement. The favorable response is usually more pronounced with Type I than with Type II infection. The temperature falls, the pulse rate is lower, the toxemia lessens, the area of consolidation ordinarily ceases to extend, and a previously positive blood culture may become negative. In a majority of the early treated cases following the initial dosage recommended, there is a fall of two, three, or more degrees in temperature, beginning eight or more hours after treatment is begun.

Patients treated early in the course of the disease may not require additional antiserum. The additional dosage which may be necessary cannot be definitely stated and must be determined in each case. The behavior of the temperature and pulse and the results of blood cultures are important guides for the administration of more serum.

If the first blood culture is positive or if progress is unsatisfactory, it is important to continue to take blood cultures at intervals of twenty-four hours or more often.

Additional Dosage and Guides to Subsequent Treatment

Additional individual doses of 40,000 to 60,000 units are recommended at intervals of every three to four hours in severe cases, and in any case if

1. The temperature does not fall below 102° F. by rectum within eighteen hours of beginning serum treatment, or if
2. Having fallen below 102° F. by rectum it again rises above this level, or if
3. Bacteriemia is demonstrated by blood culture, regardless of the clinical course, or if
4. There is evidence of a spreading lesion.

Adherence to the above recommendations regarding amounts of the initial dosage and the use of additional doses as indicated is known to yield good results. Failure to adhere to such recommendations contributes to in-

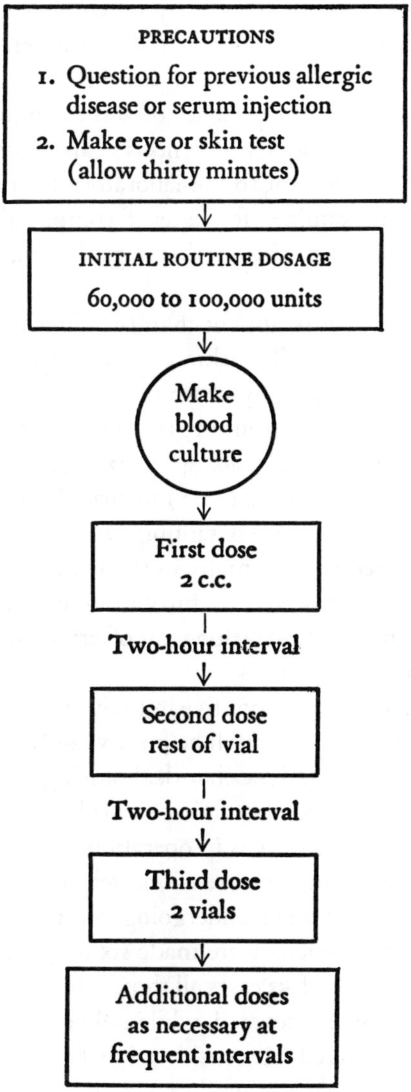

Figure 12. Usual procedures undertaken in the course of initiating serum therapy

different results, as experience has clearly shown. The general tendency of most physicians is to use too little serum in the treatment of individual cases.

Failure to improve after the serum has been given PERSISTENTLY for seventy-two hours suggests the presence of some complication, such as empyema. A mistake in bacteriologic diagnosis is also possible. Another specimen of sputum should be sent to the laboratory for typing, blood culture taken, and the patient examined for signs of complications. A mixed infection or a successive infection with another organism may be responsible (see pages 11–16).

More reliable guides for treatment than the clinical aspects are desirable but are not as yet available. The skin test with specific capsular polysaccharide of homologous type may prove of value. The use of this test was mentioned earlier (see pages 166 and 170), and its merit has been considered by numerous workers (1311, 485, 486, 459, 477, 12, 444, 1, 448). The test was introduced by Tillett and Francis (1311) in 1929. In the performance of the test 0.1 cc. of a saline dilution containing 0.01 mgm. of specific capsular carbohydrate is injected intradermally in the usual manner and the site of the injection observed for twenty to thirty minutes. The test is regarded as positive in the presence of the development of erythema, edema, wheal, and pseudopodia (477).

Though the explanation of a positive test with this substance is uncertain, it has been assumed that the test will be positive only in consequence of the interaction of type-specific polysaccharide, homologous antibody, and tissue activity. To demonstrate activity of tissue cells by this means may indicate that the mechanism for recovery is in operation.

Francis (477) studied the occurrence of reactions of this nature in patients with Type I pneumonia undergoing specific unconcentrated horse antiserum treatment. The tests were made six to eight hours following the administration of serum. Of 53 cases all those who developed a positive skin reaction to SSS (45 cases) recovered, while only one of those with negative reactions (8 cases) recovered. He considered that a positive reaction in serum treated cases predicates recovery, while a negative test calls for further serum therapy. Finland and Sutliff (460), however, observed a positive skin test with the homologous SSS in a patient treated with concentrated serum who died. They also made a similar observation in a patient treated with specific human convalescent serum (see page 813). Nevertheless, positive skin reactions were usually followed by recovery and negative reactions by death. In addition, these workers note that in two patients (Type I, and Type II pneumonia) treated with concentrated horse antiserum positive skin reactions occurred for the homologous SSS but no protective substance or agglutinins were present in the patient's serum.

In 25 serum treated Type I cases reported by Abernethy (1) an initial test with Type I SSS was performed before serum was given and repeated at intervals of four hours immediately preceding the next injection of serum. Concentrated horse antiserum, with an estimated potency of 3,000 units per cubic centimeter in most lots used, was administered in doses of 30 cc. every four hours until the skin test to Type I SSS became positive. All cases recovered. Finland (448) notes that in serum treated Type I cases a positive reaction to SSS of homologous type is an indication that sufficient antibody has been given, provided that the test is not carried out until six hours or more after the last injection of antiserum. He further mentions that in many instances a negative test may be obtained when additional doses will serve no useful purpose, such as in the presence of complications or mixed infections. In addition, Cole (305) mentions that the test is not always accurate and that additional serum is occasionally required in patients showing a positive test. Further experience with this test is desirable before its merit in the control of dosage can be regarded as established.

Tests for the presence of agglutinins in the blood or serum of patients treated with antiserum have been developed by Noble (957), Sutliff (1263), Sabin (1146, 1147), and Bullowa (176, 177) and used in the control of serum dosage (1148, 990, 989, 1001, 444, 184, 190). The slide agglutination technic, similar to that used in the Sabin method of typing (see page 630), as described by Bullowa (190), consists in obtaining a drop of blood from the patient in a capillary tube. Following separation of the serum from the resulting clot a small drop of it is mixed on a slide with a small drop of a suspension of killed pneumococci of homologous type and a similar drop is mixed with saline solution as a control. The smears are air dried and any red cells present are laked by the addition of glacial acetic acid. The preparations are then stained with alkaline methylene blue and examined for agglutination under the oil immersion lens.

Bullowa (177, 176, 184, 190) considers that usually when marked agglutination occurs in test preparations it is unnecessary to give further serum treatment. There is not complete agreement on the value of this test in the control of antiserum dosage in pneumonia, and some evidence in animals (Goodner, 532) and man (Lord and Nesche, 815) suggests that agglutinin determinations are unreliable as a measure of dosage. Though the presence of agglutinin may indicate the presence of protective antibody, one may precede or be present in the blood without the other. Finland (448) points out that this test is satisfactory only when agglutination is marked. He further mentions that minor degrees of clumping have been observed in some instances before the required amount of serum had been given and even before the blood stream had been completely sterilized.

Another test was mentioned by Park and his associates (992, 195) who suggested that by determining the amount of SSS in the blood of patients the dose of antibody solution required for its neutralization might be estimated and administered. The method has been little investigated and offers technical difficulties of some degree.

Use of Unconcentrated Serum

Where unconcentrated serum is used the individual doses are necessarily large and usually comprise 100 cc. of serum diluted in an equal volume of freshly prepared sterile physiologic saline solution. Such doses are repeated at intervals of about eight hours until the desired effect is obtained.

The precautions outlined earlier (see pages 836–842) are taken prior to the use of whole immune serum. A blood culture is made as described above before the first serum injection and subsequently as desirable.

Inasmuch as the amounts of diluted serum to be injected are large, a special intravenous outfit, while not necessary, is of aid in administering unconcentrated serum. Such an apparatus is described and illustrated in Monograph No. 7 of the Rockefeller Institute for Medical Research, *Acute Lobar Pneumonia* (33), published in 1917. Briefly it consists of a large glass bottle to hold the diluted serum which can be inverted and hung at a convenient height above the patient. A glass tube with rubber connections joins the bottle with a three-way stopcock. Short lengths of rubber tubing connect the second and third arms of the stopcock to a 20 cc. syringe and to the intravenous needle. The entire apparatus with one 2 cc. and at least two 20 cc. syringes with suitable needles is sterilized dry or by boiling. The outfit is arranged conveniently close to the patient, care being taken to maintain asepsis.

If physiologic saline solution is not available to dilute the serum, it may be given undiluted. The bottles containing the serum and saline solution are immersed in warm water at body temperature to heat them. Following this, by pouring the serum from its container or by the use of a sterile pipette, the serum and an equal volume of saline are transferred to the bottle of the intravenous outfit which may be surrounded with hot water bags at slightly above body temperature to keep the mixture warm.

One of the 20 cc. syringes is attached to the appropriate end of the tube leading to the stopcock, the system filled with serum, and air bubbles expelled. The apparatus, except for the serum container, is arranged on a sterile sheet close at hand. Blood for an initial culture is taken; the free end of the tube attached to the stopcock is connected with the needle in the vein, and by the use of the syringe attached to the system, the injection of the serum is begun. The first 10 or 15 cc. are injected slowly at a rate not to exceed 1 cc. per minute. During the injection of this amount the patient is observed for any change, such as a rapid increase in pulse rate, respiratory difficulty, pallor, cyanosis, or urticaria. If any of these appear Cole (297) states the administration of serum is stopped for ten or fifteen minutes, and if the symptoms quiet down during this interval, the treatment is then slowly continued. During the period of waiting the needle may be kept clear by the injection of saline. In the absence of further reaction the remainder of the serum is slowly run in by gravity over a period of thirty to fifty minutes. Doses are given in this fashion at intervals of about eight hours.

If apparatus as described is not available, two or more 50 cc. syringes may be used to give the serum, alternating the syringes as necessary.

In contrast to the method used for the administration of whole serum as just described, that used for the injection of the concentrated product mentioned earlier is relatively simple.

In the use of unconcentrated serum the dosage indications are similar to those for concentrated serum, as mentioned above (pages 856 and 858), and the occurrence of factors recognized as unfavorable are an indication that a larger total amount of serum than usual should be administered.

SERUM REACTIONS AND THEIR TREATMENT

General discussions of the adverse reactions in man which may occur following the initial and other injections of a foreign protein have been given by numerous workers (801, 802, 283, 762, 1220, 986, 996, 842, 668, 889, 1456, 1426, 1140, 1427, 490, 403). The reactions in animals have also been investigated (802, 1180, 471, 672, 573, 692, 586). The three general types of adverse reaction which may occur after the injection of an alien serum are (a) the immediate, allergic, or anaphylactic reaction, (b) the chill or thermal reaction, and (c) serum sickness or serum disease. No effort will be made here to consider the mechanism of these reactions in detail.

Following the injection of specific horse antiserum in the treatment of pneumonia or other diseases, two of these types of reaction may occur at once or within a short interval after the injection. These are the immediate or allergic reaction and the chill or thermal reaction; but certain symptoms are common to both and at times it may be difficult or impossible to make a distinction between them. Because such reactions may possibly occur, the physician should be present or immediately available for at least thirty and preferably forty-five minutes or more after each injection.

Allergic Reactions

An allergic reaction manifests itself as flushing of the face, dyspnea, cyanosis, lumbar or abdominal pain, rapid weak pulse, apprehension, and a feeling of substernal oppression in various combinations. Sweating, nausea, and vomiting, and less often involuntary urination or defecation may occur. When they occur such symptoms ordinarily appear within thirty minutes and are usually transient and of mild or moderate severity. Their occurrence in cases treated with whole immune serum was studied by Cole (297) and in cases given concentrated serum has been noted by numerous investigators (223, 245, 991, 897, 1265, 444, 184, 557). After intravenous treatment they were reported as occurring in about 4 to 10 per cent of cases in adults. In infants and children such reactions developed in 33 per cent of a few cases after intravenous treatment but were absent following intramuscular treatment (Kereszturi and Hauptmann, 710). Mild or moderate reactions occurred in 7.1 per cent, or 122 of 1,719 cases* in the Massachusetts Pneumonia Series given concentrated antiserum intravenously. Treatment consists in the subcutaneous, intramuscular, or intravenous injection of 0.5 to 1.0 cc. of a 1:1,000 dilution of epinephrine (adrenalin solution).

In a second type of allergic reaction the symptoms in the above group may be combined with urticaria and an acute asthmatic attack. Reactions of this type have occurred in patients who give a history of previous serum administration. They are termed "accelerated" reactions and are regarded as a form of serum sickness. Epinephrine repeated at intervals of a few minutes should be given to such patients.

It is well recognized that in rare instances an acute allergic reaction may lead to immediate death after an injection of foreign protein regardless of the precise nature of the inciting agent. Lamson (762), Mackenzie and

* In 36 other cases in the series no statement was made on the records relating to such reactions.

Hanger (842), and Freedman (490) have collected from the literature reports of at least 78 fatalities of this kind developing after the injection of one kind of foreign protein or another. Among the 41 cases collected by Lamson (762) about one-third had a history of previous asthma or hay fever. Attention was called earlier to the possible danger of treating patients with a history of these conditions (see page 837).

The exact cause of death in these instances is uncertain. It has been attributed to a protein-anti-protein antibody combination (842) or to a sudden release of histamine-like substances into the blood stream (649). Intense prolonged contractions of smooth muscle are known to occur which variously affect the vascular system and produce a marked constriction of the bronchi.

An immediate or allergic reaction of an acute, fatal, shocklike type may come on at once or within a few minutes after the injection of horse serum when patients are extremely sensitive to horse protein. It is probable that reactions of this type can be almost entirely eliminated by observing the precautions previously outlined (see pages 836–842).

Four such deaths have been reported following the use of whole antipneumococcic horse serum. Cecil (219, 220) reported the case of a patient given 100 cc. of serum who recovered from his illness but, seventeen days later, had a relapse. A small so-called desensitizing dose of serum was given at this time and three hours later administration of the regular dose was begun. When 50 cc. of serum had been given, sudden dyspnea and cyanosis occurred, followed by death within a few minutes. Henson (634) reported one death from acute anaphylaxis but made no other statement about the case. A case similar to that of Cecil's above was reported by Wadsworth (1365). The patient was given four doses of whole serum, following which an interval of eleven days elapsed without more specific treatment. At that time 60 cc. of serum were given and death occurred from anaphylaxis. Cole (299) reported the fatal case of a patient given 80 cc. of serum who had a mild immediate reaction from which he apparently recovered, but who one hour later had a chill of moderate severity, became delirious, pale, began to sweat, and died at the end of two hours. Cole was uncertain whether or not this response represented an anaphylactic reaction. As described it seems more likely it might be attributed to a thermal reaction.

Of the many thousands of patients treated with concentrated antiserum, death from allergic reactions, or what appear to be allergic reactions, has been reported in sixteen instances. The death of one child was reported by Burgess (202) and of another by Nemir (930), and the death of a child from what may have been an allergic reaction was reported by Keresztúri and Hauptmann (710). Two deaths were reported by Bullowa (190) out of 205 cases in children (1 per cent) treated. There were three deaths (0.2 per cent) out of 1,755 cases in adults in the Massachusetts Pneumonia Series and eight deaths (0.2 per cent) out of 3,250 cases in Bullowa's (190) series.

The patient reported by Burgess (202), a fourteen-year-old girl, received 5 cc. of serum and by mistake another 15 cc. fifteen minutes later. The history was negative for protein sensitivity. Urticaria with a weak pulse, dyspnea, and coma occurred and one and one-half hours later asthmatic wheezing developed. Epinephrine in repeated doses was of little aid. Death occurred a little over three hours after the initial dose was given. In Nemir's (930) case the skin and eye tests were negative and death occurred within three to five minutes of the intravenous injection of 2 cc. of serum. Keresztúri and Hauptmann's (710) patient died one hour after treatment but they were uncertain whether death resulted from a reaction or from the illness. The cause of death in the two children reported by Bullowa (190) was apparently an allergic reaction, death occurring a few minutes after injection in each instance. One of these patients had received five doses of serum totaling 45 cc. prior to the fifth and fatal dose of 5 cc. which was from a new lot.

Of the fatal allergic reactions in patients in the Massachusetts series the first occurred in a patient treated early in the Pneumonia Study (869) before the Neufeld method of typing was generally available and serum was administered before typing. There was no history of asthma or hay fever or the previous injection of serum, and the eye test was reported negative. An attempt was made to give 30 cc. of serum as the initial injection. After 17 cc. had been given explosive cough appeared, followed by vomiting, cyanosis, sweating, and progressive dyspnea, ending in death within four or five minutes. The necropsy showed acute otitis media, pulmonary infarction, and no pneumonia. As noted on page 854 the first dose is a test injection and should consist of only a small amount of serum. The second fatality occurred in a patient with Type I pneumococcus pneumonia complicated by hypertension, diabetes, and chronic alcoholism. No history of previous allergic manifestation was obtained. The eye test was negative. No skin test was made. There was no allergic reaction after the first injection of 2 cc. of serum or the second of 10 cc. Death occurred shortly after the third dose of 10 cc. Necropsy showed "acute bronchopneumonia, acute myocardial degeneration, acute fatty degeneration of the liver, and early parenchymatous nephritis." In a third case with Type I pneumonia, the patient was treated with 57 cc. of serum in the usual manner over a period of a few hours. Empyema developed and a rib resection was made. On the twenty-third day after beginning specific treatment it was decided to try serum again. The skin test was repeated and was negative. After the injection of 2 cc. the patient collapsed while the needle was still in the vein and died in a few minutes. As there had been spells of collapse during the previous week with symptoms similar to those following the injection, death may not have been due to the serum. As noted on pages 838 and 842, however, serum should not be given to patients who have received horse serum within a period of about seven days to three months previously. A fourth patient already in extremis died following the administration of serum but probably not in consequence of it.

In the eight fatal cases in adults reported by Bullowa (190), death occurred within a period of a few minutes to more than an hour after the injection of serum. In three patients it occurred after the initial dose. One patient treated with serum recovered, developed empyema, and was given another dose of serum of 0.5 cc. twenty-two days later, with death within ten minutes.

In reactions of extreme severity with collapse, epinephrine should be injected, heat applied, oxygen given, and artificial respiration instituted.

The milder immediate reactions of an allergic type without urticaria or asthma are not ordinarily a contraindication to further serum treatment, but subsequent individual doses should be smaller than usual. The occurrence of urticaria or an asthmatic attack is, however, a contraindication to further injections.

Chill or Thermal Reactions

A chill or thermal reaction may occur within a period of twenty minutes to one hour and a half after serum injection. A reaction of this type is probably not due to sensitiveness as an allergic manifestation but to some peculiarity of the serum or of the patient or of both. Such reactions are not ordinarily serious. There may be chilliness or, in the more severe cases, a general shaking chill lasting up to twenty to thirty minutes, with cyanosis, dyspnea, and apprehension. The temperature usually rises one to two degrees or more and falls with an accompanying sweat within one to two hours. Such reactions are more commonly observed after the first or second injection, but may follow any injection. They may occur after only one of a number of injections of serum of the same lot. Reactions are less common, however, with certain lots than with others, and are less common with concentrated antibody solution than with whole serum. Rapid administration, failure to warm the serum, or the presence of a precipitate may be responsible.

Reactions of this type frequently follow the intravenous injection of vaccines and are thought under such circumstances to be beneficial. Cole (297) has remarked that there is no evidence that such reactions are of aid to patients with pneumonia. This is borne out by figures relating to the serum treated Type I cases studied during the Massachusetts Pneumonia Study (869, 615). The fatality rate of 75 such cases who had chill reactions during treatment was 9.3 per cent, while that of 325 similar cases who did not have chills during treatment was 9.8 per cent, or very much the same.

From 20 to 60 per cent of cases treated with whole immune horse antiserum may experience chill or thermal reactions (1299, 986). When concentrated serum is used, such reactions may occur in from 10 to 20 per cent of adult patients (245, 986, 195, 897, 442, 1269, 930, 184, 186) or be somewhat more common in children (710). Among 1,718 cases in adults in the Massachusetts Pneumonia Series treated with concentrated antiserum, reactions of this nature occurred in 339 or 19.7 per cent.

The treatment of the ordinary thermal reaction is symptomatic. During the chill hot drinks, hot water bottles, and extra blankets may be used. Following this, when the temperature is elevated a degree or more, cold drinks, ice bags, cold sponges, or alcohol rubs may be helpful. Epinephrine is of no value in the treatment of thermal reactions. Bullowa (190) considers that epinephrine prolongs the chill. For aborting the chill he recommends the inhalation of amyl nitrite as soon as it appears. If the fever is extremely high, the patient should be treated as in heatstroke: ice bags or ice packs and sheets wrung out of ice water should be applied and enemas of ice water administered. Venesection may be of service with pulmonary edema.

Fatal chill reactions have occurred. Leys (779) reported a death attributed to such a reaction in an adult given 75 cc. of serum. A mild immediate reaction occurred and an hour later a slight chill, followed by sweating, symptomatic relief, and sleep. Within two hours stertorous breathing developed and the patient was comatose. His temperature was then 108° F. and a few minutes later was 110° F. The pulse was almost imperceptible. Respiration soon failed, then heart action. Necropsy showed pneumonia in the stage of red hepatization but no other lesions in other organs, including the brain.

Among the 1,755 cases in the Massachusetts Pneumonia Series an acute fatal thermal reaction occurred in three patients after an initial dose of 5 cc. of concentrated antiserum. There was a chill within eighty minutes, hyperthermia (108° F. and over), and death in one hour and forty minutes to six hours and thirty-five minutes. One patient had no history of previous serum injections and the eye test had been negative. The second had a history of the injection of 75 cc. of serum for pneumonia two years before and the eye test was negative. In neither of these was the skin test made. In only one was the infection amenable to specific therapy, and in this case with Type I pneumococcus the eye test was doubtful, the skin test markedly positive, and serum should not have been given. The reactions in these three cases occurred in the early part of the Massachusetts Pneumonia Study (869) and before the development of the monkey test (see page 831) for the chill-producing activity of concentrated antipneumococcic serum.

The milder thermal reactions need not modify the usual régime with respect to serum therapy. If the reaction is severe, however, it is best at the next injection to diminish the dose and postpone its administration for three or four hours after the chill. In any instance it is not advisable to administer a subsequent dose while the temperature is elevated from a previous reaction. The laboratory where the serum is manufactured should be notified of the lot number of the serum causing the reaction and, if possible, serum from a different lot should be obtained. If the reaction should be alarming, with excessive fever, pronounced cyanosis, delirium, and collapse, no further serum should be given.

Attempts to eliminate the chill-producing factor from immune horse serum have been only partially successful, as earlier described (see page 830). In view of the possibility that chill-free serums may develop reactive properties on aging, serum should not be used if the expiration date on the vial has passed. It is desirable to warm the serum and inject it slowly and to reject serums containing a precipitate.

Serum Sickness or Serum Disease

Following the injection of alien serum, serum sickness or serum disease not infrequently develops. The usual symptoms are mild, consisting of joint pains, urticarial or erythematous skin rashes, edema of the skin, fever, and general glandular enlargement. These manifestations may appear singly or in combination. Joint involvement is the commonest when concentrated horse antiserum is used. The temporomandibular joint is frequently involved, causing great annoyance. The attack usually comes on between the seventh and the tenth day after the first injection of serum, but in some cases certain manifestations, especially the skin rashes, may come on at once, and in others the onset of the disease may be delayed for as long as four weeks. Single attacks usually last only from a few hours to a day or two, but may be more severe and prolonged when whole serum is used. Repeated attacks may occur.

Evidence of an impaired kidney function is not uncommon but is always temporary. Edema of nephritic distribution may occur, accompanied by water and chloride retention, a decrease of the power to excrete various dyes in the urine, and albumin and casts may appear. Abdominal pain, vomiting, diarrhea, headache, conjunctivitis, and sore throat have been described (842). Wilson and Hadden (1426) and Young (1456) report that neuritis and multiple neuritis may be an infrequent development, lesions involving the shoulder girdle being commonest (see also page 611).

Apparently about 10 per cent of patients treated with horse serum never get serum sickness (802, 283, 842). The condition may be more frequent and severe in white than in colored persons (985, 283, 842) and be unaffected by age variations (283, 842, 668). In animals and man Longcope (802) demonstrated the appearance of humoral precipitins for the protein of the serum toward the end of serum disease, accompanied by a disappearance of horse serum from the blood. He attributed the termination of serum sickness to the fact that the horse serum is used up in combining with the precipitins and disappears. Using rabbits, Jones and Fleisher (692) were unable to confirm this observation. Recurrent attacks have been attributed to the development of sensitivity to the various protein components of horse serum at different times, sensitivity to the globulins appearing first and that to the albumins a few days later (842, 668).

In severe cases the temperature may reach 104° or 105° F. and raise the question as to the occurrence of some septic complication. Physical and roentgen-ray examination of the chest will aid in ruling out complications such as delayed resolution or fluid as a cause of the fever. The ears should be examined for otitis media. Patients generally look ill with the occurrence of a septic complication, while they seldom do with serum sickness, and their appetite usually remains fairly good. A total and differential leucocyte count may be of value at times in differentiating this condition from a septic complication. During serum sickness the total count may or may not be increased to 15,000 to 20,000 leucocytes. Usually there is a relative lymphocytosis of 30 or 40 per cent and frequently a slight eosinophilia of from 3 to 7 per cent is also present.

In cases treated with unconcentrated antipneumococcic serum Cole (297) found that the severity of serum disease was not directly proportional to the total dose used. After the use of concentrated serum Cecil and Sutliff (245) found a definite relationship between the volume of serum given and the occurrence of this condition. Of patients receiving 50 cc. or less of serum, only 4.9 per cent had serum sickness, as compared with 27.2 per cent of those given more than 50 cc. In general the manifestations of serum sickness are likely to be more severe, and as shown in the Massachusetts cases (615) in Table 165, are of increasing frequency with increasing amounts of serum. As seen in this table, serum sickness occurred in 22.1 per cent of 653 recovered cases. It was present in only 4.8 per cent of cases receiving 15 cc. or less of serum but occurred with increasing frequency as larger doses were used and was found in 30.2 per cent of patients receiving 151 cc. or more of serum.

TABLE 165. LOBAR PNEUMONIA. NUMBER OF RECOVERED CASES AND NUMBER AND PERCENTAGE OF CASES DEVELOPING SERUM SICKNESS AFTER TREATMENT WITH CONCENTRATED HORSE ANTISERUM, BY DOSE ADMINISTERED*

DOSE OF SERUM USED	NUMBER OF RECOVERED CASES	CASES WITH SERUM SICKNESS REPORTED	
		Number	*Per cent*
1–15 cc.	21	1	4.8
16–45 cc.	98	17	17.3
46–75 cc.	350	74	21.1
76–105 cc.	83	24	28.9
106–150 cc.	58	15	25.9
151 cc. and over	43	13	30.2
Total	653	144	22.1

* Cases were taken from those investigated in the early part of the Massachusetts Pneumonia Study (869).

Among a grand total of 1,423 recovered cases treated with concentrated antipneumococcic serum in the Massachusetts Pneumonia Series, serum sickness was noted in 282, or 19.8 per cent. In most other series similarly treated the incidence has varied from about 12 to 33 per cent (245, 195, 442, 326, 1269, 995, 446, 190). Of 82 infants and children treated by Nemir (930) this condition developed in only one. In a series of 25 cases, presumably all adults, studied by Abernethy (1) some signs of the disease (joint involvement, fever, skin lesions, or lymphadenopathy) were found in 17, or 68 per cent. Joint involvement was the commonest symptom and urticaria was mild. As suggested by Abernethy, particular attention to the occurrence of mild symptoms may be responsible for the finding of a relatively high incidence of serum disease in his series. Serum sickness of any severity usually occurs in only about 10 per cent of patients.

In patients treated with whole unconcentrated antiserum, serum sickness is frequently more severe and has occurred in from about 50 to 95 per cent or more of such cases (985, 297, 1299, 283, 986, 842, 190, 658).

Serum sickness is annoying and not serious. Various calcium salts, calcium gluconate, milk, and sodium thiosulphate have been given as preventive measures with variable but usually little success (668, 337). Ephedrine by mouth given over a period of several days as a prophylactic measure seems of little use. After the condition has developed, the itching may be allayed by the external application of calamine lotion (white wash) containing one per cent of phenol or of dilute vinegar or alcohol or hot sodium bicarbonate solution. Ephedrine by mouth in doses of 1/3 to 3/4 grain may also be helpful. If itching is especially troublesome the injection of 0.5 to 1.0 cc. of epinephrine subcutaneously may be expected to give temporary relief. Calcium gluconate, 20 cc. of a 10 per cent solution given at a rate of 0.5 cc. per minute intravenously, or 10 cc. of a 10 per cent solution injected intramuscularly at twelve-hour intervals as needed, may help. Salicylates may likewise be useful in allaying itching. Acetylsalicylic acid 5.0 grams, ephedrine sulphate 0.5 gram, and phenobarbital 0.5 gram can be mixed and made up into 15 capsules and one given every two to four hours as needed to promote sleep (403). A warm alkaline bath prepared by adding a cup of baking soda to a tub of warm water, and followed by free dusting of the skin with talcum powder to which 0.25 per cent menthol has been added, may also be of value in overcoming itching. Salicylates, if necessary, may be given for the relief of joint pains.

TREATMENT WITH IMMUNE RABBIT SERUM

Specific antipneumococcic rabbit serum has recently been introduced for the treatment of pneumococcus pneumonia. It has long been known that rabbits, stimulated by appropriate injections of pneumococcal antigens, respond to the stimulus by elaborating specific antibodies to pneumococci, and that these antibodies are to be found in the blood of the animals so immunized. The application of this knowledge to the production of therapeutic antiserum, however, is of recent origin. Rabbits were often used in the early experimental studies on the pneumococcus and it was observed that the injection of pneumococci or their growth products or derivatives induced in these animals specific humoral immune bodies capable not only of precipitating various components of the organisms but of protecting experimentally infected animals from an otherwise fatal infection due to their inoculation with virulent cultures of the same strain or type.

That differences exist between antibody produced in the rabbit and that produced in the horse was mentioned earlier (see pages 172–173). Some of these differences, such as the smaller size of the rabbit antibody, at least for Type I, suggested that it might have advantages over horse antibody in the treatment of pneumonia and that it might penetrate more readily into inflammatory processes.

In 1934 Barnes and White (77), in an experimental study of the immunizing value of formalinized and heat killed pneumococci, demonstrated that serum of much higher antibody content could be obtained from rabbits than from horses (see also page 421). It was, however, Horsfall and his colleagues, Goodner, MacLeod, Harris, and Dubos (657, 659, 545, 658) at the Hospital of the Rockefeller Institute for Medical Research, who were the first to prepare specific antipneumococcic serum from rabbits for therapeutic purposes and they and Bullowa (190, 189) put the serum to clinical test.

Methods of Preparation and Standardization

The details of the procedures carried out in the preparation of specific immune rabbit serum for therapeutic purposes, as described by Goodner, Horsfall, and Dubos (545) are, in the main, as follows.

Pneumococci of the different specific types, in the smooth or virulent phase, are maintained in rabbit-blood broth at 37.5° C., planted and grown for eighteen hours in beef heart infusion broth, then centrifuged from the culture medium and suspended in saline solution. The suspended cocci are killed by immediate exposure to a temperature of 70° C. for thirty minutes, or to one per cent formalin in the cold for twenty-four hours, or first treated with formalin and heated to 80° C. for thirty minutes. The suspensions are then standardized.

Rabbits, preferably of the New Zealand Red or Chinchilla breeds and weighing between 1,600 and 2,800 grams, are immunized according to the so-called "four-week complete" system, that is, a series of daily intravenous injections is given for four days each week and continued for three weeks, followed by a rest. After a rest period of eleven days following the last injection of the third course, the animals are bled from the heart and then put on a schedule of a regular series of three daily injections of antigen for three days and a rest, followed by a bleeding.

The serum is drawn from the clot and filtered through a Berkefeld V candle. "Merthiolate" is added as a preservative to a final concentration of 1:10,000. Inasmuch as immune serum from rabbits in the raw state is almost invariably toxic for man, the serum is heated at 56° C. for thirty minutes, then adsorbed with sterile kaolin. The serum is freed from kaolin by centrifugation, again run through a bacteria-proof filter, and once more heated to 56° C. for thirty minutes. The serum thus processed is then assayed by a modified Heidelberger and Kabat (620) method, which is based upon the determination in milligrams of the specific antibody content. Tests are then performed to ensure the sterility of the finished product.

In its essentials the process of standardizing the serum consists in carrying out an absorption test with pneumococci of homologous type and determining the amount of nitrogen removed from the serum, the latter having been shown to represent the amount of antibody present. Comparison is made of the total nitrogen content of the serum before and after such absorption and the amount of nitrogen removed by the organisms determined. As a check on this method of standardization, the results obtained were compared with the findings of numerous protection tests. It was possible, by immunizing rabbits with Type I pneumococci, to produce in as short a time as four weeks serum containing about 2,000 mouse protective units per cubic centimeter. Goodner and his associates (545) state:

> With type I antipneumococcic rabbit serum it has been determined that on the average 1 mgm. of specific agglutinin-*nitrogen,* or 6.25 mgm. of specific agglutinin-*protein,* is equivalent to 1100 mouse-protective units, in comparison with standard sera. Since the relationship between protective potency and the content of specific antibody of antipneumococcic rabbit serum appears to be constant, it is suggested that for rabbit sera this relationship be used for all types.

These workers anticipate being able to measure serum dosage in milligrams of antibody rather than in terms of the somewhat unsatisfactory unit, and remark:

> With the present knowledge as to the properties of antipneumococcic antibodies of the rabbit it seems as rational to use a definite number of milligrams of antibody therapeutically as it is to use quantitative amounts of any therapeutic agent.

In addition to the above method of "processing" rabbit antiserum, concentrated immune rabbit serums for many types have also been prepared by several manufacturers and are available on the market.

The requirements of the National Institute of Health in the standardization of rabbit antipneumococcic serums are that for Types I, II, V, VII, and VIII, comparative mouse protection tests, using the standard serums for these types mentioned elsewhere (page 828), should be used. For rabbit antiserums of other than these five types, antibody-nitrogen tests are permissible, although mouse protection tests are considered preferable when they can be carried out satisfactorily. For the time being, 1 mgm. of antibody-nitrogen is regarded officially as equivalent to 750 units.

Processed rabbit antiserum may be tested *in vivo* to identify those lots likely to cause chills or thermal reactions when used clinically. For this purpose the temperature of a normal rabbit is taken, after which the animal is injected intravenously with 2 cc. of the serum. On the basis of their experience, Goodner and his co-workers (545) state that if serum processed by their method is used, and if the animal's temperature an hour after the injection has risen more than 1.2° F., the serum is likely to produce chills in patients, and if the mean rabbit thermal reaction exceeds 2° F., the serum frequently produces such severe chills that it should not be distributed for human use.

Clinical Use of Rabbit Antiserum

Rabbit antipneumococcic serum offers important possibilities with respect to the production of a concentrated antibody solution of higher potency in small volume than is the case with horse antiserum. It may possibly cost less to produce than antipneumococcic horse serum. Accumulating evidence suggests that rabbit antiserum is as useful therapeutically as horse antiserum. Data are still too meager, however, to define clearly its possible advantages or disadvantages. The administration of rabbit antiserum may give rise to allergic reactions or at times to a severe thermal reaction leading to death (658), and in consequence caution should be exercised in its use.

PRECAUTIONS IN THE USE OF RABBIT ANTISERUM. Care should be taken not to use rabbit antiserum in the treatment of patients who may be sensitive to the product. To what extent toxicity of rabbit serum for man may enter into the problem is at present uncertain and needs further investigation. It may be presumed, however, until evidence is presented to the contrary, that as an alien serum it presents hazards at least equal to those of horse serum.

It is desirable, therefore, to take the precaution of inquiring, as in the use of horse serum, whether the patient has a history of allergic manifestations and especially whether he has known sensitivity to emanations, dander, or fur of rabbits.* Inquiry should also be made concerning any previous administration of rabbit serum and direct tests made for sensitiveness to this material.

Before injecting rabbit serum intravenously for therapeutic purposes, Horsfall, Goodner, MacLeod, and Harris (659) tested all patients for sensitiveness in a routine way by three methods:

Method 1: The intradermal test. The test was made with a 1:10 dilution of normal rabbit serum in physiologic sodium chloride solution, and controlled by a preliminary injection of physiologic salt solution as in the test for horse serum sensitivity (page 840). All patients in the experience of the investigators cited reacted positively to the test, with the development, in many, of a small and transient erythematous patch and, in a few, a blanched wheal with surrounding erythema. None of these positive reactions was regarded as significant of sensitivity to rabbit serum injected intravenously.

Method 2: The eye test. This test for sensitivity was made by instilling a drop or two of a 1:10 dilution of normal rabbit serum in physiologic saline solution into one conjunctival sac. The results were negative in the patients tested; hyperemia of the conjunctival vessels, itching, and lacrymation did not develop.

Method 3: The intravenous test. In this test Horsfall and his associates (659) first used 0.1 cc. of type-specific antipneumococcic rabbit serum diluted to 5 cc. with physiologic saline solution. With further experience (658) they regarded it safer as a routine slowly to inject 0.05 cc. of rabbit antiserum similarly diluted. They also stated that in cases with a suggestive history of allergy or where sensitiveness to the serum of an animal of another species is demonstrated, it would seem wise to inject not more than 0.01 cc. of rabbit antiserum diluted to 5 cc. It was stated that a positive reaction with this test consists in a fall in arterial systolic blood pressure of 15 mm. of mercury or more and an increase in the cardiac rate of fifteen beats per minute or more, both occurring within five minutes or less after the injection of the test dose of antiserum. The reaction was negative and no symptoms suggesting sensitiveness to rabbit serum developed during or after the administration of the full therapeutic dose in 65 of 67 cases. In two cases the test was markedly positive, with symptoms of mild shock accompanied by a sharp fall in arterial pressure and a marked rise in cardiac rate.

ADMINISTRATION OF ANTIPNEUMOCOCCIC RABBIT SERUM. In considering a departure from the use of horse antiserum to the use of rabbit antiserum, it is

* Felt, in many instances, contains rabbit hair.

desirable to proceed with care as already noted. Of the direct tests for sensitiveness, special importance should be attached to the eye test with rabbit serum.

Brief mention may be made of the method of injecting this antiserum for therapeutic purposes used by Horsfall, Goodner, MacLeod, and Harris (659). Following a negative reaction to the intravenous test with unconcentrated processed rabbit antiserum, the administration of serum was begun. In the first few cases an initial injection of 2 cc. of serum diluted to 20 cc. with saline solution was given. The volume of serum was then doubled every two hours until from 30 cc. to 40 cc. of undiluted serum were given at each injection. It was later found that larger amounts could be used at shorter intervals and that administration at intervals of forty minutes produced a more rapid drop in temperature. In the more recent experience of Horsfall, Goodner, and MacLeod (658), one-half hour after the intravenous test for sensitiveness, as described above, was found to be negative, the injection of rabbit antiserum was begun. The rate of injection was quite rapid in most instances. They find that 120 cc. may be injected in ten minutes and a dose as large as 300 cc. has been given during this short period without producing discomfort. Such a procedure would appear too hazardous for general use. An effort was made in the last fifty cases to give an adequate amount of serum in a single injection.

Of the 67 cases treated with rabbit antiserum by the above workers, 13 were of Type III in which the average dose of serum given was 320 cc., while the remaining 54 cases, due to pneumococci of one or another of eight different types (Types I, II, V, VI, VII, VIII, XIV, and XVIII), received an average of 165 cc. per case. The average total amount of serum administered to the 25 Type I cases in the series was 134 cc., while the average amount in 10 Type II cases was 225 cc., and in one Type V case the dose was 190 cc. In the 6 Type VII and 7 Type VIII cases an average dose of 160 cc. was given. The average interval from the time of onset to the beginning of serum therapy was 77 hours for the Type I cases, 68 hours for the Type II cases, 13 days for the Type V case, and 55 and 35 hours respectively for the Type VII and Type VIII cases.

For 22 of the Type I cases treated, the average time elapsing between the intravenous test for sensitiveness and the completion of serum therapy was only 5 hours.

The average total dose of whole processed rabbit antiserum for Type I cases in this series (134 cc.) is considerably smaller than the average total dose of 420 cc. of unconcentrated horse antiserum used in the Type I cases reported by Cole, as already mentioned (see page 847). The administration of specific rabbit serum which has been concentrated may permit a further reduction in the volume of serum necessary to inject.

REACTIONS AND THEIR TREATMENT. The reactions occurring after the administration of rabbit serum are similar to those which may follow the injection of horse serum, as above described (see pages 863–872).

It is advisable with severe allergic reactions to discontinue serum therapy. The occurrence of urticaria or an asthmatic attack accompanying an immediate allergic type of reaction is probably also a contraindication to further injections. Epinephrine is used in the treatment of these reactions, as elsewhere mentioned (see page 864).

With respect to chill or thermal reactions, Horsfall and his associates (659, 658) find that immune rabbit serum frequently contains sufficient chill-producing substances to cause severe reactions. Though these reactions are not usually dangerous, death occurred in one instance three hours after the onset of an extremely severe chill reaction. Heating the serum and adsorbing it with sterile kaolin, as mentioned above (see page 874), and the elimination of those lots which produce chills or fever on intravenous injection into normal rabbits (see page 875), were considered to render processed rabbit antiserum safe for general use. Fourteen lots of untreated antipneumococcic rabbit serum were used in the treatment of 31 patients, of whom 24, or 78 per cent, had one or more chills. Twenty-six lots of treated serum, used in treating 51 patients, produced one or more chills in 19, or 37 per cent. Eleven lots of treated serum tested in rabbits with negative results were used in treating 26 patients, none of whom had chills.

As with chill reactions following the injection of horse serum, such reactions following the use of rabbit antiserum should have symptomatic treatment, as described on page 868. It is also desirable in such instances to stop the injections when an alarming reaction occurs, as excessive fever, pronounced cyanosis, delirium, and collapse, and to use smaller doses, where divided dosage is given, at longer intervals than usual in the presence of the milder reactions.

Serum sickness may also occur after treatment with rabbit antiserum. Horsfall and his colleagues (658) found evidence of serum sickness in 40 per cent, or 24, of their 59 cases recovering after rabbit serum therapy. The symptoms were mild in 16 cases and moderately severe in 8. In 75 per cent of those with serum sickness following rabbit antiserum, the manifestations were almost entirely cutaneous, that is, urticaria, transient rashes, and so forth. In the limited experience of these workers, the development of the disease was unrelated to the quantity of rabbit antiserum administered. The treatment of this condition has been described on page 872.

CHAPTER NINETEEN

RESULTS OF SERUM TREATMENT

Effect of Treatment on the Patient 882
Clinical Picture 882
Appearance of Antibodies in the Blood and Sterilization of the Blood Stream 885
Pulmonary Extension 886
Resolution 887
Incidence of Complications 887
Effect of Treatment on Case Fatality Rate: Variation with Type 888
Type I Cases 890
Relation of Early Treatment to Fatality Rate 894
Relation of Other Factors to Fatality Rate 897
Type II Cases 899
Relation of Early Treatment to Fatality Rate 901
Cases Due to Other Types 903
Type V Cases 903
Type VII Cases 904
Type VIII Cases 904
Type XIV Cases 905
Cases of Pneumococcus Pneumonia of Various Types 905
Infants and Children with Pneumococcus Pneumonia 906
Effect of Treatment on Case Fatality Rate: Variation with Type and Other Factors 909
Age 909
Sex and Place of Treatment 911
Bacteriemia 912
Season 916
Rabbit Antipneumococcic Serum and Results with Treatment 917
Analysis of Deaths Occurring Despite Serum Treatment 918
Unavoidable and Avoidable Causes of Failure of Specific Treatment 920

RESULTS obtained by the treatment of patients with pneumococcus pneumonia with specific antiserum have been reported by many investigators. Summaries of much of the available information were presented by Lord and Heffron (813, 814) and the following discussion is an amplification of the recent review of the matter in their handbook on *Pneumonia and Serum Therapy* (814).

For the continued and productive study of lobar pneumonia and the early, persistent, and successful application of horse serum therapy, we are largely indebted to Cole and his associates, as earlier mentioned (see page 807). Following the favorable report in 1913 by Cole and Dochez (306) on the specific treatment of Type I pneumonia, equally favorable reports from this source have from time to time been presented on an increasingly large number of cases. By 1936 Cole's (302) treated series numbered 462 cases with a fatality rate of only 10.5 per cent. In addition to the low fatality rate in the treated group, such important supporting evidence as the cessation of spread, rapid appearance of protective antibodies in the blood, and the prevention or disappearance of blood invasion in consequence of specific therapy has been presented. In spite of these brilliant therapeutic results, the advantage of specific treatment was not generally recognized for some time. This was due in part to the failure to determine the fatality rate in large series of cases treated without serum. The average fatality rate from a small early series of untreated Type I pneumonias was estimated at 25 to 30 per cent and, convinced of the effectiveness of antiserum, Cole did not feel justified in withholding the treatment from a control series. Also partly responsible for the failure to recognize the merit of specific therapy was the frequent and often unavoidable use at an early period by some workers of unsatisfactory serum of low potency which was given in small amounts at any time during the illness. Among others, Spooner and his associates (1222, 1221) brought this matter into sharp relief by pointing out the poor results they obtained in 1918 with an unsatisfactory serum of low potency and by contrasting these results with those obtained at a later period when good potent serum was used. Even today continued emphasis on the use of only serums of high potency is desirable.

The fatality rates of cases treated with and without specific therapy in Cole's series have since been confirmed, but only after a long period of uncertainty on the part of the general medical profession. Topley (1317) has pointed out in discussing similar matters that the period of trial of any form of treatment may be unduly prolonged by the difficulty of obtaining adequate reports and states that, "Any student who cares to master the history of the use of antipneumococcal serum will find a case in point." Unfortunately others had less striking success than Cole, and Locke's (793) report in 1923 of a fatality rate of 17.2 per cent in 145 serum treated Type I cases (only 12 of which were treated in the first three days) and practically the same fatality rate, 16.9 per cent, in 71 untreated control cases, raised serious doubts in the minds of many regarding the value of the procedure. These doubts were resolved by further determination of the comparative results with and without antiserum in contemporaneous series and an analysis of the treated group according to the time when specific treatment was begun. In Boston and New York, Lord; Cecil and Sutliff; Park, Bullowa, and Rosenblüth; Finland; Cecil and Plummer; and Sutliff and Finland furnished evidence of marked reduction in the fatality rate of cases treated with serum and showed that this reduction depended largely on its application early in the course of the disease. These favorable results in controlled experiments dealing, all told, with large series of cases, were an indispensable preliminary to the more general acceptance of the method. Without this assurance of the merit of specific therapy its more general application, as in organized pneumonia programs, such as the Massachusetts Pneumonia Study and Continuing Program, would not have been possible.

It should be appreciated that the results of specific serum therapy in the Massachusetts series presented in this chapter are based only on patients treated within the first four days of illness.* As earlier mentioned, this restriction in the use of antipneumococcic horse serum supplied by the Department of Public Health was imposed throughout the Pneumonia Study and Service (1931–1935) and during the Continuing Program until March 1937 (see page 833).

EFFECT OF TREATMENT ON THE PATIENT

The general effects on the patient of specific serum treatment will be mentioned. There seems no reason to go into exhaustive detail as to each of the effects noted. Those interested in the matter may refer to the many reports cited where discussion of a large number of cases is given individually (see also pages 175–177). With adequate treatment the results are similar whether unconcentrated or concentrated serum is used.

Clinical Picture

For several hours after the administration of the initial dosage of antiserum, no change in the patient is likely to be observed, but within eight to twenty-four hours after the first dose there is usually a marked improvement. The favorable response is usually more pronounced when patients are treated early, particularly within the first seventy-two hours of illness. The patient becomes clearer mentally and begins to take an interest in his sur-

* These and other treated Massachusetts cases are summarized in Appendix A, page 937.

roundings (297, 238, 444, 813, 814). Concurrent with this improvement there is generally a marked alleviation of the acute symptoms (297, 245, 830, 156, 930, 190). Symptoms such as cyanosis, dyspnea, chest pain of the more severe type, delirium, and toxemia are largely or wholly relieved (1269, 444, 1272, 446, 1051).

In a large majority of the cases the temperature drops two or three degrees or more and does not again reach its former level (297, 245, 238, 442, 176, 930, 813, 814; see Figure 13). At the same time, though less rapidly, there is a fall in the rate of the pulse and respiration, the whole picture resembling that of natural crisis. In patients not treated with serum Sutliff and Finland (1272) found that a much smaller proportion show symptomatic improvement and a sharp drop in temperature during the course of the disease. Following this initial fall in the temperature of serum treated cases, there may be a continued low-grade fever and lesser complaints for several days. During this period patients may feel relatively well, though by physical signs and roentgen-ray examination little or no change in the size and density of the consolidated area may be demonstrated. In such instances, however, the progress of the disease is ordinarily stopped (297).

Where specific treatment is begun on or before the fourth or fifth day of illness the duration of the acute symptoms is shortened, as Cole (292, 297) and others have demonstrated (60, 245, 176, 238, 442, 1269, 24, 463, 557, 1088, 1272, 184, 339, 447). In a few instances where late treatment was given (793, 1450) or only a few cases were observed (830), no shortening of the course was reported. Similar results were obtained in some infants and children (710), while in others (930) definite shortening of the course was demonstrated. Studies by Sutliff and Finland (1269, 1272) on a series of serum treated Type I cases in adults compared with others not so treated indicate that the average duration of the *more acute symptoms* measured from onset to a persistent lowering of the temperature is shortened by about thirty hours in the serum treated group. The average duration of the low-grade fever following the relief of the more acute symptoms, however, is about the same in both groups. The disease runs a milder course following serum therapy.

An even more marked shortening of the acute illness in the treated as compared with control cases is reported in Great Britain by Armstrong and Johnson (24) and the Therapeutic Trials Committee of the Medical Research Council (557). They find, on the average, that crisis occurred two and one-half days earlier in the treated than in the control Type I cases and

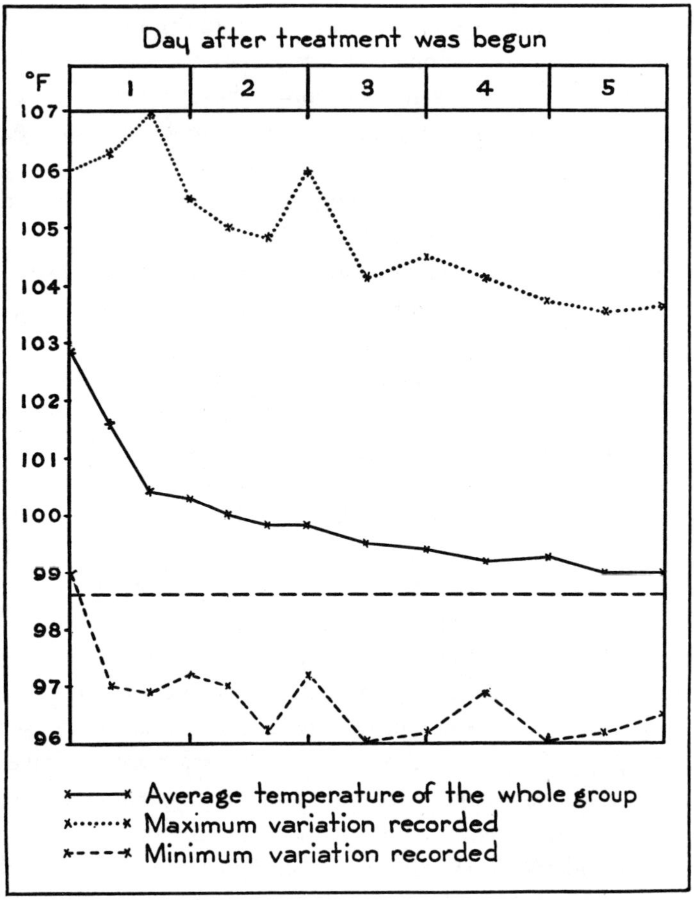

Figure 13. Composite temperature chart of 320 recovered Type I cases in which treatment with concentrated serum was begun within 96 hours of onset

Temperatures are shown at eight-hour intervals for the first forty-eight hours after the beginning of treatment and then twice daily.

For 27 of the 320 cases treatment was begun on the first day of illness; for 101 on the second day; for 120 on the third day; for 72 on the fourth day.

Cases are taken from the series studied during the Massachusetts Pneumonia Study, 1931–1935. An additional 128 recovered cases investigated during that period are not included as their temperature charts are not available or are inadequate for the purpose.

about two days earlier in the treated than in the control Type II cases. In other instances where the progress of cases was analyzed in a different way, they note that, compared with the control cases, from four to seven times as many treated Type I cases show defervescence on or before the fifth day of illness and from three to six times as many Type II cases.

Earlier and more regular symptomatic improvement is almost invariably seen when specific treatment is begun within the first seventy-two hours than when it is begun later. Serum therapy has no special influence on the electrocardiographic findings in pneumonia and does not appear to influence the incidence of abnormalities of cardiac rate, rhythm, or conduction, as DeGraff, Travell, and Yager (349) have found.

Appearance of Antibodies in the Blood and Sterilization of the Blood Stream

Antibodies such as those ordinarily encountered only shortly before or at the time of recovery promptly become demonstrable in the blood in a large proportion of cases following serum therapy, as Avery, Chickering, Cole, and Dochez (33) and other investigators have shown (295, 297, 61, 60, 1263, 245, 815, 1275, 820, 761, 1088). Much individual variation is seen, however, and humoral immune substances may become demonstrable after the injection of only a few thousand units of antibody in some cases and yet be absent after the administration of several hundred thousand units in others. The sudden appearance of antibodies under such circumstances makes it probable that the demonstrable immune substances have come from the serum injected (61, 1263, 820). If serum administration is stopped, such antibody tends to decrease in amount or disappear from the blood in the usual instance, presumably through its combination with the organisms and the specific capsular polysaccharide (295, 33, 992, 1088). In Type I cases positive urine precipitin reactions for the homologous capsular polysaccharide were found by Dochez and Avery (363) and Avery and his colleagues (33, 297) to become negative following specific serum treatment, suggesting that the antibody injected had combined with the SSS and stopped its excretion.

The administration of antipneumococcic horse serum does not appear to decrease or alter the number of platelets in the blood (Reimann, 1062).

The antibody administered markedly enhances the efficiency of the blood-clearing mechanism and assists in removing organisms from the circulation. As Cole and his associates (306, 292, 293, 33, 297) and several additional workers have demonstrated (794, 61, 60, 245, 991, 299, 1269, 183, 1088, 190), the blood stream is rapidly sterilized in this way, and, with adequate treatment, reinvasion of the blood is prevented (306, 33, 297, 1269, 813, 190, 814). Though this action of antibody is difficult to determine with accuracy, it is possible that it is the most important result of the use of antiserum in pneumonia and its effectiveness is far greater in the early stages of the disease than it is after three or four days have passed. Drinker, Enders, Shaffer, and Leigh (377) demonstrated that the blood of rabbits infected intravenously was promptly cleared of organisms by treatment with specific serum. They also found that when such animals had a heavy blood-stream infection, organisms were present in the lymphatics and serum treatment had little if any effect in clearing the organisms from these vessels. If sufficient serum was not used to keep the blood clear of organisms, those continually entering from the lymph stream soon caused a reinfection of the blood.

In general, specific serum therapy has a marked effect in preventing blood invasion and far less serum is usually necessary to maintain sterility of the blood than is required to overcome bacteriemia after it has developed. Blood cultures previously positive usually become negative within a few to twenty-four hours or more if adequate amounts of serum are used. With an especially heavy bacteriemia, showing more than twenty or thirty colonies of organisms per cubic centimeter of blood, death nearly always occurs (see page 691) unless specific treatment is given, and under such circumstances repeated large doses should be administered beginning at the earliest possible moment. Bullowa (183) has reported recovery in patients having several hundred pneumococci per cubic centimeter in their blood where large amounts of serum were given within the first five days of illness.

The evidence is clear that RECOVERY CANNOT OCCUR IN THE PRESENCE OF PERSISTENT BACTERIEMIA and that thus far the only treatment of demonstrated value is THE ADMINISTRATION OF AN ADEQUATE AMOUNT OF SPECIFIC SERUM. Failure to give more than the usual amounts of serum to bacteriemic patients may result in unnecessary loss of life. The literature indicates that insufficient attention has been paid this matter in the past.

Pulmonary Extension

With few exceptions following suitable specific serum treatment the area of lung involvement ceases to spread, as was shown by Cole and his associates (292, 293, 33, 297) and by Sutliff and Finland (1269, 444, 1272) and other workers (24, 1088). If extension occurs it takes place slowly. By contrast, extension is frequent in those not treated with antiserum. With early treatment the consolidation may be confined to a small part of one lobe. Similar findings were reported by Helm, Ferguson, and Noble (629) in a few cases specially investigated by serial roentgenograms.

Where treatment is begun early, within the first day or two of illness, and when few signs of consolidation are present in roentgenograms, crisis and recovery may be brought about abruptly, yet evidence of more extensive consolidation be apparent in roentgenograms taken a day or so later (629, 341). Such an occurrence doubtless represents an instance where exudate continues to accumulate in response to the initial stimulus in the lung even though the acute phase of the infection is terminated.

Resolution

Resolution appears to be primarily unrelated to immunity factors and is not obviously affected by serum treatment (297, 793, 245, 176, 897, 341, 813, 814). In a few instances where specific therapy was instituted during the first twenty-four hours of illness, rapid cessation of the acute symptoms and of the spread of the process occurred, followed by rapid resolution (629, 1088). In such instances it is likely the full-blown lesion never developed, thus probably simplifying the process of resolution.

Incidence of Complications

Observing that infection is most likely to be localized in experimental animals having some immunity, whether it be actively or passively acquired, Cole and his associates (33, 297, 299) have stated that one might possibly expect as a consequence of serum therapy in man to find an increase of focal septic complications and that severely infected patients given an insufficient amount of serum might be expected to recover but to have some variety of focal infection during recovery. Finland (444) remarked that this might well apply to bacteriemic patients who, without the use of serum, would probably otherwise have died, and Bullowa (190) has presented evidence supporting such an assumption. The latter worker studied a group of bacteriemic Type I cases and found a larger proportion with empyema among cases treated with specific serum (20 per cent of 150 cases) than in similar bacteriemic cases not receiving such treatment (12.5 per cent of 24 cases). In a review of a few cases studied, Davies and his associates (339) also suggested that the use of serum might increase the occurrence of empyema. These workers, however, ascribed its occurrence to the operation of mechanical rather than immune factors. Aside from somewhat inconclusive evidence such as this, there is no indication that serum administration has any significant effect in increasing the incidence of complications in pneumonia.

In the past it was commonly stated that specific therapy probably had no effect in lowering the incidence of complications (297, 793, 245, 176, 442, 897, 238, 24, 1450). Beginning in 1933, however, occasional reports have appeared suggesting that the incidence of complications may be reduced by specific treatment, as Nemir (930) found in the antiserum treatment of infants and children. This view has been supported by Hamilton (592) and Finland (446), and Robertson and his colleagues (1088) point out that the immune substances injected during treatment appear to confine the organism to the pulmonary lesion.

In addition, observations in Great Britain by the Therapeutic Trials Committee of the Medical Research Council (557) and in this country by Bullowa and Mayer (193) suggest that the incidence of empyema may be reduced in early treated cases. In the British series (treatment begun within ninety-six hours of onset) of Type I cases, empyema occurred in 5.5 per cent of 256 control cases not given serum and in 2.4 per cent of 166 cases receiving such treatment, and in Type II cases in the two groups it was present in 2.7 per cent of 223 control cases and in 0.8 per cent of 131 treated cases. Analysis of the Massachusetts series suggests that the incidence of empyema in Type I cases rises with the lapse of time from the onset of the disease to the day when specific treatment is begun. This complication occurred in 5.3 per cent, or 8, of 152 cases treated on the first day; in 7 per cent, or 18, of 257 cases treated on the second day; in 7 per cent, or 11, of 157 cases treated on the third day; and in 11.3 per cent, or 8, of 71 cases treated on the fourth day. Statistical analysis, by subjecting the Massachusetts figures to the usual formula for detecting the sampling error as given by Yule (1457), has shown, however, that the groups are too small and the percentages too nearly alike to justify any definite conclusion. Judging from the limited data available, antiserum does not appear to reduce the frequency of such complications as endocarditis and meningitis.

EFFECT OF TREATMENT ON CASE FATALITY RATE: VARIATION WITH TYPE

The crucial test of the value of antiserum is its effect on the case fatality rate. Sufficient evidence is now at hand, at least for Type I cases, and to a lesser extent for Type II cases, in the form of large series treated without and with specific horse antiserum to demonstrate the value of the method. Evidence is also accumulating relating to the treatment of cases due to a number of the higher types. The results obtained with the use of rabbit antipneumococcic serum are discussed later (see page 917).

In considering the fatality rate of pneumococcus cases of various types treated without specific therapy, recourse will be had to the large series given in the chapter on Prognosis (page 655) as most of the series there listed were reported as control cases in studies of the value of specific serum treatment for the corresponding type. In numerous instances the alternate case system of treatment was employed until the merits of such treatment were considered established, after which specific treatment was not withheld from a control series. This applies particularly to Type I and Type II cases. Additional data are needed on the results obtained in cases of the higher types treated with and without specific antiserum.

Though the effect on the fatality rate of cases given specific serum treatment is the same whether whole or concentrated serum in equivalent dosage is used, it will simplify tabulation, at least in the instance of the treated Type I cases, to list those treated chiefly with unconcentrated serum first and to consider those given concentrated serum separately, following which the two groups will be combined. In a number of instances Type I cases occurring in various military camps and hospitals throughout the country during and shortly after the War were treated with unconcentrated specific serum. These cases are considered below as a separate group. All other cases at hand are from civilian sources. The results obtained in the serum treatment of infants and children with pneumococcus pneumonia are likewise considered separately (see page 906).

From time to time general reviews of the literature summarizing or discussing the results in serum treated cases have appeared (1299, 324, 793, 223, 195, 990, 225, 92, 1368, 813, 814). In the present review every available series of cases of known type given specific horse serum therapy is included in the cases listed. A few small series of cases have been omitted (1424, 1003a, 1423, 84, 592) as the data given were not sufficient to determine the identity of the organism causing the cases or the nature of the serum used in their treatment. Also, cases receiving Huntoon's antibody solution or any serum except specific antipneumococcic horse serum have been excluded in the following discussion; cases treated with many of these other serums were considered in the previous chapter (see pages 809–822).

For cases receiving specific serum treatment, the fatality rate is usually lower than for untreated cases and varies markedly with the way the serum is used. Moreover, the outcome in many instances is affected by such factors as the time of instituting treatment, the dosage administered, the interval in hours or days over which all doses are given, the age of the patient, the presence of bacteriemia, the season of the year, and the presence of the parturient state or of some general chronic illness.

Type I Cases

To facilitate the remaining discussion in this chapter, the Type I cases treated with specific antiserum in various military camps and hospitals throughout the United States during and shortly after the War may be considered first (Table 166). These cases are chiefly of historical interest, although at the time of treatment a lively controversy was carried on as to whether or not the results obtained were indicative of a specific therapeutic effect. Unconcentrated antiserum was used, in some instances was hurriedly produced and of low or unknown potency, and probably at times of little value. It is presumably for these reasons that the results obtained were by no means uniformly successful. Despite this handicap the findings are in general suggestive of the favorable effect of treatment. In other series treated with the Type I serum then available etiologic diagnosis was not always carried out, so presumably a number of cases were given Type I serum for pneumonia due to pneumococci of some other type. No cases of this description are included in Table 166.

The reports of many physicians treating Type I cases, both of military and civilian origin, at this period were summarized by Thomas (1299), Locke (793), and Wadsworth (1365). Locke (793) viewed the results obtained from the use of specific whole immune serum in Type I cases with some pessimism. He collected from the literature up to 1923 the reports of all available treated cases of Type I lobar pneumonia and found that of 358 such cases treated in military hospitals there were 34 deaths, or 9.5 per cent. This fatality rate he compared with the 10.7 per cent rate reported by the Surgeon General of the United States Army for 1918, for 6,964 cases of lobar pneumonia with 747 deaths. These figures are not strictly comparable, however, as the series reported by the Surgeon General was not made up merely of Type I cases but consisted of all cases of pneumonia in the lobar form and doubtless the largest proportion of them were due to pneumococci of other types and probably some were due to other organisms as well.

TABLE 166. TYPE I LOBAR PNEUMONIA IN MEN IN AMERICAN MILITARY CAMPS OR HOSPITALS, 1917–1924. SOURCE, NUMBER OF CASES TREATED WITH UNCONCENTRATED SPECIFIC ANTISERUM, AND NUMBER AND PERCENTAGE OF DEATHS

SOURCE	CAMP OR HOSPITAL AND DATE	NUMBER OF CASES	DEATHS *Number*	DEATHS *Per cent*
Nichols (952)	Mobilization (Texas), 1917	63	5	7.9
McClelland (829)	Beauregard (La.), 1918	15*	–	–
Cecil (219)	Upton (N.Y.), 1918	20	2	10.0
Cole and MacCallum (307)	Fort Sam Houston (Texas), 1918	8	–	–
Stone, Phillips, and Bliss (1251)	Fort Riley (Kansas), 1918	27	4	14.8
Vaughan and Schnabel (1351)	Sevier (S.C.), 1918	10	2	20.0
Medalia and Schiff (879)	MacArthur (Texas), 1918	3	–	–
Leopold (774)	Dix (N.J.), 1918	24	2	8.3
Thomas (1295)	Meade (Md.), 1918	50	3	6.0
Spooner, Sellards, and Wyman (1222)	Devens (Mass.), 1918	51	20	39.2
Greenway, Boettiger, and Colwell (566)	Bowie (Texas), 1918	125	5	5.6
Park and Chickering (985)	Jackson (S.C.), 1919	34	2	5.9
Tenney and Rivenburgh (1289)	Upton (N.Y.), 1919	61	9	14.8
Henson (634)	Johnston (Fla.), 1920	22	3	13.6
McGuire (839)	Chelsea Naval Hospital (Mass.), 1922	35†	2	5.7
Wadsworth (1365)	Several camps, 1924	168	7	4.2
Total		716	66	9.2

* Sixteen other Type I cases were treated with a "polyvalent" serum of unknown characteristics with four deaths.

† Treatment with serum begun within seventy-two hours of the onset.

The generally low fatality rate for pneumonia in men in military organizations was pointed out in the chapter on Prognosis (page 699). In Table 141 (page 701) of that chapter it was seen that death occurred in 19.4 per cent, or 18 of 93 cases of Type I lobar pneumonia in men in American army camps in this country during and shortly after the War. This rate may be contrasted with that of 9.2 per cent for 716 other Type I cases of lobar pneumonia (66 died) occurring in the same or similar camps and hospitals at the same period in patients given specific serum treatment, as seen in Table 166. The difference in the rates in the two groups strongly suggests that the fatality rate was reduced by such treatment.

TABLE 167. TYPE I LOBAR PNEUMONIA IN THE UNITED STATES, 1913–1936. SOURCE, NUMBER OF CASES TREATED WITH UNCONCENTRATED SPECIFIC ANTISERUM, AND NUMBER AND PERCENTAGE OF DEATHS

SOURCE	PERIOD OF INVESTIGATION	NUMBER OF CASES	DEATHS *Number*	DEATHS *Per cent*
Alexander (9)	1913–1917	11	2	18.2
Bloomfield (134)	1916–1917	11	3	27.3
Hartman and Lacy (604)	1917	5	3	60.0
Christian (266)	1917	53	10	18.9
Hart (600)	1917–1918	30	7	23.3
Thomas (1299)	1917–1921	50	9	18.0
Locke (793)	1919–1922	145	25	17.2
Wadsworth (1365)	1915–1923	277	50	18.1
Wadsworth (1366)	1931	89	10	11.2
Cole (302)	1913–1936	462*	48	10.4
Total		1,133	167	14.7

* Apparently at least thirty of these cases received concentrated antiserum (see Abernethy, 1).

For civilians, the expected case fatality rate without specific therapy may be estimated, as shown in Table 117 (page 664), as 29 per cent for 2,314 Type I cases in the United States and Canada; as 18.5 per cent for 655 cases (Table 118, page 665) in Great Britain and Denmark; and as about 23.5 per cent for 119 cases from elsewhere in the world. The fatality rate in the untreated cases seems appreciably lower in the British and Danish series. Combining these series treated without specific antiserum, there is a grand total of 3,088 Type I cases almost wholly of lobar pneumonia, of which 820, or 26.6 per cent died.

In contrast to these figures death occurred in 14.7 per cent, or 167, of 1,133 American Type I cases shown in Table 167. The cases in this table received specific serum and nearly all were treated with unconcentrated serum. Further, Table 168 lists a large number of similar cases treated chiefly with con-

TABLE 168. TYPE I LOBAR PNEUMONIA IN THE UNITED STATES, CANADA, GREAT BRITAIN, GERMANY, AND CHINA. SOURCE, NUMBER OF CASES TREATED WITH CONCENTRATED SPECIFIC ANTISERUM, AND NUMBER AND PERCENTAGE OF DEATHS

SOURCE	PERIOD OF INVESTIGATION	NUMBER OF CASES	DEATHS	
			Number	*Per cent*
United States				
Park, Bullowa, and Rosenblüth (991)	1926–1928	109	18	16.5
Cecil and Plummer (238)	1924–1929	239	48	20.1
Finland (442)	1924–1929	80	17	21.3
Baldwin (59)	1926–1930	19	1	5.3
Bigelow (104)	1928–1930	86	18	20.9
Sutliff and Finland (1269)	1929–1930	28	7	25.0
Chickering (258)	1930	52*	12	23.1
Lord (809)	1917–1931	99*	20	20.2
Ryland (1144)	1930–1932	3	–	–
Kohl and Reitzel (734)	1932–1935	19†	9	47.4
Price (1051)	1935	27‡	5	18.5
Finland (449)	1930–1936	289	52	18.0
Bullowa (190)§	1928–1936	752†	100	13.3
Benjamin, Blankenhorn, Ruegsegger, and Senior (94)	1935–1937	73‡	3	4.1
Rogers (1102)	1935–1937	1,402	248	17.7
Total		3,277	558	17.0
Canada				
Howard and Fullerton (663)	1929–1931	24	5	20.8
Brown (156)	1931	14	2	14.3
Total (United States and Canada)		*3,315*	*565*	*17.0*
Great Britain				
Physicians to Royal Infirmary, Edinburgh (1023)	1929–1930	12	–	–
Leys (779)	1932–1933	15	4	26.7
Therapeutic Trials Committee of Medical Research Council (557) ..	1931–1933	184*‖	18	9.8
Davies, Hodgson, and Whitby (339)	1932–1933	19	2	10.5
Total		230	24	10.4
Germany				
Lichtenstein (781)	1928	21*	2	9.5
China				
Wu and Chiu (1450)	1922–1931	45*	5	11.1
Total (Great Britain, Germany and China)		*296*	*31*	*10.5*
Grand total		*3,611*	*596*	*16.5*

* Some cases treated with unconcentrated serum.

† Cases of pneumococcus pneumonia (lobar pneumonia and bronchopneumonia together).

‡ Serum treatment begun within the first four days of illness.

§ See also Table 175 (page 906).

‖ Only patients twenty to sixty years of age having their serum treatment begun within the first four days of illness are included. All patients dying within twenty-four hours of admission to hospitals were omitted.

centrated serum. The fatality rate of 3,315 American and Canadian treated cases is 17 per cent (565 died). Together the treated American and Canadian cases in these two tables total 4,448, of which 732 or 16.5 per cent died. Comparison of this fatality rate with that for the untreated Type I cases (29 per cent) from these countries, as mentioned above, indicates a reduction in the rate for the treated cases of 43.1 per cent.

Of 230 treated cases in the British series in Table 168 death occurred in only 24, or 10.4 per cent. Most of the British cases were selected as indicated in the table and their specific treatment was begun within the first four days of illness. Although the series of untreated Type I cases from British and Danish sources, referred to above, which were almost wholly British cases, had a fatality rate of 18.5 per cent, which is considerably lower than the death rate for untreated cases of this type in the United States and Canada, the proportional reduction of the fatality rate for cases treated with specific antiserum appears about the same in each instance, 43.1 per cent for the American and Canadian series, as already noted, and 43.8 per cent for the treated as compared with the untreated British cases.

In a total of 296 treated Type I cases in Table 168 from Great Britain, Germany, and China, 31, or 10.5 per cent, died. Together all the Type I cases treated with concentrated antiserum in Table 168 total 3,611, of which 596, or 16.5 per cent, died.

Table 169 gives a summary of the cases from Tables 167 and 168. In all there is a grand total of 4,744 treated Type I cases, with a fatality rate of 16.1 per cent (763 deaths), which is considerably lower* than the total rate of 26.6 per cent for 3,088 untreated Type I cases mentioned above.

The case fatality rates in these large series of collected Type I cases may be compared with the fatality rates in the following groups.

RELATION OF EARLY TREATMENT TO FATALITY RATE. The earlier specific treatment is begun the more favorable are the results. Observations suggestive of such an effect were obtained in a number of the earlier studies (797, 793, 1365, 223, 195, 991, 245, 442, 809, 238, 183). The greatest measure of success in a large series of serum treated Type I cases is reported by Cole (302). In his 462 cases with 48 deaths, or 10.4 per cent, the fatality rate in cases treated during the first three days was only 4.8 per cent, during the first four days 8.2 per cent, during the first five days 8.6 per cent, and after the fifth day 19.5 per

* The proportional reduction of the fatality rate in the treated as compared with the untreated cases amounts to 39.5 per cent.

cent. Benefit from serum obtains throughout, but the results are progressively less favorable with the lapse of time between onset and inauguration of specific therapy. The low case fatality rate in the series as a whole shows what may be expected from serum treatment under highly favorable circumstances.

Cecil's (227) finding of a fatality rate of 5 per cent (8 deaths) for a collected series of 160 Type I cases, treated with serum within the first twenty-four hours of illness, serves further to emphasize the importance of early specific therapy. This series includes 37 of Cecil's cases with two deaths; 13 of Bullowa's with no deaths; 87 cases from the Massachusetts Pneumonia Series with five deaths; and 23 cases contributed by Rogers from the New York State Department of Health Pneumonia Control Series with one death.

TABLE 169. TYPE I LOBAR PNEUMONIA. NUMBER OF CASES TREATED WITH EITHER UNCONCENTRATED OR CONCENTRATED ANTISERUM, AND NUMBER AND PERCENTAGE OF DEATHS

SOURCE	NUMBER OF CASES	DEATHS *Number*	DEATHS *Per cent*
Total of cases in Table 167	1,133	167	14.7
Total of cases in Table 168	3,611	596	16.5
Total	4,744*	763	16.1

* The Massachusetts Pneumonia Series of treated Type I cases is not included as many of Finland's (449) cases in Table 168 are included in the Massachusetts series. If Finland's 289 cases with 52 deaths are omitted and the 1,043 Massachusetts cases (all received specific treatment within ninety-six hours of onset) with 145 deaths are added to the remaining total, there is a grand total of 5,498 cases with 856 deaths, or 15.6 per cent.

Bullowa (190) in a series of serum treated Type I cases (lobar pneumonia and bronchopneumonia together) reports a fatality rate of 8.6 per cent (25 died) for a series of 290 cases in which specific treatment was begun during the first four days of illness. In contrast to this, 424 similar cases treated later in their illness had a fatality rate of 15.3 per cent (65 died).

The results in the Massachusetts Pneumonia Series were obtained by nearly 1,100 physicians in all parts of the state in the course of the program to make specific serum generally available throughout the state. In this series of 1,043 cases of Type I lobar pneumonia treated with concentrated antiserum within the first four days (ninety-six hours) of the illness, 145, or 13.9

per cent, died. This fatality rate may be compared (see Figure 14) with that of the 29 per cent rate for 2,314 cases (671 deaths) collected from the American and Canadian literature and not treated with serum, as already described (see Table 117, page 664).

The importance of time is emphasized by the figures shown in Table 170. Of 861 Type I cases in which treatment with serum was begun within the first three days of illness 108, or 12.5 per cent, died. The apparently higher rate (14.2 per cent) on the first day is not statistically significant and it is not

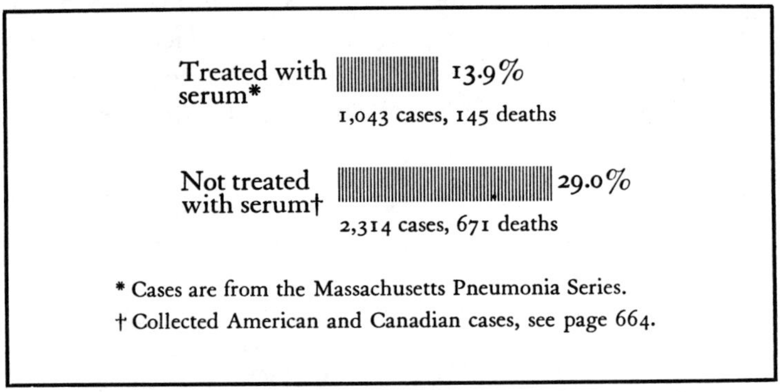

Figure 14. Type I pneumonia. Number of cases in which serum treatment was begun within 96 hours of onset and number of cases not given serum, and number and percentage of deaths in each group

to be expected that it will obtain with a larger number of cases. It cannot be regarded as a violation of the well-established principle of a larger measure of success in specific therapy the earlier in the course of the disease it is instituted. Vagaries of diagnosis and difficulties in dating the time of onset are believed at least partly responsible for the apparently high fatality rate on the first day.

The fatality rate rises abruptly in cases treated on the fourth day of the disease. Of 182 cases in the Massachusetts series treated on this day, 37, or 20.3 per cent, died.

In the New York State Pneumonia Control Series Rogers (1102) reports that of 1,402 Type I serum treated cases 248, or 17.7 per cent, died (see Table 168). Of 1,023 cases in which treatment was started within the first four days 143, or 13.9 per cent, died.

Evidence has accumulated which indicates that no time limit can be set beyond which serum is ineffective and that in consequence patients should not be deprived of the benefit of specific treatment even though it is begun late in the course of the disease. Out of 711 Type I cases* collected by Lord (814), which were treated after the fourth day, there were 140 deaths, or 19.7 per cent, and out of 558 controls not treated with serum there were 181 deaths, or 32.4 per cent, a finding which indicates that the fatality rate falls when the treatment is begun after the fourth day of illness. The restriction by the Massachusetts Department of Public Health of the use of antiserum

TABLE 170. TYPE I LOBAR PNEUMONIA. NUMBER OF CASES TREATED WITH CONCENTRATED ANTISERUM AND NUMBER AND PERCENTAGE OF DEATHS, BY DAY ON WHICH SERUM TREATMENT WAS BEGUN

SERUM TREATMENT BEGUN	NUMBER OF CASES	DEATHS *Number*	DEATHS *Per cent*
On first day	183	26	14.2
On second day	384	42	10.9
On third day	294	40	13.6
In first three days	861	108	12.5
On fourth day	182	37	20.3
Total	1,043	145	13.9

Cases from the Massachusetts Pneumonia Series

to patients who had not been ill longer than four days was removed in March 1937, as already mentioned. In the New York State Pneumonia Control Program and in several other programs of like nature no restriction as to time is set on the use of specific serum, though in all instances the striking success of early therapy is emphasized.

RELATION OF OTHER FACTORS TO FATALITY RATE. In appraising the results in the serum treated Type I cases in the Massachusetts series, it is encouraging to note that there has been a reduction from the expected fatality rate of 29 per cent to 13.9 per cent, a decrease of 52.1 per cent. In comparison with a case fatality rate of 8.2 per cent for cases treated within the first four days in Cole's series, mentioned above, the results in Massachusetts may be assumed to fall short of an attainable goal. There is one significant difference in the two series. Though the average dosage in units in Cole's series cannot be stated

* Collected from the American literature.

(see page 847), it was obviously larger than in the Massachusetts cases. The fatality rate in the latter series during the first three years (see Table 163, page 847) encouraged the hope that the dosage then used might prove adequate, but the lower fatality rate in Cole's series and less favorable results in the Massachusetts series during the last four years made it desirable to recommend an increase in dosage (see pages 848 and 856) over that previously suggested.

The fatality rate of cases treated with optimum dosage and at the earliest possible moment is obviously unknown but it is clear that the size of the total dose, the time of administration of antiserum, and variation in dosage according to the need of the individual case are important factors (see page 856). In this connection the influence of age (see pages 703–710) and of bacteriemia (see pages 681–693) on the outcome demands serious consideration, and some attention should also be given the season of the year the case occurs (see page 680).

When specific serum is to be administered in the treatment of a case due to any type, the estimated dosage needed should be given as rapidly as is consistent with safety. As nearly as possible the total dosage used should be given over a period not to exceed forty-eight hours in the usual instance. An interval of less than twenty-four hours is preferable. Particularly is this true in the presence of bacteriemia, as the findings of Finland (448) and of Finland and Dowling (452) suggest. Unnecessary prolongation of the intervals between doses or the use of small doses given in haphazard fashion should be avoided. Under such circumstances poor results are usually obtained, a larger total amount of serum is frequently required, and life may be unnecessarily lost.

Observations of similar significance are reported by Bullowa (190) who analyzed the results of specific treatment of a series of Type I cases. His findings indicate the value of giving the required dosage within a period of less than thirty-six hours. Of 287 Type I cases so treated 36, or 12.5 per cent, died, as compared with 25.4 per cent, or 44, of 173 similar cases in which treatment was protracted over a period of more than thirty-six hours. Analysis of these cases with respect to the presence or absence of bacteriemia and the period over which treatment was given revealed findings somewhat similar. Among 221 non-bacteriemic Type I cases whose specific treatment was completed within a period of thirty-six hours after its inauguration, death occurred in 10, or 4.5 per cent, while in 102 cases treated over a longer period 13, or 12.7 per cent, died. In the bacteriemic cases in the two groups there was less difference, however, and there were 66 whose treatment was completed within thirty-six hours with 26 deaths, or 39.4 per cent, in contrast with 40.3 per cent, or 31, of 77 (71?) cases in which treatment was extended over a longer period. The cases were also divided into those receiving total doses up to 120,000 units of serum and those receiving more than this amount within the shorter or the longer period. In 235 cases given the smaller amount of serum within a thirty-six-hour interval there were 29 or 12.3 per cent of deaths and in 76 cases receiving similar amounts of serum given over a longer period 16, or 21.1 per cent died. Where more than 120,000 units of antibody was administered death occurred in 7, or 13.5 per cent, of 52 patients in which treatment was completed within a thirty-six-hour interval and in 28, or 28.9 per cent of 97 patients treated over a longer period. It was shown that less serum is required when treatment is given over the shorter period and results were particularly good in bacteriemic cases when large amounts of serum were used in the space of less than thirty-six hours.

Factors such as those above mentioned which influence the fatality rate of treated cases have a bearing on the specific serum treatment of cases due to pneumococci of any type.

Type II Cases

The Type II cases at hand and all available cases due to pneumococci of other types mentioned later are from civilian sources. Among 1,753 collected Type II cases treated without serum in the United States and Canada, as shown in Table 119 (page 667), there were 651 deaths, a fatality rate of 37.1 per cent (Figure 15). The rate for 627 similar cases from foreign sources, including Great Britain, as shown in Table 120 (page 668), is 29 per cent (182 deaths). Combining these two series there is a grand total of 2,380 Type II cases not given serum with 833 deaths, or 35 per cent.

In contrast to these figures the serum treated Type II cases seen in Table 171 show a fatality rate of 32.7 per cent for 893 cases with 292 deaths occurring in the United States and Canada and a rate of 21 per cent (38 deaths) for 181 treated Type II cases in Great Britain. Most of the British cases, as indicated in the table, were selected and treated in the first four days of illness. Together there are 1,074 treated Type II cases with 330 deaths, or 30.7 per cent. The difference between the fatality rates for all the treated Type II cases (rate 30.7 per cent) and all the untreated cases (rate 35 per cent) of this type indicates a proportional reduction of the rate in the treated cases of 12.3 per cent, which is considerably less striking than the results for the total

TABLE 171. TYPE II LOBAR PNEUMONIA IN THE UNITED STATES, CANADA, AND GREAT BRITAIN. SOURCE, NUMBER OF CASES TREATED WITH CONCENTRATED ANTISERUM, AND NUMBER AND PERCENTAGE OF DEATHS

SOURCE	PERIOD OF INVESTIGATION	NUMBER OF CASES	DEATHS *Number*	DEATHS *Per cent*
United States				
Cole (291)	1912	8*	2	25.0
Baldwin and Rhoades (63)	1925–1926	12†	4	33.3
Park, Bullowa, and Rosenblüth (991)	1926–1928	56	13	23.2
Cecil and Plummer (239)	1924–1929	252‡	102	40.5
Finland (442)	1924–1929	39	11	28.2
Baldwin (59)	1926–1930	35	9	25.7
Bigelow (104)	1928–1930	14	3	21.4
Ryland (1144)	1930–1932	3	–	–
Kohl and Reitzel (734)	1932–1935	7§	2	28.6
Price (1051)	1935	29‖	7	24.1
Bullowa¶ (190)	1928–1936	159§	54	34.0
Finland (449)	1930–1936	129	32	24.8
Benjamin, Blankenhorn, Ruegsegger, and Senior (94)	1935–1937	26‖	8	30.8
Rogers (1102)	1936–1937	95	42	44.0
Canada				
Howard and Fullerton (663)	1929–1931	21	2	9.5
Brown (156)	1931	8	1	12.5
Total (United States and Canada)		*893*	*292*	*32.7*
Great Britain				
Physicians to Royal Infirmary, Edinburgh (1023)	1929–1930	17	5	29.4
Therapeutic Trials Committee of Medical Research Council (557)	1931–1933	164**†	33	20.1
Total (Great Britain)		*181*	*38*	*21.0*
Grand total		*1,074*††	*330*	*30.7*

* Eight cases treated by Cole (291) received unconcentrated serum.

† Some cases may have received unconcentrated serum.

‡ Patients dying within twenty-four hours of admission to hospital are omitted.

§ Cases of pneumococcus pneumonia (lobar pneumonia and bronchopneumonia together).

‖ Serum treatment begun within the first four days of illness.

¶ See also Table 175 (page 906).

** Only patients twenty to sixty years of age having their serum treatment begun within the first four days of illness are included. All patients dying within twenty-four hours of admission to hospitals were omitted.

†† The Massachusetts Pneumonia Series of treated Type II cases is not included as many of Finland's (449) 129 cases with 32 deaths in the table are included in the Massachusetts series. If Finland's cases are omitted and the 281 Massachusetts cases (all received specific treatment within ninety-six hours of onset) with 63 deaths are added to the remaining total, there is a grand total of 1,226 treated cases with 361 deaths, or 29.4 per cent.

series of Type I cases shown above. Much better results with the specific serum treatment of Type II cases are obtained when treatment is instituted early in the illness, as shown below.

Rogers (1102) reports that of 95 Type II serum treated cases in the New York State Pneumonia Control Series 42, or 44 per cent, died (Table 171). The unduly high fatality rate may be explained by the small size of the series and the inclusion of a group of 17 cases with 13 deaths, or 76.4 per cent, from

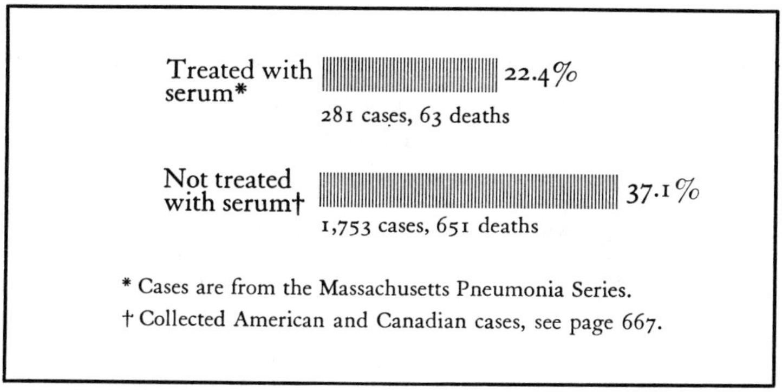

Figure 15. Type II pneumonia. Number of cases in which serum treatment was begun within 96 hours of onset and number of cases not given serum, and number and percentage of deaths in each group

one source. In view of the favorable experience in the treatment of Type II pneumococcus pneumonia in several series reported in literature and in the Massachusetts cases, the apparent lack of success in the small New York series probably has no special significance.

RELATION OF EARLY TREATMENT TO THE FATALITY RATE. Of 281 cases of Type II lobar pneumonia in the Massachusetts series treated with concentrated antiserum within four days (ninety-six hours) of onset, 63 died, a fatality rate of 22.4 per cent (Figure 15). By contrast the fatality rate of 1,753 untreated collected American and Canadian Type II cases is 37.1 per cent, as noted above. These figures indicate a reduction in the proportion of deaths in the Massachusetts treated cases of 39.6 per cent.

Separation of the Massachusetts Type II cases into groups according to the day on which specific treatment was begun is shown in Table 172. Owing to the small numbers in the different groups no special importance can be ascribed to the fatality rates by groups for comparative purposes. The total of 229 cases treated within the first three days with 44 deaths, or 19.2 per cent, however, is large enough to be significant and emphasizes the importance of early specific treatment.

In cases of Type II pneumococcus pneumonia (lobar pneumonia and bronchopneumonia together) Bullowa (190) finds a fatality rate of 23.6 per cent for 55 cases (13 deaths) in whom serum treatment was begun before the end of the fourth day and of 40.4 per cent for 62 cases (25 deaths) when treatment was instituted at a later period.

TABLE 172. TYPE II LOBAR PNEUMONIA. NUMBER OF CASES TREATED WITH CONCENTRATED ANTISERUM AND NUMBER AND PERCENTAGE OF DEATHS, BY DAY ON WHICH SERUM TREATMENT WAS BEGUN

SERUM TREATMENT BEGUN	NUMBER OF CASES	DEATHS	
		Number	*Per cent*
On first day	56	8	14.3
On second day	97	21	21.6
On third day	76	15	19.7
In first three days	229	44	19.2
On fourth day	52	19	36.5
Total	281	63	22.4

Cases from the Massachusetts Pneumonia Series

Analysis of the Massachusetts series of serum treated Type II cases with respect to the average dosage administered (see Table 164, page 849) shows a fatality rate of 24.6 per cent for 126 cases (31 deaths) treated during the Massachusetts Pneumonia Study (1931–1935) with an average of 59,700 units of antibody. During the Continuing Program in 1936 and the first half of 1937, however, the average dose was increased to 123,996 units of antibody and the fatality rate for 133 treated cases decreased to 19.6 per cent (26 deaths). Finland and Dowling (452) have also presented evidence of a lowered fatality rate in Type II cases receiving a larger as compared with a smaller amount of serum, as elsewhere mentioned (see page 849). With Type II infections particularly, it is desirable to administer the estimated dosage required in a short interval and especially if bacteriemia is present. With bacteriemia the administration of one or two doses of serum daily for several days, even though fairly large, usually accomplishes little. Success is often obtained in such cases, however, where repeated doses of large amounts of antibody are given at intervals of a few hours.

Cases Due to Other Types

Specific treatment has thus far been applied to only a limited number of cases of pneumonia due to the recently classified higher types of pneumococci. As elsewhere noted, Types I, III, II, V, VIII, and VII, in the order named, are the most common types and together account for about 76 per cent of cases of pneumococcus lobar pneumonia (see page 52). In pneumococcus pneumonia in general (lobar pneumonia and bronchopneumonia together), these same six types, along with Type IV, are responsible for approximately 72 per cent of cases (see page 54). A satisfactory horse antiserum has never been developed for Type III cases. Such information as is available with respect to the results of specific treatment in Types V, VII, VIII, XIV, and a few other types is briefly reviewed in the following discussion (see also Table 175). Using serums for several of the higher types introduced by Cooper and her associates (318, 320) with Park (991, 990), Bullowa and his co-workers have led the attack on the higher types (Type V, 199; Type VII, 179, 180, 183; Type VIII, 183, 184, 186; Type XIV, 187; these and other types, 190).

Type V Cases

The expected fatality rate for Type V cases of pneumococcus pneumonia without or with specific therapy may be estimated from the results reported by several investigators and the findings in a limited number of cases studied during the Massachusetts Pneumonia Study and in the Continuing Program. Nearly all cases were in adults.

As shown in Table 123 (page 672), of 472 Type V cases treated without specific serum 154, or 32.6 per cent, died. In contrast to this the fatality rate for 210 cases treated with serum, as seen in Table 173, was 16.2 per cent (34 deaths). The number of cases in these collected series treated with or without serum appears to be large enough and the results of specific therapy sufficiently definite to warrant the conclusion that serum treatment is of benefit in Type V pneumococcus pneumonia. The clinical response obtained is often striking. It is of interest that among the cases treated with serum there were at least 54 in which such treatment was begun before the end of the fourth day of illness, as indicated in Table 173. In this group only 7, or 12.9 per cent, died. In addition, Bullowa (190) reports a fatality rate of 14.3

per cent for 21 cases (3 deaths) of Type V pneumococcus pneumonia (lobar pneumonia and bronchopneumonia together) receiving specific treatment before the end of the fourth day and of 20 per cent in 65 cases (13 deaths) treated later in their illness. These series are included in Bullowa's cases in Table 173.

TABLE 173. TYPE V PNEUMOCOCCUS PNEUMONIA. SOURCE, NUMBER OF CASES TREATED WITH SPECIFIC ANTISERUM, AND NUMBER AND PERCENTAGE OF DEATHS

SOURCE	NUMBER OF CASES	DEATHS	
		Number	*Per cent*
Finland and Tilghman (466)	26*	4	15.4
Massachusetts Pneumonia Series	17†*	1	5.9
Benjamin, Blankenhorn, Ruegsegger, and Senior (94)	11†*	2	18.2
Bullowa (190)	117	17	14.5
Rosenblüth and Block (1113)	39	10	25.6
Total	210	34	16.2

* Specific treatment begun within ninety-six hours of the onset.
† Cases of lobar pneumonia.

Type VII Cases

The expected death rate for Type VII cases of pneumococcus pneumonia without or with specific serum treatment may be estimated from the results reported by various investigators. Nearly all cases were in adults. It is seen in Table 124 (page 673) that of 383 cases treated without antiserum 94, or 24.5 per cent, died. Among a group of 154 cases shown in Table 174 which received specific treatment, however, there were but 20 deaths, or 13 per cent. Not only was the fatality rate in the serum treated cases much less than in those not treated with serum, but the duration of the acute illness was apparently curtailed. All of the 18 cases reported by Benjamin and his colleagues (94) were known to have had their specific therapy begun within ninety-six hours of the onset and all recovered.

Type VIII Cases

For 520 Type VIII cases of pneumococcus pneumonia treated without specific serum the fatality rate is shown in Table 125 (page 674) to be 22.9 per

TABLE 174. TYPE VII PNEUMOCOCCUS PNEUMONIA. SOURCE, NUMBER OF CASES TREATED WITH SPECIFIC ANTISERUM, AND NUMBER AND PERCENTAGE OF DEATHS

SOURCE	NUMBER OF CASES	DEATHS Number	Per cent
Finland, Ruegsegger, Dowling, and Tilghman (456)	30	3	10.0
Benjamin, Blankenhorn, Ruegsegger, and Senior (94)	18*	–	–
Bullowa (190)	106	17	16.0
Total	154	20	13.0

* Cases of lobar pneumonia. Serum treatment was begun within ninety-six hours of onset in these cases.

cent (119 deaths). Relatively few cases treated with specific antiserum are available. Benjamin, Blankenhorn, Ruegsegger, and Senior (94) report treating 8 cases of Type VIII lobar pneumonia within ninety-six hours of onset without a death. Bullowa (190) treated 94 cases of Type VIII pneumococcus pneumonia with 10 deaths, or 10.6 per cent. Together these two series of treated cases total 102 cases with 10 deaths, or 9.8 per cent. As yet the evidence of the value of serum treatment for this type is less obvious than for cases due to some other types.

Type XIV Cases

The expected fatality rate for Type XIV cases in adults was shown earlier (page 674) to be 35.6 per cent for 180 cases (64 deaths). Bullowa (190) has treated adults with pneumococcus Type XIV pneumonia with specific serum. Among 27 treated cases death occurred in 8, or 29.6 per cent. The results of specific treatment of Type XIV pneumonia in infants and children are considered later. Additional observations are necessary to demonstrate the value of specific serum therapy for infections due to this type.

Cases of Pneumococcus Pneumonia of Various Types

In 1937 Bullowa (190) reported his results with specific serum treatment in a total of 1,498 cases of pneumococcus pneumonia in adults due to one or another of sixteen different types (Table 175). The Type I, II, V, VII, VIII, and XIV cases were referred to or included in the appropriate sections and tables already mentioned. Untreated cases of corresponding type presented by Bullowa in the same report are listed in Table 127 (page 676). In the case of the types in the treated group above Type II, none of the individual series due to a given type appears large enough to permit satisfactory conclusions from the figures alone, as to the value of specific serum for the different types. It is desirable that investigations of this nature be continued and that suitable data be obtained on large series of treated and untreated cases due to those types concerning which there may be uncertainty as to the efficacy of specific serum in treatment.

TABLE 175. PNEUMOCOCCUS PNEUMONIA (LOBAR PNEUMONIA AND BRONCHOPNEUMONIA TOGETHER) IN ADULTS. NUMBER OF CASES TREATED WITH SPECIFIC ANTISERUM AND NUMBER AND PERCENTAGE OF DEATHS, BY TYPE*

PNEUMOCOCCUS TYPE	NUMBER OF CASES	DEATHS	
		Number	*Per cent*
I	752	100	13.3
II	159	54	34.0
III	94	43	45.8
IV	70	23	32.9
V	117	17	14.5
VI	16	4	25.0
VII	106	17	16.0
VIII	94	10	10.6
IX	20	7	35.0
X	4	2	50.0
XIII	4	1	25.0
XIV	27	8	29.6
XVIII	19	1	5.2
XIX	10	5	50.0
XX	5	1	20.0
XXII	1	–	–
Total	1,498	293	19.6

From Bullowa (190)

* Possibly a few of the included cases were treated with rabbit antiserum.

Infants and Children with Pneumococcus Pneumonia

Such information as is available relating to the effect on the case fatality rates obtained from the use of specific serums in the treatment of pneumonia in infants and children, due to pneumococci of any one of a number of types, appears inconclusive in most instances with respect to showing a reduction of the fatality rate in the treated cases. The number of cases due to any individual type in the treated series is still small, however (Tables 176 and 177).

TABLE 176. PNEUMOCOCCUS LOBAR PNEUMONIA IN INFANTS AND CHILDREN. NUMBER OF CASES TREATED WITH SPECIFIC ANTISERUM AND NUMBER AND PERCENTAGE OF DEATHS, BY AGE GROUP AND BY TYPE

PNEUMOCOCCUS TYPE	UNDER 2 YEARS OF AGE			2 TO 12 YEARS OF AGE		
	NUMBER OF CASES	DEATHS *Number*	DEATHS *Per cent*	NUMBER OF CASES	DEATHS *Number*	DEATHS *Per cent*
I	–	–	–	22	–	–
II	–	–	–	4	–	–
IV	–	–	–	1	–	–
V	–	–	–	3	–	–
VI	5	1	20.0	5	–	–
VII	4	1	25.0	1	–	–
XIV	17	2	11.8	8	–	–

From Nemir (930)

Attention was called earlier (see page 704) to the expected fatality rate in untreated cases due to various types of pneumococci in infants and children. It was also noted that the fatality rate for all pneumonias in infants under two years of age was much higher than for pneumonias in older children and this is likewise true for the serum treated cases.

Nemir's (930) findings in a group of cases of lobar pneumonia in infants under two years of age and in children over this age due to pneumococci of one or another of seven different types (Types I, II, IV, V, VI, VII, and XIV) and given specific serum treatment are shown in Table 176. All the treated cases (44 cases) in the older children recovered. Among 22 treated Type I cases in children in the older group there were no deaths and in 30 similar cases not given serum Nemir (930) had one death (3 per cent). In Type XIV cases in infants there were 2 deaths (11.8 per cent) in 17 cases treated, and in 22 similar untreated cases this investigator also reported 2 deaths (9 per cent). In addition to the cases of lobar pneumonia in Table 176, Nemir (930) treated a few cases of pneumococcus bronchopneumonia without any special success, though at times lysis and recovery occurred. Kereszturi and Hauptmann (710) likewise treated a few cases of pneumococcus pneumonia in children with specific serum but were not impressed with the results.

Table 146 (page 707) gives the fatality rate for cases of pneumococcus pneumonia (lobar pneumonia and bronchopneumonia together) due to pneumococci of some one of a number of types in infants and older chil-

TABLE 177. PNEUMOCOCCUS PNEUMONIA (LOBAR PNEUMONIA AND BRONCHOPNEUMONIA TOGETHER) IN INFANTS AND CHILDREN. NUMBER OF CASES TREATED WITH SPECIFIC ANTISERUM AND NUMBER AND PERCENTAGE OF DEATHS, BY AGE GROUP AND BY TYPE*

PNEUMOCOCCUS TYPE	UNDER 2 YEARS OF AGE			2 YEARS OF AGE AND OVER		
	NUMBER OF CASES	DEATHS *Number*	DEATHS *Per cent*	NUMBER OF CASES	DEATHS *Number*	DEATHS *Per cent*
I	10	3	30.0	78	3	3.9
II	2	1	50.0	2	–	–
III	5	2	40.0	3	–	–
IV	3	2	66.7	5	–	–
V	7	3	42.9	14	–	–
VI	16	2	12.5	6	–	–
VII	3	2	66.7	1	–	–
VIII	–	–	–	1	–	–
IX	2	1	50.0	–	–	–
X	1	–	–	–	–	–
XIV	22	2	9.1	17	2	11.8
XV	–	–	–	1	–	–
XVIII	2	–	–	2	–	–
XIX	–	–	–	1	–	–
XX	1	1	100.0	–	–	–
Total	74	19	25.7	131	5	3.8

From Bullowa (190)

* Possibly a few of the included cases were treated with rabbit antiserum.

dren not given serum treatment. Bullowa's (190) findings in a number of similar cases treated with specific serum are listed in Table 177. Of the untreated Type I cases in infants under two years of age in Table 146 there are 26 with 26.9 per cent of deaths (7 deaths) as compared with 30 per cent (3 deaths) for 10 treated cases in Table 177. Among the older children with Type I pneumonia in these two tables the fatality rate for 116 untreated cases is 1.7 per cent (2 deaths) as compared with 3.9 per cent for 78 treated cases (3 deaths). Obviously these series are too small to mean much, but the results suggest that, as carried out, the treatment given produced little if any favorable effect on the fatality rate.

The best results apparently were obtained in the specific treatment of Type XIV cases in infants and the fatality rate for 125 untreated cases in Table 146 is 16.8 per cent (21 deaths) in contrast to the rate of 9.1 per cent for 22 treated cases (2 deaths) in Table 177 (see also page 693). Bullowa (190) attributes the absence of striking reduction in the fatality rate for the pneumonias in infants and children following specific treatment to the lower incidence of bacteriemia in such patients (see also page 557).

EFFECT OF TREATMENT ON CASE FATALITY RATE: VARIATION WITH TYPE AND OTHER FACTORS

Age

Advancing age is, in general, one of the most important factors in unfavorably modifying the outlook with pneumonia (see pages 703–710). As shown in Figure 16, the case fatality rate for Type I cases from the Massachu-

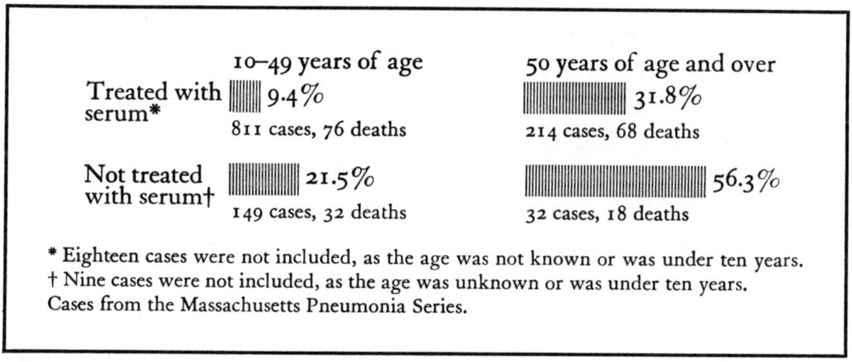

Figure 16. Type I lobar pneumonia. Number of cases treated and not treated with antiserum, and number and percentage of deaths, by age group

setts series is 21.5 per cent without and 9.4 per cent with specific treatment in patients from ten to fifty years of age, and 56.3 per cent without and 31.8 per cent with such treatment in patients fifty years of age and over. Benefit was obtained by specific serum treatment in both the younger and the older groups though the most marked lowering of the fatality rate occurred in the younger patients. The advisability of the routine use of larger amounts of serum in the older than in the younger patients was mentioned earlier (see page 856).

In the serum treated Type II cases in the Massachusetts Pneumonia Series death occurred in 15.8 per cent, or 32, of 201 cases in patients from ten to fifty years of age,* while in those fifty years of age and over, 39 per cent, or 30, of 77 cases died. The results in suitably analyzed untreated Type II cases of American origin are not available for comparison with the findings in the treated cases.

In Great Britain, the Therapeutic Trials Committee of the Medical Research Council (557) studied the fatality rates of treated and untreated Type I and Type II cases in patients in different age groups. Only patients twenty to sixty years of age were included in the cases analyzed and all patients dying within twenty-four hours of admission to the hospitals included in the study† were omitted from the tabulation. In addition, all treated cases had their specific treatment begun within the first four days of illness. In short, the series comprise selected groups of cases.

The results of this study are shown in Table 178. With Type I infections the fatality rate in patients twenty to forty years of age was 5.7 per cent for the treated group and 11.2 per cent for the untreated group, and in patients forty to sixty years of age the rates were 22.7 per cent for the treated and 26 per cent for the untreated cases. With Type II infections the fatality rates in the younger patients were 12.6 per cent for the treated and 22.7 per cent for the untreated, while in the older group the rates were 35.8 per cent for the treated and 34.2 per cent for the untreated. The findings indicated that the fatality rates for the treated Type I and Type II cases in patients under forty years of age were lower than for the untreated cases in this age group, but that in patients over forty the fatality rate was only slightly lower for the treated Type I cases than for the untreated cases and about the same for the treated and untreated Type II cases. It is not possible, however, to draw correct conclusions concerning the significance of these findings in the older patients, as the serum dosage used in the treatment of these cases must be considered inadequate. Doses totaling from 50,000 to 120,000 units, averaging about 80,000 units per case, were ordinarily employed. Although these amounts may be adequate for many Type I and some Type II cases in the younger patients, it is obvious that they are too small to produce satisfactory results in the older patients.

In Bullowa's (190) series of cases of Type I pneumococcus pneumonia (lobar pneumonia and bronchopneumonia together), divided by age groups

* One recovered case is omitted as it occurred in a patient under ten years of age, and two other cases, one of which recovered, are omitted as the age was unknown.

† Certain hospitals in Aberdeen, Edinburgh, Glasgow, and London cooperated in supplying cases for this study.

from twelve to forty years of age and forty years of age and over, data are available as to the fatality rates for cases having their specific treatment inaugurated before the end of the fourth day or at a later period in their illness. In patients in the younger age group the fatality rate for 225 cases was 4.9 per cent (11 deaths) when treatment was begun within four days and 11.7 per cent for 299 cases (35 deaths) when treatment was begun later. In

TABLE 178. TYPE I AND TYPE II LOBAR PNEUMONIA. NUMBER OF CASES TREATED AND NOT TREATED WITH ANTISERUM AND NUMBER AND PERCENTAGE OF DEATHS, BY AGE GROUP

	20–40 YEARS OF AGE			40–60 YEARS OF AGE		
	NUMBER OF CASES	DEATHS *Number*	DEATHS *Per cent*	NUMBER OF CASES	DEATHS *Number*	DEATHS *Per cent*
			Type I			
Treated with serum	140	8	5.7	44	10	22.7
Not treated with serum	224	25	11.2	77	20	26.0
			Type II			
Treated with serum	111	14	12.6	53	19	35.8
Not treated with serum	194	44	22.7	111	38	34.2

From the report of the Therapeutic Trials Committee of the Medical Research Council (557).

similar fashion in patients forty years of age and over the fatality rate for 65 early treated cases was 21.5 per cent (14 deaths) and 24 per cent for 125 cases (30 deaths) in patients in the same age group treated later (after the fourth day) in their illness. In these series, as is usual, early treatment produced a greater proportional reduction of the fatality rate in the younger than in the older cases.

Sex and Place of Treatment

There seems to be no significant relation between fatality rates and sex in the Massachusetts series of Type I and Type II cases receiving specific antiserum treatment, though the fatality rate was slightly higher in the males with Type I pneumonia and in the females with Type II.

In a total of 724 Type I cases in males, 107, or 14.8 per cent, died, while of 319 cases in females 38, or 11.9 per cent, died. Among the Type II cases death occurred in 21.5 per cent, or 48, of 223 cases in males and in 25.9 per cent, or 15, of 58 cases in females.

As seen in Appendix A (page 939), about one-quarter of the Massachusetts Type I cases and one-fifth of the Type II cases occurred in patients given specific serum treatment in their homes. The resulting fatality rates obtained in these cases and in the others treated in hospitals may be considered.

With the Type I cases the proportion of deaths was the same in each instance and 13.9 per cent, that is, 108 of 777 cases treated at hospitals throughout the state died, as did 37 of 265 cases treated at home.* With the Type II

TABLE 179. TYPE I LOBAR PNEUMONIA. SOURCE, NUMBER OF BACTERIEMIC CASES TREATED WITH SPECIFIC ANTISERUM, AND NUMBER AND PERCENTAGE OF DEATHS

SOURCE	NUMBER OF CASES	DEATHS *Number*	DEATHS *Per cent*
Avery, Chickering, Cole, and Dochez (33)	50	13	26.0
Chickering (258)	31	8	25.8
Bullowa, Rosenblüth, Park, and Cooper (195)	28	11	39.3
Bullowa (183)	96	37	38.5
Therapeutic Trials Committee of Medical Research Council (557)	28	5	17.9
Finland (448)	69†	25	36.2
Total	302	99	32.8

† A number of these cases are also included among those in the Massachusetts Pneumonia Series (Figure 18).

cases death occurred in 24.1 per cent, or 54, of 224 cases treated in hospitals and in a somewhat smaller proportion, 15.8 per cent, or 9, of 57 home treated cases. All of 4 Type V cases treated at home recovered, while one, or 7.7 per cent, of 13 cases treated in hospitals died.

Bacteriemia

Attention was called in Chapter XII to the occurrence of bacteriemia in the following approximate proportion of cases: 28 per cent of Type I cases (page 551), 43 per cent of Type II cases (page 552); and, with pneumococcus pneumonia due to the higher types, 28 per cent of Type V cases, 11 per cent of Type VII cases, 21 per cent of Type VIII cases, and 30 per cent

* There was in addition one recovered case which is not included here as the place of treatment is unknown.

of Type XIV cases (see Table 97, page 556). Further, in the chapter on Prognosis it was pointed out that in the absence of specific serum treatment a much higher death rate obtained in patients with bacteriemia than without it (pages 681–693). The fatality rates for patients with bacteriemia are usually three to eight times as high as the rates for patients with negative blood cultures. The analysis in Figure 17 relates to the outcome of collected Type I and Type II cases having bacteriemia and treated with or without specific serum.

With Type I lobar pneumonia the fatality rate for 351 bacteriemic cases collected from the literature and not given serum was 58.1 per cent (204 deaths), as seen in Table 131 (page 683). The fatality rate for a number of

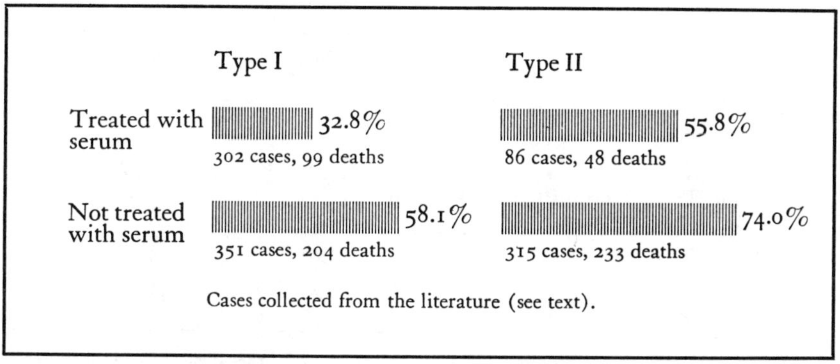

Figure 17. Type I and Type II lobar pneumonia. Number of bacteriemic cases treated and not treated with antiserum and number and percentage of deaths

similar cases which received specific treatment has been determined by various workers, as seen in Table 179. Of 302 bacteriemic Type I treated cases in the table, 99, or 32.8 per cent, died (see also Figure 17).

With Type II lobar pneumonia the fatality rate for 315 bacteriemic cases collected from the literature and not given specific treatment was 74 per cent (233 deaths), as shown in Table 132 (page 684). Among 86 similar cases treated with antiserum, as seen in Table 180, death occurred in 48, or 55.8 per cent.

As shown in Figure 17, based on these summaries of cases in the literature, the fatality rate in bacteriemic cases is much reduced by specific treatment and with Type I infections shows a decrease from the expected rate of 58.1 per cent to 32.8 per cent, and with Type II infections from 74 per cent to 55.8 per cent.

Bullowa's (190) experience with the specific treatment of bacteriemic cases of pneumococcus pneumonia (lobar pneumonia and bronchopneumonia together) in adults is very similar. His untreated cases are shown in Table 136 (page 688). He reports a fatality rate in bacteriemic Type I cases of 79.3 per cent (19 deaths) for 24 untreated cases and of 46 per cent (69 deaths) for 150 similar cases given specific antiserum. With his bacteriemic Type II cases death occurred in 78.5 per cent (47 deaths) of 60 untreated cases and in 68.4 per cent (41 deaths) of 60 treated cases. With cases due to

TABLE 180. TYPE II LOBAR PNEUMONIA. SOURCE, NUMBER OF BACTERIEMIC CASES TREATED WITH SPECIFIC ANTISERUM, AND NUMBER AND PERCENTAGE OF DEATHS

SOURCE	NUMBER OF CASES	DEATHS *Number*	DEATHS *Per cent*
Bullowa, Rosenblüth, Park, and Cooper (195)	13	5	38.5
Bullowa (183)	26	18	69.2
Therapeutic Trials Committee of Medical Research Council (557)	18	7	38.9
Finland and Dowling (452)	29*	18	62.1
Total	86	48	55.8

* A number of these cases are also included among those in the Massachusetts Pneumonia Series (Figure 18).

the higher types the results were usually less marked. In each instance, however, the series was so small that it is doubtful if the results obtained can be given any weight at this time. The need for further data on additional series of cases is obvious. With bacteriemic Type V cases death occurred in 59 per cent (23 deaths) of 39 untreated cases and in 53.7 per cent (15 deaths) of 28 treated cases. With bacteriemic Type VII cases there was a fatality rate of 77.4 per cent (17 deaths) for 22 untreated cases and of 61.6 per cent (8 deaths) for 13 treated cases. With Type VIII cases having bacteriemia death occurred in 41.7 per cent (15 deaths) of 36 untreated cases and in 28.6 per cent (6 deaths) of 21 treated cases.

With Bullowa's (190) Type XIV cases in adults with bacteriemia 75 per cent (21 deaths) of 28 cases in the untreated group died, as did 50 per cent, or 2, of 4 treated cases. His Type XIV cases in children were divided into those occurring in patients under and over two years of age. With the bacteriemic cases of this type in the younger patients 3 of 4, or 75 per cent, died without serum treatment and one of 2, or 50 per cent, with specific treatment. In the older children with Type XIV bacteriemia the groups are also small and one of 4, or 25 per cent, died without serum therapy and one of 2, or 50 per cent, with such treatment.

Figure 18 presents an analysis of the results of serum treatment of Type I and Type II cases of lobar pneumonia in the Massachusetts Pneumonia Series with and without bacteriemia. Out of 112 bacteriemic Type I cases treated within the first four days of the illness 32, or 28.6 per cent, died, while

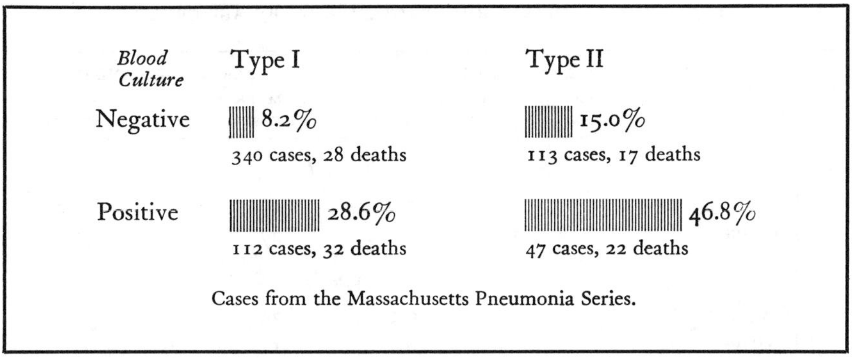

Figure 18. Type I and Type II lobar pneumonia. Number of cases with and without bacteriemia treated with antiserum and number and percentage of deaths

of 340 with negative blood cultures only 28, or 8.2 per cent, died. The corresponding figures for the bacteriemic Type II cases are 47 cases with 46.8 per cent of deaths (22 deaths) and 113 non-bacteriemic cases with 15 per cent of deaths (17 deaths).

Analysis of the serum treated Type I and Type II cases in the Massachusetts series with respect to the incidence of bacteriemia in patients fifty years of age and over and in those under fifty years old suggests, as already mentioned (see page 557), that bacteriemia occurs more often in the older than in the younger age group. It has seemed desirable, in consequence, to analyze serum treated bacteriemic and non-bacteriemic Type I and Type II cases with respect to the fatality rates obtained in a younger and in an older age group.

As shown in Table 181, of 290 serum treated Type I cases in patients under fifty years of age with negative blood cultures, only 5.9 per cent, or 17, died, while of 85 with positive cultures in this age group 21.2 per cent, or 18, died. These results in the younger age group may be contrasted with those in the older age group. Of 49 serum treated Type I cases in patients fifty years of age and over with negative blood cultures, 22.4 per cent, or 11, died and of 27 with positive cultures, 51.8 per cent, or 14, died. Thus, the fatality rate for specifically treated Type I cases in the younger age group is about four times as high for those with bacteriemia as for those without bacteriemia, and in the older age group over twice as high.

TABLE 181. TYPE I AND TYPE II LOBAR PNEUMONIA. NUMBER OF CASES TREATED WITH SPECIFIC ANTISERUM AND NUMBER AND PERCENTAGE OF DEATHS IN CASES WITH AND WITHOUT BACTERIEMIA, BY AGE GROUP

BLOOD CULTURE	0–49 YEARS OF AGE			50 YEARS OF AGE AND OVER		
	NUMBER OF CASES	DEATHS *Number*	DEATHS *Per cent*	NUMBER OF CASES	DEATHS *Number*	DEATHS *Per cent*
			Type I			
Negative	290	17	5.9	49	11	22.4
Positive	85	18	21.2	27	14	51.8
			Type II			
Negative	87	8	9.2	25	9	36.0
Positive	34	13	38.2	13	9	69.2

Cases from the Massachusetts Pneumonia Series

The results in serum treated Type II cases with and without bacteriemia according to age are also shown in Table 181 and are much the same as in Type I cases. In the younger age group the fatality rate for serum treated cases is about four times as high with positive as with negative cultures and in the older age group nearly twice as high.

The figures are of interest in showing the unfavorable influence of bacteriemia on the fatality rate in specifically treated cases in both the younger and the older age groups. Though the fatality rate to be expected in the absence of specific treatment is reduced by serum therapy, it still remains high and is an obvious indication for the intensive use of serum in the treatment of bacteriemic cases and particularly in the older patients, as previously mentioned (see pages 855 and 856).

Season

In the chapter on Prognosis the effect of season on the fatality rate of cases treated with or without the use of specific antiserum was discussed (see page 679). It is apparent from the results obtained in the serum treated Massachusetts Type I and Type II cases shown in Table 129 (page 681), that higher fatality rates obtain in the late winter and early spring than at other times of the year. As a consequence of this observation, particular attention should be given cases treated at that period of the year and it seems advisable to administer as a routine procedure more than the usual amounts of serum to such cases (see also page 856).

As seen in Table 129, analysis of the Massachusetts cases shows that for 299 Type I cases treated during the late spring and summer months the low fatality rate of 9.4 per cent (28 deaths) was obtained. In 217 similar cases treated during the early fall and winter 26, or 12 per cent, died, while for 527 Type I cases treated during the late winter and early spring with 91 deaths, the fatality rate was 17.3 per cent, or much higher. Results were somewhat the same with Type II, although the individual groups of cases are still too small to yield significant findings.

RABBIT ANTIPNEUMOCOCCIC SERUM AND RESULTS WITH TREATMENT

Attention has already been called (page 876) to the use of unconcentrated type-specific antipneumococcic rabbit serum in the treatment of pneumonia by Horsfall and his co-workers (659, 658). Their series comprises 67 unselected cases due to pneumococci of one or another of the nine types, Types I, II, III, V, VI, VII, VIII, XIV, and XVIII.

In the rabbit as in the horse it is difficult to produce potent antiserum against Type III pneumococcus. Of 13 Type III pneumonias treated with Type III antipneumococcic rabbit serum 6, or 46 per cent, died. As there was no evidence of a favorable result in these cases they are excluded from further consideration.

Excluding the Type III cases there were 54 cases, the type distribution of which was as follows:

Pneumococcus type	*Number of cases*
I	25
II	10
V	1
VI	2
VII	6
VIII	7
XIV	2
XVIII	1
Total	54

Only one case with Type I infection and one case with Type II infection died, a fatality rate of 3.7 per cent for the group of 54 cases. The small size of the series, however, makes it difficult to judge the merit of rabbit antiserum on the basis of the fatality rate alone, but there are other significant aspects which add weight to the observations. Thirteen patients were fifty years of age or over. There was consolidation of two or more lobes in 18 cases. Pneumococcus bacteriemia was present in 17 cases. Pleural exudates, infected with pneumococci, occurred in 7 cases. Two of these 7 had empyema before serum therapy was instituted and 2 developed it later. In the 3 remaining cases, following specific treatment, type-specific antibody of rabbit origin was demonstrated in the exudates and subsequently the pneumococci disappeared.

Rapidity of recovery after the administration of an adequate amount of rabbit antiserum was a striking feature. The average interval from the inauguration of specific therapy to the disappearance of the acute signs of the disease was only twenty-seven hours. In 18 patients to whom an adequate quantity of antiserum was given in a single injection, the crisis was completed in an average interval of seven and one-half hours after beginning treatment.

Bullowa (190, 189), also, has successfully used specific immune rabbit serum in the treatment of pneumococcus pneumonia. Detailed analysis of his treated cases was not presented in his reports.

The high mouse protective potency of immune rabbit serum as compared with that of immune horse serum, absence of the prozone phenomenon, and the smaller size of the antibody produced in the rabbit (at least for Type I) must be taken into consideration in estimating the value of the product.

Rabbit antiserum gives promise of being a valuable therapeutic agent for pneumococcus pneumonia and is now being rather widely used, at least in this country. It is desirable that detailed studies of the efficacy of the agent be made available.

ANALYSIS OF DEATHS OCCURRING DESPITE SERUM TREATMENT

With respect to the use of specific immune serums for the treatment of pneumonia due to pneumococci of a given type, complete success is seldom achieved. Numerous studies have been made to determine the apparent reasons for the failure of serum to bring about recovery in treated cases which have terminated fatally. Analysis of the deaths occurring after specific treatment in Type I infections was made by Wadsworth (1365) in 33 fatal cases, by Cole (299) in 39 fatal cases, by Cecil and Plummer (238) in 48 fatal cases, by Leys (779) in 4 fatal cases, by Parsons and Myers (1000) in one such case, by Sutliff and Finland (1272) in 12 fatal cases, and by Price (1051) in 5 fatal cases. Similar analyses were made of the deaths following specific treatment of 9 Type II cases by Finland and Sutliff (463) and of 7 Type II cases by Price (1051). In addition, efforts were made to determine the cause of death in a number of fatal Type I and Type II cases treated with specific antiserum during the course of the Massachusetts Pneumonia Study and Continuing Program (869, 813, 814). The findings in all these investigations are very similar. General discussions of the apparent failure of specific serum to bring about recovery in some treated cases of pneumonia are given by Finland (444, 446) and by Robertson, Graeser, Coggeshall, and Sia (1088).

Studies such as these indicate that in about one-half of the cases which fail to recover even though serum treatment is given, the presence of complications of one sort or another appears responsible for the fatal outcome. Septic complications such as empyema, marked bacteriemia, endocarditis, and meningitis are common in these cases. Mixed infections (see pages 11–16) or relapse (see pages 532–533) due to infection with a pneumococcus of another type or with a different organism such as the hemolytic streptococcus are occasionally responsible. Other complications which were present before treatment was instituted, such as cardiovascular collapse or auricular fibrillation with signs of cardiac decompensation or other chronic disease, either in the lungs or in other parts of the body, are present in some of these cases.

Of the remaining half of the fatal cases a large proportion are in patients given late, insufficient, and inadequate serum treatment. Many are chronic alcoholics and a history of delirium tremens is not uncommon in this group. Most deaths are in patients over fifty years of age and in a number of instances two or more lobes are involved and in some the infection appears overwhelming from the start.

As Finland (444) points out, most deaths in treated cases given adequate amounts of serum may be attributed to associated factors rather than to the presence of pneumonia alone, while in cases not receiving specific treatment death is usually due to the pneumonia. However, death may occur in untreated cases (see pages 545–546), or in treated cases in a few instances, in the absence of demonstrable complications or bacteriemia and with a well-localized and relatively small pulmonary lesion which is apparently confined to one lobe, as Robertson and his colleagues (1088) have mentioned. Instances of this nature in treated cases were reported by Cole (299); and

Cecil and Plummer (238) had two unexplained fatalities, as did Sutliff and Finland (1272). Possibly a few of Price's (1051) cases also fall into this category.

As pointed out in Chapter IV (page 176), in the absence of adequate and positive knowledge concerning the role of specific antibodies in bringing about recovery, the conclusion appears inescapable with the limited information at hand, that there is a small proportion of cases, possibly in the neighborhood of two or three per cent, in which specific therapy alone in presumably adequate amounts is ineffective in bringing about recovery. It is desirable that further studies of this matter be made.

Unavoidable and Avoidable Causes of Failure of Specific Treatment

The analyses mentioned above permit classifying the reasons for obtaining unsatisfactory results with specific therapy in some instances as unavoidable causes or avoidable causes. These may be briefly reviewed, the unavoidable causes being considered first. The presence of complications, and especially empyema, is not infrequent. Mixed infections with more than one type of pneumococcus, the streptococcus, or other organism may be present. Lastly, the infection may be so severe that specific treatment is ineffectual, or the infection may be overcome, but the patient, exhausted by the struggle, succumbs.

Chief among the avoidable causes of failure is the delay before beginning treatment. In suitable cases specific therapy should be instituted at the earliest possible moment. Second in importance is the time required for the determination of the type of infection, previously often unavoidably long and now greatly reduced by the use of the Neufeld method. A third factor is the possibility that in Type I or II cases bacteriologic examination of the sputum may fail to show the infecting type because at the first typing some other type is identified and the typing is not repeated. Failure to retype under these circumstances is responsible for an error of about 10 per cent. Other causes may be insufficient antiserum, low potency, or too long intervals between doses. In connection with insufficient dosage, failure to appreciate the importance of the administration of more than the usual amount of antibody in severe cases—as when treatment is begun after the third day of the disease, in patients over forty years of age, in pregnancy or in the first week of the puerperium, with involvement of more than one lobe, with a spreading lesion or with bacteriemia, and in cases occurring in the late winter and early spring of the year—may also be responsible.

CHAPTER TWENTY

CONTINUING PROBLEMS

General Statement 921
Suggestions for Future Endeavor 923
Standardization of Typing Serums and Culture Collection 923
Standardization of Therapeutic Serums 924
Production of Therapeutic Serums 925
Prophylactic Vaccination Against Pneumonia 925
Epidemiologic Studies 925
Study of Pneumonia Incidence 927
Study of the Etiology and Treatment of Pneumococcus Pneumonia .. 927
Chemotherapy 927
Pneumonia Statistics 927
Application of Specific Serum Therapy to Pneumococcus Pneumonia 928
Pneumonia Programs 929
Outline of Pneumonia Programs 932

GENERAL STATEMENT

THE content of the foregoing chapters will serve to indicate the progress made in our understanding of pneumonia. The situation in the United States and to some extent in many other areas throughout the world has been discussed. Prominent among matters relating to an advance of knowledge concerning pneumonia must be a more adequate understanding of the pneumococcus, which is the etiologic agent in the majority of cases. The pneumococcus recognizes no political or geographic boundaries and in consequence the cooperation of national governments and of responsible medical and health organizations through the appropriate sections of the Health Organization of the League of Nations is essential to progress in combating this organism.

Despite the extensive investigations carried out on pneumonia and matters related to it, particularly in the past two or three decades, the disease continues to rank high among the common causes of death in this and many other countries. Thus far administrative and other measures designed to prevent pneumonia have met with little success. In consequence efforts at control have been directed chiefly to therapeutic measures. In the past few years medical history has been made by the extension of previous bacteriologic and immunologic studies and, as a result, a rapid and accurate method of pneumococcus typing has been developed, and therapeutic serums of generally accepted effectiveness against pneumococci of several types have been produced. Further, epidemiologic investigations have afforded information on the mode of spread of the pneumococcus in the population at large. Certain recently introduced chemicals have been shown to exert a variable bacteriostatic or bactericidal power against this organism. The future holds great promise for subsequent research, as is indicated in numerous places throughout the preceding chapters.

One of the greatest advances in recent years has been the introduction of generally available facilities for rapid pneumococcus typing and the provision of specific therapeutic serums by several states and a number of large cities in the United States. These enterprises are saving lives in the communities where they are being carried on, and it is desirable that similar activities be undertaken elsewhere. Among other important problems relating to pneumonia that demand serious consideration, possibly the most pressing is the need for more data relating to the epidemiology of the disease, and for improved serums and a suitable chemotherapeutic agent for use in pneumococcus infections.

White, with Robinson and Barnes (1417), in their masterly discussion of the pneumococcus, have outlined a number of problems immediately concerning the biology of the organism and the production, concentration, and standardization of antipneumococcic serums for therapeutic purposes which constitute a challenge to interested workers. Additional comments concerning some of the points these investigators mentioned, as well as statements relating to certain other problems at hand, are desirable. Many of these matters were surveyed by the Advisory Committee on Pneumonia* of the United States Public Health Service (1340) designated by Dr. Thomas Parran, Surgeon General of that service. The committee was formed to review the current pneumonia problem in this country and to make recommendations designed to assist in developing pneumonia control work for the country as a whole. A number of the following points mentioned are cited in the Committee's General (1343) and Special (1342) Reports to Surgeon General Parran.

* The following are members of the United States Public Health Service Advisory Committee on Prevention of Pneumonia Mortality:

Dr. Donald B. Armstrong
Dr. David P. Barr
Dr. Russell L. Cecil
Dr. Lloyd D. Felton
Dr. Alfred Friedlander
Dr. Roderick Heffron
Dr. Ernest E. Irons
Dr. Roger I. Lee
Dr. George H. Ramsey

SUGGESTIONS FOR FUTURE ENDEAVOR

Excluding for the moment the question whether healthy persons carrying pneumococci in their nose and throat may be considered infected, the commonest pathologic state produced by the pneumococcus is pneumonia. Means of lessening the toll on mankind from this disease are increasing. Such progress has resulted from years of painstaking investigation on the part of many workers in many lands. The discovery of new facts has broadened the horizon of search for a more adequate understanding of the pneumococcus and the infections it produces but much additional investigation is needed. A number of matters requiring further extended study will be mentioned. In addition, it is necessary for the preservation and general application of the advances thus far made that certain steps be taken to consolidate the gains of the past.

Standardization of Typing Serums and Culture Collection

The classification of pneumococci into the types from Types I to XXXII inclusive has been invaluable as a means of studying many of the problems presented by pneumococcus infections and of attempting to evolve procedures directed at the solution of some of them. In the foreign literature these types are commonly referred to as the "American" types. Their distribution, however, appears to be world-wide. Diagnostic serums produced by various laboratories in this country for many, if not all, of these types, have been used throughout the United States and, to a lesser extent, in several other places throughout the world (see pages 31–41).

Progress in the study and treatment of pneumonia has depended almost wholly on the development of this important and valuable classification. There are difficulties in the production of diagnostic serums for pneumococcus typing, however, as is apparent to all who have had experience with such work. Through changes in the biologic characteristics of laboratory strains of these types, the varying response of animals to immunization with them, and the influence of other factors, alterations in the specificity of diagnostic serums may occur from time to time, and in such instances cross agglutinations and other confusing serologic reactions may appear. It is necessary that meticulous care be exercised in the preparation of these serums.

As several laboratories (city, state, and commercial) are producing diagnostic serums for varying numbers of the recognized types, the possibility that undetected errors may creep into such work is very great and the potential significance of these errors is enormous. To safeguard progress thus far made it is essential that all typing serums produced be uniform in specificity, and to achieve this it is desirable that some governmental agency ensure by appropriate tests and other necessary means the strict specificity of all diagnostic serums. This task might be suitably carried out by the Public Health Service in this country, and the Commission of the League of Nations concerned with the standardization of biologic agents should be requested to cooperate in this matter.

As an important corollary of standardization procedures it is advisable that a collection be maintained of cultures of each of the types of pneumococci for which diagnostic serum is now available. Cultures of any other pneumococci encountered should be investigated and if the organisms do not belong to any of the recognized types, they should be classified as new types. The matter of pneumococcal variants and of type transformation calls for further study.

When typing is carried out for all types it is customary to use various pools of diagnostic serum (see page 626). Inasmuch as some types of pneumococci are encountered more frequently than others, time may be saved in the examination of specimens if the pools of typing serum include certain combinations of types. Additional investigation is necessary to define the most satisfactory combinations of types for this purpose. In this country Type I is perhaps the only type to occur *regularly* in more than 15 per cent of specimens from patients with pneumonia and it seems likely that tests should be made for this type separately and that Type I serum should not be included in any of the pools. The next most common types should be so grouped in pools that the use of two or perhaps three pools will include diagnostic serums for all of the commoner types. Combinations of types suitable for use in the United States may have to be altered to achieve the best results in other countries, depending upon the frequency with which the various types are found in such regions.

Standardization of Therapeutic Serums

Standardization of specific therapeutic antipneumococcic serum is important for, when the potency of such a serum can be uniformly measured, reliable recommendations can be made as to the size of the minimum dose usually needed in treatment. As was mentioned elsewhere (page 827), official standard antiserums have been developed for Types I, II, V, VII, and VIII. The desirability of having available standard antiserums for certain other of the types most commonly causing pneumonia, such as Type XIV, may be mentioned. In addition, uniform methods of testing the potency of therapeutic serum of types, such as those mentioned above, should be rapidly developed. Tests for the standardization of the potency of serums of other types should be considered.

Such problems should naturally come under the jurisdiction of the United States Public Health Service in this country. It is desirable also to cooperate with the League of Nations Commission for the standardization of biologic products in an effort to establish reliable international potency standards and methods of testing for all antipneumococcic serums used for therapeutic purposes.

Production of Therapeutic Serums

Attention should be directed to the improvement of materials, methods of administration, and schedules of dosage used in immunizing animals so as to increase the quantity of antibody produced. The higher antibody output per animal would result in a lowering of the cost of therapeutic serum. Methods of serum concentration and refinement also need to be perfected. It is of immediate practical importance to devise satisfactory methods by which chill-free antiserum may be produced and by which lots of serum likely to give rise to a chill reaction may be detected. Additional studies of the chemical and physical characteristics of antibody with a view to determining the nature and structure of the portion of the molecule which permits the specific union of the antibody with its antigen are desirable.

Prophylactic Vaccination Against Pneumonia

Comment has been made elsewhere concerning the use of vaccines and other agents for prophylactic inoculation against pneumonia. Further efforts should be made to prepare a relatively stable vaccine or other suitable agent of high antigenic value that may be used for the prevention of pneumonia.

The preliminary findings resulting from the experimental inoculation of many thousands of men in various Civilian Conservation Corps camps in this country with derivatives of certain types of pneumococci suggest that this material may aid in reducing the incidence of pneumonia among the immunized (see page 474). Continuation of this investigation is advisable and there is need of carrying out the experimental immunization of a selected civilian population of considerable size in similar fashion in an effort to determine the usefulness of these preparations under the conditions of ordinary life.

Epidemiologic Studies

Great need exists for more extensive and continued epidemiologic investigation of pneumonia. The somewhat limited studies of normal persons indicate that at a given time pneumococci of some type may be found in the nasopharynx of about 40 to 50 per cent of normal people. A much larger proportion of all normal people carry pneumococci of some type in the nose or throat at some time during each year. The proportion of persons carrying these organisms is known to increase during the colder months of the year. Most of the strains carried, however, are representatives of types least often found in pneumonia.

A few studies of a small number of families suggest that when pneumonia due to one of the more invasive types, such as Type I, occurs in an individual, approximately 20 per cent of the other members of the family will also be found harboring that same type. Where acute upper respiratory infections such as colds are prevalent among the family contacts, the incidence of homologous type carriers may approach 70 to 80 per cent. The influence of these minor infections upon the carrier state needs extensive investigation.

The evidence suggests that a pneumococcus of a given type may be carried by a healthy individual into the family group, where it rapidly spreads to several members of the family and that at times some one or more persons within the group may subsequently develop pneumonia due to that organism. As a consequence, it would appear to do little good to insist upon the strict isolation and quarantine of the case in an effort to prevent the patient from spreading the organism to other members of the family, for many of the latter individuals have *already* become carriers of the homologous type by the time the case develops. It is important to bear this in mind when plans are made to control the prevalence of pneumonia by administrative procedures and the matter should be further studied to determine the usual means by which infection is spread both inside and outside the family group.

At various times outbreaks of pneumonia and other infections due to pneumococci of a single type have been studied in a few localities and in several institutions. Evidence suggests that similar localized epidemics occur with considerable regularity in various population groups generally. Such outbreaks may be studied with profit as little is known of their ordinary course. Some evidence has appeared suggesting that the general immunization of the exposed population in institutional epidemics may be of use in aborting the outbreak (see page 473). Further study of this matter is desirable. One of the additional problems encountered in efforts to stop such epidemics is the difficult one of handling healthy carriers who are harboring the type of pneumococcus responsible for the infections. Attention might well be paid to means of curing or eradicating the carrier condition in these individuals, as elsewhere mentioned (see page 404). The practical importance of identifying the factors which influence the carrier rate of pneumococci in man is great.

Study of Pneumonia Incidence

The true frequency of pneumonia due to pneumococci and other organisms, either of a primary or secondary nature, in city, county, or larger political unit, has never been accurately determined.* Such information is desirable and might be obtained through special studies. The influence of host factors on the pathogenesis of pneumonia requires further investigation, as does the role of minor respiratory infections such as the common cold.

Study of the Etiology and Treatment of Pneumococcus Pneumonia

Data should be gathered on the incidence of the various types of pneumococci and other organisms in pneumonia in various geographic sections of the United States and elsewhere throughout the world. A comparative study should be made of the fatality rates of large series of cases due to pneumococci of various types treated with and without specific serum. Decision as to the merit of antiserum in the treatment of cases due to any one of a number of types will be difficult or impossible until such information becomes available.

Chemotherapy

The desirability of more intensive study of the chemotherapeutics of pneumococcus infections has already been mentioned (see pages 775–795). Numerous investigations of this matter are under way and it is advisable that they be continued and extended. There is greater hope today than ever before of finding a chemical agent of outstanding clinical effectiveness against the pneumococcus. It is also advisable that further work on the use of enzymes in the treatment of pneumococcus infections be carried out.

Pneumonia Statistics

Pneumonia should be made a reportable disease and physicians stimulated to report all cases. Case reporting systems should be developed so that it would be possible to specify the type of pneumococcus or other infecting organism. All deaths from pneumonia should be reported and, as soon as practicable, the etiologic agent should be stated on death certificates and in the listing of deaths in various communities. With more adequate reporting, the extent of the problem of controlling this disease will become more

* Certain data relative to this point are mentioned in the footnote on page 258.

apparent and will almost surely be followed by a marked increase in efforts directed toward this end.

APPLICATION OF SPECIFIC SERUM THERAPY TO PNEUMOCOCCUS PNEUMONIA

It has been recognized for many years that pending the development of reliable measures for controlling morbidity from pneumonia, efforts should be directed toward improving the treatment of current cases with a view to decreasing mortality from the disease. The adequate use of specific antipneumococcic serum in appropriate cases was demonstrated to reduce the fatality rate in numerous instances and yielded better results than any other form of treatment. As a consequence, New York City in 1911 (1101), New York State in 1915 (1101), and Massachusetts in 1917 (104) undertook to supply antipneumococcic serum, at least for Type I infections, for the treatment of suitable cases. In addition, commercially prepared therapeutic serum was obtainable in practically all parts of the country. As mentioned later, numerous factors operated to restrict the general use of specific serum and only a small number of cases received the benefit of this form of treatment, even in those communities where antiserum was more or less freely available to physicians wishing to use it and where extensive investigations of pneumonia and its specific treatment were being carried out.

Pneumonia should be regarded as a medical emergency and physicians should no longer be satisfied with the diagnosis until the identity of the infecting organism is known. It is essential that any pneumococci found be typed. Approximately 90 per cent or more of all the lobar pneumonias and one-half or more of the bronchopneumonias are due to pneumococcus infection. In pneumococcus cases success in treatment may depend on the early adequate use of specific serum. The distinction between lobar pneumonia and bronchopneumonia is immaterial from the point of view of antiserum treatment. In suitable cases serum should be given at frequent intervals, whether by day or by night, until the desired response is obtained.

Difficulties in obtaining early bacteriologic diagnosis, cost of serum, lack of familiarity with the technic of administration, undue fear of reactions, and uncertainty as to the merit of the procedure have delayed the wider adoption of the method. Specific treatment in the United States is, in consequence, chiefly confined to large medical centers and general hospitals, as Lord and Heffron (814) have mentioned. As a result of this restriction only a small proportion of those with the disease have the benefit of serum treatment and patients are often admitted to hospitals too late to be successfully treated. In a series of 2,670 cases of lobar pneumonia admitted to the Bellevue and Harlem Hospitals, New York City, Cecil (226) in 1935 reported that 55.1 per cent were admitted on the fourth day or later in the disease.

The situation is improving with respect to the extent to which specific serums are used, but in the country as a whole provision for specific treatment has not been generally made.

The departments of health of New York City and State, of Massachusetts, and of Michigan manufacture and distribute antipneumococcic serum. There are in addition more than a half dozen commercial organizations in the United States which produce antipneumococcic serum under federal license.

PNEUMONIA PROGRAMS

Organized investigations of pneumonia, enlisting the cooperation of numerous physicians, are not new in this country and the Medical Commission for the Investigation of Acute Respiratory Diseases of the Department of Health of the City of New York was appointed as early as 1904 (648, 235). Other groups formed for a similar purpose were later organized in other cities as well. In addition, the work of the Influenza Commission of the Metropolitan Life Insurance Company, which has been in existence since 1919 (235), has successfully fathered numerous findings of great importance relating to the pneumococcus, to means by which the organism was spread, and to the specific treatment of pneumonia. The Massachusetts Pneumonia Study, however, was unique in that it embraced a relatively large geographic area and enlisted the cooperation of many groups of workers. By the time this Study was completed at the end of 1935, general interest in the problem of pneumonia was being aroused.

The Massachusetts Pneumonia Study and Service (869) was conducted for the five years of 1931–1935 under the auspices of the State Department of Public Health and the guidance of a Pneumonia Advisory Committee. It was financed by the Commonwealth Fund. Information concerning the details of that work has been made available in a final report of the Study* (615). The Pneumonia Study demonstrated that patients can be successfully treated with antipneumococcic serum by physicians in general practice (813, 1170, 868, 506, 814). During the course of the Study and in the Continuing Program, more than 1,700 patients with lobar pneumonia were treated by nearly 1,100 physicians in all parts of the state. Details regarding the treated

* A copy of the *Final Report of the Massachusetts Pneumonia Study and Service 1931–1935*, by Heffron and Robinson (615), may be obtained by application to the Department of Public Health, State House, Boston, Massachusetts.

cases are given in the chapter on the Results of Serum Treatment (see page 880) and in Appendix A (see page 937).

A pneumonia control program was inaugurated in November, 1935, in New York State as a cooperative enterprise of the State Department of Health, the State Medical Society, the State Association of Public Health Laboratories, the Metropolitan Life Insurance Company, and the Commonwealth Fund, the last two rendering financial assistance (226, 1101, 235, 677, 678). By the end of May, 1937, Rogers (1102) reported that 1,402 Type I and 95 Type II cases had been treated.

It is the accepted policy of the departments of health of New York City and State, Massachusetts, and Michigan to furnish pneumonia serum free of charge for the treatment of all patients needing it.

Interest in the application of specific therapy to pneumococcus pneumonia is rapidly spreading and pneumonia programs are in operation or under consideration in states (1030, 554, 608, 1032, 1355, 1034, 943, 791, 1033, 1288, 1171) and cities (212, 1043, 1040, 1042) in many parts of the United States. The general report of the United States Public Health Service Advisory Committee on Pneumonia (1343) includes data obtained* from the 48 states, indicating that the health departments of 10 have pneumonia control programs, 11 more have definite plans for programs, and 12 others are contemplating programs, as seen in the accompanying summary.

State health departments having or planning therapeutic programs for the prevention of pneumonia mortality

STATES WITH PROGRAMS	STATES WITH DEFINITE PLANS FOR PROGRAMS	STATES WITH INDEFINITE PLANS FOR PROGRAMS
Connecticut	Georgia	Alabama
Delaware	Iowa	Colorado
Maine	Kentucky	Indiana
Maryland	New Hampshire	Kansas
Massachusetts	New Jersey	Louisiana
Minnesota	New Mexico	Michigan
New York	North Carolina	Ohio
Oklahoma	Rhode Island	Tennessee
Pennsylvania	Vermont	Utah
South Carolina	Virginia	Washington
	Wyoming	West Virginia
		Wisconsin

* As of January, 1938. A number of the states listed in the accompanying summary as having plans for programs have subsequently begun their projects.

According to the above report, pneumonia programs are in operation in 23 of the 93 cities of 100,000 population or more in the United States. In 17 other cities definite plans have been made, and in 5 others the matter is under consideration. Considerable difference exists in the scope of the programs in operation in both the cities and states.

It is pointed out in the same report (1343) that a belt of states with high mortality from this disease may be found along the eastern border of the country and another group of states with excessive pneumonia death rates in the southwest (this was mentioned earlier, pages 269–274); and that, in general, fewer typings were carried out and facilities for such diagnostic work were less generally available in the southwestern and southeastern states with high pneumonia mortality rates than in the northeastern states (1039).

A survey of the typing facilities of more than 2,500 hospitals throughout the United States was made by the American Medical Association for the committee report referred to (1343). It showed that such facilities were available in November 1937, in at least 1,850 hospitals in various sections of the land. In most states from 30 to 70 per cent of the hospitals had facilities for pneumococcus typing.

In some states and cities where antipneumococcic serums are available for therapeutic use in suitable cases, serum is supplied free. In other communities the distribution of free serum is restricted to patients who are indigent or to those in whom payment would involve a hardship, and in still other areas serums are available through health departments at cost and none is distributed free.

In large-scale programs where therapeutic antipneumococcic serums have been supplied through a department of health, the prevailing cost of immune horse serum has been approximately $35 for the average case of pneumococcus Type I pneumonia and about $50 for the average Type II case. The available evidence suggests that the cost of serum for the usual case due to pneumococci of Type V, VII, or VIII is somewhere between these two figures. Costs are generally higher, however, where serums are purchased by individual hospitals or physicians. When laboratories manufacturing serum are better able to plan advance production schedules it is likely that a substantial lowering of the cost of serum per case may result (1098). The certainty of a large and stable demand for such serums and the accumulation of more data on the incidence of the various types of pneumococci in pneumonia throughout the United States and elsewhere in the world would be of material assistance in attaining this desirable goal. There is a possibility that antipneumococcic rabbit serum may be more economical than specific horse antiserum.

Outline of Pneumonia Programs

To obtain the maximum utilization of valuable information already at hand relating to pneumonia, experience has shown the desirability of developing sound pneumonia programs (813, 814, 1102). A comprehensive program to make specific antiserum available to all can ordinarily be most advantageously planned as a community project on a state-wide basis, and involves the cooperation of health departments, the medical profession, nurses, laboratory workers, and hospitals. Programs of this nature support and assist the practicing physician and make generally available to him, usually for the first time, adequate facilities for the bacteriologic diagnosis, as well as specific serum for the treatment of many cases of pneumonia. Such programs should be initiated by departments of health and the medical profession and carried on as cooperative enterprises. Certain important activities must be undertaken, and to initiate them new precedents must frequently be established.

In planning and conducting the program, the formation of a local advisory committee, composed of representatives of the department of health, the medical society, and the association of laboratory workers, and at times, of members of other related professional groups, is desirable. The successful functioning of the advisory committee is of particular value in securing the desired cooperation of professional groups in the formation of a suitable plan of pneumonia control designed to meet the needs of the individual community. The program outlined should be sufficiently flexible to allow alterations in procedure from time to time, as the adoption of new advances in the control of pneumonia becomes advisable. It is important that some worker within the health department be appointed to supervise the pneumonia work in the community and wherever possible a pneumonia control unit should be established within the department.

On the official agencies falls the responsibility of administering the project. For its general acceptance, reliance must be placed on the medical profession and chief responsibility rests on physicians in general practice.

On the member of the health department appointed to supervise the pneumonia service should fall the responsibility for administering the project under the guidance of the advisory committee—the care and analysis of the records of treated cases, follow-up for additional data as necessary, response to inquiries from physicians, and other matters. The complexity and technical nature of the problem make it desirable that such supervision be entrusted only to a physician adequately trained in matters pertaining to the laboratory and clinical aspects of pneumonia and specific serum therapy.

If necessary, sufficient funds to carry out the program should be made available by special appropriation to be administered by departments of health.

Provision should be made to have adequate facilities for free bacteriologic diagnosis, with the typing of any pneumococci found, generally available in local laboratories to all physicians at any time during the twenty-four hours. Even in sparsely populated areas arrangements should be made by which sputum and blood cultures can be sent to an approved laboratory and a report received by telephone or telegraph. Technicians should be trained in methods of typing in a well-equipped laboratory where many specimens are examined. The work of technicians in laboratories approved for typing should be under competent supervision. Accuracy in bacteriologic diagnosis is essential if success is to accrue to attempts to control mortality from pneumococcus pneumonia by specific serum therapy. Laboratory technicians are frequently unaware of the importance of the role they play in pneumonia work. Every effort should be made to acquaint them with the facts.

Typing should be carried out in the approved laboratories for as many of the known types as possible, and in every case for those types for which specific therapeutic serums of generally accepted effectiveness are available. Diagnostic serums, at least for the latter number of types, can be supplied to the laboratories at relatively small expense.

Specific therapeutic serum should be equally available for all. Due to its expense it will not be available to those of limited means unless its cost is met by public funds. Local conditions may determine whether serum should be manufactured by the local department of health or purchased from a commercial laboratory. In a few communities where suitably equipped department of health laboratories have already been established for the production of therapeutic serums, antipneumococcic serum may be manufactured with little or no further capital outlay. The population served and the annual number of pneumonia cases must be considered in estimating the per capita cost. It is unlikely that serum can be economically produced by local health department laboratories in communities of less than several million inhabitants. To set up a new laboratory for the production of antipneumococcic horse serums requires skilled personnel as well as equipment. Two or three years may be required before the quality and volume of the serum produced are adequate. A high standard of performance and low cost of production are essential.

Centers for the distribution of therapeutic serum to physicians may be established in the approved laboratories where typing is done. The establishment of too many depots of serum supply in a single community should be avoided, however, as it involves needless duplication of resources and unnecessary expense, for in many instances serum may be stored until its dated period of usefulness, as marked on the label of the vial, has passed. Each of the distributing centers must be supplied with sufficient serum for the commoner types to anticipate the expected demand. The distribution of serums for other types may well be limited to a smaller number of strategically located laboratories.

In every instance where serum is used, typing should be carried out first to ensure that the serum given is of the proper type. In return for the typing service rendered and the serum supplied, physicians should be required to fill out and send to some central office in the community a record of each case treated.

A blood culture should be taken in all cases prior to serum administration and at intervals thereafter if the initial culture is positive or the progress of the case is not satisfactory (see pages 855 and 858). Outfits which can be easily transported without contamination for obtaining blood cultures from patients at home should be available through the typing laboratories (see page 618).

Printed instructions concerning the selection of patients to be treated, directions for the avoidance of the use of serum in sensitive patients, dosage advised, and the treatment of any untoward reactions which may occur should be prepared and distributed with the therapeutic serum.*

As typing facilities and therapeutic pneumonia serum become available in the community, circulars should be sent to physicians acquainting them with the facts. Subsequently similar notices may be sent by health departments for the next few years to each physician who reports a case or a death from pneumonia.

Many physicians are unfamiliar with the procedure of serum therapy for

* Copies of the instruction sheets or fliers included with each package of pneumonia serum dispensed by the Antitoxin and Vaccine Laboratory of the Massachusetts Department of Public Health may be seen in Appendix A (pages 940 and 943).

pneumonia. As a means of supplying them with assistance when such aid is requested, several suitably trained physicians in practice in various parts of the community may be designated as consultants or assistants to render such aid as needed.

The need for suitable publicity among professional groups on matters relating to pneumonia is considerable and urgent. For this purpose the publication of articles in medical journals, the distribution of circulars and pamphlets, and the use of charts, slides, moving pictures, and exhibits at medical meetings are of value. Graduate courses and symposiums on pneumonia at medical meetings have proved an important means of acquainting physicians with the more recent developments in the epidemiology, the clinical and bacteriologic diagnosis, and the treatment, particularly the specific serum treatment, of pneumonia. Such meetings should be held periodically in suitable locations throughout the community. Meetings devoted to discussions of pneumonia by medical societies, medical groups, and hospital staffs are helpful. At meetings and exhibits the technic of intravenous serum administration, of the conjunctival and intradermal tests for sensitivity, and of methods of pneumococcus typing can be demonstrated or illustrated by motion pictures.

Interest in the program and familiarity with it should be aroused in public health nursing groups by addresses on pneumonia at meetings of state and district nursing associations. Extension courses for nurses on the care and treatment of pneumonia are of value. A *Handbook on the Nursing Care of Pneumonia* prepared by the Bureau of Pneumonia Control of the New York State Department of Health (945) and containing valuable information for the nurse is available.*

The extent to which serum treatment is accepted depends to a considerable degree on an enlightened public opinion. Educational activities may well be directed to the spread of information to the laity by the distribution of official circulars and pamphlets and addresses by authorized speakers at public meetings. Health exhibits, radio addresses and plays, the release of articles and editorials to the press, and motion pictures (1035) are of value (813, 1248, 1101, 814, 250, 1041). It is desirable that the importance of the proper care of colds or other minor respiratory infections be stressed, as well

* A copy of the *Handbook on the Nursing Care of Pneumonia* (945), prepared by the New York State Department of Health, and reprinted by the Metropolitan Life Insurance Company, may be obtained by application to the Metropolitan Life Insurance Company, New York, New York.

as the value of prompt medical assistance in the event that serious symptoms or signs develop. The advantages of suitable nursing care can be brought out, as may the fact that for some pneumonias a helpful serum is available. It is advisable that great emphasis be placed upon the need of getting pneumonia patients under medical care at the earliest possible moment in the illness.

Numerous other activities may also be entered into. Wherever opportunity offers, special clinical, laboratory, and epidemiologic studies should be carried out with a view to adding to the existing knowledge of pneumonia.

The findings of programs such as have been described should be reported at intervals in some suitable medical journal.

It may be noted that the United States Public Health Service is initiating special studies to determine the incidence of all the recognized types of pneumococci in pneumonia in several places in the country. Investigations of healthy carriers of these organisms are also contemplated. In addition, an advisory service to health departments wishing to develop pneumonia control programs is now available through the Public Health Service (1341).

APPENDIX A

INFORMATION RELATING TO THE MASSACHUSETTS PNEUMONIA STUDY AND CONTINUING PROGRAM

I

THE Massachusetts Pneumonia Study was begun in 1931. From that date up to the latter part of 1934, in order to save time, it was advised that serum treatment should be begun on all cases as soon as the clinical diagnosis of lobar pneumonia could be made. The initial doses of serum could thus be given while the typing was being done. As a result of this policy many cases later proving to be caused by organisms other than pneumococcus Type I or II received varying amounts of serum.

During 1934 the Neufeld method of rapid typing was adopted as a routine procedure. This usually afforded a great saving of the time required for type determination. Since then, typing has been required before the specific serum available from the Department of Public Health was dispensed.

The Massachusetts Pneumonia Study, financed by the Commonwealth Fund, terminated on December 31, 1935. With its completion, the Massachusetts Department of Public Health assumed financial responsibility and has continued the manufacture and distribution of antipneumococcic serum (864, 814, 6, 506, 252).

From 1931 to the present, concentrated Type I and Type II antipneumococcic horse serum has been prepared and distributed by the Department of Public Health. The distribution of concentrated antipneumococcic horse serum for Type V was begun in 1937 and for Type VII and Type VIII in 1938.

Restriction of the use of antiserum to the first four days of the illness was imposed during the Pneumonia Study and the Continuing Program until March 1937.

Cases occurring during the Pneumonia Study and the Continuing Program are referred to as the Massachusetts Pneumonia Series.

The analysis of cases by type and period of study (Table A) and by type and Special Groups (Tables B and C) follows. These same data are reported by Lord and Heffron (814).

To ensure accuracy as well as to simplify the task of analyzing the findings in the treated cases, the essential data on the records were transferred to 80-column punch cards which were sorted mechanically.

MASSACHUSETTS PNEUMONIA SERIES

TABLE A. SERUM TREATED CASES BY TYPE AND BY PERIOD OF STUDY, FROM RECORDS RECEIVED FROM JANUARY 1, 1931, TO AND INCLUDING JUNE 30, 1937

	1931–35 PNEUMONIA STUDY	1936–37 CONTINUING PROGRAM	TOTAL
Type I	484	700	1,184
Type II	117	208	325
Type V	–	29	29
Type III	28	1	29
Group IV	127	3	130
Miscellaneous and organism not stated	42	16	58
Grand total	798	957	1,755

TABLE B. SERUM TREATED CASES BY TYPE AND BY CHARACTER OF TREATMENT, FROM RECORDS RECEIVED FROM JANUARY 1, 1931, TO AND INCLUDING JUNE 30, 1937

Type I			
1. Special Group (specific serum treatment within four days [ninety-six hours] of onset). Dosage administered cases treated in 1931–1935 was 16 cc. or more and dosage of this amount or of 20,000 units or more was given those treated from January 1, 1936—June 30, 1937.			
Number of cases treated with serum			
Of known potency	956		
Of unknown potency	87		
		1,043	
2. Others given less serum or treated later than above		141	
Total			1,184
Type II			
1. Special Group (specific serum treatment within four days [ninety-six hours] of onset). Dosage administered cases treated in 1931–1935 was 16 cc. or more and dosage of this amount or of 20,000 units or more was given those treated from January 1, 1936—June 30, 1937.			
Number of cases treated with serum			
Of known potency	259		
Of unknown potency	22		
		281	
2. Others given less serum or treated later than above		44	
Total			325

Type V			
1. Special Group (specific serum treatment within four days [ninety-six hours] of onset). Dosage administered was 16 cc. or more, or 20,000 units or more.			
Number of cases treated with serum			
Of known potency	17		
Of unknown potency	–		
	—	17	
2. Others		12	
		—	
Total			29
Type III			29
Group IV			130
Miscellaneous and organism not stated			58
			—
Grand total			1,755

TABLE C. PLACE OF TREATMENT OF TYPE I, II, AND V SPECIAL GROUP CASES

	HOSPITAL		HOME		
	Number	*Per cent*	*Number*	*Per cent*	TOTAL
Type I	777	74.6	265	25.4	1,043*
Type II	224	79.7	57	20.3	281
Type V	13	76.5	4	23.5	17
Total	1,014	75.7	326	24.3	1,341*

* The place of treatment was unknown for one case.

II

ON the following pages are copies of the instruction sheets or fliers distributed to physicians by the State Department of Public Health in Massachusetts. The first, Form A, relates to the precautions advisable to take in the administration of serums and antitoxins. The treatment of any untoward reactions which may develop is also described. Such instructions are changed from time to time as necessary. This flier was released for use March, 1937.

The second, Form B, contains information as to the selection of cases for treatment, dosage of concentrated antipneumococcic horse serum to be used in pneumonia, and serum administration. The treatment of allergic and of thermal reactions is described. Instructions of this nature are changed from time to time as becomes desirable. This flier was released for use February, 1938.

Form A

The Commonwealth of Massachusetts

THE DEPARTMENT OF PUBLIC HEALTH
DIVISION OF BIOLOGIC LABORATORIES

PRECAUTIONS ADVISABLE IN THE ADMINISTRATION OF SERUMS AND ANTITOXINS

Reactions of various types may follow the parenteral administration of a foreign protein, such as horse serum, if the person has a natural or acquired hypersensitivity to the protein injected. Therefore, serum therapy should be employed only when definitely indicated and only by those equipped to combat such reactions as may occur.

I. Acute Anaphylactic Type of Reaction. These reactions, although infrequent, are of the utmost importance, because they may prove fatal. They may follow the administration of even minute amounts of serum in extremely hypersensitive persons and may occur following the injection of serum by any route. The symptoms are dyspnea, cyanosis, urticaria, lumbar or abdominal pain, and collapse, any or all of which may begin within a few moments to an hour or more after the injection. Treatment is discussed below in paragraph F.

Such reactions may usually be avoided by observance of the following precautions which are designed to detect hypersensitive persons and lessen the dangers of serum administration.

A. *History*. Before the injection of serum, patients should be asked whether they have had asthma, hay-fever, eczema, urticaria, or angioneurotic edema. A positive history of these conditions is of importance only in suggesting the need for caution because such individuals probably have an allergic tendency. The method of serum administration described in paragraph C. 4 below is recommended for these patients.

A history of previous serum treatments (diphtheria, tetanus, or other antitoxin, antimeningococcic or antipneumococcic serum, diphtheria toxin-antitoxin mixture, etc.) and their sequelae should also be obtained. One injection of serum sometimes sensitizes to a succeeding injection of serum. If rapid or severe reactions followed earlier administrations of serum, similar reactions may or may not occur again, but preparations should be made to combat them if serum is given.

Note: Bacterial vaccines and diphtheria toxoid do not contain horse serum.

B. *Tests for Hypersensitivity*. Tests are of more importance than history; and at least one such test should be done on each patient who is to receive serum. (Material for testing is available at places supplying other biologic products.) Tests are not infallible but they give us the best information obtainable with our present knowledge. The ophthalmic test, in suitable cases, is probably a more reliable indicator of those individuals who may have severe reactions than is the intradermal test, because the latter apparently is capable of detecting degrees of hypersensitivity below the level of clinical importance. Although occasionally hypersensitive persons may not react to either test, such individuals appear to be rare. Tests should not be done nor any serum administered unless fresh epinephrine solution is at hand, preferably in a syringe.

1. Ophthalmic Test. Observe both eyes carefully for any evidence of inflammation of the conjunctivae. Then put a drop of horse serum diluted 1:10 (if available; if not, use the serum it is planned to inject) in the conjunctival sac of one eye, leaving the other eye as the normal control. A positive reaction is indicated by itching, watering, and a diffuse reddening of the eye within 30 minutes. Severe reactions may be controlled by the instillation of a few drops of epinephrine, 1:1000 dilution. The test is of no value in young children, for they may wash out the serum by

crying. In adults with marked injection of the conjunctivae it may prove difficult of interpretation.

2. Skin Test. If only one syringe is available, first make a control injection by injecting enough physiological saline solution *into* (not under) the skin of the anterior surface of one fore-arm to give a small elevation. In the corresponding location on the other arm, inject a similar amount of a 1:100 dilution of normal horse serum, having previously ejected some of the diluted serum from the needle to rid it of any water which may have remained from the sterilizing process. (The elevations caused by the injections tend to disappear within a few minutes if the test is negative, but the one produced by the serum may not disappear quite so quickly as the other.)

In hypersensitive patients the elevation at the site of serum injection rapidly enlarges within 5 to 20 minutes, becomes urticarial in appearance and is surrounded by a zone of erythema. Pseudopodial extensions of the central wheal are considered evidence of the higher and more dangerous degrees of sensitivity. Reactions usually subside within an hour or two.

C. *Use of Information Derived from Tests.*

1. Negative Test. Serum may be administered by any route to persons who do not react to these tests (or to either test, if only one is done). If serum is given intravenously, the first dose should not exceed 5 cc. and should be given very slowly, taking several minutes to administer the first cubic centimeter and at least one minute more for each additional cubic centimeter.

2. Positive Eye Test.

a. This is so nearly an absolute contra-indication to intravenous serum therapy that no serum should be given by this route except after consultation. Intravenous serum administration probably should not be undertaken at all in these patients, except possibly in a hospital, for severe reactions may be expected.

b. A positive eye test is also a sufficient contra-indication to the administration of serum by any other route to warrant the precautions (consultation and hospitalization) advised in the preceding paragraph.

3. Positive Skin Test. The import of positive skin tests is probably less than that of positive eye tests, but the same precautions are advised, particularly if the skin test is strongly positive.

4. Doubtful Tests. If the tests give doubtful reactions or if the administration of serum is decided upon in spite of positive tests, the subcutaneous injection of a dose of epinephrine (5–15 minims of 1:1000 dilution) given a measured six minutes before the serum, is a procedure which has been used with success and which appears to be rational. Smaller initial doses than usual should be given at a very slow rate.

D. *Desensitization.* The practice of desensitizing hypersensitive patients by the administration of repeated graduated doses of serum, starting with minute amounts (0.005 cc. more or less) subcutaneously and giving increasing doses at intervals of approximately one-half hour, is no longer recommended.

E. *Observation.* All patients receiving serum should be kept under close observation for not less than 30 minutes and preferably at least 45 minutes, during which time a physician should be immediately available.

F. *Treatment.* Fresh epinephrine solution, ready for administration, should be at hand in a syringe whenever serum is administered. The dose is 1 cc. (15 minims) for an adult, correspondingly less for a child. It should be given if the patient complains of lumbar or abdominal pain or shows evidence of urticaria, dyspnea, cyanosis or collapse. The dose may be repeated within a few minutes if necessary, and may be given intravenously. Artificial respiration may be required and measures to combat shock (the application of heat, etc.) instituted if collapse occurs.

II. Thermal or "Chill" Reactions. These occur after the intravenous administration of serum and are seen most frequently with antipneumococcic serum, possibly because it is given intravenously more often and in larger doses than other serums. If the patient develops a chill, which when it appears at all usually begins within twenty minutes to one and one-half hours after any dose, the advent of hyperpyrexia should be watched for. Should hyperpyrexia develop, immediate treatment is essential. Epinephrine is of no use at such a time, but procedures advocated for the treatment of heat stroke are indicated, such as the use of ice packs, the application of sheets wrung from ice water, and ice water enemas.

Venesection may be of use should pulmonary edema develop.

III. Serum Sickness. This is characterized most often by urticaria, but fever, enlarged glands, and joint pains are other common signs. It may come on any time up to four weeks after serum therapy, most commonly between the fourth and tenth days. Although this complication is disagreeable for the patient, it is not serious. Epinephrine may be given to allay discomfort, but its effect is of short duration. Cold applications lessen the annoyance of the urticaria. Large doses of salicylate have also been recommended.

IV. Arthus Phenomenon. A local reaction not incited by infection but going on to necrosis, at the site of subcutaneous or intramuscular injections occurs rarely. Serum injected within a period of several days to a few weeks or months after a previous injection is more likely to cause such reactions than is serum given either a few hours or days or some months or years after an injection. Such reactions are said to be most likely to occur if the patient shows signs of serum sickness at the time of injection. The possibility of such reactions should be kept in mind to avoid confusing them with local abscesses.

Inquiries concerning the use of serum should be made to either of the following:

The Director
Division of Communicable Diseases
Department of Public Health
State House, Boston, Mass.
Tel. Capitol 4660

The Director
Division of Biologic Laboratories
Antitoxin and Vaccine Laboratory
375 South Street,
Jamaica Plain Station, Boston, Mass.
Tel. Jamaica 4127

Form B

The Commonwealth of Massachusetts

THE DEPARTMENT OF PUBLIC HEALTH
DIVISION OF BIOLOGIC LABORATORIES

ANTIPNEUMOCOCCIC SERUM, CONCENTRATED

Prepared at the Antitoxin and Vaccine Laboratory, Forest Hills, Mass.

Pneumonias due to certain types of pneumococci are amenable to treatment with appropriate specific serums. Serums specific for pneumococci of Types 1, 2, 5, 7 and 8 are now or will be presently furnished by the Department of Public Health to physicians provided that (1) an examination in an approved laboratory of sputum or other material from the patient shows pneumococci of one of these types and (2) the physician agrees to fill out and return to the Department the questionnaire furnished with the serum. A list of the hospitals through which serum may be obtained will be sent on request.

Selection of Patients to be Treated.

Every patient with pneumococcus pneumonia should receive treatment with serum specific for the type causing the infection unless the patient is sensitive to horse serum or is in extremis. Directions for detecting hypersensitiveness to horse serum are given in the accompanying circular. A summary of the conditions under which the administration of antipneumococcic serum may be hazardous is as follows:

I. *Serum should NOT be given to:*

1. Those with a history of asthma or vasomotor rhinitis under exposure to emanations from horses.
2. Those giving a positive reaction to an eye test or a strongly positive reaction to an intradermal test.
3. Those in extremis.
4. Those who have received horse serum several days to several months previously. No strictly accurate limits can be placed on this period, but roughly it may be defined as seven days to three months.

II. *Serum treatment should be discontinued* in those who have had a severe, shock-like reaction, an asthmatic attack or urticaria, or alarming thermal reaction following any injection.

Dosage.

No hard and fast rule for dosage will hold for every patient, but the following suggestions are dictated by experience. Successful serum therapy is usually dependent upon *early* and *adequate* dosage. Delay in beginning treatment may expose the patient to additional risk of death and usually will necessitate the time-consuming administration of extra doses of serum.

For Type 1 infections administer *at least* 60,000 units, for Types 2, 5, or 8 *at least* 100,000 units, and for Type 7 *at least* 60,000–90,000 units in accordance with the scheme outlined below (See Serum Administration). Give *at least double* these doses of serum in the initial course of injections if

1. Treatment is begun after the third day of the disease;
2. The patient is over 40 years old;
3. The patient is pregnant or in the first week of the puerperium;
4. There is involvement of more than one lobe; or
5. Pneumococcus bacteriemia is known to be present.

The majority of patients so treated will respond well but some will require more than the amounts given in the initial course of injections. The dosage which may be necessary in addition to this basic dosage can not be definitely stated and must be decided by the physician for each case. The behavior of the temperature and the results of blood cultures are at present the most reliable guides for the use of more serum. Additional individual doses of 40,000 to 60,000 units are recommended at intervals of every three to four hours in severe cases and in any case if

1. The temperature does not fall below 102°F. by rectum within 18 hours of beginning serum treatment, or

2. Having fallen below 102°F. by rectum it again rises above this level; or

3. Bacteriemia is demonstrated by blood culture, regardless of the clinical course, or

4. There is evidence of a spreading lesion.

If the first blood culture is positive, or if negative, and the progress of the case is unsatisfactory, blood cultures should be taken at intervals of twenty-four hours, or more often.

Failure to improve after the serum has been given *persistently* for 72 hours suggests the presence of some complicating factors such as empyema or a mistake in the bacteriologic diagnosis. Another specimen of sputum should be typed, blood culture taken and the patient examined for signs of complications.

SERUM ADMINISTRATION.

Before giving this serum, patients to be treated should be questioned and tested for evidence of sensitivity to horse protein, as directed on the accompanying sheet.

A blood culture should be taken just before giving the first dose of serum.

The type and number of units of antibody per vial are stated on the labels. The volume of serum per vial depends upon the potency of the particular batch but does not exceed 15 cc. The total dose to be administered is determined by the number of units of antibody, but the amount to give in any one injection is determined by volume.

Serum is usually administered at two hour intervals until the dose decided upon has been given unless reactions severe enough to warrant discontinuing serum intervene. The customary first dose is 2 cc., the second the remainder of the contents of the vial, the third the contents of two vials and subsequent doses the contents of three or more vials; but no dose should exceed 45 cc. If the response to the initial course is not adequate and more serum is required, doses should be injected at intervals of three to four hours.

All doses of serum are given intravenously. Because of the possibility of allergic or chill reactions the first dose of serum should be small (2 cc.). Warm the serum to body temperature and inject at a rate not faster than 1 cc. per minute. Use only dry syringes and needles, preferably those that have been sterilized by dry heat. After injecting serum, note the appearance of any symptoms of allergic reaction, such as flushing of the face, dyspnea, cyanosis, lumbar or abdominal pain, rapid weak pulse, or a feeling of substernal oppression. The milder immediate reactions of this sort without urticaria or wheezing are not ordinarily a contra-indication to further serum treatment, but subsequent individual doses should be smaller than usual. The occurrence of urticaria or an asthmatic attack is, however, a contra-indication to further injections. At the appearance of any symptoms of allergic reaction give immediately a subcutaneous injection of 1 cc. (16 minims) of a 1:1000 dilution of epinephrine (adrenalin) and repeat this if necessary. If shock occurs, supply heat to the patient and give oxygen and artificial respiration by the prone pressure method.

If the patient develops a chill, which when it appears at all usually comes on within twenty minutes to one and one-half hours, the advent of hyperpyrexia should be watched for; and should it develop, immediate treatment is essential. Epinephrine is of no use at such a time, but procedures advocated for the treatment of heat stroke are indicated, such as the use of ice packs, the application of sheets wrung from ice water, and ice water enemas. Venesection may be of use should pulmonary edema develop. If the thermal reaction is alarming, no further serum should be given.

If reactions occur, the symptoms and the lot number of the serum used should be reported to the Antitoxin and Vaccine Laboratory, 375 South Street, Jamaica Plain, Mass. (telephone Jamaica 4127).

Records of all patients treated with this serum are to be prepared on a form supplied by this Department and when completed, immediately after the discharge of the patient, are to be sent to the Director of the Antitoxin and Vaccine Laboratory, 375 South Street, Jamaica Plain Station, Boston.

The Department of Public Health, under U. S. License No. 64, prepares and distributes antitoxins, serums, vaccines and other biologic products to the boards of health, health officers and physicians of the Commonwealth. All products are supplied free and under no circumstances are they to be sold.

After the expiration date stamped on the container the products should be returned to the Antitoxin and Vaccine Laboratory, 375 South Street, Jamaica Plain Station, Boston, Mass.

Inquiries concerning the use of concentrated antipneumococcic serum should be made to

THE DIRECTOR,
DIVISION OF COMMUNICABLE DISEASES
Department of Public Health, State House,
Boston, Mass., Tel. Capitol 4600

or

THE DIRECTOR,
DIVISION OF BIOLOGIC LABORATORIES
Antitoxin and Vaccine Laboratory,
375 South Street,
Jamaica Plain Station, Boston, Mass.
Tel. Jamaica 4127

APPENDIX B

INFORMATION RELATING TO TYPES OF PNEUMOCOCCI IN SOUTH AFRICA

FOLLOWING the completion of the manuscript for this book, a recent report from South Africa became available (see Ordman, D., *Pneumococcus Types in South Africa: A study of their occurrence and distribution in the population and the effect thereon of prophylactic inoculation,* South African Institute for Medical Research, 9:1, April 1938). In this article Ordman gives the relationship of the South African groups of pneumococci to the types in the so-called American or Cooper classification, as shown below:

South African and American (Cooper) Classifications Compared

SOUTH AFRICAN	AMERICAN	SOUTH AFRICAN	AMERICAN
A	V	Delta	XXIII
B	II	Epsilon	VI
C	I	Zeta	XXVII
E	III	Eta	XIX
K	VII	Theta	VIII
N	XXII	Lambda	XXI
R	XII	Mu	XXIX
S	XIV	Nu	XI
T	–	Xi	XVI
V	–	Omicron	IX
W	XV	Pi	XXIV
Y	X	Rho	XXVIII
Z	XXV	Sigma	XVII
Alpha	XX	Tau	XIII
Beta	IV	–	XXXI
Gamma	XVIII	–	XXXII

– = not represented.

It will be seen that the South African Groups D, F, G, H, J, L, and P are not shown in the table. These may or may not have corresponded with certain of the American types. These organisms were infrequently found and were isolated years ago. Apparently cultures of them have not been available for some time, for Ordman states that owing to the exhaustion of the supply of diagnostic serum for them it has not been possible to again identify these types even if they had reappeared.

Further, Groups M and C/M are not shown in the table as they were found to be identical with, or closely related to, Group C. Lastly, Types XXXI and XXXII have not yet been identified in South Africa and similarly, Groups T and V are not represented in the Cooper classification.

BIBLIOGRAPHY

As far as possible the system adopted for the abbreviation of journal titles is that used in the *Quarterly Cumulative Index Medicus.* With few exceptions, notably a number of older articles in the foreign literature, rather complete abstracts of which were kindly supplied by Drs. White, Robinson, and Barnes (1417), the original articles, or translations of them, have been read, and names, titles, and dates have been taken directly from the original publication. In the remaining few instances this information has been taken from the *Quarterly Cumulative Index Medicus.*

1. Abernethy, T. J. Concentrated antipneumococcus serum in Type I pneumonia; control of dosage by skin tests with type-specific polysaccharide. New York State J. Med., 36:627, Apr. 15, 1936.
2. Abernethy, T. J. Studies on somatic C polysaccharide of pneumococcus. II. Precipitation reaction in animals with experimentally induced pneumococcic infection. J. Exper. Med., 65:75, Jan. 1937.
3. Abernethy, T. J., and Francis, T., Jr. Studies on somatic C polysaccharide of pneumococcus. I. Cutaneous and serological reactions in pneumonia. J. Exper. Med., 65:59, Jan. 1937.
4. Adams, F. D., and Berger, B. J. Differential diagnosis of lobar pneumonia and appendicitis in children. J.A.M.A., 79:1809, Nov. 25, 1922.
5. Adler, H. Über Pneumokokkentypen und Pneumokokkenimmunität. Ztschr. f. Hyg. u. Infektionskr., 101:140, 1923.
6. Advances in the specific treatment of pneumonia (editorial). New England J. Med., 215:1248, Dec. 24, 1936.
7. Albert, J., and Abad, M. Lobar pneumonia in children under three years old. J. Philippine Islands M.A., 15:29, Jan. 1935.
8. Alexander, H. L. Asthma complicating the serum treatment of pneumonia. Arch. Int. Med., 20:636, Oct. 1917.
9. Alexander, H. L. Observations at the Peter Bent Brigham Hospital on cases of pneumonia in relation to types of pneumococci and the serum treatment of Type I cases. Boston M. & S. J., 177:874, Dec. 20, 1917.
10. Alloway, J. L. Transformation in vitro of R pneumococci into S forms of different specific types by use of filtered pneumococcus extracts. J. Exper. Med., 55:91, Jan. 1932.
11. Alloway, J. L. Further observations on the use of pneumococcus extracts in effecting transformation of type in vitro. J. Exper. Med., 57:265, Feb. 1933.
12. Alston, J. M., and Lowdon, A. S. R. Studies of skin reactions to the specific soluble substances of the pneumococcus Types I and II. Brit. J. Exper. Path., 14:1, Feb. 1933.
13. Alston, J. M., and Stewart, D. Incidence of serological types of pneumococcus in lobar pneumonia. Brit. M. J., 2:860, Nov. 22, 1930.
14. Amoss, H. L., and Craven, E. B. Serum treatment of hemolytic streptococcus pneumonia. J. Clin. Investigation, 12:885, Sept. 1933.
15. Amoss, H. L., Persons, E. L., and Hansen-Prüss, O. C. Serum in the treatment of streptococcus pneumonia. Tr. A. Am. Physicians, 46:208, 1931.
16. Anders, J. M. Serum treatment of pneumonia (535 cases). J.A.M.A., 43:1777, Dec. 10, 1904.
17. Anderson, G. W., and Heffron, R. Present status of pneumonia problem. Pub. Health Nursing, 27:633, Dec. 1935.

18. Antipneumococcus serum containing Type II antibodies (Council on Pharmacy and Chemistry of American Medical Association). J.A.M.A., 101: 1968, Dec. 16, 1933.
19. Archer, V. W., Blackford, S. D., and Wissler, J. E. Pulmonary manifestations in human tularemia; roentgenologic study based on 34 unselected cases. J.A.M.A., 104:895, Mar. 16, 1935.
20. Arkwright, J. A. Variation in bacteria in relation to agglutination both by salts and by specific serum. J. Path. & Bact., 24:36, Jan. 1921.
21. Armstrong, R. R. Serological characters of disease-producing pneumococci. Brit. M. J., 1:259, Feb. 19, 1921.
22. Armstrong, R. R. Swift and simple method for deciding pneumococcal "type." Brit. M. J., 1:214, Feb. 7, 1931.
23. Armstrong, R. R. Immediate pneumococcal typing. Brit. M. J., 1:187, Jan. 30, 1932.
24. Armstrong, R. R., and Johnson, R. S. Treatment of lobar pneumonia by antipneumococcal serum. Brit. M. J., 2:662, Oct. 8, 1932.
25. Aschoff, L. Lectures on pathology (delivered in the United States, 1924). New York, Paul B. Hoeber, Inc., 1924, 365 p.
26. Ashton, T. G., and Landis, H. R. M. Croupous pneumonia. Analysis from clinical observation of 991 cases occurring in Philadelphia General Hospital from May 1, 1897 to October 1, 1904. Am. J. M. Sc., 129:952, June 1905.
27. Atchley, D. W., and Benedict, E. M. Serum electrolyte studies in normal and pathological conditions: pneumonia, renal edema, cardiac edema, uremic and diabetic acidosis. J. Clin. Investigation, 9:265, Oct. 1930.
28. Auenbrugger, L. Inventum novum. *As seen in* Major, R. H., Classic Descriptions of Disease, p. 525. Springfield, Ill., Charles C. Thomas, 1932.
29. Austregesilo, A. Pneumonia in Rio de Janeiro und Pneumococciae bastardae. Ztschr. f. klin. Med., 76:423, 1912.
30. Avery, O. T. The distribution of the immune bodies occurring in antipneumococcus serum. J. Exper. Med., 21:133, Feb. 1915.
31. Avery, O. T. Further study on biologic classification of pneumococci. J. Exper. Med., 22:804, Dec. 1915.
32. Avery, O. T. Determination of types of pneumococcus in lobar pneumonia. A rapid cultural method. J.A.M.A., 70:17, Jan. 5, 1918.
33. Avery, O. T., Chickering, H. T., Cole, R., and Dochez, A. R. Acute lobar pneumonia: prevention and serum treatment. New York, Rockefeller Institute for Medical Research, 1917, 110 p. (Monographs of the Rockefeller Institute for Medical Research, No. 7.)
34. Avery, O. T., and Cullen, G. E. Hydrogen-ion concentration of cultures of pneumococci of the different types in carbohydrate media. J. Exper. Med., 30:359, Oct. 1919.
35. Avery, O. T., and Cullen, G. E. Studies on the enzymes of pneumococcus. I. Proteolytic enzymes. J. Exper. Med., 32:547, Nov. 1920.
36. Avery, O. T., and Cullen, G. E. Studies on the enzymes of pneumococcus. II. Lipolytic enzymes, esterase. J. Exper. Med., 32:571, Nov. 1920.
37. Avery, O. T., and Cullen, G. E. Studies on the enzymes of pneumococcus. III. Carbohydrate-splitting enzymes; invertase, amylase and inulase. J. Exper. Med., 32:583, Nov. 1920.

38. Avery, O. T., and Dubos, R. The specific action of a bacterial enzyme on pneumococci of Type III. Science, 72:151, Aug. 8, 1930.
39. Avery, O. T., and Dubos, R. Protective action of a specific enzyme against Type III pneumococcus infection in mice. J. Exper. Med., 54:73, July 1931.
40. Avery, O. T., and Goebel, W. F. Chemoimmunological studies on conjugated carbohydrate-proteins. V. Immunological specificity of an antigen prepared by combining capsular polysaccharide of Type III pneumococcus with foreign protein. J. Exper. Med., 54:437, Sept. 1931.
41. Avery, O. T., and Goebel, W. F. Chemoimmunological studies on soluble specific substance of pneumococcus. I. Isolation and properties of the acetyl polysaccharide of pneumococcus Type I. J. Exper. Med., 58:731, Dec. 1933.
42. Avery, O. T., Goebel, W. F., and Babers, F. H. Chemoimmunological studies on conjugated carbohydrate-proteins. VII. Immunological specificity of antigens prepared by combining a and b glucosides of glucose with proteins. J. Exper. Med., 55:769, May 1932.
43. Avery, O. T., and Heidelberger, M. Immunological relationships of cell constituents of pneumococcus. J. Exper. Med., 38:81, July 1923.
44. Avery, O. T., and Heidelberger, M. Immunological relationships of cell constituents of pneumococcus. J. Exper. Med., 42:367, Sept. 1925.
45. Avery, O. T., and Morgan, H. J. Occurrence of peroxide in cultures of pneumococcus. J. Exper. Med., 39:275, Feb. 1924.
46. Avery, O. T., and Morgan, H. J. Immunological reactions of isolated carbohydrate and protein of pneumococcus. J. Exper. Med., 42:347, Sept. 1925.
47. Avery, O. T., and Neill, J. M. Studies on oxidation and reduction by pneumococcus. I. Production of peroxide by anaerobic cultures of pneumococcus on exposure to air under conditions not permitting active growth. J. Exper. Med., 39:347, Mar. 1924.
48. Avery, O. T., and Neill, J. M. Studies on oxidation and reduction by pneumococcus. II. Production of peroxide by sterile extracts of pneumococcus. J. Exper. Med., 39:357, Mar. 1924.
49. Avery, O. T., and Neill, J. M. Studies on oxidation and reduction by pneumococcus. III. Reduction of methylene blue by sterile extracts of pneumococcus. J. Exper. Med., 39:543, Apr. 1924.
50. Avery, O. T., and Neill, J. M. Studies on oxidation and reduction by pneumococcus. IV. Oxidation of hemotoxin in sterile extracts of pneumococcus. J. Exper. Med., 39:745, May 1924.
51. Avery, O. T., and Neill, J. M. Antigenic properties of solutions of pneumococcus. J. Exper. Med., 42:355, Sept. 1925.
52. Avery, O. T., and Tillett, W. S. Anaphylaxis with the type-specific carbohydrates of pneumococcus. J. Exper. Med., 49:251, Feb. 1929.
53a. Bachmann, A., and Miravent, J. M. Classification des pneumocoques isolés en Argentine. Compt. rend. Soc. de biol., 88:385, Oct. 1923.
53b. Bahia. Relatorio da Secretaria de Saúde e Assistencia Publica, anno de 1928.
54. Bail, O. Untersuchungen über Typhus- und Cholera-immunität. Arch. f. Hyg., 52:272, 1905.

55. Bailey, G. H., and Shorb, M. S. Heterophile antigen in pneumococci. Am. J. Hyg., 13:831, May 1931.
56. Bailey, G. H., and Shorb, M. S. Chemical and immunological properties of pneumococci and other heterophile antigens. Am. J. Hyg., 17:329, Mar. 1933.
57. Bailey, G. H., and Shorb, M. S. Immunological relationships of pneumococci and other heterophile antigens and biological significance in pneumococcus infections. Am. J. Hyg., 17:358, Mar. 1933.
58. Bakst, H. J., Hazard, J. B., and Foley, J. A. Pulmonary moniliasis. J.A.M.A., 102:1208, Apr. 14, 1934.
59. Baldwin, H. S. Specific therapy of pneumococcus Type I and Type II pneumonia. Am. J. M. Sc., 181:788, June 1931.
60. Baldwin, H. S., and Cecil, R. L. Rationale of specific therapy in pneumococcus pneumonia. J.A.M.A., 87:1709, Nov. 20, 1926.
61. Baldwin, H. S., and Rhoades, D. R. Studies on pneumococcus immunity. VII. Protective substance in pneumococcus pneumonia with special reference to bacteriemia and specific treatment. Hygienic Laboratory Bulletin, No. 141:43, Apr. 1925.
62. Baldwin, H. S., and Rhoades, D. R. Studies on pneumococcus immunity. Use of optochin base in the treatment of lobar pneumonia. Hygienic Laboratory Bulletin, No. 141:69, Apr. 1925.
63. Baldwin, H. S., and Rhoades, D. R. Specific therapy of pneumococcus Type II pneumonia. Am. J. M. Sc., 174:191, Aug. 1927.
64. Banzhaf, E. J. Distribution of the immune bodies occurring in Types I, II, and III antipneumococcus serum. Proc. Soc. Exper. Biol. & Med., 22:329, Mar. 1925.
65. Banzhaf, E. J., and Curphey, T. J. Modified method for the production of antipneumococcus serum in horses. Proc. Soc. Exper. Biol. & Med., 28: 279, Dec. 1930.
66. Banzhaf, E. J., and Klein, A. J. A practical method for concentrating chill free pneumococcus antibodies from sera without use of salt precipitation. Proc. Soc. Exper. Biol. & Med., 28:276, Dec. 1930.
67. Barach, A. L. Methods and results of oxygen treatment in pneumonia. Arch. Int. Med., 37:186, Feb. 1926.
68. Barach, A. L. Rate of development of pneumococcus immunity. Proc. Soc. Exper. Biol. & Med., 25:558, Apr. 1928.
69. Barach, A. L. Factors involved in production of immunity with pneumococcus vaccine. I. Active and passive immunity during the first seven days after injection of antigen. J. Exper. Med., 48:83, July 1928.
70. Barach, A. L. Oxygen therapy in pneumonia. New York State J. Med., 29:985, Aug. 15, 1929.
71. Barach, A. L. Factors involved in production of immunity with pneumococcus vaccine. II. Induction of active immunity during the course of lobar pneumonia. J. Exper. Med., 53:567, Apr. 1931.
72. Barach, A. L. Immune transfusion in lobar pneumonia. Am. J. M. Sc., 182:811, Dec. 1931.
73. Barach, A. L. Analysis of 376 consecutive oxygen-treated cases from a study made at the Presbyterian Hospital, New York, from 1929 to 1932. New York State J. Med., 34:41, Jan. 1, 1934.
74. Barker, M. H., Parker, D. M., and Wassel, G. Nasal catheter administration

of oxygen: with observations on alveolar saturation. J.A.M.A., 103:244, July 28, 1934.

75. Barnes, L. A., and Kramer, S. D. A test for reaction-producing substances in concentrated antipneumococcic serum. Am. J. Pub. Health, 23:616, June 1933.

76. Barnes, L. A., and Robinson, E. S. Monkey test for chill-producing activity of concentrated antipneumococcic serum. Am. J. Pub. Health, 26:51, Jan. 1936.

77. Barnes, L. A., and White, B. Antibody response of rabbits during prolonged immunization with Type I pneumococcus vaccines. Am. J. Hyg., 21:35, Jan. 1935. *Abstract in* J. Immunol., 26:335, Apr. 1934.

78. Barnes, L. A., and Wight, E. C. Serological relationship between pneumococcus Type I and an encapsulated strain of Escherichia coli. J. Exper. Med., 62:281, Aug. 1935.

79. Barnes, L. A., and Wight, E. C. Spontaneous transformation of pneumococcus Type V to Type II. J. Bact., 32:557, Nov. 1936.

80. Barreto, A. L. C. A. de B. Relatorio da Secretaria de Saúde e Assistencia Publica, anno de 1928. Bahia, Imprensa official do estado, 1929.

81. Baumgartner, L. Age and antibody production. I. Qualitative changes in antisera associated with age. J. Immunol., 27:407, Oct. 1934.

82. Baumgartner, L. Age and antibody production. II. Further observations on qualitative changes in antisera associated with age. J. Immunol., 27:417, Oct. 1934.

83. Bazán, F. El púrpura en las neumococcias. La Semana Médica, 28:209, Aug. 18, 1921.

84. Becker, V. H. Beitrag zur Serumbehandlung der Pneumonie. München. med. Wchnschr., 81:1487, Sept. 1934.

85. Beckler, E. Pneumococcus type determination. Commonhealth (Massachusetts Department of Public Health), 18:162, July–Aug.–Sept. 1931.

86. Beckler, E., and MacLeod, P. The Neufeld method of pneumococcus type determination as carried out in a public health laboratory: a study of 760 typings. J. Clin. Investigation, 13:901, Nov. 1934.

87. Beckler, E. A., Marden, K., and Gillette, H. H. Pneumococcus type determination by Avery's cultural method. J.A.M.A., 70:836, Mar. 23, 1918.

88. Beebe, R. T., and Sutliff, W. D. Treatment of lobar pneumonia with homologous convalescent serum. New England J. Med., 203:823, Oct. 23, 1930.

89. Beecher, H. K., Bradshaw, H. H., and Lindskog, G. Effect of laparotomy and abdominal distention on lung volume. J. Thoracic Surg., 2:444, June 1933.

90. Behrend, A., and Cowper, R. B. G. Artificial pneumothorax in the treatment of lobar pneumonia. J.A.M.A., 102:1907, June 9, 1934.

91. Belk, W. P. Pulmonary infections by Friedländer's bacillus. J. Infect. Dis., 38:115, Feb. 1926.

92. Belk, W. P. Specific treatment of lobar pneumonia: a statistical review. J.A.M.A., 105:868, Sept. 14, 1935.

93. Belk, W. P., and Sharpe, J. S. Pneumococcus antibody solution in the treatment of lobar pneumonia. Results in 130 cases. Am. J. M. Sc., 187:844, June 1934.

94. Benjamin, J. E., Blankenhorn, M., Ruegsegger, J. M., and Senior, F. A.

Study of diagnosis and treatment of lobar pneumonia according to types and specific serum therapy. Ann. Int. Med., 11:437, Sept. 1937.
95. Bermuda: Medical and Health Department. Medical report on the health and sanitary conditions of Bermuda for the year 1935, by Henry Wilkinson.
96. Berry, F. B. Lobar pneumonia: analysis of 400 autopsies. M. Clin. North America, 4:571, Sept. 1920.
97. Besredka, A., and Steinhardt, E. Du mécanisme de l'anti-anaphylaxie. Ann. Inst. Pasteur, 21:384, May 1907.
98. Bethea, O. W. Treatment of pneumonia. J.A.M.A., 95:925, Sept. 27, 1930.
99. Bezançon, F., and Griffon, V. Pouvoir agglutinatif du sérum dans les infections expérimentales et humaines à pneumocoques. Compt. rend. Soc. de biol., 49:551, June 1897.
100. Bhatnagar, S. S., and Singh, K. Bacteriological studies in acute lobar pneumonia due to pneumococcus and *B. pneumoniae* Friedlander. Indian J. M. Research, 23:337, Oct. 1935.
101. Biach, A. Statistische Studien über die Pneumonie in den drei Krankenhäusern Wiens (allgem. Krankenhaus, Rudolfstiftung, Wiedener Spital) im Decennium 1866–1876. Med. Jahrb., 2nd series, 9:1, 1879.
102. Bie, V. Prognosis of broncho-pneumonia. Acta. med. Scandinav., 55 (6): 589, 1921.
103. Bigelow, G. H. Intracutaneous reactions in lobar pneumonia. Arch. Int. Med., 29:221, Feb. 1922.
104. Bigelow, G. H. Serum treatment of pneumonia. New England J. Med., 205:242, June 30, 1931.
105. Bigler, J. A., Clifton, W. M., and Werner, M. The leukocyte response to sulfanilamide therapy. J.A.M.A., 110:343, Jan. 29, 1938.
106. Binger, C. A. L. Anoxemia in pneumonia and its relief by oxygen inhalation. J. Clin. Investigation, 6:203, Oct. 1928.
107. Binger, C. A. L., and Christie, R. V. An experimental study of diathermy. I. Measurement of lung temperature. J. Exper. Med., 46:571, Oct. 1927.
108. Binger, C. A. L., and Christie, R. V. An experimental study of diathermy. II. Conditions necessary for production of local heat in the lungs. J. Exper. Med., 46:585, Oct. 1927.
109. Binger, C. A. L., and Christie, R. V. An experimental study of diathermy. III. Temperature of the circulating blood. J. Exper. Med., 46:595, Oct. 1927.
110. Binger, C. A. L., and Christie, R. V. Diathermy in pneumonia. J.A.M.A., 91:367, Aug. 11, 1928.
111. Birge, E. G., and Havens, L. C. Comparison of bacteriology of pneumonia, antemortem and postmortem. Based on study of recent epidemic at Camp Wadsworth, S. C. New York M. J., 109:544, Mar. 29, 1919.
112. Blacklock, J. W. S., and Guthrie, K. J. Pneumococcal infections in infancy and childhood. J. Path. & Bact., 36:349, May 1933.
113. Blackman, S. S., Jr. Pneumococcal lipoid nephrosis and the relation between nephrosis and nephritis. I. Clinical and anatomical studies. Bull. Johns Hopkins Hosp., 55:1, July 1934.
114. Blackman, S. S., Jr. Pneumococcal lipoid nephrosis and the relation between nephrosis and nephritis. II. Experimental studies. Bull. Johns Hopkins Hosp., 55:85, Aug. 1934.

115. Blackman, S. S., Jr., Brown, J. H., and Rake, G. Production of acute nephritis by means of a pneumococcal autolysate. Bull. Johns Hopkins Hosp., 48:74, Feb. 1931.
116. Blackman, S. S., Jr., and Rake, G. Acute pneumococcal nephritis. Bull. Johns Hopkins Hosp., 51:217, Oct. 1932.
117. Blake, F. G. Methods for the determination of pneumococcus types. J. Exper. Med., 26:67, July 1917.
118. Blake, F. G. Antigen-antibody balance in lobar pneumonia. Arch. Int. Med., 21:779, June 1918.
119. Blake, F. G. Diagnosis and treatment of pneumonia. New England J. Med., 202:991, May 22, 1930.
120. Blake, F. G. Observations on pneumococcus Type III pneumonia. Ann. Int. Med., 5:673, Dec. 1931.
121. Blake, F. G. Observations on active immunity to pneumococcal pneumonia. Tr. A. Am. Physicians, 47:153, 1932.
122. Blake, F. G., and Cecil, R. L. Studies on experimental pneumonia. I. Production of pneumococcus lobar pneumonia in monkeys. J. Exper. Med., 31:403, Apr. 1920.
123. Blake, F. G., and Cecil, R. L. Studies on experimental pneumonia. II. Pathology and pathogenesis of pneumococcus lobar pneumonia in monkeys. J. Exper. Med., 31:445, Apr. 1920.
124. Blake, F. G., and Cecil, R. L. Studies on experimental pneumonia. III. Spontaneous pneumonia in monkeys. J. Exper. Med., 31:499, May 1920.
125. Blake, F. G., and Cecil, R. L. Studies on experimental pneumonia. IV. Results of prophylactic vaccination against pneumococcus pneumonia in monkeys. J. Exper. Med., 31:519, May 1920.
126. Blake, F. G., and Cecil, R. L. Studies on experimental pneumonia. VIII. Experimental streptococcus hemolyticus pneumonia in monkeys. J. Exper. Med., 32:401, Oct. 1920.
127. Blake, F. G., and Cecil, R. L. Studies on experimental pneumonia. IX. Production in monkeys of an acute respiratory disease resembling influenza by inoculation with bacillus influenzae. J. Exper. Med., 32:691, Dec. 1920.
128. Blake, F. G., Howard, M. E., and Hull, W. S. Artificial pneumothorax in the treatment of lobar pneumonia. J.A.M.A., 105:1489. Nov. 9, 1935.
129. Blake, F. G., and Trask, J. D. Pneumococcus variants intermediate between the S and R forms. J. Bact., 25:289, Mar. 1933.
130. Blanton, W. B., and Irons, E. E. Recent epidemic of acute respiratory infection at Camp Custer, Mich. J.A.M.A., 71:1988, Dec. 14, 1918.
131. Bliss, E. A., and Long, P. H. A second note on the communicability of colds. Proc. Soc. Exper. Biol. & Med., 31:31, Oct. 1933.
132. Bliss, E. A., and Long, P. H. Observations on mode of action of sulfanilamide. J.A.M.A., 109:1524, Nov. 6, 1937.
133. Bliss, E. A., McClaskey, W. D., and Long, P. H. A study of pneumococcus carriers. J. Immunol., 27:95, July 1934.
134. Bloomfield, A. Effects of serum therapy in acute lobar pneumonia. Bull. Johns Hopkins Hosp., 28:301, Oct. 1917.
135. Bloomfield, A. L. The dissemination of bacteria in the upper air passages. III. The relation of bacteria to the mucous membranes. Bull. Johns Hopkins Hosp., 33:252, July 1922.

136. Bloomfield, A. L. Therapeutic value of Type I antipneumococcus serum. J.A.M.A., 81:1437, Oct. 27, 1923.
137. Boothby, W. M. Oxygen therapy. J.A.M.A., 99:2026, Dec. 10, 1932.
138. Boothby, W. M., and Haines, S. F. Oxygen therapy. J.A.M.A., 90:372, Feb. 4, 1928.
139. Bordet, P. Qualités propres aux sérums de diverses espèces animales par rapport au pneumocoque. Ann. Inst. Pasteur, 51:503, Oct. 1933.
140. Borrel, A. Pneumonie et tuberculose chez les troupes noires. Ann. Inst. Pasteur, 34:105, Mar. 1920.
141. Bosman, J. R. Pneumonia. South African M. J., 6:257, Apr. 23, 1932.
142. Boston Health League, Pneumonia Committee. Specific treatment for lobar pneumonia (notice). New England J. Med., 214:219, Jan. 30, 1936.
143. Boston Health League, Pneumonia Committee. Specific treatment for lobar pneumonia (notice). New England J. Med., 215:890, Nov. 5, 1936.
144. Bourn, J. M. Hemophilus influenzae in upper respiratory disease and in health, 1928–1930. Am. J. Hyg., 15:64, Jan. 1932.
145. Brainard, D. H., and Noble, W. C., Jr. Studies of acute respiratory infections. V. Attempts to demonstrate bacteriophage for pneumococci and influenza bacilli. Am. J. Hyg., 21:58, Jan. 1935.
146. Branch, A., and Stillman, E. G. Pathology of experimental pneumococcus pneumonia in mice. J. Exper. Med., 40:743, Dec. 1924.
147. Brem, W. V., Bolling, G. E., and Casper, E. J. Pandemic "influenza" and secondary pneumonia at Camp Fremont, Calif. J.A.M.A., 71:2138, Dec. 28, 1918.
148. Bristol, L. D. Vaccines against the common cold. Are they of value in the industrial health program? Am. J. Pub. Health, 27:987, Oct. 1937.
149. Brooks, C. Non-specific protein antigens prepared from hemo-proteins. Science, 49:196, Feb. 21, 1919.
150. Brooks, C. The effect of shattered hemoprotein on the colorless blood corpuscles. Am. J. Physiol., 49:127, June 1919.
151. Brooks, C. The treatment of pneumonias with a deuteroproteose. South. M. J., 31:534, May 1938.
152. Brooks, C., Pack, G. T., and Goode, H. Further studies on the physiological action of non-specific antigens prepared from shattered hemo-proteins. Proc. Soc. Exper. Biol. & Med., 21:321, Mar. 1924.
153. Brooks, H. Cause of death in pneumonia. J.A.M.A., 103:1192, Oct. 20, 1934.
154. Brown, A. L., and Debenham, M. W. Postoperative pulmonary complications. A study of their relative incidence following inhalation anesthesia and spinal anesthesia. J.A.M.A., 99:209, July 16, 1932.
155. Brown, E. G., Gottlieb, S., and Laybourn, R. L. Dust storms and their possible effect on health: with special reference to the dust storms in Kansas in 1935. Pub. Health Rep., 50:1369, Oct. 4, 1935.
156. Brown, M. H. The treatment of pneumonia with concentrated serum—with a preliminary report of 22 cases. Canad. Pub. Health J., 22:109, Mar. 1931.
157. Brown, M. H. Recent observations on pneumonia. Canad. Pub. Health J., 23:429, Sept. 1932.

158. Brown, R. Observations on induction of anaphylactic shock by the specific carbohydrates of Type I pneumococcus. Proc. Soc. Exper. Biol. & Med., 31:699, Mar. 1934.
159. Brown, R. Failure of antipneumococcus horse serum to sensitize guinea pigs to anaphylactic shock with specific carbohydrates. Proc. Soc. Exper. Biol. & Med., 31:700, Mar. 1934.
160. Brown, W. E. Vaccine in prevention of the common cold. Experiment. Am. J. Hyg., 15:36, Jan. 1932.
161. Brundage, D. K. Mortality of coal miners. Washington, Government Printing Office, 1933. 17 p. (Public Health Bulletin No. 210).
162. Brundage, D. K., and Bloomfield, J. J. Pneumonia problem in steel industry. J. Indust. Hyg., 14:345, Dec. 1932.
163. Brundage, D. K., Russell, A. E., Jones, R. R., Bloomfield, J. J., and Thompson, L. R. Frequency of pneumonia among iron and steel workers. Washington, Government Printing Office, 1932. 51 p. (Public Health Bulletin No. 202).
164. Buchanan, J. A., and Ashley, F. The scientific results of neglect in the treatment of pneumonia. M. Rec., 141:21, Jan. 2, 1935.
165. Buckler, T. H. On the etiology, pathology, and treatment of fibro-bronchitis and rheumatic pneumonia. Philadelphia, Blanchard and Lea, 1853, 150 p.
166. Buerger, L. Studies of the pneumococcus and allied organisms with reference to their occurrence in the human mouth. J. Exper. Med., 7:497, Aug. 1905.
167. Bulkley, K. Pneumococcic arthritis. Ann. Surg., 59:71, Jan. 1914.
168. Bull, C. G. Mechanism of curative action of antipneumococcus serum. J. Exper. Med., 22:457, Oct. 1915.
169. Bull, C. G. Immunity factors in pneumococcus infection in the dog. J. Exper. Med., 24:7, July 1916.
170. Bull, C. G., and Bartual, L. Pneumococcus cultures in whole fresh blood. I. The retardative effect of the blood of immune animals and mechanism of the phenomenon. J. Exper. Med., 31:233, Mar. 1920.
171. Bull, C. G., and McKee, C. M. Antipneumococcus protective substances in normal chicken serum. Am. J. Hyg., 1:284, May 1921.
172. Bull, C. G., and McKee, C. M. Respiratory immunity in rabbits. VI. The effects of immunity on the carrier state of the pneumococcus and *Bacillus bronchisepticus*. Am. J. Hyg., 8:723, Sept. 1928.
173. Bull, C. G., and McKee, C. M. Respiratory immunity in rabbits. VIII. Rabbits immunized with pneumococcus Types II, III, and IV resist intranasal infection with Type I. Am. J. Hyg., 10:229, July 1929.
174. Bull, C. G., and Tao, S. M. Method for determining the anti-pneumococcal properties of whole blood and the protective power of immune serum. Am. J. Hyg., 7:648, Sept. 1927.
175. Bullowa, J. G. M. The pneumococcus pneumonias and their serum treatment. Med. & Surg. Year-book, Physicians Hospital of Plattsburg, 1:3, 1929.
176. Bullowa, J. G. M. Serum treatment and its evaluation in lobar pneumonia. Bull. New York Acad. Med., 5:328, Apr. 1929.

177. Bullowa, J. G. M. Serum treatment of the pneumococcus pneumonias. M. Clin. North America, 13:625, Nov. 1929.

178. Bullowa, J. G. M. Use and abuse of therapeutic inhalations of oxygen. International Clinics, 4:262, Dec. 1931.

179. Bullowa, J. G. M. Therapeutic value of pneumococcus Type VII (Cooper) serum. Proc. Soc. Exper. Biol. & Med., 29:343, Dec. 1931.

180. Bullowa, J. G. M. Therapeutic value of specific Type seven (Cooper) antipneumococcic serum. *In* Contributions to the Medical Sciences in Honor of Dr. Emanuel Libman by his Pupils, Friends and Colleagues, 1:283. New York, The International Press, 1932.

181. Bullowa, J. G. M. Pulmonary edema occurring in the course of lobar pneumonia treated with intravenous, hypertonic, fifty per cent glucose solution and insulin. Report of a case. M. Clin. North America, 15:1115, Mar. 1932.

182. Bullowa, J. G. M. Two cases of pneumococcus pneumonia with concurrent paratyphoid fever. M. Clin. North America, 15:1127, Mar. 1932.

183. Bullowa, J. G. M. Studies in the serum treatment of pneumonia. New York State J. Med., 33:13, Jan. 1, 1933.

184. Bullowa, J. G. M. Therapeutic pneumococcus Type VIII (Cooper) serum. J.A.M.A., 102:1560, May 12, 1934.

185. Bullowa, J. G. M. Simple method for calibration of clinical oxygen regulators. J. Lab. & Clin. Med., 20:526, Feb. 1935.

186. Bullowa, J. G. M. Pneumonias due to pneumococcus Type VIII. Am. J. M. Sc., 190:65, July 1935.

187. Bullowa, J. G. M. Pneumonia due to pneumococcus Type XIV (Cooper) and its treatment with specific antiserum. J. Clin. Investigation, 14:373, July 1935.

188. Bullowa, J. G. M. Reliability of sputum typing and its relation to serum therapy. Reprinted with additions from J.A.M.A., 105:1512, Nov. 9, 1935.

189. Bullowa, J. G. M. Discussion on the prophylaxis and serum treatment of pneumonia. Abstract of Sectional Proceedings *in* Report of Proceedings of Second International Congress for Microbiology, p. 502, London, 1937.

190. Bullowa, J. G. M. Management of the pneumonias. New York, Oxford University Press, 1937, 508 p.

191. Bullowa, J. G. M., and Greenbaum, E. Pneumococcic pneumonia in infants and children. Am. J. Dis. Child., 53:22, Jan. 1937.

192. Bullowa, J. G. M., and Greenbaum, E. Pneumonia due to pneumococcus Type VII (Cooper). Specific serum treatment. Arch. Int. Med., 60:179, Aug. 1937.

193. Bullowa, J. G. M., and Mayer, E. The hazards of the induction of pneumothorax in the treatment of lobar pneumonia. J.A.M.A., 105:191, July 20, 1935.

194. Bullowa, J. G. M., Rosenblüth, M. B., and Merkin, A. K. Studies on leukocytes in lobar pneumonia. I. Changes produced by refined antiserums (Felton and Banzhaf) on polymorphonuclear leukocytes in the treatment of lobar pneumonia and their relation to chills. II. Relation of total leukocytes and active polymorphonuclear leukocytes to prognosis in lobar pneumonia. Tr. Sect. Path. & Physiol. A.M.A., p. 106, 1927.

195. Bullowa, J. G. M., Rosenblüth, M. B., Park, W. H., and Cooper, G. Use of antipneumococcic refined serum in lobar pneumonia (Bullowa). J.A.M.A., 90:1354, Apr. 28, 1928. Relation of bacteremia in lobar pneumonia to prognosis and therapy (Rosenblüth). J.A.M.A., 90:1351, Apr. 28, 1928. Antipneumococcus serum in lobar pneumonia (Park and Cooper). J.A.M.A., 90:1349, Apr. 28, 1928.

196. Bullowa, J. G. M., and Schuman, A. H. Rapid method of using Sabin slide microscopic test for determining types of pneumococci. Am. J. Pub. Health, 20:878, Aug. 1930.

197. Bullowa, J. G. M., and Wilcox, C. Pneumococcus chain formation: its relation to virulence in mice, occurrence and distribution by pneumococcus types in human respiratory infections, and its relation to prognosis in lobar pneumonia. J. Lab. & Clin. Med., 19:1156, Aug. 1934.

198. Bullowa, J. G. M., and Wilcox, C. Incidence of bacteriemia in the pneumonias and its relation to mortality. Arch. Int. Med., 55:558, Apr. 1935.

199. Bullowa, J. G. M., and Wilcox, C. Therapeutic serum for pneumococcus Type V (Cooper) pneumonia. J. Clin. Investigation, 15:711, Nov. 1936.

200. Bundesen, H. N. Chicago Pneumonia Commission. Preliminary report. J.A.M.A., 84:884, Mar. 21, 1925.

201. Bunim, J. J., and Trask, J. D. Familial studies on lobar pneumonia: epidemiologic studies on families of children with pneumococcic lobar pneumonia. Am. J. Dis. Child., 50:626, Sept. 1935.

202. Burgess, A. M. Sudden death following the administration of concentrated pneumococcus serum. J.A.M.A., 93:768, Sept. 7, 1929.

203. Burgess, A. M. Oxygen therapy; modification of box method for giving 95 per cent oxygen. New England J. Med., 216:467, Mar. 18, 1937.

204. Burgess, A. M., and Burgess, A. M., Jr. New method of administering oxygen; preliminary note. New England J. Med., 207:1078, Dec. 15, 1932.

205. Burhans, C. W., and Gerstenberger, H. J. Protective power of infants' and maternal serum against pneumococci. Am. J. Dis. Child., 28:415, Oct. 1924.

206. Burn, C. G., Chandler, C. A., and Hartshorn, M. The production of streptococcus hemolyticus bacteremia in non-specifically sensitized animals. J. Exper. Med., 60:1, July 1934.

207. Cabot, R. C. Diagnostic pitfalls identified during a study of 3000 autopsies. J.A.M.A., 59:2295, Dec. 28, 1912.

208. Cahn-Bronner, C. E. Zehn Jahre Chininbehandlung der kruppösen Pneumonie. Therap. d. Gegenw., 29:97, Mar. 1927.

209. Calder, R. M. Microscopic method of typing pneumococci by the use of stained organisms. J.A.M.A., 97:698, Sept. 5, 1931.

210. Callomon, V. B., and Ungar, J., Jr. Treatment of pneumonia with serum containing type-specific, heterophile, and neutralizing antibodies. Ann. Int. Med., 9:1664, June 1936.

211. Camac, C. N. B. Clinical report upon cases of lobar pneumonia treated with antipneumococcus serum observed at General Hospital No. 6, Fort McPherson, Georgia, October, 1917, to May, 1918. Am. J. M. Sc., 156: 887, Dec. 1918.

212. Campaign against pneumonia in Detroit (news item). J.A.M.A., 106:303, Jan. 25, 1936.

213. Canada Year Book (official statistical annual of Canada), 1927–1928, p. 177; and 1932, p. 133.

214. Capps, J. A. An experimental and clinical study of pain in the pleura, pericardium, and peritoneum. New York, The Macmillan Co., 1932, 99 p.

215. Capps, J. A., and Coleman, G. H. Influence of alcohol on prognosis of pneumonia in Cook County Hospital: a statistical report. J.A.M.A., 80: 750, Mar. 17, 1923.

216. Carbonell, A., and Cook, E. L. Pneumococcus meningitis, report of a case treated with ethylhydrocuprein and Huntoon's antibody solution with recovery. Mil. Surgeon, 63:718, Nov. 1928.

217. Castellani, A., and Chalmers, A. J. Manual of tropical medicine, p. 1875. 3rd Edition, New York, Wm. Wood & Co., 1929.

218. Catron, L. Studies on bacterial localization. Effects of specific immunization and of a gum acacia medium on localization of Type I pneumococci in mice. J. Exper. Med., 61:735, June 1935.

219. Cecil, R. L. Pneumonia and empyema at Camp Upton, N. Y. M. Clin. North America, 2:567, Sept. 1918.

220. Cecil, R. L. Classification and serum treatment of pneumonia at Camp Upton. New York State J. Med., 18:414, Oct. 1918.

221. Cecil, R. L. Biologic therapy. XI. Pneumococcus vaccine. J.A.M.A., 76: 178, Jan. 15, 1921.

222. Cecil, R. L. Immunization against pneumonia. Medicine, 4:395, Nov. 1925.

223. Cecil, R. L. The specific treatment of lobar pneumonia. Arch. Int. Med., 41:295, Mar. 1928.

224. Cecil, R. L., *editor*. A textbook of medicine, p. 15. 2nd ed., Philadelphia and London, W. B. Saunders Co., 1930.

225. Cecil, R. L. Remarks on serum treatment of pneumonia. Brit. M. J., 2:657, Oct. 8, 1932.

226. Cecil, R. L. Campaign to reduce the death rate of pneumonia in New York State. New York State J. Med., 35:1123, Nov. 15, 1935.

227. Cecil, R. L. Effects of very early serum treatment in pneumococcus Type I pneumonia. J.A.M.A., 108:689, Feb. 27, 1937.

228. Cecil, R. L., and Austin, J. H. Results of prophylactic inoculation against pneumococcus in 12,519 men. J. Exper. Med., 28:19, July 1918.

229. Cecil, R. L., and Baldwin, H. S. The treatment of lobar pneumonia with subcutaneous injections of pneumococcus antibody solution. J. Pharmacol. & Exper. Therap., 24:1, Aug. 1924.

230. Cecil, R. L., Baldwin, H. S., and Larsen, N. P. Clinical and bacteriologic study of 2000 typed cases of lobar pneumonia. Tr. A. Am. Physicians, 41:208, 1926. Also: Arch. Int. Med., 40:253, Sept. 1927.

231. Cecil, R. L., and Blake, F. G. Studies on experimental pneumonia. V. Active immunity against experimental pneumococcus pneumonia in monkeys following vaccination with living cultures of pneumococcus. J. Exper. Med., 31:657, June 1920.

232. Cecil, R. L., and Blake, F. G. Studies on experimental pneumonia. VI. Active immunity following experimental pneumococcus pneumonia in monkeys. J. Exper. Med., 31:685, June 1920.

233. Cecil, R. L., and Blake, F. G. Studies on experimental pneumonia. VII. Treatment of experimental pneumococcus Type I pneumonia in monkeys with Type I antipneumococcus serum. J. Exper. Med., 32:1, July 1920.
234. Cecil, R. L., and Blake, F. G. Studies on experimental pneumonia. X. Pathology of experimental influenza and of bacillus influenzae pneumonia in monkeys. J. Exper. Med., 32:719, Dec. 1920.
235. Cecil, R. L., Bullowa, J. G. M., Chickering, H. T., and Corwin, E. H. L. Community provision for the serum treatment of pneumococcic pneumonias. Report of the Committee on Public Health Relations of the New York Academy of Medicine by a special sub-committee. J.A.M.A., 109:1323, Oct. 23, 1937.
236. Cecil, R. L., and Larsen, N. P. Clinical and bacteriologic study of 1000 cases of lobar pneumonia. J.A.M.A., 79:343, July 29, 1922.
237. Cecil, R. L., and Plummer, N. Motorless oxygen therapy apparatus. J.A.M.A., 95:1263, Oct. 25, 1930.
238. Cecil, R. L., and Plummer, N. Pneumococcus Type I pneumonia. Study of 1161 cases with especial reference to specific therapy. J.A.M.A., 95: 1547, Nov. 22, 1930.
239. Cecil, R. L., and Plummer, N. Pneumococcus Type II pneumonia. A clinical and bacteriologic study of 1000 cases, with especial reference to serum therapy. J.A.M.A., 98:779, Mar. 5, 1932.
240. Cecil, R. L., and Steffen, G. I. Studies on pneumococcus immunity. I. Active immunization of monkeys against pneumococcus Type I pneumonia with pneumococcus Type I vaccine. J. Exper. Med., 34:245, Sept. 1921.
241. Cecil, R. L., and Steffen, G. I. Vaccination of monkeys against pneumococcus Type I pneumonia by means of intratracheal injection of pneumococcus Type I vaccine. Pub. Health Rep., 37:2735, Nov. 3, 1922.
242. Cecil, R. L., and Steffen, G. I. Studies on pneumococcus immunity. II. Active immunization of monkeys against pneumococcus Types II, III, and IV pneumonia with the homologous pneumococcus vaccine. J. Exper. Med., 38:149, Aug. 1923.
243. Cecil, R. L., and Steffen, G. I. Studies on pneumococcus immunity. IV. Active immunization of monkeys against pneumococcus pneumonia by means of intratracheal injection of pneumococcus vaccine. Hygienic Laboratory Bulletin, No. 141:1, Apr. 1925.
244. Cecil, R. L., and Steffen, G. I. Studies on pneumococcus immunity. V. The treatment of experimental pneumococcus pneumonia in monkeys with pneumococcus antibody solution. Hygienic Laboratory Bulletin, No. 141:19, Apr. 1925.
245. Cecil, R. L., and Sutliff, W. D. Treatment of lobar pneumonia with concentrated antipneumococcus serum. J.A.M.A., 91:2035, Dec. 29, 1928.
246. Cecil, R. L., and Vaughan, H. F. Results of prophylactic vaccination against pneumonia at Camp Wheeler. J. Exper. Med., 29:457, May 1919.
247. Ceylon: Colombo. Report XXVII of the Acting Medical Officer of Health for the year 1932. Colombo, Municipal Printing Office, 1933.
248. Chadwick, H. D. Diseases of the inhabitants of the Commonwealth. (Shattuck Lecture.) New England J. Med., 216:1003, June 10, 1937.

249. Chadwick, H. D. Distribution of antipneumococcus serum in Massachusetts (letter to the editor). J.A.M.A., 109:1926, Dec. 4, 1937.
250. Chadwick, H. D. Lay publicity concerning serum treatment of pneumonia in Massachusetts (letter to the editor). New England J. Med., 218:136, Jan. 20, 1938. *See also 1041.*
251. Chadwick, H. D. Pneumococcus-typing and serum-distribution service in Massachusetts (letter to the editor). New England J. Med., 218:242, Feb. 3, 1938.
252. Chadwick, H. D. Serum treatment of pneumonia in Massachusetts (letter to the editor). New England J. Med., 218:366, Feb. 24, 1938.
253. Chapman, E. M. Acute silicosis. J.A.M.A., 98:1439, Apr. 23, 1932.
254. Chatard, J. A. An analytical study of acute lobar pneumonia in the Johns Hopkins Hospital from May 15, 1889 to May 15, 1905. Johns Hopkins Hosp. Rep., 15:55, 1910.
255. Chatard, J. A. Leucocytes in acute lobar pneumonia. Johns Hopkins Hosp. Rep., 15:89, 1910.
256. Chatard, J. A. An analytical study of terminal pneumonia. Johns Hopkins Hosp. Rep., 15:99, 1910.
257. Chickering, H. T. Agglutination phenomena in lobar pneumonia. J. Exper. Med., 20:599, Dec. 1914.
258. Chickering, H. T. Prognosis and treatment of lobar pneumonia. South. M. J., 23:112, Feb. 1930.
259. Chickering, H. T. Acute bacterial pneumonic infection. M. Clin. North America, 14:1463, May 1931.
260. Chickering, H. T., and Park, J. H., Jr. Staphylococcus aureus pneumonia. J.A.M.A., 72:617, Mar. 1, 1919.
261. Chile: Dirección general de estadística. Anuario estadístico de la Republica de Chile, años 1929–30, v. 8.
262. Chile: Dirección general de estadística. Estadística anual, v. 1, Demografía y asistencia social, año 1930.
263. Chow, B. F., and Goebel, W. F. Purification of antibodies in Type I antipneumococcus serum, and chemical nature of the type-specific precipitin reaction. J. Exper. Med., 62:179, Aug. 1935.
264. Christensen, S. Studies on pneumococcus types. Communications de l'Inst. Sérothérap. de l'État Danois. Extraits. 14 (5), 1923.
265. Christensen, S. Pneumococcus types and prognosis in pneumonia crouposa. Acta. path. et microbiol. Scandinav., 2:1, 1925.
266. Christian, H. *Quoted in* E. A. Locke, Treatment of Type I pneumococcus lobar pneumonia with specific serum. *See reference 793.*
267. Christie, I. M. Epidemiological significance of the serological types of pneumococci. Lancet, 2:39, July 7, 1934.
268. Christie, R. V., and Binger, C. A. L. An experimental study of diathermy. IV. Evidence for penetration of high frequency currents through the living body. J. Exper. Med., 46:715, Nov. 1927.
269. Christie, R. V., Ehrich, W., and Binger, C. A. L. An experimental study of diathermy. V. Elevation of temperature in the pneumonic lung. J. Exper. Med., 47:741, May 1928.
270. Churchill, E. D., and McNeill, D. Reduction in vital capacity following operation. Surg. Gynec. & Obst., 44:483, Apr. 1927.
271. Churchman, J. W., and Emelianoff, N. V. Bacterial structure with par-

ticular reference to the capsule. Proc. Soc. Exper. Biol. & Med., 29:996, May 1932.

272. Claiborn, L. N. The ophthalmic test for sensitivity to horse serum. J.A.M.A., 98:1718, May 14, 1932.

273. Clark, H. C. The pneumococci, by types, in cultures from 71 autopsies. *In* United Fruit Company, Medical Department, 16th annual report, 1927, p. 247.

274. Clausen, S. W. Influence of nutrition upon resistance to infection. Physiol. Rev., 14:309, July 1934.

275. Clifford, R. The sputum. Its examination and clinical significance, p. 123. New York, The Macmillan Co., 1932.

276. Clinical applications of heterophile antigens and antibodies (editorial). New England J. Med., 213:1038, Nov. 21, 1935.

277. Clough, M. C. A study of incidence of types of pneumococci isolated from acute lobar pneumonia and other infections, and an analysis of the cases classified by types in regard to mortality, complications, associated diseases, bacteremia, and leucocytosis. Bull. Johns Hopkins Hosp., 28:306, Oct. 1917.

278. Clough, P. W. The development of antibodies in the serum of patients recovering from acute lobar pneumonia. Bull. Johns Hopkins Hosp., 24: 295, Oct. 1913.

279. Clough, P. W. Some observations on hypersensitiveness to pneumococcus protein, with special reference to its relation to immunity. Bull. Johns Hopkins Hosp., 26:37, Feb. 1915.

280. Clough, P. W. Phagocytosis and agglutination in the serum in acute lobar pneumonia, the specificity of these reactions and the regularity of their occurrence. Bull. Johns Hopkins Hosp., 30:167, June 1919.

281. Clough, P. W. The protective power of normal human serum against pneumococcus infection. Bull. Johns Hopkins Hosp., 35:330, Oct. 1924.

282. Coburn, R. C. Minimizing early postoperative pneumonia. J.A.M.A., 100:1392, May 6, 1933.

283. Coca, A. F. Studies in specific hypersensitiveness. VII. Age incidence of serum disease and of dermatitis venenata as compared with that of natural allergies. J. Immunol., 7:193, Mar. 1922.

284. Coca, A. F. Immunity in human beings to the pneumococcus. Proc. Soc. Exper. Biol. & Med., 29:1042, May 1932.

285. Coggeshall, L. T. Tests for pneumococcus hypersensitiveness in dogs after recovery from experimental pneumococcus lobar pneumonia. J. Exper. Med., 61:235, Feb. 1935.

286. Coggeshall, L. T., and Robertson, O. H. Study of repeated attacks of experimental pneumococcus lobar pneumonia in dogs. J. Exper. Med., 61: 213, Feb. 1935.

287. Coghlan, J. J. Treatment of acute lobar pneumonia by artificial pneumothorax. Lancet, 1:13, Jan. 2, 1932.

288. Cohn, A. E., and Lewis, W. H., Jr. Lobar pneumonia and digitalis. Am. J. M. Sc., 189:457, Apr. 1935.

289. Cole, R. I. Toxic substances produced by pneumococcus. J. Exper. Med., 16:644, Nov. 1912.

290. Cole, R. I. Treatment of pneumonia by means of specific serums. J.A.M.A., 61:663, Aug. 30, 1913.

291. Cole, R. I. Pneumococcus infection and lobar pneumonia. Harvey Lectures 1913–1914, p. 118.
292. Cole, R. I. Pneumococcus infection and lobar pneumonia. Arch. Int. Med., 14:56, July 1914.
293. Cole, R. I. Specific treatment of acute lobar pneumonia. Pennsylvania M. J., 20:345, Feb. 1917.
294. Cole, R. I. Present status of serum therapy. New York State J. Med., 17:347, Aug. 1917.
295. Cole, R. I. Neutralization of antipneumococcus immune bodies by infected exudates and sera. J. Exper. Med., 26:453, Oct. 1917.
296. Cole, R. I. Prevention of pneumonia. J.A.M.A., 71:635, Aug. 24, 1918.
297. Cole, R. I. Acute lobar pneumonia. *In* Nelson's Loose-Leaf Living Medicine, 1:203. New York, Thomas Nelson & Sons, 1920–28.
298. Cole, R. I. Acute pulmonary infections. De LaMar Lectures, Johns Hopkins Univ. School of Hygiene and Pub. Health, 1927–1928.
299. Cole, R. I. Serum treatment in Type I lobar pneumonia. J.A.M.A., 93: 741, Sept. 7, 1929.
300. Cole, R. I. Nature of pneumonia (Pasteur Lecture). Proc. Inst. Med. Chicago, 9:2, Jan. 15, 1932.
301. Cole, R. I. The outlook for overcoming pneumonia. Canad. M.A.J., 30: 237, Mar. 1934.
302. Cole, R. I. Treatment of pneumonia. Ann. Int. Med., 10:1, July 1936.
303. Cole, R. I. Pneumonia. Prevention, management and serum treatment. New York State J. Med., 36:1699, Nov. 15, 1936.
304. Cole, R. I. Recent advances in the control of pneumonia. Am. J. Pub. Health, 26:1191, Dec. 1936.
305. Cole, R. I. Serum therapy of pneumococcic pneumonia. J.A.M.A., 109: 2059, Dec. 18, 1937.
306. Cole, R. I., and Dochez, A. R. Report of studies on pneumonia. Tr. A. Am. Physicians, 28:606, 1913.
307. Cole, R. I., and MacCallum, W. G. Pneumonia at a base hospital. J.A.M.A., 70:1146, Apr. 20, 1918.
308. Cole, R. I., and Moore, H. F. Production of antipneumococcic serum. J. Exper. Med., 26:537, Oct. 1917.
309. Collins, K. R. Application of the reaction of agglutination to the pneumococcus. J. Exper. Med., 7:420, Aug. 1905.
310. Collins, L. H., Jr. Chronic pulmonary infection due to the Friedländer bacillus. Arch. Int. Med., 58:235, Aug. 1936.
311. Collins, S. D., and Gover, M. Age and seasonal incidence of minor respiratory attacks classified according to clinical symptoms. Am. J. Hyg., 20: 533, Nov. 1934.
312. Colombia: Departamento de Contraloria Estadística General. Anuario estadístico, 13:50, 1923; and 16:196, 1924.
313. Connecticut State Department of Health. Report for the year ended June 30, 1934, p. 205.
314. Conner, L. A. Experiences in New York Hospital with treatment of lobar pneumonia by a serum-free solution of pneumococcus antibodies. Am. J. M. Sc., 164:832, Dec. 1922.
315. Contraindicated vaccines (editorial). J.A.M.A., 100:1773, June 3, 1933.
316. Cooke, R. A. Studies in specific hypersensitiveness. III. On constitutional

reactions: the dangers of the diagnostic cutaneous test and therapeutic injection of allergens. J. Immunol., 7:119, Mar. 1922.
317. Cooper, F. B., Gross, P., and Mellon, R. R. Action of p-aminobenzenesulfonamide on Type III pneumococcus infections in mice. Proc. Soc. Exper. Biol. & Med., 36:148, Mar. 1937.
318. Cooper, G. M., Edwards, M., and Rosenstein, C. Separation of types among pneumococci hitherto called Group IV and the development of therapeutic antiserums for these types. J. Exper. Med., 49:461, Mar. 1929.
319. Cooper, G. M., Mishulow, L., and Blanc, N. E. Studies on acute respiratory infections. II. A study of the serological relationships of pneumococci from the upper respiratory tract with special reference to common colds and influenzal conditions. J. Immunol., 6:25, Jan. 1921.
320. Cooper, G. M., Rosenstein, C., Walter, A., and Peizer, L. Further separation of types among pneumococci hitherto included in Group IV and development of therapeutic antisera for these types. J. Exper. Med., 55:531, Apr. 1932.
321. Cooper, G. M., and Walter, A. W. Application of the Neufeld reaction to identification of types of pneumococci. Am. J. Pub. Health, 25:469, Apr. 1935.
322. Coryllos, P. N. Bronchoscopic findings in lobar pneumonia. Preliminary note. Am. J. M. Sc., 178:8, July 1929.
323. Coryllos, P. N., and Birnbaum, G. L. The size of the consolidated lung in lobar pneumonia. Am. J. M. Sc., 178:15, July 1929.
324. Cotoni, L., Truche, C., and Raphael, A. Pneumocoques et affections pneumococciques. Paris, Masson et Cie, 1922, 224 p. (Monographies de l'Institut Pasteur.) *English edition.* Page, D. S., and Morton E. Pneumococcus and pneumococcal affections. London, John Bale Sons & Danielsson, Ltd., 1924, 218 p.
325. Couvy and Popoff. Note sur le traitement de la pneumonie par le salicylate de soude en injections intraveineuses. Bull. Acad. de méd., Paris, 105: 163, Feb. 3, 1931.
326. Cowan, J., Cruickshank, R., Cuthbertson, D. P., Fleming, J., and Harrington, A. W. Treatment of lobar pneumonia by Felton's serum. A preliminary report based on 58 cases. Lancet, 2:1387, Dec. 27, 1930.
327. Cowan, J., Harrington, A. W., Cruickshank, R., Cuthbertson, D. P., and Fleming, J. Treatment of lobar pneumonia by Felton's serum. Lancet, 2:8, July 2, 1932.
328. Cowan, S. T. Pneumococcal haemolysin; its extracellular nature, production and properties. J. Path. & Bact., 38:61, Jan. 1934.
329. Crone, N. L., and Chapman, E. M. Epidemic pleurodynia. New England J. Med., 209:1007, Nov. 16, 1933.
330. Cross, F. B. Principles and applications of numoquin-base (ethylhydrocupreine) in the treatment of lobar pneumonia. M. J. & Rec., 126:271, Sept. 7, 1927, and 126:354, Sept. 21, 1927.
331. Cruickshank, R. Pneumococcal infections (Milroy Lectures, 1933). Lancet, 1:563, Mar. 18, 1933; 621, Mar. 25, 1933; and 680, Apr. 1, 1933.
332. Cruz, J. Z. S. Pathological incidence of lobar pneumonia in the Philippine Islands. J. Philippine Islands M. A., 7:162, May 1927.
333. Cunningham, A. R. Results of open air treatment of pneumonia in chil-

dren. An analysis of 1500 cases of lobar pneumonia from the records of the Children's Hospital, Boston. Boston M. & S. J., 174:753, May 25, 1916.

334. Cunningham, J., Cruickshank, J. A., and Ramakrishnan, S. Note on types of pneumococci found in cases of pneumonia in Madras, Southern India. Indian J. M. Research, 12:479, Jan. 1925.

335. Curphey, T. J., and Baruch, H. B. The titration of pneumococcus "exudate" antisera. Proc. Soc. Exper. Biol. & Med., 28:280, Dec. 1930.

336. Curphey, T. J., and Baruch, H. B. Therapeutic value of intramuscular dosage of Type I pneumococcus antisera. J. Exper. Med., 55:925, June 1932.

337. Curphey, T. J., and Solomon, S. Therapeutic value of calcium salts in serum sickness. New England J. Med., 214:150, Jan. 23, 1936.

338. Curtis, A. H., *editor*. Obstetrics and gynecology, 1:972. Philadelphia and London, W. B. Saunders Co., 1933.

339. Davies, D. T., Hodgson, H. G., and Whitby, L. E. H. A study of pneumococcal pneumonia. I. Lancet, 1:791, Apr. 6, 1935.

340. Davies, D. T., Hodgson, H. G., and Whitby, L. E. H. A study of pneumococcal pneumonia. II. Lancet, 1:849, Apr. 13, 1935.

341. Davies, D. T., Hodgson, H. G., and Whitby, L. E. H. A study of pneumococcal pneumonia. III. The radiology of pneumonia. Lancet, 1:919, Apr. 20, 1935.

342. Davies, J. A. V. Response of infants to inoculation with Type I pneumococcus carbohydrate. J. Immunol., 33:1, July 1937.

343. Davis, J. S. Effect of morphine on the respiration in pneumonia. J. Clin. Investigation, 6:187, Oct. 1928.

344. Dawson, M. H. Interconvertibility of "R" and "S" forms of pneumococcus. J. Exper. Med., 47:577, Apr. 1928.

345. Dawson, M. H. Bacterial variation in pneumococcus and streptococcus hemolyticus. Proc. Soc. Exper. Biol. & Med., 31:590, Feb. 1934.

346. Dawson, M. H., and Sia, R. H. P. In vitro transformation of pneumococcal types. I. Technic for inducing transformation of pneumococcal types in vitro. J. Exper. Med., 54:681, Nov. 1931.

347. Dawson, M. H., and Warbasse, A. Further observations on transformation of type-specific pneumococci by in vitro procedures. Proc. Soc. Exper. Biol. & Med., 29:149, Nov. 1931.

348. Dean, H. R. Mechanism of the serum reactions. (Horace Dobell Lecture.) Lancet, 1:45, Jan. 13, 1917.

349. DeGraff, A. C., Travell, J. G., and Yager, J. A. Electrocardiographic study of the heart in lobar pneumonia. J. Clin. Investigation, 10:633, Aug. 1931.

350. DeLee, J. B. The principles and practice of obstetrics, p. 529. 6th Edition, Philadelphia & London, W. B. Saunders Co., 1933.

351. Dennis, E. W., and Berberian, D. A study on the mechanism of invasiveness of streptococci. J. Exper. Med., 60:581, Nov. 1934.

352. Denys, J. Recherches sur le sérum antipneumococcique. Ann. Soc. méd.-chir. d'Anvers, 2:51, Feb. 1897.

353. Dernby, K. G., and Avery, O. T. The optimum H-ion concentration for the growth of pneumococcus. J. Exper. Med., 28:345, Sept. 1918.

354. Diehl, H. S. Medicinal treatment of the common cold. J.A.M.A., 101: 2042, Dec. 23, 1933.
355. Dingle, J. H. The serological specificity of bacterial carbohydrates, with especial reference to Type II pneumococcus and a heterophile strain of bacterium lepisepticum. Am. J. Hyg., 20:148, July 1934.
356. Dochez, A. R. The presence of protective substances in human serum during lobar pneumonia. J. Exper. Med., 16:665, Nov. 1912.
357. Dochez, A. R. Coagulation time of blood in lobar pneumonia. J. Exper. Med., 16:693, Nov. 1912.
358. Dochez, A. R. Acute infection of the respiratory tract. Tr. Am. Clin. & Climatol. Assn., 49:245, 1933.
359. Dochez, A. R. A limited consideration of certain aspects of acute infection of the respiratory tract. Medicine, 12:245, Sept. 1933.
360. Dochez, A. R., and Avery, O. T. Varieties of pneumococcus and their relation to lobar pneumonia. J. Exper. Med., 21:114, Feb. 1915.
361. Dochez, A. R., and Avery, O. T. Occurrence of carriers of disease producing types of pneumococcus. J. Exper. Med., 22:105, July 1915.
362. Dochez, A. R., and Avery, O. T. Antiblastic immunity. J. Exper. Med., 23:61, Jan. 1916.
363. Dochez, A. R., and Avery, O. T. Elaboration of specific soluble substance by pneumococcus during growth. J. Exper. Med., 26:477, Oct. 1917.
364. Dochez, A. R., and Gillespie, L. J. A biologic classification of pneumococci by means of immunity reactions. J.A.M.A., 61:727, Sept. 6, 1913.
365. Dochez, A. R., Mills, K. C., and Kneeland, Y., Jr. Studies of the mechanism of upper respiratory infection. Lancet, 2:547, Sept. 5, 1931.
366. Dochez, A. R., Mills, K. C., and Kneeland, Y., Jr. Variation of H. influenzae during acute respiratory infection in the chimpanzee. Proc. Soc. Exper. Biol. & Med., 30:314, Dec. 1932.
367. Dochez, A. R., Mills, K. C., and Kneeland, Y., Jr. Disease of the upper respiratory tract. Problems concerned with the etiology and prophylaxis. J.A.M.A., 101:1441, Nov. 4, 1933.
368. Dochez, A. R., Mills, K. C., and Kneeland, Y., Jr. Filterable viruses in infection of the upper respiratory tract. J.A.M.A., 110:177, Jan. 15, 1938.
369. Dochez, A. R., Shibley, G. S., and Mills, K. C. Study of acute infection of respiratory tract in the ape. Proc. Soc. Exper. Biol. & Med., 26:562, Apr. 1929.
370. Dochez, A. R., Shibley, G. S., and Mills, K. C. Studies in the common cold. IV. Experimental transmission of the common cold to anthropoid apes and human beings by means of a filtrable virus. J. Exper. Med., 52:701, Nov. 1930.
371. Dold, H. Die bakterizide Wirkung des Blutes, Plasmas und Serums auf Pneumokokken und ihre Bedeutung für die Immunität. Arb. a. d. k. Gsndhtsamte., 36:419, Apr. 1911.
372. Domagk, G. Ein Beitrag zur Chemotherapie der bakteriellen Infektionen. Deutsche med. Wchnschr., 61:250, Feb. 15, 1935.
373. Doull, J. A., Harmon, G. E., and Fisher, B. The sex ratio of pneumonia mortality and its possible relation to occupation. Am. J. Hyg., 20:628, Nov. 1934.
374. Downie, A. W. Specific capsular polysaccharide of pneumococcus Type I

and immunity which it induces in mice. J. Path. & Bact., 45:131, July 1937.

375. Downie, A. W. Experiments with type-specific pneumococcus polysaccharides in rabbits. J. Path. & Bact., 45:149, July 1937.

376. Downing, J. G., and Cousins, S. M. Exhibit of fungi pathogenic to man shown at the one hundred and fifty-third anniversary of the Massachusetts Medical Society. New England J. Med., 211:963, Nov. 22, 1934.

377. Drinker, C. K., Enders, J. F., Shaffer, M. F., and Leigh, O. C. Emigration of pneumococci Type III from the blood into the thoracic duct lymph of rabbits, and the survival of these organisms in the lymph following intravenous injection of specific antiserum. J. Exper. Med., 62:849, Dec. 1935.

378. Dubos, R. Factors affecting the yield of specific enzyme in cultures of the bacillus decomposing the capsular polysaccharide of Type III pneumococcus. J. Exper. Med., 55:377, Mar. 1932.

379. Dubos, R. Studies on mechanism of production of specific bacterial enzyme which decomposes capsular polysaccharide of Type III pneumococcus. J. Exper. Med., 62:259, Aug. 1935.

380. Dubos, R., and Avery, O. T. Decomposition of capsular polysaccharide of pneumococcus Type III by a bacterial enzyme. J. Exper. Med., 54:51, July 1931.

381. Dubos, R., and Bauer, J. H. Use of graded collodion membranes for concentration of bacterial enzyme capable of decomposing the capsular polysaccharide of Type III pneumococcus. J. Exper. Med., 62:271, Aug. 1935.

382. Duckwall, B. F. Protective value of pneumococcus vaccine against respiratory disease. Mil. Surgeon, 47:593, Nov. 1920.

383. Dunham, E. K. Empyema. Washington, Government Printing Office, 1924. 392 p.

384. Ecuador. Informe que presenta el director general de sanidad publica al señor ministro de instrucción pública y sanidad sobre los trabajos sanitarios correspondientes, año 1923.

385. Ecuador. Boletin general de estadistica: organo trimestral de la direccion general del ramo, 3 (6), Nov. 1933.

386. Eddy, N. B. Dilaudid (dihydromorphinone hydrochloride). J.A.M.A., 100:1032, Apr. 1, 1933.

387. Egbert, J. H. Epidemic pneumonia in the tropics. New York M. J., 103: 1125, June 10, 1916.

388. Eggers, H. E. On the antipneumococcal powers of the blood in pneumonia. J. Infect. Dis., 10:48, Jan. 1912.

389. Egypt: Ministry of Finance, Statistical Department. Annual return of births, deaths and infectious diseases, 1925 and 1933.

390. Elwyn, H. Pneumonia at Camp Greene: a few considerations from a clinical standpoint. South. M. J., 11:780, Dec. 1918.

391. Emmerich, R. Ueber die Infection, Immunisirung und Heilung bei croupöser Pneumonie. Ztschr. f. Hyg. u. Infektionskr., 17:167, 1894.

392. Enders, J. F. A type specific substance distinct from the specific carbohydrate in pneumococcus Type I. J. Exper. Med., 52:235, Aug. 1930.

393. Enders, J. F. Note on specific agglutination of pneumococcus Types I, II, and III. J. Exper. Med., 55:191, Feb. 1932.

394. Enders, J. F., and Shaffer, M. F. Studies on natural immunity to pneumococcus Type III. I. Capacity of strains of pneumococcus Type III to grow at 41° C. and their virulence for rabbits. J. Exper. Med., 64:7, July 1936.
395. Enders, J. F., and Wu, C. J. An immunological study of the A substance or acetyl polysaccharide of pneumococcus Type I. J. Exper. Med., 60: 127, Aug. 1934.
395a. Evans, G. M., and Gaisford, W. F. Treatment of pneumonia with 2-(p-aminobenzenesulphonamido)-pyridine. Lancet, 2:14, July 2, 1938.
396. Eyre, J. W. H., and Washbourn, J. W. Further experiments with Pane's antipneumococcus serum. Brit. M. J., 2:1247, Nov. 4, 1899.
397. Eyre, S., and Stovall, W. D. Antigenic similarity of 2 strains of non-capsulated methemoglobin-producing organisms to Type XXIX pneumococcus. J. Infect. Dis., 58:190, Mar.–Apr., 1936.
398. Faber, H. K. Use of rabbits as substitute for white mice in pneumococcus type differentiation. J.A.M.A., 70:1459, May 18, 1918.
399. Fabyan, M. Pathological analysis of 195 cases of lobar pneumonia. Johns Hopkins Hosp. Rep., 15:81, 1910.
400. Falk, K. G., McGuire, G., Valentine, E., and Whitney, E. Studies on antibodies. II. Antipneumococcus serum. J. Immunol., 21:199, Sept. 1931.
401. Falk, K. G., Valentine, E., McGuire, G., and Whitney, E. Studies on antibodies. V. Use of green bananas in media for culture of pneumococci. J. Bact., 23:235, Mar. 1932.
402. Fantus, B., *editor*. Therapy of Cook County Hospital. Therapy of disturbances due to heat. J.A.M.A., 103:990, Sept. 29, 1934.
403. Fantus, B., *editor,* in collaboration with Feinberg, S. M. Therapy of Cook County Hospital; therapy of (horse) serum reactions. General rules in administration of therapeutic serums. J.A.M.A., 107:1717, Nov. 21, 1936.
404. Farley, D. L., St. Clair, H., and Reisinger, J. A. Normal filament and non-filament polymorphonuclear neutrophil count: its practical value as a diagnostic aid. Am. J. M. Sc., 180:336, Sept. 1930.
405. Faulkner, W. B., Jr., and Faulkner, E. C. Postoperative massive collapse of the lung: its cause, prevention and treatment. Northwest Med., 32:87, Mar. 1933.
406. Feinblatt, H. M. Analysis of one hundred and eighty necropsied cases of pneumonia, with reference to anatomic complications and bacterial causes. Boston M. & S. J., 189:136, July 26, 1923.
407. Felton, L. D. Isolation and concentration of specific antibodies of anti-pneumococcus sera. Boston M. & S. J., 190:819, May 15, 1924.
408. Felton, L. D. Protective substance in antipneumococcic serum. I. Type I serum. J. Infect. Dis., 37:199, Sept. 1925.
409. Felton, L. D. Protective substance in antipneumococcic serum. II. Effect of certain chemical manipulations on the stability of the protective substance in Type I antipneumococcus serum. J. Infect. Dis., 37:309, Oct. 1925.
410. Felton, L. D. Protective substance in antipneumococcus serum. IV. A separation of phosphorous and some inert protein from the water-insoluble precipitate of antipneumococcus serum. J. Infect. Dis., 42:248, Mar. 1928.

411. Felton, L. D. Protective substance in antipneumococcus serum. V. Febrile reaction from intravenous injection. J. Infect. Dis., 42:256, Mar. 1928.

412. Felton, L. D. Units of protective antibody in antipneumococcus serum and antibody solution. J. Infect. Dis., 43:531, Dec. 1928.

413. Felton, L. D. Concentration of pneumococcus antibody. J. Infect. Dis., 43:543, Dec. 1928.

414. Felton, L. D. Concentration of antipneumococcus serum. J.A.M.A., 94: 1893, June 14, 1930.

415. Felton, L. D. The variables in the mouse. Protection test of antipneumococcus serum. J. Immunol., 19:485, Dec. 1930.

416. Felton, L. D. Study of neutralizing substance of the pneumococcus. J. Immunol., 19:511, Dec. 1930.

417. Felton, L. D. Correlation of protective value with titers of other antibodies in Type I antipneumococcus serum. J. Immunol., 21:341, Nov. 1931.

418. Felton, L. D. Use of ethyl alcohol as a precipitant in the concentration of antipneumococcus serum. J. Immunol., 21:357, Nov. 1931.

419. Felton, L. D. Dissociation of specific protein precipitate of antipneumococcus horse serum, and comparison with protein isolated by chemical means from this immune serum. J. Immunol., 22:453, June 1932.

420. Felton, L. D. Studies on virulence. IV. Influence on virulence of pneumococci of growth on various media. J. Exper. Med., 56:13, July 1932.

421. Felton, L. D. Studies on virulence. V. The effect of oxygen, nitrogen, and carbon dioxide on virulence of growing pneumococci. J. Exper. Med., 56:27, July 1932.

422. Felton, L. D. Active immunization of white mice by non-polysaccharide and probably non-protein derivative of pneumococcus. J. Immunol., 23: 405, Nov. 1932.

423. Felton, L. D. Pneumococcus antibodies—what are they? Science, 79:277, Mar. 23, 1934.

424. Felton, L. D. Studies on the immunizing substances in pneumococci. II. Separation of organism into acid soluble and acid insoluble fractions. J. Immunol., 27:379, Oct. 1934.

425. Felton, L. D. Discussion on the possibility of prophylaxis against pneumococcus infections. Abstract of Sectional Proceedings *in* Report of Proceedings of Second International Congress for Microbiology, p. 502, London, 1937.

426. Felton, L. D., and Bailey, G. H. Biologic significance of the soluble specific substances of pneumococci. J. Infect. Dis., 38:131, Feb. 1926.

427. Felton, L. D., and Bailey, G. H. The specific precipitates obtained from antipneumococcus serum and antibody solution by the soluble specific substances of pneumococci. J. Infect. Dis., 38:145, Feb. 1926.

428. Felton, L. D., and Kauffmann, G. Action of enzymes on protective antibody of pneumococcus. J. Immunol., 13:219, Mar. 1927.

429. Felton, L. D., and Kauffmann, G. Pyrogenic reaction to concentrated antipneumococcus serums, with respect to certain serum constituents. J. Infect. Dis., 49:337, Oct. 1931.

430. Felton, L. D., Kauffmann, G., and Stahl, H. J. Precipitation of bacterial polysaccharides with calcium phosphate; pneumococcus. J. Bact., 29: 149, Feb. 1935.

431. Felton, L. D., and Prescott, B. Studies of the immunizing substances in pneumococci. V. Effect of alkalis on the immunizing properties of a Type I pneumococcus polysaccharide. Bull. Johns Hopkins Hosp., 59: 114, Aug. 1936.

432. Felton, L. D., and Stahl, H. J. Standardization of antipneumococcus horse sera and concentrates. National Institute of Health, Bull. No. 169, Feb. 1937. 58 p.

433. Felton, L. D., Sutliff, W. D., and Steele, B. F. Antigenic characteristics in man of certain products of the pneumococcus. J. Infect. Dis., 56:101, Mar.–Apr., 1935.

434. Ferguson, D. A reinvestigation of the value of active pneumococcus immunity (preliminary report). U. S. Nav. M. Bull., 30:409, July 1932.

435. Ferguson, D. The human response to immunization with Type I pneumococcus vaccine. U. S. Nav. M. Bull., 32:155, Apr. 1934.

436. Ferguson, F. R., Davey, A. F. C., and Topley, W. W. C. Value of mixed vaccines in prevention of common cold. J. Hyg., 26:98, Mar. 1927.

437. Ferguson, F. R., and Lovell, R. Investigation of primary lobar pneumonia in Manchester, 1925–7. Quart. J. Med., 22:73, Oct. 1928.

438. Ferrell, J. A. Health problems peculiar to the southern states. Am. J. Pub. Health, 23:441, May 1933.

439. Ferry, N. S., and Blanchard, E. Preparation and standardization of polyvalent antipneumococcic serum. J. Lab. & Clin. Med., 6:23, Oct. 1920.

440. Ferry, N. S., and Fisher, L. W. Production of immunity with soluble antigen of pneumococcus. J. Lab. & Clin. Med., 10:817, July 1925.

441. Finkle, P. Metabolism of S and R forms of pneumococcus. J. Exper. Med., 53:661, May 1931.

442. Finland, M. Serum treatment of lobar pneumonia. New England J. Med., 202:1244, June 26, 1930.

443. Finland, M. Immunological reactions of pneumonic pleural fluids. J. Exper. Med., 55:169, Feb. 1932.

444. Finland, M. Rationale and practical aspects of serum treatment in pneumonia. International Clinics, 4:45, Dec. 1933.

445. Finland, M. Significance of mixed infections in pneumococcic pneumonia. J.A.M.A., 103:1681, Dec. 1, 1934.

446. Finland, M. Use of serum in the treatment of pneumonia. M. Clin. North America, 18:1093, Jan. 1935.

447. Finland, M. The modern treatment of pneumonia. Am. J. Nursing, 36: 24, Jan. 1936.

448. Finland, M. Adequate dosage in specific serum treatment of pneumococcus Type I pneumonia. Am. J. M. Sc., 192:849, Dec. 1936.

449. Finland, M. Significance of specific pneumococcus types in disease, including Types IV to XXXII (Cooper). Ann. Int. Med., 10:1531, Apr. 1937.

450. Finland, M., Brown, J. W., and Ruegsegger, J. M. Anatomic and bacteriologic findings in infections with specific types of pneumococci, including Types I to XXXII. Arch. Path., 23:801, June 1937.

451. Finland, M., and Dowling, H. F. Cutaneous reactions and antibody response to intracutaneous injections of pneumococcus polysaccharides. J. Immunol., 29:285, Oct. 1935.

452. Finland, M., and Dowling, H. F. Dose of antibody effective in treatment of pneumococcus Type II pneumonia. Am. J. M. Sc., 191:658, May 1936.
453. Finland, M., and Dowling, H. F. Pneumococcus Type II and Type V infections. Arch. Int. Med., 58:598, Oct. 1936.
454. Finland, M., and Loverud, H. I. L. Massive atelectatic collapse of the lung complicating pneumococcus pneumonia. Ann. Int. Med., 10:1828, June 1937.
455. Finland, M., and Ruegsegger, J. M. Immunization of human subjects with the specific carbohydrates of Type III and related Type VIII pneumococcus. J. Clin. Investigation, 14:829, Nov. 1935.
456. Finland, M., Ruegsegger, J. M., Dowling, H. F., and Tilghman, R. C. Infections with pneumococcus Type VII. Am. J. M. Sc., 193:48, Jan. 1937.
457. Finland, M., Ruegsegger, J. M., and Felton, L. D. Heterophile antibodies in pneumonia. J. Clin. Investigation, 14:683, Sept. 1935.
458. Finland, M., Ruegsegger, J. M., and Felton, L. D. Should heterophile antibody be used in the treatment of pneumococcic pneumonia? J.A.M.A., 105:1180, Oct. 12, 1935.
459. Finland, M., and Sutliff, W. D. Specific cutaneous reactions and circulating antibodies in the course of lobar pneumonia. I. Cases receiving no serum therapy. J. Exper. Med., 54:637, Nov. 1931.
460. Finland, M., and Sutliff, W. D. Specific cutaneous reactions and circulating antibodies in the course of lobar pneumonia. II. Cases treated with antipneumococcic sera. J. Exper. Med., 54:653, Nov. 1931.
461. Finland, M., and Sutliff, W. D. Specific antibody response of human subjects to intracutaneous injection of pneumococcus products. J. Exper. Med., 55:853, June 1932.
462. Finland, M., and Sutliff, W. D. Immunity reactions of human subjects to strains of pneumococci other than Types I, II, and III. J. Exper. Med., 57:95, Jan. 1933.
463. Finland, M., and Sutliff, W. D. Specific serum treatment of pneumococcus Type II pneumonia. J.A.M.A., 100:560, Feb. 25, 1933.
464. Finland, M., and Sutliff, W. D. Infections with pneumococcus Type III and Type VIII: Characterization of pneumonia caused by pneumococcus Type III and that associated with a biologically closely related organism, pneumococcus Type VIII. Reprinted with additions from Arch. Int. Med., 53:481, Apr. 1934.
465. Finland, M., and Tilghman, R. C. Bacteriological and immunological studies in families with pneumococcic infections: development of type-specific antibodies in healthy contact carriers. J. Clin. Investigation, 15:501, Sept. 1936.
466. Finland, M., and Tilghman, R. C. Clinical and immunologic observations in cases of pneumococcus Type V pneumonia treated with specific antibody. New England J. Med., 215:1211, Dec. 24, 1936.
467. Finland, M., Tilghman, R. C., Ruegsegger, J. M., and Dowling, H. F. Clinical and immunological observations in cases of pneumococcus Type VII pneumonia treated with concentrated type-specific antibody. Am. J. M. Sc., 193:59, Jan. 1937.
468. Finland, M., and Winkler, A. W. Antibody response to infections with

Type III and the related Type VIII pneumococcus. J. Clin. Investigation, 13:79, Jan. 1934.

469. Finland, M., and Winkler, A. W. Antibody response to infections with Type II and the related Type V pneumococcus. J. Clin. Investigation, 13:97, Jan. 1934.

470. Finland, M., and Winkler, A. W. Recurrences in pneumococcus pneumonia. Am. J. M. Sc., 188:309, Sept. 1934.

471. Fleisher, M. S., and Jones, L. Serum sickness in rabbits. I. Manifestations of serum sickness. J. Exper. Med., 54:597, Oct. 1931.

472. Foà, P., and Bordoni-Uffreduzzi, G. Ueber Bakterienbefunde bei Meningitis cerebrospinalis und die Beziehungen derselben zur Pneumonie. Deutsche med. Wchnschr., 12:249, Apr. 15, 1886.

473. Foà, P., and Bordoni-Uffreduzzi, G. Sulla eziologia della meningite cerebro-spinale epidemica. Arch. per le sc. med., 11:385, 1887. *Abstract in* Deutsche med. Wchnschr., 15:506, June 20, 1889.

474. Foà, P., and Bordoni-Uffreduzzi, G. Ueber die Aetiologie der "Meningitis cerebro-spinalis epidemica." (Translation.) Ztschr. f. Hyg. u. Infektionskr., 4:67, Apr. 1888.

475. Fox, F. W. Some investigations into the vitamin A content of livers of native mine labourers. South African M. J., 6:689, Nov. 12, 1932.

476. Francis, T., Jr. Identity of mechanisms of type-specific agglutinin and precipitin reactions with pneumococcus. J. Exper. Med., 55:55, Jan. 1932.

477. Francis, T., Jr. Value of skin test with type specific capsular polysaccharides in serum treatment of Type I pneumococcus pneumonia. J. Exper. Med., 57:617, Apr. 1933.

478. Francis, T., Jr. Antigenic action of the specific polysaccharide of pneumococcus Type I in man. Proc. Soc. Exper. Biol & Med., 31:493, Jan. 1934.

479. Francis, T., Jr. Recent advances in the study of influenza. J.A.M.A., 105: 251, July 27, 1935.

480. Francis, T., Jr. Studies in influenza. Health News (New York State Department of Health) 13:159, Oct. 5, 1936.

481. Francis, T., Jr. Studies in influenza. Pennsylvania M. J., 40:249, Jan. 1937.

482. Francis, T., Jr., and Magill, T. P. Immunological studies with the virus of influenza. J. Exper. Med., 62:505, Oct. 1935.

483. Francis, T., Jr., and Terrell, E. E. Experimental Type III pneumococcus pneumonia in monkeys. I. Production and clinical course. J. Exper. Med., 59:609, May 1934.

484. Francis, T., Jr., Terrell, E. E., Dubos, R., and Avery, O. T. Experimental Type III pneumococcus pneumonia in monkeys. II. Treatment with an enzyme which decomposes the specific capsular polysaccharide of pneumococcus Type III. J. Exper. Med., 59:641, May 1934.

485. Francis, T., Jr., and Tillett, W. S. Cutaneous reactions in pneumonia. Development of antibodies following the intradermal injection of type-specific polysaccharide. J. Exper. Med., 52:573, Oct. 1930.

486. Francis, T., Jr., and Tillett, W. S. Cutaneous reactions in rabbits to the type-specific capsular polysaccharides of pneumococcus. J. Exper. Med., 54:587, Oct. 1931.

487. Fraenkel, A. Die Genuine Pneumonie. Verhandl. d. Cong. f. innere Med., Wiesb., 3:17, 1884.

488. Fränkel, A. (1) Bakteriologische Mittheilungen. Ztschr. f. klin. Med., 10:401, 1886. (2) Bakteriologische Mittheilungen. II. Die Mikrococcen der Pneumonie. Ztschr. f. klin. Med., 10:426, 1886.

489. Fraenkel, A. Weitere Beiträge zur Lehre von den Mikrococcen der genuinen fibrinösen Pneumonie. Ztschr. f. klin. Med., 11:437, 1886.

490. Freedman, H. J. Acute anaphylactic shock following intracutaneous test for sensitivity to horse serum: report of a fatal case. New England J. Med., 212:10, Jan. 3, 1935.

491. Freeman, W. T., and Hoppe, L. D. The intravenous use of mercurochrome-220 soluble in the treatment of pneumonia in children. Am. J. Dis. Child., 28:310, Sept. 1924.

492. Fremmel, F., Henrichsen, K. J., and Sweany, H. C. Pulmonary infections by Friedländer's bacillus (Bac. mucosus capsulatus). Ann. Int. Med., 5:886, Jan. 1932.

493. French, J. M. The vaccine treatment of pneumonia. Clin. Med. & Surg., 35:107, Feb. 1928.

494. Freund, J. Reaction of young and adult rabbits to pneumococci injected into the skin. J. Exper. Med., 54:171, Aug. 1931.

495. Fried, B. M. Allergic lobar pneumonia. J. Exper. Med., 57:111, Jan. 1933.

496. Fried, B. M. Allergic inflammation of the lungs: pathogenesis of lobar pneumonia. Arch. Path., 18:865, Dec. 1934.

497. Friedberger, E., and Mita, S. Ueber eine Methode, gröszere Mengen artfremden Serums bei überempfindlichen Individuen zu injizieren. Deutsche med. Wchnschr., 38:204, Feb. 1, 1912.

498. Friedemann, U. Ueber Behandlung der akuten Lungenentzündung mit künstlichem Pneumothorax. Deutsch. med. Wchnschr., 47:443, Apr. 21, 1921.

499. Friedlander, A., McCord, C. P., Sladen, F. J., and Wheeler, G. W. Epidemic of influenza at Camp Sherman, Ohio. J.A.M.A., 71:1652, Nov. 16, 1918.

500. Friedländer, C. Ueber die Schizomyceten bei der acuten fibrösen Pneumonie. Virchows Arch. f. path. Anat., 87:319, Feb. 1882.

501. Friedländer, C. Die Mikrokokken der Pneumonie. Fortschr. d. Med., 1: 715, Nov. 15, 1883.

502. Friedlander, M., Sobotka, H., and Banzhaf, E. J. Precipitin reaction of antipneumococcus sera. II. Ratio of precipitin to protective antibody. J. Exper. Med., 47:79, Jan. 1928.

503. Frissell, L. F., and Famulener, L. W. A report of a series of pneumococcic pneumonias, classified according to the group of type of pneumococcus present. St. Luke's Hosp. (New York City) Med. & Surg. Rep., 4:23, 1917.

504. Fussell, M. H. Acute dilatation of the stomach in pneumonia. Am. J. M. Sc., 142:794, Dec. 1911.

505. Gafafer, W. M. Eye color and disease of upper respiratory tract (common cold). Am. J. Hyg., 16:880, Nov. 1932.

506. Gains in the study and control of pneumonia (editorial). New England J. Med., 216:1088, June 17, 1937.

507. Garnham, P. C. C., and deSmidt, F. P. G. Preliminary note on pneumonia in Nairobi with particular reference to type-incidence of pneumococcus. Kenya & East African M. J., 8:150, Sept. 1931.
508. Gaskell, J. F. Experimental pneumococcal infections of the lung. J. Path. & Bact., 28:427, July 1925.
509. Gaspari, E. L., Sugg, J. Y., Fleming, W. L., and Neill, J. M. Influence of heating the immunization material upon the antibody-invoking effectiveness of the type-specific and species-specific antigens of Type II pneumococcus cells. J. Exper. Med., 47:131, Jan. 1928.
510. Gautier, R. Tropical pneumonia. Quart. Bull. Health Organ., League of Nations, 1:64, Mar. 1932.
511. Gay, F. P., and Chickering, H. T. Concentration of the protective bodies in antipneumococcus serum by means of specific precipitation. J. Exper. Med., 21:389, Apr. 1915.
512. Gelarie, A. J., and Sabin, A. B. Study of the therapeutic mechanism of antipneumococcic serum on experimental dermal pneumococcus infection in rabbits. III. Influence of non-specific factors. J. Exper. Med., 58: 237, Aug. 1933.
513. Genesis and control of epidemics (editorial). J.A.M.A., 105:968, Sept. 21, 1935.
514. Gibson, C. L. Note on the diagnosis of pneumococcus peritonitis from the blood picture. Am. J. M. Sc., 180:344, Sept. 1930.
515. Gilbert, R., and Davenport, C. K. Failure of mouse test to demonstrate presence of Type I pneumococcus in sputum. Unusual instance. J. Lab. & Clin. Med., 12:944, July 1927.
516. Gill, C. A. Genesis of epidemics and natural history of disease. An introduction to the science of epidemiology based upon the study of epidemics of malaria, influenza, and plague. London, Baillière, Tindall and Cox, 1928, 538 p.
517. Gilmour, J., *editor*. Report on an investigation into the sanitary conditions in Persia: undertaken on behalf of the Health Committee of the League of Nations at the request of the Persian Government. Geneva, League of Nations, Health Organisation, 1925, 64 p.
518. Gleich, M. Aputrid pulmonary necrosis. A complication of pneumonia. Report of case. Arch. Pediat., 49:258, Apr. 1932.
519. Globus, J. H., and Kasanin, J. I. Pneumococcus (Type IV) meningitis. J.A.M.A., 90:599, Feb. 25, 1928.
520. Glynn, E. E., and Digby, L. Bacteriological and clinical observations on pneumonia and empyemata, with special reference to the pneumococcus and to serum treatment. London, His Majesty's Stationery Office, 1923, 167 p. (Medical Research Council, Special Rept. Series No. 79.)
521. Goebel, W. F., and Avery, O. T. A study of pneumococcus autolysis. J. Exper. Med., 49:267, Feb. 1929.
522. Goebel, W. F., and Avery, O. T. Chemo-immunological studies on conjugated carbohydrate-proteins. IV. Synthesis of the p-aminobenzol ether of soluble specific substance of Type III pneumococcus and its coupling with protein. J. Exper. Med., 54:431, Sept. 1931.
523. Goebel, W. F., Avery, O. T., and Babers, F. H. Chemo-immunological studies on conjugated carbohydrate-proteins. IX. The specificity of

antigens prepared by combining the p-aminophenol glycosides of disaccharides with protein. J. Exper. Med., 60:599, Nov. 1934.

524. Goebel, W. F., Babers, F. H., and Avery, O. T. Chemo-immunological studies on conjugated carbohydrate-proteins. VI. Synthesis of p-aminophenol, a-glucoside and its coupling with protein. J. Exper. Med., 55:761, May 1932.

525. Goebel, W. F., Babers, F. H., and Avery, O. T. Chemo-immunological studies on conjugated carbohydrate-proteins. VIII. The influence of the acetyl group on the specificity of hexoside-protein antigens. J. Exper. Med., 60:85, July 1934.

526. Gohar, M. A., and Abboud, M. A. The causative organisms of pneumonia in children in Egypt. J. Lab. & Clin. Med., 19:751, Apr. 1934.

527. Goldstein, H. I., and Goldstein, H. Z. Endocarditis and meningitis (pneumococcic). M. Times, 55:200, Sept. 1927; 229, Oct. 1927; and 259, Nov. 1927.

528. Gonzalez, P. Essais de classification des pneumocoques au Chili. Compt. rend. Soc. de biol., 105:244, Oct. 24, 1930.

529. Goode, J. P. Goode's School Atlas: physical, political, and economic; for American schools and colleges. Revised and enlarged. New York, Rand McNally & Co., 1933, 287 p.

530. Goodman, A. R. Pneumonia in high altitudes. Summary of one hundred and one cases of lobar pneumonia treated at American Hospital, Mexico City, from 1890 to 1904. M. Rec., 67:56, Jan. 14, 1905.

531. Goodner, K. Experimental intradermal pneumococcus infection in rabbits. J. Exper. Med., 48:1, July 1928.

532. Goodner, K. Further experiments with the intradermal pneumococcus infection in rabbits. J. Exper. Med., 48:413, Sept. 1928.

533. Goodner, K. Experiments on concentration of antipneumococcic and antimeningococcic horse sera. J. Immunol., 19:473, Nov. 1930.

534. Goodner, K. Development and localization of dermal pneumococcic lesion in the rabbit. J. Exper. Med., 54:847, Dec. 1931.

535. Goodner, K. Effect of pneumococcus autolysates upon pneumococcus dermal infection in the rabbit. J. Exper. Med., 58:153, Aug. 1933.

536. Goodner, K. Studies on host factors in pneumococcus infections. I. Certain factors involved in the curative action of specific antipneumococcus serum in Type I pneumococcus dermal infection in rabbits. J. Exper. Med., 60:9, July 1934.

537. Goodner, K. Studies on host factors in pneumococcus infections. II. The protective action of Type I antipneumococcus serum in rabbits. J. Exper. Med., 60:19, July 1934.

538. Goodner, K., and Dubos, R. Studies on quantitative action of specific enzyme in Type III pneumococcus dermal infection in rabbits. J. Exper. Med., 56:521, Oct. 1932.

539. Goodner, K., Dubos, R., and Avery, O. T. Action of specific enzyme upon dermal infection of rabbits with Type III pneumococcus. J. Exper. Med., 55:393, Mar. 1932.

540. Goodner, K., and Horsfall, F. L., Jr. Protective action of Type I antipneumococcus serum in mice. I. Quantitative aspects of the mouse protection test. J. Exper. Med., 62:359, Sept. 1935.

541. Goodner, K., and Horsfall, F. L., Jr. Properties of the type specific pro-

teins of antipneumococcus sera. I. Mouse protective value of Type I sera with reference to precipitin content. J. Exper. Med., 66:413, Oct. 1937.

542. Goodner, K., and Horsfall, F. L., Jr. Properties of type specific proteins of antipneumococcus sera. II. Immunological fractionation of Type I antipneumococcus horse and rabbit sera. J. Exper. Med., 66:425, Oct. 1937.

543. Goodner, K., and Horsfall, F. L., Jr. Properties of type specific proteins of antipneumococcus sera. III. Immunochemical fractionation of Type I antipneumococcus horse and rabbit sera. J. Exper. Med., 66:437, Oct. 1937.

544. Goodner, K., Horsfall, F. L., Jr., and Bauer, J. H. Ultrafiltration of Type I antipneumococcal sera. Proc. Soc. Exper. Biol. & Med., 34:617, June 1936.

545. Goodner, K., Horsfall, F. L., Jr., and Dubos, R. J. Type-specific antipneumococcic rabbit serum for therapeutic purposes; production, processing, and standardization. J. Immunol., 33:279, Oct. 1937.

546. Goodner, K., and Miller, D. K. Protective action of Type I antipneumococcus serum in mice. II. Course of the infectious process. J. Exper. Med., 62:375, Sept. 1935.

547. Goodner, K., and Miller, D. K. Protective action of Type I antipneumococcus serum in mice. III. Significance of certain host factors. J. Exper. Med., 62:393, Sept. 1935.

548. Goodner, K., and Stillman, E. G. Evaluation of active resistance to pneumococcus infection in rabbits. J. Exper. Med., 58:183, Aug. 1933.

549. Gorgas, W. C. Recommendation as to sanitation concerning employees of the mines on the Rand made to the Transvaal Chamber of Mines. J.A.M.A., 62:1855, June 13, 1914.

550. Graeser, J. B. Specific soluble substance of pneumococcus in lungs of dogs recovered from experimental lobar pneumonia. Proc. Soc. Exper. Biol. & Med., 32:386, Nov. 1934.

551. Graeser, J. B., and Harrison, M. C. Changes in the titer of antipneumococcal humoral immunity in adult human beings. J. Exper. Med., 58:245, Aug. 1933.

552. Graeser, J. B., Wu, C., and Robertson, O. H. Physical signs and roentgenographic findings in lobar pneumonia in adults. Arch. Int. Med., 53:249, Feb. 1934.

553. Grant, M. H. Pneumonias in Glasgow and their pneumococcal types. Glasgow M. J., 98:193, Sept. 1922.

554. Grant for research in pneumonia control in Michigan (news item). J.A.M.A., 107:219, July 18, 1936.

555. Gray, A. W. Antipneumococcus serum (Kyes) in the treatment of pneumonia. Am. J. M. Sc., 159:885, June 1920.

556. Great Britain: Medical Research Council. The pneumococcus, by W. Mair, J. W. McLeod, F. Griffith; with sections by C. H. Browning and W. Bullock. *In* A system of bacteriology in relation to medicine, 2:164. London, His Majesty's Stationery Office, 1929.

557. Great Britain: Medical Research Council. Report of Therapeutic Trials Committee. Serum treatment of lobar pneumonia. Lancet, 1:290, Feb. 10, 1934.

558. Great Britain: Medical Research Council and Department of Scientific and

Industrial Research. Report no. 5 of the Industrial Fatigue Research Board: Fatigue and efficiency in the iron and steel industry. (Metal trade series, No. 4.) p. 78. London, His Majesty's Stationery Office, 1920.

559. Great Britain: Registrar General. Annual report of births, deaths and marriages in England and Wales (abstracts of 1875–1910). *Continued as* Registrar General's statistical review of England and Wales for the years 1921–1931 (new annual series, Nos. 1–11). London, His Majesty's Stationery Office.

560. Great Britain: Registrar General. Decennial supplement, England and Wales, 1921. Part II. Occupational mortality, fertility and infant mortality. London, His Majesty's Stationery Office.

561. Great Britain: War Office. Reports on the health of the army for the years 1922–1931, v. 58–67. London, His Majesty's Stationery Office, 1924–1933.

562. Greece: Statistique générale de la Grèce. Annuaire statistique de la Grèce, 1931.

563. Greenberg, D. Meteorological conditions and prevalence of pneumonia. J.A.M.A., 72:252, Jan. 25, 1919.

564. Greene, M. R. Effects of vitamins A and D on antibody production and resistance to infection. Am. J. Hyg., 17:60, Jan. 1933.

565. Greenwald, I. Metabolism in pneumonia. III. The excretion of anions and of total base in pneumonia. Arch. Int. Med., 48:440, Sept. 1931.

566. Greenway, J. C., Boettiger, C., and Colwell, H. S. Pneumonia and some of its complications at Camp Bowie. Arch. Int. Med., 24:1, July 1919.

567. Greenwood, M., Jr., and Candy, R. H. Fatality of fractures of lower extremity and of lobar pneumonia. A study of hospital mortality rates, 1751–1901. J. Royal Statistical Soc., 74:365, Mar. 1911.

568. Griffith, F. Serological types of pneumococci in lobar pneumonia: study of 100 cases. Lancet, 2:226, July 30, 1921.

569. Griffith, F. Types of pneumococci obtained from cases of lobar pneumonia. *In* Great Britain, Ministry of Health, Rep. on Pub. Health & Med. Subjects, No. 13, p. 20. London, His Majesty's Stationery Office, 1922.

570. Griffith, F. Bacteriological studies: I. The influence of immune serum on the biological properties of pneumococci. *In* Great Britain, Ministry of Health, Rep. on Pub. Health & Med. Subjects, No. 18. London, His Majesty's Stationery Office, 1923, 13 p.

571. Griffith, F. Significance of pneumococcal types. J. Hyg., 27:113, Jan. 1928.

572. Gross, P., and Cooper, F. B. Efficacy of p-aminobenzenesulfonamide in experimental Type III pneumococcus pneumonia of rats. Proc. Soc. Exper. Biol. & Med., 36:225, Mar. 1937.

573. Grove, E. F. Studies in anaphylaxis in the rabbit. I. Study of factors concerned in establishment of maximal hypersensitiveness in rabbits to egg white and horse serum. J. Immunol., 23:101, Aug. 1932.

574. Grulee, C. G., and Mulherin, P. Lobar pneumonia in infants and young children. J. Pediat., 1:593, Nov. 1932.

575. Gudger, J. R. Tularemic pneumonia: report of a case. J.A.M.A., 101:1148, Oct. 7, 1933.

576. Gundel, M. Zur Frage einer Behandlung der Pneumonia crouposa mit Rekonvaleszentenserum. Klin. Wchnschr., 10:728, Apr. 18, 1931.
577. Gundel, M. Immunbiologische Studien über Pneumokokkeninfektionen. Ztschr. f. Immunitätsforsch. u. exper. Therap., 73:193, Jan. 1932.
578. Gundel, M. Bakteriologische und epidemiologische Untersuchungen über die Besiedlung der oberen Atmungswege Gesunder mit Pneumokokken. Ztschr. f. Hyg. u. Infektionskr., 114:659, Feb. 1933.
579. Gundel, M., and Linden, H. Über die Verbreitungsweise der menschlichen Pneumokokkeninfektionen. Ztschr. f. Hyg. u. Infektionskr., 112:1, Jan. 15, 1931.
580. Gundel, M., and Okura, G. Untersuchungen über das gleichzeitige Vorkommen mehrerer Pneumokokkentypen bei Gesunden und ihre Bedeutung für die Epidemiologie. Ztschr. f. Hyg. u. Infektionskr., 114:678, Feb. 1933.
581. Gundel, M., and Schwarz, F. K. T. Studien über die Bakterienflora der oberen Atmungswege Neugeborener (im Vergleich mit der Mundhöhlenflora der Mutter und des Pflegepersonals) unter besonderer Berücksichtigung ihrer Bedeutung für das Pneumonieproblem. Ztschr. f. Hyg. u. Infektionskr., 113:411, Jan. 1932.
582. Gundel, M., and Schwarz, F. K. T. Über die Typendifferenzierung und Epidemiologie der Gruppe X der Pneumokokken. Ztschr. f. Hyg. u. Infektionskr., 113:498, Jan. 1932.
583. Gundel, M., and Seitz, L. Experimentelle Untersuchungen über die Chemotherapie von Pneumokokkeninfektionen mit neuen, noch nicht in die Therapie eingeführten Chininpräparater. Ztschr. f. Immunitätsforsch. u. exper. Therap., 80:240, Oct. 5, 1933.
584. Gundel, M., and Wasu, C. Die Bedeutung der Virulenz des Erregers für die Pathogenese menschlicher Pneumokokkenerkrankungen. Ztschr. f. Hyg. u. Infektionskr., 112:436, May 1931.
585. Hadley, P. Microbic dissociation. Instability of bacterial species with special reference to active dissociation and transmissible autolysis. J. Infect. Dis., 40:1, Jan. 1927.
586. Hagebusch, O. E., Robben, F. J., Fleisher, M. S., and Jones, L. Serum sickness in rabbits. III. Reactions of body temperature and leucocytic curves. J. Immunol., 22:373, May 1932.
587. Haldane, J. S. Symptoms, causes and prevention of anoxemia. Brit. M. J., 2:65, July 19, 1919.
588. Hall, J. N., Stone, M. C., and Simpson, J. C. Epidemic of pneumonia following influenza at Camp Logan, Texas: preliminary report. J.A.M.A., 71:1986, Dec. 14, 1918.
589. Hallermann, A., and Kähler, H. Über die Typeneinteilung der Pneumonie und ihre Behandlung mit Serum. Klin. Wchnschr., 9:650, Apr. 5, 1930.
590. Haman, W. A. Influenzal bronchopneumonia: its prophylaxis and jugulation. Hahnemannian Monthly, 55:540, Sept. 1920.
591. Hamburger, W. W., and Fox, H. Study of epidemics of pneumococcus and streptococcus infections, and measles, at Camp Zachary Taylor, Kentucky, autumn, 1917, to summer, 1918. M. Clin. North America, 2:321, Sept. 1918.

592. Hamilton, R. L. Treatment of pneumonia: comparative results obtained with and without serum. M. Rec., 140:298, Sept. 19, 1934.
593. Hare, R. Two cases of influenzal pneumonia treated by injection of convalescent serum. Lancet, 2:293, Aug. 5, 1933.
594. Harkavy, J. Pneumococcus meningitis recovery with serum therapy. J.A.M.A., 90:597, Feb. 25, 1928.
595. Harley, D. Study of pneumococcal allergy, anaphylaxis and immunity. J. Path. & Bact., 41:491, Nov. 1935.
596. Harloe, R. F. Empyema: report of 351 cases treated by a closed negative pressure method. Am. J. Surg., 26:231, Nov. 1934.
597. Harrington, A. W. Serum treatment in pneumonia. Glasgow M. J., 1:148, June 1933.
598. Harris, A. H., and Varley, F. M. Preservation of sputum for pneumococcus-type differentiation. J. Lab. & Clin. Med., 23:164, Nov. 1937.
599. Hart, A. L. The postpneumonic lung: critical review. Am. J. Roentgenol., 26:371, Sept. 1931.
600. Hart, T. S. Lobar pneumonia. A year's experience in the Presbyterian Hospital with special reference to the use of antipneumococcus serum. M. Rec., 95:895, May 31, 1919.
601. Hartley, P., Parish, H. J., Petrie, G. F., and Smith, W. Provisional stable standard for antipneumococcus serum, Type I, and its practical application. Lancet, 2:91, July 8, 1933.
602. Hartley, P., and Smith, W. A proposed international standard for antipneumococcus serum (Type I). Quart. Bull. Health Organ., League of Nations, Special Number, p. 48, Jan. 1935.
603. Hartley, P., and Smith, W. A proposed international standard for antipneumococcus serum (Type II). Quart. Bull. Health Organ., League of Nations, Special Number, p. 65, Jan. 1935.
604. Hartman, C. C., and Lacy, G. R. The biologic classification in pneumococcic infections. J.A.M.A., 69:2165, Dec. 29, 1917.
605. Hatcher, R. A. Indispensable uses of narcotics in treatment of coughing. J.A.M.A., 96:1383, Apr. 25, 1931.
606. Hay, J. Treatment of acute lobar pneumonia. I. Prophylaxis: specific treatment: symptomatic treatment. Brit. M. J., 2:477, Sept. 17, 1927.
607. Haythorn, S. R., and Meller, H. B. Necropsy evidences on the relation of smoky atmosphere to pneumonia. Am. J. Pub. Health, 28:479, Apr. 1938.
608. Heathman, L. S., McDaniel, O., and Chesley, A. J. Pneumonia in Minnesota. What can be done about it? Minnesota Med., 20:1, Jan. 1937.
609. Heffron, R. The Massachusetts pneumonia plan. Commonhealth (Massachusetts Department of Public Health), 18:172, July–Aug.–Sept. 1931.
610. Heffron, R. Massachusetts pneumonia program. New England J. Med., 206:328, Feb. 18, 1932.
611. Heffron, R. A study of lobar pneumonia in Massachusetts. New England J. Med., 207:153, July 28, 1932.
612. Heffron, R. Pneumonia death rate (letter to the editor). New England J. Med., 213:1049, Nov. 21, 1935.
613. Heffron, R. Campaign against pneumonia (letter to the editor). New England J. Med., 214:222, Jan. 30, 1936.

614. Heffron, R., and Anderson, G. W. Two years' study of lobar pneumonia in Massachusetts. J.A.M.A., 101:1286, Oct. 21, 1933.
615. Heffron, R., and Robinson, E. S. Final report of the Massachusetts Pneumonia Study and Service, 1931–1935. Commonhealth (Massachusetts Department of Public Health), 24:2, Jan.–Feb.–Mar. 1937.
616. Heffron, R., and Varley, F. M. A study of lobar pneumonia in Massachusetts: methods and results of type determination, 1931–1932. Am. J. Pub. Health, 22:1230, Dec. 1932.
617. Heidelberger, M., and Avery, O. T. Soluble specific substance of pneumococcus. J. Exper. Med., 38:73, July 1923.
618. Heidelberger, M., and Avery, O. T. Soluble specific substance of pneumococcus. J. Exper. Med., 40:301, Sept. 1924.
619. Heidelberger, M., Goebel, W. F., and Avery, O. T. Soluble specific substance of pneumococcus. J. Exper. Med., 42:727, Nov. 1925.
620. Heidelberger, M., and Kabat, E. A. Chemical studies on bacterial agglutination. I. A method. J. Exper. Med., 60:643, Nov. 1934.
621. Heidelberger, M., and Kabat, E. A. Quantitative studies on antibody purification. II. Dissociation of antibody from pneumococcus specific precipitates and specifically agglutinated pneumococci. J. Exper. Med., 69:181, Feb. 1938.
622. Heidelberger, M., and Kendall, F. E. Specific and non-specific polysaccharides of Type IV pneumococcus. J. Exper. Med., 53:625, May 1931.
623. Heidelberger, M., and Kendall, F. E. Studies on the precipitin reaction. Precipitating haptens; species differences in antibodies. J. Exper. Med., 57:373, Mar. 1933.
624. Heidelberger, M., and Kendall, F. E. Precipitin reaction between Type III pneumococcus polysaccharide and homologous antibody. II. Conditions for quantitative precipitation of antibody in horse sera. J. Exper. Med., 61:559, Apr. 1935.
625. Heidelberger, M., and Kendall, F. E. Precipitin reaction between Type III pneumococcus polysaccharide and homologous antibody. III. A quantitative study and a theory of the reaction mechanism. J. Exper. Med., 61:563, Apr. 1935.
626. Heidelberger, M., Sia, R. H. P., and Kendall, F. E. Specific precipitation and mouse protection in Type I antipneumococcus sera. J. Exper. Med., 52:477, Oct. 1930.
627. Heintzelman, J. H. L., Hadley, P., and Mellon, R. R. Use of p-aminobenzenesulphonamide in Type 3 pneumococcus pneumonia. Am. J. M. Sc., 193:759, June 1937.
628. Heist, G. D., and Solis-Cohen, S. Bactericidal action of the whole blood of rabbits following inoculations of pneumococcus bacterins. J. Immunol., 4:147, July 1919.
629. Helm, J. B., Ferguson, D., and Noble, H. J. X-ray observations of pneumonia treated with specific antisera. U. S. Nav. M. Bull., 32:147, Apr. 1934.
630. Henderson, Y. Acapnia as a factor in post-operative shock, atelectasis and pneumonia. J.A.M.A., 95:572, Aug. 23, 1930.
631. Henderson, Y. Reasons for the use of carbon dioxide with oxygen in the treatment of pneumonia. New England J. Med., 206:151, Jan. 28, 1932.

632. Henderson, Y., Haggard, H. W., Coryllos, P. N., and Birnbaum, G. L. The treatment of pneumonia by inhalation of carbon dioxide. I. The relief of atelectasis. Arch. Int. Med., 45:72, Jan. 1930.
633. Henry, J. E. Study of bacteriology of recent epidemic of influenza at the U. S. Naval Training Camp, Seattle, Wash. Northwest Med., 18:46, Mar. 1919.
634. Henson, G. E. Serum therapy in lobar pneumonia, with report of 67 cases. South. M. J., 13:178, Mar. 1920.
635. Herrold, R. D., and Traut, E. F. Skin reactions with pneumococcal and other bacterial filtrates and extracts. J. Infect. Dis., 40:619, May 1927.
636. Herzog, B. M. Die in der Schweiz bei croupöser Pneumonie vorkommenden Pneumokokkentypen. Schweiz. med. Wchnschr., 5:573, June 19, 1924.
637. Hess, F. O. Einiges zur Behandlung der kruppösen Pneumonie. München. med. Wchnschr., 78:2078, Dec. 4, 1931.
638. Heuer, G. J. Acute empyema. J. Thoracic Surg., 1:461, June 1932.
639. Hickling, R. A. Monocytes in pneumonia. Clinical and hematologic study. Arch. Int. Med., 40:594, Nov. 1927.
640. Hickling, R. A., and Sutliff, W. D. Pneumonia in a case of chronic lymphatic leukemia. Am. J. M. Sc., 175:224, Feb. 1928.
641. Hill, J. H., and Martin, L. A review of experimental studies of nonspecific inhibition of anaphylactic shock. Medicine, 11:141, May 1932.
642. Hill, L. "Nose-opening" rays. Am. J. Hyg., 22:183, July 1935.
643. Hines, L. E. Artificial pneumothorax in the treatment of acute lobar pneumonia (note). J.A.M.A., 104:149, Jan. 12, 1935.
644. Hippocrates. The genuine works of Hippocrates, 1:324. Translated from the Greek with a preliminary discourse and annotations by Francis Adams. London, Sydenham Society, 1849.
645. Hippocrates. Empyema. *In* The genuine works of Hippocrates, 1:248. Translated from the Greek with a preliminary discourse and annotations by Francis Adams. London, Sydenham Society, 1849. *As seen in* Major, R. H., Classic Descriptions of Disease, p. 531. Springfield, Ill., Charles C. Thomas, 1932.
646. Hirano, H. Studies on diplococcus pneumoniae, especially pneumococcus mucosus. Abstract in English (unpublished) by Y. Miyagawa, Government Institute for Infectious Diseases of the Tokyo Imperial University. Shirokane-Daimachi, Shiba-Ku, Tokyo, 1925.
647. Hirsch, A. Handbook of geographical and historical pathology, 3:116. Translated from the 2d German ed. by Charles Creighton. London, The New Sydenham Society, 1886.
648. Hiss, P. H., Jr. Comparative study of pneumococci and allied organisms. Report from the Central Laboratory to the Medical Commission for investigation of acute respiratory diseases of the Department of Health of the City of New York. J. Exper. Med., 7:547, Aug. 1905.
649. Histamine factor in anaphylaxis (editorial). J.A.M.A., 98:2143, June 11, 1932.
650. Hoffman, F. L. Cancer in Mexico. Newark, The Prudential Insurance Company of America, 1927, 70 p.
651. Hoge, V. M. Psittacosis in the United States: incidence, scientific aspects,

and administrative control measures. Pub. Health Rep., 49:451, Apr. 6, 1934.

652. Hong Kong: Medical Department. Medical & sanitary reports for the years 1932 and 1933, by A. R. Wellington.

653. Hong Kong: Medical Department. Medical & sanitary report for the year 1934, by W. B. A. Moore.

654. Hooker, S. B., and Follensby, E. M. Influence of hypersensitiveness to horse serum on duration of local passive antitoxic immunity in man. J. Immunol., 20:269, Apr. 1931.

655. Hoover, C. F. Moisture in the air spaces of the lungs and oxygen therapy. J.A.M.A., 71:880, Sept. 14, 1918.

656. Horsfall, F. L., Jr., and Goodner, K. Lipoids and immunological reactions. I. Relation of phospholipins to type-specific reactions of antipneumococcus horse and rabbit sera. J. Exper. Med., 62:485, Oct. 1935.

657. Horsfall, F. L., Jr., Goodner, K., and MacLeod, C. M. Type specific antipneumococcus rabbit serum. Science, 84:579, Dec. 25, 1936.

658. Horsfall, F. L., Jr., Goodner, K., and MacLeod, C. M. Antipneumococcus rabbit serum as therapeutic agent in lobar pneumonia. II. Additional observations in pneumococcus pneumonias of nine different types. New York State J. Med., 38:245, Feb. 15, 1938.

659. Horsfall, F. L., Jr., Goodner, K., MacLeod, C. M., and Harris, A. H., 2nd. Antipneumococcus rabbit serum as therapeutic agent in lobar pneumonia. J.A.M.A., 108:1483, May 1, 1937.

660. Howard, C. P. Pneumococcus arthritis. Johns Hopkins Hosp. Rep., 15: 229, 1910.

661. Howard, C. P. The diagnosis and treatment of pneumonia. New York, Oxford University Press, 1931, 373 p.

662. Howard, C. P. The rheumatic lung. Ann. Int. Med., 7:165, Aug. 1933.

663. Howard, C. P., and Fullerton, C. W. Treatment of lobar pneumonia. Canad. M.A.J., 27:367, Oct. 1932.

664. Hoyle, L. Production of pneumonia in mice by bacteria and filterable viruses. J. Path. & Bact., 41:163, July 1935.

665. Huber, E. G. Control of the communicable diseases prevalent in Massachusetts, with study of mortality due to them during past 75 years. Boston M. & S. J., 195:122, July 15, 1926 and weekly through Nov. 11, 1926.

666. Hunnicutt, T. N., Jr. Early diagnosis and specific treatment of lobar pneumonia. Virginia M. Monthly, 62:448, Nov. 1935.

667. Hunnicutt, T., and Sutliff, W. D. Penetration of antipneumococcic horse serum into the consolidated lung in lobar pneumonia. Proc. Soc. Exper. Biol. & Med., 29:635, Feb. 1932.

668. Hunt, L. W. Recent observations in serum disease. J.A.M.A., 99:909, Sept. 10, 1932.

669. Huntoon, F. M. Antibody studies. I. Reversal of the antigen-antibody reaction. J. Immunol., 6:117, Mar. 1921.

670. Huntoon, F. M., and Etris, S. Antibody studies. II. Recovery of antibody from sensitized antigens: technic. J. Immunol., 6:123, Mar. 1921.

671. Huntoon, F. M., Masucci, P., and Hannum, E. Antibody studies. III. Chemical nature of antibody. J. Immunol., 6:185, Mar. 1921.

672. Hurwitz, S. H., and Wessels, A. L. Reaction of perfused isolated lung of

sensitized guinea pig to horse serum. Proc. Soc. Exper. Biol. & Med., 29: 120, Nov. 1931.

673. India: Mysore Department of Health. Annual report with the Government review thereon, January 1 to December 31, 1930.

674. India: Public Health Commissioner with the Government of India. Annual report for 1930, v. 1, with appendices.

675a. Ireland, M. W., and Bancroft, W. D., and associates. *See reference 1344.*

675b. Ireland, M. W., Callender, G. R., and Coupal, J. F. Medical Department of United States Army in the World War. Vol. XII. Pathology of acute respiratory diseases, and of gas gangrene following war wounds. Washington, Government Printing Office, 1929. 583 p.

676. Ireland, M. W., and Weed, F. W. Medical Department of the United States Army in the World War. Vol. V. Military hospitals in the United States. Washington, Government Printing Office, 1923. 857 p.

677. Irving, P. Reduction of mortality from pneumococcus pneumonia. Preventive Medicine (New York Academy of Medicine), 6:3, Feb. 1937.

678. Irving, P. A state medical association's part in a pneumonia control program. Organization section of J.A.M.A., 110:86B, Feb. 12, 1938.

679. Irwin, M. R., and Hughes, T. P. Differences in bactericidal power of the blood within an inbred strain of rats. Proc. Soc. Exper. Biol. & Med., 29:295, Dec. 1931.

680. Ishida, I. Studies on influenzas and pneumonias of infants and children. I. Bacteriological research with special references to occurrence of various types of pneumococci. Orient. J. Dis. Infants, 8:29, Nov. 1930.

681. Ishida, I., Nagai, H., and Saito, T. Study of pneumococcus in throat of healthy infant, especially on its type occurrence. Orient. J. Dis. Infants, 10:21, July 1931.

682. Jacobson, M. A. Studies on respiratory diseases. XXX. Epidemiology of lobar pneumonia. J. Prev. Med., 1:259, Jan. 1927.

683. Jamieson, W. A., and Powell, H. M. Further studies on immunology of pneumococcus. Am. J. Hyg., 13:823, May 1931.

684. Joannides, M. Insufflation of compressed air in the treatment for pneumonia. Arch. Int. Med., 47:196, Feb. 1931.

685. Joannides, M., and Steinman, F. H. Mechanism of pneumonia. Arch. Int. Med., 47:24, Jan. 1931.

686. Johnston, J. M. Therapy in pneumococcus pneumonia: a critical review. Pennsylvania M. J., 38:67, Nov. 1934.

687. Jones, F. S. Effects of the intratracheal administration of foreign serum. J. Exper. Med., 40:63, July 1924.

688. Jones, F. S. Permeability of the lining of the lower respiratory tract for antibodies. J. Exper. Med., 40:73, July 1924.

689. Jones, F. S., and Little, R. B. Changes in bacterial volume as result of specific agglutination. J. Exper. Med., 57:721, May 1933.

690. Jones, F. S., and Little, R. B. Significance of changes in antigenic volume as result of specific agglutination. J. Exper. Med., 57:729, May 1933.

691. Jones, H. W. Report on a series of cases of acute lobar pneumonia. Therap. Gaz., 3rd series, 34:846, Dec. 1918.

692. Jones, L., and Fleisher, M. S. Serum sickness in rabbits. II. Precipitinogen

and precipitins in relation to appearance of reaction. J. Exper. Med., 55:79, Jan. 1932.

693. Jordan, E. O., and Sharp, W. B. Influenza studies. IV. Effect of vaccination against influenza and some other respiratory infections. J. Infect. Dis., 28:357, Apr. 1921.

694. Juergensen, T. Croupous pneumonia, catarrhal pneumonia, hypostatic processes in the lungs, and pneumonia from embolism. Translated by A. B. Ball, E. Frankel, and E. W. Schauffler. *In* Cyclopaedia of the practice of medicine, H. V. Ziemssen, *editor,* 5:3. New York, Wm. Wood & Co., 1875.

695. Julianelle, L. A. Biological classification of encapsulatus pneumoniae (Friedländer's bacillus). J. Exper. Med., 44:113, July 1926.

696. Julianelle, L. A. Immunological relationships of encapsulated and capsule-free strains of encapsulatus pneumoniae (Friedländer's bacillus). J. Exper. Med., 44:683, Nov. 1926.

697. Julianelle, L. A. Immunological relationships of cell constituents of encapsulatus pneumoniae (Friedländer's bacillus). J. Exper. Med., 44:735, Dec. 1926.

698. Julianelle, L. A. Reactions of rabbits to intracutaneous injections of pneumococci and their products. I. The antibody response. J. Exper. Med., 51:441, Mar. 1930.

699. Julianelle, L. A. Reactions of rabbits to intracutaneous injections of pneumococci and their products. II. Resistance to infection. J. Exper. Med., 51:449, Mar. 1930.

700. Julianelle, L. A., and Morris, M. C. Reactions of rabbits to intracutaneous injections of pneumococci and their products. VIII. Inter-relationships of hypersensitiveness to pneumococcus and streptococcus. J. Exper. Med., 55:867, June 1932.

701. Julianelle, L. A., and Reimann, H. A. Production of purpura by derivatives of pneumococcus. I. General considerations of the reaction. J. Exper. Med., 43:87, Jan. 1926.

702. Julianelle, L. A., and Rhoads, C. P. Reactions of rabbits to intracutaneous injections of pneumococci and their products. VII. Relation of hypersensitiveness to lesions in lungs of rabbits infected with pneumococci. J. Exper. Med., 55:797, May 1932.

703. Katz, L. N., Hamburger, W. W., and Rubinfeld, S. H. Observations on effects of oxygen therapy. II. Changes in the circulation and respiration. Am. J. M. Sc., 184:810, Dec. 1932.

704. Kaufmann, E. Pathology for students and practitioners, 1:388. Translated by S. P. Reimann. Philadelphia, P. Blakiston's Son & Co., 1929.

705. Keefer, C. S. Jaundice—its clinical significance. M. Clin. North America, 15:929, Jan. 1932.

706. Kelley, E. R., and Hamblen, A. D. Trend of pneumonia in Massachusetts. Pub. Health Rep., 40:1631, Aug. 7, 1925.

707. Kelley, W. H. Antipneumococcus properties of normal swine serum. J. Exper. Med., 55:877, June 1932.

708. Kelly, F. B. Observations on 6500 cases of lobar pneumonia at the Cook County Hospital, Chicago. J. Infect. Dis., 38:24, Jan. 1926.

709. Kelly, F. B., and Gussin, H. Studies on respiratory diseases. XVIII. Rela-

tive reliability of throat swabs for isolating causative pneumococcus type. J. Infect. Dis., 35:323, Oct. 1924.

710. Keresztúri, C., and Hauptmann, D. The serum treatment of pneumonia in children. J. Pediat., 4:331, Mar. 1934.

711. Kerr, W. J., and Lagen, J. B. Transmissibility of the common cold. Exposure of susceptible individuals under controlled conditions. Proc. Soc. Exper. Biol. & Med., 31:713, Mar. 1934.

712. Kessel, L. Clinical aspect of aputrid pulmonary necrosis. Arch. Int. Med., 45:401, Mar. 1930.

713. Kessel, L., and Hyman, H. T. The treatment of lobar pneumonia in a general hospital. J.A.M.A., 88:1703, May 28, 1927.

714. Kibbey, C. H. Relative pneumonia fatality among surface workers and miners. Study of 2603 cases of pneumonia and 238 deaths from tuberculosis in the experience of the Tennessee Coal, Iron and Railroad Company, 1925 to 1930, inclusive. Am. J. Pub. Health, 22:360, Apr. 1932.

715. Kibbey, C. H. Pneumonia and tuberculosis among industrial workers and their dependents. Am. J. Pub. Health, 27:555, June 1937.

716. King, D. S. Postoperative pulmonary complications. I. A statistical study based on two years' personal observation. Surg., Gynec. & Obst., 56:43, Jan. 1933.

717. King, D. S. Postoperative pulmonary complications. II. Carbon dioxide as a preventive in a controlled series. J.A.M.A., 100:21, Jan. 7, 1933.

718. King, D. S. Postoperative pulmonary complications: part played by anesthesia, as shown by a two-years' study at the Massachusetts General Hospital. Anesth. & Analg., 12:243, Nov.–Dec., 1933.

719. King, H. H. Analysis of Captain Malone's results in vaccination against pneumonia. Indian J.M. Research, 12:571, Jan. 1925.

720. Kirchner. Types of pneumococcus in the Dutch East Indies (foreign letter). J.A.M.A., 100:834, Mar. 18, 1933.

721. Kirkbride, M. B., Hendry, J. L., and Murdick, P. P. Concentration and standardization of Type I antipneumococcus serum. Am. J. Hyg., 23:187, Jan. 1936.

722. Kitagawa, K. J. On the mechanism of pneumococcic immunity (preliminary note). Proc. Soc. Exper. Biol. & Med., 12:213, May 1915.

723. Klemperer, G. Die Beziehungen verschiedener Bakteriengifte zur Immunisirung und Heilung. Ztschr. f. klin. Med., 20:165, 1892.

724. Klemperer, G., and Klemperer, F. Versuche über Immunisirung und Heilung bei der Pneumokokkeninfection. Berl. klin. Wchnschr., 28:833, Aug. 24, 1891.

725. Klemperer, G., and Klemperer, F. Versuche über Immunisirung und Heilung bei der Pneumokokkeninfection. Berl. klin. Wchnschr., 28:869, Aug. 31, 1891.

726. Kline, B. S. Experimental study of organization in lobar pneumonia. J. Exper. Med., 26:239, Aug. 1917.

727. Kline, B. S., and Meltzer, S. J. The effect of previous intravenous injection of pneumococci upon experimental lobar pneumonia produced by the method of intrabronchial insufflation. Proc. Soc. Exper. Biol. & Med., 12:185, May 1915.

728. Kline, B. S., and Winternitz, M. C. Studies upon experimental pneumonia

in rabbits. VII. The production of lobar pneumonia. J. Exper. Med., 21:304, Apr. 1915.
729. Kline, B. S., and Winternitz, M. C. Studies upon experimental pneumonia in rabbits. VIII. Intra-vitam staining in experimental pneumonia, and the circulation in the pneumonic lung. J. Exper. Med., 21:311, Apr. 1915.
730. Kneeland, Y., Jr. Studies on the common cold. III. The upper respiratory flora of infants. J. Exper. Med., 51:617, Apr. 1930.
731. Kneeland, Y., Jr. The protection afforded by vaccination against secondary invaders during colds in infancy. J. Exper. Med., 60:655, Nov. 1934.
732. Kneeland, Y., Jr., and Dawes, C. F. Studies on the common cold. V. The relationship of pathogenic bacteria to upper respiratory disease in infants. J. Exper. Med., 55:735, May 1932.
733. Koch, K. R. Prognostic value of repeated blood cultures in pneumococcus lobar pneumonia. Am. J. M. Sc., 184:364, Sept. 1932.
734. Kohl, C., and Reitzel, R. J. Type specificity in pneumonia and pneumococcic infections: a preliminary report. J.A.M.A., 106:1557, May 2, 1936.
735. Kolmer, J. A. Principles and practice of chemotherapy with special reference to the specific and general treatment of syphilis, p. 156. Philadelphia, W. B. Saunders Company, 1926.
736. Kolmer, J. A. Intracarotid method of treatment for meningitis with recoveries. J.A.M.A., 96:1358, Apr. 25, 1931.
737. Kolmer, J. A., and Rule, A. M. Oral immunization of rabbits against pneumococcus pneumonia and septicaemia. Proc. Soc. Exper. Biol. & Med., 30:107, Oct. 1932.
738. Kolmer, J. A., and Rule, A. M. Vaccination of monkeys against pneumococci with special reference to oral immunization. Proc. Soc. Exper. Biol. & Med., 31:243, Nov. 1933.
739. Kolmer, J. A., and Rule, A. M. Vaccination of rabbits against pneumococci with special reference to oral immunization. Proc. Soc. Exper. Biol. & Med., 31:245, Nov. 1933.
740. Kolmer, J. A., and Rule, A. M. Vaccination of rabbits against intradermal pneumococcus infection. Proc. Soc. Exper. Biol. & Med., 32:86, Oct. 1934.
741. Kolmer, J. A., and Rule, A. M. Chemotherapy of intradermal pneumococcus infection of rabbits. Effects of optochin and other quinine compounds. Proc. Soc. Exper. Biol. & Med., 32:89, Oct. 1934.
742. Kramár, E., and Gyüre, D. Untersuchungen über die Immunbiologie der Lungenentzündung. Erste Mitteilung. Einleitung. Pneumokokkentypen und Hautreaktion. Arch. f. Kinderh., 89:73, Dec. 13, 1929.
743. Kramár, E., and Gyüre, D. Untersuchungen über die Immunbiologie der Lungenentzündung. Dritte Mitteilung. Mechanismus und immunbiologische Bedeutung der Pneumokokkenhautprobe. Arch. f. Kinderh., 89:88, Dec. 13, 1929.
744. Kramár, E., and Gyüre, D. Untersuchungen über die Immunbiologie der Lungenentzündung. Vierte Mitteilung. Die experimentelle Pneumonie. Arch. f. Kinderh., 91:278, Oct. 21, 1930.
745. Kreidler, W. A. Treatment of pneumococcal infections in rabbits with sulfanilamide. Proc. Soc. Exper. Biol. & Med., 37:146, Oct. 1937.

746. Krumwiede, C., Jr., and Valentine, E. Determination of the type of pneumococcus in the sputum of lobar pneumonia. J.A.M.A., 70:513, Feb. 23, 1918.
747. Kubie, L. S., and Retan, G. M. Forced drainage of the cerebrospinal fluid: its experimental basis, the technic of clinical application, and the indications and contraindications. J.A.M.A., 101:354, July 29, 1933.
748. Kyes, P. Production of antibodies to pneumococci in an insusceptible host. J.A.M.A., 56:1878, June 24, 1911.
749. Kyes, P. The natural resistance of the pigeon to the pneumococcus. J. Infect. Dis., 18:277, Mar. 1916.
750. Kyes, P. Treatment of lobar pneumonia with an antipneumococcus serum. J. M. Research, 38:495, July 1918.
751. Kyes, P. Pneumococcus meningitis treated with immune chicken serum. Personal communication, Dec. 1932.
752. Kyes, P., and Carey, E. S. Elimination of serum shock. J. Immunol., 14:123, Aug. 1927.
753. Kyes, P., and Carey, E. S. Preparation of fibrinogen-free fowl serum. J. Immunol., 17:529, Dec. 1929.
754. Lacy, G. R., and Hartman, C. C. Specific reactions of the body fluids in pneumococcic infections. J. Immunol., 3:43, Jan. 1918.
755. Laënnec, R. T. H. A treatise on the diseases of the chest and on mediate auscultation, p. 210. Translated from the 3d French ed. by J. Forbes, with notes of Prof. Andral from the 4th ed. New York, S. S. & Wm. Wood, 1838.
756. Laënnec, R.-T.-H. Signs and symptoms of peripneumony: a treatise on the diseases of the chest and on mediate auscultation, p. 211. Translated by John Forbes. New York, Samuel E. Wood and Sons, 1930. *As seen in* Major, R. H., Classic Descriptions of Disease, p. 527. Springfield, Ill., Charles C. Thomas, 1932.
757. Lamar, R. V., and Meltzer, S. J. Experimental pneumonia by intrabronchial insufflation. J. Exper. Med., 15:133, Feb. 1912.
758. Lamb, F. H., and Brannin, E. B. Epidemic respiratory infection at Camp Cody, N. M. J.A.M.A., 72:1056, Apr. 12, 1919.
759. Lamb, W. L. Treatment of lobar pneumonia, with special reference to the use of nuclein and of vaccines. Edinburgh M. J., 36:593, Oct. 1929.
760. Lambert, A. Use of mixed stock vaccines in pneumonia. Tr. A. Am. Physicians, 41:225, 1926.
761. Lambert, A. Some effects of vaccines on antibodies in pneumonia. Tr. A. Am. Physicians, 48:73, 1933.
762. Lamson, R. W. Sudden death associated with the injection of foreign substances. J.A.M.A., 82:1091, Apr. 5, 1924.
763. Langley. Pneumonia types (editorial). M. Officer, 53:259, June 29, 1935.
764. Langley, G. J. Serum treatment of pneumonia. Brit. M. J., 2:1139, Dec. 19, 1931.
765. Langley, G. J. Some problems of lobar pneumonia. Lancet, 2:70, July 8, 1933.
766. Lauche, A. Über die lobäre Pneumonie der Neugeborenen. Ein Beitrag zum Studium der Beziehungen zwischen Entzündungsablauf und Immunitätslage. Ztschr. f. Geburtsh. u. Gynäk., 91:627, Sept. 1927.

767a. League of Nations. Report of permanent commission on biological standardization. Session held at Copenhagen from Aug. 28th to 30th, 1934. Quart. Bull. Health Organ., League of Nations, Special Number, p. 4, Jan. 1935.
767b. League of Nations, Health Organisation. Report on an investigation into the sanitary conditions in Persia. *See reference 517.*
768. League of Nations: Health Section of the Secretariat. Monthly epidemiological report. 8: R.E. 124, p. 120, Mar. 15, 1929; R.E. 129, p. 349, Aug. 15, 1929; 9: R.E. 135, p. 93, Feb. 15, 1930; R.E. 139, p. 273, June 15, 1930; 10: R.E. 147, p. 83, Feb. 15, 1931; R.E. 152, p. 291, July 15, 1931.
769. League of Nations: Health Section of the Secretariat. Monthly epidemiological report. 11: R.E. 159, p. 74, Feb. 15, 1932; 12: R.E. 166, p. 114, Mar.–Apr. 1933; 13: R.E. 173, p. 147, May–June 1934; 14: R.E. 179, p. 200, July–Sept. 1935.
770. League of Nations: Health Section of the Secretariat. Notes on vital statistics in Africa (continued). IV and V. Central, East, and South Africa. Epidemiol. Rep., League of Nations, 11:167, July–Aug. 1932.
771. League of Nations International Health Year-Book. 1927, 1928, and 1930.
772. Leake, C. D., Vickers, J. L., and Brown, T. K. Observations on blood reaction in experimental pneumonia. J. Exper. Med., 39:393, Mar. 1924.
773. Lejeune, E. Importance du pneumocoque dans la morbidité des troupes noires pendant la campagne d'Afrique 1915–1918. Conclusions pratiques à en déduire pour notre Congo. Ann. Soc. belge de méd. trop., 1:313, Dec. 1921.
774. Leopold, S. S. Pneumonia and empyema at Camp Dix: résumé of cases which occurred at base hospital during year 1918. New York M. J., 110: 578, Oct. 4, 1919.
775. Levi, M. Ricerche sui tipi di diplococco nella polmonite lobare. Policlinico (sez. med.), 40:38, Jan. 1933.
776. Levine, S. A. Medical aspects of pericarditis. New England J. Med., 208: 773, Apr. 13, 1933.
777. Levy, R. L. The size of the heart in pneumonia. A teleroentgenographic study, with observations on the effect of digitalis therapy. Arch. Int. Med., 32:359, Sept. 1923.
778. Lewis, J. H. Slow intravenous injection of antiserum to prevent acute anaphylactic shock. J.A.M.A., 72:329, Feb. 1, 1919.
779. Leys, D. Serum treatment of Type I lobar pneumonia. Lancet, 2:748, Sept. 30, 1933.
780. Li, K. H. Artificial pneumothorax treatment for lobar pneumonia. A report of six cases. Chinese M. J., 46:886, Sept. 1932.
781. Lichtenstein, H. Die Serumbehandlung der croupösen Pneumonie. Med. Klin., 25:1966, Dec. 20, 1929.
782. Lieberman, L. M., and Leopold, S. S. Therapeutic pneumothorax in experimental lobar pneumonia in dogs. Am. J. M. Sc., 187:315, Mar. 1934.
783. Lindau, A. Studies on varying response to pneumococcal infections, especially lobar pneumonia. Acta path. et microbiol. Scandinav., 10:1, 1933.
784. Lister, F. S. Specific serological reactions with pneumococci from different sources. Publ. South African Inst. Med. Res., 1(2), Dec. 1913.
785. Lister, F. S. An experimental study of prophylactic inoculation against

pneumococcal infection in the rabbit and in man. Publ. South African Inst. Med. Res., 1(8), Oct. 1916.

786. Lister, F. S. Prophylactic inoculation of man against pneumococcal infections, and more particularly against lobar pneumonia; including a report upon results of experimental inoculation, with a specific group vaccine, of native mine labourers employed upon the Premier (Diamond) Mine and Crown (Gold) Mines in the Transvaal and the De Beers (Diamond) Mines at Kimberley covering period from November 1, 1916 to October 31, 1917. Publ. South African Inst. Med. Res., 1(10), Nov. 1917.

787. Lister, S. Note on aetiology of epidemic influenza and secondary pneumonia. J.M.A. South Africa, 3:179, Apr. 13, 1929.

788. Lister, S., and Ordman, D. Epidemiology of pneumonia on the Witwatersrand goldfields and prevention of pneumonia and other allied acute respiratory diseases in native labourers in South Africa by means of vaccine. Publ. South African Inst. Med. Res., 7(37), Apr. 1935.

789. Litchfield, L. Pneumococcus meningitis. J.A.M.A., 72:1345, May 10, 1919.

790. Livingstone, D. Missionary travels and researches in South Africa; including a sketch of sixteen years' residence in the interior of Africa, and a journey from the Cape of Good Hope to Loanda on the west coast; thence across the continent, down the river Zambesi, to the eastern ocean, p. 143. New York, Harper & Bros., 1858.

791. Lobar pneumonia serum (special article). Conn. Health Bulletin (Connecticut State Department of Health), 52:4, Jan. 1938.

792. Locke, A. Lack of fitness as predisposing factor in infections of the type encountered in pneumonia and in common cold. J. Infect. Dis., 60:106, Jan.–Feb. 1937.

793. Locke, E. A. Treatment of Type I pneumococcus lobar pneumonia with specific serum. J.A.M.A., 80:1507, May 26, 1923.

794. Locke, E. A. The serologic treatment of lobar pneumonia. Boston M. & S. J., 190:196, Feb. 7, 1924.

795. Locke, E. A. Acute empyema. New England J. Med., 203:391, Aug. 28, 1930.

796. Locke, E. A. Prophylaxis and treatment of lobar pneumonia. Commonhealth (Massachusetts Department of Public Health), 18:141, July–Aug.–Sept. 1931.

797. Locke, E. A., Thomas, H. M., and O'Hara, D. Acute respiratory infections at the Boston City Hospital from the Pneumonia Service. Boston M. & S. J., 183:480, Oct. 21, 1920.

798. Loeschcke, H. Untersuchungen über die kruppöse Pneumonie. Beitr. z. path. Anat. u. z. allg. Path., 86:201, Jan. 3, 1931.

799. Logan, W. R., and Smeall, J. T. Direct method of typing pneumococci. Brit. M. J., 1:188, Jan. 30, 1932.

800. Lombard, H. L., and Doering, C. R. Influenza in Massachusetts. Boston M. & S. J., 195:405, Aug. 26, 1926.

801. Longcope, W. T. Serum disease, protein intoxications, urticaria, and angioneurotic edema. *In* Nelson's Loose-Leaf Living Medicine, 2:631, New York, Thomas Nelson & Sons, 1920–28.

802. Longcope, W. T. Protein hypersensitiveness and its importance in the etiology of disease. J.A.M.A., 77:1535, Nov. 12, 1921.
803. Longcope, W. T., and Fox, W. W. Comparative study of pneumococci and streptococci from mouths of healthy individuals and from pathological conditions. J. Exper. Med., 7:430, Aug. 1905.
804. Lord, F. T. Personal communication, 1935.
805. Lord, F. T. Factors influencing recovery and resolution in lobar pneumonia. With special reference to the chemistry of the pneumonic exudate. J.A.M.A., 73:1420, Nov. 8, 1919.
806. Lord, F. T. The bearing of the evolution of pneumonic exudate on local chemical factors influencing recovery and resolution in lobar pneumonia. Tr. A. Am. Physicians, 36:61, 1921.
807. Lord, F. T. Diseases of the bronchi, lungs and pleura, p. 281. 2nd Edition, Philadelphia and New York, Lea and Febiger, 1925.
808. Lord, F. T. Diagnosis of lobar pneumonia. Commonhealth (Massachusetts Department of Public Health), 18:134, July–Aug.–Sept. 1931.
809. Lord, F. T. Immunity factors in recovery from lobar pneumonia and results of specific treatment in Type I pneumococcus pneumonia. New England J. Med., 205:854, Oct. 29, 1931.
810. Lord, F. T. Pneumococcus endocarditis. New England J. Med., 207:767, Nov. 3, 1932.
811. Lord, F. T. Pulmonary collapse. *In* The Cyclopedia of Medicine, Geo. M. Piersol, *editor,* 8:364. Philadelphia, F. A. Davis Co., 1933.
812. Lord, F. T. Certain aspects of the common cold. M. Clin. North America, 19:1499, Mar. 1936.
813. Lord, F. T., and Heffron, R. Lobar pneumonia and serum therapy: with special reference to the Massachusetts Pneumonia Study. New York, The Commonwealth Fund, 1936, 91 p.
814. Lord, F. T., and Heffron, R. Pneumonia and serum therapy. Revised edition of Lobar pneumonia and serum therapy. New York, The Commonwealth Fund, 1938, 148 p.
815. Lord, F. T., and Nesche, G. E. Antibody and agglutinin in pneumococcus pneumonia. J. Exper. Med., 50:449, Oct. 1929.
816. Lord, F. T., and Nye, R. N. Studies on pneumococcus. I. Acid deathpoint of the pneumococcus. J. Exper. Med., 35:685, May 1922.
817. Lord, F. T., and Nye, R. N. Studies on pneumococcus. II. Dissolution of pneumococci at varying H-ion concentrations. Effect of temperature, previous killing of the organisms, and fresh human serum on the phenomenon. Behavior of other organisms. J. Exper. Med., 35:689, May 1922.
818. Lord, F. T., and Nye, R. N. Studies on pneumococcus. III. Dissolution of pneumococci in pneumonic cellular material at varying H-ion concentrations. Resistance of certain other organisms to dissolution. J. Exper. Med., 35:699, May 1922.
819. Lord, F. T., and Nye, R. N. Studies on pneumococcus. IV. Effect of bile at varying H-ion concentrations on dissolution of pneumococci. J. Exper. Med., 35:703, May 1922.
820. Lord, F. T., and Persons, E. L. Certain aspects of mouse protection tests

for antibody in pneumococcus pneumonia. J. Exper. Med., 53:151, Feb. 1931.

821. Lyon, A. B. Bacteriologic studies of one hundred and sixty-five cases of pneumonia and post pneumonia empyema in infants and children. Am. J. Dis. Child., 23:72, Jan. 1922.

822. Lyons, C. Immunotransfusion and antitoxin therapy in hemolytic streptococcus infections. J.A.M.A., 105:1972, Dec. 14, 1935.

823. Macaulay, T. S. Treatment of pneumonia. Malayan M. J., 1:7, Jan. 1926.

824. MacCallum, W. G. Pathology of epidemic streptococcal bronchopneumonia in army camps. J.A.M.A., 71:704, Aug. 31, 1918.

825. MacCallum, W. G. Pathology of pneumonia following influenza. J.A.M.A., 72:720, Mar. 8, 1919.

826. MacCallum, W. G. Text-book of pathology, p. 542. 3rd Edition, Philadelphia, W. B. Saunders Co., 1925.

827. M'Cartney, J. E. The pathogenesis of primary pneumococcal peritonitis. J. Path. & Bact., 26:507, Oct. 1923.

828. McClellan, J. H. Antipneumococcus serum (Kyes) in the treatment of lobar pneumonia. J.A.M.A., 72:1884, June 28, 1919.

829. McClelland, J. E. Determination of type and serum treatment in pneumococcus infections. Cleveland M. J., 17:226, Apr. 1918.

830. MacCordick, A. H. A statistical review of 525 cases of lobar pneumonia. Canad. M.A.J., 25:704, Dec. 1931.

831. McCoy, G. W., Hasseltine, H. E., Wadsworth, A., and Kirkbride, M. B. A report on pneumococcus inoculation in New York State institutions. J.A.M.A., 79:1128, Sept. 30, 1922.

832. McCrae, T. Empyema in acute lobar pneumonia. Johns Hopkins Hosp. Rep., 15:167, 1910.

833. McCrae, T. Delayed resolution in lobar pneumonia. Johns Hopkins Hosp. Rep., 15:277, 1910.

834. McDaniels, H. E. Leucocyte counts and bacteriemia studies in rats orally immunized against pneumococci. Proc. Soc. Exper. Biol. & Med., 29:897, Apr. 1932.

835. McDowell, C. The effect of different temperatures and humidities on the resistance of rats to a pneumococcus infection. Am. J. Hyg., 3:521, Sept. 1923.

836. McEnery, E. T., and Brennermann, J. Aspiration in treatment of empyema in children with critical evaluation based on 94 cases. Am. J. Dis. Child., 44:742, Oct. 1932.

837. Macgregor, A. S. M. Some epidemiological features of the pneumococcus and its types. Pub. Health, 46:117, Jan. 1933.

838. McGuire, G., Valentine, E., Whitney, E., and Falk, K. G. Studies on antibodies. IV. The carbohydrate content as criterion of the suitability of broth for culture of pneumococci. J. Bact., 23:223, Mar. 1932.

839. McGuire, L. W. Serum treatment of lobar pneumonia. Boston M. & S. J., 186:389, Mar. 23, 1922.

840. McGuire, L. W., and Redden, W. R. Treatment of influenzal pneumonia by the use of convalescent human serum; second report. J.A.M.A., 72:709, Mar. 8, 1919.

841. Mackenzie, G. M. Significance of anaphylaxis in pneumococcus immunity. J. Exper. Med., 41:53, Jan. 1925.
842. Mackenzie, G. M., and Hanger, F. M. Serum disease and serum accidents. J.A.M.A., 94:260, Jan. 25, 1930.
843. Mackenzie, G. M., and Woo, S. T. Production and significance of cutaneous allergy to pneumococcus protein. J. Exper. Med., 41:65, Jan. 1925.
844. McLachlan, D. G. S. Immunological types of pneumococcus in their relation to prevention and treatment of pneumococcal infections. J. Roy. San. Inst., 46:112, Sept. 1925.
845. Maclachlan, W. W. G. Problem of chemo-therapy in pneumonia. Scient. Monthly, 45:105, Aug. 1937.
846. Maclachlan, W. W. G., Kastlin, G. J., and Lynch, R. Use of dextrose in pneumonia. Am. J. M. Sc., 179:93, Jan. 1930.
847. Maclachlan, W. W. G., Kastlin, G. J., and Lynch, R. Further observations on use of dextrose in pneumonia. Am. J. M. Sc., 184:511, Oct. 1932.
848. Maclachlan, W. W. G., Permar, H. H., Johnston, J. M., and Kenney, J. R. Some effects of quinin derivatives in experimental pneumococcus studies. Am. J. M. Sc., 188:699, Nov. 1934.
849. McLean, C. C. Incidence of respiratory infections during first five years of life. Arch. Pediat., 49:279, May 1932.
850. McLean, C. C. Influence of age factor on the frequency and monthly seasonal incidence of respiratory infections. J. Pediat., 1:729, Dec. 1932.
851. McMeans, J. W. Incidence of pneumococcus types in pneumonia in Pittsburgh. Atlantic M. J. 30:499, May 1927.
852. Macnalty, A. Memorandum on pneumonia. M. Officer, 54:167, Oct. 19, 1935.
853. McSwan, D. M. Foci of pulmonary necrosis in lobar pneumonia. Malayan M. J., 2:56, June 1927.
854. Malloch, A. Study of pneumonias and types of pneumococci. Quart. J. Med., 15:103, Jan. 1922.
855. Mallory, F. B. Principles of pathologic histology, p. 473. Philadelphia & London, W. B. Saunders Co., 1914.
856. Mallory, T. B. Rheumatic pneumonia. Case records of Massachusetts General Hospital: case 21392. New England J. Med., 213:626, Sept. 26, 1935.
857. Malone, R. H. Note on the types of pneumococcus found in the Punjab and Northwest Frontier Province of India. Indian J. M. Research, 11:947, Jan. 1924.
858. Malone, R. H. Note on a series of cases of pneumonia treated with pneumococcus vaccine. Indian J. M. Research, 12:105, July 1924.
859. Malone, R. H. Report on prophylactic inoculation of Indian troops in Baluchistan district against pneumonia. Indian J. M. Research, 12:565, Jan. 1925.
860. Marginesu, P., and Corda, L. Studi sui Pneumococchi. Frequenza ed importanza dei vari tipi di Pneumococco. Policlinico (sez. med.), 30:610, Dec. 1923.
861. Marshall, E. K., Jr., Emerson, K., Jr., and Cutting, W. C. Para-aminobenzenesulfonamide; absorption and excretion: method of determination in urine and blood. J.A.M.A., 108:953, Mar. 20, 1937.

862. Marvin, H. M., and Soifer, J. D. The value of camphor in oil as a cardiac stimulant. J.A.M.A., 83:94, July 12, 1924.

863. Mason, J. M. Acute empyema in children. J.A.M.A., 105:1114, Oct. 5, 1935.

864. Massachusetts Commissioner of Public Health and the Public Health Council. Report for the year ending November 30, 1936.

865. Massachusetts Department of Public Health. Annual reports for the years 1921–1930.

866. Massachusetts Department of Public Health: Division of Communicable Diseases. Reported cases of lobar pneumonia (unpublished data).

867. Massachusetts: Office of the Secretary, Division of Vital Statistics. Annual reports on the vital statistics of Massachusetts: births, marriages, divorces and deaths, 1920–1930.

868. Massachusetts pneumonia campaign (editorial). New England J. Med., 214:489, Mar. 5, 1936.

869. Massachusetts Pneumonia Study. Data obtained during the Pneumonia Study and Service, 1931–1935, in Massachusetts. *See references 104, 611, 616, 75, 614, 77, 86, 76, 813, 615, 814, and 1417.*

870. Massachusetts Pneumonia Study. 1931 to 1935 inclusive. Unpublished observations. All types, I to XXXII, have been obtained from patients with pneumonia. *For details of Study see reference 869.*

871. Massachusetts Pneumonia Study: Epidemiologic Investigation. Investigation carried out in conjunction with the Pneumonia Study. *See references 869 and 615.*

872. Mathers, G. Varieties of pneumococci causing lobar pneumonia, with especial reference to their biologic differences. J. Infect. Dis., 17:514, Nov. 1915.

873. Matsuda, S. I. Comparative studies in bactericidal action of ethylapoquine and ethylhydrocupreine (optochin) on type strains of pneumococci; in vivo experiments. Jap. J. M. Sc. Tr., IV, Pharmacology, 8:30*, Aug., 1934.

874. Maynard, G. D. Enquiry into the etiology, manifestations, and prevention of pneumonia amongst natives on the Rand, recruited from "tropical areas." Publ. South African Inst. Med. Res., 1 (1), Nov. 1913.

875. Means, J. H., and Barach, A. L. Remarks upon the symptomatic treatment of pneumonia. Tr. A. Am. Physicians, 36:39, 1921.

876. Means, J. H., and Barach, A. L. Symptomatic treatment of pneumonia. J.A.M.A., 77:1217, Oct. 15, 1921.

877. Means, J. H., Bock, A. V., and Woodwell, M. N. Studies of the acid-base equilibrium in disease from the point of view of blood-gases. J. Exper. Med., 33:201, Feb. 1921.

878. Means, J. H., Newburgh, L. H., and Porter, W. T. On the state of the respiratory mechanism in pneumonia. Boston M. & S. J., 173:742, Nov. 11, 1915.

879. Medalia, L. S., and Schiff, N. S. Lobar pneumonia at a base hospital. J.A.M.A., 71:1821, Nov. 30, 1918.

880. Mehlman, J., and Seegal, B. C. Comparison of the sensitizing and therapeutic effect of rabbit and horse antipneumococcus Type I serums in albino mice. J. Immunol., 27:81, July 1934.

881. Mendel, F. Die Behandlung der Pneumonie mit Optochin basicum und Milchdiät. Deutsche med. Wchnschr., 42:537, May 4, 1916.
882. Menetrier, M. P. Relevé statistique de 400 autopsies de pneumonie. Bull. et mém. Soc. méd. d. hôp. de Paris, 3rd series, 43:679, July 10, 1919.
883. Menkin, V. Studies on inflammation. IV. Fixation of foreign protein at site of inflammation. J. Exper. Med., 52:201, Aug. 1930.
884. Mennes, F. Das Antipneumokokken-Serum und der Mechanismus der Immunität des Kaninchens gegen den Pneumococcus. Ztschr. f. Hyg. u. Infektionskr., 25:413, 1897.
885. Menten, M. L., Bailey, S. F., and DeBone, F. M. Pneumonia in children. J. Infect. Dis., 51:254, Sept. 1932.
886. Metropolitan Life Insurance Company. The two pneumonia belts. Statistical Bull., 15:2, Dec. 1934.
887. Mexico: Departmento de Salubridad Pública. Boletin del Instituto de Hygiene. Nos. 3 and 4, 1926; Nos. 1 and 3, 1927; and Nos. 1 and 2, 1928; No. 5, 1929.
888. Meyer, H. Weitere Untersuchungen über die Bedeutung des Reticulo-Endothels für die Immunität. Ztschr. f. Hyg. u. Infektionskr., 106:124, Mar. 1926.
889. Meyers, H. R. A contribution to the study of the etiology of serum disease. J. Immunol., 22:83, Feb. 1932.
890. Middleton, R., and Gibbon, J. H., Jr. Prognostic value of initial leukocyte and differential count in lobar pneumonia. Am. J. M. Sc., 180:31, July 1930.
891. Miller, H., Piness, G., Feingold, B. F., and Friedman, T. B. Allergic bronchopneumonia. J. Pediat., 7:768, Dec. 1935.
892. Miller, J. L., and Lusk, F. B. Epidemic of streptococcus pneumonia and empyema at Camp Dodge, Iowa. J.A.M.A., 71:702, Aug. 31, 1918.
893. Miller, W. S. Structure of the lung. J. Morphol., 8:165, Apr. 1893.
894. Miller, W. S. Studies on tuberculous infection. II. Description of plastic models (reconstructions) of a conglomerate tubercle and the surrounding structures in a human lung. Am. Rev. Tuberc., 3:65, Apr. 1919.
895. Miller, W. S. The lung. Springfield, Ill., Charles C. Thomas, 1937, 209 p.
896. Millett, J. Intrathecal use of prontosil soluble; report of case of Type III pneumococcus meningitis and septicemia treated with prontosil soluble, with complete autopsy report. J.A.M.A., 109:2138, Dec. 25, 1937.
897. Mills, E. S. Serum treatment of pneumonia. Canad. M.A.J., 22:488, Apr. 1930.
898. Mills, K. C., Shibley, G. S., and Dochez, A. R. Studies in the common cold. II. Study of certain gram-negative filter-passing anaerobes of the upper respiratory tract. J. Exper. Med., 47:193, Feb. 1928.
899. Mitchell, A. G. The types of pneumococci in infants and children. Pennsylvania M. J., 20:343, Feb. 1917.
900. Monserrat, C. Types of pneumococcus in the Philippines: preliminary report. J. Philippine Islands M. A., 10:424, Oct. 1930.
901. Moor, H. D., and Brown, I. L. The occurrence of diplococcus pneumoniae in infections of the urinary tract. J.A.M.A., 108:1594, May 8, 1937.
902. Moore, H. F. Note on types of pneumococci causing acute lobar pneumonia in Dublin. Irish J. M. Sc., Ser. 5 (13):1, Mar. 1923.

903. Moore, H. F., and Chesney, A. M. A study of ethylhydrocuprein (optochin) in the treatment of acute lobar pneumonia. Arch. Int. Med., 19: 611, Apr. 1917.
904. Moore, H. F., and Chesney, A. M. A further study of ethylhydrocuprein (optochin) in the treatment of acute lobar pneumonia. Arch. Int. Med., 21:659, May 1918.
905. Moorman, L. J. Artificial pneumothorax in the treatment of pneumonia. South. M. J., 27:233, Mar. 1934.
906. Morgan, H. J. Correlation of certain phenomena occurring during the growth of pneumococcus. J. Exper. Med., 39:565, Apr. 1924.
907. Morgan, H. J., and Avery, O. T. Growth-inhibitory substances in pneumococcus cultures. J. Exper. Med., 39:335, Mar. 1924.
908. Morgan, H. J., and Neill, J. M. Methemoglobin formation by sterile culture filtrates of pneumococcus. J. Exper. Med., 40:269, Aug. 1924.
909. Morgan, W. T. J., and Petrie, G. F. Titration of antipneumococcus serum (Type I) in mice. Brit. J. Exper. Path., 14:323, Oct. 1933.
910. Morgenroth, J., and Levy, R. Chemotherapie der Pneumokokkeninfektion. Berl. klin. Wchnschr., 48:1560, Aug. 21, 1911.
911. Mosny, E. Recherches expérimentales sur la vaccination contre l'infection pneumonique et sur sa guérison. Arch. d. méd. expér. et d'anat. path., 4:195, 1892.
912. Müller, E. F. Über das Auftreten und die Bedeutung von bactericiden Schutzstoffen des Blutes im Verlauf der croupösen Pneumonie. Ztschr. f. Hyg. u. Infektionskr., 97:26, Nov. 1922.
913. Muller, G. P. Mortality of operation for acute empyema. J. Thoracic Surg., 1:15, Oct. 1931.
914. Muller, G. P., Overholt, R. H., and Pendergrass, E. P. Post-operative pulmonary hypoventilation. Arch. Surg., 19:1322, Dec. 1929.
915. Müller, O. Zur Behandlung der Lungenentzündung. Deutsche mil.-ärztl. Ztschr., 29:353, July 1900.
916. Murphy, R. V. Collosol iodine in the treatment of the pneumonias. Irish J. M. Sc., Ser. 6:563, Oct. 1934.
917. Musser, J. H. The treatment of pneumococcic infection of the lung, or croupous pneumonia. Internat. Clin., 13th series, 4:13, 1904.
918. Musser, J. H., and Norris, G. W. Lobar pneumonia. *In* Modern Medicine: its theory and practice in original contributions by American and foreign authors, Wm. Osler, *editor,* 2:537. Philadelphia and New York, Lea Brothers & Co., 1907.
919. Mutual antagonism of bacterial variants (current comment). J.A.M.A., 103:494, Aug. 18, 1934.
920. Myers, J. A. Artificial pneumothorax. J.A.M.A., 103:1299, Oct. 27, 1934.
921. Naish, A. E. The rheumatic lung. Lancet, 2:10, July 7, 1928.
922. Nakajima, H. Experimental studies on pathogenesis and resolution of pneumococcus pneumonia in rabbits. Scient. Rep. Gov. Inst. Infect. Dis. (Tokyo), 5:1, 1926.
923. Nakajima, H. Experimental studies on the mechanism of development of pneumonia by pneumococcus residue substances. Japan. J. Exp. Med., 14:239, June 20, 1936.

924. Napier, L. E., and Dharmendra. Incidence of pneumococcal types in pneumonia in Assam. Indian M. Gaz., 70:181, Apr. 1935.
925. Neale, A. V. The kidneys in pneumococcal infections. Brit. M. J., 2:891, Nov. 17, 1928.
926. Nedzel, A. J. Exposure to cold as a factor in the etiology of a lobar pneumonia. Illinois M. J., 68:340, Oct. 1935.
927. Neill, J. M., and Avery, O. T. Studies on oxidation and reduction by pneumococcus. V. Destruction of oxyhemoglobin by sterile extracts of pneumococcus. J. Exper. Med., 39:757, May 1924.
928. Neill, J. M., and Avery, O. T. Studies on oxidation and reduction by pneumococcus. VI. Oxidation of enzymes in sterile extracts of pneumococcus. J. Exper. Med., 40:405, Oct. 1924.
929. Neill, J. M., and Avery, O. T. Studies on oxidation and reduction by pneumococcus. VII. Enzyme activity of sterile filtrates of aerobic and anaerobic cultures of pneumococcus. J. Exper. Med., 40:423, Oct. 1924.
930. Nemir, R. L. Treatment of pneumonia in infants and children with antipneumococcus serum. J. Pediat., 3:827, Dec. 1933.
931. Nemir, R. L., Andrews, E. T., and Vinograd, J. Pneumonia in infants and children; bacteriologic study with special reference to clinical significance. Am. J. Dis. Child., 51:1277, June 1936.
932. Neufeld, F. Ueber die Agglutination der Pneumokokken und über die Theorieen der Agglutination. Ztschr. f. Hyg. u. Infektionskr., 40:54, 1902.
933. Neufeld, F., and Etinger-Tulczynska, R. Nasale Pneumokokkeninfektionen und Pneumokokkenkeimträger im Tierversuch. Ztschr. f. Hyg. u. Infektionskr., 112:492, May 1931.
934. Neufeld, F., and Etinger-Tulczynska, R. Versuche einer spezifischen Behandlung von Pneumokokken-Keimträgern. Ztschr. f. Immunitätsforsch. u. exper. Therap., 74:160, Mar. 1932.
935. Neufeld, F., and Etinger-Tulczynska, R. Untersuchungen über die Pneumokokkenseuche des Meerschweinchens. Ztschr. f. Hyg. u. Infektionskr., 114:324, Aug. 1932.
936. Neufeld, F., and Händel. Ueber Herstellung und Prüfung von Antipneumokokkenserum und über die Aussichten einer spezifischen Behandlung der Pneumonie. Ztschr. f. Immunitätsforsch. u. exper. Therap., 3:159, July 1909.
937. Neufeld, F., and Händel. Ueber die Entstehung der Krisis bei der Pneumonie und über die Wirkung des Pneumokokkenimmunserums. Arb. a. d. k. Gsndhtsamte., 34:166, June 1910.
938. Neufeld, F., and Händel. Weitere Untersuchungen über Pneumokokken-Heilsera. III. Mitteilung. Über Vorkommen und Bedeutung atypischer Varietäten des Pneumokokkus. Arb. a. d. k. Gsndhtsamte., 34:293, Aug. 1910.
939. Neufeld, F., and Meyer, H. Über die Bedeutung des Retikulo-Endothels für die Immunität. Ztschr. f. Hyg. u. Infektionskr., 103:595, Sept. 1924.
940. Neufeld, F., and Rimpau, W. Ueber die Antikörper des Streptokokken- und Pneumokokken-immunserums. Deutsche med. Wchnschr., 30:1458, Sept. 29, 1904.

941. Neufeld, F., and Rimpau, W. Weitere Mittheilungen über die Immunität gegen Streptokokken und Pneumokokken. Ztschr. f. Hyg. u. Infektionskr., 51:283, Sept. 1905.
942. Neufeld and Ungermann. Ueber experimentell erzeugte Pneumonien und ihre Beeinflussung durch Antipneumokokkenserum. Centralbl. f. Bakt. 1 Abt. Ref. Beilage, 54:71,* Aug. 22, 1912.
943. New Hampshire State Board of Health. Announcement regarding availability of pneumonia serums. New England J. Med., 218:198, Jan. 27, 1938. *See also 1171.*
944. New York City Department of Health. Pneumonia services available to the physician from the New York City Department of Health. Health Examiner (New York Academy of Medicine), 5:19, Mar. 1936.
945. New York State Department of Health. Handbook on the nursing care of pneumonia. Circular 19, issued by Bureau of Pneumonia Control, Division of Communicable Diseases and Division of Public Health Nursing, 1936, 35 p. *Also in* New York State J. Med., 36:1989, Dec. 15, 1936.
946. New York State Department of Health. Clinical aspects of pneumococcus pneumonia. Circular 20, issued by Bureau of Pneumonia Control, Division of Communicable Diseases, 1936. 15 p. *Also in* New York State J. Med., 37:80, Jan. 1, 1937.
947. New York State Department of Health. Additional sera for diagnosis and treatment of pneumonia distributed by State Laboratory (note). Health News (New York State Department of Health), 14:185, Nov. 15, 1937.
948. Newburgh, L. H., Means, J. H., and Porter, W. T. A second statement regarding the respiratory mechanism in pneumonia. Boston M. & S. J., 174:464, Mar. 30, 1916.
949. Newburgh, L. H., Means, J. H., and Porter, W. T. Respiratory mechanism in pneumonia. J. Exper. Med., 24:583, Nov. 1916.
950. Newburgh, L. H., and Porter, W. T. Heart muscle in pneumonia. J. Exper. Med., 22:123, Aug. 1915.
951. Nichol, E. S. Rheumatic fever and lobar pneumonia: notes on occurrence in southern Florida. J. Florida M. A., 17:366, Feb. 1931.
952. Nichols, H. J. Lobar pneumonia problem in the army from viewpoint of the recent differentiation of types of pneumococci. Mil. Surgeon, 41:149, Aug. 1917.
953. Niles, W. L., and Wyckoff, J. Studies concerning digitalis therapy in lobar pneumonia. Am. J. M. Sc., 180:348, Sept. 1930.
954. Nishikawa, N. Study on the history of bacteria artificially introduced into body and factors of infection. IV. Effect of cooling of body on pneumonias experimentally produced by diplococcus pneumoniae. J. Orient. Med., 22:63, Apr. 1935.
955. Nobécourt, P., and Mathieu, R. Le purpura dans les pneumococcies des nourrissons. Arch. de Méd. des Enfants, 23:689, Dec. 1920.
956. Nobécourt, P., and Paraf, J. Étude des pneumocoques isolés dans une crèche d'hôpital. Bull. et mém. Soc. méd. d. hôp. de Paris, 3rd series, 43:687, July 10, 1919.
957. Noble, A. A rapid method for the macroscopic agglutination test. J. Bact., 14:287, Nov. 1927.

958. Noble, J. F., and Kibler, F. E. Heterophile pneumococcic serum in therapy of lobar pneumonia. Minnesota Med., 19:205, Apr. 1936.
959. Noble, W. C., Jr., and Brainard, D. H. Studies of acute respiratory infections. IV. Filter-passing anaerobic bacteria from cases of epidemic influenza in New York City 1928–1929. Am. J. Hyg., 20:181, July 1934.
960. Noble, W. C., Jr., and Brainard, D. H. A note on the suggested etiological relationship of certain strains of green streptococci to epidemic influenza. Am. J. Hyg., 20:191, July 1934.
961. Norris, G. W., and Landis, H. R. M. Diseases of the chest and the principles of physical diagnosis, p. 460. 4th Edition, Philadelphia and London, W. B. Saunders Co., 1931.
962. Nye, R. N. Studies on the pneumonic exudate. V. The relation of pneumonic lung protease activity to hydrogen ion concentration, and a consideration of the origin of the enzyme. J. Exper. Med., 35:153, Feb. 1922.
963. Nye, R. N., and Harris, A. H., 2nd. Viable pneumococci and pneumococcic specific soluble substance in lungs from cases of lobar pneumonia. Am. J. Path., 13:749, Sept. 1937.
964. Odell, H. R. Observations on the standardization of antipneumococcus serum by the protection test. J. Immunol., 18:73, Jan. 1930.
965. O'Keefe, E. S. Analysis of three hundred cases of asthma in children. New England J. Med., 214:62, Jan. 9, 1936.
966. Olcott, C. T. Pneumonia due to Friedländer's bacillus. Arch. Path., 16: 471, Oct. 1933.
967. Operation in pneumococcal peritonitis (annotations). Lancet, 1:1072, May 19, 1934.
968. Opie, E. L. Enzymes and anti-enzymes of inflammatory exudates. J. Exper. Med., 7:316, June 1905.
969. Opie, E. L., Blake, F. G., Small, J. C., and Rivers, T. M. Epidemic respiratory disease: the pneumonias and other infections of the respiratory tract accompanying influenza and measles. St. Louis, C. V. Mosby Co., 1921, 402 p.
970. Ordman, D. Pneumonia in the native mine workers of the Witwatersrand goldfields. A bacteriological and epidemiological study. J.M.A. South Africa, 5:108, Feb. 28, 1931.
971. Ordman, D. Pneumonia in the native mine labourers of the Northern Rhodesia copperfields with an account of an experiment in pneumonia prophylaxis by means of a vaccine on the Roan Antelope Mine. Publ. South African Inst. Med. Res., 7 (37), Apr. 1935.
972. Ordman, D. Some aspects of the local application of recent work in experimental medicine: (a) cerebrospinal meningitis, (b) pneumonia, (c) influenza, (d) typhoid fever, (e) typhus fever. Proceedings of the Transvaal Mine Medical Officers' Association, 15:77, Mar. 1936.
973. Orenstein, A. J. Vaccine prophylaxis in pneumonia. A review of fourteen years' experience with inoculation of native mine workers on the Witwatersrand against pneumonia. J.M.A. South Africa, 5:339, June 13, 1931.
974. Orenstein, A. J. Vitamin A in treatment of pneumonia. South African M. J., 6:685, Nov. 12, 1932.

975. Osgood, E. E. Culture of human marrow: studies on the mode of action of sulfanilamide. J.A.M.A., 110:349, Jan. 29, 1938.
976. Osler, W. The principles and practice of medicine, p. 81. 10th Edition, revised by T. McCrae. New York, D. Appleton & Co., 1926.
977. Palmer, R. S. Oxygen therapy in the treatment of pneumonia and postoperative pulmonary complications. New England J. Med., 200:330, Feb. 14, 1929.
978. Palmer, W. W. Acidosis and acid excretion in pneumonia. J. Exper. Med., 26:495, Oct. 1917.
979. Panama Canal Health Department. Annual report for 1929, by J. F. Siler.
980. Panama Canal Health Department. Annual report for 1934, by O. G. Brown.
981. Pane, N. Ueber die Heilkraft des aus verschiedenen immunisierten Tieren gewonnenen antipneumonishen Serums. Zentralbl. f. Bakt. 1 Abt. Orig., 21:664, May 29, 1897.
982. Pappenheimer, A. M., Jr., and Enders, J. F. Specific carbohydrate of Type I pneumococcus. Proc. Soc. Exper. Biol. & Med., 31:37, Oct. 1933.
983. Parish, H. J. Titration of antipneumococcus serum. J. Path. & Bact., 33: 729, July 1930.
984. Park, F. E. Treatment of influenza by an apparently specific method. M. Rec., 97:66, Jan. 10, 1920.
985. Park, J. H., Jr., and Chickering, H. T. Type I pneumococcus lobar pneumonia among Porto Rican laborers at Camp Jackson, South Carolina. J.A.M.A., 73:183, July 19, 1919.
986. Park, W. H. Deleterious effects from serum injections. Am. J. Pub. Health, 18:355, Mar. 1928.
987. Park, W. H. Types of pneumococci in adults and children and their significance (Harben Lectures, 1930. Pneumonia, Lecture I). J. State Med., 38:621, Nov. 1930.
988. Park, W. H. Epidemic of pneumonia and colds caused by pneumococcus. Pneumococcus vaccine as a prophylactic. Refining pneumococcus antiserum (Harben Lectures, 1930. Pneumonia, Lecture II). J. State Med., 39:3, Jan. 1931.
989. Park, W. H. Use of pneumococcus vaccine in the treatment of lobar pneumonia (Harben Lectures, 1930. Pneumonia, Lecture III). J. State Med., 39:125, Mar. 1931.
990. Park, W. H. Use of pneumococcus vaccine in the treatment of lobar pneumonia (Harben Lectures, 1930. Pneumonia, Lecture III). J. State Med., 39:187, Apr. 1931.
991. Park, W. H., Bullowa, J. G. M., and Rosenblüth, M. B. Treatment of lobar pneumonia with refined specific antibacterial serum. J.A.M.A., 91: 1503, Nov. 17, 1928.
992. Park, W. H., and Cooper, G. The possibility of rendering the blood of cases of Types I and II lobar pneumonia antibacterial by injections of antibody solution. Tr. Sect. Path. & Physiol. A.M.A., p. 117, 1927.
993. Park, W. H. and Cooper, G. Method of administration and dosage of antipneumococcus serum in lobar pneumonia. Bull. New York Acad. Med., 4:347, Mar. 1928.
994. Park, W. H., and Williams, A. W. Study of pneumococci: comparison between pneumococci found in throat secretions of healthy persons living

in both city and country and those obtained from pneumonic exudates and diseased mucous membranes. J. Exper. Med., 7:403, Aug. 1905.
995. Park, W. H., and Williams, A. W. Pathogenic microörganisms: a practical manual for students, physicians and health officers. 10th Edition, Philadelphia, Lea & Febiger, 1933, 867 p.
996. Park, W. H., Williams, A. W., and Krumwiede, C. Pathogenic microorganisms, p. 301. 9th Edition, Philadelphia, Lea & Febiger, 1929.
997. Parker, J. T. Production of skin necrosis by certain autolysates of pneumococcus (Types I and II). J. Exper. Med., 47:531, Apr. 1928.
998. Parker, J. T. Experimental pneumonia in guinea pigs. II. Effect of anti-autolysate sera on pneumococcus pneumonia in guinea pigs. J. Exper. Med., 50:161, Aug. 1929.
999. Parker, J. T., and McCoy, M. V. S. The production and titration of potent horse antipneumotoxin. J. Exper. Med., 50:103, July 1929.
1000. Parsons, J. W., and Myers, W. K. Streptococcic sepsis complicating recovery from pneumococcic pneumonia. Report of three cases. J.A.M.A., 100:1857, June 10, 1933.
1001. Parsons, J. W., and Sutliff, W. D. Specific serum treatment of Type I lobar pneumonia. Regulation of dosage by observation of circulating agglutinins with the stained slide agglutinin test (Sabin). Am. J. M. Sc., 186:52, July 1933.
1002. Pasteur, L. Sur une maladie nouvelle, provoquée par la salive d'un enfant mort de la rage. Compt. rend. Acad. d. sc., 92:159, Jan. 24, 1881.
1003a. Patterson, S. W. Prognosis of lobar pneumonia and the influence of serum in treatment. M. J. Australia, 2:115, July 29, 1922.
1003b. Patterson, S. W., and Williams, F. E. Studies in respiratory infections in southern Australia. III. Pneumococcus and other members of viridans group of micrococci. J. Path. & Bact., 25:450, Oct. 1922.
1004. Paul, J. R. Pneumococcus variants. I. Intermediate forms and the influence of environment in their production during in-vitro S to R and R to S transitions. J. Bact., 28:45, July 1934.
1005. Paul, J. R., and Lawrence, J. A. Occurrence of pneumococcus variants in lobar pneumonia. J. Clin. Investigation, 12:986, Sept. 1933.
1006. Peabody, F. W. Carbon dioxide content of the blood in pneumonia. J. Exper. Med., 16:701, Nov. 1912.
1007. Peall, P. A. Prophylactic inoculation against pneumonia and other acute respiratory diseases with vaccine on the Randfontein Estates Mine. Publ. South African Inst. Med. Res., 7(37), Apr. 1935.
1008. Pearson, A., and Mouchet, R. Practical hygiene of native compounds in tropical Africa: being notes from experience of first eighteen years of European work in the Katanga. London, Baillière, Tindall & Cox, 1923, 188 p.
1009. Penfold, W. J. Developments in the production of therapeutic sera in Australia. M. J. Australia, 1:245, Mar. 26, 1921.
1010. Pepper, D. S. Urinary excretion of S substance in lobar pneumonia. Yale J. Biol. & Med., 7:13, Oct. 1934.
1011. Perlzweig, W. A., and Keefer, C. S. Immunizing antigen of the pneumococcus. III. Purification of water-soluble antigen. J. Exper. Med., 42:747, Dec. 1925.
1012. Perlzweig, W. A., and Steffen, G. I. Studies on pneumococcus immunity.

III. The nature of pneumococcus antigen. J. Exper. Med., 38:163, Aug. 1923.

1013. Permar, H. H. Pathogenesis of experimental pneumonia in the rabbit. J. M. Research, 44:1, Sept. 1923.

1014. Permar, H. H. The mononuclear phagocytes in experimental pneumonia. J. M. Research, 44:27, Sept. 1923.

1015. Perry, C. B. Peripheral circulation in acute lobar pneumonia. Quart. J. Med., 27:273, April 1934.

1016. Petersen, W. F., and Levinson, S. A. The therapeutic effect of venesection with particular reference to lobar pneumonia. J.A.M.A., 78:257, Jan. 28, 1922.

1017. Peterson, W. Nursing care of the pneumonia patient. Commonhealth (Massachusetts Department of Public Health), 18:168, July–Aug.–Sept. 1931.

1018. Petrie, G. F., and Morgan, W. T. J. Curative action of anti-pneumococcus serum (Type I) in mice. Brit. J. Exper. Path., 13:96, Feb. 1932.

1019. Phelps, B. M. Lobar pneumonia. *In* United Fruit Company, Medical Department, 16th annual report, 1927, p. 179.

1020. Philippine Islands: Philippine Health Service. General statistics. Monthly Bull. of the Philippine Health Service, v. 7, Jan.–Nov. 1927.

1021. Philippine Islands: Philippine Health Service. Report for fiscal year from January 1 to December 31, 1926, by J. Fajardo.

1022. Philippine Islands: Philippine Health Service. Report for fiscal year from January 1 to December 31, 1929, in two volumes. Vol. 2. Statistical tables, by J. Fajardo.

1023. Physicians to the Royal Infirmary, Edinburgh. Report on lobar pneumonia: treatment by concentrated antiserum. Lancet, 2:1390, Dec. 27, 1930.

1024. Pierson, J. W. Pneumonia due to the aspiration of lipoids. J.A.M.A., 99:1163, Oct. 1, 1932.

1025. Pisek, G. R., and Pease, M. C. A preliminary report on pneumonia in children, with special reference to its epidemiology. Am. J. M. Sc., 151:14, Jan. 1916.

1026. Pittman, M., and Falk, I. S. Studies on respiratory diseases. XXXIV. Some relations between extracts, filtrates and virulence of pneumococci. J. Bact., 19:327, May 1930.

1027. Plummer, N. Laboratory methods in the treatment of pneumonia. J. Lab. & Clin. Med., 17:594, Mar. 1932.

1028. Plummer, N. Antipneumococcic serum Types I and II containing heterophile antibodies—Lilly not acceptable for N.N.R.: Heterophile antibody in treatment of pneumonia (Council on Pharmacy and Chemistry of American Medical Association). J.A.M.A., 107:499, Aug. 15, 1936.

1029. Plummer, N., Raia, A., and Shultz, S. Pneumonia in children. Bacteriologic study. Am. J. Dis. Child., 40:557, Sept. 1930.

1030. Pneumococcus typing stations established in Maine (news item). J.A.M.A., 106:1399, Apr. 18, 1936.

1031. Pneumonia among Filipinos traveling in the steerage (editorial). J.A.M.A., 96:2039, June 13, 1931.

1032. Pneumonia and venereal disease control commissions appointed in Pennsylvania (news item). J.A.M.A., 108:483, Feb. 6, 1937.

1033. Pneumonia control program in Essex County, N. J. (news item). J.A.M.A., 110:293, Jan. 22, 1938.
1034. Pneumonia control program in Iowa (news item). J.A.M.A., 110:52, Jan. 1, 1938.
1035. Pneumonia film "A New Day" (current comment). J.A.M.A., 110:514, Feb. 12, 1938.
1036. Pneumonia in Malaya (editorial). Malayan M. J., 4:108, Sept. 1929.
1037. Pneumonia in Northern Argentina (foreign letter). J.A.M.A., 71:989, Sept. 21, 1918.
1038. Pneumonia in the gold mines (foreign letter). J.A.M.A., 97:336, Aug. 1, 1931.
1039. Pneumonia mortality and pneumococcus typing facilities (editorial). J.A.M.A., 109:1910, Dec. 4, 1937.
1040. Pneumonia program in New York City widened (news item). J.A.M.A., 110:54, Jan. 1, 1938.
1041. Pneumonia publicity in Massachusetts (editorial). New England J. Med., 218:132, Jan. 20, 1938. *See also 250.*
1042. Pneumonia serum for indigent hospital patients in Baltimore (news item). J.A.M.A., 110:516, Feb. 12, 1938.
1043. Pneumonia serum provided by the City of Pittsburgh (news item). J.A.M.A., 108:401, Jan. 30, 1937.
1044. Pontano, T. Tipi di pneumococchi in Italia. Ann. d'ig., 32:525, July 1922.
1045. Potts, W. H. Oxygen therapy—a critical résumé. Am. J. M. Sc., 184:616, Nov. 1932.
1046. Powell, E. V. Roentgen therapy of lobar pneumonia. J.A.M.A., 110:19, Jan. 1, 1938.
1047. Powell, H. M., Jamieson, W. A., Bailey, G. H., and Hyde, R. R. Comparative study of antipneumococcus serum containing heterophile antibody. Am. J. Hyg., 17:102, Jan. 1933.
1048. Powell, J. P., Atwater, R. N., and Felton, L. D. Epidemiology of pneumonia. A study of pneumococcus carriers among four groups of persons over a period of months. Am. J. Hyg., 6:570, July 1926.
1049. Pratt, J. H. The histology of acute lobar pneumonia. Johns Hopkins Hosp. Rep., 9:265, 1900.
1050. Preble, H. B. Pneumococcus endocarditis. Am. J. M. Sc., 128:782, Nov. 1904.
1051. Price, A. E. Serum treatment of lobar pneumonia: report on use of Felton's serum in Detroit from February 25 to June 1, 1935. J. Michigan M. Soc., 34:757, Dec. 1935.
1052. Pritchett, I. W. Enhancement of the opsonizing and agglutinating powers of antipneumococcus serum by specific precipitating serum. J. Exper. Med., 32:283, Sept. 1920.
1053. Przesmycki, F., Kolago, J., Stankiewicz, R., and Zmigryder-Konopka, L. Flore bactérienne dans les affections pulmonaires chez les enfants. Compt. rend. Soc. de biol., 111:93, Oct. 3, 1932.
1054. Quigley, W. J. The precipitin reaction in the urine in pneumonia. J. Infect. Dis., 23:217, Sept. 1918.
1055. Rabinovitch, J., and Lederer, M. Lipoid pneumonia. Arch. Path., 17:160, Feb. 1934.

1056. Rackemann, F. M. Clinical allergy, particularly asthma and hay fever; mechanism and treatment. New York, The Macmillan Co., 1931, 617 p.
1057. Raia, A., Plummer, N., and Shultz, S. New types of pneumococci in the pneumonias of children. Am. J. Dis. Child., 42:57, July 1931.
1058. Rake, G. Pathology of pneumococcus infection in mice following intranasal instillation. J. Exper. Med., 63:17, Jan. 1936.
1059. Rake, G. Pathogenesis of pneumococcus infections in mice. J. Exper. Med., 63:191, Feb. 1936.
1060. Rappaport, H., and Brescia, M. A. Pneumococcus peritonitis: report of a case with recovery: review of literature with especial reference to treatment. Arch. Pediat., 52:766, Nov. 1935.
1061. Ratnoff, H. L., and Litvak, A. M. Pneumococcus meningitis treated with Morgenroth's optochin hydrochloride. Recovery. Arch. Pediat., 43: 466, July 1926.
1062. Reimann, H. A. Blood platelets in pneumococcus infections. J. Exper. Med., 40:553, Oct. 1924.
1063. Reimann, H. A. Serological relationships of type-specific and degraded pneumococci. J. Exper. Med., 43:107, Jan. 1926.
1064. Reimann, H. A. Occurrence of degraded pneumococci in vivo. J. Exper. Med., 45:807, May 1927.
1065. Reimann, H. A. Reversion of R to S pneumococci. J. Exper. Med., 49: 237, Feb. 1929.
1066. Reimann, H. A. Allergy and pneumococcus lobar pneumonia. Minnesota Med., 14:898, Oct. 1931.
1067. Reimann, H. A. Primary staphylococcic pneumonia. J.A.M.A., 101:514, Aug. 12, 1933.
1068. Reimann, H. A. Contagiousness of Types I and II pneumococcus pneumonia. Minnesota Med., 17:714, Dec. 1934.
1069. Reimann, H. A., and Julianelle, L. A. Production of purpura by derivatives of pneumococcus. II. Effect of pneumococcus extract on the blood platelets and corpuscles. J. Exper. Med., 43:97, Jan. 1926.
1070. Reisman, D. Chronic non-tuberculous bronchopneumonia. J.A.M.A., 102:673, Mar. 3, 1934.
1071. Reitzel, R. J. Lobar pneumonia in negroes: influence of syphilis as a co-existing disease. South. M. J., 21:469, June 1928.
1072. Reveno, W. S., and McLaughlin, N. Pneumococcic meningitis: recovery with Felton's serum. Ann. Int. Med., 7:1026, Feb. 1934.
1073. Reznikoff, P. Immature white blood cell counts in infectious diseases. J.A.M.A., 93:963, Sept. 28, 1929.
1074. Reznikoff, P. White blood cell counts in convalescence from infectious diseases. Am. J. M. Sc., 184:167, Aug. 1932.
1075. Rhoades, D. R. Studies on pneumococcus immunity. VI. Fate of pneumococcus protective bodies when injected into normal animals and man. Hygienic Laboratory Bulletin, No. 141:31, Apr. 1925.
1076. Rhoads, C. P., and Goodner, K. Pathology of experimental dermal pneumococcus infection in the rabbit. J. Exper. Med., 54:41, July 1931.
1077. Rich, A. R. Mechanism responsible for prevention of spread of bacteria in the immune body. Bull. Johns Hopkins Hosp., 52:203, Mar. 1933.

1078. Rich, A. R., Jennings, F. B., Jr., and Downing, L. M. The persistence of immunity after the abolition of allergy by desensitization. Bull. Johns Hopkins Hosp., 53:172, Oct. 1933.
1079. Richardson, R. Pneumococcus types in rural districts. J.A.M.A., 72:863, Mar. 22, 1919.
1080. Richardson, R. Types of pneumococcus in lobar pneumonia. J. Lab. & Clin. Med., 4:484, May 1919.
1081. Rischbieth, H. On pneumococcal peritonitis. A paper based upon a series of fifty-seven cases in children and one in an adult. Quart. J. Med., 4:205, Jan. 1911.
1082. Robertson, O. H. Instance of lobar pneumonia acquired in the laboratory. J. Prev. Med., 5:221, May 1931.
1083. Robertson, O. H., Coggeshall, L. T., and Terrell, E. E. Experimental pneumococcus lobar pneumonia in the dog. II. Pathology. J. Clin. Investigation, 12:433, Mar. 1933.
1084. Robertson, O. H., Coggeshall, L. T., and Terrell, E. E. Experimental pneumococcus lobar pneumonia in the dog. III. Pathogenesis. J. Clin. Investigation, 12:467, Mar. 1933.
1085. Robertson, O. H., and Cornwell, M. A. Study of resistance of normal human beings to recently isolated strains of pathogenic pneumococci. J. Exper. Med., 52:267, Aug. 1930.
1086. Robertson, O. H., Graeser, J. B., Coggeshall, L. T., and Harrison, M. A. The relation of circulating antipneumococcal immune substances to the course of lobar pneumonia. I. Natural immune substances. J. Clin. Investigation, 13:621, July 1934.
1087. Robertson, O. H., Graeser, J. B., Coggeshall, L. T., and Harrison, M. A. The relation of circulating antipneumococcal immune substances to the course of lobar pneumonia. II. Acquired immune substances. J. Clin. Investigation, 13:633, July 1934.
1088. Robertson, O. H., Graeser, J. B., Coggeshall, L. T., and Sia, R. H. P. The relation of circulating antipneumococcal immune substances to the course of lobar pneumonia. III. Injected immune substances (antipneumococcus serum, Types I and II). J. Clin. Investigation, 13:649, July 1934.
1089. Robertson, O. H., and Sia, R. H. P. Studies on pneumococcus growth inhibition. II. Method for demonstrating the growth-inhibitory and bactericidal action of normal serum-leucocyte mixtures. J. Exper. Med., 39:219, Feb. 1924.
1090. Robertson, O. H., and Sia, R. H. P. Studies on pneumococcus growth inhibition. III. Influence of specific antipneumococcus serum on the growth-inhibitory and bactericidal action of normal serum-leucocyte mixtures. J. Exper. Med., 40:467, Oct. 1924.
1091. Robertson, O. H., and Sia, R. H. P. Studies on pneumococcus growth inhibition. VII. Relation of opsonins to natural resistance against pneumococcus infection. J. Exper. Med., 46:239, Aug. 1927.
1092. Robertson, O. H., Sia, R. H. P., and Cornwell, M. A. Activating effect of fresh normal serum on pneumococcidal-promoting action of antipneumococcus serum, Type I. J. Immunol., 19:429, Nov. 1930.
1093. Robertson, O. H., Sia, R. H. P., and Woo, S. T. Studies on pneumococcus

growth inhibition. I. Protective action of gelatin for pneumococci in suspension. J. Exper. Med., 39:199, Feb. 1924.

1094. Robertson, O. H., Terrell, E. E., Graeser, J. B., and Cornwell, M. A. Relation of natural humoral antipneumococcal immunity to the inception of lobar pneumonia. J. Exper. Med., 52:421, Sept. 1930.

1095. Robertson, O. H., and Uhley, C. G. Changes occurring in the macrophage system of the lungs in pneumococcus lobar pneumonia. J. Clin. Investigation, 15:115, Jan. 1936.

1096. Robertson, O. H., Woo, S. T., and Cheer, S. N. Studies on pneumococcus growth inhibition. IV. Simplified agitator for growth inhibition tests with serum-leucocyte mixtures; and certain modifications in the technique of the test. J. Exper. Med., 40:487, Oct. 1924.

1097. Robertson, O. H., Woo, S. T., Cheer, S. N., and King, L. P. Study of the mechanism of recovery from experimental pneumococcus infection. J. Exper. Med., 47:317, Feb. 1928.

1098. Robinson, E. S. The antiserum treatment of pneumonia from the standpoint of public health. New England J. Med., 216:459, Mar. 18, 1937.

1099. Robinson, J. E. Result of sputum typing in pneumonia for season of 1919–1920. Texas State J. Med., 16:345, Dec. 1920.

1100. Rockwell, G. E., and Tyler, R. Antipneumococcus serum containing heterophile antibody; laboratory and clinical report. J. Lab. & Clin. Med., 21:721, Apr. 1936.

1101. Rogers, E. S. The New York State program for the control of pneumococcus pneumonia. Am. J. Pub. Health, 27:133, Feb. 1937.

1102. Rogers, E. S. Report of the meeting of the Advisory Committee on Pneumonia Control of the New York State Department of Health, Saratoga Springs, June 23, 1937 (unpublished).*

1103. Rogers, L. Relationship between pneumonia incidence and climate in India. Lancet, 1:1173, June 6, 1925.

1104. Rokitansky, C. Inflammations of the lungs (pneumoniae). *In* Manual of Pathological Anatomy, 4:71. London, Sydenham Society, 1852.

1105. Rolleston, H. D. Pneumococcic peritonitis. Clin. J., 31:319, Feb. 26, 1908.

1106. Römer, P. Experimentelle Grundlagen für klinische Versuche einer Serumtherapie des Ulcus corneae serpens nach Untersuchungen über Pneumocokkenimmunität. Arch. f. Ophth., 54:99, Apr. 1902.

1107. Römer, P. Wertbestimmung des Pneumokokkenserums mit Demonstration von Tieren. Ber. ü. d. Versamml. d. ophth. Gesellsch., 32:325, Aug. 1905.

1108. Rood, A. D. Clinical study of influenza pneumonia. New York M. J., 109:493, Mar. 22, 1919.

1109. Rosenau, M. J. Preventive medicine and hygiene, p. 233. 5th Edition, New York, D. Appleton & Co., 1927.

1110. Rosenau, M. J. Epidemiology of pneumonia. Commonhealth (Massachusetts Department of Public Health), 18:132, July–Aug.–Sept. 1931.

1111. Rosenau, M. J., Felton, L. D., and Atwater, R. M. Epidemiologic study of pneumonia and its mode of spread. Am. J. Hyg., 6:463, May 1926.

* Permission to cite figures from this report in Lord and Heffron (814) was kindly granted by Dr. Rogers.

1112. Rosenblüth, M. B., and Block, M. Three uncommon complications of lobar pneumonia. M. Clin. North America, 14:1359, May 1931.
1113. Rosenblüth, M. B., and Block, M. Pneumonia due to Type V pneumococcus. Arch. Int. Med., 60:567, Oct. 1937.
1114. Rosenow, E. C. The blood in lobar pneumonia—with remarks concerning treatment. J.A.M.A., 44:871, Mar. 18, 1905.
1115. Rosenow, E. C. The rôle of phagocytosis in the pneumococcidal action of pneumonic blood. J. Infect. Dis., 3:683, June 1906.
1116. Rosenow, E. C. Human pneumococcal opsonin and the antiopsonic substance in virulent pneumococci. J. Infect. Dis., 4:285, June 1907.
1117. Rosenow, E. C. Pneumococcus anaphylaxis and immunity. J. Infect. Dis., 9:190, Sept. 1911.
1118. Rosenow, E. C. Partially autolyzed pneumococci in the treatment of lobar pneumonia. J.A.M.A., 70:759, Mar. 16, 1918.
1119. Rosenow, E. C., and Sturdivant, B. F. Studies in influenza and pneumonia. IV. Further results of prophylactic inoculations. J.A.M.A., 73:396, Aug. 9, 1919.
1120. Rosenthal, L., and Sternberg, B. Rapid method for determining type of pneumococcus in sputum. J. Lab. & Clin. Med., 15:78, Oct. 1929.
1121. Rosenthal, M. Pulmonary lesions associated with intrauterine asphyxia. J. Pediat., 6:71, Jan. 1935.
1122. Rosenthal, S. M. Studies in chemotherapy. I. The action of sodium formaldehyde sulphoxylate in bacterial infections. Pub. Health Rep., 49:908, Aug. 3, 1934.
1123. Rosenthal, S. M. Studies in chemotherapy. II. Chemotherapy of experimental pneumococcus infections. Pub. Health Rep., 52:48, Jan. 8, 1937.
1124. Rosenthal, S. M. Studies in chemotherapy. III. The effect of p-aminobenzene sulphonamide on pneumococci in vitro. Pub. Health Rep., 52:192, Feb. 12, 1937.
1125. Ross, A. H. Atelectasis of the lung and lobar pneumonia: their etiologic identity. Northwest Med., 32:93, Mar. 1933.
1126. Ross, V. Immunity to pneumococcus produced in rats by feeding tissues of animals killed by the same organism. J. Immunol., 12:219, Sept. 1926.
1127. Ross, V. Immunity to pneumococcus produced in rats by feeding them the germ. J. Immunol., 12:237, Sept. 1926.
1128. Ross, V. Response of orally immunized rats to second injection of pneumococcus and minimum duration of immunity. J. Immunol., 12:323, Oct. 1926.
1129. Ross, V. Oral immunization against the pneumococcus. Use of bile salt dissolved organisms, etc., time of appearance of immunity and dosage. J. Exper. Med., 51:585, Apr. 1930.
1130. Ross, V. Fate of orally administered specific polysaccharide of pneumococcus. Proc. Soc. Exper. Biol. & Med., 28:274, Dec. 1930.
1131. Ross, V. Oral immunization against pneumococcus Types II and III and normal variation in resistance to these types among rats. J. Exper. Med., 54:875, Dec. 1931.
1132. Ross, V. The role of the soluble specific substance in oral immunization against pneumococcus Type I. J. Exper. Med., 54:899, Dec. 1931.

1133. Ross, V. The role of soluble specific substance in oral immunization against pneumococcus Types II and III. J. Exper. Med., 55:1, Jan. 1932.
1134. Ross, V. Fate of orally administered soluble specific substance of pneumococcus, Types I, II, and III. J. Exper. Med., 55:13, Jan. 1932.
1135. Ross, V. Duration of the immunity produced in rats by feeding the pneumococcus, Type I. J. Immunol., 27:235, Sept. 1934.
1136. Ross, V. Protective antibodies following oral administration of pneumococcus Type I to rats. J. Immunol., 27:249, Sept. 1934.
1137. Ross, V. Protective antibodies following oral administration of pneumococcus Types 2 and 3 to rats, with some data for Types 4, 5, and 6. J. Immunol., 27:273, Sept. 1934.
1138. Ross, V. Oral immunization of humans against the pneumococcus. J. Immunol., 27:307, Sept. 1934.
1139. Roubakine, A. Psittacosis. Epidemiol. Rep., League of Nations, 9:141, Apr. 15, 1930.
1140. Rudolph, J. A., and Cohen, M. B. Types of human hypersensitiveness: their relation to the liability to serum reactions. J.A.M.A., 102:900, Mar. 24, 1934.
1141. Ruegsegger, J. M., and Finland, M. Influence of dosage and route of injection on antibody response of human subjects to the specific carbohydrate of Type VIII pneumococcus. J. Clin. Investigation, 14:833, Nov. 1935.
1142. Ruffer, M. A. Studies in the palaeopathology of Egypt, p. 15. Edited by R. L. Moodie. Chicago, Ill., University of Chicago Press, 1921.
1143. Russell, A. E., Britten, R. H., Thompson, L. R., and Bloomfield, J. J. The health of workers in dusty trades. II. Exposure to siliceous dust (granite industry). Washington, Government Printing Office, 1929, 206 p. (Public Health Bulletin, No. 187).
1144. Ryland, C. P., Jr. Some results of serum therapy in lobar pneumonia. Virginia M. Monthly, 60:272, Aug. 1933.
1145. Ryle, J. A., Waterfield, R. L., and others. Pneumococcal infections. Guy's Hosp. Rep., 83:389, Oct. 1933.
1146. Sabin, A. B. "Stained slide" microscopic agglutination test. Application to (1) rapid typing of pneumococci, (2) determination of antibody. Proc. Soc. Exper. Biol. & Med., 26:492, Mar. 1929.
1147. Sabin, A. B. "Stained slide" microscopic agglutination test. Application to (1) rapid typing of pneumococci, (2) determination of antibody. Am. J. Pub. Health, 19:1148, Oct. 1929.
1148. Sabin, A. B. Microscopic agglutination test in pneumonia. Its application to rapid typing and control of serum therapy. J. Infect. Dis., 46: 469, June 1930.
1149. Sabin, A. B. On the presence in antipneumococcus serum of type-specific protective antibody not neutralized by homologous specific soluble substance. J. Exper. Med., 53:93, Jan. 1931.
1150. Sabin, A. B. Role of certain anaerobic toxins in pneumococcus infection. Proc. Soc. Exper. Biol. & Med., 28:457, Jan. 1931.
1151. Sabin, A. B. Study of therapeutic mechanism of antipneumococcic serum on the experimental dermal pneumococcus infection in rabbits. I. Presence in antipneumococcic serum of non-antibacterial therapeutic factor. J. Exper. Med., 56:531, Oct. 1932.

1152. Sabin, A. B. Study of therapeutic mechanism of antipneumococcic serum on the experimental dermal pneumococcus infection in rabbits. II. Comparison of therapeutic effect of unrefined antipneumococcic serum with that of its various protein fractions: role of non-antibacterial factor. J. Exper. Med., 57:139, Jan. 1933.
1153. Sabin, A. B. Immediate pneumococcus typing directly from sputum by the Neufeld reaction. J.A.M.A., 100:1584, May 20, 1933.
1154. Sabin, A. B., and Wallace, G. B. A method for determining the chill-producing properties of antipneumococcic serum. Proc. Soc. Exper. Biol. & Med., 27:198, Dec. 1929.
1155. Sailer, J., Hall, M. W., Wilson, R. L., and McCoy, C. A study of pneumococcus carriers. Arch. Int. Med., 24:600, Dec. 1919.
1156. Saklad, M. Oxygen and carbon dioxide therapy. New England J. Med., 207:1132, Dec. 22, 1932.
1157. Salvador (Central America): Dirección general de estadística. Anuario estadístico, correspondiente al año de 1928, p. 36.
1158. Sante, L. Lobar pneumonia. A roentgenological study (a correlation of Roentgen-ray findings with clinical and pathological manifestations). New York, Paul B. Hoeber, Inc., 1928, 137 p.
1159. Schattenberg, H. J., and Harris, W. H. Intraperitoneal injections of pneumococcus in animals primarily receiving leucocytic stimulating antigens. Proc. Soc. Exper. Biol. & Med., 29:1052, June 1932.
1160. Schiemann, O., and Casper, W. Sind die spezifisch präcipitablen Substanzen der 3 Pneumokokkentypen Haptene? Ztschr. f. Hyg. u. Infektionskr., 108:220, Oct. 1927.
1161. Schmidt, L. H. Use of sulfanilamide in treatment of Type XIV pneumococcus infections in mice. Proc. Soc. Exper. Biol. & Med., 37:205, Oct. 1937.
1162. Schöbl, O., and Sellards, A. W. Experimental pneumonia in monkeys. Philippine J. Sc., 31:1, Sept. 1926.
1163. Schorer, E. H., Clark, F. D., Sanderson, R., Dickson, J. D., and Huntoon, F. M. Pneumonia and empyema in the late winter of 1917–1918. M. Rec., 95:673, Apr. 26, 1919.
1164. Schottstaedt, W. E. R. Lobar pneumonia: an attempt to evaluate various methods of treatment. California & West. Med., 41:244, Oct. 1934.
1165. Schroder, M. C., and Cooper, G. Epidemic of colds, bronchitis and pneumonia due to Type V pneumococci. J. Infect. Dis., 46:384, May 1930.
1166. Scott, T. F. McN., and Finland, M. The cytology of pleural effusions in pneumonia studied with a supravital technique. Am. J. M. Sc., 188:322, Sept. 1934.
1167. Scott, W. J. M., and Cutler, E. C. Postoperative massive atelectasis. J.A.M.A., 90:1759, June 2, 1928.
1168. Sears, G. G., and Larrabee, R. C. Analysis of nine hundred and forty-nine cases of pneumonia. Med. & Surg. Rep. Boston City Hosp., Series 12, p. 1, 1901.
1169. Seegal, D. Acute glomerulonephritis following pneumococcic lobar pneumonia: analysis of seven cases. Arch. Int. Med., 56:913, Nov. 1935.
1170. Serum treatment of lobar pneumonia (editorial). New England J. Med., 214:848, Apr. 23, 1936.
1171. Serum treatment of pneumonia in New Hampshire. Announcement re-

garding availability of pneumonia serums. New England J. Med., 218: 364, Feb. 24, 1938. *See also 943.*
1172. Sevag, M. G., and Maiweg, L. The respiration mechanism of pneumococcus. III. J. Exper. Med., 60:95, July 1934.
1173. Shanghai Municipal Council, Public Health Department. Annual report, 1929.
1174. Sharp, E. A., and Blake, F. G. Host factors in the pathogenesis of pneumococcus pneumonia. J. Exper. Med., 52:501, Oct. 1930.
1175. Sharp, W. B., and Urbantke, E. Influenza studies. XX. Identification of fixed type pneumococcus carriers: a study of technical methods. J. Infect. Dis., 37:473, Nov. 1925.
1176. Shattuck, F. C., and Lawrence, C. H. Acute lobar pneumonia. Boston M. & S. J., 178:245, Feb. 14, 1918.
1177. Shattuck, L. Bills of Mortality, 1810–1849, City of Boston. With an essay on the vital statistics of Boston from 1810 to 1841. Boston, Printed for the Registry Department, 1893, 87 p.
1178. Shaw, F. W., and Bigger, I. A. Necrobacillosis of the lung. J.A.M.A., 102:688, Mar. 3, 1934.
1179. Shearer, M. C. "Plateau R-T" in a case of lobar pneumonia. Am. Heart J., 5:801, Aug. 1930.
1180. Sherwood, N. P., and Stoland, O. O. Anaphylaxis. XII. The pulmonary permeability in normal and sensitized dogs and its relation to anaphylactic shock. J. Immunol., 20:101, Feb. 1931.
1181. Shibley, G. S., Hanger, F. M., and Dochez, A. R. Studies in the common cold. I. Observations of normal bacterial flora of nose and throat with variations occurring during colds. J. Exper. Med., 43:415, Mar. 1926.
1182. Shibley, G. S., Mills, K. C., and Dochez, A. R. Further consideration of transmissibility of human upper respiratory infection (common cold) to the ape. Proc. Soc. Exper. Biol. & Med., 27:59, Oct. 1929.
1183. Shibley, G. S., Mills, K. C., and Dochez, A. R. Studies of etiology of common cold. J.A.M.A., 95:1553, Nov. 22, 1930.
1184. Shibley, G. S., and Rogers, E. S. Occurrence of rough pneumococci in lungs of patients with lobar pneumonia. Proc. Soc. Exper. Biol. & Med., 30:6, Oct. 1932.
1185. Shibley, G. S., and Spies, T. D. Effect of vitamin A on the common cold. J.A.M.A., 103:2021, Dec. 29, 1934.
1186. Shuller, E. H. Pneumonia—differential typing and treatment. J. Oklahoma M. A., 27:153, May 1934.
1187. Shultz, S. M. A study of certain epidemiological factors in the pneumonia of children. Am. J. Hyg., 15:80, Jan. 1932.
1188. Shwartzman, G. Phenomenon of local skin reactivity to pneumococcus. J. Immunol., 23:429, Dec. 1932.
1189. Sia, R. H. P. Studies on pneumococcus growth inhibition. VI. Specific effect of pneumococcus soluble substance on the growth of pneumococci in normal serum-leucocyte mixtures. J. Exper. Med., 43:633, May 1926.
1190. Sia, R. H. P. Antipneumococcus protective substances in normal pig serum. Proc. Soc. Exper. Biol. & Med., 26:284, Jan. 1929.
1191. Sia, R. H. P. Susceptibility of hamsters and white mice to pneumococcus infection. Nat. M. J. China, 16:65, Feb. 1930.

1192. Sia, R. H. P., and Chung, S. F. Use of dog blood agar for differentiation of "S" and "R" pneumococci. Proc. Soc. Exper. Biol. & Med., 29:245, Dec. 1931.

1193. Sia, R. H. P., and Dawson, M. H. In vitro transformation of pneumococcal types. II. The nature of the factor responsible for the transformation of pneumococcal types. J. Exper. Med., 54:701, Nov. 1931.

1194. Sia, R. H. P., Robertson, O. H., and Woo, S. T. A study of the mechanism of recovery from lobar pneumonia. J. Exper. Med., 48:513, Oct. 1928.

1195. Sia, R. H. P., and Zia, S. H. Effect of Type II pneumococcus soluble specific substance on infectivity of pneumococcus Type II. Proc. Soc. Exper. Biol. & Med., 29:791, Apr. 1932.

1196. Siam: Ministry of Finance, Department of General Statistics. Statistical year book of the Kingdom of Siam, B. E. 2473 (1930–31). English edition, p. 507.

1197. Sickles, G. M. Comparative potency of concentrated and unconcentrated antipneumococcus serum. J. Infect. Dis., 45:490, Dec. 1929.

1198. Sickles, G. M., and Shaw, M. Micro-organisms which decompose the specific carbohydrate of pneumococcus Types II and III. J. Infect. Dis., 53:38, July–Aug. 1933.

1199. Sickles, G. M., and Shaw, M. Action of microorganisms from soil on type-specific and nontype-specific pneumococcus Type I carbohydrates. Proc. Soc. Exper. Biol. & Med., 31:443, Jan. 1934.

1200. Singapore Municipality. Administration report for 1920.

1201. Sloan, L. H., Freedberg, A. S., and Erlich, J. C. Tularemic pneumonia. J.A.M.A., 107:117, July 11, 1936.

1202. Small, A. A. Pneumonia at a base hospital: observations on one thousand one hundred cases at Camp Pike, Ark. J.A.M.A., 71:700, Aug. 31, 1918.

1203. Smillie, W. G. Field studies of acute respiratory disease. Porto Rico J. Pub. Health and Trop. Med., 5:1, Sept. 1929.

1204. Smillie, W. G. An epidemic of influenza in an isolated community—Northwest River, Labrador. Am. J. Hyg., 11:392, Mar. 1930.

1205. Smillie, W. G. Common colds. Personn. J., 9:470, Apr. 1931.

1206. Smillie, W. G. Epidemiology of lobar pneumonia. Study of the prevalence of specific strains of pneumococci in the nasopharynx of immediate family contacts. J.A.M.A., 101:1281, Oct. 21, 1933.

1207. Smillie, W. G. Study of an outbreak of Type II pneumococcus pneumonia in Veterans' Administration Hospital at Bedford, Massachusetts. Am. J. Hyg., 24:522, Nov. 1936.

1208. Smillie, W. G. The common cold. Edited by the National Health Council. New York, Funk & Wagnalls Company, 1937, 77 p. (National Health Series).

1209. Smillie, W. G., and Caldwell, E. L. A study of pneumonia in a rural area in southern Alabama. J. Exper. Med., 50:233, Aug. 1929.

1210. Smillie, W. G., and Leeder, F. S. Epidemiology of lobar pneumonia. Am. J. Pub. Health, 24:129, Feb. 1934.

1211. Smillie, W. G., Warnock, G. H., and White, H. J. Study of a Type I pneumococcus epidemic at the State Hospital at Worcester, Mass. Am. J. Pub. Health, 28:293, Mar. 1938.

1212. Smith, C. H. Pneumonias of childhood. Proceedings of the International Assembly of the Interstate Postgraduate Medical Association of North America, October 1935, p. 23.
1213. Smith, C. M. Some notes on pneumonia statistics in Glasgow with special reference to children under five years of age. J. Hyg., 27:328, Mar. 1928.
1214. Smith, W., Andrewes, C. H., and Laidlaw, P. P. A virus obtained from influenza patients. Lancet, 2:66, July 8, 1933.
1215. Smith, W., Fischer, W., and Smith, M. L. Provisional stable standard for antipneumococcus serum Type II, and its practical application. Lancet, 2:155, July 21, 1934.
1216. Snyder, F. F., and Rosenfeld, M. Intra-uterine respiratory movements of the human fetus. J.A.M.A., 108:1946, June 5, 1937.
1217. Solomon, S. Primary Friedländer pneumonia. J.A.M.A., 108:937, Mar. 20, 1937.
1218. Solomon, S., and Curphey, T. J. Streptococcic septicemia complicating pneumococcic lobar pneumonia. J.A.M.A., 108:187, Jan. 16, 1937.
1219. South African Institute for Medical Research (Johannesburg). Annual report for the year ended 31st December, 1931, p. 7.
1220. Spicer, S. Ophthalmic test for horse serum sensitivity contrasted with intradermal. Performed on 353 patients. J. Immunol., 15:335, July 1928.
1221. Spooner, L. H. Specific diagnosis and treatment of acute lobar pneumonia. Boston M. & S. J., 182:224, Feb. 26, 1920.
1222. Spooner, L. H., Sellards, A. W., and Wyman, J. H. Serum treatment of Type I pneumonia. J.A.M.A., 71:1310, Oct. 19, 1918.
1223. Stadie, W. C. The oxygen of the arterial and venous blood in pneumonia and its relation to cyanosis. J. Exper. Med., 30:215, Sept. 1919.
1224. Steiner, W. R. Peripheral venous thrombosis in pneumonia with report of three cases and a review of those previously recorded. Johns Hopkins Hosp. Rep., 15:189, 1910.
1225. Steinke, C. R. Bilateral empyema: report of 8 cases. J. Thoracic Surg., 2:287, Feb. 1933.
1226. Stengel, A. On the use of serum and blood of convalescent patients in the treatment of lobar pneumonia and influenzal pneumonia. M. Clin. North America, 4:937, Jan. 1921.
1227. Sternberg, G. M. A fatal form of septicaemia in the rabbit, produced by subcutaneous injection of human saliva; an experimental research. *In* National Board of Health annual report, 1881, p. 87. Washington, Government Printing Office, 1882.
1228. Stewart, C. C. Five-year review of pulmonary complications following operation. Canad. M.A.J., 26:55, Jan. 1932.
1229. Stewart, F. W. Local specific therapy of experimental pneumococcal meningitis. I. Experimental pneumococcal meningitis in rabbits. J. Exper. Med., 46:391, Sept. 1927.
1230. Stewart, F. W. Local specific therapy of experimental pneumococcal meningitis. II. Production, pathology, and treatment of Type I pneumococcal meningitis in dogs. J. Exper. Med., 46:409, Sept. 1927.

1231. Stewart, F. W. Local specific therapy of experimental pneumococcal meningitis. III. Incidental myelitis, abscess, and organization of exudates. J. Exper. Med., 47:1, Jan. 1928.
1232. Stewart, F. W. Local specific therapy of experimental pneumococcal meningitis. IV. Type II pneumococcal meningitis in dogs. J. Exper. Med., 47:515, Apr. 1928.
1233. Stewart, H. E. Diathermy in the treatment of pneumonia. Brit. J. Phys. Med., 8:133, Jan. 1934.
1234. Stillman, E. G. A contribution to the epidemiology of lobar pneumonia. J. Exper. Med., 24:651, Dec. 1916.
1235. Stillman, E. G. Further studies on the epidemiology of lobar pneumonia. J. Exper. Med., 26:513, Oct. 1917.
1236. Stillman, E. G. A study of atypical Type II pneumococci. J. Exper. Med., 29:251, Mar. 1919.
1237. Stillman, E. G. Persistence of inspired bacteria in the lungs of alcoholized mice. J. Exper. Med., 40:353, Sept. 1924.
1238. Stillman, E. G. Production of immunity in mice by inhalation of pneumococci. J. Exper. Med., 40:567, Oct. 1924.
1239. Stillman, E. G. Susceptibility of rabbits to infection by the inhalation of Type II pneumococci. J. Exper. Med., 52:215, Aug. 1930.
1240. Stillman, E. G. Development of agglutinins and protective antibodies in rabbits after inhalation of Type II pneumococci. J. Exper. Med., 52:225, Aug. 1930.
1241. Stillman, E. G. Duration of demonstrable antibodies in the serum of rabbits immunized with heat-killed Type I pneumococci. J. Exper. Med., 54:615, Oct. 1931.
1242. Stillman, E. G. Duration of demonstrable antibodies in the serum of rabbits immunized with heat-killed Type II and Type III pneumococci. J. Infect. Dis., 57:223, Nov.–Dec. 1935.
1243. Stillman, E. G., and Branch, A. Experimental production of pneumococcus pneumonia in mice by the inhalation method. J. Exper. Med., 40:733, Dec. 1924.
1244. Stillman, E. G., and Branch, A. Localization of pneumococci in lungs of partially immunized mice following inhalation of pneumococci. J. Exper. Med., 54:623, Oct. 1931.
1245. Stillman, E. G., and Goodner, K. Resistance to pneumococcus infection in rabbits following immunizing injections of heat-killed pneumococcus suspensions. J. Exper. Med., 58:195, Aug. 1933.
1246. Stillman, E. G., and Schulz, R. Z. Reaction of partially immunized rabbits to inhalation of Type I pneumococci. J. Infect. Dis., 57:233, Nov.–Dec. 1935.
1247. Stillman, E. G., and Schulz, R. Z. Reaction of normal and partially immunized rabbits to intranasal instillation of Type I pneumococci. J. Infect. Dis., 57:238, Nov.–Dec. 1935.
1248. Stoll, H. F. Eavesdropping on the doctor: a case of pneumonia. Hygeia, 14:1021, Nov. 1936.
1249. Stoltenberg, L. Combating of catarrhal hospital infections with anticatarrhal vaccines. Experiences in children's department of the University Hospital, Oslo. Acta Paediat., 12 (4):169, 1932.

1250. Stone, W. J. Pericarditis as a complication in pneumonia: based on three hundred necropsies. J.A.M.A., 73:254, July 26, 1919.
1251. Stone, W. J., Phillips, B. G., and Bliss, W. P. Clinical study of pneumonia based on eight hundred and seventy-one cases. Arch. Int. Med., 22:409, Oct. 1918.
1252. Strøm, A. Epidemic of croupous pneumonia caused by pneumococcus Type I. J. Infect. Dis., 50:430, May–June 1932.
1253. Strouse, S. Experimental studies on pneumococcus infections. J. Exper. Med., 11:743, Sept. 1909.
1254. Strouse, S. Phagocytic immunity in pneumococcus infections, and in pneumonia with relation to the crisis. J. Exper. Med., 14:109, Aug. 1911.
1255. Struthers, R. R. Pneumococcal peritonitis. Canad. M.A.J., 14:955, Oct. 1924.
1256. Stryker, L. M. Variations in the pneumococcus induced by growth in immune serum. J. Exper. Med., 24:49, July 1916.
1257. Stuart-Harris, C. H., Andrewes, C. H., and Smith, W., with Chalmers, D. K. M., Cowen, E. G. H., and Hughes, D. L. A study of epidemic influenza: with special reference to the 1936–7 epidemic. London, His Majesty's Stationery Office, 1938, 151 p. (Medical Research Council, Special Report Series No. 228).
1258. Stuppy, G. W., Cannon, P. R., and Falk, I. S. Nature of immunity in lungs of rabbits following immunization with pneumococci. J. Prev. Med., 5:97, Mar. 1931.
1259. Stuppy, G. W., and Falk, I. S. Experimental pneumonia in rabbits produced by intrabronchial insufflation of pneumococci. J. Prev. Med., 5:89, Mar. 1931.
1260. Stuppy, G. W., Falk, I. S., and Jacobson, M. A. Intratracheal inoculation of monkeys with pneumococci. J. Prev. Med., 5:81, Mar. 1931.
1261. Suárez, R. M. Study of lobar pneumonia in Porto Rico. Preliminary report. Porto Rico J. Pub. Health & Trop. Med., 6:294, Mar. 1931.
1262. Sunderman, F. W. Studies of serum electrolytes. VII. Total base and protein components of serum during lobar pneumonia with note on gastric secretion. J. Clin. Investigation, 9:615, Feb. 1931.
1263. Sutliff, W. D. Agglutinins and protective bodies in pneumococcus immunity and application to the control of specific therapy. Proc. Soc. Exper. Biol. & Med., 25:292, Jan. 1928.
1264. Sutliff, W. D. Investigation of reliability of sputum typing for pneumococcus by mouse method. J. Infect. Dis., 42:485, May 1928.
1265. Sutliff, W. D. Constitutional reactions immediately after injection of concentrated serum. J. Allergy, 1:156, Jan. 1930.
1266. Sutliff, W. D. Serum therapy in Type I lobar pneumonia. Commonhealth (Massachusetts Department of Public Health), 18:152, July–Aug.–Sept. 1931.
1267. Sutliff, W. D. Cases illustrating interpretation of positive blood cultures. M. Clin. North America, 15:1041, Jan. 1932.
1268. Sutliff, W. D., and Davies, J. A. V. Study of origin of naturally occurring immune bodies for pneumococci in infants. J. Immunol., 32:43, Jan. 1937.

1269. Sutliff, W. D., and Finland, M. Type I lobar pneumonia treated with concentrated pneumococcic antibody (Felton). Clinical course. J.A.M.A., 96:1465, May 2, 1931.
1270. Sutliff, W. D., and Finland, M. Antipneumococcic immunity reactions in individuals of different ages. J. Exper. Med., 55:837, June 1932.
1271. Sutliff, W. D., and Finland, M. The significance of the newly classified types in disease, Types IV to XX inclusive. Reprinted, with additions, from the J.A.M.A., 101:1289, Oct. 21, 1933.
1272. Sutliff, W. D., and Finland, M. Type I pneumococcic infections with especial reference to specific serum treatment. New England J. Med., 210:237, Feb. 1, 1934.
1273. Sutliff, W. D., Finland, M., and Hunnicutt, T. N. Direct comparison between specific and non-specific serum therapy for Type I lobar pneumonia. Arch. Int. Med., 51:435, Mar. 1933.
1274. Sutliff, W. D., and Rhoades, D. R. The pneumococcidal power of whole blood. I. Description of method. Results in individuals with no history of lobar pneumonia. J. Clin. Investigation, 9:43, Aug. 1930.
1275. Sutliff, W. D., and Rhoades, D. R. The pneumococcidal power of whole blood. II. Estimations in lobar pneumonia. J. Clin. Investigation, 9:55, Aug. 1930.
1276. Sutliff, W. D., and Steele, B. F. Relationship of infection to postoperative pulmonary complications. Arch. Surg., 30:14, Jan. 1935.
1277. Sutton, A. C., and Sevier, C. E. Study of bacteriaemia in lobar pneumonia. Bull. Johns Hopkins Hosp., 28:315, Oct. 1917.
1278. Sutton, D. C. Vaccine therapy in pneumonia. Preliminary report. Illinois M. J., 53:280, Apr. 1928.
1279. Sutton, D. C., Kendall, A. I., and Rosenblum, A. Clinical observations of the immunizing value of "natural bacterial antigens." I. Pneumococci. Am. J. M. Sc., 182:454, Oct. 1931.
1280. Swartout, H. O. Ante mortem and post mortem diagnoses. New England J. Med., 211:539, Sept. 20, 1934.
1281. Swift, E. V., and Smith, H. L. Complete heart block associated with pneumonia and peritonitis. Review of literature and report of case in which a lesion was demonstrated histologically. J.A.M.A., 109:2038, Dec. 18, 1937.
1282. Sydenstricker, V. P. W., and Sutton, A. C. Epidemiological study of lobar pneumonia. Bull. Johns Hopkins Hosp., 28:312, Oct. 1917.
1283. Szenti, J. Ueber die Optochinbehandlung der kruppösen Pneumonie im Kindesalter. Fortschr. d. Med., 45:403, Mar. 25, 1927.
1284. Tchistovitch, N. Études sur la pneumonie fibrineuse. Ann. Inst. Pasteur, 4:285, May 1890.
1285. Tchistovitch, N. Contribution à l'étude de la pathogénie de la crise dans la pneumonie fibrineuse. Ann. Inst. Pasteur, 18:304, May 1904.
1286. Tchistovitch, N., and Yourevitch, V. Sur les opsonines et les antiphagines dans l'infection pneumococcique. Ann. Inst. Pasteur, 22:611, July 1908.
1287. Tebbutt, A. H. On pneumococci in pneumonia in Sydney. M. J. Australia, 1:228, Mar. 19, 1921.
1288. Technicians trained for pneumonia control in Ohio (news item). J.A.M.A., 110:294, Jan. 22, 1938.

1289. Tenney, C. F., and Rivenburgh, W. T. Group of sixty-eight cases of Type I pneumonia occurring in thirty days at Camp Upton: with special reference to serum treatment. Arch. Int. Med., 24:545, Nov. 1919.
1290. Terrell, E. E. Changes in humoral immunity occurring during the early stages of experimental pneumococcus infection. Proc. Soc. Exper. Biol. & Med., 27:353, Feb. 1930.
1291. Terrell, E. E. Changes in humoral immunity occurring during the early stages of experimental pneumococcus infection. J. Exper. Med., 51:425, Mar. 1930.
1292. Terrell, E. E., Robertson, O. H., and Coggeshall, L. T. Experimental pneumococcus lobar pneumonia in the dog. I. Method of production and course of disease. J. Clin. Investigation, 12:393, Mar. 1933.
1293. Thjøtta, T. Pneumonia with pyemia due to leptothrix. (Abstract.) J.A.M.A., 101:1440, Oct. 28, 1933.
1294. Thjötta, T., and Hanneborg, O. Pneumonia death rate and types of pneumococci in Norway. J. Infect. Dis., 34:454, May 1924.
1295. Thomas, H. M. Pneumonia at Camp Meade, Maryland. J.A.M.A., 71: 1307, Oct. 19, 1918.
1296. Thomas, H. M., Jr. Recurrent Type I pneumonia: serum treatment of two attacks one month apart. Am. J. M. Sc., 161:103, Jan. 1921.
1297. Thomas, H. M., Jr., and O'Hara, D. Pneumococcus Type I vegetative endocarditis. Bull. Johns Hopkins Hosp., 31:417, Nov. 1920.
1298. Thomas, H. M., Jr., and Parker, F., Jr. Results of antemortem lung punctures in lobar pneumonia. Their bearing on the mechanism of crisis. Arch. Int. Med., 26:125, July 1920.
1299. Thomas, W. S. Type I pneumonia and its serum treatment. J.A.M.A., 77:2101, Dec. 31, 1921.
1300. Thompson, L. D., and Kelly, E. Pneumococcus serum to which heterophile antibody (Forssman) has been added. J.A.M.A., 106:324, Jan. 25, 1936.
1301. Thompson, L. R., Russell, A. E., Bloomfield, J. J., Brundage, D. K., Frasier, E. S., Dreessen, W. C., Goddard, J. C., and Britten, R. H. The health of workers in dusty trades. General statement and summary of findings. III. Exposure to dust in coal mining. IV. Exposure to dust in a textile plant. V. Exposure to the dusts of a silverware manufacturing plant. VI. Exposure to municipal dust (street cleaners in New York City). Washington, Government Printing Office, 1933, 37 p. (Public Health Bulletin No. 208.)
1302. Thompson, R. L. Electrophoresis of organisms belonging to pneumococcus group. Am. J. Hyg., 14:244, Sept. 1931.
1303. Thomsen, O., and Christensen, S. Contributions to the characterization of pneumococcus types. Acta med. Scandinav., 54:501, May 1921.
1304. Thomson, D., and Thomson, R. Influenza: with special reference to the complications and sequelae. Bacteriology of influenzal pneumonia, pathology, epidemiological data, prevention and treatment. Ann. Pickett-Thomson Research Lab., 10:641, May 1934.
1305. Thomson, St. C., and Hewlett, R. T. The fate of micro-organisms in inspired air. Lancet, 1:86, Jan. 11, 1896.
1306. Tilghman, R. C., and Finland, M. Pneumococcic infections in families. J. Clin. Investigation, 15:493, Sept. 1936.

1307. Tilghman, R. C., and Finland, M. Availability of specific pneumococcus antibody after intravenous, intramuscular, and subcutaneous injection, including study of the cutaneous reactions to type-specific polysaccharides following serum injection. J. Immunol., 31:239, Sept. 1936.

1308. Tilghman, R. C., and Finland, M. Clinical significance of bacteriemia in pneumococcic pneumonia. Arch. Int. Med., 59:602, Apr. 1937.

1309. Tillett, W. S. Studies on immunity to pneumococcus mucosus (Type III). III. Increased resistance to Type III infection induced in rabbits by immunization with R and S forms of pneumococcus. J. Exper. Med., 46: 343, Aug. 1927.

1310. Tillett, W. S. Active and passive immunity to pneumococcus infection induced in rabbits by immunization with R pneumococci. J. Exper. Med., 48:791, Dec. 1928.

1311. Tillett, W. S., and Francis, T., Jr. Cutaneous reactions to polysaccharides and proteins of pneumococcus in lobar pneumonia. J. Exper. Med., 50: 687, Nov. 1929.

1312. Tillett, W. S., and Francis, T., Jr. Serological reactions in pneumonia with a non-protein somatic fraction of pneumococcus. J. Exper. Med., 52: 561, Oct. 1930.

1313. Tillett, W. S., Goebel, W. F., and Avery, O. T. Chemical and immunological properties of a species-specific carbohydrate of pneumococci. J. Exper. Med., 52:895, Dec. 1930.

1314. Tomanek, E., and Wilson, E. B. Pneumonia in Pittsburgh. Proc. Am. Philosophical Society, 63:279, 1924.

1315. Tomanek, E., and Wilson, E. B. Is pneumonia increasing? Proc. Nat. Acad. Sc., 10:161, May 1924.

1316. Toomey, J. A. Infection and immunity (critical review). J. Pediat., 4: 529, Apr. 1934.

1317. Topley, W. W. C. Outline of immunity. Baltimore, Wm. Wood & Co., 1933, 415 p.

1318. Townsend, C. W. Acute lobar pneumonia in children. Arch. Pediat., 6: 148, Mar. 1889.

1319. Townsend, C. W., and Coolidge, A., Jr. Mortality of acute lobar pneumonia, from a study of all the cases of this disease treated at the Massachusetts General Hospital from the first case, in 1822, up to the present day. Tr. Am. Climatological Assn., 6:22, 1889.

1320. Townsend, J. G., and Sydenstricker, E. Epidemiological study of minor respiratory diseases: progress report II: based on records for families of medical officers of Army, Navy, and Public Health Service and of members of several university faculties. Pub. Health Rep., 42:99, Jan. 14, 1927.

1321. Trask, J. D., O'Donovan, C., Jr., Moore, D. M., and Beebe, A. R. Studies on pneumonia in children. I. Mortality, blood cultures, and humoral antibodies in pneumococcus pneumonia. J. Clin. Investigation, 8:623, June 1930.

1322. Treatment for empyema in infancy (editorial). Lancet, 2:783, Oct. 12, 1929.

1323. Trinidad and Tobago. Health conditions 1923. Administration report of Medical Inspector of Health for the year 1923. Laid before the Legislative Council on the 16th May, 1924. Port-of-Spain.

1324. Truesdale, P. E. Low pericardiotomy for acute suppurative pericarditis. New England J. Med., 208:671, Mar. 30, 1933.
1325. Tuft, L. Serum sensitiveness after toxin-antitoxin. Clinical and laboratory study. J. Allergy, 3:235, Mar. 1932.
1326. Tureen, L. L. Tularemic pneumonia. J.A.M.A., 99:1501, Oct. 29, 1932.
1327. Turkey: Office Central de Statistique. Annuaire statistique, 1934–35.
1328. Tuttle, W. M., and Cannon, P. R. Passage of bacteria from lungs into blood stream. J. Infect. Dis., 56:31, Jan.–Feb. 1935.
1329. Ude, W. H. Roentgenologic studies in early lobar pneumonia. Am. J. Roentgenol., 26:691, Nov. 1931.
1330. Ungermann, E., and Kandiba, L. Über quantitative Verhältnisse bei der Antikörperwirkung. Arb. a. d. k. Gsndhtsamte., 40:24, May 1912.
1331. United Fruit Company. Medical Department, 16th annual report, 1927, p. 22.
1332. United Fruit Company. Medical Department, 19th annual report, 1930.
1333. United Fruit Company. Medical Department, 20th annual report, 1931.
1334. United States Bureau of Animal Industry. Special report on diseases of the horse. Revised edition, 1923, pp. 113, 521. Washington, Government Printing Office, 1923.
1335. United States Bureau of the Census. Mortality statistics, 1920–1933. Annual reports, 21–34. Washington, Government Printing Office, 1922 1936.
1336. United States Bureau of the Census. Manual of the International List of Causes of Death: based on the fourth decennial revision by the International Commission, Paris, October 16 to 19, 1929. Washington, Government Printing Office, 1931. 342 p.
1337. United States Bureau of the Census. Fifteenth census of the United States, 1930. Population, v. 2, general report, statistics by subjects. Washington, Government Printing Office, 1933.
1338. United States Public Health Service. Potency of antimeningococcic and antipneumococcic serums. Pub. Health Rep., 34:2657, Nov. 21, 1919.
1339. United States Public Health Service. Regulations for the sale of viruses, serums, toxins, and analogous products. Approved February 25, 1935, U. S. Pub. Health Service, Miscellaneous Publication No. 10, U. S. Pub. Health Service Decision No. 7, Revision as of January 1, 1937, of section 63, paragraph 72.
1340. United States Public Health Service, Advisory Committee on Pneumonia (news item). J.A.M.A., 109:1997, Dec. 11, 1937.
1341. United States Public Health Service. Plan for pneumonia control studies. Health Officer, 2:606, Apr. 1938.
1342. United States Public Health Service. Special Report of Pneumonia Advisory Committee to Surgeon General, United States Public Health Service. J.A.M.A., 110:1701, May 14, 1938.
1343. United States Public Health Service. Pneumonia mortality and measures for prevention. Report of Advisory Committee on Prevention of Pneumonia Mortality. Pub. Health Rep., Supplement No. 142, 1938, 32 p.*

* The author is indebted to Dr. Thomas Parran, Surgeon General, United States Public Health Service, for permission to cite certain unpublished data assembled for this report.

1344. United States, Office of the Surgeon General. Medical Department of the United States Army in the World War. V. 14. Medical aspects of gas warfare; prepared under the direction of M. W. Ireland, by W. D. Bancroft and associates. Washington, Government Printing Office, 1926. *See also references 675b and 676.*

1345. United States, Office of the Surgeon General. Annual reports of the Surgeon General, U. S. Army, to the Secretary of War, 1926–1935. Washington, Government Printing Office, 1926–1935.

1346. Urquhart, A. L. Serological and morphological characteristics of the pneumococcus: An analysis of organisms isolated from 77 cases of pneumococcal infection. Lancet, 2:1313, Dec. 24, 1921.

1347. Valentine, E., McGuire, G., Whitney, E., and Falk, K. G. Studies on antibodies. III. Agglutinin and precipitin reactions of dried antipneumococcus preparations after storage under various conditions. J. Immunol., 21:221, Sept. 1931.

1348. Van Volkenburgh, V. A., and Frost, W. H. Acute minor respiratory diseases prevailing in group of families residing in Baltimore, Md., 1928–1930. Prevalence, distribution and clinical description of observed cases. Am. J. Hyg., 17:122, Jan. 1933.

1349. Vaucel, M., and Salaün, G. Contribution à l'étude du pneumocoque en Afrique Equatoriale Française. Bull. Soc. path. exot., 25:58, Jan. 1932.

1350. Vaughan, W. T. Type determination of pneumococcus infection: as practiced in the field with Avery's new cultural method. J.A.M.A., 70:431, Feb. 16, 1918.

1351. Vaughan, W. T., and Schnabel, T. G. Pneumonia and empyema at Camp Sevier. Arch. Int. Med., 22:440, Oct. 1918.

1352. Vaux, C. J. (1) Rules and regulations concerning quarantine of all patients with pneumonia of any form. Official publication of Department of Health of Pittsburgh. n.d. (2) Pneumonia from a public health point of view, with especial reference to pneumonia quarantine. J.A.M.A., 87:1980, Dec. 11, 1926.

1353. Viktorow, L. K., Semzowa, O. M., and Oettinger, I. G. Epidemiologie der kruppösen Pneumonie. I. Mitteilung: Die Bedeutung der Bazillenträger in der Epidemiologie der kruppösen Pneumonie. Zentralbl. f. Bakt. I. Abt. Orig., 131:162, Apr. 5, 1934. *Abstract in* Bull. Hyg., 9: 460, July 1934.

1354. Vinograd, J., Nemir, R. L., and Park, W. H. Rapid typing of pneumococci by Neufeld reaction directly from laryngeal swabs from infants and children. Am. J. Dis. Child., 51:792, Apr. 1936.

1355. Virginia Pneumonia Commission Report. Virginia M. Monthly, 64:406, Oct. 1937.

1356. Viswanathan, R. Treatment of pneumonia by artificial pneumothorax (letter to the editor). Lancet, 2:760, Oct. 1, 1932.

1357. Vitug, W., and Hizon, J. Statistical studies on pneumonia. J. Philippine Islands M. A., 8:461, Nov. 1928.

1358. Von Oettingen, W. F., Calhoun, O. V., Badertscher, V. A., and Pickett, R. E. Comparative studies on mercurochrome and other antiseptics (Council on Pharmacy and Chemistry of American Medical Association). J.A.M.A., 99:127, July 9, 1932.

1359. Von Sholly, A. I., and Park, W. H. Studies on acute respiratory infections. VII. Report on the prophylactic vaccination of 1536 persons against acute respiratory diseases, 1919–1920. J. Immunol., 6:103, Jan. 1921.
1360. Wadsworth, A. B. Agglutination of the pneumococcus with certain normal and immune sera. J. M. Research, 10:228, Oct. 1903.
1361. Wadsworth, A. B. Experimental studies on the etiology of acute pneumonitis. Am. J. M. Sc., 127:851, May 1904.
1362. Wadsworth, A. B. Studies on pneumococcus infection in animals. J. Exper. Med., 16:54, July 1912.
1363. Wadsworth, A. B. Studies on pneumococcus infection in animals. J. Exper. Med., 16:78, July 1912.
1364. Wadsworth, A. B. Experimental organizing pneumonia. J. M. Research, 39:147, Nov. 1918.
1365. Wadsworth, A. B. Review of recently published reports on the serum treatment of Type I pneumonia, together with a report of 445 additional cases. Am. J. Hyg., 4:119, Mar. 1924.
1366. Wadsworth, A. B. Recent advances in the serum therapy of pneumonia, meningitis, scarlet fever and other streptococcus infections. Tr. A. Am. Physicians, 47:161, 1932.
1367. Wadsworth, A. B. Serum therapy: Its value in pneumonia, meningitis, scarlet fever and other streptococcus infections. J.A.M.A., 99:204, July 16, 1932.
1368. Wadsworth, A. B. Practical limitations of vaccine and serum therapy. New England J. Med., 213:1285, Dec. 26, 1935.
1369. Wadsworth, A. B., and Brown, R. Chemical and immunological studies of the pneumococcus. I. Specific antigenic carbohydrate of Type I pneumococcus. J. Immunol., 21:245, Sept. 1931.
1370. Wadsworth, A. B., and Brown, R. Chemical and immunological studies of the pneumococcus. II. The ether-soluble fraction of Type I pneumococcus. J. Immunol., 21:255, Oct. 1931.
1371. Wadsworth, A. B., and Sickles, G. M. A study of pneumococci isolated from horses undergoing pneumococcus immunization. J. Exper. Med., 45:787, May 1927.
1372. Waldbott, G. L. Prevention of anaphylactic shock: with a study of nine fatal cases. J.A.M.A., 98:446, Feb. 6, 1932.
1373. Waldbott, G. L., and Snell, A. D. Pulmonary lesions resembling pneumonia as the result of allergic shock. J. Pediat., 6:229, Feb. 1935.
1374. Walker, E. L. Lobar pneumonia and its treatment. New Orleans M. & S. J., 84:369, Nov. 1931.
1375. Wallfield, M. J. Experimental vaccination against colds in an infants' home. J. Pediat., 10:69, Jan. 1937.
1376. Walravens, P. Etude sur le pneumocoque. Ann. Soc. belge de méd. trop., 1:241, 1920–21.
1377. Wámoscher, L. Infektionsversuche mit einzelnen Pneumokokken. Ztschr. f. Hyg. u. Infektionskr., 106:421, June 1926.
1378. Wang, T. T., and Van Allen, C. M. Concentration of congo-red in blood after absorption from pneumonic lung. Proc. Soc. Exper. Biol. & Med., 30:814, Mar. 1933.

1379. Ward, H. K. Observations on the phagocytosis of pneumococcus by human whole blood. I. Normal phagocytic titre and antiphagocytic effect of specific soluble substance. J. Exper. Med., 51:675, May 1930.
1380. Ward, H. K. Observations on the phagocytosis of pneumococcus by human whole blood. II. Neutralization of the antiphagocytic action of the specific soluble substance by antiserum. J. Exper. Med., 51:685, May 1930.
1381. Ward, H. K. Examination of mechanism of pneumococcus immunity by means of bactericidal measurements. I. Reaction between anticarbohydrate antibody and purified specific carbohydrate. J. Exper. Med., 55:511, Apr. 1932.
1382. Ward, H. K. Examination of mechanism of pneumococcus immunity by means of bactericidal measurements. II. Reaction between anticarbohydrate antibody and type-specific products of organism. J. Exper. Med., 55:519, Apr. 1932.
1383. Ward, H. K., and Enders, J. F. An analysis of the opsonic and tropic action of normal and immune sera based on experiments with the pneumococcus. J. Exper. Med., 57:527, Apr. 1933.
1384. Warfield, L. M. Treatment of circulatory failure. J.A.M.A., 106:892, Mar. 14, 1936.
1385. Warr, O. S., and Alperin, J. Lobar pneumonia. A report of 2039 cases. Ann. Int. Med., 6:1474, May 1933.
1386. Warwick, M. Pneumonia in newborn infants. Am. J. Path., 9:961, Nov. 1933.
1387. Warwick, M. Pneumonia in newborn and stillborn infants. New York State J. Med., 37:2075, Dec. 15, 1937.
1388. Washbourn, J. W. Experiments with the pneumococcus, with especial reference to immunity. J. Path. & Bact., 3:214, 1894–1895.
1389. Washbourn, J. W. Antipneumococcic serum. Brit. M. J., 1:510, Feb. 27, 1897.
1390. Watson, E. L., and Cooper, G. Production of infection with pneumococci in rabbits by intradermal inoculation of Type III pneumococci, treatment with specific antiserum, and comparison with Type I infections. J. Exper. Med., 52:849, Dec. 1930.
1391. Webster, L. T., and Clow, A. D. Association of pneumococcus, hemophilus influenzae and streptococcus hemolyticus with coryza, pharyngitis and sinusitis in man. J. Exper. Med., 55:445, Mar. 1932.
1392. Webster, L. T., and Clow, A. D. Intranasal virulence of pneumococci for mice. J. Exper. Med., 58:465, Oct. 1933.
1393. Webster, L. T., and Hughes, T. P. Epidemiology of pneumococcus infection. Incidence and spread of pneumococci in nasal passages and throats of healthy persons. J. Exper. Med., 53:535, Apr. 1931.
1394. Webster, R. Study of incidence of various serological types of pneumococci in pneumonia of childhood: observations on serum therapy. M. J. Australia, 1:129, Feb. 9, 1924.
1395. Webster, R. Note on mode of transmission of pneumococcal infection. M. J. Australia, 1:591, June 14, 1924.
1396. Weichselbaum, A. Ueber die Aetiologie der acuten Lungen- und Rippenfellentzündungen. Med. Jahrb., 3rd series, 1:483, 1886.

1397. Welch, A. D., Jr. Pharmacologic basis for sufanilamide therapy. J. Pediat., 11:159, Aug. 1937.

1398. Weld, J. T., and Gunther, A. Effect of anaerobically prepared pneumococcus autolysate toxin on mice and evaluation of pneumococcus autolysate antitoxin in mice. J. Exper. Med., 62:119, July 1935.

1399. Wells, E. F. Introduction to study of pneumonic fever. II. Epidemics. J.A.M.A., 12:258, Feb. 23, 1889.

1400. Wells, E. F. Introduction to study of pneumonic fever. III. Nature. J.A.M.A., 12:332, Mar. 9, 1889.

1401. Wells, E. F. Introduction to study of pneumonic fever. V. Geography. J.A.M.A., 12:582, Apr. 27, 1889.

1402. Wells, E. F. Introduction to study of pneumonic fever. VI. Prevalence and meteorology. J.A.M.A., 12:802, June 8, 1889.

1403. Wells, E. F. Introduction to study of pneumonic fever. VII. Prevalence. J.A.M.A., 12:869, June 22, 1889.

1404. Wells, E. F. The mortality and management of pneumonia. J.A.M.A., 43:866, Sept. 24, 1904.

1405. Wells, E. F. Prevalence and prophylaxis of pneumonia. J.A.M.A., 44:361, Feb. 4, 1905.

1406. Wells, H. G. The chemical aspects of immunity. 2nd Edition, New York, Chemical Catalog Co., Inc., 1929, 286 p. (American Chemical Society Monograph Series).

1407. Wells, J. R., and Heinbecker, P. Respiratory flora of Eskimos in remote northern regions. J. Infect. Dis., 50:281, Apr. 1932.

1408. Wells, W. F. Effect of polluted waters for purposes of humidification. *In* Massachusetts Department of Public Health, Annual Report, 1934, p. 166.

1409. Wells, W. F. On air-borne infection. II. Droplets and droplet nuclei. Am. J. Hyg., 20:611, Nov. 1934.

1410. Wells, W. F., and Stone, W. R. On air-borne infection. III. Viability of droplet nuclei infection. Am. J. Hyg., 20:619, Nov. 1934.

1411. Wells, W. F., and Wells, M. W. Air-borne infection. Reprinted with additions from the J.A.M.A., 107:1698, Nov. 21, 1936; and 107:1805, Nov. 28, 1936.

1412. Westlund, R. E. Incidence of pneumococcus types in pneumonias of children. J. Infect. Dis., 38:514, June 1926.

1413. Wetherbee, W., Jr., Foley, J. A., and Resnik, J. Diathermy in lobar pneumonia: preliminary report. New England J. Med., 213:796, Oct. 24, 1935.

1414. Whipple, A. O. A study of postoperative pneumonitis. Surg., Gynec. & Obst., 26:29, Jan. 1918.

1414a. Whitby, L. Chemotherapy of pneumococcal and other infections with 2-(*p*-aminobenzenesulphonamido) pyridine. Lancet, 1:1210, May 28, 1938.

1414b. Whitby, L. Chemotherapy of bacterial infections (Bradshaw Lecture). Lancet, 2:1095, Nov. 12, 1938.

1415. White, B. Personal communication, 1938.

1416. White, B. Antipneumococcic serum. Commonhealth (Massachusetts Department of Public Health), 18:164, July–Aug.–Sept. 1931.

1417. White, B., with the collaboration of Robinson, E. S., and Barnes, L. A. The biology of pneumococcus. The bacteriological, biochemical, and immunological characters and activities of diplococcus pneumoniae. New York, The Commonwealth Fund, 1937, 799 p.
1418. White, P. D. Heart disease, p. 275 and 375. New York, The Macmillan Co., 1931.
1419. Whitehead, N. T. Some investigations on thirty-five cases of pneumonia in Khartoum. J. Roy. Army M. Corps, 49:440, Dec. 1927.
1420. Whitney, J. S. Death rates by occupation. Based on data of the United States Census Bureau, 1930. New York, National Tuberculosis Association, 1934, 32 p.
1421. Whittle, C. H. Virulence of pneumococci in pneumonia. Brit. M. J., 2: 134, July 23, 1927.
1422. Whittle, C. H. Relation of virulence in pneumococci to disease, with comparison of virulence of different types of pneumococci in various pathological conditions. J. Hyg., 27:412, June 1928.
1423. Williams, C. S. Serum treatment of pneumonia. New Zealand M. J., 23:56, Feb. 1924.
1424. Williams, W. R. Twenty-three cases of pneumonia treated with antipneumococcus serum. Arch. Int. Med., 13:978, June 1914.
1425. Wilson, E. B. Some statistical aspects of pneumonia. Am. J. Pub. Health, 14:931, Nov. 1924.
1426. Wilson, G., and Hadden, S. B. Neuritis and multiple neuritis following serum therapy. J.A.M.A., 98:123, Jan. 9, 1932.
1427. Wilson, J. R., Wyatt, T. C., Bennett, J., Chapman, O. D., and Knowlton, C. Serum sickness. Clinical and experimental study. Preliminary report. New York State J. Med., 34:915, Nov. 1, 1934.
1428. Winchester, J. W. Observations on incidence of lobar pneumonia among Tamils and Chinese in Malaya. Malayan M. J., 4:75, June 1929.
1429. Winkler, A. W., and Finland, M. Antibody response to infections with the newly classified types of pneumococci (Cooper). J. Clin. Investigation, 13:109, Jan. 1934.
1430. Winslow, C.-E. A., and Greenburg, L. Vasomotor reactions to localized drafts. Am. J. Hyg., 15:1, Jan. 1932.
1431. Winslow, C.-E. A., Greenburg, L., and Herrington, L. P. The influence of heat and light upon nasal obstruction. Am. J. Hyg., 20:195, July 1934.
1432. Winternitz, M. C., and Kline, B. S. Studies upon experimental pneumonia in rabbits. IX. The part of the leucocyte in the immunity reaction. J. Exper. Med., 21:320, Apr. 1915.
1433. Winternitz, M. C., Smith, G. H., and Robinson, E. S. An unrecognized pathway for bacterial invasion of the respiratory tract. Bull. Johns Hopkins Hosp., 31:63, Mar. 1920.
1434. Wittes, S. A., and Bullowa, J. G. M. Gastric aspiration in children with pneumonia to obtain material for pneumococcus typing. Am. J. Dis. Child., 50:1404, Dec. 1935.
1435. Wollstein, M. Types of pneumococci found in pneumonia of infants and young children. New York State J. Med., 23:148, Apr. 1923.
1436. Wollstein, M., and Benson, A. W. Types of pneumococcus found in

pneumonias of infants and young children. Am. J. Dis. Child., 12:254, Sept. 1916.

1437. Wollstein, M., and Meltzer, S. J. Pneumonic lesions made by intrabronchial insufflation of non-virulent pneumococci. J. Exper. Med., 17:353, Mar. 1913.

1438. Wollstein, M., and Meltzer, S. J. The reaction of the lungs to the intrabronchial insufflation of killed virulent pneumococci and of plain sterile bouillon. J. Exper. Med., 17:424, Apr. 1913.

1439. Woo, S. T. Studies on pneumococcus growth inhibition. V. Relation of virulence to the pneumococcidal activity of normal rabbit serum-leucocyte mixtures. J. Exper. Med., 43:623, May 1926.

1440. Wood, F. C. Viability of the pneumococcus after drying: study of one of the factors in pneumonic infection. J. Exper. Med., 7:592, Aug. 1905.

1441. Woodford, L. G. Diagnosis and treatment of lobar pneumonia: a review of recent advances. Northwest Med., 32:97, Mar. 1933.

1442. Wright, A. E., and Douglas, S. R. An experimental investigation of the *rôle* of the blood fluids in connection with phagocytosis. Proc. Royal Soc. London, 72:357, July 29, 1903.

1443. Wright, A. E., and Douglas, S. R. Further observations on the *rôle* of the blood fluids in connection with phagocytosis. Proc. Royal Soc. London, 73:128, Mar. 7, 1904.

1444. Wright, A. E., and Douglas, S. R. On the action exerted upon the *Staphylococcus pyogenes* by human blood fluids, and on the elaboration of protective elements in the human organism in response to inoculations of a staphylococcus vaccine. Proc. Royal Soc. London, 74:147, Sept. 28, 1904.

1445. Wright, A. E., Morgan, W. P., Colebrook, L., and Dodgson, R. W. Observations on the pharmaco-therapy of pneumococcus infections. Lancet, 2:1633, Dec. 14, 1912.

1446. Wright, A. E., Morgan, W. P., Colebrook, L., and Dodgson, R. W. Observations on the pharmaco-therapy of pneumococcus infections. Lancet, 2:1701, Dec. 21, 1912.

1447. Wright, A. E., Morgan, W. P., Colebrook, L., and Dodgson, R. W. Observations on prophylactic inoculation against pneumococcus infections, and on the results which have been achieved by it. Lancet, 1:1, Jan. 3, 1914, and 1:87, Jan. 10, 1914.

1448. Wright, H. D. Experimental pneumococcal septicaemia and anti-pneumococcal immunity. J. Path. & Bact., 30:185, Apr. 1927.

1449. Wright, S. Applied physiology. London, Oxford University Press, 1926, 418 p.; 4th edition, 1931, 552 p.

1450. Wu, C. J., and Chiu, T. Y. Pneumococcal lobar pneumonia. Clinical study of 242 typed cases. China M. J., 47:545, June 1933.

1451. Wu, C. J., and Sia, R. H. P. Simplified technique for study of pneumococcus growth inhibition. Proc. Soc. Exper. Biol. & Med., 29:786, Apr. 1932.

1452. Wyckoff, J., DuBois, E. F., and Woodruff, I. O. Therapeutic value of digitalis in pneumonia. J.A.M.A., 95:1243, Oct. 25, 1930.

1453. Wynn, W. H. The vaccine treatment of acute pneumonia. Brit. M. J., 2:480, Sept. 17, 1927.

1454. Yens, D. S. Nursing care of the pneumonia patient. Am. J. Nursing, 34: 106, Feb. 1934.
1455. Yens, O. C. Pneumonia. Am. J. Nursing, 34:101, Feb. 1934.
1456. Young, F. Peripheral nerve paralyses following the use of various serums: report of a case and review of the literature. J.A.M.A., 98:1139, Apr. 2, 1932.
1457. Yule, G. U. An introduction to the theory of statistics, p. 269. 2nd Edition, London, Chas. Griffin & Co., Ltd., 1912.
1458. Zander. Ausgedehnte Endemie von Lungenentzündungen durch Infektion mit Friedländerschen Pneumobazillen unter Zivilarbeitern. Deutsche med. Wchnschr., 45:1180, Oct. 23, 1919.
1459. Ziegler, E. E. Specific effect of bile salts on pneumococci and on pneumococcus pneumonia. Arch. Int. Med., 46:644, Oct. 1930.
1460. Zinsser, H. Essential identity of the antibodies. J. Immunol., 6:289, Sept. 1921.
1461. Zinsser, H. The study of immunity in its relation to the problem of practical medicine (Shattuck Lecture). Boston M. & S. J., 192:1191, June 18, 1925.
1462. Zinsser, H. Immunological consideration of pneumonia and a discussion of the rational basis for vaccine therapy. New England J. Med., 200: 853, Apr. 25, 1929.
1463. Zinsser, H., and Grinnell, F. B. Further studies on bacterial allergy: the antigen involved in pneumococcus allergy. J. Bact., 14:301, Nov. 1927.
1464. Zinsser, H., and Mallory, T. B. Observations on bacterial anaphylaxis with pneumococcus. J. Immunol., 9:75, Mar. 1924.
1465. Zinsser, H., and Parker, J. T. Further studies on bacterial hypersusceptibility. II. J. Exper. Med., 37:275, Feb. 1923.
1466. Zolov, B. Transient hemiplegia accompanying lobar pneumonia. New England J. Med., 216:206, Feb. 4, 1937.
1467. Zozaya, J. Fermentation of "Levan" by pneumococci. Proc. Soc. Exper. Biol. & Med., 29:26, Oct. 1931.
1468. Zozaya, J., Boyer, J., and Clark, J. Standardization of antipneumococcic serum Types I and II. J. Exper. Med., 52:471, Oct. 1930.
1469. Zozaya, J., and Clark, J. Active immunization in human cases with polysaccharide of pneumococcus Type I. Proc. Soc. Exper. Biol. & Med., 30: 44, Oct. 1932.
1470. Zozaya, J., and Clark, J. Active immunization of mice with the polysaccharides of pneumococci Types I, II, and III. J. Exper. Med., 57:21, Jan. 1933.
1471. Zozaya, J., and Medina, L. Immunological reactions between agar-agar and some bacterial antisera. J. Exper. Med., 57:41, Jan. 1933.

INDEX

A substance, 117
Abortive pneumonia, 511, 512
Abscesses, 3, 10, 505, 593, 603, 604
  lung. *See* Lung abscess
Acetyl polysaccharide, 22, 117
Acidosis, 500
  alkali treatment, and, 768
Actinomycosis, and pneumonia, 17
Active immunity. *See* Immunity, pneumococcus, acquired; Immunization, active; Immunization, active, against pneumonia
Age:
  allergy to pneumococcus, and, 241
  antibody response, in pneumonia, and, 515, 731
  antibody response, variations in acquired immunity, 177, 187
  antibody titer, variations in natural immunity, 186–192
  bacteriemia, and, 515, 557, 558, 580
  cellular response to infection, variations with, 177, 178
  colds, incidence, and, 237, 238
  complications, and, 515, 549
  crisis and lysis, relation to, 529
  death, and, 305, 306
  death rates, and, 274, 301–305, 310–312
  differential diagnosis, and, 648
  empyema, and, 515, 571, 572
  fatality rates, and, 702–710
  fatality rates, digitalis treatment, and, 751, 752
  fever, duration, and, 492
  heart rate, abnormalities, and, 495
  immunity, acquired, weight, and, 178, 179
  immunity, and, 129, 186–192, 557
  incidence of pneumonia, and, 299–307
  lesion developed, nature of, and, 513–515
  leucocytosis, variation of, and, 497
  necropsy studies, and, 91
  pneumococcus carrier rate, influence of, and, 373, 377
  prognosis, and, 703–710
  prognosis, in Type III cases, and, 669
  prognosis, with alcoholism, and, 718, 719
  prognosis, with cardiovascular disease, and, 702
  prognosis, with empyema, and, 579, 580
  recovery, limited by, 737
  resolution, and, 540
  resolution, delayed, and, 515, 543
Age (*cont.*):
  respiratory infections, minor, incidence of, and, 237, 238
  serum dosage, and, 850, 856
  serum dosage with bacteriemia, and, 916
  serum sickness, incidence variations, and, 870
  serum treatment, and, 835
  serum treatment, results:
    and advanced age, 919
    and variation of fatality rate, 907–911
    by age and bacteriemia, 915, 916
  type incidence in pneumonia, and, 60–64, 74–89, 616, 617
  type incidence in pneumonia, by sex and, 66, 67
  Type I and II lobar pneumonia, average age in, 62, 63
Agglutinins. *See under* Antibody(ies), pneumococcus
Air-borne infection, 295–297
Alcohol(ism):
  delirium, and prognosis, 727
  delirium tremens, and, 504
  Friedländer's bacillus pneumonia, and, 7
  host resistance, depression of, and, 157, 158, 203, 217, 333, 334
  incidence of pneumonia, and, 327, 333, 334
  predisposing factors, and, 333, 334
  prevention, and, 398
  prognosis, and, 702, 718, 719, 727
  serum treatment, results, and, 919
  treatment of pneumonia with, 754, 759
Allergic reactions:
  after horse serum, 836, 864–867
  after rabbit serum, 875, 878
  prevention with adrenalin, 838, 841
  prevention with atropine, 841
Allergy, pneumococcus:
  acquired, 184, 185
  age variations, 241
  animals, normal, sensitized, immunized, and after infection, and, 241–245
  antibody, immobilizing action of, and, 123
  antibody, and, 182–184
  colds, and, 241, 245
  crisis, and, 528
  immunity, and, 182–185
  lobar pneumonia, and, 240–245
  meningitis, and, 594, 595
  natural, 184, 185

Allergy, pneumococcus (*cont.*):
- recurrence, and, 538, 539
- repeated attacks in animals, and, 242, 243
- skin tests for immunity, and, 126, 127
- skin tests for, with pneumococcus products, 182–185, 241–245
- spread of lesion, and edema fluid, 254

Allergy, serum reactions, and, 836–842, 875, 878

American Drug Manufacturers Association, 828

American Medical Association:
- Council on Pharmacy and Chemistry, 820, 827
- survey of typing facilities in United States hospitals, 931

Amino compounds, treatment with, 783–790

p-Aminobenzenesulfonamide. *See* Chemotherapy, sulfanilamide

2-(*p*-Aminobenzenesulphonamido)-pyridine. *See* Chemotherapy, sulfapyridine

Anaphylactic reactions:
- after horse serum, 836, 864–867
- after rabbit serum, 875, 878
- in animals sensitized with SSS, 134, 173, 182, 184

Anemia, during course of pneumonia, 498, 499

Anesthesia pneumonia, 519, 520, 524

Angioneurotic edema, importance of history of, 838, 842

Animal parasites, and pneumonia, 17

Animals:
- experimental infections. *See* Experimental infections
- immunity, natural, 27, 120, 121, 137–143, 186
- immunity, natural, specificity, 135
- immunity, non-specific, 136
- immunity, variations with breed, 120, 158, 177, 186
- immunization:
  - against contact infection, 214, 446
  - against pneumonia, 440–446
  - immunity, and, 196–198
  - response, duration of, 437–440
  - response, factors affecting, 412–425, 429–434
  - response, time of appearance, 434–437
  - with SSS and related agents, 28, 134, 198, 412, 414, 415, 417, 418, 429–431
- pneumonia, experimental. *See* Experimental pneumonia
- pneumonia, spontaneous in horses, 142

Animals (*cont.*):
- pneumonia, spontaneous in monkeys, 244, 316, 387

Anoxemia:
- cyanosis, and, 496, 499, 761, 762
- death, and, 545, 546, 761
- during course of pneumonia, 499, 760–762
- morphine in treatment, and, 755
- prognosis, and, 726, 761
- symptoms and altitude, and, 717

Anthracosis:
- as factor in organizing pneumonia, 101, 544
- incidence of pneumonia, and, 338, 340

Anti-SSS antibody, 117, 134, 137

Antibody(ies):
- causative agent in pneumonia determined by studies of, 11, 14–16, 50
- in Friedländer's bacillus cases, 6
- in mixed infections, 11, 12, 14, 16
- in streptococcus cases, 5

Antibody(ies), heterophile. *See* Heterophile antibody

Antibody(ies), influenza virus, failure to find after pneumococcus pneumonia, 237

Antibody(ies), pneumococcus:
- abortive pneumonia, and, 511
- actions, 27, 28, 114–125, 171, 172, 832, 885, 886
  - agglutination, 115, 116
  - antitoxic, 124, 125
  - bactericidal, 117–120, 171, 172
  - biologic changes in organism produced by, 123, 124
  - complement-fixing, 120, 124, 172
  - curative, 120, 121, 168, 169, 174–177
  - extraction of phospholipins, and, 173
  - horse and rabbit antibody, 172, 173
  - immobilizing and localizing, 122, 123, 164
  - in infected animals, 169
  - opsonic or tropic, 116–120
  - precipitins, and, 116
  - protective, 120, 121, 168
  - reaction with surface antigen of cell, 115
  - relative importance, 172
  - SSS and, 25, 121, 122, 131, 132
  - sensitization of organisms, 116, 117, 152, 162, 172
  - unity of, 136, 137
- age and antibody response, 177, 187, 515, 731
- age and variations in natural antibody, 186–192
- agglutinins, 115, 116

Antibody(ies), pneumococcus (*cont.*):
allergy to organism, and, 182–184
antagonistic substances, 131, 132, 256
anti-protein, 25, 134, 166
anti-SSS, 117, 134, 137
antitoxins, and immunity, 124, 125, 128
bactericidal:
effect of heat on, 116–120
effect of SSS on, 116–120
sensitivity of test for, 127
bacteriemia, effect of acquired antibody on, 169, 175, 176, 561, 563, 732, 832, 881, 885, 886, 902, 903
bacteriemia, relation of natural antibody to, 153, 154
blood-clearing mechanism, and acquired antibody, 163, 169, 175, 885, 886
C substance precipitins, and immunity, 125, 128, 129
causative agent in pneumonia, determined by studies of, 11, 14–16, 50
complications, effect of acquired antibody on occurrence, 176, 732, 887, 888
concentration methods, 808, 809, 825
course and outcome of infection, relation of acquired antibody to, 173–177
course and outcome of infection, relation of natural antibody to, 153, 154
course, appearance during, 125, 160, 161, 174–177, 584, 729–733
curative power of acquired antibody, 121, 168, 169, 174–177, 806, 832, 833
death of organism, and, 117–120, 124, 151, 152, 162, 172
death, relation of acquired antibody to, 174–177, 733, 919
formation, mode of, 155–157
formation, site of, 136, 137
globulins, and, 825
growth changes in pneumococcus, and, 123, 124
heterophile, and immunity, 125, 128
horse and rabbit, compared, 172, 173
immunity:
correlation with, 127–131
cross, and, 135, 136
natural, correlation with, 128–131, 137, 138, 143, 150–155
physiologic variables and acquired antibody, 178
relation of acquired antibody to, 168–171, 178
immunization, appearance after, 159–162, 196–199, 408–440
in animals, natural, 137–143

Antibody(ies), pneumococcus (*cont.*):
in infants, natural, 147, 187–192
in man, natural, 143–150
in susceptible animals, for strains of low virulence, 139
incidence of pneumonia, and natural antibody, 154, 155
infections, experimental, appearance in, 160, 181, 205, 218
integrity of organism, and, 28, 133, 134, 136, 198, 414
macrophage reaction in recovery, relation to, 736
meningitis, experimental, appearance after, 596
nature of, in immune serum, 137
nature of, need for further study, 925
nucleoprotein antibody, 25, 134, 166
opsonins, 116–120
effect of heat on, 116–120
effect of SSS on, 117–119
natural immunity, and, 151–154
pneumococcus carrier rate, and antibody in convalescence, 378
pneumococcus carriers, antibody production, and, 156, 157, 200, 201
pneumonia, appearance of, in recovery from, 160, 161, 174–176, 729–733
pneumonia in children, appearance of, during course, 177, 515, 731
pneumonia, occurrence in presence of antibody, 129, 153–155, 234, 511
pneumonia, post-operative, and natural antibody, 517
pneumonia, post-operative, appearance during, 522
precipitins, 116
protective substance and tests, 120, 121, 168, 179, 180, 826–828
recovery, and:
absence in, 174, 730, 732
amount at, 177, 515, 730, 731
appearance in, 14, 16, 160, 161, 174–176, 181, 729–733
appearance in pleural fluid during, 566
bronchopneumonia, appearance in, 68
duration in blood after, 537, 737–740
heterologous antibody in, 731, 739
heterophile antibody, and, 125, 733, 734, 820
relation of acquired antibody to, 173–177, 732
resolution, relation to, 542, 887
respiratory infections, minor, antibody variations caused by, 199, 200

Antibody(ies), pneumococcus (*cont.*):
respiratory infections, minor, appearance during, 157
SSS:
antibody and, in blood, 122
effect on antibody in serum treatment, 175, 885
excretion in urine, and, 122, 695
immunization with, and antibody appearance in animals, 134, 198, 412, 415, 417, 430, 431
immunization with, and antibody appearance in man, 198, 199, 415, 418, 431, 432, 474
neutralization of antibody by, 25, 131, 132
skin tests with, and acquired antibody, 126, 127, 166, 167, 170, 171, 738–740, 813, 847, 860, 861
sensitization of organisms, and, 116, 117, 152, 162, 172
serum treatment:
agglutinin reaction as guide to dosage, 861, 862
appearance in blood after, 175, 843, 844, 881, 885, 886
appearance in pleural fluid after rabbit antiserum, 918
disappearance from blood after, 175, 885
persistence in blood after, 739, 740
routes of, and antibody appearance, 843, 844
size, 173
skin sensitivity to pneumococcus products, and acquired antibody, 166, 167
skin tests for immunity, correlation with, 126, 127
species-specific, immunity, and, 25, 133–135, 155
species-specific, recovery, and, 125, 135, 166, 733, 734
specificity of acquired antibody, 50
specificity of natural antibody, 135
spread of lesion, effect on, 153, 154, 174–177, 570, 732, 881, 883, 886–888
tests for antibody nitrogen, and, 874, 875
tests for natural antibody, correlation between, 148, 149
tests for, sensitivity of, 127, 130
time, variations of acquired antibody with, 194, 195, 437–440
time, variations of natural antibody with, 195, 196
toxemia, and, 732
type, and antibody response, 161, 162, 432–434, 730, 731

Antibody(ies), pneumococcus (*cont.*):
type-specific, and immunity, 134, 135
unitarian conception, 137
unusual findings with natural antibody of pig, 141, 142
utilization of, factors in, 178–180
vaccine treatment, appearance after, 797–799, 804
virulence variations of organism, and, 27, 28
Antigenic relationship of pneumococcus types to pneumonia, 50, 68, 69
Antigenicity, pneumococcus, 27, 28, 125, 133, 134
C substance, and, 135
character of agent used for immunization, and, 24, 25, 27, 28, 410–415
condition of organism for optimum response, 28, 133, 410, 411
disrupted organisms, and, 28, 133, 134, 198, 414
early studies of, 807
intact organisms, and, 28, 133, 134, 136, 412–414
live organisms, and, 196, 197, 411, 442
nucleoprotein, and, 24, 25, 28, 133, 134
R forms, and, 133, 136
SSS, and. *See* Specific capsular polysaccharide(s), antigenicity
serum treatment, effect on, 167, 537, 739
type, and, 161, 162, 432–434, 730, 731
virulence, and, 27, 28
Apical pneumonia, 111, 510, 511
cough, and, 501
delirium, and, 504
pain at onset, 489
prognosis, 511, 698
Appendicitis, differentiation of lobar pneumonia from, 654
Arthritis, septic, 598–600
diagnosis, 599, 600
treatment, 600
Aspiration pneumonia, 340–342, 514
Asthma, horse, importance of history, 837, 842
Asthma, importance of history, 837, 838, 842, 865
Asthmatic attack:
after serum, as contraindication to further treatment, 842, 867, 878
in allergic reaction, 864, 878
Atelectasis:
complicating pneumonia, 252, 493, 525, 649

Atelectasis (*cont.*):
differentiation of lobar pneumonia from, 651
experimental pneumonia, and, 230, 250–253
heart displacement, and, 493, 525, 651
massive, in pneumonia, 252, 525
massive pneumonia, and, 512
nursing care, and, 745
pathogenesis, and, 250–253
physical signs with, 518, 649, 651
pneumothorax treatment, and, 769–772
post-operative pneumonia, and, 252, 515–520, 523, 524
sputum in, 651
symptoms, and, 651
x-ray findings, and, 250–253, 493, 651
Atypical pneumonia. *See* Bronchopneumonia
Avery broth, 636
Azo dyes, treatment with, 783–790

Bacillus Friedländeri. See Friedländer's bacillus
Bacillus influenzae. See Influenza bacillus
Bacillus mallei in bronchopneumonia, 68
Bactericidal antibody. *See under* Antibody (ies), pneumococcus
Bacteriemia, 549–563
abscesses, and, 603
alcohol and, in experimental infections, 333
antibody, acquired, effect on, 169, 175, 176, 561, 563, 732, 832, 881, 885, 886, 902, 903
antibody, natural relation to, 153, 154
arthritis, septic, and, 599
blood-clearing mechanism, and, 162–164, 548, 561
blood cultures, frequency of, and, 550
complications, and, 549, 560, 561
death, and, 544, 545, 560–562, 690
diagnostic importance, 50
empyema, and, 567, 570, 578
empyema incidence, and, 560, 561, 887
endocarditis, and, 591, 592
experimental infections, and, 205, 212–231, 549
Friedländer's bacillus cases, 7
Group IV cases, 553, 554, 556
immunity variations with age, and, 557
incidence, 549–560
incidence variations:
age, and, 515, 557–559, 580
duration of illness, and, 559–561
factors affecting, 555–560

Bacteriemia (*cont.*):
incidence variations (*cont.*):
mixed infections, and, 560
season and year, and, 559
site of lesion, and, 559
infants and children, 515, 557, 558, 580
and adults, compared, 557
prognosis, and, 693
results of serum treatment, and, 907–909, 914, 915
influenza bacillus cases, 9
intensity, and duration of illness, 560, 561
leucocyte count, and, 724
lobar pneumonia, 549–563
lobar pneumonia and bronchopneumonia together, 50, 551–556
Massachusetts Pneumonia Series, 551–554, 557–561
mixed infections, and, 14, 560
pericarditis, and, 560, 561
pneumococcus carriers in animals, and, 156
pneumococcus cases, 50, 549–563
pregnancy, and, 713
prevention of, 563
prognosis, and, 681–693, 886
prognosis, with or without cyanosis, and, 726
recovering cases, and, 561, 562
recurrence, and, 536, 538, 539
SSS, and extent of, 731, 732
septicaemia, and, 561, 562
staphylococcus cases, 10
streptococcus cases, 4
treatment, 562, 563
enzyme, of experimental Type III infections, and, 792–794
glucose therapy and toxemia, 768
non-specific, and, 821, 822
optochin, 563, 780
pneumothorax, and, 771
serum, bacteriemia as cause of failure, 919
serum, dosage and intervals between, 898, 899, 902
serum, dosage, influence on, 850, 851, 855, 856, 858, 886, 916
serum, effect on, 169, 175, 176, 562, 563, 832, 881, 885, 886, 902, 903
serum, effect on incidence of empyema, 887
serum, fatality rates with or without bacteriemia, 898, 899, 912–916
serum, in infants and children, 835, 909
serum, results and length of treatment, 898, 899, 902, 903

Bacteriemia (*cont.*):
  treatment (*cont.*):
    serum, results by age groups in presence or absence of, 915, 916
    serum, results compared with untreated cases, 912–915
    serum, results in infants and children, Type XIV, 907–909, 914, 915
    serum, routes of, 843, 844
    sulfanilamide, 563, 784–786
    sulfapyridine, 787–789
    with or without digitalis, fatality rates, and, 751, 752
  tympanites, association with, 756
  Type I, 551, 552, 556
  Type I, by age group, 558, 559
  Type I, septic complications, and, 560, 561
  Type I, II, III, and Group IV, compared, 554
  Type I–XXXII, 555, 556
  Type II, 552, 556
  Type II, by age group, 558, 559
  Type III, 552, 553, 556, 561
  Type IV, 555, 556
  Type IV–XXXII, 556
  Type V, 554, 556
  Type V, by age group, 558, 559
  Type VII, 554, 555, 556
  Type VIII, 555, 556, 561
  Type XIV, 555, 556
  types, failure of certain ones to cause, 50, 553, 556
  urogenital infection, and, 604
Bacteriologic study, 50, 614–645
  arthritis, septic, 600
  blood cultures, 641, 642
  causal relation of pneumococcus types to pneumonia, 49–51, 67, 68
  collection of specimens for, 617–620
  differential diagnosis, and, 614
  double infections, 11–16
  early investigations, xiii, xiv
  empyema, 577, 582
  epidemics in families, and, 388
  facilities for, in United States hospitals, 931
  Friedländer's bacillus, 6
  gastric aspiration, technic, 618
  importance, 615, 616, 834
  Krumwiede test for Friedländer's bacillus, 6
  laryngeal cultures, 642
  lung puncture, technic and complications, 619
  lung puncture material, 11, 14, 15, 50, 619, 620, 644
  lung puncture material, at necropsy, 734
Bacteriologic study (*cont.*):
  lung puncture material, at recovery, 528, 734, 735
  Massachusetts Pneumonia Study, and, 54–56, 622, 937
  meningitis, 595
  mixed infections, 11–16
  Neufeld test for Friedländer's bacillus, 6
  organisms, mixed, in sputum, and, 12, 13
  pathologic exudates, 644
  peritonitis, septic, 602, 603
  pleural fluids, 643, 644
  pneumococcus typing. *See* Pneumococcus typing
  pneumonia programs, and facilities for, 932–934
  post-operative pneumonia, 522–524
  prevention of pneumonia, and, 400, 453–468, 471, 473–476
  pus, 644
  routine procedures, 614, 615
  serum treatment, failure of, due to errors in, 860, 920
  spinal fluids, 644, 645
  sputum, 620–637, 639–641
  throat cultures, 14, 642, 643
  type incidence, 42–89
    bronchopneumonia, 67–74
    bronchopneumonia in infants and children, 84–89
    lobar and bronchopneumonia together, 51–57, 71–79
    lobar pneumonia, 42–54, 89
    lobar pneumonia in infants and children, 79–84
    pneumonia in infants and children, 74–89
  types, commonest in Massachusetts, by season, 381–385
  types, found at necropsy, 51
  types, in sputum, significance, 12, 49–51, 623, 624
  typing methods. *See* Pneumococcus typing
  United States, facilities for, in hospitals, 931
Bile and bile salts:
  dissolution of pneumococci by, 20, 21
  organisms insoluble in bile, 21
  treatment with bile salts, 783
Biology of Pneumococcus, The, 19, 114
Blood:
  antibody, appearance in, after serum treatment, 175, 843, 844, 881, 885, 886
  antibody, disappearance from, after serum treatment, 175, 885
  antibody, persistence in, after serum treatment, 739, 740

Blood (*cont.*):
changes in, 497–500, 759–762
coagulation time, 499
hemoproteose, for treatment, 773–775
oxygen and carbon-dioxide content, 499, 759–762
platelets, 499
pneumococcus growth in media, and, 20
pneumococcus in. *See* Bacteriemia
pressure, during course, 496
pressure, prognosis, and, 722, 723
SSS in, during course, 26, 131, 497
SSS in, during serum treatment, 122
sulfanilamide levels in, 784
sulfapyridine levels in, 787–789
treatment with:
blood from convalescent patients, 773
human immune blood, 813, 814
intrapulmonary blood, 773
transfusion in staphylococcus cases, 11
transfusion in streptococcus cases, 5
Blood-clearing mechanism:
immunity, and, 162–164, 167–169, 885, 886
serum treatment, and increased efficiency of, 163, 169, 175, 886
Blood cultures:
agar pour plates, and, 20, 550
amount of blood needed, 618
at death, 560–562
bacteriemia, and repetition of, 550
bacteriologic study, 641, 642
equipment for, and pneumonia programs, 855, 934
equipment for, in home treated cases, 618, 619, 854, 855
equipment for, in hospitalized cases, 618, 855
examination of, routine, 614, 615, 624
importance in serum treatment, 855, 856, 858
Massachusetts Pneumonia Series, and, 619, 855
prior to serum treatment, 856, 857, 862, 863
typing of, 641, 642
See also Bacteriemia
Bronchiectasis:
complicating empyema, 584
Friedländer's bacillus, and, 6
influenza bacillus pneumonia, and, 9
organized lesions, and, 543, 544
Bronchitis:
associated lesion at necropsy, 112
capillary, and bronchopneumonia, xv
Bronchitis (*cont.*):
death rates, trend, 284–286
in lobar pneumonia, 112
incidence peaks, with minor respiratory infections, 293–295
post-operative pneumonia, and, 515–519
predisposing factors, and, 235, 236
rales with, and differentiation of consolidation from, 509
Type III, and, 112
Bronchopneumonia:
aspiration of noxious substances, and, 340, 341
associated lesion in lobar pneumonia, 111
atelectasis during, 252, 493, 525, 649
bacteriologic study, 67–74, 614–645
capillary bronchitis, and, xv
causative organisms, xiii, 2–17, 67–74
causative organisms, in infants and children, 84–89
causative organisms unknown, 16
chronic disease, and, 513
colds, and, 339
colds, frequency after, 238
complications, 566, 568, 569, 571, 575
confluent, differentiation of lobar pneumonia from, xiii, 649
confluent, in Friedländer's bacillus cases, 7
confluent, in staphylococcus cases, 10
death in, 544, 545
deaths from all causes, proportion from, 265, 266
definition, xiii
diagnosis, 648, 649
diagnosis, accuracy, 613
differentiation of lobar pneumonia from, 612
experimental. *See* Experimental pneumonia
Friedländer's bacillus, 5–8
immunity, and, 234
in childhood, 514, 515
in infants and children, 84–89, 514, 515, 704, 705
in newborn infants, 305
in old age, 514, 515
incidence increasing in South Africa, 457
influenza, and, 4, 68, 72–74, 339, 386
influenza bacillus, 8, 9, 663
influenzal, pregnancy and prognosis, 713
interstitial lesions, and, 3
lesion in, xiii, 649
measles, and, 4, 72, 73
mixed infections in, 10–16, 67–69
necropsy studies, 3
onset, symptoms at, 649

Bronchopneumonia (*cont.*):
organized, 543
physical signs, 649
pneumococcus in, xiii, 67–74, 84–89
post-operative pneumonia, and, 515, 517, 522, 523, 767
primary, causative organisms, 68–72
psittacosis, and, 16
recovery in, 68, 649
relapse, 649
scarlet fever, and, 72
secondary, 4, 6, 9, 15, 68, 72–74, 513
secondary, causative organisms, 4, 6, 9, 15, 72–74
secondary, necropsy studies, 72, 73
staphylococcus, 9, 10, 67–69
streptococcus, 3–5, 471, 648, 649
streptococcus, epidemic, 3, 68
synonyms, xv
terminal, 471, 513
treatment:
deuteroproteose, 774
oxygen, in post-operative cases, 767
serum. *See* Serum treatment; Serum treatment, results
sulfapyridine, 788
vaccine, 799–803
vitamin, 790
x-ray, 773
See also Treatment; Oxygen treatment
tularemia, and, 16
x-ray findings, 649
Bronchopneumonia, pneumococcus:
antibody at recovery, 68
antibody response during, specificity, 50
bacteriemia, and, 68
crisis in, 530
diagnosis, 612
recurrence, and, 535–537
symptoms at onset, 649
type incidence, in children and adults, 87–89
type incidence, in various countries, 68–74
types:
causal relation to, 49–51, 68, 69, 72
commonest in, 71, 72, 84–89
found at necropsy, 68, 69

C substance of pneumococcus, 24, 25, 125, 135, 733
Capsule of Friedländer's bacillus, 6
Capsule of pneumococcus, 20, 22
Carbohydrate fractions of pneumococcus. *See* Specific capsular polysaccharide(s); Pneumococcus, C substance
Carbohydrate in media for pneumococcus growth, 20
Cardiovascular system:
blood pressure, and, 496, 722, 723
care of bowels, and, 750
convalescence, symptoms in, 547
cyanosis, and, 493
death, changes at, 544–546
dicrotic pulse, and, 494
embolism, pulmonary, and sudden death, 546
endocarditis, 10, 589–592
heart and pulse, during course, 492, 493
heart disease, association of pneumonia with, 525
heart irregularities, during course, 494–496
heart muscle and experimental pneumonia, 493
heart, hypertrophy at necropsy, 112
myocarditis, 608
pericarditis, 4, 10, 586–589
pericarditis, bacteriemia, and, 560, 561
pericarditis, delayed resolution, and, 543, 588
peripheral vascular dilatation, 545, 546, 748, 750
phlebitis, thrombosis, and embolism, 610
post-operative pneumonia and vascular stasis, 516
prognosis, and, 702, 720–723
pulmonary infarct, differentiation of pneumonia from, 650
pulse, during course, 494
pulse rate, prognosis, and, 720–722
serum reactions, and symptoms in, 864, 865, 868
shock, and, 750
thrombosis, pulmonary, and sudden death, 546
toxemia, and, 544–546, 748, 750
treatment, 749–755, 758, 759
treatment, serum, and, 883, 885, 888, 919
treatment, venesection, and, 769
Carriers of pneumococci. *See* Pneumococcus carriers
Causative organisms:
bronchopneumonia, xiii, 2–17, 67–74, 84–89
infants and children with pneumonia, 2, 3, 74–89
lobar pneumonia, xiii, 1–17, 41–54, 79–84, 89
mixed infections, 1–3, 11–16, 74, 111
pneumococcus, significance in sputum, 12, 49–51, 623, 624

Causative organisms (*cont.*):
pneumonia, xiii, 1–17, 40–89, 457, 458, 927
post-operative pneumonia, 516, 517, 522, 523
type incidence. *See* Pneumococcus tvpe incidence
Cellulitis, 604
Central pneumonia, 512
dullness in, 508
tactile fremitus, and, 507
x-ray findings, 646, 647
Chemical constituents of pneumococcus. *See* Specific capsular polysaccharide(s); Pneumococcus, C substance; Pneumococcus, nucleoprotein
Chemotherapy, 775–795
amino compounds, and, 783–790
azo dyes, and, 783–790
bile salts, 783
colloidal silver solutions, 783
creosote, 782
Dagenan, 786
drug fastness to optochin, 780
drug fastness to sulfapyridine, 789
empyema, 585
endocarditis, 592
enzymes, 736, 791–795
destruction of Type I SSS, 795
destruction of Type II SSS, 795
destruction of Type III SSS, 736, 791, 792, 794
in experimental Type III infections, 736, 792–795
ethylapocupreine, 781
ethylhydrocupreine. *See below under* Chemotherapy, optochin
formaldehyde sulphoxylate, 783
hydroxyethylapocupreine, 781, 782
M. & B. 693, 784, 786–790
meningitis, 595–597
mercurochrome, 782
miscellaneous chemicals, 782, 783
Nuclein, 783
Numoquin-base, 779
optochin:
bactericidal effect, 778–781
bacteriemia, and, 563, 780
blindness from, 780, 781
dosage, 778–782
drug fastness to, 780
empyema, and, 585, 778
failure of, reasons for, 780
fatality rates with, 780, 781
meningitis, and, 595–597, 778
Chemotherapy (*cont.*):
optochin (*cont.*):
pneumococcus carriers, and, 404, 405, 778
quinine treatment combined with, 777
related compounds, and, 778–782
serum treatment combined with, 781
toxic effects, 779–782
pneumococcus carriers, treatment of, 404–406, 778, 926
potassium permanganate, 782
Prontosil, 784–786
Prontosil soluble, 784, 786
Prontylin, 784
Proseptasine, 786
quinine:
bactericidal effect, 775–777
derivatives, 775–782
dosage, 776, 777
endocarditis, and, 592
fatality rates with, 776
results, compared with optochin, 777
value in animals, compared with serum, 776
recovery, and, 737, 775–795
serum treatment combined with, 595–597, 737, 742, 781, 789
sodium salicylate, 782, 783
Soluseptasine, 786
sulfanilamide, 783–786, 789, 790
absorption and elimination, 784, 786
agranulocytosis from, 785, 786
allied agents, and, 783–790
allied agents, classification, 786, 787
bacteriemia, and, 563, 784–786
dosage, 785, 786
endocarditis, and, 592
experimental infections, and, 784, 785
meningitis, and, 597, 786
pneumococci, effect on, 784, 785, 787
serum treatment combined with, 789
streptococci, effect on, 784, 785, 790
streptococcus pneumonia, 5, 790
toxic effects, 785, 786
Type III cases, 785, 786
value of, conclusions, 789
sulfapyridine, 784, 786–790
absorption and elimination, 787–789
bacteriemia, and, 787–789
dosage, 787–789
drug fastness to, 789
experimental infections, and, 787, 789
fatality rate with, 788
immunity, effect on, 789
in infants and children, 788

Chemotherapy (*cont.*):
sulfapyridine (*cont.*):
pneumococci, effect on, 784, 787, 789
serum treatment combined with, 789
streptococci, effect on, 787, 790
toxic effects, 787, 788
value of, conclusions, 789
sulphone compounds, 787
Uleron, 787
unsolved problems, 775, 777, 781, 789, 790, 794, 927
vitamins, and, 790, 791
Children, pneumonia in. *See* Infants and children with pneumonia
Chill, 488, 514
arthritis, septic, and, 599
bronchopneumonia, and, 649
empyema, and, 575
endocarditis, and, 591
phlebitis, and, 610
pleurisy with effusion, and, 652
pulmonary infarct, and, 650
reactions after serum treatment. *See* Reactions after . . .
terminal pneumonia, and, 513
tuberculous pneumonia, and, 651
Chronic disease:
bronchopneumonia, and, 513
Friedländer's bacillus in chronic lung lesions, 6
incidence of pneumonia, and, 335, 336
lobar pneumonia, and, 336, 513, 525
predisposing factors, and, 201, 335, 336, 338
prognosis, and, 701, 702
serum treatment, failure of, due to, 919
staphylococcus cases, and, 9
Type III cases, and, 335, 336
Type III cases, and prognosis, 669
Cinchona derivatives, treatment with, 775–782
Climate and pneumonia, 47–49, 288, 289, 297–299, 312, 313, 330–332, 337
Clinical Study of Pain, A, 489
Clinical varieties of pneumonia, 510–524
Colds, common:
allergy to pneumococcus, and, 241, 245
antibody appearance during, 157
distribution, world-wide, 339
epidemic, and cold weather, 337
filterable virus, as cause, 237, 239, 375
incidence of, 238
and eye color, 186
seasonal, 237, 238, 293–295
seasonal, and pneumococcus carriers, 237, 294, 295, 379–385
Colds, common (*cont.*):
incidence of (*cont.*):
variation with age, 237, 238
incidence peaks of, 237, 294, 295
lung, damage to protective mechanism, and, 257
organisms in respiratory tract, activity of, and, 200, 238, 239, 337, 375–377
pneumococcus carriers, influence on, 362, 374–377
pneumonia, frequency after, 238
pneumonia, route of infection, and, 247
predisposing factors, and, 236–240, 339
prevention of, by active immunization, 406–408
prevention of pneumonia, and, 397, 403
spread of organisms in community, and, 239, 397
systemic reaction to, 237, 238, 295
virus of, effect on pneumococcus virulence, 200, 239
Vitamin A, and, 334, 335
See also Respiratory infections, minor
Collapse, 546, 753, 759
Commonwealth Fund, The, 929, 930, 937
Complement, pneumococcus immunity, and, 117, 120
Complement-fixing antibody(ies), 124, 172
Complications, 3–5, 7, 8, 10, 111, 112, 515, 525, 548–611
incidence of, factors influencing, 175, 176, 549, 570–573, 888
organisms other than pneumococci in, in pneumococcus cases, 111, 112
See also under particular complication by name
Concurrent infection(s), 12, 15, 16
Confluent pneumonia, xiii, 649
Friedländer's bacillus cases, 7
staphylococcus cases, 10
Conjunctivitis, 607
Consecutive infection(s), 12, 15, 16, 532, 533
Contusion pneumonia, 340
Convalescence, 546, 547
antibody in, 117, 120, 125, 729, 730
antibody in, and mixed infections, 11, 14–16
antibody in, persistence during and after, 537, 737–739
cardiovascular changes in, 547
death, sudden, in, 546, 610
leucocyte count in, 498
lung abscess, simulated appearance in, 541, 606, 607
mixed infections, and, 16

Convalescence (*cont.*):
neuritis, peripheral, in, 611
phlebitis in, 610
physical signs, and, 507
platelet count in, 499
pneumococcus carriers in, 366, 367, 369–372, 547
antibody studies of, 378
recurrence of pneumonia, and, 535, 539
respiratory tract pathology, and, 376
treatment of, 404
unclassified strains in nasopharynx, 366, 367
SSS in urine during, 504, 695
urinary findings in, 503
x-ray, for follow-up, in, 546
Convalescent blood, transfusions with, in treatment, 5, 11, 773, 813, 814
Convalescent serum:
pneumococcus, activity inhibited by, 124
treatment with, 5, 9, 809, 812–814
treatment with, and skin sensitivity to SSS, 171, 813
Cooper types, 29–31, 946
Cough, 490, 501
apical pneumonia, and, 501
bronchopneumonia, and, 649
death, and, 544
diagnosis, and, 613
empyema, and, 575
in infants and children, 514
massive pneumonia, and, 512
post-operative pneumonia, and, 517
pulmonary exudate, removal of, and, 97
serum reactions, and, 866
spread of lesion, and, 255
treatment, 749
Crisis, 527–531
age, and, 529
antibody, relation to, 729, 733
definition, 528
factors affecting occurrence, 528, 529
monocytosis, and, 100
onset, mode of, and, 530
organisms, death of, and, 528, 734
organisms in lung, and, 528, 734
physical signs, after, 507
pneumococcus types, and, 530
pneumococcus typing at, 617
resolution, and, 528, 540
SSS in urine, and, 504
time of, in control and serum treated cases, 883
toxic products, and, 528, 734
varieties, 531
Crisis (*cont.*):
vasomotor paralysis, and, 545, 547
Cross immunity, 135, 136, 731, 739
Croupous pneumonia. *See* Lobar pneumonia
Cyanosis:
anoxemia, and, 496, 499, 761, 762
cardiovascular symptoms, and, 493
diathermy treatment, and, 772
during course, 496, 497
extent of lesion, and, 496
jaundice, and, 503
mechanism of, 496, 497, 759–762
prognosis, and, 726
pulmonary infarct, and, 650
rheumatic pneumonia, and, 653
serum reactions, and, 815, 864, 865, 867, 878
staphylococcus cases, 10
streptococcus cases, 4
sulfanilamide treatment, and, 786
sulfapyridine treatment, and, 788
tuberculous pneumonia, and, 651

Dagenan, 786
Death(s):
age groups, and, 305, 306
anoxemia, and, 545, 546, 761
antibody, and, 174–177, 733, 919
bacteriemia, and, 544, 545, 560–562, 690
cause, 546
cause, war gases, and, 341
clinical observations at, 544–546
complications, and, 544–546
economic factors, and, 267, 268
Friedländer's bacillus cases, 7, 8
from pneumonia in relation to deaths from all causes, 264–269
in hospitals, by age group, 306
in hospitals, by sex, 308, 309
lobar cases:
seasonal distribution of, 290–293
seasonal distribution, compared with pneumococcus carriers, 385
yearly variations, 293
lung puncture studies at, 734, 735
myocarditis, and, 608
pulmonary embolism, and, 610
reported in Massachusetts, with cases, 290–293, 299, 300, 306–309, 383, 385
reporting of, 258–260, 927
serum treatment:
and analysis of cause of, 918–920
presumably adequate, and, 176, 177, 920

Death(s) (*cont.*):
  serum treatment (*cont.*):
    reactions from, and, 815, 817, 818, 820, 836, 864–869, 875, 878
  sudden, in convalescence, 546, 610
  symptoms at, 544, 545
  terms included in International List of Causes, xv, xvi, xvii
  time of, 544
  toxemia, and, 544–546
  Type I and II cases without bacteriemia, 545
Death rate(s):
  age and sex, and, 310–312
  age groups, and, 274, 301–305
  altitude, and, 298, 332, 333
  American Indians, and, 274
  army troops, and, 465
  climate, and, 288, 289, 298
  computation over long periods, caution in, 259
  crowding, and, 317, 318
  diet, and, 317
  dust, and, 319–325, 327, 329
  dust and chronic interstitial pneumonia, and, 321
  environmental change, and, 313, 330
  excessive in males:
    and age, 193, 310, 311, 328
    and occupation, 193, 310, 311, 328, 329
    and urbanization, 193, 311, 312, 328
  for cities with a large steel industry, 327, 328
  for foreign cities with highest rates, and altitude, 283, 284
  for foreign countries, 264–266, 268, 277–284
  for groups of states, by age and sex, 193
  for large and small cities, 276, 277, 279, 284
  for largest foreign cities, 284
  for North America, 269–277
  for pneumonia of various forms, 271–273
  for states with highest rates, availability of typing facilities, and, 931
  for states with highest rates, by age groups, 302, 303
  for United States, 264–268
    average, 269–273
    bronchopneumonia by states, 276
    by cities and states, 269–277
    cities with highest rates, 277
    largest cities, 276, 277
    lobar pneumonia by states, 276
    rural areas and small cities, 288
    states with highest rates, 269–274
Death rate(s) (*cont.*):
  for urban and rural areas, 279, 288
  highest in world, geographic groups, 283
  immunization, active, and, 454–456, 457, 458, 460–463
  immunization of Negroes, and, 468, 469
  industry, and, 319–329
  influenza and pneumonia, by age, sex, and urbanization, 193, 310, 311, 328, 329
  lobar and bronchopneumonia, by age groups, 301, 303, 304
  local conditions, influence on, 288, 289
  meteorological factors, and, 297, 298
  Mexicans, and, 274
  miners, underground and surface, 329, 448, 463
  mines, African, variations in, 288, 289
  Negroes, and, 312–316
  Negroes in population, and, 271–273
  Negroes in South Africa, and, 456, 462, 463
  occupation, and, 193, 310, 311, 318–329
  pneumonia belts, and, 269–274, 283
  race, and, 312–316
  sex, and, 308–312
  sex ratio of, and occupation, 193, 310, 311, 328, 329
  social condition, and, 288
  social condition in males, and, 319–323
  temperature variations, and, 319–323, 329
  trend, 284–287, 395, 396
  tropics, and, 283
  tuberculosis and pneumonia, 274, 319, 324
  weather variations, and, 321
  zinc oxide fumes, and, 319
  See also Fatality rate(s)
Definitions:
  bronchopneumonia, xiii
  lobar pneumonia, xiii, xvii
  pneumococcus pneumonia, xvii
  unit of antiserum, 826, 827
Delayed resolution. *See* Resolution, delayed
Delirium:
  alcohol, and, 504, 727
  apical pneumonia, and, 504
  during course, 504, 505
  nursing care, and, 745
  prognosis, and, 727
  serum reactions, and, 865, 878
  serum treatment, effect on, 883
  treatment, 756
Departments of health:
  appropriations for serum by, 933
  availability of typing facilities, and, 834, 933, 934

Departments of health (*cont.*):
manufacture of serum by, 829, 928, 929, 933, 934
Massachusetts:
dosage recommendations for serum treatment, 848, 850–852, 856, 858, 943, 944
instruction sheets for dosage and administration of horse antiserum, 939, 943–945
instruction sheets for precautions in use of serums, 939–942
lobar pneumonia:
reported cases by age, 299, 300, 306, 307
reported cases by month, 290–293
reported cases by season, 383, 385
reported cases by sex, 308, 309
reported deaths by season, 383, 385
manufacture of serum by, 829, 929
provision of serum by, 829, 851, 928–930, 937
removal of time restriction on distribution of serum, 833, 882, 897, 937
serum, conditions under which provided, 833
types of antiserum distributed, 829, 851, 937
typing at state laboratory without animals, 622
See also Massachusetts Pneumonia Series; Massachusetts Pneumonia Program
Michigan, manufacture of serum by, 929
Michigan, provision of serum by, 929, 930
New York City:
commission for study of respiratory disease, 929
manufacture of serum by, 929
provision of serum by, 928–930
types of antiserum distributed, 830
New York State:
handbook on nursing care, availability, 935
manufacture of serum by, 929
provision of serum by, 829, 928–930
types of antiserum distributed, 829
See also New York State; New York State Pneumonia Program; New York State Pneumonia Series
pneumonia programs, 928–936
pneumonia programs, advisory service for, of United States Public Health Service, 936
provision of serum by, 829, 830, 851, 928–934, 937
Departments of health (*cont.*):
provision of serum by, cost per case, 931, 932
purchase of serum by, 933
Diagnosis, 612–647
accuracy, 612, 613
bacteriologic. *See* Bacteriologic study
central pneumonia, 512
clinical, changes over long periods, 259
differential, 647–654
age, and, 648
appendicitis, and, 654
atelectasis, and, 649, 651
bronchopneumonia, and, xiii, 612, 648, 649
confluent bronchopneumonia, and, xiii, 649
first differentiation of lobar from bronchopneumonia, xiii
meningitis, and, 654
pleural effusion, and, 652
pulmonary infarct, and, 650
rales, character of, and, 509
rheumatic pneumonia, and, 652, 653
tuberculous pneumonia, and, 650, 651
early, 613
early, and urine typing, 621, 637
Friedländer's bacillus cases, 7, 614
herpes, and, 507, 613
history, and, 613
influenza bacillus cases, 9, 614
leucocytosis, and, 515, 613, 645
mixed infections, 11–16
physical signs, and, 506–509, 613
post-operative pneumonia, 518
rusty sputum, and, 613
special features, with various organisms, and, 613, 614
sputum, character of, and, 613, 614
staphylococcus cases, 10
streptococcus cases, 4
x-ray, and, 613, 645–647, 649
Diagnosis and Treatment of Pneumonia, 19
Diplococcus lanceolatus, 20
Diplococcus pneumoniae, 19, 20
Diplococcus pneumoniae. See Pneumococcus
Dissociation of pneumococci. *See* Pneumococcus, variants
Dochez and Gillespie's classification of pneumococci, 22, 23
Double infection, 11–16
Double pneumonia, 109, 110, 512
Droplet infection, 295–297, 316
prevention, and, 396
sneezing, and, 392, 393

Droplet nuclei infection, 296, 316, 392
Dust:
  alkaline silica, and acute silicosis, 340
  chronic interstitial pneumonia, and, 321
  danger from, and quartz (silica) content, 297, 325
  death rates, and, 319–325, 327, 329
  high silica content and death rates, 320, 321, 324, 325
  incidence, and, 324, 325, 327, 329, 340
  irritating, and prevention of pneumonia, 398
  pneumococcus in, 341, 392, 396
  pneumococcus types, homologous, in room dust, 341
  spread of infection, and, 295–297, 316

Eczema, importance of history of, 838, 842
Edema fluid:
  early lesions, pathology, and, 103–106
  experimental pneumonia, and, 219, 220, 222, 227–232
  initial lesion, and, 250
  pathogenesis, and allergy to pneumococcus, and, 254
  SSS in, antagonism to antibody, 256
  spread of experimental pneumonia, and, 219, 220, 222, 227–232, 255, 256
  spread of lesion, and, 254–256
  spread of lesion, effect of gravity on, 212, 220–222, 255, 256
Edema of skin and serum sickness, 869, 870
Edema, pulmonary:
  death, and, 544, 545
  prognosis, and, 727
  restriction of fluids with, 747, 758
  salt in diet, and, 746
  treatment, 746, 747, 758, 767
Emphysema, subcutaneous in staphylococcus cases, 10
Empyema:
  abscess, sub-pleural, and origin, 606
  arthritis, septic, and, 599
  bacteriemia, and, 567, 570, 578
  bilateral, 573, 574, 581, 582
  bronchopneumonia, 566, 568, 569, 571, 575
  bronchopneumonia and pericarditis, and, 566
  causative organisms, 574, 575
  chest tap for diagnosis, 577
  chronic, 583
  complicated cases, 566, 567, 574, 575, 577–579, 582
Empyema (*cont.*):
  complications of, 566, 567, 575, 578, 582, 584, 585
  diagnosis, 576, 577
  diagnosis, bacteriologic, 577, 582
  during World War, 567, 574, 581, 582
  encapsulated, 573, 576, 577
  fatality rates, 4, 575, 578–581
  furunculosis, and, 604
  immunity and, 566, 573
  incidence, 566–573
    age, and, 515, 571, 572
    bacteriemia, and, 560, 561, 887
    effect of serum treatment on, 570, 887, 888
    factors affecting, 570–573
    side involved, and, 574
  infants and children, 515, 568, 571, 572, 574, 576, 579, 580, 585
  influenza epidemic, and, 566, 567, 582
  lesion in, 573–575
  lesion, nature of, and causative organism, 574, 575
  leucocyte count in, 576
  leucocytes in pleural fluid, 564, 577, 643
  lobar pneumonia, 566–573
  Massachusetts Pneumonia Series, and, 568–570
  measles epidemic, and, 567
  mechanism of development, 564, 566
  meningitis, and, 567, 578
  pericarditis, and, 566, 575, 588, 589
  physical signs, 575, 576
  pneumococcus, 568–575, 578–582, 584
  pneumothorax treatment complicated by, 770, 771
  prevention of, 566
  prognosis, 577–582
    factors affecting, 582
    seasonal variation, 581, 582
    time of onset, and, 578
  pyopneumothorax, and, 611
  SSS in pleural fluids, and, 566, 584
  skin sensitivity to SSS, and, 170
  staphylococcus, 10, 574
  staphylococcus, fatality rates, 579, 580
  streptococcus, 4, 5, 567, 571, 573–575, 582, 584, 589
  streptococcus, fatality rates, 4, 579–581
  symptoms, 575
  treatment, 582–585
    infants and children, 583, 585
    optochin, 585, 778
    serum, 584
      effect on incidence, 175, 176, 570, 887, 888

Empyema (*cont.*):
treatment (*cont.*):
serum (*cont.*):
failure of, due to, 860, 919
rabbit, 918
tuberculosis, and, 583, 584
Type I and II cases at necropsy, 567
Type I, II, III, and Group IV cases, 568–570
x-ray, and, 576, 577
Endocarditis, 10, 589–592, 888
arthritis, septic, and, 599
diagnosis, 591, 592
meningitis, and, 591, 594
pericarditis, and, 588
treatment, 592
treatment, serum, effect on incidence, 592, 888
Enzyme(s):
anti-enzyme balance in resolution, and, 98, 100
for splitting Type I or II SSS, 795
for splitting Type III SSS, 736, 791–794
for splitting Type III SSS, reactions from treatment with, 794
pneumococcal, 21, 97, 98, 100, 763
recovery, and, 736
soil bacillus, and, 791
treatment with, in experimental Type III infections, 736, 792–795
treatment with, need for further study, 794, 927
Ephedrine:
for serum sickness, 872
treatment with, 755
Epidemic(s), 260, 386–390
abortive pneumonia, and, 511
crowding, and, 316–318
factors controlling, 389, 390
families, and, 387, 388
Friedländer's bacillus cases, 6–8
immunization against, 404, 406, 454, 465, 473, 474, 477, 478
isolated population, and, 195
localized, 386–389
monkeys, lobar pneumonia in, 316
natural history of, 474
need for further study, 474, 926
Negroes, and, 386
pneumococcus:
Group IV, in monkeys, 387
Type I, 386–388
Type I, homologous type carriers, and, 369, 386, 387
Type II, 387
Epidemic(s) (*cont.*):
pneumococcus (*cont.*):
Type II, homologous type carriers, and, 387, 393, 394, 473
Type II, immunization against, 473, 474
Type V, 387
type transformation, and, 393, 394
types, commonest in, 58
pneumococcus carriers, and, 369, 376, 386–388, 393, 394, 404, 473, 926
pneumococcus carriers, isolation in, 404, 926
pneumonic plague, and, 386
respiratory infection in families, and pneumonia, 377, 392
staphylococcus cases, 10
streptococcus cases, 3, 68
termination, by immunization, 404, 406
theory of, 389, 390
See also under Friedländer's bacillus pneumonia; Influenza; Measles; Scarlet fever; Staphylococcus pneumonia; Streptococcus pneumonia
Epidemiological Reports of the Health Section of the Secretariat of the League of Nations, 260
Epidemiology of pneumonia, 258–394
air-borne infection, and, 295–297
autogenous and exogenous infection, and, 16, 355, 391, 392
contact infection in animals, 219
death rate(s). *See* Death rate(s)
droplet and droplet-nuclei infection, 295–297, 316, 392, 393, 396
dust, and, 295–297, 316, 319–325, 327, 329, 398
environmental change, and, 330–332
epidemics. *See* Epidemic(s)
incidence. *See* Incidence; Prevalence
infection from cases or carriers, 391, 392
isolated population, and, 195
lobar or bronchopneumonia, in temperate regions, 259
need for further study, 390–394, 396, 922, 925–927
pneumococcus carriers, and. *See* Pneumococcus carriers
pneumonia belts, 269–274, 283
predisposing factors. *See* Predisposing factor(s)
prevalence. *See* Prevalence; Incidence
prevention. *See* Prevention; Immunization, active, against pneumonia
reported cases and deaths, unreliability of statistics, 258–260

Epidemiology of pneumonia (*cont.*):
  reported cases and deaths in Massachusetts, 290–293, 299, 300, 306–309, 383, 385
  reporting of cases or deaths, 258–260, 927
  respiratory infections, minor, and, 235–240, 392
  respiratory infections, minor, in families, and, 377, 392
  sex, and exposure, 310
  significance of certain types, and, 351, 353–355, 357, 361, 390, 391
  similarity of, with meningococcus meningitis, 394
  spread of organisms, and crowding, 298, 316, 318, 389, 392, 394
  spread of pneumococci, and, 239, 295–297, 316, 330, 366, 374, 392–394, 397
  transmission and spread of pneumonia, 342–394
  Type I and II, possible differences in, in America and Great Britain, 360, 361
  Type I or II infections, compared with Type III and Group IV, 351, 353
  type transformation, and, 393, 394
  virus infections, and, 236–240
Epidemiology of minor respiratory infections, 293–295
Epinephrine:
  availability before testing and treating with serum, 839
  treatment of allergic reactions with, 864, 867, 878
  treatment of positive eye test with, 840
  treatment of serum sickness with, 872
  treatment with, 750, 754, 755, 759
  use prior to serum treatment, 838, 841
  valueless in chill reaction, 868
Epithelial tissues, penetration by pneumococci, 232, 549
Ethylhydrocupreine treatment, 778–781
Etiology of pneumonia. *See* Causative organisms
Experimental infection(s), 204–232, 248–256
  alcohol, effect on, 157, 158, 333, 334
  allergy and immunity, role in, 183, 184
  antibody appearance during, 160, 181, 205, 218
  bacteriemia in, 205, 212–231, 549
  bacteriemia in, and leucocyte count, 724
  blocking experiments in mice, for detection of multiple types in sputum, 368
  breed of animals, and variations in, 177, 186, 212–216
  course and outcome, miscellaneous factors influencing, 201–203
Experimental infection(s) (*cont.*):
  eye, anterior chamber of, and, 211, 231
  immunity, and, 204–232
  immunity, passive, and host variables, 178–180
  immunization against, 214, 440–446
  inhalation of sprayed organisms, and, 209, 210, 217, 218
  intrabronchial, 210, 211, 224–231
  intradermal, 205–207, 212, 843
  intranasal instillation of organisms, and, 209, 214–217
  intraperitoneal, 207–209, 213
  intrapleural or intrapulmonary, 211, 231
  intratracheal, 210, 218–224
  intravenous, 207, 212, 213
  kidney lesions, and, 212, 216, 609
  meningitis, 209, 213, 214, 596, 597
  meningitis, and immunity, 596
  mixed infection, and spread, 212
  pathology, 212–232
  peritonitis, from vaginal infection in the monkey, 602
  pneumonia. *See* Experimental pneumonia
  prognosis, and mobilization of leucocytes, 151, 179
  prognosis with mixed infection, 199
  relapse in, 532
  routes employed, 205–232
  spread, and autolysates, 131, 132, 212
  spread, effect of gravity on edema fluid, 212, 220–222, 255, 256
  subarachnoid, 209, 213, 214, 596, 597
  subcutaneous, 19, 205, 206
  treatment:
    enzyme, of Type III infections, 736, 792–795
    gold salts and serum combined, 736
    non-specific, 821
    of meningitis, 596, 597
    optochin, 778
    optochin and serum combined, 781
    quinine, 776, 777
    serum:
      and bacteriemia, 821, 843, 886
      curative effect, 121, 168, 169, 821
      importance of time begun, 169, 832, 833
      route of, with intradermal infections, 843
    sulfanilamide, 784, 785
    sulfapyridine, 787, 789
  type of pneumococcus and predictable lesions, 216

Experimental infection(s) (*cont.*):
virulence, and, 27, 139, 193, 194, 205, 212–232, 511
Experimental pneumonia:
allergy, and, 241–245
antibody in recovery in dogs, 181
associated lesions, 213, 215, 216
atelectasis in, 230, 250–253
bronchopneumonia, 3, 214, 219–222, 225, 226
contact infection, 214, 219
course, 214–231
death in, cause, 546
development, 219–231
diaphragm, elevation of, 251, 252
dogs, immunity, and, 141
dosage of organisms used, compared with cases in man, 249
edema fluid in, and spread, 219, 220, 222, 227–232, 255, 256
Friedländer's bacillus, 7
heart muscle, and, 493
immunization against, 214, 440–446
immunization against, and fate of organisms in lungs, 441, 442
influenza bacillus, 8, 9
inhalation of organisms, and, 217
intrabronchial infection, and, 224–231
intranasal infection, and, 214–216
intravenous infection, and, 212, 213
kidney lesions in mice, and, 609
lesion:
development of, 219–231
initial, nature of, 249, 250
initial, site of and route of infection, 247, 248
lobar, 140, 216, 217, 219, 220, 222, 225–231
lobar, conditions controlling development, 257
lobar, relation to route of infection, 246
lobular, 216, 223, 225, 226, 228
lung, defense barriers of, and, 217, 218, 225, 232
macrophage reaction in resolution, 181, 227–229
mediastinal displacement in, 230, 251, 252
mixed infections in, 101, 111, 220, 227, 532
monkey, species of, and, 139, 140
morphine, effect on pathogenesis, 202
organized lesions and mixed infections, 101, 220, 227
pathogenesis, 202, 219–231
pericarditis, and, 588

Experimental pneumonia (*cont.*):
pleurisy in Type I infections, 564
prognosis, and dose of organisms, 219, 221, 226, 227
prognosis, and mixed infections, 111
recovery, SSS in lungs after, 541
relapse, and mixed infections, 532
repeated attacks, 181, 182, 230, 231
repeated attacks, and allergy, 242, 243
repeated attacks, character of disease and immunity, 538
resolution:
delayed, production of, in dogs, 100
large mononuclear cells in, 98, 99
macrophage reaction, and, 227–229
respiratory centers, sensitivity, and, 501
respiratory tract, protective mechanism in, 225, 232, 235, 257
spread of lesion, and edema fluid, 219, 220, 222, 227–232, 255, 256
staphylococcus, 9
streptococcus, 3
temperature of body, and, 202
treatment:
compressed air, 767, 768
diathermy, 772
enzyme, of Type III infections, 793, 794
Huntoon's antibody solution, 814, 815, 843
non-specific, 821
pneumothorax, 769
serum, curative effect, 169, 821
sulfanilamide, 785
virulence, and, 193, 194, 215, 216, 219, 221, 225, 511
virus infection preceding, 232, 240
Eye test:
fallibility, 840
interpretation, 840, 841
in young children, 840
positive:
as contraindication to serum treatment, 841, 842
importance, 841, 842, 877
use of epinephrine for, 840
sensitivity to horse serum, and, 839–842
sensitivity to rabbit serum, and, 876, 877
technic, 839, 840, 876

Fatality rate(s), 656–727
age, and, 702–710
albuminuria, and, 727
alcoholism, and, 702, 718, 719
altitude, and, 717, 718

Fatality rate(s) (*cont.*):
apical lesions, and, 698
army troops during Civil War, 700
army troops during World War, 663, 700, 890
bacteriemia, and, 681–693, 886
and day of development, 690, 691
and digitalis treatment, 751, 752
and intensity, 691, 692
in infants and children, and, 693
bronchopneumonia, 663
by type, 666, 668, 675
during World War, 663
infants and children, 704, 705
Canada, 657, 658
cardiovascular disease, and age, 702
chill reaction from serum treatment, effect on, 868
chronic disease, and, 701, 702
comparison of, in areas with high or low attack rates, 338, 660, 662
comparison of, in Boston City Hospital with Harlem Hospital, 670–672
complications, and, 695, 696
cyanosis, and, 726
empyema, 4, 575, 578–581
environment, and, 717, 718
extent of lesion, and, 696–698
foreign countries, 658–662
Friedländer's bacillus cases, 8, 677
heart rate, and, 721–723
home treated cases, 715–717
hospital and home treated cases compared, 715–717
hospital cases, and variations in, 657–663, 670–672
infants and children, 515, 703–707
infants and children, and pneumonia not due to pneumococci, 707
infants and children, by type, 704–707
influenza bacillus cases, 8, 9
influenza epidemics, and variations in, 9, 582, 811, 812
influenzal bronchopneumonia, 663
leucocyte count, and, 723, 724
military organizations, 663, 699–701, 810, 890
miners, surface and underground, 662
mixed infections, and, 11, 15, 16, 677
need for further study, 927
Negroes, 678
occupation, and, 692, 713, 714
organisms other than pneumococci, and, 4, 5, 8–11, 677, 707

Fatality rate(s) (*cont.*):
organisms other than pneumococci, and bacteriemia, 689
physical condition, and, 699–702
pregnancy, and, 713
pulse rate, and, 720–722
race, and, 710–712
recurrence, and, 539, 696, 698
respiration rate, and, 725, 726
SSS in urine, and, 693–695
season, and, 679–681
sex, and, 712, 713
social condition, and, 671, 672, 714–717
staphylococcus cases, 10, 11
streptococcus cases, 4, 5, 677
streptococcus empyema, 579–581
temperature, and, 719, 720
treatment:
chemicals, miscellaneous, and, 782
deuteroproteose, and, 774
diathermy, and, 772
digitalis, and, 751, 752
enzyme, in experimental infections, and, 792–794
optochin, and, 780, 781
oxygen, and, 767
quinine, and, 776
serum, and. *See* Serum treatment, results
sulfanilamide, and, 785, 786
sulfapyridine, and, 788
vaccine, and, 798–803
vitamin, and, 790
x-ray, and, 773
tropical regions, 659–662
type, and. *See* Fatality rate(s) by type
United States, 657, 658
United States and Canada, compared with other countries, 658–660, 666–669, 684–686
year, and, 677–679
Fatality rate(s) by type, 663–677
bacteriemia, incidence of, and, 692
bronchopneumonia, 666, 668, 675
Group IV, 671, 672
Group IV, bacteriemia, and, 686, 687, 688
infants and children, 704–707
pneumococcus pneumonia, 674–677, 706, 707
pneumococcus pneumonia, and bacteriemia, 687–689
season, and, 679–681
Type I, 664–666, 675, 676, 881
Type I, army troops during World War, 700, 701

Fatality rate(s) by type (*cont.*):
Type I, bacteriemia, and, 683–685, 687, 688
Type I, II, III, and Group IV, and bacteriemia, 687, 688
Type II, 666–669, 675, 676
Type II, and bacteriemia, 684, 685, 687, 688
Type III, 669–672, 675, 676
age, and, 669
bacteriemia, and, 685–688
experimental infections, and enzyme treatment, 792–794
Type V, 672, 673, 675, 676
Type V, bacteriemia, and, 687, 688
Type VII, 673, 675, 676
Type VII, bacteriemia, and, 688, 689
Type VIII, 673–676
Type VIII, bacteriemia, and, 688, 689
Type XIV, 674–676
Type XIV, bacteriemia, and, 688, 689
Type XIV, infants and children, and, 693, 706, 707
year, and, 678, 679
Felton's antibody solution, 808, 809, 825
Friedländer's bacillus, 5–8
classification, serologic, 6
discovery, 6, 19
in bronchopneumonia, 5–7, 67–69
in lobar pneumonia, 1, 2, 5–7
in mixed infections, 6, 13
in post-operative pneumonia, 523
in secondary pneumonia, 6
in sputum, 6, 7
Krumwiede test for, 6
mixed vaccines, and, 458–461, 472
Neufeld test for, 6
pathogenicity, 7
relation to pneumonia, 19
specific capsular polysaccharides of, 6
types, 6
virulence and capsule, 6
Friedländer's bacillus pneumonia, 1, 2, 5–8, 457
alcoholism, and, 7
animals, and, 7
bacteriemia in, 7
bronchopneumonia, 5–8
consolidation in, 5–8
course, 7, 8
diagnosis, 7, 614
epidemic, 6–8
fatality rates, 8, 677
immune response to, 6
incidence, 1, 2, 5, 6
Friedländer's bacillus pneumonia (*cont.*):
leucocyte count in, 7
lobar pneumonia, 1, 2, 5–7, 19
necrosis of lung tissue in, 7, 8
pulmonary tuberculosis, resemblance to, 8
symptoms, 7, 8
treatment, 8
x-ray, 7
Fungus diseases, and pneumonia, 17
Furunculosis, 604

Gangrene and lung abscess, 10, 604–607
Gastrointestinal tract:
bowels, care of, 747, 748, 750
lesions in, 607, 611, 748
peritonitis complicating pneumonia, 4, 601–603
stomach, acute dilatation, 611, 748
sulfanilamide absorption from, 784
sulfapyridine absorption from, 787
symptoms:
at onset, 490, 491, 653, 654
during course, 502, 503
in infants and children, 491, 514
treatment, 747, 748, 750, 756–758
with serum reactions, 864, 870
tympanites. *See* Tympanites
vomiting, 490, 491, 502, 514, 611, 748, 761, 780, 786, 864, 866, 870

Handbook on the Nursing Care of Pneumonia, 935
Hapten, 134
Hay fever, importance of history of, 837, 838, 842, 865
Health departments. *See* Departments of health
Heart. *See under* Cardiovascular system
Hemophylus influenzae. *See* Influenza bacillus
Hemoptysis, 501
Herpes:
as diagnostic aid, 507, 613
during course, 505
prognosis, and, 726, 727
Heterophile antibody:
immunity, and, 125, 128
prognosis, and, 125, 733, 734
rabbit serum, and, 820, 821
recovery, and, 125, 733, 734, 820
treatment with, 809, 820, 821
Histiocytes. *See* Macrophage; Macrophage reaction

Horse asthma:
as contraindication to serum treatment, 837, 842
importance of history, 837, 838, 842, 865
Horse serum:
immune. *See* Serum, horse, antipneumococcic; Serum treatment; Serum treatment, dosage; Serum treatment, results; Reactions after horse serum
normal, diluted for skin test, 840, 853
previous injection, importance of history, 837–839, 842, 864, 865, 867
sensitiveness to, 838, 839, 865, 867
Horse vasomotor rhinitis as contraindication to serum treatment, 837, 842
Host factors:
in acquired immunity, 177–180
in natural immunity, 157, 158
Host resistance:
acute or chronic disease, and, 199–201, 335, 336, 338
alcohol, and depression of, 157, 158, 203, 217, 333, 334
bacteriemia, and, 559, 690
comparison of, in United States and Canada, with other countries, 669
comparison of, with Type I or II infections, in America and Great Britain, 360, 361
compound life, in Negroes, and, 312, 313
development of pneumonia, and, 257
diet, and, 334, 335
environment, and, 312, 313
exposure to wet, cold, and temperature changes, and, 336
factors depressing, and pneumonia, 393, 394
immunization of special groups against pneumonia, and, 465, 478
immunization results, and, 433, 466
influenza, and, 465
inhalation of irritating substances, and, 340–342
of animals, to pneumococcus, 137–143, 186
of man, to pneumococcus, 27, 143–150, 186, 195
Negroes, and, 312–316, 399, 462, 463
pathogenesis of pneumonia, and, 233–235, 392, 393
pneumococcus carriers, animals, and, 378
pneumococcus carriers, pneumonia in, and, 392
population, and epidemics, 389
post-operative pneumonia, and, 516, 517
prevention of pneumonia in special groups, and, 399–401, 465, 477, 478
Host resistance (*cont.*):
race, and, 47, 312–316
recurrence, and, 538
rickets and scurvy, and, 334
seasonal variation, 203, 680, 681
and bacteriemia, 559
and pneumococcus carriers, 378, 380, 385
and prevention, 398
variations, factors affecting, 177–180, 185–203, 393, 394
See also Immunity, pneumococcus
Humoral antibody(ies). *See* Antibody(ies); Antibody(ies), pneumococcus; Heterophile antibody
Huntoon's antibody solution. *See under* Serum, horse, antipneumococcic; Serum treatment
Hydroxyethylapocupreine treatment, 781, 782

Immunity:
alcohol, and, 157, 158, 203, 217, 333, 334
diet, and, 334, 335
empyema, and, 566, 573
environmental factors, and, 330–332
environmental factors, and acquired immunity in Negroes, 312, 313
environmental factors, and sex, 311
inhalation of irritating substances, and, 340–342
lesion developed, character of, and, 232–235, 257, 392, 393, 514, 515
local, in lung, 99, 180–182, 735, 736
population, and, 330–332
recovery, and, 528, 728–737
vitamins, and, 335
Immunity, pneumococcus, 113–203
acquired. *See* Immunity, pneumococcus, acquired
age variations, 129, 186–192, 557
alcohol, and, 157, 158, 217, 333, 334
allergy, and, 182–185
allergy, separation of immunity from, 183, 184
antibody:
actions, and. *See* Antibody(ies), pneumococcus, actions
circulating, and, 115–125
correlation with, 127–131, 739
mode of formation, 155–157
site of formation, 136, 137
antitoxins, and, 124, 125
C substance, and, 25
C substance precipitins, and, 125, 128, 129, 773

Immunity, pneumococcus (*cont.*):
cellular:
factors in, 114
skin tests with pneumococcus products, and, 126, 127, 735
tests for, 125–127
complications, and, 548, 549, 570
cross immunity, 135, 136, 731, 739
death of organism, and, 117–120, 124, 151, 152, 162, 172
experimental infections, and, 204–232
factors affecting, 185–203
genetic factors, and, 177, 186
heterologous, 135, 136
heterophile antibody, and, 125, 128
immunization, and. *See* Immunization, active; Immunization, active against pneumonia; Immunization, passive
macrophage reaction, and, 99, 100, 181, 735, 736
measurement by antibody determinations, 115–125
mechanism of, and allergy, 241–245
natural. *See* Immunity, pneumococcus, natural
nature of, 114–137
non-specific, mechanism of, 136
nucleoprotein, and, 24, 25
pregnancy, and, 203
race, and, 186
recovery, and, 173–175, 728–740
recurrence, and, 537–540
respiratory infections, minor, and, 157, 199–201
SSS, and, 25, 26, 131, 132, 731, 732
sex, and, 192, 193
skin tests, correlation with, 126, 127
specificity, 133–136
substances neutralizing SSS, and, 121, 122
tests for, sensitivity of, 127
time, variations with, 194–196
treatment:
deuteroproteose, and, 774, 775
oxygen, and, 767
sulfapyridine, and, 789
type-specific, 134, 135
virulence and type, and, 193, 194
vitamins, and, 203, 335, 790
Immunity, pneumococcus, acquired, 158–180
age and weight, and, 178, 179
age, variations of antibody titer with, 177, 187, 515, 731
allergy to pneumococcus, and, 182–185
altered reactivity in, 159–168
anti-autolysate serum, and, 446
Immunity, pneumococcus, acquired (*cont.*):
antiblastic, 729
antibody:
absence of, and, 136
relation to, 168–171, 178
relation of, to course and outcome of infection, 173–177
bactericidal power in, 119, 120
blockade of, 167, 168
blood-clearing mechanism, and, 162–164, 167–169, 885, 886
cellular status, and, 167, 168, 178–180
course of infection altered with, 164, 165, 173–177
death, and, 174–176
differentiation from natural, 119
host factors in, 177–180
immobilization of organisms, and, 164
immunization, 196–199, 406–482
duration after, 194, 195, 408, 437–440, 450, 460, 461, 473, 476, 477
with autolysates, and kidney lesions in animals, 609
with live organisms, and, 196, 197, 411, 442
with SSS and related agents in animals, 28, 134, 198, 412, 414, 415, 417, 418, 429–431
with SSS and related agents in man, 134, 198, 199, 412, 418, 430–432, 474, 475
leucocytes, and, 167, 178, 179
localization of infection, and, 164
lung resistance, and, 99, 180–182, 735, 736
macrophage reaction in recovery, 181, 735, 736
mechanism, 158–182
mechanism, comparison of, in animals and man, 409
meningitis, experimental, and, 596
negative phase, and immunization, 482, 798
Negroes, environmental factors, and, 317, 318
passive:
antibody action in, 171, 172
curative power and antibody, 120, 121, 168, 169, 174–177, 882–920
duration, 166, 167, 537, 739, 740
protective power and antibody, 120, 121, 168
skin sensitivity to SSS, and, 126, 127, 166, 167, 170, 171, 739, 740, 813, 860, 861
physiologic variables in, 177–180
pneumococcus carrier rate, and, 156, 157, 195, 214, 377, 378, 385

Immunity, pneumococcus, acquired (*cont.*):
pneumococcus carriers, development of immunity in, 156, 157, 200, 201
prevention of infection in animals, and, 164, 165, 440–446
prevention of pneumonia in man, and, 446–483
recovery, 173–175, 728–737
cross immunity, 731, 739
duration after, 538, 737–740
in local lung areas, and, 99, 180–182, 735, 736
macrophage reaction, and, 181, 735, 736
recurrence, and, 537–540
resolution, and, 542
SSS, development of immunity hindered by, 132, 731, 732
skin sensitivity to SSS in actively acquired immunity, 126, 166, 185, 735, 738
tests for, variability of, 410
treatment, serum, and, 120, 121, 167–172, 174–177, 882–920
treatment, serum, duration after, 739, 740
treatment, vaccine, and, 795–804
type, variation of response with, 161, 162, 193, 194, 432–434, 730, 731
vitamins, and, 790
Immunity, pneumococcus, natural, 137–158
abortive pneumonia, and, 511, 512
age and lung lesion in man, 513–515
age variations, 129, 186–192, 557
age variations, and bacteriemia, 557
allergy to pneumococcus, and, 182–185
animals, and, 137–143, 186
animals of beef group, and, 142
antibody:
correlation with, 128–131, 137, 138, 143, 150–155
in animals, and, 137–143
mode of production, 155–157
relation to course and outcome of infection, 153, 154
relation to incidence of pneumonia, 154, 155
type-specific in animals, 141, 142
antibody titer, age variations, 186–192
at birth, 187–192
at birth, and allergy, 241, 243
bactericidal power in, 119, 120
blood-clearing mechanism, and, 162, 163
breed of animals, and experimental infections, 212–216
breed of animals, variation with, 138, 158, 177, 186
cats, and, 140
Immunity, pneumococcus, natural (*cont.*):
cellular factors in, 157, 158
chickens, and, 142
comparison of, in man and animals, 27, 144
differentiation from acquired, 119
dogs, and, 140, 141
epidemics, and, 389
guinea pigs, and, 139
horses, and, 142
immunization with vaccine, reactions to, and, 481
incidence of pneumonia, and, 154, 155, 394
incidence of pneumonia by age, and, 299, 307
leucocytes, and, 150–152, 167, 179, 180
man, and, 27, 143–150, 186, 195
man, variation in different countries, 669
mechanism of, 150–158
mice, and, 27, 138
mice, variability in, 120, 121
migratory pneumonia, and, 513
monkeys, and, 139, 140
Negroes, and, 236, 312, 313
pathogenesis of lobar pneumonia in animals, and, 219, 220, 222, 225–232, 257
pathogenesis of lobar pneumonia in man, and, 233–255, 257, 393, 514
pigeons, and, 143
pigs, and, 141, 142
pneumococcus carriers, and, 156, 157, 200, 201
prevalence of pneumonia in natives in tropics, and, 299
prognosis, and, 656
rabbits, and, 27, 138, 139
rats, and, 141
respiratory infections, minor, and variations of, 156, 157, 199–201
seasonal variation of, 203
seasonal variation and pneumococcus carriers, 378, 380, 385
sheep, and, 142
skin sensitivity in man, and, 149, 150, 184, 185
species of animal, variation with, 186
species-specific, and incidence of pneumonia, 155
time, variation with, 195, 196
Immunization, active, 196–199, 408–482
against contact infection in animals, 214, 446
against minor respiratory infections, and vaccine composition, 406–408

Immunization, active (*cont.*):
against pneumonia. *See* Immunization, active, against pneumonia
agents used, 28, 196–199, 407, 408, 410–415
agents used and response, 410–415, 441, 442
allergy and immunity from, and extent of pulmonary lesion in pneumonia, 241–245
altered reactivity from, 159–168
animals and man, comparison of response, 409
antibody appearance, 159–162, 196–199, 408–440
antibody appearance, variation with type, 161, 162, 194, 432–434
antibody produced, actions of, 28, 114–125, 171, 172
antibody response, specificity, 133–136
antitoxin production in animals, 125
condition of pneumococcus for optimum response, 28, 133, 410, 411
dosage, and response, 418–434, 441–445
duration of response, 194, 195, 408, 437–440
factors affecting response, 409–434, 441–445
horses, for antiserum production, 823, 824
individual variation of response, 409, 419
live organisms, and, 196, 197, 411, 442
negative phase, and, 482, 798
non-specific immunity, and, 136
prevention of pneumonia, and. *See* Immunization, active, against pneumonia
prevention of respiratory infections, and, 406–408
rabbits, for antiserum production, 873, 874
reactions to vaccine, 427, 478–481
reticulo-endothelial system, blockade of, and immunity, 167, 168
route of administration, and response, 415–418, 441–445
SSS and related agents:
dosage, and, 429–432
in animals, and, 28, 134, 198, 412, 414, 415, 417, 418, 429–431
in man, and, 134, 198, 199, 412, 418, 430–432, 474, 475
reactions from, 481, 482
response, duration, 438, 440
response, time of appearance, 436, 437
route, and, 417, 418
route and dosage, and, 430–432
SSS and vaccine, comparison of response, 414, 415, 418, 430

Immunization, active (*cont.*):
serum production, and, 823, 824, 873, 874, 925
specificity of response, 135, 408, 409, 413, 415
splenectomy, in mice, and, 167, 168
tests for response, variability of, 410
time of appearance of response, 434–437
treatment by. *See* Treatment, vaccine
type of pneumococcus, and response, 161, 162, 194, 432–434, 442–445
vaccines:
and dosage, 418–429
and dosage in man, 425–429
and route, 416, 417
and route and dosage, 419–429
factors in preparation of, 410–415
reactions to, 427, 478–481
variability of response, tests for, 438
virulence of pneumococcus, and, 28, 194, 411, 441–443
Immunization, active, against pneumonia, 197, 198, 401, 446–483
animals, 214, 440–445
army camps, 463–469
CCC camps, 474, 475
community autogenous vaccine, and, 458–463
contraindications to, 482
control groups, benefit to, 453
countries other than South Africa or Rhodesia, 449, 463–475
death rates, and, 454–456, 457, 458, 460–463, 465, 468, 469
duration of effects, and predisposing factors, 462, 478
duration of immunity, and, 450, 460, 461, 473, 476, 477
epidemics, and, 404, 406, 454, 465, 473, 474, 477, 478
factors affecting results, 450, 463, 475–478
host resistance, and, 466
incidence of pneumonia, decrease, in absence of antibody, 130
incidence of pneumonia, effect on, 447–478
incidence of pneumonia, increase of, 452, 482
incidence of respiratory diseases, effect on, 450, 461, 469, 470, 472, 473
influenza death rates, and, 460
influenza incidence rates, and, 461, 468
mixed vaccines, and, 448, 458–464, 468, 470, 472, 473
need for further study, 475–478, 925, 926
negative phase, and, 482

Immunization, active, against pneumonia (*cont.*):
- procedure, 448–475
- prognosis, effect on, 450, 451, 454, 466
- reactions to SSS, 481, 482
- reactions to vaccine, 477–481
- results, and severity of predisposing factors, 462, 478
- results, discussion of, 475–478
- Rhodesia, 449, 462–464
- route, choice of, 417
- SSS or related agents, and, 474, 475, 481, 482
- selection of groups for, 401, 477, 478
- South Africa, 197, 447–462
- South Africa, changing etiology of cases, and results, 457, 458
- South Africa, results questioned, 461, 462
- spontaneous, in Negroes, 313
- vaccines, 425–429, 448–482
- vaccines, community autogenous, and, 458–463
- vaccines, mixed, 448, 458–464, 468, 470, 472, 473

Immunization, passive:
- of animals, against contact infection, 446
- of animals, and induced infections, 445, 446
- of man, for prevention of pneumonia, 483
- of man, for treatment. *See* Serum treatment
- of mice and rabbits, variables in recovery from infection, 178, 179

Incidence, 258–260
- acute infections, and, 335
- age, and, 299–307
- age, and immunity variations, 129
- alcohol, and, 327, 333, 334
- altitude, and, 299, 332, 333
- annual, in United States, 258, 259
- anthracosis, and, 338, 340
- antibody, natural, relation to, 154, 155
- army troops, recruits and seasoned, 332
- aspiration of noxious substances, and, 340–342
- chilling, and, 319, 326–329
- chronic disease, and, 335, 336, 513, 525
- climate, and, 288, 289, 297–299, 312, 313, 337
- climatic factors in, and environmental change, 330–332
- control and immunized groups, incidence in, 450–478
- countries other than North America, variations in, 277–284

Incidence (*cont.*):
- crowding, and, 298, 299, 316–318
- crowding and epidemics, 389
- diet, and, 334, 335
- dust, and, 324, 325, 327, 329, 338–340
- economic status, and, 316
- environmental change, and, 329–332
- epidemics, and, 386–390
- estimated for England and Wales, 266
- estimated for South African Negroes, 456
- estimated for United States, 266
- factors influencing, 299–342, 394
- fatigue, and, 327, 335
- gases, exposure to, and, 327, 338, 339, 341
- hospitals over world, incidence in, 264
- humidity, and, 297–299, 337
- immunity, natural, and, 154, 155, 394
- immunization, effect on. *See under* Immunization, active, against pneumonia
- large and small cities, 276, 277, 279, 284
- local conditions, and variations of, 288, 289
- lung, damage to, and, 202, 203, 217, 218, 225, 230, 236, 257, 340–342
- meteorological factors, and, 289, 290, 295–299, 332
- miners, underground and surface, 328, 329, 337, 338, 448
- need for further study, 927
- Negroes, and occupation, 328, 329
- Negroes, tropical, 330–332
- North America, variations in, 269–277
- occupation, and, 318–329, 337, 338, 448
- personal condition, and, 333–336
- pneumococcus carriers, and, 366, 374, 393, 394
- pneumoconiosis, and, 338
- pneumonia belts, 269–274, 283
- post-operative pneumonia, 520, 521
- race, and, 312–316
- rates, comparison of, in areas with low fatality rates, 338, 660, 662
- rates, trend, 395, 396
- recurrence, and, 339, 340, 533, 534, 538, 539
- reported cases and deaths in Massachusetts, 290–293, 299, 300, 306–309, 383, 385
- reporting of cases or deaths, 258–260, 927
- respiratory infections, minor, and, 235–240, 339
- respiratory infections, minor, and family epidemics, 392
- rickets or scurvy, and, 334
- seasonal distribution of lobar cases, compared with pneumococcus carriers, 385
- seasonal factors, and, 289–295, 297, 298, 394

Incidence (*cont.*):
sex, and, 307–312
silicosis, acute, and alkaline silica dust, 340
silicosis, and, 324
smoke, exposure to, and, 327, 338, 339
social status, and, 316–333
starvation, and, 334
steel workers, and season, 295
systemic disease, and, 335, 336, 513, 525
temperature variations, exposure to, and, 297, 299, 318–323, 326–329, 336–339
transmission and spread of pneumonia, 342–394
trauma, and, 340
tuberculosis, and, 274
Type III infections and chronic disease, 335, 336
unreliability of figures for, 258–260
urban and rural areas, 279, 288
variations, 269–284
virus infections, and, 236–240
wet and cold, exposure to, and, 336–339
yearly variations, of lobar cases, 293
Incidence of causative organisms in pneumonia. *See* Causative organisms; Pneumococcus type incidence
Incubation period:
experimental infections, 487
lobar pneumonia, 486, 487
of sensitiveness to serum, 838, 839
of serum sickness, 838, 869
Indurative pneumonia, 101, 220, 227, 543, 544
Industrial Fatigue and Research Board of Great Britain, 318
Infants and children with pneumonia, 2, 3, 74–89, 513–515
abdominal pain at onset in lobar pneumonia, 653, 654
allergy, role in lobar pneumonia in infants, 241, 243
antibody appearance, 177, 515, 731
aspiration of amniotic fluid by infants, 341
at birth, 241, 243, 305
bacteriemia in, 515, 557, 558, 580, 693
bronchopneumonia, 305, 514, 515, 704, 705
causative organisms, 2, 3, 74–89
causative organisms in bronchopneumonia, 84–89
causative organisms in lobar pneumonia, 79–84
complications, 515, 557, 558, 568, 571, 572, 574, 576, 579, 580, 585
crisis in lobar pneumonia, 529
Infants and children with pneumonia (*cont.*):
empyema in, 515, 568, 571, 572, 574, 576, 579, 580, 585
fatality rates, 515, 693, 703–707
leucocyte count, 515
lobar pneumonia, 514, 529, 653, 654
lobar pneumonia, commonest types in, 79–84, 515
lobar pneumonia, symptoms and physical signs, 514, 515
mediastinal displacement in children, 253
meningismus at onset in lobar pneumonia, 654
mixed infection in, 74
organisms other than pneumococci in bronchopneumonia, 84–86
organisms other than pneumococci in lobar pneumonia, 79–82
otitis media in, 515
physical signs, 514, 515
pneumococcus in, 2, 3, 74–89
pneumococcus in bronchopneumonia, 84–89
pneumococcus in lobar pneumonia, 79–84
prognosis, 515, 703–707
prognosis, bacteriemia, and, 693
respiratory infections, epidemic in family, and, 377, 392
SSS in urine, 643, 695
serum treatment, 835, 844, 845, 852, 853
dosage, 852, 853
fatality rates by type, 906–909
fatality rates, with bacteriemia, 909, 914, 915
Huntoon's antibody solution, 818, 819
reactions from, 864–866, 868, 871
routes of, 844, 845
sputum, and, 514, 617, 618
staphylococcus cases, 11
symptoms, 491, 514, 515
treatment, other than serum. *See* Treatment; Oxygen treatment; Chemotherapy
type incidence, 74–89, 515
age variations, 76–79
bronchopneumonia, 84–89
bronchopneumonia compared with bronchopneumonia in adults, 87–89
lobar and bronchopneumonia, compared, 87, 89
lobar pneumonia, 79–84
age variations, 80–84
compared with adults, 83, 84, 89
compared with type incidence in noncontact carriers, 350, 351
Type XIV, incidence, 74–77, 82, 83, 88, 89, 515

Infants and children with pneumonia (*cont.*):
types, commonest:
in bronchopneumonia, 84–89
in bronchopneumonia in infants, 88
in infants, 76–79
in lobar pneumonia in children, 83, 84
in lobar pneumonia in infants, 82–84
in pneumococcus cases, 75–79, 515
Infarction, pulmonary, 610
differentiation of lobar pneumonia from, 650
Influenza:
as cause of antibody variation, 200
bacillus as cause, 8
death rates:
and occupation, 325
with pneumonia, by age, and sex, 310
with pneumonia, in immunized man, 460
distribution, world-wide, 339
epidemics:
bronchopneumonia, and, 4, 15, 68, 72–74, 339, 386
empyema, and, 566, 567, 582
in army camps, 15, 465, 467
influenza bacillus pneumonia in, 9
mixed infections, and, 15
prognosis of pneumonia, variations during, 9, 582, 811, 812
treatment of pneumonia with chicken serum during, 810, 811
treatment of pneumonia with convalescent serum during, 812
incidence of pneumonia, and, 339
incidence rates, after immunization against pneumonia, 461, 468
isolation of, and prevention of pneumonia, 400
mixed infections during, 13, 15
occupation factors, and, 310
prevention of, by immunization, 468, 469
type incidence in lobar pneumonia, variations during, 60, 466
virus:
as cause, 8
failure to find antibody for, after pneumococcus pneumonia, 237
infection, preceding pneumococcus pneumonia, 237
transformation of R pneumococci to S forms, and, 239
Influenza bacillus:
as cause of influenza, 8
carriers of, and minor respiratory infections, 375
Influenza bacillus (*cont.*):
in bronchopneumonia, 67–69
in lobar pneumonia, 1, 2, 8
in mixed infections, 13
in pneumonia, 8, 9
mixed vaccines, and, 458–461, 470, 472
pathogenicity, 8, 9
transformation of R to S forms by cold virus, 239
viability in air, 296
Influenza bacillus pneumonia, 1, 2, 8, 9, 457
bacteriemia in, 9
bronchopneumonia, 8, 9, 663
bronchopneumonia, fatality rates, 663
bronchopneumonia in animals, 8, 9
diagnosis, 9, 614
in influenza epidemics, 9
in military camps, 9
pathology, 9
prognosis, 8, 9, 663
treatment with convalescent serum, 9
Inhalation pneumonia, 341, 524
Interstitial pneumonia, 3, 111, 321
Intradermal tests. *See* Skin tests for sensitiveness to serum; Skin tests with pneumococcus products
Intravenous test for sensitivity to rabbit serum, 876, 877
Inulin, fermentation by pneumococci, 20

Jaundice:
during course, 502, 503
prognosis, and, 727

Kidney lesions, 608–610
experimental infections, and, 212, 216, 609
immunization of animals with autolysates, and, 609
See also Urine
Kupffer cells, and antibody formation, 137
Kyes immune chicken serum. *See* Serum, chicken, antipneumococcic

Laboratory technicians:
role in pneumonia programs, 930, 932, 933
training for typing, 933
Larval pneumonia, 512
Laryngitis, 607
Latent pneumonia, 512
League of Nations:
epidemiologic reports of, 260, 277–284
report on race of African Negroes, 313

League of Nations (*cont.*):
serum:
diagnostic, standard, 624
diagnostic, standardization by, 924
therapeutic, standard, 827
therapeutic, standardization by, 924, 925
unsolved problems, and, 921, 924, 925
Leucocyte count:
age variations, 497
bacteriemia, and, 724
convalescence, 498
delayed resolution, and, 542
diagnosis, and, 515, 613, 645, 654
differential, during course, 498
differential, prognosis, and, 724, 725
differentiation of serum sickness from complications, and, 870
during course, 497, 498
empyema, and, 576
Friedländer's bacillus cases, 7
host reactivity and outcome, and, 178–180
in children, 515
influenza bacillus cases, 9
peritonitis, and, 602
prognosis, and, 498, 723–725
pulmonary infarct, and, 650
serum sickness, and, 870
severity of illness, and, 498
staphylococcus cases, 10
treatment:
deuteroproteose, and, 773, 775
Huntoon's antibody solution, and, 817
serum, and outcome in animals, 178, 179
sulfanilamide, and, 785, 786
Leucocyte(s):
action, effect on, of various substances, 132
blood-clearing mechanism, and, 162–164, 167
count. *See* Leucocyte count
death of pneumococcus, and, 116–120, 124, 151, 152, 162, 167, 172, 724, 731
empyema fluids, cells in, 577, 643
immunity, acquired, and, 167, 178, 179
immunity, natural, and, 150–152, 167, 179, 180
meningitis, and, 594, 595, 597
pleural fluids, cells in, 564, 577, 643
prognosis, and degenerate forms, 724
prognosis in experimental infections, and mobilization of, 151, 179
protection tests, inhibition of action in, 180
recovery, and, 735, 736
resolution, and, 98–101, 106, 541, 542
SSS, effect on, 132, 180
Lipoid pneumonia, 341
Lipoids, serum:
agglutination reaction, and, 115
chill reactions, and, 830
effect on phagocytic activity, 132
precipitin reaction, and, 116
Lister's classification of pneumococci, 22, 23, 30, 51, 453, 946
Lobar pneumonia:
alkali tolerance during, 500
allergy, and, 240–245
antibody, presence at onset, 129, 153–155, 234, 511
aspiration of noxious substances, and, 340, 341
associated lesions, 111, 112
association with other diseases, 111, 524, 525
at birth, 514
at birth, and allergy, 243
bacteriologic study. *See* Bacteriologic study
bronchopneumonia, associated with, 111
causative organisms, xiii, xvii, 1–17, 41–54, 79–84, 89
characteristic features, 613
clinical varieties, 510–524
complications. *See* Complications; Resolution, delayed
congenital, 305
consolidation, maximum, time of, 96
course, special features in, 526–547
definition, xiii, xvii
differentiation from bronchopneumonia, xiii, 612, 648, 649
duration, 526–532
duration, factors affecting, 511
duration of red and gray stages, 96
electrocardiograms in, 494–496
experimental. *See* Experimental pneumonia
exudate, disappearance in resolution, 96–100
fibrosis, massive, in, 544
Friedländer's bacillus cases, 1, 2, 6, 7, 19
gas warfare, and, 341
incubation period, 486, 487
infants and children. *See* Infants and children with pneumonia
in old age, 514, 515
lobes involved, incidence of, 107–111
lung involved, incidence of, 107–110
organized lesions, 101, 543, 544
organized lesions in animals, 101, 220, 227
pneumococcus. *See* Lobar pneumonia, pneumococcus
pneumococcus, discovery of organism as usual cause, 19

Lobar pneumonia (*cont.*):
pneumococcus in, xiii, xvii, 1–3, 19, 42–54, 79–84
predisposing factors. *See* Predisposing factor(s)
prolongation of illness in, 531, 532
pulmonary circulation, impairment of, 95, 96
reportable disease, 259, 260, 290
reported cases in Massachusetts
by age, 299, 300, 306, 307
by month, 290–293
by season, 383, 385
by sex, 308, 309
reported deaths in Massachusetts, by season, 383, 385
severity and density of consolidation, 646
spread of lesion, 253–256
staphylococcus cases, 1, 2, 9
streptococcus cases, 1–5
synonyms, xiv, xv, xvi
time of admission to hospital, 928, 929
toxic changes in organs, at necropsy, 112
toxicity, and vasomotor paralysis, 545–547
toxin, and crisis, 528
vascular failure, peripheral, in, 545, 546
Lobar pneumonia, pneumococcus, 612, 648, 649
accidental infection, 240, 486
allergy to organism, and, 240–245
antibody, and. *See* Antibody(ies), pneumococcus
bacteriologic study. *See* Bacteriologic study
causal relation of various types to, 49–51
complications. *See* Complications; Resolution, delayed
development, factors controlling, 257
diaphragm, elevation in, 251, 253
duration, by types, 527
experimental. *See* Experimental pneumonia
hilar lesions, 256
infants and children. *See* Infants and children with pneumonia
initial lesion, site of, 247–250, 256
mediastinal displacement, and, 251, 253
predisposing factors. *See* Predisposing factor(s)
route of infection, 245–247, 257
silent lesion in adjacent lobe, 647
spread of lesion, 253–256
transmission and spread of, 342–394
types, and. *See under* Pneumococcus types; Pneumococcus type incidence
Lobes involved in pneumonia, 108–111
Loeschcke's views of pathology of lobar pneumonia, 101–106
Lung:
condition of uninvolved tissue in lobar pneumonia, 106, 111, 112
consolidation in, 3–5, 7, 9, 10, 92–96, 103–107, 228
consolidation, duration of red and gray stages, 96
defense barriers, damage to, by colds, 257
defense barriers, in experimental pneumonia, 217, 218, 225, 232
elasticity, comparison of, in dogs and man, 228, 253
Friedländer's bacillus in chronic lesions of, 6
immunity, local, in, 99, 180–182, 735, 736
lesion in recurrence, 536–539
lymph flow in, 250
macrophage in exudate, in animals, 98, 99, 167, 180, 181, 227, 228
macrophage in exudate, in man, 98–101, 106, 167, 181, 542, 735, 736
mixed infections, and, 12–16
necrosis, aputrid, 541, 606, 607
necrosis, in Friedländer's cases, 7, 8
pulmonary circulation, impairment of, 95, 96, 496, 499, 743, 755, 759–762
repair of tissue in recovery, 604, 606, 607
resistance of, and contact with irritating substances, 202, 203, 217, 218, 225, 230, 235, 236, 257, 340–342
SSS in, 26, 541
Lung abscess:
empyema, and, 578
gangrene, and, 10, 604–607
organized lesions, and, 543
simulated appearance in resolution, 541, 606, 607
Lung involved in pneumonia, 107–110
Lung puncture:
findings at necropsy, 734
findings at recovery, 528, 734, 735
material for bacteriologic study, 11, 14, 15, 50, 619, 620, 644
mixed infections, and, 11, 14, 15
technic and complications of, 619
typing, and, 644
Lymphatics, infection in, and prognosis, 163, 169, 886
Lyons' immuno-transfusion method, in treatment of streptococcus pneumonia, 5
Lysis, 529, 531
age, and, 529
complications, and, 531
definition, 531
factors affecting occurrence, 529, 531
pneumococcus types, and, 531

M. & B. 693, 784, 786–790
Macrophage:
  antibody formation, and, 137
  blood-clearing mechanism, and, 162
  in acquired immunity, 167
  in allergic meningitis, 594
  in lung exudate in animals, 98, 99, 167, 180, 181, 227, 228
  in lung exudate in man, 98–101, 106, 167, 181, 542, 735, 736
Macrophage reaction, 181, 182
  delayed resolution, and, 101
  local lung resistance, and, 99, 180–182, 735, 736
  pneumonia in dogs, and, 181, 227–229
  recovery, and, 181, 735, 736
  recurrence, in animals, and, 538
  resolution, and, 98, 101, 181, 227–229, 542
Manual of the International List of Causes of Death, xv
Manual of Tropical Medicine, 17
Massachusetts Department of Public Health. *See* Departments of health, Massachusetts; Massachusetts Pneumonia Series; Massachusetts Pneumonia Program
Massachusetts Pneumonia Program, 937–945
  advisory committee, 929
  bacteriologic diagnosis in, and epidemics, 388
  blood culture outfits, and, 619, 855
  chill-producing factor in serum, monkey test for, 831
  duration of, 929, 937
  interest aroused by, 929
  laboratories for typing, 54
  mixed infections in, 16
  physicians treating cases in, 929
  pneumococci, prevalence by season, 381–385
  pneumococci, strains classified, 29
  report, final, of, 929
  respiratory disease, death rates by age and sex, 311, 312
  respiratory disease, hospitalization rate in, 308–310
  serum distribution, removal of time restriction on, 833, 882, 897, 937
  serum treatment, success with, 808
  serums distributed, 829, 851, 937
  sputum, character observed in, 502
  sputums typed, 29, 54–57
  treatment, non-specific in, 822
  type incidence, variations during, 59, 60
  types obtained from patients with respiratory infections, 29, 54–57, 381–385
Massachusetts Pneumonia Program (*cont.*):
  typing errors in, 628
  typing methods illustrated, 625
  typing, Neufeld method, adoption as routine, 937
  See also Massachusetts Pneumonia Series
Massachusetts Pneumonia Series:
  analysis, method of, 937
  bacteriemia:
    in Type I cases, 551, 557–561
    in Type II cases, 552, 557–559
    in Type III and Group IV cases, 553
    in Type V cases, 554, 558, 559
  blood cultures, and, 619, 855
  cases included, nature of, 882, 937–939
  deaths, from serum reactions, 836, 866–869
  empyema in, 568–570
  empyema incidence, by day of serum treatment, 888
  fatality rate of home and hospital treated cases, 715–717
  Group IV cases, fatality rate, 671
  home treated cases, proportion in, 912, 939
  mediastinitis, 604
  pulmonary necrosis, aputrid, in, 607
  serum reactions:
    allergic, 864
    allergic, death from, 866, 867
    chill, and fatality rate, 868
    chill, death from, 868, 869
    serum sickness, 871
  serum treatment:
    dosage, minimum, 938, 939
    dosage, relation to serum sickness, 871
    fatality rate variations, with season, 680, 681, 917
    patients with history of asthma or hay fever, 838
    physicians, and, 808, 895
    results in home and hospital treated cases, 912
    time of treatment of cases included, 882
  Type I:
    average age, 62, 63
    fatality rate, 664, 716, 909
    fatality rate by age groups, with and without serum treatment, 909
    serum treatment:
      composite temperature curve, 884
      dosage, average, 846, 847
      dosage, need for larger, 847, 898
      dosage recommended, 848, 856
      failure of, analysis of cause, 919
      fatality rate, 895–898

Massachusetts Pneumonia Series (*cont.*):
  Type I (*cont.*):
    serum treatment (*cont.*):
      fatality rate by age, 909
      fatality rate by season, 680, 681, 917
      fatality rate by sex, 911
      results by day of illness, 896, 897
      results by year and average dose, 846, 847
      results with and without bacteriemia, by age, 915, 916
  Type I and II, proportion in males, 65
  Type I, II, and V, serum treatment, fatality rate of home and hospital cases, 912
  Type II:
    average age, 63
    fatality rate, 667
    serum treatment:
      dosage, average, 848, 849
      dosage, need for larger, 849
      dosage, recommended, 850, 856
      failure of, analysis of cause, 919
      fatality rate, 900, 901
      fatality rate by age, 909, 910
      fatality rate by season, 680, 681, 917
      fatality rate by sex, 911
      results by day of illness, 901, 902
      results by year and average dose, 848, 849, 902
      results with and without bacteriemia, by age, 915, 916
  Type III, fatality rate, 670
  Type V:
    fatality rate, 672
    serum treatment:
      dosage, average, 850
      dosage, recommended, 850, 851, 856
      fatality rate with and without serum, 903, 904
  Type VII, fatality rate, 673
  Type VIII, fatality rate, 674
  Type XIV, fatality rate, 674
  See also Massachusetts Pneumonia Program
Massive pneumonia, 509, 512
Measles:
  bronchopneumonia, and, 4, 72, 73
  bronchopneumonia, fatality rates, 663
  epidemic, empyema, and, 567
  epidemic, pneumonia, and, 15, 72, 73
  isolation of, and prevention of pneumonia, 400
  mixed infections in pneumonia, and, 15
Media for cultivation of pneumococci, 20, 550, 618, 636
Mediastinitis, 604
Medical profession:
  Massachusetts Pneumonia Program, and, 808, 895, 929
  role of, in pneumonia programs, 929–932
  serum treatment, results by physicians in general practice, 808, 895, 896, 929
Meningitis, 10, 592–599
  allergy, and, 594, 595
  arthritis, septic, and, 599
  diagnosis, 595
  empyema, and, 567, 578
  endocarditis, and, 591, 594
  experimental, in animals, 209, 213, 214, 596, 597
  meningococcus, similarity of epidemiology with pneumococcus pneumonia, 394
  prognosis, 595, 596
  treatment, 595–598, 888
    optochin, 595–597, 778
    serum, 595–597
    serum, combined with optochin, 595–597, 781
    serum, effect on incidence, 888
    sulfanilamide, 597, 786
Mercurochrome, 782
Metabolic changes during course, 500
Metropolitan Life Insurance Company, 269, 271, 929, 930
  handbook on nursing care, availability, 935
  Influenza Commission of, 929
Michigan Health Department. *See* Departments of health, Michigan
Micrococcus catarrhalis:
  in bronchopneumonia, 67
  mixed vaccines, and, 458–463, 472
Micrococcus of pneumonia, 19
Migratory pneumonia, 513
Mixed infection(s), 1–3, 11–16, 74, 111, 533
  antibody in convalescence, 14, 16
  bacteriemia in, 14, 560
  bacteriologic diagnosis, 11–16, 642, 643
  causative organisms, 1–3, 11–16, 74, 111
  clinical study, 11–16
  complications, and, 11
  contact infection, and, 16, 392, 403
  convalescence, and, 16
  diagnosis, 11–16
  fatality rates, 11, 15, 16, 677
  infants and children, 74
  influenza, and, 13, 15
  lung abscess or gangrene, and, 606
  lung lesions with, 12–16
  lung puncture in, 11, 14, 15
  Massachusetts Pneumonia Study, and, 16
  measles, and, 15

Mixed infection(s) (*cont.*):
- military camps, and, 15, 16
- necropsy study, 11, 15, 16
- organisms other than pneumococci in, 3, 8–10, 13, 15, 16
- organized lesions, relation to, 101
- pneumococcus in, 12–16
- predisposing factors, 16
- prevention of, 16
- prevention of pneumonia, and cross infection, 403
- prognosis in, 11, 15, 16, 111, 199, 533
- prolongation of illness, and, 532
- relapse, and, 16, 532, 533
- repeated invasions in, 12
- secondary infection, and, 15
- serum treatment, failure of, due to, 11, 15, 533, 860, 919
- simultaneous invasions, and, 12, 15, 16
- South Africa, 457
- spread, and, in experimental infections, 212
- super-infections in, 12, 15, 16
- throat cultures, and, 642, 643
- yearly variation of, 13

Monocyte, immunity mechanism, and, 179, 180

Morbidity. *See* Incidence; Prevalence; Epidemiology

Mortality. *See* Death rate(s); Fatality rate(s)

Mucin, 785

Multiple infections. *See* Mixed infections

National Institute of Health, 826–829, 874

Natural immunity. *See* Immunity, pneumococcus, natural

Necropsy:
- arthritis, septic, at, 598
- associated lesions at, 111, 112
- bacteriemia at, 562
- bacteriologic study at, 614
- death, study of cause, 544–546
- diagnosis, accuracy of, and, 612, 613
- differentiation of lobar from bronchopneumonia at, 612
- empyema and pericarditis at, 566, 575
- empyema at, 566, 567, 573
- empyema, bilateral, at, 574
- endocarditis at, 590, 591
- gas, pneumonia from, and, 341
- lobar pneumonia at, 3, 7, 90–112
  - age, sex, and race, and, 91
  - at birth, 514
  - incidence at, 90, 91
- lung abscess or gangrene at, 604–606

Necropsy (*cont.*):
- lung puncture findings at, 734
- mediastinitis at, 604
- meningitis at, 592, 593
- mixed infections, and, 11, 15, 16
- myositis at, 112
- nephritis at, 608
- organized lesions, incidence, at, 543
- otitis media and sinusitis at, 585
- parotitis at, 600
- pericarditis at, 586–588
- peritonitis at, 601
- pleura after pneumonia, 564, 565, 771
- pulmonary embolism, or thrombosis, at, 610
- rheumatic pneumonia at, 652, 653
- types found at, 50, 51, 68, 69
- *See also* Pathology

Negroes:
- arthritis, septic, in, 599
- Bantu race, 313
- bronchopneumonia, and, 457
- causative organisms in, 3, 4, 453, 456–459, 462
- complications, and, 312
- crisis, time of, 529
- crowding, and incidence and death rates, 317, 318
- death, importance of pneumonia as cause, 268
- death rates, 271–273, 315, 316, 318, 456, 462, 463
- death rates, trend, 287
- delayed resolution, and, 543
- diet, and incidence, 334
- duration of disease, 527
- empyema in, 566, 572, 573
- empyema in, and prognosis, 581
- epidemics in, 386
- etiology, changes of, in Africa, 457
- fatality rates, variation of, 678
- immunity, natural, and, 236, 312, 313
- immunity, natural, and reactions to vaccine injections, 481
- immunization, 447–469
  - antibody response to, 425, 426
  - prevention of minor respiratory infections, and, 406, 407
  - reactions to vaccine injection, 480, 481
- incidence:
  - alcohol, and, 333
  - climate, and, 312–316
  - environmental change, and, 330–332
  - estimated in South Africa, 456
  - occupation, and, 328, 329

Negroes (*cont.*):
incidence (*cont.*):
season, and, 290, 331
incidence and death rates, and, 312, 313
incidence and death rates, in control and immunized groups, 468, 469
incubation period in, 486, 487
lobar pneumonia:
at necropsy, 91, 106
lung involvement in, 108
pneumococcus, 42–49, 453, 456–459, 462
meningitis, and, 592, 593
pericarditis, and, 586
pleural effusions, and, 564
pneumococcus infections, and, 312, 313
predisposing factors, upper respiratory infections, and, 236
predisposing factors, virus infections, and, 457
prognosis in, 330, 710–712
recurrence in, 534, 535, 539
streptococcus pneumonia in, 3, 4, 457, 462, 573
susceptibility, 312–316, 399, 462, 463
treatment:
sodium salicylate, 782, 783
vaccine, 798, 799
vitamin, 790
type incidence, and, 42–49, 453, 456, 457
Nephritis, 212, 216, 608–610
See also Urine
Nervous system:
aphasia or aphonia, 505, 607
brain abscess or hemorrhage, 593
hemiplegia, 505
meningismus at onset, 654
meningitis, 10, 592–599
empyema, and, 567, 578
in animals, 209, 213, 214, 596, 597
treatment, 595–598, 778, 781, 786, 888
neuritis, 611
pachymeningitis, 593
psychosis, toxic, in convalescence, 547
symptoms:
at onset, 491, 514, 654
delirium. *See* Delirium
during course, 504, 505, 510
hydrotherapy, and, 756, 758
in convalescence, 546, 547
prognosis, and, 547, 727
sedatives, and, 755, 756
Neufeld and Händel's classification of pneumococci, 22, 23
Neufeld *Quellung* phenomenon, 172, 626, 627
New York City Department of Health, 830, 928–930
New York State:
association of Public Health Laboratories, 930
Medical Society, 930
New York State Department of Health, 829, 928–930, 935
See also New York State Pneumonia Program; New York State Pneumonia Series
New York State Pneumonia Program:
handbook on nursing care, 744, 935
nursing care, and, 744
provision of therapeutic serum in, 829, 929, 930
serum treatment:
dosage recommended in Type I and II cases, 856
duration of illness, and, 897
success with, 808
New York State Pneumonia Series:
Type I, serum treatment, fatality rate, 896
Type I and II, serum treatment, number of cases treated, 930
Type II, serum treatment, fatality rate, 901
Nuclein, 783
Nucleoprotein(s) of pneumococcus, 24, 25, 133–135, 149
Numoquin-base, 779
Nurse:
nursing care, 743–746
nursing care, handbook on, 744, 935
nursing technic and prevention of pneumonia, 400, 402
oxygen treatment, and, 746
pneumonia programs, and, 932, 935, 936
serum treatment, and, 746

Onset:
abdominal pain at, 653, 654
antibody at, 129, 153–155, 234, 511
bronchopneumonia symptoms at, 649
chill at, 488
cough at, 490
fever at, 490
Friedländer's bacillus cases, 7
meningismus at, 654
mode of, 487
and crisis, 530
and type, 487–489, 616, 649
in Type III and VIII cases, 649
nervous system symptoms at, 491, 514, 654
pain at, 488–490
and initial lesion, 250

Onset (*cont.*):
pain at (*cont.*):
and type, 489
in apical pneumonia, 498
physical signs at, 506
pneumococcus carriers in family at time of, 392, 403, 926
prognosis, and symptoms at, 486
respiratory distress at, 490
respiratory infections, minor, and, 235–240
sputum at, 486, 490
staphylococcus cases, 10
streptococcus cases, 4
symptoms at, 4, 7, 10, 485–491, 498, 514, 649, 653, 654
symptoms at, and pneumococcus type, 488, 489, 616
vomiting at, 490, 491
Operations. *See* Post-operative pneumonia
Opsonins. *See under* Antibody(ies), pneumococcus
Optochin treatment. *See under* Chemotherapy
Organisms in pneumonia. *See* Causative organisms; Pneumococcus type incidence
Organisms insoluble in bile, 21
Organized pneumonia, 101, 220, 227, 543, 544
Otitis media, 515
mastoiditis, and, 585, 586
sinusitis and meningitis, and, 594
Oxygen treatment, 759–768
anoxemia and morphine, and, 755
carbon-dioxide treatment, and, 768
commercial oxygen, and, 764
complications of, 766, 767
compressed air, and, 768
cost, 766
face mask, 762, 763
face mask, for pulmonary edema, 758
fatality rate, and, 767
indications for, 762
methods, 762–768
morphine, and, 749, 755
nasal catheter, 762, 765, 766
nasal inhaler, 762, 763, 765, 766
oxygen box, 764
oxygen chamber, 762, 764–766
oxygen tent, 762, 763, 765, 766
post-operative pneumonia, and, 524, 767
pulmonary edema, and, 758, 767
rationale, 759–762
rebreathing apparatus, 762, 763
results, 766, 767
tube and funnel, 762, 763
tympanites, relief of, and, 757
Pain, 488–490, 498
abdominal, at onset, 653, 654
abdominal, with serum reactions, 864, 870
apical pneumonia, and, 498
atelectasis, and, 651
initial lesion, and, 250
pleurisy, and mechanism of, 250
pleurisy with effusion, and, 652
referred, 488–490
serum sickness, and joint pains, 869, 872
terminal pneumonia, and, 513
treatment, 749, 750, 755, 772
treatment by artificial pneumothorax, 749
treatment, serum, effect on, 883
Panophthalmitis, 607
Parotitis, 600, 601
Passive immunization. *See* Immunization, passive; Serum treatment
Pathogenesis, 232–257
allergy, and, 240–245
atelectasis, and, 250–253
chilling, and organisms in lung, and, 247
colds, and, 236–240
defense barriers of lung, in animals, and, 217, 218, 225, 232
defense barriers of lung, in man, and, 235, 236
edema fluid:
and allergy to pneumococcus, 254
in experimental infections, 212, 219, 220, 222, 227–232
in initial lesion, 250
experimental pneumonia, 202, 219–231
factors affecting, 233–235, 257
immunity, and character of lesion developed, 232–255, 257, 392, 393, 514, 515
influenza, and, 237
initial lesion, site and nature, 247–250, 256
lobar pneumonia, 232–257
lobar pneumonia, virus infections as primary cause in pneumococcus cases, 232, 239, 240
lung, local injury, and, 217, 218, 230, 246, 247, 257
mixed infections, 16
origin, bronchiogenic, 245–247
pneumococci in upper respiratory tract, and, 393
pneumococcus cases, 232–257
post-operative pneumonia, 516, 517, 522
protective mechanism, in respiratory tract, and, 225, 232, 235, 246, 257
respiratory infections, minor, and, 235–240
route of infection, 245–247, 257

Pathogenesis (*cont.*):
spread of experimental pneumonia, and edema fluid, 219, 220, 222, 227–232, 255, 256
spread of lesion, 253–256
autolyzed organisms, and, 212
cough, and, 255
effect of gravity on edema fluid, 212, 220–222, 255, 256
mixed infections, and, 212
transformation of pneumococcus type, and, 393, 394
virulence, and, 200, 233–235, 257, 393
virus infections as primary cause, 3, 9, 232, 239, 240
Pathogenicity of pneumococcus. *See* Virulence, pneumococcus
Pathology, 90–112
allergic meningitis in animals, 594, 595
allergic pneumonia in animals, 241–243
bronchopneumonia, pneumococcus types found at necropsy, 68, 69
bronchopneumonia, secondary, bacteriologic findings, 72, 73
delayed resolution, macrophage reaction, and, 101
delayed resolution, production in dogs, 100
experimental infections, 212–232
experimental pneumonia, edema fluid in, 219, 220, 222, 227–232, 255, 256
experimental pneumonia, organized lesions in, 101, 220, 227
Friedländer's bacillus cases, 7, 8
gas pneumonia, 341
immunity, local in lung, and, 181, 182
influenza bacillus cases, 9
lobar pneumonia, 90–112
associated lesions, 111, 112
bronchial lymph glands, swelling of, 112
bronchitis, and, 112
consolidation:
duration of red and gray stages, 96
stages found at necropsy, 106, 107
stages of, 92–95, 103–105
time of maximum, 96
edema in early phase, 103–106
engorgement, 92, 93
gray hepatization, 94
gross and microscopic findings, 91–106
heart, hypertrophy or dilatation, 112, 545, 546
initial lesion, site and nature, 248–250
liver necrosis, 112
lobes involved, 109–111
Loeschcke's views, 101–106
Pathology (*cont.*):
lobar pneumonia (*cont.*):
lung, condition of uninvolved tissue in, 106, 111, 112
myositis, 112, 543
organized, 101
pulmonary circulation, impairment of, 95, 96
red hepatization, 93, 94
resolution:
decrease in number of pneumococci during, 99, 100
enzyme-anti-enzyme balance in, 98, 100
histiocytes or macrophage cells in, 98–101
large mononuclear cells in, 98–101, 106
macrophage reaction in, 98–101, 181
spleen enlargement, 112
toxic changes in organs, 112
viability of pneumococci from consolidated areas in different stages, 95
organized lesions, relation to anthracosis, 101
staphylococcus cases, 10
streptococcus cases, 3
types found at necropsy in pneumococcus cases, 50, 51, 68, 69
See also Necropsy
Pericarditis, 586–589
arthritis, septic, and, 599
bacteriemia, and, 560, 561
bronchopneumonia and empyema, and, 566
delayed resolution, and, 543, 588
diagnosis, 589
empyema, and, 566, 575, 588, 589
endocarditis, and, 588
staphylococcus cases, 10
streptococcus cases, 4
treatment, 589
Peritonitis, 601–603
diagnosis, 603
experimental, in the monkey, 602
streptococcus cases, 4
treatment, 603
Physical signs, 506–509
abortive pneumonia, and, 511
absence of, with lesion of adjacent lobe, 647
after crisis, 507
atelectasis and pneumonia, 518, 649, 651
at onset, 506
auscultation, 508, 509
central pneumonia, and, 512
confluent bronchopneumonia, and, 649

Physical signs (*cont.*):
correlation with x-ray findings, 613
delayed resolution, and, 542
diagnosis, and, 506–509, 613
diaphragm, elevation of, and, 252, 253
early:
and breath sounds and rales, 508
and dulness, 508
and x-ray diagnosis, 613
empyema, 575
friction rubs, and, 507
Friedländer's bacillus cases, 7
infants and children, 514, 515
inspection, 507
massive pneumonia, 512
mensuration, 507
palpation, 507
percussion, 508
pleurisy with effusion, and, 652
post-operative pneumonia, 518
pulmonary infarct, 650
resolution, and, 540, 647
staphylococcus cases, 10
tuberculous pneumonia, 651
typical, 506–509
Platelets, 499
Pleurisy with effusion, 564–566, 652
diagnosis, 565, 576, 577
differentiation of lobar pneumonia from, 652
incidence, 564, 565
treatment, 566
Pneumococcidal antibody. *See* Antibody(ies), pneumococcus, bactericidal
Pneumococcus, 18–41
A substance, 117
acid formation during growth, 20
activation by colds, 200, 238, 239, 337, 375–377
air-borne infection, 245–247
allergy. *See* Allergy, pneumococcus
antibodies. *See* Antibody(ies), pneumococcus
antigen, 115, 133
antigen, integrity of cell, and, 28, 133, 410, 411
antigenicity. *See* Antigenicity, pneumococcus
antiphagines, 131
autolysates:
anaerobic, 22
immunization with, 198, 414
skin sensitivity and allergy, 594, 595
spread of experimental infection, and, 131, 132, 212
Pneumococcus (*cont.*):
autolysates (*cont.*):
toxicity, 22, 609
autolysis, 20, 21
Avery broth, 636
bile solubility, as means of differentiating from streptococci, 20, 21
bile solubility, test for, 634
biologic alterations from growth in antibody, 123, 124
biology, 19–28
biology, alterations in, at recovery, 734, 735
blood broth, 20, 618
C substance, 24, 25
antigenicity, 135
precipitins in blood during pneumonia, 125, 733
relation to pneumonia, 25
capsule and relation to virulence, 20, 22
capsule and SSS, 24–26, 133
carriers. *See* Pneumococcus carriers
causal relation to pneumonia, 19, 49–51, 67, 68
cell components, 24–26
cell structure, 133
chain formation, 20, 698
chemical fractions, 24–26
colony appearance, 20
culture collection, need for making, 924
cultures, and their preservation, 20, 21
death:
antibody action, and, 117–120, 124, 151, 152, 162, 172
at crisis, 734
in cultures, 20
leucocyte action, and, 116–120, 124, 151, 152, 162, 167, 172, 724, 731
discovery of, 18
discovery of relation to disease, 19
distribution, world-wide, xiv
drug fastness, 780, 789
early studies of, 18, 19
edema fluid:
and spread of lesion, 253–256
in early lesions, 250
in experimental infections, 212
in experimental pneumonia, 219, 220, 222, 227–232
enzymes, endocellular:
action on proteins, fats, and carbohydrates, 21
and recovery, 736
and resolution, 97, 98, 100
epithelial tissues, penetration by, 232, 549
experimental infections, 204–232, 248–256

Pneumococcus (*cont.*):
formaldehyde sulphoxylate, effect on, 783
Friedländer's bacillus, similarity to, 6
Gram-positive and Gram-negative forms, 20
growth:
Avery broth for, 636
blood-agar plates for, 20, 550
blood broth for, 20, 618
changes from antibody contact, 123, 124
in media, 20
SSS, and, 25, 26
hapten, 134
hemolysin, 20, 21
hemolytic power, and anemia, 498, 499
heterophile antigen in, 125
immunity. *See* Immunity, pneumococcus; Immunity, pneumococcus, acquired; Immunity, pneumococcus, natural
immunization with. *See* Immunization, active; Immunization, active, against pneumonia
in air, 296, 392, 396
in bronchopneumonia, xiii, 67–74, 84–89
in consolidated areas, viability of, 95
in dust, 341, 392, 396
in initial lesions, 247–250, 253–256
in lobar pneumonia, xiii, xvii, 1–3, 19, 42–54, 79–84
in mixed infections, 12–16
in pneumonia, xiii, 1–3, 42–89
in pneumonia in infants and children, 2, 3, 74–89
in sputum:
and prevention of pneumonia, 396, 401
dried, 392
etiologic significance, 12–14, 49–51, 623, 624
inulin fermentation, 20
isolation. *See* Bacteriologic study; Pneumococcus typing
lesion most commonly produced by, 923
macrophage reaction, and, 181, 182, 227–229, 735, 736
methemoglobin formation, and cyanosis, 496
morphology, 20
need for more knowledge of, 921, 922
neutralizing substance in, 131
non-carriers, 367, 368
non-carriers, and minor respiratory infections, 375, 376
nucleoprotein, 24, 25
antigenicity, 24, 25, 133, 134
relation to pneumonia, 25, 135

Pneumococcus (*cont.*):
nucleoprotein (*cont.*):
skin sensitivity to, in normal man, 149
specificity, 25
optochin, effect on, 778–781
organisms resembling, 21
pH for optimum growth, 20
parasitism with, xiv, 390
pathogenicity. *See* Virulence, pneumococcus
platelets, effect of pneumococcus extracts on, 499
prevalence, and season, xiv, 378–385
protection tests, and, 120, 121
protein. *See* Pneumococcus, nucleoprotein
purpura-producing substance, effect on mice, 22
quinine preparations, effect on, 775–777
resolution, decrease in number of organisms during, 99, 100
SSS. *See* Specific capsular polysaccharide(s)
secondary invasion with, 236–240
skin sensitivity in active immunity, and, 165–167
skin sensitivity in normal man, and, 149, 150
solutions, immunization and immunity, 198, 414
somatic carbohydrate. *See* Pneumococcus, C substance
spherules, 123
spread:
colds, and, 239, 397
crowding, and, 298, 316, 318, 389, 392, 394
economic status, and, 316
environmental change, and, 330
in droplets, 296
in droplets and droplet-nuclei, 316
in dust, 295–297, 316
means of, 366, 392–394
traced from carriers, 366, 374, 393, 394
stability of, 385
strains, serum production, and, 823
strains, virulence variations in, 27, 139, 193, 372
substances from, antagonistic to antibody, 131, 132
sulfanilamide, effect on, 784, 785, 787, 789
sulfapyridine, effect on, 784, 787, 789
tests for antibody against, 115–125
tests for cellular immunity against, 125–127
toxemia:
antibody, and, 732
cardiovascular system, and, 544–546, 748, 750

Pneumococcus (*cont.*):
toxemia (*cont.*):
effects on smooth muscle, 546, 748, 756
recovery, and, 528, 734, 737
toxic substances in cultures, 21, 22
toxin:
and antitoxins, 125
changes attributed to, in cases at necropsy, 112
failure to find, 21, 22
place in clinical picture of pneumonia, 21
symptoms, and, 485
transformation. *See under* Pneumococcus, variants
types. *See* Pneumococcus types
typing. *See* Pneumococcus typing
vaccine(s):
condition of cells for optimum response to, 28, 133, 410, 411
immunization with. *See* Immunization, active; Immunization, active, against pneumonia
treatment with, 795–804
variants:
agglutination tests, and, 116
animal passage, and, 27
at recovery or death, 734, 735
M, S, and R, 26, 27
need for study, 924
pneumonia, and, 26, 200, 393, 394
transformation of:
R to S forms, and influenza virus, 239
R to S forms by natural antibody, 155
S to R forms, 124
viability, at different stages of consolidation in pneumonia, 95
viability in air, 296, 392
virulence. *See* Virulence, pneumococcus
virulins, 131
Pneumococcus carriers, 40–42, 342–386, 390
animals, normal, 244, 361
antibody production in, 156, 157, 200, 201
as infected individual, 375
bacteriemia, in animals, 156
chronic, 367, 368, 372
chronic, pathologic conditions of upper respiratory tract, and, 375, 376
chronic, seasonal variations and respiratory infections, 380
classification by persistence of carrier state, 367, 368
colds, and increased activity of organisms carried, 200, 238, 239, 337, 375–377
Pneumococcus carriers (*cont.*):
contacts, 351–365
carriers of type to which exposed, 353–362
duration of carrier state, 368, 369
epidemic Type I pneumonia, and, 369
family members, 353–362, 377, 391, 392
family members, at onset of pneumonia, 392, 403, 926
family members, duration of carrier state, 369
in hospitals, 359–362
length of contact, and, 362
proportion who are carriers, 351–353, 359, 360, 362–365
proportion who are carriers, compared with non-contacts, 352, 353
seasonal variations, and, 379–381, 385
type incidence, among strains found, 352–362, 364
type incidence in, compared with non-contacts, 352, 353
types carried, 351–365
with other carriers, 365–367
convalescence, carrier state after, 366, 367, 547
convalescent, 366, 367, 369–372, 547
antibody, and, 378
duration, 369–372
pathologic condition of upper respiratory tract, and, 376
recurrence of pneumonia, and, 535, 539
strains in nasopharynx, alteration of biologic character, 366, 367
detection, methods for, 342, 343, 368
duration of carrier state, 156, 367–372
epidemic pneumonia, and isolation of, 404, 926
epidemics of pneumonia, and, 369, 376, 386–388, 393, 394, 404, 473, 926
estimated numbers, 364, 365, 390, 391
experimental, in animals, 156, 200, 217, 244
immunity, and, 156, 195, 214, 378
pneumonia, and, 232
virulence of strain, and, 215, 216
experimental, in man, 374, 375
factors affecting, 362, 373–385, 927
family members, at onset of pneumonia, 392, 403, 926
from contact with cases or carriers, compared, 366
immunity, and occurrence of, 156, 157, 195, 214, 377, 378, 385

Pneumococcus carriers (*cont.*):
immunity, development in, 156, 157, 200, 201
immunization against spread of infection by, 446, 473
immunization, passive, and, 483
in community, 362–365
comparison with number of cases, 402, 403
estimated, in Massachusetts, 364, 365
immunity, and, 378
minor respiratory infections, and, 339
types carried, compared with occurrence in cases, 390, 391
Types I and II, estimated for United States, 390, 391
infants, and natural immunity, 157
isolation and treatment, 403–406, 926
mixed infections, and, 392
multiple strains in, 344, 351, 368
need for further study, 926, 927
non-carriers, 367, 368, 375, 376
non-contacts, 343–351, 360, 362–365
duration of carrier state, 367, 368
proportion who are carriers, 343–348, 360, 362–365
repeated examinations of, 347–349
seasonal variation, and, 379–381, 385
type incidence, among strains found, 346, 348–351, 364
type incidence, comparison of, with types in lobar pneumonia, 350, 351
types carried, 343–351, 360, 362–365
periodic, 367, 368
post-operative pneumonia in, 516, 522, 523
prevention of pneumonia, and, 396, 397, 400, 402–406, 926
recurrence of pneumonia, and, 535, 539
respiratory infections, minor, and, 238, 239, 294, 337, 362, 375–377, 379, 380, 926
respiratory tract, pathology of, and, 366, 375, 376
seasonal variations, xiv, 374, 378–385, 390
compared with cases and deaths from lobar pneumonia, 385
peaks of minor respiratory infection, and, 294, 379, 380
prevalence of pneumococci in infections, and, 380, 383, 385
secondary, 365–367
sinus and respiratory infections in, 375
spread of infection in animals, and, 446
spread of infection traced from, 366, 374, 393, 394

Pneumococcus carriers (*cont.*):
spread of organisms, importance in, 390–394
spread of organisms in persons in close contact, 298, 316, 318, 389, 392, 394
strains from healthy carriers, alteration of biologic character, 367
transient or intermittent, 367, 368
treatment, 404–406, 926, 927
treatment, optochin, 404, 405, 778
type, homologous:
during Type II epidemic, 473
in convalescence, 366, 367, 369–372, 547
to which exposed, 353–362, 365, 369, 374, 377, 386–388, 392, 394
to which exposed, proportion of cases or households producing, 358, 359
type transformation, and, 393
Type I and II, comparison with number of cases due to same types, 391
Type III, incidence among strains found, and in lobar and bronchopneumonia, compared, 390
types associated with serious disease, and ease of spread, 361
types in cases and carriers, compared, 350, 351, 390, 391
types, multiple, biologic means of detecting, 368
United States Public Health Service, studies of, 936
virulence of strains from, 216, 217, 372, 373, 378
Pneumococcus mucosus, relation to Type III, 23
Pneumococcus pneumonia. *See* Pneumonia, pneumococcus; Lobar pneumonia, pneumococcus; Bronchopneumonia, pneumococcus
Pneumococcus type incidence:
bronchopneumonia, 68–74
climatic factors, and, 47–49
estimated number of Type I and II cases in the United States, 391
Europe, high incidence of Types I and II in lobar pneumonia, 48
higher types in pneumonia, 51–54, 68–72, 74–77, 82, 83, 88, 89
infants and children:
with bronchopneumonia, 84–89
with lobar pneumonia, 79–84
with pneumonia, 74–89
with pneumonia, age variations, 76–84
lobar and bronchopneumonia together, 54–57, 74–79

Pneumococcus type incidence (*cont.*):
- lobar pneumonia, 42–54, 89
  - age and sex variations, 66, 67
  - age variations, 60–64, 80–84, 89
  - and non-contact carriers, compared, 350, 351
  - in children and adults compared, 83, 84, 89
  - in colored races, 42–49, 51, 52
  - in rural or urban areas, 59, 60
  - monthly variations, 58, 59
  - seasonal variations, 58, 59
  - sex variations, 64–67, 616, 617
  - temperate zones and tropics, 47–49
  - variation:
    - during influenza, 60, 466
    - with factors other than geographic, 57–67
    - with geographic factors, 43–49
    - with place, 57, 58
    - with social class, 59
  - yearly, 57, 58, 60
- Negroes, and, 42–49, 453, 456, 457
- United States Public Health Service, studies of, 936

Pneumococcus types, 22–24, 924
- American, 22–24, 946
- American and South African, compared, 946
- anemia, and, 499
- antibody response to, amount in recovery, 177, 515, 730, 731
- antibody response to, in pneumonia, 160, 161, 174–176, 729–733
- associated with serious disease, and ease of spread, 361
- Avery's subtypes, 23
- bacteriemia, failure of certain ones to cause, 50, 555, 556
- carriers of. *See* Pneumococcus carriers
- causal relation to pneumonia, 49–51, 68, 69
- chill at onset, and, 488
- classifiable strains, 29–31, 51, 52, 946
- classification, 22–24, 946
  - importance, 342, 923
  - Lister's, 22, 23, 30, 51, 453, 946
  - Lister's and American, compared, 946
- commonest:
  - at necropsy, 51
  - in bronchopneumonia, 71, 72, 84–89
  - in epidemics, 58
  - in infants and children, 74–89, 515
  - in lobar or bronchopneumonia in children and adults, compared, 89
  - in lobar pneumonia, 52–54, 79–84, 89

Pneumococcus types (*cont.*):
- commonest (*cont.*):
  - in Massachusetts, 55–57, 381–385
  - in pneumococcus pneumonia, 54–57, 74–79, 515
- consolidation, density of, and, 647
- Cooper and South African, compared, 946
- Cooper types, 23, 24, 946
- crisis, and, 530
- cross reaction between, 24, 134, 625
- culture collection, 924
- degradation, 24
- discovery, 22–24
- distribution, world-wide, 31–41
- Dochez and Gillespie's classification, 22, 23
- dust in patients' rooms, and, 341
- epidemics, and. *See under* Epidemics
- epidemiology, significance in, 351, 353–355, 357, 361, 390, 391
- errors in diagnosis of, 617, 620, 621, 623, 624, 628, 629
- fever, duration of, and, 492
- fixed, 24
- "Franz" strain, 23
- Group IV. *See below under* type
- "Groups," 22, 23
- higher types identified in various countries, 24, 31–41
- immunity, variation of response with, 161, 162, 193, 194, 432–434, 730, 731
- immunization, and. *See* Immunization, active
- in cases and carriers, compared, 350, 351, 390, 391
- in minor respiratory infections, and prevention, 396, 397
- in mixed infections, 11–16
- in sputum, as causative agent, 12, 49–51, 623, 624
- incidence in pneumonia. *See* Pneumococcus type incidence
- interconvertibility, 24
- invasive power, unusual, 355, 391
- invasive power, unusual, and prevention, 397, 400
- leucocytosis during course, and, 498
- Lister's classification, 22, 23, 30, 51, 453, 946
- lobar pneumonia, types obtained from, 1, 2, 42–54, 79–84, 89
- lobe involved in lobar pneumonia, and, 108, 109
- lysis, and, 531
- miscellaneous group, 23
- need for further study, 927

Pneumococcus types (*cont.*):
- Neufeld and Händel's classification, 22, 23
- nucleoprotein, and, 24
- onset, mode of, and, 487, 489, 649
- pneumonia, clinical aspects, and, 616, 617
- pneumonia, duration of, and, 527
- post-operative pneumonia, and, 522, 523
- prevalence, and season, 379–385
- prognosis, and. *See* Fatality rate(s) by type
- recovery, duration of immunity after, and, 538, 737–740
- recurrence, and, 534–539
- relapse, and, 532, 533
- resolution, and, 540
- SSS, and, 25, 26, 663
- SSS in urine, and, 503, 504, 694
- serologic differences, 22–24
- serum treatment, and. *See* Serum treatment; Serum treatment, dosage; Serum treatment, results
- sputum, character of, and, 502
- strains, and immunity, 194
- subtypes, 24
- symptoms at onset, and, 488–489, 616, 649
- symptoms during course, and, 236, 492, 498, 499, 502–504
- terminal pneumonia, and, 513
- transformation, 26, 27
  - growth characteristics, and, 26
  - influenza virus infection, and, 200
  - pathogenesis, and, 393, 394
- Type I:
  - average age in lobar pneumonia, 62, 63
  - death in lobar pneumonia in absence of complications, 545
  - etiologic significance in pneumonia, 12, 49–51, 623, 624
  - in lobar pneumonia, 1, 2, 43–54, 79–84, 89, 924
  - in lobar pneumonia, in patients under 50 years old, 60–63
- Type I and II:
  - America and Great Britain, differences in, in lobar pneumonia, 361
  - colds, as factor producing carriers of, 362
  - carriers of homologous type, proportion of cases producing, 358, 359
  - commonest in males with lobar pneumonia, 64–66
  - lobar pneumonia, proportion of cases in males, 65
  - primary peritonitis, and, 602
- Type I, II, III, and Group IV, in lobar pneumonia, 42–49

Pneumococcus types (*cont.*):
- Type II:
  - aputrid pulmonary necrosis in recovery, and, 607
  - atypical strains, 23, 24
  - average age in lobar pneumonia, 63
  - death in lobar pneumonia, in absence of bacteriemia, 545
  - etiologic significance in pneumonia, 12, 49–51, 623, 624
  - in lobar pneumonia, 1, 2, 43–54, 79–84, 89
  - in lobar pneumonia, in patients under 50 years of age, 63
- Type III:
  - bronchitis and tracheitis, and, 112
  - chronic disease, and, 335, 336
  - etiologic significance in pneumonia, 12, 49–51, 623, 624
  - in lobar pneumonia, 1, 2, 43–54, 79–84, 89
  - in lobar pneumonia, in patients over 50 years of age, 60–64
  - lung abscess, and, 605
  - relation to *Pneumococcus mucosus,* 23
  - SSS-splitting enzyme, effect on, 792
- Type III and VIII, form of pneumonia, and, 649
- Type III and VIII, otitis media and mastoid infections, and, 585
- Group IV, 23, 24
- Group IV, etiologic significance in pneumonia, 12, 49–51, 623, 624
- Group IV, in lobar pneumonia, 1, 2, 43–54, 79–84
- Type IV–XXXII, in lobar pneumonia, 51–54, 89
- Type V, etiologic significance in pneumonia, 12, 49–51, 623, 624
- Type V, in lobar pneumonia, 51–54, 82, 83, 89
- Type VII, in lobar pneumonia, 51–54, 82, 83, 89
- Type VIII, in lobar pneumonia, 51–54, 89
- Type XIV:
  - in pneumonia in adults, 53, 54
  - in pneumonia in infants and children, 74–77, 82, 83, 88, 89, 515
  - urogenital infection with, 604
- unclassified strains, 23, 24, 29–31, 51, 52, 617, 621, 946
- unclassified strains, in respiratory tract following convalescence, 366, 367
- unclassified strains, need for study of, 924

Pneumococcus types (*cont.*):
virulence, and. *See* Virulence, pneumococcus
X group, 23
Pneumococcus typing:
artificial mouse method, 622
Avery cultural method, technic, 635–637
Calder method, 641
collection of specimens for, 617–620
diagnostic serums, and, 134, 624, 625
pooled, 626, 632
pooled, need for study of, 924
standardization needed, 923, 924
during World War, 635
errors in, 617, 620, 621, 623, 624, 628, 629
facilities:
availability, 931
need for, 614, 834
recent extension of, 921, 922
failure of strains to type, 617, 621
Group IV, desirability of retyping cases, 920
Group IV, errors in diagnosis, 623, 624
importance, 615, 616, 834, 923
importance in both lobar and bronchopneumonia, 928
Krumwiede method, technic, 629–631
laboratories approved for, 933, 934
methods, 620–641
methods, merits of, 620–625
mixed infections, and, 11–16
mouse inoculation, technic, 630
need for, before serum treatment, 834
Neufeld method:
adoption as routine, by Massachusetts, 937
errors with, 628, 629
failure, 621
rapidity, 622, 625
reliability, 624
technic, 625–629
of bile dissolved organisms, 636, 637
of blood cultures, 641, 642
of dead organisms, 628
of laryngeal cultures, 642
of lung puncture material, 644
of old sputum, 628
of organisms mixed with disinfectants, 628
of pleural fluids, 643, 644
of pus, 644
of spinal fluids, 644, 645
of sputum, reliability, 624
of stored cultures, 635
of throat cultures, 642, 643
physicians' responsibility, and, 928
Pneumococcus typing (*cont.*):
pneumonia programs, and, 932–934
precipitin borax method, 640, 641
precipitin method, technic, 631, 633–635
precipitin test with Avery method, 636, 637
Quellung effect, 626, 627
rabbit antiserum for, 625
Rosenthal and Sternberg method, 640, 641
Sabin method, and agglutination test as guide to treatment, 861
Sabin method, technic, 630–633
supervision of, 933
technicians, training for, 933
tube agglutination method, technic, 631, 633–635
Type I or II, errors in diagnosis, 920
Type II and V, differentiation, 625
Type III and Group IV, desirability of retyping cases, 920
Type III or V, errors in diagnosis, 628, 629
Type III and VIII, differentiation, 625
Type VI and XXVI, cross reaction between, 24
Type VIa and VIb, 24
Type XV and XXX, cross reaction between, 24
types to examine for, 616, 933
urine precipitin methods, technic, 637–639
without animals, 620–622, 635
See also Pneumococcus types
Pneumonia:
antiquity, xiii
as a group of diseases, xiii, 390
at birth, 241, 243, 305
bacteriologic study. *See* Bacteriologic study; Pneumococcus typing
causative organisms, xiii, 1–17, 40–89, 457, 458, 927
causative organisms, changes in, in South Africa, 457, 458
causative organisms, evidence certain types may not cause, 50, 51
clinical aspects, and pneumococcus type, 616, 617
clinical knowledge, origin of, xiii
clinical varieties, 510–524
complications. *See* Complications; Resolution, delayed
consolidation, comparison of, in animals and man, 228
control programs. *See* Programs, pneumonia control
course, effect of mixed infections on, 11
course, special features in, 526–547
diaphragm, elevation in, 251, 253

Pneumonia (*cont.*):
differentiation of lobar from bronchopneumonia, xiii, 612, 648, 649
duration, factors affecting, 511
estimated number of pneumococcus cases in the United States, 391
experimental. *See* Experimental pneumonia
gas warfare, and, 341
hilar lesions in, 256, 646
immersion in water, and, 341
in mummies, xiii
in old age, 514, 515
in old age, allergy and lobar lesions, 241
initial lesion, site and nature, 247–250, 256
lobes involved, 108–111
lung involved, 107–110
massive collapse in, 252, 525
mediastinal displacement, and, 251, 253
mixed infections from contact with cases or carriers, 16, 392, 403
mixed infections in, 2, 11–16
organized lesions, relation of anthracosis to, 101
pneumococcus in, xiii, 1–3, 19, 42–89
pulmonary circulation, impairment during, 95
reporting of, need for more adequate, 927
spread:
air-borne infection, and, 295–297
crowding, and, 298
of lesion, 253–256
of lesion, relation of antibodies to, 153, 154, 174, 176, 570, 732, 881, 883, 886–888
synonyms, xiv, xvi, xvii
toxicity and vasomotor paralysis, 545–547
transmission and spread, 342–394
unsolved problems concerning, 921–936
vascular failure, peripheral, in, 545, 546, 748, 750
Pneumonia and Serum Therapy, 880
Pneumonia, pneumococcus:
as a group of diseases, xiii, 390
definition, xvii
duration, 527
mixed infections in, 11–16
toxin, and, 21, 22
types:
causal relation to, 49–51, 68, 69
commonest in, 54–57, 74–79, 515
obtained from, 40, 41, 50, 51
Pneumonias, The, 17
Pneumonic plague, pneumonia epidemics, and, 386
Pneumonitis and post-operative pneumonia, 515, 517–520
Pneumothorax:
artificial treatment by, 749, 769–772
complicating pneumonia, 611
Polysaccharide-splitting enzymes. *See* Enzymes, for splitting SSS
Post-operative pneumonia, 515–524
anesthesia, and, 519, 520, 524
atelectasis, and, 252, 515–520, 523, 524
bad risk group, and, 520, 521
causation, factors in, 516–520, 522, 523
causative organisms, 516, 517, 522, 523
diagnosis, 518
incidence, 520, 521
lobar pneumonia, 515, 522
operation, variety of, and, 519–521
origin and nature, 515–519
pneumococcus carriers, and, 516, 522, 523
prevention, 523, 524
prognosis, 521, 522
respiratory infections, pre-operative, and, 519
sepsis, and, 519
sex, and, 519–521
signs and symptoms, 517, 518
staphylococcus in, 9
streptococcus in, 523
treatment, 523, 524
treatment, oxygen, 524, 767
treatment, serum, 524
virulence of pneumococcus, and, 27, 518, 522, 523
Potency test(s), for serum standardization, 116, 120, 121, 826–829, 874, 875, 924, 925
need for standard serum in, 924, 925
Precipitins. *See under* Antibody(ies), pneumococcus
Predisposing factor(s):
acute and chronic disease, 199–201, 335, 336, 338
alcohol, 333, 334
alcohol, and Friedländer's bacillus pneumonia, 7
altitude, and, 332, 333
anthracosis, 338, 340
aspiration of foreign substances, 340–342
aspiration of foreign substances, and site of lesion, 248
atelectasis, 250–253
atelectasis, and post-operative pneumonia, 252, 515–520, 523, 524
chilling, 201, 202, 337
colds. *See* Colds, common

Predisposing factor(s) (*cont.*):
crowding, 316–318
diet, 334, 335
environmental change, 329–332
epidemics in families, and, 388, 389
gas, smoke, and dust, 338, 339
host resistance, factors affecting, 185–203, 393, 394
humidity, 201
immunization against pneumonia, and, 482
incidence, control of, and, 394
influenza, 339
lobar lesions in animals, and, 225, 232
mechanism of development of pneumonia, and, 257
mixed infections, carriers and cases as source of organisms, 16, 392, 403
occupation, 318–329
pathogenesis, and, 232–240
pneumococci in upper respiratory tract, and, 393
pneumoconiosis, 338
post-operative pneumonia, and, 516–519, 522, 523
recurrence, and, 538, 539
respiratory infections, minor. *See* Respiratory infections, minor
rhinitis, tonsillitis, or laryngitis, and, 607
season, and, 394
severity of, and immunization against pneumonia, 462, 478
severity of, and prognosis, 656
staphylococcus cases, and, 9
streptococcus cases, and, 3, 4
temperature variations, 201–203, 336–339
trauma, 202, 203, 340
virus infections, 3, 4, 9, 200, 236–240, 457
wet and cold, 201, 336–339
See also Pathogenesis
Pregnancy:
bacteriemia, and, 713
immunity, and, 203
prognosis, and, 713
serum treatment, dosage, and, 850, 856, 920
Prevalence:
acute and chronic disease, and, 199–201, 335, 336, 338
age and sex, and environment, 310–312
air-borne infection, and, 295–297
alcohol, and, 333
aspiration of foreign substances, and, 340–342
climatic factors, and, 288, 289, 297–299
Prevalence (*cont.*):
countries other than North America, 277–284
crowding, and, 298, 299, 316–318
diet, and, 334, 335
dust, and, 295–297
environmental change, and, 329–332
epidemics, and, 386–390
factors controlling, 394, 395
geographic, 260–269
humidity, and, 297–299
local conditions, influence on, 288, 289
meteorological factors, and, 289, 290, 295–299
North America, 269–277
occupation, and, 318–329
pneumococcus carriers, and, 366, 374, 376, 390–394
preceding respiratory infection, and, 235–240, 339, 392
temperate zones, seasonal factors, and, 290–295
temperature changes, and, 297–299, 336–339
trauma, and, 340
tropical zones, 261, 263, 264, 268, 269
tropical zones, seasonal factors, and, 289, 290
wet and cold, and, 336–339
See also Incidence; Epidemiology
Prevention, 395–483
alcohol, and, 398
army camps, and, 399, 400
aspiration of foreign substances, and, 398, 399
bacteriologic study, and, 400, 453–468, 471, 473–476
care of patients, and, 401, 402
chilling, and, 397, 398, 400
cleaning of patients' rooms, and, 401
community hygiene, and, 398–401
concurrent sterilization, and, 401
contact with infectious diseases, and, 397
contact with pneumococci of certain types, and, 397, 400
contact with respiratory infections, and, 396, 397
cross infection, and, 403
crowding, and, 397–400
diet, and, 398, 400
droplet infection, and, 396
dust, and, 398
exposure, and, 397, 398, 400
gowns and masks, wearing of, and, 400, 402

Prevention (*cont.*):
host resistance, and, 398
immunization:
and minor respiratory infections, 406–408
of animals, and, 214, 440–446
of man, and. *See* Immunization, active, against pneumonia
isolation and treatment of pneumococcus carriers, and, 403–406
isolation of cases, and, 400, 401–403, 926
isolation of cases, and pneumococcus carriers in community, 365
isolation of cases from children, and, 403
isolation of patients with infectious disease, and, 400
isolation of persons with minor respiratory infections, and, 397, 398, 401, 403
measures for, methods of determining success of, 400
mixed infections, carriers and cases as source, 16, 392, 403
nursing technic, and, 400, 402
occupational hazards, and, 398–401
pathologic conditions of upper respiratory tract, care of, and, 400
personal hygiene, and, 396–398
physical condition, and, 401
pneumococcus carriers, and, 402–406, 926
post-operative pneumonia, 523, 524
respiratory tract discharges, spread of, and, 396, 397
spitting, and, 396, 400
sputum, disposal of, and, 401
steel mills, and, 399
streptococcus carriers, and, 400
susceptible populations, and, 399–401, 465, 477, 478
temperature changes, marked, and, 398
unsolved problem, 921
visitors to patients, and, 744
wetting, and, 398
See also Immunization, active, against pneumonia; Programs, pneumonia control
Previous attacks. *See* Recurrence; Relapse
Primary pneumonia. *See* Lobar pneumonia; Infants and children with pneumonia, lobar pneumonia
Prognosis, 655–727
age, and, 703–710
albuminuria, and, 727
alcoholism, and, 702, 718, 719, 727
altitude, and, 717, 718
anoxemia, and, 726, 761
Prognosis (*cont.*):
anthracosis, and, 338
antibody:
acquired, and, 173–177
appearance, and, 173–177, 732, 733
natural, and, 153, 154
antitoxins, and, 125
apical lesions, and, 511, 698
apical lesions, necropsy findings, and, 111
areas with high incidence rates, and, 338, 660, 662
arthritis, septic, 598, 600
bacteriemia, and, 560, 681–693, 886, 912–916. *See also* Bacteriemia
bilateral lesions, and, 109, 110, 512
blood-clearing mechanism, and, 163, 690, 886
blood pressure, and, 722, 723
C substance precipitins and, 125
chain-forming pneumococci, and, 698
chronic disease, and, 701, 702
complications, effect on, 111, 112, 549, 695, 696
cyanosis, and, 726
dehydration, and, 727
delirium, and, 727
diarrhea, and, 727
digitalis, and, 751, 752
empyema, and, 577–582
empyema and pericarditis, 575
endocarditis, 592
environment, and, 717, 718
environmental change, in Negroes, and, 330
experimental pneumonia, dosage of organisms, and, 219, 221, 226, 227
extent of lesion, and, 696–698
factors affecting, 656
fatality rates. *See* Fatality rate(s); Serum treatment, results
Friedländer's bacillus cases, 7, 8
furunculosis, and, 604
heart, and, 702, 720–723
herpes, and, 726, 727
heterophile antibody, and, 125, 733, 734
home treatment, and, 715–717
immunity, and, 656
immunization for prevention of pneumonia, effect on, 450, 451, 454, 466
infants and children, 515, 703–707
infants and children with bacteriemia, 693
influenza bacillus cases, 8, 9
influenza epidemic, variations during, 9, 582, 811, 812
jaundice, and, 727

Prognosis (*cont.*):
leucocyte count, and, 498, 723–725
leucocytes:
degenerate forms, and, 724
differential count, and, 724, 725
in pleural fluids, nature of, and, 643
mobilization of, in experimental infections, and, 151, 179
lymphatics, organisms in, and, 163, 169, 886
macrophage reaction, and, 181
mediastinitis, and, 604
meningitis, 595, 596
mixed infections, 11, 15, 16, 111, 199, 533
Negroes, 710–712
occupation, and, 713, 714
oxygen want, and, 726
pericarditis, 575, 589
peritonitis, 603
physical condition, and, 178, 179, 699–702
physical condition and, with empyema, 581
pneumoconiosis, and, 338
post-operative pneumonia, 521, 522
predisposing factors, severity of, and, 656
pregnancy, and, 713
pulmonary edema, and, 727
pulse rate, and, 720–722
race, and, 710–712
recurrence, and, 539, 696, 698
relapse, and, 532, 533
repeated attacks, in dogs, and, 230
respiratory rate, and, 725, 726
SSS, and, 26, 663
SSS in urine, and, 693–695
season, and, 679–681
secondary infections, effect on, 199
sex, and, 712, 713
social condition, and, 671, 672, 706, 714–717
staphylococcus cases, 10, 11
streptococcus cases, 4, 5
symptoms, and, 486, 719–727
temperature, and, 719, 720
terminal pneumonia, and, 9, 10, 513, 515, 701, 702
toxicity, and, 545–547
trauma and shock, effect on, 340
treatment, and. *See* Treatment; Chemotherapy; Oxygen treatment; Serum treatment, results
tympanites, and, 727
type of pneumococcus, and. *See* Fatality rate(s) by type; *and under* Serum treatment, results
year, variation with, 677–679

Prognosis (*cont.*):
See also Fatality rate(s); Recovery
Programs, pneumonia control, 929–936
administration of, 932, 933
advisory committee, 932
advisory committee, Massachusetts, 929
advisory committee, United States Public Health Service, 922, 930
advisory service for, of United States Public Health Service, 936
blood cultures, and, 855, 934
consultants, and, 935
diagnosis, bacteriologic, and, 932–934
educational activities in, 935, 936
extension of, 922, 930, 931
funds for, 929, 930, 933
health departments, and, 928–936
laboratories approved, and, 933, 934
laboratory workers, and, 930, 932, 933
medical meetings, and, 935
nurses, and, 932, 935, 936
outline, 932–936
physicians, and, 929–932, 934, 935
publicity, 935, 936
records of treated cases, and, 934
serum:
availability and production, 929–934
cost per case, 931–933
distribution centers, and, 934
free, provision for, 930, 931, 933
manufacture or purchase, 933
sensitiveness to, instructions concerning, 934, 939–942
serum treatment, and, 882, 929–936
dosage recommendations, 848, 856, 858, 943, 944
duration of illness, and, 897
instruction sheets concerning, 934
states and cities having or planning programs, 930, 931
studies, special, in, 936
types to examine for, in, 616, 933
typing, and, 932–934
See also Departments of health; Massachusetts Pneumonia Series; Massachusetts Pneumonia Program; New York State Pneumonia Program; New York State Pneumonia Series; Prevention
Prontosil, 784–786
Prontylin, 784
Protection tests, 120, 121
excess antibody, and, 121, 180, 856
in mice, variables affecting, 121, 179, 180, 826
in rabbits, variables affecting, 178, 179

Protection tests (*cont.*):
leucocytes, and, 179, 180
SSS, and, 180
serum standardization, and, 120, 121, 826
serum standardization, standard serums for, 827, 828
serum standardization, standard test for, 828
variability of, 120, 121, 826
Protective substance. *See under* Antibody(ies), pneumococcus
Prozone effect, 121
serum dosage, and, 856
Psittacosis and pneumonia, 16
Pulmonary infarct, 610
differentiation of lobar pneumonia from, 650
Pulse rate, 494, 720–722
Purpura:
during course, 505
in mice from injection of pneumococcus extracts, 22
Pyopneumothorax, 611

Quellung reaction, 172, 626, 627
Quinine treatment. *See under* Chemotherapy

Rabbit serum, immune. *See* Serum, rabbit, antipneumococcic; Serum treatment, rabbit antiserum; *under* Serum treatment, results; Reactions after rabbit serum
Reactions:
from enzyme treatment of experimental Type III infections, 794
to injection of derivatives of pneumococci, 481, 482
to vaccine injections, 478–481
Reactions after chicken serum, chill, 811
Reactions after convalescent serum, chill, 813, 814
Reactions after horse serum, 836, 863–872
accelerated, 864
allergic, 836, 864–867
accelerated, and serum sickness, 864.
cause, 836, 864, 865
death from, 836, 864–867
dosage, influence on, 867
in children, 864–866
incidence, 864
prevention, 838, 841
symptoms, 864–867
treatment, 864, 867
unconcentrated serum, and, 864, 865
Reactions after horse serum (*cont.*):
anaphylactic type, 836, 864–867
chill, 836, 855, 867–869
avoidance, 869
cause, 867
death from, 836, 868, 869
dosage, influence on, 869
fatality rate, influence on, 868
in children, 868
incidence, 868
lipoids, and, 830
lot of serum, and, 867, 869
precipitated serum, and, 855
prevention, 869
symptoms, 867–869
tests for factor producing, 830, 831, 925
treatment, 868
unconcentrated serum, and, 868
death from, 836, 864–869
discontinuance of serum treatment after, 842, 867, 869
immediate, 864–867
instructions concerning, distributed by Massachusetts Department of Health, 939–942
nursing care, and, 746
peripheral neuritis, and, 611
serum sickness, 869–872
accelerated development, 839
accelerated reaction, and, 864
dosage, relation to, 870, 871
in children, 871
incidence, 870–872
skin test negative during, 838
symptoms, 869–871
treatment, 872
unconcentrated serum, and, 870, 872
thermal, 836, 867–869
Reactions after Huntoon's antibody solution, chill, 815, 817–820
Reactions after rabbit serum, 878, 879
allergic, 875, 878
allergic, influence on dosage, 878
allergic, treatment, 878
chill, 875, 878
death after, 875, 878
influence on dosage, 878
processed serum, and, 875, 878
test for factor producing, 875
treatment, 878
discontinuance of serum treatment after, 842, 878
serum sickness, 878, 879
thermal, 875, 878

Recovery, 728–740
  antibody:
    absence in, 174, 730, 732
    acquired, relation to, 173–177, 732
    amount in, 177, 515, 730, 731
    appearance in, 14, 16, 160, 161, 174–176, 181, 729–733
      and vaccine treatment, 797
      in experimental infections, 160, 181, 205, 218
    cellular reaction in lung, and, 181
    children and adults, compared, 177, 515, 731
    duration in blood after serum treatment, 740
    duration in blood after spontaneous recovery, 537, 737–739
    for influenza virus, failure to find, 237
    heterologous, and, 731, 739
    heterophile, and, 125, 733, 734, 820
    in pleural fluids during, 566
    natural, relation to, 153, 154
    post-operative pneumonia, and, 522
    response to different types in, 161, 162, 730, 731
    species-specific, at, 125, 135, 166, 733, 734
  bronchopneumonia, 68, 649
  carrier state in, 366, 367, 369–372, 547
  cellular factors in, 736, 737
  cellular status, and, 178–180
  enzymes, and, 736
  factors influencing, 173–177, 728–737
  immunity, and, 728–737
    cross immunity after, 731, 739
    development of, and, 528, 728, 737
    duration after, 538, 737–740
    specificity in, 135
  leucocytes, and, 498, 724, 735, 736
  local, in lung, 181, 182
  lung puncture studies at, 528, 734, 735
  lung tissue, repair in, 604, 606, 607
  macrophage reaction, and, 181, 735, 736
  organisms, biologic changes in, 734, 735
  organisms, decrease in number in lung, and, 528, 734
  physiologic variables, and, 178–180
  recurrence after, interval between attacks with same type, 536, 739
  relapse after, 533, 650
  resolution, and, 540–543
  SSS, and, 731, 732
  SSS in lungs of dogs after, 541
  SSS in urine, duration of excretion after, 504, 695
Recovery (*cont.*):
  skin tests with pneumococcus products at time of, 166, 167, 170, 171, 735, 739, 740, 813, 860, 861
  skin tests with SSS after, 738
  skin tests with SSS, and immunity in, 126, 166, 167, 170, 171, 735
  skin tests with SSS at time of, 166, 167, 735
  skin tests with SSS at time of, after serum treatment, 166, 167, 170, 171, 739, 740, 813, 860, 861
  toxemia, and, 528, 734, 737
  treatment:
    chemotherapy, and, 737, 775–795
    enzyme, and, 791–795
    oxygen, and, 766, 767
    pneumothorax, and, 769–772
    serum, and, 176, 737, 832, 882–918
    vaccine, and, 795–804
    x-ray, and, 773
    See also Prognosis; Fatality rate(s)
Recurrence, 533–540
  accidental infection, and, 240, 486
  allergy, and, 242, 243, 538, 539
  antibody of homologous type, presence at, 739
  bacteriemia in, 536, 538, 539
  bronchopneumonia, and, 535–537
  experimental pneumonia in dogs, 181, 182, 230, 231, 242, 243
  immunity, and, 537–540
  immunity, local in lung, and, 181, 182
  incidence of, 339, 340, 533, 534
  incidence of pneumonia, and, 339, 340, 533, 534, 538, 539
  interval between attacks, 534–536, 739
  macrophage reaction, in animals, and, 538
  pneumococcus carriers, and, 535, 539
  prognosis, 539, 696, 698
  pulmonary lesion in, 536–539
  susceptibility, and, 538
  treatment, serum, and, 535, 537–539, 740
  type, homologous, after serum treatment, 740
  type, homologous, interval between attacks, 536, 739
  types, and, 534–539
Relapse, 532, 533
  in bronchopneumonia, 649
  migratory lesions, and, 513
  mixed infections, and, 16, 532, 533
  streptococcus in, 3, 4, 533, 650
Repeated invasions, 12–16, 532–540
  in animals, 181, 182, 230, 231, 242, 243

Resistance. *See* Host resistance; Immunity, pneumococcus; Immunity, pneumococcus, natural
Resolution, 96–100, 540–542
age, and, 540
antibody, and, 542, 887
aputrid pulmonary necrosis, and, 541, 606, 607
bronchopneumonia, 649
chemical nature of, 97–100, 542
crisis, and, 528, 540
delayed, 100, 101, 542, 543
in children, 515
macrophage reaction, and, 101
pericarditis, and, 543, 588
enzyme-anti-enzyme balance in, 98, 100
factors governing, 100
failure of, 101, 543, 544
hilar glands, and, 99, 541
loss of lung tissue as accident of, 604–607
lung abscess, simulated appearance in, 541, 606, 607
macrophage reaction, and, 98, 101, 181, 227–229, 542
mononuclear cells, and, 98–101, 106, 541, 542
pneumococci, decrease in number during, 99, 100
rales in, 508
recovery, and, 542
sequence of, 541
spread, and, 541
time required, 540
treatment, serum, effect on, 887
tuberculosis, simulated appearance in, 541
types, and, 540
x-ray evidence of, early, 647
x-ray findings, 540, 541
Respiratory infection(s):
cause of disability and mortality, 259
contact with, and prevention of pneumonia, 396, 397
contraindication to immunization against pneumonia, 482
control or prevention, 395, 396
death rates, trend, 285–287
deaths, by age and sex, in Massachusetts, 311
hospitalization rates for, in Massachusetts, 308–310
incidence rates, and immunization against pneumonia, 450, 461, 469, 470, 472, 473
occupation, and, 318–321, 324–326, 329
Respiratory infections, minor:
allergy to pneumococcus, and, 241, 245
antibody appearance during, 157
antibody variations caused by, 199, 200
complications of, prevention by immunization, 407, 408
epidemic, and pneumonia in families, 377, 392
epidemiologic studies of, 293–295
immunity, and, 157, 199–201
incidence, 238, 339
in patients developing pneumonia, 236, 339
seasonal, 237, 238, 293–295, 379, 380
variation with age, 237, 238
variation with eye color, 186
variation with sex, 193
influenza bacillus carriers, and, 375
isolation of, and prevention of pneumonia, 397, 398, 401, 403
Negroes, and, 236
organisms in respiratory tract, activation by, 200, 238, 239, 337, 375, 380
pathogenesis of pneumonia, and, 235–240
pneumococci in, and prevention of pneumonia, 396, 397
pneumococcus carriers:
need for study of relation to, 926
occurrence in, 375, 376, 390
rate, influenced by, 374–377
seasonal peaks, and, 294, 379, 380
Type I and II, caused by, 362
pneumonia:
in infants, and, 236
mechanism of, and, 257
route of infection, and, 247
post-operative pneumonia, and, 519
predisposing factor in lobar pneumonia, 236, 238, 339
prevention of, 397
prevention of, by active immunization, 406–408
prevention of pneumonia, and, 396–398, 401, 403
spread of organisms in community, and, 239
streptococcus carriers, and, 239, 375
symptoms of, at onset of pneumonia, 487
symptoms of pneumonia, and, 235–240
systemic reaction to, 237, 238
See also Colds, common; Virus
Respiratory tract:
discharges of, and prevention of pneumonia, 396, 397
irritation by dust, 297, 341

Respiratory tract (*cont.*):
irritation by temperature changes, 297, 298
irritation by war gases, 341
nasal mucus, growth-inhibiting properties of, 246
pathology of, and carrier rate of organisms in nasopharynx, 366, 375, 376
pathology of, and prevention or cure of carrier state, 400, 406
protective mechanism of, 225, 232, 235, 246, 257
protective mechanism of, and alcohol, 334
Reticulo-endothelial system:
antibody formation, and, 136, 137
blockade of, 167, 168
immunity, and, 162–164, 167, 168
Rheumatic lesions, differentiation of lobar pneumonia from, 652, 653
Rhinitis, 607
Roentgenograms or Roentgen-ray. *See* X-ray

SSS. *See* Specific capsular polysaccharide(s)
Scarlet fever:
epidemic, and bronchopneumonia, 72
isolation of, and prevention of pneumonia, 400
lobar pneumonia, and, 525
Schwellenwert, 121
Season:
bacteriemia, and, 559
cases and deaths compared with pneumococcus carriers, and, 385
cases and deaths in Massachusetts, and, 383, 385
colds and pneumococcus carriers, variations with, 237, 294, 379–385
colds, incidence variations with, 237, 238, 293–295
complications, and, 549
crowding during cold weather, and epidemics, 389
deaths from pneumonia, and, 290–293, 383, 385
empyema, and, 571, 581, 582
fatality rate, variations with, 679–681
Friedländer's bacillus cases, and, 6
host resistance:
variation with, 203, 559, 680, 681
variation with, and pneumococcus carriers, 378, 380, 385
variation with, and prevention, 398
incidence, and, 289–295, 297, 298, 337, 394
incidence, Friedländer's bacillus cases, 6
Season (*cont.*):
incidence, in Negroes, and, 290, 331
pneumococcus carriers, variations with, xiv, 294, 374, 378–385, 390
post-operative pneumonia, and, 521
predisposing factor, 394
prevalence of pneumonia in the tropics, and, 289, 290
prevalence of pneumonia in temperate zones, and, 290–295
prognosis, and, 679–681
prognosis with empyema, and, 581, 582
respiratory infections, minor, incidence variations with, 237, 238, 293–295, 379, 380
serum dosage, variations with, 856
serum treatment, results, and, 680, 681, 846, 847, 916, 917
temperature variations, and incidence, 337
type incidence, variations with, 58, 59
types, commonest, in Massachusetts, and, 381–385
virulence, pneumococcus, and, 385
Secondary pneumonia. *See* Bronchopneumonia, secondary
Sensitiveness to serum, 875, 876
chill reaction, and, 867
consultation concerning, 837
contraindication to serum treatment, 835, 836, 841, 842, 875–877
decrease after lapse of time, 839
desensitization, uncertainty of, 841, 842
development, after serum injection, 838, 839, 865, 867
eye test, positive, importance of, 841, 842, 877
incubation period, 838, 839
instructions concerning, distributed by Massachusetts Department of Health, 939–942
intravenous test, for sensitiveness to rabbit serum, 876, 877
reactions from. *See* Reactions after horse serum; Reactions after rabbit serum
recognition of, 837–842, 875, 876
relation to history of:
allergic diseases, 837–839, 842, 875, 876
allergy to rabbit dander or fur, 875, 876
angioneurotic edema, 838, 842
asthma, 837, 838, 842, 865
asthma, horse, 837, 842
eczema, 838, 842
hay fever, 837, 838, 842, 865
horse vasomotor rhinitis, 837, 842

Sensitiveness to serum (*cont.*):
  relation to history of (*cont.*):
    previous injection of horse serum, 837–839, 842, 864, 865, 867
    previous injection of rabbit serum, 876
    previous vaccine injection, 838
    sensitiveness to felt, 876
    serum injection seven days to three months previously, 838, 839, 842
    urticaria, 838, 842
  skin test:
    negative during serum sickness, 838
    positive, mildly, 840, 842
    positive, strongly, 841, 842
  tests for, equipment, 839, 840, 853, 854
  tests for, limitation of, 836, 837
  tests for sensitiveness:
    to horse serum, eye, 839–842
    to horse serum, skin, 840–842
    to rabbit serum, eye, 876, 877
    to rabbit serum, intravenous, 876, 877
    to rabbit serum, skin, 876
Septicaemia. *See* Bacteriemia
Serum, anti-autolysate, and passive immunity, 446
Serum, antipneumococcic:
  animals, as source, 807, 822, 823
  antibodies in:
    actions, 115–125, 137, 151, 171, 172, 832, 885, 886
    most important actions, 175, 176, 886
    specificity, 28, 134–136
  antitoxins and curative power, 124, 125
  blocking tests in mice, for detection of multiple types in sputum, 368
  chill-producing substances, need for study of tests for, 925
  commercial, availability, 928, 929
  concentrated, first preparations of, 808
  concentrated, methods of preparation, 808, 809, 825
  cost per case, 931–933
  course and outcome of infection, effect on, 175–177
  curative power in animals, 121, 168, 169, 821, 832, 833
  diagnostic:
    availability, 624
    cross agglutination, and, 134
    pools of, 626, 632, 924
    standardization, need for, 923, 924
  distributing stations, 934
  growth of pneumococci in, 123, 124
  history of development, 806–809
Serum, antipneumococcic (*cont.*):
  horse and rabbit, comparison of properties, 172, 173
  leucocytes, inhibition of, in protection tests, 180
  passive immunization for prevention of pneumonia, 445, 446, 483
  production, 28, 823–826, 873–875
  production and concentration, need for study, 925
  programs, to make available, 929–936
  protection tests, and, 120, 121, 178–180, 826–828
  protective value, comparison with quinine and optochin, 776
  provision by departments of health, 829, 830, 851, 928–934, 937
  SSS, precipitation by, 122
  standardization, 826–830, 873–875
    League of Nations, and, 924, 925
    need for standard serums for, 924, 925
    need for standard tests for, 924, 925
    United States Public Health Service, and, 826–829, 874, 875, 924, 925
  treatment with. *See* Serum treatment; Serum treatment, dosage; Serum treatment, results
Serum, antiprotein, 25
Serum, antistaphylococcus, treatment with, 11
Serum, antistreptococcus, treatment with, 5, 584
Serum, antitoxic, 125, 809
Serum, chicken, antipneumococcic:
  preparation, 809, 810
  reactions from, 811
  treatment of meningitis with, 596
  treatment and results, 809–812
Serum, convalescent:
  antibodies in, in mixed infections, 14, 16
  treatment and results, 5, 9, 171, 809, 812–814
Serum disease. *See* Serum sickness
Serum, heterophile, treatment and results, 809, 820, 821
Serum, horse, antipneumococcic, 822–872
  advantages and disadvantages of, 822
  bivalent, 823
  chill-producing substances, lot of serum, and, 867, 869
  chill-producing substances, tests for, 830, 831, 925
  coagulation by heat, 855
  commercial, dosage with, 857
  concentrated:
    Avery's, 825

Serum, horse, antipneumococcic (*cont.*):
concentrated (*cont.*):
Banzhaf's, 825
by various methods, 808, 809, 825
dilution with saline, 841
expiration date, 828
Felton's, 808, 809, 825
Gay and Chickering's, 814
Huntoon's, 814
in skin test, 840
potency, 829
production, 823–826
danger in use of, in certain patients, 835–839, 841, 842, 867, 869, 875–878
dosage. *See* Serum treatment, dosage
exudate antiserum, 824
Felton's antibody solution, 808, 809, 825
first use of, 807
heterophile antibody and, in treatment, 820, 821
Huntoon's antibody solution:
preparation, 814, 818
treatment and results, 814–820
treatment of animals with, 814, 815, 843
treatment of meningitis with, 595, 597
monovalent, 823
Neufeld typing method, and, 625
potency:
compared with whole serum, 826
minimum requirements, 829
of standard test serums, 828
variations, 828, 829
preparation, and dosage of organisms, 421
production, 823–826
production, and pneumonia control programs, 933, 934
properties, compared with rabbit antiserum, 172, 173
provision by health departments, 829, 830, 851, 928–934, 937
prozone effect, and, 121, 856
reactions to. *See* Reactions after horse serum
standardization, 826–830
standard serums for, 827, 828, 924, 925
standard serums for, and League of Nations, 827
standard test for, 826–829
treatment with. *See* Serum treatment; Serum treatment, dosage; Serum treatment, results
unconcentrated:
dilution with saline, 841
disadvantages of, 824
production, 823, 824

Serum, horse, antipneumococcic (*cont.*):
unconcentrated (*cont.*):
use in military camps during World War, 808, 889–892
unit:
definitions of, 826, 827
standard, 826, 827
standard, and dosage, 845–852
Serum, horse, antistaphylococcus, treatment with, 11
Serum, horse, antistreptococcus, treatment with, 5
Serum, human, immune, treatment of streptococcus cases with, 5
Serum-leucocyte mixtures, in bactericidal tests, 117–120
Serum lipoids:
agglutination, and, 115
chill reactions, and, 830
phagocytosis, effect on, 132
precipitin reaction, and, 116
Serum, non-specific:
action, 25
treatment and results, 809, 821, 822
Serum, rabbit, antipneumococcic, 872–879
antibody content compared with horse serum, 172, 173, 809
antibody nitrogen tests with, 874, 875
antibody size, in horse and rabbit compared, 173, 873
chill-producing substances, test for, 875, 878
concentrated, 874, 878
dilution with saline, 876, 877
dosage, 877, 878
first use of, 806, 807
heterophile antibody, and, 820, 821
Neufeld typing method, and, 625
potency for Type III, 917
preparation, 873, 874
preparation, and dosage of organisms, 420–422
processed, 874, 875
properties, compared with horse antiserum, 172, 173
reactions to. *See* Reactions after rabbit serum
results with, 917, 918
standardization, 874, 875
treatment with, 874–879, 917, 918
types, less frequent, and, 830
Serum, rabbit, heterophile, and treatment, 820, 821
Serum reactions. *See* Reactions after . . .
Serum sickness:
accelerated development, 839

Serum sickness (*cont.*):
after horse serum, 869–872
after rabbit serum, 878, 879
Serum treatment, 805–879
advantage of, failure to recognize, 881
advantage of high potency serum, 881
animal serums for, 806–809
animals. *See under* Experimental infection(s); Experimental pneumonia
antibody, most important action, 175, 176, 886
antitoxic serum, and, 125, 809
blood culture prior to, 856, 857, 862, 863
blood cultures, importance in, 855, 856, 858
chemotherapy combined with, 595–597, 737, 742, 781, 789
chicken serum, immune, 809–812
chicken serum, immune, and meningitis, 596
children, 835
children, with Huntoon's antibody solution, 818, 819
community problem, 922, 928–936
contraindications, 835, 836, 841, 842
convalescent serum, and, 809, 812–814
convalescent serum, and skin sensitivity to SSS, 170, 171, 813
cost per case, 931–933
dangers of, in certain cases, 835–839, 841, 842, 867, 869, 875–878
delay in general use, reasons for, 928
discontinuance after severe reactions, 842, 867, 869, 878
divided doses, desirability of, 841, 842, 853
dosage. *See* Serum treatment, dosage
during World War, 808, 889–892
early, advantage in animals, 169, 832, 833
early, advantage in man, 176, 177, 823, 882, 883, 885, 887, 888, 894–897, 901, 902
empyema, with horse antiserum, 584
endocarditis, with horse antiserum, 592
equipment for, 853–855
failure of:
associated lesion as cause, 111
causes, 176, 177, 860, 881, 898, 899, 902, 918–920
causes, avoidable, 920
causes, unavoidable, 176, 177, 909, 920
mixed infections as cause, 11, 15, 533, 860, 919
secondary infection as cause, 15
staphylococcus infection as cause, 10
Friedländer's bacillus cases, 8

Serum treatment (*cont.*):
gold salts and, in animals, 736
health departments, and. *See under* Departments of health; Programs, pneumonia control
heterophile serum, and, 809, 820, 821
history, 806–809
horse antiserum, 822–872
Huntoon's antibody solution, 814–820
Huntoon's antibody solution, and meningitis, 595, 597
infants and children, 844, 845, 852, 853
influenza bacillus cases, with human serum, 9
instructions concerning dosage and technic, distributed by Massachusetts Department of Health, 939, 943–945
limited use of, 928
lobar and bronchopneumonia, together, 834, 893, 895, 900, 902–911, 914, 915, 928
lobar or bronchopneumonia, 834, 928
Massachusetts Pneumonia Series. *See* Massachusetts Pneumonia Series
meningitis, 595–597
combined with optochin treatment, 595–597, 781
Huntoon's antibody solution, and, 595, 597
immune chicken serum, and, 596
mild cases, 833
miscellaneous serums, and, 807, 809–822
mixed infections, and, 11
need for greater use, 928, 929
non-specific serum, and, 809, 821, 822
nursing care, and, 746
optochin treatment combined with, 781
patients in extremis, and, 835, 842
patients with family history of allergy and negative sensitivity tests, 838
pericarditis, with horse antiserum, 589
peritonitis, 603
physicians, responsibility for, 932
physicians, successful use by, in general practice, 895, 896, 929
plan of, 853–855, 859, 877
pneumococcus carriers, 404, 405
pneumonia programs, and. *See under* Programs, pneumonia control
post-operative pneumonia, 524
precautions prior to, with horse serum, 836–842
precautions prior to, with rabbit serum, 875–877

Serum treatment (*cont.*):
prevention of pneumonia, and, 445, 446, 483
previous serum treatment, and, 838, 839, 842
pulmonary edema, and, 758
rabbit antiserum, 872–879
recovery, and, 176, 737, 832, 882–918
recurrence, and, 535, 537–539
recurrence with homologous type, after, 740
relapse after, 533
results. *See* Serum treatment, results
risks increased, in certain cases, 842, 875–877
route, and, 843–845
and bacteriemia, 843, 844
in infants and children, 844, 845
intramuscular, with chicken serum, 810
intramuscular, with Huntoon's antibody solution, 818, 819
intratracheal, in monkeys, with Huntoon's antibody solution, 815
intravenous, risks of, 836
subcutaneous, in monkeys, with Huntoon's antibody solution, 815, 843
subcutaneous, with Huntoon's antibody solution, 817, 818, 843, 844
SSS and antibody in blood during, 122
selection of cases for, 832–842, 875–877
sensitiveness to serum, and. *See* Sensitiveness to serum
severe cases, 835, 842, 848
skin tests with SSS, and, 166, 167, 170, 171, 739, 740, 813, 847, 860, 861
staphylococcus cases, 11
streptococcus cases, with human serum, 5
sulfanilamide treatment combined with, 789
sulfapyridine treatment combined with, 789
technic, 856–859
time limitation of, removal in Massachusetts, 833, 882, 897, 937
type, and dosage. *See* Serum treatment, dosage
type determination before, need of, 834
types against which effective, 834, 903, 927
unconcentrated serum, and, 862, 863
unconcentrated serum, dosage, 845, 847, 862, 863
unsolved problems in use of, 927–929
Serum treatment, dosage, 845–863
age, and, 850, 856
age and bacteriemia, and, 916
allergic reaction, influence on, 867, 878
average in Type I, 846–848
Serum treatment, dosage (*cont.*):
average in Type II, 848–850
average in Type V, 850
average in Type VII, 851
average in Type VIII, 851
average in Type XIV, 851, 852
bacteriemia, and, 850, 851, 855, 856, 858, 886, 916
bacteriemia and interval between doses, 898, 899, 902
chill reaction, influence on, 869, 878
commercial serum in syringes, and, 857
continuing, 858, 859
day of disease, and, 856
early treatment, and, 855, 856
extent of lesion, and, 856, 858
guides to, 856, 858, 860–862
agglutinin test, 861, 862
skin test with SSS, 847, 860, 861
test for SSS in blood, 862
in infants and children, 852, 853
increase of, indications for, 856, 858, 860–862, 920
initial, 853, 855–858
insufficient, as cause of poor results, 881, 919, 920
intervals between, 857–859
intervals between, effect of shortening, 898, 899, 902, 903
lobes involved, and, 856, 858
physiologic variables, and, 178, 179
pregnancy, and, 850, 856, 920
prozone phenomenon, and, 121, 856
recommended:
for any type, 856
in pneumonia programs, 848, 856, 858, 943, 944
in Type I, 848, 856, 943, 944
in Type II, 850, 856, 943, 944
in Type V, 850, 851, 856, 943, 944
in Type VII, 851, 852, 856, 943, 944
in Type VIII, 851, 852, 856, 943, 944
in Type XIV, 852, 856
relapse, and, 533
season, effect on, 856
serum sickness incidence, effect on, 870, 871, 879
severe cases, and, 848
spread of lesion, and, 851, 858
standard unit, and, 845–852
temperature, and, 858
unconcentrated serum, 845, 847, 862, 863
Serum treatment, rabbit antiserum, 875–879
advantages, 875, 918
dosage, 877, 878

Serum treatment, rabbit antiserum (*cont.*):
dosage, in milligrams of antibody nitrogen, 874, 875
dosage, standard unit, and, 875
precautions prior to, 875–877
reactions to, 875, 878, 879
results, 917, 918
technic, 877
Serum treatment, results, 880–920
acute symptoms, effect on, 882–885
after fourth day, evidence of benefit, 897
age, advanced, and, 919
age, and fatality rate with or without bacteriemia, 915, 916
alcoholism, and, 919
animals. *See under* Experimental infection(s); Experimental pneumonia
antibody:
appearance in blood, 175, 843, 844, 881, 885, 886
appearance in pleural fluid after rabbit antiserum, 918
disappearance from blood, 175, 885
antigenicity of attack lessened, 167, 537, 739
bacteriemia:
fatality rate, 898, 899, 912–916
fatality rate, comparison with untreated cases, 898, 899, 912–915
in infants and children, and, 909, 914, 915
prevention or disappearance, 169, 175, 176, 561, 563, 832, 881, 885, 886, 902, 903
rabbit antiserum, and, 918
bacteriemia present or absent, fatality rate by age, 915, 916
bacteriemia present or absent, fatality rate by length of treatment, 898, 899
blood-clearing mechanism, efficiency increased, 163, 169, 175, 886
cardiac abnormalities, and, 885
chill reaction, effect on fatality rate, 868
chronic disease, and, 919
clinical condition, 858, 882–885
comparison of, with whole or concentrated serum, 882, 889–892
complications, and, 919
complications, effect on incidence of, 175, 176, 570, 592, 887, 888
death, analysis of cause, 918–920
death from reactions, 815, 817, 818, 820, 836, 864–869, 875, 878
duration of disease, 176, 177, 883–885

Serum treatment, results (*cont.*):
duration of immunity, 166, 167, 537, 739, 740
early treatment, 882, 883, 894–899, 901–905
electrocardiogram, and, 885
empyema, and rabbit antiserum, 918
factors affecting, 178, 179, 890, 898, 899, 902, 903, 918–920
fatality rates:
by age, 909–911
by age, infants and children, 907–909
by type, 888–918
by type, infants and children, 906–909
by type, need for further study, 927
home treated cases, 912
hospital treated cases, 808, 912
infants and children, by type, 906–909
lobar and bronchopneumonia together, 834, 893, 895, 900, 902–911, 914, 915, 917, 918
lymphatics, infection in, and, 886
Massachusetts series. *See* Massachusetts Pneumonia Series
mixed infections, and, 919
peripheral neuritis, and, 611
physicians in general practice, and, 808, 895, 896, 929
pneumococcus pneumonia of various types, 893, 895, 900, 902–911, 914, 915, 917, 918
poor, caused by insufficient dosage, 881, 919, 920
rabbit antiserum, and, 917, 918
resolution, and, 887
SSS:
cessation of urinary excretion, 122, 885
skin sensitivity to, after recovery, 166, 167, 740
skin sensitivity, and, 126, 127, 166, 167, 170, 171, 739, 740, 813, 860, 861
season, and fatality rate, 680, 681, 846, 847, 916, 917
serum potency, and, 881, 919, 920
spread of lesion, and, 176, 177, 570, 881, 883, 886–888
temperature, and, 883–885
toxemia, and, 737
Type I:
bacteriemia:
empyema incidence increased, 887
fatality rate, 913–916
length of treatment, and, 898, 899
Cecil's series of early cases, 895
Cole's series, 881, 894

Serum treatment, results (*cont.*):
Type I (*cont.*):
comparison with untreated cases, 881–883, 885, 888–896, 909–911
dosage considerations, and, 846, 847, 897–899
dosage considerations, and age, 910, 911
empyema, effect on incidence, 887, 888
empyema, incidence by day of treatment, 888
fatality rate, 881, 888–899, 906
age groups, and, 909–911
age groups, and day of treatment, 910, 911
age groups, comparison with untreated cases, 909–911
age groups, with or without bacteriemia, 915, 916
bacteriemia, comparison with untreated cases, 913, 914
bacteriemia present or absent, 915, 916
cases from various countries, 891–894
concentrated serum, and, 893–899
day of treatment, and, 894–897
in home and hospital cases, 912
interval between doses, and, 898, 899
proportional reduction, 894, 897
season, and, 680, 681, 917
sex, and, 911
unconcentrated serum, and, 889–892
year and average dosage, and, 846, 847
in military camps, during World War, 889–892
Locke's series, 881
Lord's series of late treated and untreated cases, 897
rabbit antiserum, and, 917, 918
SSS, disappearance of, from urine, 122, 885
Type I and II, age variations, and, 909–911
Type II:
bacteriemia, fatality rate, 913–916
comparison with untreated cases, 899–901, 910, 911
dosage considerations, and, 848, 849, 902, 903
dosage considerations, and age, 910, 911
empyema, effect on incidence, 888
fatality rate, 899–903, 906
age groups, and, 909–911
age groups, comparison with untreated cases, 910, 911
age groups, with or without bacteriemia, 915, 916

Serum treatment, results (*cont.*):
Type II (*cont.*):
fatality rate (*cont.*):
bacteriemia, comparison with untreated cases, 913, 914
bacteriemia present or absent, 915, 916
cases from various countries, 899, 900
day of treatment, and, 901, 902
in home and hospital cases, 912
interval between doses, and, 902, 903
proportional reduction, 899, 901
season, and, 680, 681, 917
sex, and, 911
year and average dosage, and, 848, 849, 902
rabbit antiserum, and, 917, 918
Type III, fatality rate, 903, 906
Type III, rabbit antiserum, and, 917
Type V:
bacteriemia, fatality rate, comparison with untreated cases, 914
comparison with untreated cases, 903, 904
fatality rate, 903, 904, 906
fatality rate, in early cases, 903, 904
fatality rate, in home and hospital cases, 912
rabbit antiserum, and, 917
Type VII:
bacteriemia, fatality rate, comparison with untreated cases, 914
fatality rate, 904, 906
rabbit antiserum, and, 917
Type VIII:
bacteriemia, fatality rate, comparison with untreated cases, 914
fatality rate, 904–906
rabbit antiserum, and, 917
Type XIV:
bacteriemia in adults, comparison with untreated cases, 914
bacteriemia in infants and children, comparison with untreated cases, 914, 915
fatality rate, in adults, 905, 906
fatality rate, in infants and children, 907–909
rabbit antiserum, and, 917
variables, physiologic, and, 178, 179
Sex:
death rates, and, 308–312
delayed resolution, and, 543
empyema, and, 572, 573
hospitalization rate, and, 308
immunity, and, 192, 193
incidence, and, 307–312

Sex (*cont.*):
necropsy studies, distribution of cases by, 91
pneumococcus carrier rate, influence on, 373, 374
post-operative pneumonia, and, 519–521
prognosis, and, 712, 713
respiratory infections, minor, and, 193
serum treatment, results, and, 911
type incidence in pneumonia, variations with, 64–67, 616, 617
Simultaneous infection(s), 12, 15, 16
See also Mixed infection(s)
Sinusitis:
at necropsy, 585
Friedländer's bacillus in, 6
meningitis, and, 594
pneumococcus carriers, and, 375
streptococcus cases, and, 4
Skin tests for sensitiveness to serum, 840–842, 876
concentrated antiserum in, 840
danger of, 840
dilute normal horse serum in, 839, 840, 853
dilute normal rabbit serum in, 876
fallibility, 840
interpretation, 840, 841, 876
negative during serum sickness, 838
physiologic saline in, 839, 840, 853, 876
positive, 840–842, 876
strongly positive, a contraindication to serum treatment, 841, 842
technic, 840, 876
See also under Sensitiveness to serum
Skin tests with pneumococcus products:
age variations in response, 192
allergy, and, 182–185, 241–245
animals, and, 165, 166, 170, 171, 182–184, 241, 242, 594, 595
cellular immunity, and, 126, 127, 735
SSS:
after recovery, 738
at recovery, 166, 167, 735
at recovery after serum treatment, 126, 127, 166, 167, 170, 171, 739, 740, 813, 860, 861
in normal man, 126, 149, 150
relation of immune factors to reaction, 126, 127, 170, 171, 860
serum treatment, convalescent serum, and, 171, 813
serum treatment, guide to dosage, 847, 860, 861
Sodium salicylate, 782, 783
Soluble specific substance (SSS). *See* Specific capsular polysaccharide(s)
Somatic carbohydrate of pneumococcus, 24, 25, 125, 135, 733
Somatic protein of pneumococcus, 24, 25, 133–135, 149
Special features in the course of pneumonia, 526–547
Specific capsular polysaccharide(s), 24–26
A substance identical with, 117
acetylated preparations, 22, 117
agglutinin absorption, and, 115
anaphylaxis in sensitized animals, and, 134, 173, 182, 184
antibody:
disappearance in serum treatment, and, 175, 885
effect on, 25, 121, 122, 131, 132
of horse and rabbit, reaction with, 172, 173
antigenicity, 28, 133, 134, 198, 199
compared with vaccine, 414, 415, 418, 430
dosage, and, 429–432
type, and, 432, 433
chemical analysis, 25
conjugated preparations, specificity of antibody response to, 134
dominant antigen, 133, 134
enzymes for splitting of, 736, 791–795
fate of, in body, 566
Friedländer's bacillus, 6
hapten, 134
immunity, effect on, 132, 731, 732
immunity, for heterologous types, and, 135, 136
immunization:
adsorbed preparations, 430
dosage, and, 429–432
reactions from, 481, 482
related agents, and, in animals, 28, 134, 198, 412, 414, 415, 417, 418, 429–431
related agents, and, in man, 134, 198, 199, 412, 418, 430–432, 474, 475
response, duration, 438, 440
response, time of appearance, 436, 437
route, and, 417, 418, 430–432
type, and, 432, 433
in blood, 26, 131, 497
in blood, during serum treatment, 122, 862
in body fluids, 25, 26
in edema fluid, and antagonism to antibody, 256
in infected exudates, 26, 131, 566, 584

Specific capsular polysaccharide(s) (*cont.*):
in lung, 26
in lungs of dogs after recovery, 541
in pleural fluids, 566, 584
in spinal fluid, 26
in sputum, 26, 629
in urine, 25, 26, 503, 504
cessation of excretion after serum treatment, 122, 885
duration of excretion after recovery, 504, 695
in children, 695
in children and adults, compared, 643
precipitin tests for, 116, 637–639
presence of antibody, and, 122, 695
prognosis, and, 693–695
with empyema, 566
Krumwiede typing, and, 629
leucocytes, effect on, 132, 180
opsonins, and, 117–119
precipitin absorption, and, 116
precipitin typing methods, and, 620, 637–639
prognosis, and, 26, 663
purpura-producing properties, 22
recovery, and, 731, 732
skin tests:
age variations of sensitivity, 192
as guide to serum dosage, 847, 860, 861
for allergy, 184, 185
in actively acquired immunity, 126, 166, 185, 735, 738
in blood, and serum dosage, 862
in normal man, 126, 149, 150
in passive immunity, 126, 127, 166, 167, 170, 171, 739, 740, 813, 860, 861
in pleural fluids, 643, 644
in spinal fluids, 644
in urine, 116, 637–639
toxicity, 22
transformation of type, and, 24
type, and amount produced, 663
type specificity, relation to, 25
types for which isolated, 25
typing errors with Type III, and, 629
virulence, relation to, 25, 131, 132
Specific treatment. *See* Serum treatment
Spinal fluid, typing with, 595, 644, 645
Sputum:
anchovy sauce appearance, in staphylococcus cases, 10, 614
atelectasis, and, 651
at onset, 486, 490
bacteriologic diagnosis, and, 614, 617, 618, 620–637, 639–641
Sputum (*cont.*):
blood in, 501
blood in, and pulmonary infarct, 650
blood in, and trauma, 340
character, and pneumococcus type, 502
diagnosis, and, 613, 614
disposal of, 745, 746
disposal of, and prevention, 401
dry, pneumococcus in, 392
during course, 501, 502
examination of, routine, 614
Friedländer's bacillus in, 6, 7
in infants and children, 514, 617, 618
in the very old, 617
influenza bacillus in, 8
lung abscess, and, 605, 606
mixed flora in, 12–14
multiple types in, detection by blocking tests in mice, 368
organisms found at repeated examinations, 11–16
organisms in, in mixed infections, 11–16
organisms in, significance, 11–16, 49–51, 623, 624
pneumococcus in, and prevention, 396, 401
rusty, as symptom, 485
rusty, diagnosis, and, 613
salmon pink, in staphylococcus cases, 10, 614
SSS in, 26, 629
tuberculous pneumonia, and, 651
typing of pneumococci in. *See* Pneumococcus typing
Staphylococcus:
associated lesions in lobar pneumonia, and, 111
empyema, and, 10, 574, 606
empyema, fatality rate, 579, 580
in bronchopneumonia, 9, 10, 67–69
in mixed infections, 15, 16
in pneumonia, 2, 9, 10
relapse, and, 533
vaccines, mixed, and, 458–463, 468, 472
Staphylococcus pneumonia, 1, 2, 9–11
bronchopneumonia, 9, 10
epidemic, 10
in South Africa, 457
lobar pneumonia, 1, 2, 9
sputum in, and diagnosis, 10, 614
Statistics, vital. *See* Death(s); Death rate(s); Incidence; Prevalence
Streptococcus:
associated lesions in lobar pneumonia, and, 111

Streptococcus (*cont.*):
carriers, and minor respiratory infections, 239, 375
carriers, and prevention of pneumonia, 400
empyema, 4, 5, 567, 571, 573–575
character of exudate, 574, 582
fatality rates, 4, 579–581
influenza epidemic, and, 582
pericarditis, and, 575, 589
prevention of, 5
symptoms, 575
treatment, 574, 575, 582, 584
in bronchopneumonia, 3–5, 67–69, 471, 648, 649
in lobar pneumonia, 1–5
in mixed infections, 15, 16
in post-operative pneumonia, 523
infections, isolation of, and prevention of pneumonia, 400
relapse, and, 3, 4, 533, 650
sulfanilamide, effect on, 784, 785, 790
sulfapyridine, effect on, 787, 790
vaccines, mixed, and, 458–463, 468, 470, 472
Streptococcus pneumonia, 1–5, 457, 462, 573
bronchopneumonia, 3–5, 68, 471, 648, 649
complicating pneumococcus cases, 533, 650
epidemic, 3, 68
fatality rates, 4, 5, 579–581, 677
in Negroes, 3, 4, 457, 462, 573
treatment, 5, 574, 575, 582, 584
Huntoon's pneumococcus antibody solution, 816, 817
serum, failure of, due to, 533, 919
sulfanilamide or sulfapyridine, need for study, 790
Sulfanilamide and allied agents. *See under* Chemotherapy
Sulfapyridine. *See under* Chemotherapy
Susceptibility. *See* Host resistance
Symptoms, 484–505, 649, 653, 654
allergy in lobar pneumonia, and, 240
anoxemia, 499, 717, 760–762
at onset, 4, 7, 10, 485–491, 498, 514, 649, 653, 654
at onset, in bronchopneumonia, 649
at onset, pneumococcus type, and, 487–489, 616, 649
at time of death, 544, 545
atelectasis, and, 651
cardinal, 485
convalescence, and, 546, 547
cough, and spread of lesion, 255
delayed resolution, and, 542
Symptoms (*cont.*):
during course, 491–505, 760–762
pneumococcus type, and, 236, 492, 498, 499, 502–504
toxemia, and, 748
tympanites, association with bacteriemia, 756
Friedländer's bacillus cases, 7, 8
incubation period, 486, 487
infants and children, and, 491, 514, 515
influenza bacillus cases, 9
nucleoprotein, relation to, 25
pain, referred, 488–490
pleurisy with effusion, and, 652
prognosis, and, 486, 719–727
pulmonary circulation, impairment of, and, 496, 499, 743, 755, 759–762
pulmonary infarct, and, 650
rheumatic pneumonia, and, 653
severity, and extent of consolidation, 486
staphylococcus cases, 10
streptococcus cases, 4
toxemia, antibody, and, 732
toxic products, neutralization at recovery, 734
toxic psychosis in convalescence, 547
toxicity, and, 485
tuberculous pneumonia, 651
typical, and diagnosis, 613
variability, 486
See also particular symptom by name
Synonyms, xiv–xvii
System of Bacteriology, 19

Temperature, 490–492
body, and experimental pneumonia, 202
death rates, and climatic variations of, 319–323, 329
duration, age, and, 492
incidence of pneumonia and exposure to variations of, 297, 299, 318–323, 326–329, 336–339
pathogenesis, and variations of, 233, 235
prevention of pneumonia, and variations of, 398
prognosis, and, 719, 720
serum reactions, and, 811, 813, 815, 818, 867–870, 878
treatment:
chemotherapy, effect on, 776, 783, 794
oxygen, effect on, 766, 767
pneumothorax, effect on, 770
serum, effect on, 883–885
x-ray, effect on, 773

Terminal pneumonia, 9, 10, 27, 513, 515, 701, 702
Thermal or chill reactions, from serum treatment. *See under* Reactions after . . .
Throat swabs:
for detection of pneumococcus carriers, 342, 343
organisms on, and mixed infections, 11, 13, 14
typing from, 614, 617, 618, 642, 643
Tonsillitis, 607
Torulosis and pneumonia, 17
Toxemia:
abortion or delivery, and, 748
antibody, and, 732
antibody, and symptoms, 732
arthritis, septic, and, 599
bacteriemia, and glucose treatment, 768
cardiovascular complications, and, 544–546, 748, 750
death, and, 544–546
during course, 748
recovery, and, 528, 734, 737
serum treatment, results, and, 737
smooth muscle, effects on, 546, 748, 756
stomach, acute dilatation, and, 611, 748
symptoms, and, 748
treatment, 746
tympanites, and, 611, 748, 756
vascular dilatation, peripheral, and, 545, 546, 748, 750
Tracheitis, 112
Transformation of pneumococcus types. *See* Pneumococcus, variants; *and under* Pneumococcus types
Transfusions:
of convalescent blood, for treatment, 773
with human immune blood, for treatment, 5, 11, 813, 814
Traumatic pneumonia, 340
Treatment, 741–804
alcohol, 754, 759
alkali, 768
anoxemia, and morphine, 755
auricular fibrillation or flutter, 750, 752, 753
bowels, care of, 747, 748, 750
caffeine, 753, 759
camphor, 753, 754
carbon-dioxide, 768
cardiovascular system, and, 749–755, 758, 759
chemotherapy. *See* Chemotherapy
codeine, 749, 756
cold air, 743, 744
Treatment (*cont.*):
collapse, 753, 759
compressed air, 768
cough, 749
decompensation, cardiac, and, 752
delirium, 756
deuteroproteose, 773–775
diathermy, 749, 772
diet, 746, 747, 756
diet and vitamins, 790, 791
digitalis, 750–753
dilaudid, 755
enemas, and, 747, 757
enzymes, and, 736, 791–795, 927
ephedrine, 755
ephedrine, for serum sickness, 872
epinephrine, 750, 754, 755, 759
epinephrine, use in connection with serum treatment, 838–841, 864, 867, 868, 872, 878
expectorants, 749
fluid intake, 747, 756
general care, 742, 743
glucose, 747, 758, 759, 768
heart failure, 752
hemoproteose, 773–775
hemotherapy, 773
historical note, 741, 742
home care, 743, 744
hospital care, 743
humidity, and, 744
hydrotherapy, 750, 758
morphine, 749, 755, 756
mouth and nose care, 745
nursing care, 743–746
of complications. *See particular complication by name*
oxygen. *See* Oxygen treatment
pain, 749, 750, 755, 772
pituitrin, and, 750, 757
pneumothorax, 749, 769–772
complications of, 770–772
contraindications, 771
results, 769–772
technic, 769–771
post-operative pneumonia, 523, 524
pulmonary edema, and salt in diet, 746
pulmonary edema, restriction of fluids for, 747, 758
respiratory stimulants, 753, 754
sedatives, 750, 755, 756
serum. *See* Serum treatment; Serum treatment, dosage; Serum treatment, results
serum reactions, 864, 867, 868, 872, 878
sodium chloride, and, 746, 750, 756

Treatment (*cont.*):
strophanthin, 753, 759
strychnine, 750, 754
toxemia, 746
turpentine stupes, 757
tympanites, 746, 747, 756–758
unsolved problems of, 927
vaccine, 795–804
antibody appearance after, 797–799, 804
autolyzed vaccine for, 798
bacteriemia, 563
clinical use and results, 798–804
dangers with, 804
fatality rates, 798–803
mixed vaccine for, 799–803
natural bacterial antigen for, 802, 803
rationale, 796
value, discussion of, 795–797, 803, 804
venesection, 769
visitors, and, 744
vitamins, and, 790, 791
x-ray, 772, 773
Tropins. *See under* Antibody(ies), pneumococcus
Tubercle bacillus, in mixed infections, 13
Tuberculosis, empyema, and, 583, 584
Tuberculosis, pulmonary:
bloody sputum, and, 501
contraindication to immunization against pneumonia, 482
death rates of, and pneumonia, 274, 319, 324
differentiation of delayed resolution from, 542
differentiation of lobar pneumonia from, 650, 651
Friedländer's bacillus cases, resemblance to, 8
incidence of pneumonia, and, 274
lipoid pneumonia confused with, 341
pneumonia associated with, 274, 525
pneumonia, tuberculous, sputum in, 651
simulated appearance in resolution, 541
Tuberculous pneumonia, differentiation of lobar pneumonia from, 650, 651
Tularemia and pneumonia, 16
Tympanites:
bacteriemia, and, 756
oxygen treatment, and, 757
prognosis, and, 727
toxemia, and, 611, 748, 756
treatment, 756–758
treatment, diet, and, 746, 747, 756
Type determination, pneumococcus. *See* Bacteriologic study; Pneumococcus typing
Type(s), of Friedländer's bacillus, 6
Type(s), of pneumococcus. *See* Pneumococcus types
Typhoid pneumonia, 525

Ulcers, 607
Uleron, 787
Unclassified strains of pneumococci, 29–31, 51, 52
United States Public Health Service:
Advisory Committee on Pneumonia, 922, 930
advisory service to health departments undertaking pneumonia programs, 936
National Institute of Health, 826–829, 874
pneumococcus incidence and carrier rate, special studies of, 936
pneumonia programs, and, 922
potency tests, standard serums for, 827, 924, 925
potency tests, standardization, 924, 925
serum, diagnostic, standardization, 924
serum, therapeutic, standardization, 826–829, 874, 875
unsolved problems, and, 922, 924, 925, 936
Unsolved problems, 921–936
antibody, nature of, 925
causative organisms, 927
chemotherapy, 775, 777, 781, 789, 790, 794, 927
chill reactions, 925
enzyme therapy, 794, 927
epidemics, 474, 926
epidemiologic studies, 390–394, 396, 922, 925–927
fatality rates, 927
League of Nations, and, 921, 924, 925
pneumococcus, and, 921, 922
pneumococcus carriers and minor respiratory infections, 926, 927
potency tests, standardization of, 924, 925
prevention of pneumonia by immunization, 475–478, 925, 926
prevention of respiratory diseases, 395, 396
reporting methods, 927
serum:
diagnostic, pooled, need for study of, 924
diagnostic, standardization, 923, 924
production and concentration, 925
therapeutic, standardization, 924, 925
suggestions for study, 923–928
treatment, 927–929
types, new, classification, 924

Unsolved problems (*cont.*):
United States Public Health Service, and, 922, 924, 925, 936
Unspecified pneumonia, synonyms, xvi, xvii
Urine:
acid in, 500
albumin and casts in, 503, 608, 609
albuminuria, and prognosis, 727
chlorides in, 500
chlorides in, and pneumothorax therapy, 769
collection of, for typing, 619
findings in, with nephritis, 609
pneumococci in, with urogenital infection, 603, 604
SSS in, 25, 26, 503, 504
antibody, and, 122, 695
disappearance after serum treatment, 122, 885
duration of excretion after recovery, 504, 695
empyema, and, 566
in children, 695
in children compared with adults, 643
precipitin tests for, 116, 637–639
prognosis, and, 693–695
sulfanilamide excretion in, 784
sulfapyridine excretion in, 788, 789
typing, 116, 637–639
typing, and early diagnosis, 621, 637
typing, merits of, 621
Urticaria:
after serum treatment, a contraindication to further treatment, 867, 878
importance of history of, 838, 842
in allergic reaction, 864, 878

Vaccine(s):
immunization, and, 196–198, 406–482, 823–826, 873, 874
previous injection, in relation to sensitiveness to serum, 838
treatment with, 563, 795–804
Variants of pneumococcus. *See* Pneumococcus, variants
Vascular system. *See* Cardiovascular system
Vasomotor rhinitis, horse, importance of history of, in relation to sensitiveness to serum, 837, 842
Virulence, pneumococcus:
abortive pneumonia, and, 511
animal passage, and, 27
antigenicity, and, 27, 28
blood-clearing mechanism, and, 163, 164
Virulence, pneumococcus (*cont.*):
C substance, and, 25
capsule, and, 20, 22
carrier state in animals, and, 216, 217, 378
comparison of, for mice and man, 27
determination, 27
experimental infections, and, 27, 139, 193, 194, 205, 212–232, 511
immunity, and, 28, 193, 194
immunization response, and, 28, 194, 410, 411, 441–443
increase of, by SSS or autolysates, 131, 132
intrabronchial infection in animals, and, 225
intranasal infection in animals, and, 215, 216
intraperitoneal infection in animals, and, 215, 216
intratracheal infection in animals, and, 219, 221
M forms, 26
nucleoprotein, and, 24
pathogenesis of pneumonia, and, 200, 233–235, 257, 393
pneumococcus carriers, and, 216, 217, 372, 373, 378
post-operative pneumonia, and, 27, 518, 522, 523
R forms, 26
recovery, changes at, 734, 735
S forms, 26
SSS, and, 25, 131, 132
seasonal variation, 385
stability, 385
strains, identical, in different animals, 27
strains, variations in, 27, 139, 193, 372
susceptibility of animals, and, 138–143
terminal pneumonia, and, 27
type, and, 49, 194, 372, 373
type, transformation, and, 26, 27
Type III, for rabbits, and, 139
variations of, and tests for immunity, 410
virus of colds, effect on, 200, 239
virus of influenza, effect on, 200
Virus:
common cold, 237, 239, 375
common cold, and activation of organisms in upper respiratory tract, 200, 239
influenza:
antibody for, failure to find after pneumococcus pneumonia, 237
effect on pneumococcus, 200
infection, preceding pneumococcus pneumonia, 237

Virus infections:
experimental pneumonia in animals, and, 232, 240
pneumonia in Negroes, and, 457
predisposing factor in pneumonia, 3, 4, 9, 200, 236–240, 457
primary agent:
in influenza bacillus cases, and, 9
in pneumococcus cases, and, 232, 239, 240
in streptococcus cases, and, 3
route of infection in pneumonia, and, 247
Vitamins:
colds and vitamin A, 334, 335
immunity, and, 203, 335, 790
treatment with, 790, 791
Vomiting:
acute dilatation of stomach, and, 611, 748
anoxemia, and, 761
at onset, 490, 491
during course, 502, 514
optochin treatment, and, 780
serum reactions, and, 864, 866, 870
sulfanilamide treatment, and, 786

X-ray:
aputrid pulmonary necrosis and, 541, 606, 607
atelectasis, differentiation of lobar pneumonia from, 651
atelectasis, in pneumonia, and, 250–253, 493
bronchopneumonia, and, 649
central pneumonia, and, 646, 647
X-ray (*cont.*):
convalescence, for follow up, 546
diagnosis, and, 613, 645–647, 649
diaphragm, elevation of, and, 251, 253
differential diagnosis, and, 647, 649
differentiation of lipoid pneumonia from pulmonary tuberculosis, and, 341
early findings, 646, 647
empyema, diagnosis, and, 576, 577
Friedländer's bacillus cases, 7
heart size, and, 492, 493
lesions:
confluent, and, 649
course of, in serum treated cases, and, 883, 887
hilar, and, 256
in adjacent lobe, and, 647
initial, and, 256
organized, and, 543
spread of, and, 255, 256
lobar pneumonia, and, 646, 647
lung abscess, and, 604, 606, 607
mediastinal displacement, and, 251, 253
mediastinitis, and, 604
pericarditis, and, 589
physical signs, correlation with, 613
pleural effusions, and, 565, 576, 577, 652
pneumococcus type, and findings, 647
pneumothorax treatment, and, 770
resolution, and, 540, 541
resolution, beginning, and, 647
resolution, delayed, and, 542
spread of lesion, and, 255, 256
staphylococcus cases, 10
treatment, 772, 773
tuberculous pneumonia, and, 651

THE BIOLOGY OF PNEUMOCOCCUS

This volume is published as part of a long-standing cooperative program between the Harvard University Press and the Commonwealth Fund, a philanthropic foundation, to encourage the publication of significant scholarly books in medicine and health.

THE BIOLOGY OF PNEUMOCOCCUS

THE BACTERIOLOGICAL, BIOCHEMICAL, AND IMMUNOLOGICAL CHARACTERS AND ACTIVITIES OF DIPLOCOCCUS PNEUMONIAE

BENJAMIN WHITE, Ph.D.

with the collaboration of

ELLIOTT STIRLING ROBINSON, M.D., Ph.D.

AND LAVERNE ALMON BARNES, Ph.D.

A COMMONWEALTH FUND BOOK
Harvard University Press
Cambridge, Massachusetts
London, England

Printed in the United States of America

Library of Congress Cataloging in Publication Data

White, Benjamin, 1879-
The biology of pneumococcus.

"A Commonwealth Fund book."
Reprint of the ed. published by the Commonwealth Fund, New York.
Bibliography: p.
Includes index.
1. Streptococcus pneumoniae. 2. Streptococcus pneumoniae—Bibliography. 3. Immunity. 4. Immunity—Bibliography. I. Robinson, Elliott Stirling Andrew, 1894- joint author. II. Barnes, Laverne Almon, 1901- joint author. III. Title. [DNLM: QW142.5.C6 W582b 1938a]
QR201.P7W5 1979 616.01'4'5 78-10453
ISBN 0-674-67444-8

Second Printing, 1979

Affectionately dedicated to the memory of

GEORGE HOYT BIGELOW, M.D.

who gave to the Massachusetts Pneumonia Study and Service an inspiring guidance, and who, by his gallantry, set us an enduring and ennobling example of scientific fellowship

FOREWORD TO THE SECOND PRINTING

The republication of *The Biology of Pneumococcus* by Benjamin White makes readily available once again to students of bacteriology, immunology, infectious disease, and internal medicine a classic monograph concerned with a major pathogen of man. Because of the morbidity and high mortality of pneumococcal pneumonia, termed "captain of the men of death" by Sir William Osler, probably no bacterium was subjected to more intensive scrutiny in the early years of this century than the pneumococcus, as biologists and physicians attempted to control the diseases it causes. That so much was learned in an era of relatively unsophisticated technology is a tribute to the workings of the human mind and the ingenuity of man.

This remarkable volume is a repository of knowledge gleaned about the pneumococcus in the first six decades following its discovery, and deals with all aspects of the organism. In it can be found the history of the organism's discovery and descriptions of its cultural requirements, morphologic properties, biochemical constitution, pathogenic properties, and immunologic attributes. The accounts of the development of the treatment of pneumonia with type specific antiserum and of the exploration of the therapeutic potential of enzymes splitting pneumococcal capsular polysaccharides make fascinating reading, as do the accounts of the work leading to the polyvalent polysaccharide vaccine recently made available for protection against pneumococcal disease. It may come as a surprise also to some to see reference to drug fastness (resistance) and to the beginnings of bacterial genetics and modern immunochemistry in a work published originally in 1938.

Scientists are humans, however, and subject to the frailties of human behavior. The discovery, first of the sulfonamides, and then of penicillin was followed by a precipitous drop in interest in the pneumococcus by the majority of biologists and the medical profession. Despite the extraordinary amount of knowledge accumulated about the pneumococcus that provided a broad base from which to extend future studies, relatively little work has been done on it since the introduction of safe and effective chemical and antibiotic drugs with which to treat pneumococcal infection. The recognition in the past decade that the morbidity and mortality of pneumococcal disease are still significant has rekindled interest in the intriguing organism that causes it. The development of prophylactic vaccination takes its departure from work described in this text. Other problems remain to be solved, perhaps none more important than the means whereby the pneumococcus injures its mammalian host. Clues to the solution of this fundamental question may lie within the confines of this work and its extensive bibliography. Its republication with the financial support of the Commonwealth Fund and under its auspices can be welcomed only with enthusiasm and gratitude.

Robert Austrian, M.D.
John Herr Musser Professor of
Research Medicine, School of
Medicine, University of
Pennsylvania, Philadelphia,
Pennsylvania
July 1978

FOREWORD

In the introduction to one of his *Lectures and Lay Sermons*, Huxley used an analogy aptly illustrating his subject, and singularly fitting the purposes of the present undertaking: "Merchants occasionally go through a wholesome, though troublesome and not always satisfactory, process which they term 'taking stock.' After all the excitement of speculation, the pleasure of gain, and the pain of loss, the trader makes up his mind to face facts and to learn the exact quantity and quality of his solid and reliable possessions. The man of science does well sometimes to imitate this procedure; and, forgetting for the time the importance of his own small winnings, to re-examine the common stock in trade, so that he may make sure how far the store of the bullion in the cellar—on the faith of whose existence so much paper has been circulating—is really the solid gold of truth."

The present undertaking is not an inventory of small personal winnings, but rather a re-examination of the circulating paper and an attempted appraisal of the quantity and quality of the stored bullion, done with a sense of humility before the importance and magnitude of the task. Nor is this an original enterprise. There are the familiar Rockefeller Institute *Monograph, Number Seven*, the ample summary of Neufeld and Schnitzer, and the later symposium in the British *System of Bacteriology*, but since their publication more gold has been mined, vastly enriching the common stock. In drawing upon this stock for the purpose of learning better ways of applying our knowledge to the discovery of means for mitigating the ills inflicted upon man by Pneumococcus, the whole storehouse has been ransacked for hidden or forgotten goods. To sort out the accumulation of more than fifty years, to convert old specie into modern currency, and finally to set a value on the whole store has been a troublesome task which it is hoped may be spared others by the presentation of this re-examination and appraisal.

The present review of the literature on the biology of Pneumococcus forms a part of the Pneumonia Study and Service carried on during the years 1931 to 1935 by the Massachusetts Department of Public Health under a grant from the Commonwealth Fund.

The labor of preparing the manuscript has been lightened and made an agreeable occupation by the help so graciously given by many friends. An added pleasure, now that the work has come to completion, is to record grateful acknowledgments to the officers and members of the staff of the Commonwealth Fund for their sympathetic interest and liberal support; to Professor Doctor Fr. Neufeld for permission to reproduce original drawings from his publications and for aid in securing some of the portraits included in the text; to Dr. Rufus Cole and colleagues at the Hospital of the Rockefeller Institute for Medical Research for many courtesies; to Dr. O. T. Avery for the rich benefits of his counsel; to Dr. M. A. Dawson for the generous loan of unpublished illustrative material; to Miss L. M. D. Trask, librarian of the Rockefeller Institute, for her able assistance in searching the literature; to Miss E. C. Campbell of the Publication Division of the same Institute for the loan of original electrotypes from the *Journal of Experimental Medicine;* to Miss Emily Jackson and associates at the Massachusetts Antitoxin and Vaccine Laboratory for their competent and willing services; to many of the authors quoted for criticism and suggestions; and to Mrs. Helen M. Boynton for her intelligent and discriminating digest of the whole story of Pneumococcus.

B. W.

Boston, 1937

CONTENTS

I. HISTORY OF PNEUMOCOCCUS 1

1875–1890: inoculation of rabbits with human sputum (Pasteur and Sternberg); isolation, cultivation, and animal inoculation (Friedländer); pneumococci in dust and air (Emmerich and Pawlowsky); Fraenkel's experiments; acquired resistance to infection; Weichselbaum's contributions; artificial active immunity. 1890–1900: passive immunity (Klemperers); dissociation (Kruse and Pansini); agglutination (Metchnikoff and others); type differentiation; tropins (Denys). Summary.

II. BIOLOGY OF PNEUMOCOCCUS 30

Morphology: staining methods; the capsule; staining the capsule. Isolation of Pneumococcus: animal inoculation; direct cultures. Cultivation: accessory substances; vegetable accessory substances; appearance of growth; differential media. Viability. Autolysis. Bile solubility. Sensitiveness to germicides and other chemical substances.

III. BIOCHEMICAL FEATURES 65

Proteolysis, lipolysis, and carbohydrate fermentation. Acid production. Oxidation and reduction: methemoglobin production; peroxide formation. Hemolysin and hemotoxin. Purpura production. Virulin, leucocidin, and analogous substances. So-called toxins. Summary.

IV. CLASSIFICATION OF PNEUMOCOCCI 103

Serological classification, 1898–1932: first differentiation by agglutination reaction; differentiation by immunological reactions; *Pneumococcus mucosus;* two groups; typical and atypical strains; four groups; five groups; subgroups of Type II; Group IV differentiated into twelve groups; further differentiation of subgroups of Type II; further differentiation of subgroups of Group IV. Classification according to electrophoretic potential. Type determination: mouse protection test; culture agglutination; urine precipitation test; sputum precipitinogen; sputum digestion; bile-solution of sputum; slide agglutination; *Quellung* phenomenon. Summary.

V. PNEUMOCOCCAL DISSOCIATION AND TRANSFORMATION 134

Early observations of dissociation, 1891–1921. Later observations of dissociation: smooth and rough forms of Pneumococcus; modifications A, B, and C; composite cultures; species-specificity of rough forms; electrophoretic potential of variants; effect of charcoal, yeast, optochin; *in vivo* variation; details of colony formation; antigenicity of rough forms; respiratory capacity of variants; intermediate forms; reversal of dissociation; reversion by means of pneumococcal vaccine. Transformation of type: transformation by vaccine and animal inoculation; isolation of the transformative principle. Dawson classification. Transmutation of species. Summary.

VI. PATHOGENICITY OF PNEUMOCOCCUS: EXPERIMENTAL ANIMALS 179

Susceptibility of the animal host: the rabbit; the guinea pig; the mouse; the rat; the monkey; the cat; the dog; the horse; birds. Virulence of the organism: freshly isolated strains; numbers of cocci required to infect; avenue of inoculation; determination of virulence; substances that enhance virulence; cultural conditions and virulence; strain variations in virulence; virulence in respect to animal species; artificial exaltation of virulence; degradation of virulence; dissociation and virulence. Summary.

VII. PATHOGENICITY OF PNEUMOCOCCUS: MAN 214

Etiology of pneumonia: pneumococcal types in lobar pneumonia; pneumococcal types in bronchopneumonia; pneumococcal types in pneumonia in infants and children. Serological types and fatality-rates. Localized epidemics of pneumococcal infection. Infectious processes other than pneumonia. Pneumococcemia. Excretion of pneumococci. The carrier state. Summary.

VIII. CHEMICAL CONSTITUENTS OF PNEUMOCOCCUS 238

Work of earlier investigators. First description of the pneumococcal carbohydrate. Isolation of carbohydrate fractions. Isolation of C Fraction. Relation of the pneumococcal carbohydrate to carbohydrates isolated from other organisms. Function of sugars in determining antigenic specificity and conjugated proteins. Isolation of "A substance." Comparison of various cellular carbohydrates. Type VIII carbohydrate. Isolation of an unidentified constituent of the pneumococcal cell. Cause of differences in carbohydrates isolated from Pneumococcus. Relation of the acetyl group to the immunological activity of Pneumococcus. Recent methods of preparing capsular polysaccharide. Other physicochemical properties of the capsular polysaccharide. Summary.

IX. SPECIFIC POLYSACCHARIDE-SPLITTING ENZYMES 301

First isolation of polysaccharide-splitting enzyme: SIII bacillus. Effect of the enzyme on the cell capsule. Protective action of enzyme in mice. Philosophical aspect of the action of the enzyme. Methods of production. Effect of enzyme on infection induced in rabbits. Effect on infection induced in monkeys. Isolation and study of other bacteria possessing polysaccharide-splitting enzymes. Differences in susceptibility of polysaccharides to enzymatic action. Summary.

X. ANTIGENICITY OF PNEUMOCOCCUS 323

Antigenic spectrum. First observations of immunity. Influence of virulence on immunological response. Dead cultures: heat-killed antigens; other devitalized antigens. Sensitized pneumococci. Filtrates and extracts: culture filtrates and bacterial extracts; tissue extracts and exudates. Toxins and hemotoxins: so-called toxins; hemotoxins. Methods of administering antigens: intradermal injection; inhalation and intrabronchial insufflation; oral administration. Host response. Antagonistic action of soluble specific substance. Summary.

XI. ANTIBODIES TO PNEUMOCOCCUS 355

Agglutinins: history; agglutinins in the blood of pneumonia patients; agglutination and serological classification; agglutinability of pneumococcal variants; agglutinins in the blood of animals; additional data. Precipitins: history; antiprotein precipitins; somatic carbohydrate (C Fraction); the mechanism of specific precipitation; correlation of precipitins with other antibodies. Complement-fixing antibodies. Bactericidins. Antihemotoxin. Antitoxin. Heterophile antibodies. Phagocytosis: history; sensitization of pneumococci; normal tropins or opsonins; antiopsonins; opsonins in pneumonia; the mechanism of phagocytosis. Protective antibodies: specificity; relation to other antibodies; additional data;

chemical nature of protective antibodies; the separation of antibodies from immune serum; the estimation of protective antibodies. Other immunological phenomena: growth of pneumococci in specific immune serum; antiblastic immunity; immunological relationships between Pneumococcus and other microbic species and unrelated substances. Summary.

XII. HOST RESPONSE TO ANTIGENIC ACTION OF PNEUMOCOCCUS 427

Natural immunity: in animals; in man. Naturally induced immunity: specific antibodies in the blood during pneumonia; immune substances in sputum; antagonistic substances in pneumococcal exudates. Artificially induced immunity: active immunity; passive immunity. Allergy and anaphylaxis: actively induced sensitization; passive sensitization; relation of pneumococcal allergy to pneumococcal immunity. Dermal allergy: skin reactions in experimental animals; skin reactions in lobar pneumonia; active and passive skin allergy; the mechanism of dermal allergy; the Shwartzman phenomenon. Summary.

XIII. PNEUMOCOCCAL VACCINES 479

Experiments on monkeys. Types of vaccines employed. Dosage. Special constituents of Pneumococcus. Potency tests on vaccines. Route and spacing of injections. Local and systemic reactions. Appearance and duration of vaccinal immunity. Results following vaccination in man. Prophylaxis. Vaccine treatment of pneumonia.

XIV. CHEMOTHERAPY 507

Chemical agents other than cinchona derivatives: bile; soap; coal-tar dyes; metals and metallic salts; other medicinal agents. Cinchona derivatives: effect of the various quinine derivatives on pneumococci; effect on various pneumococcal types; effect on pneumococcal infection; adjuvant action of cinchona compounds with specific serum; effect on virulence of Pneumococcus. Summary.

XV. PRODUCTION OF ANTIPNEUMOCOCCIC SERUM 522

Immunization of the horse: selection of horses; selection and standardization of the immunizing antigen; injections; bleedings. The production of therapeutic serum: reasons for and against the use of unconcentrated serum;

avian serum; polyvalent serum; methods of concentrating serum. Physical properties. Chill-producing factors. Potency tests: *in vivo* tests; *in vitro* tests; correlation between *in vitro* and *in vivo* tests. Safety tests: routine safety test; tests on mice. Final processing of serums: total solids; filtration; bulk sterility and potency tests; dispensing and labeling; sterility tests on final containers; safety and identity tests; identity test; records; regulations governing antipneumococcic serum. The production of diagnostic serum: immune horse serum; immune rabbit serum; preservatives, bottling, and labeling. Summary.

XVI. SERUM TREATMENT OF LOBAR PNEUMONIA 598

The rationale of serum therapy. Problems and limitations of serum therapy. The results of serum therapy. Summary.

XVII. UNSOLVED PROBLEMS 613

Toxins. Serological types. Dissociation. Chemical constituents of pneumococci. Virulence. Methods for the production of active immunity. Chemotherapy. Immunological response. Antibodies and animal species. Skin reactions. The nature of pneumococcal antibody. Concentration of antipneumococcic serum. Potency tests on therapeutic serum. Summary.

APPENDIX. SPECIAL METHODS USED IN THE STUDY OF PNEUMOCOCCUS AND IN THE PREPARATION OF ANTIPNEUMOCOCCIC SERUM 623

I. MEDIA. Pneumococcus broth for all general purposes. Nutrient broth for mass cultures for the production of soluble specific substances: preparation of infusion; preparation of medium; growing the pneumococci. Blood broth. Inulin serum water. 623

II. ISOLATION OF PNEUMOCOCCUS. Mouse method: mouse inoculation; mouse necropsy. Plating methods: preparation of blood agar; use of blood agar. Blood cultures. 626

III. TYPE DETERMINATION. Mouse method. Krumwiede method. Neufeld *Quellung* method. Urine test: unconcentrated urine; concentrated urine for precipitin test. 628

IV. ISOLATION OF SEVERAL COMPONENTS OF PNEUMOCOCCUS. Medium for the production of culture of standard maximal density, virulence, and polysaccharide content. Pneumococcal protein. Somatic carbohydrate or C Fraction. Capsular polysaccharide: preparation of the specific polysaccharide of Type I Pneumococcus; preparation of the specific polysaccharide of Type II Pneumococcus; preparation of the specific polysaccharide of Type III Pneumococcus. 634

V. PREPARATION OF BACTERIAL ENZYMES CAPABLE OF DECOMPOSING CAPSULAR POLYSACCHARIDES. 640

VI. SEROLOGICAL REACTIONS. Agglutination. Precipitation: optimal proportions; nitrogen determination; modified routine; combining equivalents. Complement fixation. Bactericidal tests. 641

VII. POTENCY TESTS ON ANTIPNEUMOCOCCIC SERUM. United States Hygienic Laboratory, now National Institute of Health: culture; serum; the test. League of Nations: animals; culture; serum. American Drug Manufacturers' Association: unit of serum; test dose of culture; the test; interpretation of test; records and reports. Massachusetts Antitoxin and Vaccine Laboratory: culture; serums; the test; interpretation of the test; protocols and records. 648

VIII. STERILITY TESTS ON ANTIPNEUMOCOCCIC SERUM. Bulk sterility tests. Sterility tests on final containers. 662

IX. PREPARATION OF DIAGNOSTIC ANTIPNEUMOCOCCIC RABBIT SERUM. Massachusetts Antitoxin and Vaccine Laboratory method: vaccine; injection of rabbits; bleeding of rabbits; testing of serum; dilution of serum. 663

BIBLIOGRAPHY 665

INDEX 771

INTRODUCTION

Pneumococcus is altogether an amazing cell. Tiny in size, simple in structure, frail in make-up, it possesses physiological functions of great variety, performs biochemical feats of extraordinary intricacy and, attacking man, sets up a stormy disease so often fatal that it must be reckoned as one of the foremost causes of human death. Furthermore, living or dead, whole or in part, on entering the animal body Pneumococcus starts a train of impulses, stimulating all the reactions grouped under those inclusive phenomena known as immunity.

Digesting foreign proteins, Pneumococcus rebuilds the fragments into a new protein common to all types of the species; splitting and consuming carbohydrates, from the simplest sugars to the starch-like substances, inulin and glycogen, the cell synthesizes the cleavage products of these same sugars into complex polysaccharides. These polysaccharides, chemically distinct and immunologically specific for the type, are built into a morphological structure which forms a defensive armor against the destructive forces of the animal body, and in a highly selective fashion determines the precise nature of the immunological response each separate type calls forth.

Man has not been content to allow Pneumococcus to destroy human life in an unrestrained way. The sanitarian has sought hygienic and prophylactic measures to curb the incidence of acute respiratory infections; the pathologist has studied the anatomical distribution and histological nature of pulmonary lesions in order to gain fuller knowledge of the portal of entry and the pathway of infection through the living tissues; the epidemiologist has attempted to track the mode of dissemination of the infectious agent in the hope of breaking the vicious cycle of transmission from man to man; pending the discovery of specific therapy, the physician has ameliorated suffering by symptomatic treatment and contributed to recovery by instituting supportive measures until the natural capabilities of living tissue have repaired the injuries inflicted by the invading microorganisms.

The bacteriologist has persisted in the pursuit of information, and as a result the positive identification, the growth needs, and much of the physiological behavior of Pneumococcus are now common knowledge. The immunologist, by serum reactions, has found that pneumococci are not all alike; that they may become degraded and even transmuted into strange forms, and that on this degradation or exaltation depend certain vital processes within the cell related to virulence and the morbid effects produced in the animal economy. With this information he has devised ways of identifying types among the species, and of using the cocci for his own purposes.

In time the chemist joined forces with his colleagues in the field of medical science, and as a result of their combined efforts the answer has been found to some of the riddles which the bacteriologist alone could not solve. Breaking down Pneumococcus into its component parts, the chemist found the expected protein, and then discovered the new sugars which have so altered our ideas about pneumococci in general, and which are bringing a solution to the cryptic working of the immunological mechanism.

The chemist, laboring with the bacteriologist and immunologist, has given us a new conception of the significance of chemical constitution and molecular arrangement in determining the power of proteins and of carbohydrates, either alone or combined, to call into activity those reactions which spell the fate of the infected host or the fate, not only of Pneumococcus, but of other bacteria and even of non-living alien substances that gain entrance to the animal body. New biological principles have been disclosed, explaining many of the functions of the living bacterial cell amidst both natural and artificial surroundings and opening fresh and inviting paths of investigation.

The study of the members of this small group of microorganisms in a subordinate branch of biology is bringing light into some of the obscure realms of the related sciences. The peculiarities of Pneumococcus are yielding a generous return to the investors and speculators who have cast in their resources with its lot, resulting in the accumulation of a store of solid bullion for the scientist and for mankind.

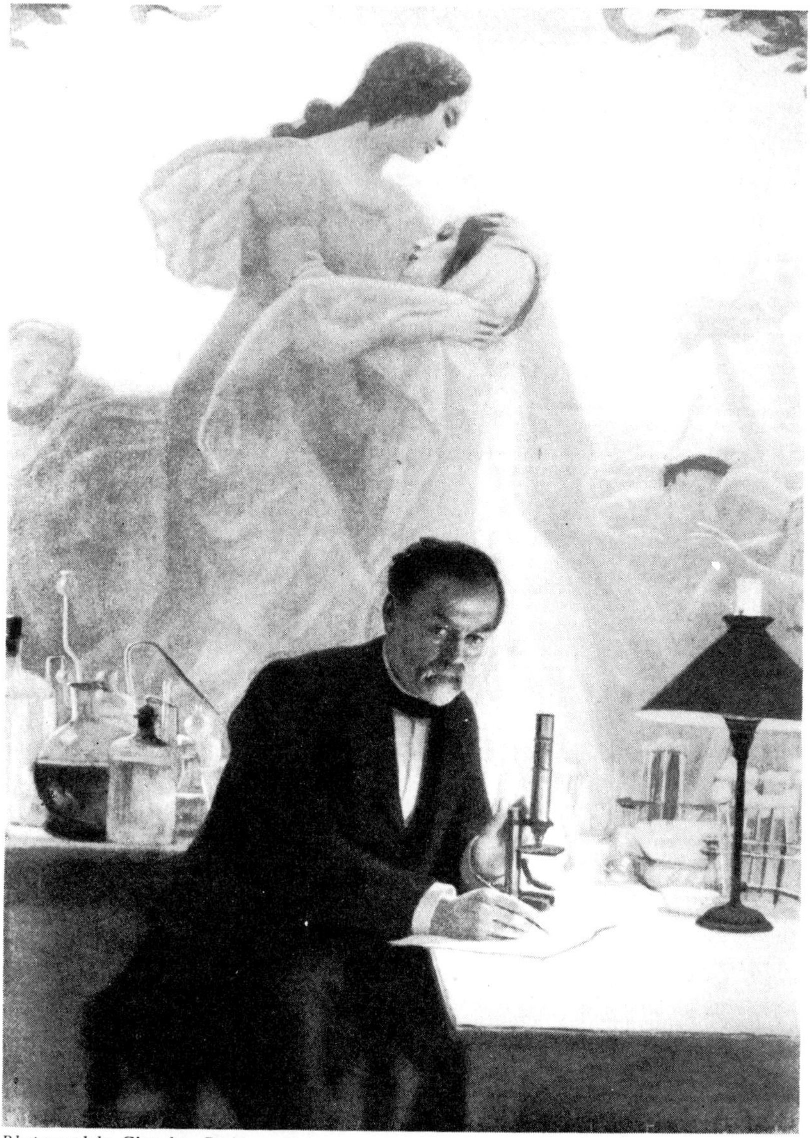

Photograph by Giraudon, Paris

LOUIS PASTEUR 1822–1895

By Louis Edouard Fournier, Ecole Normale Supérieure, Paris

CHAPTER I

HISTORY OF PNEUMOCOCCUS

A chronological account of the early observations of the coccus in tissues, saliva, and other body fluids; first isolation and cultivation, and description of effects on animals; separation into types; variation; and attempts to produce immune serum.

THE lanceolate, Gram-positive diplococcus, now known as the chief etiological agent in lobar pneumonia and commonly called Pneumococcus, has the species name *Diplococcus pneumoniae*, genus *Diplococcaceae*, tribe *Streptococcaceae* of the family *Coccaceae*.[104] During the years in which the organism has been the subject of investigation, it has received many appellations which are given below in chronological order.

Monas pulmonale (Klebs)[718]	1875
Microbe septicémique du saliva (Pasteur)[1066]	1881
Pneumoniekokken (Mátray)[869-70]	1883
Coccus lancéolé de la pneumonie (Talamon)[1377]	1883
Pneumoniemikrokokken (Friedländer)[487]	1883
Pneumonie-Micrococcen (Friedländer)[490]	1884
Micrococcus Pasteuri (Sternberg)[1319]	1885
Pneumoniemikrococcus (Fraenkel)[469]	1886
Pneumococcus (Fraenkel)[469]	1886
Bacillus septicus sputigenus (Flügge)[495]	1886
Diplokokkus lanceolatus pneumoniae (Flügge)[495]	1886
Diplococcus pneumoniae (Weichselbaum)[1497]	1886
Bacillus salivarius septicus (Biondi)[117]	1887
Micrococcus pneumoniae crouposae (Sternberg)[1320]	1887
Streptococcus lanceolatus Pasteuri (Gamaléia)[498]	1888
Diplococcus lanceolatus (Foà, Bordoni-Uffreduzzi)[462]	1888
Virus pneumonico (Gabbi)[497]	1889
Bacterium pneumoniae (Migula)[901]	1900
Diplococcus pneumoniae Weichselbaum (Bergey)[104]	1930

In giving proper credit for the discovery of an organism it usually becomes necessary to decide which special events constitute a discovery. Is it the report of the first sight of the organism in the fluids or tissues of the infected animal; is it the first formal association of the virus with a disease; is it the setting up of a specific infection in an alien animal species; or must one await the complete fulfilment of all the postulates of Koch's law?

It is not essential to our purpose to be too exacting in asking or answering these questions. It should suffice to describe the observations of early pioneers and their successors in the order of their happening.

1875–1890

In 1875, Klebs[718] was probably the first to see—or at least the first to tell about seeing—Pneumococcus. Searching for proof of the infectious nature of pneumonia, he examined fluid from the lungs of men dying of the disease and found non-motile, sometimes linked monads in astonishing numbers. Growing these cocci on egg albumen, he thought they developed motility when grouped in chains, but their true identity escaped him. In 1880, Eberth[347] was undoubtedly looking at pneumococci when he examined the exudate from a gray-hepatized lung and the subarachnoid fluid of a pneumonia patient with a secondary meningitis. His description of the organisms as non-motile, slightly oval, almost round bodies, occasionally occurring singly but more often in pairs, taken with their source, makes it seem more than likely they were pneumococci, but Eberth thought they were only varieties of diphtheria or pyemia micrococci. Mátray,[869-70] in the same year, gave the name *Pneumoniekokken* to the cocci which he found in the sputum of pneumonia patients and in normal sputum as well. Had animal inoculation been tried by either Eberth or Mátray their find would have preceded the real discovery by Pasteur and Sternberg by over a year; but it was not tried.

In 1881, these two authors, Pasteur and Sternberg, independently inoculating rabbits, the former with the saliva of a child dead from rabies, the latter with normal saliva, isolated Pneumococcus for the first time through animal passage. Pasteur, contrary to the subsequent opinions of others, thought that he had discovered a new disease.* Sternberg reported that the fatal septicemia which normal saliva produced in rabbits was due to an organism that later, upon microscopic examination, appeared to agree exactly with the description given by Pasteur.

Pasteur[1065-6] passed his virus from infected to normal rabbits, producing infection each time, recovered the organism from the blood by cultivation in bouillon and other media, and with these cultures induced a similar fatal septicemia in other rabbits. On microscopic examination he found the bacteria to be very short rods, somewhat depressed in the center, with a visible aureola due, as he thought, to mucin.

Sternberg[1316-8] ascertained that the ability to incite fatal rabbit septicemia was a peculiarity of the saliva of some normal individuals but not of others, and that normal blood, putrid urine, liquid feces, and bouillon undergoing spontaneous putrefaction failed to produce a similar infection. In a later study appearing after the publication of Pasteur's paper, using aniline violet as a stain and making a permanent record by photomicrographs, Sternberg confirmed Pasteur's and his own findings. Here the dates are worth noting. Pasteur announced his discovery before the French Academy of Sciences in December, 1880, the report appearing in the Academy's *Comptes Rendus* in January, 1881. Sternberg began his experiments in the summer of 1880, and made his report which was first published in April, 1881.

There then arose a misconception of Pasteur's claims which was to persist for a long time. By his fellow countryman, Colin,[269] he was gratuitously credited with the claim that he had isolated the microbe of rabies. Pasteur emphatically replied, *J'ignore absolument les relations de cette nouvelle maladie avec la rage.* Pasteur

* The original communication was presented by Pasteur, but the work was done with the collaboration of Chamberland and Roux.

also stated that this new disease was not a septicemia, and this mistake undoubtedly contributed to the confusion of ideas. Disturbed by this false imputation, Pasteur, in March, 1881, in a letter to Parrot[1064] who had, like Sternberg, produced a fatal infection in rabbits with normal saliva, again stated positively that his organism bore no relation to rabies. Pasteur, by the way, showed his great perspicacity in a paragraph which was included in that letter. It bears repeating: *J'y vois, pour ma part, un symptôme nouveau de grand avenir pour la connaissance étiologique des maladies dont la cause doit être attribuée à la présence et au développement d'organismes microscopiques.* Again, in a communication read at the May 31st session of the *Académie de Médecine,* Pasteur sharply protested against the claims ascribed to him.

In this connection, the originals of Pasteur's and of Sternberg's later papers (1885 and 1887)[1319-20] are well-worth reading. In these days of petty priority claims it is refreshing to read of these two gentlemen of the eighteen-eighties, of whom one, Pasteur, frankly acknowledged his ignorance, while the other granted precedence and magnanimously named the organism after Pasteur. Sternberg's statement (1885) ran as follows:

> In attaching to this micrococcus the name of the illustrious French chemist I have no desire to perpetuate the memory of the mistake he made in supposing for a time that it was the germ of hydrophobia. Having found that this was a mistake, he did not fail to correct it. . . . It is easy to make mistakes in this field of investigation; easier, perhaps, than to acknowledge them.* And believing, as I do, in human fallibility, I have no hesitation in questioning the conclusions of the most illustrious workers in the field of microbiology, if they are in conflict with my own observations. On the other hand, if, upon fuller investigation, I am convinced that I have been mistaken in regard to this or any other question, I shall feel no hesitation in following the example of Pasteur in making a public announcement of my error.

Here is material for a Hippocratic oath for the biologist or any other fellow of science.

* Sternberg was prominent among those who had given an entirely erroneous interpretation to Pasteur's claims, and this statement, gracious though it was, served to foster the unfortunate misconception.

Vulpian,[1453] at the March (1881) meeting of the French Academy, said that he regretted that he had not been present at a former session when the letter from Pasteur to Parrot had been read, because he also might have reported that he had caused the death of a rabbit by the subcutaneous injection of normal saliva, while the blood of that animal killed another rabbit within the space of two days. The blood of the animals contained a number of "microbes," the majority having the same characteristics as those described by Pasteur. Here was the link between the work of Pasteur and that of Sternberg, but Vulpian, besides failing to appreciate the connection, was tardy in his announcement. Claxton (1882),[237] too, found normal human saliva infectious for rabbits. Believing in Pasteur's idea, he however confirmed Sternberg's results, with the added observation that human saliva varied in its infecting power, that of individuals from such tropical countries as Cuba and Brazil being extremely virulent.

In 1881, Osler[1039] spoke of finding "micrococcus balls" in four cases of endocarditis complicating pneumonia. He was not willing to assert they were the cause of the disease, but called attention to the frequency with which this condition and meningitis accompany pneumonia. Osler's comment recalls the earlier description by Koester (1878)[736] of "bullet-like masses of micrococci" in embolic endocarditis, which may or may not have been pneumococci.

The year 1881 was an eventful one. If one examines the photomicrographs accompanying Robert Koch's[735] paper on pathogenic organisms, there is little difficulty in identifying these lance-shaped diplococci, but to Koch they were that and nothing more. Poincaré[1102] was nearer the truth when he spoke of finding "prodigious numbers of little spheres of double contour" in pneumonic lung tissue, but he lacked the support of positive animal experiments to justify a claim that these organisms were responsible for pneumonia.

Shortly after the preliminary announcements of Pasteur and of Sternberg, Friedländer (1882)[486] presented a communication which takes high rank in the history of Pneumococcus. He reported that in September, 1881, in the fibrinous exudate and in hardened sections of lung and pleural tissue, stained by the Weigert-Koch method, from eight cases of acute pneumonia and in the fluid withdrawn from living pneumonia patients by lung puncture, he had observed spherical and ellipsoidal cocci, occurring mostly in pairs, and sometimes in longer chains made up of diplococci.

In 1882, Günther,[579] at a meeting of the *Verein für innere Medizin* in Berlin, had reported that the microscopic examination of stained preparations of purulent, bloody matter from lung puncture showed numerous diplococci. He gave a demonstration of his preparation and exhibited a drawing which caused Fraenkel to remark that the cocci seemed to be surrounded by an unstained rim. Günther replied that the rim was really a hull. Early in the same year, Colomiatti,[271] who was familiar only with the work of Klebs, reported finding *Monas pulmonale* in a growth on the heart valve and in the subarachnoid fluid in a case of croupous pneumonia complicated with endocarditis and meningitis.

In 1883,* Friedländer[487-8] announced that he had found the same micrococci in the alveolar exudate in all but a few of fifty cases of pneumonia. Stained by the method of his colleague, Gram, these cocci took an intense color, which was not extracted by treatment with alcohol, and exhibited a well-defined capsule. The capsule, which a short time before had been observed by Günther, could be clearly demonstrated by fixing the preparations with acetic or mineral acids and staining with gentian violet, fuchsin, Bismarck brown, or methylene blue. The capsular substance was insoluble in alcohol, ether, or chloroform, and was best shown by preliminary staining with aniline gentian violet, a short exposure to alcohol, and counterstaining with eosin. The contour was brought out by osmic acid but there was no blackening of the capsule or cell. Friedländer observed that the capsules were most characteristic at the highest stage of the cells' development, and con-

* A greater part of this work was done with the collaboration of Frobenius, who, because he did not remain until the completion of the study, declined the inclusion of his name in the authorship of the paper!

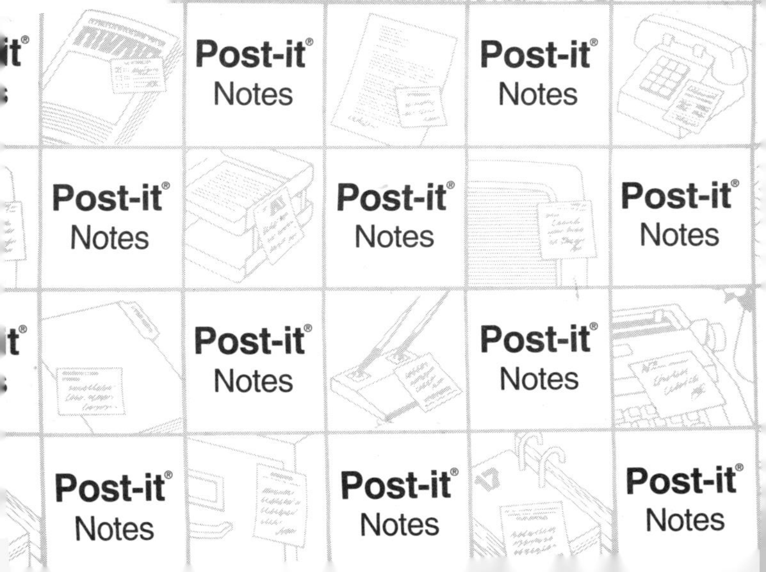
Post-it® Notes
Post-it® Notes
Post-it® Notes
Post-it® Notes
Post-it® Notes
Post-it® Notes
Post-it® Notes
Post-it® Notes
Post-it® Notes
Post-it® Notes

sidered them not as a passive precipitate, but as a product of the vital action of the coccus. Applying several microchemical tests to the capsular material, he felt justified in concluding that it consisted of mucin or an allied substance. When one remembers that mucin is a protein-carbohydrate complex in which the saccharide yields on hydrolysis two glucosamin, one acetic acid, and two hexose molecules, one appreciates the value of this observation in anticipating the discovery of the soluble specific substance or capsular polysaccharide by Heidelberger and Avery. Friedländer cultivated these organisms on Koch's coagulated blood serum, upon which they grew as round and elliptical cocci. His descriptions of the colonies on this medium corresponded with the appearance of the colonies of typical pneumococci. He also said that he had carried the cultures through eight transfers in meat-infusion peptone gelatin. In this medium the coccus lost its capsule and grew in "nail-form" colonies.

When one-half to one cubic centimeter of aqueous suspensions of the gelatin cultures was injected into the lungs of rabbits no infection resulted. Guinea pigs inoculated in this way were more susceptible, six of nine becoming infected. Mice were far more susceptible, all dying of infection. From the pleural and lung exudate of the infected animals Friedländer isolated typical diplococci. In four of twelve mice he succeeded in producing infection by inhalation. One of four dogs succumbed to the injection of cultures into the lung, and this animal at necropsy showed red and gray hepatization of the lung. From these areas, from the blood, and from the right pleural cavity, Friedländer recovered typical organisms. He noted variations in the capsule of the organisms depending upon their propagation in mice, guinea pigs, dogs, and man.

At that time, Friedländer was unable to demonstrate cocci in the blood of pneumonia patients, but in 1884[489-90] reported that he had cultivated typical micrococci from the blood of one of six patients. The cocci were encapsulated and virulent for mice, but by the method tested were avirulent for rabbits. It was in his first communication that, after giving credit to Klebs for the first reference to Pneumococcus and to Eberth and Koch for previous reports, Friedländer gave the name *Pneumoniemikrokokken* to the organisms. He believed that the capsule and the nail-form colony were not distinctive diagnostic characters, but that the whole cycle of phenomena must be observed, namely, the effect on animals and recultivation of the cocci from the artificially infected animals. He agreed that it was impossible to obtain this complete series of events in all cases of pneumonia, and suggested that there might be several forms of pneumonia, one of which was caused by the *Pneumoniemikrokokken,* or that the organisms while present at one stage of the disease were either not present or dead at other stages. He inclined to the first viewpoint.

Salvioli and Zäslein (1883)[1217] examined the sputum, cantharides blister fluid, and the blood of pneumonia patients. Here the same cocci, less frequent in the sputum than in the other fluids, could be cultivated in broth and in Pasteur's solution and rendered visible with Bismarck brown and methyl violet.

In 1883, Strassmann[1843] also found diplococci in pneumonic sputum.

In the same year, before the Berlin Medical Society, von Leyden demonstrated in blood and exudate aspirated from the hepatized lung of a pneumonia patient diplococci, largely oval in form, occasionally in longer chains. He added that similar cocci could be seen, without staining, in small masses scraped from the affected lung at necropsy. He surmised that Klebs had seen the same organisms.

Considering the meagerness of information in his time (1882), Bozzolo[145] contributed some sound ideas. He concluded from his studies that pleurisy, pericarditis, endocarditis, and cerebrospinal meningitis were frequently associated with lobar pneumonia; that this association, whether the disease occurred in epidemic or sporadic form, was caused by the action of a single infecting agent;

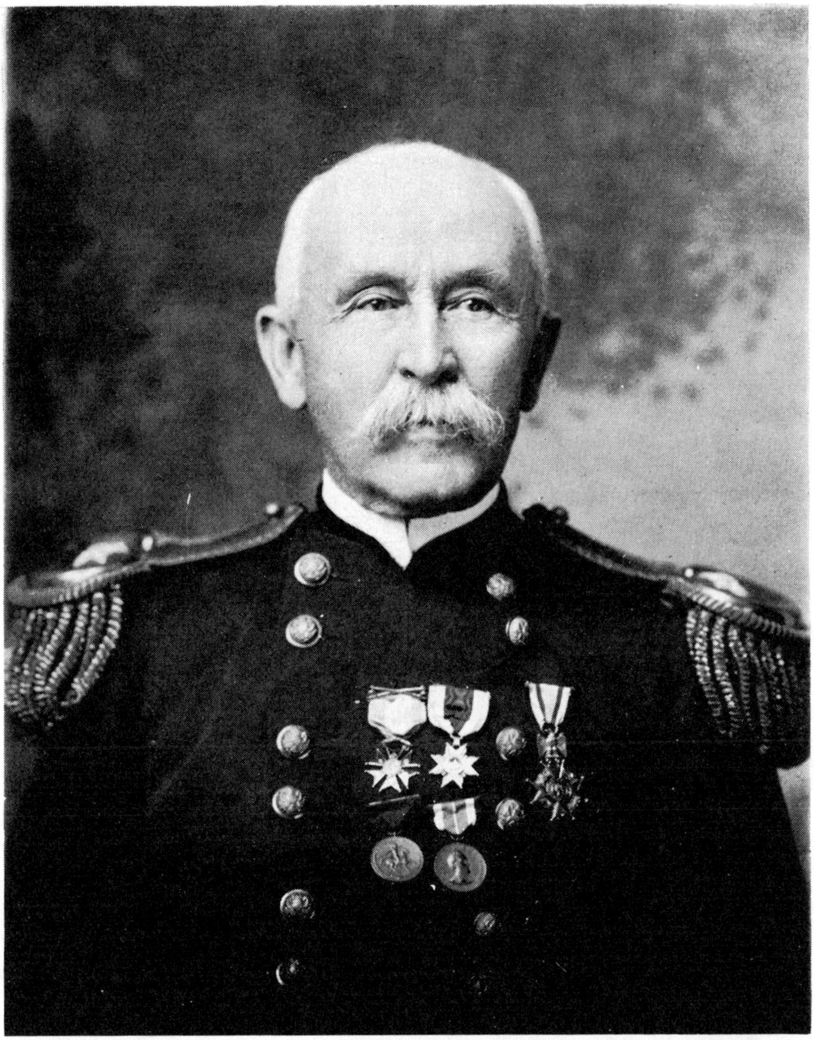

Courtesy of the Journal of the American Medical Association

GEORGE MILLER STERNBERG 1838–1915

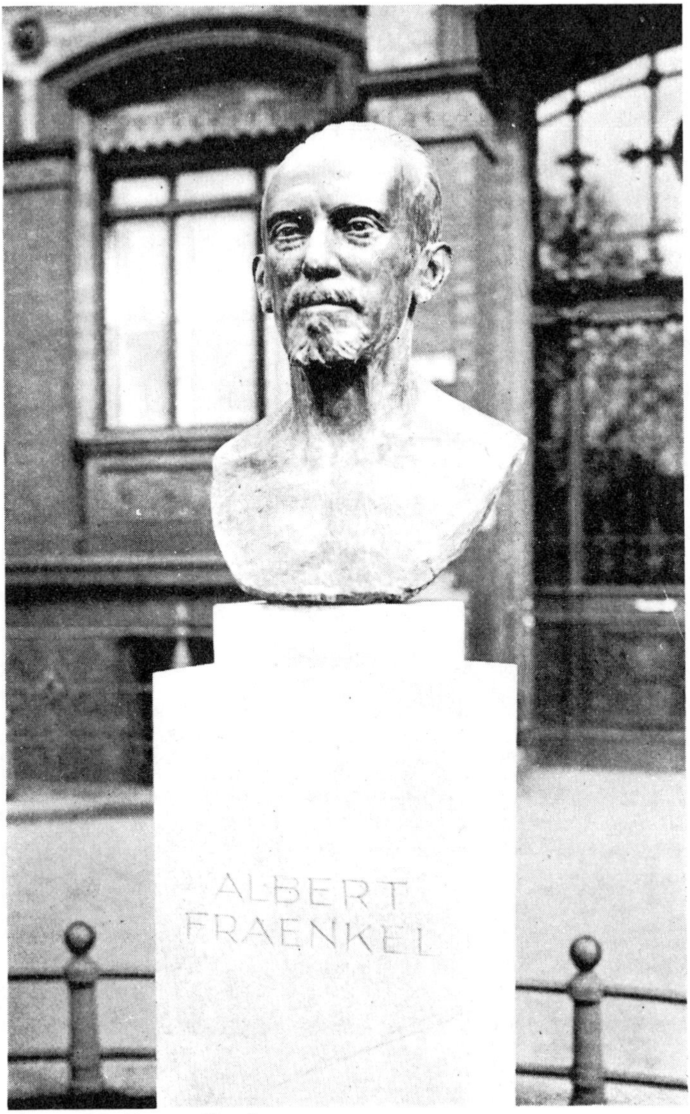

Photograph by Keystone View Co.

ALBERT FRAENKEL 1848–1916

By Alexander Oppler, Städtisches Krankenhaus, Berlin

and that the agent, as demonstrated by sufficient scientific facts, could be said to be a species of *Schyzomycetes.*

Ziehl,[1574] familiar with the work of Klebs, Eberth, Friedländer, and von Leyden, sought bacteria in the sputum of two pneumonia patients. He saw ellipsoidal cocci in the early stages of the disease, and the same organism mixed with many other bacterial forms in the later stages. Peiper[1076] reported the presence of large numbers of diplococci in lung-puncture fluid. That primary sporadic cerebrospinal meningitis could be caused by Pneumococcus was first discovered by von Leyden[810] but, because the oval diplococci appeared to be slightly larger than those found in pneumonia, he was in doubt as to their true nature.

Late in 1883, Talamon,[1377] although lacking conclusive experimental data, felt justified in stating that lobar, fibrinous pneumonia was an infectious disease produced by a specific microbe with a characteristic form, and he named the organism, *Coccus lancéolé de la pneumonie.* He found this coccus in the pulmonary exudate taken by lung puncture, and once in the blood during life. Since only a fluid medium was used, the cultures were seldom pure. Talamon failed to infect guinea pigs or dogs with this mixed growth, but sixteen out of twenty rabbits succumbed to inoculation, although none developed pleuritis, pericarditis, or pneumonia. Notwithstanding the fact that his experimental results did not fulfill all the requirements of Koch's law, the claim was correct, and the statement that pneumonia is a localized disease, principally pulmonary, and susceptible of becoming generalized in other organs, was true.*

During the year 1884, interest in Pneumococcus spread and fresh information came from various sources. Gram[545] himself gave the details of the indispensable stain which now bears his name, and described how the capsule first took the dye and then gave it

* Mendelsohn (1884)[892] gave an excellent review of the current ideas on the epidemiology and infectiousness of pneumonia.

up to alcohol, while the coccus retained the violet color. Then Emmerich,[355] after hunting bacteria in air, water, dust, and dirt, recovered encapsulated diplococci from the filling between the floors of a prison in Augsburg, notorious for over twenty-five years as a breeding place of pneumonia. He cultivated the cocci on meat-infusion peptone gelatin, separated them from accompanying bacteria, injected the purified culture into rabbits with indifferent success, but obtained a higher fatality rate when he used mice. He identified the coccus as that described by Friedländer, and gave to the report the title, *Die Auffindung von Pneumoniecoccen. . . .* Emmerich's discovery, confirmed several decades later by the work of Stillman,[1326] furnished one of the first epidemiological clues to the origin of some cases of pneumonia.

Somewhat analogous to Emmerich's discovery of pneumococci in the floor filth of a pneumonia-infected prison was the apparent success of Pawlowsky (1885)[1072] in isolating, on solid media, Pneumococcus-like organisms from the air of various rooms. Influenced by the teaching of Friedländer, Pawlowsky, because his cocci were slightly smaller (they were also associated with larger cocci) and because they were pathogenic for rabbits, was not sure of his ground. The infectiousness of these cocci for rabbits, guinea pigs, and dogs indicates that among the bacteria described by Pawlowsky there were pneumococci. Cornil and Babes[278] added a note to the effect that they had found lancet-shaped bacteria in the tonsils and from the endocardium of pneumonia patients, but they made no cultures.

Exudates from the pleura and pericardium of two pneumonia patients yielded, in Salvioli's[1215] hands, encapsulated cocci which, while fatally infective for guinea pigs, rabbits, and dogs, failed to cause the typical lesions of pneumonia. Thinking that he had overwhelmed the animals with the virulence of the fluids injected, he introduced the infectious material intratracheally into four guinea pigs, two of which died. Platonow,[1095] in a detailed and critical review of the existing literature, concluded from the evidence and his own experimental experience that neither the capsule nor the nail-form colony was a differential character and that bacteriological examination of the blood of pneumonia patients was not of diagnostic value. From Platonow's notes it would seem that he used mixed cultures of bacilli and cocci, so his doubts were well founded.

In April of that year (1884), Fraenkel[466] presented the first of a series of studies that were to make the name Fraenkel and Pneumococcus almost inseparable. In a discussion of the cause of pneumonia before the *Kongress für innere Medizin* in Berlin, Fraenkel displayed a human trait that at least enlivens the sober literature if it does not always bring the desired personal reward. Fraenkel complained that he should receive some of the credit for the discovery of Pneumococcus. He had begun experiments six months before Friedländer's report was made public, and had only delayed the announcement because his results differed from Friedländer's and because he wished to recheck them! He had scored on his fellow countryman by infecting rabbits with the coccus where Friedländer failed, but his further observations had not been so positive. There was a difference in the pathogenicity of some of the materials which he used; colony appearance and capsule formation were not constant characters and, moreover, other bacterial species had capsules. Apparently unaware of Sternberg's experiments, Fraenkel[468] had missed the meaning of his success in producing a fatal septicemia in rabbits with normal sputum and the subsequent recovery by cultivation on coagulated blood serum of encapsulated diplococci from the blood of the animals. He had hesitated to draw any comparison between the diplococci from pneumonic material and his "sputum septicemia coccus." Likewise, he had ventured no outright statement that his and Friedländer's organisms were separate species; in fact, he gave the impression that they were different forms of the same organism. Friedländer, in the discussion of Fraenkel's paper, suggested that there might be several organisms causing pneumonia, so he, for the while, had the last word.

Here began a controversy, fomented principally by Fraenkel,

despite the conciliatory attitude of Friedländer, which led to confused conceptions which endure to the present day and which can never be clarified. Fraenkel, in a paper published in 1885,[467] virtually acknowledged that the coccus described by Friedländer and the one described by himself were identical, but complained that he saw it first. It has long been the verdict that the organism described by Friedländer in 1882 and 1883 was not Pneumococcus but the bacillus which later came to bear his name. This verdict would deprive Friedländer of any credit for the original isolation of Pneumococcus from lobar pneumonia and bestow it on Fraenkel who, without it, still has the honor of giving the first complete descriptions of Pneumococcus and whose studies proved for the first time the etiological relationship between this coccus and lobar pneumonia in man.

The facts given in Friedländer's first and second papers admit of more than one interpretation. The organism which Friedländer first described was an elliptical, or round, encapsulated coccus occurring principally in pairs. It was isolated from nearly all of fifty cases of acute pneumonia and was Gram-positive. It need scarcely be pointed out that these are characters of Pneumococcus and not of *B. friedländeri.** The culture was exquisitely virulent for mice. However, the lack of pathogenicity for rabbits, its ability to grow on gelatin at room temperature with the formation of nail-like colonies are not characteristic of typical pneumococci. Perhaps Friedländer, in the face of strong opposition, weakened his position by acknowledging that the cycle of isolation of the coccus from man, the production of infection in animals, and its subsequent recovery could not be accomplished in every case of pneumonia. Possibly another factor tending to detract from the true import of his discovery may have been his suggestion that there might be different forms of Pneumococcus, or that pneu-

* Inasmuch as the earlier name, *Bacillus friedländeri,* occurs in the great majority of the original publications reviewed, it, rather than the newer name, *Klebsiella pneumoniae,* will be used in this text.

monia might be caused by other organisms; ideas that we now know are true but which were scouted at the time. A careful reading of Friedländer's original communications makes it difficult to escape the conviction that he, in 1881, saw in the secretions and tissues of pneumonia patients the organism we know as Pneumococcus and, in the next two years, accomplished its isolation and cultivation. It seems likely, however, that Friedländer isolated at the same time the bacillus which later came to bear his name.

One seems justified in assuming as a cause of the divergent opinions which have so long persisted in the literature, the statement in Friedländer's communication of 1886[492] that the micrococcus so thoroughly studied by Fraenkel was the coccus he had originally described, but that the organism upon which he was then reporting was neither a coccus nor a bacillus* but a bacterium which he called *Kapselbacterium.* In addition to short elements, it existed in rod-like and thread-like forms and, furthermore, it was found only in a minority of the pneumonia cases studied—both characters of the Friedländer bacillus. Therefore, in view of all the evidence, and with due deference to the opinion of distinguished authorities, it would seem that the credit for first indicating that a diplococcus—*Diplococcus pneumoniae*—might be the cause of pneumonia should be given to Friedländer. To him, also, should go the honor of discovering another etiological agent of pneumonia, *Bacillus friedländeri.*

Afanassiew,[4] in 1884, added suggestive, if somewhat doubtful, information to the question. He, too, obtained ovoid cocci from six cases of pneumonia, but the cultures were not pure and this fact led to uncertainty. Klein,[719] on the contrary, apparently succeeded not only in growing pure cultures of Pneumococcus and in infecting mice and rabbits with them, but in recovering the organisms from the test animals and in transmitting the infection in series to

* It should be borne in mind that, at the time, the criterion for judging whether an organism was a bacillus or a bacterium was the presence of motility in the former and its absence in the latter.

other rabbits and mice. The infection was a septicemia and never a localized process as claimed by Friedländer. Klein had no hesitation in using the name *Pneumokokkus*, in the title of his paper.

Maguire (1884),[855] in England, presented before the British Medical Association three preparations to illustrate the micrococcus of pneumonia. One was a section of a pneumonic lung, another a section of kidney from a case of pneumonia, and the third, sputum from a similar patient. Employing both methylene blue and the Gram stain, he found capsules on the cocci, although they were not always present. Maguire exhibited the specimens as illustrating Friedländer's micrococcus but, lacking cultural or inoculation experience, showed caution in saying that the question of the role of Pneumococcus must remain in abeyance until more data were forthcoming.

In the same year, Foà and Rattone,[464] working with a pure culture of Friedländer's "Pneumococcus" obtained from his colleague, Frobenius, duplicated Friedländer's observations even to the resistance of rabbits to its invasion. They confirmed the results with cultures isolated from the lung of a pneumonia patient, and were the first to succeed in producing meningeal infection in guinea pigs by inhalation, recovering "capsule-cocci" from the exudate on the pia mater.*

By 1885, Sternberg[1319] was ready to state that the pneumonia-coccus of Friedländer, the *Microbe septicémique du saliva* of Pasteur, and the organism he himself had isolated from normal saliva were not only the same but were probably the cause of pneumonia.† His conclusion bears quoting: "It seems extremely probable that this micrococcus is concerned in the etiology of croupous pneumonia, and that the infectious nature of this disease is due to its presence in the fibrinous exudate into the pulmonary alveoli." Its

* Jürgensen[699] reviewed the literature up to his time (1884) and concluded, "True pneumonia is an infectious disease, which principally but not exclusively, affects the lungs."

† Sternberg, after seeing the Friedländer culture in Koch's laboratory in 1885, changed his mind, and in 1887[1320] said he was in error in thinking that this and his saliva-coccus were identical. He then tentatively changed the name to *Micrococcus pneumoniae crouposae*.

presence in normal human saliva seemed to Sternberg to indicate that some other factor was necessary for the development of an attack of pneumonia. It was possible that some condition, such as "alcoholism, sewer-gas poisoning, crowd-poisoning or any other depressing agency" might render the individual vulnerable, while a "reflex vaso-motor paralysis, induced by cold, might affect a single lobe of the lung." It was at this time that Sternberg graciously gave the name *Micrococcus Pasteuri* to the coccus.

Fraenkel (1886),[468] now reassured by his experiments but still conservative, issued another note, preliminary to a more positive statement to appear later, to the effect that diplococci were sometimes, but not always, found in normal human saliva, more often in the saliva of a sick person, and still more frequently in the rusty sputum of pneumonia patients. He called the disease produced by this organism in rabbits and mice, "sputum septicemia." The organisms failed to grow on gelatin at room temperature, but on congealed blood serum or on agar at body-heat developed characteristic veil-like or dewdrop-like colonies. A similar coccus was present in two cases of empyema following pneumonia, but in some cases of empyema other organisms were to be found in the pus. Fraenkel then went so far as to say that these facts would make it seem highly probable that the microbe of sputum septicemia and Pneumococcus were identical.

In the following year (1886), more positive in his convictions, Fraenkel[469] was ready to grant that his coccus—that of sputum septicemia—the sputum coccus of Pasteur and that of Sternberg, as well as the organisms described by Talamon and by Salvioli, were identical, and then to state definitely that this coccus was the cause of true fibrinous pneumonia. With new assurance Fraenkel became somewhat caustic in his comment about Friedländer's claims and flatly avowed that his organism and that of Friedländer were not the same. He then named it *Pneumoniemikrococcus,* calling it also Pneumococcus. Here, more so than previously, Fraenkel's experiments are impressive for their care and thoroughness.

He grew the cocci on liquid and solid media, studied the most favorable reaction for growth, and found that while the organisms retained their virulence on coagulated blood serum or meat-infusion agar, they lost it rapidly in broth because of its changed reaction during incubation. Young cultures were highly pathogenic for mice and rabbits, less so for guinea pigs, and avirulent for dogs, pigeons, and chickens.

Fraenkel was able to isolate the diplococcus from all cases of true fibrinous pneumonia, grew it in pure culture, produced a fatal septicemia in susceptible animals, again recovered from them the organism in a pure state, and then further transmitted the infection to other test animals. His results therefore met all the requirements of Koch's law, and it would seem that Fraenkel was the first to establish the fact beyond a reasonable doubt that Pneumococcus was the causative agent in lobar pneumonia.

Fraenkel[468] made another important and original contribution when he reported that rabbits, recovering from a subcutaneous infection of the ear, resisted a subsequent inoculation with the same coccus. Although Foà and Bordoni-Uffreduzzi had independently discovered the same phenomenon (1884), this is probably the first controlled observation that pneumococcal infection may induce immunity.

Fraenkel also found Pneumococcus in the exudates in the pia mater from a case of meningitis accompanying pneumonia, but was unable to decide which lesion was primary. Senger (1886)[1255] had seen these diplococci in amazing numbers in fluid from the subarachnoid and ventricular spaces in similar cases and, in addition, in the lesions of endocarditis, pericarditis, pleuritis, and nephritis of pneumonia patients. He was, of course, correct in supposing that these and other metastases might be expected to arise from a pulmonary lesion. Netter,[962-3, 965] and also Lancereaux and Besançon,[778] reported the same findings in two corresponding cases of meningitis, pericarditis, and endocarditis. Lebashoff,[795] in Russia, at this time announced similar observations on the occurrence of

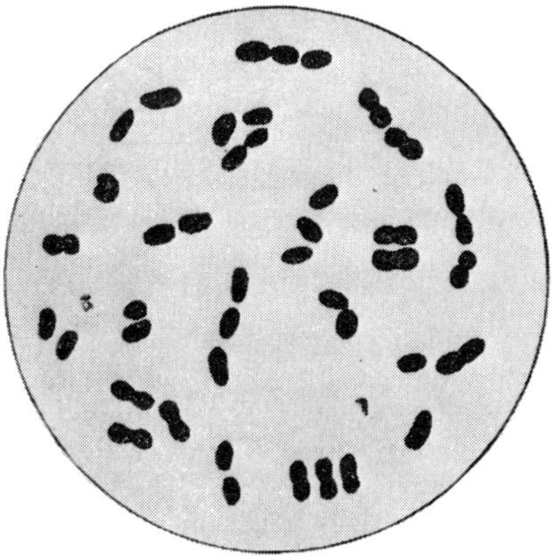

Figure 1

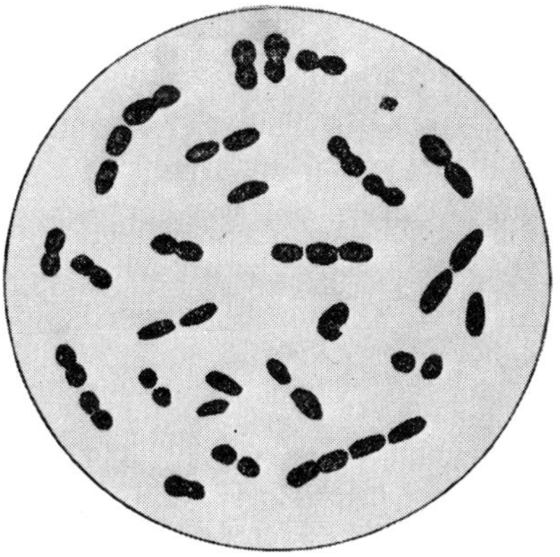

Figure 2

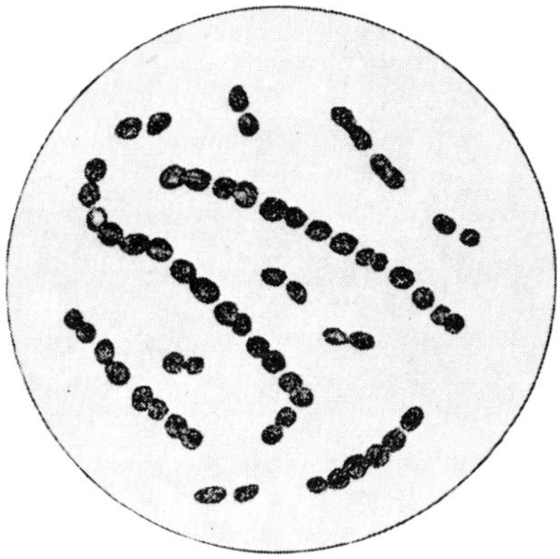

Figure 3

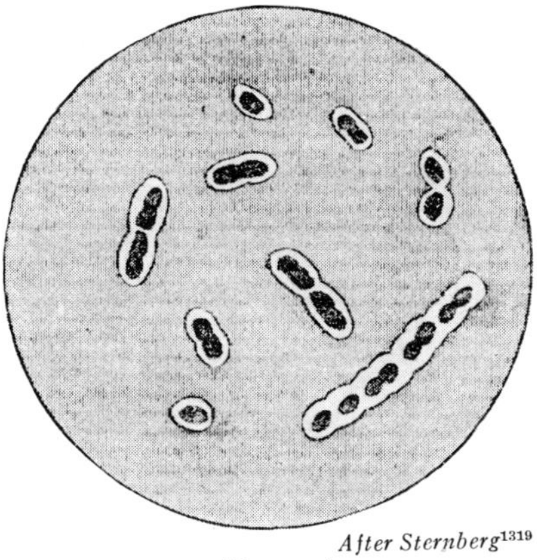

After Sternberg[1319]

Figure 4

MICROCOCCUS PASTEURI, 1885

Figure 1. *Micrococcus Pasteuri* from blood of rabbit inoculated subcutaneously with normal human saliva (Dr. S.). Stained by the method recommended by Friedlander. Magnified 1000 diameters. Figure 2. *Micrococcus Pasteuri* from blood of rabbit inoculated subcutaneously with fresh pneumonic sputum from a patient in the seventh day of the disease. Same staining and amplification as Figure 1. Figure 3. Surface culture of *M. Pasteuri,* showing development of long chains. Same staining and amplification. Figure 4. Surface culture of *M. Pasteuri* from blood of rabbit injected with pneumonic sputum, showing the so-called "capsule" of Friedlander. Same staining and amplification.

these diplococci in other organs as well as in lung tissue but, evidently being ignorant of Fraenkel's work, he described the organisms as Friedländer's cocci.

In France, Gamaléia (1886),[498] after isolating, cultivating, and inoculating into several different species of animals, cocci obtained from lungs and fluids from meningitis and endocarditis complicating pneumonia, announced that the encapsulated lancet-form diplococcus derived from these sources was the same as the organism originally described by Pasteur. As a compliment to his chief, but deceived by the occasional chain formation, Gamaléia named it *Streptococcus lanceolatus Pasteuri.* In offering an explanation for the resistance of man to its invasion, he drew attention—an original observation—to the possible part played by leucocytes in the body's defense.

Pneumococcal infection of the kidneys was first reported by Nauwerck[944-6] in 1886. Among 550 cases of croupous pneumonia there were thirteen complicated with acute nephritis and in these instances he found in the kidneys cocci which he said were identical with those described by Friedländer. Nauwerck stated that the infection was specific and was caused by "pneumonia cocci" carried to the kidney by the blood.

At this time the differentiation began between Fraenkel's Pneumococcus and the bacillus of Friedländer. Weichselbaum, and Foà and Bordoni-Uffreduzzi sharply distinguished between the two organisms, although it may be again emphasized that Friedländer's first descriptions were those of a diplococcus and not of a bacillus. Some of the credit usually given to Fraenkel's contributions may be granted to Foà and Bordoni-Uffreduzzi[460] whose work was done independently of Fraenkel's and was actually made public somewhat earlier.

A full confirmation of Fraenkel's work, if not of his conclusions, came from Weichselbaum.[1497-8] Beginning his studies shortly after Friedländer's first announcements, Weichselbaum covered the ground gone over by the earlier investigator, found the diplococci in a percentage of cases sufficiently high to promise diagnostic value, and gave clear and detailed descriptions of their isolation, cultivation, and animal pathogenicity. He added the gums, tonsils, accessory sinuses, cerebrospinal fluid, and joints as sites of pneumococcal infection. The organism differed, as in Fraenkel's experience, from Friedländer's in that it failed to grow on gelatin, while the author emphatically differed from Fraenkel in the belief that this coccus was the sole cause of pneumonia.

Weichselbaum (1886)[1498-1500] separated pneumonic affections into lobar, croupous, lobular, and hypostatic pneumonias, fixed on Pneumococcus the guilt of causing the lobar type, and on streptococci, staphylococci, and a bacillus (*Bacillus pneumoniae*—probably the Friedländer bacillus) that of producing the other types. He presented new data concerning the morphology and growth characters of Pneumococcus; from the infected lung tracked the organism through the lymphatics to the cerebral ventricles; and suggested the blood stream as a further avenue of its spread. To the organism Weichselbaum gave the name *Diplococcus pneumoniae.* In the next year (1887), Weichselbaum repeated Sternberg's work and, in addition, by the subcutaneous injection of dried spleens from animals succumbing to the diplococcal infection, and of post-pneumonic pleural exudate containing attenuated pneumococci, immunized mice and rabbits. He, like Fraenkel, called the organism Pneumococcus.

In the same year, confirmation of the diversity of organisms involved in pneumonia came from Wolf,[1529] while Meyer[895] offered further proof of the presence of pneumococci in the lungs, heart, and cerebrospinal exudates in infections secondary to pneumonia. Netter,[965] finding these same cocci in the nasal fossae, sinuses, and tympanic cavity, then made the original observation that a local process, such as pneumococcal meningitis, could arise without a contributing lung infection.

Sternberg, not yet entirely convinced that the lanceolate diplococcus was the true cause of pneumonia, but hoping for a better understanding of his work by the German bacteriologists, presented his views (1887) in a paper[1320] in the *Deutsche medizinische Wochenschrift.* He first admitted his original error in thinking that his saliva-coccus and the organism of Friedländer were the same; then went on to say that if this diplococcus could finally be proved to be the cause of true pneumonia, it should be called *Micrococcus pneumoniae crouposae,* but until that time the name he originally proposed should stand. This statement aroused Fraenkel,[471] and a month later, again feeling that he had been slighted, he took issue in print with the American, and made another plea for priority. Fraenkel characterized Sternberg's work as incomplete, made capital out of the confusion of the Sternberg coccus with Friedländer's bacterium, and disposed of Sternberg's objection to Fraenkel's name, *Pneumoniemikrococcus.*

Foà and Bordoni-Uffreduzzi[460-2] put in a bid for credit as being the first to report (1886) the discovery of the organism to which they gave the name *Diplococcus lanceolatus* in a case of primary cerebrospinal meningitis. They also reported the isolation of the organism from every case in an epidemic of the disease,* as well as from cases of polyarthritis and from the blood of the placenta in a patient aborting during pneumonia. Ortmann,[1037] too, isolated pneumococci from meningeal infections, and in so doing felt that he should be acclaimed as the first to obtain "capsule-cocci" on artificial media. Infection of the parotid glands was another manifestation of the invasiveness of Pneumococcus, two instances in which parotitis occurred being reported by Testi,[1388-90] who also noted subcutaneous abscesses as a further complication of pneumonia.

More important than the priority claim of Foà and Bordoni-Uffreduzzi, however, was their achievement in immunizing rabbits by subcutaneous injection at three or four-day intervals, first with attenuated material, then with cultures of increasing virulence. The animals thus treated became resistant to inoculation with

* It is probable that the epidemic was one of meningococcal meningitis.

virulent cultures or infected blood. Encouraged by these results, the authors applied the procedure to human beings but without success. Incidentally, Foà and his colleague were among the first to maintain virulence of the cocci by preserving the cultures in infected blood in the cold and the dark. So also, Biondi,[117] in experiments with *Bacillus salivarius septicus* (the Fraenkel or Sternberg diplococcus in spite of the name), by chance noticed that rabbits recovering from inoculation with weakened cultures became immune. Biondi looked upon such attenuated cultures as true vaccines. Netter[971] accomplished the same result with the dried spleens of animals dying from pneumococcal infection and with "old" pleural exudate containing this organism.

Zaufal (1888)[1568-9] contributed otitis media to the list of primary infections due to Fraenkel's diplococcus, and sharply differentiated this coccus and the Friedländer bacillus, which was also found to be responsible for a similar condition. Then Gamaléia,[498] harking back to the Pasteur organism, told of its constant presence in fibrinous pneumonia, and insisted that the Friedländer bacillus was a saprophyte.

In 1889, Foà and Bordoni-Uffreduzzi[461] introduced a confusing note with the isolation of a monococcus from some mild cases of fibrinous pneumonia. They suggested the possibility of there being two types of organisms, but the descriptions are too incomplete to warrant a decision.

The names of Fraenkel and Weichselbaum had now become practically hyphenated when applied to Pneumococcus. Arustamow (1889)[24] found this organism in every one of fifty cases of pneumonia, but failed in the examination of the saliva of fifteen normal persons and the sputum from a like number of bronchitis patients. Gabbi[497] isolated in pure culture the *Virus pneumonico* (*Microbio capsulato del Fraenkel*) from a peritonsillar abscess without pneumonia; while Monti,[905] after finding Pneumococcus in an arthritic joint of the hand, induced a localized infection experimentally in a rabbit with the strain he isolated from the joint.

The decade of the eighties saw the first important chapter in the history of Pneumococcus written, edited, and given to the medical world. Its causative association with pneumonia, meningitis, and certain localized infections was accepted as established despite some confusion concerning its various identities. Fraenkel, and not Friedländer, was now looked upon as its true sponsor. The early and necessarily crude and incomplete immunization experiments were to encourage a closer study of this phase of the activity of Pneumococcus. The next ten years were to be less fruitful, but here and there facts were disclosed which, with a better understanding, were to take on a new significance.

1890–1900

In the second decade, Foà and Carbone[463] used soluble products of Pneumococcus to stimulate the immune response in rabbits, and sought by chemical means to refine and concentrate the antigenic principle—believed to be a poison or toxin—elaborated during pneumococcal growth. The authors went no further than to say that while the refined substance, which had been precipitated by ammonium sulfate and refined by dialysis, failed to kill the animal, it produced marked physiological changes—a statement which is scarcely descriptive of any specific action.

The Klemperers (1891)[723-5] might justly be looked upon as the forefathers of antipneumococcic serum therapy. They immunized rabbits with sputum obtained from pneumonia patients after recovery, with purulent, but bacteria-free, pleural exudate, with heated glycerol extracts of pneumococci, and with heated whole and filtered broth cultures. They introduced the intravenous route of injection, finding that the immunity to subsequent infection appeared far more rapidly than after subcutaneous injection—in two to three days against fourteen days. They found that duration of immunity varied from twenty-one days to more than six months. Their greater contribution was the observation that the young of immunized mother rabbits were usually passively protected, and this observation naturally led the authors to test the curative value of the serum of actively immunized rabbits. The direct injection of such serums into the blood stream of the rabbit was effective against a lethal dose of pneumococci injected twenty-four hours later.

The Klemperers presented an array of new facts which, disregarding certain misinterpretations, have withstood the test of time and supply a rational basis for the treatment of human beings with immune serum. They observed that the serum of pneumonia patients after crisis conferred protection upon rabbits, that the protective substance came into action at the beginning of crisis, and that it neutralized the harmful properties of Pneumococcus without destroying the antigenicity of the organism. Having tested the harmlessness of immune serum on themselves, they treated six pneumonia patients with subcutaneous injections of only four to six cubic centimeters, obtaining a fall of temperature within six to twelve hours after injection, the temperature in two cases remaining normal. The Klemperers sought to explain the action of serum on an antitoxic basis, but in the light of our present knowledge it would seem doubtful if the effect was a specific one.

From bacteria-free bouillon cultures of virulent organisms, by repeated alcohol precipitation and re-solution of the precipitate in water, they isolated a protein substance, thought by them to be a pneumotoxin, which was poisonous for rabbits, withstood a temperature of 60°,* and in proper doses was capable of raising the resistance of the animals above the normal threshold of infection. In the blood of the immune animals they detected a substance not there previously, which it was conjectured must have been formed in the interval between the act of injection and the appearance of immunity, and which must be dependent upon the action of the injected albumen. The newly found substance in blood had no killing effect on living pneumococci but inhibited their toxic action. In an

* Throughout this text the figures given for temperatures represent degrees on the Centigrade scale, and the initial "C" will be omitted.

attempt to isolate this new curative substance, the Klemperers progressed far enough to be able to say that it also was a protein. They believed that they had found an antitoxin for Pneumococcus, but that mistake is of no importance in view of the value of their major contribution.

The work of the Klemperers gave new impetus to investigation. Here was an alluring and promising field; there loomed the possibility of a biological cure for pneumonia. Emmerich and Fowitzky,[357] still using the subcutaneous route for the injection of attenuated pneumococci, obtained only partial immunity in rabbits. However, when they injected diluted, fully virulent cultures intravenously, the resistance appeared to be complete. Instead of using the serum of these animals for protective or curative experiments, they used the filtered juices expressed from the tissues. The fluids so obtained were claimed to possess *idealer Heilkraft* but, although Emmerich and Fowitzky considered their use justifiable for human therapy, they employed the immune tissue extracts only in animal tests. Bonome (1891)[137] tried sterile filtrates of bouillon cultures injected every other day subcutaneously, intravenously, and intraperitoneally into rabbits and found that immunity appeared as early as two or three days after the final injection. The toxicity of the filtrates was directly related to the virulence of the strain, some animals showing local reactions, others none. He employed, with like effect, blood and spleen from mice killed by a culture insufficiently virulent to kill rabbits. The defibrinated blood of the treated rabbits injected into the peritoneum of other rabbits protected them against lethal doses of the toxic filtrate, but only when the blood was administered just prior to the injection of the filtrate or culture.

Kruse and Pansini[763] likewise produced immunity with daily injections of sterile filtrates of broth cultures. They attributed the protective properties of the blood of the immune rabbits to bactericidins, and although they observed phagocytosis, this was held to be a secondary factor. In their paper, apart from the immunological data, there is the account of a phenomenon, the meaning of which the authors failed to realize, but which much later was to assume wide biological significance. Studying forty-six strains of diplococci of pneumonic origin under varying cultural conditions, Kruse and Pansini noticed that the organisms when subjected to unfavorable media, with succeeding generations began to differ from the parent strain in morphology and colony formation. The variations ran the gamut from typical *Diplococcus lanceolatus* to *Streptococcus pyogenes*. Along with the changes in form there took place loss of capsule and of virulence, although animal passage restored the original characters. Because of the loss of capsule, diminution of virulence, and the appearance of chain formation, Kruse and Pansini concluded that they had effected a mutation of Pneumococcus into Streptococcus, and that both species arose from a common saprophytic, streptococcal form. Whatever may have been their conclusions, it seems certain that they were observing the phenomenon of bacterial dissociation.

A notation of Metchnikoff's[894] was undoubtedly the first record of the agglutination of pneumococci by immune serum. He wrote that the microbe of pneumonia formed very long plaquettes of "streptococci" in the serum of vaccinated rabbits.

Foà and Carbone (1891),[463] continuing their work with alcohol and ammonium sulfate precipitates from culture filtrates, learnt that the immunity induced by their preparations was less enduring than that evoked by the untreated filtrates. Foà's later studies (1893)[459] were, in a way, less productive, since, unknowingly, he was apparently dealing with both pneumococci and meningococci. He did show, however, that these two cocci differed from each other in biological characters, and that the serum of animals immunized against the one species was inactive against the other.

Here, in the matter of time and because of its bearing on the discussion in some of the preceding pages, there may be interpolated the final description which Sternberg (1892)[1321] gave to Pneumococcus under the title, *Micrococcus pneumoniae crouposae:*

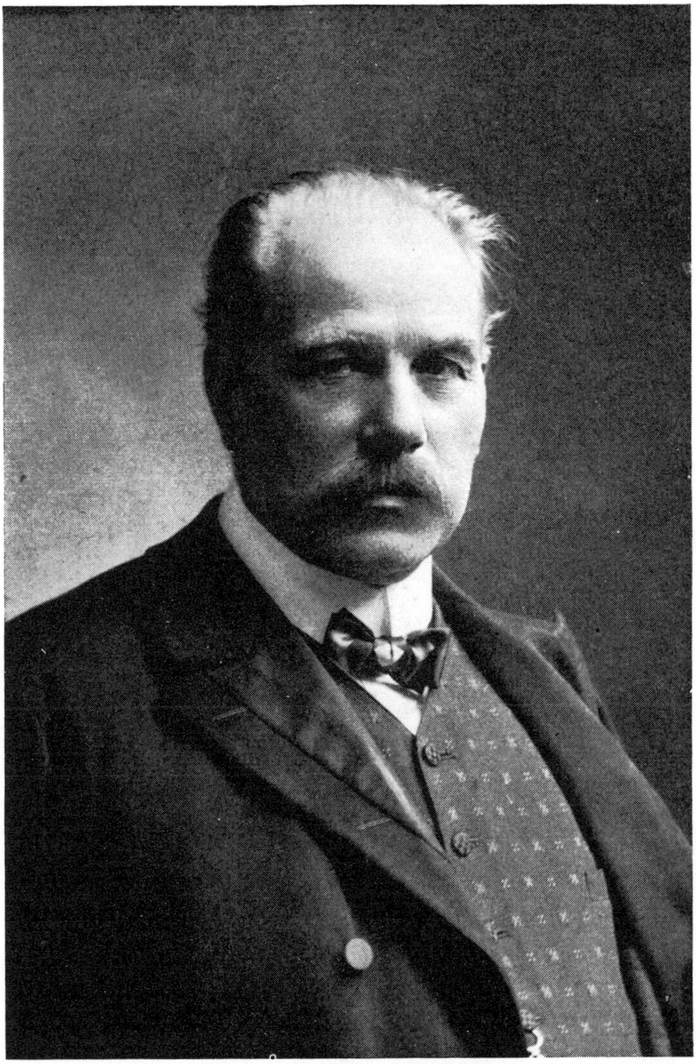

Courtesy of Wiener Medizinische Wochenschrift

ANTON W. WEICHSELBAUM 1845–1920

Discovered by the present writer in the blood of rabbits inoculated subcutaneously with his own saliva in September, 1880; by Pasteur in the blood of rabbits inoculated with the saliva of a child which died of hydrophobia in one of the hospitals of Paris in December, 1880; identified with the micrococcus in the rusty sputum of pneumonia, by comparative inoculation and culture experiments, by the writer in 1885. Proved to be the cause of croupous pneumonia in man by the researches of Talamon, Salvioli, Sternberg, Fraenkel, Weichselbaum, Netter, Gamaléia, and others.

Mosny (1892),[932] unconcerned about priority, turned his attention to immunological experiments. He grew virulent pneumococci in broth, heated the cultures at 60°, and then filtered them. The subcutaneous or intravenous injection of the filtrates into rabbits brought about immunity four days later, but the immunity was of a low order. The serum of the rabbits so treated gave protection only when injected before or at the same time with the inoculated culture. Mosny could detect no bactericidal action of the immune serum. The cocci, on the contrary, grew fully as well in immune as in normal serum. In watching the growths he noted a change in the physical appearance of the immune serum-culture mixture which we now know must have been agglutination. Mosny, like Klebs, and more particularly Metchnikoff, saw something new and told of it, unconscious that he had made a discovery.

The toxin idea was then current, and Issaeff,[673] using sterilized broth cultures of virulent pneumococci and chloroform and glycerol extracts of infected blood, interpreted the effects following their intravenous injection as being due to a toxin, but frankly confessed that the immune serum so obtained had no antitoxic properties; neither did it show any bactericidal action. The serum did, however, promote phagocytosis, and Issaeff quite rightly concluded that phagocytosis played a most important part in immunity to Pneumococcus. Emmerich[856] also entertained the toxin idea, but instead of heating or filtering broth cultures, injected them in diluted state. He stressed the desirability of using virulent strains, as well as the necessity of taking blood only from highly immunized animals. Failure to do this would explain the unsatisfactory results of Foà and the Klemperers. Emmerich looked upon the action of the immune serum as antibacterial rather than antitoxic, and came near the truth when he explained the action as a combination of two proteins, globulin from the blood combining with a poisonous substance, probably also protein from the bacterial cell. He, like Fraenkel and Sternberg, made a bid for precedence, objecting to Foà's claim of being the originator of serum therapy.

In 1896, Washbourn,[1486] apparently unaware of Mosny's original observation, thus described the effect of adding pneumococci to specific immune serum: "When protective serum is inoculated it appears perfectly clear at the end of twenty-four hours, but at the bottom a sediment is seen. The sediment consists of pneumococci staining well and grouped in masses."

Metchnikoff's, Mosny's, and Washbourn's unnamed phenomenon was verified in 1897 by Bezançon and Griffon[108-9] and called by them "agglutination." They found that the serum of patients during pneumococcal infections acquires agglutinative power, and from their experiences they drew the conclusion, "that from the standpoint of agglutination there exist several races of pneumococci, which behave as though different microbes." Here was the basis for a method of serological classification, neglected for thirteen years until Neufeld and Haendel made it their own.

Eyre, with Washbourn (1896),[373] like Kruse and Pansini, was also close to the phenomenon of bacterial dissociation.

> In old broth cultivations the majority of cocci are dead, but a few resistant forms remain living; and, by transplanting a sufficient quantity into fresh media, growth occurs and a new generation arises. We have, moreover, found that this second generation differs in morphology, biology and pathogenic properties from the parent stock. It in fact represents a distinct variety, possessing practically no virulence, and growing luxuriantly, even at 20° C., on all the usual media.

Their first attempts to bring about reversion failed, mainly because they passed the strain through eggs. Finally, however, passage through a rabbit restored the degenerated forms to the original state of the parent strain. Without venturing an explanation, Eyre and Washbourn concluded, "Our experiments are in favor of the theory . . . that the individual cocci or their descendants actually alter in character under varying conditions," or, to use the modern term, dissociate.

The quest for a potent immune serum was continued by Denys (1897),[312] who met with greater success than did his predecessors. Denys first raised the virulence of pneumococcal cultures by serial passage of infected blood through rabbits, then administered both heated and filtered cultures to normal animals, at first rabbits, then goats, and later horses. After this preliminary treatment, Denys gave a series of injections of unheated cultures, then of the blood of infected rabbits, and finally of living, virulent pneumococci. The serum thus obtained prevented infection, was curative, and neutralized in rabbits the alleged "toxins" of Pneumococcus. The results of controlled experiments convinced Denys that the immune serum so prepared was not bactericidal, but that it contained a substance which stimulated the white corpuscles to phagocytosis, or as he phrased it, *L'immunité du lapin contre le pneumocoque, a sa source dans une modification de son sérum;* and, *L'élément immunisant primordial est le sérum et le leucocyte par lui-même n'est rien.*

Pane,[1044] in the same year, not only obtained potent serums from rabbits, cows, and asses, but tested their curative action on human beings. Of twenty-three pneumonia patients treated by intravenous injection, only two died. Pane, incidentally, noted definite agglutination in the test tube and phagocytosis in the blood and therefore was inclined to accept Metchnikoff's theory as affording an explanation for the therapeutic action of the serum.

Mennes[893] fully agreed with Denys' idea that it was the immune serum and not the normal or immune leucocyte which stimulated phagocytosis. He, also, immunized horses, gave the serum intravenously to pneumonia patients, and favored large doses. In the same year, a few months earlier as a matter of fact, Washbourn[1487] had injected ponies with a culture of exalted and constant virulence, and after proving to his satisfaction the favorable action of the serum on rabbits, administered it to six pneumonia patients. All, although severely ill with the disease, recovered. He made another advance by standardizing the serum, and set as a unit the smallest amount of serum which, when mixed with ten times the least fatal dose of pneumococci and injected into the peritoneum, would bring about the survival of the test rabbit. Washbourn emphasized the necessity of early treatment and advised injections of at least six hundred "units" twice daily. By himself, and in the following year with Eyre,[376] he examined immune horse serum for protective properties, and concluded that there was no parallelism between agglutinative, bactericidal, and protective power. In their papers (1899–1900),[375, 377] these two authors gave further reports on the results of potency tests made on antipneumococcic serum, including two samples of Pane's product. By this time they had modified their method, and now injected the serum intravenously and then the culture intraperitoneally into rabbits. The serums, in one cubic centimeter amounts, usually protected rabbits against a thousand or more fatal doses of pneumococci, but in a few instances failed to protect against strains from another source, owing, as we now know, to a lack of type correspondence.

Summary

At the turn of the century the results of Pneumococcus investigations could be inventoried as follows: Pneumococcus was accepted as the causative agent in lobar pneumonia; it could be grown outside the body, and some of its habits and metabolic activities were becoming known; Pneumococcus or its products were found to raise the resistance of some experimental animals to homologous infection; these animals could be made to yield a serum capable of conferring passive protection on vulnerable or stricken creatures; and such a serum gave an early promise of mitigating pneumococcal affections in man.

The first glimpses of the vagaries of microbic behavior under varying environment were later to expand into broader views of that instability of bacterial characters which result in dissociation into varied and distinct forms or possible mutation into alien species. These discoveries were to clarify our ideas concerning virulence and the consequent infectiousness of a bacterium for a susceptible host. The fact that the serum from animals treated with Pneumococcus or some of the derivatives of Pneumococcus possesses the property of clumping this organism was, at the hands of Neufeld, Dochez, and Gillespie, and later of Cooper and her associates, to form the basis for a method of separating the members of a supposedly homogeneous species into thirty or more clearly defined and serologically specific types. This biological classification was to give a new aspect to the problems perplexing the epidemiologist, the bacteriologist and immunologist, and the clinician.

For a time Pneumococcus investigation was to lag, and then, stirred by the contributions of Neufeld and of the Cole school, it was to receive a new impetus, and to bring the vital activities of this amazing cell more clearly into sight. The facts that have been disclosed in this new and closer view, their bearing on general biological problems, and their application to the development of preventive and curative agents will be related in subsequent chapters.

CHAPTER II

BIOLOGY OF PNEUMOCOCCUS

The morphology of Pneumococcus in tissues and in cultures; isolation, cultivation, and preservation; viability and fragility, and sensitiveness to bile, soaps, and other chemical substances.

For the student of Pneumococcus there is no lack of reliable descriptions of its general or detailed biological features. In order, however, that the student may not be obliged to go beyond the covers of this volume for information about the organism, its intimate features will be presented here. The more important points have been freely taken from the clearest and most accurate accounts in current text and reference books, and acknowledgement is made to the respective authors.*

Morphology

The anatomy of Pneumococcus is simple and distinctive. It is best studied in preparations made from body fluids of man or animals suffering from infection. Next best are young, vigorous cultures grown on proper culture media containing blood, serum, or other body fluids. When typical, the organism consists of a pair of oval or lance-shaped cocci, their somewhat flattened proximal ends in apposition and their distal portion pointed. Sometimes single cocci are seen, while at other times single or paired cocci may be arranged in short or even long chains, resembling a string of beads —the *chapelet* originally described by Pasteur. There may be many variations from this characteristic form even when the environment is favorable. The individual cocci may be round and of

* The sources consulted, besides original papers, are the article by Neufeld and Schnitzer in the third edition of the Kolle-Kraus-Uhlenhuth *Handbuch der Pathogenen Mikroorganismen;*[740] Zinsser and Bayne-Jones, *Textbook of Bacteriology,*[1579] *Acute Lobar Pneumonia* (Rockefeller Institute Monograph, No. 7[36]); and *A British System of Bacteriology in Relation to Medicine.*[552]

varying size (0.5 to 1.25μ), or they may be so elongated as to resemble bacilli. One authority describes the cells as "small," another as "rather large," but the actual size varies with the circumstances under which the organism is observed. In any given preparation, along with typical forms, other members displaying every degree of involution or degeneration may be present, while in aged cultures aberrant forms may be the rule.

Pneumococcus has no spores, no vacuoles, no visible granules, no flagella, and is non-motile. It reproduces by the primitive method of transverse fission.

The most distinctive morphological feature of the organism is the capsule. The capsule is more prominent when the cocci are examined in the body fluids of infected animals, or in media enriched with body fluids, becoming faint or disappearing when the strain is grown on less rich substrates. The capsule envelops the single, paired, or chained cocci, frequently with a uniform periphery, although sometimes it shows indentations between the twin cells or between the paired individuals in chains.

STAINING METHODS

Pneumococcus is readily stained with the usual aniline dyes and is Gram-positive. Exposure to the action of specific immune serum, or even to acidulated pepsin or alkalinized trypsin mixtures fails to rob the cocci of this property (Wilke[1520]). Only when they are subjected to the digestive action of leucocytes, or after death and partial disintegration in old cultures, do they give up the dye to decolorizing agents. For peritoneal fluids, sputum, and cultures the Gram stain is generally used. The authors prefer Burke's modification[191] to that of Sterling* or to the original formula.[545]

Dold[324-5] recently devised a staining method by which he claimed to be able to divide Gram-positive cocci into four groups and to demonstrate tinctorial differences between pneumococci and streptococci. He treated preparations made from cultures on solid me-

* Original reference unknown.

dia, stained by an aniline dye, phenol, and iodine, with a mixture of one part 40 per cent aqueous solution of urea and nine parts absolute alcohol. Organisms which retained the dye were called positive; those from which the dye was extracted were negative; a third class exhibited fluctuations in their ability to retain the aniline color; while the fourth group displayed periodic changes from positive to negative and vice versa. He reported that all strains of streptococci tested were without exception negative, while *Streptococcus mucosus* and thirty-nine strains of pneumococci showed a change from positive to negative or vice versa. Some of the latter gave predominantly positive results while some were usually negative with only an occasional positive reaction. These latter he considered as transition forms between the predominantly positive pneumococci and the uniformly negative strain of Streptococcus.

For demonstrating pneumococci in tissues the method described by Wadsworth* may be used to advantage, while the Gram stain is to be preferred to the Gram-Weigert technique.†[1506]

THE CAPSULE

Modern chemical study of the capsular material has given a rational basis for the serological classification of all pneumococci into definite and specific types. It is this peculiar and complex component of the pneumococcal cell that determines its specific antigenic stimulus and its immunological behavior in the presence of antibodies. This knowledge enables us to utilize in a far more intelligent way Pneumococcus or its components in the induction of active immunity and consequently in the production of immune serums, and furnishes us with a delicate reagent for measuring the body's response to various immunizing procedures, and for determining the potency of antipneumococcic serums.

The capsule interested and perplexed many of the earlier investigators. Described first by Pasteur[1066] as an *auréole*, and by Fried-

* Zinsser and Bayne-Jones.[1579]

† Neufeld prefers the Gram technique; Zinsser the Gram-Weigert technique.

länder[486-7] as a *Kapsel,* it was later called a rim, or a hull, and its presence undoubtedly contributed to the confusion between the cocci first described by Friedländer and the well-known bacillus that bears his name. Because of the inconstancy of its appearance particularly under different conditions of artificial cultivation, the belief arose that it was not a diagnostic feature of the species. Pane[1045] went so far as to assert that it was a degenerative and not a developmental phenomenon. Friedländer had always contended, however, that the capsule was the product of a vital function of the cell.

Aoki[16] noticed that capsule formation proceeded more rapidly at body than at lower temperatures, and that the capsules were larger and more distinct when the cocci were grown in immune serum or in media containing such serum. This was the *Quellung* effect utilized by Neufeld and Etinger-Tulczynska[988] in their recently published method for type determination. The capsule was often described as gelatinous but, since the time of Pasteur and Friedländer, it had been more generally believed to consist of mucin. It was Preisz[1108] who, acting upon this assumption, was the first to demonstrate capsular material in the blood and other body fluids of animals succumbing to pneumococcal infection. He believed that a general, fatal invasion of the body by these cocci could occur only when the accumulation of mucin—now soluble specific substance—in the body had reached a certain level.

STAINING THE CAPSULE

Many methods have been devised for demonstrating the capsule of Pneumococcus. The first record of a capsule stain for Pneumococcus is that by Friedländer (1885)[491] who, after fixing the preparation in the flame, dipped it for a few minutes in one per cent acetic acid. After blowing off the acid he dried and then stained the film by a few seconds' exposure to a saturated aniline-water gentian violet solution. MacConkey (1898)[843] recommended staining with dahlia, methyl green, and a saturated alcoholic solution of fuchsin. The method, he claimed, gave a clear image suitable for photography. Hiss[650] in 1902 gave two procedures, the first, a gentian violet-potassium carbonate method, the other, and a better one, a preliminary treatment with gentian violet or fuchsin followed by washing with 20 per cent copper sulfate solution. The Welch* formula of glacial acetic acid, followed by aniline-water gentian violet gives clear pictures of the capsule. These methods are widely used and give satisfactory results.

Buerger (1905)[168] described a different and also reliable procedure, but the intricacy of the technique prevented general adoption. Malone,[860] after a preliminary staining with Congo red, treated the film with dilute hydrochloric acid in alcohol, counterstaining with methyl violet. Malone claimed that by this technique he was able to demonstrate capsules when the Hiss method failed. Wherry[1515] mixed a suspension of pneumococci in diluted serum with an equal amount of 0.05 normal hydrochloric acid, spread the mixture in a thin film, fixed the film with heat, and stained it quickly with carbol gentian violet. Leifson[797] applied to films a mixture of a saturated aqueous solution of ammonia or potassium alum, tannic acid in water, 95 per cent ethyl alcohol, and saturated alcoholic solution of basic fuchsin. He followed this treatment with methylene blue in aqueous borax solution. This method never came into general use. The Huntoon* technique is suitable only for cultures and not for animal exudates. India ink is the choice of some bacteriologists. It is a negative stain, in that the medium on the slide is colored black, while the cells and the capsule are unstained. Lévy-Bruhl and Borin,[805] however, reported that this stain outlined the capsules on Type III organisms when no albuminous substances were present in their "T" medium, but failed with other types of pneumococci grown on this special substrate. For general purposes, however, the Burke or Sterling modifications of the Gram stain suffice, while the Gram stain, the Gram-Weigert, or the

* Zinsser and Bayne-Jones.[1579]

method described by Wadsworth* may be used to demonstrate capsules in tissue sections.

The capsules are indicative of the vigor and virulence of the strain. They may best be seen "in the blood, serum and inflammatory exudate of the infected rabbit and white mouse. They are equally well marked in the fresh sputum of pneumonia patients, especially in the early stages of the disease, and in the exudate accompanying such pneumococcus infections as meningitis, otitis media and empyema."*

The addition of blood, serum, milk, or other body fluids to nutrient media favors the development of the capsule under artificial cultivation.

Isolation of Pneumococcus

ANIMAL INOCULATION

One of the simplest ways of isolating pneumococci from infected material is by mouse inoculation. If the source material is sputum, a small portion can be washed in sterile broth or saline solution in a Petri dish to remove the majority of accompanying mouth organisms. The washed sputum together with a small quantity of broth is emulsified by grinding in a sterile mortar and the suspension in amounts of 0.5 to one cubic centimeter injected into the peritoneal cavity of a white mouse. Just before or shortly after death of the animal, the heart is exposed and, under sterile precautions, punctured with a capillary pipette or hypodermic needle, and the blood aspirated and planted in broth and on blood-agar plates. In this way a pure culture can usually be obtained at the first trial. Pieces of lung or other infected material may be treated in the same manner as sputum. When it is suspected that few pneumococci are present, the tissue may be macerated in broth and given a preliminary incubation before the mouse injection.†

* Zinsser and Bayne-Jones.[1579]
† For complete details of the method see Appendix.

DIRECT CULTURES

Instead of the practice of animal inoculation, washed sputum, blood, or broth suspensions of infected material may be streaked on plates poured with fresh blood agar or serum-dextrose agar. For the cultivation of organisms directly from the circulating blood, the blood withdrawn by venous puncture may be added to a fairly large volume of dextrose broth in flasks, or mixed with molten dextrose agar and poured into Petri dishes. Pneumococcus, being facultative in its oxygen needs, grows on the surface as well as in the depths of the medium.

From agar plates single colonies of pneumococci may be picked and replanted on agar, seeded on serum or blood-agar slants or in serum or glucose broth. These media serve for the further propagation of the original broth cultures when pure. Small inoculums grow more successfully on solid than on liquid media. Incubation should be carried on at a temperature of about 37.5° ; 25° and 41° represent the lower and upper limits favorable to growth. A rarity were the strains isolated from blood and exudates by Eaton* in Zinsser's laboratory, which grew only at 25°. At 37.5° the organisms failed to grow unless incubated in an atmosphere containing about 10 per cent of carbon dioxide. A somewhat similar strain was that previously reported by Kindborg.[712] Isolated from rusty sputum by mouse inoculation, the organism displayed all the characters of a typical pneumococcus, yet it grew readily at 22° and rapidly and energetically liquefied gelatin. While pathogenic for mice, it was avirulent for rabbits.

Cultivation

Pneumococcus, being a strict parasite, is somewhat fastidious in nutritional requirements, as well as sensitive to the physical and chemical conditions of its surroundings. The essential ingredients of culture media are meat extractives prepared from fresh muscle

* Quoted by Zinsser and Bayne-Jones.[1579]

tissue, protein of comparatively small molecular size in the form of peptone, a small amount of sugar, mineral salts, and a suitable concentration of hydrogen ions. All media should be subjected to the least degree of heat necessary to effect extraction of the meat, to render the ingredients soluble, and to ensure final sterility.

The earlier bacteriologists employed the only media known in their time, such as egg albumen (Klebs[718]), veal or beef broth (Pasteur), then broth with the addition of gelatin or agar (Friedländer[487]) and later of blood (Nissen,[1013] and Gilbert and Fournier,[513] among others), serum, or other body fluids. Fraenkel[469] employed milk, but finding the cocci lost virulence on this medium, turned to coagulated blood serum and then to meat-infusion agar. Eggs, both in the shell (Bunzl-Federn[186]), inspissated, and as a base with broth (Gaskell[499]) have been employed for the maintenance of virulence, while Grawitz and Steffen[547] preferred coagulated sputum as a favorable medium for capsule formation. Schmidt[1236] also recommended sputum as a medium on which Pneumococcus developed clear, well-formed capsules, and which also would restore capsules to cocci that had lost them after cultivation on agar. Gilbert and Fournier[513] found defibrinated blood of man and other animals to be suitable for the propagation of pneumococci. Carnot and Fournier[200] noted constancy of virulence and capsule formation of strains grown in broth and on agar containing brain tissue, but the fluid medium could be employed only for the carrying on of pure cultures.

Among the great variety of nutrient materials recommended, time and experience have shown the essential ones, and these are now incorporated into a few formulas which meet all the needs of the student of Pneumococcus.* While Pneumococcus can be grown within a fairly wide range of cultural conditions, the most vigorous and viable individuals are obtained when careful attention is given to the needs peculiar to this organism. Fresh beef, veal, or

* See Appendix.

horse muscle, freed from fat, furnish a better base than the commercial meat extracts. Peptone preparations containing the higher proportion of proteose nitrogen, mainly because of the stronger buffering action, are to be preferred to preparations in which the bulk of the nitrogen is in the form of peptones and amino acids. The latter, however, because of their lower cost may be substituted for routine purposes. In different formulas the amount of peptone varies from 0.1 to 2 per cent, depending upon the proteose nitrogen content of the preparation. Felton and Dougherty[425] claimed that 2 per cent of peptone preserves and increases virulence.

Kruse and Pansini[763] first drew attention to the fact that certain preparations of peptone hindered full growth, a problem later studied by Wright[1549] in 1933, who pointed out the fact that one of the difficulties in preparing suitable broth was largely due to incomplete reduction of peptone. This obstacle could be overcome by adding the peptone to the broth before heat is applied, thus exposing it to the reducing action of meat or meat infusion during the steaming process. The inhibitory action of peptone may be further diminished by the reducing action of sugars and an alkaline reaction (Wright). Dubos[333-4] also found that some commercial peptones contain bacteriostatic substances. These may be removed by precipitation with acid and acetone, or their inhibitory action may be neutralized by the addition of reduced thiol compounds (0.0003 per cent thioglycollic acid). Reduced cysteine increases the rate of growth.

A small amount of sodium chloride, usually 0.5 per cent, appears to be a necessary ingredient, although sodium phosphate may be substituted. An excess of salt retards or prevents the growth of Pneumococcus (Wright[1548]), and its concentration, whether as chloride or phosphate, should not exceed 0.1 molar (Dernby and Avery[313]). Glucose stimulates and enhances initial growth, and quantities ranging from 0.1 to 4.0 per cent have been advised, while Turro[1430] preferred 8 per cent! Amounts higher than one per cent, because of the glycolytic action of Pneumococcus with the resulting acid production, may produce retardation or complete inhibition of growth and bring about autolysis (Wright[1548]). The presence of muscle sugar in the meat base must be reckoned as an additional sugar factor when fermentation reactions are to be quantitatively measured. McGuire, Valentine, Whitney, and Falk[879] advised titration of the fermentable reducing sugar in muscle (beef heart) infusion and, taking the equivalent of 0.5 milligram of glucose per cubic centimeter as the lower limit, then added glucose to the desired concentration. Glycerol may replace glucose or other sugars as a source of carbohydrate material, but glycerol, like the other sugars, is susceptible to the fermentative action of Pneumococcus and yields acid on enzymatic cleavage.

The acid formed in broth by the action of Pneumococcus may be neutralized either by the addition of sterile, powdered calcium carbonate (Wurz and Mosny,[1554] and Hiss[650]), or of small pieces of marble, washed and placed in the test tubes before filling and sterilization (Bolduan[135]).

The initial hydrogen ion concentration of the medium and the changes occurring during growth are vital factors in the proper cultivation of the organism. According to Dernby and Avery,[313] culture media should have an initial reaction represented by a pH of 7.8 to 8.0 with an optimal pH of 7.8. They gave the limiting hydrogen ion concentration for initiation of growth for the various types of Pneumococcus as pH 7.0 to 8.3. Strains will live but will not actively multiply in substrates having a degree of acidity or alkalinity greater than those represented by these figures. Lord and Nye[829] have given further information regarding the relation of hydrogen ion concentration to the life, growth, and death of Pneumococcus. As the medium becomes more acid (pH 7.4 to 6.8) the organism may live many days; between 6.8 and 5.1 death begins to take place—the greater the acidity, the more rapid the death, while at 5.1 the cocci die within a few hours. In cloudy suspensions of washed pneumococci dissolution is most marked within the range pH 5.0 to 6.0. Some disintegration occurs toward the alkaline side but none at the most acidic end of the scale.

For the successful initiation of growth in broth, once a pure culture is obtained, a fairly heavy amount of inoculum is advisable. Cole used 0.1 cubic centimeter for every cubic centimeter of broth. These amounts are obviously impossible when cultures are to be planted from single colonies or from mouse-hearts' blood and similar materials. When original infectious material is used as inoculum a small amount usually suffices. A generous planting, however, favors multiplication.

The cycle of pneumococcal growth in broth has been studied by Chesney.[220] When broth is inoculated with a culture that has passed the stage of maximal growth, there ensues a latent period before growth appears in the freshly seeded broth. When, however, inoculation is performed with cultures at their maximal rate of growth, there is no delay in multiplication. This initial latent period or lag—that is, the interval between the time of seeding and the time at which maximal rate of growth begins—is followed by a phase of rapid growth, during which the organisms are dividing regularly. This stage is followed by a stationary period, in which the organisms cease to multiply at maximal rate so that the increase in number becomes slower and finally ceases and, although they remain viable, the number of cells present in a unit volume remains approximately constant for an appreciable length of time. Finally the period of decline sets in, in which the number of living organisms begins to decrease. Chesney believed that this lag is an expression of injury which the bacterial cell sustains from previous environment.

The failure of pneumococci to continue to grow and multiply after the stationary period is due to the production of acid or possibly of other inhibiting substances. Morgan and Avery[915] listed the inhibiting factors as the accumulation of acid products, the exhaustion of nutritive substances, and the formation and accumulation, under certain cultural conditions, of peroxide in the medium. Hager,* by daily neutralizing the newly formed acid has succeeded in prolonging the period of growth and, therefore, in obtaining unusually heavy yields of pneumococci from a single lot of broth.

Felton and Dougherty[423-4] contrived an ingenious apparatus for delivering a continuous supply of pneumococci at the stage of most active growth. By an automatic device, an inoculum of vigorous, young culture was removed from the exhausted medium and planted in a flask containing a fresh food supply of milk. The transfers were made at two, four, and eight-hour intervals. Propagation by this method at eight-hour intervals raised the virulence of the strain to a degree unprecedented in any former *in vitro* experiments. Methods for obtaining large amounts of living pneumococci for chemical study as well as for other purposes have been described by Felton and Huntoon,[667] while that of Hager has not yet come to publication.†

These media, varying in their constituents, all require heavy inoculation with a vigorous culture (Gillespie[515]), careful initial adjustment or subsequent correction of the reaction and, of course, incubation at a constant temperature of about 37.5° if they are to give a large yield. Dubos[331] explained the necessity for large amounts of inoculum in seeding broth as being based on the establishment of a proper reduction potential in the medium. This condition is brought about by the large inoculum owing to the reducing properties of the bacterial cells.

ACCESSORY SUBSTANCES

Optimal growth conditions, that is, as far as rate of growth, number, and viability of the organisms are concerned, can be provided beyond those already mentioned by the addition of a variety of substances. Autoclaved gelatin, by its buffering action in addition to its nutritive elements, has been found by Platt[1096] to induce

* Personal communication. † See Appendix.

and sustain growth of Pneumococcus in otherwise unsuitable media. Robertson, Sia, and Wood[1149] ascertained that the protective action of gelatin lies largely in shielding pneumococci against physical injury—possibly the toxic action of electrolytes—which occurs during dilution in solutions of crystalloids. Furthermore, gelatin exerts a well-marked preservative action of unknown nature in protecting the organisms against early dissolution.

One of the most commonly used substances is blood, of either man, rabbit, horse, or sheep. Pasteur, Sternberg, and Levy and Steinmetz[802] early recognized its value. Citrated, laked, or, better, defibrinated blood augments the growth-promoting value of the substrate. It is best used in a ratio of one part or less to ten to twenty parts of medium. Normal serum, transudates, and ascitic and hydrocele fluids similarly supply elements favorable to the growth of Pneumococcus, and are common ingredients in many media formulas (Fraenkel,[468] Behring and Nissen,[98] Mosny,[933] Levinthal,[800] and many others).

In a study of the growth-promoting properties of serum from a variety of animal species, Bezançon and Griffon[112] found that, in general, growth was more rapid and abundant in the serum of animals susceptible to pneumococcal infection. However, in these serums cell death took place rapidly after maximal growth had been reached. In the serum of resistant animals, on the other hand, growth was meager, although the organisms remained viable and virulent for a longer period of time. The serum of young animals, whether of a sensitive or refractory species, possessed the growth-promoting properties of susceptible species, whereas the serum of older animals was less favorable to growth.

Bordet[139] has recently described an unexplained and as yet unconfirmed cultural and morphological appearance of cultures in rabbit serum. The growth of pneumococci had a milky appearance, and at the bottom of the tube a sediment formed which consisted of a clustered mass of large round elements. These bodies failed to take well the basic stains but were readily stained by neutral dyes. They were variable in size and had fairly regular outlines and a granular structure. Inasmuch as these bodies did not appear in serum media previously heated at 56° for one-half hour, but did appear when the temperature was no higher than 50°, Bordet thought that their production was due to alexin, although they were not present in broth containing serum from rabbits vaccinated against Pneumococcus, either of homologous or heterologous type.

Blood and serum, in addition to contributing some nutritive substances, act as buffers in controlling the reaction and, being colloids, arrest any toxic action of inorganic salts. Blood, because of its oxidation-reduction system, tends to maintain a proper oxygen balance, while the iron in the hemoglobin seems to act as a catalase. In studying the supposed necessity for hemoglobin for the growth of *Bacillus influenzae*, Thjötta[1391] discovered that this substance could be omitted if extracts of mucoid bacilli or of *Bacillus proteus* were substituted. Thjötta looked upon the accessory substance in such extracts as a vitamin which, in many ways, corresponded to Wildier's "Bios" of yeast, the "auxomones" of Bottomly, or the hormones. Then Thjötta and Avery[1392-3] learnt that these substances—the "V" factor—alone would not support the growth of hemophilic bacteria through several generations, but that another substance, the so-called "X" factor, contained in red corpuscles was essential. This X factor is heat-stable and acts in minute amounts. Both the V and X factors are required for the continued and complete development of Pneumococcus as well as for the growth of hemophilic organisms.

Baudisch and Dubos[89] investigated the influence of iron compounds on the viability of pneumococci. Small amounts of iron oxide prolong the life of avirulent strains but are less favorable to virulent strains. Iron may be stimulating or harmful depending upon the particular chemical radical with which it is combined.

Another accessory substance of animal origin, recommended by Quiroga,[1115] is liver. The addition of an extract of beef liver to peptone broth or Martin bouillon gives early growth with less production of acid than that which occurs when glucose is used. In such a medium it is probably the glycogen or other sugars which supply the stimulus, while the tissue itself and the hemoglobin furnish the other growth-promoting factors. The protective action of muscle tissue is exemplified in the hormone-blood agar and hormone-gelatin broth of Bailey.[67] The formula is a modification of that of Huntoon[664] for the preparation of original hormone medium, and both methods, and also that of Douglas for making tryptic digest medium, yield substrates well suited not only for the prolific growth of pneumococci but for conservation of essential biological characters of the organism.

Still another factor to be considered is the oxygen requirement of Pneumococcus. The organism is a facultative anaerobe, and grows both in the presence and absence of oxygen. Examples of anaerobic strains of pneumococci have been encountered by Avery and his associates,* while two similar strains which apparently constitute two new serological types have recently been described by Smith.[1296] Because of its action in elaborating toxic peroxides in the surrounding medium, as first demonstrated by McLeod and Glovenlock[885] and later proved by McLeod and Gordon[881-4] to be hydrogen peroxide, Pneumococcus may hinder or entirely prevent its own growth. The inhibiting effect of the peroxide may be overcome by the addition of plant tissues or other substances exerting an oxidizing-reducing action (Avery and Morgan[52]).

VEGETABLE ACCESSORY SUBSTANCES

Avery and Morgan[51, 53] found that the addition to broth of sterile, unheated plant tissue, such as yellow and white turnip, carrot, beet, parsnip, white and sweet potato, and banana,† not only caused acceleration of pneumococcal growth, but served to induce abundant multiplication even when the seeding was too minute to

* Personal communication.

† Falk, Valentine, McGuire, and Whitney[388] have more recently (1932) recommended the use of the green banana as enriching material in the place of

initiate growth in the medium. With potato broth the beginning period of growth was prolonged and cell death delayed. Moreover, in plant-tissue medium, the zone of hydrogen ion concentration within which growth could be initiated was considerably extended beyond the optimal range in ordinary bouillon. Fresh plant tissue, that is tissue which has not been subjected to heat or oxidation, was necessary for this effect, and this fact explains the action of the tissues in promoting the growth of certain anaerobic bacteria in the presence of oxygen. In the case of Pneumococcus, the action of the oxidizing-reducing system of the V and the X factors* leads to the destruction of toxic peroxides.

Yeast, in the form of autolysate, in combination with clotted horse blood, peptone, agar, glucose, and maltose was found by Hitchens[654] to be a favorable medium for promoting the growth of pneumococci.

APPEARANCE OF GROWTH

In a suitable broth, the first evidence of growth is a faint, uniform clouding of the medium. There is a slow deposition of a light, flocculent sediment at the bottom of the container. On further incubation there is a gradual clearing of the medium with the accumulation of a heavier deposit, while some of the falling particles may adhere to the side of the vessel. There is no pellicle formation. Growth is more rapid and luxuriant when glucose, the accessory substances already mentioned, or some sterile body fluid are added.

In milk, Pneumococcus thrives and develops capsules, and if transfers are made at six or eight-hour intervals, the vigor and virulence of the organism are maintained. Prolonged cultivation in this medium without frequent transplants, however, is detrimental to the cocci owing to the acid produced. Milk is coagulated by

fresh blood in beef-heart broth for the cultivation of pneumococci, while Larson and Thompson[786] employ broth containing sterile, fresh, unheated potato extract for growing pneumococci for type determination and bile-solubility tests. The latter medium has the advantage over serum or blood broth of being free from extraneous substances which might interfere in these tests.

* See p. 43.

practically all strains. Pneumococci will grow in gelatin at 37° but, because gelatin melts, it is not a useful medium for propagating pneumococci.

On agar, Pneumococcus grows in very small, round, water-clear, non-confluent colonies, resembling in many respects those of streptococci, but differing from them in being more transparent, more moist, and flatter. Under the microscope, colonies of Pneumococcus are seen to be finely granular, with dark centers fading to lighter zones nearer the periphery, which is regular, sometimes slightly wavy, but never showing the intertwined convolutions such as those seen in colonies of Streptococcus. In agar stab cultures and sub-surface agar plate cultures, the colonies appear within twenty-four to thirty-six hours, are smaller, sometimes almost invisible, and indistinguishable from colonies of Streptococcus. Under low magnification they show partly as yellowish-brown, partly as bright, oval, lenticular or whetstone-like forms.

On blood-agar plates the colony may be surrounded by a zone of methemoglobin formation with an exterior zone of greenish color after twenty-four or more hours of incubation. Later a zone of hemolysis may appear at the margin fainter than that encircling streptococcal colonies, and this appearance may lead to error in the differentiation of the two organisms. When grown on "mixtures of whole rabbits' blood and agar, the pneumococcus grows well, and forms, after four or five days, thick, black surface colonies, not unlike sun blisters on red paint. These colonies are easily distinguished from those of streptococci, and are of considerable differential value (Hiss)."*

"Upon potato, thin, moist growth appears, scarcely visible and indistinguishable from an increased moisture on the surface of the medium," making this an unsuitable substrate. "Upon Loeffler's coagulated blood serum, the pneumococcus develops into moist, watery, discrete colonies which tend to disappear by a drying out

* Paraphrase and direct quotation from Zinsser and Bayne-Jones.[1579]

of colonies after some days, differing in this from streptococcus colonies."*

DIFFERENTIAL MEDIA

In addition to the diagnostic features of pneumococcal colonies grown on Loeffler's medium and on the rabbit blood-agar mixture, other media have been recommended as serving to develop characters that distinguish pneumococci from streptococci. Hiss,[650] for this purpose, devised a medium consisting of one part of beef serum and two parts of distilled water, to which was added one per cent of inulin (C.P.) and enough litmus to render the medium a clear, transparent blue. By fermentation of the inulin, Pneumococcus acidifies the mixture, causing coagulation of the serum. The method is useful except in the case of those rare strains of pneumococci which are not inulin fermenters. A similar, but solid, medium for the same purpose was that recommended by Ruediger.[1195] To sugar-free broth, containing one per cent of Witte peptone and 1.5 per cent of agar, he added approximately 1.5 per cent of pure inulin and a small amount of Merck's highest purity litmus. One cubic centimeter of ascites fluid heated to 65° was added to each tube of melted agar. Pneumococci are distinguished by the formation of red colonies on this medium.

Buerger[163] claimed that the ring type of colony on serum, or better serum-glucose agar, was distinctive of Pneumococcus when compared with colonies of Streptococcus on the same medium. The method required a close inspection of the growth under transmitted and reflected artificial light. When viewed from the side or by transmitted light, the pneumococcal colony shows a distinct milky ring enclosing a transparent center, while the streptococcal colony has a prominent periphery and a definite nucleus. These and other physical characters serve to differentiate these two species of cocci.

* From Zinsser and Bayne-Jones.[1579]

Bieling,[114] by the use of laked blood agar, laked blood-optochin agar, and boiled blood agar, could differentiate pneumococci, and the *longus* and *mitior* types of streptococci. Presting[1109] used the Bieling method in studying some sixty carefully identified strains of pneumococci and streptococci, and concluded that boiled blood agar was a suitable aid in differentiating pneumococci and green-growing and hemolytic streptococci. On the laked blood agar the hemolytic streptococci exhibited such marked variation that *viridans* could not be distinguished from the hemolytic types, nor from pneumococci. Koch,[731] after one year's favorable experience with Bieling's blood-optochin agar, recommended the medium for the differentiation of pneumococci and streptococci.

The "polytrope" medium of Lange—a special lactose-mannite-peptone bouillon—as reported by Haendel and Lange,[585] develops a diffuse orange-yellow coloration when pneumococci of long artificial cultivation are grown on it, but remains uncolored when the strains are cultivated directly from infected animal material. This latter fact renders this medium unsuited to the differentiation of bacterial species, because streptococcal strains of long cultivation, and other bacterial species as well, cause no color change. Dog-blood agar plates, according to Sia and Chung,[1270] give colony differences sufficiently pronounced to enable one to distinguish between colonies of smooth and rough strains of pneumococci. For the same purpose, the authors, in a later communication,[1271] reported that a medium consisting of one per cent dextrose-beef-infusion agar with a reaction equal to pH 7.8 containing type-specific antipneumococcic serum served to identify the pneumococcal type strain. In poured plates, the colonies under the surface, when illuminated from the side on a dark background, showed an annular opacity which was claimed to be type-specific.

Thomson and Thomson,[1400] by means of photomicrographs of colonies of pneumococci grown on plasma-testicular agar, claimed that it was possible to detect significant species and even type differences. Their excellent photographs repay study.

Viability

The factors already described, along with temperature conditions, determine not only the speed and mass of growth but the span of life of Pneumococcus. In highly buffered fluids such as blood, blood serum, or media containing these body tissues, Pneumococcus can be preserved alive and virulent for long periods of time. Arkharow (1892)[17] found that blood from infected mice and rabbits retained its virulence if kept in sealed tubes in the dark at room temperature. Foà and Bordoni-Uffreduzzi (1888)[462] incubated the blood of an infected rabbit for twenty-four hours and then stored it in the dark in the cold. Vitality was preserved for fifty to sixty days. Rymowitsch[1199] accidentally noted that hemoglobin in the medium would conserve viability and virulence for an equal length of time at 36° to 38°. Yourevitch[1566] proposed a method, based on the protective action of blood and tissue, for preserving pneumococci in latent culture. Blood is aspirated by a pipette and expelled into the bottom of tubes of glucose or serum broth, or a whole heart or fragments of clotted rabbit blood may be added. After planting, the cultures are hermetically sealed and kept in the ice-box. In such cultures both viability and virulence remain unimpaired for several months.

Römer[1155] preserved pneumococci by mixing the heart-blood of a rabbit dead from pneumococcal infection with sterile saline solution and storing the infectious material in sealed tubes in a cool, dark place. He maintained the virulence of the stock material by weekly passage through rabbits.

Washbourn,[1486] dissatisfied with these methods, preserved stock cultures as long as fifty days by covering the growth on agar cultures with a thin layer of rabbit blood. Gilbert and Fournier[518] kept strains viable for two months by simple inoculation in fluid, defibrinated blood. The cocci still showed capsules and were virulent for mice. Bezançon and Griffon[112] modified Gilbert and Fournier's procedure by injecting a proteose solution in dogs, then mixing their blood with ascitic or pleuritic fluids before seeding with pneumococci. Incubated continuously at 37.5°, the pneumococci survived for four months. Truche and Cotoni[1422] added two volumes of 15 per cent gelatin in physiological salt solution to cultures grown at 37.5° in the "T" medium, sealed the tubes, and kept them in the ice-box. In this way viable stock cultures could be maintained for at least six months. Ungermann[1435] cultivated pneumococci in concentrated rabbit serum and then protected the cultures with a layer of sterile paraffin oil, with incubation at 37.5°. Later, Truche[1421] modified Ungermann's method by first growing strains on blood or serum agar, and then covering the surface with formalinized serum. Preservation continued for a year, yielding virulent material for inoculation. In a semi-fluid medium consisting of one part of nutrient agar and five parts of sterile ascitic or pleuritic fluids, with short incubation and storage at 8° to 10°, Wadsworth (1903)[1454] preserved cultures in a viable condition for three or more months. In these exudates without agar, the period of viability was even greater. A similar medium with the addition of glucose was described in 1930 by Vélicanoff and Mikhailova.[1450]

Dehydration is an excellent physical method for the preservation of cultures of Pneumococcus, particularly in those cases in which experiments continued over a long period of time require that the characters of the strain be held uniform and constant. Nissen (1891)[1013] first applied this principle to the drying of sterile silk threads saturated with broth and serum-broth cultures, but the results were only indicative of the success which was to attend Heim's[631] efforts fourteen years later. Similar threads, soaked in the blood of a cat dying of pneumococcal septicemia and dried over calcium chloride in a desiccator, fourteen and sixteen months later yielded in broth a growth of pneumococci possessing a virulence equal to that of the original material.

In the year of Nissen's publication, Bordoni-Uffreduzzi,[142] not seeking a method of preservation, reported that pneumonic sputum when dried on linen rags gave growth after twelve days' exposure to direct sunlight, and as late as after fifty-five days of exposure to diffuse daylight. They concluded that the blood and proteins in the sputum formed a protective coating for the cocci. Wood[1542] studied the longevity of Pneumococcus in sputum when subjected to varying temperatures. In moist sputum, kept in the dark at room temperature, the average life of Pneumococcus is eleven days, while at 0° it is, as a rule, thirty-five days. When the sputum is kept in strong light at room temperature the life span is less than five days. In dried sputum Pneumococcus lives, on an average, thirty-five days in the dark, thirty days in diffuse daylight, and less than four hours in sunlight. In powdered sputum, death is a matter of a few hours. Pneumococci in sprayed, moist sputum rarely survive for more than an hour, and often die in less time. The material upon which the sprayed particles fall has little influence on the life of the organism. On the contrary, Emmerich[355] and more recently Stillman,[1326] have demonstrated the longevity and continued virulence of pneumococci in a dried condition. Stillman* recovered viable organisms from pneumonic sputum dried in test tubes and exposed for three months or more to diffuse daylight at room temperature. Germano,[511] too, found pneumococci resistant to drying, but the details of his experiments are lacking. Hintze[646] kept blood-agar cultures alive for thirty-two months by storage in tubes stoppered with cotton plugs. For the purpose of keeping pneumococci viable and virulent, Savino and Acuna[1220] placed the blood of mice or rabbits infected with Pneumococcus in one arm of an H tube with phosphoric anhydride in the other arm and then sealed the tube after evacuating the air.

The thermal death-point for Pneumococcus as given by Sternberg[1321] is 52° for ten minutes.

For practical purposes, however, such as the maintenance of virulent stock cultures or of other infectious pneumococcal material, in addition to refrigeration of inoculated blood in sealed tubes and the devices already described, the rapid drying of cultures, infected organs, blood, or sputum presents many advantages.

* Personal communication.

Swift's[1370] method is a successful example. The culture is scraped from the surface of the solid medium, spread in thin layers on plates or in tubes, and quickly frozen. The frozen material is then placed in a chilled Hempel desiccator containing phosphorus pentoxide in the bottom and sulfuric ether in the moat. The drawing of a high vacuum dissipates the frozen moisture, and the resulting dry powder, if kept anhydrous, is found to contain viable organisms after many months of storage. Later, Otten,[1040] using a similar method for drying thick suspensions of pneumococci in salt solution, reported their recovery in living condition after long periods of preservation. Desiccated cultures, unlike those on moist media, can be shipped over distances involving many days' exposure to wide temperature variations.

The reader who desires further details concerning the preservation of bacterial cultures is referred to the communication of Flosdorf and Mudd[454] who, after reviewing the literature on the subject, described an apparatus for the rapid drying and preservation of bacteria, serum, and other biological substances. The method consists in applying a high vacuum to the material to be dried rapidly and freezing it by immersion in a bath chilled to —78° by the use of Dry-Ice and Methyl Cellusolve.

Another practical method for having virulent cultures at hand is that devised by Neufeld[1000] based on the principle earlier established by Heim. Pieces of spleen or heart or the whole organs of mice dead of experimental pneumococcal infection are placed in open Petri dishes or in small tubes loosely plugged with cotton and dried in a vacuum desiccator over calcium chloride or concentrated sulfuric acid. To recover the pneumococci, generous pieces of the dried organs are ground in a mortar with broth, and the suspension injected intraperitoneally into a mouse. The heart's blood of the dead or dying mouse usually yields a pure, virulent culture.

Autolysis

Pneumococcus is a delicate organism and may rapidly disintegrate under certain physical conditions of the medium which favor the action of its own lytic ferments. Bürgers[187] was among the first to study the self-dissolution of pneumococci. He reported that autolysis, while favored by the addition of chloroform, was prevented by heating the organisms to 60° or above. One of the environmental conditions which influence dissolution is the degree of acidity of the substrate. Mair[552] gave the range of hydrogen ion concentration within which autolysis occurs as from pH 8.5 to 6.0, with an optimum of pH 6.8. Lord and Nye[829] observed the dissolution of suspended living pneumococci of Types I and II in isotonic standard solutions and in approximately isotonic bouillon having reactions between pH 4.0 and pH 8.0. Lysis took place with a reaction higher than pH 5.0 and was most marked in the range pH 5.0 to 7.0. It was still observable on the alkaline side, but was absent when the acidity was greater than pH 5.0. This phenomenon takes place at ice-box, room, and incubator temperatures. Mair found the rate of lysis increased to a maximum at 42°, and stated that this maximum was due to partial destruction of the autolytic ferment at higher temperatures, and also that the autolysin was more sensitive to heat when the reaction was alkaline. Exposure of pneumococci to 47° for one hour diminishes the degree of dissolution, while an exposure of thirty minutes at 56° or five minutes at 100° completely arrests the action. Inasmuch as Sternberg[1321] determined the thermal death-point as 52° for ten minutes, if the observation was correct, the lower temperature should suffice to prevent self-lysis, but such is not the case.

The addition of fresh human serum to suspensions of the cocci at varying reactions prevents autolysis. Solutions of lysed pneumococci added to fresh suspensions of pneumococci in standard solutions of the same hydrogen ion concentration increase autolysis. Cultures of *S. viridans*, *S. haemolyticus*, and *Staphylococcus aureus* do not undergo dissolution under similar conditions. Extracts prepared by treating minced pneumonic lung tissue with chloroform, toluene, and saline solution, or the sediment from such extractions, when added to pneumococci at pH 5.5 to 6.95, dissolve the cells, but no action takes place if the reaction is as acid as pH 4.5. From this observation Lord and Nye concluded: "An enzyme derived from the bacteria themselves or from the cellular material may be the cause of the dissolution." Avery and Cullen[38-41] supported this hypothesis. Autolysates and sterile solutions of pneumococci, when added to suspensions of pneumococcal cells in phosphate solutions of known pH previously heated to 60° for thirty minutes, or 120° for twenty minutes, caused lysis of dead pneumococci and, to a less extent, disintegration of closely allied organisms such as *S. viridans*, but they had no effect on *Staphylococcus aureus*. The enzyme was most active in a substrate with a reaction between pH 6 and pH 8; it was destroyed by heating for thirty minutes at 60° and was not type-specific in its action. The bacteriolytic action was proportional to the concentration of enzyme. Avery and Cullen expressed doubt whether lysis of pneumococci under these circumstances was the result of a single enzyme or the product of the interaction of more than one. The matter was left undecided by their saying that "whether the enzyme or group of enzymes concerned in autolysis of pneumococci play any part in this form of lysis are questions at present undecided."

In 1929, Goebel and Avery[520] were able to state that:

> 1) Autolysis of Pneumococcus is accompanied by proteolysis, which results in an increase in amino and non-coagulable nitrogen; 2) autolysis of Pneumococcus is accompanied by lipolysis during which there is a liberation of ether-soluble fatty acids; 3) when extracts containing the active intracellular enzymes are added to heat-killed pneumococci, lysis of the cell occurs and there is an increase in the non-coagulable and amino nitrogens, comparable to the changes accompanying spontaneous autolysis; 4) when extracts containing the active intracellular enzymes are added to emulsions of the alcohol-soluble lipoids extracted from pneumococci an increase in the ether-soluble fatty acid occurs.

In spite of the earlier belief of Jobling and Strouse (1913)[680] that lysis of pneumococci may be independent of ferment action and the statement of Pauli[1071] that this autolysis is due to the self-production of peroxide, it would now seem wise to conclude that the self-dissolution of this organism is caused by the action of its own intracellular ferments.

Bile Solubility

The biochemical reaction taking place in the autolysis of pneumococci is also involved in the solvent action of bile on the pneumococcal cell. It was Neufeld[972] who, in 1900, first discovered that bile possessed this unusual property, a property which became of great diagnostic value in differentiating Pneumococcus from Streptococcus and other organisms, and which has since been known as the "Neufeld phenomenon." He found that rabbit bile in a ratio of 1 to 50, or often of 1 to 200 or 300, added to fresh bouillon cultures of living pneumococci, within a fairly wide range of temperature of the fluids, rendered them clear and transparent in the space of a few minutes. The microscope failed to reveal any formed elements, for there was rapid and complete dissolution of the pneumococcal cells. The bile of other animal species and of man, despite considerable variation in the content of bile-acid salts and mucus, exhibited the same property. Bile from rabbits was the most active, and clear, limpid bile was to be preferred to that which was more viscous or cloudy. Its action was not altered by previous heating, but no lysis took place if the cocci had first been killed by heat. Neufeld thought this action was attributable to cholic acid in combination with glycocol and taurin, since glycocol and taurin alone are inactive.

Nicolle and Adil-Bey (1907)[1007] preferred rabbit bile to that of the ox because of its greater solvent action on pneumococci, but better still were sodium cholate and sodium choleate. The authors found that this property was shared, although to a somewhat less degree, by quinolate, taurocholate, glycocholate, and least of all, hypocholate. Bile-solubility was looked upon as a salient character of Pneumococcus.

The advantages of sodium taurocholate over whole bile, claimed by Levy,[803] were denied by Mandelbaum,[865] who maintained that while the former dissolved strains of Pneumococcus and *Streptococcus mucosus* as against a negative action on other streptococci, dissolution was not so complete as that produced by bile. The partial failure of sodium taurocholate may have been due, as pointed out by Levy, to lack of uniformity in commercial preparations of the salt. A pure preparation of this bile-salt is to be preferred to whole bile, because solutions of constant concentration may be prepared, sterilized, and kept in stock for quantitative or repeated tests.

Malone[861] would further refine the test by always using the same strength of sodium taurocholate (10 per cent), keeping the density of the bacterial suspension uniform, employing cultures from solid rather than from liquid media, holding both time and temperature constant, and taking precautions that the mixtures are always alkaline in reaction. For routine identification tests such refinements seem to be superfluous.

Neufeld at first held the view that only freshly isolated and virulent strains of pneumococci were susceptible to the solvent action of bile, but Levy,[803] using sodium taurocholate in a 5 to 10 per cent solution, believed that the method afforded a clear-cut differentiation between all pneumococci and streptococci and other bacterial species. It was Levy who, in 1907, with this confirmatory test, definitely established *Streptococcus mucosus* as a pneumococcus, and called it *Pneumococcus mucosus*.

Neufeld's view concerning the correlation between virulence and bile-solubility was upheld by Truche, Cotoni, and Raphael[1425] who, after an experience of several years, reported that high virulence always accompanied complete solubility and total avirulence went with insolubility, whereas strains of slight virulence showed partial or varying solubility. All thirty-one strains of streptococci tested were insoluble in bile. Malone[861-2] also observed that pathogenic strains and members of fixed types tended to fall into a sodium taurocholate soluble group, while the so-called "normal" strains and cocci of Group IV fell into either soluble or insoluble groups, with some strains intermediate between the two.

Schiemann's* observations did not agree with those of Neufeld. He found completely avirulent strains which were still bile-soluble, as well as mouse-virulent strains which were insoluble. Cocci in the blood and peritoneal exudate of freshly dead mice resisted dissolution, while transitional forms were only incompletely dissolved. Cotoni* described some virulent, typical pneumococci as insoluble. In marked contrast to these results were those of Falk and Jacobson[381] who could find no relation between virulence and bile-solubility, since avirulent strains appeared to be as sensitive to the lytic action of bile as were virulent cultures. Kelly,[702] too, noted a variation in the susceptibility of different strains to lysis, but added that specimens of bile differed in solvent power, and that the presence of sugar in the medium containing the pneumococci had an inhibitory action on the lytic action of bile. Human blood serum, on the contrary, according to Ziegler,[1570] does not interfere with this power.

Differing in their experience from that of Neufeld, Cole and his colleagues[36] found all of several hundred strains of Pneumococcus isolated from lobar pneumonia to be bile-soluble. There are rare exceptions to this rule, an example being the strain of *Pneumococcus mucosus* reported by Dochez and Gillespie.[322] It seems safe to say, with Mair,[552] that "different strains of Pneumococcus show varying sensitiveness to the action of bile, just as they vary in the readiness with which they undergo autolysis in culture, but with a satisfactory technique one is very seldom in doubt as to whether a particular strain should be classed as bile-soluble or not, and strains which have been kept on culture media for long periods retain the property."†

* Quoted by Neufeld and Schnitzer.

† Sellards[1254] also stressed the importance of the characters of the cultures and the alkalinity of the medium in solubility tests. In place of bile Sellards substituted 0.01N to 0.2N solutions of sodium hydroxide, which even in the stronger concentration failed to dissolve streptococci. He thought that old strains of pneumococci were more soluble than young strains.

Harkins[590] contributed the interesting but unexplained observation that the bile of animals in which an artificial cholecystitis had been set up by intracystic injections of organisms other than Pneumococcus (*B. coli communior* excepted), was devoid of any lytic ability. The absence of this property was not due to absorption as shown by the fact that the addition of the infecting bacteria (*S. mitis, Staphylococcus aureus,* and *B. coli communior*) to normal bile failed to rob it of this lytic action.

Kozlowski[751] further elucidated the action of bile-solubility by demonstrating that the higher unsaturated fatty acids in bile were even more powerful than cholic acid. The sodium salt of one of these fatty acids with an iodine number of 174, in dilutions of approximately 1 to 50,000, inhibited the growth of pneumococci and, in a dilution of 1 to 5,000, completely killed and dissolved the cells. The soaps were active in higher dilutions and in a shorter time than were the corresponding salts of taurocholic and glycocholic acids. Ziegler[1571] reported that the cytolytic action of sodium dehydrocholate was comparable to the action of sodium taurocholate.

Downie, Stent, and White[327] tested the solvent action of saponin, cholic, dehydrocholic, dehydro-oxycholic, apocholic, and desoxycholic acids, as well as a group of choleic acids which are addition compounds of desoxycholic acid. Of the substances tested, saponin and the sodium salts of all the bile-acids except dehydrocholic and dehydrodesoxycholic acids, brought about lysis. The similarity of the action of the sodium salts of the various choleic acids to that of sodium desoxycholate indicated to the authors that the former owed their activity to the desoxycholic fraction.

Ziegler[1572] found that sodium dehydrocholate and dehydrodesoxycholate would dissolve pneumococci, thus disagreeing with Downie, Stent, and White, who used cultures grown on artificial media. Ziegler employed strains obtained directly from infected animals without any intervening cultivation. He candidly remarked that his paper created more problems than it solved.

In studying the combined action of alkaline oleates and linoleates and immune serum on the lysis of pneumococci, Lamar[773] noted that the oleates rendered the cocci more susceptible to serum lysis. In normal serum their action was incomplete, but in immune serum there was no multiplication of the organism and lysis was complete. As an explanation, Lamar suggested that the action of the soap was exerted upon the lipoidal portion of the bacterial cell, through which it was rendered more pervious to serum constituents and brought under their deleterious and dissolving influence.

In another paper, Lamar[774] reported that sodium linoleate and sodium linolenate killed and dissolved pneumococci more rapidly and in higher dilutions than did sodium oleate. Furthermore, in the experiments it was seen that blood serum inhibited the bacteriolytic action of the unsaturated soaps, partly or completely, depending upon the quantitative ratio between serum and soap. Lamar concluded that the action was probably caused in part by the avidity of the unsaturated fatty acids for protein and not wholly by their ability to dissolve lipids.

In 1926, Falk and Yang[385] compared the solvent action of sodium oleate, sodium hydroxide, tribasic sodium phosphate, and saponin on washed pneumococci, and learnt that all these substances in the concentrations tested, with the exception of saponin, were as specific in their action as is bile.

In another communication, Falk and Yang[384] described the influence exerted by certain electrolytes and non-electrolytes on bile-solubility. Chlorides with monovalent cations when present in relatively low concentrations inhibited the solution of washed pneumococci by bile, but in higher concentrations possibly accelerated solution. Chlorides with divalent cations acted in reverse fashion, inhibiting more effectively in high than in low concentrations. Of the anion series tested, sodium hydroxide and tribasic sodium phosphate were cytolytic to pneumococci, whereas dibasic and acid sodium phosphate, sodium sulfate, and sodium nitrate were not. Peptone, gelatin, and ovalbumin appeared to inhibit cytolysis by bile in the same manner as calcium or barium chloride. Falk and

Yang's observation on saponin does not agree with that of Downie, Stent, and White.

Klein and Stone[721] made the interesting observation that while pneumococci were not dissolved by saponin when tested in plain broth culture, preliminary treatment of the cocci with cholesterol rendered them susceptible to complete and rapid lysis by this substance. An excess of saponin inhibited the sensitization by cholesterol and, conversely, an excess of cholesterol inhibited lysis by saponin. The authors thought, on apparently good evidence, that the action of such body fluids as blood and ascitic and pleural fluids in sensitizing pneumococci to saponin lysis was attributable to the cholesterol content. Klein[720] later reported that ergosterol effected a similar sensitization.

In 1930, Neufeld and Etinger-Tulczynska[983] explained more details of the process of bile-lysis. Using bile, sodium taurocholate, and sodium linolenate, it was found that bile and bile-acid salts possessed the greatest solvent action for pneumococci, although soap and bile action were not always parallel. It was further observed that the same antiseptics (one per cent phenol, one per cent formalin, weak ammonium sulfide, acetone, and 0.05 per cent mercuric chloride), which interfere with bile-solubility, in general also inhibited spontaneous autolysis as well as the solution of heat-killed pneumococci by the bacteriolytic enzyme shown by Avery and Cullen[41] to exist in Pneumococcus. Neufeld and Etinger-Tulczynska stated that "the effect of antiseptics would indicate that bile-solubility and action of autolytic ferments are related," but opposed to the concept of parallel bile-solubility and autolysis there is still evidence that the bile-salts have a lytic action of their own, independent of autolytic ferments. The evidence is furnished by the study of Goebel and Avery[520] on autolysis of Pneumococcus. In addition to finding that autolysis was accompanied by definite proteolysis and lipolysis, they observed that while sodium desoxycholate in excess inhibited the action of pneumococcal protease, it did not inhibit the action of the lipase. Goebel and

Avery found, furthermore, that when suspensions of pneumococci were cooled at 0°—a temperature at which the rate of enzyme action is greatly retarded—the organisms went into solution rapidly when sodium desoxycholate was added, and the process was not accompanied by lipolysis or proteolysis. These authors concluded that it did not seem probable, therefore, that the bile solution of Pneumococcus was identical with the phenomenon of autolysis as ordinarily understood and measured. Unpublished work by Dubos would, on the contrary, seem to indicate that bile solution occurs only under conditions when cell ferments remain active.

There can be no doubt, however, that the intracellular enzymes may act as adjuvants in cell dissolution. The action of extracts of living pneumococci in dissolving dead pneumococci (Avery and Cullen[41]) with an increase in non-coagulable and amino nitrogen and in ether-soluble fatty acids (Goebel and Avery[520]) favor this view, a view which has received additional support by the experiments of Wollman and Averbusch,[1535-36] who were able to cause bile solution of killed non-soluble, virulent, and avirulent pneumococci by the addition of a small amount of a living, avirulent culture to the bile-culture mixture. This phenomenon they called *autolyse transmissible.*

Atkin[29] made the original observation that organisms comprising the papillae which frequently arise as secondary growths on autolyzed colonies of pneumococci on serum agar were quite insoluble in bile. It was evident that the organisms of which the papillae consist were devoid of autolysin since they showed no tendency to undergo dissolution or self-digestion even after several weeks of incubation. The organisms thus derived, when subcultured on fresh serum agar, regained autolytic power and at the same time became bile-soluble. Atkin made the statement that "bile solubility of pneumococcus is due to an acceleration of the normal autolytic process by this substance, and that no solution of the organism occurs except in the presence of the autolysin."

Another observation which contributed to the question was that of Lord and Nye,[835-7] who found that more rapid dissolution of pneumococci occurred in bile than in standard buffer solutions and that lysis proceeded at a more rapid rate when the reaction of the mixture was slightly alkaline. The authors attributed the effect to the more rapid death of the organisms in bile and, hence, to the liberation of a larger amount of enzyme at the optimal hydrogen ion concentration.

Whatever may be the facts regarding the exact nature of bile solution of Pneumococcus, it cannot be gainsaid that this phenomenon and that of autolysis bear striking similarities. Whether or not they are due to entirely separate mechanisms, bile may be regarded as an accelerator of natural autolysis.

Sensitiveness to Germicides and Other Chemical Substances

Pneumococcus is highly vulnerable to the usual antiseptics and germicides. The problem of killing pneumococci and of rendering infectious material harmless is a simple one, and can be dismissed with scant discussion. As an example of the effective concentrations of two common germicides, Schiemann and Ishiwara[1230] gave for the growth-inhibiting strength of phenol and mercuric chloride 1 to 600 and 1 to 100,000, respectively. These figures were obtained by adding a small quantity of a twenty-four-hour broth culture of pneumococci to 5 per cent ox-serum containing varying dilutions of the two substances.*

Simon and Wood[1288-9] investigated the action of a large number of dyes and concluded that the majority of the basic type, especially those of the triphenylmethane series, in a concentration of 1:100,000 in agar were inhibitory for pneumococci as tested by making a stroke culture on the medium. Acriflavine (trypaflavine) acts powerfully both on virulent and non-virulent pneumococci (Schiemann and Baumgarten, 1923). Norton and Davis (1923) found that organisms belonging to the *S. viridans* and Pneumococcus groups were inhibited by dyes to the same extent, so that none could be used for the purpose of differentiating between them.

* Quoted from Browning.[159]

For killing cultures to be used as antigens for the production of active immunity 0.5 per cent phenol and 0.3 per cent formalin are commonly used. Sodium ricinoleate was first used for this purpose by Larson and Nelson,[791] because of its rapid lethal effect on pneumococci and the absence of any impairing action on the antigenicity of the treated cells. Barnes and Clarke[81] determined that sodium ricinoleate and sodium oleate were pneumococcidal in concentrations of 0.04 and 0.004 per cent respectively, which, in conjunction with Lamar's results on the action of sodium lanolate, give us definite figures for these soaps.

In discussing the effect of various chemical substances on the vitality of Pneumococcus, mention may be made of the method developed by Schnabel[1238-9] for measuring such effects. Based on the reducing power of pneumococci, he determined the ability of the organism in contact with varying strengths of the test chemicals to produce significant color changes in methylene blue, litmus, neutral red, indigo blue, and other dyes. Since the reducing power of pneumococci is a variable one, this factor must be carefully controlled by proper observance of time, temperature, and hydrogen ion concentration. The method enabled Schnabel to study both the inhibiting and the sensitizing action of quinine, optochin, mercuric chloride, formaldehyde, phenol, and silver nitrate on Pneumococcus. The method holds possibilities for the study of drug-fastness of the coccus and Schnabel claimed that by the use of this technique he could determine the presence of optochin in a 1 to 1,000,000 dilution and that it can be applied to the quantitative measurement of the amounts of analogous substances in solution.

The discovery by Morgenroth and Levy[926] that quinine and some of its derivatives, especially optochin, possess bactericidal powers for Pneumococcus, both *in vitro* and *in vivo*, has led to investigations on the therapeutic effect of this class of substances on pneumococcal infection. The results of the studies will be discussed in the chapter on Chemotherapy.

To summarize our knowledge of the bactericidal action of various chemicals upon Pneumococcus, it suffices to say that no substance or class of substances have as yet been found which exert any selective lethal action on the cell with the exception of bile-acids and certain derivatives of quinine.

CHAPTER III

BIOCHEMICAL FEATURES

The behavior of Pneumococcus toward proteins, fats, and carbohydrates; acid production; oxidizing and reducing action; and the formation of peroxide, methemoglobin, hemolysin, hemotoxin, and alleged endotoxin.

THE pneumococcal cell is charged with a complement of enzymes capable of destroying it as well as certain extracellular substances upon which they are allowed to act. The living organism and sterile extracts made from it can digest proteins, split lipids, and invert and ferment carbohydrates.

Proteolysis, Lipolysis, and Carbohydrate Fermentation

PROTEOLYSIS

Rosenow[1169] was probably the first to express the opinion, based on experimental evidence, that Pneumococcus contained a proteolytic enzyme capable of splitting its inherent protein into a highly poisonous substance and to demonstrate the proteolytic action of Pneumococcus. Extracts of virulent pneumococci made in sodium chloride solution and filtrates of broth cultures hydrolyzed the proteins contained in heated ascites-meat broth and, to a lesser degree, those of heated serum. The extracts did not attack egg-white or pure casein. The enzyme appeared to be more resistant to heat and to long standing in broth filtrates than in salt solution. Heating at 60° reduced the enzymatic action of the filtrates by 50 per cent, and almost completely destroyed the activity of the saline extracts.

In 1920, Avery and Cullen[38] gave a still more detailed demonstration of the proteolytic action of Pneumococcus. By dissolving living cocci in bile or sodium cholate, or by allowing them to autolyze under alternate freezing and thawing in phosphate solutions with a reaction of pH 6.2, or by filtering sterile broth cultures, the authors obtained cell-free extracts capable of hydrolyzing casein and fibrin but not albumin and gelatin. The extracts digested proteoses and peptones even more rapidly, converting them into peptides and amino acids. The enzyme or enzymes were designated by the authors as protease and peptonase, although it was stated that these names might merely represent different activities of the same ferment. The activity of the enzyme was favored by a reaction of pH 7.0 to 7.8, but was suspended at pH 5.0. The enzyme, however, was not destroyed by relatively short exposure to this acid reaction, since its activity was restored when the pH of the solution was readjusted to 7.8. The rapidity of hydrolysis was proportional to the concentration of enzyme. Heating diminished the digestive action, which was lost after ten minutes' exposure to 100°. The ability of active extracts to digest the protein of heat-killed pneumococci was later shown by Goebel and Avery[520] by demonstrating an increase in the non-coagulable and amino nitrogen after contact of the extract with the killed cocci.

LIPOLYSIS

The presence of an esterase in the pneumococcal cell has also been demonstrated by Avery and Cullen.[39] Extracts of pneumococci, prepared in the manner employed for obtaining proteases, split tributyrin. Heating for ten minutes at 70° destroyed the activity of the lipase. While bile and bile-salts accelerated lipolysis, they were not essential to the reaction, since pneumococcal extracts prepared in other ways exhibited the same enzymatic activity. In the study of Goebel and Avery it appeared that on the addition of extracts containing the active intracellular enzymes of the pneumococcal cell to the ether-soluble lipids of pneumococci, an increase in ether-soluble fatty acid occurred. Falk and McGuire[386] recently reported that strains of Pneumococcus, Types I and II, in suitable broth, hydrolyzed phenylacetate, glyceryl tri-acetate, methyl n-butyrate, and benzylacetate. While different degrees of hydrolysis were shown for the four esters, the comparative ratio of the action of the two types of organisms on these esters was of the same order in different lots of broth, although the absolute values were not the same. As a rule, Type I organisms showed a greater action than those of Type II, except in the case of phenylacetate.

CARBOHYDRATE FERMENTATION

Important from a practical standpoint is the content in Pneumococcus of carbohydrate-splitting enzymes, since the selective action of the latter serves in the bacteriological differentiation of this species from other species and genera of the family *Coccaceae.*

Invertase, amylase, and inulase were first demonstrated in Pneumococcus by Avery and Cullen (1920).[40] Finding that bile solutions of pneumococci were unsuited to the purpose, the authors used sterile extracts made by alternately freezing and thawing suspensions of cells in balanced phosphate solutions at a pH of 6.2. The enzymes were active within the limits pH 5.0 to 8.0, with an optimum of 7.0. The acid death-point of pH 5.0 may be reached in carbohydrate media, even when buffered with phosphates, if the content of glucose exceeds 0.3 per cent (Avery and Cullen, Lord and Nye[829]). These authors agreed in ascribing carbohydrate fermentations to intracellular or endoenzymes. The saccharolytic ferments of Pneumococcus have a lower thermal death-point than the protease or lipase, being destroyed at 55° in ten minutes.

The enzymatic preparations freed of living cells hydrolyze sucrose, starch, and inulin but, strange to say, fail to ferment glucose, although in culture media the cleavage of this sugar into acid is a definite and constant activity of the growth of Pneumococcus. According to Hewitt,[643] the breakdown of glucose by Pneumococcus is a less complex process than in the case of many other organisms. Of the glucose constantly disappearing from such cultures, about 78 per cent was recovered by Hewitt as lactic acid.

There appeared to be marked and characteristic divergences in the behavior of different types of pneumococci toward this sugar, the variant RIII being first and SI second in order of glycolytic activity. It was Hewitt's belief that inorganic phosphorus played an essential part in the fermentation of glucose and that this part was independent of its buffering action. The full benefit to Pneumococcus from phosphates was only obtained when media containing these salts were sterilized by filtration and not by autoclaving.

The cleavage of maltose and lactose, unlike that of glucose, is due respectively to a maltase and a lactase in the pneumococcal cell (Fleming and Neill[452]), while Neill and Avery[954] have demonstrated a raffinase.

A significant and distinctive enzymatic property of Pneumococcus is its ability to ferment inulin, a polyose from dahlia bulbs. It was Hiss[649] who first in 1902 discovered that, by means of this property, it was possible to differentiate pneumococci from the closely related members of the tribe *Streptococcaceae.* Serum-water containing one per cent inulin supported growth of Pneumococcus, resulting in the development of acidity and coagulation, while streptococci, although growing, failed to form appreciable acid or to coagulate the medium. It was the use of this method which, with other biological characters, indicated that the so-called *Streptococcus mucosus* was in reality a pneumococcus.

Duval and Lewis[342] overcame the variations encountered in various batches of serum-water by using inulin broth. They found that in its fermentative ability *Streptococcus mucosus* closely resembled Pneumococcus, but decided that the inability to ferment inulin did not necessarily exclude an organism from the species, since some pneumococci failed to show this character. Dochez and Gillespie[322] described a strain of *Pneumococcus mucosus* that did not ferment inulin. Berry[106] also observed the pneumococcal characters of *S. mucosus,* and her results agreed with those of Duval and Lewis in that she encountered other strains of pneumococci that failed to attack inulin, as well as variations in this respect in strains that had undergone changes in morphology and virulence induced by longer or shorter cultivation on artificial media. Berry drew attention to the lack of uniformity in the serum-water medium and in commercial preparations of inulin. With a reliable lot of inulin serum-water, however, some non-inulin-fermenting strains acquired or regained this fermentative property after animal passage.

In a more recent paper, Berger and Silberstein[103] reported the results of a study on strains of pneumococci, of the "B" modification* of this species, and of green-producing and hemolytic streptococci. The hemolytic streptococci, none of which affected inulin, were the only group with constant behavior toward this carbohydrate. Of the typical pneumococci, four strains showed reddening without coagulation of the medium and two had no inulin-fermenting power. These two strains were found to be modification "A"* when tested with optochin. Of nine strains of modification "B" obtained from Pneumococcus, but behaving otherwise as green streptococci, two retained the inulin-fermenting property. Of thirty green streptococci, five gave marked inulin fermentation, while four others showed slightly positive reactions. Other authors to report strains incapable of fermenting inulin among the pneumococci are Hiss; Park and Williams; Levy; Avery; and Bürger and Ryttenberger.†

In addition to inulin, the polysaccharide, glycogen, is equally susceptible to the saccharolytic action of Pneumococcus. First reported by Hiss,[649] this reaction has been quantitatively studied by Barnes and White,[85] who compared the fermentative reactions of strains of Type I, II, III, and V pneumococci on glucose, inulin, mammalian glycogen, and glycogen obtained from scallops. The authors decided that, on the whole, the four type strains used fermented glycogen to essentially the same degree as they did glucose and inulin.

Pneumococcus attacks still other carbohydrates, but no specific

* To be described in Chapter V.

† Quoted by Neufeld and Schnitzer.

enzymes have been demonstrated for these reactions. In addition to glucose, galactose and levulose are actively fermented with the formation of lactic acid, as well as the trisaccharide, trehalose, and the glucoside, salicin. The fermentation of alcohols is much less marked. Slow acid production takes place in media containing glycol, glycerol, and erythritol; some strains slowly produce acid from mannitol, but there is no action on dulcitol or sorbitol. The pentoses, arabinose and xylose, are slowly attacked (Mair[552]). Zozaya[1586] added levan, obtained from *B. mesentericus* and *B. subtilis,* to the list of substances fermentable by Pneumococcus. Dextran, obtained from *Leuconostoc mesenteroides* was not affected. Although the change in levan was less than that in inulin, the acidity in both cases seemed to be mainly due to lactic acid.

Acid Production

Supplementing the brief mention that has already been made of the formation of acid from saccharides by Pneumococcus, some of the factors that condition that reaction are as follows: The amount of sugar present in the medium determines the degree of acidity attained. If sufficient carbohydrate is present, growth ceases at an acid reaction of pH 5.0. If there is less than 0.4 per cent of sugar, growth ceases at a lower hydrogen ion concentration, apparently because of exhaustion of carbohydrate. If no carbohydrate is present save that extracted from the meat from which the broth is made, growth initiated at pH 7.8 ceases at about pH 7.0. If the reaction of bacteria-free filtrates of plain broth cultures in which growth has ceased is readjusted to pH 7.8 and the medium reinoculated with Pneumococcus, no growth occurs unless carbohydrate is added. However, if bacteria-free filtrates of dextrose-broth cultures in which growth has ceased are readjusted to pH 7.8 and reinoculated with Pneumococcus, growth is resumed. Cultures of Pneumococcus, with maltose, saccharose, lactose, galactose, raffinose, dextrose, and inulin give identical results in the rate of reaction change and the final hydrogen ion concentration (pH 5.0) attained. Such are the conclusions of Avery and Cullen[37] in their 1919 study. Jones,[683] a year later, explained the failure of these authors to produce an acidity greater than a final pH of 7.0 by the fact that they did not add glucose to their beef-infusion medium, but it would seem that this failure had already been accounted for in other parts of their report.

The degree of acid production by pneumococci appeared to Gundel[569] to be correlated with pathogenicity. He grew strains isolated from human mouths in lactose bouillon (pH 7.0) and in this medium noted only a slight acid formation by pathogenic strains, whereas non-pathogenic pneumococci produced marked acidity with transition forms between the extremes. No confirmation of Gundel's results appears to have been published.

The addition of normal human serum to suspensions of living pneumococci in isotonic bouillon, while preventing cell dissolution, does not inhibit acid production (Lord and Nye[834]). In rabbit serum, according to Bordet,[139-40] the pneumococcidal hydrogen ion concentration is pH 6.2 for Types I, II, and III, and here the acidity is due to formic and acetic acids.

Oxidation and Reduction

Pneumococcus, under varying degrees of oxygen tension, manifests the phenomena of oxidation and reduction. With the activities of its oxidases are correlated, either directly or indirectly, synthesis and hydrolysis of pneumococcal protein and carbohydrates, changes in the hydrogen ion concentration, the formation of peroxide, the conversion of hemoglobin into methemoglobin, the lowering of the oxygen capacity of blood cells, and the death of the organism itself.

METHEMOGLOBIN PRODUCTION

In 1913, Butterfield and Peabody,[194] seeking an explanation for the reduction of the O_2 capacity of the blood in human lobar pneumonia, discovered that upon incubating pneumococcal cultures with washed rabbit corpuscles, there ensued a diminution of the oxygen-carrying capacity of the cells, owing to the formation of methemoglobin, or some derivative of hemoglobin with identical optical constants for these regions of the spectrum. The substance which induced this change was also present in sterile filtrates of autolyzed cultures. The authors concluded that the mechanism of the reduction of the O_2-carrying capacity of the blood in human lobar pneumonia was, in part at least, of the same nature. In rabbits with a severe experimental bacteriemia it was found that the O_2-combining power of the venous blood fell progressively up to the time of death. Coincidentally, there was an even more marked fall in the O_2 content of the arterial blood. The changes in the blood of infected animals appeared to be analogous to those seen when Pneumococcus was grown in blood *in vitro*, the oxygen-carrying capacity of the cells in both instances being due to the conversion of hemoglobin into methemoglobin.

In the next year (1914), Cole[253] reported conclusions which, because of their importance, may be summarized here: Pneumococci in contact with hemoglobin transform this substance into methemoglobin, and the reaction occurs only when the pneumococci are living; it is not induced by the culture fluid or by extracts of the bacteria, differing in this respect from the results of Butterfield and Peabody. The reaction does not occur when hemoglobin is added to an emulsion of washed pneumococci in salt solution. However, if minute traces of dextrose be added to the mixture, the transformation occurs quickly. Dextrose may be replaced by any one of a number of other sugars, and also by some organic compounds, if the latter are added in large amounts. Certain other organic substances were unable to replace dextrose, but it was impossible to determine any special molecular configuration upon which this property depends. The formation of methemoglobin by pneumococci probably resembles the changes induced in the blood by such chemical substances as amino phenol. It seems not unlikely that the transformation is always a reaction of oxidation. In the presence of reducing agents, the latter are first oxidized, the action occurring more readily in the presence of oxyhemoglobin. In some instances an alternate oxidation and reduction of the transformative agent occurs, so that the reaction is continuous. The effect of the presence or absence of free O_2 on the changes in blood pigment induced by chemical agents of known composition suggests that the reaction with Pneumococcus follows similar lines. The reaction does not occur in the absence of O_2. If the free O_2 be first removed and then replaced, the reaction takes place more rapidly than if the O_2 had not been removed. The presence of free O_2 in excess slightly delays the reaction, possibly because of the inhibition of the reduction process which forms the first part of the reaction.

In 1924, Morgan and Neill,[916] as a result of their experiments, concluded that:

Sterile filtrates of aerobic cultures of Pneumococci containing H_2O_2, were capable of converting catalase-free solutions of oxyhemoglobin into methemoglobin. In catalase-containing solutions of hemoglobin from laked corpuscles, the actual methemoglobin-forming system of Pneumococcus involves a labile constituent of the bacterial cell, which is itself susceptible to oxidizing agents and may be rendered inactive if exposed to peroxide or similar substances previous to its introduction into oxyhemoglobin solutions. The activity of this function, in the case of sterile filtrates, depends, therefore, upon the liberation of cell constituents into the medium and upon the protection of those cellular substances from the oxidizing agents which are formed when Pneumococcus cultures are freely exposed to air. When these cultural conditions are fulfilled, sterile culture filtrates of Pneumococcus convert oxyhemoglobin into methemoglobin independent of the presence of blood catalase.

In 1921, Stadie,[1311] in studying the blood changes in pneumococcal infections, found that methemoglobin disappeared rapidly from the blood stream, whether introduced by injection or formed within the circulation by pneumococci or by the action of chemicals (potassium ferricyanide and sodium nitrate). He concluded: "In the occasional cases of pneumonia which show a decrease in the oxygen capacity of the blood, the decrease is probably due to the formation of methemoglobin. The latter is removed from the circulation, however, as rapidly as it is formed, so that it can seldom be detected even qualitatively, and is probably never the cause of cyanosis." The practical impossibility of demonstrating methemoglobin in the circulating blood was also experienced by Schnabel.[1239]

The explanation of the phenomenon of methemoglobin production is of importance not only in so far as this special reaction is concerned, but also because it suggests a mechanism by which pathological effects may be produced by bacteria which apparently elaborate no soluble toxin.

PEROXIDE FORMATION

The work of McLeod and Govenlock,[885] of McLeod and Gordon,[881-3] and of McLeod, Gordon, and Pyrah[884] was confirmatory of Cole's results and amplified our knowledge of the property possessed by pneumococci to form peroxide during growth. The authors ascribed the greenish or yellowish discoloration produced on heated blood media to an accumulation of peroxide, showed that the death of pneumococci in cultures was brought about by an excess of the same product, and demonstrated that the substance was not organic peroxide but hydrogen peroxide. It was not formed in cultures deprived of oxygen, nor in cultures that contained abundant catalase.

Penfold[1077] disclosed another manifestation of the oxidizing action of pneumococci. According to him, all pneumococci and probably all streptococci acting on certain aromatic amines, notably aniline, benzidine, and the toluidines, produce pigment. When pneumococcal and streptococcal cultures were grown on citrated horse-blood agar containing benzidine, the colonies appeared black by transmitted light and metallic blue by reflected light with dark discoloration extending far into the medium around the colony. This pigment production from the amines is a peculiarity shared only by pneumococci and streptococci and, according to Penfold, is due to the peroxide produced by these organisms.

In the next year, Felton[395] studied the oxidase reaction of bacteria by means of the oxidation of *p*-amino leuco-malachite green, and found that the conditions most suitable for the reaction were the presence of a slight amount of hemoglobin and of dextrose, an acid reaction, the presence of fresh serum heated for thirty minutes at 56°, and a plentiful supply of oxygen. In order of decreasing suitability for promoting oxidation were rat, guinea pig, rabbit, horse, human, cat, and chicken serum. Of the organisms tested by Felton, only Pneumococcus, *S. viridans*, and *S. haemolyticus* exhibited oxidative power, the first named giving the most intense reaction. That this power was not an exclusive character of the three species was shown in the same year (1923) by McLeod, Gordon, and Pyrah,[884] who added *B. bulgaricus* and *B. acidophilus* to the group of peroxide-producing bacteria.

Directly opposed to the conclusions of McLeod and Gordon and of Cole, but somewhat analogous to those of Felton, were the views of Barnard and Gowen.[80] These two authors discounted the possibility that the green disintegration product of hemoglobin referable to the growth of pneumococci is methemoglobin, since methemoglobin will not exist in the presence of hydrogen peroxide. A green pigment, identical in all respects with that produced by the growth of pneumococci on hemoglobin, was prepared by Barnard and Gowen by the action of peroxide and certain nitrogenous compounds on blood pigment. A chemical study of this artificial green pigment indicated to the authors that it was not methemoglobin but a xanthoprotein compound. Without more complete information it is impossible to judge the correctness of the claim, but studies from the Hospital of the Rockefeller Institute seem to prove the case for methemoglobin. It is, however, possible that the appearance of xanthoprotein may be an additional effect of peroxide.

Avery and his colleagues published a series of papers that materially amplified our knowledge of this phenomenon of peroxide production by bacteria. Avery and Morgan[52] noted the early appearance of peroxide in cultures of pneumococci and of non-hemolytic streptococci, with a somewhat retarded development in cultures of some but not all strains of *S. haemolyticus* and *S. mucosus*. Peroxide was not detected at any time during the growth of two strains of *Staphylococcus aureus*. The factors influencing peroxide formation were free access of air, and the absence of a catalase, peroxidase, or other catalyst capable of decomposing H_2O_2. Under favorable conditions peroxide production continued during the logarithmic phase of growth and persisted for at least six to twelve days. According to Avery and Morgan the aerobic growth of anaerobic bacteria in broth containing sterile, unheated plant tissue may be related to the action of oxidizing-reducing systems of plant tissue in the destruction of toxic peroxides formed during bacterial growth. These assumptions were supported by subsequent experiments by Avery and Neill,[55] in which it was found that anaerobically grown pneumococci rapidly form peroxide on exposure to molecular oxygen. The peroxide-forming properties of pneumococci varied with different strains and with the age of the cells, and were active under conditions of reaction and temperature that did not permit active cell growth and multiplication—a range of pH 5.0 to 8.5—and at lower temperatures than those that favor growth.

Avery and Neill,[56] employing sterile, filtered extracts prepared by freezing and thawing pneumococcal cells or by dissolving them in bile, proved that the peroxide-forming ability of Pneumococcus is a function not dependent upon the presence of living, intact cells. Sterile extracts of unwashed pneumococci promptly formed peroxide on exposure to air; its formation was almost as active in extracts aerated at 2° as in those exposed to air at room temperature. The optimal zone was on the alkaline side of pH 6.0, but peroxide was detectable in the range pH 5.0 to 9.0. The peroxide-forming activity of the cells was gradually diminished by prolonged exposure to 55° and was destroyed by heating for five minutes at 65°. Moreover, cells and extracts of cells thoroughly washed before extraction with salt or phosphate solution showed no peroxide-producing activity, but such extracts could be activated by the addition of cell washings, yeast extract, or muscle infusion.

In a subsequent paper, Avery and Neill[57] reported that sterile broth extracts of unwashed pneumococci, entirely free from living or intact cells, actively reduced methylene blue, whereas sterile extracts of washed pneumococci in phosphate buffer solution were unable by themselves to reduce the dye. As in the case of peroxide formation, the reducing action was restored by the addition of meat infusion or yeast extract to extracts prepared from washed cells. Platt[1097] reported that meat extract augments the amount of peroxide formed as do also lactic acid and glucose. Gelatin, on the contrary, delays its formation, and in gelatin broth no appreciable amounts of peroxide are present until near the end of the period of logarithmic increase of bacteria.

The system or systems responsible for methylene blue reduction are destroyed by exposure to temperatures practically identical with those which had previously been found to destroy the peroxide-forming activity of the same extracts. Avery and Neill[57] suggested that peroxide formation and methylene blue reduction by pneumococcal extracts are functions of the same or closely related systems, the particular reaction induced depending upon whether molecular oxygen or methylene blue serves as hydrogen acceptor or oxygen donator.

In 1930, Hewitt[641] supplied further confirmatory data concerning the phenomena of oxidation and reduction by pneumococci and streptococci. In aerobic cultures of both species there is a rise in potential after the logarithmic phase of growth, while in the case of diphtheria bacilli and staphylococci, the potential remains at a low level long after the cessation of active cell proliferation. In a second paper, Hewitt[642] reported the use of liver, blood, or bacteria in culture media as a means of inhibiting peroxide formation and of permitting the study of other oxidation-reduction phenomena. In aerated cultures under these conditions, the potential fell to much lower levels and growth was much more luxuriant. In similar cultures without catalase the potential first declined, then rose to the level at which peroxide can be detected chemically. In the presence of catalase, however, the potential fell, then rose very slowly, and finally reached the level corresponding to peroxide accumulation only after the effective catalase had been destroyed by the active oxidizing system. If fresh catalase was then added an immediate drop in potential occurred.

Lieb[812] did not agree that the oxidation phenomenon had to do with the formation of hydrogen peroxide but thought that it was due to another mechanism operated by an unknown oxygen-carrying factor, possibly a ferment, acting in the same oxygen concentration as hydrogen peroxide. Such a conclusion would appear to be no more than conjecture.

Pauli's work (1927–8)[1071] was more or less a repetition of that of the American school. He explained the fact that Pneumococcus rapidly undergoes autolysis in cultures by assuming that lysis was due to the production of hydrogen peroxide in the absence of catalase. When he grew pneumococci, respectively, in the presence of air, under an atmospheric pressure of thirty millimeters of mercury, or under complete anaerobic conditions, the cells grew well, but autolysis took place rapidly in the first, slowly in the second, and was still absent in the third after a month's incubation. Pauli ascribed the advantage of adding any of the many growth-stimulating substances to culture media to the content of catalase which decomposes hydrogen peroxide at the time of its formation.

Another effect of the oxidizing agents formed when sterile extracts of pneumococci are exposed to air is the destructive action they exert on the saccharolytic enzymes, sucrase, raffinase, inulase, and amylase, of the cell. Aerated extracts, however, have no inactivating effect on pneumococcal protease or lipase.

The relative resistance of the enzymes of Pneumococcus to heat is consistent with their resistance to the action of hydrogen peroxide. Neill and Avery[953] found, furthermore, that sterile extracts of autolyzed anaerobic cultures of pneumococci contained much higher concentrations of active endocellular enzymes than did filtrates of autolyzed aerobic cultures. The difference may be explained by a destruction of the formed enzymes by oxidative reactions analogous to the destruction observed during oxidation of sterile broth extracts of unwashed pneumococcal cells. The more complete destruction of enzymatic activity in autolyzed aerobic cultures than in oxidized sterile cell extracts is probably due to the longer exposure to oxidation products. More recently Finkle (1931),[440] in a study of the metabolism of pneumococcal variants, confirmed the fact that oxidation may have an inhibitory effect on sugar fermentation. Under anaerobic conditions saccharolysis is approximately the same for organisms of Types I, II, and III, while, under aerobic conditions, only Type I cells are capable of this action. The difference may be explained by the relatively feebler respiratory capacity of Type I organisms. The capacity of these cells is only 56 per cent of that of Type III pneumococci, which in turn is 71 per cent of that of Type II strains.

In a later paper, Neill and Avery[956] reported further details of the oxidation-reduction system of Pneumococcus. The thermostable components of the oxidation-reduction system were still active in oxidized extracts, while the thermolabile cellular constituent was destroyed not only by products formed during oxidation, but also by molecular oxygen itself. The labile component of the system was more susceptible to the action of reagent hydrogen peroxide than any other known intracellular substance of pneumococcal origin. Neill and Avery designated the thermostable substances as

*R*H, the actual source of the oxidizing agents, and the thermolabile cellular constituent as *C*, serving as a catalyst in accelerating the reaction, which they formulated thus:

1) $C + RH + O_2 \rightarrow$ oxidizing agent
2) Oxidizing agent $+ C \rightarrow$ inactive *C*.

*R*H then represents substances that are not present in Pneumococcus after thorough washing; they are relatively stable, resisting boiling for prolonged periods, and are present in water or alcohol extracts of muscle, yeast, and vegetable tissue. *C* represents a labile cellular component, inactivated in ten minutes at 65°. By itself it is non-reactive with O_2 and possesses no reducing power, being apparently catalytic in nature.

Neill[948] observed that both living pneumococci and sterile extracts prepared from unwashed cells were capable of oxidizing hemoglobin to methemoglobin, and that the action was a reversible one, the equilibrium being shifted in either direction by regulation of the oxygen tension. Neill[947] also found quantitative evidence of the reduction of methemoglobin to hemoglobin by sterile animal tissues, such as kidney, testicle, and liver from an exsanguinated rabbit. He concluded, therefore, that "the accumulation of large amounts of methemoglobin in the circulating blood is probably an indication not only of the formation of large amounts of this pigment, but also of a poisoning of the normal reducing mechanism of the animal tissues." This statement is difficult to reconcile with that of Stadie (p. 73, *ante*) that in man, at least, methemoglobin is removed from the circulation as rapidly as it is formed.

In another note, Neill[949] added that in the presence of air the oxidizing activity of pneumococci was much stronger than their reducing activity in the absence of air, while the reverse was true for anaerobic bacteria. From subsequent studies, Neill[950] was able to elaborate the graphic representation of the oxidation-reduction reaction to include the production of methemoglobin:

$$a)\ \begin{cases} \underbrace{C}_{\substack{\text{Thermolabile}\\ \text{cellular}\\ \text{substance}}} + \underbrace{RH}_{\substack{\text{Thermostable}\\ \text{easily oxidized}\\ \text{substance}}} + O_2 \rightarrow \underbrace{ROOH}_{\text{Oxidizing agent}} \\ \text{or} \\ C + 2\,RH + O_2 \rightarrow 2\,R + H_2O_2 \end{cases}$$

$$b)\quad ROOH\ (\text{or } H_2O_2) + \text{Hb} \rightarrow \text{MetHb}$$

For comparison, Neill developed another formula to represent the process of methemoglobin formation during the auto-oxidation of other substances:

$$a)\ \begin{cases} RH + O_2 \rightarrow ROOH \\ 2\,RH + O_2 \rightarrow 2\,R + H_2O_2 \end{cases}$$

$$b)\ ROOH\ (\text{or } H_2O_2) + \text{Hb} \rightarrow \text{MetHb}$$

and for the spontaneous formation of methemoglobin in pure hemoglobin solutions, in which the iron of the hemoglobin may serve as a catalyst, as:

$$\text{Hemoglobin} + \text{x}\ (O_2) \rightarrow \text{Methemoglobin}$$

The reactivation of the bacteriolytic activity of oxidized pneumococcal extracts, according to Neill, Fleming, and Gaspari[958] appears as still another effect of the oxidation-reduction phenomenon. When oxidized and therefore inactive pneumococcal extracts were treated with bacterial reducing agents (anaerobic bacteria), the extracts regained their lytic power, and showed a species-specificity which argues for their identity with the original bacteriolytic agent. It was held that this agent is an integral part of the pneumococcal cell, and that its action is reversible and susceptible of being represented by a graphic formula similar to those already given.

Further evidence concerning the reversibility of the action involved in the transformation of oxyhemoglobin to methemoglobin was supplied by the reports of Schnabel,[1238] and of Schnabel and Ninamiya.[1243] Although few new facts were given in these papers, the authors found that the activity was not lessened by the addition of high concentrations of optochin or sodium glycocholate to broth cultures, while, on the other hand, the alkaline reaction and reducing power of blood serum and of tissue cells interfered with its operation.

Another effect of oxygen consumption by Pneumococcus is the relation between respiration and virulence as described by Sevag and Maiweg,[1258] who presented the following facts in support of their theory: Virulent pneumococci on being transformed into the avirulent forms consume much larger amounts of oxygen than do the parent organisms, but this gain in activity is only temporary. After a time, the avirulent organisms degenerate into forms which consume very much less oxygen than do either the virulent or the avirulent cells recently derived from the parent strain.

The phenomenon of oxidation-reduction by Pneumococcus is given here in considerable detail because of its important bearing on the metabolic process of the cell and because of the thoroughness with which this activity has been studied. It involves the life of Pneumococcus; it affects by inhibition or destruction the lytic and synthetic ferments of the bacterial cell; it is responsible for the conversion of the vitally necessary hemoglobin into methemoglobin and for the lessened oxygen-carrying capacity of the red blood corpuscles; it may play a part in determining virulence of a strain; and it is undoubtedly concerned in the production of hemotoxin and hemolysin and possibly of other substances harmful to the human economy.

Hemolysin and Hemotoxin

Pneumococcus, upon lysis, whether natural, or artificially induced, yields a substance or principle that is actively hemolytic for sheep, guinea pig, and human erythrocytes. The substance is labile, much of its activity is lost on passing through a filter, and it is destroyed by the action of trypsin. In its properties the hemolysin corresponds to the substance contained in the lytic extracts of pneumococci that cause the death of guinea pigs on intravenous injection. Its activity is prevented by the presence of minute amounts of cholesterol. Following the injection of autolysates into rabbits and sheep, the serum of the animal acquires increased power of inhibiting the hemolytic action and therefore Cole (1914),[252] whose conclusions these are, believed that the hemolysin has antigenic properties; that it is not simply a product of autolysis but undoubtedly exists preformed in the pneumococcal cell; it is not given up to the surrounding fluid so long as the bodies of the cocci are intact and, accordingly, is to be considered as a hemolytic endotoxin.

Previous as well as subsequent to the work of Cole, there have been isolated observations of a zone of hemolysis about the colonies of pneumococci on blood agar. Libman,[811] in 1905, demonstrated an organism, probably a pneumococcus, isolated from the blood of a pneumonia patient on the fifth day of the disease, which on blood plates produced a peculiar hemolysis. Later (1922) Hewitt and Famulener[640] described the production of a zone of hemolysis immediately around a colony on blood agar of an organism, beyond doubt a pneumococcus, isolated from the blood in a fatal case of septicemia with meningitis following mastoiditis. From their study, Hewitt and Famulener inferred that pneumococci of all serological groups, under certain cultural conditions, may hemolyze human erythrocytes, and that this property apparently is not influenced by the reaction of the medium within the growth limits of the organism nor by prolonged refrigeration of the developed colonies on blood-agar plates. The authors also expressed the opinion, later substantiated by Avery and Neill, that the hemolysin was an intracellular product liberated from the autolyzed organisms, which diffuses from the colony into the surrounding blood agar. In contradistinction to the hemolysis of *Streptococcus haemolyticus*, Hewitt and Famulener called the pneumococcal effect "pseudo-hemolysis."

Takami[1372] described a zone of hemolysis about the colonies of all the sixty strains of pneumococci plated on blood agar. This zone was separated from the periphery of the colony by a greenish zone; it appeared on standing at room or ice-box temperature and in time might spread over the whole plate.

Avery and Neill[58] made further studies on this property of Pneumococcus. Extracts of pneumococci prepared in broth, or from washed pneumococci made with phosphate solution and filtered through Berkefeld candles, were actively hemolytic for rabbit erythrocytes. The hemolysin was destroyed by ten minutes' heating at 55°. The conclusions of the authors were:

> When pneumococcus extracts are exposed to air, the hemotoxin is destroyed only in those extracts capable of undergoing auto-oxidation. The active agent responsible for this destruction is probably a peroxide formed by the union of molecular oxygen with some other easily oxidizable constituents of the extracts.

In another study, Neill[951] mixed pneumococcal extracts, in which the hemotoxin had previously been inactivated by oxidation, with *B. coli* and anaerobic *Bacillus T*, sealed and incubated the extracts thus treated for several hours. Titration of the bacteria-free supernatant fluid obtained by centrifuging this mixture showed that the inactive oxidation product of pneumococcal hemotoxin was reconverted to an actively hemolytic substance by the action of those bacteria, which were not themselves hemolytic. The reduction was also accomplished by sodium hyposulfite. The active lysin, or hemotoxin, produced by the reduction of the inactive oxidized extracts was shown to be identical with the original active hemotoxin, since it possessed the same degree of thermolability and was neutralized by the same specific antibody. Pneumococcal hemolysin or hemotoxin is, therefore, not an artificial cleavage product but a natural substance originating within the cell. Normal serum, egg albumen, cholesterol, and peptone, according to Weiss,[1509] inhibit hemolytic activity.

Returning to the original observation of Cole that active or reduced pneumococcal hemotoxin is antigenic, Neill[952] in 1927 reported that "a neutralizing antibody may be produced by immunization with the hemolytically inactive hemotoxin present in oxidized solutions as well as by immunization with the active toxin. The antibody is a species-specific antihemotoxin neutralizing the hemotoxin from all types of pneumococci." Neill also showed that the hemotoxin is independent of the bacteriolytic enzyme present in pneumococcal cells. In the next year, Cotoni and Chambrin[282] confirmed the data reported by Cole and by Avery and Neill, and described a simple method for the quantitative measurement of the hemolytic power of Pneumococcus. While Cotoni and Chambrin were able to make satisfactory determinations on a number of strains, they reported that the quantity of hemoglobin liberated did not follow the law of multiple proportions and that strains varied in their hemolytic action. To the authors there appeared to be no difference in the susceptibility of the blood cells of man, rabbit, guinea pig, cow, pig, horse, or sheep to pneumococcal hemolysin. They also gave a method for titrating the antihemolytic power of immune serum.

Sickles and Coffey[1280] published a paper on a hemolytic substance in pneumococcal culture broth. No proof was presented that this substance is not the same as the hemolysin already discussed, but Sickles and Coffey, like Neill, and Cotoni and Chambrin, found that pneumococcal immune serum had a marked inhibitory effect on hemolysis, giving complete inhibition in a 1 to 1,000 dilution, whereas normal horse serum was effective only in a 1 to 400 dilution.

The belief of Cole and his associates that hemolysin is an intracellular constituent of Pneumococcus was not shared by Cowan.[287] On the contrary, this author stated positively that the principle is extracellular and arises during the growth of the organism in fluid media. Its highest titer occurred immediately after the maximal period of multiplication—phase of logarithmic growth—while the curves of hemolytic titer and growth seemed to Cowan to denote that hemolysin production was not essentially the result of autolysis. Hemolytic power diminished in old cultures, due to oxidation, but could be restored by reducing agents. The hemolysin was not type-specific nor was it related to virulence. It filtered readily, was rapidly destroyed at 56°, was antigenic, and was produced by all but two of twenty-eight strains. The observation that the substance appears in broth cultures agrees with that of Sickles and Coffey, but it would seem that Cowan had not sufficiently ruled out the factors of autolysis to justify the conclusion that the hemolysin is extracellular in origin.

While Neill[952] found that pneumo-antihemolysin was without effect on the hemotoxins of tetanus and Welch bacilli, Todd[1412] reported that he was able, to a certain extent, to neutralize pneumococcal hemolysin and tetanolysin with the serum of horses hyperimmunized against streptococci, the action being ascribable to the content of highly active antistreptolysin in the immune serum. Todd added that the degree of neutralization was not necessarily correlated with the antistreptolytic titer and that the different hemolysins were distinguishable by quantitative serological methods. This partial antigenic overlapping of hemolysins could only be demonstrated by the use of hyperimmune serum.

Purpura Production

Somewhat analogous to the effects of the hemolysin and hemotoxin produced by Pneumococcus, but probably not a direct consequence of their action, is the purpuric condition seen in both natural and experimental pneumococcal infections. Claude[236] in 1896 was among the first to note the occurrence of purpura in an infant dying of pneumonia. The lesions tended to have black central nodes leading to ulcerative necrosis. But, more important still, the causal relation between Pneumococcus and purpura was demonstrated by the isolation by Claude of pneumococci both from the blood and from the center of the purpuric lesions. A similar case was that described by Morse[931] in 1898, in which purpura accompanied a general pneumococcal infection in a twelve-month-old girl.

A case somewhat similar to Claude's was reported in 1914 by Rolland and Buc.[1154] The patient was an infant dying of a pneumococcal meningitis without lung involvement. Necropsy revealed intense visceral purpura, and cultures taken post mortem from the meningeal pus and from serous fluid in the purpuric lesions yielded pneumococci identical with a strain isolated from the blood during life. Reh[1123] described the case of an infant with bluish-red discoloration of the right side, left elbow, and the four extremities. Bacteriological tests showed that the infection was caused by pneumococci.

Purpura, therefore, is an occasional concomitant of pneumococcal infections, and the three cases cited are sufficient to illustrate the similarity between this change in the blood with the accompanying capillary permeability and the hemotoxic effects of Pneumococcus. The experimental facts are more pertinent to the present discussion.

In 1899, Carnot[199] observed the development of a *teinte violacée* in the nose and ears of a rabbit injected with a pneumococcal "toxin." No details of the preparation of the toxin were given but Carnot stated that it was sterile. It is probable that he employed cell-free broth cultures as did Heyrovsky.[644] The latter, by injecting culture filtrates into white mice, induced hemorrhagic dermatoses and hemorrhages of the mucous membranes and other tissues. The condition was severe and affected the internal organs as well as the skin.

Julianelle and Reimann[694] quoted Neill as having observed hemorrhagic purpura in white mice injected with an extract of Pneumococcus. The authors, by injecting extracts of both virulent and avirulent strains into white mice induced a purpuric condition manifested after four to six hours as a dark-blue discoloration of the skin of the feet, tail, ears, snout, and genitals. Unless the amount of extract was large there was no intoxication and the animals recovered. The lesions reached maximal intensity within twenty-four to forty-eight hours and disappeared in five to seven days. Extracts prepared by the Avery-Neill method were more potent than filtrates of pneumococcal cultures. Neither cultures younger than eight to sixteen hours nor those that were very old were active. Whole, unfiltered cultures rarely caused a reaction, while bile-dissolved cultures produced no purpura, although bile was shown not to inhibit this activity. The extracts induced purpura in rabbits and guinea pigs as well as in white mice. Extracts of *Staphylococcus aureus*, *Streptococcus viridans* and *B. coli* did not exhibit this property.

The purpura-producing principle withstands heating to 100° for ten minutes; it resists oxidation; it is filter-passing; its activity is destroyed by digestion with trypsin; and the substance can be obtained from pneumococcal extracts by full saturation with ammonium sulfate after the acetic acid-precipitable substances have been removed. The principle is common to various pneumococci and apparently bears no relation to virulence, nor is it associated with the hemotoxin of Pneumococcus, since the hemolytic activity of an extract may be destroyed without affecting the purpurigenic property.

Julianelle and Reimann concluded that the substance is a degradation product of Pneumococcus. The authors had in previous studies of experimental purpura found that excessive diminution of blood platelets, due either to direct destruction of the cells or damage to the seat of their origin, was a causative factor. In another paper, Reimann and Julianelle[1130] reported variations in the number of blood platelets in white mice injected with pneumococcal extracts. The platelets were greatly diminished after injection, the greatest decrease taking place after twenty-four hours. With a count of less than 500,000 platelets per cubic millimeter of blood, the mice usually developed purpura. A regeneration—an over-regeneration—was accomplished by the fourth to the ninth day, with a return to normal in about two weeks. The red cells were also greatly reduced in number, but the rate of destruction and regeneration was somewhat slower than that of the platelets, while leucocytes were slightly, if at all, affected. Reimann and Julianelle emphasized the differences between the hemolysin and the purpurigenic principle in pneumococcal extracts. Both the thrombolytic and hemolytic properties were destroyed by heating *in vitro*, although such heated extracts still were able to produce purpura but not a severe anemia in mice. Extracts adsorbed with either blood platelets or erythrocytes showed a marked diminution in thrombolytic and hemolytic activity *in vitro*. Adsorbed extracts, however, caused purpura as well as severe anemia and thrombopenia in mice.

In a further study, Julianelle and Reimann[695] offered the following additional conclusions:

> The purpura-producing principle of Pneumococcus is non-antigenic in the sense that it does not stimulate the formation of antibodies; white mice acquire an increased resistance to purpura as a result of repeated injections of toxic doses of the purpura substance; the serum of rabbits immunized with the purified purpura principle, with smooth and rough strains of Pneumococcus or with cell extracts, autolysates or the nucleoprotein fraction of the organism, does not confer upon white mice protection against purpura; the purpura principle does not exist preformed in the cell, but is rather an autolytic derivative, since it is formed only when pneumococci undergo autolysis, and it is not found when the autolytic ferments are inactivated; the purpura substance is associated with the proteose fraction of active pneumococcus extracts.

Pittman and Falk,[1092] still more recently, substantiated the results of Julianelle and Reimann by causing purpura in white mice with extracts of pneumococci made by alternate freezing and thawing. This extract also protected mice against an infection with pneumococci of low virulence when the extract was injected twenty-four hours prior to inoculation, but when both extract and culture were given simultaneously death ensued. The effect has some resemblances to the action of Bails' aggressin. The strange selective affinity of bacterial proteins for blood cells reminds one of the hemagglutinative action of some vegetable proteins, especially the globulins and the proteoses of beans.

Mair,[856] differing from Julianelle and Reimann, believed that the purpura-producing principle was an intracellular substance and that the cell must be disintegrated by autolysis or other means before the active substance could be absorbed in sufficient amount to produce purpura. Another difference reported by Mair was the accelerating action of the pure bile-salts, sodium desoxycholate or sodium choleate, in releasing the purpurigenic principle. By running parallel experiments with untreated pneumococcal suspensions, some bile-treated and others containing sodium desoxycholate, Mair obtained equally good reactions. He inferred from his experiments that:

> It may be that solution of the bacterial bodies is all that is required, a preformed constituent of the cell thus being set free and rendered capable of absorption from the peritoneal cavity of the mouse. On the other hand, the delayed reactions obtained with pneumococci which had been subject only to slight autolysis, and with pneumococci dissolved in bile and immediately heated, suggest the possibility that proteolytic changes which may occur in the body of the mouse are required for the development of the substance.

Moreover, Mair found that mice varied in susceptibility to the purpura-producing substance or, perhaps, in their ability to effect proteolytic changes in the substance. By selecting for breeding mice that were sensitive to the purpura reaction, Mair discovered that this trait was hereditary, and developed a strain of mice with increased susceptibility.

That the purpura-producing principle might be associated with the carbohydrate constituents of Pneumococcus was claimed by Wadsworth and Brown[1468] and by Sickles and Shaw.[1283] The injection of the cellular carbohydrate intravenously, intraperitoneally, or subcutaneously into mice induced a purpuric condition. Notwithstanding these observations, there is a reason to believe that the effects are ascribable to small amounts of degraded protein in the preparations of cellular carbohydrate. This substance, whatever might have been its nature, in addition to being heat-stable, was neutralized by Type I antipneumococcic serum even when the latter had been adsorbed with either the homologous soluble specific substance or the cellular carbohydrate. Sickles and Shaw reported that this purpura-producing activity of the polysaccharide was destroyed when the carbohydrate was subjected to the action of its appropriate carbohydrate-decomposing enzyme, but there is no evidence to be found in the communication that the presence of proteolytic ferments in the enzymatic extract had been excluded.

The weight of evidence favors the view that the substance responsible for the purpuric manifestations is a cleavage product of pneumococcal protein, arising in the lysis of the bacterial cell and that purpura production is not a property of any of the components of Pneumococcus as they exist in the normal bacterial cell.

Virulin, Leucocidin, and Analogous Substances

Poisoning and dissolution of red blood corpuscles and the elaboration of purpurigenic substances are not the only ways in which Pneumococcus attacks body tissues. Saline extracts of the coccus, prepared by Rosenow's method, were reported by Pittman and Falk[1092] to decrease phagocytosis of avirulent organisms, to reduce the opsonic content of serum, and only slightly to increase the virulence of a borderline culture after it had been transferred several times in the presence of the extract. The extracts failed to influence the virulence of an avirulent Pneumococcus. The principle contained in the extract, prepared by incubating dense suspensions of pneumococci in small volumes of isotonic sodium chloride solution with subsequent heating and centrifuging, the authors named "Virulin." Considering the feeble action of the substance in raising the virulence of pneumococci, the name would seem to be too specific a designation for an unidentified substance.

Another toxic principle of Pneumococcus is the "Leucocidin" described by Oram,[1032] who reported that in actively growing cultures of Pneumococcus a toxin was produced that, as demonstrated by the Neisser and Wechsberg method, destroyed leucocytes. Leucocidin was present in aerobic and anaerobic cultures of both virulent and avirulent strains of Types I, II, and III. It was easily oxidized, but was not injured by exposure to 70° for one hour. The toxin in the preparation was not destroyed by evaporation in a vacuum at 5°, and its action could be enhanced three to four times by the addition to the culture of laked red blood cells. Apparently the same cultural conditions governed the production and preservation of both the hemotoxin and leucocidin, although the latter was distinguishable by its greater thermostability and its appearance in cultures where no hemotoxin could be demonstrated. The filtrates containing active leucocidin were not toxic for mice in two cubic centimeter amounts injected intraperitoneally, and repeated doses of the filtrate gave only slight protection. Simultaneous injections of the extract and avirulent pneumococci did not raise the virulence of the strain, so that the leucocidin does not share this alleged action of the so-called virulin. Sterile supernatant fluids of phenolized exudates of rabbits with empyema, while in themselves not toxic, upon repeated intravenous injection produced an antileucocidin. Normal rabbit serum did not neutralize the pneumococcal leucocidin, whereas the majority of human serums tested possessed neutralizing properties.

One more morbid effect elicited by pneumococcal extracts or autolysates deserves attention and that is the necrotizing principle reported by Parker.[1059-60] This principle is a filtrable substance, is extremely thermolabile, is sensitive to oxidation, and can be separated from hemotoxin by adsorption with red blood cells, since the necrosis-producing principle remains unaffected after removal of the hemotoxin. The necrotizing substance or substances obtained from both Types I and II pneumococci are neutralized by Type I antipneumococcic serum, and hence the necrotizing substance is not type-specific.

The virulin, leucocidin, and, to coin a name, the necrotin have been described in some detail as representing one of the recent trends in the investigation of Pneumococcus and to draw attention to still unstudied possibilities of this remarkable cell and its properties.

So-Called Toxins

The severe intoxication that so frequently accompanies pneumococcal disease naturally led early investigators to search for a soluble toxin. Profoundly impressed, as they must have been, by the discoveries by von Behring and Kitasato and by Roux of diphtheria and tetanus toxins and of the dramatic efficacy of the corresponding antitoxins, there came a vision of a new and similar agent for the treatment of pneumonia.

Foà,[458] in 1890, thought that he had found a poison in pneumococcal cultures. He isolated the supposed principle by precipitation with ammonium sulfate, dialysis, and subsequent concentration. The extract thus prepared produced marked biological changes in rabbits, but failed to kill the animals. Repeated injections raised the resistance of the test animals to later inoculation with a virulent culture, but it seems safe to infer that Foà was merely dealing with the deleterious degradation or lytic products of Pneumococcus. In the next year, Bonome[137] succeeded in preparing filtrates that were lethal for rabbits. The toxicity was directly related to the virulence of the culture, and the more poisonous extracts, after repeated doses given subcutaneously, intravenously, and intraperitoneally, rendered rabbits resistant to infection. But the subsequent effects were neither toxic nor antitoxic in the true sense of the terms. Issaeff,[673] at the Pasteur Institute, reported similar experiments with comparable results. The serum of rabbits treated with broth cultures of low toxicity possessed therapeutic but no antitoxic power. Issaeff, therefore, had not demonstrated the existence of a toxin. Bunzl-Federn[186] also tested in a similar way heated broth cultures but found that their toxicity and antigenicity were feeble. Cole[250] was able to elicit more severe and fatal toxic or poisonous effects with saline extracts and bile solutions of pneumococci. The intravenous injection of the latter materials into guinea pigs initiated a train of symptoms terminating in a type of death resembling that seen in acute anaphylaxis.

In the same year, Rosenow[1166] published a series of four papers, in which he described observations similar to those of Cole, accompanied by an explanation of the observed phenomena. In the first article Rosenow reported that a single injection of saline autolysates of Pneumococcus, Pneumococcus-leucocyte mixtures, pneumococcal exudates, and mixtures of the organism with normal or immune serum, all produced identical symptoms in normal guinea pigs, and that the symptoms were those of acute anaphylaxis. The serum of animals sensitized to Pneumococcus when allowed to act on the organisms produced this toxic substance more rapidly than did normal serum, and this toxin production as measured by the polariscope was accompanied by a more rapid proteolysis. Morphine, ether, urethan, atropin, and adrenalin protected normal guinea pigs against the poisonous action of the preparations just as they protected sensitive pigs on re-injection. Rosenow's conclusions are significant:

> The behavior of normal and sensitized guinea pigs toward unautolyzed extracts of pneumococci, which are non-toxic to the former and very toxic to the latter, toward partially autolyzed extracts which are very toxic to the former, and slightly or not at all to the latter, and toward more completely autolyzed extracts, which are non-toxic to both, speaks strongly in favor of the view of a rapid parenteral digestion into toxic cleavage products in sensitized animals.

He added that the cleavage products formed *in vivo* were identical with the toxic substances obtained *in vitro*, and that the appearance and disappearance of toxicity seemed to be definitely related to proteolysis. Rosenow also reported that a single intravenous injection of non-fatal doses of extracts before they had become toxic, or while highly toxic, and especially after the toxic stage had been passed, or of autolyzed pneumococci, rendered guinea pigs insusceptible to subsequent injections of toxic pneumococcal autolysates. Although the duration of this protection was not mentioned, the statements point to a refractory state or temporary tolerance so characteristic of degraded proteins and not to an immune condition.

In a second communication, Rosenow[1167] described other characters and properties of the poisonous substance. It was destroyed when the clear autolysate was heated for twenty minutes at 60°, as well as by weak solutions of hydrochloric acid; it was adsorbed by animal charcoal from which it could be recovered by ether. From its chemical behavior the author decided that the toxin was probably a base containing amino groups. He concluded by saying, "Indications have been obtained showing that during pneumococcus infections toxic substances are produced which do not call forth any immunizing response."

In a third paper, Rosenow[1168] ascribed the production of the toxic material to the action of a proteolytic enzyme present in extracts and autolysates of the pneumococcal cell, and in a concluding report[1169] described the action of various pneumococcal products on dogs. The symptoms and lesions were strikingly like those observed in immediate canine anaphylactic shock. The hemorrhages, especially those in the intestines, the effect on the respiration, the extreme degree of cyanosis, the delayed coagulation of the blood, and the presence of carbon dioxide in the stomach indicated to Rosenow that the chief effects of the toxic substances were due to an interference with normal oxidative processes. The action of the autolysates closely resembled that of protein cleavage products and, according to Rosenow's view, it made no essential difference whether the poisonous substances were formed *in vitro*, in the consolidated lung in man, or at once in sensitized dogs, since they were all of the same general nature and their effects differed only in degree and not in kind.

The anaphylactoid shock seen after the intravenous injection of pneumococcal extracts into guinea pigs has also been reported by

Weiss,[1509] who obtained an analogous reaction in rabbits. He saw no parallelism between the toxicity and hemolytic power of the extracts, nor any neutralizing action by antipneumococcic serum. Weiss, like Rosenow, found a similar toxic principle in lung exudates of patients suffering from acute lobar pneumonia. Clough's[241] paper (1915) contained similar observations. In the same year, Boehncke and Mouriz-Riesgo[134] failed to isolate the toxic substance from young cultures or from sodium taurocholate solutions of virulent strains. Contrary to earlier reports, these two authors found that the serum of rabbits treated with these preparations displayed antitoxic action but did not affect the infective process. There followed a paper by Weiss[1509] on "Pneumotoxin," in which he repeated Cole's observations on the anaphylactoid reaction caused by sodium choleate solutions of living, virulent, washed pneumococci. The description of the properties of the preparations agrees with previous accounts of the characters of pneumococcal hemotoxin.

Chesney and Hodges[221] departed from the idea that the intoxication in pneumonia was due to a toxin, believing that it was more reasonable to associate the phenomenon with the growth of the organisms, rather than with their death and dissolution. The authors' attempts to detect toxic substances in fluid cultures of pneumococci during the period of active growth proved entirely negative.

The demonstration of a toxin was claimed by Olson[1029] who experimented with sterile sodium ricinoleate solutions of pneumococci. He also claimed that the intraperitoneal injection of such preparations produced cutaneous reactions in animals and caused clinical and pathological symptoms of pneumonia. An antiserum against this substance appeared to prevent to a high degree both pulmonary and cutaneous reactions. Olson stated without qualifications that a toxin had been demonstrated, that the action of the immune serum was antitoxic, and that "indications are that the toxin may be of value in the production of active immunity to pneumococcus infections." In the light of later events this claim and hope would seem to be premature. Larson,[787] with pneumococcal filtrates supplied by Olson, found the same congestion of the lungs in white mice injected intraperitoneally. Of skin tests performed with the filtrates, those on pneumonia convalescents were of possible significance in being uniformly negative. Larson voiced the same conviction that the filtrates contained a soluble toxin.

In a second paper, Olson,[1030] after describing the lesions produced by pneumococcal filtrates in mice, went so far as to say that the toxin was an exotoxin and not an autolytic product or endotoxin, and gave as his reason that eight-hour culture filtrates possessed marked toxicity but contained little hemotoxin. The toxic principle was relatively thermostable, but was completely destroyed by boiling for one hour. While unpreserved lots lost activity, 0.3 per cent cresol served to maintain the toxicity for several months regardless of the temperature. Active immunization of mice by serial injections of the toxin resulted in protection against 1,000 to 10,000 fatal doses of pneumococci, while the specificity of the immunity induced bore no relation to the serological type of the organism from which the so-called toxin was obtained. The stability of the toxic principle in the presence of heat, the stabilizing action of cresol, and the lack of specificity are, as we know, characters not shared by true exotoxins.

The report of Parker and Pappenheimer[1063] takes us back to the toxic action of autolysates. Solutions were prepared by allowing a suspension of pneumococci, sealed in tubes under vaseline, to stand in the dark at 22° to 24° for two to five days and then in the ice-box. The autolysates were centrifuged in the cold, the seals opened, and the clear supernatant fluid passed through a well-iced Berkefeld filter. The filtrate injected intratracheally in a dose of 0.2 cubic centimeters was highly toxic for guinea pigs, death taking place either within a few hours or within three days. In animals succumbing early, there was intense hemorrhagic edema of the lungs with beginning inflammatory reaction; in animals surviving for eighteen hours or longer, extensive areas of pneumonia were found. As a control, the authors made intratracheal injections of living, virulent pneumococci which were followed by a transient, slight lesion and recovery, or later by death from septicemia without pneumonic lesions. The addition, however, of a sublethal dose of toxic autolysate to the living pneumococci altered the reaction of the animal so that an extensive pneumonia developed associated with unrestrained multiplication of the organism. This synergistic property was far more pronounced than that of the virulin of Pittman and Falk and was more like that of an aggressin.

Yamamoto (1929)[1557] listed unheated pneumococcal filtrate, heated filtrate, and "standard pneumococcus vaccine" (?) according to toxicity in a ratio of 1 to 2 to 6, but none of the three was notably toxic, not less than 6.0 cubic centimeters of the last-named preparation being required to kill a rabbit.

In 1929, Parker[1060] returned to a study of the necrotizing substance of Pneumococcus in comparison with the lung-toxic principles in autolysates. She found both substances to be sensitive to heat and to oxidation, and both were neutralized by the same anti-autolysate serums. The lung-toxic principle, however, was absorbed or inactivated by red blood cells, whereas the necrotizing principle was not. In the discussion, Parker wrote:

> Since pneumococcus hemotoxin is present in the anaerobic autolysate and is also absorbed by red cells, it seemed possible that it was this substance in the autolysates which caused the diffuse lung lesions and death of guinea pigs. However, it was found that the intratracheal injection of pneumococcus hemotoxin prepared by the method of Avery and Neill only occasionally produced the characteristic reaction caused by the intratracheal injection of the anaerobic autolysates. From these experiments we believe, therefore, that the necrotizing and lung-toxic principles, and probably the pneumococcus hemotoxin also, are all separate entities in the anaerobically produced autolysates described.

Pittman and Southwick[1093] were also attracted by this problem. In their experiments, the injection into mice of extracts produced by repeatedly freezing and thawing pneumococci was followed by marked hemorrhagic lesions on all or a part of the external surface that was free from hair, and at necropsy hemorrhagic areas could be found in practically every tissue of the mouse. The adjuvant action of the extract was seen when mice, dying after injection with extract followed several hours later by culture inoculation, developed more marked hemorrhagic lesions than any other group of mice studied. Fresh filtrates of virulent pneumococci produced slight pathological reactions in mice but, when the filtrates were injected with a culture of low virulence, 71 per cent of the mice at necropsy showed a fibrino-purulent pleuritis. The results might be interpreted as pointing to the production of an aggressin-like substance in the early stages of pneumococcal growth with the development of a more violent poison as growth continues and the cells undergo autolysis.

Jamieson and Powell[676] also described a skin-reacting substance in pneumococci. To them its properties were comparable to those of the toxins of some streptococci. The alleged success in developing a neutralizing antiserum led the authors to believe that the present type of antibacterial immune serum would be more valuable if it contained these antiskin-toxic elements. Sabin (1931),[1203] investigating the part anaerobic autolysates of Pneumococcus play in the course of natural infection, came to conclusions diametrically opposed to those of Parker and the other students sharing her ideas. Sabin wrote: "The only conclusion that may be drawn, however, is that the anaerobically produced toxins probably do not play any part in the causation of death of mice infected with very large doses of pneumococci." The failure of "antipneumotoxic" serum to modify the course of pneumococcal infection led Sabin to conclude that: "It seems fair to assume that the anaerobically produced toxins are probably products primarily of the enzymatic changes occurring in *in vitro* autolysis, and play no part in natural infections." The idea of producing an immune serum capable of neutralizing the poisonous principles of Pneumococcus still persists. Coca,[246] after continuing the investigation of the toxic principle in Pneumococcus, announced additional data in 1936. When the pneumococcal cultures were grown in the presence of oxygen a toxic substance was formed but it was devoid of antigenic properties. When, however, carbon dioxide was supplied to the growing cultures, the sterile filtrates were not only toxic but antigenic. According to Coca, the pyrogenic toxin seemed to be type-specific and was not the same as the type-specific polysaccharide. Evidence was presented purporting to show that the injection of the toxic filtrates into the human body or pneumococcal disease in human subjects provoked neutralizing substances in the serum for filtrates of the homologous type, which the author believed were specific antitoxins.

A careful reading of original papers dealing with the subject of toxin production by Pneumococcus fails to bring conviction that the substances or extracts described should be looked upon as true soluble toxins. The principle involved in their formation or preparation, that is, disintegration of the pneumococcal cell by self-proteolysis, bile solution, or freezing and thawing; the nature of the local and systemic reactions the materials evoke; the acute anaphylactoid death produced in guinea pigs; and the feeble antigenic powers, all argue for the classification of the so-called toxins with the proteins of smaller molecular size formed in the hydrolysis of whole proteins. One has only to recall the work of Vaughan[1447] and of others on the effects of the cleavage products of bacterial and of pure proteins, and the many studies on proteoses and peptones, to be impressed by the similarity between the alleged pneumococcal toxins arising from the autodigestion of the somatic protein of Pneumococcus and protein poisons. The slight antigenic power of the pneumococcal derivatives and their seeming lack of specificity is easily explained when one remembers that the hydrolysis of proteins is not always an orderly, step-by-step process. Along with the formation of proteoses and peptones, or polypeptids and amino acids there may be traces of proteins of larger molecular size, even to whole unsplit proteins, remaining in digestion mixtures. Traces of intact proteins acting as antigens may be responsible for the weak neutralizing power of the serum of animals treated with extracts, filtrates, and autolysates of Pneumococcus or, what is more probable, such feeble and transient resistance as these antigens induce is merely the tolerance established by degraded proteins and not immunity.

While it is possible that a true toxin may be a constituent of the pneumococcal cell or a product of its metabolic processes, until more convincing evidence is presented, it would seem reasonable to look upon these so-called "toxic" effects as being referable to the action of bacterial protein poisons.

Summary

It may assist the reader to gain a clearer conception of the relation of the biochemical phenomena manifested by this bacterial cell to the morbid processes induced by the living organism to select from the mass of data the more significant discoveries and to weave them together into a summary. Pneumococcus is a fragile body and contains within itself enzymatic forces that lead to its disruption and disintegration, rob the substrate in which it lives of nutrient substances, and from these substances evolve chemical agents that arrest further growth, cause the death of the organism, and affect the cells of the animal body into which the microbe may find its way.

Intracellular proteases break down the proteins of the cell and of the substrate upon which the cell feeds into smaller fragments, which in turn are still further reduced in size by the same ferment or possibly by a peptidase. This proteolysis reduces the food supply in the medium, and the products of the digestive action may induce purpura and cause other more or less violent toxic effects in the animal host. The poisonous principles, as far as can be learned, are not true toxins, but resemble degraded proteins in their physiological action. Pneumococcus is also endowed with saccharolytic enzymes, capable of attacking starch, inulin, and glycogen; invertases that convert complex saccharides into simpler sugars, and other ferments that split these sugars into acids, while the acid so formed arrests further proliferation of the bacterial cell. Intracellular lipids are converted into fatty acids by pneumococcal lipases and therefore the self-destruction of the cell may be complete. Furthermore, the ingredients of the medium in which the organisms grow are largely replaced by a new order of constituents. The action of all these enzymes may be reversible and by their action or that of some similar agents Pneumococcus is able to build protein, lipids, and somatic and capsular polysaccharides from substances present in the substrate.

In the operation of these vital processes, oxygen plays an important part. The element is essential to the hydrolysis and synthesis of protein, lipid, and sugar but it may act in a variety of ways. Some of the products of oxidation are inimical to the normal functioning of the bacterial cell and some affect changes in the respiratory mechanism of the blood. Pneumococcus utilizes oxygen to form peroxide that is toxic to the cell. Peroxide destroys the labile constituents of the pneumococcal cell, which with the easily oxidizable intracellular substance continue to form an oxidizing substance responsible for the conversion of oxyhemoglobin into methemoglobin.

Pneumococcus, therefore, by the action of its intrinsic enzymes may destroy itself and by the operation of its oxidation-reduction system and its extracellular derivatives or products may, through the dissolution of red cells, the conversion of oxyhemoglobin into methemoglobin, and the lowering of oxygen capacity of the blood, wreak serious damage to the tissues and pervert the normal physiological functions of the body of the infected host.

CHAPTER IV

CLASSIFICATION OF PNEUMOCOCCI

The separation of the members of the species into specific types by immunological reactions, with a description of methods for the determination of these serologically specific types.

By tinctorial and cultural methods it is a relatively simple task to differentiate pneumococci from other bacterial species but it is impossible by these methods, except in the case of Type III organisms, to distinguish pneumococci of one serological type from those of another.

The lance-shaped form, with the presence or development of a capsule, and the appearance of the colonies on blood agar, with their zone of greenish discoloration, are presumptive signs of the identity of these cocci. Solubility in bile, fermentation of inulin, marked pathogenicity for mice and rabbits, and sensitiveness to optochin are all characters which make possible a positive identification of the species. The possession of these characters has definitely placed the former bile-soluble *Streptococcus mucosus* among the pneumococci, and its mucoid growth, thick capsule, and greater virulence serve to separate it from pneumococci of some of the other types. However, it is by their serum reactions that the separation of pneumococci into definite immunological types has been accomplished.

Serological Classification: 1898–1932

It was undoubtedly Bezançon and Griffon[108-10] who, in 1897, were the first to report a discovery that later was to establish differences in the serological behavior of pneumococci as a basis for an invaluable aid in all phases of research on Pneumococcus. While Metchnikoff[894] and later Mosny[933] had previously observed the agglutinative action of antipneumococcic serum, it was Bezançon and

Griffon who announced that from the standpoint of agglutination there existed several races of pneumococci that behaved serologically as though they were different microbes.

At about the same time, Mennes (1897),[893] with a highly potent serum prepared by the immunization of goats and horses with a single strain of Pneumococcus, was able to demonstrate wide agglutinative coverage for other strains irrespective of their origin, whether from cases of pneumonia or from normal mouths. Kindborg* took the view that pneumococcal antibodies, whether agglutinins or protective antibodies, were strictly strain-specific. Two years later, Eyre and Washbourn[376] confirmed Bezançon and Griffon's discovery by means of another immunological reaction. When they tested the protective action of a specific immune serum against five strains of pneumococci, they obtained excellent protection in mice against four of the strains, but none against the fifth. From the experience, the authors concluded, "There exist varieties of pneumococci which at present are only distinguished by the action of antipneumococcic serum."

In the next year, Bezançon and Griffon,[113] continuing their study of the agglutination reaction, noted that the serum of a pneumonia patient was most active against the particular strain causing the infection. Among the experimental data was included the description of a strain that must have been a Type III pneumococcus, since its unusually large capsule and the white, viscous peritoneal exudate it caused in white mice were characteristic of that type. The authors said that the strain was also distinctive in its serum reactions, but unfortunately did not specify in what respect. In a separate paper a year later (1901), Eyre[371] reported that agglutinability of pneumococci depended upon an optimal reaction of the medium in which the organisms were grown. This observation was partly confirmed by Yoshioka[1564] in 1923.

The contribution of Collins (1905)[270] to the serological differentiation of pneumococci seems to have been overlooked by some

* Quoted by Neufeld and Schnitzer.

authors and reviewers. She prepared agglutinative serum by immunizing rabbits with repeated doses, first of killed, then of living, and finally of killed broth cultures of pneumococci. The strain used as an antigen must have belonged to a type other than I or II, since the serum agglutinated only a few of the seventy strains tested. Collins' results may be summarized as follows: Pneumococci by reason of their agglutinating properties exhibit a tendency to separate into numerous groups; *Pneumococcus mucosus* forms a distinct and consistent race, and the resistance of the agglutinins produced by it to absorption by streptococci indicates a nearer relation to Pneumococcus than to Streptococcus. There was considerable uniformity of reaction of the various strains in low dilutions, but this uniformity was not continued as the animal became more highly immunized, and it was not possible for Collins to establish a definite relationship between the agglutination reaction and the other characters of Pneumococcus except in the case of *Pneumococcus mucosus*.

In 1906, Eyre, Leathem, and Washbourn[372] suggested the separation of pneumococci into two groups according to the reaction of rabbit tissue to infection, that is, a fibrinous type and a cellular type, but this idea apparently was never pursued.

It remained for Neufeld and Haendel[991] in 1910 to demonstrate the full significance and the differential value of these phenomena. With a collection of pneumococcal strains isolated from a series of pneumonia patients the authors obtained, by the immunization of rabbits, asses, and horses, monovalent serums of high potency. With a culture isolated in 1909 a serum was prepared that protected mice against the majority of the other strains, and this strain was called "Pneumococcus I." All the pneumococci against which the serum protected mice were classed as "typical," and all others as "atypical." Among the latter was one strain, "Franz," that was later found to be Type II. The "typical" antiserum had no effect on the "Franz" strain, and a "Franz" antiserum failed to protect mice against the Type I culture. Neufeld and Haendel found that the results obtained by protection experiments agreed with those of the agglutination reaction. On the basis of these discoveries Neufeld and his colleague were the first to recommend that serums should be developed for all types, since it was thought that there were probably many types and that a given serum always exhibited type-specificity. For the serum treatment of pneumonia the authors suggested that the agglutination test be employed to determine the type of the infecting organism before administering the specific serum.

The next impetus to serological classification of pneumococci came in 1913 from the work of Dochez and Gillespie.[322] These authors, by the methods of protection and agglutination, divided the species into four groups. Groups I and II included over 60 per cent of the strains tested, Group III consisted of organisms of the *Pneumococcus mucosus* type, and Group IV was a heterogeneous collection of strains that fell into none of the first three divisions and that reacted only with strictly homologous, that is, individual, strain-specific serum. When fourteen different cultures were tested against eleven serums for these heterologous strains, no cross-protection was seen, except in one instance.*

Dochez and Gillespie's Type I Pneumococcus corresponded to the strain originally isolated by Neufeld and Haendel in 1909 and sent by the latter authors to the Rockefeller Institute. The American Type II was identical with Neufeld and Haendel's "Franz" culture, which was a representative of the most commonly occurring of the atypical strains. Group IV of the American authors Neufeld preferred to call Group X, and this designation is often found in the German literature.

The typical and atypical strains of Neufeld and Haendel had, therefore, now been sorted into three definite and specific types and a heterogeneous group of wide immunological diversity.

* Wirth,[1524] in a study (1927) of pneumococci from infections of the ears, sinuses, and throat, found strains of the *mucosus* type which, irrespective of the presence or absence of slimy growth on blood agar, agreed in their agglutinative characteristics with those of the American Type III. Wirth recommended that the name *Streptococcus mucosus* therefore be abandoned.

Lister (1913),[815] studying pneumococci recovered from native laborers in South Africa, was struck by the comparative rarity with which recently isolated pneumococci were opsonized even by serum of pneumonia patients. He succeeded however in obtaining opsonic preparations which showed massive agglutination and marked phagocytosis. Tests on his first four cases suggested the "existence of groups of pneumococci, having distinct serological reactions," and the "presence of specific agglutinins in 'critical' sera from pneumonic patients." Serum from a Group I case failed to react with cultures of Group II, III, or IV pneumococci, and serum for Groups II, III, and IV failed to react with a Group I culture, but any of the Group II, III, and IV serums reacted typically with any of the cultures of Groups II, III, and IV. The numerals are Lister's and bear no relation to the designations used by Dochez and Gillespie. It was not until the completion of his work that Lister learnt of the earlier classification. He immediately compared his groups with those of the American authors, and divided his twenty cultures into five groups, A, B, C, D, and E, of which Group A could not be identified with any of the American types, while Group C corresponded to Type I, and Group B to Type II. Lister's E group was later found to be the same as Type III.

A year later, Lister[816] was able to clarify the apparent confusion existing between his classification and that of Dochez and Gillespie. He sent to the American workers dried spleens of mice infected with cultures representing his groups and received from them in return samples of Type I, II, and III serums. This mutual investigation showed that Lister's C and B groups corresponded respectively with the American Types I and II. Since Lister had no E cultures at the time, he could not correlate it with any of the American groups. At the Hospital of the Rockefeller Institute, however, the identification of the E strain as Pneumococcus III was made. In regard to Dochez and Gillespie's Group IV, Lister stated that it was at this point that his classification departed widely from that of the workers at the Rockefeller Institute. In the Transvaal there were a number of additional groups, and Lister's A was of great importance, since its members were more prevalent than those of any of the groups C, B, or E, and caused a higher case fatality. His unclassifiable groups D, F, G, and X Lister considered of less importance, because of the fluctuation in their prevalence and low case mortality. The pneumococci in these groups showed strain-specificity with no cross-reactions in agglutination. Lister's A and D Group cultures were placed by Dochez and Gillespie in Group IV.

Dochez and Avery,[319] in their 1915 paper, explained that pneumococci of Groups I, II, and III were found principally in association with disease and were distinctly parasitic in type, while Group IV comprised a heterogeneous series of strains, not related antigenically, which caused a minority of cases of pneumonia, and from which the pneumococci occurring in the normal mouth were indistinguishable. Then Avery,[33] by means of agglutination and protection tests, further divided Type (originally Group) II pneumococci into three subgroups, designated by him as "IIA," "IIB," and "IIX." Protection tests showed that organisms of any subgroup were not protected against by the serum of other subgroups, nor did the strains absorb from Type II antipneumococcic serum the specific immune bodies of the other subgroups. Avery stated that the organisms of the three subgroups were biologically related to Type II Pneumococcus, that organisms of subgroups IIA and IIB were characterized by immunity reactions identical within the respective subgroup, but that subgroup IIX consisted of heterogeneous strains which did not cross with other strains or with Types IIA or IIB.

In 1916, Olmstead[1027] after testing the agglutinative reaction of over two hundred strains of pneumococci isolated from normal and infected human beings against fifteen serums, including Type I and Type II serums, against which all those strains failed to react, confirmed the validity of the classification of pneumococci into

Types I, II, and III and then divided the members of Group IV into at least twelve groups, some of which contained subgroups. In a subsequent report, Olmstead[1028] suggested that some members of these groups served as connecting links between Type II and Group IV, and, because of a closer relationship with the latter, should be classed as Pneumococcus IV rather than as IIX. The same proposal was made by Clough,[238] who after identifying strains of Avery's subgroups IIA and IIB among 121 cultures isolated from cases of lobar pneumonia, suggested that, since members of these two subgroups possessed relatively low virulence for animals and had been recovered from the mouths of normal persons, the strains would be found epidemiologically to resemble Group IV organisms more closely than those of Types I or II.

Nicolle, Jouan, and Debains[1011] did not accept Group IV and the American classification, claiming that a large number of pneumococci studied by them were not agglutinated by their own or American serums, except when treated with dilute hydrochloric acid according to the method of Porges. The authors recommended that the conception of Type IV—a purely negative type—ought then to be abandoned henceforth.

Nicolle with Debains[1009] again studied by the agglutination reaction a large number of pneumococci from varied sources. They used the American classification and their results showed that the strains, as studied, varied in agglutinability from a complete absence of this property to spontaneous clumping in normal horse serum.

In a review of various immunological reactions, Nicolle and Debains (1920)[1010] concluded that races of Pneumococcus—"antigenic races"—could not be determined by agglutination alone. Their work is, in one respect, reminiscent of Gillespie's[516] data on the acid agglutination of pneumococci. Tested by this method, strains belonging to Types I and II had, as a rule, narrow zones of agglutination. Other pneumococci had broad zones, or in a few cases, narrow zones not coincident with those occupied by organisms of the fixed types. The acid-agglutination of the majority of pneumococci of Types I and II was extremely susceptible to the inhibiting action of salts, but this was not true of other pneumococci. These influences, with the variations they cause, while of a certain philosophic interest, have little bearing on the practical application of agglutination to the classification of members of this bacterial species.

Following the lead developed by Avery, Stillman[1327] further subdivided Type II strains into twelve distinct groups. These were designated as IIa to IIm. Groups IIb–c–f–m originated in human mouths. Groups IIa and IIh were encountered largely in connection with disease, while the general fatality of acute lobar pneumonia due to these atypical Type II pneumococci was fairly high. Stillman's tables, showing the percentage of incidence and of mortality of strains of these subgroups, offer an interesting comparison with those given later by Cooper and her associates. They serve to emphasize the close relation which exists between some members of the Type II and those of the new types formerly included in Group IV.

In conformity with Stillman's and Olmstead's investigations, Christensen proved that Type IVm of Stillman also constituted a heterogeneous group which could be further divided into subordinate groups. Christensen[228-9] carried out comparative tests by means of agglutination, agglutinin-absorption, and complement fixation and gave preference to the simple agglutination technique as being the most convenient and efficient method for serological differentiation.

The splitting of Type II into separate groups was apparently unknown to Hintze,[646] who found anomalies in the American Type II and was not convinced that it was a clear-cut group. He, among others, also classified *Streptococcus mucosus* as Type III Pneumococcus, although strains of this organism were encountered that gave atypical reactions.

Yu,[1567] studying fifty-one strains by the agglutination method, found at least three subgroups in Type II. Sugg, Gaspari, Fleming, and Neill[1354] in 1928 described a peculiar strain which, while possessing a partial antigenic relationship to typical Type III Pneumococcus, had distinct immunological properties of its own. In a later study of this same strain, Harris, Sugg, and Neill[595] ascertained that in rabbits this culture, related to but not identical with Type III, evoked better antibody (agglutinin) response than did Type III organisms, but in mice the Type III strain gave rise to a higher degree of protection against the homologous organism.

Other serological variants were found by Clough (1919).[239] Her nine strains were agglutinated by Type I, II, and III antiserums. From the I and II serums, by absorption, two strains removed the agglutinins and tropins for the homologous cultures only and not for typical I or II organisms or for other atypical pneumococci. Absorption of the serums with homologous cultures removed agglutinins and tropins for all the atypical strains. The phagocytic and agglutinative reactions of the atypical organisms in monovalent serums indicated that, in general, the strains were serologically distinct, although in a few cases they exhibited some interrelation. The special atypical monovalent serums showed no activity with Type I, II, or atypical Type II pneumococci.

Another atypical strain of the heterogeneous Group IV was described by Pockels,[1101] who thought that its growth was sufficiently individual to warrant his calling the strain *Pneumococcus planus.* This organism has not been further identified. Gordon,[543] testing fifteen strains of Group IV by cross-agglutination and agglutinin-absorption, sorted them into three groups and eight separate heterologous strains.*

In England, Armstrong[19] was able to identify subgroups among Type II pneumococci which corresponded to Avery's IIA and IIB and, by means of agglutinin-absorption, divided Types I and III into subordinate groups of limited specificity within the main type

* For a review of serological classification as it stood in the year 1922, and for a very readable discussion of the theory of antigens and antibodies, the reader is referred to Eastwood's[343-4] two papers published in that year.

to which they belonged. Armstrong regretted the use of the American designation Type IV for the unclassified strains as being too narrow. Yu[1567] found Types I and III to be uniform and definite.

In 1921, Cooper, with Mishulow and Blane,[273] published the first of a series of studies which were to bring a new order out of the confusion regarding the proper serological classification of Group IV pneumococci, and to establish many of the atypical subgroups as separate and definite types. By the agglutination method, checked by absorption tests when cross-agglutination occurred, the authors placed their fifty-three cultures in six small groups with thirteen unrelated strains—a total of nineteen types.

In the next few years there were additional reports on the serological classification of pneumococci, but only a few were of major importance. In 1921, Griffith[558] compared strains of his own isolation with standard type strains sent him from America by Flexner. To a 1 to 10 dilution of the monovalent type rabbit serums he had prepared was added an equal amount of the supernatant fluid from centrifuged peritoneal washings from mice inoculated with pneumococcal strains. It was found that the agglutination test was sufficient for the identification of the first three specific types and the author considered that the method of absorption of agglutinins was unnecessary. Group IV was separated into six types, including the American Types IIA and IIB, but these did not complete his classification. Griffith, by the way, like others, noted that agglutinating serum from horses was less selective than that of rabbits.

Yoshioka (1922 and 1923),[1560-1] using strains of the American Types I, II, and III from the Hospital of the Rockefeller Institute, and a Type I strain of German origin, was not always able to obtain type-specific protection in mice actively immunized with these cultures. The serum of immunized rabbits was type-specific in protection experiments, but fresh normal serum in fairly high dilutions sometimes also agglutinated heterologous types. Yoshioka attributed these variations in normal specificity, such as marked decrease in agglutinability with homologous serum and the appearance of agglutinability with heterologous serum, to serological modification brought about by growth of the organisms on unfavorable media.

Takami (1925)[1373, 1375] had even less success in efforts to classify Japanese strains according to the American scheme, and said that all such attempts had completely failed in Japan. It seems highly improbable that specific types of pneumococci are not to be found in that country. The various modifications which the American strains underwent on artificial media may explain the unusual results. Takami offered this fact as an explanation when he concluded that "for serological grouping of pneumococci one must work only with strains which have become virulent through animal passage, or strains which have been cultivated directly from the human body and have not undergone variation on artificial mediums." Megrail and Ecker,[888] on the contrary, presented definite evidence that Pneumococcus possesses a type stability under conditions in which typhoid bacilli and other organisms show variability in agglutination. The reliability of the methods for the serological typing of pneumococci is further supported by the results of Christensen[229] and of Griffith,[558] who demonstrated the complete specificity of the mouse-protection test.

In 1929, Cooper, with Edwards and Rosenstein,[272] tested 120 strains of pneumococci isolated from cases of lobar pneumonia that either did not agglutinate or else reacted atypically with diagnostic antiserums for Type I, II, and III pneumococci. These authors included Avery's IIA and IIB strains, representatives of various types from Pittsburgh, and the atypical III strain described by Sugg, Gaspari, Fleming, and Neill.[1354] Cooper and her associates prepared monovalent serums from rabbits and horses, and with serum divided the 120 strains into ten groups containing four or more strains each, and a miscellaneous group comprising strains differing from the others, which at that time could not be further subdivided. These ten groups were designated as Types IV to and including XIII.

Finding that therapeutic antiserums for Types I, II, and III had little protective power against Types IV to XIII, the authors prepared from rabbits monovalent antiserums of high agglutinative and protective titer for each type. The Cooper Type IV included an "Antitoxin" strain from the Lilly Laboratories, Robinson's Group IVB strain, and one that corresponded to Griffith's 10. These strains were highly virulent for mice, and of the nineteen human cases of lobar pneumonia from which pneumococci were isolated, sixteen were rated as severe. Type V included Avery's IIA and Robinson's IVE strains. All showed a tendency to hemolyze red cells in blood broth, and had a high initial virulence for mice, which however was rapidly lost. Type VI strains were usually less virulent for mice and their hemolytic action less marked than that of Type V, but more pronounced than that of the majority of other strains. Type VI corresponded to the largest group separated by Griffith from Group IV and found by him to be second in prevalence to Types I and II. The Type VI strains had such a low virulence for mice that they were not suitable for protection tests, nor could their virulence be sufficiently increased for this purpose. Type VIII included Robinson's Group IVA organism and the atypical Type III strain described by Sugg and his associates. These strains agglutinated with Type III serum to such a marked degree that they might easily have been identified as belonging to this original type. All Type IX cultures showed low virulence for mice. The Type X strains possessed slight or moderate virulence. The four strains designated as Type XI exhibited moderate hemolytic action and were of average to high virulence for mice, which however was quickly lost. The Type XII strains were moderately virulent for mice. The virulence of the Type XIII strains was similar to that of Type XI.

In 1932, Cooper, with the collaborators Rosenstein, Walter, and

Peizer,[274] expanded the classification to include twenty-nine types in addition to the first three original types of Dochez and Gillespie, making a total of thirty-two specific types. To show how the new types compared with atypical strains described by other authors, the following list taken from the paper by Cooper and her associates may be repeated here:

Type IV—Pneumococcus 10 (Griffith), Group IVB (Robinson)
Type V—Sub IIA (Avery), Group IVE (Robinson)
Type VI—Sub IIB (Avery)
Type VIII—Group IVA (Robinson), atypical III (Sugg, Gaspari, Fleming, and Neill)
Type XV—Pneumococcus 98 (Griffith)
Type XXI—Pneumococcus 160 (Griffith)
Type XXII—Pneumococcus 41 (Griffith)

The majority of the thirty-two types showed only slight cross-reactions; Types II and V; III and VIII; VII and XVIII; and XV and XXX being exceptions. Only a small percentage of strains isolated in New York City could not be serologically identified by Cooper and her co-workers.

In the study just cited, from the majority of horses immunized for a period of more than a year serums with 500 to 1,000 units were obtained, and by the concentration of serum of lower potency, Cooper and her associates obtained preparations equal to or stronger than high-grade unconcentrated serums. In addition, the authors developed potent bivalent serums for those types which gave marked cross-agglutinative reactions.

The original publication should be consulted for full information concerning the incidence and severity of cases due to the different types, their presence in normal individuals and in spinal meningitis, and their virulence for mice. The original serological classification of Dochez and Gillespie as amplified and extended by the additions discovered by Olmstead and by Cooper and her colleagues covers practically all strains that have been studied and is now tentatively accepted as standard.

The occurrence of many of these pneumococcal types in Germany has been reported by Silberstein (1933),[1287] who found twenty-one of the new types, while there were only three strains which could not be classified. Types XVI, XXI, XXIII, XXVIII, XXX, and XXXII which had not before been reported in Germany were among those identified by Silberstein. Of all the types, XVIII and XIX seemed to be among the more common, as had earlier been noted by Gundel and Schwartz.*

That there may possibly be types beyond the present serological classification is suggested by the report of Christie (1934).[231] Of one hundred Group IV strains tested, forty-seven failed to react with specific serum for any of the thirty-two known types. Nineteen of thirty-six cultures from healthy persons, sixteen of thirty-six strains obtained from convalescent carriers, and twelve of twenty-eight organisms isolated from patients with acute pneumococcal pneumonia could not be identified by Christie with any of the type-specific serums. In India, Napier and Dharmonda[943] encountered among the pneumococci isolated from forty-five cases of lobar pneumonia and from fifteen cases of bronchopneumonia, strains that failed to correspond to any of the recognized types. Forty-six per cent of the strains studied apparently belonged to two types found only locally.

Recently two strains of pneumococci were described by Smith[1296] which the author claims constitute two new serological types. The organisms were isolated on separate occasions from the respiratory tract of a man suffering from "chronic bronchitis." A third but similar strain was found to be present in pure culture in the lungs of an individual dying of pneumonia. The strains grew anaerobically and were virulent for mice but, under the conditions tested, were not infectious to guinea pigs. The three strains appeared to represent two distinct serological varieties both of which differed from the thirty-two known types. There was no cross-

* Quoted by Silberstein.

agglutination between the two varieties and, with the exception of one strain, that agglutinated with Type XVI immune serum in a dilution of 1 to 32, the two varieties failed to be agglutinated with any of the thirty-two type serums.

Strains of pneumococci which failed to correspond to any of the thirty-two known types were encountered in China by Wu and Zia,[1552] who reported that among a total of 162 strains tested, four failed to agglutinate with any of the thirty-two type serums. The unclassifiable strains possessed typical cultural characteristics and were virulent for mice.

It may be expected that other types of pneumococci will in time be added to Cooper's list. There were still a few strains which did not fit into any of the thirty-two groups, and the work of the two Japanese bacteriologists, while leaving doubts as to the soundness of their conclusions, and the results obtained in England, India, and China present the possibility that more heterogeneous strains may be encountered which will be found to form additional serological types.

There is the further question of the pneumococci causing infections in animals other than man. Grenier (1912)[555] described cultures from three sources, namely, guinea pigs, rabbits, and horses. The first two cultures from guinea pigs and rabbits were isolated from animals undergoing experiments with other toxic or infectious agents. The pneumococcus infecting the guinea pig was moderately virulent for mice and usually led a saprophytic existence in the respiratory and digestive tracts. The culture from infected horses did not originally kill mice but acquired virulence on animal passage. The observations of Grenier suggest that in veterinary bacteriology there may be strains, or even types, which might be found to have interesting pathogenic and serological relationships with pneumococci of human origin. The authors of the present volume disclaim any acquaintance with the literature of that branch of bacteriology, so far as it concerns Pneumococcus, but studies on this phase of the biology of Pneumococcus, if they have not already been made, should be undertaken because of the additional information which may accrue.

Classification According to Electrophoretic Potential

Another criterion for classification, other than agglutination or protection tests, was advanced by Thompson (1931).[1396] By determining the electrophoretic rate of migration, he grouped the sixty-seven strains studied into five groups. The A group included typical Type III's and one Group IV strain. Group B consisted of typical Type I strains and a few Group IV strains. C took in Group IV strains, an atypical III, and two atypical II organisms. D was represented by a typical Type II, a few of Group IV, and one atypical Type I strain, while E was represented by only two Group IV strains. Since Groups C and D were shown not to be definitely distinct from each other and since the number of strains comprising Group E was too small to be significant, there remain only three large electrophoretic groups. In a second paper, Thompson[1397] presented data on the rate of migration in the electrophoretic field and the isoelectric points of various pneumococcal strains, but made his classification somewhat unwieldy by the addition of intermediary groups. While knowledge of the differences in the electrophoretic potential of different strains of pneumococci may be of scientific interest, the method has no advantage over the serological classification.

We are now learning of yet wider deviations from special specifications than those we have already discussed. At first sight they seem to confuse the definite lines of demarcation that have been drawn between bacterial species and the still finer distinctions that have been established on both chemical and serological grounds for types within the species. Pneumococcal cells possess polysaccharides peculiar to each type, and the carbohydrate is looked upon as the factor that determines the exact place of a Pneumococcus within the species. Lately it has been found that other and apparently unrelated bacteria also elaborate complex carbohydrates, and that these carbohydrates both as antigens and as haptens exhibit immunological similarities to the polysaccharides of Pneumococcus. Puzzling as these new developments are at present, they, like the discovery of the transformative processes, will only lead to the disclosure of new biological principles.

There is no doubt that the members of other microbial species and materials of vegetable origin contain polysaccharides which may be found to possess chemical and immunological relations analogous to the capsular carbohydrates of Pneumococcus but, as Heidelberger and Avery concluded, this type of immunological correspondence in no way invalidates the systematic classification of bacteria based on the more usual and general methods of species determination, and it is of greater immediate significance in connection with the study of problems dealing with bacteria as disease-producing agents than in the study of bacteria in their generic relationships.

Type Determination

The immunity reactions which form the basis of serological methods for the bacteriological differentiation of pneumococci are of inestimable importance to students of Pneumococcus and to clinicians. They aid in defining the relations and interrelations of members of this bacterial species; they afford clues in tracing the spread of pneumococcal infection; they reveal the influence of chemical constitution in determining antigenic specificity and immune response; and have an eminently practical bearing on serum treatment.

Whatever benefit is to be derived from the use of antipneumococcic serum depends on the rapid and accurate determination of the type of Pneumococcus causing the infection. While the potency of serum and the judgment directing its administration are of great importance, it is the use of the immunologically appropriate serum and the promptness of treatment which in many cases may determine the issue for the patient. The major effort, therefore, besides increasing the accuracy of these tests, has been expended in devising ways of shortening the time elapsing between the collection of the specimen and the identification of the serological type of the infecting Pneumococcus.

MOUSE PROTECTION TEST

It was Neufeld and Haendel[991] who, in 1910, realizing the importance of the delay involved in the isolation, cultivation, and identification of pneumococci from infected material, saw in Ungermann's[1433] suggestion of testing cultures on the basis of phagocytic action, possibilities for reducing the time factor. Ungermann's plan was to inject a mouse intraperitoneally with sputum, then several hours later to inject immune serum, and after a further interval of an hour and a half, to kill the mouse and make stained smears of the exudate from the surface of the liver. When the serum corresponded immunologically with the culture, marked phagocytosis of the cocci took place.

The use of the mouse as a vital differential medium cut short the time usually required by plating and subculturing and became the foundation of the protection test developed by Cole and his associates.[36] This method, which is given in detail in the Appendix, immediately came into general use, and while in the routine examination of pneumonic material it has given place to the more rapid presumptive tests, it still remains the method of choice for the ultimate determination of pneumococcal types. There are certain difficulties encountered in the practice of this method, such as the occurrence of pneumococci of more than one type in the specimen, the overgrowth of Pneumococcus by other organisms in the peritoneal cavity of the mouse, the occurrence of cross-agglutination when undiluted or slightly diluted immune horse serum is used, and the complication arising from a latent mouse-typhoid infection in the test animals.*

Sutliff's[1359] experience emphasized the apparent errors which may occur when the testing of sputum by the mouse method is taken as the only diagnostic criterion. He compared the results of the protection test with those obtained by other cultural methods or, in other words, checked the type of Pneumococcus found in the sputum with the type or types isolated from the same patient by means of blood cultures, from post-mortem lung cultures, and from miscellaneous exudates. Among eighty-one cases in which Group IV strains were found in the sputum, twelve showed the presence of pneumococci of one of the fixed types in cultures obtained from the blood or lung. This error of 14.8 per cent is significant. Sutliff demonstrated the advantage in performing a type determination on cultures isolated from the hearts' blood of the test mice as well as on those from the peritoneal exudates. In 1,326 such examinations, the outcome was positive in fifty-five instances with the hearts' blood where the peritoneal exudate was negative. Moreover, Sutliff at times recovered two types of pneumococci from the same mouse. Of 339 cases where the peritoneal exudate showed a fixed type, the hearts' blood of the same test animals in fifteen, or 4.4 per cent of these instances, yielded an organism of Group IV and, in five, or 1.5 per cent of cases, pneumococci of a different specific type. In 862 cases in which the peritoneum of the mouse yielded a Type IV organism, the hearts' blood showed fixed types in thirty-one cases, or 3.6 per cent. Sutliff then, in all cases showing Group IV pneumococci in the sputum, collected and examined a second specimen by the mouse method and here the same discrepancy held. Of 145 cases, twenty-two gave results on the second determination inconsistent with those of the first. Sutliff's experience prompted him to advise that "When a specific type of

* Faber,[378] feeling that a substitute for mice was needed, recommended rabbits, but it is feared that he failed to appreciate the economic aspects of such a substitution.

pneumococcus is obtained from the sputum by mouse test, it may safely be considered the cause of the disease, but when a pneumococcus which does not react specifically (type 4) is found in the sputum, a second examination will in approximately 15 per cent of the cases yield a specific reaction for one of the fixed types."

Gundel[568] pointed out the various sources of error in the bacteriological diagnosis of pneumococcal infections. He recommended the examination of successive specimens of sputum, mentioned the difficulty presented by the presence of more than one type of Pneumococcus in sputum, and explained the replacement of organisms of the fixed types by those of the heterogeneous "X" (American Group IV) by assuming that virulent Type I and II organisms disappeared from the sputum as the pneumonic disease progressed, thus allowing a predominance of pneumococci from the upper respiratory tract.

The reports cited above are introduced to emphasize the need for thoroughness and care in the examination of infected material submitted for pneumococcal diagnosis. In some specimens, a single type of organism may be present and may so predominate that its identification by any one of the methods is a simple matter. When, however, pneumococci are few in number, or when variable results occur, the sputum should be examined by other methods and controlled by serological tests on cultures derived from single colonies.

In 1917, Blake[123] devised a method for obviating the difficulties in the mouse test. He injected the mouse with sputum and, when infection had sufficiently progressed, washed out the peritoneal cavity with sterile saline solution, centrifuged the washings at high speed, and to one part of the sterile supernatant fluid added an equal part of diluted immune serum. When the organism was of the same serological type as that of the serum a precipitate formed immediately. Used with a large number of strains, Blake found this test to be consistently positive and specific for Types I, II, and III. The principle of the method lay in the liberation of soluble specific substance, or precipitinogen, from the pneumococcal cells during growth in the peritoneum of the test animal.

CULTURE AGGLUTINATION

In 1918, two rapid methods were announced. The urgency of war-time needs, the lack of laboratory facilities in the hastily improvised army camps, and the shortage of mice, all called for a simplification and speeding up of the methods for pneumococcal type determination. Taking advantage of the more rapid growth of pneumococci in sugar broth, Avery[34] planted washed sputum in bouillon containing one per cent glucose and after five hours' incubation, that is, in the period of active growth of pneumococci and before accompanying bacteria had multiplied to any conflicting extent, the broth was used as an agglutinating antigen with the three type serums. This procedure gave a high percentage of successful results, besides being simple, inexpensive, and speedy of execution. Oliver[1026] later made the suggestion that the Andrade indicator be added and that inulin be substituted for dextrose in the Avery medium, because these modifications yielded better results and were successful in cases when dextrose broth failed.

An exception to the general experience with the Avery method was that reported by Beckler, Marden, and Gillette,[97] who had a number of failures with this test as compared with mouse inoculation. Since they had no control over the collection of the specimens, the work being done in a state diagnostic laboratory, the sputum was often mixed with saliva, which the authors thought might account for their unsatisfactory experience. Those readers desiring to learn of the operation of the Avery rapid cultural method in the field should consult Vaughan[1448] who gave (1918) a description of laboratory requirements and satisfactory results in army base hospitals.

URINE PRECIPITATION TEST

Another diagnostic, or more exactly prognostic, aid of the same nature was the urine test of Dochez and Avery,[321] who had observed that *in vivo* as well as *in vitro,* Pneumococcus produced a soluble specific substance, and that with an appropriate immune serum its presence could easily be detected. Type III organisms formed the largest amount of the substance, Type II somewhat less and Type I the least. The majority of patients who failed to show the precipitable substance in the urine recovered, whereas the mortality was high among cases in which its presence was demonstrable. A positive test was also of diagnostic significance.

SPUTUM PRECIPITINOGEN

A rapid method depending upon the demonstration of pneumococcal precipitinogen was that of Mitchell and Muns (1917).[904] They ground sputum with fine sand to disrupt the cells and release the soluble substance, extracted the mixture with salt solution, centrifuged the extract until clear, and then added immune serum to the supernatant fluid. The test required only an hour for its completion and gave clear-cut results for Type I, II, and III pneumococci. Those sputums which gave no reactions were classed as Group IV. The success of the method depends on obtaining a specimen rich in pneumococci.

SPUTUM DIGESTION

Krumwiede and Noble,[761] also responding to the demands of the time, sought by digesting sputum with antiformin to bring the precipitinogen into solution, but difficulties were experienced in applying this technique to all specimens, and the final results were often unsatisfactory. In a second paper, Krumwiede with Valentine,[762] abandoned the use of antiformin and, instead, coagulated the sputum with heat. They broke up the coagulum and extracted the soluble antigen with saline solution in a boiling water-bath, cleared the extract by centrifugation, and then layered or floated the antigen over the type serums. The authors incubated the tubes at 50°

to 55°, and observed a more or less opaque contact ring when the antigen and antiserum were of the homologous type. Here again there were some failures due to the quality of the sputum, but with the majority of specimens the method gave a rapid and accurate type diagnosis.

The Krumwiede method was given a trial by Kohn[737] with a limited number of cultures. The results, in the main, agreed closely with those obtained by the mouse-protection test. Because of accuracy, simplicity, and the saving of time and mice, Kohn advised its more general adoption.

A somewhat unusual case was reported by Gilbert and Davenport[514] which called attention to the complication presented by the occurrence in sputum of pneumococci of more than one fixed type. The Krumwiede test was negative with the three type serums. The culture in the Avery medium showed a faint reaction with Type I serum but none with that of Types II and III. A mouse inoculated with the sputum was dead at the end of forty-eight hours and the agglutination, precipitation, and cultural tests all showed the sole presence of Type III Pneumococcus. Direct planting of the sputum and of the Avery culture on blood plates yielded a predominance of green-producing cocci, which culturally proved to be Type I organisms and *S. viridans*. Serologically the growth agglutinated with both Type I and III serums.

Another avenue of approach was that reported by Loewe, Hirschfeld, and Wallach.[821] Instead of searching for precipitinogen in the excretions of pneumonia patients, they sought precipitin in the blood. The blood was drawn into potassium oxalate, laked with ether, and added to saline suspensions of type strains of pneumococci grown on glucose-serum agar. The mixtures were incubated until a color change due to alteration of the hemoglobin appeared. Inasmuch as immune substances do not usually appear in the blood stream in the very early stages of pneumonia, it is difficult to see how this method could possess any advantage over those aimed to detect the presence of precipitinogen in the urine or blood.

BILE-SOLUTION OF SPUTUM

In 1920 and 1921, Oliver[1025-6] reported a method by which the precipitable substance of the pneumococci in pneumonic sputum was brought into solution by bile and the filtered material then set up against known antiserums. With incubation at 42° to 45°, when the serum and the specific substance derived from the organisms were of the same serological type, immediate clouding and flocculation appeared, the whole procedure requiring only about thirty minutes for completion. Checked against the mouse-protection method there was full agreement in the results obtained.

The Oliver technique had advocates in Sharp and Urbantke.[1261] These authors in a study of forty cases found that when pneumococci of fixed types were intermingled with streptococci and Group IV organisms, the presence of the former was often obscured and identification difficult. The Oliver method appeared to be more successful than the classic mouse method with such specimens. Direct type determination of the infecting strain in pneumococcal meningitis was rendered feasible by slightly modifying Oliver's scheme. The sediment from centrifuged spinal fluids was treated with sodium taurocholate, the mixture shaken, and after being allowed to stand, centrifuged at high speed. The supernatant fluid was then mixed with type serums. A positive outcome was indicated by the rapid formation of a precipitate. The procedure could also be carried out on a microscope slide with equally definite results.

Rosenthal and Sternberg[1175] proposed another rapid procedure for type determination, which consisted in digesting sputum in a borax-boracic acid solution and adding to the clear supernatant fluid of the centrifuged mixture, in separate sections on a slide, specific antiserums. The results by this method agreed in the majority of instances with those obtained by the mouse inoculation test.

Instead of utilizing the presence of precipitin as a therapeutic control, Noble[1017] described a simple, though not particularly original, method for determining the presence of agglutinins in the blood. The patients' serum was added to heavy suspensions of pneumococci. These materials used in small quantities and in concentrated form gave a rapid end result, and because of its reliability Noble used the method to measure agglutinins in the blood of pneumonia patients during serum treatment.

SLIDE AGGLUTINATION

In 1929, Sabin[1201] introduced his simple rapid "Stained Slide" microscopic agglutination test. Briefly, the test consisted in injecting the sputum into the peritoneal cavity of a mouse, then a few hours later puncturing the abdominal wall, withdrawing a small amount of peritoneal exudate, mixing it with the diagnostic serums of the various types in separate drops on the same slide, and finally smearing, fixing, and staining the mixtures. The slide was examined under an oil immersion lens for evidences of agglutination. Sabin also applied this method to the determination of antibody in the blood of pneumonia patients for the control of serum administration, as proposed by Park and Cooper.[1057] A drop or more of the patient's blood was withdrawn into a capillary tube, and after coagulation and contraction of the clot, the tube was centrifuged and a minute amount of the extruded serum spread with a loopful of a saline suspension of a heat-killed culture of the type for which agglutinins were sought. The film was air-dried, stained for one-half minute with fuchsin, and examined microscopically. When checked against the Noble and macroscopic agglutinin methods, this test was found by Sabin to be two and one-half to three times more sensitive when standard diagnostic type serums were used for comparison. In a paper published in 1930, Sabin[1202] gave further details and refinements of the technique. In addition to using the method for the control of serum administration, he found it to be of service in detecting the presence or absence of active infection in man.

Armstrong (1931),[22] giving Sabin credit for originating the method, introduced a slight modification of Sabin's technique by mixing with droplets of peritoneal exudates from mice previously injected with pneumonic sputum loopfuls of diluted Type I, II, and III agglutinating serums. Instead of spreading and fixing the film, the material was immediately examined under a cover-slip. The differences in the two methods are minor and the selection of one or the other is a matter of personal choice. The important observation of Armstrong's was that an increase in the size of the cocci appeared after the addition of homologous serum—the significant *Quellung* effect first observed by Neufeld and later made the basis by Neufeld and Etinger-Tulczynska[987] for their rapid type-determination method. A year later, Armstrong[23] published a supplemental report on the results obtained by his method. In every case the type determinations were confirmed by mouse inoculation and other methods not specified. He also reported its applicability to cerebrospinal fluids, pus from empyemata, aural discharges, and exudates from various sources.

Logan and Smeall[823] slightly changed the Armstrong modification of the Sabin method, but the change was insignificant and the satisfactory results the authors obtained with it might well be credited to the original procedure.

Calder[196] devised another slight modification of the Sabin technique. The cultures grown in Avery's medium were dried on a cover-glass, stained with a drop of gentian violet solution, and after the addition of diluted type serums, the preparation was examined as a hanging drop.

Valentine,[1444] in 1933, introduced yet another variation of the Armstrong-Logan and Smeall modification of the original Sabin method. Here again, sputum and serum samples were mixed, although in a somewhat different manner, smears made and stained first with carbol-fuchsin and then carbol-thionin. The bodies of the cocci, when the immune serum was homologous for the strain, stained black while everything else on the slide was red, including the capsule. It is difficult to discover any advantage in this technique over the simpler methods.

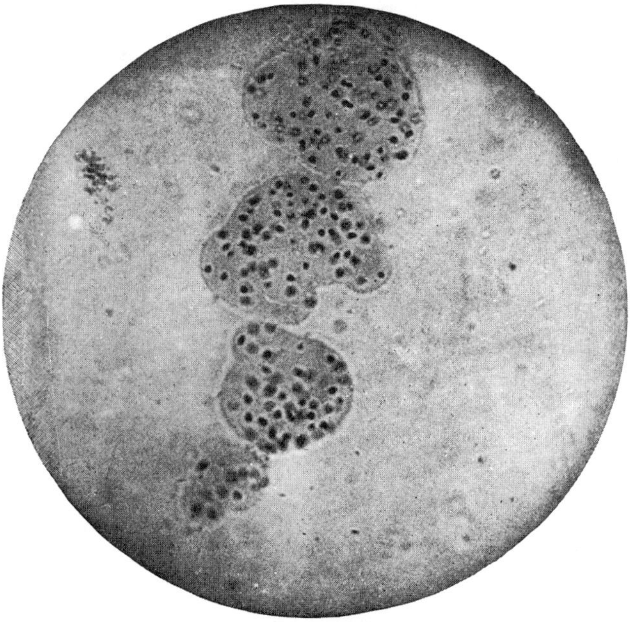

Figure 1

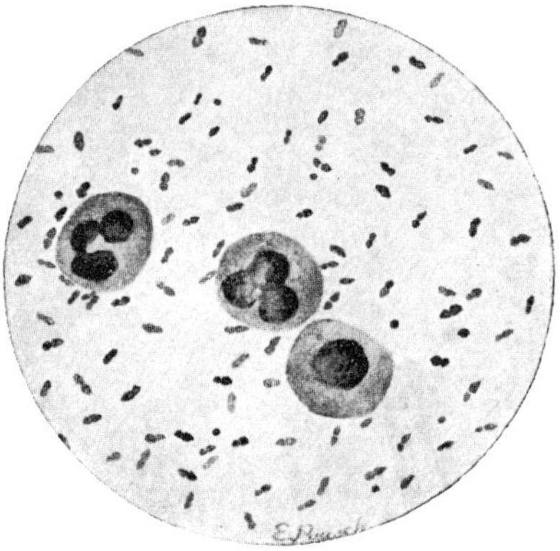

After Neufeld and Schnitzer[1000]

Figure 2

THE QUELLUNG PHENOMENON

Figure 1. Agglutination and *Quellung* of pneumococci by immune serum *in vitro.* Figure 2. Pneumococci from the peritoneal cavity of a mouse mixed with concentrated heterologous immune serum (control).

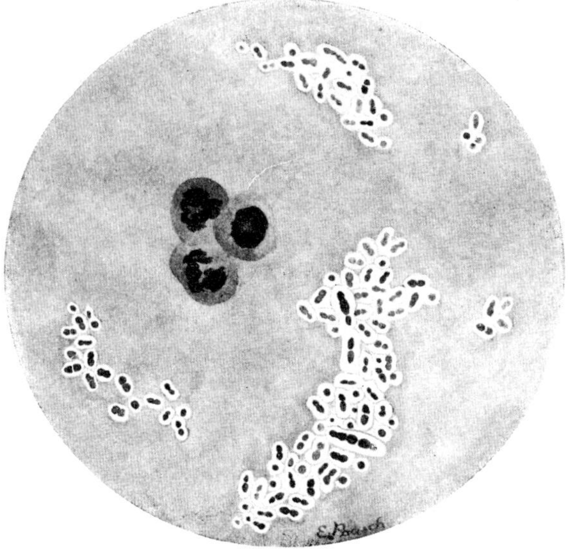

Figure 3

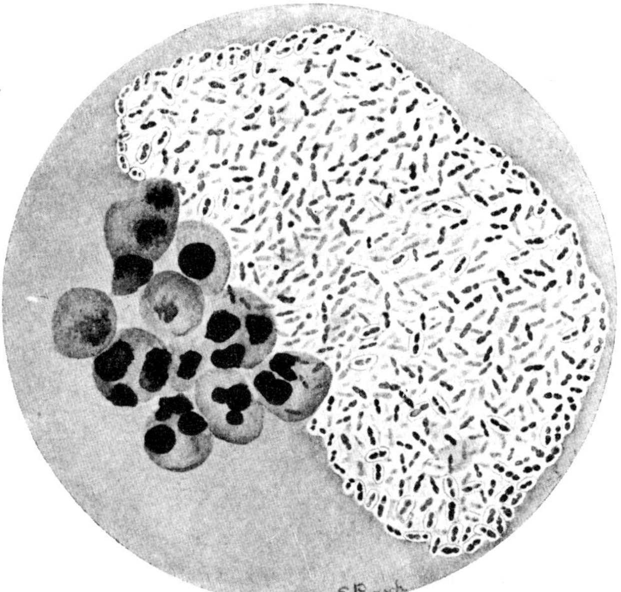

After Neufeld and Schnitzer[1000]

Figure 4

THE QUELLUNG PHENOMENON

Figure 3. Pneumococci from the peritoneal cavity of a mouse mixed with concentrated homologous immune serum. Figure 4. Pneumococci from the peritoneal cavity of a mouse mixed with concentrated homologous immune serum; particularly marked *Quellung* and mass formation.

The Sabin method, either in its original or modified form, was for some time the one of preference. Among the many satisfied users of the original technique was Brown[151] of the Connaught Laboratories. Heffron and Varley,[602] reporting in 1932 the experience of the Bacteriological Laboratory of the Massachusetts Department of Public Health with the Krumwiede, Sabin, and macroscopic agglutination methods, preferred the Sabin procedure for routine examinations because of the greater number of positive results and the shorter time required. The types as determined by the Sabin method were in all cases checked by agglutination of the culture from the hearts' blood of infected mice. The simple technique was so readily learned by laboratory technicians that Heffron recommended its adoption by diagnostic laboratories.

Bullowa and Schuman,[185] for the purpose of still further reducing the time factor when a determination of any of the thirty-two types was desired, proposed the pooling of type serums other than I, II, and III. For example, combined lot A comprised Types IV through VIII, while B, C, D, and E included Types IX through XXIII.* With these lots, diluted with saline solution in a ratio of 1 to 10, 1 to 15, and 1 to 25, Bullowa and Schuman made preliminary tests and, obtaining a positive result in any group, then tested the strain separately against the monovalent type serums included in that group. These groups may be arranged to fit the prevalence of the various types in different communities or seasons.

At about the same time, Amoss[13] described another method. A sample of the patient's blood was defibrinated, the serum filtered through celloidin in a Coor's filter, and the filtrate centrifuged at high speed. The filtrate was then concentrated on a steam-bath under diminished pressure. To aliquot portions of the concentrate containing the soluble specific substance of Pneumococcus were added equal amounts of specific serum of the three fixed types, and during incubation at 37° in a water-bath readings were made in a

* Two other lots, F and G, could, of course, be added to include the remaining types.

beam of light at five-minute intervals. In some cases definite precipitation was noted in the homologous mixtures after five minutes' incubation. To the remainder of the filtrate eight volumes of 95 per cent alcohol were then added, and, after mixing, the tubes were set in the ice-box over night. The flocculent precipitate was collected by centrifugation, the residue dried by heat under a stream of air, and after salt solution was added, the solution was distributed into tubes for the addition of serum. The author tried still another method for demonstrating the presence of precipitinogen in patient's blood. To the serum collected as in the first procedure distilled water and 0.2M sodium acetate-acetic acid buffer solution with a pH of 4.6 was added. The mixture was then boiled until coagulation was complete. The filtrate from the coagulum was evaporated to dryness over a free flame, and heated carefully until the odor of acetic acid was no longer present. The resulting dry concentrate was extracted with sterile distilled water, the solution cleared by centrifugation or by filtering through paper and the resulting liquid used as a precipitating antigen against type serums I, II, and III. The delicacy of this method was shown by the fact that precipitinogen could be detected in the blood when blood culture remained negative.

To repeat Amoss' conclusion: "The method requires less time than the sputum culture or mouse method, but has no advantage over the sputum extract method. It is useful for typing in cases in which neither sputum nor urine can be obtained"; to which might be added, it furnishes to those who are not content with negative or doubtful results one more aid in arriving at a type diagnosis. Amoss also saw in this method, by detection of the soluble specific substance in the blood, a means of judging the amount of serum necessary and for following more closely the results of serum therapy in lobar pneumonia. The intricacy of the procedure would bar its use in the busy routine of the average hospital laboratory, but it would be of service, where time and the facilities permitted, in estimating the degree of absorption, distribution, and neutralization of injected pneumococcal antibodies.

Another variation of the precipitin method was that described by Sia and Chung (1932).[1271] They seeded cultures into poured plates of dextrose-beef-infusion agar containing, in separate Petri dishes, type-specific serums. After incubation, when the type of organism and serum corresponded, a well-defined annular opacity surrounded each colony, an appearance which proved to be type-specific. The method is obviously somewhat limited in value. It requires discrimination in the quantity of inoculum as well as in the amount of serum to be added and since, with these disadvantages, it also requires twenty-four hours' incubation and large supplies of immune serum, there is no reason for selecting it instead of the less complicated and more rapid methods. In the same year, Petri[1084] described a procedure which he used in the study of pneumococcal dissociation, but which, because of the recent development of simpler techniques, has not been adopted.

QUELLUNG PHENOMENON

The latest method to be generally used is based on the *Quellung* effect first described by Neufeld[974] in 1902. It promises to supersede all the previous rapid precipitation and agglutination methods. The technique as reported by Neufeld and Etinger-Tulczynska[988] consists in placing on a slide, separately, three loopfuls of the sputum to be examined, with two loopfuls of undiluted type-agglutinating rabbit serum on each drop of sputum, and then the same amount of Loeffler's methylene blue. Each drop of the mixture is covered with a cover-glass, and examined at intervals for five to thirty minutes through an oil immersion lens. When the type of the serum and of the pneumococcus are the same, the cocci, stained blue, are seen surrounded by swollen capsules. The capsules are a pale greenish-gray with a characteristic ground-glass appearance, and are distinctly outlined by a thin, dark line around which appears a halo of light. When the serum and organisms are of different types, the pneumococci are of their usual size and are barely visible. This *Quellung* or swelling phenomenon is a distinct and specific reaction between the capsular substance of the pneumococcal cell and antibody of the same type. In the same year as that of Neufeld and Etinger-Tulczynska's publication, Sabin[1207] applied the method in the examination of sputum of one hundred cases of lobar pneumonia. The results with Type I and II organisms were found to correspond exactly to those of the mouse test. In two cases Sabin was able to identify Type I organism, whereas the results by older methods were negative. Furthermore the test was sometimes positive in purely salivary specimens.

In the next year (1934), after an experience of sixteen months, including two months in which they extended the use of the Neufeld test to all types including those from IV through XXXII, Beckler and MacLeod[96] confirmed the results by other methods in 96 per cent of the examinations. They unqualifiedly recommended this method because of its accuracy, simplicity, rapidity, and the small amount of sputum required.

Summary

The species *Diplococcus pneumoniae* has been divided by means of agglutination and other immunological methods into thirty-two separate and distinct serological types. There is evidence at hand that points to the existence of pneumococci that may belong to types other than those already established. Further investigation may reveal some new type identities, but the present list comprises the great majority of the members of this bacterial species. On the basis of cross reactions, there appears to be some relation between organisms of Types II and V, III and VIII, VII and XVIII, and XV and XXX, but the resemblances are not sufficiently close to invalidate the current classification. In nature there appears to be a stability of the types, although, as will be shown in the succeeding chapter, transformation of a strain of one type into an organism of another type can be accomplished by appropriate treatment of the culture.

The particular serological type to which a pneumococcus belongs may be determined in several ways. The agglutination, precipitation, complement-fixation and mouse-protection tests, or combinations and modifications of these tests, may be applied to disclose the type identity of a strain, but it is safe to conclude that for routine needs the Neufeld method for determining specific types of Pneumococcus should be the one of choice. It gives an answer in the shortest time, possesses a high degree of accuracy, and is simple to perform. It makes for a saving in expense and eliminates the necessity of using mice. Whenever the results are not clear or when any doubt exists as to the type to which the organisms belong, the mouse-heart-blood or mouse-protection test should always be carried out for confirmation. Before hope of type identification is abandoned, the more refined methods such as that of Amoss should be tried. The usual cultural procedures, carbohydrate fermentations—especially of inulin—and bile-solubility tests are always to accompany the bacteriological diagnosis when uncertainty arises. For clinical diagnosis and for the direction of serum administration, as well as for epidemiological studies, laboratories should be prepared to run their cultures through the series of the thirty-two known serological types. The procedure requires a supply of potent, monovalent type-specific immune serums, preferably prepared by the immunization of rabbits with standard type strains. With type-specific serums, accurately prepared reagents, healthy laboratory animals, and careful bacteriological manipulations, there should be few cultures that cannot be serologically classified within the known fixed types.

CHAPTER V

PNEUMOCOCCAL DISSOCIATION AND TRANSFORMATION

Changes in the morphological, cultural, pathogenic, and immunological characters of pneumococci caused by various physical, chemical, and serological conditions in their environment; the transformation of the diplococci from one serological type to another; and the relation of the species to streptococci.

THE constancy of the biological characters of Pneumococcus depends on the conditions of its surroundings. When the conditions are favorable, the morphological and serological integrity of the cell remains stable. Subjected to unfavorable influences, Pneumococcus exhibits great lability of form and function. The form of the cell may pass through every stage from the typical encapsulated diplococcus to one completely denuded of capsule; pathogenicity may be diminished from full virulence to entire absence of infectivity; and antigenic and serological properties may lose strict type-specificity and retain only the broader species-specificity. With the restoration of favorable conditions, the degradation process, if it has not proceeded too far, ceases and is reversed, the cell again assuming its typical characters. But, what is still more remarkable, a degraded coccus originally derived from a fixed type may, under appropriate stimulation, develop the vital and immunological properties of a different specific type. Thus, in addition to natural occurrence of variation or dissociation, the actual transformation of pneumococcal types has been experimentally induced and, possibly, species mutation has occurred. Lack of knowledge of the existence of bacterial variants and of the factors inducing dissociation has undoubtedly caused much confusion in bacteriological diagnosis and in the interpretation of the serum reactions of Pneumococcus.

Early Observations of Dissociation: 1891–1921

Bacterial variation is not a new phenomenon. It is only the study and the explanation of the underlying causes that are recent. In 1891, Kruse and Pansini[763] first called attention to changes in morphology, cultural characters, and virulence of pneumococci under artificial cultivation. Pure cultures freshly isolated from pneumonic material were typical in appearance during early generations but, on continued cultivation on unfavorable media, the cells exhibited deviations from the normal characters. The lance-shaped, diplococcal forms became streptococcal or even bacillary, the capsule rapidly vanished, and virulence waned. The degenerated cocci, when passed through susceptible animals, regained their capsules and virulence, and when returned to favorable media, again showed normal pneumococcal morphology. Kruse and Pansini, therefore, noted many of the features of dissociation and were aware of the first causes of the phenomena.

In the next year, Arkharow[17] reported changes taking place in cultures cultivated in the serum of vaccinated animals. Growth was slow in developing and at the end of three or four days the cocci began to diminish in size, to grow in long chains, and to lose virulence. Four years later, Eyre and Washbourn[373] described the variations observed on continued cultivation of pneumococcal strains in broth. Of one strain it was said that it differed in "morphology, biology and pathogenic properties from the parent stock. It, in fact, represented a distinct variety, possessing practically no virulence, and growing luxuriantly, even at 20°C., on all the usual media." The first attempts to induce this variant to revert to its former state were unsuccessful. Then, by passage through a rabbit, the variant reverted to its original form.

Hiss, Borden, and Knapp (1905)[651] encountered organisms, indistinguishable in fermentative reactions from pneumococci, which showed variations in morphology or agglutination, and the authors considered that the cultures were temporarily or permanently modified pneumococci, *Streptococcus mucosus*, or streptococci of hitherto unrecognized types.

A suggestive communication, because of its anticipation of later discoveries, was that of Rosenow[1163] published in 1910. He presented the results of a study of seven cultures isolated from endocarditis which he believed were "modified pneumococci." All the strains fermented inulin and produced a variable amount of greenish discoloration but no hemolysis on blood-agar plates, but grew atypically with the development of involution forms on media containing the patient's blood. However, cultivation in normal serum or blood and animal passage promptly restored normal pneumococcal characters to the modified strains. Recultivation in the patients' serum brought out the modified characters. These special characters varied greatly in the strains studied; the more chronic the disease process in the patient from whom the serum was obtained, the more marked were the changes. This last observation would seem to argue for the occurrence of variation or dissociation *in vivo*—a biological process concerning which there is still some doubt.

The phenomenon of bacterial dissociation, or as it was known in the early years of this century, variation, received little attention until 1915 when Friel[494] reported that prolonged cultivation of bacteria rendered them more susceptible to phagocytosis. He called the process "Piantication" (fattening for slaughter) and observed its operation with strains of Friedländer's bacillus, *Pasteurella*, and Pneumococcus. The same effect was produced by exposing the organisms to immune serum; while the reverse process took place when "pianticated" bacteria were grown in normal serum—they regained their resistance to phagocytosis.*

In the next year, Stryker[1348] described the variations induced in

* Neufeld and Schnitzer credited the first demonstration of bacterial dissociation to Friel, although Hadley[584] ascribed the discovery to Baerthlein (1912). The phenomenon had, however, been observed much earlier by Kruse and Pansini (1891),[763] and by Arkharow (1892),[17] and had been described in some detail by Eyre and Washbourn[373] in 1897.

Pneumococcus by cultivation in immune serum. When virulent strains were grown in broth containing homologous immune serum, there developed variations in agglutinability, decrease in virulence, inhibition of capsule formation, increase in phagocytability with normal serum, and a change in absorptive power and in antigenic properties. Reversion of the changed forms to the original type took place on animal passage, the number of such passages required usually varying with the number of previous serum treatments. The immune response, as measured by agglutinins, was slower in rabbits injected with strains grown in immune serum than with those cultivated in normal serum. A spread of agglutinative action was evident in the ability of the serum of immune rabbits injected with a serum-treated Type II culture to agglutinate pneumococci belonging to both Types I and II. Type-specificity was being lost and replaced by species-specificity. Cultures grown in normal serum formed capsules upon injection into mice, whereas those grown in homologous immune serum under similar conditions showed no demonstrable capsules. This loss of the ability of Pneumococcus to synthesize the capsular substance was later to assume a new and broader significance.

Later Observations of Dissociation

SMOOTH AND ROUGH FORMS OF PNEUMOCOCCUS

Arkwright (1921),[18] in studying the colony appearance of dysentery bacilli grown on media containing immune serum, gave the designations S and R—smooth and rough—to the dissociants because of the corresponding differences in colony topography of each form. Griffith,[560] in 1923, extended Stryker's observations and applied the letters S and R to the two forms of colonies he observed when pneumococci were grown in media containing homologous immune serum. The S colonies have a smooth surface, and the cocci forming them produce the soluble specific substance in broth culture, agglutinate with specific serum of the homologous type, are virulent for laboratory animals, and on injection into rabbits stimulate the production of type-specific immune substances. The R colonies have a rough surface, and the organisms comprising them form no soluble specific substance in broth culture, agglutinate atypically, and are avirulent. Cocci of the R colonies may revert to the S form, or they may remain stable for generations. Another property of the S cells is the ability to absorb from immune serum all antibodies for both S and R forms. The R forms absorb only the anti-R bodies, and when injected into animals fail to stimulate the formation of type-specific (S) antibodies.

Griffith considered that the R form was differentiated from the S by the loss of virulence and by the ability to form capsules and to elaborate soluble specific substance, and that the R form represented a stage in the degeneration of Pneumococcus from the virulent, complex type of S cell to an attenuated form with a simpler antigenic structure. Griffith also found that degradation might not be permanent and that reversion could take place after animal passage or repeated cultivation in blood broth. The author recommended for the demonstration of variant colonies an opaque "chocolate" agar to which red blood cells treated with chloroform had been added.

Griffith looked upon the S form as the original, unchanged organism, the R form as a variant due to unusual growth conditions. The degenerative action of immune serum Griffith believed to be a double one. He suggested as an explanation of the change the view that serum might disorganize the biological functions of Pneumococcus by precipitating the capsule, thus inhibiting the secretion of antileucocytic substances and rendering the organism temporarily harmless, and that when pneumococci divided in the animal body in the presence of immune serum, the influence of the serum might cause progressive attenuation of subsequent generations. In connection with the causes for such bacterial variations, Eastwood[344] contributed an interesting theoretical discussion. It would take us too far afield to quote from it here, but the communication is recommended to those readers who desire to learn more of the philosophical aspects of the phenomenon of dissociation.

In seeking a medium that would emphasize the differences in variants, Sia and Chung,[1270-1] by the substitution of normal dog blood for rabbit or horse blood in agar for plate cultures, obtained such marked differences in the morphology of S and R colonies that differentiation, they claimed, became extremely simple. With a moderate degree of magnification (× 28), the S colonies were seen to be smooth and glossy, while the R colonies, including those derived from Pneumococcus Type IIS, revealed a wrinkled and coarsely rough surface. The R colonies also exhibited strong hemolytic properties. Sia and Chung tested the blood of guinea pig, white rat, chicken, and cat, but none was so good as dog blood. These authors believed that the property of dogs' blood resided in the cellular elements rather than in the plasma, and probably was due to hemoglobin.

MODIFICATIONS A, B, AND C

Blake and Trask (1923),[129] in conducting experiments similar to those of Stryker, also found that growth of pneumococci in homologous serum resulted in a marked loss of virulence, accompanied by constant and distinct changes in agglutinative properties with respect both to the character of agglutination and the zone of optimal reaction. The authors found the changes not to be a gradual alteration of all members of a culture but, instead, there appeared to be a comparatively rapid and complete change in individual organisms. The variants exhibited changes not only in virulence and agglutinability, but also in colony appearance, by means of which three modifications, called by the authors A, B, and C, could be distinguished.

In the same year, analogous observations were published by Yoshioka.[1564] Typical pneumococci underwent apparently regular serological modifications when maintained under unfavorable conditions, such as surface cultivation on unsuitable media, incubation at 39°, and too long-continued drying. The same conditions also led to loss of virulence. The changes noted consisted in a marked decrease in agglutinability with homologous serum and in the appearance of an enhanced agglutinability with heterologous serums. The modified strains were, at times, agglutinable by antistreptococcic serum. The changes appeared irregularly and suddenly and did not parallel the degree of decrease in virulence. An immune serum obtained after immunization with an atypical strain agglutinated only that specific variant and not the parent strain.

In the discussion which followed the presentation of papers on bacterial variability before the German Association of Microbiology at Göttingen in 1924, Neufeld[979] reported a change in bile-solubility of pneumococcal variants, as well as in their susceptibility to optochin. In the same year, Felton and Dougherty[425] observed that pneumococci when grown in plain broth in an automatic transferring device suffered a loss of virulence which was directly proportional to the change in the hydrogen ion concentration of the medium—the more acid the medium the greater the loss of virulence. Accompanying the change in virulence there was an alteration in the behavior of the organisms toward agglutinating serums. Although specific, the agglutinability of the modified strains became greater than that of the parent organism.

COMPOSITE CULTURES

Amoss[12] in 1925 published an article on the composite nature of a pure culture of virulent pneumococci from which he derived several strains by the Barber single-cell technique. These were cultivated in broth containing Type I antiserum, and the pure culture was submitted to successive transfers in bile broth and acid broth. Amoss reported that the virulent strain of Type I Pneumococcus, after being passed through 190 mice, was composed of individuals possessing characters differing from those of the original culture. A pure-line strain derived from a single cell isolated from a virulent composite culture was more virulent for rabbits and less resistant to unfavorable media than was the composite strain or other strains similarly obtained from the same source. Amoss isolated by the plating method an avirulent strain from the composite virulent culture which had been repeatedly transferred and grown in immune serum broth, bile broth, and slightly acid broth. Cultures of the virulent single-cell derivative, when grown in these media, also gave rise to the avirulent form. Heterologous immune serum and also normal serum did not favor the change from virulent to avirulent variants. The avirulent strains, however procured, were all of a single sort. They formed characteristic colonies, showed no tendency to revert to the parent type, and did not become virulent on repeated passage through mice. Serum from rabbits immunized with the avirulent variants possessed agglutinins but no protective antibodies for the parent strain. It seems clear from Amoss' experiments that he had succeeded in effecting a permanent degradation of a virulent Type I Pneumococcus, with a loss of type-specificity, but not of species-specificity.

The results of Reimann's[1125] study, published in the same month in which Amoss' publication appeared, agreed with both Amoss' and Griffith's observations. Reimann reported that cultures of pneumococci from single-cell seedings, when grown in broth containing immune serum, bile, or even normal serum, suffered a decrease in virulence and loss of type-specificity. The changes might take place when the pneumococci were repeatedly grown in plain broth or on blood agar, but were due to variations in individual cells, rather than in the cocci of the culture as a whole. Reimann preferred 2 per cent unheated blood agar to Griffith's chocolate agar, and on this medium there appeared characteristic smooth colonies along with others of the rough form. Cultures from S colonies were highly virulent, had large capsules, produced soluble specific substance, dissolved in bile, and were strictly type-specific. Strains fbom R colonies were avirulent for mice, had no capsule, produced no soluble specific substance, did not dissolve so readily in bile, and had largely lost their type-specificity. Single-cell cultures propagated from S colonies, after repeated transplants under unsuitable conditions, produced some R variants, while single-cell cultures from R colonies, under the same circumstances, remained constant in character.

SPECIES-SPECIFICITY OF ROUGH FORMS

A few months later, Reimann[1126] published these further conclusions:

Immune sera prepared with the degraded or variant forms of pneumococci (R strains) are similar in their reaction to sera prepared with the protein or cell solutions of pneumococci. They contain antibodies reactive with the protein of all types of pneumococci, but no antibodies reactive with the type-specific substances. Pneumococci of the variant or R form, regardless of type derivation, are serologically identical and have the antigenic characteristics of pneumococcus protein. They evoke the species-specific and not the type-specific antibodies. Antipneumococcic sera produced by immunization with S strains may contain species-specific antibodies in addition to those which are type-specific. Each kind of antibody can be removed separately from these sera by selective absorption with the R and S strains of pneumococci.

These fundamental observations were later to be confirmed and explained by the discoveries of Avery and Heidelberger of the antigenic chemical constituents of the pneumococcal cell.

Takami,[1373] contemporaneously with Amoss and Reimann, added a few new facts about variation. His study included certain strains that were apparently stable in their original characters, since they gave rise to no variants even after two or three years' cultivation. There were other strains that showed a strong tendency to vary, and in a short time became so changed that they no longer produced any typical colonies. In agglutinative abilities the same rule held true. There appeared to be no direct relation between decrease of agglutinability and atypical colony formation. The only two characters that were closely connected were bile-solubility and inulin fermentation. When either of these properties was lost the other disappeared.

Takami[1375] followed the *in vitro* experiments with a study of the variations displayed by pneumococci propagated in the animal body. Rabbits, guinea pigs, mice, white rats, and house rats were used for this purpose, and the variants produced in these animals differed in agglutinative characters from the forms developed on artificial media. The explanation offered was that in the body the organisms lose their old receptors and acquire new ones. Takami separated five typical strains of "culture-bacteria" (pneumococci long grown on blood agar) into colonies that were still markedly agglutinable, and into others that had lost this power. The latter were found to be highly virulent for mice, whereas the former were avirulent.

A few years later, Kimura, Sukneff, and Meyer[711] repeated the dissociation experiments, using broth containing 10 per cent homologous immune serum, with subsequent cultivation of the variants on Griffith's chloroform-blood agar and Bieling's blood-water agar, both of which have a laked-blood base. The results were similar to those reported earlier, but the authors believed that they had demonstrated the production of other variants in addition to the atypical R forms with divergent cultural and serological characters. The experimental data, however, are insufficient for judging the claim.

For determining the true character of normal strains and of dissociants, Schiemann[1225] adopted as a criterion the possession of a type-specific (dominant) hapten as a prerequisite for the formation of type-specific agglutinins and protective antibodies and also for virulence. For the recognition of type-specificity the essential considerations were, first, coarse agglutination in homologous antiserum determined by the carbohydrate nature of the hapten; second, the repression of cross-agglutination in heterologous serum; and, third, mouse virulence. According to these standards, in addition to normal and degraded R forms, Schiemann postulated intermediate variants which he claimed represented pseudo-types. The discussion was largely theoretical, and since he gave no experimental data, it is impossible to judge the validity of his claims.

ELECTROPHORETIC POTENTIAL OF VARIANTS

Falk, Jacobson, and Gussin,[383] and then Falk and Jacobson,[380] studied another criterion for variability. The authors measured the electrophoretic potential of Blake's variants A, B, and C from Type I Pneumococcus during cultivation on blood-agar slants, with weekly to bi-weekly transplants, over a period of one and one-half years. The velocities remained constant and paralleled the virulence of the strains. Although the authors believed that electrophoretic potential was related in some fundamental manner to virulence, phagocytability, agglutinability, and other serological characters of microorganisms, the particular variants studied were indistinguishable from the parent strain in these characters, and after a large number of generations on blood agar showed no evidence of spontaneous changes. The only exception to this stability of character was a single-cell strain of variant C which reverted to the A form on passage through a mouse.

EFFECT OF CHARCOAL, YEAST, OPTOCHIN

The variation in pneumococci appearing after growth in broth containing animal charcoal or dry yeast and subsequently in optochin broth, first observed by Berger and Englemann[100-1] and shortly afterward by Morgenroth, Schnitzer, and Berger,[929] was corroborated in 1927 by Amzel.[14] Cultivation in these media gave rise to rough colonies, the members of which were avirulent for mice and exhibited diminished solubility in bile. One strain developed hemolytic properties, and another became agglutinable with antiserum for the fixed types. The variations observed after cultivating the cocci in the presence of bile were the same as those occurring in the Schnitzer-Berger medium.

In Amzel's[15] next paper it was reported that pneumococci isolated from pneumonia patients before optochin injections were of the smooth type, while the organisms cultivated after injection grew as rough colonies. Untreated cases yielded only smooth colonies and, in two cases repeatedly treated with optochin, the isolated culture was persistently composed of both smooth and rough forms. Amzel attempted to convert the rough into smooth strains by mouse passage but was able to effect this reversion in only one of three trials.

During the 1920's there came abundant confirmation and expansion of the earlier observations on pneumococcal dissociation. Jacobson and Falk (1926–1927),[674-5] continuing their earlier studies, were able to degrade smooth strains of Blake and Trask's A, B, and C modifications into rough strains by growing the organisms in broth containing specific immune serum, although after twenty-three transfers the conversion was incomplete. The cultures were still mixtures of S and R varieties. The former continued to have the same virulence and electrophoretic potential, but the latter were reduced in both virulence and potential. Rough variants of the B and C strains reverted after twelve transfers in homologous immune serum broth, and showed the same virulence and potential as the original smooth organisms. In all the strains studied there were alterations in virulence accompanied by parallel alterations in electrophoretic potential and by reciprocal changes in agglutinability. Levinthal[800] also observed changes in virulence and in the cultural and serological behavior of a highly virulent Type I pneumococcus after cultivation in serum broth. He was able to effect the transformation of R to S forms by growth in broth at 25° and by subsequent mouse passage.

IN VIVO VARIATION

Similar variations apparently taking place *in vivo* were described by Wadsworth and Sickles.[1474] Cultures isolated directly from the blood stream of horses undergoing immunization, or at the necropsy of animals that had died as a result of the development of pneumococcal lesions in the heart or other organs, exhibited attenuation of virulence, loss of capsule formation, antigenic power and type-specificity, and changed susceptibility to phagocytosis. In the case of some of these variants the specific characters of the original type from which they were derived were quickly restored by one or two mouse passages. In other instances, the organism remained atypical.

Sickles,[1279] in a later study (1932) of pneumococcal strains that had become atypical in the tissues of horses undergoing immunization, in comparison with the typical cultures from which they were derived and with various other typical and atypical strains, found that all the organisms were bile-soluble. The maximal limits of growth, along with the other characters, such as limiting hydrogen ion concentration and peroxide and hemoglobin formation, were similar for the same type culture whether original, degenerated, or reverted. Sickles found only one strain which departed from the general rule and that organism grew at 42°, and survived even after incubation at 43.5°. No other pneumococcal strains studied were alive after twenty to twenty-four hours at 42°.

That Pneumococcus may, however, retain its specific type characters when growing in the animal body was proved by Megrail and Ecker[888] in 1924, who injected mice and rats with suspensions of gum tragacanth followed by a saline suspension of pneumococci. In these fixation abscesses the strains displayed no variation and no change in agglutinability. Here the conditions differed from those in the horses harboring pneumococci, as reported by Sickles,[1279] since the rats and mice had not been subjected to any immunizing treatment, and their tissues, therefore, presumably contained no antibodies which might favor variation.

Reimann[1128] found that R forms occurred *in vivo* but could discover in his experiments no positive evidence that recovery from pneumococcal infection depended upon the degradation of virulent

S forms to avirulent R forms with their subsequent destruction by phagocytosis. In a still later study[1129] it was noticed that daughter colonies frequently appeared among the R variants, and in some instances tended to replace the typical R forms. The daughter strains grew in colonies with glistening surface, morphologically indistinguishable from genuine S colonies, although the characters of the bacteria comprising the daughter colonies conformed to the R variety. Strains of R pneumococci, which had seemed irreversible, were apparently converted into the S form when treated by the method of Griffith, that is, by growth in specific immune serum. Reimann considered that recent experimental studies indicated that virulent S pneumococci might dissociate into the R form *in vivo*, that R forms occasionally could be found in the sputum of pneumonia patients, and also might live dormant *in vivo* for a considerable period of time.

The recovery of R variants from the body has recently been reported by Shibley and Rogers.[1262] Twenty-four lung punctures made in lobar pneumonia patients at the time of crisis or lysis yielded R forms of pneumococci in all but four cases.

DETAILS OF COLONY FORMATION

Dawson[299] maintained that colony morphology alone could not be considered as a final criterion of dissociation; it should be confirmed by specific agglutination and virulence tests. While it was possible, by mouse passage, to accomplish a complete reversion of Type IIR to Type IIS, it was not possible to convert the particular Type IR strain studied to the corresponding S form. In the case of a Type IIIR strain, it required twenty-eight mouse passages to restore the variant to its original S condition. Growth of the same R strains in broth containing 10 per cent anti-R serum resulted in reversion of Type IIR on the fifth transfer, of Type IIIR after eight to twelve transfers, but failed to affect the Type IR. Dawson thought that the reversion of R to S did not depend on the presence of an admixture of both forms within the culture, but rather that each individual R strain might or might not possess the ability to revert. This varying tendency of R strains was exemplified in one experiment in which one of four other strains of Type IR, obtained by growing a freshly isolated Type IS strain in 25 per cent Type I anti-R serum, reverted to Type IS after forty transfers.

The finer details of colony appearance of R and S forms interested Paul (1927),[1067] who chose a small number of standard R and S strains and studied their growth on agar under a limited number of cultural conditions. Paul described the R colonies as having a rough surface, with a gradual and progressive increase in size over a period of several days and a tendency to remain discrete. The colonies failed to undergo rapid autolysis in early generations and exhibited limited secondary colony formation. Methemoglobin formation was present but might be replaced by slight hemolysis. Paul's S strains grew in rapidly developing disc-shaped colonies with a smooth surface which later showed irregularities. The colonies tended to become confluent and exhibited marked autolysis in thirty-six to ninety-five-hour cultures. In the same period, secondary colony formation took place. Methemoglobin formation was a constant feature.

In a second paper, Paul[1068] gave further information concerning the conditions which affected colony formation. Under extreme crowding, the individual S colonies gave way to irregular, amorphous, slightly elevated masses with myriads of tiny structures having irregular and roughened surfaces, comparable to R colonies, but on transfer to less crowded conditions they developed as typical S colonies. The true R colonies tended to remain discrete, but in dense growth resembled the S colonies under similar conditions. The effect of age on the S colonies was to increase autolysis and papilla formation. With the R colonies there was no autolysis, but roughness, opacity, and compactness became emphasized, with papillae appearing on about the fourth day. When the blood content of nutrient agar fell below 5 per cent, the S colonies appeared small and rough, yet were not true R colonies. The same effect was brought about by an alkaline reaction of the medium, but the original characters were restored on transplantation to a more favorable medium.

In a study of the bile-solubility of Pneumococcus, Atkin[29] reported that pneumococci growing in papillae or secondary colonies developing on an autolyzed colony from a point inoculation on a thick serum-agar medium of proper reaction were insoluble and that susceptibility of the variants to the action of bile corresponded to the possession by the organisms of autolysin. When the insoluble cocci were subcultured on a fresh serum-agar slant, they regained autolytic properties and bile-solubility.

Grumbach[563] also studied the details of colony formation accompanying the varying degrees of pneumococcal dissociation. He differed with Atkin,[29] but agreed with Paul that daughter colonies were not identical with R forms of pneumococci, because they were never truly granular on ascitic agar, they remained bile-sensitive, were fully virulent, and on transplantation developed into "bud-carrying" S colonies. Grumbach found that the ability to produce hemolysis on blood agar and in blood bouillon in forty-eight to seventy-two hours quite commonly ran parallel with the dissociation phenomena. He described the characters of three virulent S strains isolated from pneumonic material that were not agglutinated by Type I, II, or III serums. Growing for twenty-four hours on ascitic agar the organisms produced the classical picture of pneumococcal colonies. The thickness of the peripheral ring varied, and in one case there was a "wall" formation of the type Buerger and Ryttenberg[169] claimed to have found solely in colonies of streptococci. Grumbach also described a "wing-form" colony which he believed to be similar to that supposed to be caused by phage action on streptococci, and concluded that the same colony pictures could be obtained for pneumococci as for streptococci, but was not sure how far the bactericidal action of the body fluids or how far bacteriophagic action were to be considered as the basis for the phenomena.

Faragó (1932)[390] investigated the possible participation of bacteriophagic action in the dissociative processes, but decided that it was not a factor. He objected to the designation R and S for dissociants, because secondary colonies were formed from virulent organisms, whereas Griffith's R modification arose from avirulent strains. It is difficult to follow Farago's reasoning, but it may be possible that he had in mind some of the features later described by Dawson.

ANTIGENICITY OF ROUGH FORMS

Tillett[1406] turned his attention to the antigenic properties of the dissociated R forms. When he vaccinated rabbits by repeated intravenous injections of suspensions of heat-killed R pneumococci, the animals acquired a marked degree of active immunity to infection with virulent S forms of Pneumococcus I and II. (Tillett[1404-6] had previously shown that a similar immunization treatment induced active resistance to Type III infection.) Furthermore, the whole citrated blood of the immune rabbits passively protected normal rabbits against infection with Type I and Type III pneumococci, but failed to confer a like protection on mice. According to Tillett this form of acquired resistance to pneumococcal infection elicited by R organisms devoid of type-specificity, and exemplified in animals whose serum possessed no demonstrable type-specific antibodies, presented features which strongly suggested that the underlying mechanism differed from that concerned in type-specific immunity.*

RESPIRATORY CAPACITY OF VARIANTS

Another difference in the character of S and R forms was the

* For a full discussion and bibliography of microbic dissociation up to that time the reader is referred to Hadley's[584] comprehensive article.

changed respiratory capacities of pneumococcal variants. According to Finkle's[440] measurements, the capacities of organisms of Types I and II were altered during conversion from the S to the R form. For Type I Pneumococcus it was increased 110 per cent, while for Type III it was diminished by 45 per cent. In the case of Type II there occurred a diminution of only 16 per cent in respiratory activity. At the same time, anaerobic glycolysis was increased on the average 25 per cent each for all R forms irrespective of type derivation, while Type I Pneumococcus, on being converted to the R form, lost its capacity for aerobic glycolysis. Pneumococcus III in passing to the degraded stage gained this activity, which is in accordance with the respective increase and decrease in respiratory activity of the two types. In order to appreciate the degree of the respiratory capacity of pneumococci, Finkle stated that the O_2 consumption was for Type I pneumococci thirteen times and for Type II strains thirty-four times that of the human tubercle bacillus (strain H_{37}). When compared with the oxygen consumption of animal tissues, Type II strains consumed over twenty times as much oxygen as did isolated rat kidney tissue, and almost one hundred times as much O_2 as isolated dog muscle.

A respiratory phenomenon connected with loss of virulence has been described by Sevag and Maiweg.[1258] A virulent pneumococcus on being transformed into its avirulent form consumes many times more oxygen than the parent organism, but the gain of activity is a temporary property. After a time, the avirulent variant degenerates into a form that consumes much less oxygen than either the virulent or the recently derived avirulent form. The phenomenon may be associated with the change in the structure of the enzyme responsible for carbohydrate biosynthesis during the shift from the virulent to the avirulent state and hence may be related to capsule formation. According to Sevag and Maiweg, the addition of colorless, clear, blood catalase or of a small amount of sodium pyruvate to the culture enables the organisms to carry on their respiratory functions and to maintain their reproductive capacities and virulence for a longer period of time.

Petrie (1932)[1084] suggested one more means for the identification of R and S variants. In stab cultures in agar plates containing 5 per cent immune serum the virulent S pneumococci grew with a distinct halo about the colony when the organism and immune serum corresponded in type-specificity. The halo apparently consisted of a specific precipitate formed by the interaction of the pneumococcal polysaccharide and the precipitin in the homologous serum. The R colonies, in contrast, produced only a faint and narrow halo after a considerable period of incubation. Serum from immune horses appeared to be more suitable than serum from immune rabbits for halo production.

INTERMEDIATE FORMS

In addition to the well-known S and R forms, Klumpen (1932)[730] mentioned intermediate forms growing in colonies designated as SU and RK. In other characters, however, the strains were either true S or R forms. Klumpen recognized the *Flätterformen* described by Grumbach, and noted that the organisms comprising daughter colonies were of the smooth type.

Still other variants intermediate between the S and R forms were derived from pneumococci by Blake and Trask (1933).[130] By growing Type IS pneumococci in homologous immune serum broth, the progressive appearance and disappearance of forms differing from both S and R cocci were observed. The forms were designated as a, b, c, d, and e. Two of the intermediates, Type Ib and Type Ic, were easily stabilized in pure culture. All showed an orderly change in agglutinative reactions in homologous and heterologous immune serum, and also underwent a progressive loss of virulence for mice. Blake and Trask produced only one intermediate form from Type IIS and none from Type IIIS.

The importance of recognizing intermediate variants in the dissociative process was emphasized by Paul[1069] of Blake's laboratory. He believed that two methods of inducing degradative dissociation in S forms seemed to give rise to the different patterns of variant production. Thus, when S forms were grown in homologous antiserum they became rapidly stabilized as R forms, but when S forms were cultivated in media containing bile, the S organisms displayed a greater tendency to become stabilized as c forms. Paul showed that during the reversion of c, d, and R forms, induced by growth in anti-R or plain rabbit-serum broth, intermediate variants arose in the reverse order to that in which they appeared during the degradation of S forms. The intermediate variants tended to become stabilized as b forms, which was the usual high level to which these strains reverted by this method.

A process possibly related to that studied by Blake and Trask was reported by Eaton,[345] an associate of Blake, who described the production of stable strains of Pneumococcus which underwent rapid lysis or failed to grow at 37°. For the strains he introduced the term "phantom colony" or "P–C" variants. This P–C variation, he claimed, was a change independent of the ordinary smooth-to-rough variation. Eaton, moreover, made direct isolation of these variants from cases of human infection.

Another apparent complication in the symbols employed to identify pneumococcal variants is to be found in the recent papers by Eaton (1934–1935).[345-6] In addition to the phantom colony or P–C variants, he observed smooth variants arising in the daughter-colony dissociation of stock smooth strains after incubation on blood agar at 25°. These smooth variants, called V, and the smooth parent strain, termed N, from which the former were derived, had the same virulence for mice and did not differ in antigenic composition as determined by agglutination, agglutinin-absorption, and mouse protection tests. The smooth V strains were stable, and while they, too, formed daughter colonies they dissociated to rough forms much less readily than did the N or freshly isolated strains. The N and V strains appeared to differ in their capsular staining reactions, and in the ability to form methemoglobin in blood. Without an actual visual comparison of these V variants with the principals and intermediates described by other authors it is impossible to assign them their proper place in the dissociation order.

Further study is required before giving an estimate of the significance of these possibly new forms, although there is already much evidence to support the concept of a polyphasic cycle in bacterial dissociation.*

REVERSAL OF DISSOCIATION

Griffith[562] was successful in reversion experiments in the animal body. Some R strains which had not entirely lost their soluble specific substance readily reverted to the S form when passed through the mouse. The author obtained smooth colonies, with restoration of virulence and original serological type characters, after making massive injections of R strains into the subcutaneous tissues of the mouse. The original change from S to R forms was accomplished by ageing the colonies on chocolate blood agar containing horse serum and by cultivation in broth to which specific immune serum had been added. The greater the concentration of immune serum, the more complete and permanent was the change to the R form.

The possibility of the reversal of the dissociation process attracted Dawson and Avery[304] who, by mouse passage, not only brought back to the S form seven or eight cultures of single-cell isolation, pure-line S strains of Types I, II, and III, but also succeeded in causing six pure-line R strains to revert to type-specific forms by growing the cultures in media containing anti-R serum.† The authors failed in a similar attempt with a Type IR culture. As in mouse passage, reversion by cultural methods was accompanied

* Rakieten[1119] believed that a peculiar organism obtained from the peritoneal fluid and heart's blood of a mouse after inoculation with a highly virulent Type II Pneumococcus was a pneumococcal variant. It was a Gram-positive bacillus, bile-soluble, agglutinated with Type II serum in a dilution of 1 to 400, and also to a slight extent with Type I serum. The organism was not pathogenic for mice. Rakieten's description of cultural development of the strain from the infected fluids raises doubt as to its true pneumococcal origin.

† Compare Soule's[1308] similar results with *Bacillus subtilis* (1927).

by acquisition of properties of the typical S form. In the experiments, reversion was invariably toward the specific type from which the R form was originally derived.*

REVERSION BY MEANS OF PNEUMOCOCCAL VACCINE

In Griffith's experiments on reversion he introduced a new principle, which later was to effect still more surprising and momentous changes in the biological character of Pneumococcus. He reported that the most certain method of producing reversion was to add to the R culture before subcutaneous injection into the mouse a dose of a heat-killed culture of a virulent strain of the same type. Reversion from R to the S form could occasionally be brought about by the simultaneous inoculation of a virulent culture of another type when the culture had been heated for only a short period to 60°, that is, a Type IIR strain reverted to its original condition when inoculated with a heated, virulent Type I culture. The Type I antigen appeared to lose the power to cause reversion more easily than the Type II antigen, the former becoming inactive after heating to 80°, whereas the latter was still effective after steaming at 100°. Griffith found, moreover, that the antigen of certain Group IV strains appeared to be closely related to that of Type II. Both were equally resistant to heat, and stimulated the reversion of R forms derived from Type II, but failed to bring about the reversion of the RI strain to its S form.

Transformation of Type

More surprising and important was the successful transformation by the method of an R strain derived from one specific type into the S form of the same type as that of the heated culture. The S form of Type I was evolved from the R form of Type II Pneumococcus, and the S form of Type II from an RI organism.

* Alloway (1932)[8] cited Kelley as having discovered that normal hog serum was rich in these anti-R bodies and could be substituted for anti-R serum in activating the reversion process.

From the RI variant and from the R forms of Type II, were derived the clear, mucinous colonies of Type III. The newly developed Type III strains were of relatively low virulence and frequently remained localized at the site of subcutaneous inoculation. A still wider shift which Griffith effected was that of a Group IVR strain to virulent strains belonging to Types I and II. The injection of large doses of heated cultures of R pneumococci along with small amounts of living R strains never caused a transformation of type and only rarely produced a reversion of the R form of Type II to its S form. Griffith, therefore, along with his success in changing R variants back to the original S forms with accession of virulence and specific type characters, was the first to accomplish a true transformation of one pneumococcal type into another.

To degrade a pneumococcus *in vitro* to a form devoid of its original type characters and then to exalt it to its original condition was an achievement that we had come to expect, but transforming a degenerated or dissociated culture into another form possessing entirely different type characters was a somewhat amazing performance. Even remembering the theories of earlier investigators with their claims of species mutations, and discounting possible errors in their experiments, this discovery had not been anticipated. It was, for the first time, to supply a theoretical explanation for the many baffling problems encountered in the study of the spread and the invasiveness of pneumococci, and of the clinical pathology of pneumococcal infections, not to mention the broader bearing on the many riddles of microbiology.

Neufeld and Levinthal[994] also were able to reproduce Griffith's transformation phenomena, but by another procedure. They first dissociated virulent, type-specific strains by growing the organisms in broth containing sterile animal organs (spleen, heart, kidney, and liver of rabbits). The degraded R variants were then injected subcutaneously into mice with killed S pneumococci. Neufeld and Levinthal thus converted an avirulent Type IR pneumococcus into a virulent Type IS organism, and with the addition of a killed Type IIS strain obtained a typical IIS pneumococcus. Not all the R variants could be reverted.

Somewhat less success in this respect attended the efforts of Reimann.[1129] The R strains evolved by immune serum-broth cultivation were as a rule irreversible, only one of many strains passing back to the S form of Type I or over to Type III, the reversion depending upon the type of the heated culture used. No transformations to Type II occurred, although in one instance it appeared that a heated IIS culture induced the reversion of the R strain to the Type IS prototype. Reimann obtained positive reversions of typical R forms from pneumococci of Types I or II when he inoculated the R strains subcutaneously into mice with heated S cultures of Types I, II, and III. The living IR culture plus heated Type IIS vaccine gave Type IIS pneumococci; IIR became IS or IIIS, depending upon the type of heated culture used. Both Types IR and IIR, when inoculated with heated cultures of homologous type S forms, frequently reverted to the respective prototypes. These seemingly bizarre biological changes were, therefore, becoming a routine laboratory performance.

Baurhenn's[93] efforts at reversion (1932) were more fruitful than Reimann's. By subculturing R strains with homologous and heterologous vaccines consisting of heat-killed cultures, he changed the R strains into their original S forms and to the S form of a different type. Baurhenn inclined to Griffith's view that all pneumococcal types possess a common basic form. The basic form, under the stimulation of the activating principle, responds by acquiring the properties of the activator. Baurhenn claimed to be the first to have produced transformation within Group X (Group IV) as well as the transformation of a fixed type (I, II, or III) into a specific type of Group X. This feat is, of course, entirely possible, and from what we already know of the phenomena of transformation, there is no reason to doubt that similar changes may occur in the case of all the known types of pneumococci.

Dawson (1928)[299] confirmed and expanded Griffith's observations. He found that type-specific S pneumococci could be transformed from one specific S type into another specific S type through the intermediate stage of the R form; that R forms of pneumococci, derived from any specific S type, might be transformed into S organisms of other specific types by injecting mice subcutaneously with small amounts of living R strains together with heated vaccines of heterologous S cultures. The S vaccines could be heated for fifteen minutes between 60° and 80° and still remain effective in causing R forms derived from heterologous S types to revert to the type of the vaccine; S vaccines heated fifteen minutes at temperatures between 80° and 100° were not active in causing R variants derived from heterologous S types to revert to the type of the vaccine; S vaccines heated between 80° and 100° could cause Type IIR and Type IIIR variants to revert to the original S type; S vaccines of any type, including Type I, heated for fifteen minutes at 80° to 100° would no longer cause Type IR strains to revert to their original S type; S vaccines heated for periods as long as two hours at 60° were effective in causing R forms derived from heterologous types to revert to the type of the vaccine employed. Dawson successfully converted a single-cell R strain derived from a Type IIIS pneumococcus into a Type IIIS, a Type IS, and a Group IVS organism. On the other hand, every attempt to produce transformation of type *in vivo* failed.

TRANSFORMATION BY VACCINE AND ANIMAL INOCULATION

In 1930, Dawson and Sia[305] announced the transformation of a Type IIR into a Type IIIS pneumococcus. The conditions necessary for the reversal were minimal amounts of the R culture, the addition of the heated activating culture, incubation for longer than the conventional period, and the inclusion of small amounts of anti-R serum and of blood broth. When the activating organisms were heated for fifteen minutes at 100°, they lost their capacity for inducing transformation, although suspensions heated for four hours at 60° or for fifteen minutes at 80° were still effective.

Filtrates of vigorously growing cultures and of heat-killed suspensions of S organisms were inactive, as also were suspensions of S organisms disrupted by freezing and thawing, with subsequent heating for fifteen minutes at 60°. But when suspensions of S organisms were first killed by heating for fifteen minutes at 60° and then frozen and thawed, they were highly effective. In a more detailed communication, the authors gave the additional information that transformation of type could be induced by the use of small amounts of S vaccine, and that while the transformative process was brought about most readily by employing anti-R serum in the culture medium, it might be accomplished without the presence of the serum.

Transformation of one S form to the S form of a different type without any apparent development of intermediate stages was described by Dawson and Warbasse[306] in 1931. The original culture was a virulent, single-cell isolation of Type II Pneumococcus. One drop of a 10^{-6} dilution of the culture was seeded into a medium containing homologous immune serum together with large quantities of Type III pneumococcal vaccine. The cultures were incubated at 37°, and at the end of forty-eight hours streaked plates showed, in the majority of instances, numerous Type III with some Type IIS colonies. No R colonies were observed. From the experiment Dawson and Warbasse inferred that a type-specific S pneumococcus can be transformed into other type-specific S pneumococci by growth in homologous immune serum in the presence of heterologous vaccine. Although the conditions of the experiment were unfavorable to the development of R forms, the authors thought it was probable that the organism nevertheless passed through this intermediate stage during the transformation.

In 1931, Sia and Dawson[1272] reported that R cultures possessing slight degrees of R stability were most suitable for transformation experiments *in vitro*. The authors also sought a soluble principle in cultures subjected to the action of bacterial enzymes liberated in old broth cultures and during mechanical disruption of young bacterial cells. Trials with the solutions, with the supernatant fluid from an S vaccine, the filtrate from an S vaccine, purified soluble specific substance, and the filtrates of actively growing S cultures, all gave negative results.

ISOLATION OF THE TRANSFORMATIVE PRINCIPLE

Alloway (1932)[8] evidently was more successful than his predecessors in obtaining the transformative principle from the pneumococcal cell. With filtered extracts of virulent S strains of Types I and III he converted a Type IIR strain into S organisms of the same specific type as that of the cells extracted. The author stated that the constituents of the extract supplied an activating stimulus of a specific nature in that the R pneumococci acquired the capacity of elaborating the capsular material peculiar to the organisms extracted.

In the next study (1933), Alloway[9] prepared active and specific extracts by dissolving S pneumococci in sodium desoxycholate solution. These cell-free extracts were as potent as the intact cocci in causing R forms to assume new type-specific characters. With an extract of Type III Pneumococcus he was able to convert a Type IIR variant almost regularly and abruptly into the smooth form of Type III. Alloway then purified the extracts by removing a considerable amount of inert material by charcoal adsorption and reprecipitation of the adsorbed extracts with alcohol or acetone. The stimulating principle passed through Berkefeld filters without loss of strength if the reaction of the solution was alkaline. The substance was resistant to heating at 60° for thirty minutes but was appreciably affected at temperatures of 80° or over. The purified extracts apparently had suffered no loss of potency and caused a more prompt transformation than did the original solutions. An unexplained observation was the fact that in no instance could the transformation be effected without the addition to the culture-extract mixture of blood serum or of ascitic or pleural fluid.

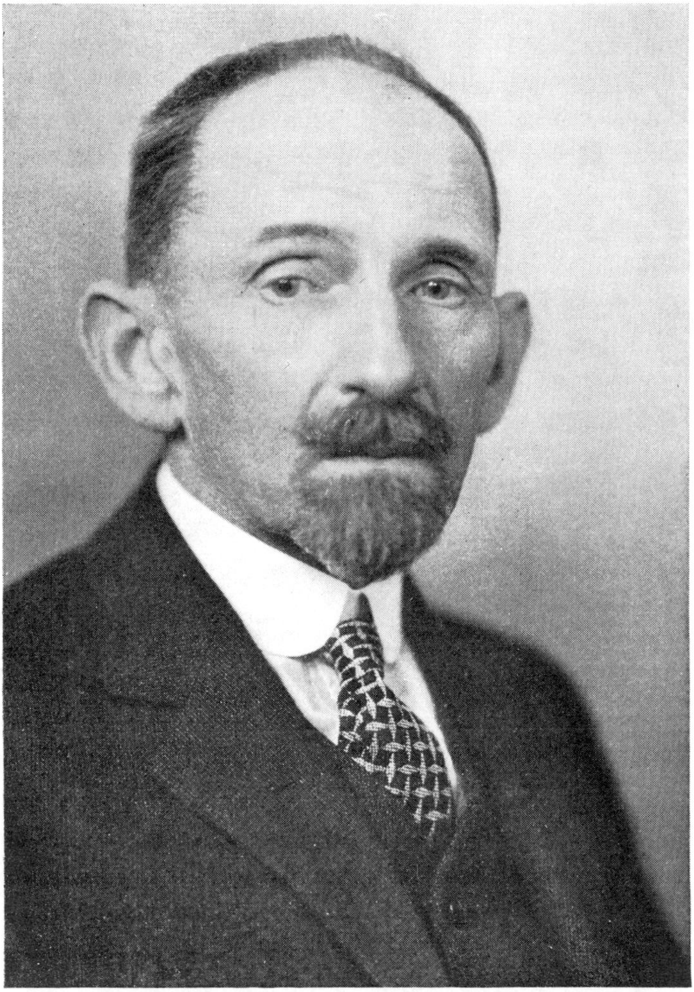

Photograph by Louis Schmidt   Courtesy of the Rockefeller Institute for Medical Research

FR. NEUFELD

Dawson Classification

A dissociation form, other than the S and R forms, was described in 1934 by Dawson.[303] It appeared to be a mucoid variant of Pneumococcus and was strikingly different from the two main, accepted variants. Dawson intimated that the terminology of bacterial dissociation should be changed to include the M form.

In later communications (1934), Dawson[302-8] gave many more details of the several stages of pneumococcal dissociation. He showed, first, that the change from the typical, virulent form to the degraded variant was not a simple direct S → R conversion, but that the dissociative process consisted of several phases. In this cycle there were three outstanding stages represented by distinct difference in colony appearance and morphology, and here he departed from the orthodox concept of the S and R forms.

At first reading, Dawson's discussion and proposals are a little bewildering. He makes the apparently radical suggestion that the old designations smooth and rough be changed and the term "mucoid" be introduced into the terminology as it applies to Pneumococcus; thus, S would become M; R would become S; and the new form would be R. His revelation of the intricacies of the dissociative phenomena and the proposed change in terminology are apt to cause some confusion in minds accustomed to the accepted order of dissociative nomenclature. But an unprejudiced and painstaking study of the facts and his recommendations serves to dispel some of the doubts raised in a cursory reading of the text. Dawson's contentions were founded on the appearance of a new variant during the cultivation of an R form of Pneumococcus originally derived from a Type IIS culture. When this strain was diluted, thinly streaked on blood-agar plates, and incubated several days at 37°, many of the colonies showed evidence of a variety of secondary growths. The following is taken from Dawson's description of the S → R transformation.

For convenience the evolution of the R variant may be described in several stages although it is emphasized that the process is both gradual and continuous. In the first stage, which may suitably be termed R^1, the colonies present more or less the general appearance of smooth (old terminology, "rough") colonies but the surface is more coarsely stippled. The constituent organisms are more or less typical pneumococci showing a tendency to staphylococcal grouping and occasional swollen or club forms may be seen. In the second stage, R^2, the colonies present a still rougher appearance and the outline may appear slightly irregular. This irregularity frequently becomes quite pronounced after several days' growth. The bacteria in this stage are much more pleomorphic and are frequently elongated in an extreme lanceolate manner. They still retain Gram's stain. In the third stage, R^3, the surface of the colony becomes exceedingly rough and the margin quite irregular. The contour of such colonies still remains convex but less so than the original S form (old terminology, R form). The organisms constituting such colonies present a bizarre morphological picture. Pointed diphtheroid elements arranged in a fashion suggesting broken twigs may be observed, with scattered long, bizarre, rod forms which are partially Gram-positive and partially Gram-negative. At this stage of development the morphological picture can scarcely be recognized as that of pneumococcus. The fourth stage, R^4, can only be defined with some difficulty. It would appear that the growth is now in a stage of considerable flux and several types of colonies and morphological elements may be produced. Some of the colonies present an appearance similar to that just described while others resemble more closely the pure R form (R^n).

The morphology of the organisms in the R^4 stage is difficult to describe because of their extreme pleomorphism. In addition to coarse and irregular coccal forms there may appear elongated Gram-negative rod-like structures exhibiting irregular Gram-positive areas. A great variety of other morphological elements may also be present.

Dawson described the R → S change in which intermediate forms of the type seen in the S → R change were not observed, and then gave a detailed description of the biological characters of this new variant. From the description a few of the more important data may be selected. The organism was bile-soluble, of low virulence for mice, agglutinated in normal saline solution, and failed to elaborate soluble specific substance. The variant was not peculiar to the

Type IIR strain, and single organisms of one individual strain also possessed the capacity to dissociate into the new form.

Dawson then pointed out certain discrepancies in the characteristic features of the S and R forms as described by Griffith for Pneumococcus and those described by Arkwright for the colon-typhoid-dysentery group, and which have been accepted by the majority of bacteriologists as the chief distinguishing features of the smooth and rough forms of many bacterial species. He further drew attention to the fact that certain attributes of Arkwright's S and R forms do not appear in Pneumococcus while other new distinctions did not have a place in Arkwright's original descriptions. Dawson has portrayed these differences in terminology in a diagram which, although as yet unpublished, was kindly loaned to the authors.

	COLON, TYPHOID, DYSENTERY		PNEUMOCOCCUS	
	ARKWRIGHT	OTHER OBSERVERS	GRIFFITHS	DAWSON
1	NOT DESCRIBED	M	S	M
2	S	S	R	S
3	R	R	NOT DESCRIBED	R

Courtesy of Dr. M. A. Dawson

RELATIONSHIPS OF MUCOID, SMOOTH, AND ROUGH COLONIES OF BACILLI OF THE COLON-TYPHOID-DYSENTERY GROUP AND PNEUMOCOCCUS

When Dawson compared the salient characters of the three pneumococcal variants (S, R, and the new M form) with the mucoid, smooth, and rough forms of members of the colon-typhoid-dysentery group and the smooth and the two rough forms of the Friedländer bacillus, the inconsistency in the use of the terms smooth and rough became convincingly apparent. On a basis of colony appearance, morphology, growth in plain broth, stability in salt solution, and of virulence and type-specificity, the smooth form of Pneumococcus and of Friedländer's bacillus conforms to the mucoid form of members of the colon-typhoid-dysentery group; the rough form of Pneumococcus and the R_1 form of Friedländer are similar to the smooth form of bacilli of the enteric group; while Dawson's new variant and Julianelle's R_2 form of the Friedländer bacillus agree with the rough form of the colon-typhoid-dysentery bacilli.

In order, therefore, to bring these terms in agreement, to conform—with an addition—to the designations of Arkwright, and to establish a uniform and logical terminology for the dissociants of all bacterial species, Dawson would change the terms now used for the variants of pneumococci as follows: Mucoid or M would replace the present smooth or S; smooth would be substituted for the former rough (R_1 form of Friedländer bacilli); while rough or R would be applied to the new variant described by Dawson and the R_2 form of Friedländer's bacillus.

There is no doubt that such a reversal of the accepted terms would cause confusion and meet with opposition. It cannot be denied that this change would be especially disturbing to the present correlation between the classification of dissociation forms and immunological behavior, but that does not necessarily preclude the possibility of a new and perhaps a deeper insight into the parallelism between the phenomena of variation and antigenic specificity. This proposed change recalls the confusion that followed the revision of the designations of blood groups, but that change has not only been endured but the new terms are now generally accepted as useful and logical. There is much to be said both for and against Dawson's proposal and so it may be permissible to turn to one who speaks with authority on this important subject of bacterial dissociation. Hadley's opinion expressed in a letter written in 1933 to Dawson was in part:*

Making a decision regarding the proper course to pursue in changing the nomenclature now employed for designating the phases of the pneumococcus, in favor of the symbolization which your studies thus far seem unquestionably to justify, might easily depend on how fully an investigator has in mind the details of dissociative variation as a phenomenon observable in all bacterial species, and how clearly he can perceive the parallel trends in such variations,—as opposed to a limited outlook on the one species in which he may be especially interested.

If bacteriology were limited to the study of a few species, or to the Pneumococcus, it would make little difference what the observed phases were called, because no generalizations would be involved, and the phase symbols would possess no significance for bacteriology as a whole. A, B and C, or X, Y and Z would serve the purpose. . . .

The desirability of adjusting the difficulty in the Pneumococcus situation, and of doing it without delay, is the more to be recommended in view of the increasingly wide recognition that the same or analogous phases exist in numerous other species. The facts are now becoming so extensive and well grounded that they are offering, for the first time in the history of bacteriology, a basis for the formulation of general laws; and for making possible a certain kind of "predictability," as I have perhaps already demonstrated to you. To this extent pure bacteriology is beginning to take on the aspects of a real science—a compliment which (to my mind) it has scarcely been appropriate to offer in the past.

To facilitate this highly gratifying trend it stands to reason that all who work with the problems of variation should keep in mind the dual significance of their results, and make possible a correlation of their own results with those of others; also to make quick and decisive corrections when such are clearly in order. To label as a smooth a Pneumococcus phase that is demonstrated to be a mucoid, or to label as a rough a phase that is clearly a smooth, may do little harm to those

* The authors appreciate the courtesy of Doctors Hadley and Dawson in granting permission to include portions of this letter here.

whose work lies chiefly in this species. But such a continued policy can only render increasingly difficult important comparisons with other species, and work havoc with the interests of those who are seriously attempting to discern some law and order in the affairs of the bacteria. Further advance in this direction can take place, according to my view, only if bacteriologists become sufficiently keen to recognize the true nature of the phases they employ, and sufficiently independent to "call a spade a spade," whenever recognized as such, regardless of politics, tradition or social etiquette. . . .

It might also be in the back of your mind that the splendid work of some of your associates on the chemical aspects of dissociation would suffer from any change in terminology made at this late date. I am absolutely convinced to the contrary. In reality I believe that the incentive to extensions of their results to many other bacterial species would be a direct and immediate outcome, through establishing a recognition of the most appropriate culture phase to be employed in such studies. . . .

It is therefore my opinion that a frank recognition of the present incongruities of the situation will not detract from, but facilitate in wide measure, researches in the important field opened up years ago by Drs. Avery, Dochez, Heidelberger and their collaborators.

Dawson believed that before making such a radical change in the accepted terminology of pneumococcal variants it would be well to ascertain if similar variants could be demonstrated in *Streptococcus haemolyticus*. From the latest study by Dawson,[303] it would seem that he succeeded in dissociating that organism into three main variants, which in their manner of colony formation and in morphology correspond closely with the three main variants of Pneumococcus. The mucoid and smooth forms appeared and, by cultivation of the streptococci on blood agar and by repeatedly picking and transplanting material from the roughest marginal areas, Dawson was able to develop the extremely rough type of colony which he had obtained with pneumococci, representing the R variant.

As Dawson said, "evidence is rapidly accumulating to show that the phenomenon of bacterial variation in a wide variety of bacterial species fits into a more or less orderly pattern." This pattern, besides fitting bacilli of the colon-typhoid-dysentery group, the types of *B. friedländeri*, and probably the streptococci, would bring order in the arrangement of the many variants of pneumococci that have been described under a wide diversity of terms. Thus, the modifications A, B, and C of Schnitzer and Berger, Blake and Trask's intermediates Type I a, b, c, d, and e, Wadsworth and Sickles' atypical strains, Reimann's daughter-colony variants, the "wall" type of Buerger, the *Flätterformen* of Grumbach, possibly the P–C or phantom colonies and the smooth N and the smooth V types of Eaton, the variants of Kimura, Sukneff, and Meyer, the atypical rough forms from budding colonies reported by Paul, the SU and RK dissociants of Klumpen, and of course the R and S forms of Griffith, and the new variant of Dawson might conceivably be arranged in accordance with the general pattern and would all either fall into the chief places designated by Dawson's M, S, and R or into the spaces between these predominating forms.

The scheme of Dawson, therefore, revolutionary as it may seem, merits further consideration and should be subjected to additional experimental trial before it is rejected or finally accepted.

These discoveries concerning the variability of Pneumococcus are full of new meaning to the bacteriologist, biochemist, immunologist, and particularly to the physiologist. They prove that Pneumococcus has the potential ability to synthesize simple sugars into diverse, complex, and highly individual polysaccharides. When the conditions of the surroundings are entirely favorable, this metabolic process operates uniformly. The end products are always of the same molecular composition and configuration, and are highly distinctive of a given serological and biochemical type. When, however, the forces of the environment are inimical, the function of carbohydrate synthesis is retarded, the cell produces less and less of the distinguishing capsular polysaccharide, and the cocci lose their capsule, virulence, and strict racial identity. If the unfavorable conditions continue, this particular metabolic activity ceases or is suppressed and the organism degenerates into a harmless coccus, devoid of any specialized earmarks—a sort of bacterial maverick. If the exposure to these untoward conditions is sufficiently protracted, the function is apparently permanently lost, but if the exposure ceases before this stage is reached, the cell retains the latent power to elaborate its original, individual capsular carbohydrate, and all that is needed to revive this power is the restoration of a satisfactory environment—either in culture or in an animal—or else the activation that comes from an encounter with immune bodies specific for its own degraded form. Living under such conditions the type-less coccus gradually returns to its former distinctive state.

These discoveries, moreover, have disclosed another and astonishing activity of the organism. When stimulated by some unknown constituent of fully functioning pneumococcal cells, this latent metabolic function of the degenerated coccus develops a new property, and instead of building up capsular carbohydrates of the former kind, the degraded cell now synthesizes polysaccharides of the same chemical constitution and specific type as those of the strains supplying the activating stimulus. The once degraded organism becomes then a virulent pneumococcus, but with all the specialized characters of its foster strain. Having lost its original features it regains a new type identity.

The cycle of degradation, regeneration, and type transformation presents so many fascinating phases that one is strongly tempted to speculate on the various factors concerned in this extraordinary evolution. The basic ability to elaborate these various specific capsular carbohydrates is always ready to respond to appropriate stimulation unless the cells have gone too far down the path of degradation, and is evidently common to all pneumococci. The direction which the transformation takes is determined wholly by the nature of the stimulus, and it is the identity of this factor which still remains unrevealed to us. It apparently exists only in cells exercising all their special functions, and seems to be a normal constituent of the cell and not a product of katabolic processes.

Whether such transformations ever take place in the animal body, in health or in disease, and if they do what causes bring them about, together with the yet broader problems of the origin of various types and the influences which established their different biological identities, are all questions that are attracting investigators in this branch of science. Whether this fundamental function of Pneumococcus can be so perverted as to bring about the transmutation of this organism into one of a different species is a problem which has been attacked in a more general way.

Transmutation of Species

The mutability of members of the bacterial tribe *Streptococcaceae* has long been a moot question. From time to time there have appeared reports of the change of a pneumococcus into a streptococcus, and even of a swing through the whole cycle from virulent Pneumococcus to *Streptococcus viridans* to *Streptococcus haemolyticus* and back to Pneumococcus. But, in these later days of refined bacteriological and immunological technique one has been inclined to look somewhat askance at such claims. The idea has, however, persisted, and what was looked upon as a mere notion is now becoming so much more than a hypothesis that there are those who would accept this metamorphosis as an accomplished fact.

There is no call to recite at any length the accounts of the early experiments. Some were based on crude, faulty methods which always raise doubts as to the purity of the cultures the pioneers studied. Disregarding claims resting solely upon morphological or cultural phenomena, it is better to confine the discussion to reports, with a few exceptions of historical interest, that have been published since the development of modern bacteriological and serological technique. In 1891, Kruse and Pansini,[763] by transplanting forty-six strains of pneumococci on media unfavorable to growth, developed eighty-four varieties that exhibited differences in character all the way from typical *Diplococcus lanceolatus* to *Streptococcus pyogenes.* The authors stated that the relation of pneumococci to streptococci was clearly evident, and that the origin of these bacterial species was a single, probably saprophytic, streptococcal form.

There the matter rested until 1907, when Buerger and Ryttenberg[169] described an organism isolated from a case of puerperal pneumococcemia which, although originally failing to ferment inulin and exhibiting streptococcal characters, developed into a typical pneumococcus after animal passage. The observation led the authors to study a number of cultures isolated from human exudates and blood, and with these strains they observed characters typical of streptococci which, however, gave way to pneumococcal characters after propagation in mice. Buerger and Ryttenberg concluded:

> The tendency of pneumococci of the streptococcus cultural type as well as those which have been converted to the normal variety, seems to be toward a gradual degeneration which manifests itself in the assumption of permanent streptococcic features. Such organisms can then no longer be differentiated from streptococci.

In 1909, Rosenow[1162] made the statement that strains of *Streptococcus viridans* isolated chiefly from the blood in cases of subacute endocarditis and obtained also from the throat and other sources might by animal passage take on the properties of typical pneumococci, and hence designated them as "modified pneumococci." Rosenow also claimed that during a study of autolysis of pneumococci in salt solution and of the effect of sodium oleate and bile on virulent pneumococci he had observed transformation of the strains into hemolytic streptococci. The statement appears to be conservative when compared to Rosenow's[1170] description in 1914 of the various transmutations accomplished within the Streptococcus-Pneumococcus group. He told of converting by cultural methods twenty-one strains originally isolated as hemolytic streptococci from cases of erysipelas, scarlet fever, puerperal sepsis, arthritis, and tonsillitis, as well as from cows' milk, into *Streptococcus viridans;* of changing three similar strains into *S. viridans* and typical pneumococci, and one into *Streptococcus mucosus* as well. Seventeen strains isolated as *S. viridans,* chiefly from the blood and tonsils in cases of chronic infectious endocarditis, and two strains from cows' milk were converted into pneumococci while two of the strains became *S. mucosus.* Ten of the *viridans* cultures were made to take on the cultural and morphological characters of hemolytic streptococci, in two of which the pathogenic powers were shown to be those of hemolytic streptococci, while one strain was converted into a hemolytic streptococcus, into *S. viridans,* and then into a pneumococcus.

Rosenow claimed to have converted into hemolytic streptococci eleven strains isolated as pneumococci from sputum, blood, and the lung in pneumonia and from human empyema fluids and Cole's Type I and II strains, while seven cultures took on the features of *S. viridans.* The streptococci derived by animal passage from three of the pneumococcal strains were alleged to acquire all the essential features of the streptococci of rheumatism, and two organisms were said to have been converted into hemolytic streptococci, the streptococci of rheumatism, *S. viridans,* and back again into Pneumococcus.

Rosenow further alleged that the transformation of some of these strains, checked in a few instances by single-cell isolations, was found to be complete by every test known. The tests included the study of morphological features, the demonstration of capsules, and observations on fermentative powers, solubility in bile and in saline solution, the behavior toward the respective broth-culture filtrates (Marmorek's test), the specific immunological response as manifested by the appearance of opsonin and agglutinin in antistreptococcic and antipneumococcic serum, and the more or less specific pathogenic powers of the various organisms.

In summary Rosenow wrote:

The changes observed have frequently the characteristics of true mutations because they appear suddenly, under conditions more or less obscure and because the newly acquired properties persist unless the organisms are again placed under special conditions. A pre-mutational stage seems to be necessary because the same strain will not yield mutants when placed under what seem to be identical conditions at different times. The underlying conditions which tend most to call forth changes are, first, favorable conditions for luxuriant growth and then unfavorable conditions—under stress and strain. This seems to call forth new or latent energies which were previously not manifest and which now have gained the ascendency and tend to persist. This may hold true *in vivo* also. This fact makes it difficult to obtain mutations outside of the body with highly virulent strains, because they die before there is opportunity for the organisms to adjust themselves to the new conditions. It explains why injection into cavities makes for greater changes than intravenous injections of moderately virulent organisms. Apparent mutations in animals have been observed almost exclusively in closed cavities, such as joints and pericardium, and here mostly when the tissues of the host were gradually getting the upper hand and the organisms were being destroyed. The mutations *in vitro* may be spoken of as "retrogressive" and those in animals as "progressive" because evidences of a vigorous vegetative life are diminished whereas in the latter they are usually increased.

The results and conclusions of Rosenow have been transcribed in some detail because they represented such a wide departure from established belief. The announcement was greeted with much skepticism. Such sudden and wide shifts from one to another supposedly fixed species appeared to violate biological laws, and it seemed that some artifact must have been responsible for the remarkable transformations. Nowhere in the literature, with the exceptions to be described, have references been found which duplicate or substantiate Rosenow's results.

Wolff (1923),[1534] in a long theoretical discussion of pneumococcal mutation, suggested that the members of the large tribe *Streptococcaceae*, from pure saprophytes to true parasites, in spite of all differences, were really linked together. He claimed to have obtained mutations by gradual adaptations of the organisms to the host. The attempts met with many failures which were explained by saying that if the organism was too weak it died in the host, and if too virulent it killed the host before any accommodation had taken place. Wolff asserted, however, that in three cases he had transformed *Streptococcus viridans* from *endocarditis lenta* into Pneumococcus. The organism became bile-soluble, optochin-sensitive, developed a capsule, fermented inulin, and was lethal for mice. Evidence of bacterial mutations of any kind coming solely from *in vivo* experiments is to be weighed with caution.

Neufeld[979] in a discussion already cited on microbic variability, recalled an observation he had made ten years previously on the original "Pneumococcus I" of Neufeld and Haendel, which had been preserved by drying and storage in a dessicator. One mouse inoculated with the culture produced a strain growing in chains, insoluble in bile, but virulent for mice, and with all typical streptococcal properties. At first Neufeld thought he had made a mistake in the material he injected, but a similar experience of Schiemann's convinced him that a mutation had actually taken place. Coming from anyone less eminent than Neufeld, this single, isolated observation would be disregarded.

In the following year, Morgenroth, Schnitzer, and Berger[929] announced that by special methods they had been able with regularity to transform pneumococci into streptococci.* Their medium contained dead yeast cells or animal charcoal which had adsorbed optochin. The altered strains became insoluble in sodium taurocholate, were avirulent for mice, and were resistant to optochin. Modification A represented the first stage in the transmutation. The organisms retained the majority of their pneumococcal characters, but were more resistant to optochin and more sensitive to

* Stanka[1312] called attention to the fact that these authors had omitted mention of similar work published by Elschnig and Ulbrich, and by Kraupa from the German Eye Clinic at Prague.

rivanol than were cocci of the original stock. In Modification B, the colonies, made up of A after growing in optochin, resembled those of *S. viridans.* The cultures contained long chains of round cocci, which were bile-insoluble and were very resistant to the pneumococcidal action of optochin. Modification C developed after further growth on artificial media or in animals, and occasionally after growth in an optochin medium. The C variants corresponded to *Streptococcus haemolyticus,* they produced more or less hemolysis on blood agar, were bile-insoluble and optochin-fast, but sensitive to rivanol. The progressive changes did not always take place or follow the A-B-C sequence. In twenty-nine experiments with fifteen strains, twenty-two trials produced modifications A and B, and of these strains seven were transformed into modification C.

Berger and Englemann[100] continued similar mutation experiments and alleged to have demonstrated Modification A in five specimens of sputum and one of pleural exudate obtained from pneumonia patients before the disappearance of fever. The strains were then converted into Modification B by allowing a fairly high concentration of optochin to act upon them. Berger and Englemann also claimed that the complete transformation could take place in the human organism. To support the claim the authors described the development of glistening Type III colonies along with a few strongly hemolytic streptococcal colonies on a blood-agar plate upon which pneumonic sputum had been spread. The organism, after the first mouse passage and three culture generations, developed into a green streptococcus; after a second direct mouse passage both pneumococci and hemolytic streptococci appeared, the latter partly reverting to Pneumococcus after two culture generations. The original hemolytic streptococci after three culture generations became green streptococci and after four culture generations reverted to pneumococci. This cycle, like Rosenow's, seems almost too rapid and direct to be credible.

In another communication, Berger and Jakob (1925)[102] returned to earlier experiments on the development of B and C modifications. During animal passage of short duration, the changes were less marked, since the authors reported only a transient loss of virulence. Berger and Englemann[101] in the next year reported the mutation of a strain of Type III Pneumococcus through the intermediary A modification to a green streptococcus. As in their former experiments, the agents necessary for the transformation were dry yeast-broth and serum-broth containing one five-thousandth part optochin. Wirth[1523] believed that *Streptococcus mucosus* represented a mutation from Pneumococcus, but he failed in his attempts to prove it.

In yet another paper Berger with Silberstein[103] described the inulin-fermentative power of the variants. The results are difficult to understand. Of ten strains of pneumococci, four showed merely a reddening of the inulin medium without coagulation, while two failed to display any action on inulin. The authors then classed the latter strains when tested with optochin with Modification A. Of the cultures of Modification B, obtained from pneumococci, but otherwise behaving as green streptococci, two retained the ability to ferment the carbohydrate. The strains were comparable in their behavior toward inulin to some thirty *viridans* strains. Of the latter, five exhibited a marked action on inulin, and four others gave slightly positive reactions.

Reimann,[1127] repeating the experiments of Morgenroth, Schnitzer, and Berger, claimed, however, that the R cultures so derived were still pneumococci, since the strains were bile-soluble and autolyzed with greater readiness than did streptococci. The immunological reactions of the variant pneumococci derived by Morgenroth's method, moreover, were identical with those of R pneumococci derived by various other means. When one considers the atypical action of the Berger strains on inulin and the author's omission of serological tests, one is inclined to accept Reimann's interpretation as the correct one.

Heim and Schlirf,[633] likewise, were unable to verify the work of

Morgenroth and his collaborators, yet Silberstein,[1286] who quoted these authors, by the aid of optochin *in vitro*, claimed to have experienced no difficulty in carrying a Group IV pneumococcus through the successive stages of Modification B (green Streptococcus) to Modification C (virulent hemolytic Streptococcus) and then from this form to a Type I pneumococcus of low virulence. Paul[1070] was another to join the newer school which believed that the gap between pneumococci and streptococci could be bridged by these methods. He produced bile-insoluble dissociants and to him they appeared to be indistinguishable from certain strains of *Streptococcus viridans.*

Görander (1930)[542] also stated that he had transmuted cultures of *Streptococcus viridans* into bacterial forms that in every respect were identical with the type-specific pneumococci of human origin, except that the strains were not agglutinated by antipneumococcic serum. The defect would seem to be a vital one. The cultural changes were accomplished by repeated cultivation on blood agar and by short mouse passages. According to Görander, after the third short (four-hour) mouse passage, hemolytic streptococci appeared. Following five twenty-four hour incubation periods in mice, the organisms resembled pneumococci. The variants had capsules, were soluble in sodium taurocholate, and were moderately virulent for mice. The pneumococci so obtained, after repeated growth of this passage culture in artificial media (alternating blood agar and broth), were retransformed "into a bacterium of perfect *Streptococcus viridans* type."

Görander claimed further to have transformed *Streptococcus viridans* and Type I and Type II pneumococci into forms which he considered to be their original state, "since they were absolutely equal culturally, biologically and serologically in all respects." The homologous antiserum agglutinated both strains, and "the bacteria absorbed not only their homologous but also heterologous agglutinins from both sera." Görander's further conclusions were so heterodox that they are quoted here:

Finally single cell cultures originating in their time from a single cell of a pneumococcus have been examined with regard to the degree of dissimilarity which such cultures can eventually show. These experiments gave the result that two pneumococcus cultures, obtained from the same cell, can show much greater dissimilarities than two cultures obtained one from a typical *Streptococcus viridans* and the other from a typical *Streptococcus lanceolatus*. . . . Thus *Streptococcus viridans* and *Pneumococcus lanceolatus* seem to be different forms of the same bacterium, and the specific agglutinability, which *Pneumococcus lanceolatus* shows when grown from the human body and which has been taken as a base for the so-called type classification, is only an occasional character.

Summary

Virulent pneumococci of all the known serological types, upon encountering unfavorable physical, nutritional, or other biochemical conditions during growth or storage, undergo marked changes in virulence, in ability to elaborate capsules, in colony development, and in their immunological characters. In studies on the dissociation phenomena displayed by pneumococci, a great variety of aberrant coccal forms have been observed which are intermediate between the typical, virulent form and the thoroughly degraded, atypical form. So many variants with such a diversity of biological characters have been described and so many designations have been given to the intermediate forms, that it is difficult to gain a clear conception of the significance of the many phases of pneumococcal dissociation. In order to bring order out of this chaos and to make the nomenclature applied to pneumococci uniform with that employed in naming the variants occurring in the case of other bacterial species, it has been proposed to change the terminology now in use. Mucoid or M would replace the present smooth or S; smooth would be substituted for rough; while rough or R would apply to a recently discovered variant. Whatever the fate of the proposal, the alterations in character which may be induced in pneumococci by appropriate means constitute one of the most important features in the biology of the species.

During the dissociative process antigenic action may vary from one of strict type-specificity to one merely of the broader species-specificity. Degraded forms may, if the degenerative process has not been complete, regain all their original morphological, cultural, and immunological characters. Regeneration can be accomplished by rejuvenating the strain by passage through a susceptible animal, by cultivation in media containing an antiserum produced by immunization with the degraded forms, or through the stimulus afforded by heat-killed virulent cultures of an homologous type. Degraded variants, moreover, can by the action of devitalized, virulent pneumococci, actually be transformed into pneumococci of types entirely different from those from which the variants were derived and identical with those of the cultures stimulating transformation. The nature of this transformative or mutative principle is still unknown, but it is probable that it is a constituent of the pneumococcal cell and not an extracellular product of its metabolism.

The broader transmutation of Pneumococcus into Streptococcus and of Streptococcus into Pneumococcus has been advanced as a biological possibility. Experiments have been described in which it was alleged that this transmutation took place. Not only has it been claimed that both virulent and degraded pneumococci were converted into avirulent *Streptococcus viridans*, but the organisms were said to have become virulent hemolytic streptococci, while the streptococcal forms have been further changed into pneumococci. Such radical departures from established theory require the closest scrutiny of the evidence advanced and of the accumulation of new and confirmatory facts before they can be accepted.

CHAPTER VI

PATHOGENICITY OF PNEUMOCOCCUS: EXPERIMENTAL ANIMALS

The ability of Pneumococcus to infect animals of different species under natural circumstances or when experimentally introduced by diverse routes into the animal body; the morbid manifestations following pneumococcal infection in animals; virulence and other factors influencing infectivity of pneumococci.

PNEUMOCOCCUS is incapable of producing disease in animals of some species, while individual creatures exhibit different degrees of resistance to pneumococcal invasion. Variations in susceptibility or in resistance may be conditioned by special differences in anatomic structure, in genetic heritage, or in physiological function, while individual differences may be due to both intrinsic and extrinsic factors affecting the physical state of the animal before or at the time of inoculation.

Susceptibility of the Animal Host

THE RABBIT

Rabbits are prone to develop spontaneous pneumococcal infection of the respiratory tract, contracting the disease from similarly affected guinea pigs or from other rabbits.* Recovery from the infection may be followed by the carrier state during which the animal may serve as a potential source of infection to other stock animals, while the presence of pneumococci in the nasopharynx may constitute a confusing factor when the animal is used for experimental pneumococcal infection.

Next to the mouse, the rabbit is the most susceptible of labora-

* This is not an uncommon laboratory experience and among the references at hand is that of Sanderson,[1218] who wrote of the spontaneous death of a rabbit from Pneumococcus following a supposedly air-borne infection in the laboratory animal room.

tory animals to pneumococcal infection. Susceptibility is greatest for strains of Type I pneumococci, less for Type II organisms, and still less for those of Type III. It should be remembered that later studies have shown that while many strains of Type III pneumococci are avirulent for rabbits, there are others of the same type that are highly pathogenic.

It will be recalled that in the early days of bacteriology, Pasteur,[1065-6] Sternberg,[1316-8] Vulpian,[1453] and Claxton[237] produced a fatal septicemia in rabbits by the subcutaneous injection of human saliva containing, as we now know, pneumococci. With the exception of the intact skin, rabbit tissues present no barriers to the invasion of virulent pneumococci; the organisms, no matter by which avenue introduced, soon reach the blood stream and, when in sufficient numbers, cause the death of the animal.

Bacteriemia is the predominant manifestation and pneumonia develops only when the organisms are implanted in the lung by way of the respiratory tract. The weakness of the rabbits' defense against subcutaneous, intraperitoneal, or intravenous pneumococcal inoculation is due, in part, to the comparative inability of the leucocytes of the animal to engulf the invading cocci (Tongs, 1922[1416]). Even when injected into the cisternal cavity of the brain, as reported by Stewart (1927),[1322] septicemia rather than meningitis ensues. As a rule, therefore, after artificial inoculation with pneumococci, infection, unless it be by the intradermal or intratracheal route, tends to become systemic and not localized.

Subcutaneous inoculation. Neufeld (1901)[973] spoke of a progressive inflammation following the injection of pneumococci into the subcutaneous tissues of the ear of the rabbit. When death did not follow, necrosis was observed, and the infection appeared to Neufeld to be similar to erysipelas, although Fraenkel, who had previously observed the same effect, had not so considered it. Cooper[276] found that the mucous membrane of the buccal surface of the rabbit's cheek was susceptible to infection, but the inoculation in reality was a subcutaneous one, since it was necessary to injure the membrane by scratching it before infection took place.

Intravenous inoculation. The rapid and frequently fatal infection resulting from the injection of pneumococci into the circulatory system has often been utilized for testing the specific resistance of rabbits after various immunizing treatments. Among the many references, there might be mentioned the observations of Tillett (1927)[1403-4] who, in attempts to stimulate the production of immune bodies, discovered differences in the pathogenicity of certain Type III strains for man and for rabbits. Some of the strains isolated from human sources, despite the possession of large capsules and high virulence for mice, exhibited low virulence for rabbits. The intravenous injection of the Type III strains avirulent for the species produced a non-fatal bacteriemia which, however, in its course differed from that caused by non-encapsulated, rough forms of pneumococci.

Intradermal inoculation. In 1928, Goodner[525-6] described the acute and often fatal infection developing in the rabbit following the introduction of Type I Pneumococcus into the skin. After the injection of a small quantity of a broth culture of the organism into the skin at the midline of the abdomen, within eight to twelve hours there appears a local lesion, consisting of a swollen, edematous area which may spread until the whole midabdominal region is involved. The development of the lesion is accompanied by an abrupt rise in temperature and invasion by the cocci of the blood stream. A varying proportion of the animals so treated spontaneously recover and, as a result of the infection, may become temporarily immune. Goodner pointed to the analogy between the nature of the localized and subsequent systemic infection arising after intradermal inoculation of the rabbit with Pneumococcus and that of lobar pneumonia in man. Since it does not come within the province of the present volume to discuss, except in a cursory way, the pathological processes caused by pneumococcal infection, the reader is referred to the original communications of Goodner,[525-7, 541] Rhoades and Goodner,[1136] and others who have described the intimate details of the phenomena.

Kolmer and Rule[748] employed the intradermal method to test the resistance of rabbits induced by previous immunization with pneumococci; Goodner, Dubos and Avery,[536] and Goodner and Dubos,[535] for studying the effect of the polysaccharide-splitting bacterial enzyme in infection with Type III Pneumococcus; while Goodner,[527] Watson and Cooper,[1492] Powell, Jamieson, Bailey and Hyde,[1105] Sabin,[1208] Gelarie and Sabin,[510] and Curphey and Baruch[293] applied the Goodner technique in determining the immunizing action of specific immune serum and other agents.

Inoculation by way of the respiratory tract. Tchistovitch (1890)[1381] was apparently the first to study the effect of Pneumococcus when introduced into the trachea of the rabbit. The diplococci caused only a feeble, local inflammatory reaction with little phagocytosis. In 1915, Kline and Winternitz[728] described the conditions necessary to produce lobar pneumonia in rabbits. The catheter must be inserted as deeply as possible into a bronchus, and the culture fluid must be injected with considerable force in order that the organisms may be introduced into the alveoli.

Permar[1082] has described in detail the manifestations appearing after the intratracheal injections of cultures of Type I Pneumococcus. He concluded that experimental pneumonia in the rabbit begins as an acute inflammatory reaction. The severity of the reaction increases from the trachea and bronchioles and is greatest in the bud-like alveoli arising from them, in the alveolar ducts, atrea, and alveoli. The process begins in the bronchus and invades other tissues by peripheral extension leading to coalescence. Acute interstitial pneumonia in the rabbit develops early as a result of acute lymphangitis arising in the peripheral lymphatics; then the process extends to both pleura and hilum. Permar suggested that septicemia might arise as the result of the direct involvement of the vascular walls, or it might possibly be due to the passage of organisms through the nodes at the hilum and thence through the thoracic duct into the circulatory system. The author believed that the process was, in its essentials, comparable to that occurring in spontaneous pneumonia in human beings, the chief difference being a more intense interstitial involvement in the experimental disease.

Through the insufflation of the lung with cultures of pneumococci of Types I, II, and III, and of Group IV, Gaskell (1925)[500] reported that organisms of Group IV possessed a greater pathogenicity for the rabbit than those of Type I which, in turn, were more invasive than those of Type II, while the Type III culture employed was the least virulent of all.

Stuppy and Falk (1931)[1352] found that intrabronchial insufflation of rabbits with cultures of pneumococci of uniformly high virulence gave rise to bronchopneumonia which, with septicemia and a generalized distribution of cocci in the lungs, usually caused the death of the animal in two to five days. In some animals there was acute inflammation of the interstitial tissue of the lung, with perivascular and peribronchial lymphangitis. Suppurative bronchitis and pleuritis were only occasionally seen. On the whole, the pulmonary lesions induced in rabbits by strains of Type I, II, and III pneumococci of the same virulence were quite similar, while individual virulence rather than the serological type of the culture employed appeared to be the important factor in establishing infection. In a study of the effects of the inhalation of pneumococci, Stillman[1336] observed that, following the spraying of rabbits with cultures of virulent Type III cultures, the organisms tended to remain in the lungs for a considerable period of time without invading the blood stream. When once the organisms had reached the blood, a fatal septicemia resulted. The course of events was in contrast to that ensuing after the similar administration of Type I and II strains. Organisms of Types I and II frequently entered the circulation, but in such instances, only a relatively small number of the animals died.

Another organ of the rabbit possessing little or no resistance to infection with Pneumococcus is the eye. Tchistovitch (1890),[1381] on introducing the organism into the anterior chamber, found that the aqueous humor, instead of being antagonistic to the cocci, served as a medium for their development. According to Neufeld and Schnitzer, injection of virulent strains of pneumococci under the conjunctiva or cornea leads to a severe infection of the eye, which is followed by systemic infection. The same result attended a similar injection of mouse blood containing pneumococci (Ginsberg and Kaufmann, 1913[517]).

Chilling and wetting, age, breed, weight, and diet as factors influencing susceptibility. The great variability in the behavior of rabbits toward pneumococcal infection, whether naturally or artificially acquired, may be due to either or both internal or external conditions. Among external causes Kline and Winternitz (1915)[728] studied the influence of cold, alcohol, ether, and bromine on rabbits infected intrabronchially with Pneumococcus. The agents appeared to predispose the animal to the development of bronchitis and even bronchopneumonia, but the results were not conclusive. In experiments in which rabbits were given intrabronchial inoculations of virulent pneumococci, Stuppy and Falk[1352] found that wetting and chilling the animals failed to lower resistance to invasion of the injected pneumococci, but exposure to cold appeared to render the test animals more susceptible to spontaneous infection.

Freund[484] observed the difference between the reactions of young and adult rabbits to intradermal inoculation with virulent pneumococci—confirming the susceptibility of immature individuals earlier reported by Kruse and Pansini.[763] In adult rabbits injected with virulent pneumococci extensive inflammation developed at the site of infection, but bacteriemia and death occurred in relatively few of the animals. Younger animals failed to develop such an extensive inflammatory process and succumbed to bacteriemia. The ability to respond to inoculation with an energetic, local reaction constitutes a barrier which apparently develops with growth of the animal.

In an investigation of the physiological variables responsible for the lack of uniformity in the behavior of rabbits to intradermal inoculation with Pneumococcus, Goodner[532] concluded that, since normal rabbits lacked any form of specific antipneumococcal antibodies, resistance to intradermal inoculation in combination with passive immunization with specific immune serum was determined by the physiological condition favorable to the utilization of passively conferred specific antibodies, which in turn depended upon the weight and white blood-cell count of the rabbits. Animals, therefore, that are physiologically mature possess an advantage over animals less mature and with a lower cell activity.

Another factor affecting the resistance of rabbits to infection is vitamin deficiency. Greene[554] reported that rachitic rabbits showed a greater morbidity and mortality from intranasal inoculation with Type I Pneumococcus than did normal controls. Differences in the susceptibility of rabbits of diverse breeds has also been noted; hence, in the selection of rabbits for comparative or quantitative tests on the virulence of strains or types of pneumococci or for measuring the potency of immune serum, consideration should be given to the breed, age, weight, and diet of the test animals.

THE GUINEA PIG

The comparatively low and variable susceptibility of guinea pigs precludes their use for many purposes in experimental studies on Pneumococcus. The susceptibility of the guinea pig to pneumococci administered by inhalation was first demonstrated by Neufeld and Ungermann[1001-2] in 1912. The inoculation, in some cases but not regularly, produced a slow pneumonic process. When the culture was injected directly into the lung, the animals developed acute infection, dying in one or two days from pleuropneumonia or bronchopneumonia.

The intrapleural injection of pneumococci into guinea pigs may cause a pleuropneumonia, as shown by Kolmer.[741] Neufeld and Ungermann[1001-2] and also Engwer[365] reported similar successful infection after the injection directly into the lung of pneumococci cultivated by several animal passages.

One objection to the use of these animals is their liability to develop spontaneous pneumococcal infection, to become carriers, and thus to transmit infection to other laboratory animals. Such an outbreak was reported in 1922 by Gheorgiu,[512] but no mention was made concerning the type to which the infecting organism belonged. The presence of pneumococci as secondary invaders in an epidemic among guinea pigs and mice caused by *B. bronchisepticus* was observed by Keegan.[700] Branch[147] in 1927 reported the presence of pneumococci of Group IV in all of thirty-six guinea pigs in a laboratory epidemic. The organism failed to agglutinate with specific immune serum for the first three fixed types, but by its protein fraction appeared to be related serologically to strains of pneumococci of human origin. The infection took the form of otitis, enlargement of the spleen, lobular and even true lobar pneumonia. According to Bruckner and Galasesco as well as to Chevrel and Ranque,* spontaneous epidemics sometimes begin with septic abortion of the guinea pigs.

The presence of pneumococci in the nares of apparently normal guinea pigs and of guinea pigs affected with snuffles, and the occurrence of natural epidemics of pneumococcal infection in animals of this species, was investigated by Neufeld and Etinger-Tulczynska[984-5] in 1931. The organisms responsible for natural infections, including those found in a previous investigation of an outbreak in another colony of animals, when tested by means of the *Quellung* phenomenon, proved to belong to Type XIX. The strain was only slightly virulent for mice and guinea pigs. The authors found further that animals surviving the intranasal implantation of pneumococci of Types I and XIX, as a rule, become carriers of the respective strains.

Neufeld and Etinger-Tulczynska also noted wide variations in the susceptibility of the animals to natural infection from pneumo-

* Quoted by Neufeld and Schnitzer.

cocci and, while cold, avitaminosis, and pregnancy had previously been shown to diminish resistance of guinea pigs, the authors concluded that higher susceptibility was apparently of a more obscure nature and was associated, as earlier suggested by Uchida,[1432] with basic or temporary variations in the disposition of individual animals. A possible explanation for some of the constitutional differences in the susceptibility of guinea pigs is to be found in the communication of Nicholls and Spaeth (1922),[1005] according to whom there is a definite correlation between pigmentation and resistance to infection. White-coated, pink-eyed guinea pigs, probably pure albinos, were found to be far more susceptible to a given Type I culture than were pigmented individuals. It seems unlikely that pigmentation of itself was responsible for the resistance, although it may well have been associated with the true cause. Uchida,[1431] who earlier had isolated pneumococci from guinea pigs suffering from spontaneous infection, noted irregularities in the results following the subsequent subcutaneous, intraperitoneal, and intravenous injection of the strains into normal guinea pigs. The author assumed that the discrepancies in the outcome of the experiments were due to varying degrees of resistance possessed by the individual animals, but offered no specific explanation for the differences.

Wámoscher (1927)[1479] observed that scurvy and chronic tuberculosis in the guinea pig were diatheses favoring spontaneous pneumococcal infection. These and similar debilitating conditions may likewise lower resistance to experimental infection. Schmidt-Weyland and Költzsch* found that scorbutic guinea pigs could easily be infected when pneumococci were introduced into the body by inhalation or feeding.

THE MOUSE

The white races of the mouse family, because of low cost, ease of handling, great susceptibility, and general uniformity of reaction,

* Quoted by Neufeld and Schnitzer.

are ordinarily chosen for the isolation of pneumococci, the preliminary testing of antigenic substances, and for the determination of type-specificity and potency of diagnostic and curative immune serums. Albino strains are preferable to strains of pigmented or wild varieties because of their lower resistance to infection. Pure-line races, with their inherited uniformity of susceptibility, would be ideal types for routine investigative purposes were it not for their present scarcity and prohibitive cost. That susceptibility or resistance to infection are transmissible characters and that the breeding of races with either high or low degrees of susceptibility can be accomplished by proper selection has been demonstrated by Irwin and Hughes[670] in the case of the rat for bacteria of the enteric group.

The extreme susceptibility of the mouse to subcutaneous, intraperitoneal, or intravenous injection of Pneumococcus is shown by the rapid invasion of the blood stream and the death of the animals without localization of the infection. Introduced by any of these routes Pneumococcus may be highly infective for mice. When the virulence of a strain of Pneumococcus has been exalted by successive mouse passage, the cultures used for intraperitoneal injection into a mouse may be so diluted that, although the amount used for inoculation may yield only one or even no colonies, infection will frequently follow. In fact, Wámoscher[1478] has demonstrated by micromechanical isolation of single cells that one pneumococcus may suffice to infect a mouse. It is for this reason, therefore, that the mouse is so admirably adapted for the detection of pneumococci in infective material, for determining virulence, for testing the immunizing action of antigens, and for measuring the protective power of specific immune serum.

An observation concerning the dominance of one type of Pneumococcus in causing general infection in the mouse following the injection of an inoculum containing pneumococci of several types was described by Etinger-Tulczynska.[368] When mixtures of equal parts of cocci of different types were administered either by the subcutaneous, intraperitoneal, or intravenous route or by all three routes simultaneously, the organisms of one type would gain the ascendancy and suppress the pneumococci of the other type even at the site of inoculation.

Webster and Clow[1494] found individual differences in mice to intranasal infection with Pneumococcus. Some mice were completely refractory, some became carriers, and others developed various forms of infection ranging from lobar pneumonia to septicemia. Animals which showed high resistance to a strain introduced through the nose might exhibit moderate or high susceptibility to the same strain injected intraperitoneally. Whether the grades of infectivity were due to differences in the virulence of the organisms or to degrees of susceptibility of the host was not ascertained.

Distinct differences in the reactivity of mice of diverse races to pneumococcal infection has been demonstrated by Rake.[1117-8] In general, reactivity was found to be influenced by the type of organism used for inoculation as well as by innate characters peculiar to the breed of the animal. For example, a single type of Pneumococcus produced in mice of the same breed lesions which were similar and predictable. Lesions differing quantitatively could be produced in various breeds of mice by inoculation of the same type of organism, but inoculation of cultures of the various types into mice of a single race produced lesions differing in quality. Experiments in which mice were infected intranasally and intravenously revealed that lesions in the lung and other organs varied with both the type of culture and the strain of mice used.

The constancy of the results obtained in infection experiments with this animal species is further conditioned by the age of the individuals employed. Moreover, there is greater regularity in the behavior of mice of approximately sixteen to twenty-one grams in weight to artificial infection, and this fact is especially significant when mice are employed for testing the potency of antipneumococcic serum. More recently, Goodner and Miller (1935),[540] extending Goodner's work on the rabbit, investigated the physiological variables responsible for the resistance of the individual mouse to pneumococcal infection by studying the capacity of animals of a single strain to utilize the protective properties of antipneumococcic serum. The authors concluded that the important variables were body-weight and the number of cells in the peritoneal cavity following the intraperitoneal injection of pneumococci and homologous immune serum, which in turn resolved itself into the number of monocytes present. The dominant factor in determining susceptibility, other factors being equal, was the relation between the number of monocytes and the number of pneumococci in the peritoneal cavity at the time of the injection of culture and serum.

The resistance of mice to infection by inhalation may be decreased by the previous administration of alcohol. Stillman and Branch (1924, 1930, 1931)[1337, 1340-1] found that inspired pneumococci rapidly disappeared from the lung of normal mice and rarely caused septicemia, but in alcoholized mice the organisms persisted in the lung for a longer period and fatal septicemia was frequent, while pulmonary localization of the infection occurred in mice previously immunized either actively with heat-killed pneumococci or passively with homologous immune serum. The observations of Branch and Stillman[148] were confirmed by Lange and Keschischian,[785] who succeeded, but only with difficulty, in inducing pulmonary infection in mice through inhalation. The latter authors also found mice to be resistant to percutaneous and peroral inoculation with pneumococci.

The frequency with which colonies of white mice are infected with the so-called mouse typhoid due to *Bacillus typhi murium* is a factor to be considered when selecting mice for experimental purposes. The disease, so often remaining latent, may not be evident, but it may nevertheless greatly alter the reaction of the animals to experimental inoculation.

THE RAT

The rat is a near zoological relation of the mouse and is highly receptive to pneumococcal infection, but it is seldom used in researches on Pneumococcus. Lamar* and also Neufeld and Haendel* proved the great susceptibility of the rat to pneumococcal infection. The subcutaneous injection of 10^{-5} cubic centimeters of a virulent strain caused septicemia which resulted two days later in death of the animal.

McDowell[878] studied the effect of high air temperatures, combined with different degrees of humidity, on resistance of rats to intraperitoneal inoculation of pneumococci. It appeared that after an exposure for two weeks to a temperature of 83°F., with the humidity varying from 44 to 72 per cent, rats exhibited greater resistance than did rats kept at medium temperatures. High or low humidity with temperatures between 65° and 72°F. were unfavorable to the survival of the test animals. However, when rats accustomed to moderate temperatures (67° to 71°F.) were inoculated intraperitoneally with Pneumococcus and then exposed to a higher temperature (83°F.) there was a lowering of resistance.

Rats, as well as mice, proved to be susceptible to pneumococcal infection when the organisms in the form of pulverized, dried, infected blood or spleens were insufflated into the trachea by Kramár and Gyüre.[757] McDaniels[876-7] employed rats in an investigation of the immunizing action of orally administered pneumococcal vaccines and found the species to be suitable for the purpose.

THE MONKEY

Monkeys in captivity are susceptible to spontaneous pneumococcal disease. Blake and Cecil (1920)[128] reported that pneumonia might occur in epidemic form, due to spread of infection from animal to animal, when conditions favoring close contact existed. The disease in monkeys, according to the authors, was identical in its clinical features, complications, and pathology, with lobar pneumonia experimentally produced in monkeys by the intratracheal injection of Pneumococcus and with lobar pneumonia in man. Two

* Quoted by Neufeld and Schnitzer.

strains of the organism isolated from the sick monkeys were pneumococci of Group IV. At that time, the authors[126-7] demonstrated that lobar pneumonia could be consistently produced in members of this animal species (*Macacus syrichtus* and *Cebus capucinus*) by the intratracheal injection of minute amounts of culture of a virulent Type I strain. When large quantities of culture were introduced into the nose or throat, no lobar pneumonia developed, but the animals became carriers of the inoculated organism and remained so for a period of at least a month.

The susceptibility of the monkey (*Macacus rhesus* and *Cercopithecus callitrichus*) to intracranial or intraspinal inoculation with Pneumococcus was demonstrated in 1912 by Lamar,[775] who described the meningitis following the injections. The experimental disease resembled pneumococcal meningitis in man but ran a more rapid course and was invariably fatal.

In studying pneumococcal infection and immunity in monkeys, Cecil and Steffen[211] found that *Macacus rhesus* was most resistant to Type I Pneumococcus and rarely developed true lobar pneumonia; *Cebus capucinus* occupied an intermediate position, occasionally showing typical lobar infection but more often interstitial or patchy lesions; while the Philippine monkey, *Macacus syrichtus,* was the most susceptible and was preferable for inoculation experiments because animals of that species develop true lobar pneumonia.

The existence of the carrier state in normal stock monkeys was also shown by Schöbl and Sellards,[1246] who recovered an avirulent strain of Pneumococcus from the Philippine monkey, *Pithecus philippinensis.* The authors also succeeded in inducing pneumonia in the animals by intratracheal inoculation with a small dose of a broth culture of Type I Pneumococcus that was highly virulent for mice.

Blake and Cecil,[126] using strains of Type I, II, III, and Group IV pneumococci, by intravenous injection failed to produce pneumonia in monkeys of the *Macacus syrichtus* species but reported that a fatal septicemia followed inoculation by that route. No greater success followed the attempts of Schöbl and Sellards, although the latter authors likewise observed fatal systemic infection after intravenous injection of a Type I culture. Cecil and Steffen[214-5] were able by injecting cultures of Types I, II, and III, and of one Group IV strain into the trachea to incite pneumonia in *Macacus rhesus*, *Macacus syrichtus*, and *Cebus capucinus*.

Among other references to the experimental production of lobar pneumonia in monkeys by the intratracheal implantation of virulent pneumococci may be mentioned the report of Francis and Terrell,[476] who were able to induce pneumonic disease in *Cynomolgos* monkeys with a Type III strain. The authors reported that the type of infection following small doses given in winter was similar to the type resulting from large doses administered in warm months. The authors also noted marked individual variations in the monkeys used. According to Stuppy, Falk, and Jacobson,[1353] *Macacus rhesus* and *Cebus capucinus* were highly resistant to intratracheal inoculation of virulent Type I Pneumococcus. None of the thirteen animals injected developed lobar pneumonia. Three monkeys died from pneumococcal infection but the lungs appeared to be normal, except for an increase in the number of polymorphonuclear leucocytes in the interstitial tissue, blood vessels, and bronchi.

THE CAT

Feline animals are unsuitable for studies on pneumococcal infection. Robertson, Woo, Cheer, and King[1152] are apparently the only authors to have reported experiments on cats in which it was possible by intrapleural injection of cultures of Type I and II pneumococci to produce lobar pneumonia. However, only one animal of those inoculated developed the disease.

THE DOG

The first reference to the use of dogs in research on Pneumococcus is probably that of Friedländer (1883),[487] who injected aqueous suspensions of gelatin cultures of cocci isolated from pneumonia patients into the lungs of four dogs, only one of which succumbed. The animal at necropsy showed red and gray hepatization of the lung, and from the areas Friedländer succeeded in recovering typical encapsulated diplococci. In the same year, Talamon[1378] failed to infect dogs with a mixed culture containing lanceolate cocci grown from the exudate of a pneumonic lung. The refractoriness of dogs was also demonstrated by Monti,[905-7] who reported that no reaction attended subcutaneous injection. However, he succeeded in producing meningitis in the dog after subdural inoculation with pneumococci.

Salvioli (1884)[1215] was more successful in infecting dogs with encapsulated cocci obtained from the pleural and pericardial exudates of pneumonia patients, but the animals so treated failed to develop the typical lesions of pneumonia. In 1912, Lamar and Meltzer,[772] by means of a catheter introduced through the larynx and bronchus, implanted pneumococci in the lungs of dogs. Of forty-eight test animals, forty-two developed lobar pneumonia with a fatality rate of 16 per cent. Wadsworth[1457] employed the method to study phagocytosis in similarly infected animals. In the next year, Wollstein and Meltzer[1539-40] in two communications described the results following the insufflation of avirulent and of heat-killed pneumococci into the lungs of this domestic animal. The injection caused pulmonic congestion with exudate but, in general, the framework of the lung was unaffected and the process was nonfatal.

Similar results were reported by Newburg, Means and Porter (1916),[1004] by Kline (1917),[726] Wadsworth (1918),[1459] Leake, Vickers and Brown (1924),[793] Christie, Ehrich and Binger (1928),[233] and by Coryllos (1929),[279] all of whom employed the same technique of using the bronchoscope for the injection of Type I culture as used by Henderson, Haggard, Coryllos, and Birnbaum (1930)[636] with a culture of Type II Pneumococcus.

With strains of both Types I and II introduced into a terminal bronchus by means of a catheter, Terrell, Robertson, and Coggeshall (1933)[1387] made fluoroscopic studies of the lobar pneumonic process which ensued in every instance when appropriate doses of culture were administered. In the experiments of the last-named authors the course of the pneumonia was short, averaging four or five days, while recovery, which took place in the majority of the animals so infected, was abrupt and simulated the crisis occurring in man. Similar experiments with pneumococci of Types I and III were described in 1934 by Lieberman and Leopold.[813] The article by Terrell, Robertson, and Coggeshall[1387] contains excellent descriptions of the pathological processes observed following intrabronchial injection of pneumococci in dogs.

Bull (1916)[173] injected dogs intravenously with pneumococci. Invasion of the blood stream appeared twenty-four to forty-eight hours after the injection. The septicemia reached a climax in four to five days, then abruptly declined, the blood becoming sterile in one to three days after the peak of the septicemia was reached. In some of the animals so injected meningitis occurred.

The results of a study of meningeal inoculation in dogs have been described by Stewart.[1323] The injection of Type I and Type II organisms into the ventricle, the cistern, and the lumbar region was followed by purulent meningitis with accompanying bacteriemia when the cultures used were of high virulence. Not all the animals infected succumbed, but those that died showed pathological changes not entirely comparable to those found in pneumococcal meningitis in man.

THE HORSE

The susceptibility of horses to infection with Pneumococcus, mentioned by Neufeld and Schnitzer, is a fact all too familiar to those engaged in the manufacture of therapeutic antipneumococcic serum. The possession of a high degree of specific, active immunity to pneumococci of a given serological type may fail to protect the horse against the subcutaneous or intravenous injection of living, virulent strains of the same type. Abscesses, pneumococcemia, endocarditis, and pneumonitis, sometimes culminating in fatal pneumothorax, may follow immunizing injections of living cultures, even when the serum of the animal under active immunization contains specific agglutinins and protective antibodies in sufficient quantity to qualify it for therapeutic use. This paradoxical phenomenon will be discussed in a later chapter.

BIRDS

Hens and doves have been found to be refractory to infection with Pneumococcus by Fraenkel,* Gamaléia,[498] and by Kyes,[766] among others. Kindborg (1905)[713] apparently was the only worker who claimed to have succeeded in demonstrating pathogenicity of Pneumococcus for pigeons. Kyes studied the cellular reaction in tissues of pigeons injected intraperitoneally with virulent pneumococci, and reported that the invading organisms were rapidly withdrawn from the blood stream and localized in the liver and spleen. Because the ultimate localization of the cocci in both of these organs was within a type of fixed phagocyte—the hemophage—common to both organs, Kyes concluded that the phagocytic destruction of pneumococci by hemophages is so extensive and so rapid as actually to constitute an important, if not indeed the determining, factor in the resistance of birds to pneumococcal infection. The natural resistance of hens and doves may, however, be lowered to the point of susceptibility through vitamin deficiency or by the administration of poisons, as reported by Strouse, by Guerrini, and by Corda.*

Virulence of the Organism

In any discussion of the pathogenicity of an organism, it should be borne in mind that virulence is a purely relative term. The factors which enter into the determination of the invasiveness of a

* Quoted by Neufeld and Schnitzer.

given strain of Pneumococcus are the serological type; the vital condition of the coccus at the time of trial as shown by the possession of a capsule; the mass of culture injected; the site chosen for inoculation; the species, and even the variety and the individual idiosyncrasies of the animals selected. There also enters the question whether the malignancy of a culture is due to a uniform virulence of all the cocci in a culture or to the presence of a few organisms of especially high virulence accompanied by other organisms possessing less or no invasive power.

Pneumococci of the various serological types as they exist in the lesions, exudates, or secretions of infected animals, or when freshly isolated from these sources, are pathogenic for other animals of the same species and, depending upon the serological type, may be virulent for animals of a different species. When a strain is passed serially through the bodies of animals of a given species it may acquire an elevated infectivity for other members of that species. Virulence may reach a permanent zenith or may decline but, virulent though an organism may be for the species used, it by no means follows that it is correspondingly pathogenic for animals of a different species.

During propagation outside the body the conditions of cultivation effect profound changes in the integrity of Pneumococcus, which, in turn, affect its pathogenic powers. Conditions that serve to maintain the organism in the highest state of metabolic activity with maximal production of capsular substance favor increase and maintenance of virulence. Conditions that, on the contrary, induce dissociation and degradation of the organism, by being inimical to capsule formation, lessen or destroy virulence.

FRESHLY ISOLATED STRAINS

In considering some of the earlier reports dealing with the pathogenicity of strains isolated from cases of lobar pneumonia and other pneumococcal infections, it should be remembered that many of the studies were conducted at a time before pneumococci were divided into serological types. Eyre and Washbourn[376] in 1899 gave descriptions of four strains of pneumococci, of which three, isolated from infections in man, were considered by the authors to be parasites, and one strain, from the normal human mouth, was looked upon as a saprophyte. The first three strains displayed great capabilities both for acquiring and for retaining a high degree of virulence, whereas the fourth culture possessed a low capacity in both respects.

The severity or lack of severity of an infection may depend on a preceding or accompanying infection with another bacterial species. For example, Sinigar (1903)[1292] described the ascending virulence of a respiratory infection among the staff and patients in the Leavesden Asylum. Beginning as a brief, indefinite illness, the disease gradually increased in severity, occasionally showing bronchial symptoms, and then developed into lobar pneumonia with a high fatality-rate. In all the cases, it was alleged that pneumococci were present in large numbers but, since there is no reference in the text to cultivation or virulence tests, it is impossible to say whether the same strain of Pneumococcus—if the organism was a pneumococcus—gradually gaining virulence, was responsible for the epidemic, or whether pneumococci of relatively low virulence were succeeded by a type having greater infectivity.

Kindborg (1905),[713] in a study of a large number of strains obtained from normal and pneumonic sputum, empyema pus, and other sources due to pneumococcal infection, observed wide limits in the pathogenicity of the different cultures. The organisms from cases of pneumonia were said usually to be the most virulent, while strains isolated from local inflammatory processes were generally avirulent. Whittle[1519] determined the virulence for mice of sixty strains of pneumococci collected at random from infections in man, and concluded from his tests that pneumococci by virtue of their pathogenic powers could be divided into at least two groups; those of high virulence were responsible for such well-recognized clinical entities as lobar pneumonia and bronchopneumonia, and those of low virulence were associated with minor illnesses or with disease occurring in persons already debilitated. Whittle denied the existence of any relation between serological type and pathogenicity.

Gundel and Wasu (1931)[578] reported that the virulence of a given type of Pneumococcus reached a maximum at the height of the disease process and that in the complications of lobar pneumonia in man, such as meningitis and otitis media, only strains of the highest virulence were found, the organisms usually belonging to the fixed serological types. Further discussion of the infectiousness for man of pneumococci of the various serological types will be found in the following chapter.

NUMBERS OF COCCI REQUIRED TO INFECT

Among reports on the quantitative determination of the infective ability of pneumococcal strains there may again be mentioned the observations of Wámoscher (1926).[1478] Using a strain of Type III Pneumococcus, counting the number of cocci in the inoculum by means of the Peterfi micromanipulator, and injecting the organisms subcutaneously into white mice, the author found that approximately one-quarter of the number of mice so treated succumbed to pneumococcal infection in two to four days after receiving an inoculation of one pneumococcus. The percentage of fatal infections rose with an increase in the number of organisms injected. Using only freshly isolated strains of pneumococci grown in broth from the culture obtained from a single mouse passage after isolation from a human source, and injecting the culture intraperitoneally into white mice, Gundel and Wasu noted marked differences in the virulence of strains within a type, although, as a rule, representatives of Types III, II, I, and IV possessed degrees of virulence in the order named, the average minimal lethal dilution for all Type III strains being 1 to 100,000,000, for Type II cultures 1 to 10,000,000, for Type I cultures 1 to 1,000,000, while for pneumococci of Type IV the killing dose varied from 1 to 100 to 1 to 1,000. One of the most virulent strains tested, a Type IV culture, was fatal in a dose of 10^{-8} cubic centimeters.

Petrie and Morgan[1085] in the same year reported the results obtained in an investigation of the factors influencing the lethal power for mice of a virulent culture of Type I Pneumococcus. Stocks of mice from different sources appeared to show some variation in susceptibility, and a small proportion—from 5 to 10 per cent—exhibited an innate resistance to small doses of pneumococci. The weight factor of the test animals failed to affect the mortality, although it modified the survival time. However, the authors decided that the density and virulence of the culture determined its lethal power, and that this power could be calculated when a reasonable number of mice were used. The criteria, by means of which the minimal fatal dose of any culture of Type I Pneumococcus could be specified, were the percentage fatality, the mean death-time, and the distribution of deaths at appropriate time intervals in a group of mice receiving a definite dose of the test culture.

AVENUE OF INOCULATION

In general, the virulence of a given organism varies with the tissue into which it is introduced. Direct inoculation into the blood stream is the most rapidly and most surely lethal route, followed in order of effectiveness by injection into the anterior chamber of the eye, into the peritoneum, under the skin, into the skin, into the lung either by direct puncture or through the bronchi, and lastly by way of the mouth.

DETERMINATION OF VIRULENCE

While the intraperitoneal injection of white mice is the preferred method for testing the virulence of pneumococcal cultures, other methods have been described. The rabbit, because of cost and individual and special idiosyncrasies, is less valuable. The relation between virulence and electrophoretic potential of different strains and serological types of Pneumococcus has been studied by Falk and his associates, Gussin and Jacobson.[379] According to the authors the highest potentials were uniformly found for Type III organisms, while the most probable sequence of decreasing potentials was from Type III to I to II and then to Group IV strains. The order corresponded to the decreasing sequence of virulence of the cultures for white mice. Washing the cultures increased electrophoretic velocities, but the order remained the same. From the results obtained with stock cultures, the authors anticipated that strains isolated from fatal cases of pneumonia might show higher potentials than would strains of the same type isolated from nonfatal cases. The experimental data confirmed the assumption for Types II and III, and Group IV, but contradicted it for Type I strains. Falk, Gussin, and Jacobson[379] concluded that electrophoretic potential was related in some fundamental manner to virulence as well as to phagocytability, agglutinability, capsule formation, and other characters of microorganisms. In a later communication, Jacobson and Falk,[675] after a study of this electrical phenomenon in pneumococcal variants, reported that in all cases studied alterations in virulence were accompanied by parallel alterations in electrophoretic potential and by reciprocal alterations in agglutinability.

The results obtained by Thompson (1931)[1396] in some respects contradict those reported by Falk and his colleagues. While the electrophoretic migration of representatives of the first three pneumococcal types was observed to decrease in the order III, I, II, as previously noted by Falk, Gussin, and Jacobson, exaltation or degradation of virulence respectively by mouse passage and by growth in increasing concentrations of ox bile were unaccompanied by any constant differences in the original velocity of migration.

Welikanow and Michailowa (1930)[1513] claimed that variation in the ability of pneumococci to ferment glucose is an indicator of the virulence of the strain, but the evidence presented is too meager to be convincing.

SUBSTANCES THAT ENHANCE VIRULENCE

In Chapter III mention was made of substances or preparations which possessed the ability to increase the invasive power of pneumococci. The virulin of Pittman and Falk,[1092] the extracts of Pittman and Southwick,[1093] the leucocidin of Oram,[1032] and the toxic autolysate of Parker and Pappenheimer[1063] are examples of substances which to a greater or less degree possess this property. A similar action was observed by Sia,[1266] who found that the addition of a very small amount of soluble specific substance or of young broth cultures of pneumococci to avirulent cultures of homologous type when mixed with rabbit or cat serum-leucocyte mixtures favored the growth of the organism. The authors interpreted the result as indicating that soluble specific substance had the power of rendering virulent an avirulent Pneumococcus of the same serological type. Sia and Zia[1275] reported that the injection of Type II soluble specific substance into rabbits depressed the resistance to such an extent that the animals succumbed to the intravenous injection of an otherwise sublethal dose of pneumococci of the same serological type. The authors left undecided the question whether the result was to be ascribed to a heightened susceptibility of the animal or to an enhanced virulence of the organism.

A somewhat similar effect was obtained by Nungester, Wolf, and Jourdonais,[1020] who added gastric mucin to twenty-four-hour broth cultures of Type II pneumococci and injected the mixture intraperitoneally into mice. Control mice received similar injections of the culture suspended in saline instead of mucin solution. At only one dose level was any marked difference noted in the percentage of survivals among the test and the control animals. The effect was not apparent when the injections were made intravenously or subcutaneously. Any action of mucin, in spite of its correspondence in chemical structure to soluble specific substance of Pneumococcus, must have been non-specific, and this surmise is strengthened by the fact that a slight adjuvant action in favoring infectivity was also noted when streptococci instead of pneumococci were the organisms so treated and inoculated.

The influence of pneumococcal autolysates on the invasiveness of pneumococci injected intradermally into rabbits was studied by Goodner. Whereas autolysates favored the pathogenicity of the culture used, they failed to alter its virulence. The evidence, taken as a whole, favors the hypothesis that the action of culture filtrates, extracts, autolysates, or specific capsular polysaccharides in increasing the infective power of pneumococci is to interfere with the natural defensive processes of the body and thereby lower the host's resistance rather than to add to the virulence of the cell itself.

CULTURAL CONDITIONS AND VIRULENCE

Influences that stimulate the anabolic processes of the pneumococcal cell make for virulence. Enrichment of the cultural medium with blood, normal serum, or other growth accessories, the proper concentration of hydrogen ions, and optimal temperature of incubation enable the organism to elaborate capsular substance, which, as will be shown in other portions of the present volume, may determine the invasive power of a given strain. Frequent transplantation in favorable media of pneumococcal cultures taken at the period of maximal growth not only maintains but increases virulence (Wadsworth and Kirkbride[1471]). Repeated transfer by means of the automatic device of Felton and Dougherty[423] of young cultures of a pure-line strain of Type I Pneumococcus into a fresh supply of sterile skimmed milk caused an avirulent strain to acquire a virulence ten million times greater than that of the original culture. Within a wide range, the hydrogen ion concentration of the milk appeared to have only a slight effect on virulence when transplants were made at two-hour intervals. However, when the reaction of the medium was adjusted to pH 8 or 9, virulence decreased; the more alkaline the reaction the more rapid the decrease.

When cultivated in broth by the same method,[425] the Type I culture lost virulence as the reaction of the medium by adjustment became more acid. Virulence fluctuated with the frequency of transfer of the organism to fresh broth. In the case of transplants made every hour, virulence immediately decreased. When the interval was two, four, or eight hours, there was first a rise and then a fall of virulence, the rise being greatest in the case of eight-hour and least with the two-hour transfers. With the hydrogen ion concentration at set points the amount of meat infusion influenced the virulence of the culture, the unfavorable action varying in inverse proportion to the concentration of meat in the substrate. The addition of glucose neutralized the action of the meat. Peptone in the broth also affected the virulence of the strain studied, Felton and Dougherty reporting that the nutrient in a concentration of 2 per cent maintained and even increased virulence of the strains studied.

In a later communication (1932), Felton[411-2] described other nutritional factors that affect the virulence of pneumococci. Media made from calf lung or heart or from the skeletal muscles of the horse maintained for a long period of time the virulence of the cultures used; conversely, media prepared from calf spleen led to a decrease in pathogenicity. Normal horse serum, or specific immune serum freed from protective antibody, preserved virulence. Media made from rabbit muscle were less suitable for the purpose than media prepared in the same way from the meat of guinea pigs. When grown in the automatic transfer device in a medium which aerobically maintained the virulence of a Type I culture, the addition of pure oxygen or pure carbon dioxide lowered virulence, but no change in infectivity was noted when the organisms were cultivated in the presence of nitrogen. Gradual increase in the temperature of incubation from 36.5° to 42° over a period of ten days, in a sample of medium otherwise suitable for maintenance of virulence, resulted in a decrease in infective power of the pneumococci studied.

According to Gaskell,[499] a medium made from beaten eggs was satisfactory for preserving the virulence of pneumococcal cultures, but the interpolation of fortnightly passages through the mouse was necessary in order to restore waning infectivity. For additional methods for assuring or preserving the virulence of cultures of Pneumococcus or of fluids or tissues containing the organism, the reader is referred to Chapter II.

STRAIN VARIATIONS IN VIRULENCE

The ability of a given strain of Pneumococcus to retain its virulence over a long period and then suddenly to lose its invasive power is too well known to require extended comment. Browning and Gulbransen (1923)[161] described a culture of Type I Pneumococcus, passed more than ninety times through mice during a period of six years, which, when preserved in the dried spleen of an infected mouse, exhibited marked variations in its ability to infect mice. The conclusions reached by Gaskell (1928)[501] in a study of the pathogenicity of single strains of pneumococci of Types I, II, and III and Group IV may be cited. The virulence of Type II strains was less than that of Type I organisms for both mice and rabbits; the pathogenicity of members of Type III was lower than that of Type I for rabbits, mice, and also man; whereas the virulence of the Group IV cultures obtained from severe infections in man was, if anything, higher than that of Type I pneumococci.

Other individual strain differences with respect to the ability of pneumococci to infect experimental animals have been reported by Webster and Clow (1933).[1494] The degree of virulence of a strain when inoculated into the nose of the mouse failed to parallel intraperitoneal virulence in 50 per cent of the strains studied—high intranasal invasiveness being accompanied by either high or moderate intraperitoneal virulence, and low intranasal by high, moderate, or low intraperitoneal virulence. Type III strains were of relatively high intranasal and intraperitoneal infectivity; Type II organisms were low in intranasal but high or moderate in intraperitoneal virulence; Type I strains were all low in intranasal but either high or moderate in intraperitoneal virulence; while the majority of strains of other types were low both in intranasal and intraperitoneal pathogenicity. Intranasal virulence of pneumococci was not enhanced by animal passage, but nasal passage reduced the intranasal virulence to zero without altering intraperitoneal virulence, colony form, or agglutinative specificity of the strains. Passage by the intraperitoneal method maintained the characteristic level of intranasal virulence for a period, increased intraperitoneal virulence in some instances, but did not affect colony form or agglutinative properties.

VIRULENCE IN RESPECT TO ANIMAL SPECIES

In addition to individual differences in pneumococci, variations in the susceptibility of various animals are factors to be reckoned with in the evaluation of the virulence of a given type or strain. An organism may possess superior virulence for animals of one species and yet fail to infect those of another species, although the animals may readily be infected with representatives of a different variety or type. Eyre and Washbourn,[874] in 1898, reported that, after increasing the virulence of a culture for guinea pigs by repeated passage through a series of these animals, there was no change in the virulence of the organism for mice. Fourteen years later, Neufeld and Ungermann[1001-2] observed that while repeated passage of a strain of Pneumococcus through the guinea pig elevated the virulence of the organism for animals of the same species, similar serial propagation in mice failed to increase the infectiousness of the strain for the guinea pig.

In 1912, Truche and Cotoni[1423] reported that strains of pneumococci isolated from human sources were rarely virulent for rabbits or guinea pigs. Strains virulent for rabbits were always infective for mice, while pneumococci that were invasive for guinea pigs possessed high virulence for both rabbits and mice. In a second paper, Truche and Cotoni[1424] described the effect of passing four strains of Pneumococcus through mice, rabbits, and guinea pigs. When strains virulent for mice were serially propagated through animals of that species the organisms maintained their high virulence but acquired no greater virulence over the original culture for rabbits or guinea pigs. The same condition held true when pneumococci were passed through rabbits, but there was no alteration in the infectiousness of the strains for guinea pigs or mice. Cultures subjected to passage through guinea pigs showed no increase in pathogenicity for animals of that species or for mice or rabbits.

Twenty strains of Type III Pneumococcus studied by Lévy-Bruhl (1927)[804] were highly virulent for guinea pigs, moderately so for mice, and very feebly or not at all virulent for rabbits. The failure of many strains of Type III Pneumococcus to infect rabbits was also reported in the same year by Tillett.[1403] Of eleven strains isolated from human sources, ten possessed low virulence for rabbits despite the fact that all the strains possessed large capsules and a high degree of virulence for mice. The odd strain was rendered highly infectious for rabbits, and since it possessed no other biological property demonstrably different from the other ten strains, Tillett concluded that its individual virulence must reside in some additional property.

The lack of virulence for rabbits of the majority of Type III pneumococci has perplexed many bacteriologists, and no explanation has been forthcoming for the disparity in virulence of Type III strains until the recent communication of Enders and Shaffer.[860] Evidence was obtained that a correlation exists between the inability of a strain to grow at 41° and virulence, since only among the thermoresistant strains were found those possessing the property of rabbit virulence. The attribute is constantly but not exclusively associated with all Type III pneumococci, and was considered by the authors as a prerequisite, but not the sole factor, in determining the virulence of an organism for rabbits. Continuing the investigation, Shaffer with Enders and Wu[1259] studied two smooth strains of the same organism, one virulent and the other relatively avirulent for rabbits. Although no antigenic differences between the two organisms were revealed by cross-absorption of agglutinins from homologous antiserum, the latter strain lost its capsule in dextrose serum-broth cultures about eight hours earlier than was the case with the rabbit-virulent organism. With the loss of capsule there was marked shrinkage in volume, alteration in the zone of acid agglutination, susceptibility to agglutination in antirough pneumococcic serum and to phagocytosis.

The results which followed the intravenous injection into rabbits of the two strains varied with the state of the capsule. A culture of either strain became susceptible to the blood-clearing mechanisms contemporaneously with the onset of capsular degeneration and the beginning of other concomitant changes at the surface of the organism which occurred much earlier with the less virulent strain. Phagocytosis by the leucocytes of the normal animal either *in vitro* or *in vivo* was observed only at such a time as the capsule had become impaired. The authors (Enders, Shaffer, and Wu)[361] concluded that virulence for rabbits of the two strains of Type III Pneumococcus does not imply that this animal possesses a defensive mechanism which is absent in other species, since it was possible to demonstrate similar differences in virulence when the organisms were injected intravenously into mice. Therefore, "the factors determining the degree of virulence of these strains are to be sought in the organisms themselves, rather than in the kind of host."

In a fourth publication of the series, Enders, Wu, and Shaffer[363] discovered that the addition of the C Fraction of Tillett and Francis[1409] to serum-leucocyte mixtures decreased the phagocytosis of both rabbit-virulent and avirulent strains of Type III by the cells and serum of both man and the normal rabbit. Furthermore, the addition of antirough pneumococcic serum to normal rabbit serum and cells resulted in increased phagocytosis of the strains that had been partially inhibited by the C Fraction; and antirough pneumococcic rabbit serum protected mice against one hundred or more minimal lethal doses of the rabbit-virulent strain, provided the organisms were injected by the intravenous route. When antirough serum was absorbed with the C Fraction, the mouse protective property was removed. In the summary and general conclusions, the authors stated:

Since there is no evidence for the occurrence of type specific antibody in the normal rabbit and since, as we have shown, the Pneumococcus Type III whether avirulent or virulent is not removed from the blood stream or destroyed when the capsule is intact, the following factors which have been revealed in the course of our work appear to represent certain essential components, if not the complete mechanism, upon which the natural immunity of the rabbit against this organism depends. (a) The elevation of the body temperature after intravenous infection to 41°C. or thereabouts and its maintenance for varying periods. (b) The ability of the phagocytic cells, both fixed and mobile, to attack any cocci which have become vulnerable through the deterioration of capsular integrity. (c) The adjuvant effect of an antibody, reacting with the somatic C carbohydrate, which enhances the phagocytosis of such organisms as no longer possess a completely intact envelope.

Conversely, the varying degrees of virulence for rabbits observed among Pneumococcus Type III strains are based upon: (a) differences in the ability of the organisms to multiply at the elevated temperatures encountered in the infected host. Strains markedly susceptible to the harmful influence of this factor fail to induce a generalized fatal infection. Not all "thermo-resistant" strains are highly virulent, however, and these may contrast sharply with regard to (b) size of the capsule and the ease with which it is impaired or completely lost. The capsules must be maintained intact for a sufficient time until multiplication of the organisms can proceed to such a degree that death of the host results. Avirulent strains even when capable of growth at 41°C. appear to be unable to satisfy this requirement.

The differences in virulence of various strains apparently conditioned by these factors are not limited solely to the case of the rabbit, since for at least two strains similar differences in virulence have been shown to exist when the intravenous route of infection is employed in mice.

The results of the studies by Enders and his colleagues were contemporaneously confirmed by the data obtained by Rich and McKee[1138] in an investigation on native immunity of the rabbit to Type III Pneumococcus. Strains of encapsulated Type III pneumococci virulent for mice, when injected intradermally into rabbits proliferate progressively in the tissues for some hours causing, with the dose used, a local lesion of considerable severity, often accompanied by bacteriemia. The proliferation of the cocci is then checked, the organisms are destroyed, and the animal completely recovers. During the first twenty-four hours of the infective process the rabbit acquires a greatly enhanced resistance to further infection and the increased resistance is due to the fever developing in the animal as a result of the infection. The encapsulated strains to which the rabbit is resistant are not phagocyted promptly either *in vitro* or *in vivo*, but after some hours' sojourn in the body of the rabbit, the organisms gradually lose their capsules and are avidly phagocyted. As in the body of the rabbit, the majority of the strains studied exhibited marked sensitivity to temperatures of 104° to 106° *in vitro*.

The work of Enders and his co-workers and of Rich and McKee, therefore, offers a striking example of one type of mechanism operating in a host-parasite relationship and again emphasizes the dependence of virulence upon a special physiological instead of a strictly immunological response on the part of a given animal species.

ARTIFICIAL EXALTATION OF VIRULENCE

There are several methods for raising the virulence of pneumococci. One is the frequent transplantation of the culture into a favorable medium, as advocated by Wadsworth and Kirkbride,[1471] and by Felton and Dougherty;[411-2, 423-4] another is serial passage through suitable animals, or by inoculation of animals with an organism of low virulence along with a killed culture of high virulence; while another method is to grow the organism in antirough pneumococcic serum of the homologous type. Propagation in the body of susceptible animals has long been practiced for the purpose of enhancing the virulence of pneumococci. Eyre and Washbourn (1898)[374] employed the guinea pig, Truche, Cramer, and Cotoni (1911)[1426] the mouse, while Neufeld and Ungermann (1912)[1001-2] increased the pathogenicity of Pneumococcus, when administered to guinea pigs by inhalation, by passage through animals of the same species.

The procedure of serial animal passage is now too well known to require extended comment. The intraperitoneal inoculation of white mice with infectious material containing pneumococci or with pure cultures, with subsequent recovery and cultivation of the organism from the heart's blood of the test animal is the method commonly used for raising and maintaining the virulence of pneumococci for experimental purposes or for the preparation of vaccines for the immunization of horses in the production of therapeutic serum as well as for testing the potency of such serums. The stimulating action of the dead bodies of virulent strains of pneumococci when injected simultaneously with living cultures of avirulent organisms of the corresponding serological type, resulting in the acquisition of higher virulence, has been discussed in the chapter on dissociation. A similar effect is produced by growth of organisms of low virulence in media containing immune serum specific for degraded variants of the homologous type.

DEGRADATION OF VIRULENCE

Pneumococci as they encounter unfavorable conditions when cultivated outside the animal body rapidly lose virulence. Insufficient nourishment, excess of alkali or acid, unsuitable incubation or storage temperatures, and infrequency of transplantation even in a favorable medium, lower the vitality of the cell, inhibit capsule formation, and consequently attenuate or destroy the pathogenic power of the organism. Furthermore, there are other and specific factors which may expedite the process.

DISSOCIATION AND VIRULENCE

Stryker[1348] in 1916 reported that virulent pneumococci when grown in homologous immune serum fail to form capsules, show a decrease in virulence, and become more susceptible to phagocytosis. By passing the altered forms through mice, reversion to the original type takes place. Normal serum has no such effect. The experiments of Stryker, therefore, constituted the first demonstration of the ability of the specific antibodies of immune serum to inhibit the elaboration of capsular substance by Pneumococcus and consequently to render the organism vulnerable to the natural defenses of the animal body. Further developments in the investigation of the action of immune serum as well as of cultural conditions on the virulence of pneumococci have already been described in such detail, that, in order to avoid needless repetition, the reader is referred to the chapter on dissociation.

Summary

To summarize the data discussed in the present chapter, it may be repeated that in the mouse and the rabbit man has at his disposal animals admirably adapted for the several purposes of the bacteriological and immunological study of Pneumococcus. The use of in-bred strains of mice, and presumably of rabbits, reduces the frequency of irregular results in experimental work, especially in quantitative estimations of specific antibodies in immune serum. The monkey, being more closely related in the biological scale to man, presents opportunity for studying the invasiveness of pneumococci and their pathological effects in the animal economy. The horse, although obviously unsuited to the study of pathogenicity, by virtue of its size and disposition, serves as the most convenient animal for the production of antipneumococcic serum. Susceptibility or resistance depends on peculiarities due to the species, on genetic factors, age, weight, environmental conditions, and the physical state of the test animal.

In addition to the variables in the host, the invasiveness of a given strain of Pneumococcus is conditioned by its serological type, the vital condition of the culture, its mass or density, the route of inoculation, and by intrinsic factors possessed by various strains of the organism. Virulence of a pneumococcus for a given animal species may be raised by serial passage through animals of the same species, and the enhanced pathogenicity can be maintained by continued animal passage or by the application of suitable *in vitro* methods of preservation. Contrariwise, the pathogenicity of a pneumococcal strain may be decreased by subjecting the organisms to unfavorable cultural conditions or by propagating the organisms in media containing increasing amounts of homologous immune serum. Pathogenicity or virulence, therefore, is only a relative term and must be interpreted in the light of the biological characters of the pneumococcal strain and of the functional variables in the animal host. As yet no *in vitro* test has been devised which equals the use of animals, particularly the mouse and the rabbit, for studying the invasive power or virulence of Pneumococcus.

CHAPTER VII

PATHOGENICITY OF PNEUMOCOCCUS: MAN

The infectiousness of pneumococci of the different serological types for human beings; incidence and lethal powers of the cocci in disease; their distribution in the body and the lesions produced; and the various phenomena of the carrier state.

PNEUMOCOCCI, if successful in passing the first defensive barriers of the human system, may become localized in a tissue or organ, mainly the lungs, whence they may invade the blood stream and under favoring conditions incite metastatic foci in other parts of the body; or, after gaining entrance, they may proceed to sites other than pulmonary tissue and there set up primary infection. The nature and severity of the infection depend on the serological type, virulence, and mass of invading cocci, the passage by which they are admitted, and on the many and varied factors which constitute natural resistance or which are involved in the creation of specific immunity in response to the presence of the invading organisms.

The epidemiology and the clinical and pathological aspects of pneumococcal infection may be left to writers competent to discuss these subjects.* Therefore, assuming that the reader of this review is more intimately interested in the vital activities of Pneumococcus as a microorganism than in the manifold morbid manifestations of the human body's response to its invasion, the present discussion is directed more particularly to the ability of pneumococci of the different serological types to incite disease in man.

Pneumococci frequently lead a vegetative existence in the normal mouth, abiding there without causing any appreciable disturb-

* A contemporary review of the literature relating to these subjects has been prepared by Heffron.[601]

ance in the host. The organisms may be virulent or avirulent and they may sometimes be found as the predominant bacterial species but, contrary to the older opinion, these so-called normal pneumococci, although possessed of full virulence, rarely cause pneumonia in the individual in whom they temporarily dwell. Since the discovery by Sternberg,[1316-8] Pasteur,[1065-6] and other early investigators that pneumococci virulent for laboratory animals were to be found in the saliva of healthy persons, many reports have appeared concerning the frequency of the occurrence. Buerger (1905),[164] by the plate method, detected pneumococci in the mouths of thirty-nine out of seventy-eight normal persons. Some of the subjects were assumed to have acquired the organisms in hospital wards and others as a result of pneumonia. In both groups, the pneumococci persisted for days and even months. In a communication published at the same time, Hiss, Borden, and Knapp,[651] from their bacteriological study of twenty-two healthy individuals, concluded that practically every person, at least during the winter season, living under such conditions as exist in New York City, acts as a host at some time or other and probably at repeated intervals for Pneumococcus. A seasonal effect on the distribution of pneumococci was suggested by Longcope and Fox[825] who observed a greater incidence of the organism in normal human beings during the winter months than during the milder seasons. The authors stated that during the winter a large percentage of healthy individuals harbor virulent pneumococci in the buccal cavity, and that it is almost certain that some persons always have virulent pneumococci in their saliva. More recently, Brown and Anderson (1932)[152] noted a correlation between the incidence of pneumococci in the throats of normal persons and periods of inclement weather.

Park and Williams,[1058] by the mouse inoculation method, found pneumococci in the sputum of 55 per cent of over two hundred healthy subjects. McLeod,[880] in reviewing these reports, gave the more conservative estimate of 20 per cent. Be that as it may, since the differentiation of the species into the many serological types, the list of publications which have appeared reveal the widespread prevalence, wherever investigated, of pneumococci of one type or another as members of the normal bacterial flora of the mouth. There is some doubt, however, as to how far down in the respiratory tract of healthy individuals pneumococci may be found in a state of saprophytism. Pneumococcus under favorable conditions may exchange this benign vegetative existence for a life of malignity for man. According to Hiss and Zinsser—who voiced a general opinion—lobar pneumonia is the type of infection most often caused by Pneumococcus. McLeod differed and expressed the belief that "the most frequent lesion produced by the organism is a catarrhal condition of the upper respiratory tract involving the larger bronchi, associated with slight or considerable pyrexia, and often popularly described as 'influenza.'" The truth of the matter is of less concern to the bacteriologist than to the clinician. On the other hand, the fact is incontestable that the great majority of cases of lobar pneumonia are caused by Pneumococcus. In addition, Pneumococcus may be the sole causative factor in bronchopneumonia, sinusitis, otitis, mastoiditis, meningitis, peritonitis, nephritis, arthritis, and infections of the eye and other tissues. Some of the manifestations may be primary in character or secondary to pneumococcal disease in the lung. In company with organisms of other bacterial species, Pneumococcus may complicate or intensify the severity of the infection.

Etiology of Pneumonia

PNEUMOCOCCAL TYPES IN LOBAR PNEUMONIA

The predominance of Pneumococcus as the causative agent in lobar pneumonia with the percentage distribution of other bacterial species is seen in the table supplied by Heffron.[601]

Organism found	*Number of cases*	*Per cent*
Pneumococcus	3,189	96.1
Streptococcus	94	2.8
Friedländer's bacillus	17	0.5
Influenza bacillus	7	0.2
Staphylococcus	6	0.2
Mixed infections	6	0.2
Total	*3,319*	*100.0*

Heffron in a searching inquiry into the part played by the various serological types in the causation of lobar pneumonia collected all the available data and presented analyses of the figures obtained. In 14,869 cases of the disease reported from many parts of the world, pneumococci of Type I occurred in 32.8 per cent; Type II in 20.6 per cent; Type III in 10.8 per cent; while all organisms listed under Group IV were found in 35.8 per cent of the cases reported. The incidence of pneumococcal types in lobar pneumonia arranged according to geographic distribution, as far as reported, may be seen in the table taken from Heffron.[601]

PERCENTAGE DISTRIBUTION BY SEROLOGICAL TYPE OF 14,869 CASES OF PNEUMOCOCCUS LOBAR PNEUMONIA IN CERTAIN GEOGRAPHIC AREAS

Geographic group	Total cases	Percentage distribution				
		Type I	*Type II*	*Types I and II together*	*Type III*	*Group IV*
United States, Puerto Rico, and Canada	10,860	31.5	19.2	50.7	11.8	37.5
Europe	3,138	38.7	28.3	67.0	7.0	26.0
Africa	230	19.1	12.2	31.3	2.2	66.5
Far East and Australia	641	41.0	15.4	56.4	6.6	37.0
Total	*14,869*	*32.8*	*20.6*	*53.4*	*10.8*	*35.8*

There occur, of course, local and seasonal variations in the prevalence of pneumococcal types in lobar pneumonia but the foregoing table furnishes a composite picture for the world at large. Since the further division of pneumococci into the present thirty-two serological types, the figures of Sutliff and Finland,[1361] and of Bullowa,[183] as tabulated by Heffron, may be taken as representative of the time and place of observation (Tables A and B).

There is no call to include in this chapter the many further detailed analyses presented by Heffron as to the percentage incidence of pneumococcal types in relation to age and sex of lobar pneumonia patients. It may suffice to include only a summary table showing the collected statistics (Table C).

A. NUMBER AND PERCENTAGE DISTRIBUTION OF CASES OF PNEUMOCOCCUS LOBAR PNEUMONIA, DUE TO TYPES I TO XX INCLUSIVE, IN ADULTS (SUTLIFF AND FINLAND'S AND BULLOWA'S SERIES)

Type	Sutliff and Finland's cases	Bullowa's cases	Total cases	Per cent
I	268	253	521	30.5
II	142	79	221	12.9
III	121	115	236	13.8
IV	14	65	79	4.6
V	38	60	98	5.7
VI	9	29	38	2.2
VII	37	69	106	6.2
VIII	42	98	140	8.2
IX	14	25	39	2.3
X	19	8	27	1.6
XI	8	6	14	0.8
XII	6	14	20	1.2
XIII	4	8	12	0.7
XIV	14	45	59	3.5
XV	3	1	4	0.2
XVI	1	4	5	0.3
XVII	1	8	9	0.5
XVIII	19	24	43	2.5
XIX	4	16	20	1.2
XX	6	11	17	1.0
Total	*770*	*938*	*1,708*	*100.0*

B. NUMBER AND PERCENTAGE DISTRIBUTION OF 1,000 CASES OF PNEUMOCOCCUS LOBAR PNEUMONIA, DUE TO TYPES I TO XXXII INCLUSIVE, IN ADULTS (BULLOWA'S SERIES)

Type	Number	Per cent
I to XX inclusive	938	77.0
XXI	13	1.3
XXII	16	1.6
XXIII	3	0.3
XXIV	3	0.3
XXV	2	0.2
XXVI	–	0.0
XXVII	2	0.2
XXVIII	9	0.9
XXIX	5	0.5
XXX	2	0.2
XXXI	3	0.3
XXXII	4	0.4
Total	*1,000*	*100.0*

C. NUMBER AND PERCENTAGE DISTRIBUTION BY AGE AND SEX OF TYPES I, II, III, AND GROUP IV CASES OF LOBAR PNEUMONIA IN ADULTS

PNEUMOCOCCUS	TOTAL CASES	UNDER 50 YEARS				OVER 50 YEARS			
		Men		Women		Men		Women	
		Cases	*Per cent*	*Cases*	*Per cent*	*Cases*	*Per cent*	*Cases*	*Per cent*
Type I	627	462	73.7	73	11.7	83	13.2	9	1.4
Type II	362	236	65.2	44	12.2	76	21.0	6	1.7
Type III	263	124	47.1	42	16.0	70	26.6	27	10.3
Group IV	615	398	64.7	86	14.0	101	16.4	30	4.9
Total	*1,867*	*1,220*	*65.3*	*245*	*13.1*	*330*	*17.7*	*72*	*3.9*

PNEUMOCOCCAL TYPES IN BRONCHOPNEUMONIA

Quoting from Heffron: "The frequency with which the various types of pneumococci are found in bronchopneumonia approximately parallels the frequency with which they are carried in the mouths of normal persons, which suggests that chance occurrence may play a large part in these infections." So short a time has elapsed since the serological classification of pneumococci has been enlarged to comprise thirty-two types that the few type analyses in bronchopneumonia can only be looked upon as suggestive. In one of Heffron's tables listing the types of organisms found in this disease in East Africa, Germany, Great Britain, India, and the United States, totalling three hundred cases, it is seen that Type I pneumococci were found in 6.3 per cent, Type II in 4.3 per cent, Type III in 14 per cent, and organisms of the fourth group (type not specified) in 75.3 per cent of all cases reported. There is a marked difference in the reported figures between the incidence of Types I and II combined (10.6 per cent) in bronchopneumonia and their incidence in lobar pneumonia (over 50 per cent).

In observations on the presence of the various pneumococcal types in bronchopneumonia, Sutliff and Finland found that the ten types occurring in a series of 174 cases were, in order of frequency, Types III, VIII, XVIII, X, V, VII, XX, II, XI, and XIV. Additional data are given in the communication of Trask, O'Donovan, Moore, and Beebe.[1417] Studying the relation of pneumococci of the first three types to pneumonia, the latter authors noted that, in patients suffering from Type I or II infections, bronchopneumonia was rare, but with Type III this form of the disease constituted one-third of the affections. Sutliff and Finland reported that 21 per cent of the Type III and 30 per cent of the Type VIII infections studied were cases of bronchopneumonia, whereas only 3 per cent of the Type I and 5 per cent of Type II affections were diagnosed as bronchopneumonia. The early studies at the Hospital of the Rockefeller Institute pointed to extrinsic infection as the cause of lobar pneumonia, whereas the few data available seem to indicate that bronchopneumonia arises more commonly from intrinsic infection or auto-inoculation.

In the case of bronchopneumonia following other affections of the respiratory tract, the infection is largely due to the bacterial species more commonly present in the air passages, among which the streptococci predominate. Pneumococci of the fourth, heterogeneous group may account for approximately 50 per cent of the cases. Streptococci of both hemolytic and non-hemolytic varieties have been found in about 31 per cent of the patients studied; the Pfeiffer bacillus and pneumococci of Types I and II were responsible for 3.3 per cent each; while Type III pneumococci appeared two and one-half times as often as did strains of either Type I or II.

PNEUMOCOCCAL TYPES IN PNEUMONIA IN INFANTS AND CHILDREN

The data presented in Heffron's analyses make it appear that, as far as reported, of pneumonia in children under twelve years of age, 9 or 10 per cent of the cases were caused by Type I pneumococci, between 2 and 4 per cent were due to organisms of Type II or III, while in approximately 75 per cent of the cases pneumococci of the remaining types appeared to be the causative organisms. Heffron placed Types I, XIV, VI, V, and VII as the order in which pneumococci are found in the pneumonias of childhood. There appears to be a conspicuous rise in the frequency of pneumococci of the first three types in pneumococcal pneumonia as age increases. Dividing the children studied into one group comprising those under three years of age and a second group in which the ages ranged from three to twelve years, the most marked increase is to be noted in the case of Type I Pneumococcus, which rose from 4.2 per cent in the first group to 20.2 per cent in the second. For pneumococci of Types I, II, and III the corresponding combined incidence was 11.1 and 25.2 per cent respectively in the two age groups. The number of cases examined is too small to allow of accurate statistical deduction, but the trend is significant and points to the greater frequency of organisms of the first three serological types in the higher age groups.

Without burdening the text with too many tables, Heffron's summary may be abridged to read: Among the 826 cases of pneumococcal lobar pneumonia in children of eleven years of age or under, Type I organisms were found in 22.4 per cent, Type II in 8.1 per cent, and Type III in 5.5 per cent, these three types together accounting for 36.0 per cent of the infections. Sixty-four per cent of the remaining cases were due to pneumococci of the other serological types. Of all the various types, XIV, I, VI, V, and VII were the more prevalent, with IV, IX, XV, and XIX of frequent occurrence.

In pneumonias of the bronchial type the picture is somewhat different. Whereas Type II Pneumococcus showed slightly greater frequency, Type I organisms fell in percentage of occurrence from 22.4 to 9.0, and Types I, II, and III combined showed a decrease of from 36.0 to 26.2 per cent. The respective rates for pneumococci other than those of the first three types were reported to be substantially the same for infants and children and for adults.

To recapitulate the enumeration so far reported of the commonest serological types of Pneumococcus in order of approximate frequency as occurring in infants, children, and adults, the following figures from Heffron are presented:

Lobar pneumonia	
Infants and children	XIV, I, VI, V, VII
Adults	I, II, III, VIII, VII, V
Bronchopneumonia	
Infants and children	VI, XIX, XVIII
Adults	III, VIII, XVIII, X, V, VII

Serological Types and Fatality-Rates

The factors making for virulence of pneumococci have been discussed in Chapter VI. In addition to the characters of individual strains dependent upon their history and immediate environment, there are variations in invasive power peculiar to the many serological types. The data so far accumulated on the fatality-rates of the different types are not extensive but enough evidence is at hand to warrant some general, if tentative, conclusions. Heffron stated that from available reports the fatality-rates, at least for lobar pneumonia due to pneumococci of Types I and II, are somewhat lower in Great Britain, and possibly in Norway, Sweden, and Germany, than in the United States and Canada. For 1,614 civilian cases receiving no serum treatment in the two American countries, Heffron calculated the death-rate as 25 per cent for Type I cases and as 41 per cent for cases due to Type II pneumococci, while of Type III infections from 45 to 60 per cent of the cases terminated fatally.

FATALITY-RATES OF LOBAR PNEUMONIA DUE TO PNEUMOCOCCI OF TYPES IV TO XXXII INCLUSIVE

Type	Cases	Deaths	Death-rate per 100
IV	43	13	30.2
V	90	27	30.0
VI	18	8	
VII	97	28	28.8
VIII	67	15	22.4
IX	25	8	
X	24	8	
XI	12	2	
XII	12	5	
XIII	17	4	
XIV	20	2	
XV	4	1	
XVI	6	–	
XVII	3	–	
XVIII	30	10	33.3
XIX	11	4	
XX	10	2	
XXI	2	1	
XXII	–	–	
XXIII	1	1	
XXIV	–	–	
XXV	–	–	
XXVI	1	–	
XXVII	–	–	
XXVIII	–	–	
XXIX	–	–	
XXX	–	–	
XXXI	–	–	
XXXII	–	–	
Total	*493*	*139*	*28.2*

NOTE: Rates are omitted where the numbers are too small to be significant.

Conning the reports published by Bullowa, Park, and Sutliff and Finland, Heffron arranged in tabular form the data representing the fatality-rate in lobar pneumonia caused by pneumococci of types other than the first three.

The above data are too few to permit statistical analysis, yet they are already guiding manufacturers in preparing antipneumococcic serum in accordance with the more prevalent types of pneumococci responsible for lobar pneumonia in this country.

The only report available on the lethal power of the different types of Pneumococcus in bronchopneumonia is that of Sutliff and Finland (1933).[1361] Here again, the data are meager, but there can be no gainsaying the fact that bronchopneumonia caused by pneumococci, with its high death-rate, is a serious affliction to man.

Localized Epidemics of Pneumococcal Infection

The infectiousness of Pneumococcus for individuals living in close association is demonstrated by the occasional outbreaks of acute disease of the respiratory tract. Sinigar (1903)[1292] described an epidemic among the staff and patients of an asylum, but inasmuch as the bacteriological study consisted merely in the microscopic examination of preparations of sputum and from the lungs of fatal cases, one is in the dark as to whether the epidemic was caused by a pneumococcus.

The presence of pneumococci of the various serological types associated with common colds has been too frequently noted to require extended discussion. The results of a study reported by Valentine (1918)[1442] may be cited as typical. From sixty-five cases of upper respiratory infections diagnosed as colds, pneumococci were recovered in forty-three instances. Of the organisms, two belonged to Pneumococcus Type I, two to Type II, four were of the third type, and the remainder fell into the heterogeneous Group IV. A more compact source of material for study was an outbreak of respiratory infection among the inmates of a children's home sheltering more than seven hundred children of both sexes between the ages of two and twelve years. In investigating the 150 cases occurring among the inmates, Schroder and Cooper (1930)[1250] isolated an organism described by them as extremely infective and which they identified as Type V Pneumococcus. All the cases save one occurred among the boys, who were in frequent and close contact, the sole exception being a girl who had assembled with the boys in a classroom.

A series of twelve cases of pneumonia and two of otitis media developing over a period of four months among eighty-seven boys in an orphanage was caused by Pneumococcus of Type I. Ström,[1344] who studied the epidemic, reported that the infection was more prevalent among the older boys and, furthermore, that of those coming in contact with the affected boys a third of the number were found to be carriers of the same organism. The strains isolated from the patients were more virulent for mice than were those recovered from the carriers.

Infectious Processes Other Than Pneumonia

Pneumococcus, during the pneumonic process, may migrate from the seat of infection in the lung to the vascular system and thereby be distributed throughout the body and create localized foci. Or, without the intermediate pulmonary lesion, the organisms may by direct or indirect routes gain access to vulnerable tissues. While, because of the abundant data, it is possible to apportion the guilt to representatives of the different serological types in lobar and bronchopneumonia, a verdict is not so easily pronounced in non-pulmonary infections of pneumococcal origin. Many of the reports appeared before the diversity of types was recognized, and since that era the comparative infrequency of non-pulmonary infections has supplied too few observations to be of any statistical value.

Meningitis as a complication or sequel of lobar pneumonia had early been reported by Fraenkel,[469] Senger,[1255] Netter,[962] Lancereaux and Besançon,[778] Gamaléia,[498] Meyer,[895] Ortmann,[1037-8] and others, but not until the report of Foà and Bordoni-Uffreduzzi[462] was any claim advanced that pneumococcal disease of the meninges could occur as a primary infection. Many references to clinical reports must necessarily be passed over in this review, but Harkavy's (1928)[589] is cited because from the one patient mentioned Type I Pneumococcus was isolated from the spinal fluid and in the case of this patient the administration of specific immune serum effected a cure.

Endocarditis and pericarditis are not unusual concomitants of pneumonia, but the condition is nearly always secondary to the pneumonic process and the same organism may be responsible for both lesions. Thomas and O'Hara (1920)[1395] described a case of endocarditis in which Type I Pneumococcus was found in a vegetation on the tricuspid valve, but the authors disclaimed that the unusual site of the infection was due to any special selective affinity of that pneumococcal type.

Such infections as sinusitis, parotitis, gingivitis, and otitis may accompany but are rarely independent of lobar pneumonia. Zaufal[1568-9] was probably the first to report primary infection of the ear by Pneumococcus. Arthritis is a metastatic manifestation of pulmonary infection and has been described by Nauwerck,[944-6] Weichselbaum,[1503-5] and Herzog,[639] but it is improbable that arthritis or nephritis occurs except as a result of pneumococcal infection elsewhere in the body. To the list of non-pulmonary infections caused by Pneumococcus, Neufeld and Schnitzer added osteomyelitis and appendicitis (Ungermann), epidydimitis and orchitis, cystitis, fibrinous enteritis (Flexner, Curlo), cholecystitis (Lenharz and others), phlegmon (Robbers), ulcus serpens and conjunctivitis (Axenfeld and others), erysipelas (v. Leube, and Reiche and Schomerus), and pyosalpinx and puerperal sepsis (Jacob).

Of the several specific complications of pneumonia, infections of the pleura and pericardium are the most common. Endocarditis and meningitis are grave sequels, while, in addition to the affections already mentioned, abscesses, retinochoroiditis, and panophthalmia may develop as secondary lesions.

Primary pneumococcal infections of the eye have been described by Mikaëljan (1931)[902] who, in a limited series of cases, found pneumococci of Types I and II in panophthalmia, ulcus cornea serpens, and purulent dacryocystitis, while organisms of Group IV were isolated from the eye in two cases of purulent conjunctivitis.

In a communication appearing in 1931, Smeall[1293] tabulated the pneumococcal types encountered in a variety of affections and stressed the fact that the organisms most commonly found in the eye and accessory sinuses belonged to Group IV and that those of Type III and Group IV were present most frequently in acute otitis media and mastoiditis. It is of course not improbable that a similar and larger series of cases investigated in another locality or country might yield different results.

Pneumococcemia

From time to time bacteriologists have alleged that virulent pneumococci as well as streptococci and other pathogens are to be found in the circulating blood of healthy persons as well as of those ill with affections to which the organisms are not related. The validity of the claims is always highly questionable, and it is problematical if Pneumococcus invades the circulatory system unless a specific focus of infection exists at some point in the body. Since the discovery by Friedländer[489-90] in 1884 of pneumococci in the blood of pneumonia patients, their presence has been recognized as a frequent accompaniment of pneumococcal disease indicating a gloomy prognosis. The literature and bedside records are replete with notes on positive blood cultures taken on pneumonia patients, but the percentage of positive cultures reported varies with the nature of the clinical material and the skill of the technician. Prochaska[1111] claimed that he found pneumococci in the blood of practically all of forty pneumonia patients; Strouse and Clough (1910)[1347] reported positive results in 56 per cent of the cases occurring in a localized epidemic in which the total mortality was only 20 per cent. Of cultures made by Lyall (1912),[840] 40.5 per cent were positive, and if those taken at the time of crisis or lysis, which were uniformly negative, are deducted, the figure rises to 53 per cent. The fatality-rate for the whole series was 26.2 per cent, while that for the patients having pneumococci in the blood was 50 per cent. The great prognostic value of blood cultures in lobar pneumonia was early pointed out by Avery, Chickering, Cole and Dochez (1917),[36] who reported positive blood cultures in 30.3 per cent of 448 cases. Of the positive cases, 55.8 per cent were fatal, whereas only 8.3 per cent of patients with no pneumococcemia died. The mortality among the patients harboring strains of Types II and III and of Group IV in the blood was above 50 per cent, and all cases in the series with Type III bacteriemia terminated fatally.

In a study made by Sutton and Sevier[1365] at Johns Hopkins Hospital in 1917 the numbers of deaths and of positive blood cultures were practically identical. The series was so small (62) that percentage figures are not of general significance. It was evident, nevertheless, that of the cases observed, positive blood cultures and deaths were far more frequent when the infecting Pneumococcus belonged either to Type I or to atypical Type II. That some organisms of Group IV may be sufficiently invasive to enter the blood stream is shown by the figure of 18.2 per cent of positive blood cultures for cases in which a Group IV pneumococcus was the causative organism.

The correlation between mortality and bacteriemia did not hold in the series reported by McClelland,[874] but pneumococci of Types I and II were responsible for the majority of the positive blood cultures and of the deaths. Here the fatality-rate for Group IV cases was only 4.2—the same as the percentage occurrence of bacteriemia. That pneumococcemia may be present in a large proportion of pneumonia cases is also apparent from the work of Christie in England (1932),[232] who found pneumococci in approximately 57 per cent of the blood samples cultured. Christie emphasized the importance of positive blood cultures as a prognostic measure, since all the fatalities in the series occurred in the positive group, whereas, in the case of the patients who had bacteriemia and recovered, convalescence was prolonged or complicated with empyema.

Heffron discusses this feature of pneumococcal infection in greater detail. For the purposes of the bacteriologist the foregoing discussion may suffice. The presence of active bacteriemia and the development of infected foci in the deeper tissues bears witness of the ability of pneumococci at times to surmount the natural obstacles in the body and to migrate to parts distant from the original site of infection.

Excretion of Pneumococci

From diseased foci pneumococci pass into the sputum in cases of sinusitis, parotitis, gingivitis, and pneumonia; into the spinal fluid in meningitis; into all purulent exudates in pericarditis, empyema, peritonitis, and arthritis. The urine in approximately 38 per cent of the cases of lobar pneumonia studied was found by Mathers (1916)[868] to contain pneumococci. The organisms appeared in the urine usually just before or immediately after crisis, and Mathers advised precautions to avoid the possible danger of passing on the infection, particularly in hospitals, by careless handling of the excreta of pneumonia patients. The intestinal tract is another exit by which pneumococci pass from the infected body. Rutz (1912)[1198] isolated virulent pneumococci from the feces of the majority of patients ill with lobar pneumonia, the organisms appearing as early as the second or third day of the disease. No pneumococci were discovered in the feces of the normal individuals tested.

In studying the distribution of pneumococci throughout the body a word of warning may be said against placing reliance on the result of cultures taken after the death of the subject. As early as 1905 Norris and Pappenheimer[1018] drew attention to the possible fallacy in making deductions from bacteriological findings at necropsy, since organisms placed in the mouth after death were conveyed to and could be recovered from the lungs by culture in over one-half of the cases in which the post-mortem implantation was made.

The Carrier State

Pneumococci abiding in the mouth and nasopharynx of healthy persons—the chief portal of entrance of Pneumococcus to the body—owe their presence either to direct or indirect contact with other persons harboring the organisms in their oral or nasal cavities, or to previous pneumococcal disease in the same individual. The mere presence of these pathogens in the body is insufficient to incite disease; it is the constitutional factors of the host which determine whether the invaders are to remain as innocuous members of the usual bacterial population or whether they are to abandon their life of saprophytism and act as malignant parasites. In the absence of such depressing conditions as alcoholism, chilling, the exhaustion of fatigue, undernourishment, avitaminosis, or the contributory influence of previous or concomitant disease, Pneumococcus may develop none of its pathogenic potentialities.

The upper respiratory passages of the new-born babe, according to Gundel and Schwarz,[575] are sterile at the time of delivery and may remain so for a few hours after birth. Then on the second or third day pneumococci may appear, the type and number depending upon the quantitative occurrence of similar organisms in the immediate environment, especially in the oral cavity of the mother. The infant as it enters and passes through childhood receives from its fellows and elders contributions from their bacterial flora. In a systematic study of the incidence of pneumococci in the upper respiratory passages of normal persons, largely schoolchildren, Gundel (1933),[569] by repeated tests made every four weeks for a year on over one hundred subjects, found that while the type of Pneumococcus usually proved to be the same in successive tests on a given individual, in many cases there were rapid and frequent changes in the types present. The relative infrequency of organisms of the first three types, so often observed in the mouth flora of healthy persons, is also to be noted in Gundel's report. Type I pneumococci occurred in 0.8 per cent, Type II in 0.4 per cent, Type III in 6.7 per cent, and organisms of Group IV (Gundel's X) were present in 60 per cent of the individuals tested successively throughout the year.

In a continuation of the study, Gundel and Okura,[573] with even more painstaking methods, investigated the occurrence of pneumococci of more than one serological type in the same subject. Thirty-eight per cent of the individuals of the series tested carried organisms of two or more types, and the frequency of occurrence was much greater among boys than among girls. The appearance of new types was attributed by the authors to infection from without or possibly to the development of a type which had been suppressed by the dominance of the first type found. Gundel and Okura did not agree with Neufeld and Etinger-Tulczinska[984] that infection of the nasal or buccal mucous membrane may lead to specific immunity against the infecting type without eliciting any apparent or at least definite morbid symptoms, since repeated serological tests failed to reveal any specific antibodies for the types carried for protracted periods. The explanation that the non-invasiveness of pneumococci existing in the normal mouth could be due to the fact that the organisms there undergo dissociation into rough and, therefore, avirulent forms was opposed by Gundel and Schwarz,[575] who encountered no such variants in their investigations. This opinion was further supported by the results of a slightly earlier series of virulence tests on pneumococci isolated from normal and pneumonic sputums, which would seem to show that virulent strains exhibit few if any signs of variation *in vivo*. Gundel and Wasu[578] concluded that the vegetative pneumococci were not culpable in causing any ensuing pneumonia but that the infection always came from without.

The disappearance of members of the first three types during convalescence and the subsequent appearance of organisms of a heterologous group was early established by Dochez and Avery (1915).[319] The authors stated that although pneumococci occur in the mouths of 60 per cent of normal individuals, the organisms are readily distinguishable from the highly parasitic types of pneumococci responsible for the severe forms of lobar pneumonia—a convincing proof that infection in that disease is, in the majority of instances, not autogenic in nature, but is derived from some extraneous source. Dochez and Avery found further that in a high percentage of instances healthy persons intimately associated with cases of lobar pneumonia harbor the disease-producing types of pneumococci. In every such instance the strain isolated from the normal subject was found to correspond in type with that of the infected individual with whom the healthy person had come in contact. In conclusion, the authors stated that the existence of the carrier state among healthy persons and among those recently recovered from pneumonia establishes a basis for understanding the mechanism by means of which lobar pneumonia spreads and maintains its high incidence from year to year.

The relative infrequency of pneumococci of the first three types in the mouths of healthy persons of varying ages who gave no history of contact with pneumonia was also observed by Meyer (1920).[899] Among one hundred normal individuals, no strains of Type I or II (excepting an atypical II), and only three strains of Type III pneumococci were found. Group IV organisms were present in seventeen instances. In the sputum of fifty tuberculous patients Lyall[841] found pneumococci in twenty cases. Excluding one patient with a history of pneumonia in the previous year, pneumococci of Type I occurred once, of Type II none were found, of Type III three subjects harbored the organism, while pneumococci of Group IV accounted for 75 per cent of the positive cultures.

The studies reported by Rosenau, Felton, and Atwater,[1157] and by Powell, Atwater, and Felton[1106] in 1926 yielded results which, while differing in some respects from those of Dochez and Avery, confirm their thesis and throw additional light on the carrier problem. Using a thoroughgoing technique for the isolation of pneumococci from the mouth and throat, the Boston authors isolated pneumococci of Type I from four times as many subjects in contact with cases of lobar pneumonia as normal persons not thus exposed. Type III organisms were recovered in twice as many instances for every one hundred cases in the first group as in the second, but there was no appreciable difference in the incidence of Type II pneumococci. Strains belonging to Group IV occurred in 83.5 per cent of the former and in 69.3 per cent of the latter subjects. The differences in the percentages representing the incidence of pneumococci of the first three types, as reported by the Boston and by the New York observers, may have been due to the broader inclusion by the Boston workers of persons in the near neighborhood of pneumonia patients.

The rarity of pneumococci of Types I, II, and III in persons far removed from centers in which pneumonia is endemic has been reported by Milam and Smillie (1931).[903] In the isolated tropical island, St. John, of the United States Virgin Islands, the pneumococci found in the nasopharyngeal flora of normal persons were avirulent, and representatives of the first three types were seldom present. Even city dwellers in a colder climate may enjoy comparative freedom from the more common disease-producing types of pneumococci. In an extended investigation, embracing monthly examinations over a period from two months to three and one-half years, of 105 children and adults living in New York City, Webster and Hughes (1931)[1495] obtained pneumococci at one time or another from the nasal passages or the throat of 80 per cent of the persons studied. Of the 500 strains isolated, 97 per cent proved to be serologically specific. The organisms formed smooth colonies and were for the most part avirulent for mice. Pneumococci of Types I and II were obtained from one and two individuals respectively on one occasion only. Type III organisms were encountered in nine subjects, Type VIII in nine, Types XVI and XVIII in three persons for varying periods in each case; and avirulent, atypical strains were isolated from thirteen persons on single and scattered occasions. The presence of the last-named organisms was considered by the authors as having no association with any type-transformation *in vivo*.

The strains isolated in successive cultures from a given carrier were, with rare exceptions, of the same serological type and similar in colony morphology, virulence for mice, and other biological characters. The persons observed differed consistently with respect to the occurrence of pneumococci. Some were Pneumococcus-free, some were transient carriers, some periodic, and some chronic carriers, and evidence was presented in the communication that these differences were due to variations in host-resistance. The incidence of pneumococci in all the individuals included in the study underwent seasonal fluctuations corresponding to changes in the prevalence of coryza and sore throats in the same persons, an observation reported by Longcope and Fox[825] in 1905.

Further data on the variety of pneumococci to be found in the nose and throat flora of individuals selected only for the nonexistence of pneumonic disease among them, are furnished by the report of Hoyle (1932)[662] who, like Webster and Hughes, carried out bacteriological observations on normal persons over periods of one, one and a half, and two years. Of the forty subjects, on one occasion—and the only one—Type I Pneumococcus appeared during an acute attack of coryza, the patient developing lobar pneumonia three or four days later. Type II organisms were never detected. Type III pneumococci were isolated on four occasions, once late in a cold, in one case persisting for fourteen days in the mouth flora of a carrier of Type IV, once in an individual free from other pathogenic bacteria, and once during an attack of mild bronchitis subsequent to a cold. The other pneumococci encountered belonged to the heterogeneous group.

Another recent report is that of Brown and Anderson,[152] who found no strains of the first three types, but only those of the remaining types—all of low virulence for mice—from a small series of normal subjects. Christie (1932),[232] in making cultures from the throats of nurses in a Glasgow hospital, isolated pneumococci from eleven of twelve nurses in the pneumonia ward but none from nurses in the control wards. Of the organisms found in the nurses exposed to pneumonia, Christie demonstrated Type I pneumococci four times and Type II seven times. Whether the organisms found corresponded to the types prevalent among the pneumonia patients was not stated in the communication.

The classification of carriers of Pneumococcus based on repeated bacteriological examinations extending over a year or more as drawn up by Webster and Hughes was slightly modified by Bliss, McClaskey, and Long (1934).[131] After a year's study of young adults, the authors divided the subjects into non-carriers and chronic carriers, the latter group including those persons who intermittently exhibited pneumococci in the throat. While the so-called intermittent carriers might or might not yield positive cultures on repeated examination, the cultures when positive were consistently of the same type of Pneumococcus in any given case, indicating to the authors a chronic condition with constant bacteriological findings only as to type. Furthermore, the authors considered that their demonstration added evidence in favor of the stability of pneumococcal types in the human body. From the foregoing discussion it would seem to be more logical to designate healthy individuals who harbor pneumococci in the nose and throat for short periods of time as temporary carriers and those in whom the organisms persist for longer periods as chronic carriers. A subdivision of the latter into continuous and intermittent carriers would define more accurately the condition and the possible menace of the chronic class.

Summary

A summary of the main facts brought out in the foregoing discussion may be presented thus:

1. The great majority of cases of lobar pneumonia (*circa* 96 per cent) are caused by Pneumococcus.

2. Pneumococci of Types I and II are accountable for approximately one-half of the cases of lobar pneumonia in all countries from which records are available, except Africa.

3. The various serological types found in lobar pneumonia, as far as at present known, are, in order of frequency, I, III, II, VIII, VII, V, IV, XIV, XVIII. In children, pneumococci of the first three types are responsible for the disease in only 36 per cent of the cases, with Types XIV, I, VI, V, VII, IV, IX, XV, and XIX occurring most frequently in the order given.

4. The fatality-rates of pneumococcal lobar pneumonia have been reported as 40 to 60 per cent for Type III cases, 41 for Type II, 25 for Type I, with Types XVIII, VII, and VIII next in order of lethal power.

5. In bronchopneumonia, the types responsible for infection in order of incidence are III, VIII, XVIII, X, V, VII, XX, II, XI, and XIV. The data are tentative pending further information.

6. Lobar pneumonia, although usually endemic, may, as is the case of other bacterial infections of the respiratory tract, appear in localized outbreaks, which are not the peculiar manifestation of any particular type of Pneumococcus.

7. As accompaniments or sequels of lobar pneumonia, infections by the pneumococcus causing the primary lesion may arise in various locations in the body, or

8. Primary lesions incited by Pneumococcus may develop in the eye, nasal, buccal, and aural cavities and adnexa, the meninges, and other tissues.

9. Healthy persons may harbor pneumococci of one or more types in the mouth and throat with no harm to themselves.

10. The carrier state may be due a) to pneumococci implanted by transference from other persons or b) to organisms arising from pneumococcal disease within the individual.

11. The organisms implanted by transference are largely of the heterogeneous types formerly classified as Group IV, except in the event that the donor is suffering or recovering from an attack of pneumonia due to the predominant types. The pneumococci that are autogenous in origin are of the type causing the pneumonia.

12. The carrier state may be brief (transient), prolonged (chronic), or sporadic (chronically intermittent).

CHAPTER VIII

CHEMICAL CONSTITUENTS OF PNEUMOCOCCUS

The preparation and properties of the protein and carbohydrate fractions of the pneumococcal cell, discussed in relation to their chemical constitution and immunological activities.

THE chemical complexity of pneumococci and the immunological significance of their constituents were never appreciated, or even suspected, until Heidelberger and Avery[606] announced the results of their study of the composition of these remarkable cells. Like many other bacteria, Pneumococcus had been neglected by chemists. Such information as we had was either based on assumption or had come from chance or collateral observations by bacteriologists. Protein, of course, was present, protein combined with phosphorus being a part of all living cells. Then fats or lipids revealed their presence by the fatty acids they yielded on autolysis of the cell. Inorganic salts were elements necessary for its vital functions, although there was no detailed knowledge of their kind or quantity. The capsule, so distinctive of the species, had been believed to consist of mucin or some allied substance. It was, therefore, the systematic study of Heidelberger and Avery (1923) which disclosed the presence of the peculiar carbohydrates that give to strains of each type their special serological characters, that spell virulence or, by their absence, lack of virulence, and that determine the exact or specific immunological response the cocci call forth. These studies, moreover, rendered a greater service in revealing a new biological principle, that is, the action of sugars as antigens per se or in orienting the antigenic stimulus of their conjugated protein, and in their exquisite action as haptens in the presence of homologous immune bodies.

Carbohydrates had always been disregarded as possessing any

immunizing properties—it was thought to be the proteins of the cells which performed this function—but now it seems that, in the case of Pneumococcus at least, the protein is merely the vehicle carrying the sugar that decides the immunological character of the saccharide-protein complex of the cell.

WORK OF EARLIER INVESTIGATORS

Before discussing the newer discoveries it may be permissible to recount briefly the observations of earlier investigators in order that their bearing on these questions may be borne in mind. The literature before 1923 is notable for its lack of reports of detailed or systematic investigations on the chemistry of Pneumococcus. Here and there one finds communications dealing with a few of the components of the cocci, some fragmentary, some pointing mostly by inference to the existence of proteins, fats, or carbohydrates. The first account was that of Friedländer[487] in 1883. His interest in the peculiar capsular material caused him to carry out a few simple tests to determine its nature. It was soluble in alkali, but insoluble in acetic or mineral acids, in alcohol, ether, or chloroform, and these properties led Friedländer to believe that the capsule was composed of mucin or some related substance.

While it was a foregone conclusion that the cell contained protein, no direct evidence had been offered proving its existence. The affinity of the cellular material for aniline dyes was presumptive evidence, as was the increase in amino nitrogen during autolysis. The work of Rosenow[1169] and of Avery and Cullen[38, 41] proved that intracellular protein must be the source of the smaller nitrogenous molecules arising in the natural self-digestion of the cell. So it was with the fats; only by their cleavage products were they recognized.

Prior to 1917, none of the constituents of Pneumococcus had been isolated or subjected to chemical study. It was in that year that Dochez and Avery[321] discovered in cell-free filtrates of broth cultures of Pneumococcus of Types I, II, and III, in human blood serum, in urine during the course of lobar pneumonia* and, at times, in the blood of experimentally infected animals, a soluble substance that gave a specific precipitate with antipneumococcic serum of the homologous type. According to the authors, the substance was present in cultures when the organisms were growing at maximal rate and undergoing little or no cell death. Consequently its presence was not dependent upon cell disintegration, but represented the extrusion of bacterial substance by the living organism. The substance was readily soluble in water, was not destroyed by boiling, was not digested by trypsin or urease, did not dialyze through parchment, and was precipitable by acetone, alcohol, ether, and colloidal iron. The substance was, of course, the now well-known soluble specific substance which has so broadened our conception of pneumococcal immunity.

From a careful reading of Perlzweig's two papers (1921)[1078-9] there seems to be no doubt that he was dealing with the same substance but in impure state. From solutions of Pneumococcus in bile-salts, by Rowland's anhydrous sodium sulfate method, and by alcohol, Perlzweig precipitated an antigenic substance which he considered was a nucleoprotein. However, on autolyzing the whole organism or digesting it with proteolytic enzymes, the antigen was found to be unimpaired. It was not injured by boiling for five minutes in neutral or slightly acid solution, but was destroyed by boiling in alkaline solution. The substance could be recovered from autolysates or digestion mixtures by extraction with alcohol in a concentration of 70 to 85 per cent, but it was not soluble in 95 to 99 per cent alcohol. Perlzweig,[1079] and Perlzweig and Steffen,[1081] described the antigen as being soluble in neutral, acid, and alkaline aqueous solutions but not in lipid solvents and, when tested antigenically on white mice, it apparently possessed the complete immunizing properties of the original pneumococcus. Because of

* The finding recalls the observation of Preisz[1108] (see Chapter II) who demonstrated the presence of this substance in the blood of pneumonia patients, but who thought it was mucin.

its physical characters and the dependence of its heat stability on the hydrogen ion concentration of the substrate, the authors suggested that this antigen might be closely related to the antineuritic water-soluble B vitamin.

In another communication (1925), Perlzweig and Keefer[1080] reported a method for purifying the antigen but gave no details of its immunological properties. From massive cultures in Huntoon's medium, after heat-killing and filtration, the antigenic substance was separated from non-antigenic material by ultrafiltration through collodion. Further purification was effected by precipitation at the isoelectric point (pH 4.1) with 0.1N acetic acid-sodium acetate buffer mixture. The precipitate was dissolved in water with the addition of a small amount of 0.1N sodium hydroxide. The preparation contained 20 milligrams of nitrogen per 100 cubic centimeters (based on the volume of the original solution), which might indicate that it was made up, in part at least, of the nitrogen-containing specific carbohydrate of Type I Pneumococcus, the organism used as source material. Since Perlzweig and Keefer gave no other details, it is impossible to judge the purity of their antigen, but Perlzweig and Steffen,[1081] in a 1923 report, considered that it existed in a loose chemical or physical union with protein. It is to be presumed, therefore, that the authors had not isolated the polysaccharide in pure form, but rather the carbohydrate-protein compound from which some of the protein had been removed.

At about the same time, Zinsser and Parker,[1583] continuing the study made by Zinsser[1575] on tuberculin, described an antigen obtained from Pneumococcus and other bacteria which was analogous to, if not identical with, the substance isolated by Dochez and Avery.[321] These "residues" or "residue antigens" were prepared in the following manner: Pneumococci were grown on agar, removed from the medium and dried, then shaken with salt solution at a pH of 9.0 to 9.4, and immediately used or neutralized and stored. The extracts were centrifuged, passed through a Berkefeld filter, and precipitated with acetic acid in the cold. After separation of the precipitate (phosphoprotein or nucleoprotein), acid was added until no more precipitate came out of solution when the precipitate was discarded. After filtration, the solution was acidified and boiled for three to five minutes, then again filtered and neutralized. The filtrate was the residue solution. It became turbid on the addition of ten volumes of alcohol, and the precipitate contained the antigenic substance, although the authors suggested that it might have been mechanically thrown down.

The residue gave a specific precipitate with homologous antiserum but no complement fixation with equine antipneumococcic serum, nor did it stimulate any immune-body production in animals injected with it. The substance, however, excited a positive reaction when injected intradermally into normal guinea pigs and, to a lesser degree, in tuberculous pigs. Its resistance to autoclaving and to boiling in alkaline solutions would seem to establish a close relationship to the soluble specific substance described by Dochez and Avery.

Two years later, Zinsser with Tamiya[1584] extended the study of pneumococcal residue and pneumococcal protein. Some rabbits were immunized with agar-grown pneumococci washed with 2 per cent formalin in saline solution, and other rabbits with Berkefeld filtrates of pneumococci dissolved in minimal amounts of bile. The serum from these animals was then tested for precipitins against the two antigens. In the discussion of the experimental results Zinsser and Tamiya expressed the opinion that the antigens consisted of two substances: the one obtained by treating pneumococci with weak alkali, the other by fractioning the extract by acid precipitation. The one was a nucleoprotein independently antigenic, inducing antibodies which reacted only with itself and not with the residue; the other was the residue material incapable of inducing any kind of antibody response but capable of reacting with antibodies formed by the injection of the whole bacteria. The two substances, therefore, although in a crude state, corresponded in their immunological reactions to the protein and carbohydrate fractions of Avery and Heidelberger.

FIRST DESCRIPTION OF THE PNEUMOCOCCAL CARBOHYDRATE

It was, however, Heidelberger and Avery who first gave definite and detailed descriptions of the carbohydrate fraction, or soluble specific substance of pneumococci. No microorganism, except perhaps the tubercle bacillus, has since that time been subjected to such thorough chemical investigation as Pneumococcus. The studies of Heidelberger and Avery and their colleagues and those coming from other laboratories have supplied a rationale for the varied immunological and pathological behavior of pneumococci and established a chemical basis for understanding many of the diverse phenomena of immunity.

In their first communication, Heidelberger and Avery (1923)[606] described the isolation of the soluble specific substance of Type II Pneumococcus, which they concluded consisted mainly of a carbohydrate, which appeared to be a polysaccharide built up of glucose molecules and which, in a dilution as high as 1 to 3,000,000, gave a specific precipitin reaction with homologous immune serum. The method of its preparation was simple. It consisted in the concentration of an eight-day autolyzed broth culture of Type II Pneumococcus, precipitation with alcohol, repeated resolution and precipitation, then a careful series of fractional precipitations with alcohol or acetone after acidification with acetic acid and, finally, repeated fractional precipitation with ammonium sulfate and dialysis of aqueous solutions of the active fractions. The product gave no biuret reaction and no precipitate with phosphotungstic acid. It contained a trace of phosphorus but no sulfur and, because 1.2 per cent of nitrogen was found to be present, the authors forebore to make any claim for the purity of the preparation.

During the next few years there came from the laboratories of the Hospital of the Rockefeller Institute a series of papers under the authorship of Avery and Heidelberger and their associates,

Goebel, Morgan, and Neill, which contained descriptions of refinements in the methods of preparing these polysaccharides and of their physical, chemical, and immunological properties. Because of their importance the data are presented here in considerable detail; and in order that the reader may be offered a full, connected, and authentic account of the results of these basic studies, the liberty is taken of quoting from and paraphrasing Heidelberger's[604-5] comprehensive discussions in 1927 of the chemical nature of the antigenic substances of Pneumococcus.

The type II Pneumococcus was first studied and the fractionation and purification of the specific substance were followed at each step by means of the precipitin test. . . . As the purification proceeded the material isolated took on more and more the properties of a polysaccharide, so that it became evident that a sugar derivative was at least the carrier of whatever might be the true specific substance itself. Attempts were made to separate this hypothetical substance from the polysaccharide by precipitation with basic lead acetate, uranyl nitrate, or safranine, by adsorption with alumina and recovery from this, and even by specific precipitation with a large quantity of Type II antibody solution (prepared by Felton's method), and recovery of the specific substance from the immune precipitate, but these failed to effect a significant change in properties, even when pneumococci themselves were used as starting material instead of the broth culture. Attempts at a separation by means of certain carbohydrate-splitting enzymes also failed since the sugar derivative proved resistant to this type of hydrolysis. Moreover, when exposed to the action of 1:1 hydrochloric acid in the cold, the substance diminished in specific activity only after reducing sugars began to appear, so that the specific substance and the polysaccharide, if not identical, appeared at least to be very closely associated. On hydrolysis the specific product yielded about 70 per cent of reducing sugars consisting mainly of glucose, as shown by the isolation of glucosazone and the formation of saccharic acid on oxidation. Other possible constituents remained unidentified.

Marked differences were found between the soluble specific substance of Type III Pneumococcus and the corresponding derivative of Type II. The former proved to be the soluble salt of an insoluble acid, far stronger than the Type II substance, and capable of being thrown out of solution by an excess of strong hydrochloric acid. This property was of great use, not only in separating the specific substance from accompanying glycogen or erythrodextrin, but also in effecting rapid purification without the use of ammonium sulfate and with fewer fractionations by alcohol. Successive lots agreed closely in their physical and chemical properties, indicating a much more definite entity than the Type II product. The Type III soluble specific substance was thus isolated as a nitrogen-free polysaccharide. No further purification could be realized either by precipitation with barium hydroxide in excess, or by adsorption on highly active alumina. The yield of this soluble specific substance was greatly increased by adding glucose to the broth.

In the case of Type I Pneumococcus, the amount of the soluble specific substance present in the culture fluid was relatively smaller than in the case of the Type II and III organisms and therefore more alcohol was required for its precipitation from the culture concentrate. Other modifications were necessitated by the insolubility of the substance at its isoelectric point (about pH 4), and advantage could be taken of its ability to form a precipitate with barium hydroxide in excess. The specific substance was reprecipitated by alcohol in the presence of hydrochloric acid and dialyzed. Being a weak base, it precipitated as the excess of hydrochloric acid was removed. The Type I soluble specific substance also appeared to be a carbohydrate, but differed in the lower percentage of sugar liberated on hydrolysis and, what is more distinctive, in containing nitrogen as an apparently essential component.

Heidelberger, Goebel, and Avery[611] arranged a comparison of the distinguishing characters of the soluble specific substances of Types I, II, and III, and included that of the Type B Friedländer bacillus (to be mentioned later) in the table which is reproduced on the following page.

The aldobionic acid, $C_{11}H_{19}O_{10}COOH$, isolated from the hydrolytic products of the specific polysaccharide of Type III Pneumococcus was shown to be a compound of glucuronic acid and glucose, combined in glucosidic linkage through the aldehyde group of glucuronic acid and one of the hydroxyl groups of glucose. The polysaccharides from the three types of pneumococci contained no sulfur or phosphorus and differed from the starch-glycogen group in giving no color with iodine and in their resistance to the usual carbohydrate-splitting enzymes. These polysaccharides, therefore, would appear to represent a new type of carbohydrate.

SOLUBLE SPECIFIC SUBSTANCES OF THE THREE FIXED ANTIGENIC TYPES OF PNEUMOCOCCUS AND OF FRIEDLÄNDER BACILLUS (TYPE B)

Type	$[a]_D$	Acid equivalent	C	H	N	Reducing sugars on hydrolysis		Highest dilution giving precipitate with homologous immune serum
			Per cent	*Per cent*	*Per cent*	*Calculated as glucose*		
I	+300°		43.3*	5.8	5.0†	28	(Galacturonic acid) (Amino sugar derivative)	1:6,000,000
II	+74°	1250	45.8	6.4	0.0	70	Glucose	1:5,000,000
III	−33°	340	42.7	5.3	0.0	75	Aldobionic acid, glucose	1:6,000,000
Friedländer bacillus B	+100°	685	44.6	6.1	0.0	73	Glucose	1:2,000,000‡

* Theory for $(C_6H_{10}O_5)_n$, C, 44.4 per cent; H, 6.2 per cent.
† Amino N, 2.5 per cent.
‡ Rabbit antiserum.
NOTE: From a determination of its diffusion coefficient, Babers and Goebel[61] calculated a molecular weight of 118,000 for Pneumococcus III specific polysaccharide, but Heidelberger and Kendall[618] later found that this was an accidental value, related only to the salt concentration at which the diffusion was carried out.

Heidelberger and Avery doubted if any of the specific substances isolated at that time (1927) represented a definite chemical compound. The three types of Pneumococcus chosen for study had, however, when grown on the same medium, yielded three distinct carbohydrates, and successive preparations of each specific substance had been quite uniform whatever methods were employed in the process of purification and whether the preparation was derived from pneumococci themselves or from autolyzed broth cultures. Furthermore, the only one of these substances investigated in detail appeared to differ in structure from that of any other known non-nitrogenous polysaccharide. It was thought by Avery and Heidelberger that these and other considerations based on the data obtained warranted the belief that the three polysaccharides isolated represented the actual specific substances, stripped of at least a large portion of accompanying impurities, and that the substances did not merely represent inert material carrying an extremely minute amount of the true specific compounds.

The studies of Heidelberger, Goebel, and Avery also included an investigation of the protein portion of the pneumococcal cell. Heidelberger, in the reviews already cited,[604-5] discussed this phase of the work as follows:

When these microbes (Pneumococci) are dissolved, either with the aid of bile, or by repeated freezing and thawing, the resulting solution yields a precipitate of so-called "nucleoprotein" on acidification with acetic acid. While probably a mixture consisting largely of nucleoprotein and mucoid, it still possesses immunological properties which differ sharply from those of the soluble specific substance. In the first place, the protein is antigenic, while the soluble specific substance, though reacting specifically with antibodies to the highest degree, is non-antigenic and unable by itself to stimulate the production of antibodies when injected into animals. Moreover, the protein isolated from the three fixed types of Pneumococcus, or from a strain of the heterogeneous group IV, appears serologically the same as that from any of the other types. Thus this portion of the pneumococcus protein is not type-specific, like the soluble specific substance, but is, rather, species-specific.

Saito[1213] also prepared nucleoprotein from Type II pneumococci which precipitated with both Types I and II serums and with which active immunity could be evoked against Type II but not against Type I Pneumococcus. Saito admitted that the preparation still contained traces of the soluble specific substance.

An apparent relationship between pneumococcal antibodies and both the protein and non-protein fractions of Gonococcus has been reported by Boor and Miller (1931).[138] The protein substance—nucleoprotein according to the authors—in a dilution of 1 to 1,000 gave definite precipitation with Types I and II antipneumococcic serum and in as high as a 1 to 10,000 dilution with Type III serum. The non-protein fraction was even more potent, reacting positively, and always more strongly with Type III serum, in ten to one hundred times the maximal dilution of the protein fraction.

Boor and Miller observed cross reactions between the gonococcal antiserum and the C Fraction of Tillett and Francis and there is good reason to believe that the non-protein fraction obtained from Gonococcus and the C Fraction of Pneumococcus are similar if not identical. The results, because of their seeming biological importance, deserve further study. There is a factor, however, which should not be overlooked and that is the participation of agar in serological reactions, as demonstrated by Sordelli and Mayer[1306] in the case of other organisms grown on agar media.

Stull (1929)[1349] furnished figures for some of the chemical constituents of Type III Pneumococcus.* A virulent strain of the organism was grown in beef-infusion peptone glucose broth for sixteen to eighteen hours and centrifuged; then the sediment was washed in distilled water, and dried at 55°. Analyses of the material gave the following results expressed in percentage amounts: Volatile matter at 105°—4.77; ash—6.48 to 8.64; nitrogen—13.00 to 13.32; acid-insoluble nitrogen and acid-soluble nitrogen

* In this connection there should be mentioned the analyses of Leineweber, Kautsky, and Famulener,[799] which were taken to indicate the comparative uniformity of pneumococci of the four types in the amount of nitrogen, and therefore of protein contained.

—each 0.2; ammonia nitrogen—1.0; total nitrogen of bases—5.5; total nitrogen in filtrate from bases—8.6; phosphorus—2.92 to 2.94; chlorine—0.71; and sulfur—0.32. An absolute alcohol extract of the dried cocci contained 6.5 per cent nitrogen and one per cent phosphorus and was claimed to be entirely free from protein. Water extraction removed material of high phosphorus content, probably of the nature of nucleoprotein, as well as the soluble specific substance. Stull's ether, alcohol, acetone, 0.1N acetic acid, and 0.1N hydrochloric acid extracts all failed to give precipitates with Type I, II, and III antipneumococcic serums. Only the dried cocci, the water extract, and the soluble specific substance precipitated with Type III serum, and here the action was specific.

It was Avery and Heidelberger's conception that, since Pneumococcus is an encapsulated organism, "The ectoplasmic layer of the cell is composed of carbohydrate material which is identical in all its biological characters with the type-specific substance. On the other hand, the endoplasm, or somatic substance, consists largely of protein, which is species- and not type-specific. This protein is possessed in common by all pneumococci, while the carbohydrate is chemically distinct and serologically specific for each of the three fixed types. The cell, therefore, may be conceived of as so constituted that there is disposed at its periphery a highly reactive substance upon which type specificity depends." It was also the authors' idea that, since this specifically reactive substance was found to be non-antigenic when separated from the other cellular constituents and was capable of inciting antibody formation only in the form in which it is present in the intact cell, it might be concluded that in the latter instance it existed not merely as free carbohydrate but also in combination with some other substance which conferred upon it specific antigenic properties.

A tabular representation of some of the immunological functions of intact pneumococci and of their principal constituents is taken from the review[605] which has been drawn upon so freely in the present discussion.*

PNEUMOCOCCUS AND CELL CONSTITUENTS		ANTIBODIES DEMONSTRABLE IN SERUM						
Material used for immunization	Effective antigen	Agglutinins	Precipitins		Complement fixation		Specificity	
			S	P	S*	P	Type	Species
Intact cells (SP)†	(SP)	+	+	−	+	−	+	−
Carbohydrate S‡	None	−	−	−	−	−	−	−
Protein P§	P	−	−	+	−	+	−	+
Solutions, extracts containing free S and free P	P	−	−	+	−	+	−	+
Suspension of intact cells and dissociated cell constituents (SP), free S, free P	(SP), P	+	+	+	+	+	+	+

* = Free S, as antigen, does not fix complement with immune horse serum; is active with immune rabbit serum.
† (SP) = Carbohydrate and protein, combined antigen of cell.
‡ S = Free carbohydrate, the soluble specific substance of cell.
§ P = Free protein of cell.

Heidelberger continued:

It was evident that morphological dissolution of pneumococci is accompanied by antigenic dissociation, for sera prepared from filtered solutions of disintegrated cells free of formed elements fail to exhibit any of the dominant type-specific properties which characterize sera obtained by immunization with whole bacteria. The injection of suspensions of pneumococci into animals induces the formation of antibodies against S [carbohydrate] alone or against both S and P [protein] separately, depending upon whether or not these suspensions contain only intact cells or a mixture of both intact and dissolved cell bodies. Since pneumococci readily undergo autolysis and dissolution, suspensions and broth cultures of these organisms almost invariably contain not only formed elements, but also more or less of dissociated cell constituents in solution. Therefore, use of suspensions of pneumococci con-

* Many of the experimental data from which the table was compiled are to be found in the original papers by Avery and Heidelberger; Heidelberger and Goebel; Heidelberger, Goebel, and Avery; Heidelberger and Avery; Avery, Heidelberger, and Goebel; Avery and Morgan; and Avery and Neill.

taining both intact cells and the soluble products of cell disintegration yields on immunization not only type-specific antibodies but antibodies reacting with the protein substance which is common to all pneumococci. While the former generally predominate it is the presence of this protein antibody with its broader zone of activity which is responsible for the confusing cross-immunity reactions occasionally encountered in supposedly type-specific sera and which has in some instances led workers to deny the existence of three distinct antigenic types of pneumococci. That the two sets of antibodies involved are separate and distinct is shown by absorption tests; the antiprotein reaction bodies in such sera can be removed by absorption with the protein of a heterologous type without diminishing the titer of specific agglutinins for the homologous culture or the precipitins for the specific polysaccharide of the corresponding type. . . .

While it had been generally assumed that only the proteins and their derivatives provided the innumerable opportunities for isomerism and subtle changes requisite for the substances exhibiting the phenomena of specificity, the discovery of carbohydrates with specific properties is not so surprising as might appear on first thought. When one considers the number of asymmetric carbon atoms in the hexoses and pentoses, the different points of attachment of the lactone bridge, the possibility of α and β-glucosidic unions at various positions in the molecule, and the addition of sugar acids, the analogs of amino acids, to the large number of sugars theoretically capable of entering into the composition of such polysaccharides, it becomes clear that perhaps only among the carbohydrates could another sufficiently large and protean group of substances be found to afford the possibility of specific manifestations.

The evidence of the lack of immunizing properties on the part of these specific carbohydrates shown in the table on page 250 was largely supplied by the experiments of Avery and Morgan.[54] Their attempts to immunize rabbits by subcutaneous and intravenous injections of the protein-free polysaccharides of pneumococci in considerable amounts and in repeated doses invariably failed to stimulate the production of any demonstrable antibodies in the serum of rabbits so treated. The isolated protein, on the contrary, was antigenic, but the antibodies it induced reacted with the nucleoprotein fraction of both homologous and heterologous types. In addition, these antiprotein serums did not agglutinate type-specific strains of Pneumococcus or react with the type-specific carbohydrate derived from them. This fact points to the capsular polysaccharide of the cell as the bearer of the type-specific determinant.

As a complement to these observations, Avery and Neill[59] added that intact pneumococci, possessing specific antigenic powers unimpaired by cultural or other procedures, gave rise to agglutinins for the homologous type and to precipitins for the type-specific carbohydrate derived from them. When, however, the cell was disrupted, the soluble cell-free constituents in the absence of formed elements failed to stimulate the formation of type-specific antibodies, but did induce the formation of antibodies reactive with pneumococcal protein regardless of the type from which the latter was derived. The data pointed to the dissociation of the carbohydrate and protein fractions during the process of cell dissolution with the subsequent change in the type-specific action of the constituents, or, put in another way, to the loss of antigenic function of the polysaccharide portion of the cell when freed from its conjugated protein.

ISOLATION OF CARBOHYDRATE FRACTIONS

From the results reported by Schiemann and Caspar,[1228] it would appear that they had isolated two carbohydrate fractions from Type II Pneumococcus. One of the protein-free substances was soluble in alcohol, gave specific precipitation with homologous serum, and was antigenic in that it immunized mice. The second fraction also gave specific precipitation but was insoluble in alcohol. The preparations were made by boiling sodium taurocholate solutions of pneumococci with acetic acid. Both substances and the one obtained from a Type III strain were evidently free from protein, since the authors could detect no nitrogen in the preparations, and yet contrary to the results of Perlzweig and Steffen and of Avery and Morgan, the non-nitrogenous fractions possessed antigenic power since they produced immunity in mice. Schiemann and Caspar noted a difference in the microscopic appearance of the precipitates produced by the carbohydrates when added to immune horse and rabbit serum. The difference in the behavior of these two kinds of serum is manifested in other reactions with pneumococci and their constituents or products. The protein fractions as a rule failed to establish protection in mice, although one such preparation from Type II Pneumococcus did induce resistance of a low order to pneumococci of both Types I and II.

Jungeblut (1927)[698] had quite a different idea concerning the chemical nature of the antigenic components of the pneumococcal cell. Pneumococci of the first three types were extracted with 95 per cent alcohol and the filtrates of these extracts were tested for specific flocculation by a modified Dujarric de la Rivière method. Antipneumococcic serums of Types I, II, and III gave flocculation of varying intensity with homologous alcoholic antigens. The reactions were species-specific and also type-specific to a high degree. From an examination of the experimental facts, and after a consideration of the data presented prior to this study, one is not inclined to go all the way with Jungeblut in concluding that this serological reaction depended upon the presence of bacterial lipids in the antigens. Remembering the activity of minute amounts of specific carbohydrates in bringing down precipitins from immune serum, one feels that emphasis should be laid on Jungeblut's comment that the method of preparing these alcoholic antigens did not preclude the possibility that "certain impurities of protein or carbohydrate character may have been carried over into the extract."

Wadsworth and Brown[1467] reported the antigenic action of the ether-soluble fraction of Type I pneumococci. The preparation, admittedly impure, was active in binding complement in the presence of antipneumococcic serum of all types but failed to stimulate the formation of agglutinins, precipitins, protective or complement-fixing antibodies in rabbits.

In 1928, Saito and Ulrich,[1214] following the lead of Heidelberger and Avery, prepared what appeared to be a protein-free carbohydrate from Pneumococcus II and which produced specific protection in mice. After dissolving the sediment from a twenty-four-hour serum-broth culture in sodium taurocholate, the authors, by a method much the same as that of Schiemann and Caspar, removed the precipitate coming down on the addition of acetic acid, and then separated the specific precipitable substance by alcohol. A concentrated watery solution of the material was then treated with a large amount of normal sodium hydroxide and the resulting sediment discarded. Upon the addition of alcohol to the clear fluid a precipitate was obtained, which in a slightly acidified solution failed to give any positive protein tests, had a dextro-rotatory power of about +30° as compared with that of +74° for the Type II carbohydrate of Heidelberger, and which on boiling with hydrochloric acid yielded reducing substances.

The carbohydrate preparation of Saito and Ulrich was strictly type-specific, giving protection to mice against a Type II culture but no protection against a Type III culture. It seems fair to assume that their carbohydrate preparation was not so pure as the corresponding preparation of Heidelberger and Avery since its dextro-rotatory power was less (+30° against +74°) and also since it contained 0.61 per cent of nitrogen.

Schiemann[1226] employed the preparations made by Saito and Ulrich in an attempt to immunize rabbits, and attributed his failure to the administration of too great dosage. In no instance was it possible to produce agglutinins, precipitins, or protective antibodies. He succeeded, however, in immunizing mice and in demonstrating protective substances in their blood.

Schiemann, Loewenthal, and Hackenthal[1231] continued the study of pneumococcal carbohydrates and retested the conclusions of Perlzweig and Steffen.[1081] From acid and alcohol precipitates of dissolved Type I pneumococci extracts were made with methyl and ethyl alcohol. The authors reported that the carbohydrate fraction contained the larger proportion of the immunizing substance and that the alcoholic extracts showed varying specific immunizing properties, which they believed might be due to the presence of small amounts of the type-specific carbohydrate carried over by the alcohol. It was found, furthermore, that watery solutions of the carbohydrate still produced immunity in dilutions which no longer gave precipitation.

The protein-free substance of Schiemann and his associates, purified by repeated alcohol precipitation in alkaline solution, showed +264°10′ angle of refraction with polarized light (compare +300° for Heidelberger and Avery's Type I polysaccharide), and with hydrochloric or nitric acids at 80° yielded no reducing sugars. The authors noticed the characteristic differences in the appearance of the precipitates obtained with specific immune horse and rabbit serum—the former appearing sooner and being coarser, while the latter were fine and formed a transparent membrane. The purified preparation actively immunized mice in doses of 0.001 to 0.0001 milligrams but failed to do so when injected in amounts greater than 0.01, or less than 0.00001 milligrams, and therefore acted in a narrower zone than the less pure fractions prepared by the method of Schiemann and Caspar.[1228]

In contrast to the immunizing action of the carbohydrate fractions of Pneumococcus in mice, as reported by Perlzweig and Steffen, Schiemann and Caspar, Saito and Ulrich, and Schiemann, Loewenthal and Hackenthal, the polysaccharides from Type I, II, and III pneumococci were devoid of any power to sensitize guinea pigs to these specific carbohydrates. When single initial doses of ten, twenty, and fifty milligrams of the preparations were injected the animals failed to react when given a shocking dose of one to ten milligrams twenty-one days later. This same shocking dose, however, produced rapid and fatal anaphylactic shock when injected into guinea pigs passively sensitized with the precipitating serum of rabbits immunized with pneumococci of the homologous type. The experiment afforded evidence of a striking difference, therefore, between the antigenic and haptenic action of preparations of specific polysaccharides. Here again there was manifested that strange difference between immune rabbit and horse serum, the latter failing to sensitize the guinea pigs to the carbohydrate. Both serums precipitate the homologous carbohydrate, but the horse serum fails to bind complement in the presence of capsular polysaccharide as well as being incapable of rendering guinea pigs hypersensitive.

ISOLATION OF C FRACTION

The existence of another and quite different carbohydrate constituent of Pneumococcus was demonstrated by Tillett and Francis.[1409] The authors used as source material a degraded, non-type-specific R strain of Pneumococcus. This particular culture was chosen in order to minimize the presence of type-specific carbohydrate. The organisms centrifuged from a full-grown broth culture were suspended in normal salt solution, the cells were frozen and thawed until dissolution was effected, and then, after the addition of acetic acid, the solution was boiled for eight to ten minutes. After removal of the heavy coagulum, acidulation and boiling were repeated in order to remove all acid- and heat-precipitable material. The final water-clear supernatant fluid contained this new substance which Tillett and Francis called "Fraction C."*

The C Fraction, although it is probably a nitrogenous sugar, is chemically distinct from both the type-specific capsular carbohydrate and the somatic nucleoprotein. It exhibits no type-specificity, but yields a precipitate with serum of individuals ill with lobar pneumonia. Following crisis the reaction is no longer demonstrable. Furthermore, the precipitation of the pneumococcal Fraction C is not limited to the serum of individuals infected with Pneumococcus, since definite reactions can be obtained in streptococcal and staphylococcal infections and in acute rheumatic fever.

In another communication appearing in the same year, Tillett

* Tillett and Francis remarked on the similarity of this substance to Lancefield's "Fraction C" which she had obtained from hemolytic streptococci.

with Goebel and Avery[1410] continued the study of the newly isolated fraction. The fraction was further purified by making the solution (the water-clear supernatant fluid described above) alkaline with sodium hydroxide and by precipitation with alcohol. The material was dissolved in water and again reprecipitated from faintly acid solution by alcohol. The procedure was repeated several times. The final precipitate was washed with alcohol and ether and freed from chlorides and was soluble in water but insoluble in organic solvents. The substance in solution showed a specific rotation of +25.0°, contained 5.07 per cent of nitrogen, and yielded 30.0 per cent of reducing sugars on hydrolysis. Unlike the type-specific polysaccharide of Type I Pneumococcus it contained no amino nitrogen, but like other pneumococcal carbohydrates was protein-free. Tillett, Goebel, and Avery also made similar preparations from S strains of Type II and Type III pneumococci.

The C Fraction was non-toxic for mice in amounts up to one milligram, it produced no purpura, and an intravenous injection of three cubic centimeters of a concentrated solution elicited no symptoms in rabbits. Three series of seven daily injections of one cubic centimeter of the concentrate, with weekly rests, failed to produce in rabbits any precipitins for the C substance. When mixed with antipneumococcic horse serum of Types I, II, and III the somatic carbohydrate precipitated each of the three, thus exhibiting a broad species coverage but no type-specificity. Tillett, Goebel, and Avery concluded from chemical studies and animal experiments that Fraction C was a common constituent of all pneumococci, and that it was distinct from the specific polysaccharide and the so-called nucleoprotein.

The isolation of the C Fraction was also accomplished by Heidelberger and Kendall (1931)[617] during an investigation of the polysaccharides of Type (not Group) IV Pneumococcus. They also obtained the C substance from Type I and Type III pneumococci. The preparations showed a higher optical rotation, higher nitrogen, and in two cases a higher reducing-sugar content on hydrolysis than reported by Tillett, Goebel, and Avery who, it should be remembered, prepared their material from rough pneumococci. An analysis of the C Fraction showed that it contained 4 per cent of phosphorus, which appeared to be firmly bound in organic combination, thus making the C Fraction the first phosphorus-containing specific polysaccharide to be encountered.

RELATION OF THE PNEUMOCOCCAL CARBOHYDRATE TO CARBOHYDRATES ISOLATED FROM OTHER ORGANISMS

In addition to the C Fraction, Heidelberger and Kendall isolated from autolyzed cultures of Type IV Pneumococcus a type-specific carbohydrate differing markedly from those of Type I, II, and III pneumococci, and representing a kind of substance hitherto not observed among specific polysaccharides. The authors also obtained a chemically similar carbohydrate without specific function. These substances were far more difficult to separate from accompanying protein degradation products than the specific polysaccharides of Type I, II, and III pneumococci. Because of the difficulty of separation, the preparations probably contained more or less of the accompanying specific carbohydrates, but were in sufficiently pure state to reveal separate identities.

The serologically inactive fraction had the lowest optical rotation and the highest carbon content of the three, was the weakest acid, the least soluble in alcohol or acetic acid, and differed from the specific Type IV carbohydrate and the C Fraction in yielding on hydrolysis crystals with the optical rotation of glucosamine. The Type IV specific substance, on the other hand, differed from the others in being the poorest in nitrogen and the richest in reducing sugars on hydrolysis, and in occupying an intermediate position as regards optical rotation, carbon content, and acidity. The species-specific C polysaccharide was highest in optical rotation and in total and amino nitrogen, and the poorest in reducing sugars yielded on hydrolysis, in carbon content, and in its proportion of acetylated nitrogen. It differed from the fully acetylated Type IV substance in being broken down by nitrous acid, and differed from all other known specific polysaccharides of Pneumococcus in containing phosphorus.

From this comparative study of the various specific carbohydrates of Pneumococcus it would seem that these substances fall into two sharply defined groups: on the one hand, the Type II and Type III type-specific polysaccharides, which are nitrogen-free, and on the other, the Type I, Type IV, and C Fractions which contain nitrogen. The two last-named examples in this group, with their content of acetylated nitrogen, are more closely related to chitin than is the Type I substance. In the nitrogenous group, the Type I substance differs sharply from the others in its high optical rotation, its pronounced amphoteric character, its insolubility at the isoelectric point, its freedom from acetyl groups, and in its high proportion of nitrogen susceptible to attack by nitrous acid. The C Fraction differs from the other members of both groups in its phosphorus content, but resembles the Type I substance in that its specificity is destroyed by nitrous acid; it is somewhat similar to the Type IV substance in that a part of the nitrogen is acetylated. The Type IV soluble specific substance, on the other hand, differs from the Type I polysaccharide and the C Fraction in containing only acetylated nitrogen and in yielding as high a percentage of reducing sugars on hydrolysis as do the nitrogen-free Type II and Type III capsular polysaccharides.

The study of the Type IV specific polysaccharide has brought to light a carbohydrate of a new type among those with specific properties. It has, moreover, again been shown that in the closely related pneumococcal types thus far studied, each polysaccharide responsible for type-specificity is different from the others in structure, composition, and properties. The study has also demonstrated the presence in Pneumococcus of a serologically inactive polysaccharide closely related to chitin. This observation points toward the cause of the still existing uncertainty as to whether chitin is a constituent of the bacterial cell wall.*

In addition to these specific pneumococcal polysaccharides, Heidelberger, Goebel, and Avery[611-2] isolated from the B strain of the Friedländer bacillus a carbohydrate closely resembling that of Type II Pneumococcus, the similarity extending even to precipitation with Type II antipneumococcic serum. But, although there was great constancy in the properties of these two substances, the absorption of agglutinins and precipitins was not reciprocal with the two organisms. It was believed that the cross-relationship was due to the occurrence in the specific polysaccharides of both microorganisms of the same or similar chemical grouping. Other strains of the bacillus showed no such reciprocal relations, nor was there any such relation between the E strains of the Friedländer group and Type I and III pneumococci.†

Heidelberger, in the review already quoted, argued that if the fact that bacteria possess mutual absorption capacity be accepted as the criterion of their antigenic identity, then the failure of the Friedländer bacilli to exhibit this property might be taken as further evidence of the lack of identity of the substances involved. The discussion continued:

However, granted a chemical difference between the two specific substances, it becomes necessary to account for their marked immunological similarity. In the absence of further evidence as to the structural relations of the two polysaccharides it seems reasonable to assume that both contain in a portion of the complex molecule the same or a closely similar configuration of atoms. The essential similarity in molecular grouping would then determine the immunological similarity of the two substances. In the case of Pneumococcus it has been shown that the polysaccharides by themselves are not antigenic, and it is believed that

* The foregoing paragraphs are based on the discussion in the paper by Heidelberger and Kendall.[617]

† In this connection it may be mentioned that in the next year Julianelle[684] classified, by their serological reactions, strains of *Encapsulatus pneumoniae* (Friedländer's bacillus) into three types, A, B, C, and one group X.

It may interest the reader to know that in 1935 Yen and Kurotchkin[1559] by means of electrolysis were able to isolate the specific carbohydrate of the Friedländer bacillus, apparently free from protein and in a highly antigenic state.

they become antigenic only when attached to some other substance, possibly the protein of the cell. The type specific character of the antigenic response, however, is dependent almost entirely upon the nature of the polysaccharide and not upon the substance to which it is attached. Therefore, since the specific carbohydrate of the Friedländer bacillus (type B) and that of Type II Pneumococcus exhibit similar chemical properties the antigenic response to each may also be similar even though the proteins or other substances with which they are combined are quite dissimilar.

In 1929, Heidelberger, Avery, and Goebel[608] described the isolation of a soluble specific substance from gum arabic (gum acacia). From this gum, which would appear to have no biological relationship to Pneumococcus, by partial hydrolysis a carbohydrate was obtained that was comparable to the specific pneumococcal polysaccharide in its precipitating activity with both Type II and Type III serum. The fraction on hydrolysis yielded galactose and two more complex sugar acids, one of which was later shown by Heidelberger and Kendall[617] to be aldobionic acid and glucuronogalactose analogous to the compounds isolated from the specific polysaccharide of Type III Pneumococcus.

Another manifestation of heterogenetic specificity was that of the encapsulated strains of *Escherichia coli*, studied by Barnes and Wight.[87] The organism, isolated from a mouse during a type-determination test on pneumonic sputum, was agglutinated by Type I antipneumococcic horse serum, but not by a similar serum produced in a rabbit. The serum from rabbits immunized with this colon bacillus agglutinated the homologous organism and precipitated the soluble specific substance, but failed to cause agglutination of Type I pneumococci or to precipitate Type I pneumococcal polysaccharide. In this case the connection was somewhat analogous to that between Type II Pneumococcus and the later Type B Friedländer bacillus of Julianelle.

Zozaya[1588] published an account of the cross and quite heterologous serological reaction with antipneumococcic serum of dextran, the synthetic polysaccharide produced from saccharose by *Leuco-*

nostoc mesenteroides. With serum produced in rabbits in response to injections of typical and rough strains of Types I and II Pneumococcus, dextran in a dilution of 1 to 5,000 gave precipitates with both anti-S and anti-R serums in low dilutions (1 to 2 to 1 to 16), showing a somewhat stronger action with the latter. When the serums were first absorbed with the type-specific polysaccharide or the C Fraction of Tillett and Francis, and then mixed with dextran, the serum precipitated to the same degree as before absorption. The outcome of the experiment would argue for the existence of a distinct antibody produced by the active group of the specific polysaccharide, which is similar to the active group of the dextran polysaccharide.

Since the discovery of the soluble specific substance in Pneumococcus by Dochez and Avery in 1917, similar complex carbohydrates have been demonstrated as components of several bacterial species. Toenniessen[1413] was the first to isolate the nitrogen-free polysaccharide from Friedländer's bacillus, which was later studied by Kramár,[753] but failed to connect it with the immunological behavior of the organism. A related substance was recovered from a strain of the same organism by Mueller, Smith, and Litarczek,[937] from yeast by Mueller and Tomcsik,[938] and from an encapsulated colon bacillus and *Bacillus aerogenes* strains by Tomcsik.[1414] A specifically precipitating, non-nitrogenous carbohydrate has been isolated from tubercle bacilli by Laidlaw and Dudley,[771] and a similar polysaccharide as well as a specifically reacting substance was derived by Mueller[936] from the same bacilli by fractionation with alcohol.

In a preliminary report of a recent study, Kulp and Borden[764] described the successful immunization of mice against Type I Pneumococcus by vaccination with a living culture of *Alkaligenes viscosus.* The authors suggested that there might be an antigenic relationship between the capsular material of these two organisms, but they had obtained no confirmation of this possibility. There is no doubt that other bacterial species contain analogous polysaccharides which may be found to possess similar chemical and immunological relationships to those of Pneumococcus but their existence in no way detracts from the soundness of our present serological classification of pneumococci. Tempting as it is, further discussion of the immunological significance of the carbohydrates from sources other than Pneumococcus would not be pertinent to the present subject.

FUNCTION OF SUGARS IN DETERMINING ANTIGENIC SPECIFICITY AND CONJUGATED PROTEINS

The newly discovered and highly important function of sugars in determining the antigenic specificity of conjugated proteins was studied by Goebel, Avery, and Tillett. The two first-named authors,[521] aiming to gain more exact information concerning this specific action of carbohydrates, set about building two isomeric carbohydrate-protein compounds. They first synthesized *p*-aminophenol β-glucoside and *p*-aminophenol β-galactoside and then coupled these hexosides with the globulin from horse serum. The two protein-sugar complexes thus obtained differed only in the carbohydrate radical of each and in the spatial configuration of the H and OH groups by a single carbon atom. In a second paper Avery and Goebel,[44] after coupling the diazophenol glucosides to crystalline egg albumin in addition to serum globulin, studied the immunological behavior of the preparations. When two chemically different carbohydrate derivatives were bound to the same protein, the newly formed antigens exhibited distinct immunological specificity. When the same carbohydrate radical was conjugated with two chemically different and serologically distinct proteins, both of the sugar-proteins thus formed acquired a common serological specificity. Therefore, simple differences in the molecular configuration of the two isomers—glucose and galactose—sufficed to orient specificity when the corresponding glucosides were coupled to the same protein. The unconjugated glucosides, although themselves not precipitable in immune serum, specifically inhibited the reaction between the sugar-protein and its homologous antibody. Furthermore, the sugar derivatives unattached to protein exhibited some of the properties of carbohydrate haptens; they were non-antigenic in that they incited no antibody production, but were specifically reactive, as shown by inhibition tests, with antibodies induced by proteins containing the homologous diazotized glucoside.

Tillett with Avery and Goebel[1407] tested these artificial, conjugated carbohydrate-proteins for other evidence of antigenic action by means of experiments in active and passive anaphylaxis. The experiments demonstrated the capacity of the synthesized sugar-proteins to produce hypersensitiveness. The fact that guinea pigs, passively sensitized with antigluco-globulin serum, or actively sensitized with gluco-globulin, could be subsequently shocked with gluco-albumin, and since the same specific relations held in the production of anaphylaxis with galacto-proteins, it was evident that the antigen-antibody specificity in these instances was directly dependent upon the carbohydrate fraction of the antigenic compounds.

In addition to the new specificity which the carbohydrate radical conferred upon the conjugated proteins, the uncombined glucosides by themselves also exerted a definite influence on the reactivity of sensitized animals. The injection of the glucosides into guinea pigs sensitized with the homologous gluco-protein immediately before the introduction of the toxigenic sugar-protein, completely but only temporarily protected the animals from shock. Tillett, Avery, and Goebel found, also, that anaphylactic shock could be induced by uncombined globulin in guinea pigs passively sensitized with either antigluco-globulin serum or antigalacto-globulin serum, thus demonstrating that the reactions elicited by globulin alone were dependent upon the common protein present in the antigens, and were manifestations only of species-specificity.

Continuing the investigations, Goebel and Avery[522] prepared the *p*-amino and *p*-nitromonobenzyl ethers of the polysaccharide of

Type III Pneumococcus, which they succeeded in coupling with serum globulin. Avery and Goebel[45] then reported the important and fundamental observation that this artificial, specific carbohydrate-protein complex was able to immunize rabbits against infection with virulent Type III pneumococci, and that the serum of rabbits thus immunized contained type-specific antibodies which precipitated the Type III capsular polysaccharide, agglutinated Type III pneumococci, and specifically protected mice against Type III infection. From the results it would seem that the antipneumococcic response produced by an antigen known to contain but a single component of the pneumococcal cell indicates the unity of the antibodies participating in the type-specific reactions of precipitation, agglutination, and protection, and relates the specificity of these antibodies to that of the capsular polysaccharide as the reactive part of the antigenic molecule.

ISOLATION OF "A SUBSTANCE"

What appeared to be a new element among the specific polysaccharides was introduced by Enders[358] in 1930. In autolytic products of Type I Pneumococcus a substance was found, thought to be other than the soluble specific substance, which reacted specifically with immune serum as determined by the precipitin reaction or, *in vivo,* by the anaphylactic behavior of appropriately sensitized guinea pigs. Enders prepared autolysates by incubating for seventy-two hours the phenolized, centrifuged sediment from twenty-four-hour dextrose broth cultures of Type I pneumococci. He obtained the nucleoprotein by precipitating with dilute acetic acid the solution derived by dissolving pneumococci with bile according to the method of Avery and Heidelberger, while the specific carbohydrate was prepared from pneumococci grown in dextrose hormone broth according to the methods described by Heidelberger and his associates.

Enders prepared a "normal" antipneumococcic serum by injecting rabbits intravenously with cultures of Type I Pneumococcus grown in broth containing rabbits' blood and killed by the addition of formalin. He obtained an immune rabbit serum by treating the animals intravenously with repeated injections of the autolysate and of the killed hormone broth-rabbit blood cultures and this serum was designated "Anti-A" serum. In addition, to other rabbits Enders gave injections of formalinized saline suspensions of agar-grown pneumococci. When the Anti-A serum was tested against SSS* no precipitate was formed, but with an autolysate from smooth Type I Pneumococcus the serum was definitely precipitating, and the reaction was type-specific. Furthermore, both the Type I autolysate and the supernatant fluid from the acetic acid precipitation of the autolysate gave precipitates with Anti-A serum but none with antipneumococcic serum prepared from rough strains.

By the method devised by Ward, Enders then added to his "normal" serum specific carbohydrate until precipitation was complete. The centrifuged supernatant fluid no longer gave any visible precipitation with SSS but, when the homologous autolysate was added, an abundant, flocculent precipitate was observed. Inasmuch as the SSS had apparently exhausted its specific antibody from the immune serum, the appearance of a precipitate on the addition of autolysate indicated to Enders the presence in the autolysate of a precipitinogen other than the specific polysaccharide and, accordingly, to this hypothetical substance he gave the name, "A Substance."

There are two other characters of the A substance of Enders which should be mentioned. One was instability when exposed to heat. Boiled for one-half hour at pH 9 its effectiveness as a precipitating antigen was reduced at least one thousandfold, while the soluble specific substance under similar treatment remained unchanged. When, however, the reaction was adjusted to pH 4 with 10 per cent acetic acid, a solution containing the A substance

* For convenience, the soluble specific substance or type-specific polysaccharides of Pneumococcus will hereafter be frequently referred to as SSS.

could be boiled for the same period of time without losing its activity. In both acid and alkaline solution, autoclaving for one hour at fifteen pounds pressure practically destroyed its effectiveness. The second character was its resistance to pepsin-hydrochloric acid mixture. The preparation probably resisted also the digestive action of trypsin, but the presence of alkali in such a substrate, by itself, tended to destroy the substance and therefore interfered with any accurate determination of its digestibility.

Enders[359] extended the investigation to embrace the carbohydrates of Type II and III pneumococci and, in addition to precipitative and anaphylactic methods, employed the agglutination and agglutinin-absorption reactions for a further comparison of his new antigen with the specific polysaccharide. He reported that type-specific agglutination of Type I, II, and III pneumococci occurred in homologous antiserum from both rabbit and horse to approximately the same titer after the antibody reacting with the purified specific carbohydrate had been removed. This fact suggested that in pneumococci there exists a type-specific agglutinogen which was to be distinguished from the specific carbohydrate. A side comment of Enders was that the presence of a specific agglutinogen in Pneumococcus Type II unrelated to the specific carbohydrate would account for the failure of this organism to remove agglutinins from *B. Friedländeri* Type B antiserum, and would add additional evidence pointing to dissimilarity of the A substance and the soluble specific substance as well as to the lack of serological identity of Pneumococcus II and Friedländer bacilli of the B type.

An effect analogous to that described by Enders was reported by Ward[1483] in 1932. In a five-day broth culture of Type III Pneumococcus he found a type-specific substance with a powerful antibactericidal action. In comparison with the soluble specific carbohydrate, its precipitating action was far greater, requiring a much larger amount of antipneumococcic serum for neutralization. A similar substance, but in higher concentration, was also found in the filtrate of a lung obtained at necropsy from a Type III pneumonia patient. Tested by his whole-blood method, Ward found that a specimen of Type III convalescent blood, though comparatively weak in anticarbohydrate antibody, was better able to neutralize the broth filtrate and lung filtrate than a corresponding mixture of normal blood and antiserum. Two other specimens of Type III convalescent blood neutralized the Type III broth filtrate. Ward attempted no isolation of this precipitinogen but concluded: "The possibility that the reacting substance in the autolysate is more complex and less stable than the carbohydrate—perhaps a substance intermediate between the antigenic carbohydrate compound in the intact pneumococcus and the carbohydrate itself—was forced on the author as the most likely explanation."

Evidence which might be taken as indicating the existence of the A substance of Enders, or of some similar principle in Pneumococcus, is to be found in the work of Sabin (1931),[1204] who, like Enders, but independently,* attempted to exhaust potent antipneumococcic horse serum of protective antibodies by preliminary saturation with homologous SSS and found that in spite of this absorptive treatment the serum still contained an appreciable quantity of the specific protective substance. There appeared to be a lack of proportionality between the quantity of SSS used for precipitation and the amount of protective antibody left in the supernatant fluid. In the reaction some of the protective antibody was evidently lost, since the sum of the precipitated and free antibody represented only from 20 to 50 per cent of the total. This large loss might be accounted for if an excess of specific carbohydrate were added since it would exert the inhibiting action observed by Felton. The same results as those obtained in the *in vitro* experiments were noted in *in vivo* tests in the rabbit.†

Sabin concluded that in antipneumococcic serum there was a

* Enders' paper was received for publication in May, 1930, and published in August of the same year, while Sabin's communication was accepted in September, 1930, and appeared in January, 1931.

† Incidentally, an observation of interest was that in the combination of SSS with its homologous precipitin there occurred a phenomenon similar to the

type-specific antibody which was not neutralized by SSS and which was apparently distinct from the anticarbohydrate precipitin. Reasoning that this non-precipitable antibody could not have been evolved in response to any antigenic stimulus from the soluble specific substance, Sabin sought an answer to the question, "Is there another type-specific antigen in the Pneumococcus in addition to the SSS?" After adding to Type I antipneumococcic serum the required amount of SSS for complete precipitation, he centrifuged the mixture after water-bath and ice-box incubation, and treated portions of the supernatant liquid with a 50 and 100 per cent excess of SSS, with a saline suspension of heat-killed Type I pneumococci, and with a similar suspension of heat-killed Type II pneumococci. The experiment showed that the residual protective antibody in the supernatant fluid was not neutralized by SSS or by absorption with Type II pneumococci, but was definitely absorbed with the homologous Type I pneumococci. Sabin assumed, therefore, that the neutralization was specific, and unless SSS in the organism was capable of neutralizing the antibody which SSS in solution could not, some other substance in Pneumococcus must be the responsible agent. This proviso, however, is all important in this connection. There is no proof that the SSS as prepared by Sobotka for Sabin, even though by his tests it was practically identical with the soluble specific substance of Heidelberger and Avery, was identical with the specific polysaccharide as it exists in the pneumococcal cell.

In 1931, Wadsworth and Brown[1466] reported the isolation of a carbohydrate which appeared to be analogous to the soluble specific substance and which yet more closely resembled the A substance of Enders. The original source material was a virulent Type I strain, and the method consisted in removing the organisms from fifteen-and-one-half hour broth cultures by means of the

Danysz effect in the combination of toxin and antitoxin. More SSS was required for complete precipitation when the total quantity was added at once, than when it was added in fractions of the total on successive days. This effect had also been observed by Heidelberger and Kendall in their studies on the precipitin reaction.

supercentrifuge and washing the sediment in distilled water. The supernatant fluid and washings were evaporated over the free flame to small volume and then used for the isolation of the specific carbohydrate by the method of Heidelberger and Avery. The preparation contained about 5 to 6 per cent of nitrogen. Its solution gave negative biuret and xanthoproteic tests, a positive Molisch test, did not reduce Fehling's solution until after hydrolysis with hydrochloric acid, and was precipitated by phosphotungstic acid. The material was more readily soluble in water than the polysaccharide of Heidelberger and Avery.

When tested against antipneumococcic serum, the dissimilarity between the substance prepared by Wadsworth and Brown and the soluble specific substance of Heidelberger and Avery and its similarity to the A substance of Enders became evident. It precipitated specifically in Type I serum in a dilution of 1 to 6,000,000, but in a dilution of 1 to 600,000 it gave an immediate ring reaction with Type I serum which had been completely absorbed with a highly purified preparation of the soluble specific substance. Wadsworth and Brown did not test the supernatant fluid from the serum precipitated with SSS for protective antibody.

Again differing in properties from the Heidelberger and Avery polysaccharide, the substance induced immunity in mice, as demonstrated by the protection test. The immunizing effect was type-specific. The substance fixed complement in the presence of Type I antipneumococcic rabbit serum and while it caused no reaction when injected intravenously in a dose of one milligram into a normal guinea pig it evoked fatal anaphylactic shock in guinea pigs passively sensitized not only with Type I antipneumococcic rabbit serum but with the same serum after removal of precipitin by absorption with the soluble specific substance. Wadsworth and Brown concluded that the substance they had isolated from the pneumococcal cell corresponded to that of Schiemann and his co-workers, and to the A substance of Enders, but was distinct from the soluble specific substance of Heidelberger and Avery.

In another communication, Wadsworth and Brown[1468] reported on chemical and immunological studies of carbohydrate fractions separated from pneumococci of the first three types and from an atypical strain as well. The cultures used were a virulent Type I Neufeld strain, a strain each of virulent Types II and III, and an attenuated Type I Pneumococcus. The carbohydrates resembled in character and action the substance described by Schiemann and his colleagues. The preparations differed in essential respects from the soluble specific substance of Heidelberger and Avery, so Wadsworth and Brown, for the purpose of distinguishing their substance from SSS, gave to it the somewhat ambiguous name, "Cellular Carbohydrate."

In a 1 to 300 dilution none of the preparations gave biuret, Millon's, or xanthoproteic tests; the Molisch test was positive and, after hydrolysis, Fehling's solution was reduced. The results of the micro-analysis of the "cellular carbohydrates" are shown in the original table taken from the paper by Wadsworth and Brown. The figures represent minimums and maximums. One specimen from each of the type preparations gave a trace of sulfur; the remainder gave none.

The apparent presence of phosphorus in organic combination in all these preparations revealed a distinct and, to the authors, possibly an important chemical difference between the antigenic and non-antigenic carbohydrate. The presence of amino nitrogen and of only small amounts of phosphorus further distinguished the cellular carbohydrates from the C Fraction of Tillett and Francis. Unlike the SSS of Types II and III, the cellular carbohydrates of these types contained nitrogen and phosphorus, although nitrogen had never been found in analogous preparations by Heidelberger and phosphorus had been shown by Heidelberger and Kendall to be a constituent only of the C Fraction. These unusual results and the wide variations in the analytical figures lead to the surmise that these preparations of cellular carbohydrates were impure.

MICRO-ANALYSIS OF THE CELLULAR CARBOHYDRATES OF THE PNEUMOCOCCUS

Type of cellular carbohydrate of Pneumococcus	Preparation number	Sulfur	Phosphorus*	Total nitrogen†	Amino nitrogen‡	Ash	Water
			Per cent	*Per cent*	*Per cent*	*Per cent*	*Per cent*
I	6		0.43	4.28		0.90	13.52
I	9		0.39	4.37	2.14	0.43	9.51
I	12	Trace	0.35	4.01	2.03	0.85	13.73
I	13		0.77	4.59	1.91	2.40	10.18
Atypical I	1			7.66		12.65	9.12
Atypical I	3		5.36	8.92		1.64	8.61
Atypical I	4		6.54	5.99		2.05	7.87
II	1		1.72	2.03		0.62	6.54
II	2	Trace	1.86	2.83		0.08	6.75
II	3		1.75	3.20		2.09	9.68
III	1		4.58	6.11		3.10	7.75
III	2		2.56	3.75		1.08	9.99
III	3	Trace	2.06	3.41		1.76	9.95

* Elek's modification of Pregl's micro method.
† Pregl micro-Kjeldahl method.
‡ Van Slyke method.

By precipitating a concentrated neutral solution of the Type I cellular substance with hydrochloric acid, Wadsworth and Brown, just as Heidelberger, Goebel, and Avery had done, obtained an acid-insoluble and an acid-soluble fraction.

When tested with homologous antipneumococcic serum, both of the fractions in a dilution of 1 to 6,000,000 gave precipitation. When a Type I rabbit serum, which had been absorbed separately with each fraction, was tested with the other, the acid-soluble fraction failed to precipitate serum absorbed by either, while the acid-insoluble fraction precipitated to a slight degree with the serum absorbed with the acid-soluble portion. Unfortunately, no protection tests were carried out with the immune serum absorbed with these fractions, so it is impossible to make a close comparison of the results with those of Enders.

Small doses of the Type I cellular carbohydrate were effective, by intraperitoneal injection, in protecting mice against a fatal dose of culture administered seven days after the immunizing dose. No data were given as to the degree of immunity established or as to its duration.

The cellular carbohydrate caused an acute inflammatory process in the lung of the rabbit when introduced into the trachea. It also induced specific anaphylactic shock in sensitized guinea pigs. The cellular carbohydrate therefore agreed in its properties and activities somewhat closely with the A substance of Enders and appeared to be a substance apart from the soluble specific substance of Heidelberger and Avery, and from the C substance of Tillett and Francis.

COMPARISON OF VARIOUS CELLULAR CARBOHYDRATES

For the purpose of comparing the properties of the various cellular carbohydrates derived from Pneumococcus, Wadsworth, Crowe, and Smith[1469] studied the absorption spectra of preparations at different stages of purification. The preparations studied were those which had been used in chemical and immunological studies previously reported from their laboratory and, in addition, a specifically reacting substance from an atypical strain of Pneumococcus, originally derived from a virulent Type I standard culture, together with a Type I soluble specific substance from the virulent culture. The absorption curves of solutions of the soluble specific substance of a virulent and of an attenuated Type I strain showed no significant differences. The curve of one preparation of a Type I cellular carbohydrate approximated that for the soluble specific substance, but that for another preparation of a Type I cellular carbohydrate approached the curve of the atypical strain of Pneumococcus.

The authors pointed out that there was considerable evidence in the literature that a large number of carbohydrates show only continuous absorption in the ultra-violet region of the spectrum but, when contaminated even slightly, yield marked absorption bands. Their work led to a contrary conclusion, since it was found that the selective absorption in the ultra-violet region was characteristic of the pure substance. In conclusion, Wadsworth, Crowe, and Smith stated, however, that the curves suggested that since their preparations were not in a pure state, the more striking differences in the curves might be attributable to substances not concerned in serological or antigenic activity or in the production of purpura.

TYPE VIII CARBOHYDRATE

Brown[157] has published a description of a preparation of the Type VIII carbohydrate isolated by the methods employed by Wadsworth and Brown. She found that the soluble specific substance was best removed from the broth concentrates of Pneumococcus by precipitation as the barium or calcium salt and by repeated alcoholic precipitation. On analysis one preparation gave a nitrogen content of 0.19 per cent, phosphorus 0.06 per cent, ash 0.70 per cent, with 3.90 per cent moisture. The specific rotation was about $+126°$, and while the substance before hydrolysis failed to reduce Fehling's solution, after boiling for four hours with 10 per cent sulfuric acid, it yielded 69.5 per cent of reducing sugars calculated as dextrose.

This VIII carbohydrate in a dilution of 1 to 4,000,000 gave a precipitate with Type VIII antiserum, and in a dilution of 1 to 2,000,000 with Type III serum. When Type VIII serum was absorbed with Type III soluble specific substance, it still precipitated with Type VIII carbohydrate in the same dilution as before absorption; but, when the same serum was absorbed with the homologous carbohydrate, it failed to precipitate with either. Also, Type III SSS removed from Type III antiserum the precipitins for both Types III and VIII polysaccharides, but Type VIII carbohydrate removed only the homologous precipitins.

This new carbohydrate produced purpura in mice but its action was partly neutralized by Types III and VIII antipneumococcic rabbit serum and was intensified by two similar antiserums from the horse. The Type VIII polysaccharide also induced fatal anaphylactic shock in guinea pigs passively sensitized with the homologous antiserum from the rabbit but not with a similar serum obtained from the horse.

Among the many methods applied to the purification of pneumococcal carbohydrate, ultrafiltration was employed by Brown.[158] By passing broth cultures of Type VIII Pneumococcus through a Sharples centrifuge and then filtering the clarified effluent through parlodion filters, or by passing broth cultures through a single nitrocellulose-coated alumina thimble, the author effected the elimination of inert material with a consequent enhancement of serological activity.

ISOLATION OF AN UNIDENTIFIED CONSTITUENT OF THE PNEUMOCOCCAL CELL

In the interval elapsing between the first and third papers of Wadsworth and Brown, Felton[413] reported the isolation of what he claimed to be yet another constituent of the pneumococcal cell. This derivative was described as a non-carbohydrate and probably a non-protein substance, possessing the ability to immunize mice against pneumococcal infection. Supplementing his preliminary announcement, Felton[417] in October, 1934, published information which, to a considerable extent, clarified the doubt concerning the true nature of his antigenic "non-polysaccharide and probably non-protein derivative" of Pneumococcus. In the earlier paper, Felton reported that this crystalline substance gave a negative biuret test, a negative Molisch reaction, and also failed to cause precipitation in antipneumococcic horse serum. Further study, however, showed "that the crystalline material lacked immunizing properties, and that in all likelihood the crystals were leucine. In addition, although the substance gave negative Molisch reaction, it was found that the difference in the reduction of copper before and after hydrolysis corresponded to from 0.25 to 0.5 per cent glucose. In other words there is present in this fraction a complex carbohydrate."*

Felton[417] amplified the study of the acid-soluble and acid-insoluble fractions of Pneumococcus on which he had already published a preliminary note.[416] The material was prepared by dehydrating broth-grown pneumococci with acetone, followed by dessication *in vacuo* over calcium chloride. Prepared by this method the organisms retained their antigenicity at least through the period of the study. Watery suspensions of the dried pneumococci were treated first with enough sodium hydroxide to make the concentration of the alkali one-tenth normal, and then after the suspensions were allowed to stand at room temperature for one-half hour, an equal volume of various mineral and organic acids was added. In this way it was possible, as Heidelberger and Avery, and Wadsworth and Brown had found, to separate the pneumococcal material into an acid-soluble and an acid-insoluble fraction. The former possessed most of the immunizing activity of the cell, and the immunity produced by injecting this fraction into white mice proved to be largely type-specific. The latter fraction, probably containing some intact cells, also possessed a small amount of the immunizing substance and evoked in mice a heterologous immunity. Precipitation of the acid-soluble fraction with ethyl alcohol or acetone yielded at least 90 per cent of the immunizing substance.

Felton's experiments, therefore, confirmed the work of Schiemann and Caspar,[1228] Saito and Ulrich,[1214] Wadsworth and Brown,[1466] and Zozaya and Clark[1590] in that active immunity can be produced in white mice by a fraction smaller than the intact pneumococcal cell. The precipitating action of the acid-insoluble

* In another part of the same paper, Felton stated that in his experience the Molisch test failed in the presence of other organic substances to indicate the presence of polysaccharide which on hydrolysis gave a glucose content of from 0.2 to 0.5 per cent, and emphasized the fact that the biuret test for protein is notably insensitive, giving a positive test with concentrations of the majority of proteins in a dilution no higher than 1 to 10,000. When one considers the extraordinary immunological activity of bacterial polysaccharides and proteins, it need scarcely be said that less reliance should be placed on these or similar tests as criteria for determining the precise chemical nature of these antigens.

fraction was also similar to that of the C Fraction of Tillett and Francis, but Felton ventured no closer comparison of the immunizing principle in the acid-soluble fraction with the soluble specific substance of Heidelberger and Avery.

Looking back on the descriptions of the properties of the original soluble specific substance of Heidelberger and Avery, this array of diverse pneumococcal carbohydrates was confusing. One wondered which, if any, of these several substances obtained from Pneumococcus actually represented the specific polysaccharide as it existed preformed in the bacterial cell, or which one most closely approached the native substance in its chemical and antigenic features. There was the possibility, of course, that Pneumococcus might contain more than one constituent of this general type, with differences in individual composition which would account for their special immunological properties.

CAUSE OF DIFFERENCES IN CARBOHYDRATES ISOLATED FROM PNEUMOCOCCUS

In the brief communication by Pappenheimer and Enders[1049] published in October, 1933, there was a definite clue to the cause of chemical and antigenic differences in some of the various carbohydrates isolated from Pneumococcus. Enders had previously observed that the immunological activity of the A substance was rapidly destroyed by heating on the alkaline side of neutrality, and so Pappenheimer and Enders surmised that in the method of Heidelberger and Avery for the preparation of soluble specific substance the A substance was destroyed at the stage where it was precipitated with barium hydroxide.* Pappenheimer and Enders, in preparing the specific polysaccharide, using the simplified method of Heidelberger and Kendall,[620] accordingly took the precaution of maintaining an acid reaction throughout the process. In this way there was obtained from Type I Pneumococcus an extremely hy-

* Dudley and Smith[840] also noted that heating with alkali destroyed the precipitating activity of a preparation of pneumococcal polysaccharide made by their method.

groscopic, white, amorphous powder, soluble in the range pH 1 to 9, and containing no sulfur or phosphorus. Its elementary analysis, amino nitrogen content, and specific rotation were practically identical with the soluble specific substance as prepared by Heidelberger, Goebel, and Avery.

The soundness of the reasoning was shown by the outcome of precipitin tests with this new preparation of the A substance and SSS. Both, in a dilution of 1 to 4,000,000, precipitated Type I immune serum. When the serum was absorbed with soluble specific substance, whereas SSS no longer gave a precipitate, the A substance produced a precipitate with the SSS-absorbed serum even when added in a concentration of 1 to 4,000,000. On the other hand, the A substance completely removed the precipitin for both itself and the soluble specific substance. The authors had, by obviating the injurious effect of alkali on the carbohydrate, succeeded in largely preserving the chemical and antigenic integrity of the specific polysaccharide of Type I Pneumococcus, and had supplied an explanation for one of the basic causes of the varied immunological behavior of the different carbohydrate preparations previously reported.

RELATION OF THE ACETYL GROUP TO THE IMMUNOLOGICAL ACTIVITY OF PNEUMOCOCCUS

The diversity of the several polysaccharides had also naturally perplexed Avery and Goebel who, quite independently of Pappenheimer and Enders and while their work was in progress,* set about the acquisition of a fuller knowledge of the nature of the relationship existing between the specifically reacting derivatives studied by other investigators and the type-specific polysaccharide formerly described by Avery and his colleagues. In a communication published in 1933 Avery and Goebel[46] presented evidence that they had isolated the soluble specific substance in a chemical form

* The paper by Pappenheimer and Enders appeared in October, 1933, and that by Avery and Goebel in December of the same year.

more closely approximating that in which it probably exists as a natural constituent of the cell capsule. They identified the type-specific carbohydrate present in the intact bacterial cells and in filtrates of autolyzed broth cultures as an acetyl polysaccharide. According to Avery and Goebel this naturally occurring acetyl polysaccharide differs chemically from the specific carbohydrate as originally isolated principally in respect to the presence of acetyl groups, which endow the native substance with additional specific properties not possessed by the polysaccharide after the removal of these labile groups by alkaline hydrolysis. Avery and Goebel claimed that, owing to the marked instability of the acetyl groups and the ease with which they are removed by treatment with alkali, the soluble specific substance as originally isolated, although still retaining the dominant type-specificity of the native substance, had, through the loss of its acetyl groups, suffered a corresponding loss of certain specific properties possessed only by the acetyl polysaccharide itself. Avery and Goebel further stated that the specific differences between the properties of the cell fractions studied by other investigators and those of the soluble specific substance as originally defined, appeared, as a result of their experiments, to be due to the presence or absence of acetyl groups in the polysaccharide molecule. They wrote: "Indeed, so distinctive are the immunological reactions of the acetyl polysaccharide and those of the deacetylated derivative, that it is now possible to clarify many of the apparently conflicting views still current concerning the nature and properties of the specific carbohydrate of Pneumococcus Type I."

By modified methods, in which treatment with alkali was purposely avoided, the soluble specific substance of Pneumococcus Type I was isolated by Avery and Goebel in the form of an ash-free, acetyl polysaccharide possessing marked acidic properties. It was readily soluble in water, and gave solutions of high viscosity which showed a specific optical rotation of about +270°. The naturally acetylated Type I polysaccharide was found to contain

4.85 per cent of nitrogen, approximately one-half of which was liberated in the amino form when the substance was treated with nitrous acid in the cold. It did not reduce Fehling's solution until after hydrolysis with dilute mineral acids. At the same time that reducing sugars appeared in the solution, the serological specificity of the acetyl polysaccharide was destroyed. In this respect its behavior was identical with that of the deacetylated polysaccharide.

The acetylated carbohydrate evidently contained uronic acids. It was soluble in water and in 80 per cent acetic acid. Aqueous solutions were precipitated by phosphotungstic acid, silver nitrate, and neutral and basic lead acetate, and were incompletely precipitated by barium hydroxide. Unlike the deacetylated product, the acetyl polysaccharide was precipitated by tannic acid but not by uranyl nitrate. It gave no color reaction with iodine-potassium iodide solution. It did not immediately decolorize weak solutions of potassium permanganate, and it gave negative reactions to the biuret, ninhydrin, sulfosalicylic, and picric acid tests. No traces of phosphorus or sulfur were detectable in the most highly purified preparations of the specific acetyl polysaccharide.

The table on page 281, copied from the article by Avery and Goebel, shows the results of the analyses of the acetyl polysaccharide of Pneumococcus Type I.

The analytical data presented in the table show that the deacetylated product (Preparation 2 A), obtained by alkaline hydrolysis of the acetyl polysaccharide (Preparation 2), contained no acetyl groups and was in all respects chemically identical with the polysaccharide that had hitherto been known as the soluble specific substance. This result agrees with that of Heidelberger and Kendall[617] who previously had found that the Type I polysaccharide (deacetylated) contained no acetyl groups.

The results of the analysis corresponded closely with the calculated composition of the acetylated polysaccharide, and this substance, therefore, approached in its chemical make-up that of the

ANALYSES OF THE ACETYL POLYSACCHARIDE OF PNEUMOCOCCUS TYPE I

Preparation No.	Source	Acid equivalent	Specific rotation	Ash	C	H	Total nitrogen	Amino nitrogen	Acetyl	Phosphorus	Reducing sugars after hydrolysis	Highest dilution of polysaccharide reacting with antipneumococcus serum
				Per cent	*Per cent*	*Per cent*	*Per cent*	*Per cent*	*Per cent*	*Per cent*	*Per cent*	
1	Bacterial cells	—	+270°	0.0	—	—	4.89	2.30	5.9	0.0	—	1:5,000,000*
2	" "	—	+265°	0.0	—	—	4.86	2.21	6.9	—	—	1:5,000,000*
3	Autolyzed broth cultures	576	+277°	0.0	42.55	6.58	4.85	2.22	6.0	0.0	32.0	1:5,000,000*
2 A, deacetylated	†	535	+297°	0.0	‡	‡	5.05	2.50	0.0	—	27.6	1:5,000,000§

* Type I antipneumococcus serum previously absorbed with Preparation 2 A (deacetylated).

† This sample of deacetylated polysaccharide was obtained by alkaline hydrolysis of Preparation 2. This material is identical with the carbohydrate formerly known as the soluble specific substance of Type I Pneumococcus.

‡ An analysis of carbon and hydrogen was made on a sample of deacetylated carbohydrate which had been reprecipitated five times at its isoelectric point. The material contained no ash, and had a carbon content of 40.33 per cent and a hydrogen content of 6.23 per cent.

§ Unabsorbed Type I antipneumococcus serum.

soluble specific substance as it probably exists in the pneumococcal cell. This hypothesis is further strengthened by the antigenic behavior of the acetylated polysaccharide when compared with that of the intact pneumococcus and with that of the soluble specific substance as it is released from the cell during natural autolysis. The experimental evidence presented by Avery and Goebel goes a long way toward reconciling the conflicting differences in some of the various carbohydrate derivatives isolated by other workers from the pneumococcal cell and its products.

The same authors found that both the acetyl polysaccharide and the deacetylated polysaccharide were precipitated by homologous immune serum in the highest dilution tested, representing a final concentration of one part in three million. When, however, the serum was absorbed with the deacetylated polysaccharide, after removal of all precipitins for this form of the specific carbohydrate, the serum still reacted with the acetyl polysaccharide in equally high dilution. On the other hand, after absorption with the acetyl polysaccharide, the serum was completely exhausted of all precipitins for both forms of the carbohydrate, as shown by the absence of reaction when tested with each substance in dilutions ranging from 1 to 20,000 to 1 to 3,000,000. The deacetylated polysaccharide, therefore, selectively removed from the serum only the precipitins for itself, whereas the acetyl polysaccharide completely removed all the precipitating antibodies for both forms of the specific substance.

Avery and Goebel discussed these results by saying:

> The specific precipitation of the acetyl polysaccharide in serum previously absorbed with the deacetylated carbohydrate, and the readiness with which the former substance is converted into the latter by heat, are similar to the relationships observed by Enders, and by Wadsworth and Brown, between the substances isolated by them and the soluble specific substance which they prepared according to methods previously described in this laboratory. Since the specific substance thus prepared is now known to be the deacetylated polysaccharide, it seems not improbable that the differences they observed, like those noted in Table II, represent the reactions not of two different carbohydrates but of a single substance in two chemically different forms; namely, the naturally acetylated and the artificially deacetylated polysaccharide.

Avery and Goebel also found that after absorbing Type I antipneumococcic serum separately with acetyl and deacetylated Type I polysaccharides, the serum absorbed with the former carbohydrate no longer agglutinated Type I pneumococci, while immune serum treated with the latter substance still contained specific agglutinins. The authors next tested the ability of the acetyl and the deacetylated polysaccharides to absorb the protective antibodies from specific immune serum and discovered that while the deacetylated carbohydrate reduced the titer of protective antibodies, it failed to remove them all, since the serum, absorbed by this substance, according to the conditions of the test, in dilutions of 1 to 10 to 1 to 100 still protected mice against virulent pneumococcal infection. On the contrary, the acetyl polysaccharide, under the experimental conditions employed, exhausted the serum of protective antibodies.

Further evidence of the specific antigenicity of the acetyl polysaccharide as compared to the incomplete antigenic action of its deacetylated derivative was furnished by Avery and Goebel's experiments on the immunizing action of the two carbohydrates on mice. Three injections of 0.5 cubic centimeters each of a 1 to 2,000,000 solution of the acetyl polysaccharide protected all the mice tested six days later against 10^{-5} cubic centimeters of a culture of Type I Pneumococcus, of which 10^{-8} cubic centimeters killed the control mice. A similar series of injections of the same amounts of the deacetylated polysaccharide, however, failed to afford any protection to the mice tested.

The outcome of the experiments just cited would explain the previous consistent failure of Avery and his associates to induce active immunity in mice and rabbits with their former preparations of the soluble specific substance, which were then used only in the deacetylated form. "This difference in antigenic action, like that already noted in the serological behavior of the two forms of the polysaccharide, is referable to known differences in chemical constitution."*

A careful examination of the chemical and immunological data presented in this communication would seem to justify Avery and Goebel's conclusion:

An analysis of the specific reactions of the acetyl polysaccharide discloses a previously unsuspected similarity between this form of the specific carbohydrate and the antigenically active fractions described by other investigators. From the chemical and immunological properties of the acetyl polysaccharide it seems highly probable that this substance in the purified state accounts for the antigenic action of the carbohydrate

* Avery and Goebel.

of Schiemann and Caspar and of Wadsworth and Brown. As in the case of these substances, the acetyl polysaccharide is antigenically effective in mice only when administered in extremely minute quantities. Although an extensive study of the purpura-producing action of the acetyl polysaccharide has not been made, in several instances purpura has been noted in mice injected with amounts of this substance ranging from 0.4 to 4.0 mg. . . . That the antigenic action of the water-soluble fraction of Perlzweig and his co-workers may have been due to the presence of traces of unhydrolyzed acetyl polysaccharide seems not unlikely from the readiness with which it lost its immunizing capacity when heated in alkaline solution.

The correspondence of the acetyl polysaccharide to the A substance of Enders and to the cellular carbohydrate of Wadsworth and Brown has already been mentioned. The exact relation of the acetyl polysaccharide to the "non-carbohydrate and probably non-protein" derivative of Pneumococcus described by Felton still remains to be determined.

Avery and Goebel had found, under the conditions of their experiment, that the acetylated polysaccharide failed to induce any immune response in rabbits. The serum of the treated animals contained no demonstrable antibodies, and the animals were not protected against subsequent infection with organisms of the homologous type. It was shown, furthermore, that the acetyl polysaccharide persisted in the circulation of the treated rabbits for considerable periods of time, was slowly excreted by the kidney, and appeared in the urine in its naturally acetylated form. This observation, particularly when compared to the immunizing action of the same substance in mice, has an important bearing on the definition of antigenicity.

In 1934, Goebel, Babers, and Avery[523] sought a better understanding of the immunological significance of the acetyl group in these complex pneumococcal polysaccharides. For this purpose the authors synthesized the *p*-aminophenol β-glucoside of glucose and its monoacetyl ester and then combined these two glucosides with horse serum globulin by means of the diazo reaction. These synthetic carbohydrate-azoproteins were employed as antigens in the production of immune rabbit serum. From the experiments, involving homologous precipitation and specific inhibition of precipitation, confirmation was obtained of the view previously expressed by Avery and Goebel that the immunological specificity of carbohydrates is determined by their stereochemical configuration, and their data lent support to the further assumption that the introduction of a simple chemical group, such as the acetyl radical, endows a carbohydrate with a new and distinct specificity which is determined by the chemical nature of the group thus introduced. The differences exhibited by these two purely synthetic carbohydrate azoproteins accurately paralleled the differences in the serological specificity exhibited by the acetylated and deacetylated polysaccharides of Type I Pneumococcus.

Additional information concerning the A substance of Enders was presented in the 1934 communication of Enders and Wu,[362] who prepared the A substance according to the procedure given by Pappenheimer and Enders and the soluble specific substance by the method of Heidelberger, Goebel, and Avery. The immune serum was obtained by the repeated intravenous injection of rabbits with Type I pneumococci in 0.3 per cent formalinized saline solution, and also of suspensions of pneumococci killed by heating at 56° and 60°. The immunological properties of the two polysaccharides were then tested by the bactericidal method of Ward and by mouse-protection tests in which the mice had been treated with antipneumococcic rabbit serum and also by active immunization with the A substance.

After the completion of the study, Enders and Wu announced that the A substance possessed greater anti-opsonic action than either the deacetylated carbohydrate obtained by boiling in alkali or the SSS of Type I Pneumococcus prepared according to the method of Heidelberger, Goebel, and Avery. The A substance practically eliminated the opsonic titer of normal human serum—an effect not observed with equivalent amounts of the deacetylated material or the soluble specific substance—while in immune serum the A substance brought about a quantitatively greater reduction in opsonic activity than its derivatives, although the authors were not able to demonstrate complete inhibition of phagocytic action by the method of absorption of antibody. The A substance by absorption lowered the mouse-protective titer of Type I antipneumococcic rabbit serum to a greater degree than did a similar treatment with the deacetylated carbohydrate. Analogous to the acetyl polysaccharide of Goebel and Avery, the A substance, administered in very small quantities, protected mice against an otherwise fatal dose of Type I Pneumococcus, although doses larger than 0.005 milligrams failed to establish protection in the animals. This particular antigenic action of the A substance was impaired by boiling in 0.02N sodium hydroxide, and was destroyed by similar treatment with 0.1N sodium hydroxide.

Enders and Wu also determined that after the injection of the A substance into mice active immunity arose within three days following the injection, reached its height in from six to twenty-five days thereafter, and became retrogressive by the forty-ninth day following vaccination. As might be expected, the injection of the A carbohydrate into immunized mice immediately before giving an infective inoculation abolished the active immunity, while the serum of mice actively immunized with the A substance conferred passive immunity on normal mice. The authors suggested that, since the evidence which had accrued in the course of their study indicated that the A carbohydrate obtained from Type I Pneumococcus and the acetyl polysaccharide of Avery and Goebel represented the same chemical substance, the designation A carbohydrate or A substance be relinquished in favor of the more accurately descriptive term, acetyl polysaccharide.

Although Enders and Wu did not include the cellular carbohydrate of Wadsworth and Brown in their comparison, taking into consideration their observations together with those of Avery and Goebel, there is good reason to believe that some of the preparations of cellular carbohydrates, though presumably in impure form, are practically identical with the A substance and the acetyl polysaccharide. There is, nevertheless, one point of difference for which as yet no explanation has been forthcoming, and that is the presence of sulfur and phosphorus reported by Wadsworth and Brown in their preparations. Heidelberger never found sulfur or phosphorus in the specific polysaccharides of Type I, II, and III pneumococci and since Avery and Goebel have stated that their highly purified preparation contained neither of these elements, it becomes difficult to reconcile these differences.

The work of Enders and Wu, taken with that of Avery and Goebel, would seem to demonstrate that the A substance and the soluble specific substance approached very closely in antigenic function the hypothetical specific polysaccharide as it exists in the intact pneumococcal cell. There developed in the latter's study one point, however, which raises a doubt as to the exact common identity of the isolated specific carbohydrate and the native capsular polysaccharide of Pneumococcus. The fact that the former, by absorption, failed to remove all the protective antibodies from the homologous immune serum might be taken to mean that in its isolation it had suffered the loss of some completing molecular group, or possibly that its full antigenic power is exerted only when it is in combination with some other constituent of the pneumococcal cell.

Another striking difference between the acetyl and the deacetylated polysaccharides of Pneumococcus was manifested in the behavior of these two derivatives toward the blood-group specific substance A. Witebsky, Neter, and Sobotka[1526] in 1935 announced that a relationship between the soluble specific substance of pneumococci and the blood-group substance A of man could be demonstrated by the inhibition of sheep-cell hemolysis by a group-specific A-antiserum, although the various types exhibited certain quantitative differences. When, however, the deacetylated carbohydrate was used, it failed to react with the group-specific A-antiserum, while the acetyl polysaccharide, under the conditions of the test, exerted an inhibitory influence on sheep-cell hemolysis by the A-antiserum up to a dilution of 1 to 1,000,000 of a one per cent solution. Furthermore, the authors could demonstrate the activity of the acetyl polysaccharide by complement fixation and by inhibition of group-specific iso-agglutination.

Witebsky, Neter, and Sobotka reported another interesting observation on the properties of the acetyl polysaccharide. When this substance was treated with the feces filtrate previously described by Schiff and Akune,[1233] by Schiff and Weiler,[1234] later by Witebsky and Satoh,[1527] and still more recently by Sievers,[1285] it lost much of its inhibitory action toward the group-specific A-antiserum, and also its ability to inhibit the iso-agglutination of Group A blood cells. Moreover, the acetyl polysaccharide of Type I Pneumococcus, after having lost its reactivity toward the group-specific A-antiserum following treatment with feces filtrate, still reacted with Type I antipneumococcic serum that had previously been absorbed with deacetylated Type I polysaccharide.

Witebsky, Neter, and Sobotka,[1526] in the introduction to their communication, mentioned the correlation between the Forssman antigen and the blood-group specific substance of human blood-group A. This fact, considered along with the relation existing between pneumococci and the blood-group specific substances A and B as reported by Bailey and Shorb,[66] and the known carbohydrate nature of the blood-group substance A as demonstrated by Landsteiner,[780] Landsteiner and Levene,[781] and by Brahn, Schiff and Weinmann,[146] and then the isolation by Freudenberg and Eichel[482] from the urine of men belonging to group A of a carbohydrate closely resembling in its chemical structure the type-specific polysaccharide of Pneumococcus of Avery, Heidelberger, and Goebel, reveals a field of investigation which yet remains to be explored.

RECENT METHODS OF PREPARING CAPSULAR POLYSACCHARIDE

The effect of alkali in impairing or destroying the antigenicity of the specific polysaccharides of Pneumococcus was tested by Felton (1934),[416] who reported that a Type I immunizing antigen, when heated at 100° in 0.1N sodium hydroxide lost 50 per cent of its antigenic strength after one hour of heating, and 94 per cent in two hours. With a Type II antigen in 0.5N sodium hydroxide, the immunizing activity remained the same as that of the control after four hours' heating. The same sample of Type I antigen heated in 0.1N acetic acid for two hours lost 50 per cent and in 0.1N hydrochloric acid 87 per cent of its immunizing power. Its precipitating action, however, remained the same. Of the samples of SSS prepared by the technique of Avery and Goebel and heated under the same condition, Type I in one test showed destruction of antigenicity and, in a second, no loss; with Type II no loss was observed. In a miscellaneous group of pneumococcal fractions with immunizing activity in dilutions of 1 to 50,000,000 to 1 to 2,000,000, and with variation of hydrolyzable sugar from 12 to 0.25 per cent, absorption end-point from 8 to 0.1 per cent, and precipitin titer from 1 to 5,000,000 to 1 to 5,000, Felton found that there was no definite correlation between acetyl group content and immunizing activity. However, acetyl groups were found in the samples studied ranging from 6.4 per cent in one sample which immunized in a dilution of 1 to 5,000,000, to 1.2 per cent in a sample which immunized in the same dilution. Inasmuch as this information was published merely in abstract form without the presentation of any experimental data, it is impossible to set a proper value upon its significance.

In 1935, Felton, with Kauffmann and Stahl,[480] gave the details of a method that had been employed in their laboratory for five years in the routine preparation of soluble specific substance of pneumococci. It had been planned to eliminate the time-consuming initial evaporation of the broth culture and to minimize any alteration of the chemical and antigenic structure of the carbohydrates. Calcium phosphate was employed as a selective adsorbent for separating the polysaccharide from the culture medium and its constituents.

Felton and his co-workers stated that the product from the first had shown characters differing from those of the soluble specific substance of Heidelberger and Avery. The new preparation precipitated more protein from a given immune serum; it consistently removed all the protective antibody from an homologous serum; and it produced immunity in white mice. The authors were not inclined to grant the validity of Avery and Goebel's explanation that this immunizing property depended upon the presence of the acetyl group in the polysaccharide. They had, it seems, in a comparative test succeeded in actively immunizing white mice not only with their preparations but also with a sample of soluble specific substance prepared by Heidelberger by his original method. Some statement as to the presence or absence of the acetyl group in their and Heidelberger's own preparation would have been helpful in arriving at a just appraisal of their contention.

In the latest paper to come from Felton's laboratory (1936), its authors (Felton and Prescott)[431] present evidence which, in their opinion, challenges the validity of the theory that the specific antigenic properties of pneumococcal polysaccharides are due to the presence of the acetyl group in the molecule. Because of the seeming heterodoxy of the claim, the summary and conclusions are here repeated practically verbatim:

A method has been indicated by which the linkage between the units in the polysaccharide of Type I pneumococcus are altered with concurrent changes in biological activity. This alteration is shown by both the high titer in bisulfite and iodine reactions in the original material and the absence in samples B* and C* of reducing sugars on hydrolysis after destruction of the aldehyde groups in hot NaOH solution.

* Sample A was a purified preparation consisting of a mixture of seven samples of Type I polysaccharide prepared by different methods both from the supernatant broth (of pneumococcal cultures) and from the bacterial cell (Pneumococcus).

Sample B was the original A dissolved at pH 7 in a concentration of 1 mg. per cc., and then made alkaline to N/10 concentration with NaOH and heated in an Arnold sterilizer at 100°C. for 30 minutes. To the alkaline solution after cooling were added 2 volumes of a 1:1 alcohol-ether mixture. The white precipitate which formed was washed thoroughly with alcohol, alcohol-ether, and dried.

Sample C was made from the foregoing fraction (B) by treating a neutral aqueous solution, containing 1 mg. per cc., with one-tenth of the volume of concentrated NH_4OH at 4°C. for 18 hours. The NH_4OH solution was precipitated

From this altered SSS, four samples were prepared by various alkaline treatments and tested both chemically and biologically in comparison with the original material. Each of the samples may be considered separately. The original material (A) gives tests for aldehyde groups, is high in "acetyl" content, and is optically as well as immunologically active. In B, a portion of A treated for 30 minutes in N/10 NaOH at 100°C., the optical activity is lost, the aldehyde groups are removed, "acetyl" content and all immunological activities are greatly reduced. In C, sample B treated with NH_4OH, there is a reduction of acid from vacuum distillation, no indication of sugar on acid hydrolysis, but an increase of the iodine reaction. Optical rotation is changed from zero to +190°, or higher than the control. Immunologically also this sample is more active than the original material (A). Sample D is the original material (A) treated with NH_4OH. There is a decrease of 90% in acid on vacuum distillation, a slight decrease in glucose number, a higher optical rotation than the original material, as well as a high titer in all immunological tests. It is significant that with a 90% decrease in "acetyl" content the immunizing activity is higher than the original. There is also a significant increase in its combining equivalent with antibody. Sample E is the NH_4OH treated control (D) further treated with hot NaOH as in sample B. The NH_4OH treatment caused a rearrangement of the molecule or stabilization, for on acid hydrolysis glucose number was 10.25 as compared to zero with sample B. Optical activity was reduced but not entirely lost. Immunological tests, although decreased, were not as low as in sample B, with the exception of the combining equivalent and that was the lowest of all samples, 0.9 unit. The acid from vacuum distillation was higher than in sample D, indicating a splitting off of the terminal carboxyl radicals.

At this stage of our investigation certain inferences may be made: (1) An antigen has been prepared from a Type I polysaccharide which in our opinion is non-protein in nature for the following reasons: (a) treatment with hot NaOH (N/10) and then NH_4OH results in a product more highly antigenic than the original preparation, and (b) all well-recognized protein tests are negative including a test for sulfur with a large sample of material. (2) This antigen may be considered

by dilution with 2 volumes of 1:1 alcohol-ether, washed repeatedly with alcohol, alcohol-ether and dried.

Sample D was made from the original material (A) by treatment with NH_4OH as in C.

Sample E was prepared from D by the same procedure as B, in other words heating at 100°C. in the Arnold sterilizer in N/10 NaOH for 30 minutes.

non-polysaccharide since both the Molisch test and the test for reducing sugars after acid hydrolysis are negative. (3) The antigens so prepared from Type I SSS produce active immunity in mice against both Type I and Type II pneumococci. (4) The restoration of the biological properties destroyed with hot NaOH by treatment with NH_4OH shows that the "acetyl" content is of no significance in determining the biological activity of the preparation studied, but conversely indicates that this property is determined by a definite molecular configuration which is readily altered by strong alkalis.

Believing that the procedures hitherto employed in the preparation of pneumococcal polysaccharides might have disrupted the molecular configuration of the carbohydrate molecule with a consequent loss of essential radicals, Sevag (1934)[1257] applied gentler measures for their isolation. Adopting the well-known action of liquid air in disintegrating bacterial cells, Sevag first froze the sediment from twelve-hour dextrose-serum broth cultures of a virulent strain of Type I Pneumococcus and then subjected the detritus to prolonged shaking in a mixture of water, chloroform, and amyl alcohol. The protein coagulated by this treatment was removed and the polysaccharide in the supernatant fluid was isolated by precipitation with alcohol. After further purification with chloroform, an alcohol-insoluble fraction was obtained which was claimed to be protein-free, gave a strong Molisch reaction, and contained between 6.60 and 6.72 per cent nitrogen, of which from 1.21 to 1.42 per cent was in the form of amino nitrogen. The specific rotation of the product was $[\alpha]\ D = +\ 218.3$* to 219.1* which after acid hydrolysis became +54.1 and showed a glucose content of 23.98 per cent. The polysaccharide thus isolated, in a dose of 0.0001 milligrams, protected mice against a thousand fatal doses of virulent Type I Pneumococcus and in high dilutions gave a high precipitation titer with homologous immune rabbit serum.

Sevag entertained some doubts concerning the validity of Avery and Goebel's claim that the capsular polysaccharide of Pneumococcus Type I was an acetylated substance and queried whether

* Typographical error in original figures gives +21.83 and 21.91.

the acetyl group might have been introduced into the carbohydrate molecule by the repeated treatment of the substance with acetic acid. Sevag accordingly excluded acetic acid from the method of preparing a special sample and found, contrary to expectations, that the polysaccharide, on analysis, had an acetyl content of 7.7 to 7.97 per cent as against the figure of 2.57 per cent obtained by Avery and Goebel.

It might reasonably be argued, therefore, that Sevag, by a less harsh treatment of pneumococcal cellular material, had succeeded in isolating a polysaccharide that more closely represented the carbohydrate as it naturally exists in the cell than did the preparation of Avery and Goebel. Apparent confirmation of the assumption came subsequently with the experimental results of Heidelberger, Kendall, and Scherp (1936).[627] In searching for a reason for the differences in the immunological behavior of acetylated and deacetylated polysaccharides and from the alkali-treated carbohydrates of Type II and Type III pneumococci, the authors devised a method of preparation in which the use of heat, strong acid, or alkali was avoided. In general the procedure consisted of the concentration of culture filtrate *in vacuo* to a convenient volume; separation of the polysaccharide from salts and protein degradation products by repeated precipitation with alcohol in the presence of sodium acetate and acetic acid; removal of proteins by denaturation with chloroform and butyl instead of amyl alcohol, as used by Sevag; and elimination of any glycogen or starch present by methods depending upon the properties of the individual polysaccharides. The products were isolated as the neutral sodium salts.

The analytical data on the polysaccharides obtained by the revised method present many points of interest when compared with results of analyses of older preparations. In the case of Type I polysaccharide the new product contained 4.62 per cent nitrogen with 2.0 per cent in the amino form, against 5.12 and 2.5 per cent for the old; showed specific rotation of +278 against +305, the acetyl content was 7.1 as compared to 3.4; it had a higher viscosity, and precipitated more antibody nitrogen from homologous antiserum from both horse and rabbit than did the earlier products. When compared with the substance isolated by Sevag, the high nitrogen, low amino nitrogen, and optical rotation indicated to Heidelberger and his associates the presence of a nitrogen-containing component not present in their products, but there was at the time no way of determining whether the component was an impurity or an integral part of the polysaccharide as it exists in the organism.

The study of Heidelberger, Kendall, and Scherp also revealed that, contrary to earlier opinion, the specific polysaccharides are not thermostable. On heating preparations from pneumococci of Types II and III there was an accompanying and marked drop in viscosity without any change in reactivity with homologous antiserum. There was a decrease in precipitating power in the case of Type I polysaccharide owing to a partial removal of acetyl. The authors suggested that unheated preparations have the largest particle size or longest chain, and that heating results in a degradation of the molecule to smaller units.

In the same communication the authors reported the actual isolation of the methyl glucoside of galacturonic methyl ester from the products of hydrolysis of the Type I polysaccharide by methyl alcoholic hydrochloric acid.

From the properties of the new preparations, Heidelberger, Kendall, and Scherp believed that while the products might be artifacts just as were the older ones, they were certainly a step closer to the native substances themselves and designated the substances as specific polysaccharides of Types I, II, and III Pneumococcus with the abbreviations SI, SII, and SIII.*

* For the purpose of obtaining a maximal yield of pneumococci with a high polysaccharide content, O'Meara and Brown[1031] devised a medium consisting of peptone, glucose, sodium chloride and sodium bicarbonate, potassium phosphate, and thioglycollic acid in water. In this medium, Type I Pneumococcus grows rapidly and abundantly. The organisms are found to be rich in capsular polysaccharide, whereas the medium contains a minimal amount of free polysac-

The susceptibility of the capsular polysaccharide to even fairly rigorous chemical treatment has been shown further in the case of the soluble specific substance of Type III Pneumococcus by Hornus and Enders.[656] By avoiding as far as possible the use of strong acids in the isolation of the carbohydrate a preparation was obtained that gave a precipitate with Type III immune serum after the serum had been absorbed by Type III SSS made by the earlier method of Heidelberger and Avery. The sample contained 0.3 per cent nitrogen and in this respect resembled the material described by Heidelberger, Kendall, and Scherp,[626] but it differed in some of its serological properties.

The gap between the polysaccharides as derived by chemical manipulation and the native substance in the pneumococcal cell is being still farther narrowed. By omitting the preliminary autoclaving of pneumococcal cultures, by leaving out alkaline treatment, and employing a method that minimized hydrolysis by acid or alkali, Chow[225] obtained a polysaccharide from Type I Pneumococcus that gave a precipitate with homologous immune rabbit serum previously absorbed with the acetyl polysaccharide. The acetyl polysaccharide failed to react with homologous immune rabbit serum after absorption by the new carbohydrate. The greater absorptive power of the new preparation as compared with that of the acetyl polysaccharide suggests its possession of a group or radical which was lacking in the acetylated derivative, but the fact that antipneumococcic serum absorbed with the new preparation was still agglutinative and specifically protected white mice against an otherwise fatal dose of Type I Pneumococcus may be taken to indicate that the carbohydrate isolated by Chow is not so com-

charide. The details of the preparation of the medium are given in the Appendix.

The use of peptone instead of meat as recommended by O'Meara and Brown, according to an unpublished personal communication of Heidelberger, greatly facilitates the preparation of both the capsular polysaccharide and the C carbohydrate. The C Fraction can be easily isolated from the supernatant fluid of such a broth after removal of the capsular polysaccharide.

plete in its antigenic or chemical constitution as the hypothetical polysaccharide existing preformed in the pneumococcal cell. While Chow's statement may be true that his polysaccharide may be the parent substance from which the acetyl polysaccharide could be obtained by appropriate treatment, there is little doubt that further search must be made in the lineage of pneumococcal carbohydrate for the original progenitor of the many derivatives which have been described.

OTHER PHYSICOCHEMICAL PROPERTIES OF THE CAPSULAR POLYSACCHARIDE

Heidelberger and Kendall[618] studied other physicochemical properties of the specific polysaccharides of pneumococci, and determined the viscosity, conductance, and behavior in diffusion of the sodium salts of Type III and other capsular polysaccharides. The high values of the equivalent conductance indicated that the sodium salt of Type III S* is a strong electrolyte characterized by a mobile negative ion of very high valence. Under varying conditions of salt concentration the authors determined the viscosities of I, II, and III S and correlated the findings with the magnitude of the charge on the anion. The experimental data indicated that at least eight or ten carboxyl groups were present in the molecule at regular intervals of every 340 of molecular weight, so the cumulative effect of the negative charges on the Type III S would be very large, which should result in large interionic or Coulomb forces. These forces were found to be strong.

The specific polysaccharide of Type I Pneumococcus showed viscosity abnormalities of a similar character, but of smaller magnitude. Although its acid equivalent was even lower than that of Type III S, Heidelberger and Kendall thought that internal compensation of negative charges by the basic groups present was the cause of the smaller effect. Further data on the specific gum arabic

* The substitution of the letter S for SSS is consistent with Heidelberger's original usage.

and Type III Pneumococcus polysaccharide showed that the viscosity effects decrease with the relative number of carboxyl groups, or negative charges in the molecule.

SUMMARY

It should by no means be assumed that the last word has been written about pneumococcal polysaccharides. Notwithstanding the fact that the presence in any appreciable percentage of what is considered the acetyl group may exert a marked influence on the antigenic properties of these substances, we should not close our minds to the many possibilities which the subject presents. We cannot as yet be sure that any of the substances isolated from Pneumococcus are truly representative of the actual components of the living cell, even though the immunological action of the acetyl polysaccharide most nearly approaches that of the unbroken Pneumococcus.

We can be sure that many of the methods employed up to the present time have led to products far from pure by any standard we set, and we can be equally certain that the majority of the procedures have caused more or less disturbance of the molecular arrangement of the cells' constituents with a consequent loss of chemical and immunological integrity. Many of the preparations hitherto derived from Pneumococcus by natural means must be looked upon as mixtures of carbohydrate, protein, and other cellular elements, and the majority of the preparations produced by chemical methods cannot be accepted as anything but artifacts containing, to be sure, a nucleus of intrinsic antigenic material but, nevertheless, representing substances which eventually may be discovered to be removed in varying degree from the native antigen.

There are chemical groups other than the acetyl radical in pneumococcal capsular polysaccharides, and until we have a more thorough analysis and more exact identification of all these substances supported by their respective immunological reactions, it would be folly to take any dogmatic stand in this highly complex question.

A careful examination of the specifications which have been given in all these reports would enable one to make a tentative and partial chemical reconstruction of the pneumococcal cell. The basic protoplasm would contain protein—a nucleoprotein—with a more or less constant composition for all pneumococci regardless of serological type. This common component would, in some respects, bear a close resemblance to the protein of other members of the genus, *Streptococcaceae*, and a more general resemblance to that of other more distantly related microorganisms. Another constituent of the protoplasm would be lipids, probably combined with the protein and conceivably loosely linked to the carbohydrate. Then the substance of the cell would also include a polysaccharide —a carbohydrate of the nature of the C Fraction of Tillett and Francis. This phosphorus and nitrogen containing carbohydrate would, like the nucleoprotein, be possessed by every Pneumococcus, whether of full virulence or degraded below the stage of any type identity. There would naturally be inorganic salts, but since little is known about them, their actual composition cannot be defined. In this viable, watery solution of colloids and crystalloids there would be enzymes—proteases, lipases, invertases, and saccharases —active in the metabolic processes of the cell and potentially able to destroy it.

This globular mass of protoplasm would be surrounded by a shielding envelope or capsule, largely carbohydrate in nature. The capsular material would be present when the cell was living in a favorable environment, in greatest amount when the surroundings were ideal, but entirely lacking when the cell had suffered from severe degenerative processes. But with or without it, these particular bacterial cells would still be pneumococci, their identity as such resting upon their somatic nucleoprotein and carbohydrate.

The normal Pneumococcus, however, would possess in its capsule a polysaccharide that would serve to distinguish the organism from many of the other members of the species. These complex carbohydrates would differ in their content of nitrogen, of phosphorus, and possibly of other elements, some being well supplied with one or the other of these elements, while others would have none. The carbon, hydrogen, and oxygen would be combined to form varying percentages of carboxyl, acetyl, or other radicals, and the presence and proportion of these groups, together with the varying sugars chemically combined, would serve to identify the special serological type to which the pneumococcus belonged. The capsular polysaccharides, furthermore, would differ in their acidic and basic affinities and in their relation to the plane of polarized light. The proportion of these carbohydrates would fluctuate in the different types, and on hydrolysis the substances would yield unequal amounts and various kinds of cleavage products such as glucosamines, sugar acids, and the simpler sugars. With the common protein and the somatic carbohydrate as a nucleus, it would be feasible, as soon as other specific polysaccharides are isolated, to hypothesize a basic reconstruction of all the thirty-two and possibly other as yet undiscovered serological types of pneumococci.

The capsular polysaccharides would be linked to some of the protein, or even to the lipids, in a combination susceptible to cleavage by the enzymes of the cell, to the disruptive effects of physical forces, to the lytic action of bile, or to the hydrolyzing action of chemical agents. Their chemical structure is frail, and to the chemist they present difficulties in the way of isolating them as they exist in their native state. They call for the utmost care in their separation lest their molecular configuration be distorted or mutilated.

While the somatic constituents are sufficient to insure the existence of the cell under ordinary circumstances, the capsular structure composed of type-specific polysaccharides is essential to the complete functioning of the cell as a pathogenic organism, and it is the latter specific complex that gives to a pneumococcus type-specificity and its individual place in the biological and immunological scheme. The capsular material conditions and is associated with the difference between a state of saprophytism and parasitism, and endows the cell with its highly specialized powers for stimulating the tissues of the animal body to the elaboration of substances antagonistic to the type-specific polysaccharide and to the cell as a whole.

The immunological properties of Pneumococcus and of its chemical constituents and derivatives will be discussed in more detail in later chapters.

CHAPTER IX

SPECIFIC POLYSACCHARIDE-SPLITTING ENZYMES

The decomposing action of bacterial enzymes on the soluble specific substance of pneumococci, with a description of the microorganisms, of the physical and biochemical properties of the enzymes and their effect on pneumococci in the test tube and in experimentally infected animals.

THE discovery of the specific polysaccharides of Pneumococcus was an incentive to a search for enzymes capable of decomposing these complex carbohydrates. During pneumococcal infections in man the soluble specific substance is present in the blood and since it is excreted unchanged by the kidneys it was reasonable to expect that none of the body tissues would be able to attack this substance. No tissue has ever been found to possess the power. Avery and Dubos[42] were the first to make a systematic hunt for a ferment possessing the ability to digest the capsular polysaccharide of Pneumococcus. The authors tested enzymes from animal and plant sources known to be active in the hydrolysis of simpler carbohydrates, but all failed to affect the polysaccharides. The similarity of these bacterial carbohydrates to hemi-cellulose led the authors to search among the molds, yeasts, actinomyces, and bacteria known to decompose substances allied to the celluloses, but here again the quest was fruitless.

FIRST ISOLATION OF POLYSACCHARIDE-SPLITTING ENZYME: SIII BACILLUS

Avery and Dubos reasoned that localities where large amounts of organic materials—especially materials belonging to the group of hemi-celluloses—accumulate and undergo decomposition were most likely to harbor the desired organism. So they tried leaf mold, composts of corn-cob, rye straw, sphagnum, oak leaves, farm manure, and soils rich in organic matter, such as peat soils and soils heavily manured, and finally came to examine a sample of soil from a cranberry bog. It seemed a far cry from a pneumococcus growing in the lung of man and, among its other vital activities, building up a complex carbohydrate, to a lowly saprophytic bacillus capable of decomposing the specific capsular polysaccharide formed by Pneumococcus. Such, nevertheless, was the case.

In 1930, Avery and Dubos announced that a mixed bacterial suspension made from bog soil was able to split the specific capsular polysaccharide of Type III Pneumococcus, and from the motley crowd of bacteria in this peat, they succeeded in isolating a pleomorphic, motile, spore-bearing bacillus that was responsible for the breaking down of the Type III polysaccharide.

In their next communication, Avery and Dubos[43] gave fuller details of the isolation, cultivation, vital characters, and enzymatic action of this curious bacillus. The authors mentioned the earlier observation of Toenniessen,[1413] who had found that when *Bacillus vulgatus* was seeded together with encapsulated Friedländer bacilli, the latter organisms grew deprived of their capsule, and then went on to describe the isolation of the new organism. The mineral medium used was based on one previously described by Dubos[329] for the isolation of cellulose-decomposing bacteria, with the addition of the capsular polysaccharide of Type III Pneumococcus in final concentrations varying from 0.001 to 0.2 per cent. The pneumococcal polysaccharide was the only source of organic carbon in the medium.

This mineral medium was selected because it contained no nutrient substances that would act as readily available sources of energy, so that the bacillus, when deprived of any other food, would attack the specific pneumococcal polysaccharide—an example of the so-called "starvation" phenomenon. By repeated transplantation and dilution, and by heating the inoculum at 70°, Dubos and Avery finally discovered the spore-bearing bacillus which they designated as the "SIII bacillus."

When grown in the synthetic medium, the organism appears as a minute Gram-negative bacillus, at times smaller than the Pfeiffer bacillus. It contains metachromatic granules; it grows diffusely in peptone solution and in this medium sedimentation of the growth occurs after several days' incubation. When cultivated in peptone solution or in plain broth the organism appears as a fairly large, actively motile bacillus, having peritrichous flagellae, the young cells measuring 2 to 3μ by 0.5μ. Short chains and diploforms are often observed. In broth the bacilli are at first Gram-positive and do not autolyze readily, but in the mineral medium the bacilli rapidly become Gram-negative and undergo almost immediate self-digestion. The spores resist heating for thirty minutes at 75° but are killed by boiling for five minutes. On plain nutrient agar free of dextrose, growth occurs in the form of small, whitish colonies, two millimeters in diameter, circular, slightly raised, umbilicated, with entire edge and fairly smooth surface.

In the media tested, the organism is strictly aerobic and exerts its saccharolytic action on Type III Pneumococcus within the range pH 6.2 to 7.8 at room temperature and at 37.5°. The isolated enzyme, however, is equally active under both anaerobic and aerobic conditions, and it is likely that this soluble principle belongs to the group of hydrolytic enzymes.

Dubos and Avery then found that the enzymatic action of the culture could be enhanced by frequent transplantation, and that the enzyme was present in filtered autolysates of the cultures. The action of the enzyme was limited, of all the substances tested, to the Type III polysaccharide, since it failed to decompose the carbohydrates of Types I, II, and VIII* Pneumococcus, and those of Types A, B, and C of Friedländer's bacillus, of *Hemophilus influenzae* Type a, and of gum arabic which, it may be recalled, gives a

* Personal communication from Dubos.

precipitin reaction with Type III antiserum. The activity of the enzyme was destroyed by heating for ten minutes at 60° to 65°. Neither normal beef nor rabbit serum had any inhibiting effect on its activity.

As a means for measuring the enzymatic strength, Dubos and Avery determined the minimal amount of a given enzyme preparation which would decompose one cubic centimeter of a 0.001 per cent solution of specific Type III capsular polysaccharide in eighteen hours at 37.5°, the decomposition of the carbohydrate being demonstrated by the disappearance of precipitating action in the presence of Type III antipneumococcic serum. As the authors stated, "The specific decomposition of the capsular polysaccharide of Type III Pneumococcus, by the organism as well as by the enzymes it produces, illustrates once more the specificity of the types of Pneumococcus, and confirms the fact that the capsular polysaccharides, and not some impurities carried along with them, are responsible for type-specificity."

EFFECT OF THE ENZYME ON THE CELL CAPSULE

Inasmuch as the capsular substance in its native state forms a morphological structure which conditions the antigenic and serological reactions of the pneumococcal cell as a whole as well as its power to invade and multiply in the animal body, it became of special interest to ascertain what effect this specific enzyme would have on the encapsulated cells growing *in vitro* and *in vivo*. To this end, therefore, Avery and Dubos performed a series of experiments the results of which revealed the fact that the enzyme by itself is neither bacteriostatic, bactericidal, nor bacteriolytic, and that, without impairing the viability of the cocci or without inhibiting the ability of the cells to synthesize polysaccharide, the enzyme, by decomposing the specific carbohydrate, merely deprives the bacteria of their capsules. It was evident that the action of the enzyme did not destroy the function of elaborating the capsular substance, since organisms decapsulated by enzyme again formed

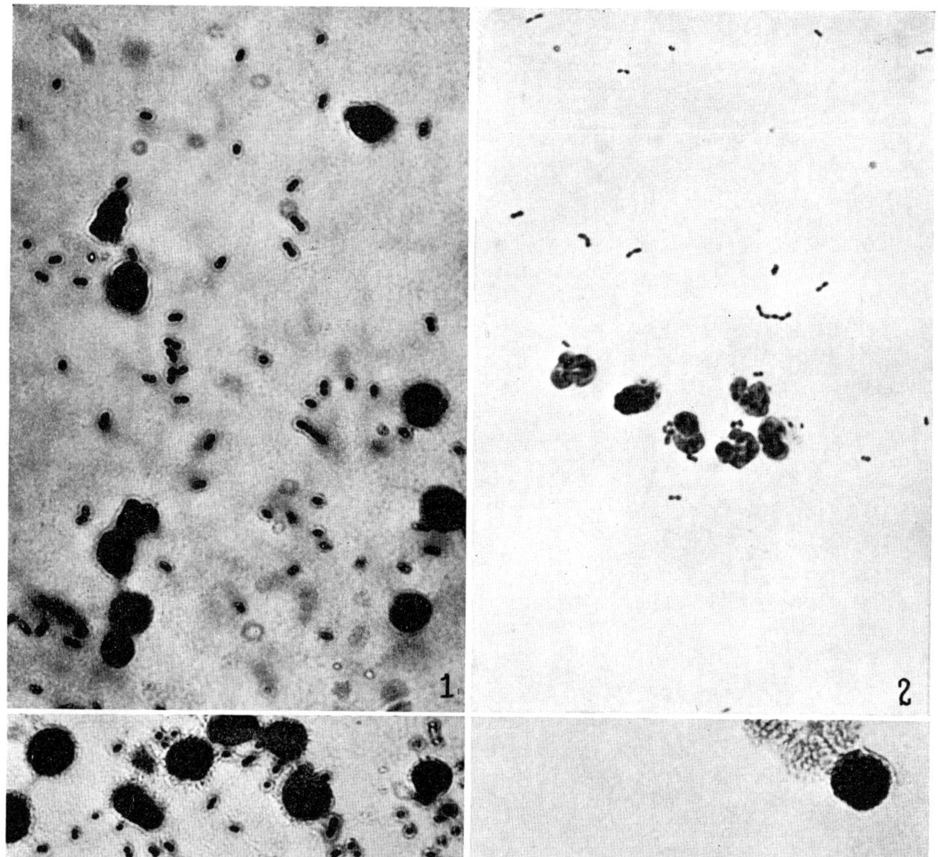

Photomicrographs by Louis Schmidt *After Avery and Dubos*[43]

ACTION OF ENZYME AGAINST TYPE III PNEUMOCOCCUS

specific polysaccharide and regained their capsule when transferred to a medium free of the enzyme.

The action of the enzyme against Type III Pneumococcus is shown in the accompanying photomicrographs, a description of which follows:

1. A stained preparation of the peritoneal exudate of a mouse two hours after the intraperitoneal injection of 0.01 cubic centimeter of a virulent culture of Type III Pneumococcus. The bacteria show well-defined capsules, and no evidence of phagocytosis is seen. Many polymorphonuclear and a moderate number of mononuclear leucocytes are present. (Gram stain. × 1000.)

2. A corresponding preparation of the exudate of a mouse two hours after receiving the same amount of culture together with 0.5 cubic centimeter of a preparation of the specific enzyme. The bacteria are devoid of capsules. Polymorphonuclear leucocytes predominate and phagocytosis is evident. (Gram stain. × 1000.)

3. A stained film of the peritoneal exudate of a mouse four hours after injection with 0.01 cubic centimeter of culture alone. The bacteria are increased in number, encapsulated, and extracellular. The cellular elements are polymorphonuclear and mononuclear leucocytes in about equal numbers. (Gram stain. × 1000.)

4. A corresponding preparation of the exudate of a mouse four hours after receiving the same amount of culture together with 0.5 cubic centimeter of a preparation of the specific enzyme. Marked phagocytosis has occurred and only an occasional organism is seen outside the accumulated leucocytes, nearly all of which are of the polymorphonuclear type. (Gram stain. × 1000.)

PROTECTIVE ACTION OF ENZYME IN MICE

Avery and Dubos then studied the protective action of the enzyme in mice against Pneumococcus Type III infection. By varying the amount of enzyme with a constant amount of culture, by keeping constant the dose of enzyme and by decreasing the quantity of culture, by giving the enzyme before and simultaneously with the infecting dose of culture, and by administering the enzyme by a single injection into mice eighteen hours after the onset of infection, the authors demonstrated that under the conditions of the experiments, 0.1 cubic centimeter of the enzyme afforded mice protection against one million times the fatal dose of virulent Type III Pneumococcus. Avery and Dubos also showed that again the action of the enzyme was specific for Type III; that the greater the activity of the enzyme *in vitro* the greater was its protective action in mice; and that the enzyme exerted a curative action since the mice receiving the enzyme eighteen hours after the onset of infection recovered. The extraordinary enzymatic principle, therefore, not only strips the capsule from Type III Pneumococcus, but renders innocuous a large multiple of the infecting dose of the organism and, what is more, under certain conditions it actually cures mice of an already active infection.

PHILOSOPHICAL ASPECT OF THE ACTION OF THE ENZYME

The possibilities presented by this and other similar enzymes in the prevention and cure of pneumococcal infection in man were strikingly promising, but before going on to experiments leading in that direction, it may be interesting and more profitable to consider first the important philosophical aspects of the action of an enzyme of this particular type on bacterial polysaccharides. It would be impossible to improve on Avery and Dubos' discussion of this phase of the subject, so it is quoted in full.

> The present study emphasizes the importance of the capsule in the biological reactions of the pneumococcus. It is, indeed, a significant fact, that no matter whether one regards this organism from the viewpoint of type-specificity, antigenicity, or its capacity to undergo variation, or whether, as in the present instance, one considers the pneumococcus with reference to its virulence and fate in the animal body, the one dominant factor influencing all these phenomena is the function of the cell to elaborate the specific capsular polysaccharide. These relationships, however, are not to be interpreted as meaning that virulence is dependent merely upon differences in the structural morphology of the bacterial cell. For it is a common observation that an encapsulated strain of Pneumococcus may be virulent for one species and not for another. However, it is equally true that the function of elaborating the

specific capsular polysaccharide is most highly developed in pneumococci that are best adapted to growth in the animal body. From this point of view, virulence and capsule formation, although not causally related, are at least intimately associated. When the function of forming the capsular substance is suppressed or inhibited, as in the case of the R variants, or when, as in the present instance, although this function is unimpaired the capsule itself is destroyed by an enzyme, the naked bacteria are thereby exposed directly to attack by the phagocytes of the host.

In this sense, the action of the enzyme may be said to result in preparing the encapsulated bacteria for phagocytosis; not as in the case of antibodies, by specific sensitization, but by the process of decapsulation. In the former instance, the reaction is an immunological one, whereby the capsular material is altered by union with the type-specific antibody; in the latter case, the reaction is a chemical one in which the capsular polysaccharide is actually decomposed by the enzyme. Although the mode of action of both these specific agents is different in each instance, the end result, so far as the fate of the microorganism is concerned, is the same in both cases.

It is of interest that although neither the enzyme nor the specific antibody is by itself bactericidal or bacteriolytic, yet each by reacting specifically with the capsular substance exposes the virulent organisms to the phagocytic action of the body tissues. The enzyme, like the specific antibody, serves merely to initiate the protective reaction, the completion of which is ultimately dependent for its successful issue upon the effective cellular response of the host.

The present study also suggests that the capsule—long recognized as a defense mechanism on the part of virulent bacteria—is a decisive factor in determining the fate of pneumococci in the animal body, and that this structure is vulnerable to attack by specific agents other than antibodies.

METHODS OF PRODUCTION

Dubos[335-6] then attempted the development of practical methods of production, purification, and concentration of the enzyme, and investigated the influence of certain factors on the potency and primary toxicity of the preparations. He first studied the growth and enzyme production of the SIII bacillus in more than fifty different media containing simple and complex saccharides, organic acids, alcohols, peptones, et cetera. Apart from the Type III specific polysaccharide he found only one other substance which caused the elaboration of the specific enzyme by the SIII bacillus and that was the aldobionic acid derived from the capsular polysaccharide of Type III Pneumococcus. When, however, he used another aldobionic acid, namely, that derived from gum arabic—a substance closely related immunologically to the Type III polysaccharide—no growth and, therefore, no enzyme could be obtained in the synthetic medium.

Dubos then learnt that the production of enzyme was also influenced by the concentration of capsular polysaccharide in the medium. The yield of enzyme rapidly increased with rising concentrations of the soluble specific substance, but decreased when the concentration exceeded 0.1 per cent and was inhibited by concentrations of 0.3 per cent or higher. Yeast extract, along with the soluble specific substance, stimulated enzyme production, but Dubos' first preparations in this medium proved to be toxic for experimental animals. Yeast extract in itself was not toxic and only when acted upon by cultures did it become so. However, Dubos was able to reduce the toxicity of the enzyme preparation by lowering the concentration of yeast extract to 0.03 per cent, the minimum compatible with good yields of enzyme.

Dubos then resumed his endeavors to produce a purer and more potent preparation of the polysaccharide-decomposing enzyme from the SIII bacillus, and in two communications (Dubos,[332] and Dubos and Bauer[338]) reported the results. It was first found that the yield of enzyme was proportional within certain limits to the amount of inoculum; that it increased with a rise in the concentration of capsular polysaccharide; and that 0.1 per cent of the carbohydrate represented the optimal amount for the purpose. After testing the influence of salt concentration in the medium on the metabolic activity of the SIII bacillus, on the basis of the collected data a method was devised which was described as follows:

The bacteria are grown in a solution of 2 per cent casein hydrolysate (pH 7.0) at 37°C. and under conditions of strict aerobiosis; the cells from the 16 hour old culture, separated by centrifugalization, are re-suspended in small amounts of distilled water.

A medium is prepared consisting of 0.1 per cent capsular polysaccharide and 0.1 per cent NaCl in distilled water. This medium is distributed in 25 cc. amounts in large Erlenmeyer flasks (1 liter capacity) to provide for aerobic conditions, and each flask is inoculated with the cells recovered from 500 cc. of the culture of the SIII bacillus in the casein hydrolysate medium. The material is incubated for 12–18 hours at 37°C. and the cultures tested to ascertain the disappearance of the specific polysaccharide and the absence of contaminants. The cultures are now frozen and thawed repeatedly to secure the release of the endocellular enzyme.

The enzyme is ultimately separated from the cell debris by filtration. However, since the cell suspension is very viscous, it is first subjected to the following treatment. The cell suspension is made alkaline to pH 10.0 by the addition of sodium borate. Equimolecular concentrations of dibasic sodium phosphate and calcium chloride are then added to bring about a heavy precipitate of calcium phosphate which facilitates the clarification of the material by centrifugalization; (it had been established previously that the enzyme is not adsorbed on the calcium phosphate at alkaline reaction). The supernatant which contains all the enzyme in solution is now passed through a Seitz filter, then through a Berkefeld (V) filter. It is important to observe that the enzyme is completely adsorbed on the asbestos pad of the Seitz filter; this, however, can be prevented by washing the filter with nutrient infusion-peptone broth previous to filtration. After this treatment, the enzyme passes through the filter without loss. The potency of this filtrate is such that 0.002–0.004 cc. are required to decompose 0.01 mg. of the capsular polysaccharide under the conditions of the test.

Dubos found that the SIII bacillus grew abundantly in casein-hydrolysate medium, but in this medium the organism did not form any appreciable amount of the enzyme responsible for the decomposition of the polysaccharide. When, however, large numbers of the bacilli grown in the casein medium were re-suspended in a solution of the capsular polysaccharide which constituted the sole source of carbon, the specific carbohydrate substrate was rapidly decomposed, and filtered autolysates of the cell suspension exhibited tremendously enhanced enzymatic activity. For a given amount of capsular polysaccharide decomposed in the new phosphate-yeast medium, the yield of enzyme obtained was much larger than that recovered by the former cultural methods. The production of the enzyme always failed when conditions in the substrate were unfavorable to cellular multiplication.

With Bauer, Dubos[338] then described an improved technique for concentrating and purifying the enzyme preparations. They filtered the solution, made in the manner just described, under fifty pounds pressure through collodion membranes of the type described by Bauer and Hughes.[90] The enzyme, under optimal conditions of filtration, passed through membranes of an average pore size of 10.6 mμ but was held back by pores having a diameter of 8.2 mμ. When the enzyme solutions were filtered to dryness through membranes of such porosity as to hold back the active principle, and when proper precautions were taken to prevent or minimize adsorption, such as the preliminary "greasing" of the collodion membrane with meat-infusion peptone broth, the enzyme could be completely recovered by immersing the membrane in distilled water or physiological salt solution.

EFFECT OF ENZYME ON INFECTION INDUCED IN RABBITS

In 1932, Goodner, Dubos, and Avery[536] studied the action of the enzyme on the dermal infection of rabbits induced with Type III Pneumococcus, employing the Type III strain virulent for rabbits previously described by Tillett. The culture was grown in rabbit-blood broth and its virulence was maintained for rabbits by frequent animal passage. Of the blood-broth culture 10^{-8} cubic centimeters given intraperitoneally sufficed to kill mice within ninety-six hours, and when given intradermally into rabbits 0.000,01 cubic centimeter caused death or a protracted disease of severe character. The enzyme preparations were, for the larger part, purified and concentrated by the method of Dubos. The intradermal infections were induced by the procedure devised by Goodner and already described in Chapter VI.

The authors found that the injection of adequate amounts of the specific enzyme twenty-four hours after infective inoculation brought about an early and complete cessation of the disease. The blood stream was freed of pneumococci and the organisms disappeared from the local lesion in the course of a few hours. Following the administration of the enzyme, the temperature at first rose, but fell within twenty-four hours to normal levels; the local lesion failed to spread and soon showed signs of healing. The results obtained by Goodner, Dubos, and Avery in a large series of infected animals indicated that in cases with severe bacteriemia large quantities of the enzyme were necessary to obtain successful results, while in animals having fewer organisms in the blood at the time of treatment smaller amounts of the enzyme would suffice.

The curative action of the enzyme was specific, at least in so far as it was tested. When given intravenously in a dose of one hundred units* twenty-four hours after inoculation with ten and one hundred minimal infective doses of Type I Pneumococcus, it failed to save the lives of the two rabbits tested. The authors found that the curative action of the enzyme was destroyed by heating at 70° for thirty minutes.

In a subsequent communication appearing later in the same year, Goodner and Dubos[535] reported the results of studies on the quantitative action of the enzyme on the dermal infection of rabbits with Type III Pneumococcus. With the same Type III culture and enzyme preparations similar to those employed in the previous experiments, using the number of pneumococci present in the blood as an indicator of the severity of the infection, Goodner and Dubos determined the amounts of enzyme required to bring about the recovery of the animal. It was ascertained that the required dose of enzyme bore a definite relation to the number of organisms circu-

* According to Dubos: "A unit of enzyme may be defined as one hundred times the smallest amount which will bring about the complete decomposition of 0.01 milligrams of the purified specific capsular polysaccharide in 18 hours at 37°C."

lating in the blood stream at the time of treatment. Thus, in animals with negative blood cultures or with a low grade bacteriemia, an amount of enzyme as small as five units might suffice to save the life of the animal; with a bacteriemia of 100 to 1,000 organisms per cubic centimeter of blood, twenty units might be necessary; with a bacteriemia of 1,000 to 10,000 organisms fifty units were required. In rabbits in which the bacteriemia exceeded 10,000 organisms per cubic centimeter a single injection of even one hundred units failed to rescue the animal, although infections of this order were successfully treated by repeated injections of large amounts of enzymes over a period of days.

Goodner and Dubos, in the discussion of their experimental data, stated that, although the quantitative relation established in the experiments was between the amount of enzyme and the number of pneumococci present in the blood, the fundamental relation was that existing between the quantity of enzyme and the total amount of specific capsular polysaccharide present in the body; and that an index of the latter was the degree of bacteriemia. The authors concluded that the enzyme is not a therapeutic agent per se, but one which, by decomposing the capsular substance of pneumococci and thus preparing the bacterial cells for phagocytosis—pianticating them, to use Friel's term—initiates a process which the body must be in condition to carry on if the animal is to recover. Hence, in the use of the enzyme, this capacity of the body must be reckoned with.

EFFECT ON INFECTION INDUCED IN MONKEYS

With this groundwork built, the next logical step was to apply the enzyme to the treatment of animals higher in the zoological scale which were suffering from experimental Type III Pneumococcus infection. Francis, Terrell, Dubos, and Avery,[477] accordingly, chose young adult monkeys—the Java monkey (*Macacus cynomolgos*)—as test animals, and infected the animals with a strain of Type III Pneumococcus virulent for rabbits. They employed the

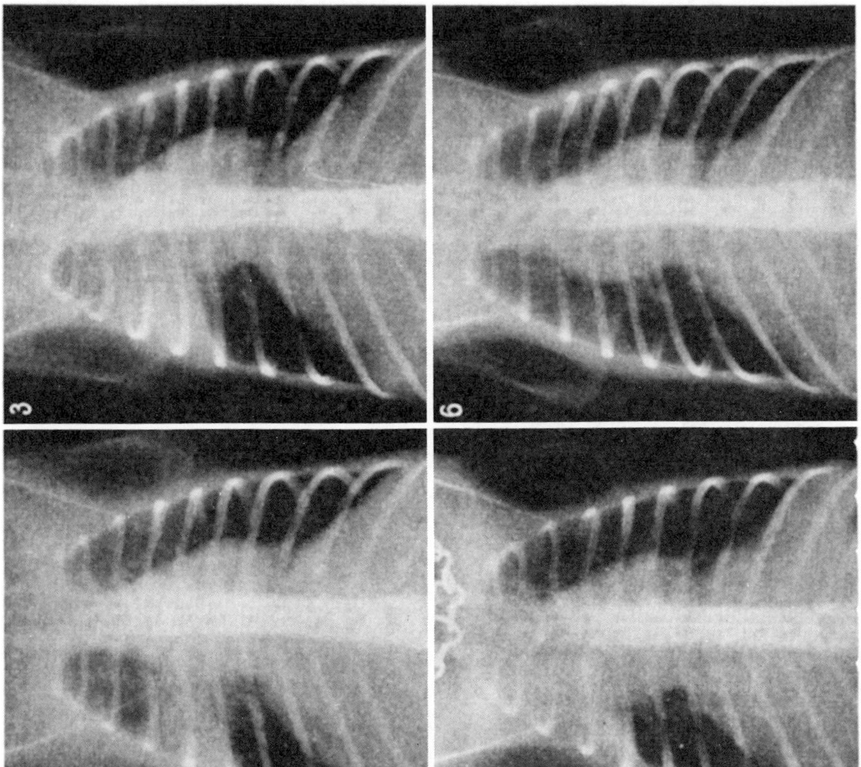

Dec. 19 Dec. 20 Dec. 21 Dec. 22 Dec. 24 Dec. 29

Photographs by Louis Schmidt *After Francis, Terrell, Dubos, and Avery*[477]

LUNGS OF A MONKEY DURING THE COURSE OF EXPERIMENTAL PNEUMONIA, TREATED THE FIRST DAY AFTER INFECTION technique developed by two of them (Francis and Terrell[476]), who had found that by intratracheal or intrabronchial inoculation of Type III cultures it was possible to produce in monkeys of the *Cynomolgos* species an experimental pneumonia, which in its clinical aspects resembled pneumococcal lobar pneumonia in man. The authors used enzyme preparations made in the manner already described, which varied in potency from two to twenty units per cubic centimeter. They began the enzyme treatment within the first three days after inoculation, administering the enzyme preparations intravenously usually in doses of ten cubic centimeters each, with additional treatments as often as three times daily, either intravenously, intraperitoneally, or by both routes simultaneously. Francis, Terrell, Dubos, and Avery purposely made no attempt to ascertain the minimal amount of enzyme required in individual monkeys but, rather, they employed the treatment intensively until the result was assured. Moreover, they selected for enzyme treatment the sickest monkeys among those infected, since this plan would reduce the factor of natural recovery from the infection as well as put the enzyme to the severest test.

The accompanying photographs show the effect of pneumonia on the lungs of a monkey that had been treated the first day after infection, as follows:

1. Control. Before inoculation (December 19).
2. Nineteen hours after infection and seven hours before the first treatment (December 20), showing well localized consolidation in lower half of the right upper lobe.
3. Second day (December 21), showing extension of pneumonia throughout right upper lobe.
4. Third day (December 22), showing increased density of the shadow over the right upper lobe, but no evidence of further spread.
5. Fifth day (December 24). Resolution of the pneumonia has begun, as shown by the decrease in density and beginning aeration of the area.
6. Tenth day (December 29), showing complete resolution of the pneumonic shadow.

THE INFLUENCE OF ENZYME THERAPY UPON MORTALITY-RATE IN EXPERIMENTAL TYPE III PNEUMOCOCCUS PNEUMONIA IN MONKEYS*

Class of infection	Untreated animals					Treated animals				
	Total	*Recovered*	*Died*	*Per cent mortality*		*Total*	*Recovered*	*Died*	*Per cent mortality*	
Pneumonia without septicemia	20	20	0	0		8	8	0	0	
Pneumonia with septicemia (1–250)†..	20	11	9	45.0	56.2	15	15	0	0	4
Pneumonia with septicemia (250–2000)†	12	3	9	75.0		9	8	1	11.1	
Pneumonia with septicemia (2000+)†	16	0	16	100.0		8	1	7	87.5	
Total	*68*	*34*	*34*	*50.0*		*40*	*32*	*8*	*20.0*	
Total for groups with septicemia	*48*	*14*	*34*	*70.8*		*32*	*24*	*8*	*25.0*	

* Classified on the basis of height of septicemia in first three days.

† The numbers in parentheses in the left-hand column equal the cocci present in one cubic centimeter of blood.

The condensed results of experiments on forty monkeys are given in the accompanying table. The figures in the table represent only the recovery or death of the monkeys, and do not give in detail the effect of the enzyme on the course of the pneumococcal infection. As Francis, Terrell, Dubos, and Avery reported, it can readily be seen that in the groups in which no invasion of the blood occurred, spontaneous recovery was to be uniformly expected, whereas in the extremely severe forms of the disease the great majority of animals were too completely prostrated to respond to any therapeutic aids. Further comment of the authors on the action of the enzyme upon the infected monkeys can best be given in their own words:

In addition to the apparently beneficial effects of specific enzyme therapy as measured by survival or death of the animals, certain other favorable influences were observed. In a high percentage of cases in which extension of the pneumonic process was occurring at the time of treatment, the spreading promptly ceased following the initial injection of enzyme. Although the density of the area of consolidation might at first appear greater than before treatment, extension did not occur and resolution of the lesion soon began. This limitation of spread of the pneumonia was not infrequently noted in the severe cases before the bacteria were completely eliminated from the blood stream. A comparison of the ultimate degree of pulmonary involvement in the treated and untreated cases reveals the fact that it was less, in general, in the former series. While in the treated cases the extension was apparently limited early, in the untreated animals extension of the pneumonia progressed, frequently with fatal results.

That the administration of enzyme promoted sterilization of the blood stream seems certain. In the milder cases this occurred quite rapidly. In animals in which the higher degrees of septicemia were present, there was rarely an increase, more regularly a prompt decrease in the number of pneumococci in the blood following the administration of enzyme. Even in cases which eventually terminated fatally, or in which extreme septicemia occurred early in the disease, cultures of the blood showed a marked reduction in the number of bacteria within 4 to 5 hours after the first treatment.

Simultaneously with limitation of the pneumonia, beginning resolution, and elimination of septicemia, a fall in temperature usually occurred. In fact, there was a tendency for the fever to subside concurrently with the cessation of pneumonic spread, even though septicemia still persisted. Although a marked leukopenia was comparatively frequent at the time treatment was begun, the number of leukocytes rose with the beginning of recovery.

In fatal untreated cases with septicemia, a high incidence of positive cultures was obtained from pleural or pericardial fluids at autopsy. In many instances frank empyema or pericarditis was present. In the treated cases with severe infections which resulted fatally, the incidence of these complications was also high. In recovered animals of the treated series, therefore, a frequency of suppurative complications equal to that of the untreated animals might be expected. The fact that the treated animals which survived recovered without suppurative sequelae suggests that enzyme therapy either prevented the development of empyema and pericarditis or was therapeutically effective even in the presence of these complications.

As previously stated, many technical difficulties have been encountered in attempting to produce enzyme preparations of uniformly high therapeutic activity and purity. The different lots of enzyme have, as a result, been inconstant in both these respects. In some instances toxic effects, attributable to impurities in the material, have been noted in animals after the administration of enzyme. These impurities may induce a febrile reaction and a decrease in the white blood count of the animal. At other times, when the animal is extremely ill with subnormal temperature and a marked leukopenia, the administration of impure preparations may produce a further depression of temperature and of the leukocytes.

The results of the present study indicate that the specific enzyme, even in its present state of purity, exerts a favorable therapeutic effect upon the course and outcome of experimental Type III pneumococcus pneumonia in monkeys. Nevertheless, the present study again emphasizes the therapeutic limitations of the enzyme. The action of the enzyme is known to be exerted upon the capsular polysaccharide of Type III Pneumococcus. By being deprived of its capsule, the bacterium is made susceptible to phagocytosis by the cells of the animal body. However, when the disease process is of extreme severity and the entire cellular mechanism of the body is markedly depressed, the animal may no longer possess the capacity to dispose of the organisms rendered vulnerable by the specific action of the enzyme.

ISOLATION AND STUDY OF OTHER POLYSACCHARIDE-SPLITTING ENZYMES

In 1933, Sickles and Shaw[1281] discovered microorganisms, other than the SIII bacillus of Avery and Dubos, capable of decomposing the capsular polysaccharide of Type III Pneumococcus and, furthermore, succeeded in obtaining from soil another organism possessing an enzymatic action on the capsular polysaccharide of Type II Pneumococcus. From decaying vegetable matter from different localities, Sickles and Shaw isolated in pure culture three strains of sporulating bacilli, which in morphology and some of their other characters differed from one another and from the SIII bacillus. The organisms were all aerobic, Gram-negative, motile rods with peritrichous flagellae, and formed oval spores wider than the vegetative cells. On beef-extract agar the organisms grew in colonies about two millimeters in diameter, which were yellowish white, smooth, and round with entire edges. On blood agar, two of the strains produced two types of colonies, one whitish and opaque and the other grayish and semi-translucent. One of the strains isolated from material from a decayed hickory stump covered with sphagnum moss appeared to utilize agar as well as the Type III polysaccharide. The cultures fermented dextrose, lactose, saccharose, maltose, dextrin, mannitol, xylose, galactose, inulin, and salicin as well as decomposing the specific polysaccharide of Type III Pneumococcus.

Sickles and Shaw made their enzyme preparations in a mineral substrate, using the yeast extract medium of Dubos only for the seed culture. The cultures were usually incubated for three days at 36°, filtered through a Berkefeld candle, and then concentrated by ultrafiltration through a 7.5 per cent pyroxyline membrane, the enzyme remaining on the membrane. In this manner a preparation was obtained with an enzymatic activity of approximately twenty units per cubic centimeter. The enzyme in a dose of 0.5 cubic centimeters, when given eighteen hours after inoculation, protected mice against infection with ten minimal fatal doses of Type III Pneumococcus and, when given seven hours after inoculation, the extract protected the animals against 1,000 fatal doses.

The organism isolated by Sickles and Shaw from soil, possessing the power to decompose Type II soluble specific substance, differed markedly from the bacillus attacking Type III SSS. It, too, was an obligate aerobe, but oval in form, resembling a yeast. It could be maintained by daily transfer on the mineral medium containing 0.01 per cent Type II soluble specific substance, but no growth could be induced in the mineral medium alone or on any of the usual nutrient solid media. No growth could be seen in meat-extract broth but microscopic examination indicated that slight multiplication had taken place. The organism grew slowly in meat-extract broth containing a fermentable carbohydrate, but did not grow in meat-infusion broth, litmus milk, or peptone water, on potato slants, or in gelatine. Growth was similarly slow on a solid medium composed of agar and the mineral medium containing Type II polysaccharide. In the mineral medium to which one per cent of carbohydrate was added, some strains of the organism fermented maltose, xylose, and dextrin, while all strains decomposed lactose and saccharose.

The cultures broke down the Type II cellular carbohydrate of Wadsworth and Brown as well as the soluble specific substance of the same type, but failed to dissolve the specific polysaccharides of Type I and III pneumococci. In the case of this organism, however, the enzyme was active only when the body of the organism was present, but Sickles and Shaw apparently did not test filtrates from the cultures. At that time no experiments were performed on the protective properties of this culture. It was observed, however, that the organism in decomposing the cellular carbohydrate robbed it of its purpura-producing property, but this effect may have been due to the digestion of admixed protein material of pneumococcal origin by a proteolytic ferment in the enzymatic preparation employed.

In a later paper, Sickles and Shaw[1283] reported the isolation from soil of another organism—a small Gram-negative bacillus—which acted on the Type I specific carbohydrate but failed to effect a complete decomposition of that substance, since it never fully lost its precipitating ability with homologous serum. Sickles and Shaw suggested that this residual reaction was due to an unused portion of the original carbohydrate or to products of decomposition, which might either be present in the original sample or be formed as a result of the action of the microorganism from the soil. Another possibility presents itself and that is that the authors' carbohydrate preparation may have contained a fraction which was not susceptible to the enzymatic action of the culture. It was impossible to obtain any soluble enzyme from this organism.

Several of Sickles and Shaw's cultures decomposed the non-type-specific carbohydrate isolated by Wadsworth and Brown (the

C Fraction) from an attenuated strain of Type I Pneumococcus. One organism was the aerobic, spore-forming bacillus that had been found to utilize the soluble specific substance of Type III Pneumococcus and agar; the other was a Gram-negative aerobic, non-motile, non-sporulating bacillus which, so far as tested, digested only this non-type-specific saccharide. From both of the strains a soluble enzyme was obtained capable, like the living cells, of splitting the non-type-specific carbohydrate and, in doing so, of abolishing its power to produce purpura.

Sickles and Shaw[1282] then undertook a systematic study of the morphological, cultural, and biochemical characters of these various polysaccharide-decomposing bacteria. The cultures had originated in the muck of swamps and in uncultivated soils of different localities, while one strain came from manure. The organisms were grown on the mineral medium of Dubos and Avery and a "Medium S" of their own concoction. To these mineral media were added the specific pneumococcal carbohydrates in concentrations varying from 0.002 to 0.01 per cent as a source of carbon.

Sickles and Shaw then subjected the strains to all the procedures required for identification, and in their communication gave a detailed account of the different biological characters of the organisms. To relate them would not be germane to the main subject but, because of the importance of this class of bacteria, a condensed description of the main characters should be recorded here. The cultures were of four distinct types:

1. Large spore-bearing rods that decompose the specific carbohydrate of Type III Pneumococcus, similar to the SIII bacillus of Dubos and Avery, and, in addition, a strain that utilizes agar. For the strains that digest only the Type III polysaccharide the authors suggested the name *Bacillus palustris,* with the sub-designation, *gelacticus,* for the variety also attacking agar.

2. Very small non-sporulating rods that attack the non-type-specific carbohydrate obtained from a degraded Type I Pneumococcus and the C Fraction from typical strains. This organism the authors called, *Flavo-bacterium ferruginum.*

3. Bacteria, oval in form, that decompose the specific carbohydrate of Type II Pneumococcus. To these organisms was given the species name of *ovale* and the designation *Saccharobacterium* was proposed for this new genus of the family *Mycobacteriaceae* including the microorganisms decomposing the specific carbohydrates of Pneumococcus of Types I and II.

4. Slender rods with tapering ends that utilize the specific carbohydrate of Type I Pneumococcus, for which the authors suggested the name *Saccharobacterium acuminatum.*

Again from soil, Sickles and Shaw[1284] isolated another strain of *Bacillus palustris,* which through the agency of a soluble enzyme decomposed the specific carbohydrate of Type VIII Pneumococcus. The enzyme was apparently without action on organisms of Types I, II, or III. Although Type VIII specific carbohydrate gave marked precipitation with Type III antiserum and, conversely, Type III carbohydrate precipitated Type VIII antiserum, it was a curious fact that the culture or enzyme that decomposed Type III carbohydrate failed to attack the polysaccharide of Type VIII, and the enzyme decomposing Type VIII carbohydrate was without action on the carbohydrate of Type III pneumococci. Here the enzymatic selectivity appears to be even greater than the overlapping serological specificity exhibited by chemically related but not structurally identical carbohydrates.

DIFFERENCES IN SUSCEPTIBILITY OF POLYSACCHARIDES TO ENZYMATIC ACTION

A possible explanation for the differences in the susceptibility of pneumococcal polysaccharides to enzymatic action and in their serological behavior is to be found in the recent study of Goebel (1935).[519] Quoting from his communication:

In the present study the specific polysaccharide of Type VIII pneumococcus has likewise been shown to be constituted from molecules of glucose and glucuronic acid. After hydrolysis with dilute mineral acid there appear in the hydrolysate of the carbohydrate from Type VIII pneumococcus a hexose, identified as glucose, and an aldobionic acid. From the actual quantities of these two constituents found in the hydrolysate, and from the value of the acid equivalent of the polysaccharide itself, it appears that this specific carbohydrate is built up from glucose and glucuronic acid approximately in the ratio of 7 molecules of hexose to 2 of uronic acid. The capsular carbohydrate of Type VIII pneumococcus represents, therefore, an entity which is chemically distinct from the specific polysaccharide elaborated by the Type III pneumococcus.

That a chemical similarity between the two substances exists, however, may be seen from the results of the experimental work in which it has been shown that the aldobionic acids appearing in the acid hydrolysates of both polysaccharides are identical. The proof of the identity of these two uronic acids was made possible through the preparation of the crystalline heptaacetyl methyl ester. Both derivatives show identical crystalline structure, melting points, and specific rotations. Furthermore, a mixed melting point of the two derivatives shows no depression. Although the actual structure of the aldobionic acid is as yet unknown, work is now in progress to establish this point.

In view of the experimental evidence which has been presented, showing that the aldobionic acids derived from the carbohydrates of Types III and VIII pneumococcus are identical, it is believed that the basis for the immunological crossing exhibited by these two specific types of pneumococcus resides in the structural and configurational identity of the uronic acid nucleus common to the encapsulating polysaccharides of both microorganisms.

Sickles and Shaw[1283] reported that the enzyme from the new soil bacillus was capable of destroying the purpura-producing action of the VIII carbohydrate and of protecting mice against several thousand minimal fatal doses of a virulent strain of Type VIII Pneumococcus. Larger amounts of the enzyme failed to protect mice against ten minimal fatal doses of Type III Pneumococcus. The observations in these two papers describing the highly selective action of the enzyme on the soluble specific substance in contrast to the cross-agglutination present another pretty problem for the chemo-immunologist.

SUMMARY

The discovery of bacteria endowed with enzymes capable of breaking down the complex polysaccharides of Pneumococcus is of more than academic interest. Here is a biological agent that in no way interferes with the vital activities of the pneumococcal cell; the cell grows, multiplies, and continues to synthesize the complex capsular carbohydrate peculiar to its serological type, but as soon as the carbohydrate is formed it is stripped from the coccus by the digestive action of the alien bacterial enzyme. The ability of a mere saprophyte to rob a pathogen of its protective covering, and thereby to deprive it of its infective power, is one of the strangely fascinating surprises of bacteriological research, but it has a much deeper meaning. The nature of this enzymatic action is in accord with the specific chemical constitution and serological behavior of the specific capsular polysaccharide of the pneumococcal type affected. By denuding the cell of its capsule through the dissolution of its polysaccharide, the enzyme exposes the cell to the destructive action of the white corpuscles of the blood, and if the tissue cells are functionally vigorous enough, the attack of the invading pneumococci is repelled and the infection aborted.

The enzymes of certain of these bacterial forms have been shown to save mice, rabbits, and monkeys from all but a massive infection from Pneumococcus and, what is more striking, the enzyme of one bacterial species directs its attack against the members of Type III, for which, as yet, no biological curative agent has been devised. The possibilities presented by these recent disclosures engage the imagination. The bacteriologist will want to search for still other microbic cells with enzymes capable of consuming the carbohydrates of pneumococci of the other serological types; the biochemist will desire to know more of the nature of the enzymatic principle existing in these bacterial cells; while the investigator in immunology will follow this inviting lead toward a resolution of some of the processes operating in infection and resistance.

CHAPTER X

ANTIGENICITY OF PNEUMOCOCCUS

The immunizing properties of Pneumococcus and of its components and derivatives; factors which operate in establishing the immune state; and the response of different animals to the antigenic action of members of this bacterial species and their constituents.

IN Chapter VIII the antigenic properties of the chemical constituents of Pneumococcus were described only in a general way in order to illustrate the similarities and dissimilarities of the protein and carbohydrate preparations which have been advanced as representing the active substances native to the cell, and to emphasize the dependence of immunological behavior on chemical constitution. No attempt was made to give any systematic account of the various antibodies or immune effects which the proteins and polysaccharides call forth, or to compare and correlate the action of the cellular fractions with that of the intact bacterial body.

Antigenic Spectrum

The antigenic spectrum of Pneumococcus can be resolved into its dominant bands in several ways. Taking the whole, living, fully virulent cell as the norm, its immunological action can be analyzed through the stimuli provided by its separate constituents or derivatives. There enter into the analysis the chemical structure of the several components of the cell, the question of their mass, and the route and spacing of their administration.

The spectral bands—or less definitely, zones or regions—appearing after the introduction of pneumococcal materials into the animal body, are represented by agglutinins, precipitins, bactericidins, tropins or opsonins—conceivably the alleged antitoxins—the complement-fixing and protective antibodies, and such manifestations of somatic reactivity as systemic or local allergy. All the phenomena depend in turn on the inherent special or racial peculiarities of the animal subject.

The resolution of the antigenic spectrum involves the study of the effects of Pneumococcus itself, of its separate constituents with their individual, chemical identification, in their relation to the parent material; the diverse serological reactions in which the whole cell or its parts participate; and the nature of the mechanism of the particular physiological response each wakens.

These ways bristle with obstacles of one kind or another. There is the tendency of Pneumococcus to digest itself or to lose its vigor; there is the danger of fracturing the molecular mosaic of the cellular substances by chemical treatment; there are all the subtle factors which influence the interaction of antigen and antibody in the test tube; and then there is the constitutional capacity or incapacity of animal tissues to function in response to the introduction of alien substances into the body. An antigen by one test may display full power; by another test it may seem to be incomplete or inert. Introduced in inappropriate quantity, an antigen may defeat its effect; administered by one route we see one set of immune bodies, by a different route some of the antibodies may appear wanting type-specificity or else be entirely absent; injected into animals of one species an antigen provides the animal with a full complement of antagonistic substances and protects it against fatal infection, while in other animals the administration of the same antigenic substance may be followed by no appreciable immune effect. Here, not only the race but the lineage, the age, and the immediate physical state of the animal all have their part in deciding the issue. Antigens and antigenicity, like virulence, therefore, are purely relative terms.

First Observations of Immunity

For a complete and orderly presentation of the manifestations of the immunological behavior of Pneumococcus it seems best to develop the subject by showing the manner in which our present knowledge has been acquired. Although it was Fraenkel[468] who first observed that rabbits surviving a subcutaneous injection of pneumococci became resistant to subsequent inoculation with the same organism, it was Foà and Bordoni-Uffreduzzi[461] who established the fact in an experimental way. By injecting rabbits subcutaneously at three or four-day intervals, beginning with attenuated cultures and then giving cultures of increasing virulence, the animals became insusceptible to inoculation with virulent cultures or infected blood. The authors applied the method to man but with no success. Then Foà[458] turned to the soluble products of Pneumococcus, and attempted the chemical isolation of the immunizing principle from broth cultures, but the experiments were inconclusive.

A great debt is owing the Klemperers,[723-5] who laid the foundation for the active immunization of animals against pneumococcal infection. As has already been told, the Klemperers used the sputum of convalescent pneumonia patients, bacteria-free pleural exudates, heated glycerol extracts, and heat-killed cultures as antigens and hence became the first to demonstrate that dead pneumococci and some of their derivatives, quite as well as the living cells, can render an animal immune. They also introduced the intravenous route for the administration of antigenic materials and proved that the serum of the immunized rabbits carried substances antagonistic to Pneumococcus. Like Foà, the Klemperers believed incorrectly that the immunizing principle in Pneumococcus was a toxin.

There then began a succession of publications dealing with the action of various pneumococcal materials in inducing immunity. There were the successful results of Emmerich and Fowitzky[357] with cultures of attenuated and then of diluted, virulent strains, and those of Bonome,[137] and of Kruse and Pansini,[763] with sterile culture filtrates, injected intravenously, subcutaneously, and intraperitoneally. Mosny[932] was another to employ sterile culture filtrates, while Foà and Carbone[463] obtained a certain degree of immunity with alcohol and ammonium sulfate precipitates from culture filtrates. The antigenic action of these agents was feeble, but Foà and Carbone demonstrated that both the intact cell, living or dead, and substances elaborated by the cell during cultivation evoke an immune response. The work of Denys[312] and of Washbourn[1486] established the fact that in order to produce immunity of high grade it was essential that pneumococci, whether used in the living or dead state or in the form of heated or filtered cultures, should be virulent.

These were the beginnings of immunizing procedures which have become routine, but there are many features of the subject that deserve more detailed discussion. The use of pneumococci taken from growths on solid media or in broth for the production of immune serum for experimental purposes has long been the common custom. For some time it was believed that for the production of a potent serum it was necessary to inject living organisms, but experience has shown that response to antigenic stimulus, that is the production of a serum with a high content of strictly type-specific antibodies, is conditioned less by the viable state of the organism than by the biological state of the culture at the time it is employed as antigen.

Influence of Virulence on Immunological Response

It is now generally accepted that for the production of a high degree of type-specific immunity the antigen, whether in a living or devitalized condition, must come from a robust, virulent culture. This conviction arises from the results of experiments on animals with strains possessing varying degrees of invasiveness, from the fully virulent, smooth forms to the degraded, rough forms, and from the experience of those workers who are engaged in the manufacture of therapeutic serum. The reason supporting the conviction is the chemical demonstration that complete antigenicity is dependent upon the maximal amount of unaltered protein and carbohydrate in the cell.

All through the literature on pneumococcal immunity, from the time of Denys and of Washbourn, there are repeated statements to the effect that virulent pneumococci are more active immunizing agents than are attenuated strains. The study of the antigenic action, especially in regard to type-specificity, of variant forms of pneumococci substantiates this fact. Neufeld, Cole, Wadsworth, and others, have always advocated the use of cultures in a virulent state for the production of immune serums. Barach[75] has shown that a highly virulent pneumococcus provokes a more marked immunity than an organism of low virulence—an observation corroborated by Meyer and Sukneff,[898] Day,[308] and many others. Therefore, whether the immunizing antigen is to be the living or killed organism or any of the separate substances isolated or derived from the cell, the evidence is wholly in favor of selecting a culture in vigorous condition and of exalted virulence.

Dead Cultures

HEAT-KILLED ANTIGENS

For a long time living pneumococci, usually after a preliminary course of injections of heat-killed cultures, were used for the vaccination of horses in the production of curative serums. The practice, however, caused a grave mortality among the animals under treatment. In 1917, the senior author of this volume, among others, desiring to prevent the depletion of his stables, substituted for living cocci, heat-killed organisms from broth cultures, and although the agglutinin titer of the horses was low, the content of the serum in mouse-protective antibodies was more than sufficient to meet standard requirements of that time.

Using cultures devitalized by heat, formaldehyde, soaps, or other means became the practice in many serum-producing laboratories, although the literature contains relatively few detailed observations on the comparative antigenic action of pneumococci when in the living and in the dead state.* In 1902, Neufeld[974] obtained satisfactory agglutinating serum by the injection of rabbits with either living or heat-killed pneumococci, but for the routine preparation of immune serum he gave the animals, first, heat-killed cultures, and then living cultures. Wadsworth,[1457] in 1912, claimed that only after immunization with living, virulent cultures did the serum acquire marked curative properties.

Cotoni and Brasie[281] made a comparative study of the immunizing effect of pneumococci heated at 56°, of cultures treated with alcohol and ether and suspended in salt solution, and of these suspensions heated for fifteen minutes at 110°. The heat-killed cocci proved to be far superior to the other antigens in protecting rabbits against infection.

The influence on antigenic action of varying exposures of pneumococci to different temperatures was investigated by Tani.[1379] According to the results obtained, cultures of Type I pneumococci incubated for a long period at 39°, when injected intraperitoneally into mice, were found to have lost virulence and were feeble immunizing agents; cocci heated for two and one-half hours and not completely killed showed poor immunizing power, whereas another specimen heated at the same temperature for an equal length of time and completely killed, and then later heated for one-half hour at 56°, gave good protection. After subjecting a similar culture to a four hours' exposure at 100°, it was still antigenic in that it afforded protection to mice. Tani's results point to virulence as an essential property of cultures used for immunization. Davidson,[298] too, tested the antigenic action of living pneumococci, of heat-killed cultures, and of detoxified and defatted vaccines. Rabbits injected with the killed cultures acquired immunity, and the serum contained protective substances. The living cultures pro-

* These facts and many similar observations by others have never been published but are widely current in the stable lore of manufacturing laboratories.

duced intoxication, while the use of acetone and other agents in removing the lipids from the vaccine destroyed its antigenic power.

In the case of Type III Pneumococcus, Tillett[1405] found that repeated injections of heat-killed cultures into rabbits were effective in producing active immunity against infection with a virulent strain of the homologous type. Even heterologous strains, devitalized by heat, were capable of affording similar protection to Type III cocci. Moreover, this form of active immunity could exist in the absence of demonstrable type-specific antibodies and apparently was unrelated to the variety of Pneumococcus used for immunization. Tillett considered that this anomalous immune state was dependent upon the exaltation of the same factors which afford normal rabbits material resistance to some strains of Type III organisms.

Employing Type II strains, Gaspari, Sugg, Fleming, and Neill[503] learnt that the continued injection of heat-killed cultures of this type led to a decrease in type-specificity and to an increase in the species-specificity of the serum of the treated rabbits. For the preparation of diagnostic serum of high type-specificity the authors preferred as an antigen the heated cells of virulent pneumococci administered over a comparatively short immunization period. A gradual shift from type-specificity to species-specificity is no uncommon occurrence in horses that have been under immunization for long periods of time with either living or dead organisms.

Day[307] reported that it was generally desirable to kill the cells with heat for the production of antibodies, but warned against the use of a temperature as high as 100° for the purpose, since such a degree of heat destroyed the antigenic properties of the culture. However, this has not been the experience of the authors of the present volume. As might be expected, Day, and also Harley,[592] found that any agent which promoted the digestion of the cell, and which consequently led to the breakdown of its constituents, weakened or finally abolished the ability to call forth type-specific antibodies. Additional evidence confirming the efficacy of heat-killed antigens is to be found in the experiments of Stillman and Goodner.[1342] Three intravenous injections at four-day intervals of saline suspensions of heat-killed cultures of Type I, II, and III pneumococci protected rabbits against an otherwise fatal infection of pneumococci of the corresponding type administered according to Goodner's intradermal technique. The results were controlled by the demonstration of agglutinins and protective antibodies in the serum of the treated animals.

In 1923, Yoshioka,[1562] finding that the successful immunization of mice was largely dependent upon the total mass as well as the spacing of the doses of antigen, devised a rapid method involving small quantities of heat-killed pneumococci injected in six half-hourly doses. In this way he obtained excellent protection in mice. In the next year, Killian[704] repeated Yoshioka's experiments with intensive serial injections and, in addition, tried injections of killed cultures with weekly intervals between each series. By this plan of three series of intraperitoneal injections at weekly intervals, it was possible to render mice immune to a fatal dose of pneumococci given three days after the completion of the immunizing treatment, but the immunity lasted only a few weeks. Killian laid stress on the proper amount of antigen to be given, because doses too small or too large yielded poorer results. The use of living, fully virulent organisms, contrary to the experience of most observers, resulted in a noticeably lower degree of immunity.

In another communication, Killian[706] gave the details of further experiments from which it appeared that by employing the intravenous route for serial injections the level of protection in mice could be elevated, and that by periodic intraperitoneal treatment of the animals with four-day intervals between injections of increasing doses of killed vaccine one could obtain a high degree of protection in a short time. In a third communication, Killian[707] described a refractory stage which lasted for several days after an immunizing injection and, in order to avoid this stage and to secure the most effective secondary stimulus, gave injections at intervals of fourteen instead of four or eight days.

The question of the effect of heat on the immunizing activity of Pneumococcus was subjected to systematic study by Barnes and White,[86] who compared the antibody response following the injection into rabbits of heat-killed and formalinized cultures of Type I Pneumococcus, administered according to different schedules over long periods—in some of the experiments for as long as eight months. As antigens, the authors used saline suspensions of the sediment from eighteen-hour broth cultures of a virulent Type I strain, subjected to 56° in a water-bath for one hour, and similar suspensions of culture sediment treated with 0.3 per cent formalin. The vaccines were standardized by the Gates[504] nephelometer and the individual doses accurately measured. The injections were given intravenously according to three different plans somewhat similar to those of Yoshioka and of Killian. The schedules consisted respectively of a single injection on each of three successive days; a single injection on each of five successive days; and a series of six injections on each of the first two days with the other four on the third day. The rest periods varied from one to three weeks, and test bleedings were usually taken seven, twelve, and, in some instances, twenty-two days after the last injection of a series. The various serum samples were titrated for agglutinins, precipitins, and mouse-protective antibodies.

Heat-killed pneumococci produced highly potent serums of strict type-specificity. The first and third named methods were equally productive, but the first was the method of choice because of its greater simplicity. The results of the study, besides confirming the value of heat-killed pneumococci in establishing a high degree of immunity, afforded a rational basis for the immunizing treatment of horses for the production of therapeutic serum.

OTHER DEVITALIZED ANTIGENS

As soon as it was found that heat-killed pneumococci were capable of calling forth a specific immune response, other attempts were made to rob the cell of the power of invasion and infection without impairing its antigenic qualities. For a long time formaldehyde in the form of formalin has been employed for the purpose of killing and preserving pathogenic organisms, but it is not clear when it was first used to prepare pneumococci for the purpose of immunization. Tao (1932)[1380] reported that the antigenic potency of formalinized cultures was greater than that of heat-killed cultures in causing the development of agglutinins and protective antibodies in rabbits and mice. Formalin in a concentration of 0.3 per cent was added to the cultures and the treatment of the animals was limited to one subcutaneous and two or three intravenous injections.

Pico and Negrete[1089] prepared immunizing antigens for horses with 0.05 per cent formalin. The authors attributed the keeping qualities of the vaccine to the action of formaldehyde in rendering the soluble specific substance insoluble in water, but it has been the experience of the writers of the present volume that concentrations of formalin as high as 0.3 per cent fail to prevent the gradual lysis of pneumococci suspended in salt solution. In Ferguson's[436] experience in actively immunizing white mice and rabbits with both heat-killed and formalinized vaccines, it appeared that the latter were only slightly superior to heat-killed cultures. Formalin was used in a strength of 0.2 per cent, and suspensions were made in salt solution containing 0.5 per cent phenol. There was a tendency of killed pneumococci to autolyze with a loss of antigenic power accompanying the disintegration of the cell. For this reason, as well as because of their better immunizing effect, Barnes and White gave their choice to heat-killed vaccines, since these vaccines undergo less deterioration than those prepared with formalin.

According to Dubos,* formalin added in a concentration of 0.3 per cent to suspensions of living pneumococci prevents multiplication but fails to inhibit the activity of intracellular enzymes. The

* Personal communication, 1936.

concentration of formalin must be raised to 0.5 per cent if enzymatic activity is to be destroyed. On the other hand, exposure of the pneumococcal suspensions to heat, when properly carried out, yields a vaccine of great stability and of high antigenic integrity. Dubos observed that exposure to temperatures that rob the cell of its ability to grow and multiply may fail to halt the action of the protease of Pneumococcus. To devitalize the organisms, to prevent autolysis, and to preserve the antigenic properties of pneumococci, Dubos heated cultures or suspensions to 75° with the least possible delay and so obtained antigens of greater stability and immunizing power than could be produced by any other method.

Confirming the claims of Barnes and White and of Dubos that immediate heating of pneumococci for use as antigens is the best method for insuring the stability of the preparation, O'Meara and Brown,[1031] during the course of an investigation on the readiness with which pneumococci disintegrate, reported that, in spite of a large number of preservatives tried, no agent except heat was found that would completely arrest autolysis of pneumococcal cultures.

Day[307] used formol, or antiformin, as a killing agent, but abandoned its use since it weakened the immunizing properties of the cultures. Truche[1419-20] favored an alcohol-ether mixture for the routine preparation of antigens in the production of equine antipneumococcic serum, and claimed that cultures so treated, dried in a vacuum, and suspended in salt solution, were tolerated better by horses than were heat-killed cultures.

There have been reported many other methods for rendering pneumococci harmless for immunizing purposes. As early as 1902, Sergent[1256] treated suspensions of agar cultures of pneumococci with crystal violet. Although the dye in the concentration used failed to kill the cocci it effected a partial attenuation, so that rabbits surviving the intravenous or intraperitoneal injection of the treated cultures were able six to eight days later to resist increased doses of the same cultures that proved fatal in animals which had not received a previous injection of the dyed cocci. Sergent's application of coal-tar dyes to pneumococci for the purpose of preparing immunizing antigens appears to be a lone observation of its kind.

Nicolle and Adil-Bey (1907)[1007] obtained immunity in rabbits by the injection of cultures treated with sodium choleate, while Meyer (1927)[897] and later Meyer and Sukneff (1928)[898] reported that Type I pneumococci dissolved in sodium taurocholate would immunize both rabbits and mice. The serum of the rabbits so treated contained a moderate amount of protective substance but, as might be expected, the serum as a rule gave some cross-protection against Type II strains. While pneumococci treated with bile-salts may induce immunity in mice and rabbits and presumably in other animals, the immunity is of a low order and is lacking in type-specificity. As late as 1933, Ziegler[1573] advocated as an immunizing agent "Pneumocholin," a substance of unknown chemical composition produced by the lysis of pneumococci in sodium taurocholate solution. The substance was stable under refrigeration and, when injected into rabbits, induced after three or four days an effective immunity to Type I infection.

Larson and Nelson[791] recommended the use of sodium ricinoleate in the preparation of pneumococcal vaccines both for prophylactic use in man and for the preparation of therapeutic serum. A virulent culture of Pneumococcus treated with ricinoleate soap in a final concentration of 0.1 per cent immediately lost its pathogenicity and, according to the authors, when injected intraperitoneally into rabbits, stimulated the production of large amounts of agglutinins within twenty-four hours. The animals resisted many multiples of the infective dose of pneumococci, and their serum protected normal rabbits against both intravenous and intraperitoneal infection. The serum of rabbits and sheep immunized with the sodium ricinoleate antigens was claimed to possess distinct curative properties for rabbits infected with Pneumococcus. The administration of the immune serum to patients suffering from lobar pneumonia was followed by a rapid drop in temperature and relief of subjective symptoms. Larson believed that the effect was due to the presence of antitoxin in the serum.

In a later communication, Larson[789] reported that the intraperitoneal injection of large amounts of soaped pneumococci of Types I, II, and III protected rabbits against infection induced by the Goodner technique, and claimed that by this method it was possible to produce both species-specific and type-specific immunity.

Sensitized Pneumococci

The use of pneumococci sensitized with homologous immune serum was described by Levy and Aoki (1910),[801] while Alexander,[7] after similarly treating and incubating the cocci with leucocytes, could immunize rabbits with the preparations. Protective substances appeared in the serum of the animals within eight to eleven days after the first injection, but the method possessed no advantages over the use of heat or formalin for the preparation of antigens. Levy and Aoki, and also Killian,[704] employed phenol as a devitalizing agent, but the latter author found that phenolized vaccines showed a definite loss of immunizing power after six weeks' preservation.

Filtrates and Extracts

CULTURE FILTRATES AND BACTERIAL EXTRACTS

Early investigators turned to culture filtrates and to other products and derivatives of Pneumococcus in a search for some principle which would increase the resistance of experimental animals and eventually of man to pneumococcal infection.

Warden (1912)[1485] claimed to have immunized rabbits with pancreatic extracts of pneumococci and made the additional observation, which apparently has never been confirmed, that similar extracts of staphylococci and pancreatic extracts alone were capable of inducing immunity in infected and non-infected rabbits, and of favorably modifying the course of pneumococcal infections in man. However, in Warden's communication no experimental data were presented to support these unusual claims. Aïtoff and Lagrange (1925)[6] stated that an injection of sterile medium T made at least twenty-four hours previous to inoculation with Pneumococcus conferred protection upon mice which was demonstrable for at least two weeks after injection of the medium.

In 1926, Horder and Ferry,[655] in a search for an ideal antigen for therapeutic immunization, measured the agglutinin content and complement-fixing titer of the serum of rabbits treated respectively with washings from agar cultures, autolysates of the residue from broth cultures, washed agar growth, and whole unwashed agar cultures. Horder and Ferry concluded that the material contained in the washings of agar cultures, because it could be prepared in watery solution and was low in protein content, as well as being practically non-toxic and high in antigenic properties, more nearly approached the ideal antigen than any preparation which had come under their observation. Barach (1928)[74-5] reported that Berkefeld filtrates of pneumococci shaken in salt solution and also filtrates of broth cultures caused in mice the development of protection which appeared on the fourth day after injection. The immunity produced was dependent upon type-specific protective substances and not upon the elaboration of the common protein antibody.

Another method of preparing antigens from broth cultures of pneumococci was that described by Maeji (1930),[850, 853-4] who employed the technique of Besredka for preparing antivirus. The supernatant fluid from centrifuged beef-serum bouillon cultures of Type I Pneumococcus, when injected subcutaneously into rabbits, gave partial protection against infection with a Type I strain. In the case of Type II Pneumococcus the protective substance appeared only when goat serum was added to the medium, while with Type III organisms no antivirus could be obtained. Maeji claimed that after the administration of Type I antivirus by inhalation, young rabbits resisted intratracheal inoculation with a virulent culture, and that resistance could be increased by repeated inhalation of the preparation. The attenuating action of filtered broth cultures of pneumococci on fresh cultures of the same organism was reported by Okischio (1932),[1023] but the use of antivirus either for the preparation of vaccines or for the treatment of pneumococcal infections has not come into general use.

There are yet other references to the use of extracts and autolysates of Pneumococcus for the purpose of inducing immunity. Among them might be mentioned those of Day (1930 and 1934)[307, 309] who reported that the intraperitoneal injection into mice of autolysates of both Type I and Type II cultures was followed one week later by protection against one thousand to ten thousand fatal doses of culture. Another communication was that of Harley (1934)[591] in which was reported the preparation of antigens by extracting Type I and II pneumococci with 0.05N hydrochloric acid at 60°.

TISSUE EXTRACTS AND EXUDATES

The possibility that products arising from the vital activities of Pneumococcus in animal tissues might exert immunizing action and that such products might be applied to the protection or treatment of animals and human beings has not been neglected. Foà and Carbone,[463] Bonome (1891),[137] and Mosny (1892)[932] were thus able to render rabbits relatively invulnerable to the injection of otherwise lethal doses of pneumococcal cultures. Hartman (1913)[598] studied the antigenic action of the principal constituents of pneumonic exudates, but the results were largely negative. Freedlander (1928)[480] employed saline extracts of organs of infected rabbits as antigens and, after three injections at five to seven-day intervals into normal rabbits, obtained a serum of high protective titer for mice against Type I Pneumococcus and a serum of somewhat less potency against a Type II culture. While the serums compared favorably in protective action with therapeutic Type I antipneumococcic serum, they were low in agglutinins, contained no precipitins, possessed no remarkable opsonic powers, and displayed no direct bactericidal action.

The idea was revived in 1930 by Banzhaf and Curphey,[71] who combined in horses intramuscular injections of phenolized pneumococcal pleural exudates with intravenous injections of the formalinized sediment from broth cultures of pneumococci. When tested by Goodner's method the therapeutic value of the serum was disproportionate to the mouse-protective action, which fact Banzhaf and Curphey interpreted as indicating the possible presence of added therapeutic substances in the serum resulting from the addition of exudate to the usual method of immunization.

Toxins and Hemotoxins

SO-CALLED TOXINS

The possible existence of toxins either in the pneumococcal cell or resulting from its metabolic processes has already been discussed in Chapter III. It is extremely doubtful if Pneumococcus possesses or produces a true toxin, but the idea still survives, and the action of some therapeutic serums, quite apart from their tropic, agglutinative, precipitative, or protective effects, in ameliorating the intoxication of pneumonia in man, has encouraged the search for a toxic principle with the hope of producing an antitoxin.

The Klemperers (1892)[725] were convinced that they had succeeded in isolating a toxic protein from Pneumococcus, which they named "Pneumotoxin," but the action of the substance can now be explained on other grounds. In 1897, Auld[30] separated an albumose and an organic acid from local lesions, lungs, and spleens of animals infected with Pneumococcus. No adequate proof could be obtained that the protein was a true toxin, but Auld intimated that a true toxin might in all probability be united with the protein. The albumose preparations had a certain immunizing value, but no evidence was advanced to show that the immunity was antitoxic in nature.

In 1912, Rosenow[1166] obtained from pneumococci a poisonous substance, similar to histamine in its action, but wholly incapable of provoking any immune response. Larson,[788] and then Olson (1926),[1029] believed that Pneumococcus contained a toxin and that by injecting animals with whole cultures of the organism treated with sodium ricinoleate, or with autolyzed broth cultures, it was possible to produce an antitoxic serum. The assumption was based solely on the physiological effect of the serum and not on any demonstration or titration of the antitoxin which the serum was supposed to contain.

The work of Parker[1061] and of Parker and McCoy (1929)[1062] is more suggestive. By allowing pneumococci of Types I, II, and III to autolyze under strict, anaerobic conditions, the authors obtained a preparation that was toxic for guinea pigs and for horses and which, when injected repeatedly into horses over a period of eight months, caused the animals so treated to develop in the serum substances capable of neutralizing *in vitro* the toxic autolysates. Parker reported that antipneumotoxic serum produced in rabbits or horses by immunization with sterile filtrates of pneumotoxin afforded heterologous protection to guinea pigs—at least as far as Type I or Type II pneumococci were concerned—against the development of pneumonia, while the serum of some of the treated horses exerted a curative action against infection with pneumococci of the homologous type, but contained little if any antitoxin for heterologous types. Furthermore, since the serums contained no specific protective antibodies against pneumococci, Parker concluded that the serum was antitoxic in action.

The experiments of Parker and McCoy, including a definite determination of the toxic power of sterile pneumococcal autolysates and of the neutralizing strength of serum produced in response to the injection of the autolysates, with evidence of the absence of specific protective antibodies, constitute the first accurately controlled observations of the kind and are sufficiently suggestive to encourage further study of pneumococcal poisons and of their antigenic properties.

Another report of a similar nature was that coming from Jamieson and Powell (1931)[676] who obtained from pneumococci toxic substances not unlike those which have been demonstrated by other workers as being produced by various streptococci. The action of the substances could be demonstrated by skin tests on human beings and on certain breeds of rabbits. By the same method, the serum of horses treated by subcutaneous injections of the toxic substances could be shown to possess neutralizing properties for the alleged toxin. The neutralizing principle could be concentrated to a moderate degree in the refinement of globulins by the usual chemical procedures and, according to Jamieson and Powell, was independent of the small amount of protective antibodies present in the serum.

HEMOTOXINS

In 1927, Neill, Fleming, and Gaspari[958] described the results of studies on the antigenic or immunizing action of various preparations of pneumococcal hemotoxin. The power of the reduced and of the reversibly oxidized forms of hemotoxin to evoke immunity were identical, but preparations in which the hemolytic principle had been rendered irreversible or destroyed by heat or by high concentrations of hydrogen peroxide were inactive in this respect. The serum of rabbits and of horses injected with active hemotoxin neutralized the substance, while the antigenic action of the hemotoxin appeared to be independent of the protein fraction of the cell.

Methods of Administering Antigens

The manner in which Pneumococcus or its several antigens are introduced into the body of an animal of any given species, other factors being constant, may determine both qualitatively and quantitatively the nature of the immunological response. In the early studies on Pneumococcus one finds references to the subcutaneous injection of the organism or its products. The introduction of the intravenous route was followed by the more rapid appearance and a higher level of immunity in the treated animals. The administration of antigens by way of the peritoneal cavity also offered advantages over the subcutaneous route both in time of development of immunity and in heightened resistance.

In 1922, Bronfenbrenner and Knights[149] published the results of a study on the comparative efficacy of the subcutaneous, intravenous, intratracheal, and intrapleural routes for the introduction of pneumococcal antigens. Rabbits were used and the immunity evoked was measured by the bactericidal, opsonizing, and protective power of the serum following the different methods of treatment. The bactericidal titer of the serum from rabbits receiving intravenous and subcutaneous injections, as determined by the Heist and Solis-Cohen[634] technique, was approximately the same and was greater than that of the serum of animals injected either by the intrapleural or intratracheal routes. Both the intratracheal and intrapleural methods induced a much higher opsonic content of the immune serum than did the other procedures, while the administration of antigen by way of the blood, or into the trachea or pleura, caused the rabbits to yield serum containing protective antibody, whereas the serum from rabbits treated subcutaneously failed to confer passive protection on mice.

In communications published in 1924, 1927, and 1930, Stillman[1330-2, 1334-5] supplied additional information concerning the nature and degree of the immune response in mice and rabbits resulting from inhalation, and from the subcutaneous, intramuscular, and intravenous application of both living and dead pneumococci. The serum of 80 per cent of rabbits injected intravenously with fixed amounts of heat-killed pneumococci and the serum of 60 per cent of the animals injected intraperitoneally with similar doses contained agglutinins and all showed protective antibodies. Of rabbits receiving intramuscular injections, the serum of only 33 per cent contained agglutinins although 86 per cent were protective. In the case of animals receiving antigen by the subcutaneous route, none produced agglutinins although protective substances could be demonstrated in 71 per cent of the individual serums.

With skin sensitivity and the presence of type-specific agglutinins and protective substances in serum as criteria for the strength and specificity of pneumococcal antigens, Harley (1935)[592] obtained a higher degree of immunity and far greater type-specificity when vaccines of smooth and rough organisms were introduced intravenously than when injected intradermally.

Killian (1924),[706] by continued subcutaneous and intraperitoneal injections—the so-called bigeminal method—obtained a higher degree of protection in mice than by the subcutaneous route alone, and he believed that the fact argued against the acceptance of the hypothesis that a purely local immunity was necessary for establishing a state of protection against pneumococcal infection. By intravenous injection, extremely small quantities of antigen sufficed to produce protection, the immune state being demonstrable in an increasing degree from the third day after injection. Killian reported that a short refractory period ensued after the administration of antigen, and accordingly, delayed further antigenic stimulation for four days until the period had passed.

It is reasonable to assume that the duration of the refractory period—or the negative phase, as Wright termed it—depends on the route employed in the injection of antigen, the ability of the body cells to respond to subsequent stimulation being contingent upon the rate of absorption of antigenic material from the site of the injection. From foci under the skin, absorption would be less rapid than that from the peritoneal cavity and, quite obviously, the utilization of antigen would be most rapid when the injection is made directly into the blood stream. Because of the slower seepage of antigenic materials from the subcutaneous tissues, that route is preferred for the production of antitoxin, but for the elaboration of antibacterial substances, the intravenous method is the one of choice.

INTRADERMAL INJECTION

The intradermal injection of pneumococci and their products may be followed by the development of the immune state. Goodner (1928),[525-6] in studying the pathogenic action of living pneumococci inoculated into the skin of rabbits, observed that the serum of animals surviving infection had acquired protective antibodies. Furthermore, within five days after a single intradermal injection of dead pneumococci, the normal rabbit developed resistance to infection. In two communications appearing in 1930, Julianelle[687-8] reported that repeated injections of small doses of suspensions of heat-killed pneumococci of Types I and III into the skin of rabbits induced species-specific but in no case type-specific antibodies for the organisms. However, animals developing only species-specific antibodies after intradermal vaccination still possessed the ability to form type-specific immune substances when subsequently given intravenous injections of pneumococci of fixed types. Despite the failure of heat-killed pneumococci when injected intradermally to evoke the formation of type-specific antibodies in the rabbit, devitalized cultures do, nevertheless, render the animal actively immune to infection with pneumococci not only of homologous but also of heterologous type. The injection into the skin of soluble derivatives of Pneumococcus in Julianelle's experiments was not followed by the production of active immunity. The destruction or inactivation in the skin of rabbits of type-specific antigen injected intradermally was later observed by Harley (1935).[593] The somatic protein, on the contrary, appeared to be unaffected and stimulated the formation of species-specific antibodies.

The observation of Julianelle was significant in that it revealed a hitherto unknown property of the epidermal cells of the rabbit.

The ability of that animal when injected intradermally to elaborate species-specific antibody, taken with the inability to manufacture type-specific antibody when similarly injected, points to a partial disruption of the molecular configuration of the pneumococcal antigen during its sojourn in the skin. The type-specific fraction of the antigen is probably destroyed and there remains only the somatic protein and carbohydrate of the bacterial cell to stimulate the immunological mechanism. That the mechanism is, nevertheless, fully capable of functioning in producing type-specific immune substances is shown by the response of the rabbit when the antigen is introduced directly into the blood stream. The hypothesis is further supported by Julianelle's observation that the intradermal injection of heat-killed R forms as well as S forms of pneumococci calls forth the production of active immunity. Julianelle therefore demonstrated that the route of administration of pneumococcal antigen, at least in the rabbit, may be a determining factor in the qualitative nature of the immune response.

An analogous process taking place in the human body was reported in the same year by Francis and Tillett.[478] The repeated injection of the specific capsular polysaccharide of pneumococci of Types I, II, and III into the skin of patients suffering from lobar pneumonia was followed in the second or third week of convalescence by the appearance of circulating antibodies for one or more heterologous types. However, in none of the normal controls was the phenomenon observed. In the next year (1931), Finland and Sutliff[446-7] confirmed the observations of Francis and Tillett. Pneumonia patients receiving repeated intracutaneous injections of soluble specific substance from Type I, II, and III pneumococci, in a week or more developed in the blood agglutinins and protective antibodies sometimes heterologous for the infecting type of organism but, unlike the effect in the rabbit, the immune bodies were homologous for the type of capsular carbohydrate injected.

In a subsequent report (1932), Finland and Sutliff[448] announced that the simultaneous intradermal injection into normal human beings of specific polysaccharide of the first three pneumococcal types and of protein and autolysates derived from organisms of Types I and II was followed by the appearance or increase of the pneumococcidal power of whole defibrinated blood and in most instances by the presence of agglutinins and protective antibodies for one or more types of pneumococci. A single intradermal injection of 0.01 milligram of the capsular polysaccharide of pneumococci of Types I, II, or III, or four similar daily injections, resulted in the development of antibodies corresponding in type only to that of the antigen injected. A single injection into the skin of autolysates obtained from virulent Type I, II, and III pneumococci gave rise to an increase in the pneumococcidal power of whole blood and the appearance of homologous type-agglutinins and protective antibodies in about one-third of the normal subjects. A similar injection of pneumococcal protein, on the contrary, failed to evoke specific antibodies to any appreciable degree.

Further evidence of the antigenic action of specific polysaccharides injected into the skin of normal individuals was presented by Zozaya and Clark[1590] who, after the intradermal injection of soluble specific substance of pneumococci of Types I, II, and III were able to demonstrate homologous precipitins and protective antibodies in the serum of human beings, who gave no history of recent pneumococcal infection. Another observation of these authors may be repeated here. It was found that by increasing the surface area of the carbohydrate by adsorption on charcoal or celloidin particles it was possible to evoke antigenic properties in preparations that otherwise appeared to lack immunizing action and to enhance the action of preparations that already possessed these properties. Francis,[474] in a still more recent paper (1934), described experiments in which he studied the antigenic action of the original and the acetylated forms of the specific polysaccharide of Pneumococcus. Weekly doses of 0.01 milligram were administered intradermally over a period of three weeks to normal individuals. The experiment showed that both the original soluble specific substance and the acetylated polysaccharide of Pneumococcus stimulated the development of type-specific agglutinins, precipitins, and mouse-protective antibodies in the serum of normal human beings.

A consideration of the work of Julianelle, of Francis and Tillett, of Finland and Sutliff, and of Zozaya and Clark demonstrates that the antigenic constituents of Pneumococcus introduced by the intradermal route may act as immunizing agents and that, while in man both type-specific immunity and corresponding type-specific antibodies may be developed, the skin of the rabbit possesses the power so to alter pneumococcal antigen that only species-specific immunity results. The difference in the epidermal and possibly the other somatic cells of animals of diverse species in their reaction to the parenteral introduction of Pneumococcus and its derivatives offers a field for study which should aid in clarifying some of the questions concerning the physiological processes involved in the development of the immune state.

INHALATION AND INTRABRONCHIAL INSUFFLATION

After giving repeated inhalations of Type I Pneumococcus, Stillman[1331-2] demonstrated agglutinins and protective antibodies in the serum of rabbits so treated. Agglutinin production appeared to remain stationary after the fifth exposure to antigen, while the protective antibody content steadily rose. Repeated inhalations of killed pneumococci by mice resulted in only a slight degree of immunity, but when living organisms were similarly administered a definite degree of active immunity could be induced in the animals.

Eguchi (1925)[351] confirmed Stillman's observation on the protection developing in mice following the inhalation of killed pneumococci, and found further that immunity could be induced by organisms of Type II as well as those of Type I. Maeji[853] also reported that, in the case of antivirus, inhalation was an effective mode of protecting young rabbits against subsequent infection with Pneumococcus, and that the degree of protection increased with the quantity of inhaled antivirus and the number of applications.

Although Cooper (1926)[276] failed in attempts to immunize rabbits to Pneumococcus by either the subcutaneous or intradermal injection of heat-killed cultures, he was able by applying the vaccine beneath the buccal membrane of the cheek to protect the majority of rabbits so treated for a period of four months against a fatal dose of the organism. Instillation of the vaccine into the eye or swabbing the nose and mouth with the agent failed to result in any effective immunity. Stuppy and Falk (1928)[1351] reinvestigated the subject presented by Cooper. Rabbits receiving ten to twenty daily injections of heat-killed Type I pneumococci into the buccal mucosa later survived inoculation with 1,000 M.L.D. of the same strain; of the animals receiving five preliminary injections three out of four lived; while all rabbits given only one or two injections died. Ten daily subcutaneous, intradermal, intravenous, and intratracheal injections or the administration of the vaccine by intratracheal insufflation or by intraocular instillation (contrary to the claims of Cooper) protected the animals against subsequent infection, although vaccination by insufflation or instillation was less reliable as an immunizing procedure than was the administration of the killed culture into the buccal submucosa or into the trachea.

Stuppy, Cannon, and Falk[1350] rendered rabbits immune to intraperitoneal infection with pneumococci of Types I and II by the daily insufflation into the nose and throat of suspensions of heat-killed cultures of homologous type, but failed in similar attempts with Type III organisms. In rabbits so treated, the insufflation of living, virulent pneumococci induced a proliferative and exudative type of reaction in the lung in which the macrophage was the predominant cell, accompanied by considerable numbers of eosinophiles. This altered reactivity of the pulmonary tissues was interpreted by the authors as affording evidence of a definite, localized type of tissue immunity in the lung. Heterologous cultures of living pneumococci induced the local immune reaction but to a lesser degree.

ORAL ADMINISTRATION

When pneumococci enter the body by way of the alimentary canal, their constituents may eventually reach the body cells responsible for the creation of immune bodies. In 1925, Eguchi[351] reported that attempts to immunize mice by feeding them Type I pneumococci met with some success when young mice were used but with none in the case of adult mice. Kimura (1927),[710] nevertheless, was able to protect a large percentage of adult mice against one hundred to one thousand lethal doses of Type I pneumococci by dropping into the mouths of the animals large amounts of heat-killed cocci of the corresponding type. A similar result attended Maeji's attempts to induce active immunity in mice by spraying the mouth with suspensions of pneumococci of Types I and II. When the effort was successful, there developed cross-protection, especially between Types I and II, with some protective action against Type III strains. Maeji[849] subsequently (1929) was able to immunize young mice, rats, and rabbits by the daily feeding of large quantities of broth cultures of highly virulent Type III organisms. Although young rabbits could be rendered resistant to infection with Type III pneumococci by the oral administration of cultures of the corresponding type, no agglutinins could be detected in the serum of the animals.

For the purpose of increasing the permeability of the intestinal mucosa for pneumococcal antigen, McDaniels (1931)[876] fed young white rats first with egg-white and then thirty minutes later with autolysates of Type I Pneumococcus. When tested after the lapse of five days by intraperitoneal inoculation with a virulent strain of Type I Pneumococcus, all the animals showed toleration of many lethal doses of culture, while the rats that had received a preliminary feeding with egg-white exhibited a greater resistance to infection than did those that had not been so fed. In a second communication (1932), McDaniels[877] reported attempts to ascertain the details of the immunological mechanism operating in orally immunized rats. Normal control rats and rats previously injected with egg-white and Type I pneumococcal autolysates were inoculated intraperitoneally with one hundred fatal doses of a virulent, homologous strain of Pneumococcus. All the normal rats died within two to four days, while 96 per cent of the vaccinated animals survived. Although the leucocyte count was subject to wide fluctuations, the immunized rats, six hours after inoculation, always showed an appreciably higher white-cell count than did the unvaccinated controls. In none of the vaccinated rats which survived infection could pneumococci be demonstrated in the blood, although pneumococcemia was present in all the animals that succumbed.

Ross (1931)[1188] described the comparative immunizing action of soluble specific substance and of whole or dissolved pneumococci when fed to rats. One feeding of Type I SSS sufficed to protect the test animals against intraperitoneal injection of virulent Type I organisms, and the increased type-specific resistance was comparable, with slight quantitative differences, to that following the oral administration of intact or dissolved pneumococci. Ross failed to immunize mice by a similar procedure and attributed the failure to some cell constituent active in the mouth of mice. In other papers (1932), Ross[1189-90] reported that the capsular polysaccharide of Type II Pneumococcus was incapable, when introduced by the oral route, of increasing the resistance of rats to infection. The soluble specific substance of Type III organisms induced protection in rats to organisms of the homologous type but the percentage of animals so protected was less than in the case of animals receiving the whole or intact cell by mouth. When the specific polysaccharide of Type I Pneumococcus was fed to rats, no immunity against Type II or Type III organisms was obtained, and the ingestion of SSS of Types II and III did not protect the animals against Type I organisms. An observation of Ross on the fate of the ingested polysaccharide was that a very large proportion of the substance, when fed to rats, appeared in the feces.

Further experiments on oral immunization against Pneumococcus, when applied to rabbits, were described in 1932 by Kolmer and Rule.[745] The antigens comprised a) pneumococci of Types I, II, and III cultivated in sterile milk for twenty-four hours and heated at 60° for one hour, b) twenty-four-hour broth cultures of the same types exposed for two hours to a N/15 concentration of hydrochloric acid, and c) sedimented cocci from twenty-four-hour broth cultures subsequently treated with sodium taurocholate. The materials were administered daily for seven days through a stomach tube, and one week after the last treatment the rabbits were inoculated intratracheally with living broth cultures. While to Kolmer and Rule the acid-killed cocci, of the three kinds of preparations used, appeared to engender the highest degree of immunity, the figures are not significant because of the lack of uniformity of the results and the low virulence of the Type II and Type III cultures employed in testing the resistance of the rabbits.

In a second report (1933), Kolmer and Rule[747] stated that the oral administration of acid-killed vaccines made from Type I, II, and III pneumococci, in doses representing 100 to 1,000 million organisms per kilo of body weight, were effective in rendering rabbits immune to subsequent intratracheal infection with pneumococci of the homologous type. Although occasionally a single dose of 1,000 million cocci produced active immunity against infection by Type I Pneumococcus, the best results were obtained with a minimum of five daily doses. The immunity thus induced was transient, decreasing after one month's time and practically disappearing in six months. Vaccines introduced by way of the mouth were inferior in immunizing action to similar agents injected subcutaneously. Using monkeys as test animals, and employing vaccines of pneumococci killed by tricresol and by hydrochloric acid, Kolmer and

Rule confirmed the superiority of the subcutaneous over the oral route of administration.

Host Response

As in all physiological processes there are periods in the development of an animal when the somatic cells function more actively in absorbing alien material and in creating and extruding immune substances into the circulating blood. This power may be lacking in very young animals, but it appears to increase as the animal grows and reaches a stage of full vigor, and then to decline as the metabolism of the body cells wanes. In addition to quantitative differences due to age in the antibody content of serum of rabbits immunized against Pneumococcus, Baumgartner (1934)[91-2] detected qualitative variations as well in the antibodies elaborated by young and older animals. The fact is sufficiently well established in immunological practice to require no detailed discussion.

Antagonistic Action of Soluble Specific Substance

In preceding chapters, mention was made of the aggressin-like action of soluble specific substance, of the zonal effect observed when this substance was used as an immunizing agent, and of its antagonistic behavior in reactions between immune serum and Pneumococcus or its derivatives. The soluble specific substance, although non-toxic in itself, can enhance the invasive power of pneumococci (Felton and Bailey[419]). The phenomenon may be an additive effect which, in turn, may be due to some interference with the natural defense mechanism of the body. Whatever the explanation of this property of specific polysaccharides, it is a fact to be reckoned with in the production of active immunity, in testing the immunity established by the administration of pneumococcal antigens, and in measuring the potency of antipneumococcic serum.

Felton and Bailey demonstrated that the immunizing action of soluble specific substance operated within certain prescribed limits. A definite minimum of the material was obviously necessary to incite the formation of antibodies, but when the dose was increased, a point was reached beyond which no immunity developed. Saito and Ulrich (1928)[1214] also observed this zone of antigenic effectiveness with a carbohydrate preparation in producing a state of protection in animals. A similar observation on the cellular carbohydrate was reported by Wadsworth and Brown (1931).[1466-7] There can be no doubt that pneumococcal antigen, particularly the capsular polysaccharide, in excess of a certain optimal amount hinders its own immunizing action.

Another manifestation of the antagonistic action of the soluble specific substance is seen in the blocking of the reaction between pneumococcal antigen and homologous antibody. Felton and Bailey[419] drew attention to the inhibiting power of SSS frequently noted in precipitin and protection tests when amounts of antigen and serum greater than the optimum are used. The authors ascribed the antagonism to the presence of precipitable residues in immune serum as well as to an excess of soluble specific substance in the antigen. The work of Felton and Bailey and that of Sickles (1927)[1277] point to at least one factor responsible for the inhibiting power of the soluble carbohydrate. Through its precipitating action, the polysaccharide removes some of the protective antibody from immune serum and at the same time (Sickles) interferes with phagocytosis, consequently robbing the serum of protective properties. The observation recalls that of Sia (1927),[1268] who found that Pneumococcus could adsorb normal opsonin from the serum of animals naturally resistant to pneumococcal infection—an observation later confirmed by Ward (1930)[1480-1] for normal human whole blood, and who also, like Sia, noted that the action was type-specific. Ward suggested that the zone of inhibition was caused by the specific precipitate formed by the antiserum and homologous capsular polysaccharide, which interfered, perhaps mechanically, with the ingestion of the pneumococci by leucocytes.

Enders and Wu (1934)[362] reported that the A carbohydrate

from Pneumococcus possessed a greater anti-opsonic action than the deacetylated polysaccharide. The opsonic titer of normal human serum was practically nullified by the addition of the A carbohydrate, while in immune serum the A carbohydrate brought about a greater diminution in opsonic activity than did its derivatives. The result was therefore a complete inhibition of the pneumococcidal action of normal serum and a partial blocking of the same action of specific immune serum. The inhibitory or antagonistic behavior of the carbohydrate fraction of Pneumococcus calls for careful discrimination in the selection of the antigenic dosage of pneumococcal materials for the production of active immunity and also for conducting serological reactions which have to do with the immune state.

Summary

The substance of the material presented in this chapter may be expressed as follows: The immunizing properties and type-specific antigenic action of Pneumococcus and its derivatives are directly proportional to the virulence of the culture employed and appear to be the same whether the organism is in a living condition or appropriately killed by heat or by formalin, the integrity of the immunizing principle being better preserved in suspensions of heat-killed than of formalinized pneumococci. Filtrates from fluid cultures and watery or saline extracts of pneumococci, representing as they do only a part of the antigenic components of the pneumococcal cell, are more limited in immunizing properties than the entire cell. Although specially prepared broth cultures may exhibit a toxic action in animals, it does not necessarily follow that the injection of the alleged toxins results in the production of pneumococcal antitoxin. To be sure, some evidence of such a possibility has been presented but at the present time it would be going beyond the facts to say that Pneumococcus contains or elaborates a true toxin or that antitoxic processes are a recognized part of the immunological mechanism against Pneumococcus.

Because of simplicity of preparation, stability, and freedom from undesirable secondary action, heat-killed vaccines are preferable to those prepared with bile, bile salts, soaps, or other solvents or devitalizing agents. Sensitized cocci present no advantages in immunizing properties over cells untreated with specific immune serum.

The route by which antigens are introduced into the animal body affects both the kind and quantity of specific antibodies called forth. Injection into the venous system is the most effective method for inducing a high degree of immunity and strict type-specificity of the antibodies. Injection into the peritoneal cavity, into the muscles, or under the skin likewise leads to the elaboration of antibodies but, owing to the respectively slower absorption of antigen, there is a broadening of the specificity of the immunological response. Injection of pneumococcal substance into the skin stimulates the formation of antibodies but type-specificity may be sacrificed for species-specificity. The introduction of antigen into the bronchi by inhalation, insufflation, or injection, and also by enteric paths, is even less effective in raising the level of resistance or in evoking demonstrable immune substances in the circulating blood.

The age of the animal treated with immunizing agents is another condition that determines the ability of animals to respond, at least in a quantitative way, to antigenic stimuli, while different species of animals display various physiological traits when injected parenterally with Pneumococcus or its derivatives.

The antagonistic effect of excessive doses of pneumococcal material, particularly of the specific capsular polysaccharide, may again be emphasized, since the amount of the soluble specific substance in a vaccine influences the development of the immune state or of immune substances.

These, then, are the several factors which condition the immunological behavior of animals toward substances of pneumococcal origin and which qualify any definition of the term antigen.

CHAPTER XI

ANTIBODIES TO PNEUMOCOCCUS

The nature of the immune substances appearing after the injection of Pneumococcus, its constituents, or products into the animal body; the detection and estimation of specific antibodies in immune serum; with a brief discussion of the factors which operate in establishing immunity to Pneumococcus.

THE introduction into animals of pneumococci, their derivatives, or their several metabolic products generates a variety of antagonistic substances which may serve to protect the animal against subsequent infection with virulent members of this bacterial species. In the present chapter there will be discussed the substances to be found in the circulating blood after active immunization and analogous substances normally present in animals, as well as changes in the somatic cells contributing to the immune state induced by parenteral injection of pneumococcal materials.

The manifestations of the physiological functions aroused by the administration to animals of different species of pneumococci in one form or another are many and varied. Furthermore, the substances evolved in the immune processes are so closely related and so intimately mingled in immune serum that a discussion of any one of the specific substances necessarily involves that of other associated antibodies. However, in reviewing the investigations of earlier workers, one finds that the various immunological effects were discovered one by one, until the mosaic of pneumococcal immunity—still incomplete, to be sure—has assumed a definite pattern which can now be recognized by improved serological and biochemical methods.

Agglutinins

The first tangible effect referable to an altered bodily state following the injection of pneumococci was that of agglutinin formation. Meager as was Metchnikoff's[894] description of the phenomenon, it was undoubtedly he who, in 1891, first observed the clumping of pneumococci in immune serum. Issaeff,[673] two years later, confirmed Metchnikoff's observation, and added that the serum of rabbits vaccinated with Pneumococcus when mixed with the organism, instead of becoming cloudy, developed a deposit. It is probable that in one of Mosny's[933] experiments (1892) agglutination took place although he interpreted the result in a different way. The incubation of a culture of Pneumococcus in normal rabbit serum was attended by a diffuse clouding of the medium with a granular sediment appearing after twenty-four hours, while in immune serum the faint cloud disappeared after eight hours due very likely to the sedimentation of agglutinated cells. In 1896, Washbourn[1486] undoubtedly observed agglutination, for he described the sediment accumulating in immune rabbit serum twenty-four hours after the addition of pneumococci as consisting "of pneumococci staining well and grouped in masses."

It was Bezançon and Griffon[108-10] who, in 1897, recognized the phenomenon as agglutination and compared the effect in the case of Pneumococcus to the Widal test for the diagnosis of typhoid infection. Although there was no difficulty in demonstrating the agglutinative properties of fluids collected from animals dying from pneumococcal infections, the results obtained with serum from patients suffering from similar infections were somewhat confusing. However, Bezançon and Griffon gave a correct interpretation to their results in concluding that from the standpoint of agglutination there existed several races of pneumococci. In the first five cases of pneumonia studied, the organisms isolated agglutinated well in immune serum and these strains were referred to by the authors as *vulgaire* pneumococci. By the agglutination method, the French workers differentiated a strain with all the characteristics of Type III Pneumococcus and were therefore the first bacteriologists to recognize the applicability of the agglutination reaction to the differentiation of Pneumococcus from related bacterial species and to the serological classification of pneumococci.

In 1902, Neufeld[974] took exception to some of his predecessors who had studied agglutination of pneumococci with specific serum. He excluded any experiments in which only thread-like growths were observed, and contended that in none of the previous studies was the serum diluted, nor were the observations made soon enough after the organisms and immune serum were mixed. It was in this communication that Neufeld first described the *Quellung* effect which appeared when homologous immune serum was added to pneumococci. Neither normal rabbit nor normal human serum agglutinated pneumococci but normal beef serum often caused clumping of the organisms. Neufeld also noted that dead as well as living pneumococci were susceptible to the clumping action of immune serum, and that in the reaction the cocci were not dissolved nor were the living organisms killed. Neufeld met with difficulties in preserving the agglutinative titer of some samples of immune rabbit serum—a difficulty later experienced by Hintze (1921)[647] and others with rabbit serum. More recently, Valentine, McGuire, Whitney, and Falk (1931)[1443] reported that the agglutination titer of dried antipneumococcic serum kept at room temperature decreased more rapidly than the mouse-protective titer. However, when the desiccated serum preparations were preserved at ice-box temperatures, the potency of the serum in this respect was not appreciably affected.

AGGLUTININS IN THE BLOOD OF PNEUMONIA PATIENTS

The serum of patients convalescing from pneumonia was in some cases found by Neufeld to contain agglutinins. Sometimes their appearance was observed shortly before crisis although the agglutinating power of convalescent serum was highest on the day after crisis. The later observation was duplicated in the same year by Huber,[663] who also reported that the agglutinative properties of convalescent serum progressively diminished and completely disappeared ten days after crisis. Similar results were obtained by Rosenow (1903),[1158] who found that when culture and serum came from the same patient agglutination was most pronounced, but in none of the serums from sixty-five cases of pneumonia when tested against twenty-five strains of Pneumococcus did agglutination fail to take place. Jehle (1903)[678] was able to demonstrate relatively high agglutinating power in the serum of all cases tested of croupous pneumonia terminating in crisis but, contrary to Huber and Rosenow, Jehle observed that only comparatively small amounts of agglutinin were demonstrable forty-eight hours after crisis and that the antibody had practically disappeared four days later.

In a second communication, Rosenow (1904)[1159] reported additional tests on the serum of pneumonia patients which confirmed his earlier results, and made the observation that pneumococci replanted from the agglutinated mass in immune serum were viable as long as thirty days after being agglutinated. Wadsworth[1455] substituted for the whole culture as antigen saline suspensions of pneumococci sedimented from twenty-four to thirty-six-hour-old broth cultures and carried out agglutination experiments with immune serum obtained from rabbits which had previously been injected with dead and later with living pneumococci. With serum from pneumonia patients in dilutions of 1 to 10 to 1 to 20 the antigen gave positive reactions in five or six hours. Wadsworth confirmed Neufeld's negative results for normal rabbit and bullock serum, but found that normal human serum in a dilution of 1 to 10 agglutinated pneumococci in less than eighteen hours. When the serum was diluted in a proportion of 1 to 30, no agglutination took place. In 1905, Longcope[824] described the sediment occurring when pneumococci were added to serum obtained from pneumonia patients, and also the accompanying swelling of the bacterial capsule, previously observed by Neufeld.

In a study of the various characters of a large number of strains of pneumococci from a variety of human sources, Kindborg (1905)[713] obtained immune rabbit and sheep serum of high agglutinin titer, but concluded that agglutination was specific only for the strain used in the preparation of the serum employed in the test. In the same year, Collins,[270] after immunizing rabbits successively with heat-killed and then with living broth cultures, tested the serum so prepared against some seventy strains of Pneumococcus. The serum of an animal immunized with one particular strain of Pneumococcus agglutinated only seven of the organisms when used in a dilution equalling that in which the homologous organism agglutinated.

Collins concluded from her study that pneumococci by reason of their agglutinative properties exhibit a tendency to separate into numerous groups, and also that by the reaction of agglutination *Pneumococcus mucosus* forms a distinct and consistent variety. The conclusions were based on results obtained by the method of agglutinin-absorption, which indicated that the agglutinating substances consist of specific and group agglutinins. Collins, appreciating that pneumococci showed marked differences in ability to undergo agglutination, and believing that there existed different types or groups as far as their agglutinative ability was concerned, was convinced that it was not possible to establish a definite relationship between the agglutination reaction and other characters of pneumococci except in the case of *Pneumococcus mucosus*.

Two other reports published before the serological classification of pneumococci was established are those of Panichi (1907),[1047-8] and of Cotoni and Truche (1912).[284] The former author, after testing the agglutinative property of a strain of Pneumococcus at different stages of growth in bouillon when added to serum from rabbits, sheep, and asses previously injected with the same culture, concluded that agglutinability of the organism was greater during the process of growth than after the cocci had attained full development. Curative serums, including one prepared by Pane, did not necessarily contain agglutinins. The experimental data suggest that the serums employed were of low potency and, hence, the results are not significant. Cotoni and Truche tested some thirty-one miscellaneous strains of pneumococci isolated from men, guinea pigs, rabbits, and horses against thirty-eight samples of serum from patients suffering from pneumococcal infections and against immune serum from horses and sheep, as well as normal serum, but the results of the agglutination reactions were confusing. For example, normal horse serum, under the conditions of the experiment, agglutinated the majority of the strains while normal sheep serum affected only a few of them. The action of the immune serums was indefinite, and Cotoni and Truche concluded that identification of pneumococci on the basis of agglutinability was uncertain.

The appearance of agglutinins in the blood during the course of lobar pneumonia was studied by Chickering (1914),[222] who found the antibody to be present in a large percentage of cases due to Groups I, II, and IV. In the most severe cases and in fatal cases, agglutinins could not be demonstrated nor could any be found, by the technique employed, in the blood of patients suffering from infection with Type III Pneumococcus. When agglutinins were demonstrable they usually appeared at the time of crisis, whereas in some cases agglutinins were present for only one day, while in others they persisted for several weeks. In infections due to pneumococci of Types I and II the reaction was always specific for the type of organism causing the infection, while in infections due to organisms of Group IV the strain was agglutinated only by a serum strictly homologous for that strain.

In an investigation of the antigen-antibody balance in lobar pneumonia, Blake (1918)[125] noted that prior to or coincident with the appearance of agglutinins, pneumococci disappeared from the blood. Patients who developed an excess of agglutinins over antigen invariably recovered; those who showed a progressive increase in the excess of antigen without the development of demonstrable antibodies invariably died. Clough[238] confirmed Chickering's findings in demonstrating pneumococcal agglutinins in approximately

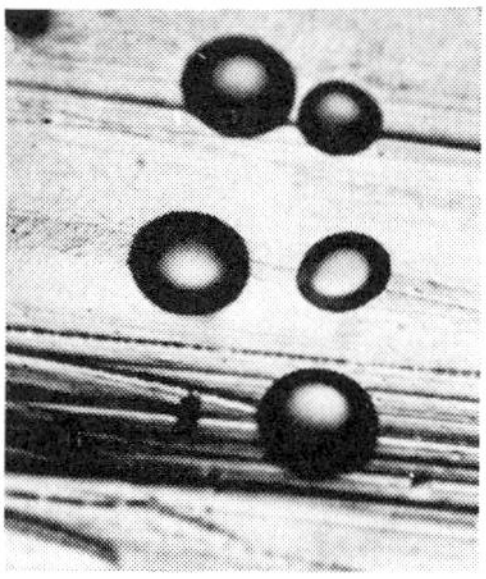

a

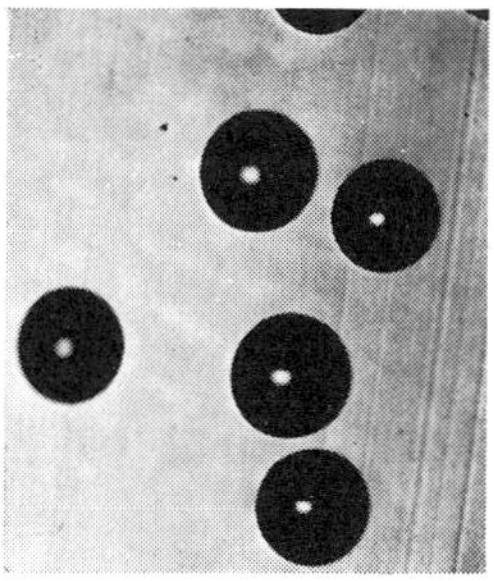

b

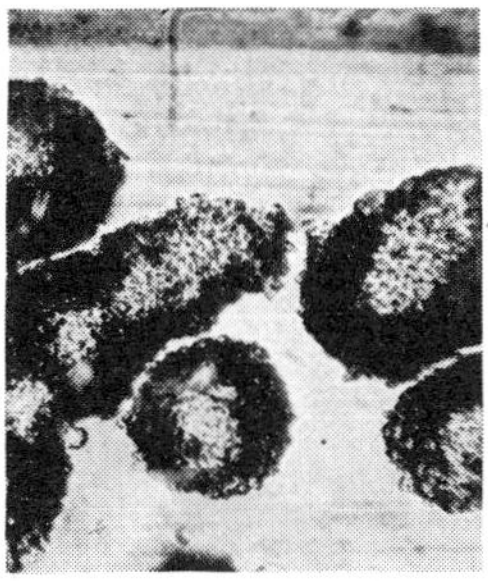

c

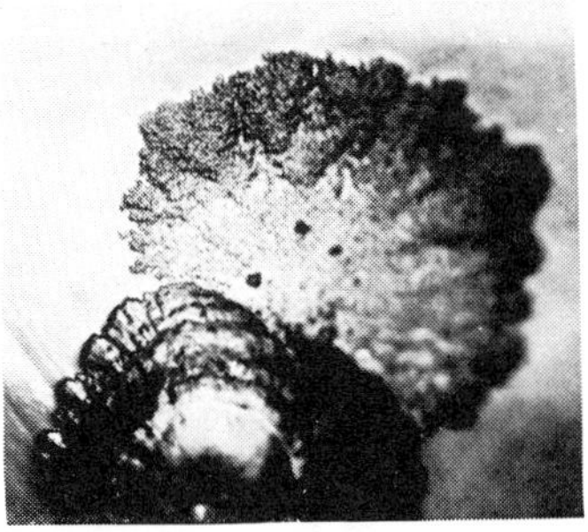

d

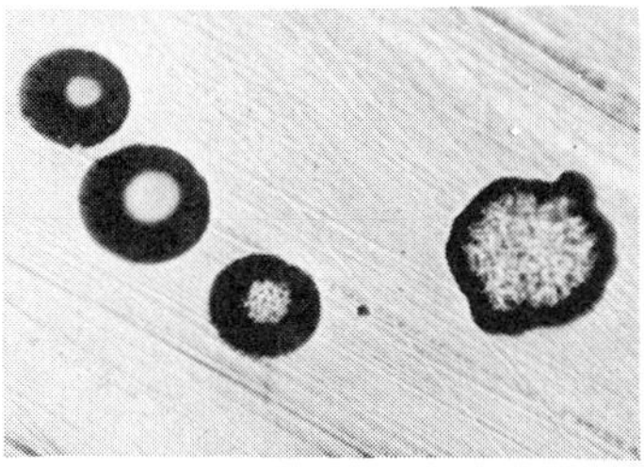

e

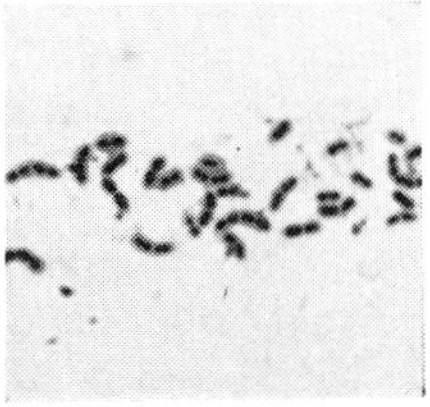

f

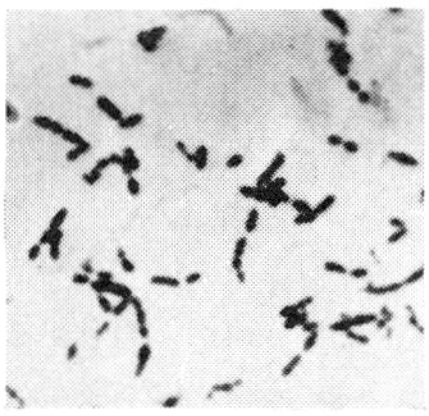

g

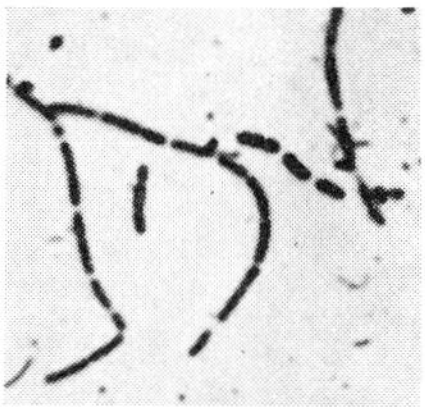

h

Courtesy of Dr. M. A. Dawson

MUCOID, SMOOTH, AND ROUGH PHASES OF PNEUMOCOCCUS

a. Mucoid colonies; twenty-four hours on blood agar. × 32. b. Smooth colonies; twenty-four hours on blood agar. × 32. c. Rough colonies; twenty-four hours on blood agar. × 32. d. Smooth colony with Rough "outbursts"; nine days on blood agar. × 32. e. Mucoid, Smooth, and Rough colonies; sixteen hours on blood agar. The Smooth colony shows a fine granulation or stippling. × 32. f. Mucoid organisms from twenty-four-hour colony on blood agar. Hiss capsule stain. × 1350. g. Smooth organisms from twenty-four-hour colony on blood agar. Gram stain. × 1350. h. Rough organisms from eighteen-hour colony on blood agar. Gram stain. × 1350.

three-fourths of the cases of lobar pneumonia tested, and substantiated Blake's observation that pneumonia patients who failed to develop demonstrable agglutinins succumbed to the infection.

The agglutination curve of the blood of pneumonia patients receiving antipneumococcic serum was employed by Cole (1917)[258] to explain variations in the curative action of the serum.

AGGLUTINATION AND SEROLOGICAL CLASSIFICATION

In studies carried on by Neufeld and Haendel[991] during the years 1909 to 1912, it was learnt that agglutination of typical and atypical pneumococci corresponded to susceptibility to the protective action of specific immune serum. In 1913, Dochez and Gillespie,[322] by the methods of mouse protection and agglutination, were able to separate strains of pneumococci isolated from cases of lobar pneumonia into four groups. The close agreement in the results demonstrated the value of the agglutination reaction in differentiating pneumococci, while the absence of cross-agglutination between the majority of representatives of the fourth group attested the heterogenicity of that class. Hanes[588] applied the method to cultures of Pneumococcus obtained from lobar pneumonia patients and, while confirming the work of Dochez and Gillespie, encountered difficulties in the serological identification of Type III organisms. In attempts to demonstrate specific agglutinins in the serum of rabbits highly immunized to cultures of the mucoid variety of Pneumococcus, the results were uniformly negative, but when the decapsulating method of Porges was used, in every instance the organisms agglutinated with homologous Type III serum, showed constant cross-agglutination within the group, and failed to react with immune serum for Types I and II and for streptococci. Hanes, therefore, suggested that henceforth the name *Pneumococcus mucosus* should be adopted for organisms of this group instead of the older designation, *Streptococcus mucosus*. With the aid of the Porges technique, Nicolle, Jouan, and Debains[1011] obtained agglutination with strains of Pneumococcus that previously had failed to agglutinate with immune serum of the authors' preparation or with samples of serum from America.

Gillespie (1914)[516] reported that strains of Type I and II pneumococci exhibited narrow zones of agglutination whereas organisms of the other types showed broad zones, and ascribed the variations to the differences in the hydrogen ion concentration of the cultures used and to the greater susceptibility of pneumococci of Types I and II to the inhibiting action of salts. Armstrong (1921–1922)[19-20] placed greater reliance on the method of agglutinin-absorption than on simple agglutination in the classification of strains of pneumococci, since he believed that the latter technique was not always sufficient for recognition of type. On the basis of agglutinability, Olmstead,[1027-8] Griffith,[558] and later Cooper and her associates[272-4] extended the serological classification of pneumococci to include the present thirty-two separate and specific types.

AGGLUTINABILITY OF PNEUMOCOCCAL VARIANTS

The experiments of Stryker[1348] in 1916 demonstrated that the biological changes produced in pneumococci by growth in homologous immune serum included alterations in agglutinative behavior. In 1923, Blake and Trask[129] found that a similar treatment of pneumococcal cultures resulted, along with loss of virulence, in constant and distinct changes in agglutinability, with respect to both the character of agglutination and the zone of optimal reaction. The changes appeared to be not a gradual alteration of all members of a culture, but to consist in a rapid and complete change in individual organisms. Three main variants developed after growth in immune serum, and all exhibited marked differences in agglutinability. Analogous changes in the agglutinability of typical pneumococci after cultivation under unfavorable conditions were reported in the same year by Yoshioka.[1564] Cultivation on unsuitable media at 39° and long drying in the desiccator brought about a marked decrease in the agglutinative ability of the cultures in the presence of homologous serum, and caused the development of agglutinability with heterologous serum. The changes appeared irregularly and suddenly. Megrail and Ecker,[888] on the contrary, claimed that Type I Pneumococcus in contact with Type I serum resisted the immunological change, as did the same organism when passed through a series of sterile abscesses artificially produced in mice and rats.

As has already been explained in Chapter V, the dissociation of typical pneumococci into degraded variants is accompanied by a loss of type-specificity and the development of species-specificity in the agglutinative properties of the organism. When the degenerative process has not extended too far and the organism is then appropriately stimulated by animal passage with the accompaniment of vaccines of typical strains or by growth in antirough serum, the organism may develop type-specific agglutinogens as it approaches the parent strain in its biological characters.

AGGLUTININS IN THE BLOOD OF ANIMALS

Bull (1915–1916)[170, 172-4] ascribed to agglutinins a decisive part in the resistance of animals to pneumococcal infection. He found that the injection of small quantities of specific antipneumococcic serum brought about almost instantaneous and specific agglutination of pneumococci in the circulation of infected rabbits. In all instances of both natural and passive immunity investigated, agglutination of the bacteria within the blood of the infected animal was followed by the rapid removal of the agglomerated cocci from the circulation and their destruction either by phagocytosis or in the capillary systems of the viscera. Unagglutinated pneumococci might remain in the blood stream and produce a progressive septicemia.

There could be found only one reference in the literature to the possible effect of an alien infection on agglutinins in the blood of immunized animals. Reimann and Wu (1930)[1132] reported that experimental typhus fever in guinea pigs vaccinated with pneumococci had no influence on the pneumococcal agglutinins.

ADDITIONAL DATA

According to Goodner,[528] agglutinins are associated with the least soluble globulins—the euglobulin fraction—of antipneumococcic horse serum. No references could be found regarding the distribution of pneumococcal agglutinins in the protein portions of specific immune serum of other animals. In a study of the changes in bacterial volume as a result of specific agglutination, Jones and Little (1933)[681-2] stated that during specific agglutination globulin from immune serum is deposited on the surface of the organism. The increase in volume of pneumococci might be ascribed to the interaction of cellular carbohydrate and immune globulin—possibly agglutinin—which results in a swelling, or *Quellung* to use the Neufeld term, of the cocci.

In the mechanism of the type-specific agglutination of Pneumococcus, Francis[472] found that when the organisms were not present in sufficient numbers to absorb completely all the antibodies from immune serum, more antibody was bound by cellular carbohydrate than was required for the process of agglutination. The excess of antibody thus fixed could then unite with additional amounts of soluble specific substance when the polysaccharide was added in soluble form to the agglutinated material. When an excess of free SSS was added to an agglutinated mass of antibody and pneumococci, the organisms were redispersed, and in the suspended state were again specifically agglutinable. Francis concluded that the reactive substance of the pneumococcal cell in type-specific agglutination is the capsular polysaccharide. The observation agrees with the observation of Avery and Goebel (1933)[46] that Type I acetyl polysaccharide in purified form absorbs from Type I antipneumococcic serum all demonstrable type-specific agglutinins as well as precipitins and protective antibodies.

Precipitins

While investigating the massing of pneumococci in the presence of immune serum, Neufeld[974] dissolved the organisms in bile, added the clear solution to the specific serum which had agglutinated the culture, and noted that a particulate substance became microscopically visible within a quarter-hour. The aggregations grew and finally formed macroscopic masses of peculiar form and with a hyaline appearance. Neufeld thus showed the close relation that exists between specific agglutination and precipitation, and the experiments indicated that both phenomena were due to the same elements in the bacterial body and in the immune serum but, owing to the physical state of the antigenic substance, differed only in the manner of manifestation. In the next year (1903), Wadsworth,[1455] applying Neufeld's technique to saline suspensions of pneumococci and using normal rabbit bile for solution of the organisms, corroborated Neufeld's observations. In order to eliminate any action of the bile, Wadsworth shook the centrifuged cultures with strong salt solution, brought the suspensions to the isotonic point, and filtered them. The filtrate precipitated with immune rabbit serum as in the case of the bile solutions of the cocci. The experiment showed that the substance precipitable by immune serum was a constituent of the normal pneumococcal cell and that it could be extracted by suitable solvents. Panichi (1907),[1047] by using filtrates of broth cultures of pneumococci, obtained precipitation with serum from rabbits, sheep, and asses previously immunized with the same organism. The reaction in the different serums varied in degree. A marked reaction was characterized by an immediate opalescence; flakes soon separated, became larger, and settled to the bottom of the fluid in the form of a membrane which did not diffuse on shaking. In milder reactions the sediment was easily dispersed.

In 1917, Dochez and Avery[321] discovered that the urine of animals experimentally infected with Pneumococcus and also the urine and blood serum of individuals ill with lobar pneumonia showed the presence of a specifically precipitable substance in almost every instance during some stage of the disease. Precipitinogen appeared as early as twelve hours after the initial chill and in some cases was demonstrable as late as five weeks following defervescence. The authors at the time presented data on the chemical nature of the soluble specific substance which showed that the substance which formed in the animal body during pneumococcal infection and passed through the kidneys into the urine was the complex carbohydrate which later was identified as the specific capsular polysaccharide.

A year later, Quigley,[1114] in following the precipitin reaction during the course of lobar pneumonia due to pneumococci of Types I, II, III, and Type (Group) IV, found that when the urine was tested at intervals of two to three days, the reaction gradually increased in intensity during a period of three or four days, persisted from two to nineteen days, and then gradually disappeared. There seemed to be no regularity as to the period in the disease when the precipitinogen appeared in the urine, nor as to the length of time it persisted. Furthermore, its presence seemed to be independent of crisis. In the same year, Blake[125] reported that there was a definite relation between the excretion of soluble pneumococcal antigen in the urine and the development of precipitin in the blood in lobar pneumonia. In patients showing an excess of precipitin in the urine over precipitinogen in the blood, recovery took place shortly after or coincidentally with the appearance of the antibody. Blake stated that daily estimation of the concentration of soluble antigen excreted in the urine, taken with the number of cocci per cubic centimeter of blood, had great prognostic value in the individual case of lobar pneumonia.

The type-specificity of the precipitin reaction was verified by Blake (1917),[123] who employed as precipitinogen the peritoneal exudate from mice infected intraperitoneally with pneumococci of Types I, II, and III, and Group IV. The method applied to a large number of strains yielded consistently positive and specific results, the precipitate forming immediately without incubation when exudate and serum were of corresponding immunological type.

There exists more than presumptive evidence that antipneumococcal precipitin and agglutinin are the same substance. In a quantitative study of the precipitation and agglutination reactions, Heidelberger and Kabat[614] obtained results which seem to prove the truth of the assumption. After removing from a combined Type I and II antipneumococcic serum the species-specific antibodies by absorption with somatic protein and the C Fraction, it developed that the application of the quantitative agglutination method of Heidelberger and Kabat and the quantitative precipitation method devised by Heidelberger, Sia, and Kendall[630] and by Heidelberger, Kendall, and Soo Hoo[628] yielded figures, within the limits of the accuracy of the methods, practically identical for anticarbohydrate precipitin and agglutinin. Heidelberger and Kabat stated that while this relation held for unconcentrated serum, in purified antibody solutions somewhat more agglutinin than precipitin was found, which they considered might be due to alteration of a portion of the antibody in the process of purification. The quantitative correspondence of type-specific anticarbohydrate agglutinin and precipitin argues for the immunological and chemical identity of the two immune substances and supports the unitarian theory of antibodies originally formulated by Zinsser.[1578]

ANTIPROTEIN PRECIPITINS

The somatic protein of Pneumococcus possesses the property of stimulating the production of precipitin and of reacting with the antibodies so formed. Since the protein is common to pneumococci of all types and to degraded variants as well as to smooth, virulent forms of the organism, its precipitinogenic activity, as might be expected, is specific only for the species and not for type. These facts were reported by Avery and Morgan (1925),[54] who found further that antiprotein serum failed to agglutinate type-specific strains of Pneumococcus or to react with the carbohydrate derived from them. A somewhat analogous reaction was described in the same year by Jungeblut.[698] When alcoholic extracts of washed, sedimented pneumococci of Types I, II, and III were mixed with tincture of benzoin, added to specific immune serum, and incubated at 40°, flocculation took place. Antipneumococcic serums of the three types with homologous antigens gave flocculation of varying intensity. The reaction was strictly specific for the bacterial species and at the same time might be highly type-specific.

SOMATIC CARBOHYDRATE (C FRACTION)

A phenomenon first discovered by Tillett and Francis[1409] and later investigated by Ash,[25] by Francis and Abernethy (1934),[475] by Abernethy and Francis,[2] and by Abernethy[1] still awaits an explanation.

It was found that the serum of individuals acutely ill with lobar pneumonia possesses the capacity of precipitating the somatic or C carbohydrate derived from pneumococci. It was further demonstrated that the precipitating action of patients' serum with the C Fraction is demonstrable in the early stages of pneumonia, sometimes within twenty-four hours of the onset, persists throughout the course of the active disease, or persists or recurs along with the development of complications, and disappears during convalescence.

In the report of the most recent experimental study available, Abernethy[1] stated that the serum of rabbits infected intradermally by the Goodner technique fails to precipitate the C carbohydrate, whereas the serum of monkeys (*Macacus cynomolgos*) given an intrabronchial infection with Type III Pneumococcus is capable of precipitating the somatic polysaccharide. The property is demonstrable within the first twenty-four hours following the experimental inoculation and persists for two or three days during the period of active infection. With the recovery of the animal the reactivity of the serum disappears almost as abruptly as it appears with the onset of the disease. Abernethy reports that the study demonstrates:

. . . the variable response of two different hosts to the same bacterial agent. In one species, the monkey, pneumococcus infection was accompanied by the demonstration of certain changes in the serum during the acute period of illness. In the other, the rabbit, these changes were not observed. These observations suggest that during infection in the monkey either some newly formed substance or some alteration occurs in the serum which renders it inactive in precipitation tests with this particular polysaccharide derived from Pneumococcus. Assuming this to be the case, then the failure to demonstrate the phenomenon in the rabbit might be explained either by the absence of or qualitative differences in the serum during infection.

The phenomenon of precipitation of the somatic or C polysaccharide of Pneumococcus cannot be explained on the basis of any of our present orthodox conceptions of immunity. The property is not limited to the serum of individuals ill with pneumococcal infection, since it is also possessed by the serum of patients suffering from rheumatic fever, bacterial endocarditis, and lung abscess, but not from other febrile diseases.

Furthermore, unlike other specific antibodies, the substance capable of precipitating the C Fraction appears in the serum of the pneumonia patient within the first twenty-four hours of the disease, and—again unlike any antibodies that we know—disappears from the serum with the beginning of recovery. Because of their importance in the body's defense against pneumococcal and other infections, the discovery of the chemical identity of the precipitating substance in the serum of pneumonia patients and of the chemical or physical processes involved in the particulation of the somatic polysaccharide is awaited with keen interest.

Jungeblut believed that lipoid substances extracted from Pneumococcus were responsible for the reaction but, as the author pointed out, the method of preparing the alcohol-soluble antigen did not preclude the possibility that certain impurities, protein or carbohydrate in character, might have been carried over into the extract. The lack of sharpness in type-specific action would denote the participation of cellular protein in the reaction.

A precipitin phenomenon described by Boor and Miller[138] in 1931 is yet to be explained. Nucleoprotein and non-protein fractions prepared from strains of Gonococcus gave precipitates when added to antipneumococcic serum of Types I, II, and III. The antigens were active in high dilutions, and displayed even greater precipitating power in the presence of antimeningococcic serum.

THE MECHANISM OF SPECIFIC PRECIPITATION

Gay and Chickering,[508-9] in 1914, found that the addition of a water-clear extract of pneumococci to homologous antiserum produces a voluminous precipitate which carries down with it agglutinins and the greater portion of protective antibodies. Subsequently, Chickering[223] found the reaction to be type-specific. In the reaction, therefore, it was evident that the precipitinogen consisted of some soluble component of the pneumococcal cell while the specific precipitin, as later shown by Goodner,[528] was a substance associated with the euglobulin of the horse serum employed.

Soluble specific substance. Heidelberger and Avery,[606] in 1923, isolated the soluble specific substance from Type II pneumococci and announced that it consisted mainly of a carbohydrate and that in as high a dilution as 1 to 3,000,000 gave positive precipitation with homologous antiserum. According to the authors, the precipitinogen was apparently a polysaccharide constituting the capsular substance of Pneumococcus. This important conclusion was the first evidence of a possible connection between the capsular material and the specific relationships of pneumococci, and accounted for the type-specificity of the precipitin reaction.

Felton and Bailey[420] fully substantiated the work of Gay and Chickering on the nature of the precipitate, and also the observation of Heidelberger and Avery[607] that a single component of

Pneumococcus—the soluble specific substance—was concerned in the particulation of type-specific antibody in immune serum.

Heidelberger, Goebel, and Avery (1925)[613] confirmed the participation of the soluble specific substance in immunological reactions and refined the methods for the isolation of the polysaccharide. The purified substance from Type I Pneumococcus gave a specific precipitin reaction with homologous Type I antipneumococcic serum and could be detected in a dilution as great as 1 to 6,000,000. Similar refined preparations from Type II and Type III pneumococci showed antigenic reactions of approximately the same magnitude, and in the precipitin reaction exhibited strict type-selectivity for the precipitins in homologous serum. The observations substantiated the view that the polysaccharides were the actual specific antigenic substances of Pneumococcus.

That the specific precipitinogen in Pneumococcus is evidently a soluble carbohydrate was shown in a different manner by Schiemann and Casper (1927),[1228] who dissolved pneumococci in sodium taurocholate, and found that the solutions gave type-specific precipitates with homologous immune serum. The authors rightly believed that the soluble carbohydrate obtained by lysis of the cocci with the bile salt was the same as the type-specific polysaccharide isolated and tested by Avery and Heidelberger.

Later (1931), Avery and Goebel[45] proved that the type-specificity of the interaction of Pneumococcus and homologous immune serum was due to the capsular polysaccharide and not to the protein of the cell. The serum of rabbits immunized with an artificial antigen, prepared by combining a specific derivative of the capsular polysaccharide of Type III Pneumococcus with globulin from horse serum, was found to contain specific precipitins for the Type III polysaccharide and, in addition, precipitins for horse globulin. It was, however, the capsular polysaccharide that was the determining factor in the specificity of the antigen as a whole. Subsequently, Avery and Goebel[46] proved that the acetyl polysaccharide, besides being antigenic in the sense of being capable of stimulating the production of specific antibodies, was also antigenic in that, in a highly purified form, it reacted specifically with homologous precipitin and completely removed precipitin from immune serum.

Balance between precipitinogen and precipitin. Morgan (1923)[912] demonstrated that a proper balance between antigen and antibody was required to bring about the phenomenon of precipitation. In order to obtain the maximal precipitate from any given quantity of antipneumococcic serum, a definite or optimal amount of precipitinogen or soluble specific substance was necessary. The ratio between the quantity of immune serum and reacting substance was found to be practically constant. Therefore, when an excess of precipitinogen was present, the resulting precipitate was not only decreased in amount, as determined by inspection and weight, but its appearance was altered. The importance of the relative proportions of antigen and antibody was also demonstrated by Dean and Webb (1926)[311] who, employing normal horse serum and its homologous antiserum, devised a method by which it was possible to determine quantitatively the amount of antigen and antibody and therefore the optimal ratio between the two components necessary for complete precipitation.

Precipitin index. Sobotka and Friedländer (1928)[1299] determined that the sensitivity of the precipitin reaction with antipneumococcic serum could be expressed by the product of the concentrations of the two reacting substances, antigen and antibody, and defined the precipitin index (P.I.) as one-millionth of the reciprocal value of the product. In investigating the zonal phenomenon and its bearing on the absolute concentration and equivalent weight of antibody, the authors found that the greater tendency toward the exhibition of a post-zone in Type III precipitation was connected with the lower acid equivalent of the homologous capsular polysaccharide. The addition of normal serum as well as an increase in pH promoted the post-zonal effect. By determining the precipitin index, it was possible to recognize and to eliminate zonal irregularities. Smith[1298] later (1932) applied the principle of optimal proportions to precipitin tests with Type I soluble specific substance and homologous antibody and reported that the method gave a true index of the protective power of the serum. More recently Felton devised a test for the combining power of antipneumococcic serum with specific polysaccharide.

In the description by Francis,[472] already cited in the discussion of agglutinins, it appeared that differences in the ratio of antigen and antibody which affect the agglutination reaction apply also to the precipitation reaction. When a solution of soluble specific substance was added in excess to homologous immune serum, a pro-zone was created in which precipitation was inhibited. As in the agglutination reaction, Francis showed that it was the capsular polysaccharide which constituted the precipitinogen.

Quantitative relations in precipitation. In 1929, Heidelberger and Kendall[616] published the first of a series of communications on a quantitative study of the precipitin reaction as related to soluble specific substance and homologous immune serum. After precipitating Type III antipneumococcic serum with Type III polysaccharide, the authors measured the amount of nitrogen in the supernatant fluid of the precipitated mixture, and then from the nitrogen content calculated the amount of protein remaining in solution. The authors then tested the experimental data by the law of mass action to determine whether the reaction showed analogies to the behavior of simpler ionic reactions. Depending on the relative amounts of the reactants, the specific precipitate appeared to be a mixture of varying proportions of two compounds, or a whole series of compounds, containing hapten and antibody in varying proportions, whose limits could be expressed by the following equilibriums, A and S being respectively equivalent amounts of antibody and Type II soluble specific substance:

(1) $A + S \rightleftharpoons AS$ (120: 1 ratio)
(2) $AS + S \rightleftharpoons AS_2$ (60: 1 ratio)

According to Heidelberger and Kendall, an inhibition-zone effect appears to be a chemical equilibrium which might be expressed by

$$(3)\ AS_2 + S \rightleftharpoons AS_3$$

In equilibrium (1) the reaction tends to proceed strongly to the right since AS is only slightly soluble. Reaction (2) will go farther to completion and more AS_2 will be precipitated (since AS_2 has an appreciable solubility and dissociation tendency) when a little S is added after equilibrium (2) has been reached. When much S is added, equilibrium (3) comes into play and the precipitate dissolves. The authors suggested as an analogy the reaction between silver and the cyanide ion, where a small amount of CN^- causes a precipitate of AgCN, and an excess of CN^- causes the formation of the silver cyanide complex which is soluble.

Heidelberger, Sia, and Kendall (1930)[630] described a rapid and simple method for the approximate determination of the specifically precipitable protein in Type I antipneumococcic serum. Inasmuch as a close parallel was found to exist between the amount of specifically precipitable protein and the number of mouse protection units, and because of the rapidity, simplicity, and economy of the method, the authors proposed its use instead of the mouse protection test as a basis for the titration of standard serum and for the comparison of other serums with the standard.

Heidelberger and Kendall (1932)[619] devised a method, based on the precipitin reaction, for the microdetermination of the specific polysaccharide of Type III Pneumococcus. By the method, as little as 0.01 milligram of Type III polysaccharide could be measured, while the procedure appeared to be applicable to any specific polysaccharide upon standardization of an homologous antiserum or antibody solution in the region of excess antibody. In another paper,[620] the authors described precipitin reactions performed with partial hydrolytic products of the specific capsular polysaccharide of Type III Pneumococcus freed quantitatively from unhydrolyzed specific polysaccharide. The fractions yielded specific precipitates, in dilutions of 1 to 1,000,000, with Type III antipneumococcic horse serum, but failed to precipitate homologous rabbit antiserum, giving rise to specific inhibition. The authors found further that aldobionic acid, the structural unit of Type III polysaccharide, did not precipitate homologous antiserum.

With Soo Hoo, Heidelberger and Kendall (1933)[628] described a method, developed from the previous work of the two last-named authors, for the microestimation of precipitin in antiserum. The technique involved the use of a deep-red protein dye, the R salt of azo-benzidene-azo-crystalline egg albumen. The procedure gave the actual weight of precipitin and could be applied to the maximal amount of precipitable antibody in any antiserum. The observation that four samples of immune rabbit serum produced in response to injection of the dye contained over one hundred times as much precipitin as the antigen injected, appeared to the authors as supplementing the growing mass of evidence against the theory that specific antigen fragments are actually incorporated into the antibody molecule.

In 1935, Heidelberger and Kendall[622] pointed out that the usual immunological technique, namely, incubation of precipitin reactions at 37° for two hours and allowing the tubes to stand in the ice-box over night, while resulting in the maximal precipitation of antibody from immune rabbit serum, in the case of antipneumococcic horse serum or purified antibody, does not permit the establishment of a true equilibrium or the precipitation of the maximal amount of antibody nitrogen. The authors recommended that analyses of antipneumococcic horse serum should therefore be carried out at 0° and the tubes containing the antigen and immune serum should be allowed to stand in the cold for at least twenty-four hours in order to ensure the completion of the reaction.

In an accompanying paper, Heidelberger and Kendall[623] reported the results of additional study of the quantitative relations in the precipitin reaction between Type III polysaccharide and homologous immune horse serum, which led the authors to the conclusion that the reaction could be accounted for quantitatively by assuming the chemical combination of the components in a bimolecular reaction, followed by a series of competing bimolecular reactions which depend on the relative proportions of the components. From the data, Heidelberger and Kendall then developed additional mathematical formulas representing the developments in the mechanism of the precipitin reaction. As the authors remarked in their 1929 communication, "Of all the reactions of immunity the precipitin test is perhaps the most dramatic and striking; while other immune reactions are more delicate, the precipitin test is among the most specific and least subject to errors and technical difficulties"; and "The isolation of bacterial polysaccharides which precipitate antisera specifically and possess powers of haptens has not only afforded one of the components of a precipitin reaction in a state of comparative purity, but has greatly simplified the analytical problem." By these exact quantitative methods, the precipitin reaction has conferred inestimable benefits on the immunologist in understanding the nature of immunological phenomena, such as the relations between antigen and antibody, in judging the purity of antigen, and in estimating the antibody content of antipneumococcic serum.

The chemical study of capsular polysaccharides and pneumococcal antibody is furnishing clues to the process which operate in the union between type-specific antigen and homologous antibody. By simple chemical experiments, Chow and Goebel[226] showed that the immunological activity of pneumococcal antibody protein is to a great extent dependent upon the presence of free amino groups in the protein molecule. With the work of Landsteiner and van der Scheer[782-3] in mind and reasoning from the results of the study on synthetic antigens made by Avery and Goebel (1929),[44] Chow and Goebel assumed that in the case of the type-specific antibody of Pneumococcus the spatial arrangements of the polar groups in the immune protein may determine its specific capacity to react with the polysaccharide of the homologous type.

In the carbohydrate of Type I Pneumococcus the authors believed, on the basis of the experimental evidence, that the carboxyl groups of the polysaccharide are the dominant groups which interact to form the immune precipitate. The questions whether the carboxyl groups of the polysaccharide actually combine with the amino groups of the antibody protein and whether the formation of an insoluble precipitate involves further chemical change in the protein molecule, such as specific denaturation, cannot be answered at present. However, Chow and Goebel concluded:

The specificity of this reaction is determined by the stereochemical relationship of the dominant polar groups in the reacting molecules, whether they be antigen or antibody. If the spatial pattern of the polar groups of both antigen and antibody is of exactly the correct order, then union occurs. If, however, this relationship is disturbed by artificial means, as has been experimentally demonstrated by covering the dominant polar group of either polysaccharide or antibody with a chemical radical, the pattern is destroyed and union between them is either greatly modified or fails to take place. When the original constitution of the reacting substances is restored, however, serological specificity is regained.

CORRELATION OF PRECIPITINS WITH OTHER ANTIBODIES

Many observations have been made on the quantitative relationships existing between precipitins and other specific antibodies in antipneumococcic serum. The discovery that the capsular polysaccharide functions as the precipitinogen in the reaction, and the development of methods for evaluating the strength of antigen and antibody, have made possible more exact determination of the amount of precipitin in a given serum in relation to the content of other immune substances. Friedlander, Sobotka, and Banzhaf (1928)[493] estimated, under known conditions, the precipitin indices of a number of monovalent and polyvalent antipneumococcic serums and found the indices to vary as did the number of protective units. The ratio of the precipitin index to protective units in monovalent serums was between 2.8 and 4.8 for Type I and about ten times greater for Type III. Lower values prevailed in polyvalent antipneumococcic horse serum and in mixtures of heterologous monovalent serums. A relative increase in precipitin activity was found in the refined and concentrated serums tested.

The experiments of Avery and Goebel (1931)[45] with the artificially conjugated Type III capsular polysaccharide-horse serum globulin would seem to argue for the unity of type-specific precipitins, agglutinins, and protective antibodies.

In a systematic study of the quantitative relations existing between the various specific antibodies in Type I and II antipneumococcic horse serum, Felton (1931)[407] determined for Type I Pneumococcus the correlation coefficient between protective and precipitin titer as 0.93; between protection and agglutination the figure was 0.80; between protection and neutralization it was 0.88; and between protection and the amount of protein precipitated with specific carbohydrate it was 0.91. From this degree of correlation it appeared to Felton that, at least for freshly drawn horse serum, the precipitin test could be used to estimate the probable therapeutic value of antipneumococcic serum.

The qualification made by Felton in respect to the freshness of the serum sample as influencing precipitation and protective titer was confirmed by Valentine, McGuire, Whitney, and Falk (1931)[1448] in experiments on the effect of ageing on antibodies in dried antipneumococcic serum. At room temperature, agglutinin and precipitin titer decreased to a greater degree than did the number of mouse-protective units, although the deterioration of the two first-named antibodies failed to take place at ice-box temperatures.

In a more recent publication (1936), Barnes, Clarke, and Wight[82] compared the unit value of serums obtained by mouse protection with a) the water test; b) agglutination test; c) the authors' routine precipitation test; d) the optimal proportions precipitation test; e) Felton's test for combining equivalents; and f) a modified precipitation test devised by the authors. The following table taken from page 131 of the authors' communication shows the correlations found between precipitation, combining equivalents, agglutination, and mouse protection.

Method of titration	Serums tested with control		Incubation		End-point = highest dilution showing	Antigen	Correlation with mouse protection
	P 11	*P 403*	*Hours at 40°*	*Ice-box*			
Agglutination	32	18	2	Over-night	Trace of aggluti-nation	Live broth culture	0.713 ±0.047
Optimal propor-tions precipita-tion	0	50	*	*	*	SSS	0.909 ±0.016
Routine precipita-tion	50	0	2	Over-night	Definite floccu-lation	SSS 1:10,000 dilution	0.866 ±0.024
Modified routine precipitation ...	50	0	2	Over-night	Definite floccu-lation	SSS 1:10,000 dilution	0.930 ±0.012
Combining equiva-lent	50	0	*	*	No un-com-bined SSS	SSS 1:10,000 dilution	0.925 ±0.014
Water test	0	50	0	Over-night	*	*	0.652 ±0.055

* Not applicable.

By closely spacing the serum dilutions in the modified test, Barnes, Clarke, and Wight succeeded in obtaining precipitin titers which agreed more closely with estimations of the mouse-protective value than with any of the other methods tested. It would seem, therefore, that the precipitin content, as determined by this method, is in close agreement with the amount of protective antibody in specific antipneumococcic serum.

Complement-Fixing Antibodies

The reaction of complement fixation is so far inferior in delicacy to that of agglutination, precipitation, or mouse protection for the serological diagnosis of pneumococcal types that the subject can be dismissed with brief mention. Hanes (1914),[588] using the method, found that strains of *Pneumococcus mucosus* were more closely related to Pneumococcus than to Streptococcus. There was a certain amount of cross-fixation between immune serum of Types I and II, and Type III antigens, whereas anti-streptococcic serums deviated complement only in the presence of antigens made from homologous strains. Christensen (1922)[228-9] employed the method of complement fixation to check type-determination of pneumococci of the first four types made by the agglutination reaction but, because the first-named method was more complicated and required a longer time for its execution, Christensen did not recommend its use in place of agglutination. In the studies made by Avery and Heidelberger (1925)[49] on the antibodies demonstrable in the serum of rabbits immunized by injection of intact pneumococci and of their carbohydrate and protein derivatives, the method of complement fixation yielded results agreeing with those obtained by specific precipitation. Bull and McKee (1929)[180] applied the method to test the production of antibodies in rabbits immunized with heat-killed broth cultures of pneumococci. Serum from animals immunized with a Type II strain fixed complement in the presence of antigens of Types I, II, and III, but the titer was always higher with the homologous antigen. The same observation held true for Type III antiserum. From rabbits injected with a Type (Group) IV organism, the serum was potent when the homologous organism was used as antigen and only slightly weaker in the presence of Type I antigen. Although the serums were low in agglutinin titer, their action was type-specific.

The mechanism of the complement-fixation reaction with the components of Pneumococcus, and the disparity between the ability of specific antipneumococcic serums produced respectively in the rabbit and horse to bind complement in the presence of homologous antigen, have been studied by Goodner and Horsfall.[538] Without retailing the experimental details, it may suffice to abstract the discussion and summary. The experiments reported supported the view that the failure to obtain complement fixation with combinations of pneumococcal capsular polysaccharide and specific immune horse serum is not due to some heterologous inhibitor in immune horse serum but is to be referred rather to some property of the horse antibody itself or some property of the immune aggregate resulting from the union of this antibody and the polysaccharide. This property is lacking in the specific antibody in immune rabbit serum which, in the presence of homologous polysaccharide, is capable under proper conditions of binding complement. Furthermore, the results support the view that the fixation of complement is a phenomenon of selective absorption. That one type of aggregate absorbs complement while another fails to do so is curious, but far from unique. Goodner and Horsfall found a close parallelism in the fact that horse antibody-polysaccharide aggregates absorb cephalin, while aggregates containing rabbit antibody selectively absorb lecithin.

The essential role of serum lipids in the demonstration of the phenomena of specific precipitation and agglutination has been described by Horsfall and Goodner.[657] The removal of lecithin from antipneumococcic horse serum and, to a lesser degree, the extraction of cephalin from antipneumococcic rabbit serum cause a loss of the visible phenomena of agglutination and precipitation. It was found that initial activity of type-specific antibody can be restored to extracted immune horse serum by the addition of lecithin, and to extracted rabbit serum by the addition of cephalin. It is therefore probable that the content of these two phospho-lipids* in the serum of the two animal species may, in part, account for

* In a recent brief communication, Horsfall, Goodner, and MacLeod[659] describe the antibody in pneumococcal immune horse serum as a lecithoprotein and that in immune rabbit serum as a cephaloprotein.

the differences in the immunological behavior of immune horse and rabbit serum.

Inasmuch as complement fixation does not occur in the absence of particulation and since particulation is a secondary phenomenon in the reaction, the authors regard complement fixation as a tertiary manifestation.

The evidence presented in the communications cited and in other reports is sufficient to demonstrate that the method of complement fixation offers no advantages over other serological methods for the identification of pneumococci or of types within the species.

Bactericidins

With the advancement of bacteriological knowledge, the pneumococcidal action of both normal and immune serum has been found to be a more complicated process than it was earlier conceived to be. Instead of being solely a function of possible bactericidins in serum, the destructive effect of blood involves the action not only of serum but of leucocytes and of fixed tissue cells. Since the pneumococcidal power of blood depends on the associated participation of tropins or opsonins and phagocytes, the special features of their combined action will be described later in the present chapter, while the nature of other inherent defenses of the animal body will be discussed in a subsequent chapter.

Antihemotoxin

Experiments on the antigenic action of pneumococcal hemotoxin reported in 1914 by Cole[252] indicated that the serum of rabbits and sheep immunized with hemolytic extracts of Pneumococcus had acquired increased power to inhibit the lytic effect of the extract on erythrocytes. In studies on the oxidation and reduction of immunological substances, Neill[952] and his colleagues[958-9] compared the immunological response to the injection into rabbits of reduced and oxidized pneumococcal extracts, and succeeded in producing a neutralizing antibody by immunizing the animal with the hemolytically inactive hemotoxin present in oxidized solutions as well as with the active hemotoxin. The antibody appeared to be a species-specific antihemotoxin neutralizing the hemotoxin from all types of pneumococci, since it was without effect on the hemotoxins of tetanus and Welch bacilli. Neill with Fleming and Gaspari determined that for the production of antihemotoxin in the rabbit or horse it was essential that the hemotoxic antigen be used in an unheated condition.

A similar antihemotoxic serum was developed by Cotoni and Chambrin (1928)[282] in rabbits, sheep, and horses after immunizing the animals with living cultures, extracts of living and dried pneumococci, as well as with dried organisms killed by alcohol and ether. The antihemotoxin was stable after heating for one-half hour and, as Neill[950] found, was devoid of type-specificity but possessed species-specificity, because when tested against the hemolysins of streptococci, tetanus bacilli, septic vibrios, and *Bacillus perfringens*, the serum displayed no neutralizing action. Doubt was cast on the species-specificity of antihemotoxins by Todd (1934),[1412] who apparently was able to neutralize, to a limited extent, the hemolysins of Type II and Type III pneumococci with antistreptolytic serum. The degree of neutralization was not necessarily correlated with the antistreptolytic titer, and the different hemolysins could be distinguished by quantitative serological methods. The partial antigenic overlapping of hemolysins could only be demonstrated by the use of hyperimmune serum.

Antitoxin

Boehncke and Mouriz-Riesgo (1915),[134] notwithstanding the fact that they were never able to obtain any very active pneumococcal toxin, believed that the curative action of some of the immune serum prepared by them was due to its antitoxic qualities. Olson (1926)[1029-30] claimed that it was possible to immunize mice by serial injections of pneumococcal toxin prepared by allowing sodium ricinoleate to act on pneumococci, but the author presented no serological evidence of the presence of antitoxin in the serum of the immune animals. In addition, serum from normal horses, sheep, rabbits, and chickens, as well as antipneumococcic serum or pneumococcic antibody solution, was found to possess little power to prevent the lung changes or cutaneous reactions evoked in mice by the toxin.

Clowes, Jamieson, and Olson (1926),[244] by injecting rabbits, sheep, and horses with progressively increasing doses of sterile toxic extracts prepared by the sodium ricinoleate method of Larson, obtained a serum that neutralized the skin-reacting substance contained in the extracts, and suggested as a provisional unit of antitoxin the amount of serum required to neutralize one million skin-test doses of toxin. Concentration of the immune serum effected the removal of 99.9 per cent of the total serum-protein without appreciable loss of antitoxin. Larson,[788] in the same year, administered an immune serum prepared and tested in the same manner to patients ill with lobar pneumonia and, because the patients showed a rapid drop in temperature and experienced relief of subjective symptoms following the administration of the serum, he believed that the serum actually contained antitoxin.

The work of Parker (1929),[1061] referred to earlier in the text, has a definite bearing on the question of the possible existence of pneumococcal antitoxin. Serum prepared by the author in rabbits and horses by using sterile filtrates of pneumotoxin as antigens, under certain conditions, protected guinea pigs against the pneumonia caused by the intratracheal injection of living pneumococci and toxic pneumococcal autolysates. The protection thus conferred was heterologous for type and appeared to be due to some immune substance other than protective antibodies, since the latter could not be demonstrated in the active serum of rabbits and horses immunized with sterile filtrates of toxic autolysates of Pneumococcus. In a second publication, Parker and McCoy (1929)[1062] described a method for standardizing the potency of antitoxic horse serum and set as the unit of toxin the amount of filtered autolysate which, when injected intratracheally, would kill a guinea pig weighing 200 to 210 grams in from four to twenty-four hours with typical symptoms and necropsy findings; while one unit of antitoxin represented the smallest amount of serum necessary to protect a guinea pig of the same weight against one unit of toxin when the test toxin-serum mixture was injected intratracheally. Neither normal horse serum nor antipneumococcic horse serum containing 500 protective units per cubic centimeter when used in a 1 to 10 dilution exerted a detoxifying action on the toxin. A sample of antipneumococcic serum concentrated by the Felton method, in a 1 to 20 dilution, neutralized the toxin but failed to do so when added in a 1 to 50 dilution.

The results obtained by Jamieson and Powell (1931)[676] were analogous to those reported by Parker and McCoy. The filtrates of young broth cultures of pneumococci of Types I, II, III, and IV, which had been found to elicit a positive reaction in the skin of rabbits and of human beings, constituted the antigen employed by subcutaneous injection for immunizing horses. The serums developed by the procedure appeared to possess neutralizing substances for the toxin, and these substances could be concentrated to a moderate degree in the refining of globulins by the usual salting-out methods. The concentrated serum contained only a small amount of protective antibody, and in neutralizing action compared favorably with the action of specific antitoxin on scarlet fever streptococcal toxin.

Employing autolysate prepared by the method of Parker, Blackman[122] produced immune serum in rabbits and horses that would protect normal rabbits not only against the toxic action of autolysate but against pneumococcal infection.

Sabin (1931)[1203] sought to determine whether antipneumotoxin influences the course of pneumococcal infection in mice. Mice were injected with large doses of Type I and II pneumococci. One series of animals was then treated with therapeutic antibacterial serum, another with antipneumotoxic serum, and a third series received both antibacterial and antitoxic serums. The results showed that the antitoxin was without effect in staying the infection. Sabin then tested the action of antipneumotoxin in rabbits infected intradermally by the method of Goodner. Rabbits were given an intradermal injection of 0.1 cubic centimeter of a 1 to 100 dilution of an eighteen-hour broth culture of virulent Type I Pneumococcus. Three groups of rabbits so injected were treated with the same serums as in the mouse experiments, some animals receiving the serum injection six or seven hours after inoculation and some twenty-four hours after inoculation. Of the untreated controls and those animals receiving antitoxin only, all died within the same time, and no beneficial effect was observed in the rabbits treated with antitoxic serum added to antibacterial serum.

The preliminary statement of Coca (1932)[245] regarding the antigenic action of a pyrogenic and skin-reacting substance in culture filtrates of Pneumococcus in raising the resistance of children to the action of the antigen has already been mentioned. Not only did the young subjects become immune to the pyrogenic substance and fail to react when the filtrate was injected into the skin, but the serum of the children so treated neutralized the action of the filtrate. Convalescent serum from patients recovering from infection with Type I and II Pneumococcus also inhibited the effect of the poisonous substance derived from pneumococci. Therapeutic antipneumococcic serum, on the contrary, in the amounts used, failed to neutralize minute amounts of the filtrate.

In a more recent report (1936), Coca[246] described further experiments with filtrates of pneumococcal cultures. The toxic principle was neutralized by the serum of young human subjects previously injected with the filtrates and by the serum of patients convalescing from lobar pneumonia. According to Coca, the neutralizing action of the human immune serum was type-specific and antitoxic in nature and not related to the type-specific polysaccharide antibody.

Heterophile Antibodies

During recent years there has developed considerable interest in the fact that the injection of pneumococci into suitable animals results in the production of heterophile antibodies. It is not necessary in this discussion to consider all the various sources and characters of heterogenetic antigens which may be used to stimulate the production of heterophile antibodies. Readers interested in the subject are referred to reviews of the subject by Davidsohn (1927),[294-7] Bull (1928),[175] and more recently and in special reference to pneumonia, by Plummer (1936).[1099] That heterogenetic antigens and heterophile antibodies may be of biological significance in pneumococcal infections has been suggested in publications by Bailey and Shorb (1931, 1933),[64-5] and by Powell, Jamieson, Bailey, and Hyde (1933).[1105] Opposed to these views are the observations of Finland, Ruegsegger, and Felton (1935).[444] It is not proposed to relate technical details of the various experiments dealing with this subject. The Council on Pharmacy and Chemistry of the American Medical Association requested Plummer to make a report on the use of heterophile antibodies and, since his conclusions appear sound, they are reproduced verbatim.

The presence of heterophile bodies in animal tissues, animal serums and bacteria is strongly suggestive that these bodies play a part in certain immune reactions. The animal experiments carried out by Bailey, Shorb, Powell, Jamieson, and Hyde do not prove that the heterophile bodies play a role in the pneumococcus immunity of the human being. Some of the results reported are open to question. The work should be repeated by an independent group of investigators before it is accepted. The study by Finland, Ruegsegger and Felton on the heterophile antibodies in the serum of patients convalescing from pneumonia and in controls leads one to believe that the heterophile bodies do not have any particular bearing on the course of pneumococcic infections in man. The clinical and statistical evidence cited by the manufacturers of the combined heterophile antibody serum is too limited and is strongly misleading. The presence of both rabbit and horse proteins in the serum will increase the incidence and the dangers of allergic reactions. This is a definite disadvantage, because with newer methods of refining serum the allergic reaction is the principal source of danger in any type of serotherapy. There is only slight experimental evidence and no clinical evidence that the combined heterophile serum gives any immunity against Type III and Group IV pneumococcic infections. There is the same lack of evidence that the combined serum produces a greater immunity for Type I and II infections than the ordinary antipneumococcus horse serum. The principal theoretical advantage of the combined heterophile serum is that it could be used for all pneumococcic pneumonias, regardless of types, and the corollary of this that pneumococcus typing would not be necessary. Serum having this advantage would be highly desirable, but because its superiority is unproved and because of the probable increase in allergic reactions it is unfair and unwise to recommend the combined heterophile serum for general distribution.

The Council on Pharmacy and Chemistry approved and adopted Plummer's report and emphasized the conclusion that, in the light of present knowledge, recommendation of the combined heterophile serum for general distribution is unwise and unwarranted.

Phagocytosis

The part played by leucocytes in checking the invasion of pneumococci and in the destruction of cocci in the infected body was apparently first suggested by Gamaléia[498] in 1888. The French author, in a study of pneumonia patients, noted large phagocytes packed with cocci in various stages of degeneration. The author also reported an observation to the effect that sheep infected intratracheally with diplococci obtained from infected cadavers, on being sacrificed, showed many phagocytes containing the organisms. Gamaléia ventured the conjecture that pulmonary phagocytes were a factor in restraining the spread of pneumococci (*Streptococcus lanceolatus Pasteuri*) in the lung. Kruse and Pansini (1891)[763] also noted phagocytosis in animals experimentally infected with pneumococci, but held that the phenomenon was of secondary importance to the bactericidal action of the serum.

At the time, opinion was divided concerning the nature of the forces which accounted for the resistance of normal and immunized animals to Pneumococcus. One school contended that immunity was due to bactericidins; the other maintained that the immunity was antitoxic in nature. The idea that mobile cellular elements—the leucocytes—might intervene in arresting pneumococcal infection came as an innovation and at first was not readily accepted. For example, Bonome[187] shared the conception that the blood of immunized animals acquired increased bactericidal power for pneumococci and although he observed both leucocytosis and phagocytosis, he did not perceive that the phenomena could be the basis of bactericidal action. It was Issaeff (1893)[673] who, as a result of his experiments, abandoned the idea that antitoxin was a factor, and emphasized the fact that phagocytosis played a most important part in acquired immunity to Pneumococcus. Mennes (1897)[893] was unable to demonstrate any effect of the white cells of normal blood on the development of pneumococcal infection. According to his views, the primary defensive element was the serum and not the leucocytes. The white cells of immune rabbits, however, exerted marked phagocytic action, and Mennes concluded that the immunity of the rabbit to pneumococcal invasion developed from a modification of the serum, and that the modification activated the phagocytic property of the leucocytes.

In 1904, Neufeld and Rimpau[997] definitely discarded bactericidins and bacteriolysins as forces operating in antipneumococcic immunity and reported that the addition of specific immune serum to normal rabbit leucocytes imparted to the cells vigorous phagocytic ability. The authors then extended the experiments to include the *in vivo* action of immune serum on virulent cultures injected into mice. When the culture alone was injected intraperitoneally, the organisms multiplied and only a few leucocytes were seen to contain cocci, but when both culture and serum were injected, a large number of pneumococci were engulfed by the white blood cells. By absorption experiments, Neufeld and Rimpau demonstrated that the serum acted on the cocci, whether living or killed, and not on the leucocytes. Complement was not necessary to render the organisms phagocytable. In a second report, Neufeld and Rimpau (1905)[998] claimed that the theory that serum was a stimulant for the leucocytes was no longer tenable, but that serum, on the contrary, caused a peculiar transformation of the bacteria. Immune serums which possessed the property of rendering bacteria susceptible to phagocytosis Neufeld and Rimpau designated by the name "bacteriotropic" to distinguish them from bacteriolytic serums.

In America, at the time when the Wright opsonic technique was arousing such general interest, Rosenow[1160] tested the susceptibility of forty strains of pneumococci to phagocytosis. All but four strains at first resisted phagocytosis in pneumonic blood, but after cultivation on artificial media the organisms became susceptible to leucocytic ingestion. While heating the cocci had no effect on susceptibility, the opsonic property of the serum appeared to be diminished after a thirty-minute exposure to a temperature of 56°. Rosenow believed that white cells from the blood of pneumonia patients possessed greater phagocytic power than did normal cells, and ascribed the pneumococcidal effect of blood to the combined action of serum and leucocytes—phagocytosis and intraphagocytic digestion. Potter and Krumwiede (1907)[1103] tested the leucocytes of pneumonia patients for phagocytic properties. While granting the inaccuracy of the method employed, the authors, contrary to Rosenow, stated that leucocytes of patients during the height of pneumonic disease were probably less active in phagocytic power than were normal leucocytes.

The principle in leucocytes responsible for the lysis of pneumococci after being phagocyted was investigated by Schneider (1910),[1244] who believed that the hypothetical substance acted directly upon the injected pneumococci. Schneider also found that specific immune serum powerfully stimulated phagocytosis, especially *in vivo*, but ascribed the action of serum to its effect on the white cells. Schneider further claimed that a serum which was lacking in this stimulating property was also lacking in precipitating, agglutinating, and complement-fixing action and displayed no protective power. Boehncke and Mouriz-Riesgo (1915),[134] who had previously corroborated the conclusion of Neufeld and Rimpau that the bacteriotropic action of antipneumococcic serum *in vitro* also participates in the action of the serum *in vivo*, were not convinced that tropins were the only factor in inducing phagocytosis. The authors had been able to rule out any participation of bactericidal and complement-fixing antibodies and, while they concluded that phagocytosis was the most important factor, the authors still inclined to the view that antitoxins might play an important part in resistance to pneumococcal infection. In 1919, Barber,[77] employing the single-cell technique, sought an explanation of the ready growth of pneumococci in immune serum. Failing to find any specific bactericidal substance in immune serum, Barber noticed that when specific serum was added to pneumococci previous to mixing with leucocytes active phagocytosis took place, and the same phenomenon occurred when the organisms were injected into the peritoneal cavity of mice passively immunized with immune serum. The author offered no explanation for the reaction.

SENSITIZATION OF PNEUMOCOCCI

Bürgers,[188] and Bürgers and Meisner (1911),[189] following the lead furnished by the work of Neufeld and Rimpau, found that while normal serum was inactive in rendering virulent pneumococci phagocytable, immune serum was highly active in this respect. Although the serum used in the experiments was evidently low in potency, the pneumococci when incubated with the serum were readily taken up by normal leucocytes. Bürgers and his colleague believed that fresh complement was necessary for phagocytosis, since they considered that the reaction was one depending upon antigen, amboceptor, and complement. Strouse (1911)[1346] also used the method of sensitizing pneumococci in studying the presence of immune opsonins in the serum of pneumonia patients. The addition of the serum accelerated the ingestion of pneumococci by the white cells.

In 1915, Friel[494] described the action of normal and immune serum on pneumococci. Cultures left in contact with normal serum for one and one-half to twenty-four hours and then washed in salt solution acquired no increased susceptibility to the action of phagocytes, but organisms similarly treated with immune serum were avidly ingested by the white cells. It will be recalled that the sensitizing effect of immune serum was called "piantication" by Friel. The term, meaning to prepare for slaughter, was in effect the same as Wright's word opsonization, meaning to prepare for the feast. In addition to the action of opsonins in rendering pneumococci susceptible to the destructive action of leucocytes, Goodner, Dubos, and Avery (1932)[536] demonstrated that organisms denuded of capsule by the action of specific bacterial enzymes became highly vulnerable to phagocytosis by tissue cells.

In an endeavor to clarify the contradictory conceptions of Neufeld and Rimpau[997] on the one hand and of Römer* on the other regarding the action of immune serum on bacterium or leucocyte, Preisz (1915),[1108] by employing normal and immune serum and leucocytes in both *in vitro* and *in vivo* experiments, concluded that the ability of immune serum to promote phagocytosis of pneumococci lay in its action on the cocci and not on the leucocytes.

A more recent report—that of Robertson and Sia (1927)[1147]—dealt with the action of the serum of both naturally resistant and susceptible animals on the phagocytability of Pneumococcus. When virulent cultures were sensitized by contact for one hour at 37° with the serum of animals resistant to Pneumococcus, the organisms were actively ingested not only by homologous leucocytes but also by the white blood corpuscles of other resistant and susceptible animals. On the contrary, when pneumococci were exposed to the action of the serum of animals normally susceptible to pneu-

* Quoted by Neufeld and Haendel.[992]

mococcal infection, the cocci were not taken up by the leucocytes of either resistant or susceptible animals. The serum of all the resistant species tested—dog, cat, sheep, pig, and horse—possessed marked opsonic properties not found in the serum of animals of susceptible species, such as the rabbit, guinea pig, and man. There appeared, however, to be no essential difference in the phagocytic activity of the leucocytes from the various animals. Heating the serum, according to Robertson and Sia, abolished the destructive power of serum-leucocyte mixtures for pneumococci. The validity of the authors' classification of resistant and susceptible animals is open to question. To group the horse with such highly resistant animals as the dog, cat, sheep, and pig, and to include species of such diverse susceptibility in the non-resistant class, may not be wholly justified. In another portion of the report, Robertson and Sia drew attention to other conditions which may influence the opsonizing property of serum on pneumococci subjected to the action of leucocytes. The strain and type of the culture employed, the age of the animals, and other factors discussed in the chapter on Pathogenicity must be taken into account in evaluating the results.

From the conclusions in an extensive report on an investigation of experimental pneumococcal septicemia and antipneumococcal immunity published by Wright in 1927,[1547] certain passages may be cited. Avirulent pneumococci of Type I inoculated intravenously into rabbits are rapidly removed and do not reappear in the blood; virulent strains of the same serological type similarly inoculated disappear for a short period and then subsequently increase in number. Previous active immunization enhances the capacity of the rabbit to remove virulent organisms and to prevent their reappearance, and in the immunity so established the outstanding effect is the increased activity of the body fluids favoring phagocytosis, although the existence of a slight degree of residual and purely cellular immunity cannot be excluded. Because leucocytes could be considerably decreased in number without interfering with the capacity of the animal to dispose of organisms introduced into the blood, taken in connection with the specific action of serum on the cocci, Wright laid particular stress on the importance of humoral immune elements in bringing about the destruction of invading pneumococci.

That circulating antibodies and not leucocytes play the dominant part in recovery from pneumococcal infection was also the contention of Robertson, Woo, Cheer, and King (1928).[1152] The blood of cats and rabbits surviving experimental pneumococcal infection possessed the ability to promote the destruction of highly virulent pneumococci in rabbit serum-leucocyte mixtures, which mixtures in themselves had no growth-inhibitory action. The bactericidal action of the serum was associated with a marked increase in acquired resistance to infection. In cats, which were studied in greater detail, the pneumococcidal promoting power of the serum as well as the opsonic, agglutinative, and mouse-protective properties, which were found to be type-specific, became demonstrable at the time of recovery, and their appearance in the serum always marked the termination of blood invasion. The animals succumbing to infection failed to develop detectable immune properties in the serum and showed persistent bacteriemia. According to the authors, the degree of leucocytosis had no constant relation to the outcome of the disease.

In two communications, Terrell (1930)[1385-6] presented the results of experiments carried out to determine the changes in humoral immunity occurring during the early stages of experimental pneumococcal infection. Using the technique of Robertson and Sia[1144-5] to determine circulating antibodies, the author, after infecting normal cats and dogs with virulent cultures of Type I and II pneumococci, found that in a generalized and overwhelming infection accompanied by early blood invasion, there was a prompt and rapid decrease in the concentration of native humoral immune bodies, which frequently disappeared entirely by the time of death. Animals surviving a moderately severe, generalized infection showed a similar early diminution of humoral immune substances, but with the onset of recovery the concentration of the immune bodies again rose. When the infection was localized, as in the case of true lobar pneumonia, the presence of humoral antibodies in quantity could be demonstrated in the blood throughout the course of an infection terminating in death.

Other evidence indicating the participation of leucocytosis in resistance to pneumococcal infections is to be found in the communication of Schattenberg and Harris (1932).[1222] The plan of the experiments was to induce leucocytosis in white mice by preliminary injections of killed cultures of typhoid bacilli or staphylococci, of detoxified suspensions of devitalized pneumococci, and of sterile milk. Six to eight hours later the animals were inoculated intraperitoneally with lethal doses of pneumococci of Types I, II, and III so measured that death of the mice could be controlled to take place at periods varying from three to twenty-four hours. The animals thus treated failed to show that stimulation of leucocytosis had any effect in preventing the development of pneumococcal peritonitis.

NORMAL TROPINS OR OPSONINS

The ability so to sensitize pneumococci that they become attractive to leucocytes and susceptible to phagocytic lysis is a character of some normal as well as of immune serums. Rosenow[1160-1] disclosed the property in normal human serum and found opsonins for streptococci, staphylococci, and tubercle bacilli, in addition to those for pneumococci.

Ungermann (1911)[1434] was unable to discover any phagocytosis of virulent pneumococci in the serum of normal mice and rabbits. Avirulent strains were readily phagocyted, and the degree of the action appeared to parallel the resistance of the particular species of animal whose serum was used. The conclusion was reached that normal resistance depended upon the phagocytic power of fresh normal serum, at least in the cases studied, and that the serum must develop this power *in vitro* in the presence of leucocytes. Woo[1541] later (1926) found, in testing the pneumococcidal activity of normal serum-leucocyte mixtures, that virulence of the cultures and the age of the test rabbit influenced the outcome of the test. Avirulent strains were readily destroyed in a mixture of normal rabbit serum and leucocytes, whereas virulent cultures resisted the destructive action of the mixture. The absence of pneumococcidal properties in the blood of very young rabbits agreed with the extreme susceptibility to pneumococcal infection of immature animals of the species.

Strouse,[1346] by both *in vitro* and *in vivo* tests, demonstrated the same quality in the peritoneal fluid of pigeons. Wright[1547] noted the rapid disappearance of virulent pneumococci injected directly into the blood stream of rabbits and the still more rapid removal of avirulent forms. Specific immunization enhanced the activity of body fluids favoring phagocytosis. Robertson and Sia,[1144] and later Sia,[1268] not only proved the existence of normal opsonins for pneumococci in the blood of cats, dogs, sheep, and pigs but, by absorption experiments, exhausted the serum of opsoninizing substance for the strain used as absorbent without removing opsonins for organisms of other types. The results suggest that there are separate type-specific opsonins for pneumococci in the serum of animals naturally resistant to pneumococcal infection.

In 1933, Ward and Enders[1484] published a communication, based on experiments with Pneumococcus, dealing with a serological analysis of the opsonic or tropic action of normal and immune serum. The authors studied the action of the anticarbohydrate substance in normal serum as an opsonic or tropic agent, and also the properties of normal and immune serum which promote phagocytosis after the anticarbohydrate substance or antibody had been removed from the serum by appropriate amounts of type-specific polysaccharide. The authors analyzed the mechanism of the phagocytosis of Pneumococcus as follows: In normal, unheated human serum virulent pneumococci may be prepared for phagocytosis by two separate antibodies acting in conjunction with complement. One of these is the type-specific anticarbohydrate antibody reacting with the carbohydrate fraction of Pneumococcus; the other is probably also a type-specific antibody, but quite distinct from the former and, therefore, reacting with a different antigenic constituent of the bacterium. In normal human serum heated to 56° these two antibodies may, after prolonged contact with the organism, promote phagocytosis of Pneumococcus without the adjuvant action of complement. The two antibodies are equally effective in the phagocytosis of twenty-four-hour cultures by normal blood, but the anticarbohydrate antibody tends to predominate as the pneumococci approach the state in which they exist in the animal body. The anticarbohydrate antibody was the only one in immune serum which could be demonstrated to induce phagocytosis. It was active by itself, but complement enhanced its effect.

To Ward and Enders it seemed that a single well-defined antibody—the anticarbohydrate antibody—might be responsible for the phagocytic action of unheated normal serum, of heated normal serum, inactivated immune serum, and immune serum activated by complement. The facts appeared to invalidate the division proposed by Neufeld of the phagocytic antibodies into bacteriotropins—antibodies, the phagocytic titer of which is not raised by the addition of complement—and opsonic antibodies—antibodies, comparable to lysins, which are only active in the presence of complement. Complement alone was found to be incapable of inducing phagocytosis of Pneumococcus and, therefore, may act merely as a catalyst in increasing the velocity of the phagocytic process. On the basis of their observations, Ward and Enders proposed that the term "tropin" be discarded, since it was misleading and unnecessary, and that the term "opsonin" be retained to denote any heat-stable antibody which prepares bacteria for phagocytosis. Contrary to current usage the latter term would not suggest a combination of antibody with complement.

ANTIOPSONINS

The existence of substances in Pneumococcus inimical to leucocytic ingestion became apparent to Rosenow (1907)[1161] who, by saline extraction or by autolysis of the cocci, obtained a substance or substances that inhibited opsonic action. It was found further that avirulent strains could absorb the inhibiting substance and then become resistant to phagocytosis, while after similar extraction virulent organisms acquired the capacity to absorb opsonin and became vulnerable to the destructive action of the white blood cells. The presence of substances in pneumococci capable of inhibiting phagocytosis was demonstrated by Tchistovitch and Yourevitch[1383] in 1908. When saline suspensions of washed, virulent pneumococci were added to serum-leucocyte mixtures, marked phagocytosis resulted, but when a small amount of the washings from the original culture was added to the combination the cocci were no longer ingested by the leucocytes. The inhibiting substances were found only in cultures of virulent strains, they were specific for the bacterial species and were thermostable. For such substances Tchistovitch proposed the name "Antiphagins."

Pritchett[1110] endeavored to develop antiopsonins in rabbits by injecting them with antipneumococcic horse serum, but could obtain no evidence of the formation of substances antagonistic to the action of immune serum. On the contrary, the serum of rabbits injected with antipneumococcic horse serum for Type I, II, or III pneumococci, when combined with antipneumococcic serum for Types I and II, increased opsonization of organisms of Types I and II but in this respect never affected strains of Type III.

Confirmation of the existence of antiopsonic principles in virulent pneumococci is to be found in the experiments of Wadsworth and Sickles,[1475] and of Sickles (1927).[1277] Intracellular substances released by sodium oleate solution of the organisms, or present in the sterile filtrates of broth cultures, prevented phagocytosis of pneumococci in immune-serum and leucocyte mixtures. There was some evidence of type-specificity in the action of the pneumococcal derivatives, since an extract of Type I Pneumococcus failed to prevent phagocytosis of Type III organisms in the presence of Type III antiserum, and vice versa. The inhibiting substance affected the organisms and not the leucocytes. Furthermore, the active principle could be absorbed from extracts by combination with specific immune serum.

Yamamoto (1929)[1557-8] studied the effect of both unheated and heated culture filtrates of pneumococci on spontaneous phagocytosis *in vivo* in the rabbit. The "Impedin," as the author called the inhibitory principle, was without action on the number of migrated leucocytes. The injection of heated filtrates affected phagocytosis in inverse ratio to the duration of previous exposure of the filtrate to heat, the antiopsonic property being completely destroyed after thirty to sixty minutes at boiling temperature.

The action of the specific capsular polysaccharide, so conspicuous in the inhibition of other serological reactions between Pneumococcus and immune serum, is manifested in its antagonistic effect on opsonins, and is referable to its function of combining with and precipitating the antibodies from serum. In studies on growth inhibition, Sia (1926),[1267] by means of normal rabbit or cat serum-leucocyte mixtures, learnt that the presence of a very small amount of purified soluble specific substance from pneumococci of both Types I and II markedly altered the conditions in the mixture so that even a small number of avirulent pneumococci were enabled to grow in the presence of serum and leucocytes of animals which ordinarily possess the power to destroy the organisms in relatively large numbers. The action of the capsular carbohydrate was type-specific, and the same neutralizing effect on the growth-inhibitory or pneumococcidal power of normal serum-leucocyte mixtures was exhibited by broth filtrates of cultures of young pneumococci.

Ward[1480-1] confirmed Sia's observations on the specific antiphagocytic action on blood of soluble specific substance, and found the action more marked in the case of Type III than Type I pneumococci. In *in vitro* phagocytic experiments with human blood, antipneumococcic serum, capsular polysaccharide, and living, virulent pneumococci, there was a zone of definite phagocytic inhibition when a strong antiserum was used. Upon dilution of the serum there appeared a zone in which phagocytosis was effective. Ward suggested that the inhibition was caused by the specific precipitate formed by the combination of soluble specific substance and precipitin, which interfered, perhaps mechanically, with the ingestion of the pneumococci by leucocytes.

In later reports, Ward[1482-3] described a type-specific substance with a powerful antibacterial action present in the filtrate of a five-day broth culture of Type III Pneumococcus. A similar substance was also demonstrated in the filtrate of a lung obtained at necropsy from a patient dying of lobar pneumonia caused by a Type III organism. Ward employed a method devised by himself for estimating the pneumococcidal action of whole blood, and found that if the precipitinogen content of the broth filtrate and the amount of soluble specific carbohydrate of Type III Pneumococcus were taken as a basis of comparison, it required approximately one thousand times as much antiserum to neutralize the antagonistic action of the broth filtrate as was necessary to neutralize the specific carbohydrate. Ward also found that a specimen of blood from a patient convalescing from Type III lobar pneumonia, though comparatively weak in anticarbohydrate antibody (precipitin), was better able to neutralize the broth filtrate and the lung filtrate than a corresponding mixture of normal blood and specific antipneumococcic serum.

Enders and Wu (1934)[362] more recently reported that the opsonic titer of normal serum could be practically abolished by the addition of the A carbohydrate. In immune serum, the A substance brought about a quantitatively greater reduction in opsonic activity than did its derivatives, but the authors were never successful in demonstrating complete inhibition of phagocytic action by the method of absorption of antibody. Enders and Wu also showed that the A carbohydrate was far more effective as an antibactericidal—that is, antiopsonic—agent than deacetylated derivatives of the capsular polysaccharide.

OPSONINS IN PNEUMONIA

Among others, Rosenow (1906)[1160] announced that the content of opsonins for Pneumococcus appeared to be less in the serum of patients succumbing to pneumonia than it was in normal human serum or in serum of patients during or after crisis. Using the Neufeld technique, Strouse (1911)[1346] could demonstrate no phagocytosis of virulent pneumococci by serum obtained from pneumonia patients after crisis, but by sensitizing the organisms with convalescent serum previous to the test, phagocytosis was observed in about one-fourth of the cases. Eggers (1912),[349] employing the plate method of cultivation, noted an increase in the pneumococcidal power of the blood of pneumonia patients at or near the time of crisis, and while he demonstrated that the action was due to phagocytosis, Eggers presented no detailed experimental evidence to prove whether the action of serum was exerted on the cocci or on the leucocytes. Clough (1913)[240] observed that the serum of approximately one-half the pneumonia patients obtained after crisis or lysis exhibited definite phagocytic activity, and that the reaction was strictly limited, under the conditions of the test, to the homologous strain of Pneumococcus isolated from the patient whose serum was being examined. Clough concluded that, since the active substances resisted heating at 56° and persisted in the serum *in vitro* for a considerable period of time, the substances must be tropins and, since phagocytic activity of the serum appeared to parallel closely the protective power for mice in incidence, time of appearance, and strain specificity, the protective action of serum was directly due to its ability to promote phagocytosis. In a second report, Clough (1919)[242] confirmed his earlier observations and added that while in 85 per cent of cases of acute lobar pneumonia the serum showed positive phagocytic activity after crisis or lysis, it lacked the property in the great majority of instances where the patient had died of the disease. The height of bacteriotropic activity of the serum of pneumonia patients was found by Adler (1923)[3] to occur at the time of crisis.

THE MECHANISM OF PHAGOCYTOSIS

The factors and processes involved in the response of rabbits to intravascular injection of pneumococci were investigated by Kitagawa (1915).[717] When the living organisms were injected directly into the blood stream of rabbits there was an immediate, initial drop in the count of circulating cocci, followed by either a slow increase or decrease in number depending upon the dosage and virulence of the injected culture. When similar injections were made into actively immunized rabbits, the cocci disappeared with great rapidity from the circulation, the blood usually becoming sterile within ten minutes after the injection. Kitagawa concluded that the speedy disappearance of the injected pneumococci from the blood stream of actively immunized rabbits was not due to destruction of the organisms by plasma or leucocytes, but rather to their mechanical removal or destruction by the fixed tissues. Kline and Meltzer (1915)[727] also noted that pneumococci promptly vanished from the pneumonic lung of dogs infected by intrabronchial insufflation after previous repeated intravenous injections of pneumococci.

The same phenomenon was studied by Winternitz and Kline (1915).[1522] In normal rabbits the reaction to inoculation was immediate and the ultimate result was bacteriemia and death; in passively immunized animals the organisms rapidly disappeared from the blood and recovery took place; in rabbits previously rendered aplastic with benzol and then injected with specific immune serum, there was an immediate effect on the injected pneumococci, but bacteriemia recurred and death ensued; in actively immunized, aplastic rabbits, the initial reaction was the same as in the passively immunized, aplastic rabbits, but the actively immunized, aplastic rabbits recovered. Winternitz and Kline accordingly concluded that the immunological response was dependent upon at least three factors, namely, immune bodies, white blood cells, and a third factor relying for its existence on the presence of white blood cells at the time of inoculation with Pneumococcus. The humoral immune bodies acted in causing the immediate disappearance of the injected organisms from the circulation, but the third factor, originating in the leucocytes, appeared to be essential to the recovery of the infected animal.

The importance of elements peculiar to immune serum for the protection of mice was shown by Tilgren (1915)[1401-2] who, by adding immune sheep serum and sheep leucocytes to an infective dose of pneumococci, protected rabbits against infection. In mice, the immune serum afforded protection but the addition of heterologous leucocytes resulted in no increase in the protective power of the serum.

More detailed information regarding the tissues concerned in resistance to pneumococcal infections is to be found in the communication of Permar (1923),[1082] who believed that the mononuclear phagocytic cells appearing in the exudate in acute experimental pneumonia in the rabbit were of vascular endothelial origin. Other cells of visceral origin possibly contributed in some degree to the total number of phagocytes in the exudate. Dust cells of similar origin already present in the alveoli also might act as phagocytes in inflammatory reactions, while interstitial dust cells could become reactivated and through liberation by inflammatory edema were enabled to appear in the exudate. The entire group of cells, therefore, including the newly produced phagocytes and the dust cells, may take part in the reaction to the invading pneumococci.

Singer and Adler (1924),[1290] after studying the response in rabbits to infection with Type III Pneumococcus, believed that the defensive factors resided in the reticulo-endothelial system, and that the histocytes of bone marrow, the capillary endothelia of the parenchymatous organs, the endothelium of serous cavities, and the biologically comparable alveolar epithelia, as well as the fixed tissue cells with phagocytic properties underlying them, must have experienced in the immune animal a specific alteration in the sense of acquiring the power to ingest pneumococci and to retain and eventually to kill the organisms. To Singer and Adler, leucocytic phagocytosis merely exerted a secondary chemotactic action, but had nothing to do with specific immunity toward a given organism. In a second communication in the same year, Singer and Adler[1291] reported analogous results obtained in experiments of the same nature with pneumococci of Types I and II. The authors maintained that in passive immunity the cellular system played the main part, the action of the serum being purely a bacteriotropic one. The phenomenon was definitely type-specific and the elements of the reaction were located in the reticulo-endothelial tissues, since functional blockade of that system caused a disappearance of the manifestations of immunity.

Tudoranu[1427] disagreed (1926) with the theory of Singer and Adler that immunity toward Type III Pneumococcus was devoid of specific humoral elements and quoted the latter's own experiments to refute the claim. Although in passively immunized rabbits injected with Type III cultures the organisms for a time multiplied in the blood, the animals eventually recovered, whereas normal rabbits similarly inoculated succumbed to infection. Tudoranu, in support of the contention, cited his success in passively immunizing rabbits by the subcutaneous, intraperitoneal, and intravenous injection of specific immune serum, and suggested that the successful result was merely a question of dosage of serum. The author concluded that the action of the serum was to neutralize the aggressins, thus permitting the production of an exudate rich in leucocytes, which modified the cocci in such a way as to render phagocytosis possible.

In the interval between the publication of the papers of Singer and Adler and of Tudoranu, Neufeld and Meyer (1924)[995] reported the results of a study of the origin of antipneumococcal immunity. According to the latter authors, actively immunized mice manifested the same specific phagocytosis as those passively immunized, but scarcely ever had demonstrable protective bodies in the blood. However, after intravenous injection of manganese salts, the protective substances appeared in the blood in large amounts. Neufeld and Meyer concluded that the active immunity depended entirely upon antibodies, that the antibodies were formed in the reticulo-endothelium and that, in a broader sense, the cells of the *Gefässbindegewebsapparat* were the sole source of antibodies.

The ability of macrophages to dispose of pathogenic bacteria was described by Nakahara (1925).[941] The method of demonstrating the action of these cells was the injection of olive oil into the peritoneal cavity of mice. The injection was followed at first by the appearance of polymorphonuclear leucocytes, which were largely replaced by mononuclear cells. When pneumococci were injected into mice during the macrophagic reaction, the organisms were destroyed more rapidly than was the case in normal animals, and the mice survived multiples of the minimal infecting dose. The macrophages were observed to phagocyte the injected cocci actively.

Meyer (1926),[896] after blocking the reticulo-endothelial system by the intravenous injection of ferric saccharate, India ink, trypan blue, and other dyes, along with the removal of the spleen, was unable, as a rule, to immunize mice by the injection of killed pneumococci of Type I. When active immunization preceded the removal of the spleen and the injection of the blocking agents, the immune condition of the animals was sometimes altered. Meyer was not able to substantiate the earlier observation of Neufeld and Meyer on the necessity of stimulating the endothelia by manganese, since protective antibodies were found to be present in the blood of the majority of mice immunized with Type I pneumococci. Inasmuch as splenectomized mice in which the reticulo-endothelial system had been blocked easily acquired passive protection after the injection of specific immune serum, Meyer argued that the effect of these measures could not be due to a decrease in the phagocytic activity of the reticulo-endothelial cells, but rather to an inhibition of antibody formation in the cells and that active as well as passive immunity depended upon specific antibodies circulating in the blood and present in the cells. The contribution of the reticulo-endothelial system to the operation of the immune mechanism was believed by Wright (1927)[1547] to be of relatively slight importance. Although he acknowledged that the possibility of a residual cellular immunity could not be overlooked, Wright considered circulating antibodies to be the prime factor in immunity to Pneumococcus.

The relationship of blood-free splenic cells of normal and immunized rabbits was investigated by Loewenthal and Micseh (1929).[822] Using the technique of tissue culture devised by the first-named author, it was found that the macrophages of the spleen of normal rabbits phagocyted avirulent pneumococci only in the presence of fresh, normal serum, and phagocyted virulent organisms only in the presence of specific immune serum. Macrophages of the spleen of immunized rabbits phagocyted both avirulent and virulent pneumococci without the addition of either normal or immune serum, when the tissue fragments were not transplanted into a fresh medium. However, when bits of spleen tissue of immunized rabbits were transplanted into fresh media during tissue culture, the macrophages behaved similarly to those of normal animals. Loewenthal and Micseh believed that the results pointed to a close relation between the mechanisms of humoral and cellular immunity.

In 1932 and 1933, Kritschewski, Rubinstein, and Heronimus[758-9] confirmed the results of Meyer on the inability of antipneumococcic serum to protect mice that had been splenectomized and had suffered artificial impairment of function of the reticulo-endothelial system. The great majority of mice so treated succumbed to intraperitoneal inoculation with Type I Pneumococcus.

Protective Antibodies

To resolve the protective action of antipneumococcic serum into the causal elements participating in the phenomenon is a difficult task. There is the innate defense mechanism of certain animal species; the functional ability of various animals to respond to antigenic stimuli, as manifested by the elaboration of antibodies of different properties; the interaction of tropins or opsonins, cocci, and white blood corpuscles; and the natural or the artificially enhanced avidity of fixed tissue cells for pneumococci. As in other aspects of antipneumococcal immunity, the communications of the Klemperers (1891)[724-5] were prophetic in suggesting that the serum of animals after being injected with derivatives of Pneumococcus developed the ability to render the cocci susceptible to the action of blood cells and body cells and, therefore, harmless to the injected animal. The authors erroneously ascribed the protective action of the serum to an antitoxic effect, but the assumption does not invalidate the observation. Eyre and Washbourn (1898),[374] by injecting mice with mixtures of varying amounts of antipneumococcic horse serum and virulent cultures of pneumococci, were the first workers to demonstrate quantitatively the protective power of specific immune serum. The authors later applied the method to the standardization of therapeutic serum and, in doing so, discovered that the method could be employed to distinguish between different varieties of the organism.*

Neufeld and Haendel (1910),[991] using the protection test for evaluating the strength of immune serum, confirmed the observations of Eyre and Washbourn on the existence of types of pneumococci with different serological affinities and thus established the protection test as a means for the classification of pneumococci into different serological types. Neufeld and Haendel at first employed 0.2 cubic centimeter of immune serum, which they in-

* Wassermann (1899)[1491] sought to locate the origin of protective substances, and from his experiments concluded that the antibodies apparently were formed in the bone marrow, and that the lymph nodes, thymus, and spleen merely served as reservoirs.

jected intraperitoneally into mice weighing 18 to 20 grams two to three hours before giving an intraperitoneal inoculation of varying amounts of virulent broth cultures. Later, when more potent serum became available, falling amounts of serum were injected into mice just previous to inoculation with one or more multiples of the minimal infecting dose. Ungermann and Kandiba[1436] applied the Neufeld and Haendel technique to a study of the quantitative relations between the protective strength of immune serum and the amount of culture used, and discovered that the action of the serum failed to follow the law of multiple proportions. When the tests were performed on rabbits, there appeared to be a definite relation between the volume of serum and the weight of the animal, called by Ungermann and Kandiba (1912) the *Schwellenwert* or threshold value. Above this value serum protected against many multiples of the minimal lethal dose of culture, but below the threshold the serum had little if any action. In their experience, Neufeld and Haendel (1912)[993] found that, in order to ensure protection with serum, it was necessary to cross the hypothetical threshold and to administer large volumes of serum.

SPECIFICITY

Some claims have been advanced concerning the lack of type-specificity in the protective mechanism. For example, Yoshioka (1923)[1561] reported that mice that had survived an intraperitoneal inoculation of pneumococci were protected against an intraperitoneal injection three or four days later of cultures of heterologous type. Furthermore, mice similarly treated were able to withstand inoculation with streptococci, while large doses of killed staphylococci produced definite protection against pneumococci. Yoshioka also noted a certain degree of cross-protection in guinea pigs and rabbits after pneumococcal infection. Kolchin and Gross (1924)[789] observed cross-protection for Type III strains in a sample of Felton's monovalent Type I antipneumococcic serum. Monovalent rabbit antiserum prepared with pneumococci of Types II and III also exhibited cross-protection between Type III serum and Type I organisms. Despite the heterologous action observed in the protection test, all the samples of immune rabbit serum tested were found to be type-specific in agglutinin content.

From the data presented in the communications of Yoshioka and of Kolchin and Gross it is difficult properly to interpret the results. However, against the claims of the occurrence of cross-protection with monovalent immune serum there is a mass of evidence attesting the specificity of the reaction when serum is prepared from carefully authenticated strains of Pneumococcus and when similarly identified strains are used for testing the protective action of immune serum. The mouse protection test, when properly executed, therefore, remains the final criterion for establishing the type-identity of pneumococcal strains.

RELATION TO OTHER ANTIBODIES

A definite relation exists between the amount of protective antibody in a given serum and its content of agglutinins and precipitins. Among the many references which might be cited, the work of Heidelberger, Sia, and Kendall (1930)[630] and the study of Felton (1931)[407] are chosen as illustrative. The former authors determined a close parallelism between the specifically precipitable protein and the number of mouse-protective units in a wide variety of Type I antipneumococcic serums. So constant were the results yielded by the simple method for determining the amount of precipitable protein in immune serum that the reaction as described in the section of the present chapter dealing with precipitins could be relied upon to measure the protective strength of the serum. Sabin (1931)[1204] was unable to precipitate the totality of protective antibody from antipneumococcic serum by the addition of homologous soluble specific substance and hence assumed the existence of a protective substance distinct from the anticarbohydrate antibody. However, Felton[407] found in samples of Type I antipneumococcic horse serum a close correlation between protection, precipitin, and agglutination titer for Type I Pneumococcus.* Similarly, Barnes, Clarke, and Wight (1936),[82] using a modified precipitin test, found that the correlation between precipitin and protective antibody content was sufficiently close to warrant the substitution of the precipitin test for the animal test in titration of the protective value of antipneumococcic serum.*

ADDITIONAL DATA

Kyes (1911)[765] employed domestic fowls for the preparation of antipneumococcic serum, giving the birds repeated inoculations of large doses of virulent pneumococci. Kyes concluded that by this method it was possible to obtain serum possessing distinct protective action against pneumococci within certain hosts. In 1920, Wadsworth,[1460] after injecting a single dose of standardized pneumococcal vaccines of Types I, II, and III into mice, found that it was possible with Type I vaccine to produce protection against Type I cultures but not against Type II or III strains. In the case of Type II vaccine there appeared to be protection exclusively against the homologous organism while, when Type III vaccine was administered, there was no protection against any of the three types. Cecil and Blake,[206] after injecting monkeys with saline suspensions of heat-killed virulent Type I pneumococci, could demonstrate protective antibodies in the serum although the animals eventually succumbed to intratracheal inoculation with the same living strains. Later, Cecil with Steffen,[213] by the intravenous and subcutaneous injection of larger doses of pneumococcal vaccine, succeeded in completely protecting monkeys against infection and made the seemingly paradoxical observation that protective substances might or might not be present in the serum of the immune monkeys.

The same authors[214] reported (1925) a similar condition in monkeys immunized by intratracheal vaccination, and decided that

* See page 378 of this chapter.

the immunity so produced was probably cellular in nature. Barach,[74] employing mice and rabbits, was able by the injection of heat-killed pneumococci of Types I and II, and of sterile culture filtrates of the organisms, to demonstrate the presence of protective antibodies in the serum of the animals three days after injection. The degree of immunity produced was greater in the case of Type I than of Type II vaccine, and Barach concluded that immunity was due to the elaboration of protective antibodies. Barach (1931)[76] obtained analogous results after injecting similar vaccines prepared from heterologous strains of pneumococci into patients suffering from lobar pneumonia. The average time of appearance of protective antibodies was between five and six days after intravenous and intradermal administration of the killed pneumococci. Similar effects followed the intradermal injection of protein-free, type-specific polysaccharide from pneumococci of Types I, II, and III into normal individuals, as reported by Finland and Sutliff (1932).[448]

In the year previous, Avery and Goebel[45] had demonstrated that the appearance of type-specific protective antibodies followed the injection into rabbits of the capsular polysaccharide of Type III Pneumococcus conjugated with horse-serum globulin, and that it was the polysaccharide which determined the type-specificity of the ensuing protective antibodies. Avery and Goebel[46] then (1933) proved that the acetyl polysaccharide could induce the development of the specific protective substance in animals. Confirmation of the formation of type-specific protective antibodies after injection of the capsular polysaccharide was forthcoming from the study of Francis (1934)[474] on the immunizing effect of the intradermal injection of small amounts of pneumococcal carbohydrate into man.

CHEMICAL NATURE OF PROTECTIVE ANTIBODIES

The work of Avery (1915)[32] yielded the first information concerning the particular protein element in antipneumococcic serum with which the specific protective antibodies are associated, and furnished the foundation for the future development of methods for the isolation and concentration of the protective substance. From the serum of horses immunized with pneumococci of Types I and II over a period of one to two years, Avery was able, by adding ammonium sulfate to 38 to 42 per cent saturation, to precipitate completely the immune bodies. The protein fraction holding the protective antibodies did not correspond to the euglobulin of the serum since the fraction was not rendered insoluble by one-third saturation with ammonium sulfate or by complete saturation with sodium chloride. In 1924, Felton,[396] by the use of water acidulated with tartaric acid, separated the bulk of protective substance from antipneumococcic serum of Types I, II, and III. The precipitate appeared to be composed largely of globulin, which in the state of purity obtained at the time by Felton had an isoelectric zone between 6.6 and 7.5.

Banzhaf,[70] by Felton's method of dialysis, separated approximately 90 per cent of the protective bodies from the fraction of globulins precipitable between the limits of 30 and 50 per cent saturation with ammonium sulfate. In further studies, Felton[397-400, 403] found that the water-insoluble globulin retained its protective power after repeated purification, and that the globulin could be largely freed from accompanying serum proteins through precipitation with appropriate concentrations of sodium sulfate and by ethyl alcohol.[408] The possible protein nature of the immune substance was suggested by the fact that its protective value was diminished by the digestive action of pepsin, trypsin, pancreatin, and papain (Felton and Kauffmann, 1927).[426]

Goodner,[528] by the addition of appropriate amounts of water, was able to precipitate the protective antibody as well as agglutinins from antipneumococcic serum. The dilution of serum, after preliminary tests to determine the proper amount of water to be added, was carried out at a temperature of approximately 4°. After carrying the precipitate through a refining process, the resulting solution was said to contain 14,000 Felton protective units per cubic centimeter.

The question arose whether the protective principle against Pneumococcus in specific immune serum is actually a protein of the globulin type representing merely an increase in the native serum globulin, whether it is a new protein substance associated with but chemically distinct from the natural globulin of serum, or whether it is a non-protein substance sharing some of the physical and chemical properties of serum pseudoglobulin. From time to time various answers have been proposed. The work of Avery, of Banzhaf, and of Felton indicated that the protective antibody is intimately associated with the pseudoglobulin fraction of immune serum, but the results do not necessarily imply that the antibody is the natural serum globulin. For example, the experiments of Felton and Kauffmann showed that the ratio of protein to protective units can be reduced by selective salting out with ammonium sulfate. A difference between immune and native serum globulin is the more alkaline isoelectric point of water-insoluble globulin containing protective antibody, as shown by Felton and by Reiner and Reiner.[1133] The unusual alkaline isoelectric point of the purified immune proteins was considered by Chow and Goebel[226] to be its most characteristic property, and the authors believed that this property might be attributed to the relatively high ratio of amino to carboxyl groups present in the protein molecule.

Chow and Goebel by repeatedly precipitating pneumococcal antibody with ammonium sulfate were able to rid the specific pseudoglobulin from much inert protein material, and then by means of potassium acid phthalate they succeeded in effecting a further purification of the pseudoglobulin antibody. Although Huntoon[666] believed that the specific protective antibody separated by him from pneumococcal antigen-antibody precipitates was non-protein in nature, Chow and Goebel were of the opinion that the circulating antibodies are in reality modified serum globulins. Confirmation of the latter hypothesis has come from the work of Heidelberger and Kendall,[625] who, by the use of strong salt concentration and proper adjustment of the hydrogen ion concentration well on the alkaline side, obtained from pneumococcal polysaccharide-homologous antiserum precipitates a protein substance of which 93 per cent of the total nitrogen was in the form of immune body nitrogen.

Heidelberger and Kendall took the precaution of removing from their source material—unconcentrated Type I, II, and III antipneumococcic serum—somatic protein antibodies and somatic carbohydrate (Fraction C) antibodies, thus reducing the antibody content of the serum to antipolysaccharide antibodies. By employing unconcentrated serum without chemical treatment, any possible denaturation of the antibody was avoided and the antibody dissociated from the specific precipitate was considered as being presumably free from artificial concomitants.

By dissociating antibody from similar antigen-antibody precipitates and then by purifying the antibody by dialysis with subsequent precipitation at its isoelectric point, Chow and Wu[227] succeeded in obtaining a protein preparation of high precipitating activity, which they considered as representing an immunologically pure protein.

The work of Wyckoff[1555] and of Heidelberger, Pedersen, and Tiselius[629] further attests the protein nature of pneumococcal antibody and points to a distinction between specific immune globulin and the globulin of normal horse serum. However, there still remain discrepancies to be explained. None of the antibody preparations so far obtained can be regarded as pure in the strict sense of the word from either a chemical or an immunological viewpoint. As Chow and Goebel remarked, no end-product ever attains a value of 100 per cent of type-specific precipitable protein. Yet the evidence that has accumulated in the past few years makes it difficult to escape the conviction that pneumococcal antibody is a protein, undoubtedly of the pseudoglobulin type, and that it is a chemical entity distinct from native serum pseudoglobulin.

Further information concerning the intimacy existing between pneumococcal antibody and immune serum globulin has come from analyses of normal and antipneumococcic serum by means of the ultracentrifuge of Svedberg[1369] and a modified machine described by Biscoe, Pickels, and Wyckoff (1936).[119] Employing the latter apparatus, Biscoe, Herčík, and Wyckoff[118] determined that in concentrates of Type I antibodies the proteins consist mainly of molecules with a sedimentation constant of about

$$16 \times 10^{-13} \text{ cm. sec}^{-1} \text{ dynes}^{-1}.$$

This finding, taken with the presence of similar molecules in unconcentrated antipneumococcic horse serum and their complete or almost complete absence from normal serum indicates that these molecules are the real bearers of antibody activity. Further support of the view is supplied by the observation of Heidelberger, Pedersen, and Tiselius[629] that after ultracentrifugation the specific antibody from serum from a horse immunized with Type I polysaccharide and a sample of concentrated Type I antipneumococcic serum (Felton) showed homogeneous sedimentation, with the following sedimentation constant:

$$s_{20} = 17.2 \times 10^{-13}$$

The sedimentation constant of normal globulin from mammalian serum is:

$$s_{20} = \text{about } 7 \times 10^{-13}$$

By applying the method to concentrated preparations of Type I antipneumococcic serum, Wyckoff[1555] found that the only protein molecules in the bottom layers of the fluid were those with

$$s = 16 \times 10^{-13}$$

Small amounts of light molecules, which in each concentrate accounted for roughly 15 per cent of the total protein content, were those of the principal serum globulin with

$$s = 7 \times 10^{-13}$$

The experiments strongly support the idea that the Type I antibody is associated with the molecule having

$$s = 16 \times 10^{-13}$$

Furthermore, Biscoe, Pickels, and Wyckoff obtained the same measurement for molecules of antibodies against other types of pneumococci. Speculating on the relation between pneumococcal antibody and specific immune protein, Wyckoff concluded: "Since this is a molecular species that appears in appreciable quantities in horse serum only when it has become antipneumococcic, two possibilities suggest themselves. It is conceivable that during immunization this globulin is made or freed in excess in order that there may be plenty of it present to fix all the antibody activity that may develop . . . and the alternate, that the globulin is the antibody." The results of investigations of this nature are highly suggestive, and the method promises to yield valuable information concerning this abstruse but important question.

Differences in the nature of the protective antibody in antipneumococcic rabbit serum and in that in antipneumococcic horse serum have been demonstrated by Chow.[224] In horse serum, the antibody in the pseudoglobulin fraction soluble at pH 5.5 was completely precipitated when the reaction of the solution was adjusted to pH 7.6. From the corresponding fraction of the immune rabbit serum no trace of precipitate was obtained. Furthermore, in the case of immune horse serum, the main portion of the antibody was concentrated in the pseudoglobulin fraction, whereas the opposite was found to be true with the immune rabbit serum, that is, the euglobulin fraction apparently contained the major portion of the antibody.*

Another difference in the antibodies present in antipneumococcic rabbit and horse serum lies in the size of the molecule of the two substances. In experiments involving the use of the ultracentri-

* A difference in the phosphatid molecules linked with the globulin in the case of antibodies from the horse and rabbit has been mentioned in the footnote on page 381 of this chapter.

fuge, Heidelberger, Pedersen, and Tiselius observed that in the case of immune rabbit serum the specific antibody was produced from the principal globulin component, while in the horse the anti-carbohydrate for Type I Pneumococcus is developed from an otherwise minor component. The isoelectric point of the protein representing the pneumococcal antibody of the rabbit was determined as approximately pH 6.6, whereas the isoelectric point of the immune protein from horse serum was as acid as pH 4.8. That the molecule of the protective antibodies as elaborated by the two animal species is of different size is also evident from the work of Goodner, Horsfall, and Bauer.[539] When Type I antipneumococcic rabbit serum was filtered through an ultrafilter of the type described by Bauer and Hughes,[90] no appreciable specifically precipitable protein passed through a membrane with an average pore diameter of one millimicron. A 13.8 millimicron filtrate contained 11.9 per cent of the total specifically precipitable protein. Slightly greater amounts were recovered as the pore sizes were increased up to 73 millimicrons, at which point the curve rose sharply until at 102.5 millimicrons the filtrate contained 86.6 per cent of the total antibody. With antipneumococcic horse serum, the smallest pore permitting the passage of antibody was 45.2 millimicrons. Between 73 and 102.5 millimicrons the curve rose steeply until at the latter porosity 76.7 per cent of the antibody was recovered. With a concentrated preparation of Type I antipneumococcic horse serum the end-point was relatively sharp, no antibody being recovered at 150.4 millimicrons, while 100 per cent was found in the filtrate at 188 millimicrons. The authors decided that in general it might be assumed that the smallest specific antibody of antipneumococcic rabbit serum corresponds to a pore size of 11 millimicrons, the smallest in horse serum to a size of 44 millimicrons, while both horse and rabbit antibodies have large specific aggregates corresponding roughly to a pore size of 88 millimicrons. Furthermore, the antibody of concentrated horse serum requires a pore size of approximately 176 millimicrons.

Goodner, Horsfall, and Bauer drew attention to the fact that the figures given are multiples of 11, which corresponds to the value of 11 to 12 millimicrons determined by Elford and Ferry[353] for the isolated form of normal horse pseudoglobulin.

Recent observations on the molecular size of pneumococcal antibody in immune rabbit serum, in immune horse serum, and in concentrated antibody solution are of importance not only in connection with differences in the characters of antibody as produced in animals of different species, but in emphasizing the range in surface area of the different types of antibody. Gram for gram, the pneumococcal antibody from the immune rabbit, because of its smaller molecular size and therefore its greater surface area, should exhibit greater combining power for homologous antigen than the antibody of the larger molecule of immune horse serum and that of the still larger aggregate present in concentrated antipneumococcic serum.

THE SEPARATION OF ANTIBODIES FROM IMMUNE SERUM

Inasmuch as the concentration and purification of pneumococcal antibodies will be described in detail in Chapter XV, only the principles involved in the separation of specific substances from immune serum will be dealt with in the present chapter. Gay and Chickering[508-9] took advantage of the particulation that takes place when cellular substances of Pneumococcus are brought into contact with homologous immune serum. From the antigen-antibody precipitates the antibody was then recovered by the use of suitable physical and chemical agents. The method was adopted, with modifications, by Huntoon and his associates[665-6, 668-9] and the use of specific precipitates has been developed as furnishing a source of pneumococcal antibody. Another basic method is founded on the relative insolubility of the immune proteins in water at their isoelectric point, as well as their insolubility in water in the absence of electrolytes. The use of protein coagulants such as ammonium and sodium sulfates, so valuable in the concentration and refinement of antitoxins, and a similar use of alcohol, have received wide application in the study of the chemical nature of immune substances against Pneumococcus and especially in the quantity concentration of antipneumococcic serum. The affinity of the immune bodies for metallic salts also affords a method for the isolation of antibody. Now ultracentrifugation and ultrafiltration promise means of separating pneumococcal antibody from the accompanying components of immune serum.

THE ESTIMATION OF PROTECTIVE ANTIBODIES

In the quantitative estimation of the content of protective antibody in antipneumococcic serum several variables are encountered in the culture, the serum, and the test animal employed. Inasmuch as methods for measuring the therapeutic potency of antipneumococcic serum will be discussed in the chapter dealing with serum production, brief mention may be made at this point of some of the factors which may influence the accuracy of the determination. Enlows[366] pointed out the necessity of using cultures in the phase of active growth or in the early stationary phase in order to avoid lag on transfer. The hydrogen ion concentration of the medium in which the pneumococci are grown should be such as to ensure the presence of cocci at the height of vitality. The virulence of the culture should be maintained at a high level. Felton[402] standardized the infecting dose of culture by plate counts and employed a dilution of culture representing 500,000 fatal doses of organisms.

Felton (1926)[399] discovered in antipneumococcic serums for Types I, II, and III, a substance that was lethal for mice. Later, Felton and Bailey[419] pointed out that from immune serum precipitable residues could be isolated that had an antagonistic action on the neutralization of protective antibody by capsular polysaccharide. Furthermore, the amount of soluble specific substance operated to cause a zonal effect in the estimation of protective action.

The mouse, on account of race, age, weight, and physical condition, presents an array of variable factors in the response to the protective action of specific antipneumococcic serum. These factors, described by Felton[405] for the mouse, and by Goodner,[532-4] and Goodner and Miller [540] for the mouse and rabbit, have already been mentioned in the chapter on antigenicity and need not be repeated.

For elimination of the variables in the animal host, for simplicity and rapidity of performance, the newer methods based on specific precipitation present many advantages over the mouse protection test for the quantitative determination of protective antibody in antipneumococcic serum.

Other Immunological Phenomena

GROWTH OF PNEUMOCOCCI IN SPECIFIC IMMUNE SERUM

The growth of pneumococci in immune serum was observed by Metchnikoff[894] in 1891, and Denys (1897)[312] reported that pneumococci grow as well in immune as in normal rabbit serum. In the experiments of Rosenow (1904),[1159] pneumonic blood was found to possess no bactericidal properties for Pneumococcus, while viable organisms could be propagated from agglutinated masses of the cocci in the serum of pneumonia patients. An initial lag in the multiplication of pneumococci planted in the serum of artificially immunized animals, followed by active proliferation of the cells, was described in 1920 by Bull and Bartual.[177] Nicolle and Césari (1926)[1008] obtained better growth in Martin bouillon containing specific homologous serum than in the same medium to which heterologous immune or normal serum had been added. The ability of pneumococci to grow in homologous anti-S and anti-R immune serum and the effects of the serum on the growth of the cocci has been described in Chapter V.

ANTIBLASTIC IMMUNITY

An action of antipneumococcic serum apparently not definitely attributable to any of the known specific antibodies was described in 1916 by Dochez and Avery,[320] who found that immune serum temporarily inhibited the multiplication of pneumococci and, at the same time, depressed the proteolytic and glycolytic functions of the bacterial cell. The retardation of growth and inhibition of metabolic activity of the cocci was ascribed by the authors to antienzymatic substances in antipneumococcic serum, and to the phenomenon they applied the term "antiblastic immunity." Blake (1917)[124] differed with Dochez and Avery in the explanation of the effect, and since it was found that the inhibitory action of serum paralleled the agglutinative power and, moreover, since serum exhausted of its agglutinins no longer interfered with the metabolic activities of the cell, Blake denied the participation of any antienzymatic principle in the phenomena. Barber (1919)[78] observed the inhibitory effect on the vital activities of pneumococci of whole fresh blood, coagulated plasma, and the serum of normal or immune horses and pigeons and, while attempting no analysis of the factors involved, believed that the action was antiblastic in nature. Bordet (1931),[140] noting the effect of normal rabbit serum on cultures of Pneumococcus, as manifested by changes in the morphology of the cocci, queried whether the disturbance in the metabolism of the organisms could be due to alexin or to the production of acid in cultures containing rabbit serum. The influences displayed by immune serum on the vital functions of pneumococci, as just described, are probably the same as those leading to the dissociation and degeneration of the pneumococcal cell.

IMMUNOLOGICAL RELATIONSHIPS BETWEEN PNEUMOCOCCUS AND OTHER MICROBIC SPECIES AND UNRELATED SUBSTANCES

Analogous to the apparent serological relations already described in Chapter VIII existing between Pneumococcus and such varied entities as gum arabic, *Bacillus coli, Leuconostoc mesenteroides,* Friedländer's bacilli, and tubercle bacilli, are the cross-reactions demonstrated by Sugg and Neill (1929)[1355] between yeast and Type II Pneumococcus. The reader may recall that

Mueller and Tomcsik (1924)[938] had described a complex carbohydrate prepared from yeast that bore certain chemical resemblances to the capsular polysaccharide of Pneumococcus. It remained for Sugg and Neill[1356] to demonstrate that the resemblance extended to the immunological behavior of these two representatives of *Schizomycetes* and *Saccharomycetes*. Pneumococci of Type II, but not of Types I or III, were agglutinated by serum from rabbits immunized by injections of a certain variety of yeast, and filtrates of young, unautolyzed broth cultures of the same type of pneumococci invariably precipitated potent antiyeast serum. The antiyeast serum, furthermore, protected normal mice against Type II pneumococci as well as the average specific antiserum produced in rabbits for this type. The reciprocal reaction of Type II antipneumococcic serum with yeast was not so definite, since serum from many normal rabbits was capable of agglutinating yeast. In a 1 to 5 dilution, Type II antipneumococcic serum gave clean-cut agglutination. The results of absorption experiments with both the antiyeast (rabbit) serum and the Type II antipneumococcic (horse) serum were the same as those usually obtained in analogous experiments with immunologically related, but not identical, species of bacteria.

The protection against infection with Type II pneumococci conferred upon mice by injection of suspensions of heated yeast cells was practically the same as that obtained by vaccination with Type II pneumococci themselves, with the exception that yeast evoked immunity to Type II and not to Type I or Type III organisms. The mutual reactions of yeast and Type II pneumococci were further demonstrated when Sugg and Neill (1931)[1356] employed semi-purified carbohydrate antigens from both yeast cell and pneumococci mixed with homologous antiserums. Antiyeast serum precipitated with, and sensitized guinea pigs to the Type II antigen but was not active with antigens from strains of Type I and III pneumococci. The Type II antigen was almost as reactive against antiyeast serum as against homologous antiserum. Conversely, Type II but not Type I or Type III antipneumococcic serum reacted with yeast carbohydrate antigen but not to the degree observed in the case of antiyeast serum and pneumococcal carbohydrate. The action of different samples of antiyeast serum of equal potency as to reactivity with yeast antigen varied greatly when tested against pneumococcal antigen.

Summary

The substance of this chapter may be recapitulated as follows: The introduction into the bodies of animals of suitable species of pneumococci and some of their natural components augments or brings into being an array of specific immune substances that serve to protect the animal against the invading cocci and that can be demonstrated by appropriate serological and other immunological reactions. The immune substances thus evoked comprise agglutinins, precipitins, opsonins or tropins, and complement-fixing and protective antibodies.

Agglutinins, arising as a result of artificial immunization or appearing in the blood of pneumonia patients at or near the time of crisis, are easily demonstrated: the specific agglutination reaction takes place between the intact pneumococcal cells, whether living or dead, and the homologous antibody in the serum used. The reaction varies from strict type-specificity to a broader species-specificity, depending upon the nature of the antigen employed in the production of the immune serum and that of the hapten participating in the reaction. The somatic protein of the cocci and of degraded or R forms of the organisms engenders agglutinins reactive with all types of pneumococci, whereas the intact, virulent forms of pneumococci or their unimpaired capsular constituents evoke agglutinable substances strictly specific for the type of antigen or component supplying the antigenic stimulus. In the latter instance the reaction is one between the specific capsular polysaccharide of the organism and its corresponding specific, immune-serum globulin. Because of the simplicity of the technique required for the detection or quantitative determination of agglutinins in immune serum, the agglutination reaction finds a wide use in the identification of members of the types within the species.

The precipitin reaction, involving as it does the interaction of hapten and immune body in solution instead of the reaction between formed microbic elements and specific serum and, moreover, being independent of the participation of the immunological factors possessed by a living, immune animal, is susceptible to the application of mathematically accurate quantitative measurements. By means of the precipitin reaction, it is possible to determine with great exactness the quantity of hapten in a given solution or the amount of immune nitrogen—that is, the amount of specific antibody in immune serum. Because of the fortunate, close parallelism existing between the content of precipitin and protective antibody in any particular serum, a quantitative estimation of the therapeutic value of antipneumococcic serum can be made in the test tube instead of in experimental animals.

The greater economy of means required in the reaction and its greater accuracy when properly performed have led to far more detailed studies of the phenomenon which, in turn, have supplied many clues to the mechanism operating in immunity to Pneumococcus. The chemist has thus been given the means of learning the very chemical radicals in the precipitinogen and the globulin fraction of immune serum which join to produce the precipitate and presumably which participate in the other immunological manifestations. The specificity of serological precipitation depends on the interaction of the capsular polysaccharide and immune globulin; and the basic process is the same as that in the phenomenon of agglutination.

The method of complement fixation offers no advantages over other serological methods for the demonstration or measurement of pneumococcal antigen and antibody. It has, however, revealed and enable one to study the striking difference in the nature of specific antibodies in immune rabbit serum and immune horse serum.

Substances that neutralize the hemotoxin of Pneumococcus have been discovered in specially prepared immune serum, and some evidence has been presented that substances capable of inhibiting the action of the poisonous products of Pneumococcus may arise in the immunization of animals with the so-called pneumococcal toxins.

In a true sense there are no specific bactericidins for pneumococci. The destructive effect on pneumococci of body tissues is referable to a more complex play of biological elements.

There exist in the normal animal body, and to a much greater degree in the body of immune animals, substances that render pneumococci susceptible to the phagocyting action of mobile leucocytes and the fixed body cells. Disregarding the confusion of terms, the opsonins or tropins act on the bacteria and not on the phagocytic cells and it is by means of the intervention of the normal or immune opsonins that, under suitable conditions, pneumococci may be destroyed in the test tube or in the body of the infected animal.

The combined phenomena of agglutination, precipitation, and opsonization are the complement of forces mustered by the animal body for protection against invading pneumococci. The assumption is supported by the close correlation found to exist between the various antibodies concerned in antipneumococcal immunity. The specific protective action of immune serum can be strikingly demonstrated in laboratory animals and the type-specificity and the degree of this protective action can be measured by *in vitro* methods. Through chemical studies, the protective antibodies have been located in the globulin fraction of immune serum and by both chemical and physical manipulations they may be isolated in relatively pure form. Recent advances in these technical procedures have made possible actual measurements of the molecular size of pneumococcal antibodies and are leading to a clearer conception of their chemical composition.

There remains to be explained the significance of the immunological relation of pneumococcal antigens and antibodies to those of alien microbic species, as well as their relation to apparently biologically unrelated substances in both animal and vegetable tissues. The solution of these problems will go far to explain dependence of immunological action on chemical composition.

CHAPTER XII

HOST RESPONSE TO ANTIGENIC ACTION OF PNEUMOCOCCUS

Normal barriers to the invasion and multiplication of pneumococci in the animal body; the immunological reaction naturally stimulated by pneumococcal infection and the reaction artificially aroused by the administration of pneumococci, their constituents, or derivatives; the somatic manifestations of the immune state; and the utilization by the body of antibodies passively acquired.

SOUND skin and healthy mucous membranes are impediments to the entrance of Pneumococcus into the animal body. Underlying these tissues, as a line of secondary defense, are the leucocytes, which with normal auxiliary elements of the blood may ingest and destroy the invading cocci. The localization or the systemic distribution of the organisms depends on the vigor of the phagocytic response and on the functional capacity of the body to elaborate specific antibodies in response to the antigenic stimulus provided by the invading microorganisms.

Total failure of the defenses means death but, with only a partial lack of antagonistic factors, the animal may pass through the rigors of pneumococcal disease and thereby acquire greater, if temporary, resistance to subsequent attacks. An analysis of the protective mechanism of the animal economy against pneumococcal infection will be attempted in the present chapter.

Natural Immunity

IN ANIMALS

A reason for the behavior of various normal animals toward pneumococcal infection was sought by Tchistovitch (1890),[1381] who subjected dogs, rabbits, and mice to subcutaneous, intratracheal, and intraocular inoculation with *Streptococcus lanceo-*

latus (Pneumococcus). The animals were killed during successive stages of infection and the lungs examined for cellular changes. The differences in the physiological response corresponded with the natural susceptibility of the animal species to infection. In non-refractory animals, the cocci caused only a feeble local inflammatory reaction with little phagocytosis, and the leucocytes neither engulfed the organisms nor inhibited their growth. In refractory animals, on the contrary, a more or less pronounced local inflammatory process developed, with leucocytic migration and accompanying phagocytosis. When the injections were made into the anterior chamber of the eye, there appeared to be no difference in the reaction of the aqueous humor of the animals of the two classes, since the fluid served as a medium for the growth of the injected cocci.

Opposed to the observations of Tchistovitch were those of Behring and Nissen,[98] published in the same year, who could find no differences in the bactericidal properties of the serum of mice, rats, and rabbits. The inability of the serum of the animals to affect pneumococci was in marked contrast to their destructive action on anthrax bacilli. Wadsworth[1455] also (1903) was unable to discover any parallelism between the action on pneumococci of serum from normal animals and the natural resistance of the animals to pneumococcal infection. When tested by agglutination and precipitation methods, the serums in low dilutions showed no significant differences.

Natural immunity of the pigeon to Pneumococcus, according to Strouse (1909),[1345] was due to high normal body temperature and not to any specific tissue reaction. Employing both *in vitro* and *in vivo* methods for studying phagocytosis, Strouse could detect no difference in the reaction of pigeons and of mice to experimental infection. Ungermann[1434] also studied the phenomenon of phagocytosis occurring after the addition of serum of various animal species to leucocytes of animals of homologous and heterologous species. While in the case of the rabbit and mouse no phagocytosis was observed when virulent pneumococci were used in the test, the destruction of avirulent strains seemed to parallel the resistance toward the particular strain possessed by the animal whose serum was tested. While Dold (1911)[323] could demonstrate no substances antagonistic to Pneumococcus in the serum, plasma, or whole blood of normal mice and rabbits, by treating rabbit leucocytes by the method of Schneider, extracts were obtained which Dold claimed had definite killing power for pneumococci.

Robertson and Sia (1923)[1144] devised an accurate method for demonstrating growth-inhibitory and bactericidal action on Pneumococcus of normal serum-leucocyte mixtures. The ingredients of the mixture were added in known quantities and mechanically agitated by rotation and oscillation. A combination of serum and leucocytes from resistant animals (cats and dogs) exerted not only a growth-inhibiting but also a bactericidal action on pneumococci. The serum-leucocyte mixtures of susceptible animals (rabbits and guinea pigs) showed no inhibitory effect. In subsequent communications, Robertson and Sia[1145-7] substantiated their earlier results. For example, the growth of pneumococci possessing low virulence for the cat was found to be markedly inhibited in mixtures of cat serum and cat leucocytes, since ten thousand times the number of pneumococci ordinarily sufficient to kill a mouse failed to infect after being exposed for twenty-four hours in the cat serum-leucocyte mixtures. Furthermore, virulent strains sensitized by contact with serum of animals resistant to Pneumococcus were actively phagocyted, not only by the homologous leucocytes, but also by the leucocytes of other resistant animals and of susceptible animals. However, pneumococci exposed to the action of serum from susceptible animals were not taken up by leucocytes of either the resistant or susceptible animals. The serum of all the resistant animals tested—dog, cat, sheep, pig, and horse

—showed marked opsonic properties which were absent from the serum of animals of such susceptible species as the rabbit, guinea pig, and man. In contrast to the activity of serum there appeared to be no essential difference in the phagocytic power of the leucocytes from the various animals. The influence of the age of the animals on the pneumococcidal properties of the blood was shown by the fact that mixtures of adult rabbit serum with either adult or young hare leucocytes exerted pronounced growth-inhibitory and coccidal action, whereas mixtures of serum from immature hares with leucocytes from either adult or young rabbits completely lacked any similar action. In the natural defense mechanism against pneumococcal infection, it appears that the serum contains the potential elements and that in a susceptible animal like the rabbit the elements develop with the growth of the animal.

The results reported by Robertson and Sia were practically duplicated by those of Woo,[1541] who found that rabbit serum-leucocyte mixtures possessed the power to kill avirulent pneumococci in relatively large numbers, but failed to inhibit growth of even minute quantities of virulent organisms, an observation also reported by Wright (1927).[1547] Woo found further that the serum of very young animals when mixed with leucocytes was powerless to affect cultures which were without virulence for mature rabbits. Bull and Tao (1927)[182] introduced citration for determining the antipneumococcic properties of whole blood. One per cent by volume of saturated, neutral sodium citrate delayed coagulation of the blood for twenty-four hours and did not inhibit the growth of pneumococci. The killing action of citrated blood was more potent than that of serum-leucocyte mixtures. When the method was applied to the blood of normal rabbits and chickens, Bull noted that it required one million times as many pneumococci to infect a given quantity of chicken blood as it did to infect the same volume of rabbit blood.

The hypothesis that it was the natural, humoral antibodies

which were responsible for the pneumococcidal action of serum-leucocyte mixtures received confirmation in a separate study by Sia (1927),[1268] in which it appeared that the active principle operative in the destruction of pneumococci in appropriate serum-leucocyte mixtures could be specifically absorbed from the serum, and that the native principle—the opsonin—was type-specific in its selective action.

It was found by Kelley (1932),[701] as Robertson and Sia had previously discovered, that normal swine serum possessed the property of protecting mice against infection with virulent pneumococci and of agglutinating both virulent smooth and avirulent rough strains of the organism. The protective action of swine serum, although slight, was evidently specific for type, since the protective antibody for one type of Pneumococcus could be absorbed by cultures of the homologous type without affecting the content of antibody for other types. Unlike the protective substances in specific immune serum, those in normal pig serum were thermolabile and disappeared after a few weeks' storage in the cold and, moreover, they could be removed from the serum by absorption with avirulent rough pneumococci. Another difference between normal swine serum and specific immune serum lay in the fact that although the former was type-specific in mouse-protective action, when mixed with soluble specific substance no precipitation took place, nor was the protective action inhibited by the carbohydrate. Kelley also confirmed Robertson and Sia's observation that swine serum shows type-specific agglutination for pneumococci, and that agglutinins for one type may be specifically absorbed, leaving agglutinins for other types undisturbed. Inasmuch as normal pig serum agglutinates avirulent, rough forms of pneumococci and the agglutinative property is not destroyed by heating at 56°, Kelley assumed that this property probably depends on factors other than those responsible for agglutination of smooth forms of Pneumococcus and for protective action in mice.

In 1929, Sia[1269] presented further evidence in support of the view that humoral defensive elements play an important part in natural immunity to Pneumococcus. Mice were given intraperitoneal injections of serum from the pig and four hours later actively growing cultures of virulent Type I pneumococci were injected into the animals. Control mice were similarly injected with serum from susceptible animals (the rabbit and guinea pig) and then inoculated with the same culture. Normal swine serum protected the mice against ten thousand minimal lethal doses of culture, whereas serum from the susceptible animals afforded no protection to the test animals. Pig serum also protected mice against virulent Type II pneumococci and to a lesser degree against Type III organisms. Moreover, absorption experiments again demonstrated that the protective substance was type-specific.

Le Guyon (1931)[796] investigated the causes of the different reactions exhibited by rabbits and guinea pigs to pneumococcal infection. The technique employed consisted in inoculating the animals intraperitoneally with a broth culture of virulent pneumococci and in examining peritoneal fluid withdrawn at various intervals after injection. Four hours after inoculation, mice developed a marked cellular reaction. Along with many cocci there were always a large number of macrophages of the clasmatocyte type. There was intense phagocytosis by the polymorphonuclear leucocytes and macrophages, but in spite of the reaction the animals developed septicemia and died within eighteen to twenty hours. In guinea pigs four hours after inoculation, the reaction was feeble. Some polymorphonuclear cells and some free pneumococci were present in the exudate, but there was only occasional evidence of phagocytosis. Sixteen hours later, the number of organisms and polymorphonuclear leucocytes had greatly increased, but lymphocytes and macrophages were rarely seen. The pneumococci, some of which were phagocyted, were clustered about the polymorphonuclear cells and appeared to be in a degenerated condition. Le Guyon therefore concluded that the initial refractory state in the guinea pig was due to the bactericidal property of the serum.

Bordet (1933)[141] believed that in addition to the leucocyte-serum complex there were other humoral factors which accounted for the unequal susceptibility of animals of different species. The action of the hypothetical factors was manifested by the altered appearance of pneumococci grown in the serum of different animals. The principles appeared to be thermolabile, could be absorbed by aluminum hydroxide, and accompanied the euglobulin when serum was separated into its protein fractions.

A type of resistance, quite independent of strictly immunological processes, is that possessed by the rabbit against the majority of strains of Type III Pneumococcus. An experimental infection can be induced in the rabbit by intradermal injection of many strains of this serological type but the infective process is aborted and the animal recovers.

In the early stages of the infection the leucocytes are powerless to engulf the cocci but, as the body temperature of the animal rises to 104° or higher as a result of the infection, the organisms lose their capsules and are avidly phagocyted. One of the determining factors in the inability of many Type III pneumococci to produce fatal infection in the rabbit is the susceptibility of the organisms to the high temperature generated in the rabbit. A detailed discussion of the experimental evidence on which the above statement is based is to be found on pages 207 to 210 in Chapter VI.

IN MAN

The presence of normal precipitin for Pneumococcus in the blood serum of man was reported by Wadsworth (1903)[1455] but its content was low, since in serum in a dilution of 1 to 10 or more the action of the native precipitin was not evident. Rosenow (1904)[1159] denied that fresh normal blood or serum had any bactericidal influence on Pneumococcus. Neufeld and Haendel (1910)[990] demonstrated the protective action of normal human serum for the mouse, while Much* reported that normal human serum, and to a still higher degree, plasma, contained thermolabile bactericidal substances for Pneumococcus.

Dold (1911),[323] testing by means of plate cultures the action of serum, plasma, and whole blood of normal human beings and of patients ill with diseases other than pneumonia, claimed to have demonstrated definite pneumococcidal effect. The action, stronger in blood than in plasma or in serum, varied from slight inhibition of bacterial growth to actual killing of the organisms.

According to Clough (1924),[243] normal human beings may possess in their serum substances capable of protecting mice against infection with pneumococci of Types I, II, and III. The degree of protection, when demonstrable, was usually slight, but in five instances was sufficient to save the animal from subsequent inoculation with 1,000 to 100,000 minimal fatal doses of pneumococci. Protective action against one type of organism was not necessarily accompanied by similar action against representatives of other types, nor was the property associated with the presence of any agglutinins or opsonins, since the latter antibodies were absent from the serums tested.

Burhans and Gerstenberger (1924)[190] tested the serum of infants and maternal parents for protective power against Type I, II, and III strains of Pneumococcus. The serum of approximately 40 per cent of the parturient mothers protected mice against inoculation with organisms of the three fixed types, while samples of serum from only about 30 per cent of the infants exhibited similar properties. The authors decided that the low incidence of lobar pneumonia during infancy was probably not due to an immunity to the fixed types of pneumococci.

Ash and Solis-Cohen (1929)[26] believed that differences in susceptibility to pneumonia among human beings could be determined by the growth-inhibitory and pneumococcidal action of

* Quoted by Neufeld and Schnitzer.

whole blood and, furthermore, that the reaction was dependent upon the presence of leucocytes.

Analogous differences in resistance were observed by Robertson and Cornwell (1930).[1143] In a study of the pneumococcidal action of normal human serum-leucocyte mixtures for freshly isolated strains of pathogenic pneumococci, the authors ascertained that human beings as a group possess in their blood well-marked destructive properties for all types of Pneumococcus studied. Individuals, however, exhibit wide variations in reaction against different types, ranging from strong killing effect for organisms of one type to no action or slight effect against strains of another type. In the light of the results of previous experiments in which actual resistance of animals to pneumococcal infection was determined, Robertson and Cornwell interpreted the findings as meaning that human beings in general possess a considerable degree of natural immunity to all types of Pneumococcus, but that some individuals may be susceptible to one or more types and at the same time be resistant to other types.

By a method employing whole blood, Ward[1480] found that the phagocytic titer against the first three types of pneumococci varied through a wide range in different normal human subjects. Similar results were obtained in the same year by Sutliff and Rhoades,[1363-4] who measured the pneumococcidal power of normal human blood by a modification of the method of Robertson and his co-workers. Whole blood, to which heparin was added in small amounts as an anticoagulant, was mixed with pneumococci and rotated in an apparatus devised by the authors. Parallel determinations of the protective power of the samples were carried out. The blood of seventeen out of twenty-seven hospital patients who had not had lobar pneumonia killed from one hundred to ten thousand virulent Type I pneumococci. When mouse-protective power and pneumococcidal power were compared, it was found that six subjects possessed both properties and that the serum of ten individuals was bactericidal but not protective, while the serum of three subjects exhibited neither property. In another communication, Sutliff with Finland[1360] reported that the incidence of pneumococcidal power and of other type-specific antibodies varied with the age of the subject as well as with the different types of Pneumococcus. The killing action of normal human serum was most frequently observed with organisms of Type II, was rarest for Type I, and was intermediate for Type III strains.

Gundel,[567] in 1932, investigated the presence of pneumococcidins, protective antibodies, and agglutinins in the blood of normal adults and of healthy nurslings and children. The blood of adults frequently showed the presence of definite amounts of antibacterial antibodies, whereas no protective or agglutinative action was observed with the serum of new-born babies and young children. Gundel concluded that antibody formation began in normal children toward the end of the second year of life. Variations in the titer of humoral immunity were manifested in a third or a fourth of the subjects, there being an increase in the case of some individuals and a decrease in others. In the majority of instances the action was specific, since the altered reactivity toward organisms of one type was not accompanied by a similar change toward other types of pneumococci.

An experimental analysis of the factors responsible for the pneumococcidal action of human serum convinced Ward and Enders[1484] that in normal human serum virulent pneumococci may be prepared for phagocytosis by two separate antibodies acting in conjunction with complement. One of the substances is probably the type-specific anticarbohydrate antibody reacting with the capsular polysaccharide of Pneumococcus; the other is probably also a type-specific antibody, but quite distinct from the former and, therefore, reacting with a different antigenic constituent of the bacterium. In normal human serum heated to 56° the two antibodies may, after prolonged contact with the organism, promote phagocytosis of pneumococci without the adjuvant action of complement. While the two antibodies are equally effective in the phagocytosis of twenty-four-hour cultures by normal blood, the anticarbohydrate antibody tends to predominate as the pneumococci approach the state in which they exist in the animal body. Enders and Wu[362] later reported (1934) that the opsonic titer of normal human serum could be practically eliminated by the addition of the A carbohydrate, that is, the acetylated capsular polysaccharide of Pneumococcus.

Naturally Induced Immunity

SPECIFIC ANTIBODIES IN THE BLOOD DURING PNEUMONIA

Pneumococcus, upon entering the animal body and inciting morbid processes in the organs and tissues, by virtue of its several components arouses or stimulates physiological functions latent or active leading to immunity, and the products of the freshly activated functions may be detected and measured by the various serological reactions. The first intimation that immune substances arise in man as a result of pneumococcal infection came from the work of the Klemperers,[725] who discovered that serum taken from pneumonia patients after crisis displayed curative properties for experimentally infected rabbits. Similar protective antibodies were observed in the serum of pneumonia patients by Römer,[1155] in some cases several days after the onset of the disease. Then Neufeld and Haendel[990] succeeded repeatedly in demonstrating not only that there was a decided increase in protective substances for the mouse in the serum of pneumonia convalescents soon after crisis, but that the action was specific for heterologous as well as for homologous strains of pneumococci. The authors, therefore, were convinced that the crisis in lobar pneumonia depended upon the formation and specific action of antibodies. Seligman (1911),[1253] on the contrary, found no difference in the degree of protective action of serum taken before or after the critical period. Strouse (1911),[1346] using the Neufeld technique, was unable to detect opsonins in heated post-critical serum. However, after sensitizing the pneumococci with the serum, as recommended by Lamar, Strouse experienced no difficulty in obtaining phagocytosis.

Eggers (1912),[349] by the plate method of determining bactericidal action, found increased antipneumococcal properties developing in the serum of pneumonia patients at or shortly after crisis and lasting for variable periods thereafter. Cases in which the apparently characteristic increase of bactericidal power did not occur presented irregularities either in course or in termination. Dochez (1912)[315] was successful in proving the presence of substances protective for mice in the serum of patients ill with lobar pneumonia. All but one of the serums tested showed the ability to protect, the reactive substance appearing in only a few instances before the time of crisis, while in some other cases the protective power appeared to persist as long as the patient was under observation. In some patients, protective antibodies either became evident at some time after crisis or could not be demonstrated at any period of the disease. Dochez concluded that the appearance of specific protective substances in the serum of patients ill with lobar pneumonia suggested that these bodies might play a part in the mechanism of recovery.

In the next year, Clough[240] reported the demonstration of protective antibodies, specific for the infecting strain of Pneumococcus, in the serum of the majority of patients after crisis or lysis. Phagocytic activity of the serum ran closely parallel with protective power for mice. In addition to protective antibodies and opsonins, Lacy and Hartmann (1918)[770] reported that specific agglutinins usually appeared in the serum of pneumonia patients during or shortly after defervescence. In a second report, Clough (1919)[242] stated that the serum of 85 per cent of the patients ill with acute lobar pneumonia whom he had studied showed positive phagocytic activity after crisis or lysis, and that the serum of 79 per cent of the cases showed agglutinative activity. In a few instances, positive results were obtained twenty-four hours or less before crisis. While phagocytic and agglutinative activity were observed for all the pneumococcal types tested, the reaction was always strictly limited to organisms homologous with those with which the patient was infected.

Müller (1923)[939] was inclined to ascribe to humoral antibodies only a minor part in recovery from pneumonia. His belief was based on negative results in tests for bactericidal power of serum from the majority of patients studied, and also on the fact that the author failed to observe any increase in the property during the course of the disease. Adler (1923),[3] on the contrary, reported that the serum of pneumonia patients developed the highest content of bacteriotropic substances at the time of crisis. However, Baldwin and Rhoades (1925)[68] contended that recovery in pneumonia is associated with the appearance of specific antibodies in the blood, and that the antagonistic action of the protective substance is revealed by the fact that pneumococci and protective antibody rarely appear simultaneously in the circulating blood. The presence of protective substance in the blood practically always precluded a concurrent bacteriemia, but it did not in every case prevent toxemia, relapse, or the development of complications. Nevertheless, protective activity of the patient's serum appeared to be an important factor in overcoming pneumococcal infection.

With refined technique for determining the antagonistic action of serum from pneumonia patients, Sia, Robertson, Woo, and Cheer (1925)[1274] found that in all cases of pneumonia studied the serum at or soon after crisis possessed the power to inhibit growth of pneumococci in rabbit serum-leucocyte mixtures. Before crisis, serum either lacked the property or exhibited it only to a slight degree. The titer reached its highest point three or four days following crisis and then gradually diminished, although in one patient recovering spontaneously from pneumonia due to Type I Pneumococcus antipneumococcic substances were still demonstrable in the blood for seventy days. In cases terminating fatally no such substances could be found at any time during the course of the disease. In a second paper, Sia with Robertson and Woo[1273] reported that the same conditions prevailed in pneumonia caused by pneumococci of Types I and II and Group IV. At the critical period, opsonins and agglutinins were also demonstrable in the blood.

Other evidence of the production of an altered condition related to the immune state developing in the body of pneumonia patients, was the abolition of reactivity of the skin to pneumococcal filtrates and extracts, as described by Herrold and Traut (1927).[637] The serum of patients failing to react to the skin test partly or completely neutralized *in vitro* the antigenic substance in the active extracts and conferred protection upon mice.

The time factor in the appearance of protective substances and agglutinins in the course of lobar pneumonia was investigated by Lord and Nesche (1929).[828] The authors were unable to find these antibodies in the blood of patients before a fall in temperature by crisis or lysis, but could demonstrate their appearance and continued presence as soon as defervescence took place. Lord and Nesche attributed importance to the action of protective antibodies in bringing about recovery, since a large proportion of pneumonia patients with these substances in the blood conquered the disease, while the majority of patients without protective antibodies in their serum died. However, that immune bodies may be present in the early stages of untreated pneumonia is indicated by the experiments of Ward,[1480] who observed that the phagocytic titer of whole human blood was comparatively high against the infecting organism. For Ward, the fact pointed to a local rather than a general lowering of resistance in infection with Pneumococcus.

In 1931, Lord and Persons,[838] continuing the study of the production of specific antibodies during pneumococcal pneumonia, reported that although in general the appearance of protective substance coincided sharply with the fall in temperature of the patient, the antibody might appear spontaneously in the blood serum as early as the third or fourth day of the disease and crisis and recovery might be delayed until the sixth to the tenth day. However, recovery might occur without demonstrable protective substance in the blood of patients whose serum later developed protective properties. According to Lord and Persons, the amount of antibody appearing in the course of pneumococcal pneumonia was small and it might be present in the blood concurrently with septicemia. The formation of protective substances by the patient gave no assurance that the infection would not progress to a fatal termination.

In empyema fluids of pneumococcal origin, Floyd (1920)[456] demonstrated the presence of specific precipitin and of much smaller amounts of agglutinin, and considered that their occurrence was generally a favorable prognostic sign. Later, Finland[441] reported (1932) that sterile pleuritic exudates from patients with lobar pneumonia contained actively acquired antibodies similar to those developing in the blood serum.

A property of the serum of pneumonia patients which had escaped previous notice was the capacity to precipitate in high titer the non-protein somatic substance—the C Fraction—derived from pneumococci. Tillett and Francis (1930)[1409] tested serum obtained from patients during illness and convalescence for antibodies specifically reactive with this chemically distinct carbohydrate of Pneumococcus. The results, when correlated with the course of the disease, demonstrated differences in the occurrence of each qualitatively distinct antibody. Strangely enough, the precipitating action of the serum on the somatic carbohydrate developed in the very early stages of the disease, only to disappear at the time of crisis. Precipitation of Fraction C was not limited to the serum of individuals ill with pneumococcal infection and, in the few cases available for comparative tests, definite reactions were obtained only in streptococcal and staphylococcal infections and in acute rheumatic fever.

IMMUNE SUBSTANCES IN SPUTUM

Lord and Nye (1921)[831-3] observed that purulent sputum collected during life and the pulmonary exudate obtained at necropsy from the later stages of lobar pneumonia commonly eroded the surface of Loeffler's blood serum and, in a separate communication, Nye[1021] reported that washed cellular suspensions of pneumonic lungs, previously preserved with chloroform and toluene, contained a proteolytic ferment, derived chiefly from the leucocytes of the exudate. Eddy (1928)[348] found that filtrates from sputum obtained after crisis from patients with lobar pneumonia conferred a certain degree of protection on mice, with sometimes only a delay in the time of death. The effect was never produced by filtrates of sputum obtained before crisis or from fatal cases, nor was the filtrate active with organisms other than those of the type infecting the patient. The sputum of two patients displayed proteolytic action, but Eddy was unable to demonstrate bacteriophage in any of the specimens of sputum. The observation recalls that of Dick (1912),[314] who by noting the optical rotation of mixtures of serum from pneumonia patients taken at the time of crisis found that a decrease in optical rotation occurred at that time and not before or after the critical period. Dick ascribed the phenomenon to proteolytic activity of the serum.

ANTAGONISTIC SUBSTANCES IN PNEUMOCOCCAL EXUDATES

Proceeding from the conception that increased acidity in pneumococcal cultures might find an analogy in the pneumonic lung, Lord (1919),[826] upon testing the hydrogen ion concentration of morbid exudates, found higher acidity in three of four cases than that in the press juice of the unaffected lung. Lord suggested that increase in acidity in the diseased pulmonary tissue might favor enzymatic action as well as inhibit pneumococcal growth.

In further studies on pneumonic exudates, Lord with Nye (1921),[830-1] demonstrated the presence of a proteolytic enzyme. The enzyme remained active after eighteen months' preservation and resisted heating at 65° for one hour, but was destroyed after heating for the same period at 75°. No dialysis of the enzyme could be demonstrated. The activity of the enzyme persisted in concentrations of sodium chloride varying from normal to thirty-two times normal. In exudates, antigenic substances were also found, evidently arising from the dissolution of pneumococci in the infected lung. The presence of specific precipitinogen was disclosed when the exudate was mixed with homologous antipneumococcic serum. After testing extracts of affected lungs, Lord and Nye[833] further concluded that the pneumonic lung contained a soluble substance inhibiting agglutination of fixed types of pneumococci by homologous serum. An analogous substance was found by Ward (1932)[1483] in the filtrate of a lung obtained at necropsy from a patient dying from pneumonia due to Type III Pneumococcus. The substance was similar to that present in somewhat lower concentration in broth cultures of Type III Pneumococcus which displayed powerful antibactericidal action.

Artificially Induced Immunity

The antigenic properties of Pneumococcus and the manifestations of the immunological reaction of the animal body to antigenic stimuli have already been treated in the text in some detail. However, in order that the presentation of the features of the animal hosts' response may be orderly and complete, a brief synopsis is made at this point of the factors that are chiefly concerned in the artificial production of the immune state.

ACTIVE IMMUNITY

The ability of pneumococcal materials, purposely introduced, to raise the resistance of susceptible animals to infection with Pneumococcus, with the accompanying elaboration of demonstrable specific immune substances or antibodies, is dependent upon the nature of the material employed and also upon the special racial and individual peculiarities of the animal treated. The more closely the state of the antigen approaches that of the vigorous, living, virulent cell, the greater the specificity and the completeness, within certain limits, of the immunity and of the antibodies evoked. The robust organism with its protein and carbohydrate constituents in fully developed and unaltered condition exerts the greatest antigenic action. The cell should be living, or devitalized at the peak of its anabolic activities by heat or by such chemical agents as rob the bacterium of the ability to propagate without disturbing its chemical integrity. The greater the mass, within certain limiting zones, the more energetic the specific antigenic stimulation; while the proper spacing of injections and the route by which the antigen enters the body may affect the specificity and the quantity of antibodies produced.

The protein of the pneumococcal cell is antigenic only in the sense that its administration by parenteral routes results in the appearance of humoral antibodies specific for the bacterial species and not for the serological type of the organism injected. The capsular polysaccharide, besides orienting the antigenic action of its conjugated protein when its molecular configuration is undisturbed, is antigenic in itself, and it is this fraction of the pneumococcal cell that determines the type-specificity of the immune response. The somatic carbohydrate—the C Fraction—if it has any antigenic action, apparently has a subordinate and as yet unknown share in the immunizing action of Pneumococcus.

In an animal of a susceptible species, unaffected by any debilitating condition, the parenteral introduction and, to a much less degree, the oral administration of properly chosen pneumococcal antigens, decreases susceptibility to pneumococcal infection and arouses physiological functions latent in the cells of the body. These functions result in the extrusion into the circulation of substances corresponding in type to the kind of antigen administered, and demonstrable and measurable by the various serological reactions. In addition to the appearance of humoral antibodies, the somatic cells undergo changes in reactivity to pneumococcal materials. Of the immune substances engendered, the agglutinins agglomerate the cocci and facilitate their removal from the circulating blood and the precipitins combine with the polysaccharide present in the capsule or released in the disintegration of the bacterial cell, while the opsonins render the organisms susceptible to the phagocytic action of the leucocytes and of certain of the fixed cells of the body.

The immunity thus established by artificial means may become apparent within the space of a few days after the administration of antigen and may persist for longer or shorter periods depending upon the total amount of antigenic material injected, the spacing and repetition of the injections, and the ability of the tissues to continue their special functions. Immunity to Pneumococcus is, at best, a transient condition, and unless the tissues are fortified by continued specific stimulation, the antibodies thus artificially induced shortly disappear from the blood and the animal again becomes vulnerable to the pathogenic action of Pneumococcus.

PASSIVE IMMUNITY

The blood or serum of an immune animal, whether transferred through the placental circulation or artificially injected into the body of a susceptible animal, carries its complement of antibodies that serve to convert susceptibility into resistance; the degree of resistance depends upon the potency of the serum in immune substances, the volume of serum, the route and frequency of administration, and the capacity of the recipient to utilize the antibodies so conferred. In the passively immunized animal, the type of immunity acquired corresponds in specificity to the immunity of the donor.

References to the inheritance of immunity to pneumococcal infection are singularly rare. By inference, it might be assumed from the work of Irwin and Hughes[670] that native resistance may be increased by selective breeding, but in that case the ability of the animals to withstand infection is due to transmitted constitutional factors unrelated to those which account for the specific immune state. The report of Eguchi (1925)[351] is one of the few communications dealing with this phase of immunity. The young of female mice which, during the period of gestation and lactation, had received repeated intravenous injections of killed Type I pneumococci were found to be immune to organisms of the same type as those employed for immunizing the mother. The ability of the mother to protect the offspring disappeared between the sixteenth and twenty-eighth day after the last immunizing injection. Eguchi believed that protection was conferred through the milk of the immune mother. The results of attempts to transmit specific immunity to the progeny by similarly treating the male parent were inconclusive.

Another natural medium for the transference of specific immune bodies is the serum of patients convalescent from pneumococcal infection. Gundel (1931)[565] studied the curative action of convalescent serum and while it was found to be inferior to the usual therapeutic serums of animal origin, yet, according to Gundel, specific therapy with human serum possesses advantages over the use of animal serum in the avoidance of anaphylaxis and serum disease. Other phases of passive immunity will be described in those sections of the text where a discussion of the mechanism is especially pertinent to the particular subject under consideration.

Allergy and Anaphylaxis

In addition to rendering a susceptible animal immune to infection by Pneumococcus, the intact pneumococcal cell and its separate or conjugated components possess the capacity to alter the reactivity of the body tissues to derivatives of the coccus when parenterally introduced. Animals so sensitized may develop acute fatal anaphylactic shock when appropriately injected with certain of the derivatives of Pneumococcus, while the uterus and the dermal tissues of animals thus treated display a newly established function when brought into contact with these products. Actively acquired hypersensitivity may be duplicated by the injection of normal animals with some forms of antipneumococcic serum.

The interaction between specific immune serum and the pneumococcal cell resulting in the formation of a substance capable of eliciting acute anaphylactic shock in the guinea pig was first demonstrated by Neufeld and Dold (1911).[981] Cocci sensitized with homologous antiserum and injected into guinea pigs regularly caused the acute death of the animals. The effect was ascribed by Neufeld and Dold to the production of anaphylatoxin.

ACTIVELY INDUCED SENSITIZATION

In 1911, Rosenow[1165] claimed that, by the subcutaneous, intravenous, intrapleural, and intraperitoneal injection of killed pneumococci or of filtered pneumococcal extracts into guinea pigs, he could so sensitize the animals that they responded with severe intoxication when the same bacterial extract was injected eight to twelve days later into a vein or into the heart. In a subsequent study, Rosenow (1912)[1166] was able to obtain highly toxic substances from Pneumococcus through autolysis, from Pneumococcus-leucocyte mixtures, and by the action of normal and of immune serum on the organisms. These toxic substances evoked in normal guinea pigs symptoms indistinguishable from the symptoms of immediate anaphylaxis. The action of the poisonous substances as well as of the preparations of Cole, Weiss, and others has been discussed in Chapter III, and undoubtedly is to be attributed to histamine-like protein-degradation products.

Clough (1915)[241] employed saline extracts of washed, dried, and ground pneumococci as sensitizing antigens and as the intoxicating agent. The extracts so prepared were sufficiently toxic to cause anaphylactoid reactions in normal guinea pigs. However, by precipitating the extracts with alcohol, Clough isolated a substance, assumed to be protein, that was antigenic in the sense that it could sensitize normal guinea pigs and specifically intoxicate animals so treated.

The allergic state produced in guinea pigs by the intraperitoneal injection of killed broth cultures of Type I pneumococci was observed by Mackenzie (1925).[844] During the course of artificially induced, active immunity, the animals at times showed anaphylactic symptoms after the injection of the immunizing antigens. Bull and McKee (1929),[180] in an investigation of sensitization of the rabbit resulting from acute experimental infection with Type I Pneumococcus, found that the animals had acquired both dermal and systemic hypersensitiveness to pneumococcal autolysate. Sensitivity appeared within forty-eight hours after infection and persisted for at least four months, apparently reaching its height shortly after recovery from infection. Rabbits immunized by the injection of killed and living cultures also became hypersensitive to autolysates but not to so high a degree as did the animals recovering from infection.

Although Avery and Tillett (1929)[60] were unable to sensitize guinea pigs with the type-specific carbohydrates of pneumococci of Types I, II, and III, Tillett, Avery, and Goebel,[1407] in the same year, demonstrated the essential function of the carbohydrate fraction in determining the specific sensitizing and anaphylactic action of the carbohydrate-protein complex. Artificially prepared gluco-globulin and galacto-globulin possessed the property of actively sensitizing guinea pigs so that the guinea pigs, when injected twenty-one days later with sugar-proteins containing carbohydrate identical with that present in the sensitizing antigen regardless of the kind of protein with which it was combined, were subject to acute anaphylactic shock. Moreover, the unconjugated glucosides, although themselves incapable of inducing shock, inhibited the anaphylactic reaction when injected immediately prior to the introduction of the toxigenic sugar-protein into the specifically sensitized guinea pig. The protective, or anti-anaphylactic action of the glucoside disappeared within two hours after injection and, in order to elicit the phenomenon, the carbohydrate had to be the same as that combined in the sugar-protein complex.

PASSIVE SENSITIZATION

From the collective experience of immunologists it becomes evident that some of the isolated constituents of the pneumococcal cell are incapable of so sensitizing the guinea pig as to render the animal susceptible to anaphylactic intoxication upon the parenteral introduction of Pneumococcus or its derivatives. However, that an animal may be rendered highly sensitive to pneumococcal substances by the injection of specific antipneumococcic serum is supported by ample evidence. Weil and Torrey[1508] passively sensitized guinea pigs by the injection of serum from pneumonia patients. When autolysates of pneumococci were added to the uterus of the treated animal, positive contractions occurred only when the serum employed originated from a case of pneumococcal pneumonia. By means of the same method, Zinsser and Mallory[1582] obtained positive reactions with the uteri of guinea pigs passively sensitized with antipneumococcic serum. More conclusive were the observations of Tomcsik (1927),[1415] who demonstrated the ability of the soluble specific substance of Pneumococcus to produce anaphylactic shock in passively sensitized guinea pigs. The purified capsular polysaccharide of Pneumococcus, though apparently devoid of sensitizing action, can induce rapid and fatal anaphylactic shock when injected intravenously into guinea pigs passively sensitized with the precipitating serum of rabbits actively immunized with pneumococci of the homologous type, the reactions induced being type-specific. Avery and Tillett,[60] who reported the observation, also drew attention to the fact that there was a complete absence of anaphylactic response to pneumococcal carbohydrate in guinea pigs similarly treated with antipneumococcic horse serum.

As in their experiments on the production of active specific sensitization with artificially prepared sugar-proteins, Tillett,

Avery, and Goebel[1407] demonstrated further the dependence of the specificity of the anaphylactic phenomenon upon the carbohydrate portion of these compounds. Guinea pigs passively sensitized with the serum of rabbits immunized with an artificial gluco-globulin exhibited typical anaphylactic shock when subsequently injected with gluco-albumin; the serum of rabbits immunized with another sugar-protein, galacto-globulin, similarly sensitized guinea pigs to galacto-albumin. The reactions, in each instance, were specific and depended for their specificity upon the carbohydrate component and not on the protein fraction of the synthesized sugar-protein. The authors found that anaphylactic shock could be induced by uncombined globulin in guinea pigs passively sensitized with either antigluco-globulin serum or antigalacto-globulin serum, and that the globulin was similarly effective in animals actively sensitized with gluco-globulin or galacto-globulin. However, the reactions provoked by globulin alone were dependent upon the common protein present in the antigens and exhibited only species specificity.

The haptenic participation of the A carbohydrate in the anaphylactic reaction was demonstrated by Enders (1930).[358] Guinea pigs injected intraperitoneally with one to two cubic centimeters of the anti-A rabbit serums used in the precipitin tests failed to develop symptoms of anaphylaxis upon intravenous injection of varying quantities of the purified specific carbohydrate. Nor was the antibody against the nucleoprotein or rough autolysate present in sufficient concentration in these serums to confer on guinea pigs anaphylactic sensitivity to the substances. Again, no anaphylaxis developed in animals treated with the serum when autolysates derived from virulent strains of either Type II or Type III pneumococci were introduced intravenously. Type I anti-A serum, however, regularly conferred upon guinea pigs a very high degree of anaphylactic sensitivity to the autolysate derived from Type I Pneumococcus. The "normal" antipneumococcic Type I rabbit serum, from which the specific anticarbohydrate antibody had been removed, also rendered guinea pigs anaphylactically hypersensitive to the A substance in the homologous autolysate. Before the removal of the anticarbohydrate antibody by precipitation *in vitro,* the serum sensitized guinea pigs to the type-specific soluble substance. After the antibody had been eliminated, animals injected with the serum failed to react to the injection of the carbohydrate, but responded typically when injected with the autolysate from virulent organisms of Type I. Furthermore, the animals showed no symptoms following the intravenous administration of autolysate derived from a rough strain of Type I or of autolysates of smooth strains of Types II and III.

The experiments in anaphylaxis showed that in the serum of rabbits receiving injections of formalinized pneumococci an antibody develops that reacts specifically with an antigen found in the autolytic products of Type I Pneumococcus. Similar autolysates of the other two types (II and III) of this organism, as well as rough strains derived from homologous or heterologous types, elicited no anaphylactic symptoms in guinea pigs. Under the same conditions, the nucleoprotein was likewise incapable of provoking specific shock. That the antigen in Type I autolysate responsible for the anaphylactic symptoms was not the specific carbohydrate appeared to Enders to be shown not only by the failure of the latter material, when pure, to produce shock in guinea pigs sensitized with anti-A rabbit serum, but also by the experiments with rabbit serum from which the carbohydrate antibody originally capable of sensitizing the animals had been removed, leaving unimpaired the power of the serum to sensitize the animals to the A substance.

The cellular carbohydrate from Type I Pneumococcus, likewise, caused immediate, lethal anaphylactic intoxication in guinea pigs previously injected with Type I antipneumococcic rabbit serum. Schiemann, Loewenthal, and Hackenthal[1231] reported a similar effect obtained with the carbohydrate preparation made by the method of Schiemann and Casper.[1228] These results, taken with further observations of Avery and Goebel (1931)[45] on the immunological action of an antigen prepared by combining the capsular polysaccharide of Type III Pneumococcus with horse serum globulin, fully justify the conclusion that it is the soluble specific carbohydrate which determines the type-specificity of the hypersensitive state and of the anaphylactic reaction.

The contrasting differences in the sensitizing properties of serum from the immune rabbit and the immune horse were studied by Mehlman and Seegal (1934).[889] In conformity with the results of Avery and Tillett, guinea pigs injected parenterally with antipneumococcic rabbit serum were thrown into anaphylactic shock by the intravenous injection twenty-four hours later of the capsular carbohydrate of pneumococci corresponding in type to that of the immune serum. Guinea pigs similarly prepared with antipneumococcic horse serum were not susceptible to an otherwise shocking dose of the homologous antigen. Uteri removed from guinea pigs sensitized passively with the immune rabbit serum contracted characteristically on contact with the homologous specific carbohydrate, whereas uteri of guinea pigs injected with immune horse serum failed to react in this manner. Tests made to determine a possible anti-alexic activity of parenterally injected antipneumococcic rabbit and horse serum failed to show any marked difference between the two serums. In a second communication, Mehlman and Seegal[890] demonstrated in mice the same difference between the sensitizing property of antipneumococcic serum from the rabbit and from the horse. The sensitizing property of immune rabbit serum appeared to be independent of protective action, since the serum of both the immune rabbit and horse were equally effective in curing mice of infection with Pneumococcus.*

The comparative inability of antipneumococcic horse serum to sensitize the guinea pig passively to Pneumococcus is also evident when sensitivity is tested by intracutaneous injection of soluble specific substance. According to Mehlman and Seegal (1934),

* Differences in the nature of antibodies in immune rabbit and horse serum have been discussed in Chapter XI.

preparations of Type I antipneumococcic serum, obtained from rabbits, sensitized the albino guinea pig so that an injection of 0.1 cubic centimeter of a 1 to 10,000 dilution of Type I polysaccharide into the skin of the ear elicited a positive reaction. However, when antipneumococcic serum from the horse was employed, the same dose of antigen gave variable results, although the injection of twice the amount evoked positive reactions. Experiments on the distribution of immune horse serum as compared with that of rabbit serum in the circulation and organs of passively immunized guinea pigs failed to disclose any explanation for the differences in the sensitizing action of the two serums.

Brown[155-6] reported similar observations on the ability of antipneumococcic rabbit serum to sensitize passively the guinea pig to the specific carbohydrate of Type I Pneumococcus. Brown found that the minimal amount of antiserum necessary to sensitize the guinea pig so that fatal shock followed the injection into the heart of the soluble specific substance was always greater than the quantity of serum required to sensitize to the cellular carbohydrate of Wadsworth. However, the minimal amount of each of the specific carbohydrates which induced fatal shock in guinea pigs previously sensitized by the injection of one cubic centimeter of immune rabbit serum was approximately the same.

The protective or inhibitory action of artificial, conjugated sugar-proteins on the anaphylactic reaction of guinea pigs passively sensitized with antipneumococcic rabbit serum, as reported by Tillett, Avery, and Goebel,[1407] was confirmed by Brown[156] in the case of the soluble specific substance and of the cellular carbohydrate. A subcutaneous injection of a suitable dose of soluble specific substance of Type I Pneumococcus given to guinea pigs twenty-four hours after passive sensitization with Type I antipneumococcic rabbit serum completely desensitized the animals to intracardial injection twenty-four hours later of capsular polysaccharide, but not to a similar injection of cellular carbohydrate. The latter substance, however, completely desensitized the guinea pigs to the anaphylactic action of the soluble specific substance and brought about partial desensitization to the cellular carbohydrate. When capsular polysaccharide prepared according to the original method of Heidelberger and Avery (probably the deacetylated carbohydrate) was added to the minimal dose of serum necessary to sensitize, and the mixture injected at once into guinea pigs, the animals failed to become hypersensitive to subsequent intracardial injection of the same preparation, but acquired sensitivity to the cellular carbohydrate. However, when cellular carbohydrate was substituted for soluble specific substances in the experiment, no sensitization to either capsular or cellular carbohydrate could be demonstrated.

The results reported by Brown were in accord with observations previously described by Wadsworth and Brown (1933).[1468] Specific immune serum, from which the precipitate, formed on the addition of SSS, had been removed, was still capable of sensitizing guinea pigs to the cellular carbohydrate but not to soluble specific substance. Antiserum, after precipitation with cellular carbohydrate, failed to sensitize the animals to either substance. The difference in the action of the two preparations of specific pneumococcal polysaccharides was undoubtedly due to the lack of molecular completeness of the preparation of soluble specific substance employed in the experiments.

RELATION OF PNEUMOCOCCAL ALLERGY TO PNEUMOCOCCAL IMMUNITY

The experiments of Mackenzie[844] suggest a lack of correlation between the hypersensitive and the immune states in guinea pigs treated with Pneumococcus or its extracts. During the course of immunity produced by the intraperitoneal injection of killed and living broth cultures of virulent pneumococci, while the animals showed high resistance to infection and possessed strong protective power in their serum, hypersensitiveness might or might not be present. Mackenzie concluded that anaphylaxis to pneumococcal protein was merely a concomitant of immunity without having any significant part in the immunological mechanism.

Sharp and Blake (1930)[1260] differed with the conclusions of Mackenzie and maintained that in rabbits a fairly close parallelism exists between cutaneous and pulmonary hypersensitiveness to pneumococcal autolysate, and that the inflammatory response of pulmonary tissue, resulting from contact with autolysate, depends on the allergic state of the animal rather than on inherently injurious substances in the autolysate. Sharp and Blake interpreted their observations as being in harmony with the theory that allergy may play a part in the pathogenesis of pneumococcal pneumonia in man.

Julianelle and Rhoades (1932),[696] in a study of the reaction of the lungs of rabbits to infection caused by intravenous injections of Pneumococcus, found that reactions occurred irregularly in the lung, and that in the lungs in which reactions did occur, the histological changes were no different in normal rabbits from the changes in rabbits made resistant by previous intravenous or intracutaneous injections of pneumococci. The authors concluded that the experiments afforded no evidence to support the view that the lesions in the lungs of rabbits, following the intravenous injection of pneumococci, were modified by any previous state of sensitivity.

Dermal Allergy

SKIN REACTIONS IN EXPERIMENTAL ANIMALS

The development of an allergic condition of the skin in guinea pigs following the intracutaneous injection of an alkaline extract of pneumococci occurred in experiments described by Mackenzie and Woo (1925).[845] About two-thirds of the animals so treated acquired cutaneous hypersensitivity but, upon the continuance of the injections, the capacity of the dermal tissues to react ceased. Neither the animals manifesting skin allergy nor those that failed to develop this type of hypersensitiveness showed any significant alteration in susceptibility to pneumococcal infection by intraperitoneal inoculation. Similarly, animals desensitized by repeated intracutaneous injection after the appearance of allergy exhibited an unaltered susceptibility to infection.

In 1927, Zinsser and Grinnell[1581] investigated the action in the skin of normal guinea pigs of various bacterial autolysates including those prepared from pneumococci. Reactions were noted only in the case of well-grown animals, whereas young guinea pigs almost invariably gave a negative reaction on the first test. On further study it was found that the cutaneous reactions were manifestations of hypersensitiveness which could be elicited by bile solutions of Pneumococcus as well as by similar autolysates. Sensitization could be induced by the previous injection of dead, intact bacteria, as well as of autolysates, but the actual skin reaction was elicited only by autolysates. When properly treated, insensitive animals could be rendered sensitive within a space of five to seven days by the daily injection of autolysate. The sensitivity thus produced was related to the bacterial species and not to pneumococcal type. Using the rabbit, Julianelle (1930),[689] after subjecting the animals to repeated intracutaneous injections of heat-killed pneumococci, demonstrated increased skin activity which reached a maximum after four to six injections had been given and then diminished. After regression of the reaction to the first injection of antigen into the skin, there frequently followed a recrudescence or exacerbation of the reaction. By injecting the serum of a highly reactive animal into a normal rabbit, the author was unable to confer the property of skin-reactivity upon the recipient.

In another paper, Julianelle[690] communicated further results obtained in rabbits during a study of actively induced skin-sensitivity to derivatives of Pneumococcus. Positive reactions were evoked in animals that had previously received repeated intracutaneous injections of heat-killed pneumococci, of the pneumococcal nucleoprotein, and of a solution of the bacterial cell from which the acid-precipitable and heat-coagulable proteins had been removed. The reaction appeared to be species-specific but not type-specific. A similar skin reaction to the protein of Pneumococcus occurred in rabbits following the repeated intracutaneous or intravenous administration of heat-killed organisms or their protein derivatives. The reactive function, although evidently related to the presence of humoral species-specific antibodies, occurred independently of resistance to infection.

A phenomenon related to skin sensitivity was the increased reactive power of the eye of rabbits immunized with heat-killed suspensions of smooth and rough pneumococci separately, as described by Julianelle.[691] Positive reactions could be elicited in immune animals by the instillation of nucleoprotein, or of a solution from which the acid-precipitable and heat-coagulable proteins had been removed. No reaction followed the similar application of living, rough cells or the protein-free, type-specific polysaccharide of Pneumococcus. Rabbits receiving intravenous injections of the intact cell or of the soluble derivatives of Pneumococcus failed to develop eye-reactivity, but acquired the property as a result of experimental infection with Pneumococcus. From the collected experimental evidence, Julianelle[692] concluded that the injection of heat-killed pneumococci into the skin created a special kind of skin and eye sensitiveness unrelated to the presence of circulating antibodies and not transferable from sensitive to normal rabbits.

In 1932, Julianelle with Morris,[693] by means of cutaneous and ophthalmic tests, disclosed another indication of a basic relation between pneumococci and streptococci and, in addition, a difference between the specificity of the reaction of the eye and of the skin of sensitized rabbits. Following repeated intracutaneous injections of heat-killed smooth and rough forms of Pneumococcus, rabbits acquired increased dermal sensitivity to both pneumococci and streptococci, while the injection of heat-killed indifferent streptococci produced skin sensitivity to both species of organisms. Injections of pneumococci into the skin were followed in some rabbits by eye sensitivity to pneumococcal protein but not to streptococcal protein or to suspensions of either living organism, whereas similar injections of indifferent streptococci were followed, in some rabbits, by eye sensitivity to suspensions of living indifferent streptococci but not to suspensions of rough pneumococci or to nucleoprotein of either organism. Measured in terms of bacterial specificity, therefore, eye sensitivity appeared to possess a degree of specificity not shared by skin sensitivity. A collateral observation of Julianelle and Morris was to the effect that the serum of rabbits injected intracutaneously with pneumococci or indifferent streptococci contained agglutinins for both rough pneumococci and indifferent streptococci, but only those rabbits which received injections of Pneumococcus acquired resistance to pneumococcal infection.

Barnes* studied cutaneous reactions to pneumococcal protein and capsular polysaccharide in rabbits both actively and passively immunized against Pneumococcus and in horses undergoing active immunizing treatment for the production of antipneumococcic serum. In rabbits actively immunized with Type II vaccine, positive skin reactions were obtained following the intradermal injection of the homologous carbohydrate. The reaction consisted of an area of swelling and erythema having an average diameter of fifteen to twenty millimeters or more, and the crest of the swollen area was raised to a height of four to five millimeters. Positive reactions usually appeared within two hours after the injection as edematous areas which, within eighteen to twenty-four hours, became indurated and then persisted for more than two weeks. Similar injections into normal rabbits or rabbits immunized with heterologous strains of pneumococci were never followed by this type of reaction, although occasionally an early, transient erythema and slight swelling would appear, only to disappear within eighteen hours. Intradermal injections of somatic protein, in the amounts used, prepared from Type III pneumococci failed to

* Unpublished observations.

elicit reactions of significance either in normal rabbits or in rabbits previously immunized with killed pneumococci of the same type.

When a mixture of equal parts of 1 to 1,000 Type II polysaccharide and undiluted homologous immune rabbit serum was injected intradermally into normal rabbits, there developed a cutaneous reaction similar to that observed in actively immunized rabbits when similarly injected with the carbohydrate alone. In the few animals tested, the reaction following the antigen-antibody mixture was not so severe or so lasting as that evoked by the injection of polysaccharide into the skin of an actively immunized rabbit.

In another experiment the precipitin titer was determined on a sample of serum from a rabbit which had been actively immunized with Type II pneumococci and which exhibited a typical cutaneous reaction to the corresponding polysaccharide. Then, on the basis of body weight, a normal rabbit was given an intravenous injection of concentrated Type II antipneumococcic horse serum in an amount calculated to establish in the serum of the rabbit so treated a precipitin titer corresponding to that of the serum of the actively immunized animal. A precipitin test on serum from a test bleeding, taken one hour after the injection of immune serum, indicated that the desired result had been obtained. Skin tests with Type II polysaccharide performed at one-half-hour, one-hour, and two-hour intervals after the serum injection yielded reactions apparently identical with those observed when the same antigen was injected intradermally into rabbits actively immunized with Type II pneumococci. A repetition of the skin tests showed that positive reactions could be elicited for at least four days after the injection of serum. It was found, however, when normal horse serum was substituted for the specific, concentrated, immune horse serum, that no reaction took place.

In horses during the course of active immunization, positive cutaneous reactions could be obtained by the intradermal injection of homologous capsular polysaccharide. The reaction tended to be larger in area but not so sharply defined as that in the actively immune rabbit. A peculiar phenomenon observed was the disappearance and subsequent recurrence of the reaction in some instances without intervening intradermal injections.* The longest period of time over which spontaneously recurring reactions were observed was slightly more than six months. The injection of pneumococcal protein into immune horses, and of type-specific polysaccharide or protein into normal horses or into horses immunized with heterologous types of pneumococci, resulted in no reaction. The experiments, though incomplete, point to a local reaction in the dermal tissues between antigen and circulating antibody or to a fixation of antigen by antibody in the dermal cells rather than to a hypersensitive state of the cutaneous tissues.

Francis and Tillett (1931)[479] succeeded in demonstrating skin reactions to capsular polysaccharides of pneumococci of Types I, II, and III in rabbits actively or, under certain conditions, passively immunized to organisms of one or another of these types. The reaction resembled that of Arthus, and was demonstrable only when type-specific precipitins for the homologous polysaccharide were present in the blood of the rabbit. A reaction was elicited in 84 per cent of actively immunized animals, the serum of which contained type-specific precipitins, and a positive result was obtained in all rabbits passively immunized with antipneumococcic horse serum. Attempts to transfer the reactive principle from immune rabbit to normal rabbit were unsuccessful. The recipients in the latter group possessed no demonstrable circulating type-specific precipitins. Francis and Tillett concluded that the reaction produced by specific capsular carbohydrates is always associated with a well-grounded type-specific immunity.

SKIN REACTIONS IN LOBAR PNEUMONIA

The value of skin reactions to tuberculin and to diphtheria

* Compare with observation of Julianelle, page 456, *ante*.

toxin in determining susceptibility or resistance to infection stimulated interest in a similar application of pneumococcal antigens. Weil (1916)[1507] employed a saline autolysate of Pneumococcus (usually of Type I) and injected the material intracutaneously in the scapular region. The injection was immediately followed at times in pneumonia patients, and in normal subjects as well, by a superficial, ill-defined, cutaneous blush. If the superficial erythema faded within a few hours, the reaction was considered to be negative. If, however, within twenty-four hours there occurred a well-circumscribed area of erythema, with infiltration and papular elevation of the skin surrounding the point of puncture persisting for twenty-four hours or more, the reaction was called positive. During the course of pneumonia, Weil found the reaction to be negative, but twenty-four hours to two weeks after crisis a considerable proportion of patients reacted positively. Normal individuals and subjects suffering from diseases due to organisms other than Pneumococcus might or might not exhibit a reaction.

Analogous results were reported by Steinfeld and Kolmer (1917),[1815] who employed saline suspensions of washed organisms of Types I, II, and III heated to 60°. A positive reaction consisted in a definite papule with an area of erythema greater than one centimeter in diameter accompanied by slight edema. Positive reactions were observed in 30 per cent of patients suffering from lobar pneumonia, but consistently negative results were obtained with normal individuals and with those afflicted with various chronic diseases. All positive reactions noted occurred after crisis or after infection had persisted for a long period of time. Steinfeld and Kolmer stated that there was no constant relation between reactions to the protein of the various types of pneumococci used and the types found in the sputum. Weiss and Kolmer (1918)[1510] employed as antigen hemolytic toxin prepared by dissolving washed, living pneumococci in sodium choleate. Among adult patients with lobar pneumonia the intracutaneous reaction was elicited as early as the fifth and as late as the thirteenth day of the disease (two days before and six days after crisis). In children the reaction was demonstrable at about the same time, but was negative immediately following crisis or within one or two days after crisis. When the pneumonia resolved by lysis, the patients reacted as late as the thirty-second day. In general, the test was positive in all active cases but was negative in all control patients whether children or adults. Weiss and Kolmer considered that the phenomenon was a manifestation of a state of allergy to toxin but, since the reactivity of the skin was present during the stage of toxemia and disappeared during convalescence, it is difficult to look upon the reaction as being strictly allergic in nature, at least in so far as toxin is concerned.

Bigelow (1922),[115] employing saline and aqueous autolysates of pneumococci as antigens, succeeded in evoking type-specific dermal reactions in some cases, while in others and in normal controls a reaction occurred differing in character from that resulting when the type of autolysate and of the infecting organism were homologous. Larson (1926)[787] also reported irregular results of skin tests obtained in normal persons and pneumonia patients injected with pneumococcal filtrates. He apparently assumed that the reaction was due to toxin since allergy was not mentioned in the communication.

The question became somewhat more confused by the observations of Herrold and Traut (1927).[637] The majority of pneumonia patients reacted negatively to filtrates of broth cultures of Pneumococcus, whereas nearly all normal individuals similarly tested also gave negative reactions. By repeated tests on pneumonia patients it was found that the condition preventing a reaction developed early in the disease and usually persisted throughout convalescence. The reactive ability of the individual corresponded to the capacity of the serum to neutralize the active principle of the filtrate, the serum of a non-reactive subject usually effecting a partial or complete inhibition of the antigen.

Comparable to the results of Herrold and Traut were those of

Kramár and Gyüre (1929).[754] Injecting intradermally suspensions of pneumococci of the different serological types, the authors noted positive skin reactions in only 18 per cent of pneumonia patients but in 50 per cent of healthy individuals. In the case of the pneumonia patients reactivity of the skin appeared in eight to sixty days after resolution of the pneumonic process. The reaction was, in general, type-specific for Types I, II, and III, as judged by the serological relation of the antigen employed to the organism isolated from the sputum of the subject tested.

Contradictory results were described by Tillett and Francis (1929),[1408] who found that pneumococcal polysaccharides, when injected intradermally into patients convalescent from lobar pneumonia, were capable of eliciting a definite response. A patient's ability to react was apparently associated with both recovery from infection and the presence of type-specific antibodies in the circulating blood. In addition to the action of the polysaccharide, the so-called nucleoprotein of Pneumococcus, when similarly injected, caused a local cutaneous reaction in subjects during convalescence from pneumonia. The local lesion resulting from the injection of protein was tuberculin-like in character, and differed from that evoked by type-specific polysaccharides in gross appearance, time of development, and duration. Although the presence of precipitins reactive with pneumococcal protein could be demonstrated in individuals acutely ill with or convalescing from pneumococcal pneumonia, the concentration of antipneumococcic antibodies in the blood serum appeared to be unrelated to the patients' capacity to react to intradermal injection of the protein.

In a second communication, Francis and Tillett[478] amplified their observations on the appearance of cutaneous reactions during lobar pneumonia. Immediate wheal formation and erythema followed the intradermal injection at the time of crisis of homologous polysaccharide in 100 per cent of Type I patients, in 55.8 per cent of those infected with Type II Pneumococcus, and in 44 per cent of those infected with pneumococci of Type III. A delayed reaction ensued after a similar injection of pneumococcal protein. The appearance of circulating antibodies for one or more heterologous types in a group of patients repeatedly tested with soluble specific substance was believed by the authors to be referable to the antigenic action of the polysaccharide introduced into the skin during successive tests.

In opposition to the conception that skin reactivity to the capsular polysaccharide of Pneumococcus is associated solely with recovery from pneumonia are the results of Alston and Lowdon (1933).[10] The majority of the individuals studied (63 per cent) who had not recently suffered from pneumococcal infection reacted positively to the intradermal injection of Type II polysaccharide, the percentage of reactions increasing in the older age groups. Retested five to twelve months later, 92 per cent of the subjects previously exhibiting a positive reaction were found to have retained the ability to react to the same antigen. The capacity to respond to similar injections decreased and in some cases entirely disappeared when the test injections were repeated at short intervals. The authors also reported that a considerable number of normal subjects, especially older persons, exhibited a delayed reaction in addition to the immediate reaction or independent of it.

The manifestation of both immediate and delayed reactions may be explained by the fact that the introduction of pure pneumococcal capsular polysaccharide into the skin of a positively reacting subject is promptly followed by a local inflammatory condition, while after the similar injection of the C Fraction or of somatic protein, an interval elapses before any local reaction occurs. Skin sensitivity to pneumococcal type-specific carbohydrates and the presence of specific antibodies in the circulating blood were found to exist independently of each other. The findings of Alston and Lowdon agree with those reported in the previous year by Sutliff and Finland,[1360] who reported that skin reactions to acetic acid-precipitable protein and autolysates of Pneumococcus were negative or rarely positive in infants, infrequently positive in childhood, and positive in a high percentage of adults.

Finland and Dowling (1935)[442] performed skin tests on patients recovering from lobar pneumonia and also on normal individuals and persons suffering from non-pneumococcal affections. The antigens employed were the capsular polysaccharides of pneumococci of Types I, II, and III, and the cellular carbohydrate of Wadsworth and Brown. Immediate cutaneous reactions, similar to those described by Tillett and Francis, were elicited in patients recovering from pneumonia. These reactions were, in general, type-specific and were associated with the homologous antibody in the serum. Similar reactions were obtained with preparations of soluble specific substance and cellular carbohydrate prepared from the same pneumococcal types by the methods of Heidelberger, Goebel, and Avery and those of Wadsworth and Brown, respectively.

Characteristic delayed reactions were seen only with the cellular carbohydrate and were not associated with type-specific antibodies. The delayed reactions were most frequently observed following the injection of the cellular carbohydrate of the atypical Type I Pneumococcus and of the analogous antigen prepared from the virulent Type I strain. Delayed cutaneous reactions to the cellular carbohydrate of an atypical Type I Pneumococcus were obtained regularly during the febrile stage of a variety of infectious diseases but could not be evoked soon after recovery in these cases. The results are similar to those obtained by Francis and Abernethy[475] with the somatic C Fraction of Tillett and Francis.

Among the non-pneumonic subjects on whom observations were made, immediate reactions in general were uncommon. They occurred most frequently with the cellular carbohydrates of Type I and atypical Type I pneumococci. Delayed reactions with soluble specific substance of any type did not occur, but they were frequent with the cellular carbohydrates of Type I and atypical Type I organisms.

In the group of subjects who gave a previous history of pneumonia, none of the eight tests done with capsular polysaccharide was positive. A higher incidence of positive, delayed reactions was, however, obtained in the small number of subjects of this group tested with the cellular carbohydrates.

ACTIVE AND PASSIVE SKIN ALLERGY

The lack of uniformity in specific cutaneous reactions occurring in normal human beings and in those ill with or convalescing from lobar pneumonia was encountered by Cecil and Austin (1918)[204] in following the administration of vaccines made from pneumococci of Types I, II, and III and used for prophylactic injection of healthy men. Small, sterile infiltrations, disappearing spontaneously, occasionally followed the injection of vaccine, and similar lesions appeared in the same individuals after subsequent injections. Subjects exhibiting these reactions rarely possessed any notable amount of agglutinative or protective antibodies in the serum after vaccination, nor was the reactive property specific for any type of Pneumococcus.

Gutfeld and Nassau (1926)[580] treated nurslings ill with bronchopneumonia with vaccines composed of heat-killed pneumococci, and injected normal children or those ill from some cause other than bronchopneumonia intracutaneously with vaccine or with watery autolysates of the same cultures from which the vaccines were prepared. The development of a reddened papule was observed at the site of puncture, appearing within eighteen or twenty-four hours and disappearing after forty-eight hours. No child under one and one-half years of age gave a positive reaction, nor did any of the young patients suffering from bronchopneumonia. The reactions occurred in more than one-half of the normal individuals tested and in a like proportion of those not afflicted with the disease. When the autolysate was mixed with serum of non-sensitive children no reaction took place, whereas the serum of sensitive children failed to neutralize or inhibit the action of the antigen. Gutfeld and Nassau assumed that individuals failing to react to the intradermal test possessed in the skin or in the serum a specific antibody similar to antitoxin, inherited in the case of young nurslings or developed during an attack of bronchopneumonia and then later lost.

Jamieson and Powell (1931)[676] believed that pneumococci produce toxic substances not unlike those obtained from various streptococci. The substances could be detected and measured by skin tests on human subjects and by similar tests performed on rabbits of a suitable breed. Serum yielded by horses that had been treated by subcutaneous injections of the toxic substance possessed the ability to neutralize the skin-reactive property of the toxic antigen. In a second paper, Jamieson and Powell reported the development of positive reactions when filtrates of pneumococci of Types I, II, III, and IV were injected intradermally into large rabbits. Similar reactions to filtrates of all four pneumococcal types were also observed in the case of twelve normal human subjects, who exhibited a degree of sensitivity approximately one hundred times that shown by rabbits. The toxic filtrates could be neutralized by the special immune serum developed in horses by the injection of the same antigen.

The work of Coca[245] bears certain resemblances to that of Jamieson and Powell.[676] Filtrates of pneumococci exhibiting toxic action for young children when injected subcutaneously also induced local inflammatory reactions in the skin at the site of puncture. In Coca's first experiments the filtrate was introduced into the child's skin and at the same time a considerably larger dose of the filtrate was injected subcutaneously. Subsequent skin tests performed with the filtrate on the children so treated were attended by a diminished reaction. Treatment of the subjects with a toxoid prepared by heating the filtrates with formalin tended to reduce the number of positive reactions. When applied to adults giving no history of previous pneumonia, the test was positive in 56 per cent of the subjects tested. In the case of individuals having a history of pneumonia in the past, 15 per cent of the subjects reacted, while in convalescent patients only 5 per cent exhibited positive reactions. Coca reported that not all filtrates tested were antigenic and, at the time, ventured no statement concerning the type-specificity of the phenomena.

Recently Coca,[246] after a further study of the alleged pneumococcal toxin, stated that the action of the toxin in the skin was type-specific and, furthermore, that the toxin was not the type-specific polysaccharide.

The application of the skin test as a guide to serum therapy and as a prognostic aid was suggested by Francis (1933).[473] All but one of the patients who had recovered from Type I Pneumococcus pneumonia (the great majority of them had received specific antipneumococcic serum) gave an immediate reaction to the Type I polysaccharide at about the time of recovery. Francis claimed:

> The test has distinct advantages over the agglutination reaction in that it is not merely an index of circulating antibodies. When positive, it invariably denotes that recovery has begun; when negative, it indicates further serum therapy. The mechanism of the positive skin test is closely related to that operative in recovery from pneumonia, and is apparently the resultant of antibody and tissue activity.

THE MECHANISM OF DERMAL ALLERGY

In addition to the foregoing discussion, two studies may be mentioned which have a direct bearing on the physiological or immunological processes operating in the production of the allergic state and in the manifestations of the hypersensitive condition as elicited by pneumococcal derivatives. Martin and Hill (1930)[866] tested the effect of an alien protein on the reactivity of dermal tissues in albino guinea pigs receiving intradermal injections of living pneumococci. One group of animals received into the skin of the left flank an injection of a suspension of washed pneumococci followed immediately by a similar injection of milk protein on the right flank. Forty-eight hours later they were given on the left side at some distance from the first puncture an injection of the same organism heated for thirty minutes at 60° and again milk protein into the skin on the right flank. The second group of guinea pigs were treated in the same manner but without the injection of milk protein. Examination of the animals of the second group revealed an area of induration and inflammation at the site of the injection of pneumococci, whereas the animals that had received milk protein in addition to the pneumococcal suspension showed only the slightest response to the bacterial antigen and none to milk protein. When intramuscular injections of milk protein were substituted for intradermal administration, with all other conditions of the experiment the same as before, the reactions of the animals so treated were less pronounced than those in the guinea pigs receiving only pneumococci, but more marked than those occurring when the protein was injected into the skin. While it is apparent that the injection of foreign protein inhibited the reactivity of the cutaneous tissues to the injected suspension of heated pneumococci, the significance of the experiments is not clear.

Kramár and Gyüre (1930)[756] sought other means for learning the manner in which the allergic manifestations of the skin take place. A comparison was made of the bactericidal, bacteriotropic, protective, and antitoxic action of the serum, plasma, and defibrinated blood of human beings who reacted either positively or negatively to an autolysate of Type II Pneumococcus. From the experiments there appeared to be no correlation between the content of humoral antibodies and the outcome of the skin tests. The authors then studied the relation of the skin reactions in man evoked by pneumococcal autolysate with the so-called "pharmacodynamic reaction" of Hecht and von Groer, which consisted in determining the maximal dose of epinephrin and caffein-sodium salicylate which, when injected alone into the skin, would produce twenty-four hours later no redness at the point of injection. For the details of the experiment the original communication of Kramár and Gyüre should be consulted. The results led Kramár and Gyüre to conclude that the cutaneous reaction to pneumococcal autolysate was similar to that produced by tuberculin and the opposite of that caused by diphtheria toxin and, therefore, that the pneumococcal skin test was an allergic reaction and was an expression of cellular immunity.

In a theoretical discussion of the mechanism of skin reactivity to Pneumococcus, Kramár and Gyüre presented the theory that allergy represents a labile condition of the animal organism, since artificial immunization causes positive reactivity to become negative reactivity, while colds, exhaustion, fatigue, massive infections, and diseases other than pneumonia, and possibly the age of the individual, change the state of allergy to one of anergy. Kramár and Gyüre presented the following schematic representation of the factors concerned in the three hypothetical states prevailing in man in relation to hypersensitivity to Pneumococcus.

I	II	III
Anergic phase—no protection	*Allergic phase—labile immunity*	*Fastness—stable immunity*
Skin test—negative	Skin test—positive	Skin test—negative
New born subjects	The majority of children and adults	The minority of children and adults
The number of negative reactors decreases with age	The number of subjects increases with age among nurslings	Those artificially immunized

The authors explain that shifts in phase to the right are influenced by increasing age of infants, by recovery from pneumococcal infection, and by repeated slight infections such as common catarrh of the upper respiratory passages. Reverse shifts to the left are brought about by the debilitating causes already mentioned.

The foregoing presentation of the subject of dermal allergy to pneumococcal products is bewildering, and from the data as presented it is difficult to gain a clear conception of the true significance of specific skin tests in health, during pneumococcal infection, and in pneumonia patients receiving specific serum therapy. The primary purpose of the authors of the present volume has been to recite the many observations as they have been reported in the literature in order that no contributions, whatever might be their value, should be neglected. It should be borne in mind that in many of the reports abstracted the materials employed for testing skin reactivity were frequently mixtures of the native constituents in more or less altered form of Pneumococcus, and of autolytic or metabolic products of the cell. It is not surprising therefore that the skin both of healthy persons and of pneumonic patients should display a diversity of reactive manifestations following the intradermal injection of bacterial suspensions in different stages of autolysis, or of extracts or filtrates of pneumococci. Observations of this nature, having been cited, may now be partly disregarded and the discussion confined to the action of the more tangible, isolated components of Pneumococcus.

To arrive at the true significance of cutaneous reactions in human beings following the intradermal introduction of pneumococcal materials it is necessary to consider the action of the separate constituents of the pneumococcal cell employed in a comparatively pure state and to determine as far as possible the experience of the subject tested in regard to past or present pneumococcal infection.

With improved methods in the preparation of bacterial protein and somatic and capsular polysaccharides, antigens are now available for an analytical study of skin tests, but it is not always possible to ascertain the immunological condition in respect to Pneumococcus of the person to be tested.

A positive cutaneous reaction to the protein fraction of Pneumococcus may be elicited by the appropriate injection of the antigen into the skin of individuals who give no history of pneumonia. In patients ill with the disease a similar injection gives a negative result during the acute stages of the disease but a positive reaction appears late in the period of convalescence (Abernethy and Francis[2]). The reaction in this case is of the delayed variety, not appearing until several hours after the injection is made, and immunologically is species-specific and not type-specific.

When the somatic C polysaccharide of Pneumococcus is employed, a positive cutaneous reaction may be obtained in the great majority of patients during the acute stages of the disease and has been demonstrated as early as twelve hours after the initial chill. The state of reactivity to the C Fraction usually persists throughout the acute febrile period. With the onset of recovery, whether associated with crisis or lysis, the reaction decreases markedly in intensity and, during an uncomplicated convalescence, in the majority of instances can no longer be demonstrated. Reactivity may persist or reappear if complications develop. If the case terminates fatally, the patient may fail to give a skin reaction to the somatic carbohydrate during some stage of the acute disease (Abernethy and Francis). The local manifestations appearing after the intradermal injection of the C Fraction occur in a positively reacting person within fifteen to twenty minutes and in their early development resemble those of the capsular polysaccharide skin test, but the zone of erythema is less intense and pseudopods extending out from the central wheal, so frequently seen in the latter, are rarely encountered. Within an hour the acute phase has usually passed and is then followed by a delayed reaction, an edematous erythema. The delayed reaction begins to appear in two to three hours, is well marked in six to ten hours, persists for eighteen to twenty-four hours, and then fades, leaving a residual brown stain (Abernethy and Francis). The C polysaccharide, being common to all pneumococci, is heterogenetic in its capacity to elicit a positive reaction in the skin of pneumonia patients and, furthermore, cutaneous reactivity to this carbohydrate component of pneumococci is not limited to patients infected with organisms of that bacterial species, since a positive reaction has been obtained in patients ill with other infectious febrile diseases.

The capsular polysaccharides of Pneumococcus, on the other hand, when injected intradermally into pneumonia patients are highly type-specific in their action, and by their action serve as an indicator of the immunological state of the individual tested. When positive, the reaction is immediate, with wheal formation and the development of erythema. Differing from the conditions observed when pneumococcal protein or somatic carbohydrate are used as test agents, reactivity of the dermal tissues is nearly always absent in normal human beings and in patients during the early stages of pneumonic infection. As the disease progresses, usually shortly before, during, or after crisis, the skin of the patient acquires the capacity to react to the capsular polysaccharide and the condition may persist for a shorter or longer time during and after convalescence. A positive reaction is regarded as evidence of definite immunological response on the part of the patient to the infection. A positive reaction denotes that recovery is taking place; a negative reaction is interpreted as indicating that the defensive forces of the body, whether natural or artificially aroused, are unequal to cope with the infection. Intradermal tests with type-specific polysaccharides, therefore, may be applied to estimate the adequacy of serum treatment.

The percentage of positive cutaneous reactions elicited by the injection of homologous capsular polysaccharide varies with the serological type of Pneumococcus responsible for the infection. Almost all patients suffering from Type I infections react to the Type I polysaccharide; approximately slightly more than one-half the number of patients with Type II disease respond to the intradermal injection of Type II polysaccharide; and in Type III infections the percentage of positive reactors is even smaller. As has been mentioned earlier in the text, the intradermal injection of pneumococcal polysaccharides into human beings may induce subsequent reactivity of the dermal cells, and this fact is to be borne in mind in studies on skin sensitivity where repeated intradermal injections of these agents are involved.

The true nature of the phenomenon of skin reactivity to Pneumococcus or its components still remains hidden. The resulting skin activity to capsular polysaccharide following the administration of homologous type-specific antipneumococcic serum has led to the hypothesis that the specific reaction is to be explained on the basis of local interaction of antigen and circulating antibody in the dermal tissues but the hypothesis fails to account for the repeated observation that a negative cutaneous reaction may be obtained even when the blood of the subject contains demonstrable antibodies. There is, to be sure, a certain parallelism between the results of serological tests and skin tests in pneumococcal pneumonia with the somatic carbohydrate C, but the correlation does not necessarily hold when the capsular polysaccharide is used as the test material.

The claim that pneumococcal toxins and their homologous antitoxins operate in this immunological reaction requires further investigation before it can be accepted. The participation of humoral antibody and the possible reactivity of the dermal cells induced by pneumococcal infections are questions shrouded in obscurity, and it would be presumptuous at the present time to venture any more definite statements regarding this interesting and important phenomenon.

THE SHWARTZMAN PHENOMENON

In 1928, Shwartzman[1263] described a dermal reaction to bacterial extracts in rabbits, which consisted in a severe local activation, by intravenous injection of the extract, of a previously inert intradermal injection of the same material. The phenomenon—since called the Shwartzman phenomenon—appeared to differ from the usual toxic or allergic cutaneous reactions in the following features: local reactivity; the short incubation period necessary to induce the local reactivity; the short duration of the state of reactivity; the ability to induce local reactivity by a single skin injection; the severity of the reaction; and the necessity of giving the second injection of the toxic agent by the intravenous route.

The phenomenon elicited by the injection of pneumococcal materials was first reported by Cope and Howell[277] in 1931. A substance obtained by dissolving pneumococci in bile evoked a local skin reaction when its intradermal injection was followed by a subsequent intravenous injection into rabbits. The reaction could not be obtained by the use of pneumococcal filtrates prepared by methods in which the cell body was not disintegrated. Type-specificity of the reaction was demonstrated in 44.4 per cent of the experiments, but positive reactions were observed in 13.8 per cent of the experiments in which heterogeneous types of pneumococci were employed for the intradermal and intravenous injections.

A wide deviation from type-specificity and even from species-specificity in the mechanism of the phenomenon was later shown by Shwartzman.[1264] Culture filtrates of Type III Pneumococcus and agar washings of *B. typhosus* were simultaneously injected at separate sites into the skin of the ear of rabbits. No reaction followed this preparatory injection. When the pneumococcal filtrates were injected intravenously twenty-four hours later, no activation at the site of the pneumococcal extract injection occurred, but in the majority of the animals a marked reaction was observed at the point where the preparatory injection of washings of the typhoid bacilli had been made. From the experiments, Shwartzman concluded that pneumococcal filtrates were devoid of the preparatory principle but were potent in reactive factors for *B. typhosus* agar-washings if not for the pneumococcal substance. There was another factor in the phenomenon, as observed under the experimental conditions, and that was the ability of pneumococcal extracts, that had lost their reactivating power for preparatory injections of *B. typhosus* agar-washings, to regain potency after being mixed with (type?) specific horse antiserum and to a lesser degree with type-specific rabbit antiserum.

In a subsequent paper, Shwartzman[1265] reported additional observations on the ability of homologous antigen-antibody combinations introduced into rabbits intravenously to render tissues vulnerable to the action of soluble products of heterologous bacterial species previously injected into the skin of the rabbit ear.

The work of Cope and Howell points to the species-specificity and, to a certain extent, to the type-specificity of the phenomenon. In following through the several communications of Shwartzman, the conviction is formed that there is no specific immunological relation between the action of the preparatory principle and that of the reactivating substance. The conditions of the experiments as conducted by Shwartzman give the impression that Pneumococcus contains no substance preparatory or activating to itself, although from the organism a substance may be obtained that causes dermal tissues to become susceptible to the local action of material present in typhoid agar-washings. It would be out of place here to enter into any detailed discussion of the factors involved in the operation of the Shwartzman phenomenon. However, from the facts available, it is difficult at present to appraise its significance in the pathology and immunology of pneumococcal infections.

Summary

Nature endows some animals with means for defending themselves against infection by pneumococci. The integument of the body and of its passages and cavities presents obstacles to the entrance of the bacteria into the deeper tissues. When, however, entrance is effected, the cocci encounter in the blood stream antagonistic forces. Among the forces may be a body temperature inimical to the proliferation of the cocci—the naturally high temperature in the case of birds, or the febrile reaction in rabbits engendered by some strains of pneumococci, varying with the species and age of the animal host. There are also normal opsonins, which prepare the invading bacteria for ingestion by the normal phagocytic cells. In addition to the opsonins protective substances are present in the serum of normal animals to ward off the attack, but these natural protective antibodies may be effective for one or more but not for all serological types of Pneumococcus. The possession or lack of these secondary, humoral defensive antibodies appears to parallel the natural susceptibility or resistance of different species of animals to pneumococcal infection. Within the species, new-born members are devoid of these circulating antibodies, but with increase in age there is a corresponding augmentation of these factors.

During pneumococcal infections in man, when native resistance is overcome, the body cells, aroused to activity by the stimulating components of the bacteria, elaborate motile immune substances, which comprise agglutinins, precipitins, opsonins, and protective antibodies. A substance, as yet of unknown nature, appears early in the serum of the pneumonia patient, which is capable of precipitating the C carbohydrate of Pneumococcus, but the true specific immune substances develop as the disease progresses, usually appearing in greatest quantity at the time of crisis, persisting in the blood stream for a while, and then disappearing during or after convalescence. The humoral antibodies thus evoked are specific for the serological type of the infecting strain, but it is conceivable that the recovered patient may possess for a time some residual immunity to organisms of a type other than that of the infecting pneumococcus. The presence of specific humoral antibodies does not always spell recovery for the patient, but their absence usually presages death. From the pneumococcal cell, as a result of its disintegration in the body, polysaccharides are introduced into the blood and, when in sufficient concentration, inhibit or block the action of the antibodies.

The humoral effects and cellular reactions taking place during pneumococcal infection may be artificially reproduced in suitable normal animals by the judicious parenteral introduction of pneumococci or of their antigenic constituents. The properties of the serum of artificially immunized animals may be transferred passively to normal animals. Owing to differences in the nature of the immune substances in the serum of animals of diverse species, the successful transference of passive immunity depends on the animal selected as the source of the immune serum.

During the development of immunity, whether evoked in a natural way or by artificial means, the tissue cells acquire a heightened sensitivity to Pneumococcus and some of its derivatives. Hypersensitivity in some animals may be manifested by an acute and fatal anaphylactic reaction, by increased contractility of the uterus, and by the inflammatory reaction of the cutaneous and pulmonary tissues arising upon the appropriate introduction of pneumococcal antigen.

The induction of the hypersensitive state and elicitation of the characteristic manifestations depend on the nature of the antigen employed. It is the capsular polysaccharide of the pneumococcal cell that orients the sensitizing stimulus and that is responsible for the type-specificity of the visible phenomena. In the case of hypersensitiveness to Pneumococcus, the allergic condition may be suspended and the specific reactions prevented temporarily by the introduction into the body of the polysaccharide homologous with that of the antigen used to induce allergy.

CHAPTER XIII

PNEUMOCOCCAL VACCINES

The preparation of vaccines from pneumococci, their components, or derivatives; the use of vaccines in the prevention and cure of pneumococcal infections; with a discussion of the theoretical and practical factors involved.

THE very nature of pneumococcal disease would seem to preclude the possibility of engendering by artificial means any secure or lasting protection against invasion of the body by pneumococci. The sudden onset, the often brief and stormy course, and the abrupt termination of the disease, so dramatically exemplified in lobar pneumonia in man, constitute a syndrome which results only in a fleeting insurance against a second attack by the same bacterial species. In diseases such as smallpox and anterior poliomyelitis, the morbid processes are caused by toxins or by living viruses, and specific stimulation of the immune mechanism usually eventuates in lasting defense. In infections by Pneumococcus, however, the struggle is between the natural forces of the body and the living cocci, and if the issue is successful on the part of the animal, the body is left almost as defenseless against these same bacteria as it was before the conflict.

Therefore, it is unreasonable to expect that the administration of pneumococci or of pneumococcal derivatives, no matter how artfully modified so as to be no longer capable of harm, would confer upon the recipient more than a short period of freedom from subsequent invasion by Pneumococcus. The attempts of immunologists to devise a suitable immunizing agent have been notable more for their ingenuity than for their success in establishing an immune state of high degree or of long duration. To be sure, there is abundant experimental evidence, as has been presented in previous chapters, that suitable antigens prepared from pneumococci and introduced into the animal body stimulate the production of specific antibodies in even less time than do true toxins or filtrable viruses; but while these specific antibodies may guard the individual against infection by Pneumococcus, the same evidence shows that the immunity so induced, when at all effective, is specific only for the serological type of the antigen employed and at best is disappointingly transient.

In the chapters on antigenicity (X), antibodies (XI), and host response to antigenic action of Pneumococcus (XII), the facts presented would seem to warrant the conclusion that antigens representing the components of the pneumococcal cell as they exist in the cell at the height of vital function are, as a rule, the most effective in establishing the immune state. With Pneumococcus as with other bacterial material, attempts by means of physical or chemical agents to rob the antigen of undesirable properties or to isolate or concentrate the antigenic principles frequently so disrupt or denature the constituents of the cell as to deprive the agent of its immunizing properties. However, the protection of the individual or of groups of individuals against pneumococcal infection is often so desirable or so urgent that, bearing in mind the limitations of the practice, the administration of vaccinal agents made from pneumococci is fully justified. The complications presented by the type-specific action of pneumococcal antigens, changes in the prevalent variety of serological types, and the temporary nature of the protection conferred only spur the immunologist to further endeavor to increase the effectiveness of pneumococcal vaccines.

Basically the antigens employed for the production of active immunity in experimental animals and man fall into four general groups.

1. Saline suspensions of pneumococci devitalized by heat, formalin, phenol, soaps, or other physical or chemical agents. Vaccines of this kind may be assumed to represent all the constituents of the cell in their natural state, making allowance for such alterations in intrinsic

properties as may have occurred in the process of preparation. In some preparations the organisms are sensitized by appropriate treatment with homologous immune serum.

2. Extracts of pneumococci made in water, saline solutions, bile or bile salts, and other solvents, freed from cellular elements and containing the substances of the bacterial cell soluble in these solutions. In the preparation of extracts, autolysis of the cocci may or may not have occurred.

3. Autolysates of pneumococci taken at different stages of self-digestion of the coccal bodies and usually cleared of formed cellular material by Berkefeld filtration or some other method for removing particulate matter.

4. Solutions of the various chemical components of the pneumococcal cell isolated from supposedly non-antigenic substances. The solutions may be composed of only one constituent or of two or more substances derived from the cell. In the case of these solutions the question should be borne in mind how closely the ingredients approach the antigens as they exist preformed in the living and fully functioning virulent bacterial body or, conversely, to what extent their molecular structure has been changed by the manipulations required in manufacture.

In the present chapter attention will be directed chiefly to the preparation and the immunizing effect of those vaccines that have been employed for prophylaxis or therapy in man. The rationale of the use of pneumococcal vaccines is based on two kinds of evidence: the result of prophylactic injection in experimental animals, and the effect of vaccines in the prevention and cure of specific infection in human beings.

EXPERIMENTS ON MONKEYS

The previous chapters of this volume are replete with references to the capacity of Pneumococcus or its derivatives to induce in mice, rabbits, and other domestic animals the formation of specific antibodies contributing to the immune state. The earlier experiences in which the monkey was the test animal, because of the closer zoological relationship of that species to man, are perhaps the most significant in estimating the probable effect of the application of the same biological agents in the case of human beings. Cecil,[202] with his associates, Blake and Steffen,[206, 212, 214-5] in a series of studies on the immunization of monkeys with different pneumococcal vaccines administered by various routes, learnt that because of the greater susceptibility of the monkey to pneumococci as compared to man, the test animals failed to respond as readily to the same amounts of vaccine. In order to induce a degree of active immunity sufficient to protect monkeys against experimental pneumonia incited with the homologous type of organism, it was necessary to employ small doses of living, virulent pneumococci, or to treat the animals by three intratracheal implantations of pneumococcal vaccines (Cecil and Steffen[214-5]). The subcutaneous injection of saline suspensions of killed pneumococci induced a greater amount of protective substances in the vaccinated animals than did lipovaccine, but in both cases the appearance of specific humoral antibodies was not always accompanied by protection against subsequent infection. By the subcutaneous, intravenous, and intratracheal route, three spaced injections of large doses of saline vaccine were required to immunize the animals against inoculation with homologous pneumococci of the four different types employed. When the immunizing treatment was carried out by way of the trachea, the immunity induced appeared to Cecil to be cellular rather than humoral in character. Large doses were required, no matter by which route given, while intravenous injection of the vaccine resulted in a higher degree of immunity than administration by the other methods tried.

Cecil concluded that immunity to Pneumococcus, like other forms of immunity, is relative and depends on the capacity of the individual to elaborate antibodies, on the virulence of the invading strain, and on the size of the dose of culture experimentally injected, to which might be added the virulence of the culture from which the vaccine is prepared, the amount, the number of injections, and the site selected for the injection of vaccine. Granting that, because of the greater susceptibility of the monkey to pneumococcal infection, the analogy between effects in the monkey and man is not a strict one, Cecil's success in protecting the more highly susceptible animal against invasion by Pneumococcus pointed to even greater possibilities of the prophylactic use of pneumococcal vaccines in man.*

TYPES OF VACCINES EMPLOYED

Saline suspensions of heat-killed pneumococci have been used by Wright, Morgan, Colebrook and Dodgson,[1543-4] Cecil and his colleagues, by Lister,[816] Maynard,[872] and others; similar suspensions mixed with heat-killed bacteria of other species by Von Sholly and Park;[1452] suspensions of the organisms in oil by Russell,[1197] Rosenow and Sturdivant,[1173] Howell,[661] McCoy, Hasseltine, Wadsworth and Kirkbride;[875] formalinized suspensions by Ferguson;[436] pneumococci devitalized by tricresol, by phenol (Levy and Aoki[801]), and by hydrochloric acid by Kolmer and Rule;[747] soaped cultures by Olson[1029-30] and by Larson;[789] cultures killed by Merthiolate by Sutton, Kendall, and Rosenblum;[1366] washings of agar cultures—the so-called "Immunogen"—by Ferry and Fisher,[438] and by Horder and Ferry;[655] extracts of pneumococci and filtrates of broth cultures by Barach;[76] autolysates by Rosenow[1171] and others; pancreatic digestion products of pneumococci by Hirschfelder;[648] neutralized alkaline extracts of pneumococci by Brotzu;[150] while Ziegler[1573] employed a hypothetical substance obtained by lysis of pneumococci with sodium taurocholate and named by him "Pneumocholin." In these later days, purified constituents of the pneumococcal cell are being studied for their immunizing action on large groups of men by Felton.

DOSAGE

Wright *et al.*,[1545-6] in 1914, gave subcutaneous doses of from 250 million to 1,000 million cocci; amounts in excess of the latter count

* The efficacy of vaccination in arresting a spontaneous outbreak of pneumonia among stock monkeys was reported by Wisner,[1525] who injected subcutaneously three doses of a saline suspension of heat-killed cultures of the strain of Pneumococcus isolated from the infected laboratory animals.

appeared to render the individual more susceptible to infection. Lister,[816] however, found that 40 billion organisms could be injected into man without eliciting any but very slight reactions. In Ferguson's[436] experimental studies on man, 150 million organisms each of Types I, II, and III were injected subcutaneously at weekly intervals. Barach's[75] studies were carried out with doses of 200 million or more cocci at each injection. Duckwall[339] administered doses as small as 500 organisms at the first injection, increasing the amount to only 1,000 cocci on two subsequent occasions. In the study made by McCoy, Hasseltine, Wadsworth, and Kirkbride,[875] the lipovaccine used contained approximately 10 billion organisms of Types I, II, and III. Howell[661] standardized his preparation on the basis of dried pneumococcal protein and found that one cubic centimeter of vaccine containing 0.83 milligram of protein was a satisfactory dose. The circulars of directions accompanying the pneumococcal vaccines supplied by some of the commercial laboratories usually recommend the initial injection, in the case of a preparation containing pneumococci of the first three types only, of an amount representing 4,500 million organisms. For second and third doses the number is increased to 9,000 million pneumococci. In the case of vaccines consisting of pneumococci mixed with other bacteria of respiratory origin, the first dose represents 50 million pneumococci combined with 75 million for the second, third, and fourth injections. It appears, therefore, that pneumococcal vaccines may be safely administered within a wide range of dosage.

SPECIAL CONSTITUENTS OF PNEUMOCOCCUS

In the chapter on antigenicity, the immunizing action of certain isolated components of the pneumococcal cell was described. It may be remembered that Francis and Tillett[478] and Finland and Sutliff[448-9] succeeded in inducing the development of specific antibodies in man by the intradermal injection of soluble specific substance. Francis,[474] by injecting two groups of normal human beings, one with the old form of capsular polysaccharide and the other with the new acetylated form, confirmed the observation that the deacetylated type of polysaccharide was antigenic for man, and ascertained that the new form possessed similar immunizing properties. More recently, Felton (1934)[417] tested the antigenic action of the acid-soluble portion of the pneumococcal cell on experimental animals and man, and reported that a small amount of the alcohol precipitate of the acid-soluble fraction immunized the test subjects to a degree approaching that possessed by patients convalescing from pneumonia. In a study with Sutliff and Steele, Felton[434] compared the immunizing effect of various fractions prepared from pneumococci with that of vaccines made from the intact cell. Although the optimal dose was not established, the injection of two milligrams of the soluble antigen produced as high a protective titer in the human subjects so treated as did the usual single dose of vaccine containing pneumococci. The authors also reported that under certain conditions the antibodies evoked by the soluble antigens prepared from pneumococci of Types I and II were heterologous as well as homologous in type.

POTENCY TESTS ON VACCINES

In order to obtain a measure of the immunizing power of pneumococcal vaccines, Bengston (1924)[99] studied the immune effects appearing in mice and rabbits after the administration of preparations obtained in the market. After testing the agglutinin, precipitin, and tropin content of the serum of the test animals as well as their ability to withstand subsequent infection with virulent pneumococci, Bengston concluded that the determination of active immunity in mice gave the best estimate of antigenic strength, particularly of polyvalent pneumococcal vaccines. The superiority of mice over rabbits could be ascribed to the fact that the virulence of the three fixed types can be maintained at a uniform level for the first-named species. In testing separately experimental vaccines prepared with organisms of Types I, II, and III, it was found that the highest degree of protection followed in the case of Type I vaccine, less was afforded by suspensions of Type II cocci, while Type III preparations induced the least protection. In testing polyvalent vaccines, Bengston observed that their use resulted in more definite protection against pneumococci of Types II and III than was noted after the use of monovalent vaccines, suggesting the production of a certain amount of cross-protection. The tests, as a whole, showed that commercial polyvalent pneumococcal vaccines afforded protection in mice against amounts of virulent cultures ranging from zero to one million fatal doses in the case of Type I organisms, from zero to ten thousand fatal doses in the case of Type II, and only from zero to one hundred fatal doses of Type III cultures.

Before employing vaccines or other immunizing agents made from pneumococci, the preparations, as is the case with other biological products, should be subjected to some suitable test or tests to determine their antigenic strength. While it is obvious that effects in animals cannot be accurately translated into effects on man, yet determinations on laboratory animals furnish information concerning the probable immunizing action of bacterial agents or derivatives in the human body.

ROUTE AND SPACING OF INJECTIONS

Animal experimentation has demonstrated that the intravenous introduction of pneumococcal antigens, as compared to other methods, stimulates a more rapid and energetic immunizing response. The technique, despite certain and largely avoidable hazards, is applicable to man. As a matter of convenience, however, the subcutaneous route, especially in the prophylactic treatment of large numbers of individuals, is to be preferred. The intradermal injection of pneumococci, as shown experimentally in rabbits by Goodner,[525-6, 529] and of soluble specific substance, as demonstrated in man, by Francis,[474] Francis and Tillett,[478] and by Finland and Sutliff,[446-7] calls forth the prompt appearance of specific antibodies. In this connection there may be also mentioned the intradermal injection in the treatment of lobar pneumonia of "natural bacterial antigens" prepared from living pneumococci by the addition of Merthiolate, as reported by Sutton, Kendall, and Rosenblum (1931).[1366] The results invite further study of the desirability of the skin as a locus for the administration of pneumococcal antigens.

That a certain degree of specific immunity in rats may follow the ingestion of pneumococcal derivatives has been shown by McDaniels,[876] among others, who, as a preparatory measure, fed egg-white to the animals thirty minutes previous to the oral administration of antigen. Animals receiving the preliminary dose of egg-white exhibited greater resistance than did the controls to a subsequent intraperitoneal injection of graded amounts of a virulent culture of pneumococci of homologous type.

In a series of communications extending over the period from 1925 to 1934, Ross[1178-94] reported the results of studies on the immunizing effect of feeding several different forms of pneumococcal material first to rats and subsequently to man. In some of the author's early experiments it was found that the ingestion of soluble specific substance from Type I pneumococci induced in the rat active immunity of homologous type, and a similar condition ensued after feeding the animals with filtrates obtained from pneumococci dissolved by bile salts. The degree of immunity following the administration of the polysaccharide appeared to be greater than that developing when suspensions of the intact cell were employed. In the case of Type II polysaccharide the animals acquired little or no immunity, but with Type III carbohydrate the effect, though slight, was type-specific. Ross noted that a large part of the polysaccharide administered orally passes through the alimentary tract practically unchanged as far as antigenicity is concerned but, strange to say, he could not detect the substance in the blood of the treated animals.

In his later publications, Ross reported the appearance of specific antibodies in the serum of man following the administration of pneumococcal vaccines by mouth. The preparations employed comprised suspensions of pneumococci freshly killed by treatment with hydrochloric acid; suspensions of the same organisms after desiccation; bile solutions, sometimes filtered, of the cocci; and dried and pulverized preparations of these solutions. In addition, in some experiments, Ross fed to the human subjects living pneumococci either dried and contained in capsules or suspended in water. The results of the later experiments on human beings reported by Ross may be epitomized thus: Vaccines administered by mouth in the case of Type I materials induced antibody formation in 74 per cent of fifty-three persons, seven of whom required two series of feeding, while in fourteen other persons no protective antibodies appeared after two series comprising ten feedings. Sixty per cent of individuals receiving Type II antigens developed antibody, while eleven of the subjects failed to react, although five were given two series by ingestion. With Type III, the results were difficult to evaluate since antibody production was slight and irregular. The content of antibody in the blood of men orally immunized was low and was similar in degree to that of convalescent blood, while variations in the amount of antibody were observed in different individuals. Ross noted heterogeneity of the antibodies appearing as a result of vaccines administered orally, especially with those derived from Type II organisms. The duration of the immunity developed after the ingestion of the various preparations was approximately seven to fourteen months, but the experimental evidence bearing on this phase of the subject is not complete. Ross recommended as a practical procedure the use of completely autolyzed cultures, because he believed that autolysates contain several times as much antigenic material as eighteen-hour cultures of cocci in broth. From all that we know of the antigenic integrity of the components of Pneumococcus, it is difficult to subscribe to this recommendation.

During the period in which Ross was prosecuting his studies,

Kolmer and Rule[746-7] were also investigating the comparative efficacy as immunizing agents of suspensions of killed pneumococci of Types I, II, and III. Vaccines containing cultures devitalized by tricresol were injected subcutaneously at intervals of five days into one series of rabbits and similar injections of organisms treated with hydrochloric acid were given through a stomach tube to animals of another series. Although the two immunizing agents were not strictly comparable, the observations led the authors to conclude that the antigenic action of the vaccines was more pronounced when administered by the subcutaneous than by the oral route. The best results were obtained with a minimum of five daily injections. The work of Ross and that of Kolmer and Rule present no evidence of the advantage, save possibly that of the ease of administration, of ingestion over injection of pneumococcal vaccines.

While intratracheal insufflation, as practiced by Cecil and Steffen,[214-5] is of interest in demonstrating the possibility of inducing immunity by local stimulation, the method obviously is scarcely applicable in the case of man.

LOCAL AND SYSTEMIC REACTIONS

Pneumococcal substance, unless in autolyzed or degraded form, is not conspicuously toxic when introduced parenterally into the tissues of man, and vaccines made from pneumococci or some of their constituents (unlike similar preparations prepared from such bacteria as the dysentery and paratyphoid bacilli, the bacillus of Pfeiffer, and *Bacillus proteus*) can be administered in the customary amounts without risk of incurring undesirable or unduly severe reactions. Cecil[201, 203] spoke of both local and general toxic manifestations following the subcutaneous injection of saline suspensions of pneumococci of the first three types when the dosage equalled several billion organisms. The subjects exhibited variations in reactivity, and the severity of the effect could be lessened by decreasing the individual dose. Malone[864] reported that less than 2 per cent of Senegalese troops reported sick after the injection of 3,000 million to 6,000 million cocci.

In the study by Von Sholly and Park,[1452] 63 per cent of the subjects vaccinated with a mixed vaccine developed after the first dose mild reactions consisting of redness and soreness of the arm; the same number had similar reactions following the second and larger dose; while the third injection elicited a comparable condition in 60 per cent of the subjects. Constitutional reactions as evidenced by headache, malaise, vertigo, chills, and general pain occurred in 19 per cent of the treated subjects after the first injection, in 27 per cent after the second, and in 23 per cent after the third dose. In a later tabulation, Park[1054-6] listed severe reactions as appearing in 3 per cent of the individuals after the first injection, 2.7 per cent following the second, and 4.1 per cent after the third dose. It should be borne in mind that the vaccine contained, in addition to pneumococci of the first three types, streptococci of the hemolytic and viridans type and the so-called influenza bacillus. One cannot say to what extent these organisms participated in the toxic action of the vaccine. Lister and Ordman,[819] also using a mixed vaccine, stated that in their experience while mild reactions were frequently noted severe reactions were uncommon. Barach (1931)[76] encountered no immediate reactions after the intravenous or intradermal administration of suspensions or filtrates of heat-killed pneumococci. A chill was later observed in one patient so treated. Although other references might be quoted, there appear no reports of reactions following the injection of pneumococcal vaccines sufficiently severe or untoward as to preclude their use.

APPEARANCE AND DURATION OF VACCINAL IMMUNITY

One of the noteworthy phenomena of artificially induced, active immunity to Pneumococcus is the early appearance of specific antibodies in the circulating blood following the parenteral injection of pneumococcal antigens. Barach (1928)[74-5] was able to detect type-specific protective substances in the serum of rabbits three days after the injection of a vaccine consisting of sterilized, intact organisms of Types I and II, while similar immune effects were demonstrable on the fourth day after the administration of filtrates of broth cultures of the cocci. In an experimental way, Goodner[525-6, 529] showed that protective and other antibodies were present in the blood of rabbits in one to two days after intradermal inoculation with living pneumococci. In immunization tests carried out on man with various antigenic preparations made from Type I and Type II pneumococci, Felton, Sutliff, and Steele[434] found that antibodies appeared in the blood stream to a slight extent on the fourth or fifth day after injection and increased up to a maximum on the fourteenth day. The literature contains many references to the early development of humoral, immune substances or of increased resistance engendered by the administration of pneumococcal antigens, but it seems scarcely necessary to relate them.

The statement was made earlier in this chapter that the duration of the immune state established by the administration of pneumococcal vaccines, as far as present evidence indicated, could not be expected to surpass that arising during an attack of pneumonia. All the experiments in which this time element was noted bear witness to the validity of the statement. Maynard,[872] basing his observations on the incidence of natural immunity in vaccinated natives in the Rand as compared to that of unvaccinated natives, reported that the protection conferred by the immunization treatment appeared to be greatest immediately or shortly after vaccination and then progressively diminished, until after a period of about four months it was lost. In the rabbit, following the intradermal injection of living pneumococci, Goodner could no longer demonstrate the existence of active immunity after a lapse of fifty to sixty days. Although the presence of demonstrable specific antibodies in the serum of a vaccinated individual may or may not be an index of resistance to pneumococci, their appearance and persistence bear witness to the fact that the physiological mechanism of the vaccinated person has been operating in the production of immunity.

On this basis, Howell[661] determined the agglutinative, complement-fixing, and protective titer of the serum of three healthy men who had received by subcutaneous injection one cubic centimeter of the American Army lipovaccine, containing 0.83 milligram of dried pneumococcal protein of Types I, II, and III. There was a definite rise in agglutinins in the second week after injection, the height being reached from the second to fourth week, although the antibody was still demonstrable from three to nine months. The complement-fixation reaction with the subjects' serum became positive from the seventh to the fifteenth day, was strongest at the twenty-fifth day, and still was positive over the period during which agglutinins were shown to endure. The content of protective antibodies in the serum more or less paralleled that of agglutinins.

When heat-killed vaccines were administered intravenously in rabbits and the animals subsequently tested by intradermal inoculation, Stillman and Goodner[1342] showed that the immune effects persisted for a somewhat longer time. In the case of Type I vaccines, the resistance induced appeared to be high ten days after the completion of the course of injections, then to become irregular in degree and generally lower during the next four months. After the seventh month, the level of resistance dropped again and was usually low. The content of protective antibodies paralleled the degree of resistance of the animals throughout the period of observation but the agglutinin titer of the treated animals' serum was high only during the first two months. With Type II vaccines, the resistance to infection was somewhat lower than that evoked by Type I vaccine, but remained moderately high for nine months with an abrupt decrease after that period. Treatment with Type III preparations resulted in a fairly marked degree of resistance during the first month, which, however, diminished sharply and remained low. None of the animals treated with Type III vaccine exhibited agglutinins or protective antibodies in the serum. While there appeared to be some correlation between the amount of humoral antibodies and the degree of resistance, the exception in the case of animals treated with Type III agents, and individual differences noted in animals as far as this parallelism was concerned, led the authors to conclude that, in addition to differences in the antigenic capacity of strains of various serological types, one must also consider the operation of cellular as well as of humoral immunity in resistance to infection.

In the experiments of Ross already cited, antibodies appearing in the serum of human beings after the ingestion of pneumococcal vaccines disappeared in some individuals within six months, and in others endured for approximately two years. Felton, Sutliff, and Steele[434] found that the presence of immune substances in the blood of human subjects, injected subcutaneously with the several preparations selected, was appreciable when the serum was tested three months after the immunizing treatment. However, the observations just quoted do not necessarily denote that resistance to infection persisted for so long a time.

There would be no object in multiplying the number of references bearing on the duration of active immunity conferred on man by the administration of vaccinal preparations made from pneumococci. Sufficient has been said to indicate that resistance, while increasing soon after injection, as far as the presence of circulating protective substances enters into the reckoning, may be naturally destroyed within the body or, at least, fail to be demonstrable. The period of active immunity is short as compared to the immunity induced by the injection of toxins or of some filtrable viruses.

RESULTS FOLLOWING VACCINATION IN MAN

In discussing the biology of Pneumococcus, it is not the intention of the authors of the present volume to invade the fields of preventive or clinical medicine. Notwithstanding this reservation, in order that the allied subjects of antigenicity and of antibody formation may be followed to their logical end, and also for the information of readers who may not have access to original source material, the results attending the use of vaccines for the prevention and cure of pneumococcal disease will be dealt with in summarized form.

PROPHYLAXIS

Because of the enormous toll exacted by pneumonia among the ranks of native workers in the diamond mines in South Africa, Maynard (1913)[872] sought whatever benefit might accrue to the men by the injection of vaccines prepared from Pneumococcus. In the beginning of the investigation, two doses of 40 to 60 million, then of 100 to 200 million, and finally of 300 million organisms given immediately upon the arrival of the natives on the Rand appeared to reduce the incidence of pneumonia for a period lasting not over four months. There was no evidence that the preventive treatment influenced case fatality, except possibly for a very short time after injection. On account of historical interest and because of the contributions of the senior author to the subject of bacterial vaccines, the work of Wright, Morgan, Colebrook, and Dodgson (1914)[1545-6] should be cited. Administering heat-killed broth cultures in subcutaneous doses representing 300 million to 600 million pneumococci to several thousand native Africans in the Rand mine, the authors reported an apparent decrease of approximately 50 to 60 per cent in the incidence of pneumonia among the vaccinated men when compared to the attack-rate among untreated controls.

During the mobilization of American troops at Camp Upton during the World War, Cecil and Austin[204] vaccinated more than twelve thousand men, giving three or four injections at intervals of five to seven days of suspensions of heat-killed cultures of Type I, II, and III pneumococci. The total dosage consisted of six to nine billion organisms of Types I and II and four and one-half to six billion of Type III pneumococci. In the ten weeks which elapsed after vaccination, no cases of pneumonia of the three specific types developed among the men who had received two or more injections, whereas there occurred twenty-six cases due to pneumococci of the same types among the nineteen thousand or more unvaccinated soldiers. The case mortality of all types of pneumococcal pneumonia among the vaccinated was 11.7 per cent against a mortality of 28.0 per cent among the unvaccinated troops.

The results following the use by Cecil and Vaughan[216] at Camp Wheeler of lipovaccine in a single dose containing approximately ten billion each of pneumococci of Types I, II, and III were not so striking as those at Camp Upton. Men representing 80 per cent of the camp strength—a total of 13,460—received the vaccine treatment and among them, during the two or three months following the injection, thirty-two cases of pneumonia caused by the first three types of Pneumococcus developed, whereas among the unvaccinated soldiers, comprising one-fifth of the whole group, there were forty-two cases in the same period. The death-rate from all pneumonias due to different types of pneumococci occurring among the vaccinated men one week or more after the single injection was 12.2 per cent, whereas among the unvaccinated control subjects the percentage was 22.3. Of the primary pneumonias among the vaccinated troops, the fatality-rate was 11.9 per cent as compared to 31.8 per cent in the case of the untreated men. In their deductions from the records, Cecil and Vaughan suggested as possible causes for the less favorable results the fact that at Camp Wheeler many of the soldiers were raw recruits, a large part of whom were Negroes of rural origin, whereas at Camp Upton the men were largely white recruits from New York City and were well seasoned at the time of vaccination. The authors made no reference to the part which the use of lipovaccine instead of saline bacterial suspension or the single injection as against two or more injections may have contributed to the less favorable experience.

In regard to the use of lipovaccines, the report of Rosenow and Sturdivant (1919)[1173] may be quoted. Three subcutaneous injections were given at weekly intervals of a vaccine in an oil menstruum containing 30 per cent of pneumococci of Types I, II, and III, 40 per cent of Group IV, 20 per cent of hemolytic streptococci, and 10 per cent of *Staphylococcus aureus*, representing individual doses of 2.5, 5.0, and 7.5 billion cocci respectively. The authors admitted that the collected data on the 93,476 individuals vaccinated were far from exact; nevertheless, the figures would seem to be significant. The average incidence of influenza and pneumonia in the group receiving three injections was one-third that of the incidence among the unvaccinated subjects, and the average mortality-rate for the treated was about one-fifth that for the untreated group.

Another Army experience was that at Camp Taylor (U.S.A.) reported in 1920 by Duckwall,[339] who employed as vaccine a saline suspension containing in each cubic centimeter one thousand organisms of heat-killed pneumococci of Types I, II, and III. For the 1,326 men receiving one, two, or three injections of vaccine at intervals of seven to ten days the annual admission-rate per thousand from pneumonia was 20.3, and for those receiving no prophylactic treatment the rate was 54. The death-rate, similarly calculated, was 2.26 for the vaccinated and 8.76 for the unvaccinated subjects. Considering the statistics for pneumonia together with those for common respiratory infections, the author stated, "The obvious conclusion is that the vaccine protects against pneumonia and the common respiratory diseases in the proportion of five to one." In comparison with the dosage employed by other observers, that used by Duckwall is conspicuously small.

In the same year, Borrell[143] described the effect of the administration of saline suspensions of pneumococci (types not given) to Senegalese troops stationed in France during the World War. When two injections of a vaccine representing 3,000 and 6,000 million cocci were injected at seven-day intervals, the morbidity-rate per thousand was thirty-six and seventy-three respectively among the vaccinated in two battalions as against one hundred thirty and eighty-five among the troops not vaccinated. The mortality-rate on the same basis was zero and seven as compared to thirty-three and eighteen. Later, when the number of injections was increased to three, consisting of doses of 0.5, 1.0, and 2.0 cubic centimeters of a suspension containing 8,000 million organisms per cubic centimeter, the results were not so satisfactory; the morbidity-rate was sixty-five among the vaccinated as compared to a rate of ninety-five among the unvaccinated soldiers and the mortality-rate was nineteen among the treated subjects and ninety-five for the controls.

In 1921, Von Sholly and Park[1452] reported their experience in vaccinating 1,536 employees of the Metropolitan Life Insurance Company in New York City. Of the employees, 1,412 received three injections of a saline suspension of pneumococci of the first three types sterilized by heat, and the other 124 were given lipovaccine prepared by Rosenow. Among 1,327 complete records there was found one case of pneumonia among those vaccinated against eleven cases among the control groups. The treatment appeared to have little effect either in preventing or in favoring respiratory infection other than pneumonia among the subjects treated.

In its chronological order there may be mentioned the note of Walravens,[1477] which stated that at Katanga in the Belgian Congo it was the routine practice in large industrial concerns to give the black employees prophylactic injections of vaccines made with cultures obtained from Lister and with other strains of local isolation.

In 1922, Field[439] communicated the results following the use of a mixed vaccine among the troops stationed at Fort Myer, Virginia. The preparation contained pneumococci of Types I and II, hemolytic streptococci, and the Pfeiffer bacillus, to a total of 6,000 million organisms per cubic centimeter, and was administered in a first dose of 0.5 cubic centimeter followed by two subsequent injections of one cubic centimeter each. The statistics presented by

Field are not highly conclusive, but it was his impression that a positive effect in lowering the incidence of pneumonia was obtained by means of the vaccine.

Of more significance is the report of the study made by McCoy, Hasseltine, Wadsworth, and Kirkbride.[875] To 17,752 inmates of various state institutions was given a single subcutaneous injection of one cubic centimeter of lipovaccine containing approximately ten billion pneumococci of the first three types, while 18,595 subjects and 7,992 newly admitted patients were reserved, untreated, as controls. Observations extended over a period of two years, and in the final analysis of the data it appeared that of the cases of pneumonia occurring among the vaccinated subjects 18.0 per cent were caused by organisms of Types I, II, and III, while in the control series the percentage was 23.6—scarcely a satisfactory degree of protection. From theoretical considerations the comparative failure of lipovaccines may be ascribed to lower antigenic potency of bacteria when suspended in oil—an opinion shared by many immunologists and expressed by Cecil in 1923.*

In a paper by Malone[864] and in one by King[714] appearing in 1925, the view was expressed, based on the results of the vaccination of 2,500 troops in India, that vaccination as practiced was probably without any protective value. The vaccine contained only pneumococci of Types I and II in such a concentration that the dose, given twice subcutaneously at an interval of a week, contained 5,000 million cocci. A case-rate among the vaccinated of 9.3 when compared to the only very slightly higher rate of 10.7 for the unvaccinated controls would justify the authors' unfavorable opinion. However, a less pessimistic view concerning the value of vaccines in the prevention of pneumococcal infections was expressed by Cole in 1920,[262] who also in 1934[266] concluded: "It is not impossible that, even with our present knowledge, something could be accomplished by vaccination." Cole, in discussing the

* A review of the prophylactic vaccine treatment of pneumonia was published by Cecil[203] in *Medicine* in 1925.

soluble specific substance of Pneumococcus, stated that possibly the polysaccharide might prove to be useful for preventive treatment of man.

Another aspect of the possible effect accomplished by the large-scale prophylactic treatment of man with pneumococcal vaccines was suggested by Lister[818] in 1929, who observed that since the influenza pandemic of 1918 the types of Pneumococcus, previously found by him to be responsible for more than 69 per cent of the cases of lobar pneumonia in the Rand, had practically disappeared, and he attributed the change in the pneumococcal flora of the native workers to the routine practice of vaccination carried on since 1918. The disappearance of the familiar types of pneumococci against which vaccine treatment had been directed and the appearance of miscellaneous types in the cases of lobar pneumonia then occurring was commented upon by Ordman[1033] in 1931. The morbidity and mortality rates from the disease decreased and there was a modification of the character of the pulmonary infection. Ordman, like Lister, believed that these changes had been brought about by the persistent vaccination of the natives. It then became the custom in the diamond mines to treat the native workers entering the mines in summer and autumn with the usual vaccines and to inject those entering in winter and spring with mixed bacterial vaccines, designated "community autogenous vaccines," containing streptococci and the influenza bacillus.

In a review of the various attempts to protect the miners in the Rand from pneumonia, Orenstein[1035] in 1931 expressed frank skepticism concerning the value of the procedure. He had doubts about the importance of the serological classification of pneumococci, he saw a serious complication presented by the multiplicity of types, and was somewhat pessimistic about the alleged immunizing action of pneumococcal antigens as shown by animal experiments. Nevertheless, in the next year, Orenstein[1036] reported on the use of mixed vaccines begun experimentally the year before, and from statistics on 40,000 natives so treated suggested that those receiving the mixed vaccine showed decreased pneumonia mortality. A fair criticism of the work of both Ordman and Orenstein would be the incompleteness of their studies of the natural bacterial flora of the natives both in the population at large and among the workers before and after prophylactic vaccination. Furthermore, as is the case in practically all studies of mass vaccination, the communications include no observations on the production of specific antibodies in the vaccinated subjects.*

Less discouraging was the experience of Peall (1935).[1075] During a three and one-half year period, over 68,000 native workers in the Randfontein mines were given, at weekly intervals, three doses of a mixed vaccine containing pneumococci—the "community autogenous vaccine"—and there occurred a prompt and marked drop amounting to 70 to 80 per cent in the incidence and fatality-rates of pneumonia and of other respiratory infections as well. Despite previous doubts, Ordman[1034] resumed his endeavors toward the prevention of pneumonia and other respiratory disease, and this time among a presumably highly susceptible class of natives—workers who had been prohibited by the South African government from working in the Rand gold fields because of the extremely high pneumonia rates prevailing among them. Previous to prophylactic vaccination, the annual attack-rate was from fifty to eighty per thousand and the mortality-rate eighteen to twenty per thousand. After the continued use of a mixed vaccine containing only one type (Type II or Group B) of Pneumococcus combined with two varieties of streptococci, *Micrococcus catarrhalis* and *Staphylococcus aureus*, administered in three weekly doses, the fatality-rate from pneumonia fell from 13.9 to 2.4 per thousand—a reduction of 82.7 per cent.

A recent historical review, summarizing the preventive work done in the Rand and neighboring mines and reporting the latest experience of the authors, was published in 1935 by Lister and

* For a general review of the many phases of the use of vaccines in warding off pneumococcal infections or in their cure, the reader is referred to Park's third Harben Lecture.[1056]

Ordman.[819] Bacteriological studies had shown the presence among the native mine population of eighteen types or groups of pneumococci other than the Lister Groups C, B, and E (the classical Types I, II, and III). The vaccine, therefore, was made to include eight groups of pneumococci and, in addition, strains of streptococci, the Pfeiffer bacillus, *M. catarrhalis*, *Staphylococcus aureus*, and the Friedländer bacillus. The cultures were suspended in salt solution, sterilized by one hour's heating at 60°, and preserved with phenol. The vaccine was injected subcutaneously in three doses at seven-day intervals. The results up to the date of the report were sufficiently encouraging to lead Lister and Ordman to believe that the practice would make possible the employment of tropical natives formerly barred from the mines because of their unusual susceptibility to respiratory infections.

Early in 1935, Felton[418] made a preliminary announcement to the effect that he had tested various water-soluble fractions of Pneumococcus for their immunizing action on man, but the nature of the preparations was not revealed. A single subcutaneous injection of two milligrams of the preparation was given, and in a group of two hundred persons antibody was found to be present in the serum of all individuals so treated fourteen days after injection. The antibody was still demonstrable in the majority of subjects after a lapse of three months and in a few tested after ten months. The amount of antibody found as compared to that originally present in the serum of the subjects varied from a seventeen-fold to a ninety-eight-fold increase. All the preparations employed were high in polysaccharide content, but Felton, at the time, had not decided whether the antigenicity of the immunizing agents was due to the polysaccharide, to the polysaccharide combined with some other substance, or to some other cell constituent or product.

In a more complete report published in the same year, Felton with Sutliff and Steele[434] presented the details of preparation of a variety of antigens derived from pneumococci of Types I and II. A single subcutaneous injection of the different agents was given to human beings and the antibody response measured by testing the protective strength of the serum of the subjects so treated. The results of the investigation proved that immunity against pneumococci may be produced in man by the injection of soluble products prepared from the microorganisms. Among the pneumococcal materials employed was a water-soluble substance that failed to give biuret and Molisch reactions,* lacked the property of precipitating immune serum, and yet immunized white mice. The substance was considered by the authors to differ from any hitherto studied fraction of Pneumococcus. All the preparations tested for antigenicity, as well as dried organisms, evoked an increase in protective antibodies in the serum of the individuals treated. The degree of immunity established from a single injection of a two-milligram dose of antigenic substance, as measured by protective antibodies in the serum, compared favorably with that found in the serum of convalescent pneumonia patients. The duration of the immunity following the use of vaccine or of the fractions employed varied in different individuals, but in some cases persisted for at least a period of three months.

Wadsworth,[1465] in a discussion of the practical limitations of the vaccinal prevention of pneumococcal infection, differing with the opinion of Lister, Ordman, and others, stated that with rare exceptions pneumonia does not yield to any form of prevention and that the protective inoculation with pneumococcal vaccine advocated by some authorities as a public health measure is not practical. Granting the soundness of the latter portion of the statement, prevention, nevertheless, as a measure for sparing the individual from an attack of pneumonia is not to be dismissed so lightly. The very definite limitations of this method of prophylaxis, such as the heterogeneity of serological types and the brief spell of immunity following vaccination are freely admitted. However, in the case of individuals debilitated by age, by the effects of

* In another part of the same paper the authors stated that the substance might contain a polysaccharide as a part of its constituency.

disturbances of nutritional function, by intercurrent or chronic disease, or by undue physical strain, to whom pneumonia may present an especially serious hazard, and in the case of large bodies of men assembled from many sections of the country and living for a time under crowded conditions, the protection, such as it is, afforded by the parenteral administration of suitable pneumococcal materials should not be disregarded. To be sure, the biological agent should be prepared with proper attention to the type or types of Pneumococcus prevalent at the time, the kind of vaccine selected should represent the best immunological practice, and the injections should be repeated at frequent intervals. The danger of pneumonia to man both individually and in masses merits the application of such preventive measures as we possess, imperfect as they are, until an antigen more closely approaching the ideal is devised.

VACCINE TREATMENT OF PNEUMONIA

The possible curative action of bacterial vaccines in pneumococcal infections more properly belongs to a discussion of the clinical features of the disease. The reader in search of this information is referred to the volume by Heffron,[601] where a more exhaustive treatment of the subject will be found. However, in order to round out the description of the many biological activities of Pneumococcus, there are included in the present chapter references to the effect of specific vaccines administered during the course of pneumococcal disease, but only a few of the many observations will be noted. The rationale of vaccine therapy in pneumonia is based on the unusually rapid development of type-specific antibodies created by the parenteral injection of suitable antigenic agents. The introduction of pneumococcal antigens into a body already infected with millions of pneumococci and therefore having its tissues permeated by the antigenic constituents of the bacteria in their native condition would, because of certain theoretical considerations, seem paradoxical. There is the possibility, however, that these stimulating substances in modified form, when introduced into the cutaneous or subcutaneous tissues or into the blood stream before circulatory invasion by the cocci has taken place, may aid in fortifying the natural defenses of the body by stimulating the rapid development of substances antagonistic to the invading bacteria.

In the clinical and statistical report published by Orenstein[1035] in 1931, the author stated that the experimental treatment of pneumonia patients with pneumococcal vaccine failed to influence favorably the mortality from the disease. Lister,[816] on the contrary, in 1916 reported that the intravenous injection of saline suspensions of killed pneumococci into seven patients suffering from lobar pneumonia caused no negative phase and apparently exerted a beneficial effect, since all the patients recovered.

Rosenow (1918),[1171] reasoning from his animal experiments that partial autolysates of virulent strains of the different types of pneumococci might better serve as auxiliaries in the mobilization of protective substances during an attack of lobar pneumonia, applied this form of treatment to pneumonia patients studied during three consecutive winters. The antigen was prepared by suspending in salt solution the sediment from cocci cultivated for eighteen to twenty-four hours in glucose broth, then allowing the suspension to autolyze at incubator temperature under a layer of ether. Self-digestion was permitted to progress until 95 per cent of the organisms became Gram-negative and five cubic centimeters of the preparation produced few or no symptoms in medium-sized guinea pigs. The dosage, in practice, was one cubic centimeter daily until the temperature became normal. The results, according to Rosenow, were surprisingly good: of ninety-five patients receiving the first injection of vaccine within forty-eight hours after onset of the disease only 3 per cent died; of one hundred five injected on the third day of the attack or later the mortality was 11 per cent. Furthermore, the administration of vaccine shortened the duration of the disease depending upon the promptness with which the treatment was begun. In the paper there was no mention of type determinations of the infecting pneumococci.

In a detailed clinical report on the use of a mixed vaccine in over two hundred pneumonia patients studied during the period 1922 to 1926, Lambert[776] published the following fatality-rates: In cases treated within the first forty-eight hours of the disease the figure was 5.8 per cent; for those patients receiving the vaccine in the first seventy-two hours the percentage was 9.8; when treatment was first instituted when the disease had been present for seventy-two hours or more 26.2 per cent of the patients died, giving a fatality-rate of 21.2 per cent for the entire series of cases treated with autolysate as against a rate of approximately 40 per cent for the untreated controls.

The significance of the results is somewhat obscured by the fact that the vaccine which Lambert employed, in addition to containing forty strains of pneumococci of the first three types and Group IV, also included four times as many other organisms such as streptococci, staphylococci, *Micrococcus catarrhalis*, and Pfeiffer bacilli. Whatever specific effect there was could be attributed to the pneumococci in the vaccine, while such influence as the bacteria of heterologous species may have had on secondary invaders might conceivably have contributed to the results. Lambert's recommendation that stock, mixed vaccines be used removes this form of therapy from the domain of scientific treatment and places it in the realm of empiricism. In Park's Harben Lecture,[1056] already quoted, he stated that a vaccine composed of several types of pneumococci and of other bacteria of respiratory origin in the treatment of lobar pneumonia was without appreciable effect.

Barach's[76] series of cases was small but his report may be included as lending some, though slight, support to the claims of advocates of vaccine treatment in pneumonia. Barach gave to twenty patients intravenous injections of monovalent vaccines representing both heat-killed cultures of pneumococci of Types I, II, and III and filtrates prepared from suspensions of the same organisms.

Two deaths occurred in the series; in one case, a vaccine of homologous type had been administered and, in the other, an heterologous preparation. Sutton and associates[1366] claimed favorable results attending the use of a "natural" pneumococcal antigen. The mortality among the treated cases was 22.5 per cent whereas 42 per cent of the untreated controls died.

Before any final appraisal can be made of the value of pneumococcal vaccines in the treatment of lobar pneumonia there must be more evidence at hand, and the evidence must be supplied by carefully controlled clinical studies in which large series of cases of which some groups are given monovalent preparations of pneumococci of a type homologous with that infecting the patient; other groups should receive vaccines of pneumococci of a variety of serological types without admixture of other bacteria; others should be given similar vaccines combined with organisms of respiratory origin; while the results in all the cases in the groups studied should be compared with the fate of a group of pneumonia patients who receive no pneumococcal antigens. Furthermore, type-determinations and blood cultures should be carried out in all cases studied. Without accurate and thorough observation of all the manifestations following the administration of the specific agent with proper bacteriological and serological controls no sound verdict can be reached.

CHAPTER XIV

CHEMOTHERAPY

The action in vitro *and* in vivo *of various organic and inorganic compounds on Pneumococcus, and their use in the treatment of pneumococcal infections.*

It would be a digression—a digression far beyond the scope of this book—to treat at any length the administration of drugs for the cure of infections due to pneumococci. It is assumed that the reader has a special interest in the effects of chemical agents on the life processes of Pneumococcus; for those whose interest extends to the more strictly therapeutic features of pneumococcal disease, Heffron's *Pneumonia*[601] will be found to contain an exhaustive discussion of the subject.

In the chemical treatment of diseases of parasitic origin, the agents usually employed fall into several main groups: arsenical preparations, modifications of alkaloids, derivatives from coal tar, metallic salts, and the usual pharmacopeial formulas. Those compounds have been chosen that exert a selective action on the invading parasite rather than those that stimulate normal physiological functions of the host; in other words, those that are specific rather than supportive. As with many other pathogenic bacteria, the great majority of chemical agents which are noxious to the pneumococcal cell are similarly injurious to the cells of animal tissues; many are too poisonous in the animal body, possess too narrow a margin of safety between therapeutic and toxic doses, or manifest such undesirable side or secondary actions that their use is precluded.

In pneumococcal infections the substances which have been studied for specific curative properties include bile and its component salts, some of the coal-tar dyes (especially the flavines), such metals as gold, silver, and iodine, and derivatives of the alkaloid, cinchona. Because of the relative unimportance of all chemical agents so far tested, with the exception of the cinchona compounds, the discussion of all but the last-named group will be presented in summarized form.

Chemical Agents Other Than Cinchona Derivatives

BILE

Powerful as is the action of whole bile or of sodium salts of the bile acids in the dissolution of the pneumococcal cell in the test tube, the lytic effect on pneumococci in the body is much less pronounced. Pneumococci, circulating in the blood or present in lesions or cavities accessible to the agent, may undergo lysis, but that is only one feature of the effect, because the physiological action of injected bile salts in a large measure offsets any benefits to be derived from the dissolution of the cocci. Barjot (1928)[79] treated a few cases of lobar pneumonia by the intravenous administration of sodium taurocholate in an artificial serum containing magnesium sulfate, but the small number of patients and the nature of the results would scarcely seem to justify the author's faith in the benefits to be derived from the treatment. Ziegler,[1570] employing saline solutions of the sodium salts of taurocholic and glycocholic acids, reported, as might be expected, a cholagogic effect along with erratic fluctuations in the temperature curves of the patients so treated. The bile salt caused damage to the vein at the point of injection, sometimes resulting in obliteration of the vessel, but its use was attended by no other appreciable toxic symptoms, although, to be sure, a slight degree of anemia was observed. In a second communication, Ziegler[1571] stated that in rabbits the intravenous injection of sodium dehydrocholate in the concentration employed was without the injurious action of the corresponding taurocholate and glycocholate on the tissues in the neighborhood of the injection, but apparently the treatment was not applied to human beings. Because of both the predictable local and systemic effects of biliary salts these substances hold little promise as medicinal agents for the treatment of pneumococcal infections.

SOAP

So, too, with soaps. According to Lamar (1912),[775] sodium oleate when added to specific immune serum and boric acid, may exhibit an adjuvant action in combating pneumococcal infection of the meninges. The combination regularly exerted a more powerful action than immune serum alone and not only prevented the occurrence of infection, but also, when administered repeatedly, arrested the progress of an already established infection and often led to the recovery of the infected animals. The treatment, however, was not applied to meningitis in man. Lauric acid was shown by Walker[1476] to be strongly germicidal for pneumococci, while Larson and Nelson[791] in their study of sodium ricinoleate found that the soap was fatal to virulent cultures of the organism. These compounds, however, were not administered to human beings.

COAL-TAR DYES

The affinities possessed by bacterial cells for dyes render the cells susceptible to the bacteriostatic action of the dye retained by the cell after treatment by the Gram technique, but the action of the dye, even when mordanted, is rarely of such a nature as to affect the organism when circulating in the blood stream. Of the many substances studied with a view to ascertaining the pneumococcidal action in the circulation, dyes of the triphenylmethane series were found by Simon and Wood,[1288] in cultivation experiments, to be strongly inhibitory to the growth of pneumococci. Because of their antiseptic or germicidal properties, the flavines have received special attention from students of Pneumococcus. Schiemann and Baumgarten[1227] reported that acriflavine exerted a powerful, selective action on both virulent and avirulent members of the species. Neufeld and Schiemann[999] showed that trypaflavine and different salts of 3–6 diamino-acridine were strongly bacteriostatic *in vitro*. *In vivo*, the compounds when administered subcutaneously rescued a certain percentage of mice infected intraperitoneally with pneumococci. The dyes were also efficacious when applied in the form of irrigations in wounds experimentally infected with pneumococci in mice and guinea pigs (Neufeld and Reinhardt,[996] and Reinhardt[1134]). From animal experiments, Schiemann,[1224] by intraperitoneal or topical application, substantiated the observation on the favorable influence exerted by trypaflavine on pneumococcal infection. Maeji[851-2] stated that trypaflavine was pneumococcidal in a dilution of 1 to 100,000. To the list of pneumococcostatic agents Schiemann added the aurophosphine and trimethane dyes, crystal violet and brilliant green. As for Mercurochrome, the few references (Freeman and Hoppe,[481] and Phelps[1088]), lacking any laboratory tests, are not significant, whereas the somewhat analogous substance, Metaphen, was reported by Kolmer and Borrow[742] to be less effective than optochin, a substance which will be discussed later. From the few references in the literature it would appear that such tinctorial substances derived from the nitrobenzines as have been studied manifest no conspicuous pneumococcidal properties when introduced into the animal body.

METALS AND METALLIC SALTS

Of metallic elements, gold in colloidal form has been tried in the treatment of pneumococcal infection in man (Gautier[505]), and as a synergist with specific serum in the treatment of experimental infection in rabbits (Gelarie and Sabin[510]). In the latter case, the survival ratio of the animals treated with serum and gold was greater than that of those receiving subeffective doses of serum alone. Schiemann and Feldt[1229] reported that gold in the form of Sanocrysin had slight if any action in protecting mice infected with pneumococci. Gautier mentioned iodine as a therapeutic agent in the treatment of pneumonia but offered little information concerning the effect in combating pneumococcal infections. Iodine in colloidal solution was administered by Murphy[940] to ninety patients ill with pneumonia; of the ninety, ten died. The report contained no account of any *in vitro* experiments with the solution.

OTHER MEDICINAL AGENTS

Many drugs have been subjected to clinical trial, not on the basis of laboratory experiment, but apparently in the hope that some selective action on Pneumococcus might follow their administration. Reports on epinephrine have come from Puscariu and Nitzulescu,[1113] and on camphor by Rosenthal and Stein[1174] and by Welch and Rueck.* According to Boehncke,[133] the subcutaneous injection of camphor dissolved in oil was able to protect mice and rabbits against intraperitoneal and intravenous inoculation with virulent pneumococci made some hours later. Formaldehyde sulfoxylate which, according to Rosenthal,[1177] was without pneumococcidal action *in vitro*, nevertheless, when injected subcutaneously into mice at the time of inoculation in three or four-hour doses repeated daily, protected the animals from an otherwise fatal infection. Rosenthal,[1176] and Powell and Jamieson[1104] have also published the results of experiments with the same drug. Schottstaedt[1249] and physicians of the United Fruit Company have used without laboratory control enemas of potassium permanganate in the treatment of lobar pneumonia with more or less favorable results which, however, indicate no specific action of the agent used. The same may be said for sodium salicylate as reported by Couvey and Popoff.[285] Hexamethyltetramine (Urotropin) was found by Maeji[851] to be capable in a concentration of 1 to 1,000 to 1 to 2,000 of killing pneumococci *in vitro*.

Any further recital of reports on other therapeutic agents would add nothing of value to the present discussion, which may now be directed to a class of substances possessing markedly specific antagonistic properties against pneumococci.

* Quoted by Neufeld and Schnitzer.

Cinchona Derivatives

EFFECT OF THE VARIOUS QUININE DERIVATIVES ON PNEUMOCOCCI

Quite different from the agents already described in their action on pneumococci are certain products prepared from the alkaloid, cinchona. In the first experiments reported by Morgenroth and Levy (1911),[926-7] quinine was found to be valueless in sparing from infection mice inoculated with a fatal dose of pneumococci. However, when the related substance, hydroquinine (methylhydrocupreine) was used, the pneumococcidal effect was marked and a yet more pronounced action was observed when the next higher homologue, ethylhydrocupreine (optochin) was employed. The two substances in the form of aqueous solutions of their respective sulfates and hydrochlorides, when injected into mice at the time of inoculation or during the course of a virulent pneumococcal infection, saved a significant number of the test animals. Ethylhydrocupreine sulfate was less toxic and more potent in protective and curative action than was the hydrochloride of methylhydrocupreine. Another homologous derivative possessing active pneumococcidal properties, as determined by Morgenroth and Bumcke,[921] was isopropylhydrocupreine. Vuzine, described by Morgenroth,[920] is also an active homologue, but its action is influenced by variations in the susceptibility of different pneumococcal strains.

A disadvantage of the watery solutions of these alkaloidal salts was their rapid absorption and excretion—a disadvantage overcome by Morgenroth and Kaufmann,[922-5] as well as by Gutmann,[582] by dissolving the optochin base in oil. The toxicity of this type of compound, according to Morgenroth and Kaufmann, could be lowered by substituting the salicylic ester of optochin, and it was found that of the homologues of hydroquinine, optochin was the most active in germicidal effect on pneumococci.

The sterilizing action of optochin on pneumococci *in vitro* was demonstrated by Wright, Morgan, Colebrook, and Dodgson,[1543-4] a result corroborated by Schiemann and Ishiwara.[1230] Optochin in concentrations of about one to one million and somewhat less inhibited the growth of pneumococci, while its bacteriostatic and pneumococcidal action was exerted in solutions of high protein content. The fact is of importance in relation to the effect of optochin on pneumococci in the blood stream—an effect demonstrated by Wright, Morgan, Colebrook, and Dodgson, as well as by Kolmer and Borrow.[742] The experiments of Moore[908] showed the highly specific action of ethylhydrocupreine hydrochloride on pneumococci and, moreover, disclosed the fact that the phenomenon took place with pneumococci of all the four groups tested. So specific was the effect that Moore saw in it a means for the identification of pneumococci.

The preeminence of ethylhydrocupreine among the quinine derivatives was established by Tugendreich and Russo,[1429] an observation confirmed by Solis-Cohen, Kolmer, and Heist[1304] among others. Felton and Dougherty[422] made a comparative study of four closely related synthetic cinchona derivatives. The first preparation was hydroquinine chloracetanilide, and the remaining three were substitution products of the first compound. The effect of the preparations was tested *in vitro* and *in vivo* against a young culture of Type I Pneumococcus. The *in vitro* tests were carried out by holding the dose of the drug constant in mixtures with varying amounts of culture, and then by injecting uniform amounts of the organism and increasing doses of the drug. In the *in vivo* experiments, a fatal dose of the culture was injected and the medicament administered in the maximal tolerated dose. All four compounds tested were found to display rapid pneumococcidal activity both in the test tube and in the peritoneal cavity of mice and to a lesser extent in rabbits. Optochin appeared to be the slowest in action, but its action was not so easily inhibited either *in vitro* or *in vivo*. The *meta* substitution product (hydroquinine *m*-chloracetylaminophenol) exerted the strongest killing action on pneumococci when injected simultaneously with the culture into the peritoneal cavity. However, optochin, notwithstanding the fact that the zone between therapeutic dose and toxic dose was narrower than in the case of the other derivatives studied, appeared to be less injurious to the natural defenses of the body.

EFFECT ON VARIOUS PNEUMOCOCCAL TYPES

Felton and Dougherty noted variability in the bactericidal action *in vivo* of the compounds on different strains of pneumococci, since the virulence of the culture contributed to fluctuations in the effect of the drug. The observation was contrary to those of Kleinschmidt,[722] of Moore, and also of Solis-Cohen, Kolmer, and Heist, whose results indicated that the germicidal power of the cinchona derivatives which they studied, possibly with the exception of some Type III strains, was apparently the same for all the types of pneumococci tested. Schiemann, and Schiemann and Ishiwara, however, had earlier reported that virulent strains were more susceptible to the effect of optochin than were attenuated strains, and that the source of the culture was also concerned in sensitivity to drug action.

According to Wright, Morgan, Colebrook, and Dodgson, and to Schiemann and Ishiwara, optochin, unlike some metallic salts, loses little of its germicidal power in the presence respectively of human serum or rabbit serum, but Solis-Cohen and his associates reported that the agent lost from one-fiftieth to one-tenth of its activity in a menstruum of serum as compared with that exhibited in isotonic salt solution.

Wright and his co-workers had early found (1912) that three hours subsequent to the administration of optochin to adults the serum of the treated subjects would kill pneumococci *in vitro*. Moore and Chesny[910] later made the same observation but stated that the effect depended upon the administration of a sufficient amount of the drug and the spacing of the doses. Similarly, Baldwin and Rhoades[69] concluded that the ethylhydrocupreine base, as employed by them, is absorbed from the gastro-intestinal tract in sufficient quantities to impart demonstrable pneumococcidal properties to the serum when tested *in vitro*.

In carrying out pneumococcidal experiments with derivatives of cinchona, the technique, the temperature of the mixture, the duration of exposure, and the vigor and virulence of the organisms employed should be considered and should always be uniform. Solis-Cohen and his colleagues advised for the best results a small number of organisms and a long exposure to the action of the drug. Kolmer and Idzumi,[743] in studying the effect of optochin on Type II pneumococci in purulent spinal fluid, found that sterilization was complete in sixty to ninety minutes when the preparation was used in a concentration of 1 to 10,000 but, in a concentration of 1 to 50,000, optochin was ineffective. In a more highly purulent empyema exudate containing Type I Pneumococcus, Kolmer and Sands[749] noted death of the organisms after a thirty-minute exposure at 37° to an equal volume of optochin in a 1 to 10,000 solution. Maeji[852] gave the following figures as representing the effective pneumococcidal strengths of the cinchona derivatives tested: optochin hydrochloride, 1:8,000 to 1:10,000; remijine, 1:8,000 to 1:10,000; quinine, 1:2,000 to 1:4,000; eucopine, 1:20,000 to 1:40,000; vuzine, 1:30,000 to 1:40,000. Mention of the curative action of the compounds was not included in Maeji's papers.

A more delicate method for determining the bacteriostatic action of optochin was that described by Schnabel.[1238, 1240] The reducing property of the bacterial cell was chosen as an indicator of the vital activities of Pneumococcus and the effect studied of the drug on the ability of the organism to reduce methylene blue. Schnabel reported that optochin in as low a concentration as one to eight million was able to inhibit the reduction of the dye by the strain of the Pneumococcus chosen for the test. The reaction could also be utilized to determine the amount of optochin in the serum of animals treated with the drug.

EFFECT ON PNEUMOCOCCAL INFECTION

More recent experience casts doubt on the effectiveness claimed for optochin in combating pneumococcal infection. Reimann and Moen,[1131] for example, employing the Goodner intradermal method for infecting rabbits, after comparative trials with large doses of quinine hydrochloride and ethylhydrocupreine in rabbits, concluded that the feeble curative action of the drugs was in no way comparable to the effect produced by specific immune serum. The skepticism felt in Germany concerning the work of the American authors led Gundel and Seitz[577] to investigate several hitherto untried quinine derivatives. As a result of their experiments on mice, the authors placed ethylapoquinine in the foremost rank. The compound in high dilution killed pneumococci in fairly large numbers both *in vitro* and *in vivo*, and in its action was to be preferred to *alpha* and *beta*-isoquinine and even to optochin.

In contrast to the report of Gundel and Seitz was that of Kolmer and Rule[748] who, like Reimann and Moen, tested cinchona preparations on rabbits suffering from "dermal pneumonia" following inoculation by the Goodner technique. Neither the optochin base, ethylhydrocupreine hydrochloride, nor quinine and urea hydrochloride, given by stomach tube and by repeated intramuscular injection, exhibited any beneficial effect on the local lesion, bacteriemia, or leucocyte count resulting from intradermal infection with Type I pneumococci. In a more extended study comprising tests on some thirty-five preparations of the quinine group, Maclachlan, Permar, Johnston, and Kenney[846] found that only three compounds of those tested possessed any conspicuous killing power for pneumococci, and these substances were ethylapoquinine, hydroethylapoquinine, and hydroxyethylhydrocupreine. The authors' preference was given to ethylapoquinine because it gave greater protection to the mice treated than did optochin. The results were not in agreement with those of Okomoto and Sogen,[1024] who found that while apoquinine exhibited strong pneumococcidal action *in vitro*, it afforded practically no protection to mice against experimental pneumococcal infection.

Other experiments that serve to substantiate the claims of Maclachlan and his colleagues are those of Butler, Nelson, Renfrew, and Cretcher.[193] The authors tested cinchona alkaloids, their hydrogenated derivatives, and some artificially prepared homologues and reported that hydroxyethylhydrocupreine was less toxic for mice than optochin and was highly efficient in protecting the test animals against pneumococcal infection. In a second communication, Butler and Cretcher[192] stated that apocupreine hydrochloride displayed fairly high pneumococcidal action *in vitro*, when compared to other members of the cinchona group, was very low in toxicity for mice, and possessed protective properties similar to those of optochin and ethylapoquinine.

Optochin and its allied compounds possess marked disadvantages. The substances do not penetrate the infected lesions and, therefore, do not affect the cocci at the point of greatest concentration. A more serious drawback is the toxic action of some of the drugs of the cinchona series. Moore and Chesny,[910] in an analysis of the manifestations observed during optochin treatment of lobar pneumonia in man, pointed out the well-known tendency of optochin to damage eyesight. The authors stated that in the literature on optochin treatment, among the patients developing serious ophthalmic disturbances with impairment of vision (4.5 per cent of those reported) there were some whose iris failed to react to light and others in whom the ophthalmoscope revealed a tortuosity of the retinal vessels with a general constriction of the arteries. Acute retinitis accompanied by temporary blindness has been observed, but interference with vision is rarely permanent. Browning[159] has stated that this complication has occurred mainly after administration of the soluble hydrochloride and may be minimized by avoiding excessive doses or by the use of relatively insoluble forms of the drug. However, the comparative insolubility of the base constitutes a disadvantage in its use. A precaution to be observed in this class of substances is to keep the compound from coming in contact with free hydrochloric acid in the stomach.

ADJUVANT ACTION OF CINCHONA COMPOUNDS WITH SPECIFIC SERUM

The first report on the combined action of optochin and immune serum on pneumococci was that of Neufeld and Engwer[982] in 1912 and of Engwer[365] in 1913, who found in guinea pigs an augmented action of the two agents when employed together. Another observation reported by Boehncke[132] in 1913 suggested that optochin may exert an auxiliary or possibly a synergistic action when administered along with specific immune serum. In tests on white mice, Boehncke[133] claimed better curative effects with a mixture of ethylhydrocupreine and immune serum than with either agent alone and that this favorable therapeutic action could be produced by the combined use of both agents in less than the curative dose of either. The observation was confirmed by Moore,[909] who concluded that a single small dose of optochin base, which by itself exerted no protective action against pneumococcal infection in mice, was capable of increasing by at least fifty times the threshold value of antipneumococcic serum. The effect occurred only when the serum and the infecting organism were of the same serological type and proportionally was many times greater than a simple summation of the protective action of the two single components of the mixture.

The phenomenon finds an analogy in the adjuvant action of sodium oleate with immune serum already quoted from Lamar[775] and that of gold as reported by Gelarie and Sabin.[510] The use of cinchona derivatives, especially ethylhydrocupreine, in combination with specific serum therapy would appear to possess the advantage of making it possible to reduce the dose of the drug well below the toxic limit as well as to enhance the curative action of the immune serum. Search has failed to reveal any record of further trials of this combined form of treatment in pneumococcal infections.

In this connection a comparison of the protective power of cinchona derivatives and of antipneumococcic serum may not be out of place. Felton[404] reported that the specific protective globulin of immune horse serum was one million times more effective against Pneumococcus than was quinine sulfate and one hundred thousand times more powerful than optochin.

EFFECT ON VIRULENCE OF PNEUMOCOCCUS

Drug-fastness. In Chapter V, the effect of optochin in inducing variation in pneumococci was described. In that biological change the bacterial cell acquires a tolerance for the drug. Morgenroth and Kaufmann[922-5] showed that the passage of a pneumococcal strain four times through animals treated with optochin caused the organisms to lose their sensitivity to the action of the drug. The observation was confirmed by Tugendreich and Russo,[1429] and by Koehne,[738] who discovered that pneumococci suffered an enormous loss of susceptibility after cultivation in the presence of optochin *in vitro.* Schnabel and Jungeblut* likewise demonstrated the acquisition by the bacterial cell of a high-grade resistance following cultivation in broth containing optochin. Koch, by growing pneumococci in artificial media, could decrease optochin sensitivity without destroying the virulence of the organisms. After a few animal passages the strains regained their normal sensitivity.

During this process of biological adaptation, according to Jungeblut,[697] the bacterial cell may lose virulence but, on the other hand, Lewy[807] was able to maintain the full virulence of strains of pneumococci by alternate passage through untreated mice and through culture media containing optochin, although the strain had become eighty to one hundred twenty times more resistant to

* Quoted from Neufeld and Schnitzer,[1000] from whose account and that of Browning[159] much of the above information is taken.

the chemical. Drug-fastness was retained for some time during cultivation in optochin-free media as well as during animal passage. Lewy noted that during the treatment just described variants of the original strain appeared (Modification B) which lacked sensitivity to optochin. The resistance or tolerance was general in nature and was not to be confused with specific optochin-fastness. In an analysis of the specificity of optochin-fastness in pneumococci, Lewy[808] found that there was a slight, specific action of quinine as well as of hydroquinine. With more marked chemical variations in the side-chain, as in the case of the higher homologues, or in the nucleus of the optochin molecule, the specific action of optochin on Pneumococcus disappears. The susceptibility of the optochin-fast strain to other compounds quite foreign to this class of substances suggested to Lewy the presence of other sensitive groups—chemoceptors—in the pneumococcal cell.

Heightened susceptibility. That the reverse of acquired tolerance by Pneumococcus may take place was shown by the experiments of Schnabel[1241] and of Schnabel and Kasarnowsky.[1242] Cultures of pneumococci injected into mice with subsequent administration to the infected animals of dilute optochin solutions caused the organisms after a twenty-four-hour sojourn in the body of the treated animals to develop a heightened susceptibility to the drug. In addition to the influence of lesser concentrations of optochin, the length of exposure of the organisms in the treated animals was a factor in increasing the sensitivity of the cocci.

Summary

In reviewing the data which have been accumulated from experiments in the test tube and in the animal body, the conviction is gained that not yet has the ideal drug been found that lends itself to the chemotherapy of pneumococcal infection. The action of cinchona derivatives in affecting the vital characters of Pneumococcus may render the bacteria more vulnerable to the natural defensive forces of the body, and this action may be a distinct aid in specific serum therapy. Failure so far to discover a satisfactory medicinal agent with pneumococcidal properties and free of undesirable side effects is tempered with the promise offered by cinchona compounds and leaves this inviting and profitable field open to renewed and extended investigation.

CHAPTER XV

PRODUCTION OF ANTIPNEUMOCOCCIC SERUM

Procedures employed in the routine manufacture of therapeutic serum, including immunization of horses, methods of concentration and purification of specific immune serum; processing, standardization, and control of the products; and the preparation of serum for diagnostic purposes.

THE early demonstration that serum from immunized rabbits and other small experimental animals exerts protective and curative effects in similar animals infected with pneumococci supplied ample warrant for extending studies to include larger domestic animals in the hope of providing serum for use in the treatment of pneumococcal infection in man. Interest in this phase of study first developed by 1897, for in that year there appeared publications by Denys,[312] Pane,[1044] Mennes,[893] and Washbourn[1487] describing the results attending the immunization of goats, asses, cows, and horses. Occasional reports on the use of other animals have been made, but where large amounts are required horses are at the present time the commonly accepted source of antipneumococcic serum.

Immunization of the Horse

SELECTION OF HORSES

Little is known as to the precise type or breed of horse most suitable for the production of antipneumococcic serum. Avery, Chickering, Cole, and Dochez[36] preferred sound, fairly heavy horses, and the same opinion is shared by some laboratories today. At the Massachusetts Antitoxin and Vaccine Laboratory experience has shown that the breed, weight, and sex of horses are less important factors than the variations in the immune response of individual animals. Not infrequently it has been observed that a horse showing poor response to injections of diphtheria and scarlet fever toxins or even of suspensions of Meningococcus may develop a high titer of specific humoral antibodies following immunization with pneumococcal vaccines. It is equally true that animals of the same general type may produce serum exhibiting considerable differences in potency. The trial-and-error method of selection of horses for immunization, while expensive and time-consuming, appears to be the most reliable procedure available at the present time. There is an impression in certain quarters at least, that the age of the horse may be of some importance. Wadsworth and Kirkbride[1470] used horses of over eleven years of age. Although it has not been proved that older horses are more readily immunized with pneumococcal vaccines, it can be said that the more mature horses respond quite as well as do younger animals and, furthermore, are likely to be more tractable.

Prior to initiation of the immunization process, the horses selected should be subjected to a rigid physical examination, with particular attention to the existence of respiratory affections. Animals exhibiting evidence of the "heaves" should not be used. A quarantine period of three weeks should be the rule, during which time a careful examination for glanders by physical means and by the mallein and complement-fixation tests is made, and the absence of other communicable diseases determined. When the animals have satisfactorily passed the quarantine period they may be stabled in permanent quarters and the immunization process begun.

SELECTION AND STANDARDIZATION OF THE IMMUNIZING ANTIGEN

The ideal pneumococcal antigen for the routine immunization of horses is yet to be found. Such questions as the degree of virulence of the cultures, whether the organism should be in a living or devitalized state (or combinations of both), and which derivatives of the pneumococcal cell possess the desired antigenic properties, along with a host of modifications in the preparation of each antigen have been considered in attempts to increase the therapeutic potency of antipneumococcic serum.

Virulence. The virulence of strains of pneumococci used for immunization was recognized as an important factor soon after immunological studies were begun. Emmerich and Fowitzky (1891)[857] found that rabbits injected subcutaneously with attenuated cultures became only partly immune, but after the intravenous administration of fully virulent cultures a "complete" immunity resulted. It should be borne in mind, however, that while the difference in the routes of injection may have played a part in the outcome of the experiments, the conclusions reached are in accord with present conceptions. A year later, Mosny[932] stated that cultures used for immunization should be virulent, and added the requirement that cultures should be heated for three hours at 60°. Emmerich,[856] and Römer[1155] both subscribed to the idea of using only virulent strains for immunization, and Landmann,[779] who worked under Römer, found that more uniform and potent serums were obtained when only highly virulent strains of pneumococci were employed. Neufeld and Haendel[989] also used only strains of exalted virulence. Wadsworth,[1458] in determining the curative and protective activity of immune serum in infected rabbits, reported that while immune serum might be protective, only after immunization of animals with living, virulent cultures did the serum acquire marked curative properties. In the same year, Dochez[316] reported the development of highly potent protective serum by immunization of the horse with large doses of virulent organisms in the living state.

In the well-known Rockefeller Monograph No. 7, Avery and his colleagues[36] emphasized the importance of using virulent strains for immunization. So, too, Raphael[1121] declared that the degree of immunizing action is dependent upon virulence, and advocated a study of the antigenicity of only virulent strains in rabbits before attempting the hyperimmunization of larger animals. In studying the response of mice and rabbits to immunization with living or killed avirulent pneumococci, Yoshioka (1925)[1565] found that only weak serums were produced. During investigations on the smooth and rough forms of pneumococci, Griffith (1923)[560] concluded that only smooth strains should be employed for the production of serum. Using Type III pneumococci, Lévy-Bruhl (1927)[804] obtained agglutinating and precipitating serums readily from horses, but protective antibody was obtained only when recourse was had to the injection of exceptionally virulent strains. Meyer and Sukneff (1928)[898] reported that the administration of sodium taurocholate solutions of virulent strains yielded serum with protective and some cross-protective powers, but the injection of solutions of avirulent strains evoked no protective antibodies. The observations are consistent with the earlier reports of Avery and Neill[59] and of Avery and Heidelberger[49] on the antigenic action of constituents of the pneumococcal cell. In studies on the response of rabbits to inhalation of pneumococci, Stillman (1930)[1334] concluded that the type-specific response of the animals, as evidenced by the appearance of specific protective antibodies and agglutinins in the serum, varies in direct proportion to the virulence of the culture used. There seems to be little dissent, therefore, from the opinion that only cultures of maximal virulence furnish satisfactory antigenic material for the production of potent antipneumococcic serum. In the opinion of the authors of the present volume, the best results are obtained by choosing cultures of exalted virulence and strong antigenicity and by maintaining high virulence by passing the strains through mice daily for at least five days a week. The various methods of maintaining the virulence of cultures in routine use have been discussed in Chapter VI.

In a study of the immunizing properties of the four groups of pneumococci classified by Dochez and Gillespie,[322] Dochez and Avery[318] found the order of virulence of the types of pneumococci for human beings to be III, II, I, and Group IV, and stated that "the degree of protective power developed in the sera of animals immunized against members of these groups varies inversely with the virulence and the amount of capsular development." The statement of Dochez and Avery just cited should not be construed as meaning that the virulence of a strain of Pneumococcus militates against its ability to provoke the elaboration of immune substances in the animal body. There are other considerations peculiar to each pneumococcal type that determine the antigenic properties of its members. The factors may be differences in the chemical constitution of the cellular components or in the manner in which the polysaccharide and other elements of the cell are joined together, which affects the lability or stability of the antigen when introduced into the body and, therefore, determines the specific immune response of the animal. Thus, it is known to be more difficult to obtain a potent serum for Type III than for Type II Pneumococcus, and easier to produce serum of higher protective value for Type I than for Type II. Investigations on the twenty-nine separate types formerly in Group IV indicate differences in antigenicity which may follow the principle established by Dochez and Avery. Attempts to produce serum effective against Type III pneumococci, possessing as they do an unusually large amount of capsular material, have been disappointing.

Filtrates of broth cultures. Much of the early work was done with filtrates of broth cultures or other agents containing the soluble, cell-free components of the pneumococcal cell. Of great importance are the investigations by Avery and Morgan (1925),[54] Avery and Neill (1925),[59] and Avery and Heidelberger (1925).[49] The results of these studies show that solutions or extracts of Pneumococcus containing free somatic protein and free capsular polysaccharide give rise only to species-specific antibodies; suspensions containing mixtures of intact cells and dissociated cellular components induce both species-specific and type-specific antibodies; preparations of intact cells containing no free pneumococcal protein stimulate the production of type-specific immunity. Confirmation of these findings came from Barach,[75] Meyer and Sukneff,[898] Ferguson,[436] and from various unreported observations made during the routine work in manufacturing laboratories. At present, therefore, the most satisfactory antigen for stimulating the production of type-specific therapeutic serum is one composed of a natural combination of the pneumococcal protein and polysaccharide as found in the intact cell, and containing a minimum of uncombined carbohydrate and somatic protein.

Exudates of infected tissues. Exudates of infected pneumonic tissue have also been tried as immunizing agents. Netter (1887)[969] obtained immunity in mice and rabbits by the injection of post-pneumonic pleural exudate, and the Klemperer brothers (1891)[724] observed similar results. Hartman (1913)[599] also described the use of the various constituents of exudative material as antigens but the results were disappointing. A vaccine prepared from pneumococci washed from the peritoneal cavity of a rabbit dead from pneumococcal infection was, according to Heist and Solis-Cohen (1919),[635] more active as an immunizing agent for rabbits than one made from the organisms grown on artificial culture media. Freedlander (1928),[480] by using saline extracts of infected tissues as antigens in rabbits, claimed to have obtained protective serum of a potency corresponding to that of antipneumococcic horse serum. In 1929, Curphey and Baruch[291] described a method of collecting and using pleural exudate from horses in the immunization of other horses against pneumococci. The authors believed that the procedure would decrease the length of time necessary to produce a potent immune serum. A year later, these investigators[292] reported the results of tests with the so-called exudate antiserum. The effects of the serum in treating intradermal infections in rabbits were compared with those of serum prepared in the usual manner, and in the opinion of the authors the exudate antiserum contained antibodies other than those of an antibacterial nature.

Viability of the organism. The question whether dead pneumococci are more or less efficient antigens than living pneumococci is still unsettled. Mosny (1892),[932] already quoted, stated that when cultures are to be used for immunization, "they must be virulent and heated for three hours at 60°," thus favoring the use of killed suspensions. Issaeff[673] reported successful immunization of rabbits by administering killed bouillon cultures and later blood from infected animals, the organisms being first killed by chloroform or heat. In immunizing horses, Denys (1897)[312] injected first heated, then unheated cultures, next the blood of a rabbit dead of pneumococcal infection, and finally living broth cultures. He thus was able ultimately to inject a large amount of an extremely virulent culture without causing any more marked symptoms than a transient rise in temperature. Mennes (1897),[893] by using methods similar to those of Denys, produced in the horse after three or four months' treatment, serum that exhibited preventive, curative, and "antitoxic" properties. Washbourn (1897)[1487] immunized ponies by the subcutaneous injection of heated broth cultures, then living agar cultures, and finally living broth cultures. After nine months of treatment, the serum was found to possess marked protective action.

Neufeld (1902)[974] recommended the use first of killed, then of living organisms. Later, however, with Haendel (1909),[989] Neufeld stated that in immunizing horses and asses there was no such marked difference between the use of living and dead organisms as was found in rabbits, although horses injected with viable cultures produced better serum. Horses proved to be more sensitive than asses to living organisms.

For developing antipneumococcic serum of high protective titer in horses, Dochez (1912)[316] employed large doses of living, virulent organisms. In an investigation of the action of immune serum on pneumococcal infection in rabbits, Wadsworth (1912)[1458] found that little or no curative effect was exerted by serum from animals immunized with washed, dead organisms or culture filtrates; only after immunization with living, virulent cultures did the serum acquire marked therapeutic properties. In a study on the distribution of immune bodies in antipneumococcic serum, Avery[32] immunized horses over periods of one or two years by injecting progressively increasing doses of dead organisms until the animals were able to tolerate the sedimented residue from one liter of living, virulent culture. Cole and Moore (1917)[268] also favored this method. Their experiments indicated that, for the most rapid production of primary immunity, several series of small doses of dead cultures should be given, but in order to produce the highest degree of immunity, living organisms were required.

In the Rockefeller Monograph, Avery, Chickering, Cole, and Dochez[36] outlined their methods for the immunization of horses. After the administration of two series of injections of heat-killed organisms, a sample of blood was obtained for agglutination and protection tests. Serum taken at this time was never found to be of satisfactory titer and, consequently, injections of living organisms were given in increasing amounts until tests on the serum samples indicated the desired potency. Cole (1917)[257] obtained potent serum from horses injected over a period of six to seven weeks with gradually increasing doses of dead organisms. Wadsworth and Kirkbride (1917)[1470] reported the development of protective serums in horses immunized first by injections of heated organisms followed by increasing doses of living pneumococci. In 1918, Alexander[7] described the use of mixtures of pneumococci and leucocytes, and of serum-sensitized organisms and leucocytes, in immunizing rabbits, and found that protective antibodies were developed within eight to eleven days.

Despite the observations and beliefs that living cultures of pneumococci induce the production of more effective therapeutic serum than do killed organisms, there has been an increasing tendency to use dead cultures. It is doubtful if any of the larger manufacturing laboratories employ living cultures for the routine immunization of horses. The writers of the present volume question whether the alleged superiority of living antigens over devitalized preparations in stimulating antibody production outweighs the hazards associated with the use of living, virulent cultures. Granting the opinion to be sound, the problem arises of choosing a method by which suspensions of pneumococci may be rendered non-infective but which will preserve a maximum of antigenicity.

Methods of devitalizing the organism: heat and formalin. Heat has long been employed as a means of devitalizing organisms to be used for immunization purposes. Mosny[932] recommended the heating of cultures for three hours at 60°. Washbourn[1487] advocated a temperature of 60°, but for a period of only one hour, and Neufeld and Haendel[989] also utilized the same temperature. In preparing killed suspensions of pneumococci, Avery, Chickering, Cole, and Dochez[36] heated the coccal suspensions in the water-bath at 56° for one-half hour. Truche (1920)[1420] preferred vaccines killed by alcohol and ether, since he stated that heat-killed suspensions were not tolerated well by horses. In a study of the effect of the degree and period of heating on the antigenicity of pneumococci, Tani[1379] obtained better immunization with vaccines subjected to 100° than with those heated at lower temperatures. The period of heating varied from ten minutes to four hours. A culture heated at 45° for two and one-half hours was found to have low immunizing value. In the investigations of Gaspari, Sugg, Fleming, and Neill,[503] in which a large number of rabbits were used as test animals, the influence of heat on the antigenic strength of the type-specific and species-specific antigens of the Type II pneumococci was studied. The temperatures varied from 55° to 120° applied for a period of one-half hour, and the results indicated that heating pneumococcal suspensions tends to decrease the effectiveness of the species-specific antigen without having any appreciable influence on the antigenic power of the type-specific complex.

Chemical agents have also been employed in preparing pneumococcal vaccines for animal immunization. The use of alcohol and ether has already been mentioned, while glycerol extracts have also been tried. Takami[1374] used carbolized cultures with rabbits, but there appear to be few adherents to the practice. By the subcutaneous injection of horses with ricinoleated cultures, or with sterile pneumococcal "toxin," Clowes, Jamieson, and Olson[244] reported the demonstration of antitoxic properties in immune serum so produced.

The methods of choice in devitalizing pneumococcal vaccines appear to have become reduced, in recent years, to treatment either with heat or with formalin. For immunizing horses, Savino, Negrete, and Acuna (1931)[1221] added 0.2 per cent formalin to cultures and then centrifuged out the organisms. Pico and Negrete[1089] added 0.5 per cent of formalin to suspensions to be used for the same purpose, and claimed that the preparations retained their antigenic power over a long period of time. Tao[1380] compared the immune response of rabbits and mice injected with heat-killed vaccines and suspensions of pneumococci killed by exposure to 0.3 per cent formalin for eight hours. He reported that formalinized vaccines stimulated the production of specific antibodies quite as well if not better than did heated suspensions, but it was observed that the immunity developed in the animal body under the stimulus from formalin-treated vaccine appeared somewhat later than that from heated vaccine. The latter observation was confirmed by the work of Barnes and White (1934)[86] during studies on the comparative antigenicity of heat-killed and formalinized vaccines in rabbits and horses but, contrary to Tao's observations, vaccines killed by one-hour exposure to 56° were at least as effective, if not more so, than the formalinized suspensions. In addition, heat-killed vaccines appeared to be somewhat less toxic than those treated with formalin.

The amount of formalin used by different workers in preparing pneumococcal vaccines has varied. In this connection, some observations by Barnes and Hager* (1932) may be cited. A culture of pneumococci was divided into four parts and to each portion there was added 0.2, 0.3, 0.4, and 0.5 per cent respectively of formalin. After storage at room temperature overnight, the cultures were centrifuged and the supernatant fluids tested for free and combined formaldehyde. In each case only about 0.05 per cent of for-

* Unpublished.

malin remained in combination with the sedimented organisms. This fact implies that when formalin is added in a concentration greater than that necessary for devitalizing pneumococci, the excess may remain uncombined, and participate in some of the disturbing reactions in animals injected with formalinized vaccines.

Results of investigations by Barnes and Wight* (1935) suggest that formalinized suspensions of pneumococci, particularly those of Type II, undergo rapid autolysis during storage in the refrigerator; vaccines killed by heat at 56° for one hour are somewhat more stable, while those heated at 100° for fifteen minutes retain their original turbidity for periods of at least four months. The antigenic potency, in rabbits and horses, of pneumococcal vaccines devitalized by heat at 100° appears to be as high, if not higher, than that of the more readily autolyzable preparations.

In the authors' experience, pneumococcal vaccines prepared by heating the cultures at 100° for fifteen minutes have yielded satisfactory results in the immunization of rabbits and horses and have been adopted in the routine immunization of the latter animals for the production of antipneumococcic serum.†

Dried antigens have also been employed, largely on an experimental basis, but the preparations have not been used routinely to a sufficient extent to warrant detailed description.

Standardization. Regardless of the method used in preparing pneumococcal antigens for the routine immunization of animals, it is desirable to standardize the vaccine. In order to obviate laborious and time-consuming bacterial counts on each preparation, many of the standardization methods have depended upon a comparison of the density of the bacterial suspensions with that of suspensions of inert materials such as silicates, fuller's earth, barium sulfate, and so forth, in which a given amount of the material chosen is made to correspond to a given bacterial count.

Gates[504] contrived a simple device for determining opacity by measuring the depth of disappearance of a wire loop when im-

* Unpublished.

† See Dubos, p. 332, Chapter X.

mersed in a column of bacterial suspension. A formula was derived by which the reading obtained can be translated into terms representing the concentration of bacteria per cubic centimeter of fluid. Once this figure is determined for the suspension chosen as a standard, it is necessary only to adjust each new preparation of vaccine to a density affording corresponding readings by the instrument.

By a method similar to the older technique of Hopkins, Krueger[760] measured the cell concentration of bacterial suspensions and reported a deviation of 2 to 5 per cent from actual counts. Feemster, Wetterlow, and Cianciarulo[393] recently compared the values obtained with suspensions of typhoid bacilli by direct counts, nitrogen determinations, and the Gates densitometer readings and found the latter two methods to be highly correlated. Since the nitrogen content is an index of bacterial mass, rather than of numbers, and hence presumably is related directly to antigenic value, determinations of density by the Gates apparatus appear to afford a simple and satisfactory means of measuring antigenic substance and therefore of standardizing bacterial vaccines. A corrected Gates reading of 2.0 centimeters on a 1 to 30 dilution of suspension of pneumococci corresponds approximately to 25 billion organisms per cubic centimeter, which furnishes a satisfactory standard suspension from which measured doses of vaccine may be made for routine injections.

INJECTIONS

Route of injection. As early as 1891, the Klemperer brothers[724] introduced the intravenous method of injecting pneumococcal preparations, having found the immunological response to be superior to that following subcutaneous injection. For stimulating the production of pneumococcal antibodies, the intravenous route for the injection of antigen is the method of choice. In the search for therapeutic serum of greater efficacy, it may prove of value to administer antigenic materials subcutaneously with the hope of stimulating the production in the horse of antibodies in addition to those commonly found in immune serum. For the purpose, the agar-agar technique of Dochez* (1924), the blood-clot method of Zinsser and Grinnell,[1580] or the procedures followed by Clowes, Jamieson, and Olson,[244] or those of Parker and McCoy[1062] may be useful.

Dosage. It is difficult to evaluate many of the earlier reports regarding the dosage of antigens used, since the descriptions referred only to the volume of cultures, extracts, solutions, or other preparations of pneumococci, without any indication of the bacterial content. There is an optimal range in the amount of vaccine which will induce satisfactory antibody production without causing harmful effects in the animal. Landmann (1908)[779] observed a greater loss of horses following increases in dosage. When living cultures are used for immunization the doses cannot be increased as rapidly as when killed antigens are used (Neufeld and Haendel, 1909[989]). Avery and his associates[36] stated that "doses should be small, as very large doses inhibit the immunity response." The authors recommended that the heat-killed suspensions used for injection should contain about 200 to 300 million organisms per cubic centimeter and the dose should represent the bacteria from 50 cubic centimeters of culture; with living organisms, the first injection consisted of the organisms from 2.5 cubic centimeters of original culture. Doses were usually doubled progressively if the reaction of the horse was favorable until the maximal dose consisting of the sediment from 300 to 400 cubic centimeters of broth culture was administered.

In a study of the immune response of rabbits to prolonged immunization with vaccines of Type I Pneumococcus, Barnes and White[86] determined the density of the bacterial suspensions as a measure for regulating dosage. Based on the experience thus gained, the present practice of the authors in immunizing horses is as follows: All vaccines are standardized by means of the Gates

* Personal communication.

apparatus to a corrected reading of 2.0 centimeters in a 1 to 30 dilution of the standard suspension—approximately twenty-five billion organisms per cubic centimeter. Formerly, the doses were given in gradually increasing amounts until "holding doses" of 9.0, 10.0, and 10.0 cubic centimeters, or a maximum of about 250 billion pneumococci, were administered. More recently, the doses have been decreased, so that the usual amounts are approximately one-fourth (2.0, 2.5, 2.5 cubic centimeters of the standard suspension) of those previously used. The content of protective substances of the serum produced under the present scheme is as great as, if not greater than, it was when larger amounts of vaccine were used. It must be noted, however, that because horses vary widely in their response to injections of bacterial suspensions it is occasionally necessary in individual instances to decrease the dose still further.

Spacing. The spacing of injections of vaccines is important. In earlier investigations, the antigens were usually administered at weekly intervals. Wadsworth and Kirkbride[1470] began the immunization process by giving injections either weekly or on three successive days. Cole[257] scheduled injections daily for seven days as a single series, with a rest interval of a week, followed by seven more daily injections. Cole and Moore[268] gave injections of dead organisms daily for six or seven days, with a rest of a week, then a series of three daily doses of live organisms with an interval of a week between each series. Avery, Chickering, Cole, and Dochez[36] recommended the following procedure: Six daily injections of heat-killed vaccines were given, followed by an interval of seven days, after which a second series of six daily doses was administered. Injections of living organisms were then made on three successive days, followed by a rest of seven days, when three consecutive daily doses were again given. This routine was followed throughout the course of immunization.

Using dried antigen, Truche[1420] gave injections on ten successive days and, after the lapse of from ten days to a fortnight, injected increasing doses on four successive days, followed by a ten-day rest period. In a comparison of results of different schedules of injections of vaccines in rabbits, Yoshioka (1923)[1562] tried three series of six daily injections at intervals of eight days, but reported better results when the same dose was given in six aliquot parts at one-half hour intervals in one day. Two years later (1925), the same author[1565] reported the results of a more extensive study in mice. One group of animals received three doses of vaccine in a period of two weeks; a second was given injections daily for three days; a third was injected six times at one-half-hour intervals in one day; and the fourth group was given one single injection. The total amount of antigen administered was the same in each group. Yoshioka decided that the best results were obtained by giving the vaccine to animals in divided doses at frequent intervals, as in the third group. Killian,[706] however, failed to confirm the observations.

Barnes and White[86] investigated antibody production in rabbits receiving intravenous injections of formalinized and heat-killed Type I pneumococci under three different schedules: 1) a single injection on each of three successive days; 2) a single dose on each of five consecutive days; and 3) a series of six injections, one on each of the first two days with the other four at one and one-half-hour intervals on the third day. Of the three plans, the first and last yielded better results than the second, and the first was at least as good as the last. The first scheme corresponds to the so-called "three-week" schedule. In the routine immunization of horses it has been found to give satisfactory results and is, moreover, convenient. According to the three-week schedule of immunization, the following plan has been used at the Massachusetts Antitoxin and Vaccine Laboratory: The horses are injected on Tuesday, Wednesday, and Thursday of one week and on Thursday, Friday, and Saturday of the following week. The animals are bled on Monday, the ninth day after the last injection in the course, and the same schedule of injections is resumed on the day following the bleeding.

Whichever schedule of injections is chosen, it has been generally customary to allow a rest period of about a week between series. It is possible that a longer interval might be used to advantage, but it seems doubtful if shorter periods would be advisable. Barnes and White[86] observed that in rabbits in which a primary immunity had been established, rest periods of three weeks instead of the usual one week between courses of injections did not lessen antibody response to subsequent injections of antigen.

The experiments of Cole (1904),[248] of Hachtel and Stoner (1916),[583] and of Feemster (1932)[392] have suggested that antibody response of animals and man to typhoid vaccine is more rapid and vigorous in both animals and man who have either had the disease or been inoculated than in those who have never been in contact with the organism. The observations of Barnes and White[86] on rabbits under immunization against Pneumococcus bear on the question. The principle involved has been applied in the immunization of horses for the production of antipneumococcic serum. Unpublished experiments at the Massachusetts laboratory serve to illustrate the results that may be expected in immune horses when subjected to delayed secondary stimulation. A group of horses under immunization for periods sufficiently long to establish primary immunity were rested for approximately three months without receiving injections of any sort. Test bleedings on this group of horses, taken prior to the resumption of immunization, showed an average decrease of 75 per cent in antibody content during the three-month rest period. After the first course of six injections following the rest period, in which the total dosage of vaccine averaged about one-fifth that of the last course, there was found to have developed in the serum of the animals so treated an average increase in antibody content (as compared with titers prior to the rest period) of approximately 25 per cent for both Types I and II. The same principle seems likely to hold true if, instead of omitting all injections during the rest period, the horses are subjected to some other form of immunization. It is open to question, however, whether the increased potency of serum from horses after such rest intervals is of sufficient value to counterbalance the loss of serum which might have been obtained had the animals been kept continuously on the routine schedule of immunization and bleeding.

Relation of method of injection to reactions of the horse. There is usually a febrile reaction in horses following each injection of pneumococcal vaccine. The rise in temperature varies with the individual animal and with the amount and kind of material injected. More severe reactions follow the administration of living cultures, dose for dose, than of killed suspensions. Thus, Avery, Chickering, Cole, and Dochez[36] referred to a body temperature of 40.5° as moderate, subsequent to the injection of living cultures. It is the custom in some laboratories to omit injections if the temperature of the horse under immunization remains above 38°. There appears to be no definite correlation between the temperature rise and the degree of antibody production, although an increase in body temperature may be related to immunological response to the substance injected.

There are reactions in horses undergoing immunization against Pneumococcus that are of a more serious nature. In some instances the animals exhibit symptoms of poor appetite and of gastrointestinal disturbances, or show abnormally high temperatures lasting for several days. Not infrequently, when the animals come to necropsy, extensive thrombus formation is observed, particularly in the blood vessels of the portal circulation. Occasionally, when respiratory disturbances are noted prior to death, thrombi are found also in the lungs. While it cannot be considered as proved, evidence has been accumulated to indicate that horses given intravenous injections of formalinized suspensions of pneumococci are more prone to develop thrombi than animals receiving vaccines devitalized by heat. In comparing the antigenic effect of heat-killed and formalinized cultures in rabbits, Barnes and White noted a smaller loss of animals in the former than in the latter group.

Another serious disturbance sometimes encountered in horses undergoing immunization is the occurrence of anaphylactoid reactions. The symptoms usually occur within a short time following an injection of vaccine and are characterized in typical cases by their abruptness, by excessive perspiration, marked respiratory embarrassment resulting in a blood-tinged, frothy exudate from the nostrils, complete collapse, and death shortly after the onset of symptoms. At necropsy, the gross pathological findings are usually negative except for marked congestion and hemorrhages in the lung tissue, and pulmonary edema. It is difficult to assign a definite cause to the reactions. A study of records at the Massachusetts laboratory showed that the majority of deaths of this nature occurred after the first injection in a series following the routine bleeding subsequent to the rest interval, and that deaths occurred most frequently in the period from two to eighteen months after initiation of the immunization process.

Because of these disturbances and the suggestion that the symptoms were indicative of a hypersensitive condition, the practice was adopted of administering subcutaneously a small dose of the vaccine on the day preceding the first of each series of three regular daily intravenous injections. These "desensitizing doses" were given to horses that exhibited unusual reactivity to the routine injections. Although the number of horses so treated has been too small to justify definite conclusions, the impression has been gained that the desensitizing treatment reduced the expected mortality rate of horses undergoing immunization. In the experience of the authors, the majority of sudden spontaneous deaths in horses have occurred when formalinized suspensions were in use and possibly may be referable, in part at least, to the more rapid lysis of these preparations as compared with vaccines killed by heating at 100°. Since the substitution of vaccines prepared in the latter manner it has not been found necessary to employ desensitizing doses. Truche[1419] claimed that death due to hypersensitivity could be avoided by diluting the organisms to be injected in a large quantity of physiological salt solution. In order to combat these immediate reactions it is advisable to have on hand a supply of epinephrine which may be injected into horses showing symptoms of possible hypersensitivity; glucose solution may also be administered intravenously to advantage.

When living cultures are used as the immunizing agent, certain complications may occur. White* observed four instances of pneumonitis, one of endocarditis, and one of spontaneous pneumothorax in a group of horses in which living cultures had been eventually substituted after a course of immunization with heat-killed organisms. The pneumococci obtained from the lesions were apparently identical with the strains routinely injected. An interesting observation was that the serum of the horses at the time the infections occurred contained sufficient protective antibody so that 0.2 cubic centimeter of serum prevented the death of mice injected with 0.1 cubic centimeter of virulent culture, either of the organisms isolated from the horse or of those used in preparing the vaccine. These apparently paradoxical phenomena may be explained in part by the investigations of Griffith,[559] who reported that in rabbits the effect of intravenous inoculations of culture into an immune animal was to abolish temporarily the protective power of the serum. Griffith thought that the transient suppression of antibodies enabled the pneumococci to become established in the tissues of the animals. It seems, however, that any alleged superiority of serums from horses immunized with living cultures, unless the dosage is very carefully controlled, would be outweighed by the loss of animals from infections of the nature just described.

BLEEDINGS

Period of immunization prior to bleeding. The period of immunization necessary for the production in horses of sufficient protective antibodies to warrant initiating routine bleedings depends on the material injected, the spacing of doses, and the response of

* Unpublished observations.

the individual animal. Barach[75] studied the rate of development of immunity in mice and rabbits following administration of vaccine prepared from intact pneumococci of Types I and II and observed that protective substances developed three days after injection. The immunity increased markedly to the fifth day and remained essentially stationary to the seventh day. Barnes and White,[86] in studying the antibody response of rabbits to vaccines of Type I Pneumococcus, determined the average protective titer in a group of animals after twelve, twenty-four, thirty-six, and forty-eight injections of vaccine. The accompanying table illustrates the results obtained.

Course of injections	*1*	*2*	*3*	*4*
Number of injections prior to bleeding	12	24	36	48
Number of weeks between start of immunization and bleeding	6	12	24	36
Average protective titers	99	449	960	1500

It is probable that the protective potency of immune serum does not develop so rapidly in horses as in rabbits, and it has been believed that a period of from eight or nine months to a year or two of immunization might be required before a serum of satisfactory potency could be obtained. For over two years at the Massachusetts laboratory, as a result of studies on the immunizing efficacy of various antigens and injection schedules, all horses used in the production of antipneumococcic serum have been placed on routine bleedings approximately two months after the initiation of the immunization process. The plan has had no apparent harmful effect on the animals and, almost without exception, the serum has been found to be sufficiently high in protective antibody content to be suitable for concentration.

The interval to be allowed between the last injection of vaccine and the bleeding is somewhat elastic. By regulation of the National Institute of Health, at least one week must elapse in order that there may be no antigen circulating in the blood stream. Avery and his associates[36] stated that bleeding ordinarily took place about ten days after the last injection of antigen. Barnes and White[86] observed that the highest titers in rabbits were usually found in seventh-day bleedings, occasionally in those on the twelfth day, and never when the blood was drawn on the twenty-second day. The authors therefore concluded that the optimal time for bleeding animals is in the period seven to ten days after the last injection of a series. According to the schedule adopted, the horses are bled on the ninth day after the last injection.

Amount of blood. The amount of blood which may be withdrawn from a horse depends on the size and physical condition of the animal. Usually from nine to twelve liters are taken.

Yield of serum. The yield of serum is subject to variation and is dependent in part upon the method used for collecting the blood, the number of bleedings to which the horse has been subjected and, apparently, to other more obscure factors. The yield obtained by using weights as an aid in expressing serum from the clot, as described by Avery and his associates, was from 50 to 55 per cent. If suitable equipment is available, the blood may be drawn directly into bottles of several liters capacity, and centrifuged after the clot has formed. In this manner the percentage of serum obtained may be slightly higher. When no special methods are employed and serum expressed by simple coagulation is drawn, the yield is likely to average only about 30 to 35 per cent of the total volume of blood.

There has been an impression in some laboratories that the amount of serum obtained from the first few bleedings was less than that from later bleedings. An analysis of results from a small group of horses under the observation of the authors of the present volume supports this belief. The data are taken from records of horses that had been bled from twenty-one to forty-six times. The average percentage yield was calculated for the first three, the middle three, and the last three bleedings, respectively, of each horse. Approximately 8 per cent more serum was obtained from the middle three bleedings as compared with the first series, and about the same increase was noted in the last three bleedings when compared with the intermediate three.

The Production of Therapeutic Serum

REASONS FOR AND AGAINST THE USE OF UNCONCENTRATED SERUM

Until relatively recent times, the feasibility of concentrating and refining the specific serum used in the treatment of lobar pneumonia found scant recognition. Avery, Chickering, Cole, and Dochez[36] in 1917 believed that the disadvantages of the concentrated product were such as to render it of little practical value. In a later publication, Cole (1929),[265] although recognizing that treatment of pneumonia with large doses of whole serum was not ideal, questioned seriously the advisability of using concentrated preparations. Cole objected to the methods used for standardization and doubted whether the small doses of concentrated antibody recommended would have any effect on the mortality rate. He concluded that unless very large doses of concentrated serum were employed or unless more accurate methods of standardization were adopted, it would be wiser to continue to treat cases of Type I pneumonia with potent, whole serum in large doses.

Sickles (1929)[1278] offered a comparison of the protective titers of unconcentrated and concentrated serums. The results led to the impression that unconcentrated serums were superior to concentrated products because of zonal phenomena in the action of the concentrates, and because, in her experience, the potencies of the two kinds of preparations were not essentially different. Much of the objection to concentrated serum voiced by Sickles was based on unsatisfactory results attending the methods of standardization employed. In 1932, Wadsworth,[1463] in discussing the question, stated that there were no clinical data to indicate that refined products were more effective in the treatment of pneumonia than whole serum of the highest potency and, furthermore, that before introducing new methods of preparation it was of importance to be certain that during the process of concentration the serum would lose no activity that might be effective in treating the disease. Wadsworth also maintained that the existing methods of standardization were inadequate, although it was acknowledged that the potency of concentrated serum approximated that of the unconcentrated product. It is difficult to concede the cogency of an argument in favor of unconcentrated serums based on difficulties in estimating the content of antipneumococcic protective antibody, since the methods for determining potency are alike for both whole and refined products.

Park,[1053] in the Harben Lectures, discussed the entire question and stressed some important points which may be included here. Park stated that in cases of pneumonia it is desirable to avoid unnecessary administration of serum, but when the use of serum is indicated, its disadvantages should be borne in mind. Large intravenous doses of unrefined serum have frequently resulted in attacks of serum sickness, and the technique of administration presents difficulties in the hands of those inexperienced with the method. By concentration methods, serum of lower potency can be utilized and a satisfactory product obtained, thus resulting in reduced cost. Five cubic centimeters of concentrate containing two thousand protective units per cubic centimeter should equal the protective value of one hundred cubic centimeters of serum containing one hundred protective units per cubic centimeter. The dose of the former, containing less foreign protein, being smaller in quantity, and easier to administer, would be superior to whole serum. Park concluded, therefore, that the refining of antipneumococcic serum provides a preparation preferable to whole serum. The Therapeutic Trials Committee of the Medical Research Council in England,[887] in a report on the serum treatment of lobar pneumonia, stated that delayed reactions were rare and slight with concentrated serum, whereas with unconcentrated serum of high titer the treatment more frequently caused rashes, swollen joints, and pyrexia. Unconcentrated serum, however, was quite as effective as concentrated serum if the same number of units were used. That the concentrated product is effective therapeutically has been amply demonstrated, and confirmatory data have been summarized by Lord and Heffron (1936).[827]

AVIAN SERUM

The therapeutic use of antipneumococcic serum produced by repeated injections of Brahma cockerels with virulent pneumococci has been reported by Kyes (1918).[767] Severe constitutional reactions followed the administration of the serum to human beings. Although later publications by Kyes and Carey (1927, 1929)[768-9] described methods for eliminating the factors believed to be responsible for the reactions, fowl serum has not been generally accepted for the treatment of lobar pneumonia. The small size of the birds used, resulting in many technical disadvantages, is an objection which, in the opinion of the authors of this volume, would discourage its routine use.

POLYVALENT SERUM

Prior to the separation of pneumococci into specific serological types, it was customary to prepare antiserums against individual strains. The serums were tested serologically against cultures from heterologous sources. Neufeld and Haendel[991] found that some of the earlier, so-called polyvalent serums reacted with only one type of Pneumococcus. Cole[249] reported that a univalent serum used by himself and colleagues protected animals against only 40 per cent of the cultures tested. Cole and Moore[268] emphasized the importance of using pneumococci of strict immunological specificity for immunization and, inasmuch as at the time the only serum of proved therapeutic value was for Type I, monovalent serum was recommended. In the same year, 1917, Avery and his associates advised against the routine manufacture of polyvalent antipneumococcic serums.

Subsequent to the division of pneumococci into types by Dochez and Gillespie,[322] Cooper, Edwards, and Rosenstein,[272] in separating Group IV pneumococci into twenty-nine types, found little cross-protection of monovalent serums against heterologous strains. For example, a concentrated Type II serum contained only ten to twenty units against a Type V culture. In 1932, however, Cooper, Rosenstein, Walter, and Peizer[274] suggested that, because of the marked cross-reactions of many Type V strains with Type II antiserums and *vice versa,* it might be advisable to prepare an antiserum potent for both types. Observations by Barnes and Wight (1936)[88] which suggested that, under stated conditions, Type V Pneumococcus might become transformed into Type II Pneumococcus, led them to make a recommendation in accord with that of Cooper and her colleagues.

Aside from such a basis for the manufacture of bivalent or polyvalent serums, there are other factors which should be taken into consideration. In some laboratories, serum bivalent for Types I and II has been produced. Since there has been no demonstration of close relationship between the types, the only justification for the custom appears to be one of economy. This explanation also holds true in the case of serums polyvalent for other pneumococcal types. Horses appear to tolerate injections of a vaccine containing pneumococci of several types as well as of an antigen made from a single strain. Antibodies active against the various strains used can thus be produced in one animal instead of using separate horses for each type serum desired. Whether the economy is real or apparent is a question which remains for the producer to determine. On the other hand, an impression, confirmed, at least in part, by Cooper and her associates,[272] has been gained, that higher protective powers are developed in monovalent immunization than is the case when strains of several types are injected into producing animals. Definite evidence to support the hypothesis is, however, lacking. With the rapid and accurate Neufeld method of typing sputum now in general use, the former practice of administering a dose of bivalent or polyvalent serum during the period required for type diagnosis is no longer necessary. In view of present-day knowledge, a logical and conservative procedure would be the production of monovalent Type I serum, bivalent Type II and V, possibly a serum combining Type III and VIII antibody, and either bivalent or polyvalent serums for other closely related types.

METHODS OF CONCENTRATING SERUM

The objectives of the processes employed in the concentration and refinement of antipneumococcic serum are to eliminate nonessential and harmful constituents and to reduce the volume of fluid while conserving specific protective substances. In a study of the distribution of immune bodies occurring in antipneumococcic serum, Avery,[32] by chemical methods, demonstrated that the antibodies in antipneumococcic serum are associated with the globulins and not with the albumin fraction. Gay and Chickering (1915),[508-9] and later Chickering (1915),[223] showed that the precipitate which forms when an extract of pneumococcal cells is mixed with homologous antiserum contains practically all the immune substances and that the antibodies can be recovered from the precipitate in a water-clear solution by treatment with dilute alkali. By a similar method, Huntoon *et al.* (1921)[665-6, 668] precipitated the specific antibody from antipneumococcic serum by treatment with heavy suspensions of pneumococci. Various procedures have since been utilized for the purpose of dissociating the antigen-antibody complex so formed and of preparing for therapeutic use solutions of the specific antibodies so released.

Biological methods. The biological methods of concentration employed by Gay and Chickering and by Huntoon are of interest in establishing immunological principles. Although, as stated in the Rockefeller Monograph, the products thus obtained were ideal in many ways, there were serious disadvantages in the method. The technical manipulations were laborious, the preparations varied in strength, were not stable, and frequently gave rise to severe reactions in patients.

Chemical methods. Chemical methods of refining antipneumococcic serum are more practicable and have received greater recognition.

Ammonium Sulfate: In the investigations made by Avery,[32] the serum used was obtained from horses immunized with cultures of pneumococci of Types I and II. Avery's work showed that the antibodies in antipneumococcic serum are absent from the albumin fraction but associated with the globulins, and while not associated wholly with pseudoglobulin, precipitation by 38 to 42 per cent saturation with ammonium sulfate offered a promising method for the practical purification of antipneumococcic serum.

Avery's experiments with ammonium sulfate were confirmed by the investigations of Banzhaf (1925),[70] which stimulated a continued interest in the method. By a modification of Avery's method, and using plasma instead of serum, Brown and Knowles (1932)[153] attempted to increase the yield of antibody and to determine the comparative protective value of the euglobulin and pseudoglobulin fractions. The percentage recovery obtained is not clear, but the results suggested that the bulk of protective antibody is to be found in the pseudoglobulin.

In studying the "non-antibacterial" factors in the therapeutic action of immune serum on dermal pneumococcal infection in rabbits, Sabin (1933)[1206] used the ammonium sulfate method of fractionation. A zonal effect was observed in the experiments, and, because of this, Sabin stated that "the 30 to 50% ammonium sulfate globulin, either total or water-insoluble, would be quite undesirable for therapeutic purposes." Felton and Kauffmann (1933),[429] on the other hand, found that the highest protective potency for mice in relation to the amount of protein was in portions precipitated by ammonium sulfate between 36 and 50 per cent saturation, thus corroborating Avery's observations.

Several different lots of antipneumococcic serum, bivalent for Types I and II, have been concentrated by ammonium sulfate at the Massachusetts Antitoxin and Vaccine Laboratory. The percentage recovery in all cases has been high, averaging approximately 90 per cent of the original antibody and, furthermore, the products have possessed the desirable physical characters. Chill-reactions have followed the administration of some of these lots, however, in a fairly high percentage of cases. Although it has been possible by reconcentration processes to render batches relatively free from this undesirable property, it is not definitely clear that the method was at fault.

Sodium Sulfate: In Banzhaf's[70] experiments it was found that solutions of precipitate obtained from antipneumococcic serum by adding 12.5 per cent dried sodium sulfate contained after dialysis only 8 to 10 per cent of the total immune bodies. If, however, a filtrate of globulins, soluble in 12.5 per cent sodium sulfate, was treated with sodium sulfate up to 18.5 per cent at a temperature of 36°, the preparation after dialysis contained about 90 per cent of the total antibody. Felton (1928)[403] reported detailed observations on the concentration of serum by the use of sodium sulfate, which method gave a product suitable for intravenous therapy. In a later publication by the same author (1931),[408] some disadvantages of the antibody solution prepared by the sodium sulfate method were acknowledged.

Banzhaf and Klein[72] made a further report on the use of sodium sulfate in a normality of about 0.05 for precipitating dialyzed antiserum. In the process, the reaction was corrected to pH 5.0 to 5.1 and the precaution was believed to result in a chill-free product. Savino, Negrete, and Acuna,[1221] using plasma instead of serum, applied a sodium sulfate method of concentration substantially the same as that of Felton. Although the method undoubtedly marked an advance in refinement procedures, it was somewhat expensive, and difficulties attended its execution particularly in the relative insolubility of the antibody at different stages of the refining process, in filtration for sterilization, and in obtaining lots consistently free from chill-producing elements.

Dialysis: The removal of crystalloids by the dialysis of serum in water was studied by Avery[32] as a means of concentrating antipneumococcic serum. The procedure resulted in an incomplete precipitation of antibody. Dialysis, however, may be utilized to advantage at some stage in processing serum by salting-out methods. Banzhaf[70] found that serum precipitated by sodium chloride or ammonium sulfate contained about 90 per cent of the immune bodies following dialysis. Later Banzhaf and Klein[72] recommended dialyzing serum until practically free from salts as the initial step in eliminating inert protein and chill-producing substances. Goodner[528] reported that it was unnecessary in dialysis to remove electrolytes completely in order to obtain a precipitate containing the majority of the agglutinins. The method of dialysis has certain advantages not possessed by other processes of concentration. It is inexpensive and frequently results in a volume concentration not readily obtained by other procedures, and it entails less harsh physical treatment of the antibody than the addition of chemicals. Some unpublished data, however, show that solutions of antibody made by the method are not stable.

Dilution with Water: Felton (1924)[396] observed that a heavy precipitate formed when antipneumococcic serum was diluted in a proportion of 1 to 10 with water, and believed that the amount of water-insoluble precipitate so obtained gave an indication of the protective strength of the serum. A higher yield of precipitate was recovered when small amounts of tartaric, citric, oxalic, or acetic acids were added to the water. Experiments on the influence of hydrogen ion concentration on the precipitation of immune substances from specific serum suggested that the isoelectric zone of the protective antibody lies between pH 6.6 and 7.5, possibly at about pH 6.8.

In later papers, Felton[400] and Felton and Bailey[421] reported additional experiments dealing with the water precipitation of pneumococcal antibody. The amount of precipitate obtained did not always parallel the protective titer of the antibody solutions. The optimal yield of precipitate varied with dilution and the serological type of the serum used. Thus dilutions of 1 to 18 and 1 to 20 for Type I, 1 to 14 and 1 to 18 for Type II, and 1 to 12 and 1 to 14 for Type III serum were recommended as yielding maxima of antibody. The amounts thrown down were, however, also dependent upon the hydrogen ion concentration of the water-serum mixture, and zones of pH 5.5 to 7.8, 5.5 to 7.8, and 6.2 to 7.8 were observed for serum of Types I, II, and III respectively.

Banzhaf[70] corroborated Felton's observations on Type I serum diluted tenfold with water containing phosphoric acid, and obtained varying results with Type II and III serum similarly treated. In 1928, Felton[403] published a further description of the characters of the water-insoluble fraction of antipneumococcic serum, and believed that the fraction, while similar in qualities to pseudoglobulin, more closely resembled euglobulin.

Felton's work received further confirmation in the experiments of Savino, Negrete, and Acuna.[1221] Reiner and Reiner,[1133] using a similar method of concentration, found that globulin can be precipitated from both normal and antipneumococcic serum by dilution with distilled water at hydrogen ion concentrations varying from pH 5.0 to 7.0. The zone of maximal precipitation was observed to lie between pH 5.5 and 6.0. By repeated precipitation at pH 5.1 and pH 6.8, respectively, two fractions were obtained, one of which was more soluble at neutral, the other at acid reaction. It was shown that the two fractions combine with each other if the solutions are mixed. The latter observation is of significance in connection with the concentration of antipneumococcic serum bivalent for Types I and II.

After experimenting with water precipitation, Goodner[528] recommended the employment of preliminary water tests for each lot of serum to determine its suitability for concentration. By observing the dilution of serum with distilled water necessary to cause opalescence—the initial point—it was possible to calculate the total amount of water necessary to obtain maximal precipitation. One of the requirements of the procedure was the maintenance of low temperatures with the materials used. Banzhaf and Klein[72] employed a somewhat similar process except that adjustments in hydrogen ion concentration were made, but the authors stated that Goodner's method probably yielded a purer form of antibody despite the presence of chill-producing agents.

There is some evidence that the percentage recovery of Type II antibody is appreciably lower than that of Type I. It has been suggested that the disparity might be due to a difference in the isoelectric points, or zones, of the two types of antibody, and that Type II immune substances might precipitate more completely at a lower hydrogen ion concentration without affecting the yield of Type I immune substances. The question of the solubility of one antibody fraction in the other has also been raised by Savino, Negrete, and Acuna. Observations by Hager, Barnes, and Wight* (1935), are pertinent to the subject. From a single, pooled lot of antipneumococcic serum of Types I and II, four different batches were concentrated by the alcohol method and the antibody precipitated at pH 5.0, 6.0, 7.0, and 8.0, respectively. Repeated mouse tests gave the following approximate percentage yield of protective substances: At pH 5.0, Type I, 83 per cent and Type II, 66 per cent; at pH 6.0, Type I, 80 per cent and Type II, 59 per cent; at pH 7.0, Type I, 98 per cent and Type II, 93 per cent; at pH 8.0, Type I, 98 per cent and Type II, 85 per cent. No acid fraction was removed from the solutions. The results suggest that, under the experimental conditions employed, antibodies of both Types I and II are precipitated more completely at pH values of 7.0 and 8.0 than at 5.0 and 6.0, with the optimum at neutrality or thereabouts. The results are also in essential agreement with the earlier observations made by Felton, and by Felton and Bailey, regarding the isoelectric points of antipneumococcal antibodies. It is possible

* 1935, unpublished.

that concentration of antipneumococcic serum by water precipitation might be developed into a practical method. Water subjects the antibody to as little physical injury, perhaps, as any of the processes employed. If modifications were made so that a high yield of antibody free from reactive substances could be obtained, the method would also possess the added advantage of being highly economical.

Carbon Dioxide: Avery reported that after diluting antipneumococcic serum with one-half its volume of water saturation with carbon dioxide resulted in an incomplete precipitation of the antibodies. Felton[396] repeated the experiment and as Avery had found, noted that the yield in protective substance was never more, and usually less than one-half the amount contained in the original serum. The method of concentration with carbon dioxide has little value from the practical standpoint.

Sodium Chloride: Avery found that saturation of serum with sodium chloride, as with carbon dioxide, resulted in a low yield of antibody, since the immune substances were apparently associated with both the euglobulin and pseudoglobulin separated by this treatment. Banzhaf (1925)[70] corroborated the observation and determined that the euglobulin so obtained contained only 8 to 10 per cent of the immune bodies.

Alcohol Precipitation: From the sodium sulfate method, Felton (1931)[408] turned to the use of ethyl alcohol as a precipitant in concentrating antipneumococcic serum. Briefly, the technique recommended is as follows: Ethyl alcohol (95 per cent) and the serum are cooled to 0°, and the alcohol is added to the serum in the proportion of 20 cubic centimeters of alcohol to 100 cubic centimeters of serum. The mixture is allowed to stand for eighteen hours in the cold, and the precipitate which forms is then recovered either by centrifugation or filtration. The precipitate is washed with one and one-half volumes of cold distilled water to remove the water-soluble protein. The insoluble fraction is dissolved to the volume desired in isotonic salt solution. The so-called acid fraction may be removed by suspending the alcoholic precipitate in water or by adding sodium chloride to effect solution, then adjusting the reaction to pH 5.0. The precipitate thus formed is separated by centrifugation. The importance of maintaining an even, low temperature during contact of the alcohol with serum is emphasized because a slight increase in temperature was believed to result in solution of the precipitate and in partial destruction of antibody. A yield of at least 80 per cent of the protective substance originally present in the serum is obtained by this method.

Felton reported that several different lots of serum concentrated by the method had been used therapeutically without causing untoward reactions. Some modifications of the original technique have been found advisable during routine practice, chiefly those directed toward avoiding denaturation of the immune globulin.

Other Methods: An objectionable feature of the antibody solutions prepared by the methods of Gay and Chickering and of Huntoon is the difficulty in separating the cellular components of Pneumococcus from the antigen-antibody precipitate. Felton and Bailey[420] found that 0.01 molar sodium carbonate was the most satisfactory of the agents tried for dissociating the polysaccharide-antibody combination. Dissociation took place on heating the specific precipitate in the presence of sodium carbonate, disodium phosphate, saccharose, or sodium chloride, and the protective substance could then be precipitated by sodium sulfate. The released antibody, however, was found to contain a substance antagonistic to specific protection, thus suggesting that not all the capsular polysaccharide had been removed.

In a later study, Felton[410] reported that calcium or strontium phosphate could also be used to dissociate specific carbohydrate-antibody precipitate yielding a water-insoluble protein that conferred protection on mice. Felton and Kauffmann[429] observed that the zone of minimal solubility of the immune fraction isolated by calcium phosphate dissociation of an SSS-antibody complex was pH 6.7 and above, corresponding roughly to the fraction of immune serum obtained by 36 to 50 per cent saturation with ammonium sulfate. The various modifications of the methods of Gay and Chickering and of Huntoon are of academic interest and afford means of studying and analyzing the immune substances, but it seems unlikely that the procedures have sufficient practical application to warrant consideration for large-scale concentration of serums. The probable presence of residual antigenic substance in preparations made by either the original or modified methods is one of the more important objections to the antibody solution obtained in this manner.

The use of metallic salts in preparing antibody solutions was introduced by Felton[410] during studies designed to increase the yield of immune substances obtained by alcohol precipitation. Treatment of the total water-insoluble protein of antipneumococcic serum with either aluminum chloride at pH 5.2 or with zinc chloride at pH 7.0 caused heavy precipitation, with the immunologically active protein remaining in solution as the metallic salt. When freed from zinc by means of a carbonate or phosphate, the water-insoluble protein was highly protective for mice. As far as can be learned, antibody solutions prepared by this or similar methods have not progressed beyond the experimental stage.

The use of ultrafiltration as a means of purifying antibody is a more recent development. Goodner, Horsfall, and Bauer (1936)[539] applied the method to rabbit serum, horse serum, and concentrated horse serum containing antibody for Type I pneumococci. With membranes having a pore diameter of 102.5 millimicrons, the filtrates of the horse and rabbit serums contained 76.7 and 86.6 per cent respectively of the total antibody, while at a pore diameter of 188 millimicrons the filtrate of concentrated horse serum contained 100 per cent of the antibody. It is possible that ultrafiltration may prove to be of practical value in the routine production of concentrated antipneumococcic serum.

The recent description by Wyckoff[1555] of ultracentrifugation as a means of concentrating antipneumococcic serum is of interest. By use of a vacuum centrifuge having a maximal field of about forty thousand times gravity it was possible to separate the serum constituents into different layers. The sedimented portion was found to contain only those protein molecules that were considered to be antibody. These observations, if confirmed, promise to be of practical value in the production of antipneumococcic serum.

Of the methods of concentrating antipneumococcic serum discussed in this section, the one employing alcohol as a precipitant is at the present time in more general use than other processes. The recovery of antibody is fairly satisfactory, the method is economical, the end product usually possesses the desired physical characters, and results following its intravenous administration are generally favorable and do not include an undue number of disagreeable reactions.

PHYSICAL PROPERTIES

Total solids. The physical characters of the product are of importance because of the fact that antipneumococcic serum is administered intravenously. By regulation of the National Institute of Health, serums intended for use in intravenous therapy should not be of excessive viscosity or have a content of total solids greater than 20 per cent. Unconcentrated serums usually contain about 8 or 9 per cent of solids, whereas the amount present in concentrated antibody preparations varies with the method of processing and with the degree of concentration attained. An ideal product in this respect would be one containing a high antibody content with the viscosity and total solids at points permitting ease in handling. Hence, from a practical standpoint it is well to maintain the total solids content of concentrated antipneumococcic serum at about 10 to 12 per cent.

Inorganic solids. Determination of the ash in antipneumococcic serum is unnecessary as a routine procedure, but is of value as a check on the amount of salt added. No concentration of salt higher than that sufficient to effect complete solution of the antibody precipitate should be used. For the majority of preparations 0.85 per cent suffices; concentrations higher than one per cent should not be required.

Reaction of the product. The buffering action of the blood is ordinarily considered sufficient to compensate for minor fluctuations in reaction from neutrality of substances introduced intravenously, but a system already strained by disease should not be required to make any unnecessary adjustment of hydrogen ion concentration in the blood. Antipneumococcic serum and concentrates used for clinical purposes, therefore, should be approximately neutral in reaction. The usual preparations for therapeutic use show hydrogen ion concentrations ranging from pH 6.0 to 7.0, with the average approaching pH 6.5, and hence require no readjustment.

Preservatives. There is no substitute for sterility in products intended for therapeutic use. It is customary, and is required by governmental agencies, to add a preservative to antipneumococcic serum. In some laboratories, the antiseptic is added when the serum is drawn from the clot. The precipitate which sometimes forms, sediments during storage in the cold. Other manufacturers prefer to add the preservative at some stage during concentration or final processing. In either case, the preservative should be added prior to final filtration. The purpose of the preservative is not to destroy contaminating organisms but to prevent the growth of any adventitious bacteria.

The choice of preservative, and the concentration of the bactericidal agent, are questions of no small moment. Investigations conducted by Hale (1913)[586] with tricresol when used as a preservative in antimeningococcic serum led him to conclude that the agent is dangerous when serum is to be introduced by a route that brings the agent into direct contact with the nervous centers. Leake and Corbitt (1917)[794] attempted to determine the toxicity of phenol, cresols, and glycerol by physiological tests on mice. It was impossible to establish a definite minimal lethal dose of the substances because of marked variations in susceptibility of the test animals. It was found, however, that tricresol and phenol exerted approximately the same germicidal effect. Voegtlein (1918)[1451] studied the effect of the addition of tricresol and phenol to antipneumococcic serum introduced intravenously into monkeys, cats, and dogs. The doses given were calculated to correspond to the amounts given in the treatment of pneumonia. Voegtlein concluded that the addition of tricresol or phenol to antipneumococcic serum in concentrations not exceeding 0.5 per cent does not seem to impart to the serum toxic properties which might give rise to serious symptoms following its intravenous administration. It was suggested, however, that serum containing phenol should not be given to patients with nephritic complications because of the injurious action of phenol on the kidney.

A mercurial preparation, Merthiolate, has been recommended as a preservative for biological products. Jamieson and Powell (1931)[677] reported that the substance is highly effective as a germicide, possesses low toxicity, and is not subject to precipitation in protein solutions. The agent has not, however, come into general use as a preservative in antipneumococcic serum.

Malcolm (1931)[857] studied the germicidal and toxic effects of various chemical substances, and found that the mercury compounds, Metaphen and Mercurophen, possessed higher bactericidal powers than phenol and tricresol, and were relatively less toxic, thus permitting a wider margin of safety when used as preservatives for biological products. Another advantage possessed by the two mercury compounds is that at their effective germicidal strength they do not precipitate proteins. Of the preservatives studied, Malcolm concluded that Mercurophen was the most satisfactory, with Metaphen second in order of effectiveness, and that both were superior to phenol or tricresol. At the present time both phenol and tricresol in final concentrations not exceeding 0.5 per cent are in general use. At the Massachusetts laboratory, 0.2 per cent phenol has been found to be satisfactory in maintaining the sterility of therapeutic antipneumococcic serum. Care must be taken that precipitation of protein does not follow the addition of phenol and tricresol.

Interest in the drying of serum as a means of preservation has recently been revived, largely through the investigations of Mudd, Reichel, Flosdorf and Eagle,[934] Elser, Thomas and Steffen,[354] and Flosdorf and Mudd (1935).[454] The methods employed are applications of familiar physical conditions, namely, the use of low temperatures and absence of moisture and oxygen. A detailed description of the equipment used for desiccating biological products, now known as the "Lyophile apparatus" may be found in the publication of Flosdorf and Mudd.[454]

CHILL-PRODUCING FACTORS

A disturbing, and as yet unsolved, problem is the occasional occurrence of a thermal reaction, or chills, in patients following the administration of some lots of antipneumococcic serum. For a discussion of the clinical manifestations and management of the reaction the reader is referred to *Lobar Pneumonia and Serum Therapy* by Lord and Heffron[827] and the more comprehensive treatise by Heffron.[601] The incidence of chills varies with different lots of serum and with the method of refinement in the case of concentrated products.

During the development of various methods of concentrating antipneumococcic serum, attempts have been made to eliminate non-essential constituents for the purpose of reducing reaction-producing propensities. Unfortunately, some of the manipulations involved are likely to result in varying degrees of denaturation of the proteins associated with the protective antibody. Denaturation may be considered as such an alteration in serum proteins that they become insoluble in solutions of neutral salts. That these changes may occur readily is shown by the work of Wu and Yen

(1924).[1553] Felton[398] observed that, in general, agents that cause denaturation of the globulins in antipneumococcic serum also result in a destruction of protective antibody. The addition of acids, alkalies, and preservatives—particularly chloroform, which coagulates the water-insoluble globulin—repeated solution in hydrochloric acid and precipitation by sodium hydroxide, or frequent solution in sodium chloride and precipitation by water at room temperature were all observed by Felton to result in a modification of the immune globulin.

Felton[403] also stated that serums which were stored for a long period of time, with or without preservative, undergo denaturation and, in describing the sodium sulfate method of concentration, listed three common causes which may be controlled, namely, bacterial contamination, maintenance of serum or precipitate at too high a temperature in acid or alkaline solution, and too high a concentration of preservative. Excessive heat also alters the solubility of the protective globulin in antipneumococcic serum (Felton[397]). Impurities and the hydrogen ion concentration of agents used as precipitants in the concentration process may also contribute to the change in the protein. In the report on the use of sodium sulfate, Felton emphasized the point that the salt may be markedly alkaline and require neutralization prior to use. Serum concentrated by ammonium sulfate, although satisfactory in many ways, frequently elicits a high incidence of thermal reactions, possibly due in part to changes in the serum protein. Observations by Cianciarulo (1935)* on the hydrogen ion concentration of ammonium sulfate offer a possible explanation for alterations in protein antibody when purified by means of the ammonium salt. The reaction of some lots of the sulfate was found to be as acid as pH 4.4 and, when used in concentrating diphtheria antitoxin, resulted in marked denaturation as evidenced by the formation of an insoluble, jelly-like precipitate. The salt, with the reaction properly adjusted, no longer caused this effect.

* Unpublished.

Aside from the resultant loss of antibody and difficulty in effecting solution occasioned by denaturation of globulins, there is the possibility that the chemical or physical alteration may be responsible for the chills following therapeutic administration of concentrated serums.

Studies designed to determine the cause of chill-reactions and methods for eliminating chill-producing principles in antipneumococcic serum have followed several directions. The reactions are not confined to the use of antipneumococcic serum, according to Rhoades.[1185] Larson and Fahr (1925)[790] observed marked chills in three of seven patients treated with antipneumococcic rabbit serum. Differences between immune horse and rabbit serums have been studied by Goodner and Horsfall (1935),[537] and by Goodner, Horsfall and Bauer (1936),[539] while Chow (1936)[224] recently reported that the major portion of antibody in antipneumococcic rabbit serum occurs in a different globulin fraction from that in horse serum. Whether these differences may explain in part the high incidence of chills following therapeutic use of untreated rabbit serums remains unknown.

A different approach to the problem was reported by Kolmer and Matsumoto (1920),[744] who studied normal and immune horse serum for the content of hemagglutinins and hemolysins to ascertain whether intravascular agglutination or hemolysis might play a part in chill reactions incident to serum therapy in pneumonia. Although it was found that practically all horse serum contains agglutinins for human erythrocytes, the authors believed that the intravenous administration of horse serum probably does not introduce sufficient amounts of hemagglutinin and hemolysin to produce ill effects referable to agglutination and hemolysis. Bullowa, Rosenbluth, and Merkin (1927),[184] as a result of an incidental observation that a chill-producing serum agglutinated red cells *in vitro* whereas a chill-free serum did not, restudied this phase of the question. No constant relation was found between erythrocyte agglutination *in vitro* and serum reactions in man, thus confirming the earlier impression of Kolmer and Matsumoto. In spite of these concurring opinions, the hypothesis should be subjected to further investigation, including a study of the effect of heterophile antibodies. Sabin and Wallace (1931)[1210] reported the results of studies on the nature of the chill-producing principle in antipneumococcic serum. They were unable to find any relation between the reaction and the presence of formed elements, fibrinogen, or lipids, but confirmed Felton's belief that the agent in the acid fraction is probably carried by the globulin through an adsorptive process.

The administration of antipneumococcic fowl serum to pneumonia patients was found by Kyes (1918)[767] to result almost invariably in severe chills. In a later report, Kyes and Carey (1927)[768] suggested that the antecedents of fibrin present in serum, by favoring the formation of fibrinous emboli in the blood stream, were responsible for serum shock. By treating the serum with calcium or cephalin and removing the resultant precipitate, the authors claimed to have rendered fowl serum free of shock-producing qualities. Meyers (1932)[900] reported a series of studies in which titrations were made of the fibrinogen content of antipneumococcic horse serum. The investigations appear to be chiefly concerned with serum disease rather than with chill-reactions, but from the results the author concluded that fibrinogen was not involved. The intravenous injection of reasonably pure fibrinogen failed to cause reactions, whereas concentrated serum, containing no detectable fibrinogen, not infrequently produced serum shock.

The acid fraction. In 1928, Felton,[403] after describing his method of concentrating antipneumococcic serum by the use of sodium sulfate, recommended the removal of a precipitate that formed when the reaction of the dialyzed material was adjusted to pH 4.6 to 4.8. The supernatant fluid, after removal of the acid fraction, was readjusted to pH 6.8 and diluted with distilled water. The white precipitate thus formed, when dissolved in salt solution, was reported to be practically free from severe chill-producing properties. In studying the possible causes of chill-production, Felton (1928) found that removal of the acid fraction from the crude, water-insoluble precipitate carried most of the phosphorus and lipids, but the author hesitated to conclude that these substances were entirely responsible for chill-production, although concentrates so prepared were reported to be essentially free from the substance provoking reactions. In 1930, Felton[404] stated that, notwithstanding the fact that elimination of the acid fraction was the most important single step in preparing chill-free concentrates, toxins due to bacterial contamination during manufacture and storage might also be a contributory factor. In comparing chill-producing concentrates with bland preparations, Felton and Kauffmann (1931)[427] found the former to contain some residual acid fraction, a higher phosphorus and lipid content, and more ammonia and non-protein nitrogen. Of these factors, the acid fraction was considered to be the most important. However, it is not always possible to obtain an acid fraction precipitate from chill-producing lots as reported by Barnes and Kramer (1933).[83] Complete reconcentration of the serum may render some, but not all, of the preparations suitable for use (Park, 1930[1053]).

Banzhaf and Klein (1930)[72] described the details of a method of preparing chill-free concentrates. After dialysis, sodium sulfate or sodium chloride is added and, after storage in the cold overnight, the reaction is adjusted to pH 5.1 to 5.3. Insoluble substances, fibrin, fibrinogen, euglobulin, and chill-producing substances flocculate and are removed. The material is filtered and the reaction of the fluid is adjusted to pH 6.8 for further precipitation, principally of fibrin. The sediment is removed by filtration and the water-insoluble precipitate prepared by the usual technique. In the alcohol method of concentration, Felton (1931)[408] advised the removal of the acid fraction at pH 5.0. Concentrates prepared by this means, particularly when precautions are taken to avoid denaturation by the alcohol, have been for the most part satisfactory, although lots that occasion reactions are sometimes encountered.

Tests for chill-producing properties. Until the nature of the chill-producing factor is known and until the substance can be removed from antipneumococcic serum, it is necessary, prior to distribution of the product, to have recourse to some means of determining the presence or absence of this property. It is not expedient to make preliminary tests on human subjects, and the smaller, more commonly used laboratory animals are unsatisfactory for the purpose. Sabin and Wallace[1209] stated that it was possible to differentiate chill-producing from satisfactory lots of serum by intravenous injection into suitable dogs. A rise in temperature of 1.5°F. or more was considered the criterion of a positive reaction, regardless of the presence or absence of a definite chill. In a later and more complete paper, Sabin and Wallace[1210] reported observations on a considerable number of serums tested by the method, and confirmed their previous results. Barnes and Kramer (1933)[83] made a preliminary report on the use of monkeys (*Macacus rhesus*) in detecting chill-producing lots of concentrated serum and found the response of the animals to correspond closely with those observed in patients with lobar pneumonia treated with the preparations. In the test animal, the presence or absence of frank chills appeared to be of more significance than elevation of body temperature.

In comparing the products obtained by the sodium sulfate and alcohol methods, Barnes and Kramer[83] tested a pooled lot of antipneumococcic serum that had been divided into two equal parts. One batch had been concentrated by sodium sulfate precipitation, the other by alcohol. The sodium sulfate concentrate gave chills in a high percentage of cases, while the batch refined with alcohol was essentially chill-free in its action.

The practical value of the method was affirmed by the observations of Barnes and Robinson (1936),[84] who found that application of the test over an extended period of time and the rejection of lots of serum eliciting chills in the test monkeys had reduced the incidence of chills by at least 50 per cent in patients undergoing antipneumococcic serum therapy.

Under existing circumstances, it is therefore advisable to utilize some method for selecting only chill-free concentrates for clinical use. Lots found by preliminary tests to possess this unwanted property may be reprocessed, with particular attention paid to solubilities at various hydrogen ion concentrations.

Potency Tests

In the manufacturing laboratory, the determination of the antibody content of antipneumococcic serum is of economic importance in measuring the response of animals during the process of immunization and in selecting serum suitable for therapeutic use. In the clinic it is essential to know the potency of the preparation being used in order to obtain more uniform dosage and to estimate its effectiveness. Standardization of antipneumococcic serum involves difficulties not encountered in the assaying of such biological products as diphtheria and tetanus antitoxins. Progress has been made, however, and, as Park and Cooper[1057-a] observed, although the unit of pneumococcal antibody cannot be so accurately estimated as the diphtheria antitoxic unit, the present standard suffices for therapeutic purposes.

IN VIVO TESTS

During the development of methods for standardizing antipneumococcic serum, both *in vivo* and *in vitro* tests have been utilized. The former have included procedures for determining the protective and the therapeutic qualities of serum, and the latter have been concerned with estimating the content of antibodies demonstrable by serological reactions.

Early animal tests. Washbourn[1487] injected intraperitoneally into rabbits mixtures of measured amounts of serum and a quantity of culture representing ten times the minimal fatal dose. A unit of antibody was defined as the smallest amount of serum that would protect rabbits under the conditions of the test. High virulence of the cultures for rabbits was maintained by special methods. Washbourn also tested the therapeutic action of serum in rabbits and gauged the dosage on the basis of units of antibody. Eyre and Washbourn[374] reported further experiments on standardization, employing mice and administering the mixtures subcutaneously. The authors stated that there was no relation between protection, agglutination, and bactericidal action of the serums—an observation that must be discounted in view of evidence obtained by more recent investigators. In a later publication, Eyre and Washbourn[377] announced the method adopted by them for standardizing antipneumococcic serum, which depended upon determining the protective power of 1.0 cubic centimeter of serum in terms of the number of fatal doses of highly virulent pneumococci injected. The serum was administered intravenously to rabbits and was followed immediately by an intraperitoneal inoculation of culture, the minimal lethal dose of which was determined by injecting various dilutions of the culture into control rabbits.

In testing the protective value of various serums, Römer (1902)[1155] made simultaneous injections of culture and of serum, using both mice and rabbits and, in 1905,[1156] he made a further report of his technique in which a series of mice were inoculated subcutaneously with decreasing doses of serum. After twelve to seventeen hours the test animals and the controls were injected with 10 to 100 lethal doses of culture. For the purpose of interpreting results, Römer termed a serum of which 0.01 cubic centimeter protected animals a "simple serum" and assumed that one cubic centimeter of simple serum constituted one "immunizing unit." If the protective dose was found to be one milligram, the serum was designated as "10 normal." It is difficult to compare the definitions of units as described by Washbourn and by Römer, but their contributions demonstrated the feasibility of standardizing antipneumococcic serum by the use of animals.

Tests of protective effect: the mouse protection test. In 1909, Neufeld and Haendel[989] described a method of testing antipneumococcic serum that was more or less generally adopted and used until comparatively recent times. Mice were injected intraperitoneally with 0.2 cubic centimeter of serum and three hours later different groups of the animals were given increasing amounts of culture by the same route. It appeared that the action of antipneumococcic serum follows the law of multiple proportions only within certain limits and under certain conditions and, furthermore, that there is a limit to the effectiveness of the serum. To this latter character was applied the term *Schwellenwert.* Ungermann and Kandiba (1912)[1436] found that when 0.2 cubic centimeter of serum protected mice against 0.1 cubic centimeter of culture, one-tenth of that amount of serum did not protect against 0.01 cubic centimeter of culture, thus substantiating Neufeld and Haendel's observations regarding multiple proportions. Neufeld and Haendel[992] reported additional technical details of their method in which varying amounts of both serum and culture were employed and recommended duplicate series of tests and the inclusion of a standard serum of known potency. Wadsworth and Kirkbride[1470] reported that more consistent results were obtained when one-half the amount of serum recommended by Ungermann and Kandiba was used, but Avery, Chickering, Cole, and Dochez[36] were in favor of adhering to the more commonly used quantity.

In 1918, as a result of a regulation requiring that control tests on antipneumococcic serums in this country be done at the United States Hygienic Laboratory (now the National Institute of Health), Wayson and McCoy[1493] reported the adoption of the Neufeld method as modified by Cole, with a serum supplied by Cole as the standard for purposes of comparison. Official control was confined to Type I serum. Because of the importance of this action in developing methods of standardization, a brief citation of the essentials of the technique is given. The test consisted in inoculating a series of mice with a fixed dose of serum and varying doses of culture. Serum and culture were injected intraperitoneally, either simultaneously or one immediately following the other. A serum was considered sufficiently potent if 0.2 cubic centimeter protected mice weighing from fifteen to twenty grams against 0.1 cubic centimeter of an eighteen to twenty-four-hour broth culture of such virulence that 10^{-6} cubic centimeter killed control mice of similar weight. Survival of mice for ninety-six hours indicated protection. There were irregularities in the results obtained by this method, but it served as a valuable means of controlling the potency of serums by establishing minimum standards. Wadsworth, Kirkbride, and Gilbert (1919)[1472] described the New York State standard method of testing antipneumococcic serum which, in its essentials, corresponded to that of the federal laboratory. In 1919, the United States Public Health Service[1439] published the details of the mouse protection test as used at the Hygienic Laboratory.*

Felton (1924)[396] experimented with varying amounts of Type I culture in protection tests in an effort to overcome the irregular results obtained by the governmental method. He defined a unit of antibody as that amount which would protect mice against 0.5 cubic centimeter of a 1 to 10 dilution of an eighteen-hour broth culture of such virulence that 10^{-7} cubic centimeter killed mice in thirty-six to forty-eight hours. This dose was calculated to contain one million minimal lethal doses. In estimating the protective power of an antibody solution, Felton tested varying dilutions of the serum against a constant inoculum of culture in duplicate series of mice, as practiced by Neufeld (1922).[977] Formerly the test depended upon titrating a constant amount of serum against varying amounts of culture; here the reverse was true, that is, a constant dose of culture was used against varying amounts of serum. In 1928, Felton[402] presented the details of the protection test developed in his investigations. The method was an improvement over those previously used, but it was subject to limitations, recognized by Felton, which will be considered later.

* See Appendix.

In 1921, at the International Conference on the Standardization of Sera and Serological Tests in London, a committee of the Health Organization of the League of Nations[506] drew up a plan for the technique to be practiced in the assay of antipneumococcic serum. At the Second International Serological Conference,[596] held in Paris in 1922, it was believed that the titration test in mice, when controlled by a standard serum, would provide a method for standardization. Emphasis was placed upon the necessity of including a control serum in every test. In 1923, a subcommittee of the Health Organization of the League of Nations[597] proposed, as a basis for international investigation, that, in performing the mouse protection test, constant volumes of culture should be mixed for five minutes with decreasing volumes of serum and the mixtures injected intraperitoneally into mice. The method* was found in some instances to be satisfactory by Christensen,[847] but it failed to receive universal recognition.

In two articles dealing with the protective action of Type I antipneumococcic serum in mice, Sickles (1927)[1276-7] stated that if broth cultures, freed from organisms, were added to dilutions of serum and the precipitate removed prior to use in the test, the protective action of the serum was diminished or neutralized. It is probable that most, if not all, of this loss of activity was due to absorption of antibody by the soluble type-specific and species-specific substances although these were not emphasized as the factors responsible for the removal of protective antibody. It was stated, however, that the reaction appeared to be associated with that by which the precipitative elements of serum are absorbed when treated with the homologous culture broth.

Felton[406] utilized the principle in developing the technical details of the neutralization method for assaying the antibody content of antipneumococcic serum and concentrates. In the test, equal amounts of a diluted, neutralizing culture and varying serum dilutions are mixed and incubated at 37.5° for one to two hours. The

* See Appendix.

neutralizing antigen is made by adding 0.4 per cent formalin to an eighteen-hour serum-broth culture of virulent pneumococci of the type desired. It is necessary to allow a sufficient period of contact with formalin to elapse in order to kill the organisms. The proper dilution of the neutralizing culture is determined by a preliminary test with the control serum. Mice are injected intraperitoneally with 0.5 cubic centimeter of the serum-neutralizing culture mixture and with 0.5 cubic centimeter of a 1 to 200 dilution of a three to six-hour culture made from an eighteen-hour transplant of a mouse passage culture. Mice used to test the virulence of the organism are also injected with 10^{-6}, 10^{-7}, 10^{-8}, and 10^{-9} cubic centimeter of the living culture, and blood-agar plates are made of these dilutions for counting the number of pneumococci present. The potency of a serum is determined by comparing the highest dilution of serum that will protect for twenty-four hours at least two of the three mice injected with the highest dilution of the control serum conferring a similar degree of protection.

One of the many difficulties encountered in mouse protection tests has been a lack of uniform results with samples of serum tested in different laboratories, and even when tested repeatedly in the same laboratory. At least one source of the discrepancies has been the fact that too few mice were used on each dose of serum or culture. Recognition of this fault resulted in various changes in the test, and the Park and Cooper[1053] modification of the Felton technique has served as a basis for the mouse protection test commonly used in this country at the present time.

In February, 1933, the Committee on Standardization of Antipneumococcic Serum of the Biological Section of the American Drug Manufacturers' Association suggested a method based on the Park-Cooper modification of the mouse protection test. The method was revised in December, 1933, and in its essentials has been approved by the National Institute of Health which supplies a standard bivalent serum for comparison in Type I and Type II protection tests. In general, the method conforms to that of Felton already described. For establishing the unit value of an unknown serum, at least two complete tests must be made, using ten mice for each serum dilution. Different laboratories have modified the details of the test, particularly with regard to the doses of serum and culture employed. It has been found that satisfactory results may be obtained by using dilutions of serum and culture higher than those proposed in the American Drug Manufacturers' Association method. The details of a similar modification which, in the experience of the authors, has proved satisfactory may be found in the Appendix, pages 651–653.

Limitations of the mouse protection test. Although the mouse protection test is generally accepted as the most satisfactory means of assaying antipneumococcic serum for therapeutic use, it has been subjected to criticism on the basis of its inaccuracy and the irregular results not infrequently obtained. Aside from the personal equation in the technical manipulations of the test, the most important variables are those connected with the cultures and the mice used and the ratio between the amounts of serum and culture injected.

Variations related to the culture may be referable to fluctuations in the virulence of the organisms, their ability to neutralize or combine with antibody, and the number of pneumococci present in the test inoculum. Following a study of the standardization of antipneumococcic serum, Enlows (1923)[366] stipulated that the culture should be used in its active or early stationary phase of growth. Felton (1925)[397] observed that the unit value of serum might vary depending upon the strain of Pneumococcus employed in the test, even though only slight differences in virulence of the cultures could be demonstrated. Variable results occurred also when the same strain of Pneumococcus was used under standard conditions. According to Felton,[402] the change from larger to smaller doses of organisms gave more satisfactory results in protection tests.

In studies dealing with the lethal power of the test culture in potency tests, Morgan and Petrie (1931, 1933)[917, 1085] concluded that some control over this factor could be obtained by choosing suitable mediums for growth and by selecting appropriate doses of culture. In considering the variables in the mouse protection test, Felton[405] placed the greatest emphasis on the culture employed and cited the killing power and antibody-neutralizing ability of the organisms as factors of first magnitude. There can be no doubt that variations in cultures contribute to lack of uniformity in the results of tests. Although many laboratories employ the so-called original Neufeld Type I strain, conditions under which cultures are maintained are certain to induce changes of greater or lesser extent in the organisms. In order to minimize variations in cultures of the various types used it would be well to have an international central supply from which representative strains could be issued and to establish standard conditions under which cultures should be maintained in different laboratories. A similar suggestion was made by Felton and is worthy of general consideration.

Variability in the outcome of potency tests on antipneumococcic serum is introduced by the mice employed. Uniformity in susceptibility, the numbers used for each determination, the age, weight, and sex of the animals are all factors to be considered. Petrie and Morgan found that the sex of the animals appears to have no significant influence on the results of titrations. Furthermore, the weight of mice had no effect on the mortality-rate, but heavier animals tended to show a longer survival time. Although little work relating to the effect of age of mice has been done, it is preferable to use young stock. Of greater importance is the degree of uniformity in susceptibility of the mice to pneumococcal infection. It has been customary in titrating serum to employ, when possible, white mice from homogeneous breeding stock. Even when this is done, some mice, or groups of mice, may exhibit unequal susceptibility to the infecting doses of culture. Petrie and Morgan found that from 5 to 10 per cent of the animals used possessed an innate resistance to small doses of pneumococci.

In attempts to decrease the discrepancies introduced by the test animal, it has become customary to increase the number of mice used per dose of serum. In the older methods where only two or three animals were used for each amount of serum or culture, chance death or survival caused confusion. Trevan (1930)[1418] found that the number of animals necessary to offset a given margin of error depends on the ratio of the increment of effect of the serum to the increment of dose of culture. As an example, it was found that if forty mice per dose are used to test two serums, the first may be estimated as equal in potency to the other, although in reality the potency of the first may be as low as 72 per cent or as high as 140 per cent of the second. Trevan suggested computing the survival time of test mice as a means of increasing the accuracy of results and believed that by this plan not more than one-half the number of mice would be required for the same determination as would be necessary if simple enumeration of the number dead on a given day were made. It was found, however, that this plan might be unduly favorable to the serum, since the distribution of survival times was not normal. Discrepancies in the results of tests were also investigated by Beard and Clapp (1932),[95] who recommended the use of at least ten mice per dose of serum and at least two independent tests on each lot of serum. Results of different tests were considered together, rather than separately. Barnes, Clarke, and Wight (1936),[82] using the method described in the Appendix, found that when two or more separate tests, each of which included thirty mice per sample of serum, were used in estimating the value of a serum as compared with a standard, it was practicable to arrange the amounts of serum in the ratio 4 to 2 to 1.

Calculations of the potency of serum were based on the following equation:

$$\text{Units per cubic centimeter in unknown serum} = a\left(\frac{Dx}{D'y}\right)$$

a = units per cubic centimeter in control serum
D = total number of mice dead on control serum
x = lowest dilution of unknown serum
D′ = total number of mice dead on unknown serum
y = lowest dilution of control serum

Although this method served to compensate for irregularities in the mortality-rate of the test animals, it has been found to be unreliable, since a different value may be obtained when the number of survivals is substituted for D and D′. A more accurate formula has been derived and is included in the Appendix, page 657.

It has been claimed that satisfactory end points may be obtained by using serum doses more closely spaced (Park, 1930;[1053] Morgan and Petrie, 1933[917]), but in the experience of the authors of the present volume this plan is not reliable under routine laboratory conditions unless an inconveniently large number of mice are used.

In a recent series of studies on the mouse protection test, Goodner and Horsfall[537] and Goodner and Miller (1935)[540] decided that the most important variable in the mouse is the number of monocytes present in the peritoneum at the time of injection of serum and culture. The mice were carefully selected from a strain inbred for several years. It seems not unlikely that the phagocytic activity of the animals used may condition the progress of the pneumococcal infection in the protection test. On the other hand, it is questionable how this factor may be controlled in selecting mice, even from an inbred stock, at the time of carrying out protection tests. Irwin and Hughes (1931)[670] found in studying the bactericidal power of the blood of rats that, when matings were made of susceptible animals, that is, those with low bactericidal powers, the offspring were all susceptible; if a low × high mating was made, two-thirds of the offspring were susceptible and the remainder resistant. The breeding of a stock of mice of uniform susceptibility to pneumococcal infection, therefore, would appear by analogy to be possible. Such a program has been initiated at the Rockefeller Institute under the direction of Webster and by Little at Bar Harbor. If the efforts are successful, it may be possible to establish a supply of mice of uniform susceptibility for titrating antipneumococcic serum.

The outcome of protection tests is also dependent upon the proportions of serum and culture employed. The so-called *Schwellenwert*, also noted by Neufeld and Haendel,[989] is another phenomenon which limits the applicability of the test. The *Schwellenwert* may be defined as the maximal amount of culture against which protection can be demonstrated with any amount of serum. Coventry (1927),[286] in measuring the protective action of serum by noting survival time of the mice, failed to obtain evidence of this threshold of effectiveness of serum. That such a relation exists, however, appears to be generally conceded although the explanation is obscure. Goodner and his colleagues[537, 540] believed the phenomenon to be due to the interrelation between serum and culture and the number and kind of phagocytic cells in the host. The authors also list certain zonal effects as referable to the variable factors in the test. Thus, the limiting zone of titration is defined as the smallest amount of serum that will protect against a given quantity of culture, and is believed to be related to the number of virulent organisms and to the antibody content of the serum. The reaction, however, is not strictly one following the law of multiple proportions. In the same general category is the so-called pro-zone which is manifested by a lack of protection when an excessive amount of serum is employed. The pro-zone is, therefore, related to the *Schwellenwert*. Goodner and Horsfall[537] found such a zone in tests with immune horse serum but not with immune rabbit serum, and others have confirmed this observation.

The fact that the zonal effect may be observed in tests with horse serum but not with rabbit serum suggests the presence of some non-protective, antagonistic substance in immune horse serum. The effect may be at least partially obviated according to Goodner and Horsfall by previous treatment of the mice with sodium nucleinate. That excessive amounts of specific polysaccharide may serve to operate against the protective action of serum is a possibility suggested by the work of Felton and Bailey (1926).[419] The interference may be due simply to a combination of polysaccharide and antibody, thus decreasing the amount of antibody available for protection. Felton[402] suggested that an action of this nature might be responsible for the zonal effects mentioned above, or it is possible that Goodner and Horsfall's explanations already cited may be nearer the truth.

Confusion in the standardization of antipneumococcic serum has been occasioned by the lack of a universally accepted control serum. The need was supplied by Cole in 1918, and Felton (1930)[405] distributed serum "F 146" to many laboratories as a standard for tests on Type I and II serum. The supply was not large, however, and efforts were made in this country and abroad to substitute other serums comparable in potency to F 146. Unfortunately, the present standard serum for the United States (as well as F 146) is supplied in liquid form and, according to Hartley and Smith (1935),[596] is subject to deterioration. It has been the experience of the authors that loss of protective power of a control serum may introduce major difficulties in standardization. Both F 146 and P 11, the present American standard serum, are for Type I and II titrations. Hartley and Smith have proposed an international standard serum, to be distributed in dry form, for Type I and another for Type II. The unit values of these standards are based on Felton's F 146. Hartley and Smith have placed their standard serums at the disposal of the Health Organization of the League of Nations. If present methods of standardization are continued in use, it follows that similar standards for types other than I and II will be required.

Tests of therapeutic effect. One of the objections to the protection test as generally employed in mice has been the fact that it is a prophylactic test rather than a means of estimating the therapeutic activity of serums. Experience has indicated that the curative value of serums in human beings may be expressed in terms of mouse protective units, yet there has been a surmise that products selected on the basis of experimentally demonstrated therapeutic efficacy might yield better results in treatment. Attempts have therefore been made to devise tests in both rabbits and mice for determining the curative properties of serum in pneumococcal infections.

Washbourn[1487] administered a single dose of serum to rabbits five to six hours following inoculation of a test dose of culture and observed protection, but when the serum was given eight to twelve hours after the culture he observed only retardation of death. Wadsworth[1458] utilized rabbits in testing the curative action of immune rabbit serum, but used the method for experimental comparison rather than for actual standardization. In a series of publications beginning in 1928, Goodner[525] reported experiments dealing with the therapeutic effect of antipneumococcic serum in rabbits following intradermal infection. By inoculating rabbits intradermally with small amounts of living, virulent pneumococci it was found that a local lesion developed and symptoms appeared somewhat analogous to lobar pneumonia. The results of intravenous treatment of animals so infected with antipneumococcic serum administered twenty-four hours after inoculation were advanced as a means of estimating therapeutic efficacy. The curative value of serum as determined by the Goodner technique did not correspond with the results of the mouse-protective test. The intradermal method was suggested (1929)[527] for the routine standardization of serum since it was based on the ability of a serum to combat a preexistent infection. Later (1933),[531] however, it was admitted that the method was too elaborate for routine use, and it was found (1934),[532-4] furthermore, that variable factors, such as the severity of the infection, the number of white cells, and the breed and weight of the test animals complicated the results. In the observations of Francis and Terrell (1934)[476] on experimental Type III intratracheal infection in monkeys, it was found that the mortality was dependent upon the presence and severity of the septicemia following inoculation. Thus, there were no deaths in animals without bacteriemia; with a low degree of blood invasion the mortality-rate was 45 per cent; with a moderate degree of septicemia 75 per cent died; and with massive septicemia all animals died.

In intradermal infections in rabbits with Type I pneumococci, it appears that similar mortality-rates may be expected. Barnes and Clarke, in investigations* (1934) on the intradermal method, observed extremely wide variations in the number of pneumococci present in blood samples taken twenty-four hours after infection. Because of the time at which serum treatment of rabbits is ordinarily begun in this method, it is impossible to base dosage on the severity of septicemia, inasmuch as this condition cannot be readily determined until twenty-four hours after taking blood samples. As a result of this and other objections (irregularity in susceptibility to infection, et cetera),[531, 533] the intradermal method of assaying antipneumococcic serum is impracticable for routine use.

Tests for the curative effects of antipneumococcic serum in mice have also been advocated. Coventry[286] reported that a majority of mice could be saved by administering concentrated serum intraperitoneally four hours after an injection of Type I culture had been given by the same route. Parish (1930)[1051] studied the therapeutic effect in mice of serum given intravenously at intervals of one and one-half to seven hours after the intraperitoneal injection of culture. It was found that serum was effective when given in this manner but, as was to be expected, the longer the interval between injections, the fewer the animals that survived. Petrie and Morgan[1086] reported investigations on the curative action of antipneumococcic serum in mice and stated that in the case of Type I recovery might take place even when a bacteriemia was present. The serum was administered intravenously up to twelve hours after inoculation. The outcome of the test was apparently conditioned by the amount of antibody injected, the time of its injection in relation to the infecting dose, and the degree of infection at the time of serum administration. The authors thought that the test might prove satisfactory as a means for standardizing therapeutic serum.

In a later communication, Morgan and Petrie[917] observed that a comparison of the curative and protective tests showed that both

* Unpublished.

were equally reliable for measuring the protective antibody, but that the prophylactic technique was more convenient. Trevan[1418] found that intravenous administration of serum did not increase the accuracy of titrations. It appears, therefore, that curative tests on mice for estimating therapeutic value of serum fail to offer any information in addition to that obtained by the usual protection tests and, because of their greater inconvenience, cannot be considered as of sufficient worth to warrant general adoption.

Tests of other effects. During the development of antipneumococcic serum therapy, investigators have sought for qualities in serum other than those of an antibacterial nature. Attempts have been made to demonstrate antitoxic properties (Klemperer brothers[724]), but no convincing evidence has yet been brought forward that pneumococcal antitoxin has been produced. The work of Clowes, Jamieson and Olson (1926),[244] of Parker and McCoy,[1062] and of Coca[246] has already been discussed in some detail in other chapters, but as yet none of the methods described has been adopted for the routine testing of therapeutic antipneumococcic serum.

With the Goodner intradermal technique, Curphey and Baruch (1930)[292] tested the therapeutic effect in rabbits of so-called exudate antiserum. When compared by mouse protection tests, the preparations showed essentially the same antibody content as serum obtained from horses immunized by formalinized vaccines. When compared in rabbits for therapeutic effect, however, it was found that 70.4 per cent of animals treated with the "exudate antiserum" survived, while only 34.7 per cent of those given the usual antipneumococcic serum lived. As a result, the authors assumed that "exudate antiserums" contain substances, other than antibacterial antibodies, which exert greater therapeutic action.

Sabin[1204-6] reported experiments which led him to conclude that the therapeutic action of antipneumococcic serum depends to a considerable extent on a non-antibacterial factor. He found type-specific protective antibody in serum after complete precipitation of the anticarbohydrate precipitins, using capsular polysaccharide prepared by the early method of Heidelberger, Goebel, and Avery.[613] The soundness of the argument appears questionable in view of the more recent experiments of Avery and Goebel (1933)[46] with acetyl polysaccharide. Ward (1932),[1483] after using the sensitive bactericidal test in determining the phagocytic power of SSS-absorbed serum, concluded that there was no necessity to predicate the presence of an additional and possibly non-antibacterial antibody in immune serum. Other evidence advanced by Sabin to support his hypothesis depended upon tests with serum prepared or utilized in different ways in treating the dermal pneumococcal infection in rabbits, but the results failed to parallel those of the mouse protection tests.

Some antipneumococcic serums are therapeutically more active than others and the differences may possibly be due to the presence or absence of antitoxic or non-antibacterial substances in addition to the mouse protective antibody. Felton,[404] however, doubted the evidence put forward in support of this hypothesis. Claims for extra-therapeutic properties of serum based on tests in rabbits infected intradermally are subject to the limitations of the method.

IN VITRO TESTS

Various means have been employed for titrating the antibody content of antipneumococcic serum without resorting to the use of animals. Thus, tests for determining the amount of water-insoluble proteins, the complement fixation and bactericidal reactions, flocculation with toxic preparations, and the *Quellung* reaction, in addition to agglutination and precipitation tests have been devised for the purpose.

Water test. The so-called water test was an outgrowth of the observation by Felton (1924)[396] that simple dilution of serum with water resulted in precipitation. It was thought that the amount of precipitate so formed was an indication of the protective strength of the serum and, furthermore, that the method could be used to determine the suitability of the serum for concentration (Goodner[528]). The method, however, has not proved to be accurate and has fallen into disuse.

Complement fixation. Although there appear to have been no systematic studies directed toward applying complement fixation as a means of serum standardization, it is a method which, at least from the theoretical standpoint, might be employed.

Bactericidal power. Tests for determining the bactericidal or phagocytic power of blood have been developed in attempts to measure natural or artificial immunity to pneumococci. However, because of irregularities in the results, tests for bactericidal action have not been adopted routinely for the standardization of therapeutic antipneumococcic serums.

It is generally assumed that defense of the body against pneumococcal infection depends on the neutralization of capsular polysaccharide, thus permitting phagocytosis of the organisms. Determination of the opsonic or tropic activity of serum should presumably offer a valuable means of estimating therapeutic effect. No *in vitro* method of this sort yet devised is superior to a satisfactory mouse protection test.

Antitoxic flocculation. If it is proved that antitoxic properties can be imparted to antipneumococcic serum and if these properties are of clinical benefit, then some *in vitro* method for estimating the antitoxic potency of the serum will be needed. In that event, the flocculation test devised by Powell* would be applicable.

Quellung reaction. Clapp, Phillips, and Stahl (1935)[234] have suggested an adaptation of the well-known Neufeld *Quellung* reaction for the titration of antipneumococcic serum. The technique requires relatively small amounts of materials and appears to be equally applicable to all types of antipneumococcic serum. Some of the difficulties involved in other methods are apparently avoided in this test, but its advantages as a routine procedure have not as yet been demonstrated.

* Mentioned by Clowes, Jamieson, and Olson.[244]

Agglutination. Agglutination tests have been utilized in the past for measuring the antibody content of antipneumococcic serum. In view of the more recent work on the subject (Heidelberger and Kabat, 1934[614]), it appears that agglutination tests may give a definite measure of the antibody response of animals but owing to uncontrollable variables the usual method does not yield sufficiently consistent results to justify its use as a routine means of standardizing serums.

Precipitation. Accumulated evidence strongly indicates that the effective therapeutic antibody in antipneumococcic serum is closely related to, if not identical with, the immune substance reacting with the type-specific capsular polysaccharide. The logical course in establishing *in vitro* methods of standardization is, therefore, to utilize tests employing the specific carbohydrate of the various pneumococcal types as precipitinogen. Although precipitin reactions between antipneumococcic serums and corresponding antigens were observed soon after the development of immune serum (Panichi, 1907[1046]), it was not until Heidelberger and Avery[606] isolated the capsular polysaccharide that efforts were made to apply specific precipitation methods in the standardization of antipneumococcic serum. With many of the tests carried out with polysaccharides similar to the original preparations of Heidelberger and Avery, the results have been decidedly promising. It is probable, however, that even more accurate and reproducible titrations may be obtained with the acetyl form of polysaccharide more recently described by Avery and Goebel (1933),[46] or better still, with the purified materials prepared according to the later methods of Heidelberger, Kendall and Scherp.[627]

In general, there have been three methods employed for determining the precipitin content of antipneumococcic serum: one using a constant amount of polysaccharide mixed with varying dilutions of serum; another utilizing the principle of optimal proportions of antigen and antibody; and, finally, one dependent upon the determination of the nitrogen content of antigen-antibody aggregates.

The first-named procedure, which may be termed a routine precipitin test, has been subjected to various modifications and interpretations. With this method, Zozaya, Boyer and Clark (1930),[1589] Felton (1931),[407] Falk, McGuire, Valentine and Whitney (1931),[387] and Barnes, Clarke and Wight[82] obtained fairly consistent results in titrating whole antipneumococcic serum. Inaccuracies are introduced by variations in spacing of dilutions of serums and in establishing end points, in addition to variations in technical manipulations. It is customary to take as the end point the highest dilution of serum affording visible precipitation with a fixed amount of antigen after incubation for two hours in a water-bath at 37.5° and storage overnight in the cold, although Zozaya, Boyer, and Clark preferred to make readings after the preliminary two-hour incubation. If the spacing of serum dilutions is too wide, the titrations will not be satisfactory for comparative purposes. On the other hand, difficulty in reading end points arises when the increment of antibody is too small. Barnes, Clarke, and Wight used the same serum dilutions employed by Sobotka and Friedlander (1928)[1299] which proved satisfactory in routine tests. The details of the method used by Barnes and his associates are given in the Appendix, page 644.

The importance of optimal proportions of serum and antigen in precipitin reactions was pointed out by Dean (1911),[310] and reported upon in detail by Dean and Webb (1926).[311] Morgan (1923)[912] studied the principle in relation to antipneumococcic serum, and further observations were reported by Smith (1932),[1298] who stated that titration by the method would fulfill the requirements placed upon an *in vitro* method of testing native serum. Unfortunately, the results with concentrated preparations were not wholly satisfactory. The method is similar in principle to the flocculation test introduced by Ramon (1923)[1120] for assaying diphtheria antitoxin, and since the technique is given in the Appendix, its details need not be described here. Smith used a small number of samples in developing this method as applied to antipneumococcic serum, but Barnes, Clarke, and Wight[82] corroborated his findings in titrations on a larger series of unconcentrated Type I and II serums.

In 1935, Felton and Stahl[432] described a method of titration by determining the combining equivalents of antibody and SSS. The method is based on the principle of optimal proportions, and the point of equivalence is measured by testing for excess antigen in a series of mixtures of antigen and antibody, rather than by determining the point at which particulation first occurs as in Smith's method. The method reported by Felton and Stahl appears to be applicable to concentrated antibody preparations as well as to native serum and this fact may favor its adoption in the event that *in vitro* methods of standardization are eventually substituted for mouse protection tests.

A different method of estimating the antibody content of serums was introduced by Heidelberger, Sia, and Kendall (1930),[630] who calculated the amount of immune nitrogen in SSS-antibody precipitates and converted this figure into terms of immune protein present in the serum. Additional details of the method and results of titrations have been reported in subsequent publications.[619, 624] The essentials of the technique may be found in the Appendix, pages 643 and 644.

CORRELATION BETWEEN IN VITRO AND IN VIVO TESTS

Much of the evidence obtained thus far concerning the relationship between laboratory tests and therapeutic efficacy of antipneumococcic serum has been based on mouse protection tests, and the correspondence has proved to be satisfactory for general purposes. If the mouse test is to be supplanted by a chemical or serological method of standardization, the correlation between the results obtained by mouse protection tests and various *in vitro* methods of assay must be determined. The best approach to this question is a study of the relation between mouse protection and the amount of polysaccharide antibody as determined by some form of precipitation test. Brown (1933)[154] found a high degree of correspondence between mouse protection and precipitation with the cellular carbohydrate, but it is difficult to concede any advantage in its use over the purified forms of capsular polysaccharide.

In a study of thirty-nine serums, Felton[407] observed correlation coefficients of 0.93 and 0.91 between protection and precipitin titer, and between protection and the amount of immune protein precipitated with polysaccharide. Barnes, Clarke, and Wight, using fifty samples of unconcentrated serum, calculated the correlation coefficients between mouse protection and their modified routine precipitin test, Felton and Stahl's combining equivalent test, and Smith's optimal proportions test. Correlation coefficients found for these three methods were 0.930 ± 0.012, 0.925 ± 0.014, and 0.909 ± 0.016, respectively, in the case of Type I preparations. Between mouse protection and the first two precipitin tests, values of 0.817 ± 0.031 and 0.739 ± 0.043 were obtained in the case of Type II serums. Felton and Stahl[432] reported correlation coefficients of 0.90 and 0.89 for Type I and Type II, respectively, between the combining equivalent test and mouse protection for both native serum and concentrates. Results of titrations by methods depending upon precipitation of antibody by SSS therefore agree closely with those of the mouse protection test. It is not unlikely that the correlation would be even higher were it not for the inherent errors of the mouse protection test.

The data on methods of standardization may be summarized thus: The mouse protection test is inconvenient, expensive, and subject to variations difficult to control. It appears likely that some *in vitro* method of titration may ultimately supplant the animal test, and of those discussed, some form of precipitin test with purified capsular polysaccharides offers the greatest promise. The adoption of any new method depends largely upon its simplicity, accuracy, and close correlation between estimated potency of the preparations tested and their therapeutic efficacy. Moreover, the method should be equally applicable to unconcentrated and concentrated products. From the theoretical standpoint, at least, some method utilizing the principle of optimal proportions appears to meet these requirements. As long as the mouse protection test remains the accepted procedure for assaying antipneumococcic serum, a stable, standard serum should be available for general use, only standard cultures maintained under uniform conditions should be employed in the test, and a technique should be adopted that would be acceptable to all engaged in the manufacture and use of the products.

Confusion has existed because of a lack of any satisfactory definition of a unit of antibody. The unit as defined by Felton (1924)[396] furnished a convenient working basis, but experience has shown that the number of lethal doses of pneumococci against which a given serum will protect is too variable a factor to serve as a criterion for establishing the unit. A stable, desiccated standard serum of which a given weight contains, by international agreement, one unit of antibody as suggested by Hartley and Smith,[596] would, for the time being, supply the need. In the event that a precipitin test is substituted for the mouse protection method of standardization, it is possible that the standard of comparison, as suggested by Felton and Stahl, should be a uniform and satisfactory preparation of type-specific polysaccharide, rather than a control serum.

A comprehensive discussion of the standardization of antipneumococcic serum and concentrates is to be found in the latest communication of Felton and Stahl (1937).[433] The report comprises the results of a restudy of the various methods advocated for determining the potency of serum. The original report should be consulted for the details of the several tests carried out in the study but, because of the pertinency of the conclusions, some of them are quoted here.

(1) When the mouse-protection test is applied by the technic described in this paper, namely by carrying out the test in the zone in which the law of multiple proportions is valid; by controlling the dose of culture by preliminary test against 0.5 unit of antibody; by using mouse strains which have been shown to be uniform in their resistance to pneumococci and by titrating the unknown serum or concentrate against the protective power of 0.5 unit of antibody of a standard control serum, reliable and reproducible assays of the protective titer of types I and II antipneumococcus serum can be made.

(2) The in vivo method described in this report termed the "combining-equivalent method" which, in principle, measures the antibody present by means of the amount of SSS with which it combines shows a high degree of correlation with the mouse-protection test described in the foregoing (in 62 samples $r = 0.94$ for type I and $r = 0.91$ for type II antibody).

(3) The use of the "combining equivalent technic" as an economical, rapid, and reliable method for the titration of antipneumococcus serum is suggested.

(4) Standardization by several different methods in 1933 of the United States National Institute of Health's standard serum P11 by comparison with serum F146 gave the following results: Mouse-protection method, 300 type I units and 131 type II units per cc; by the neutralization method, 333 type I and 150 type II units per cc; by the combining equivalent method, 322 type I and 150 type II units per cc; and by Heidelberger's method, 308 type I and 150 type II units per cc.

(5) Standardization by three different methods in 1935 of three sera—F146, Lyo P11, and the British type I and type II dried standards, with proof of the deterioration of serum F146 as compared to serum P11, gave the following results for the antibody content of the British standards as compared to serum P11: Mouse-protection method, 1,150 type I units, 750 type II units; by the combining equivalent method, 1,177 type I units, 720 type II units; by Heidelberger's method, 949 type I and 426 type II units per cc of the respective samples.

Safety Tests

Antipneumococcic serum intended for therapeutic use must be tested for the possible presence of harmful substances. The most important tests are those planned to demonstrate freedom from tetanus spores and from pathogenic bacteria, the absence of toxic or chill-producing properties, and an excess of preservative. The National Institute of Health[1440] requires that "a sample of each lot of all products shall be tested for identity if such test is applicable, otherwise for safety, after the labels have been affixed to the final containers."

ROUTINE SAFETY TEST

This test consists in the injection of 5.0 cubic centimeters of the product into the peritoneum of a normal guinea pig. The animal is observed over a period of ten days for any symptoms referable to harmful serum components or to bacterial contamination.

The possibility that the intravenous administration of antipneumococcic serum may result in more or less severe thermal reactions renders it obligatory to test each lot for this property. The tests proposed by Sabin and Wallace[1209-10] in dogs, and by Barnes and Kramer,[83] and Barnes and Robinson[84] in monkeys have been discussed in a previous section of this chapter. It would be desirable to test for this property on human subjects, but where such a course is not possible, one of the two animal tests mentioned should be employed. In addition to chill-production, other unwanted properties of the serum may thus also be detected.

TESTS ON MICE

One of the reasons advanced by Felton and Stahl for continuing the use of the mouse protection test in standardizing antipneumococcic serum is that it also serves as a safety test. The value of the test, however, is limited; mice and rabbits are unreliable animals for detecting chill-producing properties, and the usual mouse protection test is of insufficient duration to meet the requirements in other respects to ensure the safety of the serum.

Mice may be used for detecting excessive amounts of preservatives as described by Leake and Corbitt.[794] The need for such a test rarely arises, but the intraperitoneal and intravenous injection in mice affords a rapid and convenient means of detecting the presence of toxic amounts of some of the chemical preservatives used in serum.

Final Processing of Serums

After a lot of antipneumococcic serum has been selected and, as is the case in many laboratories, has been concentrated, there are routine procedures to be followed before the product is ready for distribution. A brief discussion of a convenient and approved system covering this phase of processing follows.

TOTAL SOLIDS

It is necessary to determine the total amount of solids present in concentrated preparations intended for human use, because the solids content may be too high to permit of ready filtration and ease of administration. The determination is made by drying to constant weight an accurately measured amount—at least ten cubic centimeters—of serum and calculating the percentage of dried matter in terms of the original weight of serum. Experience has shown that concentrated serum with a total solids content between 10 and 15 per cent is usually of satisfactory viscosity to meet the requirements in processing and administration to patients. Lots with a solids content above this level are diluted with an appropriate volume of salt solution.

FILTRATION

All antipneumococcic serum intended for therapeutic use must be passed through a Berkefeld or some similar filter to ensure the absence of contaminating microorganisms. Filtration of concentrated products is facilitated by first passing the serum through a high-speed centrifuge. Warming the serum to slightly above room temperature also facilitates filtration. In order to minimize subsequent testing, it is desirable to filter as large quantities of serum as possible into single containers. The usual aseptic precautions must be observed throughout the process.

BULK STERILITY AND POTENCY TESTS

As soon as the lot of serum is filtered, samples are removed for sterility and potency tests and for tests of chill-producing properties, in case the latter test is to be performed on laboratory animals. Regulations of the National Institute of Health covering the tests for sterility are included in the Appendix, page 662.

It is necessary to determine the potency of antipneumococcic serum prior to filling the final containers. These tests, as well as tests on animals for chill-producing qualities, may be done conveniently with samples taken from the bulk containers and while the tests for sterility are being made. The methods employed have been described in a previous section of this chapter. It is obvious that the product must pass these tests satisfactorily before it is dispensed into the final containers.

DISPENSING AND LABELING

After the serum has passed all the tests made on samples taken from the bulk containers, it may be dispensed into final containers for distribution. Sterile, rubber-capped vials or syringe ensembles of a capacity never greater than the maximal dose for man are used for the purpose. A convenient method of dispensing the bulk product into the vials or syringes is briefly as follows: The serum from the bulk container is forced by compressed air into a burette, equipped with a specially designed filling device, which, by means of a protecting bell or dome, covers the neck of the vial to be filled. All openings are protected against air-borne bacteria by sterile cotton air-filters. The entire filling apparatus must, of course, be sterilized before use. As soon as the vial is filled with serum, a soft rubber stopper is inserted, and sealed with a viscose cap or gelatin. The bottling process should be conducted under strict aseptic conditions in a room free from draughts and dust.

When the lot of serum has been dispensed into the final containers, approved labels, on which are recorded the lot number of the preparation, the potency for each type of antibody contained, and the expiration date set by federal regulation are affixed to the bottles.

STERILITY TESTS ON FINAL CONTAINERS

The method required by the National Institute of Health is described in the Appendix, page 662.

SAFETY AND IDENTITY TESTS

Using the serum from one of the labeled, final containers, the routine safety test in a guinea pig is made (see page 588 of this chapter).

IDENTITY TEST

For this purpose, the simple precipitin test with type-specific pneumococcal capsular polysaccharide homologous for the types of antibody contained in the product is satisfactory.

RECORDS

It is important that complete records be made of every lot of antipneumococcic serum produced. These are conveniently kept on a separate form for each lot, suitable to the needs of the laboratory, and giving in detail all essential data on each step in the process of manufacture, with the initials of the person making each entry.

In the United States, for laboratories operating under federal license, it is necessary to submit to the National Institute of Health protocols of potency tests together with two of the final containers of each lot of serum to be distributed for therapeutic use (see Appendix, page 661).

REGULATIONS GOVERNING ANTIPNEUMOCOCCIC SERUM

In the United States, control over biological products concerned in interstate commerce is maintained by the Treasury Department through the Public Health Service which, from time to time, formulates or revises and issues regulations. Antipneumococcic serum (Types I and II) is included among those products for which "the official standards of potency . . . shall be those distributed by the National Institute of Health of the United States Public Health Service."

Minimum standards for Type I serum to be submitted for official tests were established in 1919, but they need not be discussed here since they were based on methods no longer in use. In January, 1934, a regulation[1437] was promulgated to the effect that samples of all antipneumococcic serum intended for sale in interstate commerce must be submitted to and released by the United States Public Health Service before distribution. A memorandum of December, 1935,[1438] stated that after April 1, 1936, the National Institute of Health would pass for distribution only serums (Type I) showing at least 1,000 units per cubic centimeter if concentrated and at least 500 units per cubic centimeter if unconcentrated. A later memorandum effective March 1, 1937, established the same minimal potency for Type II serum.

The British Therapeutic Substances Act of 1925,[549] followed by the Statutory Rules and Orders of 1927, is similar to the United States regulations governing biological products. The Statutory Rules and Orders of 1935[551] regulate the preparation of both Type I and Type II serums.

Governmental control over therapeutic antipneumococcic serum is desirable for uniformity in standardization and in interpreting clinical results. Ideally, however, it would be preferable to secure international agreement for a set of standard regulations without interference with separate governmental requirements.

AUTHOR'S NOTE: The 1936 (11th) edition of the United States Pharmacopoeia[1087] gives official recognition only to Type I antipneumococcic serum.

The Production of Diagnostic Serum

In order that patients with lobar pneumonia may be given effective serum treatment, it is necessary first to determine the infecting type of Pneumococcus. Before the serological differentiation of pneumococci into groups was accomplished by Dochez and Gillespie, serum therapy of lobar pneumonia was purely empirical owing to the lack of exact knowledge concerning the diversity of pneumococcal strains. The separation of pneumococci into thirty-two distinct types and the recent development of the Neufeld *Quellung* reaction as a method of type determination have rendered serum therapy far more rational, effective, and economical than formerly. For many years, monovalent, immune horse serum was employed in the serological diagnosis of pneumococcal types, but now the Neufeld technique employing immune rabbit serum for the demonstration of capsular swelling yields more satisfactory results, besides being more rapid than the agglutination or other reactions involving the use of immune horse serum.

IMMUNE HORSE SERUM

Diagnostic serums may be produced by immunizing horses with type-specific strains of pneumococci by the same methods followed in the production of therapeutic serum. In laboratories where monovalent therapeutic serums are manufactured it is convenient to select bleedings, usually the earlier ones, and, if tests are satisfactory, to utilize the serum for type identification. In determining the suitability of immune horse serum for diagnostic purposes, the specific agglutinin titer, the presence of heterologous agglutinins for other pneumococcal types (particularly those of closely related types), and the velocity of the agglutination reaction are to be considered. For these tests it is essential to use organisms of maximal virulence, and preferably young, living cultures. The macroscopic method of agglutination is satisfactory, and readings should be taken at frequent intervals during the first two hours. Serums that are suitable for diagnostic use usually give clear-cut, specific agglutination in relatively high dilutions after one-half-hour's incubation in a water-bath at 37°, and exhibit no visible agglutination with representative strains of other types, although serums that show some non-specific agglutination in dilutions well below the type-specific titer may be employed. If the serums are to be used for precipitation tests, the same routine should be followed in determining the titer against homologous and heterologous polysaccharide.

It is generally conceded that antipneumococcic horse serum is unsatisfactory for use in the Neufeld *Quellung* reaction because of the non-specific effects caused by that serum (Neufeld and Etinger-Tulczynska, 1931;[984] Etinger-Tulczynska, 1933;[368-a] Sabin, 1933[1206]). The British Therapeutic Trials Committee of the Medical Research Council (1934)[887] concluded, however, that results with either immune horse or immune rabbit serum are equally reliable provided the serum has an agglutinative titer of 1 to 160 to 1 to 320. At the Massachusetts Antitoxin and Vaccine Laboratory it has been observed that, even when the same vaccines are used for immunization purposes, immune horse serum is likely to give cross-reactions, whereas immune rabbit serum is highly type-specific.

Relatively small amounts of serum are required for the Neufeld test, and, therefore, it is better to use rabbit serum because of the irregular reactions exhibited by horse serum. For routine identification tests, and for other methods involving macroscopic agglutination or precipitation, diagnostic horse serum may be found more economical to use than rabbit serum.

IMMUNE RABBIT SERUM

Various methods are employed for producing antipneumococcic rabbit serum for use in the Neufeld *Quellung* test. For the purpose, methods outlined by Barnes and White[86] have given satisfactory results. Cooper and Walter (1935)[275] published the details of the methods employed at the laboratories of the New York City Department of Health and emphasized the necessity of using scrupulously clean syringes for antigen injections, and of selecting representative strains of pneumococci for immunization. It was also found that long-continued immunization of the stock animals resulted in the acquisition by the serum of non-specific immunological properties. The latter point has been considered in the development of the so-called "rapid method" of producing rabbit typing serums, in which the animals are subjected to an intensive course of immunization and, when the titer of the serum is satisfactory, the animals are exsanguinated. Experience at the Massachusetts laboratory has shown that, with properly selected cultures killed by heating at 100°, rabbits may be immunized over a period of at least a year and bled routinely every three weeks after a course of twelve to fifteen injections. The amount of serum obtained when the plan is followed reduces the cost of production and, when the specificity of closely related strains is carefully controlled, as suggested in the paper by Barnes and Wight,[88] cross-reactions with the serum are avoided. The methods recommended by the authors are described in the Appendix, page 663.

Rabbit serum intended for use in the Neufeld method should be tested for both potency and type-specificity. Cooper and Walter (1935)[275] recommended a minimal agglutinative titer of at least 1 to 200, with freedom from cross-reactions, and that each serum be tested for its ability to cause a characteristic capsule swelling of pneumococci of the homologous type.

Some workers have maintained that rabbit serum for use in the Neufeld test must be used in undiluted state. The claim is not necessarily valid, however, for in the authors' experience completely satisfactory results are obtainable, at least with certain pneumococcal types, if highly potent serums are diluted as much as 1 to 5 to 1 to 10 with normal rabbit serum.

As in the case of therapeutic serums, it is recommended that standard methods of producing diagnostic serum for the type determination of all known pneumococcal types should be universally adopted and put into effect. A movement to bring about the fulfilment of the object has been initiated in the United States.

PRESERVATIVES, BOTTLING, AND LABELING

The choice of a preservative for diagnostic serums is not so important as in the case of therapeutic products. A satisfactory procedure is the addition of tricresol to a concentration of 0.3 per cent at the time of the collection of the serum from the clot. Any resulting precipitate or detritus may be removed by centrifugation or filtration prior to filling the serum into final containers.

Containers of diagnostic serum should be labeled with the lot number, the serological type, the dilution to be used (if any), a notation of any cross-reactions produced, and an expiration date beyond which no reliance can be placed upon the indicated potency. Serums should be retested at intervals of three to four months.

Summary

The main points developed in this chapter may be summarized as follows. For stimulation of antipneumococcal immune substances in animals, vaccines made from highly virulent, type-specific cultures, killed preferably by heating at 100°, have given satisfactory results. The so-called "three-week" schedule of injections is to be recommended, and the dosage of antigen should be as small as is consistent with satisfactory immunological response as indicated by repeated potency tests on the serum. Concentrated and refined serum is preferable to unconcentrated serum for therapeutic use; the method of Felton in which alcohol is used as a precipitant being at present the one most generally employed. Current methods for determining the potency of serums are not wholly satisfactory, but as long as the mouse protection test remains the accepted procedure, for the sake of uniformity this method should be used. A standard serum for comparative purposes should be adopted for use in the assay of antipneumococcic serum and, in the event that a precipitin test is substituted for the *in vivo* method, a standard preparation of type-specific pneumococcal polysaccharide should be available. Standard methods for preparing and testing diagnostic serums for all pneumococcal types with a central source of supply and control of the serums should also be incorporated in a plan for developing the uniformity of all antipneumococcic serum.

CHAPTER XVI

SERUM TREATMENT OF LOBAR PNEUMONIA

The theoretical basis for the administration of specific immune serum in the therapy of pneumonia; a discussion of complicating problems and of the limitations of serum therapy; with a summary of the results so far observed in the clinic.

THE intelligent employment of specific immune serum in the treatment of pneumonia has abundant factual justification. The scientific background based on precise animal experimentation and the immunological study of artificial infection in animals and natural infection in man makes it possible to predict with a considerable degree of certainty the probable effect of antipneumococcic serum in controlling infection by Pneumococcus, and to understand some of the very obvious present limitations of specific serum therapy. The results at the bedside bear out the theoretical expectations.

The Rationale of Serum Therapy

The presence of virulent pneumococci in susceptible tissues stirs the latent physiological functions of the body to elaborate substances antagonistic to Pneumococcus. The same immunological defenses may be called into being by introducing into the sound animal body parts or the whole of artificially attenuated pneumococci.

The specific immune substances elaborated in response to the antigenic stimulus are extruded from the tissue cells into the circulating blood in which they may be identified and measured. These antibodies, through the medium of the serum in which they are present, may be transferred to the blood stream of man already beleaguered by pneumococci and, by combining with the cocci, render them susceptible to the attack of the natural protective forces of the body. The chapters on antigenicity (X), antibody formation (XI), and host response (XII) enumerate the several antigenic elements of the pneumococcal cell with their common or individual characters, trace the activity of these constituents in the animal economy, and describe the nature of the antagonistic substances thus created.

Problems and Limitations of Serum Therapy

The immunologist has succeeded in raising the antibody content of the serum of experimental animals to a level high above that engendered by spontaneous pneumococcal disease in man, but specific immune serum, even though it be rich in these protective principles, cannot convey to the recipient those less tangible properties acquired by the tissues as a result of antigenic stimulation. This failure constitutes one limitation of serum treatment.

The variety of serological types of Pneumococcus presents another complication, since the serum to be effective must correspond in type to the organism causing the infection to be treated. Antipneumococcic serum, therefore, does not have the broad immunological species-specificity of diphtheria or tetanus antitoxin; its affinities are strictly specific for type. Moreover, no matter how rich in type-specific antibodies a serum may be, when the mass of infecting pneumococci exceeds a given amount—all other conditions being equal—the serum is powerless to stop the multiplication, invasion, and subsequent malignant activities of the organisms within the infected host. The interaction of antibodies and pneumococci does not operate strictly according to the law of multiple proportions, and this relation between concentration of specific antibody and living pneumococcal cells may determine the outcome of the infection. There are variations in this relation which are not yet understood. The ratio of amount of antibody to number of cocci is lower for Type I than for Type II. The utter inadequacy of Type III immune horse serum in the treatment of lobar pneumonia caused by organisms of that serological type is still one of the riddles of pneumococcal research.

The substitution of immune rabbit serum for immune horse serum in the treatment of lobar pneumonia holds promising possibilities. From the experimental standpoint, antipneumococcic serum produced in rabbits confers a greater degree of protection on mice in proportion to the content of specifically precipitable protein than does antipneumococcic serum obtained from horses. In mice, small amounts of cholesterol, cephalin, or materials rich in these lipids block the protective action of antipneumococcic horse serum but are without effect in the case of rabbit serum. In massive infections in laboratory animals there are optimal amounts of antipneumococcic horse serum which must be used in order to obtain successful results. Larger amounts are less efficacious and still larger amounts may have no protective action whatever. The prozone effect is not observed with antipneumococcic rabbit serum.

As compared with horses, rabbits almost invariably respond to pneumococcal immunization with the production of serum of good titer. If serum treatment is to be carried out in all cases due to any of the thirty or more serological types, the production of these serums would be greatly simplified by employing small animals rather than horses. It is also probable that the cost of producing immune rabbit serum may be less than the cost of producing concentrated antipneumococcic horse serum. Preliminary clinical trials with antipneumococcic rabbit serum have been sufficiently encouraging to invite further study of this seemingly important advance in the serum treatment of lobar pneumonia.*

The details of the mechanism by which immune serum overcomes pneumococcal infections are only partly known. When the immune serum is type-specific and high in antibody content, the cocci are clumped and possibly to some degree removed from the circulation

* The foregoing statements are the conclusions of Horsfall, Goodner, and MacLeod.[659]

by the filtering action of the viscera. Antibody, by combining with somatic or capsular substance of homologous pneumococci, inhibits some of the vital activities of the cells and renders them more susceptible to ingestion by leucocytes. The completeness of the phagocytosis and the ability of the body to dispose of any remaining free cocci determine whether recovery or death is to take place.

There are other unexplained aspects of serum action. Serum may bear components antagonistic to its own antibodies, creating a restricted zone of effective action. The phenomenon is involved in the question of the optimal dosage of serum—a question influenced by the potency of the particular lot of serum at hand and the type and severity of the infection to be treated. Underlying these specific immunological considerations is the non-specific factor represented by the physical ability of the patient to cope with the invading pneumococci. Debilitation from any cause detracts from the active properties of the serum, but the matter is one largely of clinical interest. There are conceivably as yet unknown qualities of human blood or human tissue cells as well as of pneumococci which may either augment or decrease the curative action of specific immune serum.

The conditions stipulated by Neufeld and Haendel[992-3] in 1912 for the successful use of antipneumococcic serum have been subject to only slight modification in the intervening years. Based on the German authors' recommendations, the following main directions should guide the physician if serum is to be administered to greatest advantage:

1. The serological type of Pneumococcus infecting the patient should be determined with minimal delay, and the serum should correspond immunologically to the infecting organism.

2. The serum should be of known high potency and injected intravenously at the earliest possible moment after diagnosis is established. It is during the incipiency of the disease before pneumonic consolidation is advanced and before invasion of the vascular system is massive that the *Schwellenwert* of the serum is theoretically at its highest. Se-

rum administered in the late stages of the disease may be harmful to the patient.

3. The dosage of serum to be given will depend on the potency of the preparation, the type of organism involved, the severity of the infection, and the presence of complications such as pregnancy.

Reliable directions for testing the patient for hypersensitiveness to serum protein, for the technique used in the actual administration of serum, and the details of the many clinical attentions to be accorded the pneumonia sufferer are to be found in Lord and Heffron's *Lobar Pneumonia and Serum Therapy.*[827]

In the array of experiences already reported in the literature, the foregoing conditions presumably have not always been fulfilled. Serum of low potency or of heterologous type has been employed; the dosage has been sometimes insufficient and at other times excessive; injections have often been delayed beyond the most favorable time in the course of the disease; and it is conceivable that the bedside care has not always been ideal. Other derogatory conditions may obscure the true value of serum treatment. Nevertheless, the accumulated statistics taken as a whole, and especially those culled from selected series of cases in which serum therapy has been applied with proper regard for the many contributing circumstances, prove the value of antipneumococcic serum as a remedial agent in some of the infections caused by Pneumococcus.

In the above summary, only those data have been selected that bear evidence of the past and present status of serum therapy. The ensuing discussion is borrowed entire from Lord and Heffron's *Lobar Pneumonia and Serum Therapy*, Chapter X, Results of Serum Treatment. The numbers given to bibliographical references have been changed to correspond with those in the present volume.

The Results of Serum Therapy

For the continued and productive study of lobar pneumonia and the early, persistent, and successful application of serum therapy, we are largely indebted to Cole and his associates at the Hospital of the Rockefeller Institute for Medical Research. Following the favorable report in 1913 by Cole and Dochez[267] on the treatment of Type I pneumococcus pneumonia, equally favorable reports from this source have from time to time been presented on an increasingly large number of cases. By 1929, Cole's[265] treated series numbered 371 with a case fatality rate of only 10.5 per cent. In addition to the low death rate in the treated group, such important supporting evidence as the cessation of spread, rapid appearance of protective antibodies in the blood, and the prevention or disappearance of blood invasion in consequence of specific therapy has been presented. In spite of these brilliant therapeutic results, the advantage of specific treatment was not generally recognized for some time. This was because the expected fatality rate in a large series of cases treated without serum had not been determined. The average fatality rate from a small early series of untreated Type I pneumonias was estimated at 25 to 30 per cent, and, convinced of the effectiveness of antiserum, Cole did not feel justified in withholding the treatment in a control series.

These fatality rates of cases treated with and without specific therapy have since been confirmed, but only after a long period of uncertainty on the part of the general medical profession. Unfortunately others had less striking success than Cole, and Locke's[820] report in 1923 of a death rate of 17.2 per cent in 145 serum treated cases (only 12 of which were treated in the first three days) and practically the same death rate, 16.9 per cent, in 71 untreated cases raised serious doubts in the minds of many regarding the merit of the procedure. These doubts were resolved by further determination of the comparative results with and without antiserum in contemporaneous series and an analysis of the treated group according to the time when specific treatment was begun. Among others, Lord; Cecil and Sutliff; Park, Bullowa and Rosenblüth; Finland; Cecil and Plummer; and Sutliff and Finland showed that successful specific treatment depends largely on its application early in the course of the disease.

For several hours after the administration of the initial doses of antiserum, no change in the patient is likely to be observed, but within eight to twenty-four hours after the first dose there is usually a marked improvement. This favorable response is likely to be more pronounced in the case of Type I than in the case of Type II infections and when patients are treated early. The patient becomes clearer mentally and begins to take an interest in his surroundings. Cyanosis and dyspnea may be completely relieved. In a large majority of the cases the temperature drops two or three degrees or more and does not again reach its former level (Figure 1). At the same time, though less rapidly, there is a fall in the rate of the pulse and respiration. In patients not treated with serum, Sutliff and Finland[1362] found that a much smaller proportion show symptomatic improvement and a sharp drop in temperature during the course of the disease. Following this initial fall in the temperature of serum treated cases, there may be a continued low-grade fever and lesser complaints for several days.

Studies by Sutliff and Finland on a series of serum treated cases compared with others not so treated indicate that the average duration of the more acute symptoms measured from onset to a persistent lowering of the temperature is shortened by about thirty hours in the serum treated group. The average duration of the low-grade fever following the relief of the more acute symptoms, however, is about the same in both groups. The disease runs a milder course following serum therapy.

An even more marked shortening of the acute illness in the treated as compared with control cases is reported in Great Britain by the Therapeutic Trials Committee of the Medical Research Council.[887] They find, on the average, that crisis occurred two and one-half days earlier in the treated than in the control Type I cases, and two days earlier in the treated than in the control Type II cases. In other instances where the progress of cases was analyzed in a different way, they note that, compared with the control cases, from four to seven times as many treated Type I cases show defervescence on or before the fifth day of illness, and from three to six times as many Type II cases.

FIGURE 1

COMPOSITE TEMPERATURE CHART OF 320 RECOVERED TYPE I CASES WHOSE TREATMENT WITH CONCENTRATED SERUM WAS BEGUN WITHIN 96 HOURS OF ONSET

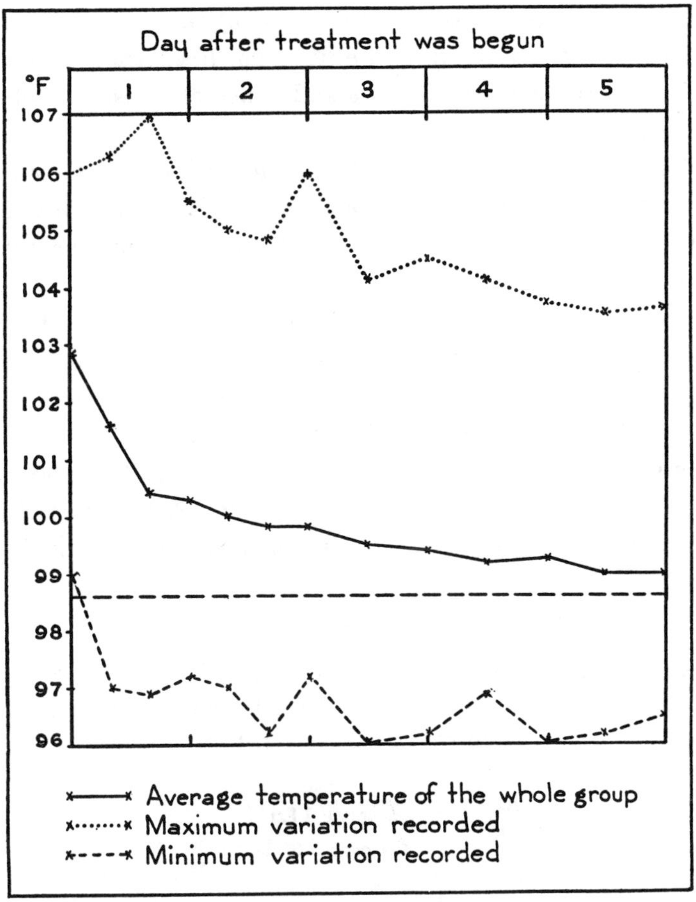

Temperatures are shown at eight-hour intervals for the first forty-eight hours after the beginning of treatment and then twice daily.

For 27 of the 320 cases treatment was begun on the first day of illness; for 101 on the second day; for 120 on the third day; for 72 on the fourth day.

Cases are taken from the Massachusetts Pneumonia Study. The remaining 128 recovered cases are not included as their temperature charts are not available or are inadequate for the purpose.

Specific serum therapy has a marked effect in preventing blood invasion, and blood cultures previously positive usually become negative within a few to twenty-four hours or more. The area of lung involvement with few exceptions ceases to spread. If extension occurs, it takes place slowly. By contrast, extension is frequent in those not treated with antiserum. Resolution appears to be unrelated to immunity factors and is not obviously affected by specific treatment.

Antiserum appears to have little or no effect in reducing such complications as endocarditis and meningitis. Observations in Great Britain[887] suggest that the incidence of empyema may be reduced.

The crucial test of the value of antiserum is its effect on the case fatality rate. The expected case fatality rate without specific therapy for Type I infections may be estimated from a large series of civilian cases, collected from the literature by Heffron, at about 25 per cent. Of 1,614 cases occurring in the United States and Canada, 403 or 25.0 per cent died (Figure 2). In Great Britain the fatality rate of Type I cases is somewhat lower than this.

FIGURE 2

TYPE I: COMPARISON OF DEATH RATES OF CASES WHOSE SERUM TREATMENT WAS BEGUN WITHIN NINETY-SIX HOURS OF ONSET AND OF CASES NOT GIVEN SERUM

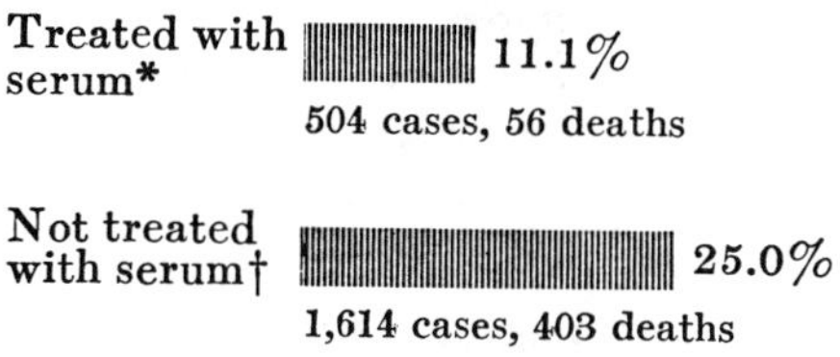

* Massachusetts Pneumonia Study cases.
† Cases collected from the literature.

With these figures for comparison, Heffron finds that of 2,458

Type I serum treated* cases in the literature, 384 or 15.6 per cent died, indicating the saving of many lives. The expected death rate of 25 per cent can be still further reduced, as shown by the results in the Massachusetts cases, when the treatment is begun within the first four days (ninety-six hours) of the onset. Of 504 cases thus treated with concentrated serum, only 56 or 11.1 per cent died (Figure 2). The importance of time is further emphasized by the figures shown in the accompanying table. Of 377 cases of Type I pneumonia treated within the first three days, only 32 or 8.5 per cent died. The death rate rises abruptly by the fourth day. Of the 127 cases treated on this day, 24 died, or 18.9 per cent.

TABLE I

TYPE I CASES TREATED WITH SERUM. NUMBER AND PERCENTAGE OF DEATHS BY DAY ON WHICH SERUM TREATMENT WAS BEGUN

Serum treatment begun	Number of cases	Deaths	
		Number	*Per cent*
In first three days	377	32	8.5
On fourth day	127	24	18.9
Total	*504*	*56*	*11.1*

NOTE: Cases were taken from the Massachusetts Pneumonia Study.

The fatality rate is, however, diminished when treatment is begun still later in the illness, but less strikingly than in the earlier period.

Similarly, Heffron has collected from the literature 992 Type II cases treated without serum in the United States and Canada, with 407 deaths, a fatality rate of 41.0 per cent (Figure 3). By contrast, he finds 670 antiserum treated* Type II infections in the literature with 205 deaths, or 30.6 per cent. Of 136 such cases in the Massachusetts series, treated with concentrated serum within four days (ninety-six hours) of onset, 37 died, a fatality rate of 27.2 per cent (Figure 3).

* With unconcentrated or concentrated serum in the United States or Canada.

Figure 3

TYPE II: COMPARISON OF DEATH RATES OF CASES WHOSE SERUM TREATMENT WAS BEGUN WITHIN NINETY-SIX HOURS OF ONSET AND OF CASES NOT GIVEN SERUM

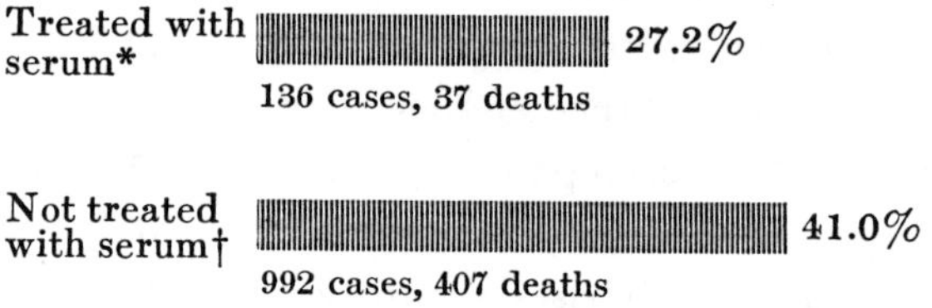

* Massachusetts Pneumonia Study cases.
† Cases collected from the literature.

The lowering of the death rate in the serum treated Type I and II cases in Massachusetts is of special importance in indicating that the method can be satisfactorily used by practicing physicians outside of large hospitals. Over one half were treated by physicians in general practice in the home or in small hospitals in the state.

Figure 4

TYPE I CASES TREATED WITH SERUM AND NOT TREATED WITH SERUM. NUMBER AND PERCENTAGE OF DEATHS BY AGE GROUP

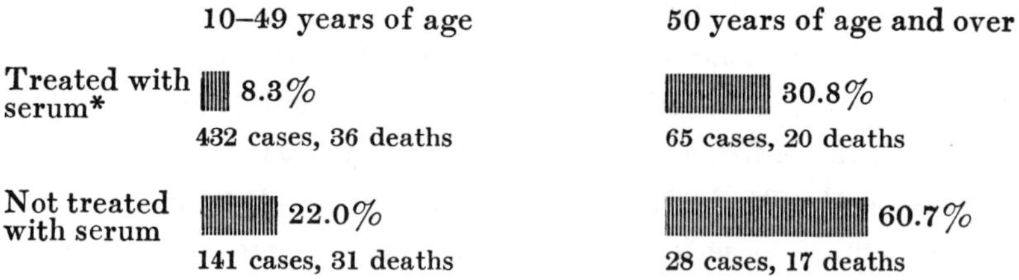

* Seven cases were not included as the age was not known.

Note: Cases were taken from the Massachusetts Pneumonia Study.

Advancing years is, in general, one of the most important factors in unfavorably modifying the outlook with lobar pneumonia. As shown in the accompanying figure (Figure 4), the case fatality rate is 22 per cent without and 8.3 per cent with specific treatment in patients from ten to fifty years of age, and 60.7 per cent without and 30.8 per cent with such treatment in patients fifty years of age and over. Analysis of the data with respect to the age of patients with and without specific therapy indicates that the favorable results of treatment cannot be ascribed to a difference in the ages of patients in the two groups.

As previously noted, bacteriemia occurs in about a quarter of Type I infections and in about a third of Type II infections. As shown in the accompanying figure (Figure 5), the occurrence of blood invasion in patients treated without antiserum greatly in-

FIGURE 5

TYPE I AND TYPE II CASES WITH AND WITHOUT BACTERIEMIA NOT TREATED WITH SERUM. NUMBER AND PERCENTAGE OF DEATHS

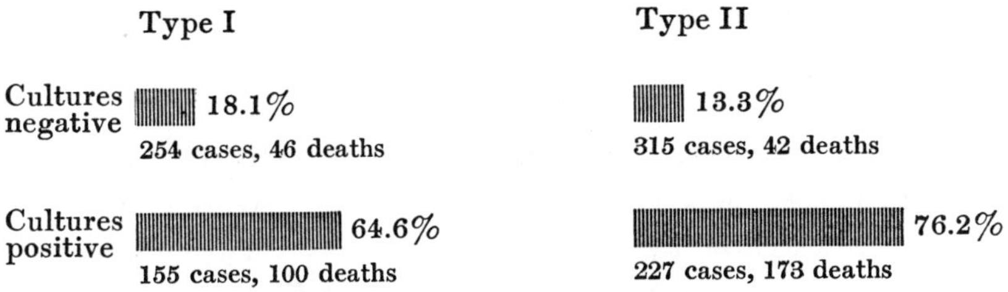

NOTE: Figures were collected from the literature. No cases of the Massachusetts Pneumonia Study were included.

creases the death rate. Thus the fatality rate in Type I cases with negative cultures is 18.1 per cent and with positive cultures 64.6 per cent. The situation is much the same with Type II infections, the death rate rising from 13.3 per cent with negative to 76.2 per cent with positive cultures. With bacteriemia, the death rate is thus about three to five times as great. The larger the number of organisms per cubic centimeter of blood, the more unfavorable the outlook.

As shown in Figure 6, specific treatment lowers the death rate in bacteriemic cases, in Type I infections from 64.6 to 31 per cent

FIGURE 6

TYPE I AND TYPE II CASES WITH BACTERIEMIA TREATED WITH SERUM AND NOT TREATED WITH SERUM. NUMBER AND PERCENTAGE OF DEATHS

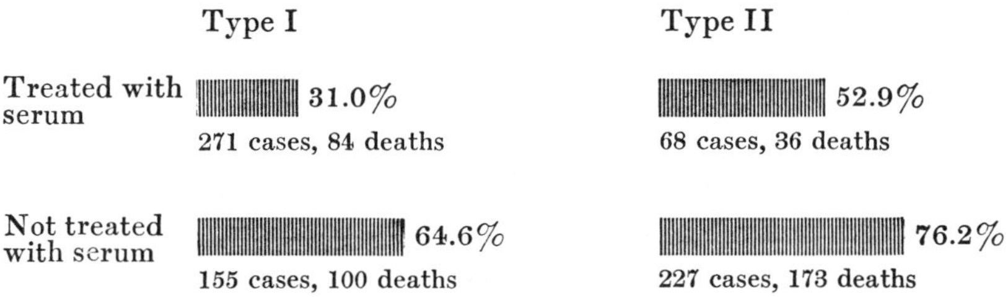

NOTE: Cases were collected from the literature. No cases from the Massachusetts Pneumonia Study were included.

and in Type II from 76.2 to 52.9 per cent. As shown in Figure 7, when serum treatment is given within the first four days (ninety-six hours) in Type I infections, the fatality rate is reduced to 26.2 per cent and in Type II to 54.2 per cent, the corresponding fatality rate with early specific treatment and negative cultures being respectively 5.2 per cent and 16.7 per cent.

With respect to the possibility that selection may have modified the case fatality rates of reported series, it may be assumed that exclusion of patients sensitive to horse serum from treated groups and their inclusion in control groups did not of itself modify the death rate. When the age has been averaged, it has been found to be approximately the same in the treated and the

Figure 7

TYPE I AND TYPE II CASES WITH AND WITHOUT BACTERIEMIA TREATED WITH SERUM. NUMBER AND PERCENTAGE OF DEATHS

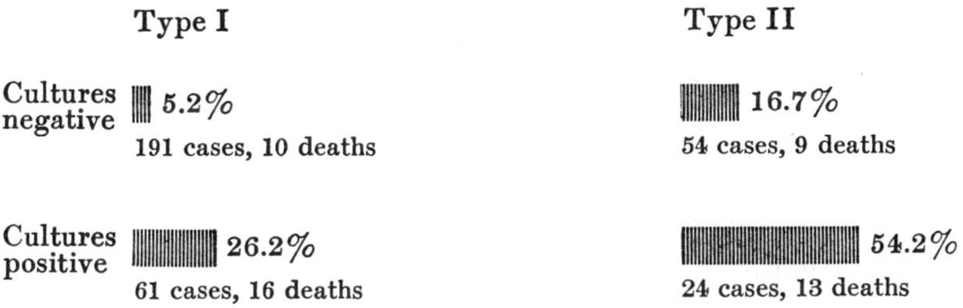

Note: Cases were taken from the Massachusetts Pneumonia Study.

untreated groups. The inauguration of treatment within the first four days makes it improbable that any important number of cases were excluded because in extremis from pneumococcus infection.

Certain avoidable causes of failure in the application of specific therapy may be briefly reviewed. Chief among these is the delay before beginning treatment. Second in importance is the lapse of time, previously often unavoidable, required for the determination of the type of infection and now largely obviated by the use of the Neufeld method. A third factor is the acceptance of other than Type I and Type II pneumococci in the sputum as the etiologic agent without repetition of the typing and a possible consequent error of about 10 per cent. Other causes may be the use of insufficient antiserum, low potency, or too long intervals between doses and failure to recognize the importance of administering more than the usual amount of antibody in severe cases and with pregnancy, during the post-partum period, and with bacteriemia.

Among unavoidable causes of failure, the presence of complications, and especially empyema, is not infrequent. Mixed infection with more than one type of pneumococcus, the streptococcus, or other organism may be present. Lastly, the infection may be so severe that specific treatment is ineffectual, or the infection may be overcome but the patient, exhausted by the struggle, succumbs.

Summary

A notable beginning has been made, but it is after all only a beginning. With the development of more potent and refined serum, possibly from an animal other than the horse, and a better knowledge of dosage, with a wider appreciation of the urgency of early diagnosis and prompt administration of serum, and with greater discrimination in the use of this biological agent, the doubts which linger in many a medical mind should be largely dissipated and specific serum treatment should advance to an even more important place than that which it now holds in the treatment of pneumonia.

CHAPTER XVII

UNSOLVED PROBLEMS

IMPRESSIVE as is the progress that has been made in Pneumococcus research, the subject holds almost endless possibilities for further investigation. Some of the metabolic activities of Pneumococcus, the processes operating in dissociation and type transformation, the exact chemical composition and precise antigenic properties of the pneumococcal cell, these are subjects, among many others, calling for continued study.

It is probable that the heights which may be achieved in the production of artificial immunity to Pneumococcus in man and in serum-producing animals have not been reached. Antipneumococcic serum, at best, leaves much to be desired in the way of purity and potency. There are many inviting leads and, with the application of rapidly developing chemical and serological methods, the years to come should be even more fruitful than those of the past.

TOXINS

The idea persists, in spite of many disappointing failures, that some of the symptoms incident to pneumococcal infection, especially those of lobar pneumonia, are caused by a soluble toxin. The idea is a reasonable one but convincing evidence to support it has never been presented. Among the varied activities of the pneumococcal cell a substance of this nature may be produced. It may exist in nascent or evanescent form or be present in such minute quantities as to escape detection. Conditions that exist in the animal body cannot be reproduced in full in lifeless media and therefore the environment supplied by artificial culture is quite different from that encountered by microorganisms in living tissues. There is the well-known influence of specific substrates on the biochemical activities and physiological processes of bacteria in revealing potential or latent functions not active or even suspected when the same cells are grown in ordinary media. Toxins as such may not be elaborated by pneumococci themselves in an artificial substrate but may possibly be a secondary product of the interaction between the bacteria and the cells of the host. The question is by no means closed.

SEROLOGICAL TYPES

The present division of pneumococci into thirty-two distinct serological types may not be all-inclusive. Further study of strains at present considered as unclassifiable and continued search of fresh material will undoubtedly add other specific types to the list, although the operation of the law of diminishing returns is inevitable.

There is increasing need for a central source of type-specific diagnostic serum to ensure the accuracy and uniformity of type-determination throughout this and other countries. The problem is largely an administrative one but the requirements come from bacteriologists, immunologists, and epidemiologists. The movement to establish such a center is to be strongly encouraged, and might well be included in the deliberations of the Health Organization of the League of Nations.

DISSOCIATION

A reconciliation of the many descriptions of pneumococcal variants is greatly to be desired. Modifications A to Zed, the bizarre forms, the mucoid, smooth, and rough variants should be sorted into a uniform, descriptive grouping, and the designations, if possible, should be made to conform to those of similar variant forms of other bacterial species.

The unknown principle in the virulent pneumococcal cell which has the remarkable ability not only to restore a degraded form to its original condition of type-specificity, but which also can actually transform the degraded variant into a member of a different serological type, invites further study.

Does dissociation of pneumococci proceed in the animal body? At present the answer is, Probably not; but the manner in which the many types of pneumococci have arisen may some day be discovered to be related to the influences that cause variation, reversion, and transformation of type.

The supposition that the close relation apparently existing between pneumococci and streptococci denotes a divergent evolution from a common progenitor does not bear analysis in a genetic sense. Bacteria are unicellular organisms reproducing by the elementary process of fission and it is far more likely that environmental influences induce or result in more or less transient physiological or protoplasmic changes that are wholly or in part reversible when the cells grow under other conditions. The recognition of the stability of biological types or species, therefore, leads rather to continued study of the cultural factors that bring about temporary modifications in bacterial characters.

CHEMICAL CONSTITUENTS OF PNEUMOCOCCI

The knowledge gained in the last score of years concerning the chemical nature of the components of the pneumococcal cell furnishes abundant material for a broad program of future biochemical and immunological studies. How closely do the proteins and polysaccharides thus far isolated correspond in molecular configuration to the parent substances as they exist in the living, intact cell? What are the relationships between chemical constitution and biological specificity? What is the exact grouping and what are the linkages of radicals that determine for a strain its type-identity? Are there actually antigenic and haptenic groups in some of the specific carbohydrates, or are antibody stimulation and antibody combination only quantitative manifestations of the same phenomenon? How can one account for the partial serological similarities or differences between the polysaccharides of the present pneumococcal types and the polysaccharides of other bacteria and non-living substances?

What is the importance of the chemical configuration of the molecule as a whole and the role of determinant groups in orienting the specificity of the immune response in animals? What is the nature of the chemical processes in the bodies of animals of different species which deal with one and the same antigenic substance in such diverse ways after it reaches the tissues? For example, it is possible that a complex antigen may be broken down to non-antigenic form or to a simple hapten-like substance, so modified by conjugation or synthesis within the tissues that it acquires new antigenic properties—the result depending not only upon the chemical nature of the substance introduced and the route of its administration, but also upon the chemical changes brought about in the particular tissue or animal species tested.

These are some of the problems that confront the chemist and the immunologist. Perhaps the isolation of specific polysaccharides from pneumococci of the remaining unstudied types, from unrelated organisms, and from other sources, and an investigation into the more minute details of the molecular mosaic of these higher carbohydrates, may provide clues to the solution of some of these problems.

The fact that bacterial enzymes capable of decomposing capsular polysaccharides of the different pneumococcal types have more avid and more discriminating selective affinities for capsular polysaccharides than homologous antibodies have for specific antigens, may lead to the clarification of some of the questions of chemo-immunological specificity.

VIRULENCE

Why a strain of Pneumococcus should be virulent for one species of animal and avirulent for another is a question that awaits answer, and the question is not a simple one. There are the elements in pneumococci that endow them with invasive powers and, among these elements, the type-specific capsular polysaccharide may be the principal determinant. The reasons for the differences in the virulence characteristic of pneumococcal types, of individual members within the types, and of variant forms may be linked with capsule formation, but that is only one element of this vital character. The unusual virulence of Type III pneumococci for man as compared with animals, and the invasiveness of some strains for rabbits and the harmlessness of others are striking examples of the problems to be studied. There are also marked differences in host response among various animal species and among animals within the species, and here the matter is largely beyond our ken.

Are the capsular polysaccharides toxic in themselves, or do they combine with tissue elements to produce poisonous effects or, as is now being discovered in the case of the polysaccharides of certain bacteria of the enteric group, do these carbohydrates, possibly linked with lipids, exist in a still more complex form than any yet isolated?

METHODS FOR THE PRODUCTION OF ACTIVE IMMUNITY

Procedures for the creation of active immunity in animals and in man are in a state of development. The ideal immunizing antigen and the most effective scheme for administering the antigen are yet to be found. The polysaccharides of Pneumococcus either alone or in a form to be discovered or invented may prove to be the sought-for agent. The possibilities are manifold.

Is it the protective antibody which must especially be striven for or are other immune substances also required to build resistance to infection? What part—if any—do heterophile antibodies contribute and, more particularly than we now know, what part do the somatic cells play in protecting the infected host, and do other physiological factors share in creating the immune state?

The serum of animals immunized by the injection of pneumococcal materials, besides bearing specific antibodies, contains substances antagonistic to the activity of the antibodies and limiting the protective action of the serum. By what means can these inhibitory substances be neutralized or eliminated?

Are the zonal effects observed in serological reactions and in protective experiments ascribable wholly to the capsular polysaccharide of Pneumococcus or may they be, in part at least, produced by serum lipids? To what extent are these effects dependent upon the quantitative relations existing at the time between antigen and antibody and the solubility of the immune complex so formed?

CHEMOTHERAPY

A suitable and harmless drug with high selective affinity for the protoplasm or capsular substance of Pneumococcus is wanting. The field of chemotherapy in pneumococcal infections, promising as it is, abounds in difficulties. The narrow limits between poisonous, untoward effects and therapeutic action in the animal body, the selective affinity of the agents for somatic protein or capsular carbohydrate of bacteria, and the action of the drug in inhibiting some essential physiological function, impairing the metabolic processes, or bringing about morphological changes in both bacterial and body cells, are problems that should entice rather than discourage the investigator.

At present, cinchona would appear to offer a promising source from which to prepare agents capable of specific pneumococcidal action. In the myriad of compounds now being synthesized in the chemical laboratory a key substance may be found.

IMMUNOLOGICAL RESPONSE

The comparative response of animals of different species to the introduction of pneumococcal antigens by diverse parenteral routes perplexes the immunologist. Antigen injected into the skin of the rabbit results in the appearance of species-specific but not of type-specific antibodies in the serum; antigen injected into a vein of the same animal evokes the formation of antibodies of strict type-specificity homologous with the type of antigen employed. If the nature of the tissue reaction in each case could be discovered, our conception of immunological processes would acquire further definition.

The local fixation of bacteria at the site of injection into the skin of rabbits may allow opportunity for the action of tissue enzymes to inactivate or dissociate capsular antigen of the bacterial cell, leading to or accounting for the diminution or loss of type-specific response. The assumption is susceptible of proof.

ANTIBODIES AND ANIMAL SPECIES

The immunological differences between antipneumococcic serum produced in rabbits and that produced in horses have been mentioned in earlier parts of the text. There may be, of course, quantitative differences in the antibody content of the two serums; the antibody may exist in one fraction of one and in another fraction of the other serum, and its affinity for antigen may be modified by its particular conjugation with some serum component. We are now learning that the molecular size of the antibody or the physical state in which antibody exists in immune serum may account for these differences in serological behavior.

SKIN REACTIONS

The history of the phenomena to be observed following the intradermal injection of pneumococcal materials is incomplete and confused. The diversity of antigenic preparations employed, and the variety of inflammatory reactions induced in the cutaneous tissues and classed as positive, largely account for the confusion. The antigens comprising somatic protein and carbohydrate and capsular polysaccharide should be prepared in accordance with the most advanced technique and should be selected as representative of the chemical and immunological individuality interpreted in terms of the specific reactions of the organisms as a whole. The local effects following the introduction of pneumococcal antigens into the skin should be more clearly defined and classified and all interpretations should be based on such definition and classification.

The problems involved in the several kinds of reactions elicited, their relation to the clinical course of infection, and their interpretation in respect to preexisting or newly developing states of hypersensitiveness and immunity are still to be studied and solved. Recent studies of the somatic C polysaccharide suggest that certain forms of reactivity, both serological and cutaneous, are not specific in an immunological sense, but are rather an expression of chemical changes in the blood associated with the acute stage of active infection.

THE NATURE OF PNEUMOCOCCAL ANTIBODY

The behavior of antibodies of immune serum in the presence of protein precipitants and the molecular size of the immune substances as determined by ultracentrifugation and ultrafiltration lead to the tentative assumption that these antibodies represent modified forms of serum proteins, having in general the chemical properties of globulins. The isolation by advanced methods of antibody or antibodies in purer form than that in which they have been previously obtained promises to be a desirable point of departure for further inquiry into the chemical nature of antibodies, the elucidation of the mechanism of immunological reaction, and for the development of a more efficient therapeutic serum.

CONCENTRATION OF ANTIPNEUMOCOCCIC SERUM

Methods for concentrating and refining antipneumococcic serum have undergone notable improvement, but it cannot be claimed that the agent approaches the perfection of diphtheria and tetanus antitoxin. Raw serum of greater potency is the first requisite, and then there must be devised chemical procedures which will make it possible to separate the desired antibody or antibodies from the immunologically inert and frequently undesirable components of serum without at the same time denaturing or unduly destroying the wanted immune substances. The economical concentration of the unimpaired curative principles of serum in small bulk in a solution of bland physiological action is the goal to be striven for. From a purely practical standpoint, if antipneumococcic serum is to render its greatest service, aside from an appreciable lowering of the cost of the product, the elimination of superfluous protein and of antagonistic or chill-producing substances constitutes a step of more immediate need.

POTENCY TESTS ON THERAPEUTIC SERUM

The early proximal or presumptive tests employed for estimating the curative value of antipneumococcic serums have gradually been supplanted by methods that ensure a greater degree of accuracy in measuring the antibody content of the product. Great as has been the effort expended in devising a technique that will at the same time be simple and exact and afford a reliable index of the curative value of the product, no method so far devised can be looked upon as ideal. The principles involved are discouragingly more complex than those met in the titration of antitoxic serums. The direction that further endeavors should take is toward economy of means and time and a closer correlation between antibody titer and therapeutic strength. It is now generally taken for granted that precipitin and protective titer are the only factors to be considered, but the possible importance of allied antibodies should not be overlooked.

The fairly successful production of specific serum for Type I infections encourages efforts to prepare a product of enhanced potency for Type II pneumonia and to attack from new angles the baffling puzzle presented by Type III Pneumococcus. The development of monovalent immune rabbit serums for these types and for the types of relatively low incidence holds promising possibilities.

SUMMARY

There are, of course, many knotty problems regarding the epidemiology of lobar pneumonia; the nature of contributory factors and altered physiological states associated with the occurrence and onset of the disease; the carrier state; the mode of dissemination of the infectious agent; the portal of entrance and pathways of infection in the body; and the mechanism of crisis and recovery. These problems, while involved in the larger domain of the biology of Pneumococcus, are of less immediate interest to the bacteriologist and immunologist than to the epidemiologist, the physiologist, the pathologist, and the clinician.

Opportunities for inquiries into the ways of Pneumococcus are by no means exhausted. The prosecution of future studies on the life activities of Pneumococcus cannot fail to bring new gold to the abundant store of solid bullion already accumulated. Those workers who are not as yet engaged in this field of biological research, as well as those who are already devoting their energies to solving the riddles presented by this amazing bacterial cell, may, it is hoped, gain some enlightenment and possibly a few prospects in the foregoing reexamination and appraisal of our gains.

APPENDIX

SPECIAL METHODS USED IN THE STUDY OF PNEUMOCOCCUS AND IN THE PREPARATION OF ANTIPNEUMOCOCCIC SERUM

I. Media

PNEUMOCOCCUS BROTH FOR ALL GENERAL PURPOSES (Rockefeller Institute. Courtesy of Miss Dorothy Sloan)

Beef heart	1 pound
Peptone (Witte or Pfanstiehl)	10 grams
Sodium chloride	5 grams
Tap water	1 liter

The beef hearts are obtained directly from the slaughter-house and after immediately removing all fat, the muscle is ground fine. For every 10 liters of water add 10 lb. of minced heart muscle and 500 cc. extra of water. Stir and skim off fat rising to the surface. Repeat stirring and skimming ten times. Place in refrigerator overnight, heat to 85° for one-half hour, then filter through Prat-Dumas No. 50 or other coarse filter paper. Add peptone and salt, reheat to boiling and add sufficient N sodium hydroxide to bring the reaction of the medium to pH 8.2. Boil for 5 minutes and filter immediately through coarse paper. Sterilize in the Arnold sterilizer for one hour on each of 3 successive days. The final reaction should be pH 7.8.

For the production of massive amounts of pneumococci, the medium in which the Pfanstiehl peptone is used is inoculated with 100 to 150 cc. of an 8-hour culture in plain broth for every 3,000 cc. of medium. The maximal growth will have occurred in 8 to 10 hours under these circumstances, but the yield of organisms is greatly increased by the addition of 0.10 per cent dextrose after 8 hours' incubation. Following the addition of dextrose, incubation is carried out for one to one and one-half hour; longer incubation will render the medium too acid and rapid autolysis will result. The resulting growth is immediately collected by means of a specially constructed Sharples centrifuge.

NUTRIENT BROTH FOR MASS CULTURES FOR THE PRODUCTION OF SOLUBLE SPECIFIC SUBSTANCES (Courtesy of Dr. F. D. Hager)

a. *Preparation of infusion.* Fresh horse meat is ground and mixed with aliquot parts of chipped ice and cold tap water. The mixture is stored in earthenware jars in the cold room for 3 to 5 days and is stirred at intervals. After most of the ice has melted, the mixture is transferred to aluminum kettles, heated to boiling, strained through cheesecloth, and the cake of coagulated meat pressed as nearly dry as possible in a meat press. The strained liquid part of the infusion is collected in 5-gallon Pyrex carboys and autoclaved at 120° for 45 minutes. Air is then forced into the autoclave to keep the pressure at 15 to 20 pounds until the temperature falls to about 80° or 90°. The crude, sterilized extract is stored in the cold room.

b. *Preparation of medium.* The crude infusion is filtered in the cold room through soft filter paper. It is siphoned from the carboy to avoid disturbing the layer of partly solidified fat which collects on the surface. Unless the infusion is to be used for producing Type III SSS, it is best to remove the glycogen as follows:

The infusion is evaporated to about one-tenth its original volume, and the glycogen precipitated by the addition of two volumes of 95 per cent alcohol to one of infusion. The glycogen is separated by centrifugation. The glycogen-free infusion is then distilled under reduced pressure in a water-bath to free it from alcohol.

The glycogen-free, alcohol-free infusion is then made up to its original volume with tap water, and to it is added peptone (Witte or Pfanstiehl) to a concentration of 1 per cent. The solution is filtered through soft paper into a 5-gallon Pyrex carboy and autoclaved as described above.

The infusion-peptone solution may be diluted with an equal volume of tap water before autoclaving and use. This step results in a higher yield of polysaccharide per volume of infusion, but requires the handling of larger amounts of fluid. Prior to inoculation, the medium is stored in the incubator room for a sufficient time in order that it may reach the proper temperature.

A 30 to 40 per cent solution of glucose is added to the medium in amounts to give a final concentration of 1 per cent. The glucose is sterilized separately to prevent the formation of colored products which are difficult to separate from the capsular polysaccharide.

The alkali solution used in neutralizing the acid formed during growth is sterilized in the Arnold sterilizer for 30 minutes in calibrated Pyrex flasks fitted with a stopper bearing an air filter and a glass tube which reaches to the bottom of the flask. The other end of the tube is fastened to a rubber tube of sufficient length to reach from the flask of alkali solution to the stopper of the carboy of medium. When half-strength medium is used or when the reaction is to be kept acid, 5 per cent NaOH is preferred; otherwise 10 per cent NaOH is more convenient.

c. *Growing the pneumococci.* There is placed in the carboy of medium a stopper which carries: (1) A mechanical stirrer of the usual sealed type; cresol solution is used as the sealing liquid. (2) An inlet tube to which the rubber tube from the flask of alkali solution can be attached. (3) An inlet tube through which can be added the glucose solution, defibrinated blood, and culture. (4) A sampling tube through which samples may be removed from the carboy without undue risk of contamination. The stirrer, stopper, and tubing are sterilized separately.

To the medium are added the glucose solution and about 50 cc. of defibrinated blood. The carboy is then placed on a stand so arranged that the stirrer can be driven by a motor and that the flask of alkali solution can be connected with the carboy. Alkali solution is then added to the medium in an amount sufficient to adjust the reaction to a pH of 7.0 or of 8.0 to 8.5 depending upon whether acetyl SSS or the ordinary SSS is to be made. The medium should be thoroughly stirred when the alkali is added.

Very late in the day about 5.0 cc. of an 8-hour culture of Pneumococcus is added to each carboy, the mixture stirred a few minutes, and the organisms allowed to grow overnight. By morning the pH will have fallen to about 4.5. The reaction is then readjusted to pH 7.0 or 8.0 to 8.5; the medium requires readjustment the same evening and both morning and evening of the second full day of growth, after which time adjustment of the reaction once a day will suffice. In the early stages of growth, a pH of 8.8 will not kill the culture. Appreciable acid production ceases after about a week.

The cultures are kept for about two weeks before starting preparation of capsular polysaccharide. The methods of Heidelberger, Avery, and their colleagues are followed in purifying the substance.

Blood Broth

Plain broth or hormone medium to which defibrinated rabbit, horse, or human blood is added to 0.05 to 5 per cent concentration when the medium is cool. Rabbit blood is preferable.

Inulin Serum Water (Rockefeller Monograph No. 7[36])

For the determination of inulin fermentation by Pneumococcus, the following medium devised by Hiss is used, a positive reaction being indicated by the production of acid and the coagulation of serum protein. Clear beef serum is added to 2 or 3 volumes of distilled water. Heat the mixture for 15 minutes in an Arnold sterilizer at 100° to destroy ferments present in the serum. Add 5 per cent aqueous litmus solution to a concentration of 1 per cent or an amount sufficient to give a deep blue color. Add inulin (C.P.) to the serum water to a concentration of 1 per cent. The inulin solution may best be sterilized by autoclaving at 15 pounds pressure for 15 minutes. Sterilize the inulin serum water by the fractional method at 100°.

Author's Note: An alcoholic solution of bromcresol purple is preferable to the litmus solution as an indicator.

II. Isolation of Pneumococcus

Mouse Method (Rockefeller Monograph No. 7[36])

a. *Mouse inoculation.* A small portion of the sputum, about the size of a bean, is selected and washed through three or four changes of sterile salt solution in sterile Esmarch or Petri dishes to remove surface contaminations. When the sputum is too friable or when the specimen is relatively free from secondary organisms, this washing process may be omitted. In either event, the kernel of sputum selected is transferred to a sterile mortar, ground up, and emulsified with about 1.0 cubic centimeter of sterile bouillon or salt solution, added drop by drop, until a homogeneous emulsion is obtained that will readily pass through the needle of a small syringe. With a sterile syringe, 0.5 to 1.0 cc. of this emulsion is inoculated intraperitoneally into a white mouse. Pneumococcus grows rapidly in the mouse peritoneum, while the majority of other organisms rapidly die off, with the exception of Friedländer's bacillus, *Bacillus influenzae,* and occasionally *Micrococcus catarrhalis,* Staphylococcus, and Streptococcus. Pneumococcal invasion of the blood stream also occurs early. *Bacillus influenzae,* if present, likewise invades the blood stream; other organisms, as a rule, do not. The time elapsing before there is sufficient growth of Pneumococcus in the mouse peritoneum for the satisfactory determination of type varies with the individual case, depending upon the abundance of pneumococci in the specimen of sputum and the virulence and invasiveness of the strain present. It may be from 5 to 24 hours, averaging 6 to 8 hours with the parasitic fixed Types I, II, and III. As soon as the injected mouse appears sick, a drop of peritoneal exudate is removed by means of peritoneal puncture with a sterile capillary pipette, spread on a slide, stained by Gram's method, and examined microscopically to determine whether there is an abundant growth of Pneumococcus present. If there is an abundant growth of Pneumococcus alone, the mouse is killed and the determination of type carried out. If the growth is only moderate, or if other organisms are present in any quantity, additional time must be allowed until subsequent examination of the peritoneal exudate shows an abundant growth of Pneumococcus. It should be emphasized that undue haste in killing the mouse is time lost in the end.

b. *Mouse necropsy.* As soon as the mouse is killed or dies, the peritoneal cavity is opened under sterile precautions and cultures are made from the exudate in plain broth and on one-half of a blood-agar plate. Films are made and stained for microscopic examination by Gram's stain and Hiss's capsule stain. The peritoneal exudate is then washed out by means of a sterile glass pipette with 4 to 5 cc. of sterile salt solution, the washings being placed in a centrifuge tube. Cultures are then made from the heart's blood in plain broth and on the other half of the blood-agar plate. The essential steps in the procedures given above are shown in the accompanying Chart 1.

PLATING METHODS (Zinsser and Bayne-Jones[1579])

Although the methods used in preparing and using blood agar vary, the following illustrate accepted procedures:

a. *Preparation of blood agar*

(1) Melt 100 cc. of meat infusion or Douglas' agar (pH 7.4 to 7.8) in a flask.

(2) Allow to cool to 45° to 50°.

(3) Add 5 cc. of sterile defibrinated rabbit or horse blood.

(4) Mix and pour into Petri dishes or transfer into tubes for slants as desired.

(5) Incubate for 24 hours at 37° to test sterility.

b. *Use of blood agar*

(1) Material to be cultured on blood agar for the isolation or preliminary identification of Pneumococcus may be streaked on the surface of blood-agar plates, either by platinum loops or wires, or by placing a drop of the material on the surface of the medium and then spreading the inoculum over the surface with a bent, sterile capillary pipette. Dilutions of the material in peptone water or broth may be made prior to streaking, depending upon the source.

(2) For colony counts and for studying the activities of pneumococcal colonies in blood agar, the usual procedure is to dilute the culture to an extent that will provide well-isolated colonies, using peptone water as a diluent; measured amounts of the diluted culture, usually 0.5 cc., are transferred to duplicate Petri dishes, and as soon as possible, liquid blood agar at a temperature of 45° to 50° is poured into the dishes. The contents are mixed by gentle rotary motions of the plates, care being taken to avoid splashing or bubbling of the medium.

Blood Cultures (adapted from Zinsser and Bayne-Jones[1579])

Blood is drawn in the usual manner, observing surgical precautions and strict aseptic technique. After the blood is drawn, it should be immediately transferred to the proper medium, for which the usual infusion agar (as referred to under blood agar) and Pneumococcus broth are equally satisfactory.

At least six tubes of agar should be melted and immersed in water at about 45°. Before blood is mixed with the medium, the agar should be cooled to about 41°. The blood is added to the tubes in varying quantities, ranging from 0.25 to 1.0 cc. each, in order that different degrees of concentration may be obtained. Mixing is accomplished by the usual dipping and rotary motion, the formation of air-bubbles being thus avoided. The mouth of each test tube should be flamed before pouring the contents into the plates.

Three flasks of broth suitable for development of Pneumococcus, each containing 100 to 150 cc. of medium, should be inoculated with varying quantities of blood—at least one of the flasks containing the blood in high dilution. It may be advisable to place in the flasks of broth, in addition to glucose, 1 gram of powdered calcium carbonate to inhibit the action of acid on the pneumococci.

For quantitative work, accurately measured amounts of blood should be seeded in blood agar, preferably placing the blood in the Petri dishes, pouring in the melted and cooled agar, and mixing with a gentle rotary motion.

III. Type Determination

Mouse Method (Sabin[1208])

One cc. of a fresh sample of sputum is injected intraperitoneally into a mouse. From 3 to 4 hours later, some of the peritoneal fluid is obtained by puncture with a glass capillary. A glass slide is marked off into four parts, and a minute drop of the peritoneal fluid is expelled on each one of the four partitions. The first is smeared with saline solution for control, and the others with a loopful of 1:10 dilution of Type I and of Type II, and a 1:5 dilution of Type III diagnostic serums, respectively. These dilutions of serum are chosen largely to eliminate group agglutinins. Thin smears are made, allowed to dry, and fixed by passing the slide through a flame; they are then stained for from 20 to 30 seconds with a fuchsin solution (10 cc. saturated alcoholic solution of basic fuchsin plus 90 cc. of water) or any other available stain. The stain is washed off in water or 20 per cent copper sulfate solution, and the smears are examined with the oil immersion lens. If a specific agglutination reaction is observed in one of the smears with diagnostic serum, the organism is of that type. If no reaction occurs in any of the smears and numerous pneumococci are clearly seen, a diagnosis of Group IV is suggested. When it is desired to know whether the organism is one of the fixed types of Group IV (especially those for which concentrated antiserums are available) a similar procedure is carried out with the homologous immune serums.

Bacteria other than pneumococci in the sputum as well as avirulent forms of pneumococci may occur in clumps in the peritoneal exudate; but these differ in appearance from those produced by specific agglutination and can be distinguished further by their occurrence in the saline control smear. Unless a fresh sample of sputum is used, many of the organisms will have undergone autolysis, and therefore more time must be allowed for growth. Since the mouse is not killed, another type determination can be made if the first should show insufficient organisms, and then after the death of the mouse, the type may be confirmed.

In the case of Type III pneumococci, sufficient organisms are usually present even two hours after injection. The appearance of the specific reaction with Type III pneumococci, primarily on account of the larger size of the capsule, differs somewhat from that obtained with pneumococci of other types; the organisms are farther apart in the agglutinated clumps which occur in mucoid strands. When diagnostic serums for pneumococci of types formerly in Group IV are used, a dilution must be chosen that fails to show any cross-agglutination with any other type.

The peritoneal exudate may contain too many organisms four hours after inoculation or after death of the mouse, so that it may be necessary to dilute the fluid in the capillary tube with saline solution in order to obtain a correct typing. This method is illustrated in Chart 1.

Krumwiede Method (Krumwiede and Valentine[762])

A small amount of sputum (3 to 10 cc.) is transferred to a test tube and placed in boiling water for a few minutes until coagulation occurs. The coagulum is broken up with a heavy platinum wire or glass rod and sufficient saline solution added to give just enough fluid after centrifuging. The suspension is again placed in boiling water for a few minutes to extract the soluble antigen from the coagulum, and is shaken several times during the heating process. The mixture is centrifuged and the clear supernatant fluid used for the test.

For the test, 0.2 cc. amounts of undiluted typing serum are placed in narrow test tubes and the antigen carefully layered over the serum. The tubes are placed in a water-bath at 50° to 55° and examined after several minutes. A definite contact ring occurs in the tube containing homologous serum if the sputum is rich in antigen. The true ring is more or less opaque and in the majority of positive reactions is evident in less than 10 minutes. The success of the test depends upon the quality of the sputum. If coagulation does not occur, there is little use in continuing the test (see Chart 1).

Neufeld Quellung Method (Beckler and MacLeod[96])

There are variations in the application of the Neufeld *Quellung* phenomenon to the determination of pneumococcal types in sputum samples. The one given here is the technique used in the Bacteriological Laboratory of the Massachusetts Department of Public Health.

Upon receipt of the sputum at the laboratory, stained liquid mounts of the specimen are mixed with undiluted rabbit antiserums (Types I to XXXII). Combinations of monovalent antiserums (rabbit) are used instead of making separate preparations of the sputum with each of the thirty-two monovalent serums. The combinations of serums used are:

Type I
A, Types II, IV, V, and VII
B, Types III and VIII
C, Types IX, XI, XIII, and XV
D, Types VIa, VIb, XVII, and XVIII
E, Types XII, XIV, XVI, and XXVIII
F, Types X, XIX, XX, and XXI
G, Types XXII, XXIII, XXIV, and XXV
H, Types XXVII, XXIX, XXX, XXXI, and XXXII

Nine loopfuls of sputum are placed approximately one inch apart on a 9 by 2 inch glass slide; to each drop are added 2 loopfuls of the anti-

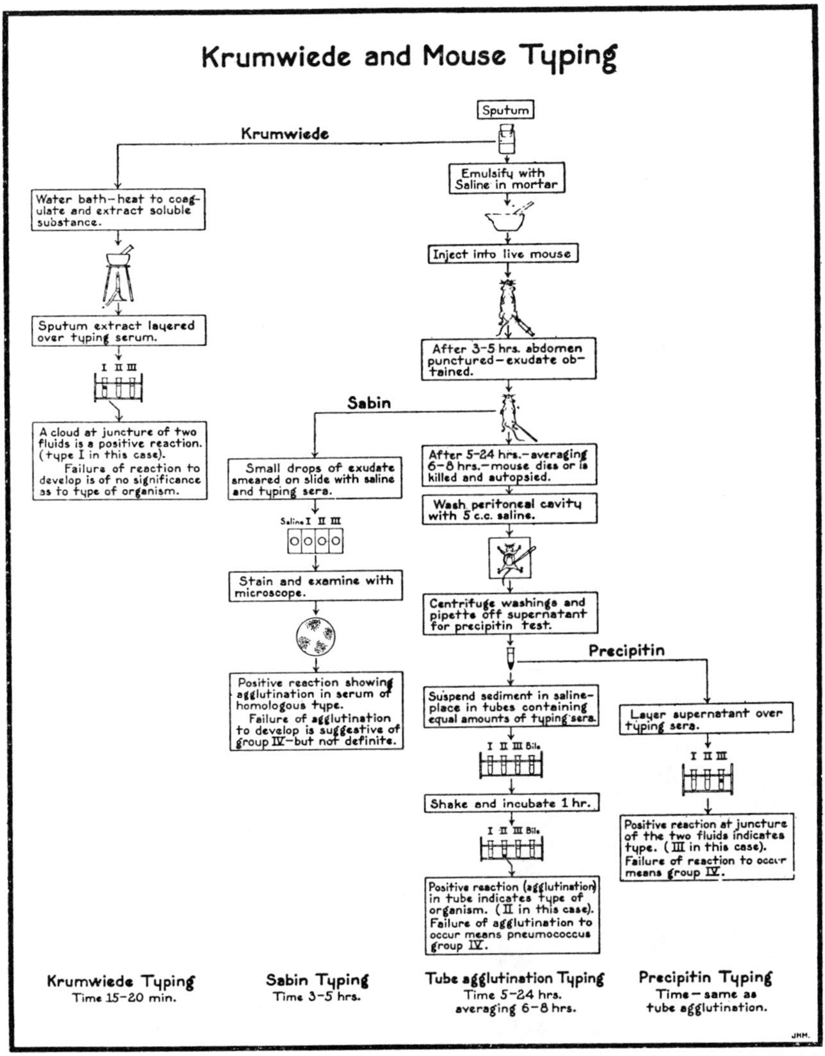

Courtesy of Massachusetts Department of Public Health

CHART I. KRUMWIEDE AND SABIN METHODS OF TYPE DETERMINATION

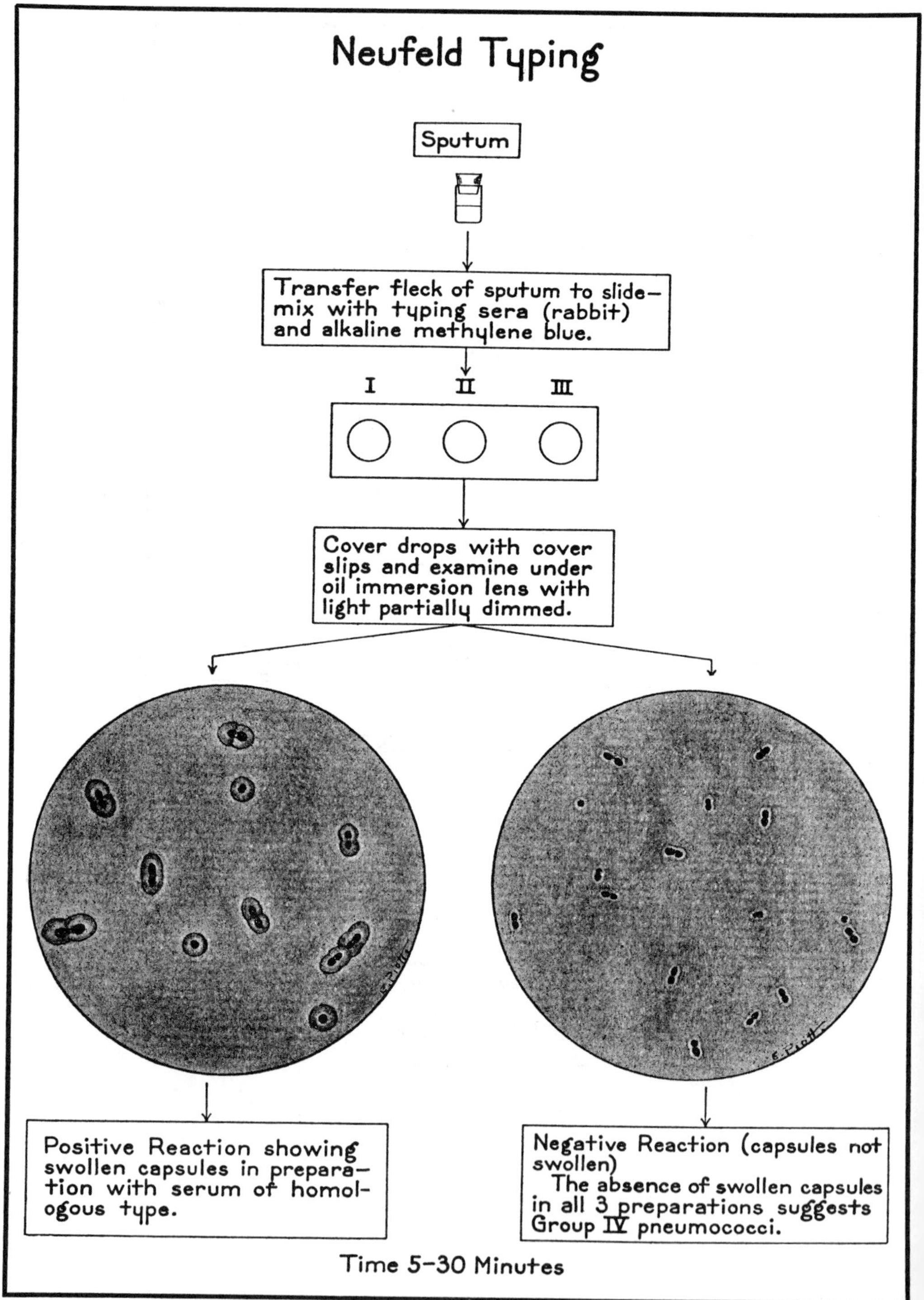

Courtesy of Massachusetts Department of Public Health

CHART 2. THE NEUFELD OR QUELLUNG METHOD OF TYPE DETERMINATION serum, that is, the first drop is mixed with Type I antiserum, the second drop with combined serum A (II, IV, V, and VII), the third drop with B, et cetera. The preparations are stained with Loeffler's alkaline methylene blue (2 drops to each mixture) and are covered at once with cover-slips to prevent drying. Examination is made with the oil immersion lens, with the light dimmed. When a positive reaction occurs, which is usually within a few minutes, there is a decided swelling of the capsule of the pneumococcus present. The swollen capsule is of a light greenish-gray color, is much less translucent than one that is not swollen, and has a definite outline which is one of the most characteristic features of a positive reaction. In the preparations in which no reaction is evident, the capsule of the pneumococcus appears as a halo of refracted light. In all preparations the body of the pneumococcus stains a definite blue. If the reaction is observed in drop 1, then the pneumococcus present is Type I and can be reported immediately; if the reaction is observed in drop 3, for example, the test is repeated using 2 drops of the sputum mixed with Type III and Type VIII undiluted monovalent rabbit serums, respectively; if the reaction is observed in drop 9, five loopfuls of the sputum are mixed with Type XXVII, XXIX, XXX, XXXI, and XXXII undiluted monovalent serums, respectively. Should no reaction be seen on the first examination, the preparations are reexamined at the end of 30 minutes.

When dealing with sputums containing many Type III organisms, it is necessary occasionally to dilute the sputum with salt solution before any *Quellung* of the pneumococcus capsule becomes evident. In such instances, when the regular Neufeld technique is used, the organisms form large masses surrounded by much precipitated material, and no definite swelling of the capsules can be seen. However, upon dilution of the sputum and repetition of the test, the individual diplococci will usually show a typical, positive reaction.

The age of the specimen of sputum makes little difference in relation to the success with which the Neufeld method is applied. Positive reactions can be demonstrated on sputum 48 hours or more after collection from the patient. Chart 2 shows the steps in the technique.

URINE TEST (Dochez and Avery[321])

a. *Unconcentrated urine.* A specimen of urine is obtained as soon as possible and cleared by centrifuging. The clear urine is mixed in quantities of 0.5 cc. each with equal amounts of antipneumococcic serum of the different types in a series of agglutination tubes.

The intensity of the reaction may vary from an almost imperceptible cloud to a heavy, flocculent precipitate. The reaction may occur in some instances immediately on mixing the urine and serum, or it may require incubation in the water-bath at 37° for one hour. Prolonged incubation, however, must be avoided, since bacterial growth may obscure the test. In the precipitin reaction it is essential that all the reagents used, including the immune serums, should be water-clear. In case the reaction is negative or so faint as to be indefinite with the whole urine, the following method of concentrating the urine may be employed:

b. *Concentrated urine for precipitin test.* Twenty-five cc. or more of a 24-hour specimen of urine, with the addition of a few drops of acetic acid, are evaporated to a volume of about 5 cc., filtered through paper to remove any precipitate of albumin that may occur, and the filtrate is added to 8 to 10 volumes of 95 per cent alcohol. The precipitate which forms is collected by centrifuging and rapidly dried to remove the excess of alcohol, and the residue extracted with 2 to 3 cc. of salt solution, which redissolves the specific substance. Any undissolved material is removed by centrifuging, and the clear salt solution extract is used for the precipitin test. Chart 3 shows the procedure.

IV. Isolation of Several Components of Pneumococcus

MEDIUM FOR THE PRODUCTION OF CULTURE OF STANDARD MAXIMAL DENSITY, VIRULENCE, AND POLYSACCHARIDE CONTENT (O'Meara and Brown[1031])

Witte peptone	10.0 grams
Difco proteose peptone, Fairchild, Parke-Davis, or Neopeptone	40.0 grams
Glucose	5.0 grams
Sodium chloride	5.0 grams
Sodium bicarbonate	5.0 grams
Potassium phosphate (K_2HPO_4)	2.0 grams
Thioglycollic acid	0.1 grams
Distilled water	to 1000.0 cc.

The Witte peptone and sodium chloride are dissolved in water and the reaction of the solution adjusted to pH 8.0. The sodium bicarbonate, glucose, potassium phosphate, and extra peptone (usually Difco proteose) are then added and when they have dissolved the broth is clarified by passing through filter paper. Thioglycollic acid is finally added and the medium sterilized by candling. During the entire course of preparation the temperature of the medium is not allowed to rise above 50°.

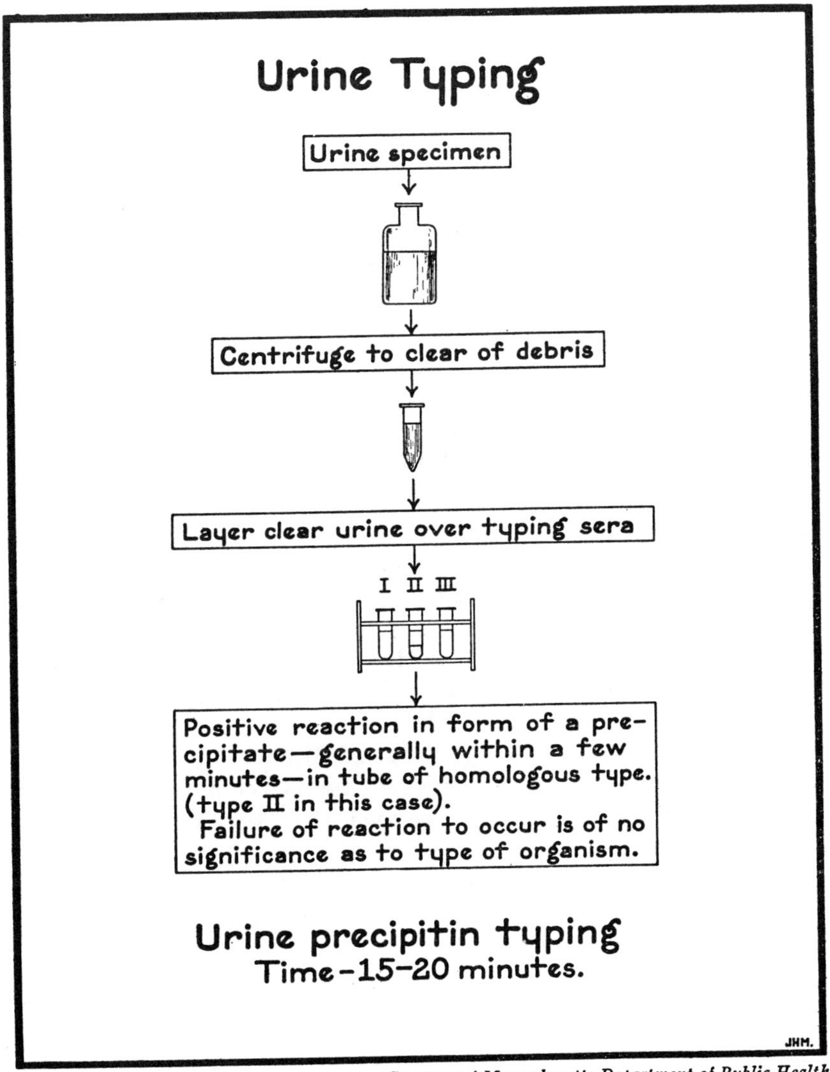

Courtesy of Massachusetts Department of Public Health

CHART 3. THE URINE METHOD OF TYPE DETERMINATION

If the medium is allowed to stand for a time, the thioglycollic acid becomes oxidized, and therefore a sterile solution of the acid should be available and an amount sufficient to give a concentration of 0.01 per cent should be added immediately before use. To obtain a culture of standard density a small inoculum from blood broth is transferred to a tube of the medium and incubated overnight. This is then subcultured into fresh medium at 37° and incubated for 5 to 6 hours.

Pneumococcal Protein (Avery and Morgan[54])

Concentrated suspensions of organisms in 0.002 N NaOH are subjected to repeated freezing and thawing to disrupt the cell bodies. This thick solution of dissolved organisms is then diluted with salt solution to one-tenth the volume of original culture fluid and passed through a Berkefeld V filter. To this filtered solution N acetic acid is added slowly and the mixture carefully shaken. Flocculation of the protein occurs promptly and completely at a reaction faintly acid to litmus. The precipitated protein is separated by centrifugation, washed several times in distilled water, and redissolved in salt solution by adding 0.1 N NaOH until the solution is faintly alkaline to litmus. Solutions of pneumococcal protein freshly prepared by this method exhibit the usual qualitative color reactions for substances of this nature: positive biuret, Hopkins-Cole, Millon, xanthoproteic, and Molisch reactions. The hydrolyzed protein gives the purine reaction with Fehling's solution. The protein solutions are standardized on the basis of their nitrogen content.

Somatic Carbohydrate or C Fraction (Tillett, Goebel, and Avery[1410])

The bacterial cells from 3 liters of broth culture of an R strain derived from Type II Pneumococcus were collected by centrifugation. The bacteria were resuspended in 50 cc. of salt solution and were repeatedly frozen and thawed to break up the bacterial bodies. To this solution of bacteria 0.5 cc. N acetic acid was added, and the mixture was then heated for 10 minutes in a boiling water-bath. The tube was cooled and the coagulated protein was separated from the clear supernatant liquid which contained the C substance. In this manner the noncoagulable material from 30 to 40 liters of culture was collected. The combined supernatant extract, after neutralization, was finally filtered through a Berkefeld candle and then concentrated *in vacuo* to 50 cc. The concentrates from 36 liters of bacteria obtained as described above were again acidified with 0.5 cc. of N acetic acid and reheated for 15 minutes at 100°. A small amount of coagulated protein was thus separated and removed by centrifugation. The clear solution was now treated with 5 volumes of alcohol and after standing overnight in the ice-box, a precipitate settled out which contained all of the so-called C substance, together with certain nitrogenous impurities. This precipitate, when redissolved in saline solution, was found to give a specific precipitin test with antipneumococcic horse serums of Types I, II, and III. The solution of the C fraction was found to contain, however, material which gave a positive biuret test, but this impurity was precipitated from solution by making the mixture alkaline with sodium hydroxide, without loss of the serologically reactive substance. The alkaline solution of the C fraction, now at a volume of 50 cc., was reprecipitated by the addition of 5 volumes of alcohol. The material was centrifuged, redissolved in 40 cc. of water, and again precipitated from faintly acid solution by alcohol. This procedure was repeated altogether four times. The carbohydrate recovered from the final alcoholic precipitation was dissolved in 15 cc. of water and was cooled to 0°. To the solution were added 2 cc. of hydrochloric acid (sp. gr. 1.09). A small amount of insoluble inactive material separated from the solution and was centrifuged off. The clear acid solution was now precipitated with five volumes of redistilled alcohol. After standing at 0° for 4 hours the C substance was separated by centrifugation. It was redissolved in 10 cc. of water and then reprecipitated with alcohol and acid. The final product was washed free from chlorides with 85 per cent alcohol, and was washed finally with redistilled alcohol and ether. The yield was about 65 milligrams from 36 liters of broth cultures.

Capsular Polysaccharide (Heidelberger, Kendall, and Scherp[627])

a. *Preparation of the specific polysaccharide of Type I Pneumococcus.* 10 liters of phosphate meat-infusion broth containing 0.3 per cent of added glucose were seeded with a highly virulent Type I pneumococcus.* After 72 hours at 37°, 1 per cent of phenol was added and the culture allowed to stand overnight. It was then centrifuged in a Sharples centrifuge and the effluent concentrated to 1 liter under reduced pressure, keeping the temperature below 35°. 100 grams of crystalline sodium acetate were dissolved in the concentrated broth and 1,250 cc.

* Recent mouse passage is necessary for good yields of the polysaccharide. After a period of 3 weeks between the last mouse passage and the preparation of the polysaccharide the yield was reduced 80 per cent.

of 95 per cent alcohol were added with constant stirring. The polysaccharide separated as a white curdy mass which settled rapidly. After standing overnight the supernatant fluid was poured off and the precipitate centrifuged. Usually a three-layer separation was obtained, but in cases in which only a single volume of alcohol was used, the phosphates and other salts were not thrown out and no syrupy layer was found. The three-layer separation was also not obtained in the absence of phosphates. If the broth used is phosphate-free, purification of the polysaccharides may often be greatly facilitated by addition of sufficient phosphate to bring about the three-layer separation. A solution of 10 grams of sodium acetate in 250 cc. of water was made acid to litmus with acetic acid and the alcohol precipitate (or middle layer) was dissolved in this and reprecipitated with 300 cc. of 95 per cent alcohol. The centrifuged precipitate was dissolved in 250 cc. of water containing 10 grams of sodium acetate and 5 cc. of glacial acetic acid, and the turbid solution was shaken with 50 cc. of chloroform and 10 cc. of n-butyl alcohol for 30 minutes. On centrifugation a semi-solid emulsion separated between the aqueous layer and the chloroform. The solution and the chloroform were poured off and the layer of emulsion was washed with two 50 cc. portions of water which were saved for washing later emulsion layers. 50 cc. of chloroform and 10 cc. of butyl alcohol were added to the aqueous layer and the shaking was repeated. On centrifugation a smaller semi-solid emulsion layer was formed and this was treated as before. Shaking with chloroform was repeated as long as an emulsion layer formed. Seven shakings were usually required. The washings of the emulsion layers were combined and shaken with fresh additions of chloroform as long as an emulsion layer formed, and were then combined with the main aqueous solution, the total volume now being 350 cc. The polysaccharide was precipitated with 500 cc. of 95 per cent alcohol, redissolved in 250 cc. of water, and the solution tested for phosphate and glycogen. Phosphate may be removed either by repeated precipitations with alcohol in the presence of sodium acetate and acetic acid or with glacial acetic acid in the presence of sodium acetate. Glycogen may be left behind by precipitating the SI from a salt-free aqueous solution with copper acetate. In the instance quoted the solution was free from phosphate but gave a strong iodine test for glycogen. 20 cc. of a saturated solution of copper acetate slightly acidified with acetic acid were added and the resulting bluish precipitate was centrifuged off. The supernatant fluid remained clear when more copper acetate was added. The precipitate was dissolved in 50 cc. of 20 per cent sodium acetate solution and 5 cc. of glacial acetic acid, and reprecipitated free from copper, after which it was dissolved in 100 cc. of water and the solution again tested for glycogen. If this is present the copper precipitation is repeated. The SI was finally precipitated with redistilled alcohol in the presence of a small amount of sodium acetate, washed with redistilled alcohol, filtered, and dried. Yield: 0.9 gram of the neutral sodium salt of SI.

b. *Preparation of the specific polysaccharide of Type II Pneumococcus.* 10 liters of a 4-day culture of Type II Pneumococcus were treated in the same way as for Type I. No differences were observed up to the point at which the copper acetate precipitation was made. However, only one-third of the SII was thrown down as the copper salt. This fraction, which was free from glycogen, was reprecipitated as the copper salt and isolated separately.

The copper-soluble fraction was freed from copper salts by several precipitations with alcohol in the presence of acetic acid and sodium acetate and was redissolved in a small volume of water. Even this concentrated solution failed to react with copper acetate. As glycogen was present in this fraction it was removed by adjusting the pH to 6.5 and adding a small amount of saliva. After a few minutes the iodine test was negative. To remove protein impurities added in the saliva, 5 grams of sodium acetate and 2.5 cc. of acetic acid were added, and the solution (volume 100 cc.) was repeatedly shaken with chloroform and a little butyl alcohol until an emulsion layer was no longer formed. Since the polysaccharide solution still contained nitrogen it was adjusted to contain 5 grams of sodium acetate per 100 cc. and was chilled and precipitated with 5 volumes of glacial acetic acid. The precipitate was centrifuged in the cold, taken up in 50 cc. of 5 per cent sodium acetate solution, and again precipitated with 5 volumes of acetic acid. This was followed by two precipitations with alcohol from 5 per cent sodium acetate solution and one precipitation with redistilled alcohol, after which the polysaccharide was washed with redistilled alcohol, filtered, and dried. One cc. of the broth contained 0.59 mg. or a total of 0.590 gm. of SII in the 10 liters used. Recovery, 78 per cent.

c. *Preparation of the specific polysaccharide of Type III Pneumococcus.* The culture filtrate was concentrated in vacuo to one-tenth its original volume. After three precipitations with 1.5 volumes of alcohol, part of the protein contained in the material was removed by 40 per cent saturation with sodium sulfate at 37°. The SIII was then precipitated by completely saturating the solution with sodium sulfate. After removing the sodium sulfate by repeated precipitations of the SIII with alcohol and acetic acid in the presence of sodium acetate the product was found to contain 2.4 per cent of nitrogen. This was removed by twice precipitating the SIII as the barium salt with barium chloride. The barium was removed by repeated precipitations from 20 per cent sodium acetate solution with acetic acid and alcohol. The SIII was isolated as the neutral sodium salt.

V. Preparation of Bacterial Enzymes Capable of Decomposing Capsular Polysaccharides (Dubos,[336] and Dubos and Bauer[338])

The bacteria are grown in a solution of 2 per cent casein hydrolysate (pH 7.0) at 37° under conditions of strict aerobiosis; the cells from the 16-hour-old culture, separated by centrifugation, are resuspended in small amounts of distilled water.

A medium is prepared consisting of 0.1 per cent capsular polysaccharide and 0.1 per cent NaCl in distilled water. This medium is distributed in 25 cc. amounts in large Erlenmeyer flasks (1 liter capacity) to provide for aerobic conditions, and each flask is inoculated with the cells recovered from 500 cc. of the culture of the SIII bacillus in the casein hydrolysate medium. The material is incubated for 12 to 18 hours at 37° and the cultures tested to ascertain the disappearance of the specific polysaccharide and the absence of contaminants. The cultures are now frozen and thawed repeatedly to secure the release of the endocellular enzyme.

The enzyme is ultimately separated from the cell débris by filtration. However, since the cell suspension is very viscous, it is first subjected to the following treatment. The cell suspension is made alkaline to pH 10.0 by the addition of sodium borate. Equimolecular concentrations of dibasic sodium phosphate and calcium chloride are then added to bring about a heavy precipitate of calcium phosphate which facilitates the clarification of the material by centrifugation. The supernatant fluid which contains all the enzyme in solution is now passed through a Seitz filter, then through a Berkefeld (V) filter. The potency of this filtrate is such that 0.002 to 0.004 cc. are required to decompose 0.01 mg. of the capsular polysaccharide under the conditions of the test.

For the purpose of further purification of the enzyme preparation, the solution is passed through collodion membranes made and calibrated according to the description given by Bauer and Hughes.[90] Membranes with a pore diameter of 5.5 to 7.5 mμ are used in a specially designed filter of stainless steel. Filtration is carried out at a pressure of 50 pounds per square inch. To minimize contamination by air bacteria and particles of dust, the air is filtered through Seitz asbestos pads inserted between the air line and each individual filter. Chloroform is used as an antiseptic during filtration. At the end of filtration (it may take 5 days to filter to dryness 600 cc. of enzyme solution), the membranes are washed several times in distilled water and all the enzymatic activity is thus recovered in solution. After filtration through Berkefeld (V) candles, the preparation is frozen and in this state evaporated to dryness in a vacuum. The final product is used dissolved in water.

VI. Serological Reactions

Agglutination

Since different lots of serum may exhibit different agglutinin titers, it is advisable to test each batch of serum in varying dilution against a culture of known type-specificity. It may occasionally be necessary, also, to employ dilutions of the material (suspensions of living or killed pneumococci) used as antigen, since zonal effects may inhibit complete agglutination. As a rule, an 18-hour broth culture, containing approximately one billion organisms per cubic centimeter serves as a satisfactory suspension for routine tests.

For the test, it is convenient to mix 0.5 cc. of serum dilutions with an equal amount of the culture. The serum dilutions may range from undiluted, for certain types, to 1 to 5 through 1 to 80 or 160. With unknown types, it may be well to perform a bile-solubility test at the same time. The mixtures are incubated in a water-bath at 37° to 40° and examined at frequent intervals up to two hours. Those tubes showing no agglutination, or an indefinite reaction, should be placed at 4° overnight, and if the reaction is still negative, the tubes are then discarded.

With cultures of strains known to be closely related, it is well to perform tests for heterologous reactions. Thus, a Type V culture should be tested with both Type V and Type II serum, and likewise a Type II serum should be tested against both Type II and Type V cultures.

Antipneumococcic rabbit serums exhibit a higher degree of type-specificity than do horse serums, and for this reason are of value in case of doubt regarding the type-specificity of recently obtained strains.

PRECIPITATION

There are various methods of titrating antipneumococcic serum based on precipitation of the antibody by the specific polysaccharide. Those listed below are given to illustrate the methods in more common use.

a. *Optimal proportions* (Smith[1298]). The test is carried out in three routine stages.

(1) Preliminary Orientation: The object is to decide upon a suitable dilution in which to use the serum in the subsequent tests, for if the serum is used insufficiently diluted, precipitation is so rapid that it becomes impossible to decide which tube is the optimal one. A suitable serum dilution is that which produces macroscopic precipitation with the equivalent amount of antigen in 20 to 30 minutes. Dilutions of serum, 1 in 5, 1 in 10, 1 in 20, are made with 0.85 per cent salt solution and 1 cc. of each mixed with 1 cc. of polysaccharide in 1 in 50,000 dilution. The tubes are placed in the water-bath at 40° and are examined at the end of 5 minutes and again at 10 minutes. The choice of the serum dilution to be used in the subsequent tests, based on the result obtained, is a matter of personal judgment, readily acquired from a few experiments.

(2) Rough Test with Widely Spaced Antigen Dilutions: A row of eight tubes is numbered from left to right and 1 cc. of buffer solution (borate buffer solution, pH 8.0) is run into each. To the first tube, 1 cc. of a stock solution of SSS, 1 in 10,000 dilution, is added by means of an accurate 1 cc. pipette, the contents are mixed thoroughly and 1 cc. of the mixture is carried over to tube 2, and so on, 1 cc. being discarded from the last tube. It is not necessary to use separate pipettes. To each tube in turn, 1 cc. of the chosen dilution of serum is added by means of a mounted syringe, care being taken to prevent the stream of serum from striking the walls of the tube. (A 2 cc. all-glass syringe is mounted vertically on a rigid stand with an adjustable screw over it, so that when the piston is raised to meet the screw, the syringe capacity is exactly 1 cc. A 23-gauge half-inch needle is fitted to the syringe, which can now be filled rapidly and accurately with serum, held in a conical centrifuge tube.) The rack of tubes is placed in the water-bath and transferred periodically for a rapid examination to a reading box, so designed that the whole series of mixtures, evenly transilluminated, can be viewed against a dead black background.

In this rough test, one tube usually shows precipitation long before any of the others; occasionally two tubes run parallel, indicating that the true optimal antigen concentration lies midway between them.

(3) Final Test with Narrow Range of Antigen Dilutions: Eight tubes are numbered and buffer solution is added from a graduated pipette; nil to tube 1, 0.1 cc. to tube 2, 0.2 cc. to tube 3, and so on. With a fresh pipette, enough antigen solution is added to each tube to bring the total content up to 1 cc. The dilution of SSS solution to be used is decided from the result of the rough test, the object being to have the optimal tube at about the middle of the series. Serum is added in 1 cc. quantities as before and the tubes are incubated. Closer observation is necessary than in the previous test because, with this narrow range of antigen dilutions, precipitation extends rapidly from the optimal tube to those on either side. A hand lens is used until one of the precipitates can be seen by the naked eye, but even so it is often impossible to be sure which tube first shows precipitation. The optimal tube, however, is distinguished more by the fact that in it the particles remain larger for some considerable time than those in any other tube and also the fluid part of the mixture looks clearer and more transparent than in any of the others. The antigen-antibody ratio is then calculated by dividing the antigen dilution of the optimal mixture by the serum dilution.

(4) Confirmation of the Precipitation Result by Tests for Excess of Antigen: Occasionally two, three, or even four tubes run so nearly parallel that it is impossible to be sure which represents the optimal; that is to say, an optimal band is produced instead of an optimal tube. In such cases it is still possible to find the optimal ratio by centrifuging the mixtures after precipitation is complete in all of them, and testing the supernatant fluids for excess of antigen. In practice it is sufficient to show that antigen remains free only in those tubes to the left of the optimal. A simple method is to layer the supernatant fluid over a potent serum suitably diluted in normal horse serum; the formation of a white ring at the junction of the fluids indicates that polysaccharide has remained in the supernatant fluid.

b. *Nitrogen determination* (Heidelberger, Sia, and Kendall[630]). If, on addition of a 1 to 10,000 saline solution of the specific polysaccharide to a portion of the immune serum, precipitation is rapid and heavy, 0.5 cc. of the serum should be used for the quantitative determination. This amount will suffice for all except very low grade serums, of which it is better to use 1 cc. The serums should be measured in duplicate with accurately calibrated pipettes into wide agglutination tubes (dimensions of 10 by 75 mm. have been found suitable). If 0.5 cc. of serum has been used, 1 cc. of saline solution is then added to each tube, followed by 0.5 cc. of a saline solution containing 1 mg. of the specific polysaccharide per cubic centimeter, to make a total volume of 2 cc. Ordinary uncalibrated pipettes are adequate for the saline and polysaccharide solutions. The tubes are plugged and the contents carefully and thoroughly mixed by a rotary motion imparted by drawing the finger tips rapidly and repeatedly in a diagonal stroke down the side of the tube. The tubes are allowed to stand 2 hours in the water-bath at 37° and overnight in the ice-box.* The plugs are then removed and the tubes centrifuged for 10 minutes at 1,000 R.P.M., either in a refrigerating centrifuge or immersed in ice-water. The supernatant liquid is then carefully drained off by inverting the tube and wiping the mouth of the tube with filter paper. The tubes are then placed in ice-water and each precipitate is washed with 2 cc. of an ice-cold, 1 to 20,000 saline solution of the specific polysaccharide, mixing the contents as before. It appears to make little difference whether the disc of precipitate is loosened from the bottom of the tube. After one-half hour in the cold, the tubes are again centrifuged and drained as before. About 0.5 cc. of water is then added to each tube, with shaking until the precipitate is loosened, after which the disc is dissolved by the addition of 2 drops of normal sodium hydroxide solution with rotation of the tube until the precipitate has disappeared. If the disc is allowed to stick to the glass, solution is much slower. The solution is then rinsed quantitatively into a micro-Kjeldahl flask or tube and the nitrogen determined by any standard procedure. The Pregl method, slightly modified, is satisfactory. Nitrogen found multiplied by 6.25 equals specifically precipitated protein.

c. *Modified routine*† (Barnes, Clarke, and Wight[82]). The test is conducted by mixing a constant amount of capsular polysaccharide with varying dilutions of immune serum and comparing the precipitin titer of the unknown serum with that of a control serum tested simultaneously.

(1) Dilution of SSS: Stock solutions of SSS are made up in 1 to

* Sterile technique should be employed up to this point. In the case of low-grade serums, identical values are obtained if the tubes are allowed to stand in the water-bath only one-half hour, followed by one-half hour in ice-water before proceeding. With more potent serums, results a few tenths of a milligram per cubic centimeter too low are obtained by shortening the process in this way.

† Suitable only for unconcentrated serums.

1,000 dilution with borate buffer solution (pH 8.0). From this stock solution, various dilutions are tested against varying dilutions of a control serum to determine the suitable dilution of the carbohydrate to be used routinely. This dilution will vary from lot to lot and according to the type of SSS. To illustrate, for Type I, the dilution 1 to 30,000; for Type II, 1 to 80,000; for Type V, 1 to 50,000; and for Type VIII, 1 to 80,000 may be found to be satisfactory.

(2) Dilution of Serums: Serums are diluted with physiological salt solution in series, 1 to 5, 10, 15, 20, 25, 30, 40, 50, 60, 80, 100, 120, 160, 200, 240, 320, 400, and so on. For the test, ten adjacent dilutions from the series are employed.

(3) The Test: 0.5 cc. of the dilution of SSS chosen is added to 0.5 cc. of the serum dilutions, and the contents mixed by shaking the racks for several minutes. The mixtures are incubated for two hours at 40° and overnight in the refrigerator at 4°.

(4) Interpretation: The end point is taken as the highest dilution of serum showing definite precipitation. By comparing the titer of the unknown serum with that of the control, the number of units in one cubic centimeter of the unknown serum can be calculated.

d. *Combining equivalents* (Felton and Stahl[433]).

(1) Preparation of SSS Dilutions: The stock solution is made in a volumetric flask from an accurately weighed sample of the dried material, dissolving it first in a small volume of saline solution with the addition of sufficient normal NaOH to maintain a neutral reaction and facilitate solution. Then salt solution is added to complete the volume for a 1 to 500 dilution. Using a volumetric flask and a quantitative delivery pipette, the dilution required for the test is prepared in such a quantity that not less than 1 cc. of the 1 to 500 stock solution need be measured.

(2) Preparation of Serum Dilutions: Physiological salt solution for the serum dilutions is measured with a burette when more than 2 cc. is required, and with a 2 cc. accurately calibrated serological pipette, graduated in tenths, when less than 2 cc. is needed. Serum for the initial dilution is drawn up to the line in a quantitative pipette calibrated to contain exactly the amount required. Excess serum clinging to the outside of the pipette is removed with a piece of cotton or gauze, and the pipette is rinsed five times in the dilution being made. Two cc. serological pipettes graduated in tenths are used in making subsequent dilutions. Each dilution should be in at least 1 cc., and preferably 2 cc. or more, volumes.

(3) Mixing the Two Components (first step): After the serum dilutions have been properly prepared, quantitative pipettes are used to deliver 1 cc. volumes into small agglutination tubes (10 cm. by 1 cm.) arranged in suitable racks. Then, with a quantitative delivery pipette, 1 cc. of the chosen SSS dilution is added to each, and the tubes are shaken separately to ensure thorough mixing. The tubes are incubated for 2 hours in a 37° water-bath, in which the water extends half-way up to the level of the mixtures in the tubes, and then stored in the cold (4°) overnight.

(4) Adding the Indicating Serum (second step): The next morning, the precipitates are separated from the supernatant fluids by centrifugation for 3 or 4 minutes, preferably in the cold or at room temperature. The supernatant fluids are drained into clean, clear agglutination tubes and to them is added the indicating serum in the amount previously found to be optimal, and each tube is shaken thoroughly. The mixtures are incubated at 37° for 2 hours, and then, without disturbing the precipitates, allowed to settle for 2 hours at room temperature before recording the end point.

(5) Reading the End Point: For consistent and reliable results, the end point is considered as that dilution next in series to the one containing a well-formed disc precipitate. With some serums and some SSS preparations, the end point is extremely definite, that is, of two adjacent tubes in a series, one contains a disc precipitate, the other contains not even a trace of flocculation. On the other hand, there are instances when the mixtures next in series to the last disc precipitate are not clear, but contain a fine sediment which becomes a swirl when the tube is shaken. These fine precipitates are disregarded, and the tube following the last disc precipitate in the series is taken as the equivalent end point.

(6) Calculating the Unit Value: The greater the unit value of any antibody preparation, the smaller is the volume required to combine equivalently with a given dilution of specific carbohydrate. Hence, an inverse proportion expresses the relationship between the antibody content of an immune serum and the percentage dilution that represents its equivalent end point. The unit value of an unknown serum is found from the proportion

$$\mathrm{A}:\mathrm{A}' = \mathrm{B}':\mathrm{B}, \text{ or } \mathrm{A} = \frac{\mathrm{A}'\mathrm{B}'}{\mathrm{B}}$$

in which A equals the unit value of the unknown serum, A′ the unit value of the standard serum, B the equivalent end point of the unknown, and B′ the equivalent end point of the standard serum.

COMPLEMENT FIXATION (Goodner and Horsfall[538])

As expressed by Goodner and Horsfall, "Complement is not fixed by immune aggregates resulting from the interaction of pneumococcus capsular polysaccharide and type-specific immune horse serum, although under proper conditions the substitution of immune rabbit serum gives positive results." The materials and methods used by these authors are as follows: Fresh guinea pig serum (complement), a 5 per cent suspension of washed sheep red blood cells, and the serum of a rabbit immunized with sheep red blood cells (amboceptor). Each reagent is used in a volume of 0.5 cc. The amboceptor is titrated with excess of complement and so diluted that 0.5 cc. contains 2 units. The complement is titrated against 2 units of amboceptor. The final volume in each tube of the titrations is 1.5 cc. The majority of the experiments were carried out with the acetyl form of Type I pneumococcus capsular polysaccharide.

For further details of the tests the reader is referred to the original article by Goodner and Horsfall.

BACTERICIDAL TESTS (Ward[1480])

In this method, a constant amount of whole blood is placed in a series of tubes, and to each of the tubes is added a decreasing number of organisms, so that—for example—the first tube is inoculated with 500,000 organisms, the second tube with 50,000 organisms, the third tube with 5,000 organisms, and so forth. The tubes are sealed and placed in a rotating box in the incubator. After some hours' incubation, the tubes are opened and the contents plated. The plates are incubated and read the next day. It is evident that the sterility of the contents of the tubes —as shown by the plates—depends on three main factors, namely, the number and virulence of the organisms, and the phagocytic power of the whole blood. As the number of organisms can easily be controlled, the method can be used to determine either the virulence of the organisms, by always using the same blood, or the phagocytic power of the blood, by always using the same organisms, providing their virulence is maintained at a constant level. The maximal number of organisms killed in the mixture is, in the one case, the direct measure of the phagocytic power of the blood and, in the other case, the indirect measure of the virulence of the organism. In other words, the more organisms that are killed, the more actively phagocytic is the blood in the former case, and the less virulent is the organism in the latter case.

The method is a modification of the one described by Todd. For further details, the reader should consult the original article by Ward.

VII. Potency Tests on Antipneumococcic Serum

United States Hygienic Laboratory, now National Institute of Health (as of January 22, 1926)

a. *Culture.* The culture of Type I pneumococcus should be of such virulence that it is fatal to mice, as a rule, in 0.00,000,001 cc. of a 3 to 6-hour beef infusion broth culture. Simultaneously with each day's tests, eight mice are inoculated with the culture alone, receiving no serum, in order to check the virulence of the culture used. These cultural check mice receive 0.00,000,1 cc., 0.00,000,01 cc., 0.00,000,001 cc., and 0.00,000,000,1 cc. of the culture, two mice on each dose. These dilutions are made as follows:

Flask or tube	*Culture*	*Sterile broth*	*Each 0.5 cc. of original culture contains*
No. 1	1 part	4 parts	0.1 cc.
No. 2	1 cc. of No. 1	9 cc.	0.01 cc.
No. 3	1 cc. of No. 2	9 cc.	0.00,1 cc.
No. 4	1 cc. of No. 3	9 cc.	0.00,01 cc.
No. 5	1 cc. of No. 4	9 cc.	0.00,001 cc.
No. 6	1 cc. of No. 5	9 cc.	0.00,000,1 cc.
No. 7	1 cc. of No. 6	9 cc.	0.00,000,01 cc.
No. 8	1 cc. of No. 7	9 cc.	0.00,000,001 cc.
No. 9	1 cc. of No. 8	9 cc.	0.00,000,000,1 cc.

Either conical flasks or tubes 28 mm. in diameter are used for making these dilutions. Thorough mixing is very essential and this is accomplished only by a rapid and vigorous blowing and sucking of the mixture with a minimal amount of air through the pipette, which is pressed against the bottom of the flask or tube. A separate pipette is used for each dilution. The culture should be checked for purity by plating on blood-agar plates previous to each test. At the Hygienic Laboratory the broth for growing the cultures is made from beef infused in the ice-box, and 2 per cent peptone is used. The hydrogen ion concentration is about pH 7.2. The culture is passed through mice weekly, 0.5 cc. of an 18-hour culture being inoculated intraperitoneally into each of three mice, which are etherized in 5 or 6 hours, about 0.5 cc. of heart's blood being obtained from each and distributed into two tubes of broth and a blood-agar plate (for purity test) which are incubated overnight. Three of the six tubes showing a good growth of Pneumococcus in pure culture are selected and stored at 15° as stock cultures; after about 3 days (the day before the test) 0.5 cc. to 1.0 cc. are transplanted from each stock culture to fresh tubes of broth, and plates are made for purity. The stock cultures are quickly put back at 15°, to be used for planting the tubes 18 hours before the next passage through mice. The first transplants are incubated 16 to 18 hours, transplanted again, and incubated 3 to 6 hours, and of these three last transplants, those showing a good growth of pure Pneumococcus, with a turbidity of 200 to 250 parts per million, silica standard, and a pH of 6.6 to 7.0 are pooled and distributed for the test. All dilutions of cultures are made in broth and should not stand diluted for more than an hour at room temperature.

0.1 cc. of the culture, diluted so that this dose is contained in 0.5 cc. volume (tube 1 in the above table), is given to each mouse, except the cultural check mice.

b. *Serum.* 0.2 cc. of each serum (including the control serum) diluted with saline solution so that this dose is contained in 0.5 cc. (2 volumes serum diluted and mixed thoroughly with 3 volumes saline) is given to each mouse, except the cultural check mice.

c. *The test.* For each serum tested, at least three mice are injected intraperitoneally with 0.2 cc. of serum, followed in less than 5 minutes by 0.1 cc. of culture intraperitoneally. Six mice should receive the control serum, three at the beginning and three at the end of each test. The mice should weigh 18 to 22 grams. If there is much variation in weight, they should be arranged in three weight groups, and a light, a medium, and a heavy mouse chosen for each serum. The mice are observed for 96 hours; all mice counted as fatalities must be proved, by smear and cultures from the heart's blood, to have died with an uncomplicated pneumococcal septicemia. Survivals of less than twelve hours should be regarded as "contaminations." Mice dying of infections or accidents other than pure pneumococcal septicemia, as revealed by necropsy, are regarded as "contaminations." Contaminations should be regarded as neither deaths nor survivals, but as if not injected. Tests are read 120 hours after injection, to allow for the obtaining of results of necropsies on mice dying on the fourth day. The control serum should, on the average, protect at least 50 per cent of the mice. The following data should be included in the protocols of tests:

Date of test, including month, day, and hour
Operator's initials
Date of last animal passage of the culture
Period of exposure of diluted culture to room temperature
Period of time necessary for injection of all mice
Hours of survival of mice dying up to 96 hours, indicated by number
Survival of mice for 96 hours, indicated by S
Contamination to be indicated by circle around the number of hours of survival

		cc. 0.1	cc. 0.1	cc. 0.1 of culture
Control serum	P1 C	72	S	S
Test serum	X	(11)	41	S
Test serum	Y	S	S	S
Test serum	Z	29	S	S
Control serum	P1 C	31	(90)	S

Date: Oct. 17, 1923
Operator: ABC

Culture checks

Millionth.	10 millionth.	100 millionth.	Billionth
29 43	39 (41)	42 43	49 S

Serum dose 0.2 cc.
Culture passed through mice Oct. 12, 1923
Dilution of culture began 11:48 A M.
Injection of serum began 12:02 P.M.
Injection of culture completed 12:09 P.M.

SAMPLE PROTOCOL OF MOUSE PROTECTION TESTS, NATIONAL INSTITUTE OF HEALTH

League of Nations (as taken from Parish[1051])

The test is intended to ascertain the amount of serum that is equivalent in protecting power to a certain dose of a standard serum, the serum and culture being mixed for 5 minutes at room temperature and injected intraperitoneally in 1.0 cc. amounts of mixture. The culture dose suggested by the League of Nations' Subcommittee is 0.001 cc. In each experiment, varying dilutions of serum in 0.9 per cent saline solution are mixed with equal volumes of the culture dilution in broth. Decreasing amounts of serum are used, such as 0.001, 0.00,05, and 0.00,025 cc.

a. *Animals.* The mice selected for the tests should weigh 18 to 22 grams. After the injections of serum and culture, the dead and sick animals should be noted morning and evening. Smears are made from the hearts' blood of the dead mice and only those animals showing the presence of large numbers of pneumococci are counted as fatalities for the purposes of the titration. Mice failing to show pneumococci in smears of hearts' blood are regarded as neither deaths nor survivals, but as if not injected.

b. *Culture.* The culture of Type I Pneumococcus should be of such virulence that it is fatal to mice in doses of 0.00,000,001 to 0.00,000,-000,1 cc. (16 to 18-hour culture in steamed Witte peptone broth at a pH of 7.5). At the beginning of each day's tests, mice are inoculated intraperitoneally with 1 cc. of 0.00,000,000,1, 0.00,000,001, and 0.00,000,1 of the culture, two mice with each dose, to check the virulence of the organisms.

For the maintenance of virulence, cultures should be passaged through the mouse monthly, being kept between passages in 50 per cent defibrinated horse or rabbit blood broth (not incubated) in 1.0 cc. vials in the ice-chest at 4°. When required for test, the cultures are incubated and used as the inoculum for 5 cc. or 10 cc. tubes of Witte peptone broth. A stock of Witte peptone broth which is known to be satisfactory should be kept for the tests, and before it is expended another supply should be prepared and tested in parallel with the stock before being adopted for use.

c. *Serum.* In every test a standard control serum should be available for purposes of comparison. Dilutions of this serum and of all serums to be tested are made in 0.9 per cent saline solution, a different pipette being used for each dilution.

Author's Note: Parish recommends the use of 0.01 cc. of an 18-hour broth culture rather than 0.001 cc. as the optimal dose for routine use.

American Drug Manufacturers' Association

The method was suggested by the Committee on Standardization of Antipneumococcic Serum of the Biological Section of the American Drug Manufacturers' Association, February 21, 1933, and revised December 29, 1933.

a. *Unit of serum.* The unit of antipneumococcic serum shall be 1/200 cc. of F–146 or its equivalent which is 1/300 cc. for Type I and 1/150 cc. for Type II of P–11. In the performance of the test, the dose of serum used is the unitage tested for. In using the control serum P–11 at a unitage of 300 units per cubic centimeter for Type I and 150 units per cubic centimeter for Type II, which is the accepted potency of this control serum, 0.5 cc. of a 1:150 dilution for Type I and of a 1:75 dilution for Type II is injected.

b. *Test dose of culture.* The test dose of culture is that amount of culture which, when drawn up in the same syringe with a unit of control serum and injected into the test mice, will on the average kill approximately 40 per cent of the mice injected. This test dose shall be not more than 0.5 cc. of a 1:100 dilution. With larger amounts of serum a higher percentage of mice is expected to live, and with smaller amounts of serum, a lower percentage of mice is expected to live. The culture to be used is one found by experience to be satisfactory for use for test with the control serum.

c. *The test.* At least two complete tests, preferably made on different days, using 10 mice on each serum dilution, must be made for each unknown serum.

(1) Mice: 16 to 20 gram white mice are used for the test. Ten mice are injected on each serum dilution.

(2) Serum: The serum is diluted, at room temperature, with physiological salt solution, never using less than 1 cc. volume in making dilutions, except if economy requires, in the first dilution of the control serum, when 0.5 cc. may be used. Accurate quantitative pipettes, with a separate pipette for each dilution, are employed.

(3) Control serum: (see Unit of serum, *ante*). It is essential that the control serum P–11 be used in at least 2 dilutions, 300 and 400 units for Type I and 150 and 200 units for Type II, namely 0.5 cc. of 1:150 and 0.5 cc. of 1:200 for Type I, and 0.5 cc. of 1:75 and 0.5 cc. of 1:100 for Type II, with each comparative test. On the average, in at least two tests, 60 per cent of the mice must survive in the 300 unit dilution and over 50 per cent die in the 400 unit dilution in Type I, and 60 per cent of the mice survive in the 150 unit dilution and over 50 per cent die in the 200 unit dilution in Type II.

The dilution of the unknown serum depends upon the relative potency. Suggestion: A primary titration may be made using mice in triplicate on dilutions representing 100, 200, 400, 800 units, etc., when testing unconcentrated serum, or 1,000, 2,000, 3,000, 4,000 units, etc., in refined and concentrated serums or globulins. After establishment of the approximate unit value of the serum, dilutions in the appropriate zone with an increment of 25 to 50 per cent are tested with ten mice to each dilution.

(4) Culture: (see Test dose of culture, *ante*).

(5) Method of Injection: In actual test, 0.5 cc. of serum dilution is drawn into a 1 cc. tuberculin syringe (fitted with a No. 23 gauge, ¾ inch needle) and then 0.5 cc. of the culture dilution is drawn into the same syringe and the mixture injected immediately (within 5 seconds). A different syringe must be used for each dilution of serum. For each dilution of serum tested a separate container shall be used

for the culture dilution. Not more than 60 minutes shall elapse between starting and finishing the injections.

(6) Length of Test: The test is terminated at the end of 96 hours and all mice living at the end of this time are counted as survivals. The hour of death is noted on mice dying before 96 hours. (Ideally, all mice dying on the test should be necropsied and the hearts' blood cultured to rule out deaths due to intercurrent infection. This may be impractical in routine testing, but certainly in each test some mice on important dilutions should be examined post mortem.)

d. *Interpretation of test.* The unit value of an unknown serum is estimated by direct comparison of the highest or end-point dilution protecting 60 per cent of mice on an average in at least two complete and separate tests with the control serum P-11 end-point dilution equalling 300 units per cubic centimeter for Type I and 150 units per cubic centimeter for Type II. Comparison should also be made of the percentage survival of other dilutions of the unknown and control serum.

e. *Records and reports.* Reports of tests shall be in the form of a summary, as outlined on page 661.

MASSACHUSETTS ANTITOXIN AND VACCINE LABORATORY

The method is a modification of the Park-Cooper technique[1054] and of the American Drug Manufacturers' Association test as revised December 29, 1933. The method herein described has been in routine use at the Massachusetts Antitoxin and Vaccine Laboratory since February, 1933.

a. *Culture.* Virulence. The virulence of the cultures used should be such that no more than 3 to 10 organisms, as determined by 24-hour blood-agar plate counts, are required to kill at least two of three mice within 48 hours after intraperitoneal inoculation. Passages of the cultures through mice are made five days each week for maintenance of virulence.

The culture used for a protection test is obtained in the following manner: A mouse is injected intraperitoneally with 0.5 cc. of an 18-hour broth culture; 6 hours later the mouse is chloroformed and a sample of the heart's blood is inoculated, by means of a sterile capillary pipette, into broth and on a blood-agar plate. After 18 hours growth, if the cultures are pure, a transfer of 1.0 cc. of the broth culture is made to 15.0 cc. of broth and a drop of defibrinated normal horse blood added. This culture is allowed to grow for 4½ hours and is the one used in the test.

(1) Virulence Test: As a part of the mouse protection test, the

virulence of the culture is checked by injecting three doses into mice in triplicate with 0.5 cc. of dilutions of the 4½ hour culture made in peptone solution. Fluctuations in the virulence and amount of growth of the culture from time to time may require variations in the dilutions, and those used in a given test are determined upon the basis of previous tests. The dilutions employed have thus varied from 1:100 million, 1:300 million, and 1:1,000 million to 1:250 million, 1:750 million, and 1:2,500 million for Type I; and 1:90 million, 1:270 million, and 1:900 million to 1:125 million, 1:375 million, and 1:1,250 million for Type II. Dilutions for other types are determined by experience. Virulence test dilutions are made in sterile test tubes.

(2) Test Dose of Culture: The test dose of culture used in determining the protective power of serums is 0.5 cc. of a dilution of the 4½ hour culture made in peptone solution. The dilution employed depends upon fluctuations in growth and virulence (mentioned above) and must be determined by experience. For Type I tests, the dilution used has varied from 1:1,000 to 1:2,500; for Type II from 1:9,000 to 1:12,500. The test dilution of culture is usually made in a sterile 125 cc. or 250 cc. Erlenmeyer flask, the amount depending upon the number of mice to be injected. A loopful of the test dilution is streaked on a blood-agar plate as a purity test and, in addition, three mice are injected with the test dose of culture alone.

Illustrations of the method of making culture dilutions in typical tests, for a total of 132 mice, are shown in the following tables:

TYPE I

Tube No.	*cc. of culture*	*cc. of sterile peptone*	*Dilution*	*cc. contained in each 0.5 cc. of original culture*
1	1	4	1:5	1×10^{-1}
2	1 of No. 1	9	1:50	1×10^{-2}
3	2 of No. 2	18	1:500	1×10^{-3}
4	15 of No. 3	60	1:2500*	2×10^{-4}
5	1 of No. 4	9	1:25,000	2×10^{-5}
6	1 of No. 5	9	1:250,000	2×10^{-6}
7	1 of No. 6	9	1:2,500,000	2×10^{-7}
8	1 of No. 7	9	1:25,000,000	2×10^{-8}
9	1 of No. 8	9	1:250,000,000	2×10^{-9}
10	2 of No. 9	4	1:750,000,000	0.66×10^{-9}
11	1 of No. 9	9	1:2,500,000,000	0.2×10^{-9}

* This is the test dilution of culture.

TYPE II

1	1	9	1:10	5 x 10-2
2	2 of No. 1	3	1:25	2 x 10-2
3	1 of No. 2	9	1:250	2 x 10-3
4	2 of No. 3	18	1:2500	2 x 10-4
5	15 of No. 4	60	1:12,500*	4 x 10-5
6	1 of No. 5	9	1:125,000	4 x 10-6
7	1 of No. 6	9	1:1,250,000	4 x 10-7
8	1 of No. 7	9	1:12,500,000	4 x 10-8
9	1 of No. 8	9	1:125,000,000	4 x 10-9
10	2 of No. 9	4	1:375,000,000	1.33 x 10-9
11	1 of No. 9	9	1:1,250,000,000	0.4 x 10-9

* This is the test dilution of culture.

b. *Serums.* All dilutions of serums are made in physiological salt solution, the amounts of diluent being drawn from an accurately graduated burette. Accurately graduated pipettes are used for mixing dilutions, using a separate pipette for each mixture. Each dilution is drawn up into the pipette 25 times to ensure thorough mixing. Excess serum adhering to the outside of the pipette after removal from the original sample is removed with a pledget of cotton. Not less than 1.0 cc. of a given serum dilution is used for making any higher dilution, and the volume of each dilution is kept as small as possible (usually 15 cc. or less) so that mixing may be thorough. (In making the first dilution of the control serum only 0.5 cc. of serum is used in order to conserve it.) The test dose of all serum dilutions is contained in a volume of 0.5 cc.

(1) Control Serum: The control serum is one supplied by the National Institute of Health and is, at present, P 11 to which have been assigned unit values of 300 and 150 units per cubic centimeter for Types I and II respectively. The dilutions used are for Type I, 1:1,000, 1:2,000, and 1:4,000; for Type II, 1:1,250, 1:2,500, and 1:5,000. These dilutions are made in the following manner:

TYPE I

0.5 cc. serum + 4.5 cc. saline = 1:10 (a)
1.0 cc. of (a) + 9 cc. saline = 1:100 (b)
2.0 cc. of (b) + 8 cc. saline = 1:500 (c)
8.0 cc. of (c) + 8 cc. saline = 1:1000 (d)
4.0 cc. of (d) + 4 cc. saline = 1:2000 (e)
2.0 cc. of (d) + 6 cc. saline = 1:4000 (f)

TYPE II

(a), (b), and (c) dilutions as above.
6.0 cc. of (c) + 9 cc. saline = 1:1250 (d)
4.0 cc. of (d) + 4 cc. saline = 1:2500 (e)
2.0 cc. of (d) + 6 cc. saline = 1:5000 (f)

In each case, only the (d), (e), and (f) dilutions are used for injecting mice.

(2) Unknown Serums: The dilutions used for injecting mice must bear the same ratio to each other as dilutions (d), (e), and (f) of the control serum. As concentrated serums are ordinarily much stronger than the control, obviously the dilutions will be much higher. For example, if a serum being tested for Type I antibody is assumed to be about 10 times as strong as the control serum, the dilutions used for injecting mice will be 1:10,000, 1:20,000, and 1:40,000, these being reached by making dilutions in steps similar to those for the control.

c. *The test.* At least two complete tests giving consistent results and preferably made on different days, using 10 mice for each dilution of serum, must be made for final estimation of the potency of an unknown serum.

(1) The Mice: It is preferable to use mice of a highly inbred, uniformly susceptible stock, in sound, healthy condition. The weights should lie between 16 and 20 grams each.

(2) Method of Injection: Serum and culture dilutions are not mixed prior to injection. Two 2 cc. vaccine syringes, fitted with 26-gauge, 3/8 inch Schick needles, are used for injecting the culture. Two ordinary 2 cc. hypodermic syringes, fitted with needles as above, are used for each serum. One operator fills the syringes, a second makes the injections, and an assistant handles the mice. The serums are always injected first, starting with the highest dilution, and followed immediately by the test dose of culture. Any mice improperly injected are discarded and replaced by others. Four serums (including the standard) and the requisite controls require 132 mice. From 30 to 40 minutes are required for injecting this number.

(3) Length of Test: Observations are made at least twice each day and the approximate hour of death is recorded for mice found dead. The test is terminated at the end of 96 hours and all mice living at this time are recorded as survivals.

(4) Necropsies: Necropsies should be performed on a sufficient

number of mice to prove death due to uncontaminated Pneumococcus infection. Streaking a sample of the heart's blood from a sterile capillary pipette on a blood-agar plate is adequate.

d. *Interpretation of the test.* In interpreting the test, no attempt is made to identify an end-point dilution, because such a procedure is statistically unsound inasmuch as it considers the fate of too small a group (10 mice). As the same number of mice is used for each serum and as the doses used for each serum are in the same ratio to each other, it is permissible to take into account the whole number (30) injected with each serum. The method of computation of potency values is, therefore, based on the equation:

$$\text{Units per cc. in unknown serum} = \frac{x}{y}\left(a + \frac{a\,(s - s')}{n}\right)$$

x = largest amount of control serum injected
y = largest amount of unknown serum injected
a = units per cc. in control serum
s = number of mice surviving on unknown serum
s′ = number of mice surviving on control serum, and
n = total number of mice injected with all dilutions of any one serum (see above).

If s is less than s′, then the part of the formula within the inner parentheses has a minus value and is subtracted from a, not added to it. The value of n will be 30, 60, 90, etc., depending upon the number of tests from which calculations are made.

The form of protocol used for reporting to the National Institute of Health does not show the value for x and y. The formula can be applied to these protocols if the following definitions are used for these values:

x = the smallest number of units tested for with unknown serum, and
y = smallest number of units tested for with control serum.

The application of the formula to the interpretation of the CP 77 B Types I and II protocols (pages 659 and 660 respectively) summarized on the attached National Institute of Health protocol (page 661), using the second definitions for x and y, is: $x = 1500$, $y = 150$, $a = 300$, $s = 14$, $s' = 15$, $n = 30$; so

$$\frac{x}{y}\left(a + \frac{a\,(s - s')}{n}\right) = \frac{1500}{150}\left(300 + \frac{300\,(14 - 15)}{30}\right) = 2900 \text{ Type I units per cc., and}$$

$$= \frac{750}{75}\left(150 + \frac{150\,(15 - 9)}{30}\right) = 1800 \text{ Type II units per cc.}$$

e. *Protocols and records.* Protocols of each protection test are kept in loose leaf notebooks for a year, after which they are filed in fireproof drawers. Samples of protocols of Type I and Type II tests appear on pages 659 and 660, and on page 661 there is a sample of the protocol for reporting to the National Institute of Health. The potencies of the various lots of serum for distribution are recorded on individual lot record cards.

Antipneumococcic Serum Potency Test - Protection Method - Type I

By L.A.B & E.C.W. Date 12-2-36

Date test begun 12-2-36 Date test finished 12-6-36
Mouse weights vary from 16 to 20 grams
Volume of test dilutions of serums injected 0.5cc.
Test dilution of culture 1:2500 Volume injected 0.5 cc
Number organisms in test dose 400,000 Number lethal doses in test dose 100,000

Serum Control No. P.11

Serum Dilutions

	1:1000	1:2000	1:4000
Dead at	67 hrs.	67	43
	67	67	43
	S	67	43
	S	92	43
	S	S	43
	S	S	48
	S	S	48
	S	S	67
	S	S	92
	S	S	S

1:2500
Culture Control:
Plate: OK
Result: Dead at
43 hrs.
43
67

Serum Lab. No. CP 77B

Serum Dilutions

	1:10,000	1:20,000	1:40,000
Dead at	43 hrs.	67	24
	67	67	43
	S	69	43
	S	92	48
	S	S	67
	S	S	67
	S	S	67
	S	S	67
	S	S	67
	S	S	92

Pneumococcus Culture Controls

Broth used 11-18-36 Seed culture used Pn I_s M 11-21-36 Volume seed used 1.0cc.
Vol. broth inoculated 15.0cc. No. hours grown 4½ Turbidity Good

Virulence Test

0.5 cc. of following dilutions injected:

	1:250 million	1:750 million	1:2500 million
No. orgs. inject.:	4	1	±1
Result Dead At	43 hrs.	S	S
	43	S	S
	67	S	S

Plate Counts

0.5 cc. of following dilutions plated:

	1:250 million	1:750 million	1:2500 million
Plate 1	3	1	1
Plate 2	5	1	0

Serum dilutions from 11:44 to 12:44 Culture dilutions from 1:56 to 2:22
Injections started 2:38 Injections finished 3:18

Interpretation of Test

CP 77B contains about 2900 Type I units per cc.

SAMPLE PROTOCOL OF A TYPE I TEST, MASSACHUSETTS DEPARTMENT OF PUBLIC HEALTH

Antipneumococcic Serum Potency Test - Protection Method - Type II

By L.A.B. & E.C.W. Date 12-8-36

Date test begun 12-8-36 Date test finished 12-12-36
Mouse weights vary from 16 to 20 grams
Volume of test dilutions of serums injected 0.5 cc.
Test dilution of culture 1:11,000 Volume injected 0.5 cc.
Number organisms in test dose 80,000 Number lethal doses in test dose 80,000

Serum Control No. P11.
Serum Dilutions

	1:1250	1:2500	1:5000
Dead at	43 hrs.	19	19
	67	24	19
	91	43	19
	S	43	19
	S	43	24
	S	43	24
	S	48	24
	S	48	43
	S	S	43
	S	S	43

1:11,000
Culture Control:
Plate: OK.
Result: Dead at
19 hrs.
19
24

Serum Lab. No. CP77B
Serum Dilutions

	1:12,500	1:25,000	1:50,000
Dead at	91 hrs.	19	24
	S	43	24
	S	67	43
	S	67	43
	S	91	43
	S	S	43
	S	S	48
	S	S	67
	S	S	72
	S	S	S

Pneumococcus Culture Controls

Broth used 11-18-36 Seed culture used PN II CW M12-1-36 Volume seed used 1.0 cc.
Vol. broth inoculated 15.0 cc. No. hours grown 4½ Turbidity Good

Virulence Test

0.5 cc. of following dilutions injected:

	1:110 million	1:330 million	1:1100 million
No. orgs. inject.:	8	1	±1
Result: Dead at	24 hrs.	19	24
	24	24	S
	43	S	S

Plate Counts

0.5 cc. of following dilutions plated:

	1:110 million	1:330 million	1:1100 million
Plate 1	11	2	1
Plate 2	5	0	0

Serum dilutions from 10:55 to 11:14 Culture dilutions from 1:40 to 2:10
Injections started 2:15 Injections finished 2:50

Interpretation of Test

CP 77B contains about 1800 Type II units per cc.

SAMPLE PROTOCOL OF A TYPE II TEST, MASSACHUSETTS DEPARTMENT OF PUBLIC HEALTH

Summary of Pneumococcus Types I and II Potency Tests

Product ________________________
(Nat. Inst. of Health Code No.)

Date of Test	Dose of Culture used 0.5 cc. of	Type I						Type II					
		Control Serum P-11						Control Serum P-11					
		150U		300U		600U		75U		150U		300U	
		S	D	S	D	S	D	S	D	S	D	S	D
12-2-36	1:2500	8	2	6	4	1	9						
12-8-36	1:11,000							7	3	2	8	0	10
Total		8	2	6	4	1	9	7	3	2	8	0	10
		Test Serum # CP 77B						Test Serum # CP 77B					
		1500U		3000U		6000U		750U		1500U		3000U	
		S	D	S	D	S	D	S	D	S	D	S	D
12-2-36	1:2500	8	2	6	4	0	10						
12-8-36	1:11,000							9	1	5	5	1	9
Total		8	2	6	4	0	10	9	1	5	5	1	9

From this summary the Potency of Lot #CP 77B is estimated to be for

Type I 2900 units per cc.

Type II 1800 units per cc.

Product - Concentrated Antipneumococcic Serum

Type - I and II

Lot No. - CP 77B

Nat. Inst. of Health Code No.

____
Name of Producing Laboratory

Signed ________________________

Date ________________________

SAMPLE PROTOCOL OF TYPE I AND TYPE II TESTS, FOR REPORTING TO THE NATIONAL INSTITUTE OF HEALTH

VIII. Sterility Tests on Antipneumococcic Serum

Bulk Sterility Tests (National Institute of Health Regulations)

For sterility tests, from each bulk container holding more than 1 liter at least 10 cc. should be planted into broth fermentation tubes; for bulk containers of less than 1 liter capacity at least 3 cc. should be planted into enough fermentation tubes so that the preservative shall not exceed 0.01 per cent of the broth used. If the bulk containers are opened at any subsequent manipulation, two 5 drop and two 20 drop fermentation tubes should be planted from each container. If contaminations appear in any of the bulk tests, the test may be repeated, but no lot shall be passed until such tests show no growth, and if the same contaminating organism appears in more than one test, the material shall be discarded or resterilized.

Inoculated tubes are incubated at 37° for seven days and should be examined on the second, fourth, and seventh days after planting, and agitated only after 48 hours incubation to ensure initial anaerobiosis; the lowest part of the bend should be examined for slight growths, as well as both arms. In case the material is turbid, transplants to fresh fermentation tubes, as well as smears, should be made on the seventh day.

Sterility Tests on Final Containers (National Institute of Health Regulations)

Of the final containers selected at random from each lot, three to ten shall be tested in accordance with the following schedule:

Total Number of Containers in the Lot	*Number of Containers to be Tested*
100 or less	3
101 to 150	4
151 to 200	5
201 to 250	6
251 to 300	7
301 to 350	8
351 to 400	9
Over 400	10

At least one 5 drop and one 20 drop fermentation tube shall be planted from each container. In the case of products to be administered in doses larger than 1 cc., the entire dose up to 5 cc. from each container tested shall be planted in fermentation tubes containing enough broth to dilute the preservative so that its concentration shall not exceed 0.01 per cent, but not more than 5 cc. need be planted from any container. In case contaminations appear in any of the tubes planted, the test may be repeated with the same number of containers but no lot shall be passed until the final test shows no growth throughout, and a lot shall be discarded if the same organism appears in more than one test.

IX. Preparation of Diagnostic Antipneumococcic Rabbit Serum

Massachusetts Antitoxin and Vaccine Laboratory Method

a. *Vaccine.* Eighteen hour broth cultures of highly virulent, type-specific pneumococci are centrifuged, the sediment taken up in physiological salt solution in quantities to give a corrected Gates reading of 2.0, and the suspension heated for 15 minutes at 100°. This results in a suspension containing approximately 25 billion organisms per cubic centimeter and is used as a stock supply of vaccine. No preservative is added. For the injection of rabbits, the stock vaccine is diluted 1 to 10 with physiological saline solution, thus giving a suspension containing about 2.5 billion organisms per cubic centimeter.

b. *Injection of rabbits.* A minimal number of six rabbits should be maintained on each type of vaccine. All injections are given intravenously, the schedule and dosages following the scheme given below:

Week	*Monday*	*Tuesday*	*Wednesday*	*Thursday*	*Friday*	*Saturday*
1	0.1	0.2	0.5			
2			0.2	0.5	1.0	
3	REST					
4	0.5	1.0	2.0			
5			1.0	2.0	3.0	
6	REST					
7	1.0	2.0	3.0			
8			1.0	2.0	3.0	
9	REST					
10					BLEED	
11	1.0	2.0	3.0			
12			1.0	2.0	3.0	
13	REST					
14					BLEED	

c. *Bleeding of rabbits.* The rabbits are bled by cardiac puncture every three weeks after routine bleedings are initiated and, with careful handling, the animals may be kept for an average of at least a year.

It has been found advisable to have available a supply of buffered glucose solution to administer intravenously to the occasional animal suffering severe systemic shock after having been bled. A minimum of 20 cc. of blood is removed from each rabbit and placed in 50 cc. centrifuge tubes, and slanted until coagulation has occurred. After standing for a few hours at room temperature, the clots are broken, and the tubes of blood stored overnight at 4°. The next morning the serum is drawn off, centrifuged, pooled, and preserved with 0.3 per cent (final concentration) of tricresol.

d. *Testing of serum.* The pooled serum of each type is tested for type-specific Neufeld reactions and for heterologous reactions with known closely related types. For these tests, mice are injected intraperitoneally with cultures of the types of Pneumococcus desired, and the peritoneal exudate washed out with saline solution about six hours after inoculation. Neufeld tests are set up in the usual manner, and if satisfactory results are obtained and no cross-reactions observed, the serum may be either filled immediately into separate containers, or added to the stock supply of serum of the respective types.

e. *Dilution of serum.* It is possible, after high titered serums are obtained, to obtain satisfactory Neufeld reactions with type-specific serums diluted with normal rabbit serum. The degree of dilution must be determined by tests, taking into consideration the amount of dilution which may occur in making the pools used in routine type determination in the diagnostic laboratory.

BIBLIOGRAPHY

The system adopted for the abbreviation of journal titles is that used in the Quarterly Cumulative Index Medicus *with any deficiencies supplied from the list prepared by the editors of the* Journal of Experimental Medicine. *The page number of the present volume on which a reference to a publication is made follows each communication cited. With few exceptions the original articles have been read and the references to them have been later compared with the originals. In spite of diligent effort in preparation, some errors undoubtedly occur in the bibliography as presented, for which the indulgence of the reader is asked.*

1. Abernethy, T. J. Studies on the somatic C polysaccharide of pneumococcus. II. The precipitation reaction in animals with experimentally induced pneumococcic infection. J. Exper. Med., 65(1): 75, Jan. 1937. 368
2. Abernethy, T. J., and Francis, T., Jr. Studies on the somatic C polysaccharide of pneumococcus. I. Cutaneous and serological reactions in pneumonia. J. Exper. Med., 65(1):59, Jan. 1937. ...... 368, 472
3. Adler, H. Über Pneumokokkentypen und Pneumokokkenimmunität. Ztschr. f. Hyg. u. Infektionskr., 101(2):140, 1923. .... 402, 439
4. Afanassiew. Note sur les micrococci de la pneumonie franche. Compt. rend. Soc. de biol., 36:356, 1884. 13
5. Aïtoff, M. Quelques observations sur la technique des cultures de pneumocoques. Compt. rend. Soc. de biol., 92(1):16, Jan. 1925.
6. Aïtoff, M., et Lagrange, E. Résistance de la souris au pneumocoque. Compt. rend. Soc. de biol., 92(18):1416, May 1925. 336
7. Alexander, H. L. A method for producing a rapid immunity to pneumococci. J. Med. Research, 37(3):471, Jan. 1918. .... 335, 529
8. Alloway, J. L. The transformation in vitro of R pneumococci into S forms of different specific types by the use of filtered pneumococcus extracts. J. Exper. Med., 55(1):91, Jan. 1932. .... 155, 160
9. Alloway, J. L. Further observations on the use of pneumococcus extracts in effecting transformation of type in vitro. J. Exper. Med., 57(2):265, Feb. 1933. 160
10. Alston, J. M., and Lowdon, A. S. R. Studies of the skin reactions to the specific soluble substances of the pneumococcus Types I and II. Brit. J. Exper. Path., 14(1):1, Feb. 1933. 464
11. Alston, J. M., and Stewart, D. Some observations on passive immunity in the normal subject produced by antipneumococcic sera. Brit. J. Exper. Path., 12(1):49, Feb. 1931.
12. Amoss, H. L. The composite nature of a pure culture of a virulent pneumococcus. J. Exper. Med., 41(5):649, May 1925. 140
13. Amoss, H. L. Specific soluble substances of the pneumococcus in the blood in pneumonia. Proc. Soc. Exper. Biol. & Med., 28(1):23, Oct. 1930. 129

14. Amzel, R. Sur la variabilité du pneumocoque, expériences de Morgenroth: Pneumocoque et Streptococcus viridans. Compt. rend. Soc. de biol., 96(18):1487, June 1927. 144
15. Amzel, R. Sur la variabilité du pneumocoque. Pneumocoque des pneumonies et des sujets sains. Compt. rend. Soc. de biol., 96(18): 1489, June 1927. 145
16. Aoki. Über Kapselbildung der Pneumokokken im Immunserum. Arch. f. Hyg., 75:393, 1912. 33
17. Arkharow, J. Recherches sur la guérison de l'infection pneumonique chez les lapins au moyen du serum des lapins vaccinés. Arch. d. méd. expér. et d'anat. path., 4:498, 1892. .... 49, 135, 136
18. Arkwright, J. A. Variation in bacteria in relation to agglutination both by salts and by specific serum. J. Path. & Bact., 24(1): 36, Jan. 1921. 137
19. Armstrong, R. R. The serological characters of disease-producing pneumococci. Brit. M. J., 1(3138):259, Feb. 19, 1921. .... 111, 362
20. Armstrong, R. R. Application of the absorption of agglutinin test to the serological study of pneumococci. Brit. J. Exper. Path., 3(6):287, Dec. 1922. 362
21. Armstrong, R. R. The correlation of clinical manifestations and serological types in pneumococcus infections. St. Barth. Hosp. Rep., 56, pt. 1(1):85, Jan. 1923.
22. Armstrong, R. R. A swift and simple method for deciding pneumococcal "Type." Brit. M. J., 1(3657):214, Feb. 7, 1931. 127
23. Armstrong, R. R. Immediate pneumococcal typing. Brit. M. J., 1(3708):187, Jan. 30, 1932. 128
24. Arustamow, M. J. Ueber Aetiologie und klinische Bakteriologie der croupösen Lungenentzündung. Woenno-M. J., (2/4):61, 1889. *Abstract in* Jahresb. ü. d. Fortschr. i. d. Lehre v. d. path. Mikroorg., 5:52 & 61, 1889. 20
25. Ash, R. Nonspecific precipitins for pneumococcic Fraction C in acute infections. J. Infect. Dis., 53(1):89, July–Aug., 1933. 368
26. Ash, R., and Solis-Cohen, M. The action of whole fresh blood on pneumococci. J. Infect. Dis., 45(6):440, Dec. 1929. 434
27. Ash, R., and Solis-Cohen, M. Influence of quinin on proliferation and autolysis of pneumococci. J. Infect. Dis., 45(6):449, Dec. 1929.
28. Ash, R.. and Solis-Cohen, M. Contrasted behavior of pneumococci toward quinin and optochin in relation to drug fastness. J. Infect. Dis., 45(6):457, Dec. 1929.
29. Atkin, E. E. The rationale of the bile solubility of pneumococcus. Brit. J. Exper. Path., 7(4):167, Aug. 1926. .... 61, 149
30. Auld, A. G. Remarks on the morphology and chemical products of the diplococcus pneumoniae, and some results of vaccination. Brit. M. J., 1(1891):775, Mar. 27, 1897. 338
31. Auld, A. G. Remarks on the toxines of the pneumococcus. Tr. Path. Soc. London, 52:108, Feb. 19, 1901.
32. Avery, O. T. The distribution of the immune bodies occurring in

antipneumococcus serum. J. Exper. Med., 21(2):133, Feb. 1915. 411, 528, 547, 548, 550

33. AVERY, O. T. A further study on the biologic classification of pneumococci. J. Exper. Med., 22(6):804, Dec. 1915. 108

34. AVERY, O. T. Determination of types of pneumococcus in lobar pneumonia. A rapid culture method. J. A. M. A., 70(1):17, Jan. 5, 1918. 123

35. AVERY, O. T. The rôle of specific carbohydrates in pneumococcus infection and immunity. Ann. Int. Med., 6(1):1, July 1932.

36. AVERY, O. T., CHICKERING, H. T., COLE, R., and DOCHEZ, A. R. Acute lobar pneumonia. Prevention and serum treatment. New York: Rockefeller Institute for Medical Research, 1917. (Monographs of the Rockefeller Institute for Medical Research, No. 7.) 30, 57, 120, 228, 522, 524, 529, 530, 534, 535, 538, 541, 543, 567, 625, 626

37. AVERY, O. T., and CULLEN, G. E. Hydrogen ion concentration of cultures of pneumococci of the different types in carbohydrate media. J. Exper. Med., 30(4):359, Oct. 1919. 71

38. AVERY, O. T., and CULLEN, G. E. Studies on the enzymes of pneumococcus. I. Proteolytic enzymes. J. Exper. Med., 32(5):547, Nov. 1920. .... 54, 65, 239

39. AVERY, O. T., and CULLEN, G. E. Studies on the enzymes of pneumococcus. II. Lipolytic enzymes: esterase. J. Exper. Med., 32(5): 571, Nov. 1920. .... 54, 66

40. AVERY, O. T., and CULLEN, G. E. Studies on the enzymes of pneumococcus. III. Carbohydrate-splitting enzymes: invertase, amylase, and inulase. J. Exper. Med., 32(5):583, Nov. 1920. .... 54, 67

41. AVERY, O. T., and CULLEN, G. E. Studies on the enzymes of pneumococcus. IV. Bacteriolytic enzyme. J. Exper. Med., 38(2):199, Aug. 1923. .... 54, 60, 61, 239

42. AVERY, O. T., and DUBOS, R. The specific action of a bacterial enzyme on pneumococci of Type III. Science, 72(1858):151, Aug. 8, 1930. 301

43. AVERY, O. T., and DUBOS, R. The protective action of a specific enzyme against Type III pneumococcus infection in mice. J. Exper. Med., 54(1):73, July 1931. 302

44. AVERY, O. T., and GOEBEL, W. F. Chemo-immunological studies on conjugated carbohydrate-proteins. II. Immunological specificity of synthetic sugar-protein antigens. J. Exper. Med., 50(4):533, Oct. 1929. .... 263, 376

45. AVERY, O. T., and GOEBEL, W. F. Chemo-immunological studies on conjugated carbohydrate-proteins. V. The immunological specificity of an antigen prepared by combining the capsular polysaccharide of Type III pneumococcus with foreign protein. J. Exper. Med., 54(3):437, Sept. 1931. .... 265, 371, 378, 411, 451

46. AVERY, O. T., and GOEBEL, W. F. Chemo-immunological studies on the soluble specific substance of pneumococcus. I. The isolation and properties of the acetyl polysaccharide of pneumococcus Type I. J. Exper. Med., 58(6):731, Dec. 1933. .... 278, 364, 371, 411, 580, 582

47. Avery, O. T., and Goebel, W. F. The chemo-immunological properties of the specific capsular polysaccharide of pneumococcus Type I. (Abstract.) J. Bact., 27(1):89, Jan. 1934.
48. Avery, O. T., and Heidelberger, M. Immunological relationships of cell constituents of pneumococcus. J. Exper. Med., 38(1):81, July 1923.
49. Avery, O. T., and Heidelberger, M. Immunological relationships of cell constituents of pneumococcus. Paper II. J. Exper. Med., 42(3):367, Sept. 1925. .... 380, 525, 526
50. Avery, O. T., Heidelberger, M., and Goebel, W. F. The soluble specific substance of Friedländer's bacillus. II. Chemical and immunological relationships of pneumococcus Type II and a strain of Friedländer's bacillus. J. Exper. Med., 42(5):709, Nov. 1925.
51. Avery, O. T., and Morgan, H. J. The effect of the accessory substances of plant tissue upon growth of bacteria. Proc. Soc. Exper. Biol. & Med., 19(3):113, Dec. 1921. 44
52. Avery, O. T., and Morgan, H. J. The occurrence of peroxide in cultures of pneumococcus. J. Exper. Med., 39(2):275, Feb. 1924. 44, 76
53. Avery, O. T., and Morgan, H. J. Studies on bacterial nutrition. V. The effect of plant tissue upon the growth of anaerobic bacilli. J. Exper. Med., 39(2):289, Feb. 1924. 44
54. Avery, O. T., and Morgan, H. J. Immunological reactions of the isolated carbohydrate and protein of pneumococcus. J. Exper. Med., 42(3):347, Sept. 1925. .... 251, 367, 526, 636
55. Avery, O. T., and Neill, J. M. Studies on oxidation and reduction by pneumococcus. I. Production of peroxide by anaerobic cultures of pneumococcus on exposure to air under conditions not permitting active growth. J. Exper. Med., 39(3):347, Mar. 1924. 76
56. Avery, O. T., and Neill, J. M. Studies on oxidation and reduction by pneumococcus. II. The production of peroxide by sterile extracts of pneumococcus. J. Exper. Med., 39(3):357, Mar. 1924. 76
57. Avery, O. T., and Neill, J. M. Studies on oxidation and reduction by pneumococcus. III. Reduction of methylene blue by sterile extracts of pneumococcus. J. Exper. Med., 39(4):543, Apr. 1924. 77
58. Avery, O. T., and Neill, J. M. Studies on oxidation and reduction by pneumococcus. IV. Oxidation of hemotoxin in sterile extracts of pneumococcus. J. Exper. Med., 39(5):745, May 1924. 84
59. Avery, O. T., and Neill, J. M. The antigenic properties of solutions of pneumococcus. J. Exper. Med., 42(3):355, Sept. 1925. 252, 525, 526
60. Avery, O. T., and Tillett, W. S. Anaphylaxis with the type-specific carbohydrates of pneumococcus. J. Exper. Med., 49(2): 251, Feb. 1929. .... 448, 449
61. Babers, F. H., and Goebel, W. F. The molecular size of the Type III specific polysaccharide of pneumococcus. J. Biol. Chem., 89 (1):387, Nov. 1930. 246
62. Bachmann, A., et Miravent, J. M. Classification des pneumocoques isolés en Argentine. Compt. rend. Soc. de biol., 88:385, Oct. 1923.

62a. Baduel, C. L'infezione diplococcica (diplococco di Fraenkel). Contributo di osservazioni cliniche e batteriologiche. Riforma med., 1(15):170, Jan. 19, 1899.

62b. Baermann, G. Ueber Pneumokokken-Pneumonie und deren Chemotherapie. Ztschr. f. Exper. Path. u. Therap., 15(3):476, March 16, 1914.

63. Baerthlein, K. Über Mutationserscheinungen bei Bakterien. Arb. a. d. k. Gsndhtsamte, 40(4):433, Sept. 1912.

64. Bailey, G. H., and Shorb, M. S. Heterophile antigen in pneumococci. Am. J. Hyg., 13(3):831, May 1931. 387

65. Bailey, G. H., and Shorb, M. S. Chemical and immunological properties of pneumococci and other heterophile antibodies. Am. J. Hyg., 17(2):329, Mar. 1933. 387

66. Bailey, G. H., and Shorb, M. S. Immunological relationships of pneumococci and other heterophile antigens and biological significance in pneumococcus infection. Am. J. Hyg., 17(2):358, Mar. 1933. 288

67. Bailey, S. F. "Hormone Mediums." Simple method of preparation and value of hormone blood agar for preserving pneumococci and streptococci. J. Infect. Dis., 36(3):340, Mar. 1925. 44

68. Baldwin, H. S., and Rhoades, D. R. Studies on pneumococcus immunity. VII. The protective substance in pneumococcus pneumonia with special reference to bacteriemia and specific treatment. Hygienic Laboratory Bulletin, No. 141:43, Apr. 1925. 439

69. Baldwin, H. S., and Rhoades, D. R. The use of optochin base in the treatment of lobar pneumonia. Hygienic Laboratory Bulletin, No. 141:69, Apr. 1925. 514

70. Banzhaf, E. J. The distribution of the immune bodies occurring in Types I, II and III antipneumococcus serum. Proc. Soc. Exper. Biol. & Med., 22(6):329, Mar. 1925. .... 412, 548, 549, 550, 551, 553

71. Banzhaf, E. J., and Curphey, T. J. A modified method for the production of antipneumococcus serum in horses. Proc. Soc. Exper. Biol. & Med., 28(3):279, Dec. 1930. 338

72. Banzhaf, E. J., and Klein, A. J. A practical method for concentrating chill free pneumococcus antibodies from sera without use of salt precipitations. Proc. Soc. Exper. Biol. & Med., 28(3):276, Dec. 1930. .... 549, 550, 552, 563

73. Banzhaf, E. J., and Klein, A. J. A practical method for concentrating chill free pneumococcus antibodies from plasma without use of salt precipitations. Proc. Soc. Exper. Biol. & Med., 28(3): 278, Dec. 1930.

74. Barach, A. L. Rate of development of pneumococcus immunity. Proc. Soc. Exper. Biol. & Med., 25(7):558, Apr. 1928. .... 336, 411, 490

75. Barach, A. L. Factors involved in the production of immunity with pneumococcus vaccine. I. Active and passive immunity during the first seven days after the injection of antigen. J. Exper. Med., 48(1):83, July 1928. .... 327, 336, 484, 490, 526, 541

76. Barach, A. L. Factors involved in the production of immunity

with pneumococcus vaccine. II. Induction of active immunity during the course of lobar pneumonia. J. Exper. Med., 53(4):567, Apr. 1931. .... 411, 483, 490, 505

77. BARBER, M. A. A study by the single cell method of the influence of homologous antipneumococcic serum on the growth rate of pneumococcus. J. Exper. Med., 30(6):569, Dec. 1919. 391

78. BARBER, M. A. Antiblastic phenomena in active acquired immunity and in natural immunity to pneumococcus. J. Exper. Med., 30(6): 589, Dec. 1919. 421

79. BARJOT, M. Sur un traitement des septicémies pneumococciques par l'injection intraveineuse de sels biliaires. Bull. Acad. de méd., Paris, 100(31), 3e sér.:898, July 31, 1928. 508

80. BARNARD, R. D., and GOWEN, G. H. The greenish discoloration produced on blood agar by the growth of pneumococcus. Proc. Soc. Exper. Biol. & Med., 29(5):521, Feb. 1932. 75

81. BARNES, L. A., and CLARKE, C. M. The pneumococcidal powers of sodium oleate and sodium ricinoleate. (Abstract.) J. Bact., 27 (1):107, Jan. 1934. 63

82. BARNES, L. A., CLARKE, C. M., and WIGHT, E. C. Comparisons of various methods for the routine titration of Types I and II antipneumococcic horse serums. J. Immunol., 30(2):127, Feb. 1936. 378, 410, 573, 583, 584, 644

83. BARNES, L. A., and KRAMER, S. D. A test for reaction-producing substances in concentrated antipneumococcic serum. Preliminary report. Am. J. Pub. Health, 23(6):616, June 1933. *Abstract in* J. A. M. A., 101(18):1423, Oct. 28, 1933. .... 563, 564, 588

84. BARNES, L. A., and ROBINSON, E. S. Monkey test for chill-producing activity of concentrated antipneumococcic serum. Am. J. Pub. Health, 26(1):51, Jan. 1936. .... 564, 588

85. BARNES, L. A., and WHITE, B. The fermentation of glycogen by pneumococci. (Abstract.) J. Bact., 27(1):106, Jan. 1934. 69

86. BARNES, L. A., and WHITE, B. The antibody response of rabbits during prolonged immunization with Type I pneumococcus vaccine. Am. J. Hyg., 21(1):35, Jan. 1935. *Abstract in* J. Immunol., 26 (4):335, Apr. 1934. .... 331, 531, 534, 536, 537, 541, 542, 594

87. BARNES, L. A., and WIGHT, E. C. Serological relationship between pneumococcus Type I and an encapsulated strain of Escherichia coli. J. Exper. Med., 62(2):281, Aug. 1935. 261

88. BARNES, L. A., and WIGHT, E. C. The spontaneous transformation of Pneumococcus Type V to Type II. J. Bact., 32(5):557, Nov. 1936. .... 546, 595

89. BAUDISCH, O., und DUBOS, R. Über Katalasewirkung von Eisenverbindungen in Kulturmedien. Biochem. Ztschr. 245(4/6):278, Feb. 1932. 43

90. BAUER, J. H., and HUGHES, T. P. The preparation of the graded collodion membranes of Elford and their use in the study of filterable viruses. J. Gen. Physiol., 18(2):143, Nov. 1934–35. .. 310, 417, 640

91. BAUMGARTNER, L. Age and antibody production. I. Qualitative changes in antisera associated with age. J. Immunol., 27(4):407, Oct. 1934. 351

92. BAUMGARTNER, L. Age and antibody production. II. Further observations on qualitative changes in antisera associated with age. J. Immunol., 27(4):417, Oct. 1934. 351

93. BAURHENN, W. Experimentelle Untersuchungen zur Variabilität und zur Analyse der R → S = Umwandlung von Pneumokokken, mit besonderer Berücksichtigung der Gruppe X. Zentralbl. f. Bakt., 1 Abt., Orig., 126(1/2):68, Oct. 25, 1932. 157

94. BAYER, G. Untersuchungen über die Gallenhämolyse. I. Über die Hemmungswirkung normaler Sera. Biochem. Ztschr., 5:368, July 1907.

95. BEARD, S. D., and CLAPP, F. L. The mouse protection test on antipneumococcic serum Type I. J. Immunol., 23(1):91, July 1932. 573

96. BECKLER, E., and MACLEOD, P. The Neufeld method of pneumococcus type determination as carried out in a public health laboratory: a study of 760 typings. J. Clin. Investigation, 13(6):901, Nov. 1934. .... 132, 630

97. BECKLER, E. A., MARDEN, K., and GILLETTE, H. H. Pneumococcus type determination by Avery's cultural method. J. A. M. A., 70 (12):836, Mar. 23, 1918. 123

98. BEHRING und NISSEN, F. Ueber bacterienfeindliche Eigenschaften verschiedener Blutserumarten. Ein Beitrag zur Immunitätsfrage. Ztschr. f. Hyg. u. Infektionskr., 8:412, 1890. .... 42, 428

99. BENGSTON, I. A. II. Studies on the potency testing of pneumococcus vaccines. Hygienic Laboratory Bulletin, No. 139:15, Nov. 1924. 485

100. BERGER, E., und ENGELMANN, B. Die Einheit der Pneumokokken und Streptokokken. Deutsche med. Wchnschr., 51(32):1317, Aug. 7, 1925. .... 144, 174

101. BERGER, E., und ENGELMANN, B. Über Änderungen des serologischen Typus bei einem Pneumokokkus. Klin. Wchnschr., 5(14): 599, Apr. 2, 1926. .... 144, 175

102. BERGER, E., und JAKUB, T. Ueber die Einheit der Streptokokken und Pneumokokken. II. Mitteilung. Ztschr. f. Immunitätsforsch. u. exper. Therap., 43(3):235, June 1925. 174

103. BERGER, E., und SILBERSTEIN, W. Die Inulinvergärung in der Streptokokken-Pneumokokkengruppe. Klin. Wchnschr., 5(49): 2307, Dec. 3, 1926. .... 69, 175

104. BERGEY, D. H. Bergey's manual of determinative bacteriology. A key for the identification of organisms of the class Schizomycetes, 48. 4th ed. Baltimore: The Williams & Wilkins Company, 1934. 1

105. BERRY, C. W., and CHICKERING, H. T. Lobar pneumonia of unusual communicability. Health News, 33(2):47, Feb. 1917.

106. BERRY, J. L. A study of the pneumococcus, with especial reference to the inulin test. J. Infect. Dis., 4(1):93, Jan. 1907. 68

107. Bessemans, A., de Potter, F., et de Geest. Sur les caractères biologiques du pneumocoque. Compt. rend. Soc. de biol., 97(24): 909, July 1927.

108. Bezançon, F., et Griffon, V. Pouvoir agglutinatif du sérum dans les infections expérimentales et humaines à pneumocoques. Part I. Compt. rend. Soc. de biol., 49:551, June 1897. .... 26, 103, 356

109. Bezançon, F., et Griffon, V. Pouvoir agglutinatif du sérum dans les infections expérimentales et humaines à pneumocoques. Part II. Compt. rend. Soc. de biol., 49:579, June 1897. ...... 26, 103, 356

110. Bezançon, F., et Griffon, V. Pouvoir agglutinatif du sérum dans les infections expérimentales et humaines à pneumocoques. Presse méd., 5²(58):25, July 17, 1897. .... 103, 356

110a. Bezançon, F., et Griffon, V. Présence constante du pneumocoque à la surface de l'amygdale. Bull. et mém. Soc. méd. des Hôp. de Paris, 15, 3ᵉ sér.:320, 1898.

111. Bezançon, F., et Griffon, V. Recherches sur le mode de développement et la vitalité du pneumocoque dans les divers sérums. Compt. rend. Soc. de biol., 50:218, Feb. 1898.

112. Bezançon, F., et Griffon, V. Milieux de culture du pneumocoque. Milieu de diagnostic; milieu de conservation. Presse méd., 6²(69):99, Aug. 20, 1898. *Also:* Compt. rend. Soc. de biol., 50:303, Mar. 1898. .... 42, 49

113. Bezançon, F., et Griffon, V. Étude de la réaction agglutinante du sérum dans les infections expérimentales et humaines à pneumocoques. Ann. Inst. Pasteur, 14(7):449, July 1900. 104

114. Bieling, R. Methoden zur Differenzierung der Streptokokken und Pneumokokken. Centralbl. f. Bakt., 1 Abt., Orig., 86(4):257, June 1921. 48

115. Bigelow, G. H. Intracutaneous reactions in lobar pneumonia. Arch. Int. Med., 29(2):221, Feb. 1922. 462

116. Bigelow, G. H., Rosenau, M. J., Lord, F. T., Locke, E. A., Sutliff, W. D., Beckler, E., White, B., Peterson, W., and Heffron, R. Lobar pneumonia. The Commonhealth, 18(3):131, July–Sept. 1931.

117. Biondi, D. Die pathogenen Mikroorganismen des Speichels. Ztschr. f. Hyg. u. Infektionskr., 2:194, 1887. .... 1, 20

118. Biscoe, J., Herčík, F., and Wyckoff, R. W. G. The size of antibodies. Science, 83(2164):602, June 19, 1936. 415

119. Biscoe, J., Pickels, E. G., and Wyckoff, R. W. G. An air-driven ultracentrifuge for molecular sedimentation. J. Exper. Med., 64 (1):39, July 1936. 415

120. Black-Milne, J., and Rogers, K. Influenzal broncho-pneumonia and pneumonia treated with the army mixed vaccine. Lancet, 2 (5017):731, Oct. 25, 1919.

121. Blacklock, J. W. S., and Guthrie, K. J. Pneumococcal infections in infancy and childhood. J. Path. & Bact., 36(3):349, May 1933.

122. Blackman, S. S., Jr. Pneumococcal lipoid nephrosis and the re-

lation between nephrosis and nephritis. II. Experimental studies. Bull. Johns Hopkins Hosp., 55(2):85, Aug. 1934. 385

123. Blake, F. G. Methods for the determination of pneumococcus types. J. Exper. Med., 26(1):67, July 1917. .... 122, 366

124. Blake, F. G. Studies on antiblastic immunity. J. Exper. Med., 26(4):563, Oct. 1917. 421

125. Blake, F. G. Antigen-antibody balance in lobar pneumonia. Arch. Int. Med., 21(6):779, June 1918. .... 360, 366

126. Blake, F. G., and Cecil, R. L. Studies on experimental pneumonia. I. Production of pneumococcus lobar pneumonia in monkeys. J. Exper. Med., 31(4):403, Apr. 1920. 192

127. Blake, F. G., and Cecil, R. L. Studies on experimental pneumonia. II. Pathology and pathogenesis of pneumococcus lobar pneumonia in monkeys. J. Exper. Med., 31(4):445, Apr. 1920. ... 192

128. Blake, F. G., and Cecil, R. L. Studies on experimental pneumonia. III. Spontaneous pneumonia in monkeys. J. Exper. Med., 31(5):499, May 1, 1920. 191

129. Blake, F. G., and Trask, J. D. Alterations in virulence and agglutination reactions of pneumococcus induced by growth in immune serum. Abstr. Bact., 7(9):353, Sept. 1923. .... 139, 362

130. Blake, F. G., and Trask, J. D. Pneumococcus variants intermediate between the S and R forms. J. Bact., 25(3):289, Mar. 1933. 152

131. Bliss, E. A., McClaskey, W. D., and Long, P. H. A study of pneumococcus carriers. J. Immunol., 27(1):95, July 1934. 235

132. Boehncke, K. E. Beobachtungen bei der Chemo-Serotherapie der Pneumokokkeninfection. München. med. Wchnschr., 50(8):398, Feb. 25, 1913. 518

133. Boehncke, K. E. Ueber die Wirkung des Camphers bei bakterieller Infektion. Berl. klin. Wchnschr., 50(18):818, May 5, 1913.

134. Boehncke, K. E., und Mouriz-Riesgo, J. Zum Mechanismus der Pneumokokkenimmunität. Ztschr. f. Hyg. u. Infektionskr., 79:355, 1915. .... 96, 383, 391, 511, 518

135. Bolduan, C. The addition of marble or other calcium compounds to nutrient broth; a reliable and convenient method for growing the pneumococcus. Proc. New York Path. Soc., 5(3), n.s.:38, Apr. 1905. 39

136. Bolognesi, G. Die Anaërobiose des Fränkelschen Diplococcus in Beziehung zu einer seiner pathogenen Eigenschaften. (Translated by Dr. Kurt Tautz, Berlin). Centralbl. f. Bakt., 1 Abt., Orig., 43(2):113, 1907.

137. Bonome, A. Der Diplococcus pneumonicus und die Bakterie der hämorrhagischen Kaninchensepticämie. Fortschr. d. Med., 9(18): 743, Sept. 15, 1891. .... 23, 93, 325, 337, 389

138. Boor, A. K., and Miller, C. P., Jr. "Nucleoprotein" and non-protein substance isolated from the gonococcus. III. Immunological reactions with anti-meningococcus and anti-pneumococcus sera. Proc. Soc. Exper. Biol. & Med., 28(9):1050, June 1931. .... 248, 370

139. Bordet, P. Morphologie du pneumocoque. Compt. rend. Soc. de biol., 108(33):707, Nov. 20, 1931. .... 42, 71
140. Bordet, P. Proprietés biochimiques du pneumocoque en rapport avec l'immunité. Compt. rend. Soc. de biol., 108(34):752, Nov. 27, 1931. .... 71, 421
141. Bordet, P. Qualités propres aux sérums de diverses espéces animales par rapport au pneumocoque. Ann. Inst. Pasteur, 51(4): 503, Oct. 1933. 433
142. Bordoni-Uffreduzzi, G. Ueber die Widerstandsfähigkeit des pneumonischen Virus in den Auswürfen. Centralbl. f. Bakt., 1 Abt., Orig., 10(10):305, Sept. 18, 1891. 50
142a. Borissoff, L. P. Examen bactériologique du sang comme moyen de diagnostic précoce de la pneumonie. Rousski Wratch, 31:609, May 16, 1908. *Abstract in* Bull. Inst. Pasteur, 6(14):638, July 30, 1908.
143. Borrell, A. Pneumonie et tuberculose chez les troupes noires. Ann. Inst. Pasteur, 34(3):105, Mar. 1920. 496
143a. Bourg. Étude sur la virulence du pneumocoque dans les affections oculaires. Thèse de Paris, 1909.
143b. Bourla, M. O. Virulence du pneumocoque dans certaines formes de congestion pulmonaire. Thèse de Paris, 1902.
144. Boyd, W. C., and Hooker, S. B. The influence of molecular weight antigen on the proportion of antibody to antigen in precipitates. J. Gen. Physiol., 17(3):341, Jan. 1934.
145. Bozzolo, C. La pneumonite lobare, la pleurite, la pericardite, la endocardite e la meningite cerebrospinale acuta considerate nei loro reciproci rapporti. Gior. d. r. Accad. di med. di Torino, 30, 3. s.:856, 1882. 8
146. Brahn, B., Schiff, F., und Weinmann, F. Über die chemische Natur der Gruppensubstanz A. Klin. Wchnschr., 11(38):1592, Sept. 17, 1934. 288
147. Branch, A. Spontaneous infections of guinea pigs. Pneumococcus, Friedländer bacillus and pseudotuberculosis (Eberthella caviae). J. Infect. Dis., 40(4):533, Apr. 1927. 186
148. Branch, A., and Stillman, E. G. Pathology of the experimental pneumonias in mice following inhalation of Streptococcus haemolyticus, of Friedländer's bacillus, and of Pneumococcus. J. Exper. Med., 41(5):631, May 1925. 190
149. Bronfenbrenner, J., and Knights, E. The value of intratracheal route of immunization with pneumococcus. Proc. Soc. Exper. Biol. & Med., 19(7):336, Apr. 1922. 341
150. Brotzu, G. Über die Herstellung einer polyvalenten Pneumokokkenvaccine. (Experimentelle Untersuchungen.) Ztschr. f. Hyg. u. Infektionskr., 103(1):139, July 1924. 483
151. Brown, M. H. A rapid method of typing pneumococci. Am. J. Pub. Health, 21(6):669, June 1931. 129
152. Brown, M. H., and Anderson, E. A further bacteriological study

of the bacterial flora of the throat of normal persons and persons with minor respiratory infections, with special reference to the pneumococcus. J. Prev. Med., 6(5):407, Sept. 1932. .... 215, 235

153. Brown, M. H., and Knowles, W. A method of concentrating the pseudoglobulins of antipneumococcus serum. Tr. Roy. Soc. Canada, 26, ser. 3, sect. 5, May 1932. 548

154. Brown, R. A specific precipitation test for the standardization of Type I antipneumococcus serum. J. Immunol., 25(2):149, Aug. 1933. 585

155. Brown, R. Observations on induction of anaphylactic shock by the specific carbohydrates of Type-I pneumococcus. Proc. Soc. Exper. Biol. & Med., 31(6):699, Mar. 1934. 453

156. Brown, R. Failure of antipneumococcus horse serum to sensitize guinea pigs to anaphylactic shock with specific carbohydrates. Proc. Soc. Exper. Biol. & Med., 31(6):700, Mar. 1934. 453

157. Brown, R. The specific carbohydrate from pneumococcus Type VIII. Proc. Soc. Exper. Biol. & Med., 32(6):859, Mar. 1935. 274

158. Brown, R. Ultrafiltration in the concentration and purification of pneumococcus specific polysaccharides. Proc. Soc. Exper. Biol. & Med., 34(5):832, June 1936. 275

159. Browning, C. H. [The pneumococcus.] Sensitiveness to antiseptics—chemotherapy. *In* Great Britain, Medical Research Council. A system of bacteriology in relation to medicine, 2:225. London: His Majesty's Stationery Office, 1929. .... 62, 517

160. Browning, C. H., and Gulbransen, R. Observations on the chemo-therapy of bacterial infections, with special reference to experimental pneumococcus infection. J. Path. & Bact., 22(3): 265, 1919.

160a. Browning, C. H., and Gulbransen, R. Alterations in morphological and biological characters in the streptococcus group brought about in vivo—(1) Streptococcus mucosus; (2) chronic pneumococcus infections. J. Path. & Bact., 26(1):121, 1923.

161. Browning, C. H., and Gulbransen, R. The effect of the individual host on the virulence of pneumococci. (Abstract.) J. Path. & Bact., 26(3):428, July 1923. 205

161a. Bruckner, J., et Galasesco, P. Sur la septicémie pneumococcique spontanée du cobaye. Compt. rend. Soc. de biol., 79:102, Dec. 2, 1916.

162. Bruns, H. Ueber die Fähigkeit des Pneumococcus Fränkel locale Eiterungen zu erzeugen. Berl. klin. Wchnschr., 34(17):357, Apr. 26, 1897.

163. Buerger, L. The macroscopic identification of colonies of the pneumococcus. Centralbl. f. Bakt., 1 Abt., Orig., 39(1):20, 1905. *Also:* Proc. New York Path. Soc., 5(3), n.s.:40, Apr. 1905. 47

164. Buerger, L. Studies of the pneumococcus and allied organisms with reference to their occurrence in the human mouth. J. Exper. Med., 7(5):497, Aug. 1905. *Also:* Department of Health, City of

New York. Report Med. Comm'n Invest. Acute Resp. Dis., Part I. Studies on pneumococcus, p. 95. New York: Department of Health, 1905. 215

165. Buerger, L. Beitrag zur Kenntnis des Streptococcus mucosus capsulatus. Centralbl. f. Bakt., 1 Abt., Orig., 41(3):314, 1906.

166. Buerger, L. Beitrag zur Kenntnis des Streptococcus mucosus capsulatus. Fortsetzung. Centralbl. f. Bakt., 1 Abt., Orig., 41(4): 414, 1906.

167. Buerger, L. Beitrag zur Kenntnis des Streptococcus mucosus capsulatus. Schluss. Centralbl. f. Bakt., 1 Abt., Orig., 41(5):511, 1906.

168. Buerger, L. A new method for staining the capsules of bacteria; being also a contribution to the morphology and differentiation of some encapsulated organisms. Mt. Sinai Hosp. Rep. (1905 & 1906), 5:513, 1907. 34

169. Buerger, L., and Ryttenberg, C. Observations upon certain properties acquired by the pneumococcus in the human body. J. Infect. Dis., 4(4):609, Nov. 1907. .... 149, 170

170. Bull, C. G. The mechanism of the curative action of antipneumococcus serum. J. Exper. Med., 22(4):457, Oct. 1915. 363

171. Bull, C. G. A method of serum treatment of pneumococcic septicemia in rabbits. J. Exper. Med., 22(4):466, Oct. 1915.

172. Bull, C. G. The agglutination of bacteria in vivo. J. Exper. Med., 22(4):484, Oct. 1915. 363

173. Bull, C. G. Immunity factors in pneumococcus infection in the dog. J. Exper. Med., 24(1):7, July 1916. .... 195, 363

174. Bull, C. G. Further observations on the agglutination of bacteria in vivo. J. Exper. Med., 24(1):25, July 1916. 363

175. Bull, C. G. Heterophile antigens and antibodies. *In* Jordan, E. O., and Falk, I. S. The newer knowledge of bacteriology and immunology, 733. Chicago: The University of Chicago Press, 1928. 387

176. Bull, C. G., and Bailey, G. H. Accessory etiologic factors of pneumonia in rabbits. I. Effect of putting brilliant green into nasal passages. Proc. Soc. Exper. Biol. & Med., 24(2):183, Nov. 1926.

177. Bull, C. G., and Bartual, L. Pneumococcus cultures in whole fresh blood. I. The retardative effect of the blood of immune animals and the mechanism of the phenomenon. J. Exper. Med., 31 (3):233, Mar. 1920. *Abstract in* Abstr. Bact., 4(1):18, Feb. 1920. 420

178. Bull, C. G., and McKee, C. M. Antipneumococcus protective substances in normal chicken serum. Am. J. Hyg., 1(3):284, May 1921.

179. Bull, C. G., and McKee, C. M. Respiratory immunity in rabbits. VI. The effects of immunity on the carrier state of the pneumococcus and Bacillus bronchisepticus. Am. J. Hyg., 8(5):723, Sept. 1928.

180. Bull, C. G., and McKee, C. M. The sensitization of rabbits to

products of the pneumococcus resulting from an acute infection with this organism. Am. J. Hyg., 9(3):666, May 1929. .... 380, 448
181. Bull, C. G., and McKee, C. M. Respiratory immunity in rabbits. VIII. Rabbits immunized with pneumococcus Types II, III, and IV resist intranasal infection with Type I. Am. J. Hyg., 10(1): 229, July 1929.
182. Bull, C. G., and Tao, S. M. A method for determining the antipneumococcal properties of whole blood and the protective power of immune serum. Am. J. Hyg., 7(5):648, Sept. 1927. 430
183. Bullowa, J. G. M. The pneumococcus pneumonias and their serum treatment. Physicians Hospital of Plattsburg, N. Y. Medical and Surgical Year Book, 1:3, July 1930. 218
184. Bullowa, J. G. M., Rosenbluth, M. B., and Merkin, A. K. Effect of antipneumococcus sera on leucocytes in vitro and on the agglutination of the red blood cells. Proc. Soc. Exper. Biol. & Med., 24(6):600, Mar. 1927. 561
185. Bullowa, J. G. M., and Schuman, A. H. A rapid method of using the Sabin slide microscopic test for determining the types of pneumococci. Am. J. Pub. Health, 20(8):878, Aug. 1930. 129
186. Bunzl-Federn, E. Ueber Immunisirung und Heilung bei der Pneumococcen-Infection. Arch. f. Hyg., 20:152, 1894. .... 37, 93
187. Bürgers. Ueber Auflösungserscheinungen an Bakterien. Centralbl. f. Bakt., Beilage zu Abt. 1, Ref., 50:*125, Sept. 1911. 53
188. Bürgers. Ueber den Bau der Opsonine und Agglutinine. Centralbl. f. Bakt., Beilage zu Abt. 1, Ref., 50:*154, Sept. 1911. 391
188a. Bürgers und Herz, H. Ueber das Vorkommen der verschiedenen Pneumokokkentypen. Centralbl. f. Bakt., 1 Abt., Orig., 91 (1):42, 1924.
189. Bürgers, T. J., und Meisner, W. Ueber den Bau der Opsonine, Bakteriotropine, und Agglutinine. Ztschr. f. Immunitätsforsch. u. exper. Therap., 1 Teil, Orig., 11(5):528, Oct. 1911. 391
190. Burhans, C. W., and Gerstenberger, H. J. The protective power of infants' and maternal serum against pneumococci. Am. J. Dis. Child., 28(4):415, Oct. 1924. 434
191. Burke, V. Notes on the gram stain with description of a new method. J. Bact., 7(2):159, Mar. 1922. 31
192. Butler, C. L., and Cretcher, L. H. Cinchona alkaloids in pneumonia. III. Apocupreines (Apoquinine). J. Am. Chem. Soc., 57 (6):1083, June 1935. 517
193. Butler, C. L., Nelson, W. L., Renfrew, A. G., and Cretcher, L. H. Cinchona alkaloids in pneumonia. I. Miscellaneous alkaloids and some hydrocupreine ethers. J. Am. Chem. Soc., 57(3): 575, Mar. 1935. 517
194. Butterfield, E. E., and Peabody, F. W. The action of pneumococcus on blood. J. Exper. Med., 17(5):587, May 1913. 71
194a. Cafiero, C. Ueber die Wirkung des virulenten Streptococcus und Pneumococcus bei verschiedenen Tierarten. Centralbl. f. Bakt., 1 Abt., Orig., 74(3/4):208, 1914.

195. Cahnbronner, C. E. 10 Jahre Chininbehandlung der kruppösen Pneumonie. Therap. d. Gegenw., 29(3), n.s.: 97, Mar. 1927.

196. Calder, R. M. A microscopic method of typing pneumococci by the use of stained organisms. J. A. M. A., 97(10): 698, Sept. 5, 1931. 128

196a. Calmette, A., Vansteenberghe, P., et Grysez. Sur l'origine intestinale de la pneumonie et d'autres infections phlegmasiques du poumon chez l'homme et chez les animaux. Presse méd., 14(70): 559, Sept. 1, 1906; Semaine méd., 26(50): 598, Dec. 12, 1906.

197. Cannon, P. R., Sullivan, F. L., and Neckermann, E. F. Conditions influencing the disappearance of living bacteria from the blood stream. J. Exper. Med., 55(1): 121, Jan. 1932.

198. Carbonell, A., and Cook, E. L. Pneumococcus meningitis. Report of a case treated with ethylhydrocuprein and Huntoon's antibody solution, with recovery. Mil. Surgeon, 63: 718, Nov. 1928.

199. Carnot, P. Reproduction expérimentale de la pneumonie fibrineuse aiguë, par la toxine pneumococcique. Compt. rend. Soc. de biol., 51: 927, Nov. 1899. 87

200. Carnot, P., et Fournier, L. Recherches sur le pneumocoque et ses toxines. Arch. d. méd. expér. et d'anat. path., 12(3): 357, May 1900. 37

200a. Cattoretti, F. Sulla siero-diagnosi de varii tipi di pneumococco. Atti d. Soc. lomb. di sc. med. e biol., Milano, 11(4): 345, Aug. 1922.

200b. Caussade, G., et Tardieu, A. Dacryocystite et conjonctivite a pneumocoques; pneumococcémie secondaire; oedème aigu du poumon et pneumonie batarde a pneumocoques consécutifs. Bull. et mém. Soc. méd. des Hôp. de Paris, 45, 3e sér.: 300, 1921.

201. Cecil, R. L. Pneumococcus vaccine. J. A. M. A., 76(3): 178, Jan. 15, 1921. 489

202. Cecil, R. L. The prevention of pneumonia by pneumococcus vaccine. Am. J. Pub. Health, 13(3): 182, Mar. 1923.

203. Cecil, R. L. Immunization against pneumonia. Medicine, 4(4): 395, Nov. 1925. .... 489, 498

204. Cecil, R. L., and Austin, J. H. Results of prophylactic inoculation against pneumococcus in 12,519 men. J. Exper. Med., 28(1): 19, July 1918. .... 466, 494

205. Cecil, R. L., Baldwin, H. S., and Larsen, N. P. Lobar pneumonia. A clinical and bacteriologic study of two thousand typed cases. Arch. Int. Med., 40(3): 253, Sept. 1927.

206. Cecil, R. L., and Blake, F. G. Studies on experimental pneumonia. IV. Results of prophylactic vaccination against pneumococcus pneumonia in monkeys. J. Exper. Med., 31(5): 519, May 1920. .... 410, 482

207. Cecil, R. L., and Blake, F. G. Studies on experimental pneumonia. V. Active immunity against experimental pneumococcus pneumonia in monkeys following vaccination with living cultures of pneumococcus. J. Exper. Med., 31(6): 657, June 1920.

208. Cecil, R. L., and Blake, F. G. Studies on experimental pneu-

monia. VI. Active immunity following experimental pneumococcus pneumonia in monkeys. J. Exper. Med., 31(6):685, June 1920.

209. Cecil, R. L., and Blake, F. G. Studies on experimental pneumonia. VII. Treatment of experimental pneumococcus Type I pneumonia in monkeys with Type I antipneumococcus serum. J. Exper. Med., 32(1):1, July 1920.

210. Cecil, R. L., and Larsen, N. P. Clinical and bacteriologic study of one thousand cases of lobar pneumonia—with special reference to the therapeutic value of pneumococcus antibody solution. Preliminary report. J. A. M. A., 79(5):343, July 29, 1922.

211. Cecil, R. L., and Steffen, G. I. Studies on pneumococcus immunity. I. Active immunization of monkeys against pneumococcus Type I pneumonia with pneumococcus Type I vaccine. J. Exper. Med., 34(3):245, Sept. 1921. 192

212. Cecil, R. L., and Steffen, G. I. Vaccination of monkeys against pneumococcus Type I pneumonia by means of intratracheal injection of pneumococcus Type I vaccine. Pub. Health Rep., 37(44): 2735, Nov. 3, 1922. 482

213. Cecil, R. L., and Steffen, G. I. Studies on pneumococcus immunity. II. Active immunization of monkeys against pneumococcus Types II, III, and IV pneumonia with the homologous pneumococcus vaccine. J. Exper. Med., 38(2):149, Aug. 1923. 410

214. Cecil, R. L., and Steffen, G. I. Studies on pneumococcus immunity. IV. Active immunization of monkeys against pneumococcus pneumonia by means of intratracheal injections of pneumococcus vaccine. Hygienic Laboratory Bulletin, No. 141:1, Apr. 1925. 193, 410, 482, 489

215. Cecil, R. L., and Steffen, G. I. Studies on pneumococcus immunity. V. The treatment of experimental pneumococcus pneumonia in monkeys with pneumococcus antibody solution. Hygienic Laboratory Bulletin, No. 141:19, Apr. 1925. .... 193, 482, 489

216. Cecil, R. L., and Vaughan, H. F. Results of prophylactic vaccination against pneumonia at Camp Wheeler. J. Exper. Med., 29 (5):457, May 1919. 495

217. Chapin, W. E. Pneumococcus infections. Their types and relation to sex, age, race, season and the course of the illness. Bull. Ayer Clin. Lab., Pennsylvania Hosp., No. 9:16, Oct. 1925.

218. Cheer, S. N. A study of the effect of sodium citrate on the antipneumococcus defense processes of the body in relation to its use in transfusion. J. Immunol., 18(3):187, Mar. 1930.

219. Chèneveau, R. Quelques résultats de vaccinations antipneumococciques à Madagascar. Bull. Soc. path. exot., 21(5):364, May 1928.

220. Chesney, A. M. The latent period in the growth of bacteria. J. Exper. Med., 24(4):387, Oct. 1916. 40

221. Chesney, A. M., and Hodges, A. B. Observations on the production of toxic substances by pneumococci. Bull. Johns Hopkins Hosp., 33(382):425, Dec. 1922. 96

221a. Chevrel, F., Ranque, A., Senez, C., et Gruat, E. Note sur une épizootie a pneumocoque chez le cobaye, jugulée par l'injection préventive de vaccin pneumococcique. Compt. rend. Soc. de biol., 82:74, Jan. 25, 1919.

222. Chickering, H. T. Agglutination phenomena in lobar pneumonia. J. Exper. Med., 20(6):599, Dec. 1914. 360

223. Chickering, H. T. The concentration of the protective bodies in antipneumococcus serum. Specific precipitate extracts. J. Exper. Med., 22(2):248, Aug. 1915. .... 370, 547

224. Chow, B. F. Distribution of precipitin in serum globulins in different species of animals. Proc. Soc. Exper. Biol. & Med., 34(5): 651, June 1936. .... 416, 561

225. Chow, B. F. Immunologic studies on new preparation of type-specific polysaccharide from pneumococcus Type I. Proc. Soc. Exper. Biol. & Med., 34(5):667, June 1936. 295

226. Chow, B. F., and Goebel, W. F. The purification of the antibodies in Type I antipneumococcus serum, and the chemical nature of the type-specific precipitin reaction. J. Exper. Med., 62(2):179, Aug. 1935. .... 376, 413

227. Chow, B. F., and Wu, H. Isolation of immunologically pure antibody. Science, 84(2179):316, Oct. 2, 1936. 414

228. Christensen, S. Sur le classement par types de pneumocoques, par fixation du complément après absorption. Compt. rend. Soc. de biol., 86(6):459, Feb. 5, 1922. .... 110, 380

229. Christensen, S. Studies on pneumococcus types. Communications l'Inst. Sérotherap. l'Etat Danois, 14, pt. 5:1, Jan. 1923. 110, 113, 380

230. Christensen, S. Pneumococcus types and prognosis in pneumonia crouposa. Acta path. et microbiol. Scandinav., 2(1):1, 1925.

230a. Christiansen, M. Diplokokkeninfektion bei Kälbern und das Verhältnis der Kälberdiplokokken zum Pneumokokkus des Menschen. (Diplococcus lanceolatus Fraenkel). Ztschr. f. Infektionskrank. der Haustiere, 14(2/3):101, Sept. 10, 1913.

231. Christie, E. M. Epidemiological significance of the serological types of pneumococci. Lancet, 2(5784):39, July 7, 1934. 116

232. Christie, I. M. Type-specific organisms in acute pneumonia and in convalescents and contacts. Lancet, 2(5700):1173, Nov. 26, 1932. .... 229, 235

233. Christie, R. V., Ehrich, W., and Binger, C. A. L. Experimental study of diathermy. V. The elevation of temperature in the pneumonic lung. J. Exper. Med., 47(5):741, May 1928. 194

234. Clapp, F. L., Phillips, S. W., and Stahl, H. J. Quantitative use of Neufeld reaction with special reference to titration of Type II antipneumococcic horse sera. Proc. Soc. Exper. Biol. & Med., 33 (2):302, Nov. 1935. 581

235. Clark, H. C. The pneumococci by types in cultures from 71 autopsies. United Fruit Co. 16th Annual Report Medical Department, 247, 1927.

235a. Clark, P. F., and Murphy, E. J. Immunity in experimental pneumonia. J. Infect. Dis., 31(1):51, July 1922.

236. Claude, H. Note sur deux cas de purpuras infectieux et toxique chez des enfants. Rev. mens. d. mal. de l'enfance, 14:143, Mar. 1896. 86

237. Claxton, C. Virulence of normal human saliva. Philadelphia Med. Times, 12(19):627, June 17, 1882. .... 5, 180

238. Clough, M. C. A study of the incidence of the types of pneumococci isolated from acute lobar pneumonia and other infections, and an analysis of the cases classified by types in regard to mortality, complications, associated diseases, bacteriemia, and leucocytosis. Bull. Johns Hopkins Hosp., 28(320):306, Oct. 1917. 360

239. Clough, M. C. A study of pneumococci reacting with antipneumococcus sera of Types I, II, and III, with an observation of a mutation of one of the strains. J. Exper. Med., 30(2):123, Aug. 1919. 111

240. Clough, P. W. The development of antibodies in the serum of patients recovering from acute lobar pneumonia. Bull. Johns Hopkins Hosp., 24(272):295, Oct. 1913. .... 401, 438

241. Clough, P. W. Some observations on hypersensitiveness to pneumococcus protein, with special reference to its relation to immunity. Bull. Johns Hopkins Hosp., 26(288):37, Feb. 1915. ..... 96, 447

242. Clough, P. W. Phagocytosis and agglutination in the serum in acute lobar pneumonia; the specificity of these reactions and the regularity of their occurrence. Bull. Johns Hopkins Hosp., 30 (340):167, June 1919. .... 401, 438

243. Clough, P. W. The protective power of normal human serum against pneumococcus infection. Bull. Johns Hopkins Hosp., 35 (404):330, Oct. 1924. 434

244. Clowes, G. H. A., Jamieson, W. A., and Olson, J. G. On a specific pneumococcus antitoxin. Proc. Soc. Exper. Biol. & Med., 23 (5):334, Feb. 1926. .... 384, 530, 534, 579, 581

245. Coca, A. F. Immunity in human beings to the pneumococcus. Proc. Soc. Exper. Biol. & Med., 29(8):1042, May 1932. .... 386, 467

246. Coca, A. F. A study of the pneumococcus toxins. J. Immunol., 30(1):1, Jan. 1936. .... 100, 386, 468, 579

247. Coggeshall, L. T., and Robertson, O. H. A study of repeated attacks of experimental pneumococcus lobar pneumonia in dogs. J. Exper. Med., 61(2):213, Feb. 1935.

248. Cole, R. I. Experimenteller Beitrag zur Typhusimmunität. Ztschr. f. Hyg. u. Infektionskr., 46:371, 1904. 537

249. Cole, R. Pneumococcus infection and immunity. J. A. M. A., 59 (9):693, Aug. 31, 1912. 545

250. Cole, R. I. Toxic substances produced by pneumococcus. J. Exper. Med., 16(5):644, Nov. 1912. 93

251. Cole, R. I. Pneumococcus infection and lobar pneumonia. Arch. Int. Med., 14(1):56, July 1914. *Also:* Harvey Lectures 1913–1914, 85.

252. Cole, R. I. Pneumococcus hemotoxin. J. Exper. Med., 20(4): 346, Oct. 1914. .... 83, 382

253. Cole, R. I. The production of methemoglobin by pneumococci. J. Exper. Med., 20(4):363, Oct. 1914. 72

254. Cole, R. I. Pneumococcus infection and immunity. New York M. J., 101(1):1, Jan. 2, 1915.

255. Cole, R. I. Pneumococcus infection and immunity. New York M. J., 101(2):59, Jan. 9, 1915.

256. Cole, R. I. Types of pneumococcus bacilli and their characteristics. Med. Rec., New York, 87(10):418, Mar. 6, 1915.

257. Cole, R. I. The specific treatment of acute lobar pneumonia. Pennsylvania M. J., 20(5):345, Feb. 1917. .... 529, 535

258. Cole, R. I. The neutralization of antipneumococcus immune bodies by infected exudates and sera. Tr. A. Am. Physicians, 32:479, May 2, 1917. 361

258a. Cole, R. Report of studies concerning acute lobar pneumonia. J. A. M. A., 69(7):505, Aug. 18, 1917.

259. Cole, R. The neutralization of antipneumococcus immune bodies by infected exudates and sera. J. Exper. Med., 26(4):453, Oct. 1917.

260. Cole, R. Prevention of pneumonia. J. A. M. A., 71(8):635, Aug. 24, 1918.

261. Cole, R. Etiology of the pneumonias. New York State J. Med., 19(7):253, July 1919.

262. Cole, R. Acute lobar pneumonia. *In* Nelson, Loose-leaf medicine. A perpetual system of living medicine, 1:203, 1920–28. New York: Thomas Nelson & Sons. 498

263. Cole, R. Antipneumococcus serum. J. A. M. A., 76(2):111, Jan. 8, 1921.

264. Cole, R. I. Acute pulmonary infections. De Lamar Lectures, 1927–28. Baltimore: Williams & Wilkins Co., 1928.

265. Cole, R. Serum Treatment in Type I lobar pneumonia. J. A. M. A., 93(10):741, Sept. 7, 1929. .... 543, 603

265a. Cole, R. The nature of pneumonia. (Twelfth annual Pasteur lecture.) Proc. Inst. Med. Chicago, 9(1):2, Jan. 15, 1932.

266. Cole, R. The outlook for overcoming pneumonia. Canad. M. A. J., 30(3):237, Mar. 1934. 498

267. Cole, R., and Dochez, A. R. Report of studies on pneumonia. Tr. A. Am. Physicians, 28:606, May 6, 1913. 603

268. Cole, R., and Moore, H. F. The production of antipneumococcic serum. J. Exper. Med., 26(4):537, Oct. 1917. .... 529, 535, 545

269. Colin. In discussion following: Raynaud and Lannelongue. Recherches expérimentales sur la transmission du virus rabique de l'homme au lapin. Bull. Acad. de méd., Paris, 10(3), 2ᵉ ser.:61, Jan. 18, 1881. 3

270. Collins, K. R. The application of the reaction of agglutination to the pneumococcus. J. Exper. Med., 7(5):420, Aug. 1905. .... 104, 359

271. Colomiatti, V. Un nuovo caso di endo-cardite acquisita acuta unilaterale destra. Gior. d. r. Accad. di med. di Torino, 30, 3. s.: 617, Mar. 10, 1882. *Also:* Arch. ital. de biol., 1:397, 1882. 6

272. Cooper, G., Edwards, M., and Rosenstein, C. The separation of types among the pneumococci hitherto called Group IV and the development of therapeutic antiserums for these types. J. Exper. Med., 49(3):461, Mar. 1929. .... 113, 362, 546

273. Cooper, G. M., Mishulow, L., and Blane, N. E. Studies on acute respiratory infections. II. A study of the serological relationships of pneumococci from the upper respiratory tract with special reference to common colds and influenza conditions. J. Immunol., 6(1):25, Jan. 1921. .... 112, 362

274. Cooper, G., Rosenstein, C., Walter, A., and Peizer, L. The further separation of types among the pneumococci hitherto included in Group IV and the development of therapeutic antisera for these types. J. Exper. Med., 55(4):531, Apr. 1932. .... 115, 362, 546

275. Cooper, G. M., and Walter, A. W. Application of the Neufeld reaction to the identification of types of pneumococci. Am. J. Pub. Health, 25(4):469, Apr. 1935. .... 594, 595

276. Cooper, M. L. Mucous membrane immunity to pneumococci in rabbits. J. Infect. Dis., 38(6):491, June 1926. .... 180, 347

277. Cope, E. J., and Howell, K. M. Local skin reactivity to "filtrates" of pneumococcus. J. Infect. Dis., 48(6):570, June 1931. 475

278. Cornil, A. V., et Babes, V. Les bacteries et leur rôle, etc. Paris: F. Alcan, 1885. 10

279. Coryllos, P. N. Bronchoscopic findings in lobar pneumonia. A preliminary note. Am. J. M. Sc., 178(1):8, July 1929. 194

279a. Costa, S., et Troisier, J. Sur l'association fréquente du pneumocoque et du B. perfringens dans les blessures de guerre, notamment dans le syndrome "gangrène gazeuse." Compt. rend. Soc. de biol., 78:283, May 29, 1915.

279b. Cotoni, L. La virulence des pneumocoques. Thèse de Paris, 1912.

280. Cotoni, L. Études sur le pneumocoque. VI. Présence du pneumocoque dans le sang des pneumoniques. Ann. Inst. Pasteur, 27(4):289, Apr. 1913.

281. Cotoni, L., et Brasie, G. Variations du pouvoir vaccinant d'un antigène pneumococcique suivant son mode de préparation. Ann. Inst. Pasteur, 38(10):937, Oct. 1924. 328

282. Cotoni, L., et Chambrin, N. Recherches sur l'hémolysine pneumococcique. Ann. Inst. Pasteur, 42(12):1536, Dec. 1928. .... 85, 383

283. Cotoni, L., et Chambrin, N. Sur l'immunité passive obtenue à l'aide du pneumocoque III. Ann. Inst. Pasteur, 45(6):706, Dec. 1930.

284. Cotoni, L., et Truche, C. Études sur le pneumocoque. IV. Agglutination des pneumocoques humains et animaux. Ann. Inst. Pasteur, 26(4):313, Apr. 1912. 359

284a. Cotoni, L., Truche, C., and Raphael, A. The pneumococcus and pneumococcal affections. English edition by Page, D. S., and Morton, E. London, John Bale, Sons & Danielsson, Ltd., 1924.

285. Couvey and Popoff. II. Note sur le traitement de la pneumonie

par le salicylate de sonde en injections intraveineuses. Bull. Acad. de méd., Paris, 105(5), 5e ser.:163, Feb. 1931. 511
286. Coventry, F. A. The protective and curative action of large doses of pneumococcus antiserum in mice. Am. J. Hyg., 7(5):515, Sept. 1927. .... 575, 578
287. Cowan, S. T. Pneumococcal hemolysin; its extracellular nature, production and properties. J. Path. & Bact., 38(1):61, Jan. 1934. 85
288. Cruickshank, R. Treatment of lobar pneumonia by Felton serum; serological typing of pneumonia. Glasgow M. J., 115(2):59, Feb. 1931. *Also:* Tr. Roy. Med.-Chir. Soc. Glasgow, 25:34, Nov. 21, 1931.
289. Cullen, G. E., and Chesney, A. M. A note on the production of acid by pneumococci. J. Exper. Med., 28(3):289, Sept. 1918.
290. Cunningham, J., Cruickshank, J. A., and Ramakrishnan, S. Note on the types of pneumococci found in cases of pneumonia in Madras, Southern India. Indian J. M. Research, 12(3):479, Jan. 1925.
291. Curphey, T. J., and Baruch, H. B. A practical method for the immunization of horses by type specific pneumococcic pleural exudates. Proc. Soc. Exper. Biol. & Med., 26(8):687, May 1929. 527
292. Curphey, T. J., and Baruch, H. B. The titration of pneumococcus "exudate" antisera. Proc. Soc. Exper. Biol. & Med., 28 (3):280, Dec. 1930. .... 527, 579
293. Curphey, T. J., and Baruch, H. B. The therapeutic value of intramuscular dosage of Type I pneumococcus antisera. J. Exper. Med., 55(6):925, June 1932. 182
294. Davidsohn, I. Heterophile antigens and antibodies. Arch. Path. & Lab. Med., 4(4):776, Nov. 1927. 387
295. Davidsohn, I. Heterophile antibodies in serum sickness. J. Immunol., 16(3):259, Mar. 1929. 387
296. Davidsohn, I. Further studies in heterophilic antibodies in serum sickness. J. Immunol., 18(1):31, Jan. 1930. 387
297. Davidsohn, I. Heterophilic antibodies in serum disease: Third report. J. Infect. Dis., 53(2):219, Sept.–Oct. 1933. 387
298. Davidson, S. Immunity to the pneumococcus. Tr. Med.-Chir. Soc. Edinburgh, 39, n.s.:67, 1924–5. 328
299. Dawson, M. H. The interconvertibility of "R" and "S" forms of pneumococcus. J. Exper. Med., 47(4):577, Apr. 1928. .... 147, 157
300. Dawson, M. H. The transformation of pneumococcal types. I. The conversion of R forms of pneumococcus into S forms of the homologous type. J. Exper. Med., 51(1):99, Jan. 1930.
301. Dawson, M. H. The transformation of pneumococcal types. II. The interconvertibility of type-specific S pneumococci. J. Exper. Med., 51(1):123, Jan. 1930.
302. Dawson, M. H. Bacterial variation in pneumococcus and Streptococcus hemolyticus. Proc. Soc. Exper. Biol. & Med., 31(5): 590, Feb. 1934. 161
303. Dawson, M. H. Variation in the pneumococcus. J. Path. & Bact., 39(2):323, Sept. 1934. .... 161, 166

304. Dawson, M. H., and Avery, O. T. Reversion of avirulent "rough" forms of pneumococcus to virulent "smooth" types. Proc. Soc. Exper. Biol. & Med., 24(9):943, June 1927. 154
305. Dawson, M. H., and Sia, R. H. P. In vitro transformations of pneumococcal types. I. A technique for inducing transformation of pneumococcal types in vitro. J. Exper. Med., 54(5):681, Nov. 1931. 158
305a. Dawson, M. H., and Sia, R. H. P. The transformation of pneumococcal types in vitro. Proc. Soc. Exper. Biol. & Med., 27(9): 989, 1930.
306. Dawson, M. H., and Warbasse, A. Further observations on the transformation of type-specific pneumococci by in vitro procedures. Proc. Soc. Exper. Biol. & Med., 29(2):149, Nov. 1931. ... 159
307. Day, H. B. The preparation of antigenic specific substance from streptococci and pneumococci (Type I). Brit. J. Exper. Path., 11 (3):164, June 1930. .... 329, 333, 337
308. Day, H. B. Species immunity to pneumococcus. J. Path. & Bact., 36(1):77, Jan. 1933. 327
309. Day, H. B. The preparation of pneumococcal species antigen. J. Path. & Bact., 38(2):171, Mar. 1934. 337
310. Dean, H. R. The relation between the fixation of a complement and the formation of a precipitate. Proc. Roy. Soc. Med., Sect. Path., 5:62, Nov. 21, 1911. 583
311. Dean, H. R., and Webb, R. A. The influence of optimal proportions of antigen and antibody in the serum precipitation reaction. J. Path. & Bact., 29(4):473, Oct. 1926. .... 372, 583
311a. Declich, M. Contributo alla diagnosi differenziale dei vari tipi di pneumococco. Biochem. e Terap. Sper., 9(10):293, Oct. 1922.
312. Denys. Recherches sur le sérum antipneumococcique. Ann. Soc. méd.-chir. d'Anvers, 2(2):51, Feb. 1897. .... 27, 326, 420, 522, 528
313. Dernby, K. G., and Avery, O. T. The optimum hydrogen ion concentration for the growth of pneumococcus. J. Exper. Med., 28 (3):345, Sept. 1918. .... 38, 39
313a. Dible, J. H. Pneumococcal infections: the bacteriological aspect. Lancet, 1:8, Jan. 5, 1924.
314. Dick, G. F. On the development of proteolytic ferments in the blood during pneumonia. J. Infect. Dis., 10(3):383, May 1912. .. 442
315. Dochez, A. R. The presence of protective substances in human serum during lobar pneumonia. J. Exper. Med., 16(5):665, Nov. 1912. 438
316. Dochez, A. R. The occurrence and virulence of pneumococci in the circulating blood during lobar pneumonia and the susceptibility of pneumococcus strains to univalent antipneumococcus serum. J. Exper. Med., 16(5):680, Nov. 1912. .... 524, 528
317. Dochez, A. R. Coagulation time of the blood in lobar pneumonia. J. Exper. Med., 16(5):693, Nov. 1912.
318. Dochez, A. R., and Avery, O. T. Varieties of pneumococcus and their relation to lobar pneumonia. J. Exper. Med., 21(2):114, Feb. 1915. 525

319. DOCHEZ, A. R., and AVERY, O. T. The occurrence of carriers of disease-producing types of pneumococcus. J. Exper. Med., 22(1): 105, July 1915. .... 108, 232
320. DOCHEZ, A. R., and AVERY, O. T. Antiblastic immunity. J. Exper. Med., 23(1):61, Jan. 1916. 421
321. DOCHEZ, A. R., and AVERY, O. T. Soluble substance of pneumococcus origin in the blood and urine during lobar pneumonia. Proc. Soc. Exper. Biol. & Med., 14:126, Mar. 1917. 124, 239, 241, 365, 633
321a. DOCHEZ, A. R., and AVERY, O. T. The elaboration of specific soluble substance by pneumococcus during growth. J. Exper. Med., 26(4):477, Oct. 1917.
322. DOCHEZ, A. R., and GILLESPIE, L. J. A biologic classification of pneumococci by means of immunity reactions. J. A. M. A., 61 (10):727, Sept. 6, 1913. .... 57, 68, 106, 361, 525, 546
323. DOLD, H. Die bakterizide Wirkung des Blutes, Plasmas und Serums auf Pneumokokken und ihre Bedeutung für die Immunität. Arb. a. d. k. Gsndhtsamte, 36(4):419, Apr. 1911. .... 429, 434
324. DOLD, H. Ein neues färberisches Einteilungsprinzip für Bakterien. Centralbl. f. Bakt., 1 Abt., Orig., 124(3/4):220, Mar. 30, 1932. 31
325. DOLD, H. Unterschiedliches Verhalten der Streptokokken- und Pneumokokkenkulturen gegenüber meiner Differentialfärbung. Ein Beitrag zur Frage der Stammesgeschichte der Strepto- und Pneumokokken. Zentralbl. f. Bakt., 1 Abt., Orig., 127(4/6):367, Jan. 30, 1933. 31
326. DOMINGO, P., et RAURICH, B. Étude sur les pneumocoques locaux. Relations entre le pouvoir antigénique et l'agglutinabilité. Compt. rend. Soc. de biol., 92:811, Mar. 20, 1925.
327. DOWNIE, A. W., STENT, L., and WHITE, S. M. The bile solubility of pneumococcus, with special reference to the chemical structure of various bile salts. Brit. J. Exper. Path., 12(1):1, Feb. 1931. 58
328. DRESCHFELD, J. Ueber Wanderpneumonie und ihre Beziehung zur epidemischen Pneumonie. Fortschr. d. Med., 3(12):389, June 15, 1885.
329. DUBOS, R. The decomposition of cellulose by aerobic bacteria. J. Bact., 15(4):223, Apr. 1928. 302
330. DUBOS, R. Observations on the oxidation-reduction properties of sterile bacteriological media. J. Exper. Med., 49(3):507, Mar. 1929.
331. DUBOS, R. The initiation of growth of certain facultative anaerobes as related to oxidation-reduction processes in the medium. J. Exper. Med., 49(4):559, Apr. 1929. 41
332. DUBOS, R. The relation of the bacteriostatic action of certain dyes to oxidation-reduction processes. J. Exper. Med., 49(4):575, Apr. 1929. 308
333. DUBOS, R. The role of carbohydrates in biological oxidations and reductions. Experiments with pneumococcus. J. Exper. Med., 50(2):143, Aug. 1929. 38

334. DUBOS, R. The bacteriostatic action of certain components of commercial peptones as affected by conditions of oxidation and reduction. J. Exper. Med., 52(3):331, Sept. 1930. 38

335. DUBOS, R. Factors affecting the yield of specific enzyme in cultures of the bacillus decomposing the capsular polysaccharide of Type III pneumococcus. J. Exper. Med., 55(3):377, Mar. 1932. 307

336. DUBOS, R. Studies on the mechanism of production of a specific bacterial enzyme which decomposes the capsular polysaccharide of Type III pneumococcus. J. Exper. Med., 62(2):259, Aug. 1935. 307, 640

337. DUBOS, R., and AVERY, O. T. Decomposition of the capsular polysaccharide of pneumococcus Type III by a bacterial enzyme. J. Exper. Med., 54(1):51, July 1931.

338. DUBOS, R., and BAUER, J. H. The use of graded collodion membranes for the concentration of a bacterial enzyme capable of decomposing the capsular polysaccharide of Type III pneumococcus. J. Exper. Med., 62(2):271, Aug. 1935. .... 308, 310, 640

339. DUCKWALL, B. F. Protective value of pneumococcus vaccine against respiratory diseases. Mil. Surgeon, 47(5):593, Nov. 1920. 484, 496

340. DUDLEY, H. W., and SMITH, W. A simple method for the preparation of the specific soluble substance of Type I pneumococcus. J. Path. & Bact., 37(3):341, Nov. 1933. 277

341. DUNCAN, J. T. Optimal agglutination: The significance of the different ratios of serum to bacteria. Brit. J. Exper. Path., 15(1): 23, Feb. 1934.

342. DUVAL, C. W., and LEWIS, P. A. Studies on the pneumococcus. J. Exper. Med., 7(5):473, Aug. 1905. *Also:* Department of Health, City of New York. Report Med. Comm'n Invest. Acute Resp. Dis., Part I. Studies on pneumococcus, p. 7. New York: Department of Health, 1905. 68

343. EASTWOOD, A. A brief review of recent bacteriological work on pneumococci. *In* Great Britain. Ministry of Health. Rep. on Pub. Health & Med. Subjects, No. 13, p. 2. London: His Majesty's Stationery Office, 1922. 111

344. EASTWOOD, A. The significance of serological differences amongst pneumococci. *In* Great Britain. Ministry of Health. Rep. on Pub. Health & Med. Subjects, No. 13, p. 46. London: His Majesty's Stationery Office, 1922. .... 111, 138

345. EATON, M. D. Studies on pneumococcus variation. I. Variants characterized by rapid lysis and absence of normal growth under the routine method of cultivation. J. Bact., 27(3):271, Mar. 1934. 153

346. EATON, M. D. Studies on pneumococcus variation. II. Smooth virulent variants produced by daughter-colony variations of smooth pneumococcus strains. J. Bact., 30(2):119, Aug. 1935. 153

347. EBERTH, C. J. Zur Kenntnis der mykotischen Processe. Deutsches Arch. f. klin. Med., 28(1):1, Dec. 1880. 2

348. EDDY, B. E. Search for protective, bacteriophagic and enzymatic agents in pneumonic sputums. J. Infect. Dis., 42(5):449, May 1928. 442

349. EGGERS, H. E. On the antipneumococcal powers of the blood in pneumonia. J. Infect. Dis., 10(1):48, Jan. 1912. 401
350. EGUCHI, C. Versuche über Infektion und Immunisierung junger und alter Mäuse und Meerschweinchen mit Pneumokokken und Streptokokken durch Fütterung und Inhalation. Ztschr. f. Hyg. u. Infektionskr., 105(1):74, Aug. 19, 1925.
351. EGUCHI, C. Versuche über Vererbung der Immunität gegen Pneumokokken. Ztschr. f. Hyg. u. Infektionskr., 105(2):265, Nov. 9, 1925. .... 346, 348, 446
352. EISLER, M., und HOWARD, A. Ueber das Forssman-Antigen der Pneumokokken. Ztschr. f. Immunitätsforsch. u. exper. Therap., 76 (6):461, Oct. 1932.
353. ELFORD, W. J., and FERRY, J. D. The ultrafiltration of proteins through graded collodion membranes. I. The serum proteins. Biochem. J., 28(2):650, June 1934. 418
353a. ELFORD, W. J., GRABAR, P., and FISCHER, W. Ultrafiltration studies with normal horse serum. Biochem. J., 30(Part 1):92, Jan. 1936.
354. ELSER, W. J., THOMAS, R. A., and STEFFEN, G. I. The desiccation of sera and other biological products (including microörganisms) in the frozen state with the preservation of the original qualities of products so treated. J. Immunol., 28(6):453, June 1935. 559
355. EMMERICH, R. Pneumoniecoccen in der Zwischendeckenfüllung als Ursache einer Pneumonieepidemie. Fortschr. d. Med., 2(5): 153, Mar. 1, 1884. *Abstract in* Deutsche med. Wchnschr., 10:181, Mar. 1884. .... 10, 51
356. EMMERICH, R. Ueber die Infection, Immunisirung und Heilung bei croupöser Pneumonie. Ztschr. f. Hyg. u. Infektionskr., 17: 167, 1894. .... 25, 524
357. EMMERICH, R., und FOWITZKY, A. Die künstliche Erzeugung von Immunität gegen croupöse Pneumonie und die Heilung dieser Krankheit. München. med. Wchnschr., 38(32):554, Aug. 11, 1891. 23, 325, 524
358. ENDERS, J. F. A type specific substance distinct from the specific carbohydrate in pneumococcus Type I. J. Exper. Med., 52 (2):235, Aug. 1930. .... 265, 450
359. ENDERS, J. F. A note on the specific agglutination of pneumococcus Types I, II and III. J. Exper. Med., 55(2):191, Feb. 1932. 267
360. ENDERS, J. F., and SHAFFER, M. F. Studies on natural immunity to pneumococcus Type III. I. The capacity of strains of pneumococcus Type III to grow at 41° C. and their virulence for rabbits. J. Exper. Med., 64(1):7, July 1, 1936. 207
361. ENDERS, J. F., SHAFFER, M. F., and WU, C.-J. Studies on natural immunity to pneumococcus Type III. III. Correlation of the behavior in vivo of pneumococci Type III varying in their virulence for rabbits with certain differences observed in vitro. J. Exper. Med., 64(2):307, Aug. 1, 1936. 208
362. ENDERS, J. F., and WU, C.-J. An immunological study of the A

substance of acetyl polysaccharide of pneumococcus Type I. J. Exper. Med., 60(2):127, Aug. 1934. .... 285, 352, 400, 437

363. Enders, J. F., Wu, C.-J., and Shaffer, M. F. Studies on natural immunity to pneumococcus Type III. IV. Observations on a non-type specific humoral factor involved in resistance to pneumococcus Type III. J. Exper. Med., 64(3):425, Sept. 1, 1936. 208

364. Engelmann, B. Weiterer Beitrag zur Frage der Einheit der Pneumokokken und Streptokokken. Centralbl. f. Bakt., 1 Abt., Orig., 98(5/6):304, May 1926.

365. Engwer, T. Beiträge zur Chemo- und Serotherapie der Pneumokokkeninfektionen. Ztschr. f. Hyg. u. Infektionskr., 73:194, 1913. 185, 518

366. Enlows, E. M. A. Factors influencing the standardization of antipneumococcic serums. Hygienic Laboratory Bulletin, No. 134: 45, May 1923. .... 419, 571

366a. Erian, A. Treatment of pneumonia by large doses of vaccine. Practitioner, 111(6):430, Dec. 1923.

367. Erös, G., Gyüre, D., und Kramár, E. Untersuchungen über die Immunbiologie der Lungenentzündung. V. Mitteilung. Die Enstehungsbedingungen der vershiedenen Pneumonietypen. Arch. f. Kinderh., 93(3):161, May 15, 1931.

368. Etinger-Tulczynska, R. Über Bakterienantagonismus. Ztschr. f. Hyg. u. Infektionskr., 113(4):762, Mar. 1932. 188

368a. Etinger-Tulczynska, R. Bakterienkapseln und Quellungsreaktion. Ztschr. f. Hyg. u. Infektionskr., 114(4):769, Feb. 1933. 594

369. Eyre, J. W. H. The neutralisation of culture media. Tr. Path. Soc. London, 51:283, June 30, 1900.

370. Eyre, J. W. H. Nutrient media of "standard" reaction for bacteriological work. Brit. M. J., 2:921, Sept. 29, 1900.

371. Eyre, J. W. H. The differentiation of strains of pneumococci. Tr. Path. Soc. London, 52:166, May 7, 1901. 104

371a. Eyre, J. W. H. The pyogenetic activities of the pneumococcus. Lancet, 1(4408):539, Feb. 22, 1908.

372. Eyre, J. W., Leathem, A. N., and Washbourn, J. W. A study of different strains of pneumococci, with especial reference to the lesions they produce. J. Path. & Bact., 11(3):246, 1906. 105

373. Eyre, J. W., and Washbourn, J. W. Resistant forms of the pneumococcus. J. Path. & Bact., 4(3):394, 1897. .... 26, 135, 136

374. Eyre, J. W., and Washbourn, J. W. Further researches upon the pneumococcus. J. Path. & Bact., 5(1):13, 1898. ..... 206, 211, 407, 566

374a. Eyre, J. W., and Washbourn, J. W. Varieties and virulence of the pneumococcus. Lancet, 1(3932):19, Jan. 7, 1899.

375. Eyre, J. W. H., and Washbourn, J. W. Experiments with Pane's antipneumococcic serum. Lancet, 1(3945):954, Apr. 8, 1899. 28

376. Eyre, J. W. H., and Washbourn, J. W. Further experiments with Pane's antipneumococcus serum. Brit. M. J., 2:1247, Nov. 4, 1899. .... 28, 104, 198

377. Eyre, J. W., and Washbourn, J. W. The standardisation of antipneumococcic serum. Tr. Path. Soc. London, 51:15, 1900. .... 28, 566
378. Faber, H. K. Use of rabbits as substitute for white mice in pneumococcus type differentiation. J. A. M. A., 70(20):1459, May 18, 1918. 121
379. Falk, I. S., Gussin, H. A., and Jacobson, M. A. Studies on respiratory diseases. XXI. Electrophoretic potential and virulence of pneumococci (Types 1, 2, 3 and 4). J. Infect. Dis., 37(6):481, Dec. 1925. 201
380. Falk, I. S., and Jacobson, M. A. Studies on respiratory diseases. XXIV. Electrophoretic potential, virulence and serum agglutination with single cell cultures of variants of Type I pneumococci. J. Infect. Dis., 37(6):507, Dec. 1925. 144
381. Falk, I. S., and Jacobson, M. A. Studies on respiratory diseases. XXVIII. The electrophoretic potentials, the dissolution and the serum agglutination of pneumococci in the presence of sodium oleate. J. Infect. Dis., 38(2):188, Feb. 1926. 57
382. Falk, I. S., Jacobson, M. A., and Gussin, H. A. Studies on respiratory diseases. XXII. Some relations between fatality in lobar pneumonia and electrophoretic potentials on pneumococci. J. Infect. Dis., 37(6):495, Dec. 1925.
383. Falk, I. S., Jacobson, M. A., and Gussin, H. A. Studies on respiratory diseases. XXIII. Electrophoretic potential and virulence of variants of Type I pneumococci. J. Infect. Dis., 37(6):499, Dec. 1925. 144
384. Falk, I. S., and Yang, S. Y. Studies on respiratory diseases. XXV. The influence of certain electrolytes and nonelectrolytes on the bile solubility of pneumococci. J. Infect. Dis., 38(1):1, Jan. 1926. 59
385. Falk, I. S., and Yang, S. Y. Studies on respiratory diseases. XXVI. The lysis of pneumococci by sodium oleate. J. Infect. Dis., 38(1):8, Jan. 1926. 59
386. Falk, K. G., and McGuire, G. Directive influences in biological systems. II. Lipase actions of Types I and II pneumococci. J. Biol. Chem., 97(3):651, Sept. 1932. 66
387. Falk, K. G., McGuire, G., Valentine, E., and Whitney, E. Studies on antibodies. II. Antipneumococcus serum. J. Immunol., 21(3):199, Sept. 1931. 583
388. Falk, K. G., Valentine, E., McGuire, G., and Whitney, E. Studies on antibodies. V. The use of green bananas in media for the culture of pneumococci. J. Bact., 23(3):235, Mar. 1932. 44
389. Famulener, L. W., and Robey, L. Pneumococcus grouping on a thousand cases. Proc. Soc. Exper. Biol. & Med., 19(8):367, May 1922.
390. Faragó, F. Untersuchungen an Pneumokokkenstämmen von verschiedenem Typus, mit besonderer Berücksichtigung der Dissoziationserscheinungen. Zentralbl. f. Bakt., 1 Abt., Orig., 125(5/6): 341, Aug. 1932. 150

391. Fowitzky, A. Ueber Farbstoffproduction durch den Pneumococcus (Fränkel). Ein Beitrag. Zur Biologie dieser Bacterienart. Deutsches Arch. f. klin. Med., 50:151, 1892.

392. Feemster, R. F. The effect of typhoid fever and of previous typhoid vaccination on the antibody response to inoculation with typhoid vaccine. J. Infect. Dis., 50(2):121, Feb. 1932. 537

393. Feemster, R. F., Wetterlow, L. H., and Cianciarulo, J. Standardization of typhoid and paratyphoid vaccines. I. The value of the Gates apparatus and total nitrogen determination. Am. J. Pub. Health, 26(12):1176, Dec. 1936. 533

394. Feinblatt, H. M. An analysis of one hundred and eighty necropsied cases of pneumonia, with reference to anatomic complications and bacterial causes. Boston Med. and Surg. J., 189(4): 136, July 26, 1923.

395. Felton, L. D. Oxidase reaction of various groups of bacteria. J. Exper. Med., 38(3):291, Sept. 1923. 75

396. Felton, L. D. A study of the isolation and concentration of the specific antibodies of antipneumococcus sera. Boston M. & S. J., 190(20):819, May 15, 1924. .... 412, 550, 553, 568, 580, 586

397. Felton, L. D. The protective substance in antipneumococcic serum. I. Type I serum. J. Infect. Dis., 37(3):199, Sept. 1925. 412, 560, 571

398. Felton, L. D. The protective substance in antipneumococcic serum. II. Effect of certain chemical manipulations on the stability of the protective substance in Type I antipneumococcus serum. J. Infect. Dis., 37(4):309, Oct. 1925. .... 412, 560

399. Felton, L. D. Studies on the protective substance in antipneumococcus serum. Study III. The protective substance in Types I, II and III antipneumococcus sera. Bull. Johns Hopkins Hosp., 38(1):33, Jan. 1926. .... 412, 419

400. Felton, L. D. The protective substance in antipneumococcus serum. 4. A separation of phosphorus and some inert protein from the water-insoluble precipitate of antipneumococcus serum. J. Infect. Dis., 42(3):248, Mar. 1928. .... 412, 550

401. Felton, L. D. The protective substance in antipneumococcus serum. 5. Febrile reaction from intravenous injection. J. Infect. Dis., 42(3):256, Mar. 1928.

402. Felton, L. D. The units of protective antibody in antipneumococcus serum and antibody solution. J. Infec. Dis., 43(6):531, Dec. 1928. .... 419, 568, 571, 576

403. Felton, L. D. Concentration of pneumococcus antibody. J. Infect. Dis., 43(6):543, Dec. 1928. .... 412, 549, 551, 560, 562

404. Felton, L. D. The concentration of antipneumococcus serum. J. A. M. A., 94(24):1893, June 14, 1930. .... 519, 563, 580

405. Felton, L. D. The variables in the mouse. Protection test of antipneumococcus serum. J. Immunol., 19(6):485, Dec. 1930. 420, 572, 576

406. Felton, L. D. A study of the neutralizing substance of the pneumococcus. J. Immunol., 19(6):511, Dec. 1930. 569

407. Felton, L. D. The correlation of the protective value with the

titers of other antibodies in Type I antipneumococcus serum. J. Immunol., 21(5):341, Nov. 1931. .... 378, 409, 583, 585
408. Felton, L. D. The use of ethyl alcohol as precipitant in the concentration of antipneumococcus serum. J. Immunol., 21(5):357, Nov. 1931. .... 412, 549, 553, 563
409. Felton, L. D. Dissociation of the specific protein precipitate of antipneumococcus horse serum, and a comparison with a protein isolated by chemical means from this immune serum. (Abstract.) J. Bact., 23(1):105, Jan. 1932.
410. Felton, L. D. Dissociation of the specific protein precipitate of antipneumococcus horse serum, and a comparison with a protein isolated by chemical means from this immune serum. J. Immunol., 22(6):453, June 1932. .... 554, 555
411. Felton, L. D. Studies on virulence. IV. Influence on virulence of pneumococci of growth on various media. J. Exper. Med., 56 (1):13, July 1932. .... 204, 210
412. Felton, L. D. Studies on virulence. V. The effect of oxygen, nitrogen, and carbon dioxide on the virulence of growing pneumococci. J. Exper. Med., 56(1):27, July 1932. .... 204, 210
413. Felton, L. D. Active immunization of white mice by a nonpolysaccharide and probably non-protein derivative of the pneumococcus. J. Immunol., 23(5):405, Nov. 1932. 275
414. Felton, L. D. Studies on the protective substance in antipneumococcus serum. Study 21. Comparison of certain characteristics of the water-insoluble proteins of antipneumococcus and normal horse serum. (Abstract.) J. Bact., 25(1):76, Jan. 1933.
415. Felton, L. D. Distribution of the immunizing antigen in the pneumococcus. (Abstract.) J. Bact., 27(1):90, Jan. 1934.
416. Felton, L. D. The effect of heat on alkaline and acid solutions of the immunizing substance of pneumococci Type I and Type II. (Abstract.) J. Immunol., 26(4):336, Apr. 1934. .... 276, 289
417. Felton, L. D. Studies on the immunizing substances in pneumococci. II. Separation of the organism into acid soluble and acid insoluble fractions. J. Immunol., 27(4):379, Oct. 1934. .... 275, 276, 485
418. Felton, L. D. The fraction of the pneumococcus antigenic for human beings. (Abstract.) J. Bact., 29(1):55, Jan. 1935. 501
419. Felton, L. D., and Bailey, G. H. Biologic significance of the soluble specific substances of pneumococci. J. Infect. Dis., 38(2): 131, Feb. 1926. .... 351, 352, 419, 575
420. Felton, L. D., and Bailey, G. H. The specific precipitates obtained from antipneumococcus serum and antibody solution by the soluble specific substance of pneumococci. J. Infect. Dis., 38(2): 145, Feb. 1926. .... 370, 554
421. Felton, L. D., and Bailey, G. H. The immunological characteristics of a water-insoluble protein in Type I antipneumococcus sera. J. Immunol., 11(3):197, Mar. 1926. 550
422. Felton, L. D., and Dougherty, K. M. Study of the action of

four aromatic cinchona derivatives on pneumococcus. A comparison with optochin. J. Exper. Med., 35(6):761, June 1922. 513

423. Felton, L. D., and Dougherty, K. M. Studies on virulence. I. An automatic transferring device: influence on virulence of growth of microorganisms during logarithmic increase phase. Bull. Johns Hopkins Hosp., 34(390):262, Aug. 1923. .... 41, 203, 210

424. Felton, L. D., and Dougherty, K. M. Studies on virulence. II. The increase in virulence in vitro of a strain of pneumococcus. J. Exper. Med., 39(1):137, Jan. 1924. .... 41, 210

425. Felton, L. D., and Dougherty, K. M. Studies on virulence. III. Influence of hydrogen ion concentration and of ingredients of plain broth on the virulence of pneumococci. J. Exper. Med., 39 (1):155, Jan. 1924. .... 38, 140, 204

426. Felton, L. D., and Kauffmann, G. The action of enzymes on the protective antibody of pneumococcus. J. Immunol., 13(3):219, Mar. 1927. 412

427. Felton, L. D., and Kauffmann, G. The pyrogenic reaction to concentrated antipneumococcus serums, with respect to certain serum constituents. Second paper. J. Infect. Dis., 49(4):337, Oct. 1931. 563

428. Felton, L. D., and Kauffmann, G. The lipoidal content of antipneumococcic horse serum. J. Immunol., 24(6):543, June 1933.

429. Felton, L. D., and Kauffmann, G. Certain characteristics of the water-insoluble protein of normal as compared with that of antipneumococcus horse serum. J. Immunol., 25(2):165, Aug. 1933. 548, 554

430. Felton, L. D., Kauffmann, G., and Stahl, H. J. The precipitation of bacterial polysaccharides with calcium phosphate. Pneumococcus. J. Bact., 29(2):149, Feb. 1935. 289

431. Felton, L. D., and Prescott, B. Studies on the immunizing substances in pneumococci. V. The effect of alkalis on the immunizing properties of a Type I pneumococcus polysaccharide. Bull. Johns Hopkins Hosp., 59(2):114, Aug. 1936. 290

432. Felton, L. D., and Stahl, H. J. A method for the standardization of antipneumococcic horse sera and concentrates. Pub. Health Rep., 50(49):1730, Dec. 6, 1935. .... 584, 585

433. Felton, L. D., and Stahl, H. J. Standardization of antipneumococcus horse sera and concentrates. Nat. Inst. of Health Bull., No. 169, Feb. 1937. .... 586, 645

434. Felton, L. D., Sutliff, W. D., and Steele, B. F. Antigenic characteristics in man of certain products of the pneumococcus. Comparison with vaccine. J. Infect. Dis., 56(2):101, Mar.–Apr. 1935. .... 485, 491, 493, 501

434a. Felty, A. R., and Keefer, C. S. Pneumococcus sepsis in the absence of pneumonia: report of case due to pneumococcus Type I. J. A. M. A., 81(19):1600, Nov. 10, 1923.

435. Fennel, E. A., and Fisher, M. B. Adjustment of reaction of culture mediums. J. Infect. Dis., 25(5):444, Nov. 1919.

436. Ferguson, D. A reinvestigation of the value of active pneumococcus immunity: Preliminary report. U. S. Nav. M. Bull., 30(3): 409, July 1932. .... 332, 483, 484, 526
437. Ferry, N. S., and Blanchard, E. Preparation and standardization of polyvalent antipneumococcic serum. J. Lab. & Clin. Med., 6(1):23, Oct. 1920.
438. Ferry, N. S., and Fisher, L. W. Production of immunity with a soluble antigen of the pneumococcus. J. Lab. & Clin. Med., 10 (10):817, July 1925. 483
439. Field, P. C. Vaccination against pneumonia. Mil. Surgeon, 51 (2):188, Aug. 1922. 497
440. Finkle, P. Metabolism of S and R forms of pneumococcus. J. Exper. Med., 53(5):661, May 1931. .... 79, 151
441. Finland, M. Immunological reactions of pneumonic pleural fluids. J. Exper. Med., 55(2):169, Feb. 1932. 441
442. Finland, M., and Dowling, H. F. Cutaneous reactions and antibody response to intracutaneous injections of pneumococcus polysaccharides. J. Immunol., 29(4):285, Oct. 1935. 465
443. Finland, M., and Ruegsegger, J. M. Immunization of human subjects with the specific carbohydrates of Type III and the related Type VIII pneumococcus. J. Clin. Investigation, 14(6):829, Nov. 1935.
444. Finland, M., Ruegsegger, J. M., and Felton, L. D. Heterophile antibodies in pneumonia. J. Clin. Investigation, 14(5):683, Sept. 1935. 387
445. Finland, M., Ruegsegger, J. M., and Felton, L. D. Should heterophile antibody be used in the treatment of pneumococcic pneumonia? J. A. M. A., 105(15):1180, Oct. 12, 1935.
446. Finland, M., and Sutliff, W. D. Specific cutaneous reactions and circulating antibodies in the course of lobar pneumonia. I. Cases receiving no serum therapy. J. Exper. Med., 54(5):637, Nov. 1931. .... 344, 486
447. Finland, M., and Sutliff, W. D. Specific cutaneous reactions and circulating antibodies in the course of lobar pneumonia. II. Cases treated with antipneumococcic sera. J. Exper. Med., 54(5): 653, Nov. 1931. .... 344, 486
448. Finland, M., and Sutliff, W. D. Specific antibody response of human subjects to intracutaneous injection of pneumococcus products. J. Exper. Med., 55(6):853, June 1932. .... 344, 411, 484
449. Finland, M., and Sutliff, W. D. Immunity reactions of human subjects to strains of pneumococci other than Types I, II, and III. J. Exper. Med., 57(1):95, Jan. 1933. 484
450. Finland, M., and Winkler, A. W. Antibody response to infections with Type III and the related Type VIII pneumococcus. J. Clin. Investigation, 13(1):79, Jan. 1934.
451. Finland, M., and Winkler, A. W. Antibody response to infections with Type II and the related Type V pneumococcus. J. Clin. Investigation, 13(1):97, Jan. 1934.

452. Fleming, W. L., and Neill, J. M. Studies on bacterial enzymes. III. Pneumococcus maltase and lactase. J. Exper. Med., 45(1): 169, Jan. 1927. 68
453. Fleming, W. L., and Neill, J. M. Studies on the oxidation and reduction of immunological substances. IX. The erythrocyte-combining property of pneumococcus hemotoxin. J. Exper. Med., 46(5):755, Nov. 1927.
454. Flosdorf, E. W., and Mudd, S. Procedure and apparatus for preservation in "Lyophile" form of serum and other biological substances. J. Immunol., 29(5):389, Nov. 1935. .... 52, 559
455. Flournoy, T. The identification of the pneumococcus in blood cultures. Proc. New York Path. Soc., 5(1/2), n.s.:20, Feb.–Mar. 1905.
456. Floyd, C. A study of the precipitin test in cases of pneumococcus empyema. J. Immunol., 5(4):321, July 1920. 441
457. Foà, P. Weitere Untersuchungen über die Aetiologie der Pneumonie. Deutsche med. Wchnschr., 15(2):21, Jan. 10, 1889.
458. Foà. Zur Biologie des Diplococcus lanceolatus. (Abstract.) Centralbl. f. Bakt., 1 Abt., Orig., 9(24):806, June 20, 1891. .... 93, 325
459. Foà, P. Ueber die Infektion durch den Diplococcus lanceolatus. Ztschr. f. Hyg. u. Infektionskr., 15:369, 1893. 24
460. Foà, P., und Bordoni-Uffreduzzi, G. Ueber Bakterienbefunde bei Meningitis cerebrospinalis und die Beziehungen derselben zur Pneumonie. Deutsche med. Wchnschr., 12(15):249, Apr. 15, 1886. 17, 19, 20
461. Foà, P., e Bordoni-Uffreduzzi, G. Sulla eziologia della meningite cerebrospinale epidemica. Arch. per le sc. med., 11(19):385, 1887. *Abstract in* Deutsche med. Wchnschr., 15(25):506, June 20, 1889. .... 19, 325
462. Foà, P., und Bordoni-Uffreduzzi, G. Ueber die Aetiologie der "Meningitis cerebro-spinalis epidemica." (Translation.) Ztschr. f. Hyg. u. Infektionskr., 4(1):67, 1888. .... 1, 19, 49, 225
463. Foà, P., e Carbone, T. Sulla natura del processo pneumonico. Gior. d. r. Accad. di med. di Torino, 54(5):251, May 1891. *Abstract in* Gior. d. r. Accad. di med. di Torino, 54(5):189, May 1891. 21, 24, 326, 337
464. Foà, P., et Rattone, G. Observations et expériences sur le pneumocoque et sur une complication grave de la pneumonite. Arch. ital. de biol., 6:366, 1884. 14
464a. Foà, P., e Scabia, E. Sulla immunità e sulla terapia della pneumonite. Gazz. med. di Torino, 43(13):245, Mar. 31; (14): 263, Apr. 7; (16):301, Apr. 21, 1892.
465. Fornet, W., und Müller, M. Zur Herstellung und Verwendung präzipitierender Sera, insbesondere für den Nachweis von Pferdefleisch. Ztschr. f. biol. Tech. u. Method, 1(3):201, Dec. 1908.
466. Fraenkel, A. Ueber die genuine Pneumonie. Verhandl. d. Kong. f. inn. Med., 3:17, Apr. 1884. 11
467. Fränkel, A. Bakteriologische Mittheilungen. Verhandl. d. Ver. f. inn. Med. Berlin, 5(7):78, July 13, 1885. 12

468. Fraenkel, A. Bakteriologische Mittheilungen. Ztschr. f. klin. Med., 10(5/6):401, 1886. .... 11, 15, 16, 42, 325
469. Fraenkel, A. Weitere Beiträge zur Lehre von den Mikrococcen der genuinen fibrinösen Pneumonie. Ztschr. f. klin. Med., 11 (5/6):437, 1886. .... 1, 15, 37, 225
470. Fränkel, A. Ueber einen Bakterienbefund bei Meningitis cerebrospinalis, nebst Bermerkungen über die Pneumoniemikrokokken. Deutsche med. Wchnschr., 12(13):209, Apr. 1, 1886.
471. Fränkel, A. Erwiederung auf die Mitteilung des Herrn Dr. Georg Sternberg über den Mikrococcus der Sputum-Septicaemie. Deutsche med. Wchnschr., 13(5):90, Feb. 3, 1887. 19
472. Francis, T., Jr. The identity of the mechanisms of type-specific agglutinin and precipitin reactions with pneumococcus. J. Exper. Med., 55(1):55, Jan. 1932. .... 364, 373
473. Francis, T., Jr. The value of the skin test with type-specific capsular polysaccharide in the serum treatment of Type I pneumococcus pneumonia. J. Exper. Med., 57(4):617, Apr. 1933. 468
474. Francis, T., Jr. Antigenic action of the specific polysaccharide of pneumococcus Type I in man. Proc. Soc. Exper. Biol. & Med., 31(4):493, Jan. 1934. .... 345, 411, 484, 486
475. Francis, T., Jr., and Abernethy, T. J. Cutaneous reactions in pneumonia to the somatic "C" polysaccharide of pneumococcus. (Abstract.) J. Clin. Investigation, 13(4):692, July 1934. .... 368, 465
476. Francis, T., Jr., and Terrell, E. E. Experimental Type III pneumococcus pneumonia in monkeys. I. Production and clinical course. J. Exper. Med., 59(5):609, May 1934. .... 193, 313, 486, 577
477. Francis, T., Jr., Terrell, E. E., Dubos, R., and Avery, O. T. Experimental Type III pneumococcus pneumonia in monkeys. II. Treatment with an enzyme which decomposes the specific capsular polysaccharide of pneumococcus Type III. J. Exper. Med., 59(5): 641, May 1934. 312
478. Francis, T., Jr., and Tillett, W. S. Cutaneous reactions in pneumonia. The development of antibodies following the intradermal injection of type-specific polysaccharide. J. Exper. Med., 52(4): 573, Oct. 1930. .... 344, 463, 484
479. Francis, T., Jr., and Tillett, W. S. Cutaneous reactions in rabbits to the type-specific capsular polysaccharides of pneumococcus. J. Exper. Med., 54(4):587, Oct. 1931. 460
480. Freedlander, B. L. The production of potent antipneumococcic serum in rabbits. J. Infect. Dis., 43(2):137, Aug. 1928. .... 337, 527
481. Freeman, W. T., and Hoppe, L. D. The intravenous use of mercurochrome-220 soluble in the treatment of pneumonia in children. Am. J. Dis. Child., 28(3):310, Sept. 1924. 510
482. Freudenberg, K., und Eichel, H. Über specifische Kohlenhydrate der Blutgruppen. Ann. Chem., Berlin, 510(3):240, May 18, 1934. 288
483. Freund, J. Reaction of young and adult rabbits to pneumococci injected into the skin. J. Exper. Med., 54(2):171, Aug. 1931.
484. Freund, R. Die Bedeutung der Disposition für Entstehung und

Verlauf von Seuchen. Epidemiologische und experimentelle Beobachtungen gelegentlich einer unter Versuchstieren herrschenden Stallseuche. Ztschr. f. Hyg. u. Infektionskr., 106(4):627, Oct. 1926. 184

485. Fried, B. M. Allergic lobar pneumonia. Experimental study. J. Exper. Med., 57(1):111, Jan. 1933.

485a. Fried, H. Prognostic importance of laboratory findings in pneumonia. Amer. Med., 30(1):25, Jan. 1924.

486. Friedländer, C. Ueber die Schizomyceten bei der acuten fibrinösen Pneumonie. Virchows Arch. f. path. Anat., 87(2):319, Feb. 1882. .... 5, 33

487. Friedländer, C. Die Mikrokokken der Pneumonie. Fortschr. d. Med., 1(22):715, Nov. 15, 1883. .... 1, 6, 33, 37, 194, 239

488. Friedländer, C. Demonstration der Pneumococcen. Verhandl. d. Ver. f. inn. Med. Berlin, 3(12):143, Nov. 16, 1883. *Abstract in* Berl. klin. Wchnschr., 20(48):752, Nov. 26, 1883. 6

489. Friedländer, C. Die genuine pneumonie. Verhandl. d. Kong. f. inn. Med., 3:31, Apr. 1884. .... 7, 227

490. Friedländer, C. Weitere Bemerkungen über Pneumonie-Micrococcen. Fortschr. d. Med., 2(10):333, May 15, 1884. .... 1, 7, 227

491. Friedländer, C. Notiz, die Färbung der Kapselmicrococcen betreffend. Fortschr. d. Med., 3(23):757, Dec. 1, 1885. 33

492. Friedländer, C. Weitere Arbeiten über die Schizomyceten der Pneumonie und der Meningitis. (Abstract.) Fortschr. d. Med., 4(21):702, Nov. 1, 1886. 13

493. Friedlander, M., Sobotka, H., and Banzhaf, E. J. The precipitin reaction of antipneumococcus sera. II. The ratio of precipitin to protective antibody. J. Exper. Med., 47(1):79, Jan. 1928. 377

494. Friel, A. R. Piantication and anapiantication. Publ. South African Inst. M. Research, No. 5:1, Jan. 26, 1915. .... 136, 392

495. Frosch, P., und Kolle, W. Die Mikrokokken. III. Diplokokken. *In* Flügge, C. Die Mikroorganismen, Auf. 3, Bd. 2:115. Leipzig: F. C. W. Vogel, 1896. 1

495a. Frost, W. D., Divine, C. B., and Reineking, C. W. The occurrence of Bacterium pneumoniae in the saliva of healthy individuals. J. Infect. Dis., Suppt. No. 1, 298, May, 1905.

496. Fukuda, J. Sterilizing function of liver against pneumococci. J. Orient. Med., 8(2):21, Feb. 1928.

497. Gabbi, U. Sopra un caso di tonsillite follicolare acuta infettiva. Contributo allo studio delle rare localizzazioni del virus pneumonico (microbio capsulato del Fraenkel). Lo Sperimentale, fasc. 4, 1889. *Abstract in* Jahresb. u. d. Fortschr. i. d. Lehre v. d. path. Mikroorg., 5:53, 80, 1889. .... 1, 20

498. Gamaléia, N. Sur l'étiologie de la pneumonie fibrineuse chez l'homme. Ann. Inst. Pasteur, 2(8):440, Aug. 1888. 1, 17, 20, 196, 225, 388

499. Gaskell, J. F. On the control of the virulence of the pneumococcus. J. Path. & Bact., 27(3):253, July 1924. .... 37, 205

500. Gaskell, J. F. Experimental pneumococcal infections of the lung. J. Path. & Bact., 28(3):427, July 1925. 183

501. Gaskell, J. F. The pathogenic values of pneumococcal types:

the lesions produced in relation to virulence. J. Path. & Bact., 31 (4):613, Oct. 1928. 205
502. Gaspari, E. L., Fleming, W. L., and Neill, J. M. Immunological properties of a typical (S-producing) and a degraded (non S-producing) strain of Type II pneumococcus with special reference to protective antibodies. J. Exper. Med., 46(1):101, July 1927.
503. Gaspari, E. L., Sugg, J. Y., Fleming, W. L., and Neill, J. M. The influence of heating the immunization material upon the antibody-invoking effectiveness of the type-specific and species-specific antigens of Type II pneumococcus cells. J. Exper. Med., 47(1): 131, Jan. 1928. .... 329, 530
504. Gates, F. L. A method of standardizing bacterial suspensions. J. Exper. Med., 31(1):105, Jan. 1920. .... 331, 532
505. Gautier, R. Tropical pneumonia. Quart. Bull. of the Health Organisation of the League of Nations, 1(1):64, Mar. 1932. 510
506. Gautier, R. Standardization of sera and bacterial products. V. Antipneumococcus sera. Quart. Bull. of the Health Organisation of the League of Nations, 4(3):512, Sept. 1935. 569
507. Gay, F. P., Atkins, K. N., and Holden, M. The resistance of dehydrated pneumococci to chemicals and heat. J. Bact., 22(4): 295, Oct. 1931.
508. Gay, F. P., and Chickering, H. T. Concentration of the protective bodies in anti-pneumococcus serum by means of specific precipitation. Proc. Soc. Exper. Biol. & Med., 12(5):115, Feb. 1915. 370, 418, 547
509. Gay, F. P., and Chickering, H. T. Concentration of the protective bodies in antipneumococcus serum by means of specific precipitation. J. Exper. Med., 21(4):389, Apr. 1915. .... 370, 418, 547
510. Gelarie, A. J., and Sabin, A. B. A study of the therapeutic mechanism of antipneumococcic serum on the experimental dermal pneumococcus infection in rabbits. III. The influence of nonspecific factors. J. Exper. Med., 58(2):237, Aug. 1933. ..... 182, 510, 518
510a. Gelera, M. Sui vari tipi di pneumococco. Gazz. d. Osp., 43 (96):1137, Nov. 30, 1922.
511. Germano, E. Die Uebertragung von Infektionskrankheiten durch die Luft. III. Mitteilung: Die Uebertragung des Erysipels, der Pneumonie und anderer Streptokokkeninfectionen durch die Luft. Ztschr. f. Hyg. u. Infektionskr., 26:66, 1897. 51
512. Gheorgiu, I. Infection à pneumocoques chez le cobaye. Vaccination antipneumococcique. Compt. rend. Soc. de biol., 87:39, 1922. 186
513. Gilbert, A., et Fournier, L. La culture du pneumocoque dans le sang défibriné. Compt. rend. Soc. de biol., 48:2, Jan. 1896. .... 37, 49
514. Gilbert, R., and Davenport, C. K. Failure of the mouse test to demonstrate the presence of Type I pneumococcus in sputum. An unusual instance. J. Lab. & Clin. Med., 12(9):944, June 1927. ... 125
515. Gillespie, L. J. The comparative viability of pneumococci on solid and on fluid culture media. J. Exper. Med., 18(5):584, Nov. 1913. 41

516. Gillespie, L. J. The acid agglutination of pneumococci. J. Exper. Med., 19(1):28, Jan. 1914. 362
517. Ginsberg, S., und Kaufmann, M. Beeinflüssung der kornealen Pneumokokkeninfektion beim Kaninchen durch Chinaalkaloide. Klin. Monatsbl. f. Augenh., 51:809, June 1913. 184
518. Goebel, W. F. The preparation of the type-specific polysaccharides of pneumococcus. J. Biol. Chem., 89(1):395, Nov. 1930.
519. Goebel, W. F. Chemo-immunological studies on the soluble specific substance of pneumococcus. II. The chemical basis for the immunological relationship between the capsular polysaccharides of Types III and VIII pneumococcus. J. Biol. Chem., 110(2):391, July 1935. 320
520. Goebel, W. F., and Avery, O. T. A study of pneumococcus autolysis. J. Exper. Med., 49(2):267, Feb. 1929. .... 54, 60, 61, 66
521. Goebel, W. F., and Avery, O. T. Chemo-immunological studies on conjugated carbohydrate-proteins. I. The synthesis of *p*-aminophenol β-glucoside, *p*-aminophenol β-galactoside, and their coupling with serum globulin. J. Exper. Med., 50(4):521, Oct. 1929. 263
522. Goebel, W. F., and Avery, O. T. Chemo-immunological studies on conjugated carbohydrate-proteins. IV. The synthesis of the p-aminobenzyl ether of the soluble specific substance of Type III pneumococcus and its coupling with protein. J. Exper. Med., 54(3):431, Sept. 1931. 264
523. Goebel, W. F., Babers, F. H., and Avery, O. T. Chemo-immunological studies on conjugated carbohydrate-proteins. VIII. The influence of the acetyl group on the specificity of hexoside-protein antigens. J. Exper. Med., 60(1):85, July 1934. 284
524. Gondolf, H. J. A rapid method for typing in pneumococcal meningitis. Proc. Soc. Exper. Biol. & Med., 24(4):295, Jan. 1927.
525. Goodner, K. Experimental intradermal pneumococcus infection in rabbits. J. Exper. Med., 48(1):1, July 1928. 181, 182, 343, 486, 491, 577
526. Goodner, K. Further experiments with the intradermal pneumococcus infection in rabbits. J. Exper. Med., 48(3):413, Sept. 1928. 181, 182, 343, 486, 491
527. Goodner, K. A method for comparison of antipneumococcus sera. J. Immunol., 17(3):279, Sept. 1929. .... 182, 577
528. Goodner, K. Experiments on the concentration of antipneumococcic and antimeningococcic horse sera. J. Immunol., 19(5):473, Nov. 1930. .... 364, 370, 412, 550, 551, 581
529. Goodner, K. The development and localization of the dermal pneumococcic lesions in the rabbit. J. Exper. Med., 54(6):847, Dec. 1931. .... 486, 491
530. Goodner, K. The effect of pneumococcus autolysates upon pneumococcus dermal infection in the rabbit. J. Exper. Med., 58(2):153, Aug. 1933.
531. Goodner, K. A test for the therapeutic value of antipneumococcus serum. J. Immunol., 25(3):199, Sept. 1933. .... 577, 578
532. Goodner, K. Certain host factors involved in the protective ac-

tion of antipneumococcus serum in experimental infections in rabbits. (Abstract.) J. Bact., 27(1):98, Jan. 1934. .... 185, 420, 577
533. GOODNER, K. Studies on host factors in pneumococcus infections. I. Certain factors involved in the curative action of specific antipneumococcus serum in Type I pneumococcus dermal infection in rabbits. J. Exper. Med., 60(1):9, July 1934. .... 420, 577, 578
534. GOODNER, K. Studies on host factors in pneumococcus infections. II. The protective action of Type I antipneumococcus serum in rabbits. J. Exper. Med., 60(1):19, July 1934. .... 420, 577
535. GOODNER, K., and DUBOS, R. Studies on the quantitative action of a specific enzyme in Type III pneumococcus dermal infection in rabbits. J. Exper. Med., 56(4):521, Oct. 1932. .... 182, 311
536. GOODNER, K., DUBOS, R., and AVERY, O. T. The action of a specific enzyme upon the dermal infection of rabbits with Type III pneumococcus. J. Exper. Med., 55(3):393, Mar. 1932. ...... 182, 310, 392
537. GOODNER, K., and HORSFALL, F. L., JR. The protective action of Type I antipneumococcus serum in mice. I. The quantitative aspects of the mouse protection test. J. Exper. Med., 62(3):359, Sept. 1935. .... 561, 574, 575
538. GOODNER, K., and HORSFALL, F. L., JR. The complement fixation reaction with pneumococcus capsular polysaccharide. J. Exper. Med., 64(2):201, Aug. 1936. .... 381, 647
539. GOODNER, K., HORSFALL, F. L., JR., and BAUER, J. H. Ultrafiltration of Type I antipneumococcal serum. Proc. Soc. Exper. Biol. & Med., 34(5):617, June 1936. .... 417, 555, 561
540. GOODNER, K., and MILLER, D. K. The protective action of Type I antipneumococcus serum in mice. III. The significance of certain host factors. J. Exper. Med., 62(3):393, Sept. 1935. .... 189, 420, 574, 575
541. GOODNER, K., and STILLMAN, E. G. The evaluation of active resistance to pneumococcus infection in rabbits. J. Exper. Med., 58(2):183, Aug. 1933. 182
542. GÖRANDER, G. On the relationship between streptococci and pneumococci. Acta path. et microbiol. Scandinav., 7(4):327, 1930. ... 176
543. GORDON, J. E. The relationship of the pneumococcus to acute infections of the upper respiratory tract in man. Influenza studies. VI. J. Infect. Dis., 29(5):437, Nov. 1921. 111
544. GRAESER, J. B., and HARRISON, M. C. Changes in the titer of antipneumococcal humoral immunity in adult human beings. J. Exper. Med., 58(2):245, Aug. 1933.
545. GRAM, C. Ueber die isolirte Färbung der Schizomyceten in Schnitt- und Trockenpräparaten. Fortschr. d. Med., 2(6):185, Mar. 15, 1884. .... 9, 31
546. GRANT, M. H. Pneumonias in Glasgow and their pneumococcal types. Glasgow M. J., 98(3):193, Sept. 1922.
547. GRAWITZ, E., und STEFFEN, W. Die Bedeutung des Speichels und Auswurfs für die Biologie einiger Bacterien. Berl. klin. Wchnschr., 31(18):419, Apr. 30, 1894. 37

548. Great Britain. Arrangement of sections. *In* Therapeutic Substances Act, 1925. [15 & 16 Geo. 5, Ch. 60.] London: His Majesty's Stationery Office, 1925.

549. Great Britain. Therapeutic substances. *In* Statutory rules and orders, No. 486. London: His Majesty's Stationery Office, 1927. 592

550. Great Britain. Therapeutic substances. *In* Statutory rules and orders (1931), No. 633. London: His Majesty's Stationery Office, 1931.

551. Great Britain. Therapeutic substances. *In* Statutory rules and orders (1935), No. 580. London: His Majesty's Stationery Office, 1935. 592

552. Great Britain. Medical Research Council. A system of bacteriology in relation to medicine, v. 2. London: His Majesty's Stationery Office, 1929. .... 30, 53, 57, 70

553. Great Britain. Medical Research Council. A system of bacteriology in relation to medicine, v. 6. London: His Majesty's Stationery Office, 1931.

554. Greene, M. R. The effects of vitamins A and D on antibody production and resistance to infection. Am. J. Hyg., 17(1):60, Jan. 1933. 185

555. Grenier, M. Études sur le pneumocoque. III. Sur quelques pneumocoques d'origine animale. (Virulence pour la souris. Conservation de cette virulence.) Ann. Inst. Pasteur, 26(1):5, Jan. 1912. 117

556. Griffini, L., e Cambria, A. Sull'eziologia della polmonite cruposa. I. Gior. internaz. d. sc. med., 4:353, 1882.

557. Griffini, L., e Cambria, A. Sull'eziologia della polmonite cruposa. II. Gior. internaz. d. sc. med., 4:462, 1882.

558. Griffith, F. Serological types of pneumococci in lobar pneumonia. A study of 100 cases. Lancet, 2(5109):226, July 30, 1921. 112, 113, 362

559. Griffith, F. Types of pneumococci obtained from cases of lobar pneumonia. *In* Great Britain, Ministry of Health. Rep. on Pub. Health & Med. Subjects, No. 13, p. 20. London: His Majesty's Stationery Office, 1922. 540

560. Griffith, F. The influence of immune serum on the biological properties of pneumococcus. *In* Great Britain, Ministry of Health. Rep. on Pub. Health & Med. Subjects, No. 18, p. 1. London: His Majesty's Stationery Office, 1923. .... 137, 525

561. Griffith, F. Inhalation experiments on mice with pneumococci. J. Hyg., 25(1):1, Feb. 1926.

562. Griffith, F. The significance of pneumococcal types. J. Hyg., 27(2):113, Jan. 1928. 154

563. Grumbach, A. Dissoziationserscheinungen an Pneumokokken. Zentralbl. f. Bakt., 1 Abt., Orig., 120(3/4):245, Mar. 1931. 149

563a. Guillain, G., et Barré, J.-A. Hémorragie méningée consécutive à une commotion par éclatement d'obus sans plaie extérieure.

Méningite à pneumocoque mortelle secondaire. Bull. et mém. Soc. méd. des Hôp. de Paris, 41, 3e sér.:898, July 20, 1917.
564. GUNDEL, M. Ueber das Vorkommen von Pneumokokken in der Mundhöhle. Centralbl. f. Bakt., 1 Abt., Orig., 95(2/4):202, June 1925.
565. GUNDEL, M. Zur Frage einer Behandlung der pneumonia crouposa mit rekonvaleszentserum. Klin. Wchnschr., 10(16):728, Apr. 18, 1931. 446
566. GUNDEL, M. Epidemiologie, Pathogenese und spezifische Therapie der Pneumonie. Zentralbl. f. Bakt., 1 Abt., Orig., 122(1/3):*112, Sept. 7, 1931.
567. GUNDEL, M. Immunbiologische Studien über Pneumokokkeninfektionen. Ztschr. f. Immunitätsforsch. u. exper. Therap., 73(3/4): 193, Jan. 1932. 436
568. GUNDEL, M. Fehlerquellen bei der bakteriologischen Diagnose menschlicher Pneumokokkeninfektionen. Zentralbl. f. Bakt., 1 Abt., Orig., 127(7/8):467, Feb. 23, 1933. 122
569. GUNDEL, M. Bakteriologische und epidemiologische Untersuchungen über die Besiedlung der oberen Atmungswege Gesunder mit Pneumokokken. Ztschr. f. Hyg. u. Infektionskr., 114(4):659, Feb. 1933. .... 71, 230
570. GUNDEL, M., und LINDEN, H. Die Bedeutung des Tierversuches für die bakteriologische Diagnose der Influenza und Pneumonie. Klin. Wchnschr., 9(30):1402, July 26, 1930.
571. GUNDEL, M., und LINDEN, H. Über die Verbreitungsweise der menschlichen Pneumokokkeninfektionen. Ztschr. f. Hyg. u. Infektionskr., 112(1):1, Jan. 1931.
572. GUNDEL, M., und LINDEN, H. Die Flora der Mundhöhle Gesunder und ihre Bedeutung für die Pathogenese der Erkrankungen der Atmungsorgane. Zentralbl. f. Bakt., 1 Abt., Orig., 121(5/6):349, July 13, 1931.
573. GUNDEL, M., und OKURA, G. Untersuchungen über das gleichzeitige Vorkommen mehrerer Pneumokokkentypen bei Gesunden und ihre Bedeutung für die Epidemiologie. Ztschr. f. Hyg. u. Infektionskr., 114(4):678, Feb. 1933. 231
574. GUNDEL, M., und SCHÄFER, O. Über das Vorkommen und über die Pathogenese von Pneumonieepidemien. Arch. f. Hyg., 108(2): 94, May 1932.
575. GUNDEL, M., und SCHWARZ, F. K. T. Studien über die Bakterienflora der oberen Atmungswege Neugeborener (in Vergleich mit der Mundhöhlenflora der Mutter und des Pflegepersonals) unter besonderer Berücksichtigung ihrer Bedeutung für das Pneumonieproblem. Ztschr. f. Hyg. u. Infektionskr., 113(2/3):411, Jan. 1932. 230, 231
576. GUNDEL, M., und SCHWARZ, F. K. T. Über die Typendifferenzierung und Epidemiologie der Gruppe X der Pneumokokken. Ztschr. f. Hyg. u. Infektionskr., 113(2/3):498, Jan. 1932.
577. GUNDEL, M., und SEITZ, L. Experimentelle Untersuchungen über

die Chemotherapie von Pneumokokkeninfektionen mit neuen, noch nicht in die Therapie eingeführten Chininpräparaten. Ztschr. f. Immunitätsforsch. u. exper. Therap., 80(3/4):240, Oct. 1933. 516

578. Gundel, M., und Wasu, C. Die Bedeutung der Virulenz des Erregers für die pathogenese menschlicher Pneumokokkenerkrankungen. Ztschr. f. Hyg. u. Infektionskr., 112(3):436, May 1931. 199, 231

579. Günther, C. [Ueber infectiöse Pneumonie.] Verhandl. d. Ver. f. inn. Med. Berlin, 2(12):123, Nov. 20, 1882. (Discussion of Leyden's paper.) 6

580. Gutfeld, von, und Nassau. Spezifische Pneumokokkenreaktionen bei Säuglingen. Centralbl. f. Bakt., 1 Abt., Ref., 82(7/8):191, Apr. 22, 1926. 466

581. Guthrie, A. C. Research work on the pneumococci and their enzymes and its significance in lobar pneumonia. London: Bailliere, Tindall & Cox, 1932.

582. Gutmann, L. Zur experimentellen Chemotherapie der Pneumokokkeninfektion. Ztschr. f. Immunitätsforsch. u. exper. Therap., 15(6):625, Dec. 1912. 512

583. Hachtel, F. W., and Stoner, H. W. Studies on acquired typhoid immunity. J. Infect. Dis., 19(3):322, Sept. 1916. 537

584. Hadley, P. Microbic dissociation. The instability of bacterial species with special reference to active dissociation and transmissible autolysis. J. Infect. Dis., 40(1):1, Jan. 1927. .... 136, 150

585. Haendel, L., und Lange, L. Beitrag zum biologischen Verhalten der Pneumokokken. Ztschr. f. Hyg. u. Infektionskr., 110(1):1, Feb. 1929. 48

586. Hale, W. The cause of death from subdural injections of serum. Hygienic Laboratory Bulletin, No. 91:5, Dec. 1913. 557

587. Hallerman, N. A., und Kähler, H. Über die Typeneinteilung der Pneumonie und ihre Behandlung mit Serum. Klin. Wchnschr., 9(14):650, Apr. 5, 1930.

588. Hanes, F. M. An immunological study of Pneumococcus mucosus. J. Exper. Med., 19(1):38, Jan. 1914. .... 361, 380

588a. Hardouin, J. Présence de la capsule dans les cultures de pneumocoque et de pneumobacille sur milieux artificiels; sa mise en évidence par le procédé de l'encre de Chine. Compt. rend. Soc. de biol., 72:298, Feb. 12, 1912.

589. Harkavy, J. Pneumococcus meningitis. Recovery with serum therapy. J. A. M. A., 90(8):597, Feb. 25, 1928. 226

590. Harkins, M. J. Studies on the pneumococcolytic activity of the bile from experimental bacterial cholecystitis of rabbits. J. Lab. & Clin. Med., 10(9):716, June 1925. 58

591. Harley, D. The immunizing action of extracts of pneumococci (Types 1 and 2) in mice and rabbits. Brit. J. Exper. Path., 15(3):161, June 1934. 337

592. Harley, D. Species immunity to pneumococcus. Brit. J. Exper. Path., 16(1):14, Feb. 1935. .... 329, 342

593. Harley, D. Study of pneumococcal allergy, anaphylaxis and immunity. J. Path. & Bact., 41(3):491, Nov. 1935. 343
594. Harris, A. B. Observations on the therapeutic value of the pneumococcus vaccine in the treatment of pneumonia and some of its complications. Brit. M. J., 1:1530, June 26, 1909.
595. Harris, A. L., Sugg, J. Y., and Neill, J. M. Studies on immunological relationships among the pneumococci. II. A comparison of the antibody responses of mice and of rabbits to immunization with typical Type III pneumococci and to immunization with a related strain. J. Exper. Med., 47(6):933, June 1928. 111
596. Hartley, P., and Smith, W. A proposed international standard for antipneumococcus serum (Type I). Quart. Bull. of the Health Organisation of the League of Nations, 4(spec. no.):48, Jan. 1935. 569, 576, 586
597. Hartley, P., and Smith, W. A proposed international standard for antipneumococcus serum (Type II). Quart. Bull. of the Health Organisation of the League of Nations, 4(spec. no.):63, Jan. 1935. 569
598. Hartman, C. C. Serum studies in pneumonia. The antigenic properties of fibrin (exudate) to serum. J. Infect. Dis., 13(1): 69, July 1913. 337
599. Hartman, C. C. The antigenic properties of the constituents of the pneumonic exudate. Serum studies in pneumonia. II. J. Infect. Dis., 13(3):499, Nov. 1913. 527
600. Hecht, A. F. Die Haut als Testobjekt. Wien: J. Springer, 1925.
601. Heffron, R. Pneumonia with special reference to pneumococcus lobar pneumonia. New York: The Commonwealth Fund. In preparation. 214, 216, 217, 503, 507, 559
602. Heffron, R., and Varley, F. M. A study of lobar pneumonia in Massachusetts: Methods and results of pneumococcus type determination. 1931–32. Am. J. Pub. Health, 22(12):1230, Dec. 1932. 129
603. Heidelberger, M. Contributions of chemistry to the knowledge of immune processes. Medicine, 12(3):279, Sept. 1923.
604. Heidelberger, M. The chemical nature of immune substances. Physiol. Rev., 7(1):107, Jan. 1927. .... 244, 247
605. Heidelberger, M. Immunologically specific polysaccharides. Chem. Rev., 3(4):403, Jan. 1927. .... 244, 247, 250
606. Heidelberger, M., and Avery, O. T. The soluble specific substance of pneumococcus. J. Exper. Med., 38(1):73, July, 1923. 238, 243, 370, 582
607. Heidelberger, M., and Avery, O. T. The soluble specific substance of pneumococcus. Second paper. J. Exper. Med., 40(3): 301, Sept. 1924. 370
608. Heidelberger, M., Avery, O. T., and Goebel, W. F. A "soluble specific substance" derived from gum arabic. J. Exper. Med., 49 (5):847, May 1929. 261
609. Heidelberger, M., and Goebel, W. F. The soluble specific substance of pneumococcus. IV. On the nature of the specific poly-

saccharide of Type III pneumococcus. J. Biol. Chem., 70(3):613, Nov. 1926.

610. Heidelberger, M., and Goebel, W. F. The soluble specific substance of pneumococcus. V. On the chemical nature of the aldobionic acid from the specific polysaccharide of Type III pneumococcus. J. Biol. Chem., 74(3):613, Sept. 1927.

611. Heidelberger, M., Goebel, W. F., and Avery, O. T. The soluble specific substance of a strain of Friedländer's bacillus. Paper I. J. Exper. Med., 42(5):701, Nov. 1925. .... 245, 260

612. Heidelberger, M., Goebel, W. F., and Avery, O. T. The soluble specific substance of Friedländer's bacillus. Paper II. Chemical and immunological relationships of pneumococcus Type II and of a strain of Friedländer's bacillus. J. Exper. Med., 42(5):709, Nov. 1925. 260

613. Heidelberger, M., Goebel, W. F., and Avery, O. T. The soluble specific substance of pneumococcus. Paper III. J. Exper. Med., 42(5):727, Nov. 1925. .... 371, 580

614. Heidelberger, M., and Kabat, E. A. Chemical studies on bacterial agglutination. I. A method. J. Exper. Med., 60(5):643, Nov. 1934. .... 367, 582

615. Heidelberger, M., and Kabat, E. A. Chemical studies on bacterial agglutination. II. The identity of precipitin and agglutinin. J. Exper. Med., 63(5):737, May 1936.

616. Heidelberger, M., and Kendall, F. E. A quantitative study of the precipitin reaction between Type III pneumococcus polysaccharide and purified homologous antibody. J. Exper. Med., 50(6):809, Dec. 1929. 373

617. Heidelberger, M., and Kendall, F. E. Specific and non-specific polysaccharides of Type IV pneumococcus. J. Exper. Med., 53(5):625, May 1931. .... 257, 260, 261, 280

618. Heidelberger, M., and Kendall, F. E. Some physicochemical properties of specific polysaccharides. J. Biol. Chem., 95(1):127, Feb. 1932. .... 246, 296

619. Heidelberger, M., and Kendall, F. E. Quantitative studies on the precipitin reaction. The determination of small amounts of a specific polysaccharide. J. Exper. Med., 55(4):555, Apr. 1932. .... 374, 584

620. Heidelberger, M., and Kendall, F. E. Studies on the precipitin reaction. Precipitating haptens; species differences in antibodies. J. Exper. Med., 57(3):373, Mar. 1933. .... 277, 374

621. Heidelberger, M., and Kendall, F. E. Quantitative studies on the precipitin reaction. (Abstract.) J. Bact., 27(1):90, Jan. 1934.

622. Heidelberger, M., and Kendall, F. E. The precipitin reaction between Type III pneumococcus polysaccharide and homologous antibody. II. Conditions for quantitative precipitation of antibody in horse sera. J. Exper. Med., 61(4):559, Apr. 1935. 375

623. Heidelberger, M., and Kendall, F. E. The precipitin reaction between Type III pneumococcus antibody and homologous anti-

body. III. A quantitative study and a theory of the reaction mechanism. J. Exper. Med., 61(4):563, Apr. 1935. 375
624. HEIDELBERGER, M., and KENDALL, F. E. A quantitative theory of the precipitin reaction. II. A study of an azoprotein-antibody system. J. Exper. Med., 62(4):467, Oct. 1935. 584
625. HEIDELBERGER, M., and KENDALL, F. E. Quantitative studies on antibody purification. I. The dissociation of precipitates formed by pneumococcus specific polysaccharides and homologous antibodies. J. Exper. Med., 64(2):161, Aug. 1936. 414
626. HEIDELBERGER, M., KENDALL, F. E., and SCHERP, H. W. Preparative changes necessitated by a quantitative study of precipitating power of pneumococcus polysaccharides. Proc. Soc. Exper. Biol. & Med., 33(1):188, Oct. 1935. 295
627. HEIDELBERGER, M., KENDALL, F. E., and SCHERP, H. W. The specific polysaccharides of Types I, II and III pneumococcus. A revision of methods and data. J. Exper. Med., 64(4):559, Oct. 1936. 293, 582, 637
628. HEIDELBERGER, M., KENDALL, F. E., and SOO HOO, C. M. Quantitative studies on the precipitin reaction. Antibody production in rabbits injected with an azo protein. J. Exper. Med., 58(2):137, Aug. 1933. .... 367, 375
629. HEIDELBERGER, M., PEDERSEN, K. O., and TISELIUS, A. Ultracentrifugal and electrophoretic studies on antibodies. Nature, London, 138(3482):165, July 25, 1936. .... 414, 415
630. HEIDELBERGER, M., SIA, R. H. P., and KENDALL, F. E. Specific precipitation and mouse protection in Type I antipneumococcus serum. J. Exper. Med., 52(4):477, Oct. 1930. ...... 367, 374, 409, 584, 643
631. HEIM, L. Die Widerstandsfähigkeit verschiedener Bakterienarten gegen Trocknung und die Aufbewahrung bakterienhaltigen Materials insbesondere beim Seuchendienst und für gerichtlich-medizinische Zwecke. Ztschr. f. Hyg. u. Infektionskr., 50:123, 1905. 50
632. HEIM, L. Zytoseroprophylaxe und Pneumonieinfektion. München. med. Wchnschr., 55(38):1995, Sept. 22, 1908.
633. HEIM, L., and SCHLIRF, K. Was ist es mit der Einheit der Streptokokken? Centralbl. f. Bakt., 1 Abt., Orig., 100(1/3):24, Oct. 1926. 175
634. HEIST, G. D., and SOLIS-COHEN, S. The bactericidal action of circulating blood upon pneumococci, with the technic of its determination. Explanation of the natural immunity of the pigeon to pneumococcic septicemia. Proc. Path. Soc. Philadelphia, 21, n.s.: 13, Apr. 1918. 341
635. HEIST, G. D., and SOLIS-COHEN, S. The bactericidal action of the whole blood of rabbits following inoculations of pneumococcus bacterins. J. Immunol., 4(4):147, July 1919. 527
636. HENDERSON, Y., HAGGARD, H. W., CORYLLOS, P. N., and BIRNBAUM, G. L. The treatment of pneumonia by inhalation of carbon dioxide. I. The relief of atelectasis. Arch. Int. Med., 45(1):72, Jan. 1930. 194

637. Herrold, R. D., and Traut, E. F. Skin reactions with pneumococcal and other bacterial filtrates and extracts. J. Infect. Dis., 40(5):619, May 1927. .... 440, 462

638. Herzog, B. M. Die in der Schweiz bei croupöser Pneumonie vorkommenden Pneumokokkentypen. Schweiz. med. Wchnschr., 5(25):573, June 19, 1924.

639. Herzog, H. Beitrag zur Kenntnis der Pneumokokkenarthritis im ersten Kindesalter. Jahrb. f. Kinderh., 63:446, 1906. 226

640. Hewitt, J. A. W., and Famulener, L. W. The hemolytic properties of the pneumococcus. Proc. Soc. Exper. Biol. & Med., 19 (8):368, May 1922. 83

641. Hewitt, L. F. Oxidation-reduction potentials of pneumococcus cultures. I. Biochem. J., 24(5):1551, 1930. 77

642. Hewitt, L. F. Oxidation-reduction potentials of pneumococcus cultures. II. Effect of catalase. Biochem. J., 25(1):169, 1931. 78

643. Hewitt, L. F. Bacterial metabolism. II. Glucose breakdown by pneumococcus variants and the effect of phosphate thereon. Biochem. J., 26(2):464, 1932. 67

644. Heyrovsky, J. Durch Bakteriengifte erzeugte Haut- und Schleimhautblutungen. Wien. klin. Wchnschr., 20(9):247, Feb. 28, 1907. 87

645. Hintze, K. 100 Pneumonien und ihre Erreger. Zugleich ein Beitrag zur Frage der Rassen- oder Typenbildung bei den Pneumokokken. Arch. f. Hyg., 94(4/6):163, 1924.

646. Hintze, K. Untersuchungen und Beobachtungen an Pneumokokken. Centralbl. f. Bakt., 1 Abt., Orig., 99(6):419, Aug. 20, 1926. .... 51, 110

647. Hintze, K., und Peter, K. Rassenbildung bei Pneumokokken. München. med. Wchnschr., 68(32):1011, Aug. 12, 1921. 357

648. Hirschfelder, J. O. The production of active and passive immunity to the pneumococcus with a soluble vaccine. A preliminary report. J. A. M. A., 59(15):1373, Oct. 12, 1912. 483

649. Hiss, P. H., Jr. A contribution to the physiological differentiation of pneumococcus and streptococcus, and to methods of staining capsules. J. Exper. Med., 6(4/6):317, Mar. 1902. .... 68, 69

650. Hiss, P. H., Jr. A method for obtaining mass cultures of bacteria for inoculation and for agglutination tests; with special reference to pneumococci and streptococci. J. Exper. Med., 7(2):223, Apr. 1905. .... 34, 39, 47

651. Hiss, P. H., Jr., Borden, J. H., and Knapp, C. B. A comparative study of pneumococci and allied organisms. The report from the Central Laboratory to the Medical Commission for the investigation of acute respiratory diseases of the Department of Health of the City of New York. J. Exper. Med., 7(5):547, Aug. 1905. *Also:* Department of Health, City of New York. Report Med. Comm'n Invest. Acute Resp. Dis., Part I. Studies on pneumococcus, p. 145. New York: Department of Health, 1905. .... 135, 215

652. Hiss, P. H., Jr., and Zinsser, H. The curative influence of ex-

tracts of leucocytes upon infections in man. 2. On the treatment of lobar pneumonia with leucocyte extract. J. Med. Research, 19 (3):455, Nov. 1908.

653. Hitchcock, C. H. Serological relationships among and between the streptococci and pneumococci. J. Exper. Med., 41(1):13, Jan. 1, 1925.

654. Hitchens, A. P. The production of yeast "vitamine" in the laboratory for the cultivation of bacteria. Abstr. Bact., 6(1):35, Jan. 1922. 45

655. Horder, T., and Ferry, N. S. A search for an ideal antigen for therapeutic immunization. Brit. M. J., 2(342):177, July 31, 1926. 336, 483

656. Hornus, G. J. P., and Enders, J. F. Soluble specific substance of pneumococcus Type III possessing properties distinct from SSS III. Proc. Soc. Exper. Biol. & Med., 34(1):102, Feb. 1936. 295

657. Horsfall, F. L., Jr., and Goodner, K. Lipoids and immunological reactions. I. The relation of phospholipins to the type-specific reactions of antipneumococcus horse and rabbit sera. J. Exper. Med., 62(4):485, Oct. 1935. 381

658. Horsfall, F. L., Jr., and Goodner, K. Lipids and immunological reactions. III. Lipid content of specific precipitates from Type I antipneumococcus sera. J. Exper. Med., 64(4):583, Oct. 1936.

659. Horsfall, F. L., Jr., Goodner, K., and MacLeod, C. M. Type specific antipneumococcus rabbit serum. Science, 84(2191):579, Dec. 25, 1936. .... 381, 600

659a. Horsfall, F. L., Jr., Goodner, K., MacLeod, C. M., and Harris, A. H., 2nd. Antipneumococcus rabbit serum as a therapeutic agent in lobar pneumonia. J. A. M. A., 108(18):1483, May 1, 1937.

660. Howard, W. T., and Perkins, R. G. Streptococcus mucosus (Nov. Spec. ?) pathogenic for man and animals. J. Med. Research, 6:163, 1901.

661. Howell, K. M. Blood changes and antibody production in human beings after injection of pneumococcus lipovaccine. J. Infect. Dis., 27(6):557, Dec. 1920. .... 483, 484, 492

662. Hoyle, L. The mouse-pathogenic bacteria (pneumococcus, B. influenzae, etc.) of the upper respiratory tract: their relation to acute infectious coryza. J. Path. & Bact., 35(6):817, Nov. 1932. 234

663. Huber, F. O. Über Agglutination des Pneumococcus. Centralbl. f. inn. Med., 23(17):417, Apr. 26, 1902. 357

664. Huntoon, F. M. "Hormone" medium. A simple medium employable as a substitute for serum medium. J. Infect. Dis., 23: 169, 1918. 44

665. Huntoon, F. M. Antibody studies. I. Reversal of the antigen-antibody reaction. J. Immunol., 6(2):117, Mar. 1921. .... 418, 547

666. Huntoon, F. M. Preparation of pneumococcus antibody solution. Tr. Coll. Physicians, Philadelphia, 45, ser. 3:617, 1923. .... 413, 418, 547

667. Huntoon, F. M. Pneumococci cultivation in large amounts. Proc. Soc. Exper. Biol. & Med., 22(5):267, Feb. 1925. 41

668. Huntoon, F. M., and Etris, S. Antibody studies. II. The recovery of antibody from sensitized antigens: Technic. J. Immunol., 6(2):123, Mar. 1921. .... 418, 547
669. Huntoon, F. M., Masucci, P., and Hannum, E. Antibody studies. III. Chemical nature of antibody. J. Immunol., 6(2):185, Mar. 1921. 418
670. Irwin, M. R., and Hughes, T. P. Differences in bactericidal power of the blood within an inbred strain of rats. Proc. Soc. Exper. Biol. & Med., 29(3):295, Dec. 1931. .... 188, 445, 574
671. Ishida, I. Studies on influenzas and pneumonias of infants and children. I. Bacteriological research with special references to the occurrence of various types of pneumococci. Orient. J. Dis. Infants, 8(3):29, Nov. 1930.
672. Ishida, I., Nagai, H., and Saito, T. A study of pneumococcus in throat of healthy infant, especially on its type occurrence. Orient. J. Dis. Infants, 10(1):21, July 1931.
673. Issaeff, B. Contribution à l'étude de l'immunité acquise contre le pneumocoque. Ann. Inst. Pasteur, 7(3):260, Mar. 1893. 25, 93, 356, 389, 528
674. Jacobson, M. A., and Falk, I. S. Influence of anti-serum and of animal passage upon virulence and electrophoresis of pneumococci. Proc. Soc. Exper. Biol. & Med., 23(8):785, May 1926. 145
675. Jacobson, M. A., and Falk, I. S. Studies on respiratory diseases. XXIX. The influence of anti-serum and of animal passage upon the virulence and electrophoresis of pneumococci. J. Bact., 13 (3):191, Mar. 1927. .... 145, 201
676. Jamieson, W. A., and Powell, H. M. Further studies on the immunology of the pneumococcus. Am. J. Hyg., 13(3):823, May 1931. .... 99, 340, 385, 467
677. Jamieson, W. A., and Powell, H. M. Merthiolate as a preservative for biological products. Am. J. Hyg., 14(1):218, July 1931. 558
678. Jehle, L. Ueber Pneumokokken-Agglutination mit dem Blutserum pneumoniekranker Kinder. Wien. klin. Wchnschr., 16(32): 917, Aug. 6, 1903. 358
679. Jobling, J. W., Petersen, W., and Eggstein, A. A. The serum ferments and antiferment during pneumonia. Studies on ferment action. XXIV. J. Exper. Med., 22(5):568, Nov. 1915.
680. Jobling, J. W., and Strouse, S. Studies on ferment action. IX. A note on the relation between lysis and proteolysis of pneumococci. J. Exper. Med., 18(5):597, Nov. 1913. 54
681. Jones, F. S., and Little, R. B. Changes in bacterial volume as the result of specific agglutination. J. Exper. Med., 57(5):721, May 1933. 364
682. Jones, F. S., and Little, R. B. The significance of changes in antigenic volume as the result of specific agglutination. J. Exper. Med., 57(5):729, May 1933. 364
683. Jones, H. M. The limiting hydrogen-ion concentration of various types of pneumococci. J. Infect. Dis., 26(6):435, June 1920. 71
684. Julianelle, L. A. A biological classification of encapsulatus

pneumoniae (Friedländer's bacillus). J. Exper. Med., 44(1): 113, July 1926. 260

685. Julianelle, L. A. Immunological relationships of encapsulated and capsule-free strains of encapsulatus pneumoniae (Friedländer's bacillus). J. Exper. Med., 44(5):683, Nov. 1926.

686. Julianelle, L. A. Immunological relationships of cell constituents of encapsulatus pneumoniae (Friedländer's bacillus). J. Exper. Med., 44(6):735, Dec. 1926.

687. Julianelle, L. A. Reactions of rabbits to intracutaneous injections of pneumococci and their products. I. The antibody response. J. Exper. Med., 51(3):441, Mar. 1930. 343

688. Julianelle, L. A. Reactions of rabbits to intracutaneous injections of pneumococci and their products. II. Resistance to infection. J. Exper. Med., 51(3):449, Mar. 1930. 343

689. Julianelle, L. A. Reactions of rabbits to intracutaneous injections of pneumococci and their products. III. Reactions at the site of injection. J. Exper. Med., 51(3):463, Mar. 1930. 456

690. Julianelle, L. A. Reactions of rabbits to intracutaneous injections of pneumococci and their products. IV. The development of skin reactivity to derivatives of pneumococcus. J. Exper. Med., 51(4):625, Apr. 1930. 456

691. Julianelle, L. A. Reactions of rabbits to intracutaneous injections of pneumococci and their products. V. The development of eye reactivity to derivatives of pneumococci. J. Exper. Med., 51 (4):633, Apr. 1930. 457

692. Julianelle, L. A. Reactions of rabbits to intracutaneous injections of pneumococci and their products. VI. Hypersensitiveness to pneumococci and their products. J. Exper. Med., 51(4):643, Apr. 1930. 457

693. Julianelle, L. A., and Morris, M. C. Reactions of rabbits to intracutaneous injections of pneumococci and their products. VIII. The interrelationships of hypersensitiveness to pneumococcus and streptococcus. J. Exper. Med., 55(6):867, June 1932. 457

694. Julianelle, L. A., and Reimann, H. A. The production of purpura by derivatives of pneumococcus. I. General considerations of the reaction. J. Exper. Med., 43(1):87, Jan. 1926. 87

695. Julianelle, L. A., and Reimann, H. A. The production of purpura by derivatives of pneumococcus. III. Further studies on the nature of the purpura-producing principle. J. Exper. Med., 45 (4): 609, Apr. 1927. 89

696. Julianelle, L. A., and Rhoads, C. P. Reactions of rabbits to intracutaneous injections of pneumococci and their products. VII. The relation of hypersensitiveness to lesions in the lungs of rabbits infected with pneumococci. J. Exper. Med., 55(5):797, May 1932. 455

697. Jungeblut, C. W. Über Festigungsversuche an Bakterien, mit besonderer Berücksichtigung der physikalisch-chemischen Veränderungen. Ztschr. f. Hyg. u. Infektionskr., 99(3):254, Apr. 1923. 519

698. JUNGEBLUT, C. W. A specific flocculation reaction occurring between alcoholic extracts of pneumococci and antipneumococcus serum. J. Exper. Med., 45(2):227, Feb. 1927. .... 253, 368

699. JÜRGENSEN. Ueber die genuine Pneumonie (Aetiologie, Pathologie, Klinik, Therapie). Verhandl. d. Cong. f. inn. Med., 3:6, Apr. 1884. 14

699a. KAKINUMA, K. Experimentelle Untersuchungen über die Pathogenese der Kreislaufsschwäche bei der Pneumokokkenpneumonie. Mitt. a. d. med. Fakult. d. K. Univ. zu Tokyo, 29:587, 1922.

699b. KAMINER. Zur Frage der Kupierung von Pneumokokkeninfektion durch Optochin. Deutsche med. Wchnschr., 48(11):357, March 17, 1922.

700. KEEGAN, J. J. The pathology of epidemic pneumonia in mice and guinea-pigs. Arch. Int. Med., 26(5):570, Nov. 1920. 186

701. KELLEY, W. H. The antipneumococcus properties of normal swine serum. J. Exper. Med., 55(6):877, June 1932. 431

702. KELLY, F. B. On the solution of pneumococci by bile. Am. J. Pub. Health, 10(9):708, Sept. 1920. 57

703. KENNISON, S. Report of research on pneumococcus. U. S. Nav. M. Bull., 12(1):150, Jan. 1918.

704. KILLIAN, H. Versuche über aktive Immunisierung von Mäusen gegen Pneumokokken und Streptokokken. Ztschr. f. Hyg. u. Infektionskr., 102(1/2):179, Apr. 1924. .... 330, 335

705. KILLIAN, H. Versuche über die Möglichkeit einer Immunisierung per os gegen Pneumokokken und Streptokokken. Ztschr. f. Hyg. u. Infektionskr., 102(1/2):279, Apr. 1924.

706. KILLIAN, H. Versuche über aktive Immunisierung von Mäusen gegen Pneumokokken und Streptokokken. II. Mitteilung. Ztschr. f. Hyg. u. Infektionskr., 103(3):607, Sept. 1924. .... 330, 342, 536

707. KILLIAN, H. Versuche über aktive Immunisierung von Mäusen gegen Pneumokokken und Streptokokken. III. Mitteilung. Ztschr. f. Hyg. u. Infektionskr., 104(3):489, Mar. 1925. 330

708. KILLIAN, H. Neuere Untersuchungsergebnisse über die Immunisierung gegen Strepto- und Pneumokokken. Klin. Wchnschr., 4 (45):2166, Nov. 5, 1925.

709. KILLIAN, H. Prüfung lyophober und lyophiler Pneumo- und Streptokokkenimpfstoffe im Tierexperiment. Ztschr. f. Hyg. u. Infektionskr., 107(1):216, Jan. 1927.

710. KIMURA, R. Weitere Versuche über aktive Immunisierung per os gegen Pneumokokken. Ztschr. f. Hyg. u. Infektionskr., 107(2): 390, Apr. 1927. 348

711. KIMURA, R., SUKNEFF, W. W., und MEYER, H. Auftreten verschiedener Varianten von Pneumokokken bei Züchtung in Immunserum. Ztschr. f. Hyg. u. Infektionskr., 109(1):51, Sept. 1928. .. 143

712. KINDBORG, A. Ein die Gelatine verflüssigender Pneumococcus. Centralbl. f. Bakt., 1 Abt., Orig., 32(8/9):573, Oct. 25, 1902. 36

713. KINDBORG, A. Die Pneumokokken. Vergleichende Untersuch-

ungen mit besonderer Berücksichtigung der Agglutination. Ztschr. f. Hyg. u. Infektionskr., 51:197, 1905. .... 196, 198, 358

714. KING, H. H. Analysis of Captain Malone's results in vaccination against pneumonia. Indian J. M. Research, 12(3):571, Jan. 1925. 498

715. KIRCHNER. Types of pneumococcus in the Dutch East Indies. Geneesk. tijdschr. v. Nederl.-Indiö, 71:990, 1931. *Abstract in* J. A. M. A., 100(11):834, Mar. 18, 1933.

716. KIRKBRIDE, M. Demonstration of methods for pneumococcus differentiation. Albany M. Ann., 37(4):158, Apr. 1916.

717. KITAGAWA, K. J. On the mechanism of pneumococcus immunity. (Preliminary note.) Proc. Soc. Exper. Biol. & Med., 12(8):213, May 1915. 402

718. KLEBS, E. Beiträge zur Kenntnis der Schistomyceten. 4. Die Monadinen. Arch. f. exper. Path. u. Pharmakol., 4(5/6):409, Dec. 1875. .... 1, 2, 37

719. KLEIN, E. Ein Beitrag zur Kenntnis des Pneumokokkus. Centralbl. f. d. med. Wissensch., 22(30):529, July 1884. 13

720. KLEIN, S. J. Studies on the solubility of pneumococcus in saponin. II. Sensitization by ergosterol. J. Bact., 26(2):215, Aug. 1933. 60

721. KLEIN, S. J., and STONE, F. M. The lysis of pneumococcus by saponin. J. Bact., 22(6):387, Dec. 1931. 60

722. KLEINSCHMIDT, H. Verschiedene Pneumokokkentypen unter Optochineinwirkung. Klin. Wchnschr., 9(8):357, Feb. 22, 1930. 514

723. KLEMPERER, G. Die Beziehungen verschiedener Bakteriengifte zur Immunisirung und Heilung. Ztschr. f. klin. Med., 20(1/2):165, 1892. .... 21, 325

724. KLEMPERER, G., und KLEMPERER, F. Versuche über Immunisirung und Heilung bei der Pneumokokkeninfection. Berl. klin. Wchnschr., 28(34):833, Aug. 24, 1891. .... 21, 325, 407, 527, 533, 579

725. KLEMPERER, G., und KLEMPERER, F. Versuche über Immunisirung und Heilung bei der Pneumokokkeninfection. Schluss. Berl. klin. Wchnschr., 28(35):869, Aug. 31, 1891. .... 21, 338, 407, 437

726. KLINE, B. S. Experimental study of organization in lobar pneumonia. J. Exper. Med., 26(2):239, Aug. 1917. 194

727. KLINE, B. S., and MELTZER, S. J. The effect of previous intravenous injection of pneumococci upon experimental lobar pneumonia produced by the method of intrabronchial insufflation. Proc. Soc. Exper. Biol. & Med., 12(8):185, May 1915. 402

728. KLINE, B. S., and WINTERNITZ, M. C. Studies upon experimental pneumonia in rabbits. VII. The production of lobar pneumonia. J. Exper. Med., 21(4):304, Apr. 1915. .... 182, 184

729. KLINE, B. S., and WINTERNITZ, M. C. Studies upon experimental pneumonia in rabbits. VIII. Intra vitam staining in experimental pneumonia, and the circulation in the pneumonic lung. J. Exper. Med., 21(4):311, Apr. 1915.

730. KLUMPEN, W. Systematische Untersuchungen über die Gewin-

nung von Varianten aus echten Pneumokokken. Zentralbl. f. Bakt., 1 Abt., Orig., 124(5/6):241, May 6, 1932. 152

730a. Knuth, P., und Sommerfeld, W. Befund von Diplococcus lanceolatus Fränkel bei einem braunen Bären. Berl. tierärztl. Wchnschr., 28(10):169, Mar. 7, 1912.

731. Koch, F. E. Optochinblutagar zur Unterscheidung von Pneumokokken und Streptokokken. Zentralbl. f. Bakt., 1 Abt., Orig., 124(5/6):258, May 6, 1932. 48

732. Koch, K. Zur Kenntnis der Pneumokokken und Streptokokken. Virchows Arch. f. path. Anat., 227(1):39, Nov. 20, 1919.

733. Koch, K. R. Quantitative determination of the bacteremia in pneumococcus pneumonia and its value as a prognostic indicator. (Abstract.) J. Bact., 23(1):106, Jan. 1932.

734. Koch, K. R. The prognostic value of repeated blood cultures in pneumococcus lobar pneumonia. Am. J. M. Sc., 184(3):364, Sept. 1932.

735. Koch, R. Zur Untersuchung von pathogenen Organismen. Mitt. a. d. k. Gsndhtsamte, 1:1, 1881. 5

736. Koester, K. Die embolische Endocarditis. Virchows Arch. f. path. Anat., 72(2):257, Feb. 1, 1878. 5

737. Kohn, L. A. Rapid pneumococcus type determination in lobar pneumonia by Krumwiede's method. J. A. M. A., 84(23):1733, June 6, 1925. 125

738. Köhne, W. Beitrag zur Kenntnis arzneifester Bakterienstämme. Ztschr. f. Immunitätsforsch. u. exper. Therap., 20(5):531, Jan. 1914. 519

739. Kolchin, B. S., and Gross, L. Observations on the cross protective power of anti-pneumococcus monovalent sera, Types I, II, and III. With a note on the cross protection afforded by so-called "antibody solution." J. Immunol., 9(6):505, Nov. 1924. 408

740. Kolle, W., Kraus, R., und Uhlenhuth, P. Handbuch der pathogenen Mikroorganismen. Dritte Auflage. Jena: Gustav Fischer; Berlin und Wien: Urban & Schwarzenberg, 1929. 30

741. Kolmer, J. A. Principles and practice of chemotherapy, with special reference to the specific and general treatment of syphilis. Philadelphia & London: W. B. Saunders Co., 1926. 185

742. Kolmer, J. A., and Borow, L. The adaptation of the Heist-Lacy method for determining the bactericidal activity of whole blood for chemotherapeutic investigations. Studies in the chemotherapy of bacterial infections. I. J. Infect. Dis., 31(2):116, Aug. 1922. 510, 513

743. Kolmer, J. A., and Idzumi, G. Chemotherapeutic studies with ethylhydrocuprein and mercurophen in experimental pneumococcus meningitis in rabbits. J. Infect. Dis., 26(4):355, Apr. 1920. 515

744. Kolmer, J. A., and Matsumoto, M. Natural antihuman hemolysins and hemagglutinins in horse sera in relation to serum therapy. J. Immunol., 5(2):75, Mar. 1920. 561

745. Kolmer, J. A., and Rule, A. M. Oral immunization of rabbits

against pneumococcus pneumonia and septicemia. Proc. Soc. Exper. Biol. & Med., 30(1):107, Oct. 1932. 350

746. KOLMER, J. A., and RULE, A. M. Vaccination of monkeys against pneumococci with special reference to oral immunization. Proc. Soc. Exper. Biol. & Med., 31(2):243, Nov. 1933. 489

747. KOLMER, J. A., and RULE, A. M. Vaccination of rabbits against pneumococci with special reference to oral immunization. Proc. Soc. Exper. Biol. & Med., 31(2):245, Nov. 1933. .... 350, 483, 489

748. KOLMER, J. A., and RULE, A. M. Chemotherapy of intradermal pneumococcus infection of rabbits. Effects of optochin and other quinine compounds. Proc. Soc. Exper. Biol. & Med., 32(1):89, Oct. 1934. .... 182, 516

749. KOLMER, J. A., and SANDS, J. R. Chemotherapeutic studies with ethylhydrocupreine hydrochloride in experimental pneumococcus pleuritis. J. Exper. Med., 33(6):693, June 1921. 515

750. KORTENHAUS, F. Zonenzyklohämolyse auf Blutagar bei Staphylokokken sowie bei Viridans-Streptokokken und Pneumokokken. Zentralbl. f. Bakt., 1 Abt., Orig., 113(7/8):499, Sept. 18, 1929.

751. KOZLOWSKI, A. Comparative studies of the action on the pneumococcus of bile acids and unsaturated fatty acids, found in bile in the form of soaps. J. Exper. Med., 42(4):453, Oct. 1925. 58

752. KRAFKA, J., JR., and ROSEN, S. F. Reticulocytes in pneumonia. South. M. J., 25(8):880, Aug. 1932.

753. KRAMÁR, E. Untersuchungen über die chemische Beschaffenheit der Kapselsubstanz einiger Kapselbakterien. Centralbl. f. Bakt., 1 Abt., Orig., 87(6):401, Dec. 30, 1921. 262

754. KRAMÁR, E., und GYÜRE, D. Untersuchungen über die Immunbiologie der Lungenentzündung. Erste Mitteilung. Einleitung. Pneumokokkentypen und Hautreaktion. Arch. f. Kinderh., 89 (1/2):73, Dec. 13, 1929. 463

755. KRAMÁR, E., und GYÜRE, D. Untersuchungen über die Immunbiologie der Lungenentzündung. Zweite Mitteilung. Pneumokokkenhautreaktion und humorale Antikörper. Arch. f. Kinderh., 89 (1/2):81, Dec. 1929.

756. KRAMÁR, E., und GYÜRE, D. Untersuchungen über die Immunbiologie der Lungenentzündung. Dritte Mitteilung. Mechanismus und immunbiologische Bedeutung der Pneumokokkenhautprobe. Arch. f. Kinderh., 89(1/2):88, Dec. 13, 1929. 469

757. KRAMÁR, E., und GYÜRE, D. Untersuchungen über die Immunbiologie der Lungenentzündung. Vierte Mitteilung. Die experimentelle Pneumonie. Arch. f. Kinderh., 91(4):278, Oct. 21, 1930. 191

758. KRITSCHEWSKI, I. L., und HERONIMUS, E. S. Ueber die Bedeutung des Retikuloendothelialsystems bei Infektionskrankheiten. X. Das Retikuloendothelialsystem als Schutzapparat bei Pneumokokkeninfektion. Ztschr. f. Immunitätsforsch. u. exper. Therap., 78(3/4): 246, Mar. 1933.

759. KRITSCHEWSKI, I. L., RUBINSTEIN, P. L., und HERONIMUS, E. S. Die Abhängigkeit des therapeutischen Effekts bei Serumbehand-

lung von der Unversehrtheit des Retikuloendothelialsystem. II. Die Behandlung mit Tetanusantitoxin und Anti-Pneumokokkenserum bei intaktem und geschädigtem Retikuloendothelialsystem. Ztschr. f. Immunitätsforsch. u. exper. Therap., 73(5/6):463, Mar. 1932.

760. Krueger, A. P. A method for the quantitative estimation of bacteria in suspensions. J. Gen. Physiol., 13(5):553, May 1930. 533

761. Krumwiede, C., Jr., and Noble, W. C. A rapid method for the production of precipitin antigen from bacteria: an attempt to apply it to the determination of the type of pneumococcus in sputum. J. Immunol., 3(1):1, Jan. 1918. 124

762. Krumwiede, C., Jr., and Valentine, E. Determination of the type of pneumococcus in the sputum of lobar pneumonia. J. A. M. A., 70(8):513, Feb. 23, 1918. .... 124, 630

763. Kruse, W., und Pansini, S. Untersuchungen über den Diplococcus pneumoniae und verwandte Streptokokken. Ztschr. f. Hyg. u. Infektionskr., 11:279, 1891. .... 23, 38, 135, 136, 169, 184, 325, 388

764. Kulp, W. L., and Borden, A. G. Further studies on immunization with heterologous antigen. (Abstract.) J. Bact., 30(2):212, Aug. 1935. 262

765. Kyes, P. The production of antibodies to pneumococci in an insusceptible host. J. A. M. A., 56(25):1878, June 24, 1911. 410

766. Kyes, P. The natural resistance of the pigeon to the pneumococcus. J. Infect. Dis., 18(3):277, Mar. 1916. 196

767. Kyes, P. The treatment of lobar pneumonia with an antipneumococcic serum. J. Med. Research, 38(3):495, July 1918. .... 545, 562

768. Kyes, P., and Carey, E. S. The elimination of serum shock. J. Immunol., 14(2):123, Aug. 1927. .... 545, 562

769. Kyes, P., and Carey, E. S. The preparation of fibrinogen-free fowl serum. J. Immunol., 17(6):529, Dec. 1929. 545

770. Lacy, G. R., and Hartmann, C. C. Specific reactions of the body fluids in pneumococcic infections. J. Immunol., 3(1):43, Jan. 1918. 438

770a. Lafforgue. Septicémies pneumococciques primitives et pneumococcies méningées parapneumoniques. Bull. et mém. Soc. méd. des Hôp. de Paris, 45, 3e sér.:264, 1921.

771. Laidlaw, P. P., and Dudley, H. W. A specific precipitating substance from tubercle bacilli. Brit. J. Exper. Path., 6(4):197, Aug. 1925. 262

772. Lamar, A. V., and Meltzer, S. J. Experimental pneumonia by intrabronchial insufflation. J. Exper. Med., 15(2):133, Feb. 1912. 194

773. Lamar, R. V. Chemo-immunological studies on localized infections. First paper. Action on the pneumococcus and its experimental infections of combined sodium oleate and antipneumococcus serum. J. Exper. Med., 13(1):1, Jan. 1911. 59

774. Lamar, R. V. Chemo-immunological studies on localized infections. Third paper. Some further observations upon the action of certain soaps on the pneumococcus and its experimental infections. J. Exper. Med., 14(3):256, Sept. 1911. 59

775. LAMAR, R. V. Chemo-immunological studies on localized infections. Fourth paper. Experimental pneumococcic meningitis and its specific treatment. J. Exper. Med., 16(5):581, Nov. 1912. 192, 509, 518

776. LAMBERT, A. The use of mixed stock vaccines in pneumonia. Tr. A. Am. Physicians, 41:225, 1926. 505

777. LANCEFIELD, R. C. The immunological relationships of Streptococcus viridans and certain of its chemical fractions. I. Serological reactions obtained with antibacterial sera. J. Exper. Med., 42 (3):377, Sept. 1925.

778. LANCEREAUX, E., et BESANÇON. Étude sur quelques cas de pneumonie observés à l'Hôpital de la Pitié au printemps de l'année 1886. Arch. gén. de méd., 17, 7e sér.: 257, Sept. 1886. .... 16, 225

779. LANDMANN, G. Ueber Pneumokokkenheilserum. Deutsche med. Wchnschr., 34(48):2062, Nov. 26, 1908. .... 524, 534

780. LANDSTEINER, K. Note on the group specific substance of horse saliva. Science, 76(1972):351, Oct. 14, 1932. 288

781. LANDSTEINER, K., and LEVENE, P. A. On the heterogenetic haptene. Fourth communication. J. Immunol., 14(1):81, July 1927. 288

782. LANDSTEINER, K., and VAN DER SCHEER, J. Serological differentiation of steric isomers. J. Exper. Med., 48(3):315, Sept. 1928. ... 376

783. LANDSTEINER, K., and VAN DER SCHEER, J. Serological differentiation of steric isomers (antigens containing tartaric acids). Second paper. J. Exper. Med., 50(4):407, Oct. 1929. 376

784. LANDSTEINER, K., and VAN DER SCHEER, J. On the specificity of serological reactions with simple chemical compounds (inhibition reactions). J. Exper. Med., 54(3):295, Sept. 1931.

785. LANGE, B., und KESCHISCHIAN, K. W. Über Versuche, weisse Mäuse durch Einatmung von Krankheitserregern zu infizieren. I. Mitteilung. Ztschr. f. Hyg. u. Infektionskr., 103(3):569, Sept. 1924. 190

786. LARSON, N., and THOMPSON, L. The use of potato extract in growing diplococcus pneumoniae for typing. (Abstract.) Proc. Staff Meet., Mayo Clin., 5(1):5, Jan. 8, 1930. 45

787. LARSON, W. P. Cutaneous reaction to pneumococcic filtrates. Proc. Soc. Exper. Biol. & Med., 23(4):295, Jan. 1926. .... 97, 462

788. LARSON, W. P. A report on the preparation of pneumococcic antitoxin. Proc. Soc. Exper. Biol. & Med., 23(6):497, Mar. 1926. 339, 384

789. LARSON, W. P. Cross protection of animals immunized with various pneumococcus types. (Read before the Am. A. Path. & Bact., 1934.) 335, 483

790. LARSON, W. P., and FAHR, G. A new anti-pneumococcus serum. Minnesota Med., 8(7):424, July 1925. 561

791. LARSON, W. P., and NELSON, E. The antigenic properties of pneumococci and streptococci treated with sodium ricinoleate. Proc. Soc. Exper. Biol. & Med., 22(6):357, Mar. 1925. .... 63, 334, 509

792. LAURINSICH, A. Ricerche batteriologiche e sierologiche sui pneumococchi nell'infanzia. Pediatria, 33(19):1029, Oct. 1925.

792a. LAVERGNE, V. DE. L'infection pneumococcique, étude épidémiologique. Ann. d'hyg., Paris, 37(5), 4e sér.:273, May 1922.

793. LEAKE, C. D., VICKERS, J. L., and BROWN, T. K. Observations on blood reaction in experimental pneumonia. J. Exper. Med., 39 (3):393, Mar. 1924. 194

794. LEAKE, J. P., and CORBITT, H. B. Toxicity of certain preservatives used in serums, viruses, and vaccines. Hygienic Laboratory Bulletin, No. 110:35, Sept. 1917. .... 557, 588

795. LEBASHOFF. The cocci of croupous and hypostatic pneumonia. Lancet, 1:753, Apr. 1886. (Abstract of article in "Russian Weekly Clinical Gazette.") 16

796. LE GUYON, R.-F. Étude comparée de la sérosité péritonéale après inoculation de pneumocoque chez un animal sensible et chez un animal à peu près réfractaire. Compt. rend. Soc. de biol., 108:45, 1931. 432

797. LEIFSON, E. A method of staining bacterial flagella and capsules together with a study of the origin of flagella. J. Bact., 20(3): 203, Sept. 1930. 34

798. LEIFSON, E. Types of bacteria on blood and chocolate agar and the immediate cause of these types. J. Bact., 24(6):473, Dec. 1932.

799. LEINEWEBER, F., KAUTSKY, R., and FAMULENER, L. W. The nitrogen content of the pneumococcus: A preliminary report. Proc. Soc. Exper. Biol. & Med., 20(8):543, May 1923. 248

799a. LESAGE. Epidémie de septicémie pneumococcique chez le nourrisson. Bull. et mém. Soc. méd. des Hôp. de Paris, 17, 3e sér.: 290, 1904.

800. LEVINTHAL, W. Umwandlung avirulenter Pneumokokken in virulente. Klin. Wchnschr., 5(43):2020, Oct. 1926. .... 42, 145

801. LEVY, E., und AOKI, K. Ueber Schutzimpfung gegen Pneumokokken mit besonderer Berücksichtigung der kombiniert aktiv-passiven Immunisierungsmethode vermittelst sensibilisierter Vaccins. Ztschr. f. Immunitätsforsch. u. exper. Therap., 1 Teil, Orig., 7(4):435, Sept. 21, 1910. .... 335, 483

802. LEVY, E., und STEINMETZ, C. Studien über den Diplococcus pneumoniae Fränkel. Arch. f. exper. Path. u. Pharmakol., 37(2/3): 89, June 2, 1896. 42

803. LEVY, R. Differentialdiagnostische Studien über Pneumokokken und Streptokokken. Virchows Arch. f. path. Anat., 187(2):327, Feb. 1907. 56

804. LÉVY-BRUHL, M. Recherches sur le pneumocoque III (Pneumococcus mucosus). Origine, caractères généraux et virulence de 20 échantillons. Ann. Inst. Pasteur, 41(4):458, Apr. 1927. .... 207, 525

805. LÉVY-BRUHL, M., et BORIN, P. Mise en évidence des capsules du pneumocoque III (Pneumococcus mucosus) en milieux liquides non albumineux. Compt. rend. Soc. de biol., 92(17):1343, May 22, 1925. 34

806. Lewkowicz, K. L'immunité et les humeurs. Infections pneumococcique, méningococcique et tuberculose. Ann. de méd., 32(5): 410, Dec. 1932.

807. Lewy, F. Ueber die spezifische Arzneifestigkeit der Pneumokokken. I. Mitteilung. Zur Methodik der Festigung gegen Optochin. Ztschr. f. Immunitätsforsch. u. exper. Therap., 43(3):196, June 1925. 519

808. Lewy, F. Ueber die spezifische Arzneifestigkeit der Pneumokokken. II. Mitteilung. Die Beziehungen zwischen chemischer Konstitution und Arzneifestigkeit. Ztschr. f. Immunitätsforsch. u. exper. Therap., 43(3):243, June 1925. 520

809. Leyden, von, E. Ueber infectiöse Pneumonie. Verhandl. d. Ver. f. inn. Med., Berlin, 2(12):121, Nov. 20, 1882.

810. Leyden, E. Die Mikrokokken der Cerebrospinal-Meningitis. Centralbl. f. klin. Med., 4(10):161, Mar. 10, 1883. 9

811. Libman, E. A pneumococcus producing a peculiar form of hemolysis. Proc. New York Path. Soc., 5(4/8), n.s.:168, May 1905—Jan. 1906. 83

811a. Libman, E., and Rosenthal, J. The action of bile on the pneumococcus, streptococcus, and Streptococcus mucosus. Proc. New York Path. Soc., 8(1/2), n.s.:40, Feb.–Mar. 1908.

812. Lieb, F. Ueber das Oxydationsvermögen der Pneumokokken. Zentralbl. f. Bakt., 1 Abt., Orig., 125(7/8):449, Sept. 21, 1932. ... 78

813. Lieberman, L. M., and Leopold, S. S. Therapeutic pneumothorax in experimental lobar pneumonia in dogs. Am. J. M. Sc., 187(3): 315, Mar. 1934. 195

814. Lindemann, E. A. Beitrag zur Kenntnis der Pneumokokkeninfektion. Arb. a. d. k. Gsndhtsamte, 38(2):233, Aug. 1911.

815. Lister, F. S. Specific serological reactions with pneumococci from different sources. Publ. South African Inst. M. Research, 1(2):1, Dec. 1913. 107

816. Lister, F. S. An experimental study of prophylactic inoculation against pneumococcal infection in the rabbit and in man. Publ. South African Inst. M. Research, 1(8):231, Oct. 1916. .. 107, 483, 484, 504

817. Lister, F. S. Prophylactic inoculation of man against pneumococcal infections, and more particularly against lobar pneumonia; including a report upon the results of the experimental inoculation, with a specific group vaccine, of the native mine labourers employed upon the Premier (Diamond) Mine and the Crown (Gold) Mines in the Transvaal and the de Beers (Diamond) Mines at Kimberley—covering the period from November 1, 1916, to October 31, 1917. Publ. South African Inst. M. Research, 1(10):1, Nov. 1917.

818. Lister, F. S. A note on the aetiology of epidemic influenza and secondary pneumonia. J. M. A. South Africa, 3:179, Apr. 13, 1929. 499

819. Lister, S., and Ordman, D. Epidemiology of pneumonia on the

Witwatersrand Goldfields and prevention of pneumonia and other allied acute respiratory diseases in native labourers in South Africa by means of vaccine. Publ. South African Inst. M. Research, 7(37):1, Apr. 1935. .... 490, 501
820. LOCKE, E. A. The treatment of Type I pneumococcus lobar pneumonia with specific serum. J. A. M. A., 80(21):1507, May 26, 1923. 603
821. LOEWE, L., HIRSHFELD, S., and WALLACH, K. A new method for typing pneumococci by the use of blood. J. A. M. A., 73(3):170, July 19, 1919. 125
822. LOEWENTHAL, H., und MICSEH, G. Phagocytose versuche mit Milzmakrophagen in der Gewebekultur. Ztschr. f. Hyg. u. Infektionskr., 110(1):150, Feb. 1929. 406
823. LOGAN, W. R., and SMEALL, J. T. A direct method of typing pneumococci. Brit. M. J., 1(3708):188, Jan. 30, 1932. 128
824. LONGCOPE, W. T. A note upon the growth of pneumococci and streptococci in blood serum. J. Exper. Med., 7(5):626, Aug. 1905. *Also:* Department of Health, City of New York. Report Med. Comm'n Invest. Acute Resp. Dis., Part I: Studies on pneumococcus, p. 224. New York: Department of Health, 1905. 358
825. LONGCOPE, W. T., and FOX, W. W. A comparative study of pneumococci and streptococci from the mouths of healthy individuals and from pathological conditions. J. Exper. Med., 7(5):430, Aug. 1905. *Also:* Department of Health, City of New York. Report Med. Comm'n Invest. Acute Resp. Dis., Part I: Studies on pneumococcus, p. 28. New York: Department of Health, 1905. .... 215, 234
826. LORD, F. T. The relation of the pneumococcus to the production of acid in fluid culture mediums and the reaction of the pneumonic lung. J. A. M. A., 72(19):1364, May 10, 1919. 442
827. LORD, F. T., and HEFFRON, R. Lobar pneumonia and serum therapy with special reference to the Massachusetts Pneumonia Study. New York: The Commonwealth Fund; London: Humphrey Milford, Oxford University Press, 1936. .... 545, 559, 602
828. LORD, F. T., and NESCHE, G. E. Antibody and agglutinin in pneumococcus pneumonia. J. Exper. Med., 50(4):449, Oct. 1929. *Also:* Tr. A. Am. Physicians, 44:189, 1929. 440
829. LORD, F. T., and NYE, R. N. The relation of the pneumococcus to hydrogen-ion concentration, acid death-point, and dissolution of the organism. J. Exper. Med., 30(4):389, Oct. 1919. .... 39, 53, 67
830. LORD, F. T., and NYE, R. N. Studies on the pneumonic exudate. I. Effect of preservation, temperature, dialysis, and salt concentration on the enzyme in the pneumonic lung. J. Exper. Med., 34(2):199, Aug. 1921. 442
831. LORD, F. T., and NYE, R. N. Studies on the pneumonic exudate. II. The presence of enzyme and antienzyme in the pneumonic lung. Local ferment-antiferment balance. J. Exper. Med., 34(2):201, Aug. 1921. 442

832. LORD, F. T., and NYE, R. N. Studies on the pneumonic exudate. III. The presence in the pneumonic exudate of a large amount of specific antigen. J. Exper. Med., 34(2):207, Aug. 1921. 442
833. LORD, F. T., and NYE, R. N. Studies on the pneumonic exudate. IV. The presence in the pneumonic lung of a soluble substance inhibiting agglutination by the homologous serum. J. Exper. Med., 34(2):211, Aug. 1921. .... 442, 443
834. LORD, F. T., and NYE, R. N. Studies on the Pneumococcus. I. Acid death-point of the pneumococcus. J. Exper. Med., 35(5): 685, May 1922. 71
835. LORD, F. T., and NYE, R. N. Studies on the pneumococcus. II. Dissolution of pneumococci at varying hydrogen ion concentrations. Effect of temperature, previous killing of the organisms, and fresh human serum on the phenomenon. Behavior of other organisms. J. Exper. Med., 35(5):689, May 1922. 62
836. LORD, F. T., and NYE, R. N. Studies on the pneumococcus. III. Dissolution of pneumococci in pneumonic cellular material at varying hydrogen ion concentrations. Resistance of certain other organisms to dissolution. J. Exper. Med., 35(5):699, May 1922. 62
837. LORD, F. T., and NYE, R. N. Studies on the pneumococcus. IV. Effect of bile at varying hydrogen ion concentrations on dissolution of pneumococci. J. Exper. Med., 35(5):703, May 1922. 62
838. LORD, F. T., and PERSONS, E. L. Certain aspects of mouse protection tests for antibody in pneumococcus pneumonia. J. Exper. Med., 53(2):151, Feb. 1931. 440
839. LORENTZ, E. Antecedentes relativos a la preparación de la vacuna antineumocóccica (mixta polivalente). Semana méd., 29(2): 60, Jan. 12, 1922.
840. LYALL, H. W. Blood cultures in pneumonia. J. A. M. A., 58 (24):1841, June 15, 1912. 228
841. LYALL, H. W. The types of pneumococci in tuberculous sputum. J. Exper. Med., 21(2):146, Feb. 1915. 232
842. LYON, A. B. Bacteriologic studies of one hundred and sixty-five cases of pneumonia and postpneumonic empyema in infants and children. Am. J. Dis. Child., 23(1):72, Jan. 1922.
843. MACCONKEY, A. Note on staining the capsules of pneumococcus and of the bacillus of Friedländer. Lancet, 2:1262, Nov. 12, 1898. 83
843a. MACFADYEN, A. Remarks upon the pneumotoxin. Brit. Med. J., 2:776, Sept. 29, 1906.
844. MACKENZIE, G. M. The significance of anaphylaxis in pneumococcus immunity. J. Exper. Med., 41(1):53, Jan. 1925. .... 448, 454
845. MACKENZIE, G. M., and WOO, S. T. The production and significance of cutaneous allergy to pneumococcus protein. J. Exper. Med., 41(1):65, Jan. 1925. 455
846. MACLACHLAN, W. W. G., PERMAR, H. H., JOHNSTON, J. M., and KENNEY, J. R. Some effects of quinin derivatives in experimental pneumococcus studies. Am. J. M. Sc., 188(5):699, Nov. 1934. ... 516

847. MADSEN, T. The occurrence of different types of pneumococci in Denmark. Based on investigations by Dr. S. Christensen on 233 patients and 1,474 healthy persons. *In* League of Nations, Health Organisation. Reports on Serological Investigations presented to the Second International Conference on the Standardisation of Sera and Serological Tests, held at the Pasteur Institute in Paris in November, 1922, p. 54. 569

848. MAEJI, Y. Studien über die Pneumokokken. I. Beiträge zur Kenntnis der Typenspezifität der Pneumokokken. Acta scholae med. univ. imp. in Kioto, 12(2):229, Aug. 1929.

849. MAEJI, Y. Studien über die Pneumokokken. II. Versuche über die orale Immunisierung junger Tiere mit dem Pneumokokken-Typ III. Acta scholae med. univ. imp. in Kioto, 12(3):295, Dec. 1929. 348

850. MAEJI, Y. Das Pneumokokken-Antivirus. I. Versuche an Mäusen und Meerschweinchen. Ztschr. f. Immunitätsforsch. u. exper. Therap., 65(1/2):35, Jan. 1930. 336

851. MAEJI, Y. Studien über die Pneumokokken. III. Wirkungen der Chemikalien auf die Pneumokokken. I. Versuche in vivo. Acta scholae med. univ. imp. in Kioto, 12(4):405, Mar. 1930. .... 510, 511

852. MAEJI, Y. Studien über die Pneumokokken. III. Wirkungen der Chemikalien auf die Pneumokokken. II. Versuche in vitro. Acta scholae med. univ. imp. in Kioto, 12(4):415, Mar. 1930. .... 510, 515

853. MAEJI, Y. Das Pneumokokken-Antivirus. II. Versuche an Kaninchen. Acta scholae med. univ. imp. in Kioto, 12(4):425, Mar. 1930. .... 336, 346

854. MAEJI, Y. Das Pneumokokken-Antivirus. III. Contribution to the study of the pneumococcus antivirus. Acta scholae med. univ. imp. in Kioto, 12(4):441, Mar. 1930. 336

855. MAGUIRE, R. The micrococcus of pneumonia. Brit. M. J., 2:1126, Dec. 1884. 14

855a. MAIR, W. Pneumococcal endocarditis in rabbits. J. Path. and Bact., 26(3):426, July 1923.

856. MAIR, W. The purpura producing substance in pneumococcus and the heritable susceptibility of mice. J. Path. & Bact., 31(2): 215, Apr. 1928. 90

857. MALCOLM, W. G. The efficiency of certain germicides in the preservation of biologic products. J. Bact., 22(6):403, Dec. 1931. .. 558

858. MALLOCH, A. A study of pneumonias and types of pneumococci. Quart. J. Med., 15(58):103, Jan. 1922.

858a. MALLOCH, A. Some aspects of experimental pneumonia. Canad. Med. Assn. J., 13(9):671, Sept. 1923.

859. MALONE, R. H. A note on the large scale production of pneumococcus vaccine. Indian J. M. Research, 9(1):63, July 1921.

860. MALONE, R. H. The demonstration of the capsules of the pneumococcus by a modification of Benian's relief stain. Indian J. M. Research, 9(4):804, Apr. 1922. 84

861. Malone, R. H. An examination of the factors concerned in Neufeld's bile solubility test. Indian J. M. Research, 11(3):867, Jan. 1924. 56
862. Malone, R. H. Degree of bile solubility as a means of differentiating pathogenic from non-pathogenic capsulated diplococci. Indian J. M. Research, 11(3):877, Jan. 1924. 56
863. Malone, R. H. A note on the types of pneumococcus found in the Punjab and north-west frontier province of India. J. Roy. Army M. Corps, 43(1):42, July 1924. *Also:* Indian J. M. Research, 11(3):947, 1924.
864. Malone, R. H. A report on the prophylactic inoculation of Indian troops in the Baluchistan district against pneumonia. Indian J. M. Research, 12(3):565, Jan. 1925. .... 489, 498
865. Mandelbaum, M. Ueber die Wirkung von taurocholsaurem Natrium und tierischer Galle auf den Pneumokokkus, Streptococcus mucosus und auf die andern Streptokokken. München. med. Wchnschr., 54(29):1431, July 16, 1907. 56
865a. Marchoux, E. Rôle du pneumocoque dans la pathologie et la pathogénie de la maladie du sommeil. Ann. Inst. Pasteur, 13(3): 193, Mar. 1899.
865b. Marginesu, P., e Corda, L. Frequenza ed importanza dei vari tipi di Pneumococco. Policl., 30(12), sez. med.:610, Dec. 1, 1923.
866. Martin, L., and Hill, J. H. III. Milk protein as an inhibitor of skin sensitization in guinea-pigs previously injected intradermally with pneumococci. Bull. Johns Hopkins Hosp., 46(3):254, Mar. 1930. 468
867. Mathers, G. The varieties of pneumococci causing lobar pneumonia, with especial reference to their biologic differences. J. Infect. Dis., 17(3):514, Nov. 1915.
868. Mathers, G. The bacteriology of the urine in lobar pneumonia. J. Infect. Dis., 19(3):416, Sept. 1916. 229
869. Mátray, M. Ueber Pneumoniekokken. Wien. med. Presse, 24 (23):733, June 10, 1883. .... 1, 2
870. Mátray, M. Ueber Pneumoniekokken. Wien. med. Presse, 24 (24):766, June 17, 1883. .... 1, 2
871. May. Ueber die Wirkung des Römerschen Pneumokokkenserums bei der kruppösen Pneumonie mit besonderer Berücksichtigung der Leukozyten. München. med. Wchnschr., 55(40):2083, Oct. 6, 1908.
872. Maynard, G. D. An enquiry into the etiology, manifestations and prevention of pneumonia amongst natives on the Rand, recruited from "tropical areas." Publ. South African Inst. M. Research, No. 1:1, Nov. 1, 1913. .... 483, 491, 494
872a. Maynard, G. D. Pneumonia inoculation experiment no. 3. Med. J. S. Africa, 11(2):36, Sept. 1915.
873. McClelland, J. E. Determination of type and serum treatment in pneumococcus infections. Cleveland M. J., 17(4):226, Apr. 1918.

874. McClelland, J. E. Importance of blood cultures in pneumonia. J. A. M. A., 71(16):1299, Oct. 19, 1918. 228
875. McCoy, G. W., Hasseltine, H. E., Wadsworth, A., and Kirkbride, M. B. A report on pneumococcus inoculation in New York state institutions. J. A. M. A., 79(14):1128, Sept. 30, 1922. 483, 484, 498
876. McDaniels, H. E. Effect of egg-white in oral vaccination against pneumococcus. Proc. Soc. Exper. Biol. & Med., 28(6):587, Mar. 1931. .... 191, 348, 487
877. McDaniels, H. E. Leucocyte counts and bacteremia studies in rats orally immunized against pneumococci. Proc. Soc. Exper. Biol. & Med., 29(7):897, Apr. 1932. .... 191, 349
878. McDowell, C. The effect of different temperatures and humidities on the resistance of rats to a pneumococcus infection. Am. J. Hyg., 3(5):521, Sept. 1923. 191
879. McGuire, G., Valentine, E., Whitney, E., and Falk, K. G. Studies on antibodies. IV. The carbohydrate content as a criterion of the suitability of a broth for the culture of pneumococci. J. Bact., 23(3):223, Mar. 1932. 39
879a. McKee, S. H. A study of the bacteriology of the normal and inflamed conjunctiva with special reference to the presence of the streptococcus and pneumococcus. Canad. Med. Assn. J., 14(3): 216, Mar. 1924. *Also* Tr. Am. Acad. Ophth., 28:192, 1923.
880. McLeod, J. W. [The pneumococcus.] Pathogenic action. *In* Great Britain, Medical Research Council. A system of Bacteriology in relation to medicine, 2:177. London: His Majesty's Stationery Office, 1929. 215
881. McLeod, J. W., and Gordon, J. Production of hydrogen peroxide by bacteria. Biochem. J., 16(4):499, 1922. .... 44, 74
882. M'Leod, J. W., and Gordon, J. On the production of peroxides by pneumococci and other bacteria. (Abstract.) J. Path. & Bact., 25(1):139, Jan. 1922. .... 44, 74
883. M'Leod, J. W., and Gordon, J. Catalase production and sensitiveness to hydrogen peroxide amongst bacteria: with a scheme of classification based on these properties. J. Path. & Bact., 26(3): 326, July 1923. .... 44, 74
884. M'Leod, J. W., Gordon, J., and Pyrah, L. N. Further observations on peroxide formation by bacteria. (Abstract.) J. Path. & Bact., 26(1):127, Jan. 1923. .... 44, 74, 75
885. McLeod, J. W., and Govenlock, P. The production of bactericidins by micro-organisms. Lancet, 1(5096):900, Apr. 30, 1921. .. 44, 74
886. McMeans, J. W. The incidence of pneumococcus types in pneumonia in Pittsburgh. Atlantic M. J., 30(8):499, May 1927.
887. Medical Research Council. Report of Therapeutic Trials Committee. The serum treatment of lobar pneumonia. Lancet, 1 (5763):290, Feb. 10, 1934. .... 544, 594, 604, 606
888. Megrail, E., and Ecker, E. E. Stability of pneumococcus types in sterile abscesses. J. Infect. Dis., 35(1):1, July 1924. ..... 113, 146, 363
889. Mehlman, J., and Seegal, B. C. Passive sensitization of the

guinea pig with rabbit and horse anti-pneumococcus Type I serums. J. Immunol., 26(1):1, Jan. 1934. 452

890. MEHLMAN, J., and SEEGAL, B. C. A comparison of the sensitizing and the therapeutic effect of rabbit and horse antipneumococcus Type I serums in albino mice. J. Immunol., 27(1):81, July 1934. 452

891. MENDEL, F. Die Behandlung der Pneumonie mit Optochinbasicum und Milchdiat. Deutsche med. Wchnschr., 42(18):537, May 4, 1916.

892. MENDELSOHN, M. Die infectiöse Natur der Pneumonie. Ztschr. f. klin. med., 7(2):178, 1884. 9

892a. MENETRIER, P., et LEVESQUE, J. Septicémie à pneumocoques primitive. Bull. et mém. Soc. méd. des Hôp. de Paris, 45, 3ᵉ sér.: 85, Jan. 28, 1921.

892b. MENETRIER, P., et TOURAINE, A. Pneumonie du foetus. Bull. et mém. Soc. méd. des Hôp. de Paris, 24, 3ᵉ sér.: 799, 1907.

893. MENNES, F. Das Antipneumokokken-Serum und der Mechanismus der Immunität des Kaninchens gegen den Pneumococcus. Ztschr. f. Hyg. u. Infektionskr., 25:413, 1897. .... 27, 104, 389, 522, 528

894. METCHNIKOFF, E. Études sur l'immunité. 4ᵉ memoire. L'immunité des cobayes vaccinés contre le vibrio Metchnikowii. Ann. Inst. Pasteur, 5(8):465, Aug. 1891. .... 24, 103, 356, 420

895. MEYER, H. Acute Endocarditis und Meningitis als Complication der croupösen Pneumonie. Deutsches Arch. f. klin. Med., 41 (4/5):433, Dec. 9, 1887. .... 18, 225

896. MEYER, H. Weitere Untersuchungen über die Bedeutung des Reticulo-Endothels für die Immunität. Ztschr. f. Hyg. u. Infektionskr., 106(1):124, Mar. 18, 1926. 405

897. MEYER, H. Über aktive Immunisierung von Mäusen durch in Natrium taurocholicum gelöste Pneumokokken. Ztschr. f. Hyg. u. Infektionskr., 107(2):416, Apr. 29, 1927. 334

898. MEYER, H., und SUKNEFF, W. W. Über die immunisierende Wirkung von avirulenten Pneumokokken und von Kulturfiltraten und Auflösungen virulenter Pneumokokken. Ztschr. f. Hyg. u. Infektionskr., 109(1):78, Sept. 1928. .... 327, 334, 525, 526

899. MEYER, J. Types of pneumococci in the throats of one hundred normal persons. J. A. M. A., 75(19):1268, Nov. 6, 1920. 232

900. MEYERS, H. R. A contribution to the study of the etiology of serum disease. J. Immunol., 22(2):83, Feb. 1932. 562

901. MIGULA, W. System der Bakterien, Bd. 2:347. Jena: Gustav Fischer, 1900. 1

902. MIKAËLJAN, R. C. Studien über den Pneumokokkus des Auges. I. Ueber Pneumokokkentypen bei einigen Augenerkrankungen. Klin. Monatsbl. f. Augenh., 87:778, Dec. 1931. 227

903. MILAM, D. F., and SMILLIE, W. G. A bacteriological study of "colds" on an isolated tropical island (St. John, United States Virgin Islands, West Indies). J. Exper. Med., 53(5):733, May 1931. 233

904. MITCHELL, O. W. H., and MUNS, W. E. A rapid method for the

determination of pneumococcus types. J. Med. Research, 37(2): 339, Nov. 1917. 124
905. Monti, A. Sull 'eziologia del reumatismo articolare acuto. Riforma med., 5(54):320, Mar. 5, 1889. *Abstract in* Jahresb. u. d. Fortschr. i. d. Lehre v. d. path. Mikroorg., 5:53; 83, 1889. .... 20, 194
906. Monti, A. Contributo allo studio della meningite cerebrospinale. Riforma med., 5(58):344, Mar. 9, 1889. *Abstract in* Jahresb. u. d. Fortschr. i. d. Lehre v. d. path. Mikroorg., 5:53, 1889. 194
907. Monti, A. Contributo allo studio della meningite cerebrospinale. Riforma med., 5(59):350, Mar. 11, 1889. *Abstract in* Jahresb. u. d. Fortschr. i. d. Lehre v. d. path. Mikroorg., 5:77, 1889. 194
908. Moore, H. F. The action of ethylhydrocuprein (optochin) on type strains of pneumococci in vitro and in vivo, and on some other microorganisms in vitro. J. Exper. Med., 22(3):269, Sept. 1915. 513
909. Moore, H. F. The chemoserotherapy of experimental pneumococcal infection. J. Exper. Med., 22(4):389, Oct. 1915. 518
910. Moore, H. F., and Chesney, A. M. A study of ethylhydrocuprein (optochin) in the treatment of acute lobar pneumonia. Arch. Int. Med., 19(4):611, Apr. 1917. .... 514, 517
910a. Morax, V. Recherches bactériologiques sur l'étiologie des conjonctivites aiguës et sur l'asepsie dans la chirurgie oculaire. Thèse de Paris, 1894.
911. Mørch, J. R. Studies on anti-meningococcus serum. I. Production of the serum. J. Immunol., 9(1):25, Jan. 1924.
912. Morgan, H. J. The inhibition zone in precipitin reactions with the soluble specific substance of pneumococcus. J. Immunol., 8(6):449, Nov. 1923. .... 372, 583
913. Morgan, H. J. The correlation of certain phenomena occurring during the growth of pneumococcus. J. Exper. Med., 39(4):565, Apr. 1924.
914. Morgan, H. J., and Avery, O. T. Studies on bacterial nutrition. IV. Effect of plant tissue upon growth of pneumococcus and streptococcus. J. Exper. Med., 38(2):207, Aug. 1923.
915. Morgan, H. J., and Avery, O. T. Growth-inhibitory substances in pneumococcus cultures. J. Exper. Med., 39(3):335, Mar. 1924. ... 40
916. Morgan, H. J., and Neill, J. M. Methemoglobin formation by sterile culture filtrates of pneumococcus. J. Exper. Med., 40(2): 269, Aug. 1924. 73
917. Morgan, W. T. J., and Petrie, G. F. The titration of antipneumococcus serum (Type I) in mice. Brit. J. Exper. Path., 14 (5):323, Oct. 1933. .... 571, 574, 578
918. Morgenroth, J. Die Chemotherapie der Pneumokokkeninfektion. Berl. klin. Wchnschr., 51(47):1829, Nov. 23, 1914.
919. Morgenroth, J. Zur Kenntnis der Beziehungen zwischen chemischer Konstitution und chemotherapeutischer Wirkung. Berl. klin. Wchnschr., 54(3):55, Jan. 15, 1917.
920. Morgenroth, J. Über chemotherapeutische Antisepsis. I. Mit-

teilung. Zur experimentellen Begründung der Vuzin-Tiefenantisepsis. Deutsche med. Wchnschr., 45(19):505, May 8, 1919. 512
921. Morgenroth, J., und Bumcke, E. Spezifische Desinfektion und Chemotherapie bakterieller Infektionen. Deutsche med. Wchnschr., 40(11):538, Mar. 12, 1914. 512
922. Morgenroth, J., und Kaufmann, M. Arzneifestigkeit bei Bakterien (Pneumokokken). Ztschr. f. Immunitätsforsch. u. exper. Therap., 15(6):610, Dec. 1912. .... 512, 519
923. Morgenroth, J., und Kaufmann, M. Zur Chemotherapie bakterieller Infektionen. Charité-Ann., 37:262, 1913. .... 512, 519
924. Morgenroth, J., und Kaufmann, M. Zur experimentellen Chemotherapie der Pneumokokkeninfektion. I. Mitteilung. Ztschr. f. Immunitätsforsch. u. exper. Therap., 18(2):145, June 1913. .... 512, 519
925. Morgenroth, J., und Kaufmann, M. Zur experimentellen Chemotherapie der Pneumokokkeninfektion. II. Mitteilung. Ztschr. f. Immunitätsforsch. u. exper. Therap., 29(3/4):217, Mar. 1920. .... 512, 519
926. Morgenroth, J., und Levy, R. Chemotherapie der Pneumokokkeninfektion. Berl. klin. Wchnschr., 48(34):1560, Aug. 21, 1911. 63, 512
927. Morgenroth, J., und Levy, R. Chemotherapie der Pneumokokkeninfektion. II. Mitteilung. Berl. klin. Wchnschr., 48(44):1979, Oct. 30, 1911. 512
928. Morgenroth, J., und Schnitzer, R. Über die Wirkung neuerer Ammoniumverbindungen des Hydrochinins und Optochins auf Pneumokokken. Ztschr. f. Hyg. u. Infektionskr., 103(3):441, July 15, 1924.
929. Morgenroth, J., Schnitzer, R., und Berger, E. Ueber die Einheit der Streptokokken und Pneumokokken. I. Mitteilung. Ztschr. f. Immunitätsforsch. u. exper. Therap., 43(3):169, June 8, 1925. .. 144, 173
930. Morrey, C. B., and Masters, V. McC. Types of pneumococci. A statistical study. Abstr. Bact., 5(1):21, Jan. 1921.
931. Morse, J. L. A case of "purpura" in an infant, probably the result of pneumococcus infection. Ann. Gynec. & Pediat., 11(5): 372, Feb. 1898. 87
932. Mosny, E. Recherches expérimentales sur la vaccination contre l'infection pneumonique et sur sa guérison. Arch. d. méd. expér. et d'anat. path., 4:195, 1892. .... 25, 325, 337, 524, 527, 530
933. Mosny, E. Sur la culture du pneumocoque. Compt. rend. Soc. de biol., 47:852, 1895. .... 42, 103, 356
934. Mudd, S., Reichel, J., Flosdorf, E. W., and Eagle, H. The preparation, properties and applications of lyophile serum proteins and complement. (Abstract.) J. Immunol., 26(4):341, Apr. 1934. 559
935. Mueller, J. H. A chemical study of the specific elements of tuberculin. I. J. Exper. Med., 43(1):1, Jan. 1926.
936. Mueller, J. H. A chemical study of the specific elements of tuberculin. II. The preparation of residue antigen from old tuberculin. J. Exper. Med., 43(1):9, Jan. 1926. 262

937. Mueller, J. H., Smith, D. E., and Litarczek, S. "Residue antigen" from a Friedländer bacillus. Proc. Soc. Exper. Biol. & Med., 22(7):373, Apr. 1925. 262

938. Mueller, J. H., and Tomczik, J. The chemical nature of residue antigen prepared from yeast. J. Exper. Med., 40(3):343, Sept. 1924. .... 262, 422

939. Müller, E. F. Über das Auftreten und die Bedeutung von bactericiden Schutzstoffe des Blutes im Verlauf der croupösen Pneumonie. Ztschr. f. Hyg. u. Infektionskr., 97(1/2):26, Nov. 1923. 439

940. Murphy, R. V. Collosol iodine in the treatment of the pneumonias. Irish J. M. Sc., (106), ser. 6:563, Oct. 1934. 511

941. Nakahara, W. The function of macrophages in local resistance to bacterial infections. J. Exper. Med., 42(2):201, Aug. 1925. ... 405

942. Nakajima, H. Experimental studies on the pneumococcus immunization by intratracheal route. Scient. Rep. Gov. Inst. Infect. Dis., Tokyo, 6:97, 1927.

943. Napier, L. E., and Dharmonda. The incidence of pneumococcal types in pneumonia in Assam. Indian M. Gaz., 70(4):181, Apr. 1935. 116

944–6. Nauwerck, C. Beiträge zur Kenntniss des Morbus Brightii. Beitr. z. path. Anat. u. z. allg. Path., 1:34, May 1886. .... 17, 226

947. Neill, J. M. Studies on the oxidation-reduction of hemoglobin and methemoglobin. I. The changes induced by pneumococci and by sterile animal tissue. J. Exper. Med., 41(2):299, Feb. 1925. .. 80

948. Neill, J. M. Studies on the oxidation-reduction of hemoglobin and methemoglobin. II. The oxidation of hemoglobin and reduction of methemoglobin by anaerobic bacilli and by sterile plant tissue. J. Exper. Med., 41(4):535, Apr. 1925. 80

949. Neill, J. M. Studies on the oxidation-reduction of hemoglobin and methemoglobin. III. The formation of methemoglobin during the oxidation of autoxidizable substances. J. Exper. Med., 41(4):551, Apr. 1925. 80

950. Neill, J. M. Studies on the oxidation-reduction of hemoglobin and methemoglobin. IV. The inhibition of "spontaneous" methemoglobin formation. J. Exper. Med., 41(4):561, Apr. 1925. .. 80, 383

951. Neill, J. M. Studies on the oxidation and reduction of immunological substances. I. Pneumococcus hemotoxin. J. Exper. Med., 44(2):199, Aug. 1926. 84

952. Neill, J. M. Studies on the oxidation and reduction of immunological substances. V. Production of antihemotoxin by immunization with oxidized pneumococcus antitoxin. J. Exper. Med., 45 (1):105, Jan. 1927. .... 85, 86, 382

953. Neill, J. M., and Avery, O. T. Studies on oxidation and reduction by pneumococcus. V. The destruction of oxyhemoglobin by sterile extracts of pneumococcus. J. Exper. Med., 39(5):757, May 1924. 79

954. Neill, J. M., and Avery, O. T. Studies on oxidation and reduc-

tion by pneumococcus. VI. The oxidation of enzymes in sterile extracts of pneumococcus. J. Exper. Med., 40(4):405, Oct. 1924. ... 68

955. Neill, J. M., and Avery, O. T. Studies on oxidation and reduction by pneumococcus. VII. Enzyme activity of sterile filtrates of aerobic and anaerobic cultures of pneumococcus. J. Exper. Med., 40(4):423, Oct. 1924.

956. Neill, J. M., and Avery, O. T. Studies on oxidation and reduction by pneumococcus. VIII. Nature of the oxidation-reduction systems in sterile pneumococcus extracts. J. Exper. Med., 41(2): 285, Feb. 1925. 79

957. Neill, J. M., and Fleming, W. L. Studies on the oxidation and reduction of immunological substances. VI. The "reactivation" of the bacteriolytic activity of oxidized pneumococcus extracts. J. Exper. Med., 46(2):263, Aug. 1927.

958. Neill, J. M., Fleming, W. L., and Gaspari, E. L. Studies on the oxidation and reduction of immunological substances. VIII. The antigenic properties of hemolytically active and hemolytically inactive modifications of pneumococcus hemotoxin. J. Exper. Med., 46(5):735, Nov. 1927. .... 81, 340, 382

959. Neill, J. M., Fleming, W. L., and Gaspari, E. L. Studies on the oxidation and reduction of immunological substances. X. Immunological distinctions between the hemotoxin and the "protein fraction" of the pneumococcus cell. J. Exper. Med., 46(5):777, Nov. 1927. 382

960. Neill, J. M., and Gaspari, E. L. Factors involved in the infection of mice after vaccination with Type II pneumococci. J. Exper. Med., 46(1):113, July 1927.

961. Nelson, J. B., and Gowen, J. W. The incidence of middle ear infection and pneumonia in albino rats at different ages. J. Infect. Dis., 46(1):53, Jan. 1930.

962. Netter. De l'endocardite végétante-ulcéreuse d'origine pneumonique. Arch. de physiol. norm. et path., 8(2), 3e sér.:106, 1886. 16, 225

963. Netter. Pericardite fibrineuse, méningite cerebro-spinale et pneumonie determinées par le pneumococcus sans pneumonie lobaire coïncidente. Bull. Soc. anat. Paris, 11, 4e sér.:188, Mar. 19, 1886. 16

964. Netter. Pleuro-pneumonie fibrineuse du cobaye, du lapin, de la souris, du rat, après inoculation des produits d'une endocardite végétante rencontrée chez une malade atteinte de pneumonie lobaire. Contribution à l'étude du pneumocoque. Bull. Soc. anat. Paris, 11, 4e sér.:269, Apr. 9, 1886.

965. Netter. De la méningite due au pneumocoque (avec ou sans pneumonie). Arch. gén. de méd., 19, 7e sér.:257, Mar. 1887. ..... 16, 18

966. Netter. De la méningite due au pneumocoque (avec ou sans pneumonie). Arch. gén. de méd., 19, 7e sér.:434, Apr. 1887.

967. Netter. De la méningite due au pneumocoque (avec ou sans pneumonie). Arch. gén. de méd., 20, 7e sér.:28, July 1887.

968. Netter. De la pleurésie purulente à pneumocoques sans pneumonie. Bull. Soc. anat. Paris, 62, 5e sér.:547, July 29, 1887.

969. NETTER. Du microbe de la pneumonie dans la salive. Compt. rend. Soc. de biol., 39(34):611, Nov. 4, 1887. 527
970. NETTER. Du microbe de Friedländer dans la salive et des réserves qu'il convient de faire au sujet de son influence pathogène chez l'homme, au moins dans les cas de pneumonie. Compt. rend. Soc. de biol., 39:799, Dec. 1887.
971. NETTER. Du microbe de la pneumonie dans la salive. (Abstract.) Centralbl. f. klin. Med., 9(18):332, May 5, 1888. 20
971a. NETTER. Microbes pathogènes contenus dans la bouche de sujets sains: maladies qu'ils provoquent: indications pour l'hygiéniste et le médecin. Revue d'hyg., 11(6):501, June 1889.
971b. NETTER. Le pneumocoque, ses caractères morphologiques, biologiques, pathogéniques, &c. Arch. de méd. exper. et d'anat. path., 2:677, 798, 1890.
971c. NETTER. Présence du pneumocoque dans les poussières d'une salle d'hôpital. Compt. rend. Soc. de biol., 4, 10e sér.:538, May 29, 1897.
971d. NETTER et SALANIER, M. Apparition de pneumocoques dans le pus des méningites cérébro-spinales en cours de traitement. Explication de cet envahissement. Emploi prophylactique du sérum antipneumococcique. Bull. et mém. Soc. méd. des Hôp. de Paris, 41, 3e sér.:394, Feb. 23, 1917.
972. NEUFELD, F. Ueber eine specifische bakteriolytische Wirkung der Galle. Ztschr. f. Hyg. u. Infektionskr., 34:454, 1900. 55
973. NEUFELD, F. Ueber die Erzeugung von Erysipel am Kaninchenohr durch Pneumokokken. Ztschr. f. Hyg. u. Infektionskr., 36: 254, 1901. 180
974. NEUFELD, F. Ueber die Agglutination der Pneumokokken und über die Theorien der Agglutination. Ztschr. f. Hyg. u. Infektionskr., 40:54, 1902. .... 131, 328, 357, 365, 528
975. NEUFELD, F. Neue Forschungsergebnisse aus dem Gebiete der Pneumonie. München. med. Wchnschr., 68(50):1635, Dec. 16, 1921.
976. NEUFELD, F. Neue Forschungsergebnisse über Pneumonie. Deutsche med. Wchnschr., 48(2):51, Jan. 12, 1922.
977. NEUFELD, F. Investigations with regard to pneumococci. *In* League of Nations, Health Organisation. Reports on Serological Investigations presented to the Second International Conference on the Standardisation of Sera and Serological Tests, held at the Pasteur Institute in Paris in November, 1922, p. 74. 568
978. NEUFELD, F. Ueber die Veränderlichkeit der Krankheitserreger in ihrer Bedeutung für die Infektion und Immunität. Deutsche med. Wchnschr., 50(1):1, Jan. 4, 1924.
979. NEUFELD. Discussion following "Die Variabilität der Mikroorganismen in allgemein-biologischer Hinsicht," by E. Gottschlich; and "Variabilität und Vererbung bei Protisten," by V. Jollos. Centralbl. f. Bakt., 1 Abt., Orig., 93 (Beiheft):*41, Oct. 1924. ... 140, 173
980. NEUFELD, F. Über den derzeitigen Stand der Pneumokokkenforschung. Klin. Wchnschr., 11(39):1632, Sept. 24, 1932.

981. Neufeld, F., und Dold, H. Ueber Bakterienempfindlichkeit und ihre Bedeutung für die Infektion. Berl. klin. Wchnschr., 48(2): 55, Jan. 9, 1911. 447

982. Neufeld, F., und Engwer, T. Zur Chemotherapie der Pneumokokkeninfektionen. Berl. klin. Wchnschr., 49(50):2381, Dec. 9, 1912. 518

983. Neufeld, F., und Etinger-Tulczynska, R. Untersuchungen zur Gallenlösung der Pneumokokken. Arch. f. Hyg., 103(1/3):107, Jan.–Mar. 1930. 60

984. Neufeld, F., und Etinger-Tulczynska, R. Nasale Pneumokokkeninfektionen und Pneumokokkenkeimträger im Tierversuch. Ztschr. f. Hyg. u. Infektionskr., 112(3):492, May 1931. ...... 186, 231, 594

985. Neufeld, F., und Etinger-Tulczynska, R. Tierversuche über Pneumokokkenkeimträger und nasale Infektion. Zentralbl. f. Bakt., 1 Abt., Orig., 122(1/3):*139, Sept. 7, 1931. 186

986. Neufeld, F., und Etinger-Tulczynska, R. Versuche einer spezifischen Behandlung von Pneumokokken-Keimträgern. Ztschr. f. Immunitätsforsch. u. exper. Therap., 74(1/2):160, Mar. 1932.

987. Neufeld, F., und Etinger-Tulczynska, R. Bakterienkapseln und Quellungsreaction. Ztschr. f. Hyg. u. Infektionskr., 114:769, 1933. 128

988. Neufeld, F., und Etinger-Tulczynska, R. Untersuchungen über die Pneumokokkenseuche des Meerschweinchens. Ztschr. f. Hyg. u. Infektionskr., 114(2):324, Aug. 1932. .... 33, 131

989. Neufeld, F., und Händel. Ueber Herstellung und Prüfung von Antipneumokokkenserum und über die Aussichten einer spezifischen Handlung der Pneumonie. Ztschr. f. Immunitätsforsch. u. exper. Therap., 1 Teil, Orig., 3(2):159, July 1909.
524, 528, 530, 534, 567, 575

990. Neufeld, F., und Haendel. Über die Entstehung der Krisis bei der Pneumonie und über die Wirkung des Pneumokkenimmunserums. Arb. a. d. k. Gsndhtsamte, 34(2):166, June 1910. .... 433, 437

991. Neufeld, F., und Haendel, L. Weitere Untersuchungen über Pneumokokken-Heilsera. III. Mitteilung. Über Vorkommen und Bedeutung atypischer Varietäten des Pneumokokkus. Arb. a. d. k. Gsndhtsamte, 34(3):293, Aug. 1910. .... 105, 120, 361, 407, 545

992. Neufeld, F., und Händel, L. Pneumokokken. *In* Kolle, W., und von Wassermann, A. Handbuch der pathogenen Mikroorganismen, 2d ed., 4:513. Jena: Gustav Fischer, 1912. .... 392, 567, 601

993. Neufeld, F., und Händel, L. Zur Frage der Serumtherapie der Pneumonie und der Wertbestimmung des Pneumokokkenserums. Berl. klin. Wchnschr., 49(15):680, Apr. 8, 1912. .... 408, 601

994. Neufeld, F., und Levinthal, W. Beiträge zur Variabilität der Pneumokokken. Ztschr. f. Immunitätsforsch. u. exper. Therap., 55 (3/4):324, Mar. 1928. 156

995. Neufeld, F., und Meyer, H. Über die Bedeutung des Retikulo-Endothels für die Immunität. Ztschr. f. Hyg. u. Infektionskr., 103 (3):595, Sept. 1924. 404

996. Neufeld, F., und Reinhardt, A. Experimentelle Untersuchungen

über die Disinfektion infizierter Wunden. Deutsche med. Wchnschr., 47(27):768, July 7, 1921. 510

997. Neufeld, F., und Rimpau, W. Ueber die Antikörper des Streptokokken- und Pneumokokken-Immunserums. Deutsche med. Wchnschr., 30(40):1458, Sept. 29, 1904. .... 389, 392

998. Neufeld, F., und Rimpau, W. Weitere Mittheilungen über die Immunität gegen Streptokokken und Pneumokokken. Ztschr. f. Hyg. u. Infektionskr., 51:283, 1905. 390

999. Neufeld, F., und Schiemann, O. Ueber die Wirkung chemotherapeutischer Stoffe auf verschiedene Bakterien in vitro und in vivo. Centralbl. f. Bakt., 1 Abt., Ref., 57 (Beiheft):183, 1913. 510

1000. Neufeld, F., und Schnitzer, R. Pneumokokken. *In* Kolle, W., Kraus, R., und Uhlenhuth, P. Handbuch der pathogenen Mikroorganismen, 3d ed., 4:913. Jena: Gustav Fischer; Berlin und Wien: Urban & Schwarzenberg, 1928.
52, 57, 69, 104, 136, 186, 187, 191, 196, 511, 519

1001. Neufeld, F., und Ungermann. Ueber experimentelle Erzeugung von Pneumonien bei Versuchstieren und ihre Beeinflussung durch spezifisches Serum. (Abstract.) Berl. klin. Wchnschr., 49 (15):717, Apr. 8, 1912. .... 185, 206, 211

1002. Neufeld und Ungermann. Weitere Heilversuche mit Antipneumokokkenserum bei experimenteller Pneumonie. (Abstract.) Berl. klin. Wchnschr., 49(21):1010, May 20, 1912. .... 185, 206, 211

1003. Neufeld und Ungermann. Ueber experimentell erzeugte Pneumonien und ihre Beeinflussung durch Antipneumokokkenserum. Centralbl. f. Bakt., Ref., 54 (Beiheft):*71, Aug. 1912.

1004. Newburgh, L. H., Means, J. H., and Porter, W. T. The respiratory mechanism in pneumonia. J. Exper. Med., 24(5):583, Nov. 1916. 194

1005. Nicholls, E. E., and Spaeth, R. A. The relation between fatigue and the susceptibility of guinea pigs to infections of Type I pneumococcus. Am. J. Hyg., 2(5):527, Sept. 1922. 187

1006. Nichols, H. J. The lobar pneumonia problem in the army from the viewpoint of the recent differentiation of types of pneumococci. Mil. Surgeon, 41(2):149, Aug. 1917. *Also:* New York M. J., 106(5):219, Aug. 4, 1917.

1007. Nicolle, M., et Adil-Bey. Action de la bile sur le pneumocoque, et diverses autres bacteries. Ann. Inst. Pasteur, 21(1):20, Jan. 1907. .... 55, 334

1008. Nicolle, M., et Césari, E. Influence des immunsérums spécifiques sur la culture des microbes pathogènes. Ann. Inst. Pasteur, 40(1):43, Jan. 1926. 420

1009. Nicolle, M., et Debains, E. Sur les races du pneumocoque, avec remarques générales sur les antigènes. Bull. Acad. de méd., Paris, 81 (25), 3e sér.:843, 1919. 109

1010. Nicolle, M., et Debains, E. Études sur le pneumocoque. XI. Races du pneumocoque. Ann. Inst. Pasteur, 34(4):177, Apr. 1920. 109

1011. Nicolle, M., Jouan, C., et Debains, E. Note sur les bactéries inagglutinables. Compt. rend. Soc. de biol., 81:839, Oct. 12, 1918. 109, 361

1012. Nissen, F. Zur Kenntnis der bacterienvernichtenden Eigenschaft des Blutes. Ztschr. f. Hyg. u. Infektionskr., 6:487, 1889.

1013. Nissen, F. Ein Vergleich des sog. Sputumsepticämiecoccus mit dem A. Fränkel'schen Pneumonieerreger. Fortschr. d. Med., 9 (16):661, Aug. 15, 1891. .... 37, 50

1014. Nobécourt, P., et Mathieu, R. Le purpura dans les pneumococcies des nourrissons. Arch. de méd. inf., 23(12):689, Dec. 1920.

1015. Nobécourt, P., et Paraf, J. Étude des pneumocoques isolés dans une crèche d'hôpital. Bull. et mém. Soc. méd. d. hôp. de Paris, 43(23), 3ᵉ sér.:687, July 10, 1919.

1016. Nobécourt, P., Paraf, J., et Bonnet, H. Recherches épidémiologiques sur les affections à pneumocoques du nourrisson. Étude des pneumocoques d'une crèche d'hôpital. Presse méd., 28(32): 313, May 19, 1920.

1017. Noble, A. A rapid method for the macroscopic agglutination test. J. Bact., 14(5):287, Nov. 1927. 126

1018. Norris, C., and Pappenheimer, A. M. A study of pneumococci and allied organisms in human mouths and lungs after death. J. Exper. Med., 7(5):450, Aug. 1905. *Also:* Department of Health, City of New York. Report Med. Comm'n Invest. Acute Resp. Dis., Part I: Studies on pneumococcus, p. 48. New York: Department of Health, 1905. 230

1019. Nukada, S., und Kako, Y. Ueber die Schwankungen der Resistenz gegen Pneumokokkeninfektion nach Immunisierung mit Heterobakterien. Ztschr. f. Immunitätsforsch. u. exper. Therap., 67(1/2):83, June 1930.

1020. Nungester, W. J., Wolf, A. A., and Jourdonais, L. F. Effect of gastric mucin on virulence of bacteria in intraperitoneal injections in the mouse. Proc. Soc. Exper. Biol. & Med., 30(2):120, Nov. 1932. 202

1021. Nye, R. N. Studies on the pneumonic exudate. V. The relation of pneumonic lung protease activity to hydrogen ion concentration, and a consideration of the origin of the enzyme. J. Exper. Med., 35(2):153, Feb. 1922. 442

1022. Odell, H. R. Observations on the standardization of antipneumococcus serum by the protection test. J. Immunol., 18(1):73, Jan. 1930.

1022a. Oettinger et Deguignand. Septicémie pneumococcique primitive avec localisation pulmonaire tardive. Bull. et mém. Soc. méd. des Hôp. de Paris, 45, 3ᵉ sér.:159, Feb. 11, 1921.

1023. Okischio, M. De l'antivirus pneumococcique et de son action sur la virulence du pneumocoque. Ann. Inst. Pasteur, 48(3):344, Mar. 1932. 337

1024. Okomoto, H., and Sogen, Y. Vergleichende Untersuchung über die lokalanästhesierende Wirkung der Apochininderivate auf die

Kaninchencornea. (Abstract.) Jap. J. M. Sc., Sect. IV. Pharmacology. 5(1):4*, Dec. 1930. 516

1025. OLIVER, W. W. A rapid method of pneumococcus typing. J. Infect. Dis., 27(4):310, Oct. 1920. 126

1026. OLIVER, W. W. Further observations on a rapid method of pneumococcus typing. J. Infect. Dis., 29(5):518, Nov. 1921. .... 123, 126

1027. OLMSTEAD, M. A preliminary report on the classification of pneumococcus IV. Proc. Soc. Exper. Biol. & Med., 14(2):29, Nov. 1916. .... 108, 362

1028. OLMSTEAD, M. An antigenic classification of the Group IV pneumococci. J. Immunol., 2(4):425, June 1917. .... 109, 362

1029. OLSON, J. G. Studies on pneumococcus filtrates. Proc. Soc. Exper. Biol. & Med., 23(4):295, Jan. 1926. .... 96, 339, 383, 483

1030. OLSON, J. G. Further studies on a specific pneumococcus toxin. Proc. Soc. Exper. Biol. & Med., 23(5):331, Feb. 1926. .... 97, 383, 483

1031. O'MEARA, R. A. Q., and BROWN, A. M. On growing the pneumococcus with a view to the production of cultures of standard maximal density, virulence and polysaccharide content. J. Path. & Bact., 42(3):679, May 1936. .... 333, 634

1032. ORAM, F. Pneumococcus leucocidin. J. Immunol., 26(3):233, Mar. 1934. .... 91, 202

1033. ORDMAN, D. Pneumonia in the native mine workers of the Witwatersrand goldfields. A bacteriological and epidemiological study. J. M. A. South Africa, 5(4):108, Feb. 28, 1931. 499

1034. ORDMAN, D. Pneumonia in the native mine labourers in the Northern Rhodesia copperfields with an account of an experiment in pneumonia prophylaxis by means of a vaccine on the Roan Antelope Mine. Publ. South African Inst. M. Research, 7(37):97, Apr. 1935. 500

1035. ORENSTEIN, A. J. Vaccine prophylaxis in pneumonia. A review of fourteen years' experience with inoculation of native mine workers on the Witwatersrand against pneumonia. J. M. A. South Africa, 5(11):339, June 13, 1931. .... 499, 504

1036. ORENSTEIN, A. J. Vitamin A in the treatment of pneumonia. South African M. J., 6(21):685, Nov. 12, 1932. 499

1037. ORTMANN, P. Beitrag zur Aetiologie der acuten Cerebrospinalmeningitis. Arch. f. exper. Path. u. Pharmakol., 24(4/5):291, Feb. 1888. .... 19, 225

1038. ORTMANN, P., und SAMTER, E. O. Beitrag zur Localisation des Diplococcus Pneumoniae (Fraenkel). Virchows Arch. f. path. Anat., 120(1):94, April 1890. 225

1039. OSLER, W. Infectious (so-called ulcerative) endocarditis. Arch. Med., N. Y., 5(1):44, Feb. 1881. 5

1040. OTTEN, L. Trockenlymphe. Ztschr. f. Hyg. u. Infektionskr., 107(3/4):677, July 1927. 52

1041. OTTENBERG, R., and STENBUCK, F. A. Studies on the purification of antibodies. III. Certain methods for the precipitation of pneumococcus protective antibody. Proc. Soc. Exper. Biol. & Med., 22 (4):211, Jan. 1925.

1042. Ottenberg, R., and Stenbuck, F. A. Studies on the purification of antibodies. IV. The removal of extraneous material from antipneumococcus extracts at an approximately neutral reaction. Proc. Soc. Exper. Biol. & Med., 22(4):215, Jan. 1925.

1043. Palier, E. On diplococci and pneumococci; their pleomorphism, virulence and mode of causing disease. An experimental study. M. News, London, 87(21):974, Nov. 18, 1905.

1044. Pane, N. Ueber die Heilkraft des aus verschiedenen immunisierten Tieren gewonnenen antipneumonischen Serums. Centralbl. f. Bakt., 1 Abt., Orig., 21(17/18):664, May 1897. .... 27, 522

1045. Pane, N. Ueber die Genesis des Pneumococcus. Centralbl. f. Bakt., 1 Abt., Orig., 24(8):289, Aug. 1898. 33

1046. Panichi, L. Ueber das Pneumokokkenpräzipitin. Centralbl. f. Bakt., 1 Abt., Orig., 43(2):188, 1907. 582

1047. Panichi, L. Biologische Wirkungen des antipneumonischen Serums. Centralbl. f. Bakt., 1 Abt., Orig., 43(6):632, 1907. .... 359, 365

1048. Panichi, L. Biologische Wirkungen des antipneumonischen Serums. Schluss. Centralbl. f. Bakt., 1 Abt., Orig., 43(7):728, 1907. 359

1049. Pappenheimer, A. M., Jr., and Enders, J. F. Specific carbohydrate of Type I pneumococcus. Proc. Soc. Exper. Biol. & Med., 31(1):37, Oct. 1933. 277

1050. Paraf, J. Le pneumocoque et les infections pneumococciques. Ann. de méd., 10(2):144, 1921.

1051. Parish, H. J. The titration of antipneumococcus serum. J. Path. & Bact., 33(3):729, July 1930. .... 578, 650

1052. Park, J. H., Jr., and Chickering, H. T. Type I pneumococcus lobar pneumonia among Porto Rican laborers. J. A. M. A., 73 (3):183, July 19, 1919.

1053. Park, W. H. The types of pneumococci in adults and children and their significance. (Harben Lectures, 1930. Pneumonia. Lecture I.) J. State Med., 38(11):621, Nov. 1930. ...... 544, 563, 570, 574

1054. Park, W. H. (Harben Lectures, 1930. Pneumonia. Lecture II.) J. State Med., 39(1):3, Jan. 1931. .... 490, 653

1055. Park, W. H. (Harben Lectures, 1930. Pneumonia. Lecture III.) J. State Med., 39(3):125, Mar. 1931. 490

1056. Park, W. H. The use of pneumococcus vaccine in the treatment of cases of lobar pneumonia. (Harben Lectures, 1930. Pneumonia. Lecture III.) J. State Med., 39(4):187, Apr. 1931. 490, 500, 505

1057. Park, W. H., and Cooper, G. Leucocytes in pneumonia. The possibility of rendering the blood of cases of Types I and II lobar pneumonia antibacterial by injections of antibody solution. Tr. Sect. Path. & Physiol., A. M. A., p. 117, 1927. 127

1057a. Park, W. H., and Cooper, G. Antipneumococcus serum in lobar pneumonia: Method of administration and dosage. J. A. M. A., 90(17):1349, April 28, 1928. 565

1058. Park, W. H., and Williams, A. W. A study of pneumococci: A comparison between the pneumococci found in the throat secretions of healthy persons living in both city and country and those obtained from pneumonic exudates and diseased mucous membranes. J. Exper. Med., 7(5):403, Aug. 1905. 215

1058a. PARK, W. H. *et al.* Introductory note to studies on the pneumococcus under the auspices of the Medical Commission for the Investigation of Acute Respiratory Diseases of the Department of Health, New York City. J. Exper. Med., 7(5):401, Aug. 25, 1905.

1059. PARKER, J. T. The production of skin necrosis by certain autolysates of pneumococcus (Types I and II). J. Exper. Med., 47 (4):531, Apr. 1928. 92

1060. PARKER, J. T. Differentiation between some toxic substances in anaerobically produced autolysates of pneumococci (Types I and II). J. Exper. Med., 49(4):695, Apr. 1929. .... 92, 98

1061. PARKER, J. T. Experimental pneumonia in guinea pigs. II. Effect of anti-autolysate sera on pneumococcus pneumonia in guinea pigs. J. Exper. Med., 50(2):161, Aug. 1929. .... 339, 384

1062. PARKER, J. T., and McCOY, M. VAN S. The production and titration of potent horse antipneumotoxin. J. Exper. Med., 50(1):103, July 1929. .... 339, 384, 534, 579

1063. PARKER, J. T., and PAPPENHEIMER, A. M. Experimental pneumonia in guinea pigs. I. The effect of certain toxic autolysates of pneumococci. J. Exper. Med., 48(5):695, Nov. 1928. .... 97, 202

1064. PARROT. L'organisme microscopique trouvé par M. Pasteur dans la maladie nouvelle provoquée par la salive d'un enfant mort de la rage. Bull. Acad. de méd., Paris, 10 2e sér.:379, Mar. 22, 1881. 4

1065. PASTEUR. Note sur la maladie nouvelle provoquée par la salive d'un enfant mort de la rage. Bull. Acad. de méd., Paris, 10, 2e sér.:94, Jan. 25, 1881. .... 3, 180, 215

1066. PASTEUR, L., CHAMBERLAND, and ROUX. Sur une maladie nouvelle, provoquée par la salive d'un enfant mort de la rage. Compt. rend. Acad. d. sc., 92(4):159, Jan. 1881. .... 3, 32, 180, 215

1067. PAUL, J. R. A comparative study of smooth and rough pneumococcus colonies. J. Exper. Med., 46(5):793, Nov. 1927. 148

1068. PAUL, J. R. The occurrence of rough pneumococci in vivo. J. Exper. Med., 46(5):807, Nov. 1927. 148

1069. PAUL, J. R. Pneumococcus variants. I. Intermediate forms and the influence of environment in their production during in vitro S to R and R to S transitions. J. Bact., 28(1):45, July 1934. 152

1070. PAUL, J. R. Pneumococcus variants. II. Dissociants of R pneumococci and their relation to Streptococcus viridans. J. Bact., 28(1):69, July 1934. 176

1071. PAULI, P. Sulla importanza dell'acqua ossigenata nel metabolismo del pneumococco. Boll. d. Ist. sieroterap. milanese, 6(3): 225, 1927. *Abstract and translation in* Zentralbl. f. d. ges. Hyg., Ref., 16(14/15):827, 1927–8. .... 54, 78

1072. PAWLOWSKY, A. Ueber das Vorhandensein der Pneumoniekokken in der Luft. Berl. klin. Wchnschr., 22(22):345, June 1, 1885. ... 10

1073. Peabody, F. W. The oxygen content of the blood in rabbits infected with pneumococcus. J. Exper. Med., 18(1):1, July 1913.

1074. Peabody, F. W. The oxygen content of the blood in lobar pneumonia. J. Exper. Med., 18(1):7, July 1913.

1075. Peall, P. A. Prophylactic inoculation against pneumonia and other acute respiratory diseases with vaccine on the Randfontein Estates Mine. Publ. South African Inst. M. Research, 7 (37):83, Apr. 1935. 500

1076. Peiper. Ein präparat von Diplokokken welche einer croupösen Pneumonie enstammen. Deutsche med. Wchnschr., 9(51):752, Dec. 19, 1883. 9

1077. Penfold, W. J. The action of the pneumococcus on aromatic amino bodies. M. J. Australia, 2(5):120, July 29, 1922. 74

1078. Perlzweig, W. A. Preliminary report on the nature of the immunizing antigen of pneumococcus Type I. Proc. New York Path. Soc., 21(6/8), n.s.:133, Oct.–Dec. 1921. 240

1079. Perlzweig, W. A. The immunizing substance of the pneumococcus. Science, 54(1401), n.s.:445, Nov. 4, 1921. 240

1080. Perlzweig, W. A., and Keefer, C. S. The immunizing antigen of the pneumococcus. III. The purification of the water-soluble antigen. J. Exper. Med., 42(6):747, Dec. 1925. 241

1081. Perlzweig, W. A., and Steffen, G. I. Studies on pneumococcus immunity. III. The nature of pneumococcus antigen. J. Exper. Med., 38(2):163, Aug. 1923. .... 240, 241, 254

1081a. Permar, H. H. The pathogenesis of experimental pneumonia in the rabbit. J. Med. Research, 44(1):1, Sept. 1923.

1082. Permar, H. H. The mononuclear phagocytes in experimental pneumonia. J. Med. Research, 44(1):27, Sept. 1923. .... 182, 403

1083. Petersen, W. F. Protein therapy and non-specific resistance. New York: The Macmillan Company, 1922.

1083a. Petit, P. Recherches cliniques et bactériologiques sur les infections aiguës de la cornée. Thèse de Paris, 1900.

1084. Petrie, G. F. A specific precipitin reaction associated with the growth on agar plates of meningococcus, pneumococcus, and B. dysenteriae (Shiga). Brit. J. Exper. Path., 13(4):380, Aug. 1932. 131, 152

1085. Petrie, G. F., and Morgan, W. T. J. A quantitative analysis of the lethal power of a strain of Type I pneumococcus. Brit. J. Exper. Path., 12(6):447, Dec. 1931. .... 200, 571

1086. Petrie, G. F., and Morgan, W. T. J. The curative action of anti-pneumococcus serum (Type I) in mice. Brit. J. Exper. Path., 13(1):96, Feb. 1932. 578

1087. Pharmacopoeia of the United States of America. Antipneumococcic serum, Type I. *In* Pharmacopoeia of the United States of America, 11th decennial revision, 332. Easton, Pa.: Mack Printing Co., [1935]. 592

1088. Phelps, B. M. Lobar pneumonia. *In* United Fruit Company. 16th Annual Report, Medical Department, 179. Boston, Mass.: United Fruit Company, 1927. 510

1088a. Picazio, A. Attenuazione della virulenza dello pneumococco in brodo vegetale. Riforma med., 40(9):195, Mar. 3, 1924.

1089. Pico, C. E., et Negrete, J. Contribution à l'étude des antigènes formolés. L'antigène pneumococcique in vitro. Compt. rend. Soc. de biol., 110(17):141, May 1932. *Also:* Rev. Soc. argent. de biol., 8(1):10, Apr. 1932. .... 332, 531

1090. Pieper, E. Streptokokken und Pneumokokken. Eine Übersicht über die neuere Literatur. Zentralbl. f. d. ges. Hyg., 3 (8):433, Apr. 25, 1923.

1090a. Pillat, A. Klinisch-bakteriologische Studien über den Pneumokokkenkatarrh. Klin. Monatschr. f. Augenheilk., 68:533, 1922.

1091. Pisek, G. R., and Pease, M. C. A preliminary report on pneumonia in children, with special reference to its epidemiology. Am. J. M. Sc., 151(1):14, Jan. 1916.

1092. Pittman, M., and Falk, I. S. Studies on respiratory diseases. XXXIV. Some relations between extracts, filtrates and virulence of pneumococci. J. Bact., 19(5):327, May 1930. .... 89, 91, 202

1093. Pittman, M., and Southwick, M. A. Studies on respiratory diseases. XXXV. The pathology of pneumococcus infections in mice. J. Bact., 19(5):363, May 1930. .... 98, 202

1094. Platonow. Über die diagnostische Bedeutung der Pneumoniecoccen. Würzburg, Stürtz, Inaugural Dissertation, 1884.

1095. Platonow, S. Ueber die diagnostische Bedeutung der Pneumoniecoccen. Mitt. a. d. med. Klin. zu Würzburg, 1:221, 1885. 10

1096. Platt, B. S. A note on the significance of gelatin for bacterial growth. Biochem. J., 21(1):16, 1927. 41

1097. Platt, B. S. Peroxide formation by pneumococcus and its relation to bacterial oxidation-reduction reactions. Biochem. J., 21 (1):19, 1927. 77

1098. Plummer, N. Laboratory methods in the treatment of pneumonia. J. Lab. & Clin. Med., 17(6):594, Mar. 1932.

1099. Plummer, N. Heterophile antibody in the treatment of lobar pneumonia. J. A. M. A., 107(7):499, Aug. 15, 1936. 387

1100. Plummer, N., Raia, A., and Shultz, S. Pneumonia in children. A bacteriologic study. Am. J. Dis. Child., 40(3):557, Sept. 1930.

1101. Pockels, W. Immunbiologische Studien bei Pneumokokkeninfektionen. Monatschr. f. Kinderh., 40(3):238, Sept. 1928. 111

1102. Poincaré. Sur l'envahissement du tissu pulmonaire par un champignon, dans la peripneumonie. Compt. rend. Acad. d. sc., 92(5):254, Jan. 1881. 5

1102a. Polettini, B. Un metodo semplice per l'isolamento del pneumococco. Policl., 30(28), sez. prat.:889, July 9, 1923.

1103. Potter, N. B., and Krumwiede, C. Some observations upon opsonins in pneumonia and in four streptococcus infections. J. Infect. Dis., 4(4):601, Nov. 1907. 390

1104. Powell, H. M., and Jamieson, W. A. The action of sodium formaldehyde sulphoxylate in experimental pneumococcus infection. Proc. Indiana Acad. Sc., 44:93, 1935. 511

1105. Powell, H. M., Jamieson, W. A., Bailey, G. H., and Hyde, R. R. A comparative study of antipneumococcus serum containing heterophile antibody. Am. J. Hyg., 17(1):102, Jan. 1933. .... 182, 387
1106. Powell, J. P., Atwater, R. M., and Felton, L. D. The epidemiology of pneumonia. A study of pneumococcus carriers among four groups of persons over a period of months. Am. J. Hyg., 6(4):570, July 1926. 233
1107. Prausnitz, C. Memoranda on the international standardisation of therapeutic sera and bacterial products. *In* League of Nations, Health Organisation. Permanent Commission on Standardisation of Sera, Serological Reactions and Biological Products. Geneva: League of Nations, 1929.
1108. Preisz, H. Untersuchungen über die Wirkungsweise des Antipneumokokkenserums. Centralbl. f. Bakt., 1 Abt., Orig., 77(1):89, Sept. 1915. ....33, 240, 392
1109. Presting, H. Zur Unterscheidung der Streptokokken und Pneumokokken. Centralbl. f. Bakt., 1 Abt., Orig., 90(6):424, July 1923. 48
1110. Pritchett, I. W. Observations on pneumococcus anti-opsonins. Abstr. Bact., 4(1):18, Feb. 1920. 398
1111. Prochaska, A. Untersuchungen über die Anwesenheit von Mikroorganismen im Blute bei den Pneumoniekranken. Deutsches Arch. f. klin. Med., 70(5/6):559, Aug. 1901. 227
1112. Prudden, T. M. Cerebro-spinal meningitis in an infant due to the Diplococcus pneumoniae of Fraenkel and Weichselbaum. Bacteriological and microscopical study of the brain and lungs. Proc. New York Path. Soc., p. 100, 1890.
1113. Puscariu, E., et Nitzulescu, I. Recherches expérimentales sur l'action de l'adrénaline sur le pneumocoque. Compt. rend. Soc. de biol., 88:540, Feb. 1923. 511
1113a. Quensel, U. Untersuchungen über das Vorkommen von Bakterien in den Lungen und bronchialen Lymphdrüsen gesunder Thiere. Ztschr. f. Hyg. u. Infektionskr., 40:505, 1902.
1114. Quigley, W. J. The precipitin reaction in the urine in pneumonia. J. Infect. Dis., 23:217, 1918. 366
1115. Quiroga, R. Milieux à l'extrait de foie pour la culture du pneumocoque. Compt. rend. Soc. de biol., 99(33):1517, Nov. 23, 1928. 43
1116. Raia, A., Plummer, N., and Shultz, S. New types of pneumococci in the pneumonia of children. Am. J. Dis. Child., 42(1):57, July 1931.
1117. Rake, G. Pathology of pneumococcus infection in mice following intranasal instillation. J. Exper. Med., 63(1):17, Jan. 1936. 189
1118. Rake, G. Pathogenesis of pneumococcus infections in mice. J. Exper. Med., 63(2):191, Feb. 1936. 189
1119. Rakieten, M. L. A variant obtained directly from pneumococcus Type II. J. Bact., 20(1):1, July 1930. 154
1120. Ramon, G. La floculation dans les mélanges de toxine et de sérum antidiphtérique. Ann. Inst. Pasteur, 37(12):1001, Dec. 1923. 583

1120a. Raphael, A. De l'immunité antipneumococcique: étude expérimentale. Thèse de Paris, 1916.
1121. Raphael, A. Études sur le pneumocoque. IX. Immunité antipneumococcique (1). Ann. Inst. Pasteur, 34(1):25, Jan. 1920. .. 524
1121a. Rasquin, É. Étude expérimentale sur la pathogénèse de la pneumonie chez le lapin. Arch. méd. exp. et d'anat. path., 22(6): 804, Nov. 1910.
1122. Ratnoff, H. L., and Litvak, A. M. Pneumococcus meningitis treated with Morgenroth's optochin hydrochloride (numoquin hydrochloride). Arch. Pediat., 43(7):466, July 1926.
1123. Reh, T. Purpura symétrique des extrémités par pneumococcémie un nouveau-né. Arch. de méd. d. enf., 23(3):179, Mar. 1920. 87
1124. Reimann, H. A. The blood platelets in pneumococcus infections. J. Exper. Med., 40(4):553, Oct. 1924.
1125. Reimann, H. A. Variations in specificity and virulence of pneumococci during growth in vitro. J. Exper. Med., 41(5):587, May 1925. 141
1126. Reimann, H. A. Serological relationships of type-specific and degraded pneumococci. J. Exper. Med., 43(1):107, Jan. 1926. ... 142
1127. Reimann, H. A. Studies concerning the relationship between pneumococci and streptococci. J. Exper. Med., 45(1):1, Jan. 1927. 175
1128. Reimann, H. A. The occurrence of degraded pneumococci in vivo. J. Exper. Med., 45(5):807, May 1927. 146
1129. Reimann, H. A. The reversion of R to S pneumococci. J. Exper. Med., 49(2):237, Feb. 1929. .... 147, 157
1130. Reimann, H. A., and Julianelle, L. A. The production of purpura by derivatives of pneumococcus. II. The effect of pneumococcus extract on the blood platelets and corpuscles. J. Exper. Med., 43(1):97, Jan. 1926. 88
1131. Reimann, H. A., and Moen, J. K. Quinine derivatives and specific immune serum in the treatment of pneumococcus infection. Arch. Int. Med., 50(2):276, Aug. 1932. 516
1132. Reimann, H. A., and Wu, C. J. The effect of experimental typhus fever on B. typhosus and pneumococcus agglutinins. J. Immunol., 18(2):159, Feb. 1930. 364
1133. Reiner, H. K., and Reiner, L. The fractional precipitation of serum globulin at different hydrogen ion activities. Experiments with globulin obtained from normal and immune (antipneumococcus) horse serum. J. Biol. Chem., 95(1):345, Feb. 1932. ...... 413, 551
1134. Reinhardt, A. Über experimentelle Wundinfektion und Wunddesinfektion (nach Versuchen an Meerschweinchen und Mäusen mit Hühnercholerabacillen, Pneumokokken und Streptokokken). Ztschr. f. Hyg. u. Infektionskr., 95(1):27, Jan. 1922. 510
1135. Rhoades, D. R. Studies on pneumococcus immunity. VI. The fate of pneumococcus protective bodies when injected into normal animals and man. Hygienic Laboratory Bulletin, No. 141:31, Apr. 1925. 561
1136. Rhoads, C. P., and Goodner, K. The pathology of experimental

dermal pneumococcus infection in the rabbit. J. Exper. Med., 54(1):41, July 1931. 182

1137. Rich, A. R. The mechanism responsible for the prevention of spread of bacteria in the immune body. Bull. Johns Hopkins Hosp., 52(3):203, Mar. 1933.

1138. Rich, A. R., and McKee, C. M. The mechanism of a hitherto unexplained form of native immunity to Type III pneumococcus. Bull. Johns Hopkins Hosp., 59(3):171, Sept. 1936. 210

1139. Richardson, R. Pneumococcus types in rural districts. J. A. M. A., 72(12):863, Mar. 22, 1919.

1140. Richardson, R. Types of pneumococcus in lobar pneumonia. J. Lab. & Clin. Med., 4(8):484, May 1919.

1141. Robertson, O. H., Coggeshall, L. T., and Terrell, E. E. Experimental pneumococcus lobar pneumonia in the dog. II. Pathology. J. Clin. Investigation, 12(2):433, Mar. 1933.

1142. Robertson, O. H., Coggeshall, L. T., and Terrell, E. E. Experimental pneumococcus lobar pneumonia in the dog. III. Pathogenesis. J. Clin. Investigation, 12(2):467, Mar. 1933.

1143. Robertson, O. H., and Cornwell, M. A. A study of the resistance of normal human beings to recently isolated strains of pathogenic pneumococci. J. Exper. Med., 52(2):267, Aug. 1930. 435

1144. Robertson, O. H., and Sia, R. H. P. A method for demonstrating growth-inhibitory and bactericidal action on the pneumococcus of a normal serum-leucocyte mixture. Proc. Soc. Exper. Biol. & Med., 20(4):223, Feb. 1923. .... 394, 396, 429

1145. Robertson, O. H., and Sia, R. H. P. Studies on pneumococcus growth inhibition. II. A method for demonstrating the growth-inhibitory and bactericidal action of normal serum-leucocyte mixtures. J. Exper. Med., 39(2):219, Feb. 1924. .... 394, 429

1146. Robertson, O. H., and Sia, R. H. P. Studies on pneumococcus growth inhibition. III. The influence of specific antipneumococcus serum on the growth-inhibitory and bactericidal action of normal serum-leucocyte mixtures. J. Exper. Med., 40(4):467, Oct. 1924. 429

1147. Robertson, O. H., and Sia, R. H. P. Studies on pneumococcus growth inhibition. VII. The relation of opsonins to natural resistance against pneumococcus infection. J. Exper. Med., 46(2):239, Aug. 1927. .... 392, 429

1148. Robertson, O. H., Sia, R. H. P., and Cornwell, M. A. The activating effect of fresh normal serum on the pneumococcidal-promoting action of antipneumococcus serum, Type I. J. Immunol., 19(5):429, Nov. 1930.

1149. Robertson, O. H., Sia, R. H. P., and Woo, S. T. Studies on pneumococcus growth inhibition. I. The protective action of gelatin for pneumococci in suspension. J. Exper. Med., 39(2):199, Feb. 1924. 42

1150. Robertson, O. H., Terrell, E. E., Graeser, J. B., and Cornwell, M. A. The relation of natural humoral antipneumococcal immunity to the inception of lobar pneumonia. J. Exper. Med., 52 (3):421, Sept. 1930.

1151. ROBERTSON, O. H., WOO, S. T., and CHEER, S. N. Studies on pneumococcus growth inhibition. IV. A simplified agitator for growth inhibition tests with serum-leucocyte mixtures; and certain modifications in the technique of the test. J. Exper. Med., 40(4): 487, Oct. 1924.

1152. ROBERTSON, O. H., WOO, S. T., CHEER, S. N., and KING, L. P. A study of the mechanism of recovery from experimental pneumococcus infection. J. Exper. Med., 47(2):317, Feb. 1928. .... 193, 394

1153. ROBINSON, G. H. The immunologic relations of Type 4 pneumococci obtained during an epidemic. J. Infect. Dis., 41(6):417, Dec. 1927.

1154. ROLLAND, J., et BUC. Forme purpurique de la septicémie à pneumocoque. Bull. Soc. de pédiat. de Paris, 16(5):276, May 12, 1914. 87

1155. RÖMER, P. Experimentelle Grundlagen für klinische Versuche einer Serumtherapie des Ulcus corneae serpens nach Untersuchungen über Pneumocokkenimmunität. Arch. f. Ophth., 54(1):99, Apr. 1902. .... 49, 437, 524, 566

1156. RÖMER, P. Wertbestimmung des Pneumokokkenserums mit Demonstration von Tieren. Ber. ü. d. Versamml. d. ophth. Gesellsch., Heidelberg, 32:325, Aug. 3, 1905. 566

1157. ROSENAU, M. J., FELTON, L. D., and ATWATER, R. M. An epidemiologic study of pneumonia and its mode of spread. Am. J. Hyg., 6(3):463, May 1926. 233

1158. ROSENOW, E. C. Blood cultures in lobar pneumonia and agglutination of the pneumococcus. Medicine, Detroit, 9(6):435, June 1903. 358

1159. ROSENOW, E. C. Studies in pneumonia and pneumococcus infections. J. Infect. Dis., 1(2):280, Mar. 1904. .... 358, 420, 433

1160. ROSENOW, E. C. The rôle of phagocytosis in the pneumococcidal action of pneumonic blood. J. Infect. Dis., 3(4):683, June 1906. 390, 395, 401

1161. ROSENOW, E. C. Human pneumococcal opsonin and the antiopsonic substance in virulent pneumococci. J. Infect. Dis., 4(3): 285, June 1907. .... 395, 398

1162. ROSENOW, E. C. Immunological and experimental studies on pneumococcus and staphylococcus endocarditis ("chronic septic endocarditis"). J. Infect. Dis., 6(2):245, Apr. 1909. 170

1163. ROSENOW, E. C. A study of pneumococci from cases of infectious endocarditis. J. Infect. Dis., 7(3):411, May 1910. 136

1163a. ROSENOW, E. C. The autolysis of pneumococci and the effect of the injection of autolysed pneumococci. J. A. M. A., 54(24):1943, June 11, 1910.

1164. ROSENOW, E. C. A bacteriological and cellular study of the lung exudate during life in lobar pneumonia. J. Infect. Dis., 8(4):500, June 1911.

1164a. Rosenow, E. C. A new stain for bacterial capsules, with special reference to pneumococci. J. Infect. Dis., 9(1):1, July 1911.
1165. Rosenow, E. C. Pneumococcus anaphylaxis and immunity. J. Infect. Dis., 9(2):190, Sept. 1911. 447
1166. Rosenow, E. C. Further studies of the toxic substances obtainable from pneumococci. J. Infect. Dis., 11(1):94, July 1912. 94, 339, 447
1167. Rosenow, E. C. Immunization in pneumococcus infections. J. A. M. A., 59(10):795, Sept. 7, 1912. 95
1168. Rosenow, E. C. On the nature of the toxic substance from pneumococci. J. Infect. Dis., 11(2):235, Sept. 1912. 95
1169. Rosenow, E. C. Of the toxicity of broth, of pneumococcus broth culture filtrates, and on the nature of the proteolytic enzyme obtainable from pneumococci. J. Infect. Dis., 11(2):286, Sept. 1912. 65, 95, 239
1170. Rosenow, E. C. Transmutations within the streptococcus-pneumococcus group. J. Infect. Dis., 14(1):1, Jan. 1914. *Also:* Wechselseitige Mutation von Pneumokokken und Streptokokken. Centralbl. f. Bakt., 1 Abt., Orig., 73(4/5):284, Mar. 1914. 170
1171. Rosenow, E. C. Partially autolyzed pneumococci in the treatment of lobar pneumonia. Results in two hundred cases. J. A. M. A., 70(11):759, Mar. 16, 1918. .... 483, 504
1172. Rosenow, E. C., and Arkin, A. The action on dogs of the toxic substance obtainable from virulent pneumococci and pneumonic lungs. J. Infect. Dis., 11(3):480, Nov. 1912.
1173. Rosenow, E. C., and Sturdivant, B. F. Studies in influenza and pneumonia. IV. Further results of prophylactic inoculations. J. A. M. A., 73(6):396, Aug. 9, 1919. .... 483, 495
1174. Rosenthal, F., und Stein, E. Zur experimentellen Chemotherapie der Pneumokokkeninfektion. Ztschr. f. Immunitätsforsch. u. exper. Therap., 20(6):572, Mar. 10, 1914. 511
1175. Rosenthal, L., and Sternberg, B. A rapid method for determining the type of pneumococcus in sputum. J. Lab. & Clin. Med., 15(1):78, Oct. 1929. 126
1176. Rosenthal, S. M. An antidote for acute mercury poisoning. Preliminary report. J. A. M. A., 102(16):1273, Apr. 21, 1934. .. 511
1177. Rosenthal, S. M. Studies in chemotherapy. I. The action of sodium formaldehyde sulphoxylate in bacterial infections. Pub. Health Rep., 49(31):908, Aug. 3, 1934. 511
1178. Ross, V. Immunity against pneumococcus afforded rats by feeding tissues of animals killed by the same germ. Proc. Soc. Exper. Biol. & Med., 23(3):183, Dec. 1925. 487
1179. Ross, V. Immunity to pneumococcus produced in rats by feeding tissues of animals killed by the same organism. J. Immunol., 12(3):219, Sept. 1926. 487
1180. Ross, V. Immunity to pneumococcus produced in rats by feeding them the germ. J. Immunol., 12(3):237, Sept. 1926. 487

1181. Ross, V. Response of orally immunized rats to a second injection of pneumococcus and the minimum duration of immunity. J. Immunol., 12(4):323, Oct. 1926. 487
1182. Ross, V. Protective power of serum of animals fed pneumococci or tissue of animals killed by pneumococcus. Proc. Soc. Exper. Biol. & Med., 24(3):273, Dec. 1926. 487
1183. Ross, V. Oral immunization of rats against pneumococcus types 2 and 3. Proc. Soc. Exper. Biol. & Med., 24(7):697, Apr. 1927. 487
1184. Ross, V. Oral immunization against the pneumococcus. Use of bile salt dissolved organisms, etc., time of appearance of immunity and dosage. J. Exper. Med., 51(4):585, Apr. 1930. 487
1185. Ross, V. Fate of orally administered specific polysaccharide of pneumococcus. Proc. Soc. Exper. Biol. & Med., 28(3):274, Dec. 1930. 487
1186. Ross, V. Oral immunization of humans against pneumococcus, determined by the increased protective antibody content of serum. Proc. Soc. Exper. Biol. & Med., 28(8):822, May 1931. 487
1187. Ross, V. Oral immunization against pneumococcus Types II and III and the normal variation in resistance to these types among rats. J. Exper. Med., 54(6):875, Dec. 1931. 487
1188. Ross, V. The rôle of the soluble specific substance in oral immunization against pneumococcus Type I. J. Exper. Med., 54(6): 899, Dec. 1931. .... 349, 487
1189. Ross, V. The rôle of the soluble specific substance in oral immunization against pneumococcus Types II and III. J. Exper. Med., 55(1):1, Jan. 1932. .... 349, 487
1190. Ross, V. The fate of orally administered soluble specific substance of pneumococcus Types I, II and III. J. Exper. Med., 55 (1):13, Jan. 1932. .... 349, 487
1191. Ross, V. Duration of the immunity produced in rats by feeding the pneumococcus, Type I. J. Immunol., 27(3):235, Sept. 1934. 487
1192. Ross, V. Protective antibodies following oral administration of pneumococcus Type I to rats. J. Immunol., 27(3):249, Sept. 1934. 487
1193. Ross, V. Protective antibodies following oral administration of pneumococcus Types 2 and 3 to rats, with some data for Types 4, 5, and 6. J. Immunol., 27(3):273, Sept. 1934. 487
1194. Ross, V. Oral immunization of humans against the pneumococcus. J. Immunol., 27(3):307, Sept. 1934. 487
1195. Ruediger, G. F. A method of isolating the pneumococcus in mixed cultures, such as throat cultures. J. Infect. Dis., 3(2):183, Apr. 1906. 47
1196. Ruegsegger, J. M., and Finland, M. The influence of dosage and route of injection on the antibody response of human subjects to the specific carbohydrate of the Type VIII pneumococcus. J. Clin. Investigation, 14(6):833, Nov. 1935.
1197. Russell, F. F. Guarding against pneumonia by vaccination. Pub. Health Rep., 33(44):1866, Nov. 1, 1918. 483

1198. Rutz, A. A. Discovery of pneumococcus in the feces; rôle of the intestine in the symptomatology and treatment of acute lobar pneumonia. New York M. J., 96(3):113, July 20, 1912. 229
1199. Rymowitsch, F. Zur Züchtung des Pneumococcus. Centralbl. f. Bakt., 1 Abt., Orig., 32(5):385, Sept. 1902. 49
1200. Sabin, A. B. The stained slide microscopic agglutination test. Application to (1) rapid typing of pneumococci, (2) determination of antibody. Proc. Soc. Exper. Biol. & Med., 26(6):492, Mar. 1929.
1201. Sabin, A. B. The "stained slide" microscopic agglutination test. Its application to (1) rapid typing of pneumococci, (2) determination of antibody. Am. J. Pub. Health, 19(10):1148, Oct. 1929. 127
1202. Sabin, A. B. The microscopic agglutination test in pneumonia. Its application to rapid typing and control of serum therapy. J. Infect. Dis., 46(6):469, June 1930. 127
1203. Sabin, A. B. Rôle of certain anaerobic toxins in pneumococcus infection. Proc. Soc. Exper. Biol. & Med., 28(4):457, Jan. 1931. 99, 385
1204. Sabin, A. B. On the presence in antipneumococcus serum of type-specific protective antibody not neutralized by homologous specific soluble substance. J. Exper. Med., 53(1):93, Jan. 1931. 268, 409, 579
1205. Sabin, A. B. A study of the therapeutic mechanism of antipneumococcic serum on the experimental dermal pneumococcus infection in rabbits. I. The presence in antipneumococcic serum of a non-antibacterial therapeutic factor. J. Exper. Med., 56(4): 531, Oct. 1932. 579
1206. Sabin, A. B. A study of the therapeutic mechanism of antipneumococcic serum on the experimental dermal pneumococcus infection in rabbits. II. A comparison of the therapeutic effect of unrefined, antipneumococcic serum with that of its various protein fractions; the rôle of the non-antibacterial factor. J. Exper. Med., 57(1):139, Jan. 1933. .... 548, 579, 594
1207. Sabin, A. B. Immediate pneumococcus typing directly from sputum by the Neufeld reaction. J. A. M. A., 100(20):1584, May 20, 1933. 132
1208. Sabin, A. B. Laboratory aids in the diagnosis and serum therapy of pneumococcus pneumonia. Am. J. Public Health, 23(9): 978, Sept. 1933. .... 182, 628
1209. Sabin, A. B., and Wallace, G. B. A method for determining the chill-producing properties of anti-pneumococcic serum. Proc. Soc. Exper. Biol. & Med., 27(3):198, Dec. 1929. .... 564, 588
1210. Sabin, A. B., and Wallace, G. B. On the nature of the chill-producing principle in antipneumococcus serum. J. Exper. Med., 53(3):339, Mar. 1931. .... 562, 564, 588
1211. Sacquépée, E. Les types pneumocoques d'avril 1919 à mars 1921. Compt. rend. Soc. de biol., 85:639, Oct. 1921.

1212. Sailer, J., Hall, M. W., Wilson, R. L., and McCoy, C. A study of pneumococcus carriers. Arch. Int. Med., 24(6):600, Dec. 1919.

1212a. Sainton, P., et Maille, J. Méningite cérébro-spinale a méningocoques et a pneumocoques chez un sujet atteint d'otorrhée ancienne. Bull. et mém. Soc. méd. des Hôp. de Paris, 39, 3e sér.:1279, Dec. 1915.

1213. Saito, T. Präcipitations- und Immunisierungsversuche mit dem Nucleoprotein aus Typ II-Pneumokokken. Ztschr. f. Hyg. u. Infektionskr., 109(1):157, Sept. 10, 1928. 247

1214. Saito, T., und Ulrich, W. Über die Gewinnung des spezifischen Kohlehydrates der II-Pneumokokken und seine chemische Eigenschaften. Ztschr. f. Hyg. u. Infektionskr., 109(1):163, Sept. 10, 1928. .... 253, 276, 352

1215. Salvioli, G. Contributo allo studio della natura infettiva della polmonite crupale. Arch. per le sc. med., 8(7):127, 1884. .... 10, 194

1217. Salvioli und Zäslein. Ueber den Mikrokokkus und die Pathogenese der croupösen Pneumonie. Centralbl. f. d. med. Wissensch., 21(41):721, Oct. 1883. 8

1218. Sanderson, E. S. Spontaneous death in a rabbit with the isolation of Type IV pneumococcus. J. Lab. & Clin. Med., 12(11): 1065, Aug. 1927. 179

1219. Satoh, T. "Blutgruppenferment" und Blutgruppensubstanz im Speichel. Klin. Wchnschr., 13(22):798, June 2, 1934.

1220. Savino, E., et Acuna, C. Conservation de la virulence du Diplococcus pneumoniae. Compt. rend. Soc. de biol., 106(5):383, Feb. 13, 1931. 51

1221. Savino, E., Negrete, J., et Acuna, C. Préparation, purification et titrage du sérum antipneumococcique. Compt. rend. Soc. de biol., 107(25):1207, Aug. 1931. .... 531, 549, 551

1222. Schattenberg, H. J., and Harris, W. H. Intraperitoneal injections of pneumococcus in animals primarily receiving leucocytic stimulating antigens. Proc. Soc. Exper. Biol. & Med., 29(9): 1052, June 1932. 395

1223. Schiemann, O. Weitere Untersuchungen über die Wirkung chemotherapeutischer Mittel in vitro. Ztschr. f. Immunitätsforsch. u. exper. Therap., 24(2):167, Sept. 14, 1915.

1224. Schiemann, O. Chemotherapeutische Versuche mit 3,6-Diaminoacridinverbindungen und anderen Farbstoffen. Ztschr. f. Hyg. u. Infektionskr., 97(1/2):280, Nov. 18, 1922. 510

1225. Schiemann, O. Die Beziehungen zwischen Typenspecifität, Virulenz und Pathogenität bei Pneumokokken. Ztschr. f. Hyg. u. Infektionskr., 110(1):175, Feb. 17, 1929. 143

1226. Schiemann, O. Weitere Untersuchungen mit dem Kohlehydrat aus Typ-II Pneumokokken. Ztschr. f. Hyg. u. Infektionskr., 110 (3):567, Oct. 12, 1929. 254

1227. Schiemann, O., und Baumgarten, W. Reagensglasversuche über die Wirkungen von Acridin- und anderen Farbstoffen auf

Bakterien. Ztschr. f. Hyg. u. Infektionskr., 97(1/2):247, Nov. 18, 1922. 509

1228. SCHIEMANN, O., und CASPER, W. Sind die spezifisch präcipitablen Substanzen der 3 Pneumokokkentypen Haptene? Ztschr. f. Hyg. u. Infektionskr., 108(1):220, Oct. 24, 1927. .... 252, 255, 276, 371, 451

1229. SCHIEMANN, O., und FELDT, A. Heilversuche an Mäusen mit Goldpräparaten. Ztschr. f. Hyg. u. Infektionskr., 106(1):83, Mar. 18, 1926. 510

1230. SCHIEMANN, O., und ISHIWARA, T. Vergleichende Untersuchungen über die Wirkung von chemotherapeutischen Präparaten und anderen Antiseptika auf Bakterien. Ztschr. f. Hyg. u. Infektionskr., 77:49, 1914. .... 62, 512

1231. SCHIEMANN, O., LOEWENTHAL, O., und HACKENTHAL, H. Über die immunisierende und shockerzeugende Wirkung von C-haltigen Fraktionen, gereinigter C-Substanz und Lipoiden aus Pneumokokken. Ztschr. f. Hyg. u. Infektionskr., 112(2):315, Mar. 18, 1931. .... 254, 451

1232. SCHIFF, F. Über die gruppenspezifischen Substanzen des menschlichen Körpers. Jena: Gustav Fischer, 1931.

1233. SCHIFF, F., und AKUNE, M. Blutgruppen und Physiologie. München. med. Wchnschr., 78(16):657, Apr. 17, 1931. 288

1234. SCHIFF, F., und WEILER, G. Fermente und Blutgruppen I. Biochem. Ztschr., 235(4/6):454, June 19, 1931. 288

1235. SCHIFF, F., und WEILER, G. Fermente und Blutgruppen II. Biochem. Ztschr., 239(4/6):489, Sept. 17, 1931.

1236. SCHMIDT, A. Über die Benutzung verschiedener Sputa als Nährböden und das Wachsthum der Pneumokokken auf denselben. Centralbl. f. klin. Med., 14(30):625, July 29, 1893. 37

1237. SCHMIDT, G. W., und MISLAP, E. G. Pneumokokkentypen in der Schweiz. Zentralbl. f. Bakt., 1 Abt., Orig., 122(6/7):409, Oct. 20, 1931.

1237a. SCHMIDT, P. Pneumokokken- und Meningokokken-Meningitis nach Schädelbasisfraktur. Deutsche med. Wchnschr., 42(5):124, Feb. 3, 1916.

1238. SCHNABEL, A. Über die Bestimmung zell- und keimschädigender Substanzen in dünnen Lösungen auf biologischem Wege. (I. Mitteilung: Optochin.) Biochem. Ztschr., 108(4/6):258, Sept. 4, 1920. .... 63, 82, 515

1239. SCHNABEL, A. Die Blutgifte der Pneumokokken. Ztschr. f. Hyg. u. Infektionskr., 93(2/3):175, Sept. 22, 1921. .... 63, 74

1240. SCHNABEL, A. Über die Bestimmung zell- und keimschädigender Substanzen in dünnen Lösungen auf biologischem Wege. II. Mitteilung. Biochem. Ztschr., 122(5/6):295, Oct. 14, 1921. 515

1241. SCHNABEL, A. Überempfindlichkeitsversuche an Bakterien. Ztschr. f. Hyg. u. Infektionskr., 96(3):351, Sept. 25, 1922.

1242. SCHNABEL, A., und KASARNOWSKY, S. Überempfindlichkeitsversuche an Bakterien im infizierten Organismus. Ein neuer Ge-

sichtspunkt für die chemotherapeutische Praxis. Klin. Wchnschr., 2(15):682, Apr. 9, 1923. 520
1243. Schnabel, A., und Ninamiya. Über den Mechanismus der Methämoglobinbildung durch Pneumokokken. Klin. Wchnschr., 3 (48):2223, Nov. 25, 1924. *Abstract in* Proc. Berliner Mikrobiologische Gesellschaft, Oct. 20, 1924. 82
1244. Schneider, R. Zur Wirkungsweise des Pneumokokkenimmunserums. Ber. ü. d. Versamml. d. ophth. Gesellsch., Heidelberg, 36:11, Aug. 4, 1910. 390
1245. Schnitzer, R., und Berger, E. Ueber die Wirkungsweise des Optochins gegenüber Pneumokokken. Centralbl. f. Bakt., 1 Abt., Orig., 93(1/4):*292, Oct. 1924.
1246. Schöbl, O., and Sellards, A. W. Experimental pneumonia in monkeys. Philippine J. Sc., 31(1):1, Sept. 1926. *Abstract in* Zentralbl. f. d. ges. Hyg., 15(7/8):352, July 10, 1927. 192
1247. Schottmüller, H. Die Artunterscheidung der für den Menschen pathogenen Streptokokken durch Blutagar. München. med. Wchnschr., 50(20):849, May 19, 1903.
1248. Schottmüller, H. Zur Aetiologie der Pneumonia crouposa. München. med. Wchnschr., 52(30):1425, July 25, 1905.
1249. Schottstaedt, W. E. R. Lobar pneumonia. An attempt to evaluate various methods of treatment. California & West. Med., 41(4):244, Oct. 1934. 511
1250. Schroder, M. C., and Cooper, G. An epidemic of colds, bronchitis, and pneumonia due to Type V pneumococci. J. Infect. Dis., 46(5):384, May 1930. 225
1251. Sée, G. De la nature parasitaire de la pneumonie. L'Union méd., 39(79):965, June 9, 1885.
1252. Seitz, A. Die Pnemokokken in der Umgebung Gesunder und Kranker. Klin. Wchnschr., 1(48):2367, Nov. 25, 1922.
1253. Seligman, E. Versuche zur Deutung der pneumonischen Krisis. Ztschr. f. Immunitätsforsch. u. exper. Therap., 1 Teil, Orig., 9(1): 78, Feb. 25, 1911. 437
1254. Sellards, A. W. Selective action of dilute sodium hydroxid on certain races of the pneumococcus. J. A. M. A., 71(16):1301, Oct. 19, 1918. 57
1254a. Selter, H. Natürliche Pneumokokkeninfektion bei Versuchstieren und experimentelle Untersuchungen über die Entstehung der Pneumonie. Ztschr. f. Hyg. u. Infektionskr., 54:347, 1906.
1254b. Selter, H. Bakterien im gesunden Körpergewebe und deren Eintrittspforten. Ztschr. f. Hyg. u. Infektionskr., 54:363, 1906.
1255. Senger, E. Bakteriologische Untersuchungen über die Pneumonie und pneumonische Metastasen. Arch. f. exper. Path. u. Pharmakol., 20(5/6):389, Jan. 20, 1886. .... 16, 225
1256. Sergent, E. Immunisation contre le pneumocoque par des cultures colorées. Compt. rend. Soc. de biol., 54:16, Jan. 1902. 333
1257. Sevag, M. G. Eine neue physikalische Enteiweissungsmethode

zur Darstellung biologisch wirksamer Substanzen. Isolierung von Kohlenhydraten aus Hühnereiweiss und Pneumococcen. Biochem. Ztschr., 273(4/6):419, Oct. 3, 1934. 292

1258. Sevag, M. S., and Meiweg, L. The respiration mechanism of pneumococcus III. J. Exper. Med., 60(1):95, July 1934. .... 82, 151

1259. Shaffer, M. F., Enders, J. F., and Wu, C.-J. Studies on natural immunity to pneumococcus Type III. II. Certain distinguishing properties of two strains of pneumococcus Type III varying in their virulence for rabbits, and the reappearance of these properties following R→S reconversion of their respective rough derivatives. J. Exper. Med., 64(2):281, Aug. 1936. 208

1260. Sharp, E. A., and Blake, F. G. Host factors in the pathogenesis of pneumococcus pneumonia. J. Exper. Med., 52(4):501, Oct. 1930. 455

1261. Sharp, W. B., and Urbantke, E. Influenza studies. XX. Identification of fixed type pneumococcus carriers: a study of technical methods. J. Infect. Dis., 37(5):473, Nov. 1925. 126

1262. Shibley, G. S., and Rogers, E. S. Occurrence of rough pneumococci in lungs of patients with lobar pneumonia. Proc. Soc. Exper. Biol. & Med., 30(1):6, Oct. 1932. 147

1263. Shwartzman, G. Studies on Bacillus typhosus toxic substance. I. Phenomenon of local skin reactivity to B. typhosus culture filtrate. J. Exper. Med., 48(2):247, Aug. 1928. 474

1264. Shwartzman, G. Phenomenon of local skin reactivity to pneumococcus. J. Immunol., 23(6):429, Dec. 1932. 475

1265. Shwartzman, G. Phenomenon of local skin reactivity to bacterial filtrates in its relation to bacterial hypersensitiveness. J. Exper. Med., 57(5):859, May 1933. 476

1266. Sia, R. H. P. The specific effect of pneumococcus soluble substance on the growth of pneumococci in normal serum-leucocyte mixtures. Proc. Soc. Exper. Biol. & Med., 22(4):262, Jan. 1925. 202

1267. Sia, R. H. P. Studies on pneumococcus growth inhibition. VI. The specific effect of pneumococcus soluble substance on the growth of pneumococci in normal serum-leucocyte mixtures. J. Exper. Med., 43(5):633, May 1926. 399

1268. Sia, R. H. P. Presence of type specific pneumococco-opsonins in sera of animals naturally resistant to pneumococcus infection. Proc. Soc. Exper. Biol. & Med., 24(7):709, Apr. 1927. ...... 352, 396, 431

1269. Sia, R. H. P. Antipneumococcus protective substances in normal pig serum. Proc. Soc. Exper. Biol. & Med., 26(4):284, Jan. 1929. 432

1270. Sia, R. H. P., and Chung, S. F. Use of dog blood agar for the differentiation of "S" and "R" pneumococci. Proc. Soc. Exper. Biol. & Med., 29(3):245, Dec. 1931. .... 48, 139

1271. Sia, R. H. P., and Chung, S. F. Use of antipneumococcus-serum-agar for the identification of pneumococcal types. Proc. Soc. Exper. Biol. & Med., 29(7):792, Apr. 1932. .... 48, 131, 139

1272. Sia, R. H. P., and Dawson, M. H. In vitro transformations of

pneumococcal types. II. The nature of the factor responsible for the transformation of pneumococcal types. J. Exper. Med., 54 (5):701, Nov. 1931. 159
1273. SIA, R. H. P., ROBERTSON, O. H., and WOO, S. T. A study of the mechanism of recovery from lobar pneumonia. J. Exper. Med., 48(4):513, Oct. 1928. 440
1274. SIA, R. H. P., ROBERTSON, O. H., WOO, S. T., and CHEER, S. N. The occurrence of antipneumococcus substances in the blood serum in lobar pneumonia. Proc. Soc. Exper. Biol. & Med., 22(7):406, Apr. 1925. 439
1275. SIA, R. H. P., and ZIA, S. H. Effect of Type II pneumococcus soluble specific substance on infectivity of pneumococcus Type II. Proc. Soc. Exper. Biol. & Med., 29(7):791, Apr. 1932. 202
1276. SICKLES, G. M. Effect of Type I pneumococcus culture broth on the protective action of Type I antiserum. J. Infect. Dis., 40 (2):369, Feb. 1927. 569
1277. SICKLES, G. M. Further observations on the effect of Type-I pneumococcus culture broth on the phagocytic action of Type-I pneumococcus serum. J. Immunol., 14(6):329, Dec. 1927. 352, 398, 569
1278. SICKLES, G. M. The comparative potency of concentrated and unconcentrated antipneumococcus serum. J. Infect. Dis., 45(6): 490, Dec. 1929. 543
1279. SICKLES, G. M. Comparison of different strains of typical and atypical pneumococci and streptococci. (Abstract.) J. Bact., 23(1):86, Jan. 1932. 146
1280. SICKLES, G. M., and COFFEY, J. M. A hemolytic substance in pneumococcus culture broth. J. Infect. Dis., 43(6):490, Dec. 1928. 85
1281. SICKLES, G. M., and SHAW, M. Micro-organisms which decompose the specific carbohydrate of pneumococcus Types II and III. J. Infect. Dis., 53(1):38, July–Aug. 1933. *Abstract in* J. Bact., 25(1):99, Jan. 1933. 316
1282. SICKLES, G. M., and SHAW, M. A systematic study of microorganisms which decompose the specific carbohydrates of the pneumococcus. J. Bact., 28(4):415, Oct. 1934. *Abstract in* J. Bact., 27(1):106, Jan. 1934. 319
1283. SICKLES, G. M., and SHAW, M. Action of microorganisms from soil of type-specific and nontype-specific pneumococcus Type I carbohydrates. Proc. Soc. Exper. Biol. & Med., 31(4):443, Jan. 1934. .... 90, 318, 321
1284. SICKLES, G. M., and SHAW, M. A microörganism which decomposes the specific carbohydrate of pneumococcus Type VIII. Proc. Soc. Exper. Biol. & Med., 32(6):857, Mar. 1935. 320
1285. SIEVERS, O. Über den Gehalt des Speichels an sog. "Blutgruppenferment." Klin. Wchnschr., 13(46):1640, Nov. 17, 1934. 288
1286. SILBERSTEIN, W. Zur Frage der Variabilität in der Streptokokken-Pneumokokkengruppe. Ztschr. f. Hyg. u. Infektionskr., 107 (3/4):725, July 18, 1927. 176
1287. SILBERSTEIN, W. Beitrag zum Vorkommen der "neuen" Pneu-

mokokkentypen (4–33). Ztschr. f. Hyg. u. Infektionskr., 115(1): 63, Apr. 8, 1933. 116

1288. Simon, C. E., and Wood, M. A. The inhibitory action of certain aniline dyes upon bacterial development. First communication. Am. J. M. Sc., 147(2):247, Feb. 1914. .... 62, 509

1289. Simon, C. E., and Wood, M. A. The inhibitory action of certain aniline dyes upon bacterial development. Second communication. Am. J. M. Sc., 147(4):524, Apr. 1914. 62

1290. Singer, E., und Adler, H. Zur Frage der Gewebsimmunität. Die Immunität gegen Pneumococcus Typus III. Ztschr. f. Immunitätsforsch. u. exper. Therap., 41(1):71, Aug. 27, 1924. 403

1291. Singer, E., und Adler, H. Zur Frage der Pneumokokkenimmunität. Ztschr. f. Immunitätsforsch. u. exper. Therap., 41(5): 468, Nov. 25, 1924. 404

1292. Sinigar, H. The variability in virulence of the pneumococcus. Lancet, 1(4142):169, Jan. 17, 1903. .... 198, 224

1293. Smeall, J. T. Types of pneumococci in relation to disease. Brit. M. J., 1(3667):661, Apr. 18, 1931. 227

1294. Smiley, H. E. Bactericidal action of blood of rabbits immunized against pneumococci. J. Infect. Dis., 33(1):88, July 1923.

1295. Smith, C. M. Some notes on pneumonia statistics in Glasgow with special reference to children under five years of age. J. Hyg., 27(3):328, Mar. 1928.

1296. Smith, F. Anaërobic pneumococcus. Brit. J. Exper. Path., 17 (4):329, Aug. 1936. .... 44, 116

1297. Smith, T. Some bacteriological and environmental factors in the pneumonias of lower animals, with special reference to the guinea-pig. J. Med. Research, 29(1):291, Oct. 1913.

1297a. Smith, T. The relation of the capsular substance of B. coli to antibody production. J. Exper. Med., 48(3):351, Sept. 1928.

1298. Smith, W. The titration of antipneumococcus serum. J. Path. & Bact., 35(4):509, July 1932. .... 373, 583, 642

1299. Sobotka, H., and Friedlander, M. The precipitin reaction of antipneumococcus sera. I. The precipitin index. J. Exper. Med., 47(1):57, Jan. 1928. .... 372, 583

1300. Sobotka, H., and Friedlander, M. The precipitin reaction of antipneumococcus sera. III. The ratio of precipitin to protective antibody in Type II. J. Exper. Med., 53(3):299, Mar. 1931.

1301. Solis-Cohen, S., and Heist, G. D. Experimental studies in immunization against pneumococcal infection, with a new method for measuring the extent of the immunity. Tr. Coll. Physicians, Philadelphia, 40, ser. 3:160, 1918.

1302. Solis-Cohen, S., and Heist, G. D. A new method for testing immunity by means of whole blood, with special reference to pneumonia and its prophylaxis by bacterination. (Abstract.) Tr. A. Am. Physicians, 34:109, 1919.

1303. Solis-Cohen, S., and Kolmer, J. A. A study of the germicidal action of quinine and urea hydrochloride, optochin, and other

cinchona derivatives upon pneumococcus cultures in vitro. (Abstract.) Tr. A. Am. Physicians, 31:375, May 9, 1916.
1304. Solis-Cohen, S., Kolmer, J. A., and Heist, G. D. Germicidal action and specific bacteriotropism of quinin and urea hydrochlorid, ethyl-hydrocuprein, and other cinchona derivatives on pneumococci in vitro. Studies in pneumonia, I. J. Infect. Dis., 20(3):272, Mar. 1917. 513
1305. Solly, R. V. The pneumococcus and some of its manifestations. Clin. J., 45(24):213, June 14, 1916.
1306. Sordelli, A., et Mayer, E. Les précipitines de la gélose. Compt. rend. Soc. de biol., 107(19):736, June 12, 1931. 248
1307. Sordelli, A., et Savino, E. Anticorps du sérum antipneumococcique. Compt. rend. Soc. de biol., 107(25):1205, Aug. 1931.
1308. Soule, M. H. Microbic dissociation in B. subtilis. J. Bact., 13(1):41, Jan. 1927. 154
1309. South African Institute for Medical Research. Research Division, Department of Bacteriology. Pneumonia. *In* Annual report for the year ended 31st December, 1931, 7. Johannesburg: The Institute, 1932.
1310. Southard, E. E., and Keene, C. W. A study of brain infections with the pneumococcus. J. A. M. A., 46(1):Jan. 6, 1906. *Reprinted in* Harvard Medical School, Neuro-Path. Papers, No. 6, 1906.
1310a. Sprunt, T. P., and Luetscher, J. A. Acute vascular lesions in mice following injections of pneumococci. J. Exper. Med., 16(4):443, Oct. 1912.
1311. Stadie, W. C. Studies on blood changes in pneumococcus infections. An experimental study of the formation and fate of methemoglobin in the blood. J. Exper. Med., 33(5):627, May 1921. 73
1312. Stanka, R. Bemerkungen über die Identität der Pneumokokken und Streptokokken. Ztschr. f. Immunitätsforsch. u. exper. Therap., 47(2):141, May 5, 1926. 173
1313. Stankiewicz, R., Przesmycki, F., Kolago, J., et Zmigryder, L. La flore bactérienne des pneumopathies (pneumonie et bronchopneumonie) de l'enfant, en considérant les différents types de pneumocoques. Rev. franç. de pediat., 8(3):324, 1932.
1313a. Stefansky, W. K. Ueber eine durch Streptococcus lanceolatus hervorgerufene Epizootie bei Meerschweinchen. Centralbl. f. Bakt., 30(5):201, Aug. 20, 1901.
1314. Steinfeld, E., and Darmstadter, H. J. Immune bodies in a Type I lobar pneumonia. Am. J. M. Sc., 162(5):696, Nov. 1921.
1315. Steinfeld, E., and Kolmer, J. A. Allergic skin reactions in pneumonia to type strains of pneumococci. Studies in pneumonia, V. J. Infect. Dis., 20(3):344, Mar. 1917. 461
1316. Sternberg, G. M. A fatal form of septicaemia in the rabbit, produced by the subcutaneous injection of human saliva. Bull. Nat. Bd. Health, 2(44):781, Apr. 30, 1881. .... 3, 180, 215
1317. Sternberg, G. M. A fatal form of septicaemia in the rabbit,

produced by the subcutaneous injection of human saliva. Ann. Rep. Nat. Bd. Health, 3:87, 1881. .... 3, 180, 215

1318. STERNBERG, G. M. A fatal form of septicaemia in the rabbit, produced by the subcutaneous injection of human saliva. Studies from the Biological Laboratory of Johns Hopkins University, 2(2):183, Mar. 1882. .... 3, 180, 215

1319. STERNBERG, G. M. The pneumonia-coccus of Friedländer (Micrococcus Pasteuri, Sternberg). Am. J. M. Sc., 90:106, July 1885. 1, 4, 14

1320. STERNBERG, G. M. Der Mikrococcus der Sputumsepticaemia (M. Pasteuri, Sternberg). Deutsche med. Wchnschr., 13(3):44, Jan. 20, 1887. .... 1, 4, 14, 19

1321. STERNBERG, G. M. Micrococcus pneumoniae crouposae. *In* his A Manual of Bacteriology, 298. New York: Wm. Wood & Co., 1892. .... 24, 51, 53

1322. STEWART, F. W. Local specific therapy of experimental pneumococcal meningitis. I. Experimental pneumococcal meningitis in rabbits. J. Exper. Med., 46(3):391, Sept. 1927. 180

1323. STEWART, F. W. Local specific therapy of experimental pneumococcal meningitis. II. The production, pathology, and treatment of Type I pneumococcal meningitis in dogs. J. Exper. Med., 46 (3):409, Sept. 1927. 195

1324. STEWART, F. W. Local specific therapy of experimental pneumococcal meningitis. III. Incidental myelitis, abscess, and organization of exudates. J. Exper. Med., 47(1):1, Jan. 1928.

1325. STEWART, F. W. Local specific therapy of experimental pneumococcal meningitis. IV. Type II pneumococcal meningitis in dogs. J. Exper. Med., 47(4):515, Apr. 1928.

1325a. STILLMAN, E. G. A contribution to the epidemiology of lobar pneumonia. J. Exper. Med., 24(6):651, Dec. 1916.

1326. STILLMAN, E. G. Further studies on the epidemiology of lobar pneumonia. J. Exper. Med., 26(4):513, Oct. 1917. .... 10, 51

1327. STILLMAN, E. G. A study of atypical Type II pneumococci. J. Exper. Med., 29(3):251, Mar. 1919. 110

1328. STILLMAN, E. G. The presence of bacteria in the lungs of mice following inhalation. J. Exper. Med., 38(2):117, Aug. 1923.

1329. STILLMAN, E. G. Persistence of inspired bacteria in the lungs of alcoholized mice. J. Exper. Med., 40(3):353, Sept. 1924.

1330. STILLMAN, E. G. Production of immunity in mice by inhalation of pneumococci. J. Exper. Med., 40(4):567, Oct. 1924. 341

1331. STILLMAN, E. G. The development of agglutinins and protective antibodies in rabbits following inhalation of pneumococci. J. Exper. Med., 45(6):1057, June 1927. .... 341, 346

1332. STILLMAN, E. G. The effect of the route of immunization on the immunity response to pneumococcus Type I. J. Exper. Med., 51 (5):721, May 1930. .... 341, 346

1333. STILLMAN, E. G. Susceptibility of rabbits to infection by the inhalation of Type II pneumococci. J. Exper. Med., 52(2):215, Aug. 1930.

1334. STILLMAN, E. G. Development of agglutinins and protective

antibodies in rabbits, after inhalation of Type II pneumococci. J. Exper. Med., 52(2):225, Aug. 1930. .... 341, 525
1335. Stillman, E. G. Duration of demonstrable antibodies in the serum of rabbits immunized with heat-killed Type I pneumococci. J. Exper. Med., 54(4):615, Oct. 1931. 341
1336. Stillman, E. G. Reaction of rabbits following inhalation of Type III pneumococci. J. Infect. Dis., 50(5/6):542, May–June 1932. 183
1337. Stillman, E. G., and Branch, A. Experimental production of pneumococcus pneumonia in mice by the inhalation method. J. Exper. Med., 40(6):733, Dec. 1924. 190
1338. Stillman, E. G., and Branch, A. Experimental pneumonia in mice following the inhalation of Streptococcus haemolyticus and of Friedländer's bacillus. J. Exper. Med., 41(5):623, May 1925.
1339. Stillman, E. G., and Branch, A. Susceptibility of rabbits to infection by the inhalation of virulent pneumococci. J. Exper. Med., 44(5):581, Nov. 1926.
1340. Stillman, E. G., and Branch, A. Early pulmonary lesions in partially immune alcoholized mice following inhalation of virulent pneumococci. J. Exper. Med., 51(2):275, Feb. 1930. 190
1341. Stillman, E. G., and Branch, A. Localization of pneumococci in the lungs of partially immunized mice following inhalation of pneumococci. J. Exper. Med., 54(4):623, Oct. 1931. 190
1342. Stillman, E. G., and Goodner, K. Resistance to pneumococcus infection in rabbits following immunizing injections of heat-killed pneumococcus suspensions. J. Exper. Med., 58(2):195, Aug. 1933. 330, 492
1343. Strassmann. Abstract of article by M. Matray. "Über Pneumoniekokken." Centralbl. f. klin. Med., 4(40):643, Oct. 6, 1883. 8
1344. Ström, A. An epidemic of croupous pneumonia caused by pneumococcus Type I. J. Infect. Dis., 50(5/6):430, May–June 1932. 225
1345. Strouse, S. Experimental studies on pneumococcus infections. J. Exper. Med., 11(5):743, Sept. 1909. 428
1346. Strouse, S. Phagocytic immunity in pneumococcus infections, and in pneumonia with relation to the crisis. J. Exper. Med., 14 (2):109, Aug. 1911. .... 391, 396, 401, 437
1347. Strouse, S., and Clough, P. W. Blood cultures in pneumonia. Bull. Johns Hopkins Hosp., 21(233):247, Aug. 1910. 228
1347a. Strumia, M. Sui tipi di pneumococchi dominanti nelle pneumoniti del 1920 a Torino. Arch. per le sci. med., 44(3/4):188, 1921.
1348. Stryker, L. M. Variations in the pneumococcus induced by growth in immune serum. J. Exper. Med., 24(1):49, July 1916. 136, 212, 362
1348a. Stuertz. Ueber Sputum-Virulenz-Prüfungen im Verlauf der croupösen Pneumonie und über die prognostische Verwertung der Virulenzcurve. Zeitschr. f. klin. Med., 52:422, 1904.
1349. Stull, A. A chemical study of Type III pneumococci. J. Biol. Chem., 82(3):641, June 1929. 248
1350. Stuppy, G. W., Cannon, P. R., and Falk, I. S. The nature of

the immunity in the lungs of rabbits following immunization with pneumococci. J. Prev. Med., 5(2):97, Mar. 1931. 347

1351. STUPPY, G. W., and FALK, I. S. The immunization of rabbits against experimental pneumococcus infections. J. Prev. Med., 2(2):175, Mar. 1928. 347

1352. STUPPY, G. W., and FALK, I. S. Experimental pneumonia in rabbits produced by intrabronchial insufflation of pneumococci. J. Prev. Med., 5(2):89, Mar. 1931. .... 183, 184

1353. STUPPY, G. W., FALK, I. S., and JACOBSON, M. A. The intratracheal inoculation of monkeys with pneumococci. J. Prev. Med., 5(2):81, Mar. 1931. 193

1354. SUGG, J. Y., GASPARI, E. L., FLEMING, W. L., and NEILL, J. M. Studies on immunological relationships among the pneumococci. I. A virulent strain of pneumococcus which is immunologically related to, but not identical with typical strains of Type III pneumococci. J. Exper. Med., 47(6):917, June 1928. .... 111, 113

1355. SUGG, J. Y., and NEILL, J. M. Studies on immunological relationships among the pneumococci. III. Relationship between a variety of Saccharomyces cerevisiae and the Type II variety of Diplococcus pneumoniae (pneumococcus). J. Exper. Med., 49 (2):183, Feb. 1929. 421

1356. SUGG, J. Y., and NEILL, J. M. Studies on immunological relationships among the pneumococci. V. Anaphylaxis and precipitation between antigens and antisera of yeast of Type II pneumococci. J. Exper. Med., 53(4):527, Apr. 1931. 422

1357. SUGG, J. Y., RICHARDSON, L. V., and NEILL, J. M. Studies on immunological relationships among the pneumococci. IV. Active immunization of mice against Type II pneumococci by vaccination with yeast. J. Exper. Med., 50(5):579, Nov. 1929.

1358. SUTLIFF, W. D. Agglutinins and protective bodies in pneumococcus immunity and application to the control of specific therapy. Proc. Soc. Exper. Biol. & Med., 25(4):292, Jan. 1928.

1359. SUTLIFF, W. D. An investigation of the reliability of sputum typing for pneumococcus by mouse method. J. Infect. Dis., 42 (5):485, May 1928. 121

1360. SUTLIFF, W. D., and FINLAND, M. Antipneumococcic immunity reactions in individuals of different ages. J. Exper. Med., 55(6): 837, June 1932. .... 436, 464

1361. SUTLIFF, W. D., and FINLAND, M. The significance of the newly classified types of pneumococci in diseases. Types IV to XX inclusive. J. A. M. A., 101(17):1289, Oct. 21, 1933. .... 218, 224

1362. SUTLIFF, W. D., and FINLAND, M. Type I pneumococcic infections with especial reference to specific serum treatment. New England J. Med., 210(5):237, Feb. 1, 1934. 604

1363. SUTLIFF, W. D., and RHOADES, D. R. The pneumococcidal power of whole blood. I. Description of method. Results in individuals with no history of lobar pneumonia. J. Clin. Investigation, 9(1): 43, Aug. 1930. 435

1364. SUTLIFF, W. D., and RHOADES, D. R. The pneumococcidal power of whole blood. II. Estimations in lobar pneumonia. J. Clin. Investigation, 9(1):55, Aug. 1930. 435
1365. SUTTON, A. C., and SEVIER, C. E. A study of the bacteriemia in lobar pneumonia. Bull. Johns Hopkins Hosp., 28(320):315, Oct. 1917. 228
1366. SUTTON, D. C., KENDALL, A. I., and ROSENBLUM, A. Clinical observations of the immunizing value of "natural bacterial antigens." Am. J. M. Sc., 182(4):454, Oct. 1931. .... 483, 487, 506
1367. SVEDBERG, T. Sedimentation of molecules in centrifugal fields. Chem. Rev., 14(1):1, Feb. 1934.
1368. SVEDBERG, T. Sedimentationsmessungen mit der Ultrazentrifuge. Naturwissenschaften., 22(15):Apr. 13, 1934.
1369. SVEDBERG, T. Die Molekulargewichtsanalyse im Zentrifugalfeld. Kolloid-Ztschr., 67(1):2, Apr. 1934. 415
1370. SWIFT, H. F. Preservation of stock cultures of bacteria by freezing and drying. J. Exper. Med., 33(1):69, Jan. 1921. 52
1371. SYDENSTRICKER, V. P. W., and SUTTON, A. C. An epidemiological study of lobar pneumonia. Bull. Johns Hopkins Hosp., 28 (320):312, Oct. 1917.
1372. TAKAMI, T. Beobachtungen über die Hämolyse von Pneumokokken. Tohoku J. Exper. Med., 4(1):1, Apr. 1923. 84
1373. TAKAMI, T. Über die Variationen der Pneumokokken. Tohoku J. Exper. Med., 6(1/2):41, June 1925. .... 113, 142
1374. TAKAMI, T. Über ein neues Verfahren, gut wirkende Pneumokokkensera herzustellen. Tohoku J. Exper. Med., 6(1/2):65, June 1925. 530
1375. TAKAMI, T. Über agglutinatorische Veränderungen der Pneumokokken im Tierkörper. Tohoku J. Exper. Med., 6(3/4):248, Sept. 1925. .... 113, 143
1376. TAKAMI, T. Über die agglutinatorische Einteilung von Pneumokokken. Tohoku J. Exper. Med., 6(3/4):260, Sept. 1925.
1377. TALAMON, C. Coccus de la pneumonie. Bull. Soc. anat., Paris, 8, 4e sér.:475, Nov. 30, 1883. .... 1, 9
1378. TALAMON, C. Note sur le coccus lancéolé de la pneumonie lobaire fibrineuse. Progrès méd., 11(51)·1030, Dec. 22, 1883. 194
1379. TANI, T. Beiträge zur aktiven Immunisierung gegen Pneumokokken und zur Veränderlichkeit der Pneumokokken. Ztschr. f. Hyg. u. Infektionskr., 103(1):204, July 1924. .... 328, 530
1380. TAO, S. M. The antigenic response and local reaction caused by formalinised pneumococcus vaccine. Chinese M. J., 46(1):12, Jan. 1932. .... 332, 531
1381. TCHISTOVITCH, N. Études sur la pneumonie fibrineuse. Ann. Inst. Pasteur, 4(5):285, May 1890. .... 182, 184, 427
1382. TCHISTOVITCH, N. Contribution à l'étude de la pathogénie de la crise dans la pneumonie fibrineuse. Ann. Inst. Pasteur, 18(5): 304, May 1904.
1383. TCHISTOVITCH, N., et YOUREVITCH, V. Sur les opsonines et les

antiphagines dans l'infection pneumococcique. Ann. Inst. Pasteur, 22(7):611, July 1908. 398

1384. Tebbutt, A. H. On pneumococci in pneumonia in Sydney. M. J. Australia, 1(12):228, Mar. 19, 1921.

1385. Terrell, E. E. Changes in humoral immunity occurring during the early stages of experimental pneumococcus infection. Proc. Soc. Exper. Biol. & Med., 27 (5):353, Feb. 1930. 394

1386. Terrell, E. E. Changes in humoral immunity occurring during the early stages of experimental pneumococcus infection. J. Exper. Med., 51(3):425, Mar. 1930. 394

1387. Terrell, E. E., Robertson, O. H., and Coggeshall, L. T. Experimental pneumococcus lobar pneumonia in the dog. I. Method of production and course of the disease. J. Clin. Investigation, 12 (2):393, Mar. 1933. 195

1388. Testi, A. Parotite doppia in seguito di polmonite. Riforma med., 5(260):1556, Nov. 8, 1889. *Abstract in* Jahresb. ü. d. Fortschr. i. d. Lehre v. d. path. Mikroorg., 5:54, 79, 1889. 19

1389. Testi, A. Di una rarissima complicazione della pneumonite fibrinosa. Riforma med., 5(281):1682, Dec. 3, 1889. *Abstract in* Jahresb. ü. d. Fortschr. i. d. Lehre v. d. path. Mikroorg., 5:54, 80, 1889. 19

1390. Testi, A. Di una rarissima complicazione della pneumonite fibrinosa. Riforma med., 5(282):1688, Dec. 4, 1889. *Abstract in* Jahresb. ü. d. Fortschr. i. d. Lehre v. d. path. Mikroorg., 5:80, 1889. 19

1391. Thjötta, T. Studies on bacterial nutrition. I. Growth of Bacillus influenzae in hemoglobin-free media. J. Exper. Med., 33(6): 763, June 1921. 43

1392. Thjötta, T., and Avery, O. T. Studies on bacterial nutrition. II. Growth accessory substances in the cultivation of hemophilic bacilli. J. Exper. Med., 34(1):97, July 1921. 43

1393. Thjötta, T., and Avery, O. T. Studies on bacterial nutrition. III. Plant tissue, as a source of growth accessory substances, in the cultivation of Bacillus influenzae. J. Exper. Med., 34(5):455, Nov. 1, 1921. 43

1394. Thjötta, T., and Hanneborg, Ö. Pneumonia death rate and types of pneumococci in Norway. J. Infect. Dis., 34(5):454, May 1924.

1395. Thomas, H. M., Jr., and O'Hara, D. Pneumococcus Type I vegetative endocarditis. Report of a case following an attack of lobar pneumonia. Bull. Johns Hopkins Hosp., 31(357):417, Nov. 1920. 226

1396. Thompson, R. L. Electrophoresis of organisms belonging to the pneumococcus group. Am. J. Hyg., 14(2):244, Sept. 1931. ...... 118, 201

1397. Thompson, R. L. Electrophoresis of the normal and chemically treated strains of pneumococci. Am. J. Hyg., 15(3):712, May 1932. 118

1398. Thomsen, O., og Christensen, S. Bidrag til Kendskabet af

Pneumococtyper. Hospitalstid., 63(47):729, Nov. 24, 1920. Contributions to the characterization of pneumococcus types. (Translation.) Acta med. Scandinav., 54(6):501, May 6, 1921.

1399. Thomsen, O., et Christensen, S. Contribution à la connaissance des types de pneumocoques. Compt. rend. Soc. de biol., 84(5): 327, Feb. 5, 1921.

1400. Thomson, D., and Thomson, R. The classification and identification of germs by microphotography. Ann. Pickett-Thomson Research Lab., 1(2):263, June 1925. 48

1401. Tillgren, J. Studien über die Pneumokokken-Immunität. II. Mitteilung. Immunserum und Leukocyten. Centralbl. f. Bakt., 1 Abt., Orig., 77(1):74, Sept. 1915. 403

1402. Tillgren, J. Studien über die Pneumokokken-Immunität. III. Mitteilung. Centralbl. f. Bakt., 1 Abt., Orig., 77(1):84, Sept. 1915. 403

1403. Tillett, W. S. Studies on immunity to Pneumococcus mucosus (Type III). I. Antibody response of rabbits immunized with Type III pneumococcus. J. Exper. Med., 45(4):713, Apr. 1927. ...... 181, 207

1404. Tillett, W. S. Studies on immunity to Pneumococcus mucosus (Type III). II. The infectivity of Type III pneumococcus for rabbits. J. Exper. Med., 45(6):1093, June 1927. .... 150, 181

1405. Tillett, W. S. Studies on immunity to Pneumococcus mucosus (Type III). III. Increased resistance to Type III infection induced in rabbits by immunization with R and S forms of pneumococcus. J. Exper. Med., 46(2):343, Aug. 1927. .... 150, 329

1406. Tillett, W. S. Active and passive immunity to pneumococcus infection induced in rabbits by immunization with R pneumococci. J. Exper. Med., 48(6):791, Dec. 1928. 150

1407. Tillett, W. S., Avery, O. T., and Goebel, W. F. Chemo-immunological studies on conjugated carbohydrate-proteins. III. Active and passive anaphylaxis with synthetic sugar-proteins. J. Exper. Med., 50(5):551, Nov. 1929. .... 264, 448, 450, 453

1408. Tillett, W. S., and Francis, T., Jr. Cutaneous reactions to the polysaccharides and proteins of pneumococcus in lobar pneumonia. J. Exper. Med., 50(5):687, Nov. 1929. 463

1409. Tillett, W. S., and Francis, T., Jr. Serological reactions in pneumonia with a non-protein somatic fraction of pneumococcus. J. Exper. Med., 52(4):561, Oct. 1930. .... 208, 256, 368, 441

1410. Tillett, W. S., Goebel, W. F., and Avery, O. T. Chemical and immunological properties of a species-specific carbohydrate of pneumococci. J. Exper. Med., 52(6):895, Dec. 1930. .... 257, 465, 636

1411. Tizzoni, G., und Panichi, L. Ueber die Zerstörung des Fränkelschen Pneumococcus im Bluteimmunisierter und hypervaccinierter Tiere. Centralbl. f. Bakt., 1 Abt., Ref., 36(1/3):25, 1905.

1412. Todd, E. W. A comparative serological study of streptolysins derived from human and from animal infections, with notes on pneumococcal haemolysin, tetanolysin and staphylococcus toxin. J. Path. & Bact., 39(2):299, Sept. 1934. .... 86, 383

1413. Toenniessen, E. Untersuchungen über die Kapsel (Gummi-

hülle) der pathogenen Bakterien. II. Die chemische Beschaffenheit der Kapsel und ihr dadurch bedingtes Verhalten gegenüber der Fixierung und Färbung. Centralbl. f. Bakt., 1 Abt., Orig., 85(4):225, Dec. 1921. .... 262, 302
1414. Tomcsik, J. A carbohydrate-like specific substance in the colon aerogenes group. Proc. Soc. Exper. Biol. & Med., 24(9):810, June 1927. 262
1415. Tomcsik, J. Anaphylactic shock produced by a soluble specific substance largely carbohydrate in nature. Proc. Soc. Exper. Biol. & Med., 24(9):812, June 1927. 449
1416. Tongs, M. S. Effects of pneumococcus Type I on leucocytes and hemopoietic organs. J. Infect. Dis., 30(3):323, Mar. 1922. 180
1417. Trask, J. D., O'Donovan, C., Jr., Moore, D. M., and Beebe, A. R. Studies on pneumonia in children. I. Mortality, blood cultures, and humoral antibodies in pneumococcus pneumonia. J. Clin. Investigation, 8(4):623, June 1930. 220
1418. Trevan, J. W. The accuracy of titration of anti-pneumococcus serum. J. Path. & Bact., 33(3):739, July 1930. .... 573, 579
1419. Truche, C. Préparation et propriétés des sérums antipneumococciques. Bull. Acad. de méd., Paris, 81(24), 3e sér.:823, June 17, 1919. .... 333, 539
1420. Truche, C. Études sur le pneumocoque. X. Préparation et propriétés des sérums antipneumococciques. Ann. Inst. Pasteur, 34 (2):98, Feb. 1920. .... 333, 530, 535
1421. Truche, C. Moyen simple et pratique de conservation des germes. Ann. Inst. Pasteur, 38(6):516, June 1924. 50
1422. Truche, C., et Cotoni, L. Études sur le pneumocoque. II. Conservation de la virulence des pneumocoques humains pour la souris. Ann. Inst. Pasteur, 26(1):1, Jan. 1912. 50
1423. Truche, C., et Cotoni, L. Études sur le pneumocoque. V. Virulence des pneumocoques, humains et animaux, pour le lapin et le cobaye. Ann. Inst. Pasteur, 26(7):530, July 1912. 206
1424. Truche, C., et Cotoni, L. Études sur le pneumocoque. VII. Passages comparés par la souris, le lapin et le cobaye (pneumocoques humains). Ann. Inst. Pasteur, 27(4):322, Apr. 1913. 207
1425. Truche, C., Cotoni, L., et Raphael, A. Études sur le pneumocoque. VIII. Action de la bile sur les pneumocoques humains et animaux. Ann. Inst. Pasteur, 27(10):886, Oct. 1913. 56
1426. Truche, C., Cramer, A., et Cotoni, L. Études sur le pneumocoque. I. Virulence du pneumocoque humain pour la souris. Ann. Inst. Pasteur, 25(6):480, June 1911. 211
1426a. Truche, C., et Gosset. Sur la morphologie du pneumocoque. Compt. rend. Soc. de biol., 70:127, Jan. 28, 1911.
1427. Tudoranu, G. Le mécanisme de l'immunité contre le pneumocoque Type III. Ann. Inst. Pasteur, 40(7):606, July 1926. 404
1428. Tuft, L., and Ramsdell, S. G. Antibody studies in serum sickness. II. Study of sera secured by serial bleeding from persons treated with immune serum. J. Immunol., 17(6):539, Dec. 1929.

1429. Tugendreich, J., und Russo, C. Ueber die Wirkung von China-alkaloiden auf Pneumokokkenkulturen. Ztschr. f. Immunitätsforsch. u. exper. Therap., 19(2):156, Aug. 1913. 513, 519
1430. Turro, R. Le glucose dans les cultures du pneumocoque. J. de physiol. et de path. gén., 6(4):718, July 1904. 38
1431. Uchida, Y. Experimentelle Infektionen von Mäusen und Meerschweinchen parenteral und von den natürlichen Eingangspforten aus. I. Mitteilung. Versuche an Mäusen mit Milzbrand und anderen Septicämieerregern. Ztschr. f. Hyg. u. Infektionskr., 106 (1):96, Mar. 1926. 187
1432. Uchida, Y. Experimentelle Infektionen von Mäusen und Meerschweinchen parenteral und von den natürlichen Eingangspforten aus. III. Mitteilung. Versuche an Meerschweinchen mit Milzbranderregern, Bacillen der hämorrhagischen Septicämie und anderen pathogenen Bakterien. Ztschr. f. Hyg. u. Infektionskr., 106(2):281, June 1926. 187
1433. Ungermann, E. Beitrag zur Kenntnis der Ursachen der Pneumokokkenimmunität, insbesondere zum Verhalten "serumfester" Pneumokokkenstämme. Ztschr. f. Immunitätsforsch. u. exper. Therap., 5(2/3):269, Mar. 1910. 120
1434. Ungermann, E. Über die Ursachen der natürlichen Pneumokokkenimmunität. Arb. a. d. k. Gsndhtsamte, 36(3):341, Feb. 1911. 395, 428
1435. Ungermann, E. Eine einfache Methode zur Gewinnung von Dauerkulturen empfindlicher Bakterienarten und zur Erhaltung der Virulenz tierpathogener Keime. Arb. a. d. Reichs-Gsndhtsamte, 51(1):180, Oct. 1918. 50
1436. Ungermann, E., und Kandiba, L. Über quantitative Verhältnisse bei der Antikörperwirkung. Arb. a. d. k. Gsndhtsamte, 40 (1):24, May 1912. 408, 567
1437. U. S. Treasury Department. National Institute of Health. Submission of samples of antipneumococcic serum. Circular Letter, dated Jan. 6, 1934. 592
1438. U. S. Treasury Department. National Institute of Health. Minimum potency of Type I antipneumococcus serum. Circular Letter, dated Dec. 30, 1935. 592
1439. U. S. Treasury Department. Public Health Service. Potency of antimeningococcic and antipneumococcic serums. Pub. Health Rep., 34(47):2657, Nov. 21, 1919. 568
1440. U. S. Treasury Department. Public Health Service. Regulations for the sale of viruses, serums, toxins and analogous products in the District of Columbia and in interstate traffic. Washington: Government Printing Office, Feb. 25, 1935. (Pub. Health Service, Misc. Pub., No. 10.) 588
1441. Urquhart, A. L. Serological and morphological characteristics of the pneumococcus. An analysis of organisms isolated from 77 cases of pneumococcal infection. Lancet, 2(5130):1313, Dec. 24, 1921.

1442. Valentine, E. Common colds as a possible source of contagion for lobar pneumonia. J. Exper. Med., 27(1):27, Jan. 1918. 224
1443. Valentine, E., McGuire, G., Whitney, E., and Falk, K. G. Studies on antibodies. III. Agglutinin and precipitin reactions of dried antipneumococcus preparations after storage under various conditions. J. Immunol., 21(3):221, Sept. 1931. .... 357, 378
1444. Valentine, F. C. O. A staining method for the direct typing of pneumococci. Lancet, 1(5706):22, Jan. 7, 1933. 128
1445. Varela, G., y Salazar, M. Titulación del suero antineumocóccico empleando el polisacárido de Zozaya, Boyer y Clarke. Bol. Inst. de Higiene, Mexico, 2(2):18, May 1932.
1446. Vaucel, M., et Salaün, G. Contribution à l'étude du pneumocoque en Afrique Equatoriale Française. Bull. Soc. path. exot., 25(1):58, Jan. 1932.
1447. Vaughan, V. C., Vaughan, V. C., Jr., and Vaughan, J. W. Protein split products in relation to immunity and disease. Philadelphia and New York: Lea & Febiger, 1913. 100
1448. Vaughan, W. T. Type determination of pneumococcus infection as practised in the field with Avery's new cultural method. J. A. M. A., 70(7):431, Feb. 16, 1918. 123
1449. Vedder, A. De veelvuldigheid der pneumococcentypes bij pneumococcoses te Amsterdam. Nederl. tijdschr. v. geneesk., 74[2](42): 5139, Oct. 18, 1930.
1450. Vélicanoff, I., et Mikhailova, Z. La perte de virulence du pneumocoque et ses rapports avec les hydrates de carbone. Compt. rend. Soc. de biol., 105(29):295, Nov. 4, 1930. 50
1451. Voegtlein, C. Phenols as preservatives of antipneumococcic serum. A pharmacological study. Hygienic Laboratory Bulletin, No. 112:5, Apr. 1918. 558
1452. Von Sholly, A. I., and Park, W. H. Studies on acute respiratory infections. VII. Report on the prophylactic vaccination of 1536 persons against acute respiratory diseases 1919–20. J. Immunol., 6(1):103, Jan. 1921. .... 483, 490, 497
1453. Vulpian, A. Inoculation de salive. Bull. Acad. de méd., Paris, 10, 2e sér.:394, Mar. 29, 1881. .... 5, 180
1454. Wadsworth, A. A convenient method for growing and storing virulent pneumococci. Proc. New York Path. Soc., 3(3), n.s.:113, Apr. 1903. 50
1455. Wadsworth, A. The agglutination of the pneumococcus with certain normal and immune sera. J. Med. Research, 10(2):228, Oct. 1903. .... 358, 365, 428, 433
1455a. Wadsworth, A. Studies on simple and differential methods of staining encapsulated pneumococci in smear and section. J. Infect. Dis., 3(4):610, June 30, 1906.
1456. Wadsworth, A. Pneumonia; a bedside and laboratory study. Am. J. Obst. & Gynec., 59(378):1080, June 1909.
1456a. Wadsworth, A. A study of the endocardial lesions developing

during pneumococcus infection in horses. J. Med. Research, 39 (3):279, Jan. 1919.

1457. Wadsworth, A. B. Studies on pneumococcus infection in animals. J. Exper. Med., 16(1):54, July 1912. .... 194, 328

1458. Wadsworth, A. B. Studies on pneumococcus infection in animals. Second paper: Action of immune sera on pneumococcus infection. J. Exper. Med., 16(1):78, July 1912. .... 524, 528, 577

1459. Wadsworth, A. B. A study of experimental organizing pneumonia. J. Med. Research, 39(2):147, Nov. 1918. 194

1460. Wadsworth, A. B. The protective value of pneumococcus vaccination in mice and rabbits. J. Immunol., 5(5):429, Sept. 1920. 410

1461. Wadsworth, A. B. Review of recently published reports on the serum treatment of Type I pneumonia, together with a report of 445 additional cases. Am. J. Hyg., 4(2):119, Mar. 1924.

1462. Wadsworth, A. Die Serumtherapie der Pneumonie des Typus I. Seuchenbekämpfung, 7(1):1930.

1463. Wadsworth, A. Recent advances in the serum therapy of pneumonia, meningitis, scarlet fever and other streptococcus infections. Tr. A. Am. Physicians, 47:161, May 1932. 543

1464. Wadsworth, A. B. Serum therapy. Its value in pneumonia, meningitis, scarlet fever and other streptococcus infections. J. A. M. A., 99(3):204, July 16, 1932.

1465. Wadsworth, A. B. Practical limitations of vaccine and serum therapy. New England J. Med., 213(26):1285, Dec. 26, 1935. 502

1466. Wadsworth, A., and Brown, R. Chemical and immunological studies of the pneumococcus. I. A specific antigenic carbohydrate of Type I pneumococcus. J. Immunol., 21(3):245, Sept. 1931. 269, 276, 352

1467. Wadsworth, A., and Brown, R. Chemical and immunological studies of the pneumococcus. II. The ether-soluble fraction of Type I pneumococcus. J. Immunol., 21(4):255, Oct. 1931. ...... 253, 352

1468. Wadsworth, A., and Brown, R. Chemical and immunological studies of the pneumococcus. III. Cellular carbohydrate fractions. J. Immunol., 24(5):349, May 1933. .... 90, 271, 454

1469. Wadsworth, A., Crowe, M. O'L., and Smith, L. A. Absorption spectra of the carbohydrates of the pneumococcus. A preliminary note. J. Immunol., 26(6):481, June 1934. 273

1470. Wadsworth, A. B., and Kirkbride, M. B. A note on the production of antipneumococcus sera. J. Exper. Med., 25(5):629, May 1917. .... 523, 529, 535, 567

1471. Wadsworth, A. B., and Kirkbride, M. B. A study of the changes in virulence of the pneumococcus at different periods of growth and under different conditions of cultivation in media. J. Exper. Med., 28(6):791, Dec. 1918. .... 203, 210

1472. Wadsworth, A. B., Kirkbride, M. B., and Gilbert, R. The standardization of antipneumococcus and antimeningococcus serums. Arch. Int. Med., 23(3):269, Mar. 1919. 568

1473. Wadsworth, A., and Quigley, J. J. Studies on the bacterial toxins. Concentration and purification of the toxin of Streptococcus hemolyticus with acetone. J. Immunol., 20(6):459, June 1931.

1474. Wadsworth, A. B., and Sickles, G. M. A study of pneumococci isolated from horses undergoing pneumococcus immunization. J. Exper. Med., 45(5):787, May 1927. 145

1475. Wadsworth, A. B., and Sickles, G. M. The effect of Type I pneumococcus culture broth on the phagocytic action of Type I pneumococcus serum. J. Immunol., 14(6):321, Dec. 1927. 398

1476. Walker, J. E. The germicidal properties of chemically pure soaps. J. Infect. Dis., 35(6):557, Dec. 1924. 509

1477. Walravens, P. Étude sur le pneumocoque. Ann. Soc. belge de méd. trop., 1(2):241, 1920–21. 497

1478. Wámoscher, L. Infektionsversuche mit einzelnen Pneumokokken. Ztschr. f. Hyg. u. Infektionskr., 106(2):421, June 1926. 188, 199

1479. Wámoscher, L. Über Pneumokokkeninfektionen bei verminderter individueller Resistenz. Ztschr. f. Hyg. u. Infektionskr., 107(1):240, Jan. 1927. 187

1480. Ward, H. K. Observations on the phagocytosis of the pneumococcus by human whole blood. I. The normal phagocytic titre, and the anti-phagocytic effect of the specific soluble substance. J. Exper. Med., 51(5):675, May 1930. .... 352, 399, 435, 440, 647

1481. Ward, H. K. Observations on the phagocytosis of the pneumococcus by human whole blood. II. The neutralization of the antiphagocytic action of the specific soluble substance by antiserum. J. Exper. Med., 51(5):685, May 1930. .... 352, 399

1482. Ward, H. K. An examination of the mechanism of pneumococcus immunity by means of bactericidal measurements. I. The reaction between the anticarbohydrate antibody and the purified specific carbohydrate. J. Exper. Med., 55(4):511, Apr. 1932. 400

1483. Ward, H. K. An examination of the mechanism of pneumococcus immunity by means of bactericidal measurements. II. The reaction between the anticarbohydrate antibody and type-specific products of the organism. J. Exper. Med., 55(4):519, Apr. 1932. 267, 400, 443, 580

1484. Ward, H. K., and Enders, J. F. An analysis of the opsonic and tropic action of normal and immune sera based on experiments with the pneumococcus. J. Exper. Med., 57(4):527, Apr. 1933. .. 396, 436

1485. Warden, C. C. Immunity in pneumococcus infections. J. A. M. A., 59(23):2085, Dec. 7, 1912. 335

1486. Washbourn, J. W. Experiments with the pneumococcus, with especial reference to immunity. J. Path. & Bact., 3:214, 1896. 26, 49, 326, 356

1487. Washbourn, J. W. Antipneumococcic serum. Brit. M. J., 1 (1887):510, Feb. 27, 1897. .... 28, 522, 528, 530, 565, 577

1487a. Washbourn, J. W. Antipneumococcic serum. Brit. M. J., 2 (1930):1849, Dec. 25, 1897.

1488. Washbourn, J. W. The Croonian lectures on the natural history and pathology of pneumonia. Lecture I. Lancet, 2(4133):1301, Nov. 15, 1902.

1489. WASHBOURN, J. W. The Croonian lectures on the natural history and pathology of pneumonia. Lecture II. Lancet, 2(4134):1378, Nov. 22, 1902.

1490. WASHBOURN, J. W. The Croonian lectures on the natural history and pathology of pneumonia. Lecture III. Lancet, 2(4135): 1439, Nov. 29, 1902.

1491. WASSERMANN, M. Pneumococcenschutzstoffe. Deutsche med. Wchnschr., 25(9):141, Mar. 2, 1899. 407

1492. WATSON, E. L., and COOPER, G. The production of infection with pneumococci in rabbits by intradermal inoculation of Type III pneumococci, the treatment with specific antiserum, and a comparison with Type I infections. J. Exper. Med., 52(6):849, Dec. 1930. 182

1493. WAYSON, N. E., and MCCOY, G. W. The potency of antipneumococcic serum. J. A. M. A., 70(23):1747, June 8, 1918. 567

1493a. WEBER, H. Ueber eine Pneumonie-Epizootie unter Meerschweinchen. Arch. f. Hyg., 39:276, 1901.

1494. WEBSTER, L. T., and CLOW, A. D. Intranasal virulence of pneumococci for mice. J. Exper. Med., 58(4):465, Oct. 1933. .... 189, 205

1495. WEBSTER, L. T., and HUGHES, T. P. The epidemiology of pneumococcus infection. The incidence and spread of pneumococci in the nasal passages and throats of healthy persons. J. Exper. Med., 53(4):535, Apr. 1931. 233

1496. WEBSTER, R. A study of the incidence of the various serological types of pneumococci in pneumonia of childhood: observations on serum therapy. M. J. Australia, 1(6):129, Feb. 9, 1924.

1497. WEICHSELBAUM, A. Ueber die Aetiologie der acuten Lungen- und Rippenfellentzündungen. Med. Jahrb., 1, N. F.:483, 1886. 1, 17

1498. WEICHSELBAUM, A. Aetiologie und pathologische Anatomie der akuten Lungenentzündungen. Wien. med. Wchnschr., 36(39): 1301, Sept. 25, 1886. .... 17, 18

1499. WEICHSELBAUM, A. Aetiologie und pathologische Anatomie der akuten Lungenentzündungen. Wien. med. Wchnschr., 36(40): 1339, Oct. 2, 1886. 18

1500. WEICHSELBAUM, A. Aetiologie und pathologische Anatomie der akuten Lungenentzündungen. Wien. med. Wchnschr., 36(41): 1367, Oct. 9, 1886. 18

1501. WEICHSELBAUM, A. Ueber seltenere Localisationen des pneumonischen Virus (Diplococcus pneumoniae). Wien. klin. Wchnschr., 1(28):573, Oct. 11, 1888.

1502. WEICHSELBAUM, A. Ueber seltenere Localisationen des pneumonischen Virus (Diplococcus pneumoniae). Wien. klin. Wchnschr., 1(29):595, Oct. 18, 1888.

1503. WEICHSELBAUM, A. Ueber seltenere Localisationen des pneumonischen Virus (Diplococcus pneumoniae). Wien. klin. Wchnschr., 1(30):620, Oct. 25, 1888. 226

1504. Weichselbaum, A. Ueber seltenere Localisationen des pneumonischen Virus (Diplococcus pneumoniae). Wien. klin. Wchnschr., 1(31):642, Nov. 1, 1888. 226

1505. Weichselbaum, A. Ueber seltenere Localisationen des pneumonischen Virus (Diplococcus pneumoniae). Wien. klin. Wchnschr., 1(32):659, Nov. 8, 1888. 226

1506. Weigert, C. Zur Technik der mikroskopischen Bakterienuntersuchungen. Virchows Arch. f. path. Anat., 84(2):275, May 1881. 32

1507. Weil, R. Note on a skin reaction in pneumonia. J. Exper. Med., 23(1):11, Jan. 1916. 461

1508. Weil, R., and Torrey, J. C. Immunological studies in pneumonia. J. Exper. Med., 23(1):1, Jan. 1916. 449

1509. Weiss, C. The properties of pneumotoxin and its probable function in the pathology of lobar pneumonia. Studies in pneumonia. IX. J. Med. Research, 39(1):103, Sept. 1918. .... 84, 96

1510. Weiss, C., and Kolmer, J. A. Studies in pneumonia. VIII. A skin reaction to pneumotoxin. J. Immunol., 3(5):395, Sept. 1918. 461

1511. Weiss, C., and Kolmer, J. A. A skin reaction to pneumotoxin. Proc. Path. Soc., Philadelphia, 21, n.s.:10, 1919.

1512. Welch, W. H. The Micrococcus lanceolatus, with special reference to the etiology of acute lobar pneumonia. Bull. Johns Hopkins Hosp., 3(27):125, Dec. 1892.

1513. Welikanow, I., und Michailowa, S. Vergärung von Kohlehydraten durch Pneumokokken als Kennzeichen ihrer Avirulenz. 2. Mitteilung. Zentralbl. f. Bakt., 1 Abt., Orig., 117(4/5):219, June 1930. 201

1514. Westlund, R. E. The incidence of pneumococcus types in pneumonias of children. J. Infect. Dis., 38(6):514, June 1926.

1515. Wherry, W. B. Action of ammonia on pneumococcus and mechanism of capsule staining. J. Infect. Dis., 34(2):124, Feb. 1924. 34

1516. Whitehead, N. T. Some investigations on thirty-five cases of pneumonia in Khartoum. J. Roy. Army M. Corps, 49(6):440, Dec. 1927.

1517. Whittle, C. H. The virulence of pneumococci in pneumonia. Brit. M. J., 2(3472):134, July 23, 1927.

1518. Whittle, C. H. On the identification of pneumococci and the tests employed for distinguishing them from streptococci. J. Hyg., 27(2):200, Jan. 1928.

1519. Whittle, C. H. The relation of virulence in pneumococci to disease, with a comparison of virulence of the different types of pneumococci in various pathological conditions. J. Hyg., 27(4):412, June 1928. 198

1519a. Widal, Lemierre, et Gadaud. Recherche du pneumocoque dans le sang des pneumoniques. Bull. et mém. Soc. méd. des Hôp. de Paris, 20, 3e sér.:415, 1903.

1519b. Widowitz, P. Ein Beitrag zur Pathogenität des Pneumokokkus bei metapneumonischen Erkrankungen in frühesten Kindesalter. Arch. f. Kinderh., 70(4):246, 1922.

1520. Wilke, W. Versuche über Gram-Festigkeit von Pneumokokken und Diphtheriebazillen. Zentralbl. f. Bakt., 1 Abt., Orig., 113 (3/4):262, July 1929. 31

1521. Winkler, A. W., and Finland, M. Antibody response to infections with the newly classified types of pneumococci (Cooper). J. Clin. Investigation, 13(1):109, Jan. 1934.

1521a. Winternitz, M. C., and Hirschfelder, A. D. Studies upon experimental pneumonia in rabbits. J. Exper. Med., 17(6):657, June 1913.

1522. Winternitz, M. C., and Kline, B. S. Studies upon experimental pneumonia in rabbits. IX. The part of the leucocyte in the immunity reaction. J. Exper. Med., 21(4):320, Apr. 1915. 402

1523. Wirth, E. Zur Kenntnis der Streptokokken. Centralbl. f. Bakt., 1 Abt., Orig., 99(4/5):266, Aug. 1926. 175

1524. Wirth, E. Die Pneumokokkentypen in der Oto-Rhinologie. Centralbl. f. Bakt., 1 Abt., Orig., 102(1/3):40, Mar. 1927. 106

1525. Wisner, B. Epidémie de pneumococcie, chez les singes inférieurs, arrêtée par la vaccination préventive. Compt. rend. Soc. de biol., 98(5):458, Feb. 10, 1928. 483

1526. Witebsky, E., Neter, E., and Sobotka, H. The relation between the type-specific carbohydrates of pneumococci and the blood group specific substance A. J. Exper. Med., 61(5):703, May 1935. 287, 288

1527. Witebsky, E., and Satoh, T. Zur Frage des Blutgruppenferments und der Ausscheidung von Blutgruppensubstanz. Klin. Wchnschr., 12(24):948, June 17, 1933. 288

1528. Wolf, S. Ein Beitrag zur Aetiologie der circumscripten Meningitis. Berl. klin. Wchnschr., 34(10):200, Mar. 8, 1897.

1529. Wolf, W. Der Nachweis der Pneumoniebacterien in Sputum. Wien. med. Bl., 10(10):295, Mar. 10, 1887. 18

1530. Wolf, W. Der Nachweis der Pneumoniebacterien in Sputum. Wien. med. Bl., 10(11):333, Mar. 17, 1887.

1531. Wolf, W. Der Nachweis der Pneumoniebacterien in Sputum. Wien. med. Bl., 10(12):366, Mar. 24, 1887.

1532. Wolf, W. Der Nachweis der Pneumoniebacterien in Sputum. Wien. med. Bl., 10(13):402, Mar. 31, 1887.

1533. Wolf, W. Der Nachweis der Pneumoniebacterien in Sputum. Wien. med. Bl., 10(14):434, Apr. 7, 1887.

1534. Wolff, E. K. Untersuchungen über die Strepto-Pneumokokken in ihren Beziehungen zueinander und zum Wirtsorganismus. Virchows Arch. f. path. Anat., 244:97, July 1923. 172

1535. Wollman, E., et Aberbuch, M. Lyse biliaire des pneumocoques. Transmission à des souches normalement non solubles. Application au diagnostic différentiel du pneumocoque. Bull. Acad. de méd., Paris, 107(4):126, Jan. 26, 1932. 61

1536. Wollman, E., et Averbusch, M. Transmission de la lyse biliaire des Pneumocoques à des formes de ces germes insolubles dans la bile. Compt. rend. Soc. de biol., 110(22):623, June 27, 1932. 61

1537. WOLLSTEIN, M. Types of pneumococci found in pneumonia of infants and young children. New York State J. Med., 23(4): 148, Apr. 1923.

1538. WOLLSTEIN, M., and BENSON, A. W. Types of pneumococcus found in the pneumonias of infants and young children. Am. J. Dis. Child., 12(3):254, Sept. 1916.

1539. WOLLSTEIN, M., and MELTZER, S. J. Pneumonic lesions made by intrabronchial insufflation of non-virulent pneumococci. J. Exper. Med., 17(3):353, Mar. 1913. 194

1540. WOLLSTEIN, M., and MELTZER, S. J. The reaction of the lungs to the intrabronchial insufflation of killed virulent pneumococci and of plain sterile bouillon. J. Exper. Med., 17(4):424, Apr. 1913. 194

1541. WOO, S. T. Studies on pneumoçoccus growth inhibition. V. The relation of virulence to the pneumococcidal activity of normal rabbit serum-leucocyte mixtures. J. Exper. Med., 43(5):623, May 1926. .... 396, 430

1542. WOOD, F. C. The viability of the pneumococcus after drying: A study of one of the factors in pneumonic infection. J. Exper. Med., 7(5):592, Aug. 1905. 51

1543. WRIGHT, A. E., MORGAN, W. P., COLEBROOK, L., and DODGSON, R. W. Observations on the pharmacɔ-therapy of pneumococcus infections. Lancet, 2(4659):1633, Dec. 14, 1912. .... 483, 512

1544. WRIGHT, A. E., MORGAN, W. P., COLEBROOK, L., and DODGSON, R. W. Observations on the pharmaco-therapy of pneumococcus infections. Lancet, 2(4660):1701, Dec. 21, 1912. .... 483, 512

1545. WRIGHT, A. E., MORGAN, W. P., COLEBROOK, L., and DODGSON, R. W. Observations on prophylactic inoculation against pneumococcus infections, and on the results which have been achieved by it. Lancet, 1(4714):1, Jañ. 3, 1914. 483

1546. WRIGHT, A. E., MORGAN, W. P., COLEBROOK, L., and DODGSON, R. W. Observations on prophylactic inoculation against pneumococcus infections, and on the results which have been achieved by it. Lancet, 1(4715):87, Jan. 10, 1914. 483

1547. WRIGHT, H. D. Experimental pneumococcal septicaemia and antipneumococcal immunity. J. Path. & Bact., 30(2):185, Apr. 1927. .... 393, 396, 406, 430

1548. WRIGHT, H. D. The effect of certain factors upon the growth of the pneumococcus. J. Path. & Bact., 32(2):203, Apr. 1929. ... 38, 39

1549. WRIGHT, H. D. The importance of adequate reduction of peptone in the preparation of media for the pneumococcus and other organisms. J. Path. & Bact., 37(2):257, Sept. 1933. 38

1550. WRIGHT, H. D. The preparation of nutrient agar with special references to pneumococci, streptococci and other Gram-positive organisms. J. Path. & Bact., 39(2):359, Sept. 1934.

1551. WU, C. J., and SIA, R. H. P. A simplified technique for the study of pneumococcus growth inhibition. Proc. Soc. Exper. Biol. & Med., 29(7):786, Apr. 1932.

1552. WU, C. J., and ZIA, S. H. The incidence of the newer types (Cooper) of pneumococcus in Peiping. Proc. Soc. Exper. Biol. & Med., 34(5):654, June 1936. 117

1553. WU, H., and YEN, D. Studies of denaturation of proteins. I. Some new observations concerning the effects of dilute acids and alkalies on proteins. J. Biochem., 4(2):345, Oct. 1924. 560

1554. WURTZ, et MOSNY. De la réaction acide des cultures du pneumocoque. Compt. rend. Soc. de biol., 46:71, Jan. 27, 1894. 39

1555. WYCKOFF, R. W. G. The ultracentrifugal concentration of pneumococcic antibodies. Science, 84(2178):291, Sept. 25, 1936. 414, 415, 556

1556. YAMAGUTI, K. Untersuchungen über die "grünen Kokken." Beitrag zur Bakteriologie der Mundhöhle. Centralbl. f. Bakt., 1 Abt., Orig., 90(5):345, June 1923.

1557. YAMAMOTO, S. Ueber den biologischen Unterschied zwischen nativem und gekochtem Antigen von Pneumokokken. III. Mitteilung. Toxizität von Normalkulturfiltrat (NF), gekochtem Kulturfiltrat (FK) und der für die Immunisierung der Tiere verwendeten Standardvakzine der Pneumokokken. Zentralbl. f. Bakt., 1 Abt., Orig., 110(4/5):151, Jan. 11, 1929. .... 98, 399

1558. YAMAMOTO, S. Ueber den biologischen Unterschied zwischen nativem und gekochtem Antigen von Pneumokokken. IV. Mitteilung: Impedinerscheinung der spontanen Phagozytose der Pneumokokken unter Mitwirkung von nativem Kulturfiltrat (NF) und gekochten Filtraten (FK) gleichnamiger Erreger. Zentralbl. f. Bakt., 1 Abt., Orig., 110(4/5):156, Jan. 11, 1929. 399

1559. YEN, A. C. H., and KUROTCHKIN, T. J. The preparation of specific bacterial carbohydrate substances by electrolysis. J. Infect. Dis., 56(3):238, May–June 1935. 260

1560. YOSHIOKA, M. Beiträge zur Pneumokokkenimmunität. I. Mitteilung. Über die Spezifität der Pneumokokkentypen und über die Grenzen dieser Spezifität. Ztschr. f. Hyg. u. Infektionskr., 96 (4):520, Oct. 1922. 112

1561. YOSHIOKA, M. Untersuchungen über Pneumokokkenimmunität. III. Mitteilung. Versuche über Schutzimpfung von Mäusen (Meerschweinchen und Kaninchen). Ztschr. f. Hyg. u. Infektionskr., 97(3/4):386, Jan. 1923. .... 112, 408

1562. YOSHIOKA, M. Beiträge zur Pneumokokkenimmunität. IV. Mitteilung. Über die Gewinnung von Antipneumo- und Antistreptokokkenserum von Kaninchen. Ztschr. f. Hyg. u. Infektionskr., 97 (3/4):408, Jan. 1923. .... 330, 536

1563. YOSHIOKA, M. Untersuchungen zur Pneumokokkenimmunität. V. Mitteilung. Beitrag zur Frage der Wertbestimmung von Pneumo- und Streptokokkensera. Ztschr. f. Hyg. u. Infektionskr., 99(2):193, Mar. 1923.

1564. YOSHIOKA, M. Untersuchungen über Pneumokokkenimmunität.

II. Mitteilung. Veränderungen der Agglutination bei Pneumokokken des Typhus I, II und III und bei Streptokokken. Ztschr. f. Hyg. u. Infektionskr., 97(1/2):232, Nov. 1923. .... 104, 139, 362

1565. Yoshioka, M. A study on the immunization against pneumococcus. Japan M. World, 5(2):23, Feb. 15, 1925. .... 525, 536

1566. Yourevitch, V. Culture latente pour la conservation des pneumocoques et d'autres microbes au point de vue de leur vitalité et de leur virulence. Compt. rend. Soc. de biol., 103(5):320, Feb. 7, 1930. 49

1567. Yu, I. Beitrag zur Differenzierung der Pneumokokken. Centralbl. f. Bakt., 1 Abt., Orig., 90(5):322, June 1923. .... 110, 112

1568. Zaufal, E. Mikroorganismen im Secrete der Otitis media acuta. Prag. med. Wchnschr., 12(27):225, July 6, 1887. .... 20, 226

1569. Zaufal, E. Weitere Mittheilung über das Vorkommen von mikroorganismen im Secrete der Otitis media acuta (genuina). Prag. med. Wchnschr., 13(8):61, Feb. 22, 1888. .... 20, 226

1570. Ziegler, E. E. The specific effect of bile salts on pneumococci and pneumococcus pneumonia. Arch. Int. Med., 46(4):644, Oct. 1930. .... 57, 508

1571. Ziegler, E. E. Sodium dehydrocholate. Its specific effect on pneumococci. II. J. Lab. & Clin. Med., 16(8):868, May 1931. .... 58, 508

1572. Ziegler, E. E. The effects on pneumococci of sodium dehydrocholate, a bile salt derivative. III. J. Lab. & Clin. Med., 17(4): 317, Jan. 1932. 58

1573. Ziegler, E. E. Some properties of pneumocholin, a biochemical antigen. J. Lab. & Clin. Med., 18(7):695, Apr. 1933. .... 334, 483

1574. Ziehl, F. Ueber das Vorkommen der Pneumoniekokken im pneumonischen Sputum. Centralbl. f. d. med. Wissensch., 21(25): 433, June 1883. 9

1575. Zinsser, H. Studies on the tuberculin reaction and on specific hypersensitiveness in bacterial infection. J. Exper. Med., 34(5): 495, Nov. 1921. 241

1576. Zinsser, H. The study of immunity in its relation to the problem of practical medicine. Boston M. & S. J., 192(25):1191, June 18, 1925.

1577. Zinsser, H. An immunological consideration of pneumonia and a discussion of the rational basis for vaccine therapy. New England J. Med., 200(17):853, Apr. 25, 1929.

1578. Zinsser, H. Note on the quantitative relations of antigen and antibody in agglutination and precipitation reactions. J. Immunol., 18(6):483, June 1930. 367

1579. Zinsser, H., and Bayne-Jones, S. A textbook of bacteriology. 7th ed. New York: D. Appleton-Century Company, 1934. 30, 32, 34, 35, 36, 46, 47, 627, 628

1580. Zinsser, H., and Grinnell, F. B. Blood clot method of immunization with observations on pneumococcus toxemia. Proc. Soc. Exper. Biol. & Med., 23(3):205, Dec. 1925. 534

1581. ZINSSER, H., and GRINNELL, F. B. Further studies on bacterial allergy. The antigens involved in pneumococcus allergy. J. Bact., 14(5):301, Nov. 1927. 456
1582. ZINSSER, H., and MALLORY, T. B. Observations on bacterial anaphylaxis with pneumococcus. J. Immunol., 9(2):75, Mar. 1924. 449
1583. ZINSSER, H., and PARKER, J. T. Further studies on bacterial hypersusceptibility. II. J. Exper. Med., 37(2):275, Feb. 1923. ... 241
1584. ZINSSER, H., and TAMIYA, T. Studies on the antigenic substance of the bacterial cell. J. Exper. Med., 42(3):311, Sept. 1925. 242
1585. ZOZAYA, J. Combination of bacterial polysaccharides and collodion particles as antigens. Science, 74(1915):270, Sept. 11, 1931.
1586. ZOZAYA, J. Fermentation of "levan" by pneumococci. Proc. Soc. Exper. Biol. & Med., 29(1):26, Oct. 1931. 70
1587. ZOZAYA, J. Carbohydrates adsorbed on colloids as antigens. J. Exper. Med., 55(3):325, Mar. 1932.
1588. ZOZAYA, J. Immunological reactions between dextran polysaccharide and some bacterial antisera. J. Exper. Med., 55(3):353, Mar. 1932. 261
1589. ZOZAYA, J., BOYER, J., and CLARK, J. The standardization of antipneumococcic serum Types I and II. J. Exper. Med., 52(4): 471, Oct. 1930. 583
1590. ZOZAYA, J., and CLARK, J. Active immunization in human cases with the polysaccharide of pneumococcus Type I. Proc. Soc. Exper. Biol. & Med., 30(1):44, Oct. 1932. .... 276, 345
1591. ZOZAYA, J., and CLARK, J. Active immunization of mice with the polysaccharides of pneumococci Types I, II, and III. J. Exper. Med., 57(1):21, Jan. 1933.
1592. ZOZAYA, J., and MEDINA, L. Adsorption isotherms of some bacterial polysaccharides. Proc. Soc. Exper. Biol. & Med., 30(1):47, Oct. 1932.
1593. ZOZAYA, J., and MEDINA, L. Immunological reactions between agar-agar and some bacterial antisera. J. Exper. Med., 57(1):41, Jan. 1933.

INDEX

A substance, blood-group specific, in relation to capsular polysaccharide, 287–288
A substance of Pneumococcus
as antiopsonin, 400
comparison with acetyl polysaccharides, 285
effect of alkali, 277
in anaphylaxis, 450
in lung filtrate, 268
interaction with immune serum, 269
isolation, 265
properties, 266–268
Abscesses, Pneumococcus in, 19, 20
Accessory substances. *See* Growth of Pneumococcus
Acetic acid in carbohydrate fermentation, 71
Acetyl carbohydrate-azoproteins, antigenicity, 285
Acetyl group
instability, 279
relation to immunological activity of Pneumococcus, 278–288
Acetyl polysaccharide(s), 277–288
A substance of Pneumococcus compared with, 285
analyses, 281
antigenicity, 283
excretion in urine, 284
in precipitation, 371
protective antibodies induced by, 411
uronic acid in, 280
Acid(s). *See* Acid formation by Pneumococcus; Agglutination; Bile solubility; Carbohydrate fermentation by Pneumococcus; Chemotherapy
Acid formation by Pneumococcus
acetic acid, 71
effect of serum on, 71
formic acid, 71
from dextrose, 70
from galactose, 70
Acid formation by Pneumococcus (*cont.*):
from glucose, 71
from inulin, 70
from lactose, 70
from maltose, 70
from raffinose, 70
from saccharose, 70
lactic acid, 70–71
Active immunity to Pneumococcus. *See* Immunization, active
Agglutination
acid, 109, 110
as potency test, 582
culture, 123
early observations, 24, 25, 27
in serological classification, 26, 103–118, 359–360, 361–362
of variants, 140, 362–363
quantitative determination, 367
slide, in type determination, 127–131
technique, 641
See also Agglutinins
Agglutinin-absorption in serological classification, 110, 111, 362
Agglutinins, 355–364
chemical nature, 364
early observations, 356
effect of alien infection, 363
identity with precipitin, 367
in blood of animals, 363–364
in blood of pneumonia patients, 357–361
in empyema fluids, 441
in lobar pneumonia, 438
in swine serum, 431, 432
natural, 423, 436
opsonins, relation to, 431
preservation, 357
See also Agglutination
Alcohol, effect on resistance, 190
Aldobionic acid
capsular polysaccharide, as constituent, 245, 246

Aldobionic acid (*cont.*):
in cultivation of SIII bacillus, 308
in precipitation, 375
Alkaligenes viscosus, immunological relation to Type I, 262
Allergy
actively induced, 447–449
dermal, 455–474
in experimental infection, 448
ophthalmic reactions. *See* Ophthalmic reactions
passive sensitization, 449–454
relation to immunity, 454–455
See also Skin reactions
Alveolar exudate, Pneumococcus in, 6
American Drug Manufacturers' Association, potency test, 570, 651–653
Amino group in precipitation, 377
Amoss' method of type determination, 129–130
Amylase in Pneumococcus, 67
Anaerobic strains of Pneumococcus, 44, 116
Anaphylaxis
A carbohydrate, 450
capsular polysaccharide, 255, 448, 449, 454
cellular carbohydrate, 270, 451, 454
conjugated carbohydrate-proteins, 264
gluco-globulins, 450, 452, 453
nucleoprotein, 451
passive sensitization, 452–453
Type VIII polysaccharide, 275
Animal host. *See* Host response; Pathogenicity of Pneumococcus
Animal inoculation and transformation of type, 158–160
Animals, experimental. *See* Pathogenicity of Pneumococcus; Skin reactions; and under particular animal
Antiblastic immunity, 420–421
Antibodies to Pneumococcus, 355–426, 436–442, 619
Antibodies to Pneumococcus (*cont.*):
agglutinins, 355–364
antihemotoxin, 382–383
antiopsonins, 398–401
antiphagins, 398
antitoxins, 383–386
bactericidins, 382
complement-fixing, 380–382
heterophile, 387–388
in blood during pneumonia, 437–442
molecular weight, 415–418
nature, 23, 364, 411–418
phagocytosis, 388–406
precipitins, 365–379
protective. *See* Protective antibodies to Pneumococcus
unsolved problems, 619–620
Antigen-antibody balance in lobar pneumonia, 360
Antigen-antibody solution, 408, 413, 418, 547
Antigenicity
and virulence, 25, 524–526
of Pneumococcus, 323–354
of polysaccharides. *See* Polysaccharides
of protein fractions. *See* Protein fraction(s)
of purpura-producing principle, 89
of rough and smooth forms of pneumococci, 150, 342, 344
of toxins, 93, 97, 338–340
See also Antigens
Antigens
administered by buccal membrane, 347
administered by inhalation, 341, 346, 348
administered by injection, 341, 342, 343–346, 347
administered by intrabronchial insufflation, 343–348
administered by intraocular instillation, 347
administered by oral route, 348–351
antivirus, 336–337, 346
bacterial extracts, 335

Antigens (*cont.*):
concentration, 21, 22
culture filtrates, 21, 22, 23, 24, 25, 27, 335–337, 526–527
cultures devitalized
by alcohol and ether, 333, 530
by antiformin, 333
by bile salts, 334
by formalin, 331–332, 531–532
by formol, 333
by heat, 327–331, 333, 530, 531, 532
by phenol, 530
by sodium choleate, 334
by sodium ricinoleate, 334
by sodium taurocholate, 334
egg white as adjuvant to, 348
exudates, 337–338, 527
fat-free, 338
glycerol extracts, 21, 25, 530
hemotoxins, 340
host response, 351, 427–478
injections in antipneumococcic serum production, 533–540
living organisms, 528–529
methods of administering, 340–351
pancreatic extracts, 335
Pneumocholin, 334, 483
polysaccharides, 251, 255, 283, 290, 292, 344–345, 349, 448
residue, 241
rough and smooth strains, 130, 328, 344
sensitized pneumococci, 335
sputum, 21
standardization, 331, 532–533
synthetic, 411
tissue extracts, 337–338
toxins, 93, 95, 338–340
virulence of cultures, 25, 326–327, 524–526
Antihemotoxin(s). *See* Antitoxin
Antiopsonins
A substance, 400–401
antiphagin, 398
capsular polysaccharide, 399, 400
Impedin, 399
Antipneumococcic serum, production, 522–597
antigens, selection and standardization. *See* Antigens
avian, 545
bleedings, 540–543
period of immunization prior to, 540–542
blood, amount drawn, 542
bottling, 596
bulk sterility and potency tests, 590
chill-producing factors, 559–563
definition of unit, 586
desiccation, 559
diagnostic serum, 592–596, 663–664
dispensing and labeling, 590–591
filtration, 589
final processing, 589–592
from asses, 522
from cows, 522
from goats, 522
from horses. *See* Horse(s)
from rabbits. *See* Rabbit(s)
governmental regulation, 591
British Statutory Rules and Orders, 592
British Therapeutic Substances Act, 592
National Institute of Health, 567, 592
United States Hygienic Laboratory, 567
identity and safety tests, 591
in vitro tests, 580–584
injections of antigen, 533–540
dosage, 534–535
reactions of horse, 538–540
route, 533–534
spacing of doses, 535–538
inorganic solids, 556–557
labeling, 590–591, 596
methods of concentration, biological, 547–548
methods of concentration, chemical, 548–556
alcohol precipitation, 553–554
ammonium sulfate, 548–549
carbon dioxide, 553

Antipneumococcic serum (*cont.*):
methods of concentration (*cont.*):
dialysis, 550
dilution with water, 550–553
dissociation of specific precipitate, 554
metallic salts, 555
sodium chloride, 553
sodium sulfate, 549–550
ultracentrifugation, 556
ultrafiltration, 555
unsolved problems, 620–621
mouse protection test. *See* Potency tests
period of immunization prior to bleeding, 540–542
physical properties, 556–559
polyvalent serum, 545–547
potency tests. *See* Potency tests
preservatives, 557–559, 588–589, 596
reaction of the product, 557
records, 591
safety tests, 587–589, 591
sterility tests on final containers, 591
therapeutic tests, 576–580
total solids, 556, 589
unconcentrated vs. concentrated, 543–545
unit defined, 28, 568, 586–587
yield of serum, 542–543
Anti-R bodies
in swine serum, 155
Anti-R serum, effect on variants, 154
Antitoxin(s), 85, 86, 96, 99, 339–340, 383–386, 561, 579
antihemotoxin, 85, 382–383
potency tests on, 579, 581
Antivirus
as antigen, 336–337, 346
effect on virulence of Pneumococcus, 337
Appendicitis, Pneumococcus in, 226
Aromatic amines, peroxide formation, 74
Arthritis, Pneumococcus in, 226
Ass(es), immune serum from, 27, 522
Aureola. *See* Capsule of Pneumococcus
Autolysates
lung-toxic principles, 98
necrotizing principle, 92–93, 98
skin reactions to, 456, 461, 462, 466
source of A substance, 265
toxic action, 94, 97, 98
virulence enhanced by, 202–203
See also Autolysis of Pneumococcus
Autolyse transmissible, 61
Autolysis of Pneumococcus, 52–55
and bile solubility, 60–62
effect of hydrogen peroxide, 78
enzymes, 54
hydrogen ion concentration and, 53
in relation to hemolysis, 86
prevention by serum, 53
temperature, 53
Automatic transfer device
in cultivation of Pneumococcus, 41
increase in virulence of cultures, 204
Auto-oxidation, effect on hemotoxin, 84
Avery's method of type determination, 123
Avian serum, 545
chill-production, 562
protective antibodies in, 410

Bacillus acidophilus, peroxide formation by, 75
Bacillus aerogenes, polysaccharide in, 262
Bacillus bulgaricus, peroxide formation by, 75
Bacillus coli
polysaccharide in, 262
relation to Pneumococcus, 261
Bacillus friedländeri, 12, 13, 18, 20
and Pneumococcus, differentiation, 17
capsular polysaccharides, 246, 260, 262
classification, 260
in lobar pneumonia, 217

Bacillus influenzae, in lobar pneumonia, 217
Bacillus mesentericus, levan from, 70
Bacillus palustris, 320
Bacillus palustris gelacticus, 319
Bacillus pneumoniae, 18
Bacillus salivarius septicus, 1, 20
Bacillus septicus sputigenus, 1
Bacillus subtilis
dissociation, 154
levan from, 70
Bacillus tuberculosis, polysaccharide of, 262
Bacillus typhi murium, as complicating factor in mouse tests, 190
Bacillus vulgatus, effect on Friedländer polysaccharide, 302
Bacteria-producing polysaccharide-splitting enzymes. *See* Enzymes, polysaccharide-splitting
Bacterial extracts, as antigens, 335–337
Bactericidal tests
for potency of serum, 581
serological reactions, 647–648
Bactericidins. *See* Pneumococcidins
Bacteriophage in dissociation, 150
Bacterium pneumoniae, 1
Bile. *See* Bile solubility; Chemotherapy
Bile salts and purpura-producing principle, 90
Bile solubility, 55–62
and autolysis, 60–62
and virulence, 56
apocholic acid, 58
bile-acid salts, 60
cholic acid, 58
dehydrocholic acid, 58
dehydro-oxycholic acid, 58
desoxycholic acid, 58
electrolytes, effect, 59
glycocholate, 55
glycocholic acid, 58
hypocholate, 55
inhibition, 60
non-electrolytes, effect, 59
Bile solubility (*cont.*):
Pneumococcus mucosus, 56, 57
quinolate, 55
rabbit bile, 55
sensitization by ascitic fluid, blood, cholesterol, pleural fluid, 60
sodium cholate, 55
sodium dehydrocholate, 58
sodium taurocholate, 60
sputum, in type determination, 126–127
Streptococcus mucosus, 56
taurocholate, 55
taurocholic acid, 58
unsaturated fatty acids, 58
variants, 140–141, 149
virulence and, 56
Biochemical features of Pneumococcus, 65–102
Biology of Pneumococcus, 30–64
Birds
natural immunity, 341, 428
susceptibility to Pneumococcus, 196
Blake's method of type determination, 122
Blood
agglutinins, 357–361, 363–367
antibodies in blood during pneumonia, 437–442
as accessory substance in promoting growth, 42
Pneumococcus in, 7, 8
precipitin in, in type determination, 125, 365–379
Blood agar as differential medium, 48
Blood cells, susceptibility to hemolysin, 85
Blood cultures
in pneumonia, 227–229
technique, 628
Blood-group specific substance A, relation to capsular polysaccharide, 287–288
Blood-optochin agar, laked, as differential medium, 48
Blood platelets as affected by purpura, 88

Bottling antipneumococcic serum, 596
British Statutory Rules and Orders, 592
British Therapeutic Substances Act, 592
Bronchopneumonia, pneumococcal types, 219–221
Broth. *See* Media
Bulk sterility and potency tests in antipneumococcic serum production, 590

C Fraction of Pneumococcus
compared to non-specific IV carbohydrate, 258
in non-type-specific R strain, 258
isolation, 256–258, 295, 636–637
precipitin reaction, 368–370, 441
precipitins in lobar pneumonia, 441
properties, 257
relation to non-protein fraction of Gonococcus, 248
relation to purpura, 257
skin reactions to, 464, 465, 471, 472
Type IV, 257
type-specificity, 257
Capsular polysaccharide(s) of Pneumococcus
acetyl group in, 277–288
administration by mouth, 349
aldobionic acid in, 245, 246
anaphylaxis, 255, 448–449, 450, 454
antagonistic action, 351–353
antigenicity, 251, 252
as antiopsonins, 399, 400
as precipitinogen in urine, 123–124, 363–365, 366, 370, 373
B. friedländeri compared with, 246, 260, 262
blood-group specific A substance, 287–288
carbohydrates from other sources, 258–263
effect of alkali and of acid upon, 295
excretion, 350
first description, 243–252
galacturonic acid in, 246

Capsular polysaccharide(s) of Pneumococcus (*cont.*):
glucose, 246
immunological behavior, 255
in agglutination, 364
injection, intradermal, 344–346
methods of preparation, 244, 288–296, 623–625, 634
microdetermination, 374
ophthalmic reaction, 457–458
optical rotation, 246, 254, 255, 257, 274, 281, 291, 292, 293
physicochemical properties, 296–297
properties, 246, 247
protective antibodies induced by, 411
relation to gonococcal polysaccharide, 248
skin reaction, 460, 463, 464, 466, 473
soluble specific substance, 243, 266, 269
thermostability, 294
Type I, 245
Type II, 244, 245
Type III, 244, 245
Type IV, 257–259
Type VIII, 274, 275
uronic acid in, 346
viscosity of, 297
See also Enzymes, polysaccharide-splitting
Capsule of Pneumococcus, 3, 6, 7, 11, 14, 31, 32–35
mucin in, 3, 7, 33, 239
stains, 33–35
substances favoring development, 35
variation during propagation, 7
Carbohydrate fermentation by Pneumococcus, 67–70
acetic acid, formation, 71
alcohols, 70
amylase, 67
arabinose, 70
dextran, 70
dulcitol, 70
erythritol, 70
exhaustion of carbohydrate, 70
formic acid, formation, 71

Carbohydrate fermentation by Pneumococcus (*cont.*):
galactose, 70
glucose, 67, 70
glycerol, 70
glycogen, 69
glycol, 70
inulase, 67
inulin, 47, 67, 68–69
invertase, 67
lactase, 68
lactic acid formation, 70
lactose, 68
levan, 70
levulose, 70
maltase, 67
maltose, 68
mannitol, 70
raffinase, 68
salicin, 70
sorbitol, 70
starch, 67
sucrose, 67
trehalose, 70
xylose, 70
Carbohydrate fractions of Pneumococcus
of Perlzweig and Steffen, 254–255
of Saito and Caspar, 254–255
of Schiemann and Caspar, 254–255
See also A substance; Acetyl polysaccharide(s); C Fraction; Capsular polysaccharide(s); Carbohydrates, cellular
Carbohydrate-proteins. *See* Conjugated carbohydrate-proteins
Carbohydrates. *See* Capsular polysaccharide(s); Carbohydrate fermentation by Pneumococcus; Carbohydrate fractions; Carbohydrates, cellular; Conjugated carbohydrate-proteins; Polysaccharide(s)
Carbohydrates, cellular, 269–275
absorption spectra, 273
anaphylaxis, 270, 272, 275, 451
antigenicity, 270, 272
comparison of types, 273–274
micro-analysis, 272
Carbohydrates, cellular (*cont.*):
purification of, 275
purpurigenic action, 90, 91, 274
skin reactions, 465, 466
Type I, 269–272
Type II, 271–272
Type III, 271–272
Type VIII, 273
Carboxyl groups in precipitation, 377
Carriers of Pneumococcus, 215, 230–236
classification of carriers, 235–236
frequency of pneumococcal types, 232–235
guinea pigs, 186
mice, 189
monkeys, 192
rabbits, 179
Cat(s)
lobar pneumonia in, 193
susceptibility to Pneumococcus, 193
Catalase, effect on peroxide, 76
Cebus capucinus, 192, 193
Cellular carbohydrates. *See* Carbohydrates, cellular
Ceropithecus callitrichus, 192
Charcoal, effect in dissociation, 144
Chemical agents in chemotherapy other than cinchona derivatives, 508–511
Chemical constituents of Pneumococcus, 238–300
fat, 239
non-polysaccharide, probably non-protein derivative, 275
unidentified constituent of pneumococcal cell, 275
unsolved problems, 615–616
See also A substance; Capsular polysaccharide(s); Carbohydrates, cellular; Conjugated carbohydrate-proteins; Isolation; Mucin; Protein fraction(s)
Chemotherapy, 507–521
bile, 508–509
salts of bile acids, 508
sodium dehydrocholate, 508
sodium glycocholate, 508
sodium taurocholate, 508

Chemotherapy (*cont.*):
cinchona derivatives, 512–520
action, adjuvant, with specific serum, 518–519
action, toxic, of some drugs, 517
alpha-isoquinine, 516
apocupreine hydrochloride, 517
beta-isoquinine, 516
dermal pneumonia in rabbits, 516
effect on virulence of Pneumococcus, 519–520
ethylapoquinine, 516, 517
ethylhydrocupreine. *See* Optochin
hydroethylapoquinine, 516
hydroquinine derivatives, 513
hydroxyethylhydrocupreine, 516, 517
isopropylhydrocupreine, 512
methylhydrocupreine, 512
optochin. *See* Optochin
pneumococcidal potency of optochin compared to antipneumococcic serum, 512, 515, 519
quinine, 512, 515
hydrochloride, 516
sulfate, 519
coal-tar dyes, 509–510
acriflavine, 509
application, 510
aurophosphines, 510
brilliant green, 510
crystal violet, 510
3–6 diamino-acridine, 510
flavines, 509
Mercurochrome, 510
trimethanes, 510
triphenylmethanes, 509
trypaflavine, 510
drug-fastness of Pneumococcus, 519–520
drugs, susceptibility of Pneumococcus, 520
medicinal agents, various, 511
camphor, 511
epinephrine, 511
formaldehyde sulfoxylate, 511
hexamethyltetramine, 511

Chemotherapy (*cont.*):
medicinal agents (*cont.*):
potassium permanganate, 511
sodium salicylate, 511
Urotropin, 511
metals and metallic salts, 510–511
colloidal gold, 510
gold as synergist, 510
iodine, 511
Sanocrysin, 510
Metaphen, 510
soaps, 509
lauric acid, 509
sodium oleate, adjuvant action of, on immune serum, 509
sodium ricinoleate, 509
unsolved problems, 618
urea hydrochloride, 516
vuzine, 512, 515
Chill-producing factors in antipneumococcic serum, 559–563
acid fraction, 562–563
in avian serum, 545, 562
tests for, 564–565
Chitin, relation to pneumococcal polysaccharides, 259
Cholecystitis, Pneumococcus in, 226
Cholesterol, effect on hemolysin, 83, 84
Cinchona derivatives. *See* Chemotherapy
Clasmatocytes in natural immunity, 432
Classification of Pneumococcus. *See* Electrophoretic potential; Serological classification
Coal-tar dyes. *See* Chemotherapy
Coccus lancéolé de la pneumonie, 1, 9
Colony formation of Pneumococcus, 46, 47, 48
in dissociation, 147–150, 152–154
nail form, 6, 7, 8, 11
Combining equivalents, precipitation tests, 645–647
Complement fixation
antibodies, 380–382
as potency test, 581

Complement fixation (*cont.*):
in serological classification, 110
technique, 647
Conjugated carbohydrate-proteins, immunological behavior, 263–265, 284–285, 448, 450, 453
Conjunctivitis, Pneumococcus in, 226, 227
Convalescent serum in treatment of pneumonia, 446
Cooper's serological classification, 113–115
Cow(s), immune serum from, 27, 522
Cross-agglutination in serological classification, 112
Cultivation of Pneumococcus. *See* Growth of Pneumococcus; Media
Culture filtrates as antigens, 21, 22, 23, 24, 25, 27, 335–337, 526–527
Cultures. *See* Dissociation; Growth of Pneumococcus; Media
Cultures, dead, as antigens. *See* Antigens
Cystitis, Pneumococcus in, 226

Dacryocystitis, Pneumococcus in, 227
Danysz effect in interaction of polysaccharide and immune serum, 269
Dawson's classification, 161–167
Death-point, thermal, of Pneumococcus, 51
Denaturation of antibody, 560
Dermal allergy. *See* Allergy; Skin reactions
Dermal pneumonia in rabbits
chemotherapy of, 516
in potency tests on serum, 182
in tests on action of polysaccharide-splitting enzymes, 182, 310–311
in tests on resistance, 182
production of, 181, 182
Dextran, 70, 261
Diagnostic serum
immune serum, horse and rabbit, 593–595
preparation, 592–596, 663–664
Differential media. *See* Media, differential
Diplococcus lanceolatus, 1, 19
Diplococcus pneumoniae, 1, 13, 18
Diplococcus pneumoniae Weichselbaum, 1
Diplokokkus lanceolatus pneumoniae, 1
Dispensing and labeling antipneumococcic serum, 590–591, 596
Dissociation of Pneumococcus
bacteriophage, 150
colony formation, 147–150, 152–154
comparison of systems, 163
composite cultures, 140–141
daughter colonies, 149
early observations, 24, 26, 27, 135–137
effect of animal organs, 156
effect of charcoal, optochin, yeast, 144–145
effect of immune serum, 137, 139, 145–147
Flätterformen, 152
forms a, b, c, d, and e, 152
in *S. haemolyticus,* 166
in vivo variation, 143, 145–147
later observations, 137–156
modifications A, B, and C, 139–140
modified pneumococci, 136
P–C variants, 153
phantom colony, 153
piantication, 136
polyphasic cycle, 154
unsolved problems, 614–615
virulence, 140–141, 212
See also Rough (R) forms; Smooth (S) forms; Transformation; Variants
Dog(s), susceptibility to Pneumococcus
inoculation, 194, 195
meningitis, 195
pathological processes, 195
septicemia, 195
Drug-fastness of Pneumococcus, 519–520
Drugs
action in relation to pneumococcal types, 514–515

Drugs (*cont.*):
susceptibility of Pneumococcus to, 520
See also Chemotherapy

Egg albumen
effect on hemolysis, 84
effect on oral vaccination against Pneumococcus, 348–349, 487
Egg white as adjuvant in oral administration of antigens, 348
Electrophoretic potential of Pneumococcus
effect of antiserum and animal passage on, 145
in classification of Pneumococcus, 118–119
of variants, 144
relation to virulence, 201
Empyema fluids, agglutinins and precipitins in, 441
Encapsulatus pneumoniae. See Bacillus friedländeri, 260
Endocarditis, Pneumococcus in, 5, 8, 16, 17, 226
Endotoxin, 97
Enteritis, fibrinous, Pneumococcus in, 226
Enzymes, pneumococcal, 65–66
amylase, 67
effect of formalin on, 332
effect of hydrogen peroxide on, 79
endocellular, in autolysates, 79
in pneumococcal exudates, 442–443
inulase, 67
invertase, 67
lactase, 68
maltase, 68
proteolytic, 65–66, 442
raffinase, 68
Enzymes, polysaccharide-splitting
action on agar, 317
action on cell capsule, 304–305
action on capsular polysaccharides
Type I, 318
Type II, 316
Type III, 302–304, 316
Type VIII, 320
Enzymes, polysaccharide-splitting (*cont.*):
action on purpurigenic principle, 321
action, protective, 306–307
bacteria-producing
B. palustris gelacticus, 319, 320
Flavo-bacterium ferruginum, 319
Mycobacteriaceae, 320
SIII bacillus. *See* SIII bacillus
Saccharobacterium, 320
differences in susceptibility of pneumococcal polysaccharides to, 320–321
effect on infection
in mice, 305–306
in monkeys, 312–316
in rabbits, 310–312
filtration, 320
methods of preparation, 307–310, 640–641
phagocytosis and, 307, 316
specificity, 308
toxicity, 308
unit defined, 311
Epidemics of pneumonia
in guinea pigs, 186
in man, 10, 224–225
in monkeys, 191, 483–484
in rabbits, 179
Epidemiology of pneumonia. *See* Carriers
Epidydimitis, Pneumococcus in, 226
Erysipelas, Pneumococcus in, 226
Escherichia coli
polysaccharide in, 262
relation to Pneumococcus, 261
Etiology of pneumonia, 9, 18, 25, 216–222
Eucopine, as germicide, 515
Exotoxin, 97
Experimental animals. *See* Pathogenicity of Pneumococcus; Skin reactions; and under particular animal
Exudates
antagonistic substances in, 442–443
antiserum, 579

Exudates (*cont.*):
as antigens, 21, 337–338, 527
Pneumococcus in, 6

Fatality-rates and serological types, 222–224
Fibrinous enteritis, Pneumococcus in, 226
Filtration of antipneumococcic serum, 589
Flätterformen, 152
Flavo-bacterium ferruginum, 319
Formaldehyde sulfoxylate in treatment of pneumococcal infection, 511
Formalin, effect on pneumococcal enzymes, 332
Formalinized cultures. *See* Antigens
Formic acid in carbohydrate fermentation, 71
Friedländer bacillus. *See Bacillus friedländeri*

Galacturonic acid, as constituent of capsular polysaccharides, 246
Gelatin
as accessory substance in promoting growth, 41, 42
growth of Pneumococcus on, 7, 12, 15, 18
Germicides
in preservation of biological products, 557, 559, 596
sensitiveness of Pneumococcus to, 62–64, 514–515
acriflavine, 62
eucopine, 515
formalin, 63
mercuric chloride, 62, 63
optochin, 63
phenol, 62, 63
quinine, 63
remijine, 515
silver nitrate, 63
soaps, 509
sodium lanolate, 63
sodium oleate, 63
sodium ricinoleate, 63, 509
vuzine, 512, 515
Gingivitis, Pneumococcus in, 226
Gluco-globulin(s). *See* Conjugated carbohydrate-proteins, immunological behavior
Glucose
as constituent of capsular polysaccharides, 246
fermentation by Pneumococcus, 67, 70
Glycerol extracts, as antigens, 21, 25
Glycogen, fermentation by Pneumococcus, 69
Goat(s), immune serum from, 27, 522
Gonococcus, immunological relations to Pneumococcus, 248, 370
Gordon's serological sub-groups, 111
Governmental regulations for antipneumococcic serum, 591–592
Gram stain, 6, 9
Burke's modification, 31, 34
Gram-Weigert, of tissues, 32, 34
Sterling's modification, 31, 34
Griffith's serological sub-groups, 112
Growth of Pneumococcus
accessory substances
ascitic fluid, 42
banana, 44
blood, 42
gelatin, 41, 42
hydrocele fluid, 42
iron, 43
liver, 43
plant tissue, 45
serum, 42
transudates, 41
V and X factors, 43, 45
vegetable, 44
X and V factors, 43, 45
yeast autolysate, 45
acid, neutralization of, 39
appearance, 45–47
automatic device for cultivation, 41
cycle of, 40
effect of hydrogen ion concentration, 39
effect of meat base, 37–38
effect of peptone, 38
effect of salt content, 37
effect of sugars, 38–39
in broth, 45

Growth of Pneumococcus (*cont.*):
in immune serum, 362, 420
in milk, 45
inhibition, 40, 42, 394, 396, 399, 429
inoculum, 41
media. *See* Media; Media, differential
on agar, 46
on blood agar, 46
on gelatin, 41, 42
on Loeffler's serum, 46
on potato, 46
peroxide formation during, 44
Guinea pig(s)
purpura in, 88
susceptibility to Pneumococcus
as carrier, 186
avitaminosis and cold, effect of, 187
epidemics in, 186
inhalation, 185
inoculation, 185, 187
pigmentation, 187
pregnancy, effect of, 187
spontaneous infection, 186
Gum arabic, polysaccharide in, 261

Health Organisation of the League of Nations, potency tests, 569, 650–651
Hemolysin, pneumococcal
lability, 82
thermolability, 84
See also Hemolysis, pneumococcal; Hemotoxin
Hemolysis, pneumococcal
effect of cholesterol, 83
effect of egg albumen, 84
effect of normal serum, 84
effect of peptone, 84
in cultures, 83, 84
in plate cultures, 46
of erythrocytes, 82, 85
pseudo-hemolysis, 83
relation to autolysis, 86
relation to purpura production, 89
See also Hemolysin, pneumococcal
Hemophilus influenzae carbohydrate, 303
Hemotoxin(s), 82–86
antigenicity, 85, 340
effect of auto-oxidation, 84
of tetanus bacilli, 86
of Welch bacillus, 86
quantitative measurement, 85
relation to necrotizing principle of pneumococcal extracts, 92
See also Hemolysis, pneumococcal
Heterophile antibodies, 387–388
Horse(s)
age as factor in selection of, 523
immune serum from, 27, 522, 593–594, 600
immunization, 522–543
paradoxical reaction to injections of vaccine, 196, 528–540
selection of, 522–523
susceptibility to Pneumococcus, 195–196
Host response
influence of virulence, 326–327
of mice in protection tests, 420, 572, 574
of rabbits to intradermal infection, 185
to antigenic action of Pneumococcus, 351
unsolved problems, 618–619
See also Pathogenicity of Pneumococcus; and under particular animal
Hydrogen ion concentration
acid death-point of Pneumococcus, 71
effect on autolysis, 53, 54
effect on enzymes, 66, 67
effect on growth of Pneumococcus, 39
in acid production by Pneumococcus, 70–71
in dissolution of Pneumococcus, 62
in media, 623, 625, 634
in pneumonic exudates, 442
in therapeutic antipneumococcic serum, 557
Hydrogen peroxide. *See* Peroxide formation
Hygienic Laboratory, United States, potency tests, 648–650

Identity test for antipneumococcic serum, 591
Immune serum
effect on dissociation, 139, 145–147
effect on phagocytosis, 392
from asses, cows, goats, 522
from horses and rabbits, 416–418, 452–453, 593–595, 600
growth of Pneumococcus in, 137, 139
separation of antibodies, 418–419
unit, 28, 568, 586–587
various animals as source, 27
See also Antipneumococcic serum, production
Immune substances in sputum, 442
Immunity to Pneumococcus
active. *See* Immunization, active
agglutinins, 355–364
antiblastic, 420–421
antibodies. *See* Antibodies to Pneumococcus
antihemotoxin, 382–383
antitoxin, 383–386
artificially induced. *See* Immunization, active
bactericidins, 382
clasmatocytes, 432
complement-fixing antibodies, 380–382
heterophile antibodies, 387–388
macrophages, 405, 432
natural, in animals, 196, 427–433
natural, in man, 433–437
naturally induced in man, 437–443
opsonins, normal, 393, 395–397
passive immunity
in rabbits, 21
inherited, 446
phagocytosis, 388–406
polymorphonuclear leucocytes, 432
precipitins, 365–379, 433
protective antibodies, 407–420, 434, 436
relation to allergy, 454–455
result of infection in rabbits, 16
tropins, normal, 393, 395–397
See also Vaccinal immunity
Immunization, active, to Pneumococcus, 433–445
antibodies. *See* Antibodies to Pneumococcus
antigens, kinds and methods of administering. *See* Antigens
by vaccines
in treatment of pneumonia, 503–506
prophylactic, 479–503
in pneumonia, 437–442
negative phase, 330, 342
unsolved problems, 617–618
See also Immunity
Immunogen, 483
Immunological response to Pneumococcus. *See* Host response
Impedin, as antiopsonin, 399
Influenza bacillus in lobar pneumonia, 217
Inhalation
in administration of antigen, 346–348
inoculation by, 183, 185, 190
Injection(s). *See* Antigens; Dermal pneumonia in rabbits; Skin reactions
Inoculum, effect in initiating growth, 40
Inulase in Pneumococcus, 67
Inulin
action of variants on, 69
agar, 47
fermentation
by Pneumococcus, 47, 67, 68–69
by Streptococcus, 68, 69
serum water, 47, 69, 625–626
Invertase in Pneumococcus, 67
Isoelectric zone of protective antibody, 412, 416, 417, 550, 551, 552, 555
Isolation
of C Fraction, 636–637
of capsular polysaccharides, 637–640, 645–647
of pneumococcal protein, 242, 636
of Pneumococcus, 626–628
by animal inoculation, 35

Isolation (*cont.*):
of Pneumococcus (*cont.*):
by blood cultures, 628, 636
by direct cultures, 36
by mouse methods, 35, 626–630
by plating method, 627–628
of protective antibodies. *See* Protective antibodies
of protein fractions, 242, 636
of somatic carbohydrate, 636–637

Kapselbacterium, 13
Koch's law, fulfilment, 2, 9, 16
Krumwiede method of type determination, 124–125, 630, 631

Labeling antipneumococcic serum, 590–591, 596
Lactase in Pneumococcus, 68
Lactic acid in carbohydrate fermentation, 70–71
Lactose, fermentation by Pneumococcus, 68
Lauric acid in chemotherapy, 509
League of Nations, Health Organisation, potency tests, 569, 650–651
Leucocidin, 91–93, 202
Leucocytes. *See* Phagocytosis
Leuconostoc mesenteroides, dextran from, 70, 261–262
Levan
from *B. mesentericus* and *B. subtilis,* 70
Lipases in Pneumococcus. *See* Lipolysis
Lipids
as antigens, 253
in agglutination, 384
in complement fixation, 381
in horse serum, 384, 563
in immune rabbit serum, 384
in precipitation, 384
Lipolysis by Pneumococcus, 66–67
esterase, 66
of benzylacetate, 67
of glyceryl tri-acetate, 66
of methyl n-butyrate, 67
of phenylacetate, 66
Lipovaccine, 483, 492, 495, 497, 498
Lister's serological groups, 107–108
Lobar pneumonia
agglutinins, 438
antigen-antibody balance, 360
associated with endocarditis, meningitis, pericarditis, pleuritis, 8
associated with various other infections, 226
C Fraction, 441
in cats, 193
in monkeys, 192, 193
mixed infections, 121, 217
opsonins, 438
percentage distribution of serological types, 217–219
pneumococcal types, 216–219
Pneumococcus in, 216–219
precipitins, 441
protective antibodies, 438, 440
serum treatment, 598–612
skin reactions in, 460–466
Streptococcus in, 217
vaccine therapy, 503–506
See also Pneumonia
Lung puncture, 6
Lungs, Pneumococcus in, 5, 14, 17, 18, 229–230
Lung-toxic principles in autolysates, 98
Lysis of Pneumococcus
by bile. *See* Bile solubility
by saponin, 58, 59, 60
by sodium hydroxide, 59
by sodium linoleate, 59, 60
by sodium oleate, 59
by tribasic sodium phosphate, 59
of variants, 153
relation to proteolysis, 54

Macacus cynomolgos, 193, 368
Macacus rhesus, 192, 193
Macacus syrichtus, 192, 193
Macrophages in natural immunity, 405, 432
Maltase in Pneumococcus, 68
Man
epidemics of pneumonia in, 10, 224–225

Man (*cont.*):
pathogenicity of Pneumococcus for, 7, 214–237, 435
Massachusetts Antitoxin and Vaccine Laboratory, potency test on antipneumococcic serum, 573–574, 653–661
Mastoiditis, Pneumococcus in, 227
Media
accessory substances. *See* Growth of Pneumococcus
blood agar, 46
blood broth, 625
broth
for general purposes, 623
for mass cultures, 41, 623
for production of polysaccharides, 623–625, 634
hormone-blood-agar, 44
hormone-gelatin broth, 44
inulin agar, 47
inulin-serum water, 69, 625
Martin bouillon, 44
milk, 37, 41
salt content, 37
sputum, 37
tryptic digest, 44
yeast as accessory substance, 45
See also Media, differential; Isolation; Growth of Pneumococcus
Media, differential
boiled agar, 48
chocolate agar, 138
inulin agar, 47
inulin-serum water, 47
laked blood agar, 48
laked blood-optochin agar, 48
plasma-testicular agar, 48
polytrope medium, 48
serum-glucose agar, 47
Medicinal agents. *See* Chemotherapy
Meningitis
accompanying pneumonia, 5, 6, 225
experimental, 14, 180, 194, 195, 509
Pneumococcus in, 8, 16, 17, 18, 19, 226
primary, 9, 18, 19, 226
Metals and metallic salts in concentration of antipneumococcic serum, 555
See also Chemotherapy
Methemoglobin, removal of, from circulation, 80
Methemoglobin formation, 71–82
by potassium ferricyanide, 73
by sodium nitrate, 73
by variants, 148
effect of catalases, 73
effect on oxygen capacity of blood, 74
in circulating blood, 73, 80
in pneumonia, 73, 80
oxidation and reduction, 71–74
relation to peroxide formation, 73–82
reversibility of action, 81
Methylene blue, oxidation and reduction, 77
Mice. *See* Mouse (mice)
Microbe septicémique du saliva, 1, 14
Microbio capsulato del Fraenkel, 20
Micrococcus Pasteuri, 1, 15
Micrococcus pneumoniae crouposae, 1, 14, 19, 24
Microphotography in identification of species, 48
Milk
as medium for Pneumococcus, 37, 41
effect on virulence of Pneumococcus, 203
protein as inhibitor of skin sensitization, 468
Mixed infections
as complicating factor in type determination, 121–122
in healthy individuals, 231
in lobar pneumonia, 121, 217
in mice, 188, 190
isolation of Pneumococcus in, 47
Modified routine in precipitation test, 644–645
Molecular weight of antibodies, 415–418
Monas pulmonale, 1, 6
Monkey(s)
enzyme therapy of pneumonia in, 314

Monkey(s) (*cont.*):
experiments on, 481–483
in tests for chill-producing properties of serum, 564–565
susceptibility to Pneumococcus
as carrier, 192
Cebus capucinus, 192, 193
Ceropithecus callitrichus, 192
epidemics in, 191, 483–484
inoculation, 191–193, 577
lobar pneumonia in, 192, 193
Macacus cynomolgos, 193, 368
Macacus rhesus, 192, 193
Pithecus philippinensis, 192
variations, individual, 193
Morphology of Pneumococcus, 30–35
Mouse (mice)
immunizing action of polysaccharides, 255
in isolation of Pneumococcus, 35, 626–630
in potency tests on antipneumococcic serum, 407–408, 567–576, 653–661
in protection tests, host response, 420, 572, 574
in safety tests for antipneumococcic serum, 588–589, 591
in serological classification, 104, 105, 106, 108, 111, 113, 114
in tests for preservatives, 588
in therapeutic tests on antipneumococcic serum, 578–579
in type determination, 120–122, 628–630, 631
protective action of enzyme in, 305–306
purpura in, 87, 89, 90
susceptibility to Pneumococcus
age, 189
as carrier, 189
Bacillus typhi murium, 190
body-weight, 189, 190
breed, 189
dose of Pneumococcus necessary to infect, 188
effect of alcohol, 190
effect of toxins, 97, 99
Mouse (mice) (*cont.*):
susceptibility to Pneumococcus (*cont.*):
inoculation, 188–190
mixed infection, 188
monocytes, 190
pigmentation, 187, 188
variation in response to infection, 187, 190, 420, 572, 574
white cells, 190
Mucin
in blood, 240
in capsule, 3, 7, 33, 239
Mucin, gastric, virulence of Pneumococcus enhanced by, 202
Mutation
in serological type, 156–169
in species, 169–177
Mycobacteriaceae, 320

National Institute of Health, potency tests, 567, 592, 648–650
Natural immunity. *See* Immunity to Pneumococcus
Necrotin, 92
Necrotizing principle of Pneumococcus
in autolysates, 92–93, 98–99
relation to hemotoxin, 92
Nephritis, Pneumococcus in, 16, 17
Neufeld *Quellung* phenomenon. *See* *Quellung* phenomenon
Nitrogen determination, precipitation tests, 643–644
Normal individuals
opsonins in, 395–397
Pneumococcus in, 215–216
See also Carriers of Pneumococcus
Nucleoprotein(s) of Pneumococcus. *See* Protein fraction(s)
Nutrient media. *See* Media

Oliver's method of type determination, 126
Olmstead's serological groups, 108–109
Ophthalmic reactions
capsular polysaccharides in, 457–458
in rabbit, 457

Ophthalmic reactions (*cont.*):
nucleoprotein in, 457
specificity, 458
Opsonins
agglutinins, relation to, 431
antiopsonins, 398–401
antiphagins, 398
Impedin, 399
in pneumonia, 401–402, 438, 439
method for demonstrating, 429, 431
normal, 393, 395–397
sensitization of pneumococci, 391–395
See also Phagocytosis
Optical rotation of polysaccharides, 246, 254, 255, 257, 273, 274, 281, 291, 292, 293
Optochin, 512–520
adjuvant action with immune serum, 518
base, 512, 516, 518
drug-fastness, 519–520
effect in dissociation, 144–145
effect on virulence, 519
germicidal action, 513, 514, 515
heightened susceptibility of Pneumococcus to, 520
specificity, 520
toxicity, 517
Oral administration of antigens, 348–351
Orchitis, Pneumococcus in, 226
Osteomyelitis, Pneumococcus in, 226
Otitis, Pneumococcus in, 20, 226, 227
Oxidation and reduction, 71–82
analysis of reaction, 80–81
B. acidophilus, 75
B. bulgaricus, 75
diphtheria bacilli, 77
effect of catalase, 78
hydrogen peroxide, 44, 74–82
methemoglobin, 71–74
methylene blue, 77
oxidases, 71, 75
peroxide, 71, 74–82
reversibility of action, 81
staphylococci, 77
streptococci, 77
Oxidation and reduction (*cont.*):
S. haemolyticus, 75
S. viridans, 75
xanthoprotein, 75

Panophthalmia, Pneumococcus in, 227
Parotitis, Pneumococcus in, 19, 226
Passive immunity. *See* Immunity, passive
Passive sensitization. *See* Sensitization, passive
Pathogenicity of Pneumococcus
for experimental animals
birds, 196
cats, 193
dogs, 7, 10, 16, 193–195
guinea pigs, 7, 185–187
horses, 195–196
mice, 7, 187–190
monkeys, 191–193
rabbits, 7, 179–185
rats, 190–191
for man, 7, 214–237, 435
See also Virulence
Peptonase, in Pneumococcus, 66
Peptone
effect on growth, 38
effect on hemolysis, 84
Pericarditis, Pneumococcus in, 8, 9, 16, 226
Peritonsillar abscess, primary, Pneumococcus in, 20
Peroxidase in peroxide formation, 76
Peroxide formation
by *B. acidophilus,* 75
by *B. bulgaricus,* 75
by Pneumococcus, 44, 74–82
by *S. aureus,* 76
by *S. haemolyticus,* 75, 76
by *S. mucosus,* 76
by *S. viridans,* 75
effect of bacteria, 78
effect of blood, 78
effect of catalase, 78
effect of cell washings, 77
effect of gelatin, 77
effect of glucose, 77
effect of lactic acid, 77

Peroxide formation (*cont.*):
effect of liver, 78
effect of muscle infusion, 77
effect of yeast, 77
effect on saccharolytic enzymes, 79
hydrogen peroxide in, 44, 74–82
in relation to methemoglobins, 71–82
optimal zone, 76
peroxidase in, 76
Phagocytosis, 388–406
antiopsonins, 398–401
antiphagins, 398
clasmatocytes, 432
early observations, 17, 23, 25, 27
in recovery from infection, 394
macrophages, 405, 432
mechanism, 402–406
normal and immune serum, 392, 393–397
opsonins in pneumonia, 401–402, 438, 439
opsonins, normal, 393, 395–397
piantication, 392
polymorphonuclear leucocytes, 432
polysaccharide-splitting enzymes and, 307, 316
sensitization of Pneumococcus to, 391–395
serum-leucocyte mixtures, 429, 430, 433, 435, 439
tropins in pneumonia, 401–402, 438, 439
tropins, normal, 393, 395–397
Phantom colony of pneumococci, 153
Phlegmon, Pneumococcus in, 226
Phosphorus in polysaccharides, 271, 287
Physicochemical properties of capsular polysaccharides, 296–297
Piantication, 392
Pigeon, natural immunity, 341, 428
Pigment formation
by aniline, 74
by benzidine, 74
by toluidine, 74
Pithecus philippinensis, 192
Plasma-testicular agar as differential medium, 48
Plating methods for isolation of Pneumococcus, 627–628
Pleural exudate as antigen, 21, 337, 339
Pleuritis, Pneumococcus in, 8, 16
Pneumocholin, as antigen, 334, 483
Pneumococcemia, 227–229
Pneumococci. *See* Pneumococcus
Pneumococcidins
analysis of action, 436
germicides, 62–64, 430, 433
in normal serum, 428, 436
in whole blood, 435–436
serum-leucocyte mixtures, 429–431, 435, 439
See also Chemotherapy
Pneumococcus
anaerobic strains, 44, 116
and *B. friedländeri,* differentiation, 17
antibodies. *See* Antibodies to Pneumococcus
antigenicity, 323–354
atypical and typical, 105, 146
autolysis. *See* Autolysis
bile solubility, 55–62
biochemical features, 65–102
biology, 30–64
C Fraction. *See* C Fraction
carbohydrates fermentable by. *See* Carbohydrate fermentation by Pneumococcus
carriers. *See* Carriers
cell wall, 260
chemical constituents. *See* Chemical constituents
classification
bacteriological, 1
serological. *See* Serological classification
colony formation. *See* Colony formation
dissociation. *See* Dissociation
drug-fastness, 519–520
epidemiology. *See* Carriers
excretion, 229–230
fatality rates, 222–224
first observation, 2

Pneumococcus (*cont.*):
Flätterformen, 152
forms a, b, c, d, and e, 152
growth. *See* Growth of Pneumococcus; Media
history, 1–29
identification by microphotography, 48
immunity to. *See* Immunity
immunization, active, to. *See* Immunization, active
immunological behavior of constituents, 250, 278–288
immunological relations to other microbic species and unrelated substances, 248, 421–423
in abscesses, 19, 20
in accessory sinuses, 18
in air, 10
in appendicitis, 226
in arthritis, 226
in blood, 7, 8
in bronchitis, 20
in bronchopneumonia, 219–221
in cantharides blister fluid, 8
in cerebrospinal fluid, 18
in conjunctivitis, 226, 227
in dust, 10
in endocarditis, 5, 8, 16, 17, 226
in endocardium, 10
in epidemics. *See* Epidemics
in exudates, 6
in feces, 229–230
in gums, 18
in the heart, 18
in infants and children, 221–222
in infections other than pneumonia, 225–227
in joints, 18, 20
in lobar pneumonia, 216–219
in lung exudate, 2, 8
in lung puncture fluid, 9
in lungs, 5, 14, 17, 18, 229–230
in meningitis, 8, 16, 17, 18, 19, 226
in nasal fossae, 18
in necropsies, 229–230
in nephritis, 16, 17
in normal individuals, 215–216
in panophthalmia, 227

Pneumococcus (*cont.*):
in parotitis, 19, 226
in pericarditis, 8, 9, 16, 226
in pericardium, 10
in phlegmon, 226
in pleura, 10
in pleural tissue, 6
in pleuritis, 16
in pneumonic exudate, 14
in puerperal sepsis, 226
in saliva, 2, 3, 4, 5, 15, 20, 25
in sinusitis, 226, 227
in sputum, 2, 8, 9, 25
in subarachnoid fluid, 2, 6, 16
in tonsils, 10, 18
in tympanic cavity, 18
in *Ulcus serpens,* 226
in urine, 229
inulase in, 67
isolation. *See* Isolation
lipolysis. *See* Lipolysis
lysis. *See* Lysis
modifications A, B, and C. *See* Dissociation
morphology, 30–35
necrotizing principle of, 92–93, 98–99
pathogenicity. *See* Pathogenicity
post-mortem cultures, 230
preservation, 49–52
protease in, 66
protein fractions. *See* Protein fraction(s) of Pneumococcus
proteolysis. *See* Proteolysis of Pneumococcus
relation to Streptococcus, 175
respiration. *See* Respiration
rough and smooth forms. *See* Rough (R) forms; Smooth (S) forms
sensitiveness to germicides. *See* Germicides
sensitization of, to phagocytosis, 391–395
sensitized as antigen, 335
susceptibility of animal host. *See* Pathogenicity; and under particular animal
synonyms, 1
thermal death-point, 51
transformation. *See* Transformation

Pneumococcus (*cont.*):
transmutation of species, 169–177
type determination. *See* Type determination
variants. *See* Variants
viability, 49–52
virulence. *See* Virulence
xanthoprotein, formation by, 75
Pneumococcus mucosus
action on inulin, 68
bile solubility, 56, 57
reclassification, 110, 361–362
serological classification, 105, 380
Pneumococcus planus, 111
Pneumokokkus, 14
Pneumonia
antibodies in blood, 437–442
associated with other infections, 5, 6, 8, 9, 16, 17, 225–229
broncho-, 219–221
dermal. *See* Dermal pneumonia in rabbits
epidemics. *See* Epidemics
etiology. *See* Etiology
in infants and children, pneumococcal types, 221–222
lobar. *See* Lobar pneumonia
methemoglobin in, 73, 80
opsonins in, 401–402, 438, 439
predisposing causes, 15
serum treatment, 598–612
skin reactions in, 440, 460–466, 468, 473
tropins in, 401–402, 438, 439
vaccine therapy, 503–506
Pneumoniecoccen, 10
Pneumoniekokken, 1, 2
Pneumonie-Micrococcen, 1
Pneumoniemikrococcus, 1, 15, 19
Pneumoniemikrokokken, 8
Pneumotoxin as antigen, 338
Poisons, protein, relation to pneumococcal toxins, 100–101
Polymorphonuclear leucocytes in natural immunity, 432
Polyphasic cycle in dissociation, 154
Polysaccharide(s)
acetyl. *See* Acetyl carbohydrate-azoproteins; Acetyl polysaccharide(s)
antigenicity, 251, 255, 283, 290, 292, 344–345, 349, 448
B. friedländeri, 246, 260, 262
B. tuberculosis, 262
C Fraction. *See* C Fraction
capsular. *See* A substance; Capsular polysaccharide(s); Carbohydrates, cellular
dextran, 70, 261
elimination, 350, 487
Escherichia coli, 262
fractions, acid-soluble and acid-insoluble, 276
gum arabic, 261
levan, 70
optical rotation. *See* Optical rotation
phosphorus in, 271, 287
production of, in broth, 623–625, 634
purpurigenic action of. *See* Purpura
relation of pneumococcal to non-pneumococcal, 258–263
sulfur in, 271, 287
Polysaccharide-splitting enzymes. *See* Enzymes, polysaccharide-splitting
Polytrope medium as differential medium, 48
Polyvalent serum, 545–547
Pooled serums in type determination, 129
Post-mortem cultures, 230
Potency tests on antipneumococcic serum, 28, 565–587
agglutination, 582
American Drug Manufacturers' Association, 570, 651–653
animal tests, early, 565–566
antitoxic flocculation, 581
antitoxin, 579
bactericidal power, 581
combining equivalents, 584
complement fixation, 581
correlation between *in vitro* and *in vivo* tests, 584–587
exudate antiserum, 579

Potency tests on antipneumococcic serum (*cont.*):
- Health Organisation of the League of Nations, 569, 650–651
- immune nitrogen, amount in SSS-antibody precipitates, 584
- *in vitro* tests, 580–584
- *in vivo* tests, 565–580
- Massachusetts Antitoxin and Vaccine Laboratory, 573–574, 653–661
- mouse protection test, 407–408, 567–576, 653–661
- National Institute of Health, 567, 592, 648–650
- precipitation, 373, 374, 375, 582, 642–647
- protocols and records, 659–661
- *Quellung* reaction (Neufeld), 581
- *Schwellenwert,* 408, 575
- tests of therapeutic effects, 576–579
- United States Hygienic Laboratory, 567, 648–650
- unsolved problems, 621
- water test, 580–581
- zonal effects, 575

Precipitation
- as potency test, 373, 374, 375, 582, 642–647
- immunological relation to Gonococcus, 248, 370
- inhibition zone, 372, 583
- mechanism, 370–377
- of soluble specific substance in urine, 123–124, 240, 633–635
- quantitative relations in, 373, 378
- specific flocculation, 253, 368
- *See also* Precipitation tests; Precipitin(s)

Precipitation tests
- combining equivalents, 645–647
- modified routine, 644–645
- nitrogen determination, 643–644
- on urine, 123–124, 633–635
- optimal proportions, 642–643

Precipitin(s), 365–379
- aldobionic acid in precipitin reaction, 375
- and precipitinogen, balance between, 372
- antiprotein, 367–368
- C Fraction, 368–370, 441
- correlation with other antibodies, 377–379, 584–585
- identity with agglutinin, 367
- in blood, 125, 365–379
- in empyema fluids, 441
- index, 372
- microestimation, 375
- natural, 428
- normal, 433
- type-specificity, 366

Precipitinogen
- and precipitin, balance between, 372
- in urine, 123–124, 366, 633–635

Preservatives for antipneumococcic serum, 557–559, 588–589, 596

Prophylaxis, vaccines in, 494–503

Protease in Pneumococcus, 66

Protection tests
- in potency determination of antipneumococcic serum, 407–408, 567–576, 653–661
- in serological classification, 104, 105, 106, 108, 111, 113, 114
- in type determination, 120–122, 626–630
- limitations, 571–576
- mice, host response of, 420, 572, 574
- rabbit in, 121, 408
- *Schwellenwert,* 408, 575

Protective antibodies to Pneumococcus, 407–420
- chemical nature, 411–418
- concentration, 547–556
- early observations, 407
- globulin, 26, 416–418
- in avian serum, 410
- in immune rabbit and horse serum. *See* Immune serum
- in lobar pneumonia, 438, 440
- induced by acetyl polysaccharides, 411
- induced by capsular polysaccharides, 411

Protective antibodies to Pneumococcus (*cont.*):
  induced by synthetic antigens, 411
  isoelectric zone, 412, 416, 417, 550, 551, 552, 555
  isolation
    by alcohol, 553–554
    by ammonium sulfate, 413, 548–549
    by carbon dioxide, 553
    by dialysis, 412, 550
    by dilution with water, 412, 550–553
    by dissociation of specific precipitates, 414, 418–419, 554–555
    by sodium chloride, 553
    by sodium sulfate, 549–550
  molecular-size, 416–418
  natural, 436
  normal serum, 434
  origin, 407
  quantitative estimation, 419–420
  relation to other antibodies, 377–379, 409–410, 584–587
  specificity, 408–409
  ultracentrifugation, 414–417, 555
  ultrafiltration, 417–418, 555
Protein fraction(s) of Pneumococcus
  antigenicity, 242, 247, 250, 253, 345, 444, 526
  antiprotein precipitins, 367–368
  in anaphylaxis, 451
  in ophthalmic reactions, 457
  in skin reactions, 456, 464, 471–472
  isolation, 242, 636
  relation to protein from Gonococcus, 248, 370
  See also Conjugated carbohydrate-proteins
Protein poisons, relation to pneumococcal toxins, 100–101
Proteolysis of Pneumococcus, 65–66
  and toxins, 94, 95
  peptonase, 66
  protease, 66
Proteolytic enzymes in Pneumococcus. *See* Enzymes, pneumococcal
Protocols and records, potency tests, 659–661
Pseudo-hemolysis, 83
Puerperal sepsis, Pneumococcus in, 226
Purpura
  and virulence, 88
  in guinea pigs, 88
  in man, 86, 87
  in mice, 87, 89, 90
  in pneumococcal infections, 86, 87
  in rabbits, 88
  produced by cellular carbohydrates, 90, 91, 274
  relation to C Fraction, 257
Purpura-producing principle
  antigenicity, 89
  characters, 88
  effect of bile salts, 90
  effect of polysaccharide-splitting enzymes on, 321
  effect of sodium choleate, 90
  effect of sodium desoxycholate, 90
  effect on blood platelets, 88
  effect on red blood cells, 88
  relation to cellular carbohydrate, 90, 91
  relation to hemolysin, 89
Pyosalpinx, Pneumococcus in, 226

Quellung phenomenon, 33
  as potency test on antipneumococcic serum, 581
  in type determination, 128, 131–132, 630, 632–633
  use of immune horse or immune rabbit serum in, 594

R forms. *See* Rough (R) forms
Rabbit(s)
  immune serum
    antibodies in, nature of, 381–382, 418–486
    in complement fixation, 380–382
    in protection tests, 121, 148
    in treatment of pneumonia, 600
    in type determination, 121
    production of, for diagnosis, 594–595

Rabbit(s) (*cont.*):
ophthalmic reactions in, 457
skin reactions in, 458
susceptibility to Pneumococcus
age, 184–185
as carrier, 179
blood-cell count, 185
breed, 184, 185
dermal pneumonia. *See* Dermal pneumonia in rabbits
diet, 184, 185
effect of chilling, wetting, 184
epidemics in, 179
erysipelas, 180
inoculation, 180–185
intrabronchial insufflation, 183
spontaneous infection, 179
spraying, 183
Type I, 180, 181
Type II, 180
Type III, 180, 207–210, 433
variation in response to infection, 187, 190, 420, 572, 574
vitamin deficiency, 185
weight, 184, 185
Raffinase, in Pneumococcus, 68
Rat(s), susceptibility to Pneumococcus, 190–191
effect of high temperatures, humidity, 191
inoculation, intraperitoneal and subcutaneous, 191
oral administration of vaccines, 191
septicemia, 191
tracheal insufflation, 191
Records and protocols, potency tests, 591, 659–661
Red blood cells as affected by purpura, 88
Reduction and oxidation. *See* Oxidation and reduction
Remijine as germicide, 515
Residue antigens, 241
Respiration of Pneumococcus
respiratory capacity of variants, 150–152
respiratory changes in relation to virulence, 82, 151
Response of host. *See* Host response
Reticulo-endothelial system in protection, 403, 405–406
Reversion of variants, 147, 153–156
by anti-R serum, 154
by mouse passage, 154
by pneumococcal vaccine, 155–156
Rough (R) forms of Pneumococcus
antigenicity, 150, 344
colony appearance, 137, 139, 148–149
differential medium, 152
in composite cultures, 141–142
in pneumonic lung, 147
in vivo variation, 146–147
respiratory capacity, 150–152
reversion to smooth (S) forms, 147, 154–155, 157
species-specificity, 142–144
stability of characters, 142
type transformation, 156–160

SIII bacillus
cultivation, 302, 303, 307–310, 640–641
isolation, 301–303, 304
S forms. *See* Smooth (S) forms
Sabin's method of type determination, 127–129, 628–631
Saccharobacterium acuminatum, 320
Safety tests for antipneumococcic serum, 587–589, 591
Saliva
pathogenesis for rabbits, 3, 4, 5
Pneumococcus in, 2, 3, 4, 5, 15, 20, 25
Salt content of media, effect on growth of Pneumococcus, 37
Sanocrysin in chemotherapy, 510
Saponin in lysis of Pneumococcus, 58, 59, 60
Schwellenwert in potency tests, 408, 575
Sensitization, passive, 449–454
differences in rabbit serum and horse serum, 452, 453
Sepsis, puerperal, Pneumococcus in, 226

Serological classification of Pneumococcus
acid agglutination, 109, 110
agglutination, 26, 103–118, 359–360, 361–362
agglutinin-absorption, 110, 111, 362
atypical and typical strains, 105, 116–117
Collin's observations, 104–105
complement fixation, 110
Cooper's classification, 113–115
cross-agglutination, 112
Dochez and Gillespie's groups, 106
electrophoretic potential, 118–119
fibrinous and cellular types, 105
Gordon's sub-groups, 111
Griffith's sub-groups, 112
Lister's groups, 107–108
Olmstead's groups, 108–109
Pneumococcus mucosus, 105, 110, 361–362, 380
protection tests, 104, 105, 106, 108, 111, 113, 114
Streptococcus mucosus, 110, 361–362
Type II, sub-groups, 108, 110
Type determination, 119–132
unidentified strains in, 116–117
unsolved problems, 614
Serological reactions, technique, 641–648
agglutination, 641
bactericidal tests, 647–648
complement fixation, 647
precipitation tests, 642–647
combining equivalents, 645–647
modified routine, 644–645
nitrogen determination, 643–644
optimal proportions, 642–643
protection tests, 648–661
Serological types of Pneumococcus. *See* Pneumococcus; Serological classification
Serum
antipneumococcic. *See* Antipneumococcic serum, production
anti-R. *See* Anti-R serum
as accessory substance in promoting growth, 42
Serum (*cont.*):
avian. *See* Avian serum
convalescent, 442
effect on acid production, 71
immune. *See* Immune serum
normal, effect on hemolysis, 84
normal, effect on phagocytosis, 392–393, 395–397
polyvalent, 545–547
protective action of normal human, 434
sterility tests, 662–663
swine. *See* Swine serum
Serum-glucose agar as differential medium, 47
Serum-leucocyte mixtures, pneumococcidal action of, 429, 430, 435, 439
Serum treatment of lobar pneumonia, 598–612
antagonistic substances, 601
duration of acute symptoms, 604
effect on temperature, 605
fatality rate, Types I and II, 607
influence of bacteriemia, 609, 610, 611
limitations, 599–602
rationale, 598–599
results, 602–612
skin reactions as guide, 468
Shwartzman phenomenon, 474–476
Sinusitis, Pneumococcus in, 226, 227
Skin allergy, active and passive, 466–468
See also Skin reactions
Skin reactions, 455–460, 471
as guide to serum treatment, 468
delayed reactions, 464, 465, 468
immediate reactions, 464, 473
in horses immunized, actively and passively, 458
in pneumonia, 440, 460–466, 468, 473
in rabbits immunized, actively and passively, 458
mechanism, 468–474
recurrence, 460
Shwartzman phenomenon, 474–476
to autolysates, 456, 461, 462, 466

Skin reactions (*cont.*):
to C Fraction, 464, 465, 471, 472
to capsular polysaccharides, 460, 463, 464, 465, 466, 473
to carbohydrates, cellular, 465, 466
to filtrates, 97, 440, 462
to heat-killed Pneumococcus, 456, 457
to nucleoproteins, 456
to proteins, 464, 471–472
to saline suspensions, 461, 463
to somatic proteins, 464, 471
to toxins, 97, 99, 461, 468, 471
unsolved problems, 619–620
Slide agglutination in type determination, 127–131
Smooth (S) forms of Pneumococcus
antigenicity, 344
colony appearance, 137–139, 147–149
differential medium, 152
in composite cultures, 141–142
in vivo variation, 145–147
respiratory capacity, 150–152
reversion of R forms to, 147, 154–155, 157
type transformation, 156–160
Smooth variants (V and N), 153
Soaps. *See* Chemotherapy; Bile solubility
Sodium choleate and purpura-producing principle, 90
Sodium desoxycholate and purpura-producing principle, 90
Sodium formaldehyde sulfoxylate in treatment of pneumococcal infection, 511
Sodium hydroxide in lysis of Pneumococcus, 59
Sodium linoleate in lysis of Pneumococcus, 59, 60
Sodium oleate
adjuvant action of, on immune serum, 509
in lysis of Pneumococcus, 59
Sodium ricinoleate
in preparation of toxins, 96
pneumococcidal action, 63, 509
Soluble specific substance (SSS)
as antigen. *See* Capsular polysaccharide(s)
media for preparation, 243, 623–625, 634
precipitation in urine, 123–124, 240, 633–635
Somatic carbohydrate(s). *See* C Fraction
Somatic protein(s). *See* Protein fraction(s)
Spleen
as inoculum, 18, 20
for preservation of Pneumococcus, 52
Sputum, 2, 8, 9, 25
as antigen, 21
as medium for cultivation of Pneumococcus, 37
immune substances in, 442
in methods of type determination
bile solution, 126–127
digestion, 124–125
Pneumococcus in, 2, 8, 9, 25
precipitinogen in, 124
SSS. *See* Soluble specific substance
Stain(s), capsule, 6, 33–35
Buerger, 34
Friedländer, 33
Gram, Burke's modification, 31, 34
Gram, Sterling's modification, 31, 34
Gram-Weigert, of tissues, 32, 34
Hiss, 34
Huntoon, 34
Leifson, 34
Lévy-Bruhl and Borin, 34
MacConkey, 33
Malone, 34
Wadsworth, of tissues, 35
Welch, 34
Wherry, 34
Staining methods, 31–35
capsule. *See* Stain(s), capsule
stain, differential, 31–32
Standardization of antigens, 331, 532–533
Staphylococcus aureus, peroxide formation by, 76

Starch fermentation by Pneumococcus, 67
Sterility tests on final containers of antipneumococcic serum, 591, 662–663
Streptococcus
  action on inulin, 69
  in lobar pneumonia, 217
  relation to Pneumococcus, 175
  transmutation of species, 169–177
Streptococcus haemolyticus
  dissociation, 106
  peroxide formation, 75, 76
  variants, 166
Streptococcus lanceolatus, 427
Streptococcus lanceolatus Pasteuri, 1, 17, 388
Streptococcus mucosus
  action on inulin, 68
  bile solubility, 56, 57
  peroxide formation, 76
  reclassification, 110, 361–362
  relation to Type III Pneumococcus, 110
  stain for, 32
Streptococcus viridans, 75
Subarachnoid fluid, Pneumococcus in, 2, 6, 16
Sucrose fermentation by Pneumococcus, 67
Sugars
  effect on growth of Pneumococcus, 39
  function in determining antigenicity, 253–265
  See also Carbohydrate fermentation by Pneumococcus; Carbohydrate fractions; Conjugated carbohydrate-proteins
Sulfur in polysaccharides, 271, 287
Susceptibility of animal host to Pneumococcus. *See* Animals, experimental
Swine serum
  agglutinins in, 431, 432
  anti-R bodies in, 155
Synergism with antipneumococcic serum
Synergism with antipneumococcic serum (*cont.*):
  cinchona derivatives, ethylhydrocupreine and optochin base, 518
  gold, 510
  sodium oleate, 518

Test(s). *See* Agglutination; Bactericidal tests; Identity test for antipneumococcic serum; Potency tests for antipneumococcic serum; Precipitation; Preservatives for antipneumococcic serum, tests for; Protection tests; Safety tests; Therapeutic tests; Type determination
Tetanus, hemotoxin, 86
Therapeutic serum, production, 543–565
Therapeutic tests for antipneumococcic serum, 576–580
Therapy. *See* Serum treatment of lobar pneumonia; Vaccine therapy
Thermal death-point of Pneumococcus, 51
Tissue extracts
  as antigens, 337–338
  in therapy, 23
Total solids, determination in antipneumococcic serum, 589
Toxin(s), 21, 27, 93–101
  adjuvant action on virulence, 98
  anaerobic, 99
  anaphylactic symptoms, 94, 95
    in guinea pigs, 95
    in rabbits, 96
  antigenicity, 93, 95, 338–340
  antitoxins. *See* Antitoxin(s)
  effect on mice, 97, 99
  endotoxin, 97
  exotoxin, 97
  in autolysates, 94, 97, 98
  in filtrates, 97, 98
  in lung exudates, 96
  in skin tests, 97, 99, 461, 467, 468
  in sodium ricinoleate solutions of Pneumococcus, 96

Toxin(s) (*cont.*):
lung-toxic principle, 98
nature, 99
necrotizing substance, 92, 98
Pneumotoxin, 338
properties, 95
relation to protein poisons, 100–101
relation to proteolysis, 94, 95
relation to virulence of Pneumococcus, 93
stability, 97
tolerance to, 95
type-specificity, 100
unsolved problems, 613–614
Transformation of Pneumococcus
by animal inoculation, 155–160
by heat-killed cultures, 157–158
by vaccines, 158–160
effect of sterile animal organs, 156
in vivo, 158
transformative principle, 160
See also Dissociation
Transmutation of species, 169–177
Tribasic sodium phosphate in lysis of Pneumococcus, 59
Tropins. *See* Opsonins; Phagocytosis
Tubercle bacilli, polysaccharide in, 262
Type determination
agglutination, 123
Amoss' method, 129–130
Avery's method, 123
Blake's method, 122
Krumwiede method, 124–125, 630, 631
mouse methods, 120–122, 628–630, 631
multiple strains, 121
Oliver's method, 126
pooled serums, 129
precipitin in blood, 125, 365–379
precipitinogen in
sputum, 124–126
urine, 123–124, 366, 633–635
protection tests, 120–122, 626–630
Quellung phenomenon, 128, 131–132, 630, 632–633
rabbit in, 121
Type determination (*cont.*):
Sabin's method, 127–129, 628–631
slide agglutination, 127–131
urine precipitation, 123–124, 633–635
See also Serological classification

Ulcus serpens, Pneumococcus in, 226
Ultracentrifugation
in determining nature of antibodies, 414–417
in purification of antipneumococcic serum, 555
in purification of cellular carbohydrates, 275
Ultrafiltration
in determining molecular size of antibodies, 417–418
in purification
of antipneumococcic serum, 555
of cellular carbohydrates, 275
Unit of immune serum, 28, 568, 586–587
Unit of polysaccharide-splitting enzymes, 311
United States Hygienic Laboratory, potency test, 567, 648–650
Unsolved problems, 613–622
active immunity, production, 617–618
antibodies and animal species, 619–620
antipneumococcic serum
methods of concentration, 620–621
potency tests, 621
chemical constituents of Pneumococcus, 615–616
chemotherapy, 618
dissociation, 614–616
immunological response, 618–619
pneumococcal antibody, nature, 620
serological types, 614
skin reactions, 619–620
toxins, 613–614
virulence, 616–617
Urine
acetyl polysaccharide in, 284
Pneumococcus in, 229

Urine (*cont.*):
- precipitation test, as method of type determination, 123–124, 633–635
- precipitinogen in, 123–124, 366, 370, 373, 633–635
- soluble specific substance in, 123–124, 240, 633–635

Uronic acid in acetylated polysaccharide, 280

Vaccinal immunity
- after ingestion, 493
- after intradermal injection, 491, 492
- after lipovaccine, 492
- after subcutaneous injection, 492, 493
- appearance and duration, 490–493, 502
- duration, 488
- water soluble fraction, 501, 502

Vaccine therapy of pneumonia, 503–506
- autolysates, 504
- killed pneumococci, 504
- mixed vaccines, 505
- rationale, 503

Vaccines, pneumococcal, 479–506
- acid-soluble portion of pneumococcal cell, 485
- antibodies evoked, 485
- as agent in reversion, 155–156
- autogenous vaccines, 499, 500
- autolysates, 481, 483, 488
- cultures
  - heat-killed, 483
  - killed by Merthiolate, 487
  - soaped, 487
  - washings of agar, 487
- dosage, 483, 484, 494, 496, 497, 498, 501
- egg-white as adjuvant, 487
- experiments on monkeys, 481–483
- extracts
  - neutralized alkaline, 483
  - of Pneumococcus, 481, 483
- filtrates, 483
- formalinized suspensions, 483

Vaccines, pneumococcal (*cont.*):
- heat-killed cultures, 483
- Immunogen, 483
- in prophylaxis, 494–503
- ingestion, 487, 488, 489, 493
- injection, route and spacing, 486–489
- intact cell, 487
- limitations, 502
- lipovaccine, 483, 492, 495, 497, 498
- mixed, 496, 497, 499, 500, 501
- Pneumocholin, 334, 483
- results in man, 493–506
- saline suspension, 496
  - devitalized, 480–481
- soluble specific substance, 484
- solutions of Pneumococcus, 481
- special constituents of Pneumococcus, 484–485
- therapy. *See* Vaccine therapy
- transformation by, 158–160
- types of, 483
- *See also* Vaccinal immunity

Variants of Pneumococcus
- action on inulin, 69
- agglutinability, 140, 362–363
- bile solubility, 140–141, 149
- effect of anti-R serum, 154
- electrophoretic potential, 144
- fermentation of glucose, 67–68
- *Flätterformen,* 152
- forms a, b, c, d, and e, 152
- intermediates, 144
- methemoglobin formation, 148
- modifications A, B, and C. *See* Dissociation
- mucoid, 161, 163, 164, 166, 167
- P–C, 153
- respiratory capacity, 150–152
- reversion by anti-R serum, 154
- reversion by mouse passage, 154
- reversion by pneumococcal vaccine, 155–156
- Smooth (V and N), 153
- type-specificity, 143
- virulence of, 82, 140–141, 212

Variation. *See* Dissociation of Pneumococcus; Transformation of Pneumococcus

Viability of Pneumococcus, 49–52
Virulence of Pneumococcus, 196–212
and antigenicity, 25, 326–327, 524–526
and antivirus, 337
and avenue of inoculation, 200
and bile solubility, 56
and dissociation, 140–141, 212
and purpura, 88
and respiratory changes, 82, 151
changes in variants, 82, 140–141, 151, 212
degradation, 211–212
determination, 200–202
electrophoretic potential, 201
mice, 200
effect of cultural conditions, 203–205
carbon dioxide, 204
cinchona derivatives, 519–520
concentration of meat in medium, 204
eggs, 205
frequency of transfer, 204, 205
glucose, 204
hydrogen ion concentration, 204
milk, 203
nitrogen, 204
oxygen, 204
peptone, 38
serum, immune and normal, 204
temperature, 204
exaltation, 27, 204
artificial, 210–211
freshly isolated strains, 197–199
in relation to toxins, 93, 98
influence on immunological response, 326–327
maintenance, 20, 648–649, 651, 653
media for growth of virulent cultures, 634
number of cocci required to infect, 199–200
Virulence of Pneumococcus (*cont.*):
relation to respiration, 82, 151
strain variations in, 205–206
substances enhancing, 202–203
autolysates, 202–203
capsular polysaccharides, 203
leucocidin, 202
mucin, 202
soluble specific substance, 203
test for, 653–654
toxins, 93, 98
virulin, 91, 98, 202
unsolved problems, 616–617
variants, 82, 140–141, 212
weight factor of animals, 200
with respect to animal species, 206–210
animal passage, 207, 210, 211
guinea pigs, 206, 207
mice, 206, 207
rabbits, 206, 207–210
Virulin, 91, 98, 202
Virus pneumonico, 1, 20
Viscosity of capsular polysaccharides, 297
Vuzine
as germicide, 515
in chemotherapy, 512

Welch bacillus, hemotoxin in, 86

Xanthoprotein, formation by Pneumococcus, 75

Yeast
as accessory substance in cultivation of Pneumococcus, 45
effect in dissociation, 144
relation to polysaccharide of Pneumococcus, 422–423